PHYSIOLOGY AND PATHOPHYSIOLOGY OF THE HEART, THIRD EDITION

Developments in Cardiovascular Medicine

S. Sideman, R. Beyar and A.G. Kleber (eds.): *Cardiac Electrophysiology, Circulation, and Transport*. Proceedings of the 7th Henry Goldberg Workshop (Berne, Switzerland, 1990). 1991. ISBN 0-7923-1145-0

D.M. Bers: *Excitation-Contraction Coupling and Cardiac Contractile Force*. 1991. ISBN 0-7923-1186-8

A.-M. Salmasi and A.N. Nicolaides (eds.): *Occult Atherosclerotic Disease. Diagnosis, Assessment and Management*. 1991. ISBN 0-7923-1188-4

J.A.E. Spaan: *Coronary Blood Flow. Mechanics, Distribution, and Control*. 1991. ISBN 0-7923-1210-4

R.W. Stout (ed.): *Diabetes and Atherosclerosis*. 1991. ISBN 0-7923-1310-0

A.G. Herman (ed.): *Antithrombotics. Pathophysiological Rationale for Pharmacological Interventions*. 1991. ISBN 0-7923-1413-1

N.H.J. Pijls: *Maximal Myocardial Perfusion as a Measure of the Functional Significance of Coronary Arteriogram. From a Pathoanatomic to a Pathophysiologic Interpretation of the Coronary Arteriogram*. 1991. ISBN 0-7923-1430-1

J.H.C. Reiber and E.E. v.d. Wall (eds.): *Cardiovascular Nuclear Medicine and MRI. Quantitation and Clinical Applications*. 1992. ISBN 0-7923-1467-0

E. Andries, P. Brugada and R. Stroobrandt (eds.): *How to Face "the Faces" of Cardiac Pacing*. 1992. ISBN 0-7923-1528-6

M. Nagano, S. Mochizuki and N.S. Dhalla (eds.): *Cardiovascular Disease in Diabetes*. 1992. ISBN 0-7923-1554-5

P.W. Serruys, B.H. Strauss and S.B. King III (eds.): *Restenosis after Intervention with New Mechanical Devices*. 1992. ISBN 0-7923-1555-3

P.J. Walter (ed.): *Quality of Life after Open Heart Surgery*. 1992. ISBN 0-7923-1580-4

E.E. van der Wall, H. Sochor, A. Righetti and M.G. Niemeyer (eds.): *What's New in Cardiac Imaging?* SPECT, PET and MRI. 1992. ISBN 0-7923-1615-0

P. Hanrath, R. Uebis and W. Krebs (eds.): *Cardiovascular Imaging by Ultrasound*. 1992. ISBN 0-7923-1755-6

F.H. Messerli (ed.): *Cardiovascular Disease in the Elderly*. 3rd ed. 1992. ISBN 0-7923-1859-5

J. Hess and G.R. Sutherland (eds.): *Congenital Heart Disease in Adolescents and Adults*. 1992. ISBN 0-7923-1862-5

J.H.C. Reiber and P.W. Serruys (eds.): *Advances in Quantitative Coronary Arteriography*. 1993. ISBN 0-7923-1863-3

A.-M. Salmasi and A.S. Iskandrian (eds.): *Cardiac Output and Regional Flow in Health and Disease*. 1993. ISBN 0-7923-1911-7

J.H. Kingma, N.M. van Hemel and K.I. Lie (eds.): *Atrial Fibrillation, a Treatable Disease?* 1992. ISBN 0-7923-2008-5

B. Ostadel and N.S. Dhalla (eds.): *Heart Function in Health and Disease*. Proceedings of the Cardiovascular Program (Prague, Czechoslovakia, 1991). 1992. ISBN 0-7923-2052-2

D. Noble and Y.E. Earm (eds.): *Ionic Channels and Effect of Taurine on the Heart*. Proceedings of an International Symposium (Seoul, Korea, 1992). 1993. ISBN 0-7923-2199-5

H.M. Piper and C.J. Preusse (eds.): *Ischemia-Reperfusion in Cardiac Surgery*. 1993. ISBN 0-7923-2241-X

J. Roelandt, E.J. Gussenhoven and N. Bom (eds.): *Intravascular Ultrasound*. 1993. ISBN 0-7923-2301-7

M.E. Safar and M.F. O'Rourke (eds.): *The Arterial System in Hypertension*. 1993 (in prep.). ISBN 0-7923-2343-2

P.W. Serruys, D.P. Foley and P.J. de Feyter (eds.): *Quantitave Coronary Angiography in Clinical Practice*. 1993 (in prep.). ISBN 0-7923-2368-8

J. Candell-Riera and D. Ortega-Alcalde (eds.): *Nuclear Cardiology in Everyday Practice*. 1993. ISBN 0-7923-2374-2

P. Cummins (ed.): *Growth Factors and the Cardiovascular System*. 1993. ISBN 7923-2401-3

K. Przyklenk, R.A. Kloner and D.M. Yellon (eds.): *Ischemic Preconditioning: The Concept of Endogenous Cardioprotection*. 1993. ISBN 0-7923-2410-2

PHYSIOLOGY AND PATHOPHYSIOLOGY OF THE HEART

Third Edition

Edited by

Nicholas Sperelakis

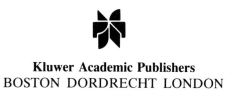

Kluwer Academic Publishers
BOSTON DORDRECHT LONDON

Distributors

for North America: Kluwer Academic Publishers, 101 Philip Drive, Assinippi Park, Norwell, Massachusetts 02061 USA

for all other countries: Kluwer Academic Publishers Group, Distribution Centre, Post Office Box 322, 3300 AH Dordrecht, The Netherlands

Library of Congress Cataloging-in-Publication Data

Physiology and pathophysiology of the heart / edited by Nicholas
   Sperelakis. — 3rd ed.
      p.   cm. — (Developments in cardiovascular medicine; 151)
   Includes bibliographical references and index.
   ISBN 0-7923-2612-1 (alk. paper)
    1. Heart — Physiology. 2. Heart — Pathophysiology. I. Sperelakis, Nick, 1930– . II. Series:
  Developments in cardiovascular medicine; v.151.
    [DNLM: 1. Heart — physiology. 2. Heart — physiopathology. W1
  DE997VME v.151 1994 / WG 202 P5787 1994]
  QP111.4.P53 1994
  612.1′7 — dc20
  DNLM/DLC
  for Library of Congress   93-39197
                                                 CIP

Dedication for 3rd Edition

This third edition is dedicated to all of my very kind Japanese colleagues, past and present. I especially want to mention Prof. Hiroshi Irisawa, who unfortunately died prematurely in November of 1991. Hiroshi was a world leader and pioneer in cellular cardiac electrophysiology. He trained many well-known scientists, including Prof. Akinori Noma, Prof. Issei Seyama, Prof. Ishio Ninomiya, Prof. Makoto Kobayashi, Prof. Shin-Ichiro Kokubun, Prof. Masaki Kameyama, Dr. Hiroko Matsuda, Dr. Nobuhisa Hagiwara, Dr. Yoshihisa Kurachi, Dr. Junko Kimura, Dr. Noritsugu Tohse, and Dr. Hiroshi Masuda. The latter two students of Prof. Irisawa came to my laboratory as visiting scientists. Other distinguished Japanese pioneers in cardiovascular electrophysiology include Prof. Toyomi Sano (now deceased), Prof. Masayosi Goto (recently retired), Prof. Kojiro Matsuda (deceased), Prof. Setsuro Ebashi, and Prof. Hirosi Kuriyama. Other distinguished Japanese scientists and leaders that I have interacted with over the years include Prof. Yoshio Ito, Prof. Michihiko Tada, Prof. Masayasu Hiraoka, Prof. Morio Kanno, Prof. Hideyo Yabu, Prof. Takashi Ban, and Dr. Atsuko Yatani. In addition, I want to acknowledge the following Japanese scientists who have spent some time in my laboratory, and with whom I have published numerous collaborative studies: Prof. Hiroto Mashiba, Prof. Koki Shigenobu, Prof. Michio Kojima, Dr. Hideaki Sada, Dr. Junichi Azuma, Dr. Akihiko Sawamura, Dr. Shunki Yoneda, Dr. Junki Goto, Dr. Shiro Ishikawa*, Dr. Yusuke Ohya*, Dr. Kazuya Fujino, Dr. Shinobu Miki, Dr. Masahiro Nozaki*, Dr. Junna Hatae, Dr. Noritsugu Tohse**, Dr. Hiroyasu Satoh, Dr. Yoshihito Inoue*, Dr. Keiichi Shimamura, Dr. Hiroshi Masuda**, Dr. Kotaro Sumii, and Dr. Masumi Kusaka. The students of Prof. Kuriyama are indicated by a single asterisk (*) and those of Prof. Irisawa by double asterisks (**). It was delightful and rewarding to have had them with me. I am especially indebted to them for their great efforts on behalf of our scientific advancement. Arigato gozai-mas!

In Memorium: Three of the contributors to the first and second editions of this book have passed away recently: Professor A. Fleckenstein, Professor L.J. Mullins, and Professor H. Irisawa. They were outstanding scientists, leaders in their fields, and men of great international stature. They will be sorely missed by the world scientific community.

Acknowledgment

The author is grateful to Rhonda S. Hentz and Heidi Short
for excellent assistance in preparation of the third edition.

Contents

Contributing Authors

ABBOUD, Francois M.
University of Iowa
College of Medicine
Iowa City, IA 52242

AKERA, Tai
MSD (JAPAN) Co., Ltd.
Kowa Bldg. 16 8F, 1-9-20 Akasaka
Minato-Ku
Tokyo 107, Japan

ARNSDORF, Morton F.
Department of Medicine
School of Medicine
University of Chicago
MC 6080
5841 S. Maryland Avenue
Chicago, IL 60637

BANAI, Shmuel
Department of Anatomy and Embryology
The Hebrew University
Hadassah Medical School
P.O.B. 1172
Jerusalem, 91010
Israel

BARNETT, Joey V.
Departments of Medicine (Cardiology) and Pharmacology
Vanderbilt University
School of Medicine
Nashville, TN 37232-2170

BASSETT, Arthur
Department of Pharmacology
University of Miami
Miami, FL 33101

BAUMGARTEN, Clive
Department of Physiology
Medical College of Virginia
Box 551
Richmond, VA 23298

BENNETT, Brian
Department of Pharmacology and Toxicology
Queen's University
Kingston, Ontario
Canada K7L-3N6

BILEZIKIAN, John
Departments of Pharmacology, Medicine, and Pediatrics
Columbia University
630 West 168th Street
New York, NY 10032

BING, Richard J.
Huntington Memorial Hospital
100 Congress Street
Pasadena, CA 91105

BLUMENTHAL, Ken
Department of Molecular Genetics
University of Cincinnati
College of Medicine
Cincinnati, OH 45267-0524

BOTTORFF, Michael
Division of Clinical and Hospital Pharmacy
University of Cincinnati
Medical Center
208-A Wherry Hall
Cincinnati, OH 45267-0004

BRADY, Allan
Department of Chemistry & Biochemistry
Welch Hall 4.230
University of Texas at Austin
Austin, TX 78712

BRAYDEN, Joseph
Department of Pharmacology
University of Vermont
Given Medical Bldg.
Burlington, VT 05405

BRETSCHNEIDER, Hans Jurgen†
Institute of Physiology
University of Gottingen
D-3400 Gottingen
West Germany

BRODY, Theodore M.
Michigan State University
Department of Pharmacology & Toxicology
B-440 Life Sciences Bldg.
East Lansing, MI 48824-0001

BUJA, Maximilian
Department of Pathology and Laboratory Medicine
University of Texas Medical School
6431 Fannin
MSB 2.136
Houston, TX 77030

COHEN, Ira
Department of Physiology and Biophysics
SUNY School of Medicine
Stony Brook, NY 11794

CORR, Peter
Department of Medicine, Biology, and Pharmacology
Washington University
School of Medicine
660 S. Euclid Avenue
Box 8086
St. Louis, MO 63110

DEMELLO, Walmor C.
Department of Pharmacology
Medical Sciences Campus
University of Puerto Rico
GPO Box 5067
San Juan, Puerto Rico 00936

DHALLA, Naranjan
Division of Cardiovascular Sciences
St. Boniface General Hospital
Research Centre
University of Manitoba
Faculty of Medicine
351 Tache Avenue
Winnipeg, Canada R2H 2A6

DOWNEY, James M.
Department of Physiology
College of Medicine
University of South Alabama
Mobile, AL 36688-0002

DRISKA, Steven
Physiology Department
Temple University
Medical School
Philadelphia, PA 19140

DROOGMANS, G.
Laboratorium voor Fysiologie
K.U.L. Campus Gasthuisberg
Herestraat
B-300 Leuven
Belgium

ELIMBAN, Vijayan
Division of Cardiovascular Sciences
St. Boniface General Hospital
Research Centre
University of Manitoba
Faculty of Medicine
351 Tache Avenue
Winnipeg, Canada R2H 2A6

ENGLAND, Sarah K.
Department of Physiology
Medical College of Wisconsin
8701 Watertown Plank Rd.
Milwaukee, WI 53226

FABIATO, Alexandre
Department of Physiology
Medical College of Virginia
Box 551
Richmond, VA 23298

FERRANS, Victor J.
Pathology Branch
National Heart, Lung and Blood Institute
Bldg. 10, Room 2N-240
National Institutes of Health
9000 Rockville Pike
Bethesda, MD 20892

FLOCKERZI, Veit
Pharmakologisches Institut
Lehrstuhl Molekulare Pharmakologic
Im Neuenheimer Feld 366
69120 Heidelberg
Germany

FORBES, Michael S.
"Merry Oaks"
Rt. 1, Box 245
Troy, VA 22974

GADBUT, Albert P.
Department of Medicine
Cardiovascular Division
Brigham and Women's Hospital
Harvard Medical School
Boston, MA 02115

GALPER, Jonas B.
Department of Medicine
Cardiovascular Division
Brigham and Women's Hospital
Harvard Medical School
Boston, MA 02115

† Deceased

GEBHARD, Martha
Institute of Physiology
Abteilung Experimentelle Chirurgie
der Chirurgischen Universitatslinik Heidelberg
Im Nevenheimer Feld 347
69120 Heidelberg
Germany

GERTZ, S. David
Department of Anatomy and Embryology
Hebrew University
Hadassah Medical School
P.O. Box 1172
Jerusalem, 91010 Israel

GINSBURG, Kenneth
Department of Medicine
Section of Cardiology
University of Chicago
MC 6080
5841 S. Maryland Avenue
Chicago, IL 60637

GORMAN, Mark W.
Department of Physiology
Michigan State University
East Lansing, MI 48824

HADDAD, George
Department of Biophysics
Faculty of Medicine
University of Sherbrooke
Sherbrooke, Quebec
Canada J1J5N4

HARDIN, Christopher
University of Washington
Department of Radiology, SB-05
Seattle, WA 98195

HARRISON, Donald
Senior Vice President and Provost for Health Education
University of Cincinnati
College of Medicine
250 Health Professional Bldg.
Cincinnati, OH 45267-0663

HE, Miao-Xiang
Department of Physiology
Michigan State University
East Lansing, MI 48824

HEINEMANN, Stefan H.
Max-Planck Gesellschaft Z.F.D.W.
AG Molekulare Und.
Zelluläre Biophysik
Drackendorfer Straße 1
D-07747 Sena
Germany

HERMSMEYER, Kent
Primate Center
Reproductive Biology/Uterus
Beaverton, OR 97006

HOFFMAN, Brian
Department of Pharmacology
College of Physicians and Surgeons of Columbia
    University
630 West 168th Street
New York, NY 10032

HOFMANN, Franz
Institut fur Pharmakologie and Toxikologie
Technische Universitat Munchen
Biedersteiner Strabe 29
D-8000 Munchen 40
Germany

HONDEGHEM, Luc
HPC N.V.
Westlaan 85
B-8400 Oostende
Belgium

HOUSER, Steven
Department of Physiology & Biophysics
Temple University
Philadelphia, PA 19140

IRISAWA, H.†
The Heart Institute of Japan
Tokyo Women's Medical College
8-1 Kawada-Cho
Shinjuku-Ku
Tokyo 162, Japan

ISENBERG, Gerrit
Department of Physiology
University of Cologne
5000 Koln 41
Germany

JOSEPHSON, Ira
Department of Physiology & Biophysics
University of Cincinnati
College of Medicine
231 Bethesda Avenue
Cincinnati, OH 45267-0576

KADOMA, Masaaki
Division of Cardiology
The 1st Department of Medicine
Osaka University
School of Medicine
2-2, Yamada-oka
Suita, Osaka 565
Japan

† Deceased

KAMOUCHI, Masahiro
Department of Pharmacology
Faculty of Medicine
Kyushu University
Fukuoka 812
Japan

KANNO, Morio
Department of Pharmacology
Hokkaido University
School of Medicine
Sapporo, 060
Japan

KARGACIN, Gary J.
Department of Medical Biochemistry
The University of Calgary
Faculty of Medicine
3330 Hospital Drive, NW
Calgary, Alberta
Canada T2N 4N1

KASS, Robert S.
Physiology Department
School of Medicine
University of Rochester
601 Elmwood Avenue
Rochester, NY 14642-8642

KATZUNG, Bertran
University of California
Department of Pharmacology
School of Medicine
San Francisco, CA 94143

KILBOURNE, Edward J.
Department of Medicine
Cardiovascular Division
Brigham and Women's Hospital
Harvard Medical School
Boston, MA 02115

KITAMURA, K.
Department of Pharmacology
Faculty of Medicine
Kyushu University 60
Fukuoka 812
Japan

KURACHI, Yoshihisa
Department of Pharmacology
Faculty of Medicine
Osaka University
2-2, Yamadaoka, Suita
Osaka 565, Japan

KURGAN, Adi
Department of Anatomy and Embryology
Hebrew University
Hadassah Medical School
P.O.B. 1172
Jerusalem, 91010 Israel

KURIYAMA, Hirosi
Kyushu University
Department of Pharmacology
Faculty of Medicine 60
Fukuoka 812; Japan

LAKATTA, Edward G.
Laboratory of Cardiovascular Science
Gerontology Research Center
National Institute on Aging
4940 Eastern Avenue
Baltimore, MD 21224

LAZZARA, Ralph
University of Oklahoma
Health Science Center
P.O. Box 26901
Oklahoma City, OK 73190-0001

LEDERER, W. Jonathan
Department of Physiology
University of Maryland
School of Medicine
600 W. Redwood St.
Baltimore, MD 21201-1541

LEVY, Matthew N.
Department of Investigative Medicine
Mount Sinai Hospital
1 Mt. Sinai Drive
Cleveland, OH 44106

LINDEMANN, Jon
Division of Cardiology, Mail Slot 532
University of Arkansas for Medical Sciences
4301 W. Markham St.
Little Rock, AR 72205

MARTIN, Paul J.
Department of Investigative Medicine
Mt. Sinai Medical Center
1 Mt. Sinai Drive
Cleveland, OH 44106

MATSUDA, H.
Kyushu University 60
Department of Physiology
Faculty of Medicine
Fukuoka 812
Japan

McHOWAT, Jane
Department of Internal Medicine
Washington University
School of Medicine
660 S. Euclid Avenue
St. Louis, MO 63110

McDONALD, Terrence F.
Department of Physiology and Biophysics
Dalhousie University
Halifax NS B3H 4H7
Canada

MIRONNEAU, Jean
Laboratoire de Physiologie
Cellulaire et Pharmacologie Moleculaire
CNRS URS 1489
Universite de Bordeaux II
3 Place de la Victoire
33076 Bordeaux
Cedex, France

MISSIAEN, Ludwig
Laboratorium voor Fysiologie
Campus Gasthuisberg
K.U. Leuven
B-3000, Leuven
Belgium

MIURA, Tetsuji
2nd Department of Internal Medicine
Sapporo Medical College
South-1 West-16
Chuo-ku
Sapporo, 060, Japan

MORKIN, Eugene
Departments of Internal Medicine and Pharmacology
College of Medicine
University of Arizona
Tucson, AZ 85724

NAGANO, Makoto
Department of Internal Medicine
Aoto Hospital
Jikei University
Tokyo, Japan

NICHOLS, Colin G.
Department of Cell Biology
Washington University School of Medicine
660 S. Euclid Avenue
St. Louis, Md 63110

NILIUS, Bernd
c/o KU Leuven
Campus Gasthuisberg
Department of Physiology
Herestraat
B-3000, Leuven
Belgium

NOMA, Akinori
Kyoto University
School of Medicine
Department of Physiology
Kyoto City
Japan

OHYA, Yusuke
Kyushu University
Second Department of Internal Medicine
Faculty of Medicine
Fukuoka 812, Japan

OPIE, Lionel H.
Heart Research Unit and
Hypertension Clinic
Department of Medicine
Medical School
University of Cape Town
Observatory 7925
Cape Town, South Africa

PATTERSON, Eugene
Department of Pharmacology
Oklahoma University
Health Science Center
P.O. Box 26901
Biomedical Sciences Bldg., Room 753
940 Stanton L. Young Blvd.
Oklahoma City, OK 73190

PAUL, Richard
Department of Physiology and Biophysics
University of Cincinnati
College of Medicine
231 Bethesda Avenue
Cincinnati, OH 45267-0576

PRATILA, Margaret G.
Memorial Sloan-Kettering Cancer Center
Department of Anesthesiology &
    Critical Care Medicine
1275 York Ave., Room C-302
New York, NY 10021

PRATILAS, Vasilios
Memorial Sloan-Kettering Cancer Center
Department of Anesthesiology and Critical Care Medicine
1275 York Avenue, Room C-302
New York, NY 10021

REEVES, John
Department of Physiology
UND-NJMS
185 S. Orange Ave.
Newark, NJ 07103-2714

ROBINSON, Richard
Departments of Pharmacology, Medicine, and Pediatrics
Columbia University
630 West 168th Street
New York, NY 10032

ROSEN, Michael
Departments of Pharmacology, Medicine, and Pediatrics
Columbia University
College of Physicians and Surgeons
630 W. 168th Street
New York, NY 10032

RUDY, Yoram
Department of Biomedical Engineering
Case Western Reserve University
505 Wickenden Bldg.
Cleveland, OH 44106-7207

RUPP, Heinz
Division of Cardiovascular Sciences
St. Boniface General Hospital
Research Centre
University of Manitoba
Faculty of Medicine
351 Tache Avenue
Winnipeg
Canada R2H 2A6

RUSCH, Nancy
Department of Physiology
Medical College of Wisconsin
8701 Watertown Plank Road
Milwaukee, WI 53226

RYAN, Una
T Cell Sciences, Inc.
38 Sidney Street
Cambridge, MA 02139-4135

SCHERLAG, Benjamin J.
Department of Cardiology
Oklahoma University
Health Science Center
P.O. Box 26901
Biomedical Sciences Bldg., Room 753
940 Stanton L. Young Blvd.
Oklahoma City, OK 73190

SCHNABEL, Philipp A.
Pathologisches Institut
Im Nevenheimer Feld 2201221
69120 Heidelberg
Germany

SHUBA, Lesya M.
Department of Physiology and Biophysics
Dalhousie University
Halifax NS B3H 4H7
Canada

SOLARO, R. John
Department of Physiology and Biophysics
University of Illinois
College of Medicine
Chicago, IL 60680

SPARKS JR, Harvey V.
Department of Physiology
Michigan State University
East Lansing, MI 48824

SPERELAKIS, Nicholas
Department of Physiology and Biophysics
University of Cincinnati
College of Medicine
231 Bethesda Avenue
Cincinnati, OH 45267-0576

STEINBERG, Susan
Departments of Pharmacology, Medicine, and Pediatrics
Columbia University
630 West 168th Street
New York, NY 10032

STUHMER, Walter
Max Planck Institut für Experimentelle Medizin
Abt. Molekulare Biologie Neuronaler Signale
Hermann-Rein-Str. 3
D-37079 Gottingen
Germany

TADA, Michihiko
Division of Cardiology
First Department of Medicine
Osaka University School of Medicine
2-2, Yamada-oka, Suita
Kukushima-ku
Osaka 565
Japan

TAKEDA, Nobuakira
Department of Internal Medicine
Aoto Hospital
Jikei University
Tokyo
Japan

TEN EICK, Robert
Department of Pharmacology
Northwestern University
Medical School
Chicago, IL 60611

TOHSE, Noritsugu
Department of Physiology
College of Medicine
Sapporo Medical University
S-1 W-17 Chuo-Ku
Sapporo 060
Japan

TORO, Ligia
Baylor College of Medicine
Department of Physiology & Molecular Biophysics
One Baylor Palza
Houston, TX 77030

TRITTHART, Helmut A.
Universitats-Institut fur Medizinische Physik und
  Biophysik
Karl Franzens-Universitat Graz
A-8010 Graz, Austria
Harrachgasse 21
Austria

VENTURINI, Catherine M.
Monsanto Company
St. Louis, MO

WALDMAN, Scott
Department of Medicine
Thomas Jefferson Medical College
1100 Walnut Street
Philadelphia, PA 19107-5563

WALSH, Michael
Department of Medical Biochemistry
University of Calgary
3330 Hospital Drive, N.W.
Calgary, Alberta T2N 4N1
Canada

WATANABE, August M.
Eli Lilly Company
7760 N. Colorado Avenue 317
Indianapolis, IN 46240

YAMADA, Kathryn A.
Department of Internal Medicine
Washington University School of Medicine
660 S. Euclid Avenue
St. Louis, MO 63110

YAN, Gan-Xin
Department of Internal Medicine
Washington University
  School of Medicine
660 S. Euclid Avenue
St. Louis, MO 63110

Foreword to the Third Edition

The title of the third edition of *Physiology and Pathophysiology of the Heart* makes a brave promise: It implies that, whatever the interest of the reader and whatever the area of inquiry, there will be an authoritative exposition on both normal physiology and also the changes therein that are causally related to or result from disease processes. Since the term *heart* here includes consideration of the coronary vasculature, the promise is broad indeed. One might wonder at the outset, because of the immense amount of information available in these fields, if any single book could make good on such a promise. As those who have read earlier editions will agree, the answer is an unqualified "yes."

In the first section, Cardiac Muscle, Dr. Sperelakis has identified a set of 41 topics that address the current major interests of basic investigators and clinicians. These chapters include consideration of cardiac structure and ultrastructure as they relate to function and our current understanding of increasingly complex subjects: the ionic basis of electrical activity and the rapidly developing area of investigation that relates ion channel function to molecular structure. Information on these topics is essential for understanding later sections on arrhythmias and the actions of antiarrhythmic and other cardiac drugs. The basic presentation on cardiac electrical activity leads to a chapter that presents current ideas on the genesis of normal and abnormal electrocardiograms.

Several chapters emphasize the crucially important role of calcium currents in electrical and mechanical activity, the regulation of those currents and their relationships to electromechanical coupling. Included are sections that provide new information on sodium-for-calcium exchange, the modulation of sarcoplasmic reticular function, and regulation of the contractile activity of cardiac myofilaments. The chapters on electrophysiology lead to sections dealing with the mechanisms for arrhythmias, and the actions and mechanisms of action of antiarrhythmic drugs; the sections on contractility are followed by consideration of the mechanical changes in hypertrophied hearts.

Several chapters present new understanding in an often neglected field: developmental changes in membrane electrical activity, cardiac receptors, and the neural regulation of cardiac performance. Also included is a presentation of the changes in cardiac electrical activity consequent to aging. After reviewing the actions of drugs, hormones, and toxic substances, this section concludes with a clear and up-to-date presentation of the effects of ischemia on electrical activity.

In the second section, Vascular Smooth Muscle and Coronary Circulation, this edition adds several new and important chapters to provide a clearer understanding of the complex behavior of blood vessels and their interactions with their environment. One can take away a full understanding of the electrophysiology of vascular smooth muscle and the many factors that contribute to the normal regulation of its mechanical activity. Also included are sections dealing with disorders of vascular function associated with disease states. These presentations are clarified by simple but full expositions on the roles of ion channels in vascular smooth muscle and endothelial cells; modifications of function caused by calcium, ATP, and pharmacologic agents, and the overall dependence of function and regulation on metabolic processes. The final chapters consider abnormalities of vascular function in hypertension, the normal control of the coronary circulation, and the consequences of myocardial infarction.

For each chapter Dr. Sperelakis has selected an author both renowned for studies in the field and expert in lucid and complete exposition. Each presentation is thorough and balanced, and each contributes to the whole. In sum, *Physiology and Pathophysiology of the Heart* does more than merely meet the needs of the reader. In addition, it provides a sense of the excitement and wonder of basic research, and the future promise of new and improved means to understand and treat cardiovascular disease.

Brian F. Hoffman
Department of Pharmacology
College of Physicians
and Surgeons of
Columbia University

Foreword to the Second Edition

The expansion of our practical knowledge in the management of cardiovascular diseases has been staggering. Few will not be awed by our ability to prolong life and reduce mortality from cardiovascular diseases. Some may argue that, at an exorbitant price, we are simply postponing death with our "halfway" technology. Our society, however, will continue to demand cardiac transplantation, artificial hearts, bypass surgery, intravenous thrombolysis with strep and TPA, balloon angioplasty, automatic defibrillation, and intracardiac pacing. We are bewildered by the effectiveness of these "clinical advances," frustrated by their complications, and often ignorant of basic concepts and mechanisms.

Parallel with this revolution in cardiovascular treatment, at a lower cost but without immediate evidence of clinical benefit, is the exciting and vital process of understanding the underlying cellular biology. This book is a repository of the state of the science with respect to function and malfunction of cardiac and vascular muscle cells. The breadth of topics covered is a prerequisite in a textbook; moreover, their depth and the expertise of the authors are indeed impressive. As anticipated from a book edited by Dr. Nicholas Sperelakis, whose contributions to electrophysiology have been nationally and internationally recognized, subjects related to electrophysiology of cardiac and vascular muscle are emphasized. For example, calcium uptake and release are discussed in three chapters: one on sodium-calcium exchange, another on calcium uptake by sarcoplasmic reticulum, and a third on calcium release by sarcoplasmic reticulum. For any "student" wishing to be introduced to a comprehensive base of knowledge on the role of this important cation in electromechanical coupling, this book is a superb reference resource. In addition, several other fundamental areas are covered with the comprehensive, analytical, and integrative approach expected from experts. Ultrastructure, pathology, energetics, metabolism, receptor regulation, and mechanics of both cardiac and vascular muscle are presented in two major parts of the book. One section on cardiac muscle encompasses 30 chapters and the other on the coronary circulation covers 10 chapters. Areas of great importance in pathophysiology of cardiovascular diseases are presented from a fundamental perspective. These include topics such as calcium injury and the calcium paradox, antiarrhythmic drugs, calcium channel blockers, cardiac hypertrophy, coronary atherosclerosis, and coronary spasm. The list of authors is a litany of the very best in each of these fields. Dr. Sperelakis takes us in his book to the frontiers of our knowledge of cellular function and pathophysiology. He impresses us by what we know and challenges us by what we do not know.

By selecting as the last chapter in his book the topic of coronary artery spasm, Dr. Sperelakis may be trying to tell us what this book is all about. The suspicion that angina represents not only an imbalance between oxygen supply and demand by the heart, but a phenomenon that can occur without an increase in demand, is about two centuries old. More than three quarters of a century ago, Osler advanced the notion of coronary spasm, but the mechanisms involved have remained a total mystery. Recently, however, the discovery that the endothelium, far from being a simple barrier, is a powerful regulator of vasomotor tone, is leading us to totally new concepts in the understanding of this and other major dysfunctions of vascular muscle. Knowledge of basic mechanisms of biological phenomena are great rewards for the biomedical scientist. These are amplified several-fold if the understanding leads to treatment and cure of disease. This chapter, and indeed the whole book, shares with us the excitement of understanding basic cellular mechanisms and the promise of the application of this new knowledge to a better understanding of pathophysiologic states and their treatment.

Francois M. Abboud, MD

Foreword to the First Edition

This book emphasizes the fundamental, functional aspects of cardiology. Within the last 30 years, the rift between clinical and investigative cardiology has widened because of the overwhelming development of new clinical procedures, both diagnostic and therapeutic. Almost forgotten is the fact that we owe most of the clinical advances to theoretical and experimental observations. I need not remind the reader of the work of Carrel, who performed the first experimental coronary bypass in 1902, or the work of the brothers Curie in 1880, both physicists, who discovered piezoelectricity, the keystone in echogradiography; of the works of Langley, who introduced the receptors concept; of Ahlquist in 1946, who first differentiated between alpha and beta receptors; of Fleckenstein, a physiologist who pioneered the field of Ca^{2+} antagonists. This list could go on for several pages. Thus the book edited by Sperelakis is a potent reminder of the almost forgotten fact that cardiology has two sites, inextricably related.

The book deals with subjects in which Dr. Sperelakis has pioneered: ultrastructure of heart muscle, electrophysiology, cardiac contractility, and ion exchange. An extension of these subjects is the chapter dealing with fundamental topics of the coronary circulation.

This book is indeed a timely reminder of the importance of the fundamental aspects of cardiology. Emphasis on clinical aspects of cardiology alone will result in a sterile and unproductive future for a field that has made such stunning advances during the last 30 years to the benefit of millions of people.

Richard J. Bing

Preface to the Third Edition

The first and second editions of *Physiology and Pathophysiology of the Heart* were quite successful for an advanced reference book of this nature. I kept on receiving kind compliments about the book, including comments such as "its the leading book in this field." It is, of course, very comprehensive and authoritative. The various chapters were written by leading researchers in their respective speciality areas of cardiovascular science.

I took the opportunity, upon embarking on the third edition, of bringing in 14 new chapters to cover topics that were not covered in the second edition. These include two new chapters on the molecular structure of ion channels and several new chapters on the ionic channels of myocardial cells, vascular smooth muscle cells, and endothelial cells. New chapters are also included on release of Ca^{2+} from the SR, and on the action of phospholipids released during ischemia on ion channels and production of dysrhythmias. These new additions make the book substantially more complete and up-to-date with respect to recent developments in cardiovascular science. The foreword to the third edition was written by Brain F. Hoffman.

As in the first and second editions, the third edition is divided into two major sections: cardiac muscle and coronary circulation. The book is multidisciplinary in approach and attempts to integrate all relevant aspects of the factors influencing the function of the heart under normal and several abnormal conditions. It also provides a foundation for understanding of the mechanism of action of various types of cardioactive drugs, including antiarrhythmic drugs and positive inotropic agents.

I trust that academic cardiologists and cardiovascular research scientists will find the third edition as valuable as were the first two editions, in addition to being updated, improved, and more complete. This book provides the foundation of the basic science aspects of cardiac function and dysfunction, and attempts to bridge the gap between basic cardiovascular science and clinical science.

The first and second editions were translated into Russian and published in the former USSR. My repeated attempts to have *Physiology and Pathophysiology of the Heart* published in Japanese, Chinese, Spanish, and Italian were not successful. Perhaps we will have more luck with the third edition.

The chapters were written by a distinguished group of experts and outstanding scientists from around the world. It has been my great pleasure and honor to work with them in the preparation of the third edition.

Nicholas Sperelakis

Preface to the Second Edition

The first edition of this book was quite successful. Several complimentary book reviews appeared soon after the first edition was published, and written and oral words of praise and appreciation were given both to the publisher and to me by quite a few individuals. It is because of such positive comments and reactions that the publisher and I decided to embark on a second edition of *Physiology and Pathophysiology of the Heart*. The second edition was long in preparation, taking over a year to complete. All chapter contributors were asked to revise, improve, and update their articles, and all have done so with enthusiasm and timeliness. A second edition not only allows for updating chapters and correcting errors and omissions, but also enables all contributors to work towards a more uniform and more didactic writing style.

In addition, a second edition enables the editor to invite other outstanding researchers of the heart to contribute articles that will help to fill in any holes or missing areas on the subject that are important and timely. A total of eight such new chapters have been added to the second edition. The new chapters are on the areas of contractile proteins of cardiac muscle (John Solaro), contractile proteins of smooth muscle (Michael Walsh), cyclic nucleotides and protein kinases in smooth muscle (Ferid Murad), calcium-activated ion currents in cardiac muscle (William Clusin), developmental changes in adrenergic modulation (M.R. Rosen, R.B. Robinson, I.S. Cohen, and J.P. Bilezikian), endothelial cell interactions with vascular smooth muscle cells (Robert High-smith), myocardial infarction and free radical effects on the heart (T. Miura, Derek Yellin, and James Downey), and extravascular coronary resistance (James Downey). In addition, a Foreword to the Second Edition was written by Frank Abboud.

Incorporating new chapters into the second edition becomes a balance between overall length and cost of the book versus completeness. The editor is usually concerned primarily with completeness, whereas the publisher establishes limits based on cost. Therefore, the final product is a compromise between these two factors.

As in the first edition, the book is divided into two major sections: cardiac muscle and coronary circulation. The book is multidisciplinary and includes membrane biophysics, electrophysiology, physiology, pathophysiology, pharmacology, biochemistry, and ultrastructure. Thus, the book attempts to integrate all relevant aspects of the factors influencing the function of the heart as a vital organ under normal and various abnormal conditions. The book also attempts to set the foundation for an understanding of the action and mechanism of action of a number of classes of cardioactive drugs.

I hope that the medical and science research community will find the second edition as useful and worthwhile as the first edition and, of course, improved, updated, and more complete. The second edition is intended for the same general audience as the first edition, namely, researchers of the heart, academic cardiologists, cardiologists and related medical specialists in private practice, resident physicians, research fellows, and graduate students. Even medical students at the better medical colleges should find the book useful as a reference volume to supplement and amplify specific points covered in lectures and broader textbooks. Many clinicians recognize the importance of basic science aspects of the heart that underlie the practice of cardiology. This book attempts to help bridge the gap between basic science and clinical science. Plans are underway to publish the second edition *of Physiology and Pathophysiology of the Heart* in several foreign languages, including Russian and Japanese.

The chapters have been written by a distinguished group of experts and outstanding researchers from around the world. It has been my great pleasure and honor to work with this distinguished group of individuals in preparation of the second edition. I trust that the reader will recognize that this multidisciplinary book is a clear, concise, up-to-date, and thorough book on the functioning of the heart in normal and pathological states.

Nicholas Sperelakis

Preface to the First Edition

The theme of this book is the physiology and function of the heart in the normal state and in various pathologic states. The two major sections are on (1) cardiac muscle and related tissues, such as nodal cell and Purkinje fiber systems, and (2) coronary circulation, including properties of the vascular smooth muscle cells. Not only are the relevant physiology and biophysics discussed, but, in addition, the ultrastructure, biochemistry, and pharmacology — that is, the book attempts to integrate all relevant aspects of the factors influencing the function of the heart as a vital organ under normal and abnormal conditions and states. The book also attempts to set the foundation for an understanding of the action of, and mechanism of action of, a number of classes of cardioactive drugs, including the calcium antagonistic drugs, antianginal drugs, antiarrhythmic drugs, and cardiac glycosides.

Each chapter is written by one or more experts in the area who have been selected from around the world. The authors were asked to aim for a clear, concise, accurate, and up-to-date summary of the topic in a didactic and textbook teaching style. It was suggested that the authors present key references only, with heavy emphasis on review-type and summary-type articles. The reader should be able to obtain the important facts, concepts, and hypotheses from the chapters and, if he or she wishes to go into greater depth and examine more of the evidence on some particular aspect, he or she can look up the appropriate reference.

This book is intended for practicing and academic cardiologists, related medical specialists, and researchers. However, resident physicians, graduate students, and medical student's should find the book useful as a reference volume to supplement and amplify specific points covered in lectures and in broader textbooks. The authors were made aware of the audience intended for the book and were requested to pitch their chapter at the appropriate level. It was suggested that they present sufficient detail, documentation, and illustrations as required for the readership that the book was aimed at. The clinican undoubtedly recognizes the importance of basic science aspects of the heart that underlie his or her practice of cardiology, and this undertaking attempts to help bridge the gap between basic science and clinical science.

As mentioned above, the chapters have been written by a distinguished group of experts and outstanding researchers in their respective fields from around the world. It has been my great pleasure in assembling and working with this distinguished group of individuals in this rather massive undertaking. I hope that the readers will recognize the merits of the book and will agree that it represents a clear, concise, up-to-date, and multidisciplinary book on the heart.

Nicholas Sperelakis

I CARDIAC MUSCLE

CHAPTER 1

Ultrastructure of Mammalian Cardiac Muscle

MICHAEL S. FORBES & NICHOLAS SPERELAKIS

INTRODUCTION

The great majority of muscle cells of the mammalian heart are superbly organized entities. It is impressive to consider that observations on these myocytes are in most cases being made on cells that are roughly the same age as the entire animal; only a scant bit of evidence is yet available to suggest that any substantial capability for regeneration is intrinsic to the myocardia of higher vertebrates (see the section, *Nuclei*). Still these venerable cells can respond admirably under trying circumstances, such as those necessitating osmotic shrinkage or hypertrophy, in which cases they adjust their sarcolemmal and myoplasmic components to maintain an extraordinarily constant surface-volume ratio {1,2}. In this chapter we provide a sketch of the fine structure of cardiac muscle cells in mammalian heart. The many electron microscopic studies of such cells have served to point out the difficulty of making generalizations when considering the numerous aspects of myocardial substructure. We will, nevertheless, describe the salient features of myocardial cells, while pointing out along the way some of the variations on these basic themes that have been discovered to date.

Myocardial cells are commonly classified either in terms of their location within the heart (i.e., atrial vs. ventricular) or according to their primary function [working (contractile) vs. conductive]. For the purposes of this description, we have chosen to deal with cardiac muscle cells primarily on the basis of the latter system of classification. *Working* cells are those that carry out the bulk of the mechanical activity of the heart, whereas cells of the atrioventricular conducting system (AVCS) are responsible for the generation and delivery of action potentials that regulate the rate and direction of heart contractions. Depending on the species being examined, the differences in morphology between working and AVCS cells may be profound, or may be scarcely appreciable.

Other comprehensive reviews of cardiac ultrastructure are available {e.g., 3–5}, and there also have been published detailed compilations addressed to one or more specific cytologic features of cardiac muscle cells, notably the membrane systems {6–8}. The efficacy of our summary sketch will be to present a picture of myocardial ultrastructure against which the results of microscopic studies — be they of normal or pathologic tissue — can be effectively compared. In addition, this study will serve, to some degree, as an anatomic reference for the remaining chapters in this book. Because of the requisite interest in the structure and function of human heart, we have weighted this chapter on the side of the myocardial cells of monkeys, which offer both the advantages of reasonably ready availability and the ethical possibility of optimum fixation by means of vascular perfusion.

SYNOPSIS OF MYOCARDIAL CELL STRUCTURE

The generalizations of microscopic appearance that can be applied to the cardiac muscle cells of mammals are briefly described in this section. The details and variations of cell structure are considered at greater length in the sections, *Working (contractile) myocardial cells* and *Conductive myocardial cells*.

Working ventricular cells

The contractile myocytes of the ventricular walls, papillary muscles, and interventricular septum are elongate, densely packed cells that are grouped into muscular rods or bands. Such cells display a distinct longitudinal polarity of the majority of their internal contents, including myofibrils, mitochondria, and nuclei (figs. 1-1 and 1-2). The closely apposed portions of cells — primarily the cell tips — contain numerous junctions, which collectively form *intercalated discs*, the extensive regions of adhesion that are obvious even with light microscopy {9,10}. Myofibrils, bundles of contractile protein filaments, constitute the majority of myocardial cell volume, followed in incidence by mitochondria, which fall into rows in the intermyofibrillar spaces and into less well-organized masses in the subsarcolemmal and nuclear pole regions (table 1-1). Ventricular myocardial cells frequently possess two or more nuclei. The two membrane systems — (1) transverse (T) and axial tubules which together comprise the T-axial tubular system (TATS), and (2) the sarcoplasmic reticulum (SR) — are well developed and frequently are arranged in patterns seemingly directed by the presence of sarcomeric segmentation of the myofibrils. Working ventricular

N. Sperelakis (ed.), Physiology and Pathophysiology of the Heart, Third Edition.
© *1995 Kluwer Academic Publishers. ISBN 0-7923-2612-1. All rights reserved.*

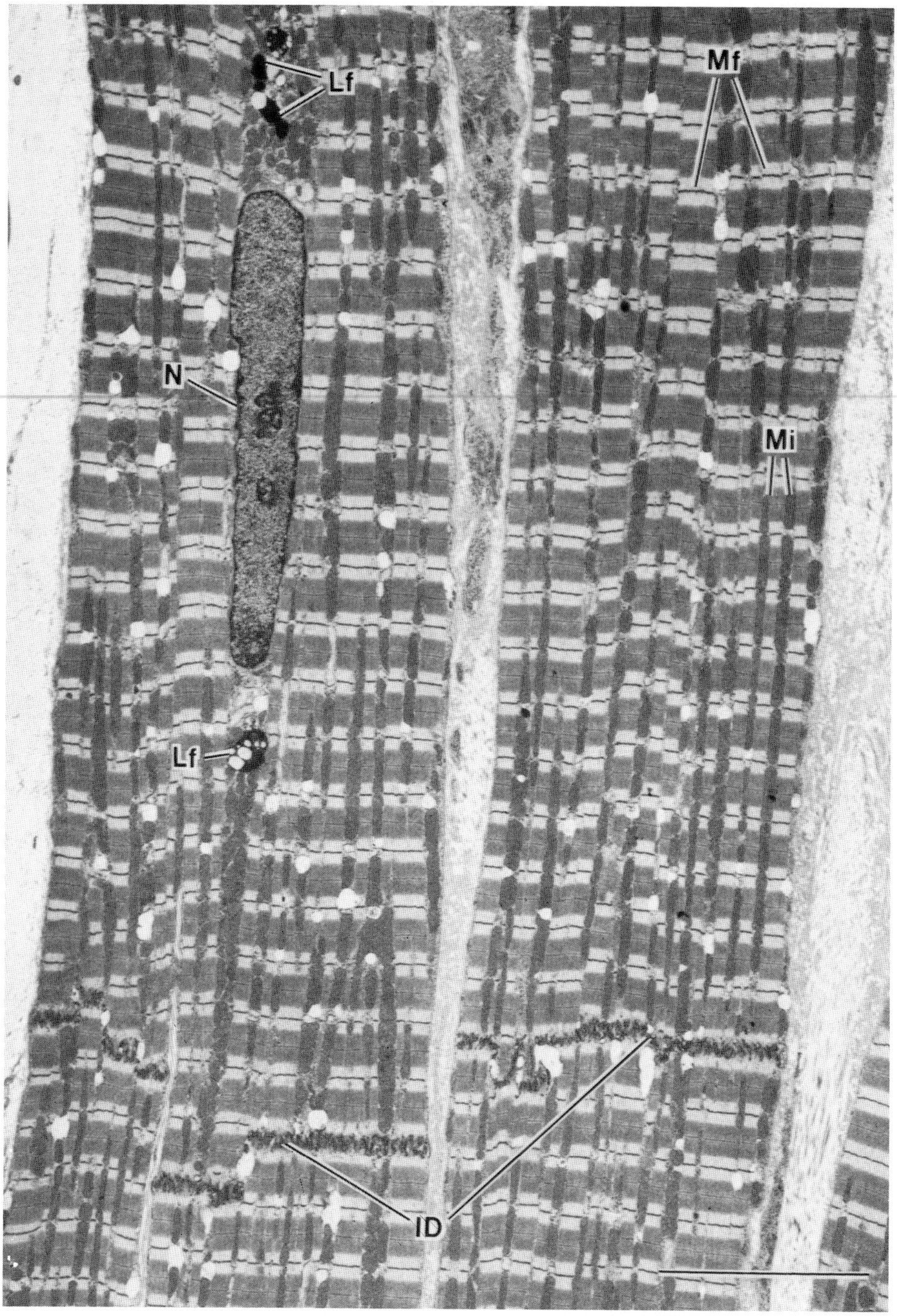

Fig. 1-1. Transmission electron micrograph. Survey of longitudinal thin section of myocardium from right papillary muscle of monkey (vervet: *Cercopithecus aethiops*). A characteristic feature of these typical cardiac muscle cells is the longitudinal alignment of their major constituents; these include the myofibrils (Mf), which frequently exhibit branched profiles; mitochondria (Mi), which are arranged in intermyofibrillar rows for the most part; and nuclei, one of which (N) appears in this field. Regions of mitochondrion-rich myoplasm extend from each pole of the nucleus; examples of lipofuscin bodies (Lf) are most often located in this "nuclear pole myoplasm." The cell tips incorporate numerous intermembranous junctions, collections of which form the intercalated discs (ID). Scale bar represents 10 μm.

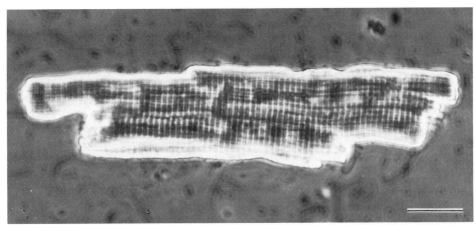

Fig. 1.2.

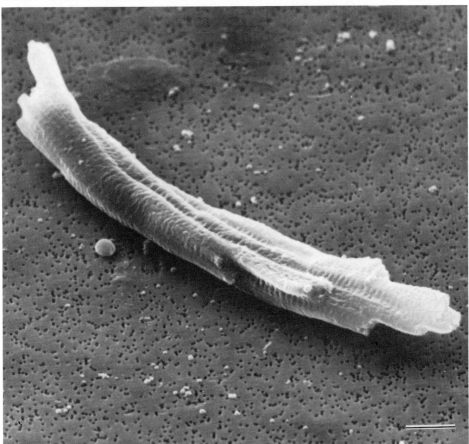

Fig. 1.3.

Fig. 1-2. Phase-contrast light micrograph of ventricular cardiac muscle cell, isolated from rat heart by means of enzymatic digestion and mechanical dispersion {13}. The longitudinal array of myofibrils is obvious, and the myofibrillar banding pattern is clearly discernible (cf. fig. 1-1). The uneven profile of the cell tips is typical, derived from the cell's content of myofibrils of different lengths. Scale bar represents 20 μm.

Fig. 1-3. Scanning electron micrograph of isolated rat ventricular myocyte. Staggered cell ends are evident; these are basis of the steplike intercalated disc profiles found in thin sections (cf. figs. 1-1 and 1-27). The transverse striations seen over the entire lateral surface are likely *Z ridges*, which probably are exaggerated by shrinkage of the sarcolemma over the Z discs of subsarcolemmal myofibrils. The curvature of this cell suggests origin from the ventricular wall. Scale bar represents 10 μm.

Table 1-1. Summary of contribution of subcellular components to myocardial cells of mouse heart[a]

Component	Parameter	Unit	Right ventricle[b]	Left ventricle[b]	Right atrium[b]	Left atrium[b]
Myofibrils	V_V	%	43.5 ± 0.9	43.2 ± 1.0	44.7 ± 1.0	44.5 ± 1.3
Mitochondria	V_V	%	38.2 ± 1.2	35.7 ± 0.9	24.7 ± 0.6	26.8 ± 0.6
Sarcoplasmic reticulum	V_V	%	6.9 ± 0.3	7.0 ± 0.3	12.2 ± 0.4	12.3 ± 0.4
Sarcoplasmic reticulum	S_V	μm^{-1}	1.87 ± 0.10	1.82 ± 0.08	2.76 ± 0.09	2.61 ± 0.14
Transverse-axial tubular system (TATS)	V_V	%	3.24 ± 0.10	3.13 ± 0.09	1.43 ± 0.11	1.61 ± 0.16
Transverse-axial tubular system (TATS)	S_V	μm^{-1}	0.50 ± 0.01	0.59 ± 0.02	0.23 ± 0.02	0.26 ± 0.03
Nuclei	V_V	%	1.35 ± 0.1	1.30 ± 0.02	2.50 ± 0.5	1.72 ± 0.3

[a] Data summarized in part from Forbes et al. {60,75,76}.
[b] Value ± SEM.

cells are thicker and more voluminous than their atrial counterparts.

Working atrial cells

Although many of their cytologic features resemble those of ventricular muscle cells, the contractile cells of the atrium are substantially thinner (figs. 1-5 and 1-36) and frequently possess a poorly developed system of T tubules (or may lack T tubules altogether). The packing of muscle cells within atrial walls and trabeculae is less dense than is the case for the ventricular musculature. Intercalated discs are less elaborate and often consist largely of side-to-side attachments (figs. 1-5 and 1-36). The hallmark of atrial myocytes is the presence of *atrial specific granules* (figs. 1-36 and 1-38), dense-cored spheroids that appear in the nuclear pole cytoplasm, between myofibrils, and in the subsarcolemmal myoplasm.

Conductive cells

Cells of the AVCS display the most varied ultrastructure among the mammalian orders, as will be further considered in the section, *Conductive myocardial cells.* For the moment it is sufficient to state that the majority of nodal cells (i.e., those of the sinoatrial and atrioventricular nodes) are small and highly interdigitated to form characteristic cell groups (fig. 1-6). Nodal cells may, however, be difficult to distinguish from adjacent atrial cells, except on the basis of the numerous specific granules of the latter and the frequent Z-disc alterations in the former. The so-called Purkinje cells, which for the most part form subendocardial networks on the inner ventricular surfaces, are in many mammals thin cells with poorly developed intercalated discs and a fair amount of myofibrillar material. However, myofibril-poor cells can be seen as well in the AVCS; in certain mammals such as ungulates, Purkinje fibers are extremely large and are occupied by great quantities of glycogen and intermediate filaments {e.g., 11,12}. There is general consensus that AVCS cells lack a system of T tubules, although they sometimes display pleiomorphic sarcolemmal invaginations (see *Nodal cells*).

WORKING (CONTRACTILE) MYOCARDIAL CELLS

Cell shape and size

The overall forms of myocardial cells are not always apparent upon inspection of their profiles in the various tissue sections utilized for light and electron microscopy (fig. 1-1). A further degree of uncertainty is imposed by the existence within the mammalian heart of several rather distinct categories of cardiac muscle cells. To date, much of the investigation of three-dimensional structure has been carried out in the working ventricular myocardial cell, the classic form of the cardiomyocyte. This has been accomplished, for the most part, by the isolation of intact individual cells and the examination of those cells by various modes of microscopy (light, scanning electron, and transmission electron {e.g., 13–15}). The shape of the "typical" cardiac muscle cell is largely the product of its internal construction: The cell appears as a fasceslike assemblage of myofibrils, about which an external covering (the sarcolemma) is wrapped. The enveloped myofibrils may assume a variety of lengths, and thus frequently create staggered cell ends, which are the basis of the steplike intercalated disc profiles (see *Intermembranous junctions* and figs. 1-1 and 1-3). In situ, the shape of the cardiac muscle cell is dictated also to some degree by its surroundings, the ventricular cell's profile in particular conforming to the contours of the numerous blood vessels of the heart (fig. 1-4). It has been pointed out that ventricular cells are not the simple cylindrical entities implied to exist by some histology texts, but in fact may be bandlike or ribbonlike, displaying in addition a good amount of branching {16,17}. There has been increasing utilization of computer-based imaging of heart cell shape {18,19}; this has been profitably used to describe the forms of both atrial and atrioventricular bundle cells {18}.

The length of the "average" mammalian ventricular myocardial cell is commonly given as ca. 100 μm, with diameters on the order of 15–20 μm. In fact, the flattened configuration of ferret ventricular cells establishes for them both major and minor "diameters" of 26.8 μm and 8.3 μm, respectively {17}. Though it cannot be stated with certainty that individual myocardial cells retain their

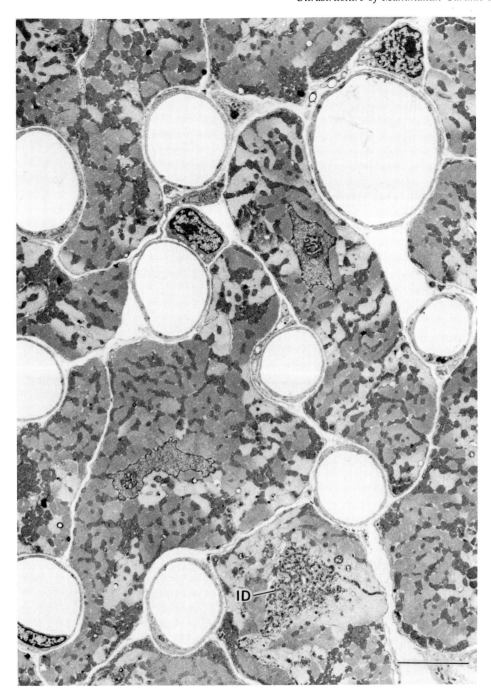

Figs. 1-4 to 1-6. Survey transmission electron micrographs of the three major categories of myocardial cells (samples taken from rhesus monkey), presented at the same magnification for comparison of the relative degrees of packing, shape, and size of the muscle cells.

Fig. 1-4. Right papillary muscle. In transverse section, these ventricular myocardial cells display extreme pleiomorphism. Profiles of cardiac myocytes are indented to accommodate the numerous blood vessels. In this field, myocardial nuclei are located in more or less central positions, and in one region a sizeable expanse of an intercalated disc (ID) is caught in section. Scale bar represents 5 μm.

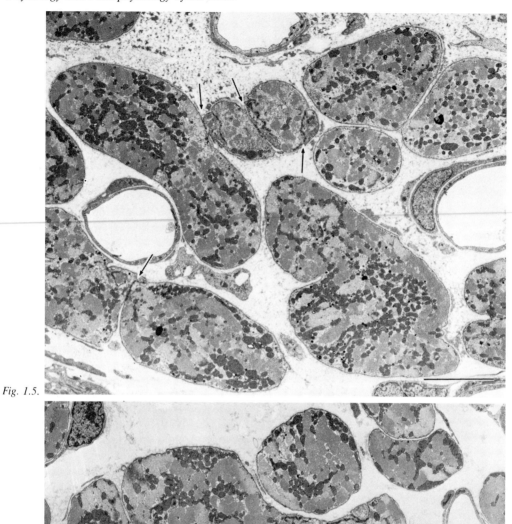

Fig. 1.5.

Fig. 1.6.

Fig. 1-5. Left atrial trabecula. Cell profiles are arranged in a loosely packed array. Although the cells vary widely in size, all are considerably smaller than ventricular cells (cf. fig. 1-4). Atrial intercellular attachments are largely invested in simple, side-to-side "spot-weld" appositions (arrows). Scale bar represents 5 μm.

Fig. 1-6. Sinoatrial node. These small cell profiles are characteristically joined together in groups by complex interdigitations (also see fig. 1-39). Scale bar represents 5 μm.

original shapes once they have become detached from one another, much of the recent data relating to cellular dimensions is derived from studies of single-cell preparations (figs. 1-2 and 1-3). There is variation between the results obtained by different investigators for similar preparations, however. Nag et al. {20} have given figures of 80 μm length and 12 μm diameter for isolated rat ventricular cells. On the other hand, Bishop and Drummond {21} record corresponding average values of 94 μm and 18 μm, but point out that two distinct cell types, mononucleate and binucleate, exist in adult rat ventricle. The binucleate cells constitute 85% of the total myocardial cell population, each possessing twice the volume of a typical mononucleate cell, and being both a third longer and a fifth again wider. Polyploidy is in fact common in ventricular cells (see *Nuclei*) and would be expected to create different populations — in terms of cell size — in a number of mammalian species.

Fibrillar components

MYOFIBRILS AND MYOFILAMENTOUS MASSES

In tonic, *fast-twitch* skeletal muscle, the discrete bundles of proteinaceous filaments (myofibrils) constitute the major portion of each cell (see table 1-1). Since a great deal of cardiac muscle terminology has been derived from the study of skeletal muscle morphology, the term *myofibrils* was automatically applied to the collections of contractile material found in heart cells (fig. 1-7). Few cardiac myofibrils attain in cross section the circular profiles and consistent small diameters of skeletal myofibrils, instead forming more massive assemblages of filaments, which in some instances partially or totally envelop the associated mitochondria (fig. 1-8). For this reason, McNutt and Fawcett {4} proposed the term *myofilamentous masses* as a more apt description of myocardial filament bundles. In this respect, myocardial cells of larger mammals are in fact reminiscent of phasic or of slow-twitch tonic skeletal muscle, whose myofibrils display a pleiomorphic *felderstruktur*, as opposed to the *fibrillenstruktur* typical of fast-twitch muscles such as frog sartorius. Conversely, *fibrillenstruktur* of a sort can be detected in smaller, fast-beating hearts, such as those of mouse and shrew (the arrangement of which apparently provides substantially greater expanses of surface upon which the system of sarcoplasmic reticulum tubules can form {fig. 1-22}). Most investigators have thus far elected to retain *myofibril* as the preeminent term for all bodies in muscle that are composed of actin, myosin, and α actinin (along with various accompanying proteins such as tropomyosin).

A longitudinally arrayed, striped pattern is obvious in cardiac myofibrils (figs. 1-1, 1-7, and 1-19). The details of this pattern are essentially the same for all mammals examined, and comprise the I bands, A bands, and Z bands (or *Z lines*, *Z discs*). These designations correspond to the terms derived from examinations of muscle with polarized light (I, isotropic; A, anisotropic) and from observations by German histologists (Z, *zwischenscheibe*, "dividing line"; H, *helle zone*, "light zone"; M, *mittellinie*,

"middle line"). The classic longitudinal unit of each myofibrils is the *sarcomere*, which contains two "half" I bands and one A band (see fig. 1-7). Strictly speaking, each sarcomere length also incorporates the transversely bisected halves of two Z bands; a more practical view is to consider a sarcomere as constituted by each region bracketed by adjacent Z bands. The construction of cardiac myofibrils has been actively studied {e.g., 4}, but exact details of structure, particularly the architecture of Z bands and of the "pseudo-H" zones at the midsection of the myocardial sarcomere, remain obscure.

In transverse view, cardiac Z bands may display an assortment of patterns, each known by a descriptive term: *basket weave*, *large square*, and *small square*. Combinations of patterns may be observed in the same transverse Z-band profile (figs. 1-8 and 1-9). The various appearances may depend on such factors as tilt of the plane of section (fig. 1-9) and the level through which the Z band has been cut {22,23}. The type of fixation used may also play a role in the generation of Z-band patterns in muscle {24}. A system containing both large axial and finer oblique "connecting" filaments makes up the Z-band latticework, which itself is likely a labile complex, judging from its coexistent variations in substructure {23}. Z bands of ventricular (fig. 1-7) and atrial (fig. 1-37) working fibers differ considerably in appearance; it remains for intensive study of the sort described above to be carried out on atrial Z discs.

Under conditions of myofibrillar relaxation, actin filaments do not project into the central zone of the sarcomere, the M-band–L-line complex (*pseudo-H zone* {4}). Three alternating striations, in the longitudinal order of L line/M band/L line, compose this region (figs. 1-7 and 1-11). The two L lines encompass those segments of myosin filaments that are neither connected by myosin-actin crosslinks (such connections, together with the overlap of actin and myosin, are the structural basis of the A band), nor by myosin-myosin crossbridges (the presence of which contributes to the opacity of the M band: figs. 1-10 and 1-11). The presence of M bands is the colophon of the mature sarcomere; in rat heart, for example, the appearance of M-band crossbridges begins only postnatally {25}. In the heart of the guinea pig, which is virtually fully developed at the time of birth {26,27}, M bands are already evident by the eighth week of gestation (unpublished observations).

The characteristic resting length of sarcomeres in mammalian ventricular cells is on the order of 2.2 μm. Approximate values for the dimensions of the various sarcomere segments are Z band, 80–160 nm; I band (each half), 0.35 μm; A band, 1.45–1.65 μm; M band, 70–90 nm; L lines, 10–20 nm. The contribution of each actin filament to the individual sarcomere is 1.25 μm or less (much of the actin filament being obscured in the relaxed sarcomere because of its overlap with myosin within the A band). It is not yet clear whether actin filaments traverse the Z band, form — or fuse with — other, thicker filament segments, or terminate in some fashion inside the Z lattice {5}.

Adjacent myocardial myofibrils often do not achieve side-to-side sarcomeric register (figs. 1-1, 1-7, and 1-36),

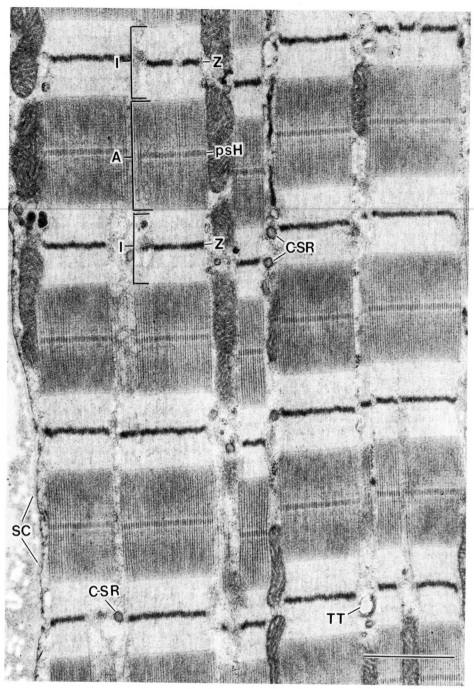

Fig. 1-7. Rhesus monkey right papillary muscle. In this longitudinally cut cell, the classic banding pattern of relaxed myofibrils is evident. Each sarcomere is delimited by Z bands (Z) and consists in addition of two "half" I bands (entire I bands are denoted I) and the opaque A band (A), which occupies much of the sarcomere length. At the center of the sarcomere there appears the M-band–L-line complex or *pseudo-H zone* (psH), which is shown in greater detail in fig. 1-11. A number of cell structures are known to be located preferentially at the Z-band level of the myofibrils {28}. Among these are transverse tubules (TT) and spheroidal expansions of the sarcoplasmic reticulum (*corbular SR*: C-SR), here seen as individual profiles (cf. figs. 1-19 and 1-26). The sarcomere pattern of the centermost myofibril is out of register with respect to the remaining myofibrils, a common occurrence in myocardial cells (also see figs. 1-1, 1-8, and 1-19). At the left of the micrograph is the cell surface (sarcolemma), which bears a lightly opaque covering (the surface coat: SC) on its extracellular side. The electron-lucent profiles near the surface coat are negatively stained collagen fibrils. Scale bar represents 1 μm.

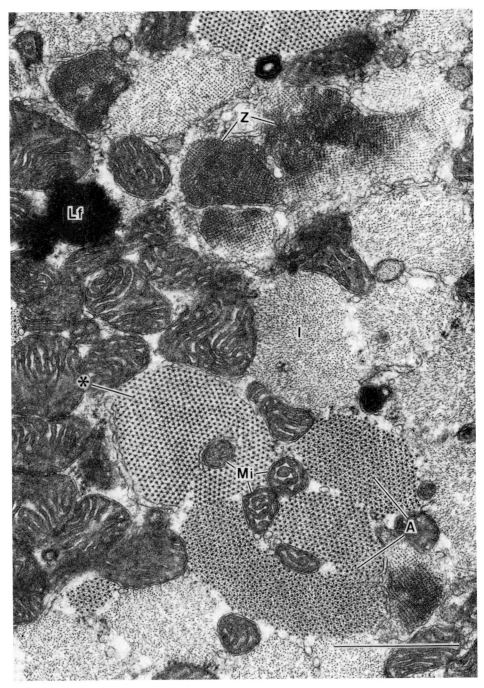

Fig. 1-8. Rhesus papillary muscle cell in transverse section. In this field all the divisions of the sarcomere appear in cross section (cf. fig. 1-7). Several areas of Z-line substance (*Z discs*) appear at the top of the field (Z); other regions contain elements of the I band (I) and A band (A). One myofibril is cut at its midlevel (*), a detail of which is shown in fig. 1-10. Note that the myofibrillar profiles are pleiomorphic, forming a *felderstruktur* similar to that of slow skeletal muscle. Mitochondria are massed between myofibrils, and some (Mi) are enveloped by them. Lf = lipofuscin body. Scale bar represents 1 μm.

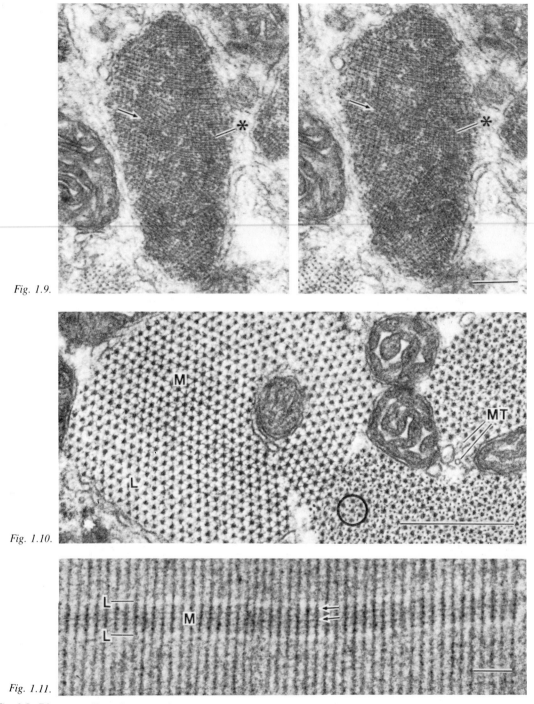

Fig. 1.9.

Fig. 1.10.

Fig. 1.11.

Fig. 1-9. Rhesus papillary. Stereoscopic pair of micrographs (20° angle of convergence) taken of a transversely sectioned Z disc. The substructure within the disc is the product of interdigitation of longitudinal and transverse filamentous components. The predominant pattern formed in this disc is that called the *small square* (exemplary region indicated by arrow); in other areas, the *basket-weave* pattern, actually the product of a negative image formed by the included fibrils, can be discerned (*). If, however, the latter region of the Z disc is compared on a "right-eye, left-eye" basis in the individual micrographs, it can be seen that the basket-weave apparent in the left-hand micrograph is converted into a pattern approaching the small-square configuration in the right-hand micrograph. Scale bar represents 0.2 μm.

Fig. 1-10. Detail of fig. 1-8. Plane of section passes through the A band of the myofibrils. At the right, the six-around-one actin-myosin configuration is seen (circled), denoting a region located to one side of the midlevel of the sarcomere. At the left, the substructure of the pseudo-H zone is revealed; at the edge of the myofibril, naked, roughly triangular myosin filaments appear (L: L-line level); and toward the center of the myofibril prominent crossbridges are present between the myosin filaments, thus indicating passage of the section through the M band (M; cf. fig. 1-11). Note the scalloped appearance of some of the mitochondrial cristae, and the transversely sectioned microtubules (MT) in the myofibrillar interstices. Scale bar represents 0.5 μm.

Fig. 1-11. Longitudinal section through the pseudo-H zone of a cardiac myofibril. Short, bare stretches of myosin filaments constitute the L lines (L), whereas the myosin segments of the broad central M band (M) are characterized by thin crossbridges (arrows). Scale bar represents 0.1 μm.

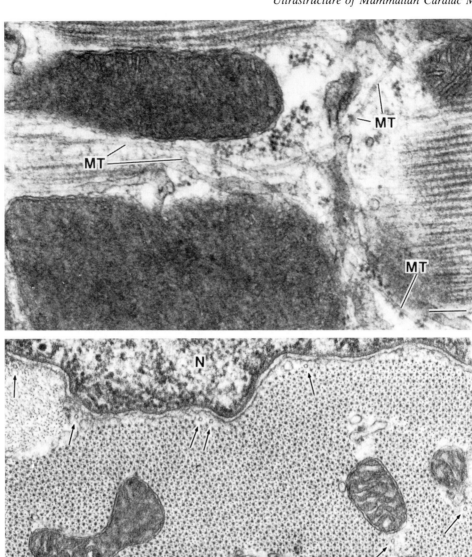

Fig. 1.12.

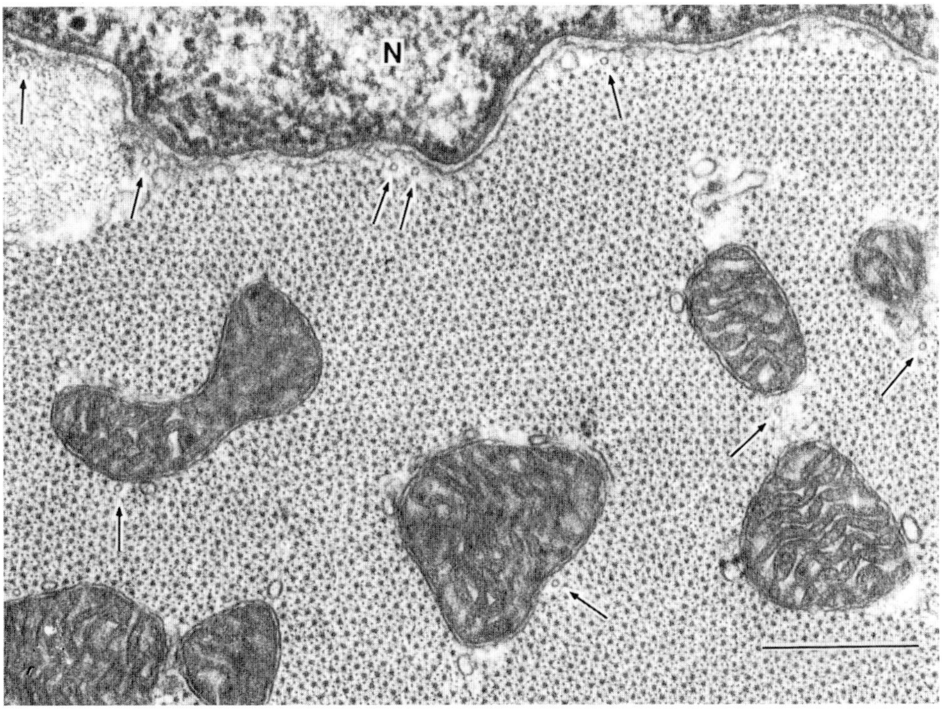

Fig. 1.13.

Fig. 1-12. Mouse ventricular myocardial cell. Microtubules (MT) run both longitudinally and obliquely in this field, the individual tubules tending to bend over the level of the I band. Scale bar represents 0.2 µm.

Fig. 1-13. Rhesus monkey papillary muscle. Cross sections of microtubules (arrows) can be found near the border of the nucleus (N), as well as in the myoplasm between the myofibrils, and thus often are located adjacent to mitochondria. Scale bar represents 0.5 µm.

and for this reason thin transverse sections of cells are found that capture examples of all basic levels of the sarcomere (fig. 1-8). Misalignment of myofibrils is related to the uneven contours of the intercalated discs at the myocardial cell tips (figs. 1-1, 1-27, and 1-37). Given that the point of each sarcomere's insertion into the intercalated disc occurs at the level at which the Z bands would be formed (figs. 1-1 and 1-27), and considering the varying lengths of excursions of the intercalated disc, the skewed alignment of adjacent myofibrils naturally follows (though the degree of individual myofibrillar growth may be involved as well).

The early formation of the myofibrils during embryony appears to influence the formation of segmented portions of sarcoplasmic reticulum, as well as the orientation of the transversely arranged components of the T-axial tubular system (TATS; see *Transverse-axial tubular system*). The Z band of the sarcomere seemingly dictates the positioning of certain myocardial cell components, among them T tubules, junctional SR saccules, *Z tubules* of SR, and intermediate filaments, most examples of which gravitate so as to be aligned parallel to the Z disc (figs. 1-14, 1-15, 1-20 to 1-22, and 1-26). Because of this preferential orientation of many cell structures, there is exclusion by them of other organelles such as mitochondria (figs. 1-1, 1-7, and 1-19), which ordinarily do not occupy the regions that constitute the *Z-level myoplasm* {28}.

MICROTUBULES

Microtubules are, in the majority of cells, the premier element of the cytoskeletal system. In the highly organized cardiac muscle cell, the system of myofibrils, whose own elements are closely packed, oriented in a predominantly longitudinal array, and securely anchored in the substance of the intercalated disc, there seems minimal need for an additional organized intracellular framework. Despite this seemingly logical conclusion, several studies have already demonstrated the presence of numerous microtubules in heart cells {e.g., 8,29,30}. Cardiac microtubules run largely in the longitudinal axis of the cell, are particularly concentrated about the nucleus (fig. 1-13), and also appear between the myofibrils — especially near mitochondria — and at the cell periphery (fig. 1-13). Goldstein and Entman {30} report, further, that microtubules in dog heart wind in helical patterns about the nuclei and myofibrils; this may account for the finding of some nearly transversely oriented microtubules near the I- or Z-band levels of heart (figs. 1-12 and 1-24; also see Forbes and Sperelakis {8,28}).

Microtubules in heart muscle range from 24 to 30 nm in diameter and may achieve lengths of at least several micrometers (fig. 1-12). In postnatal rat heart, the numerical density of microtubules reaches a peak between 5 and 9 days of age, and then rapidly decreases to a value that is maintained into the adult heart {31,32}. The perinuclear collection of microtubules remains relatively constant, and it seems therefore that it is the perimyofibrillar microtubules that drop out of the population as the myofibrils achieve maximum development {32}.

INTERMEDIATE (10-NM) FILAMENTS

These fibrils, so named because of their diameters (range of ca. 7–11 nm, average of ca. 10 nm), which are roughly intermediate between the diameters of actin and myosin, are the second major cytoskeletal component of most cells. Their contribution to the myocardial cytoskeleton occurs primarily in the transverse plane of the cell, and most particularly at the Z-band level (figs. 1-14 and 1-15) {8,28,29,33}. Such filaments may be attached to the inner sarcolemmal surface and to the nuclear membrane {29}, thus contributing in substantial part to a series of parallel strata, which apparently confer rigidity in the transverse axis to myocardial cells {8,28}. Particularly in rodents, bundles of intermediate filaments encircle the myofibrils (fig. 1-15) and may contain upward of 50 filaments. The incidence of intermediate filaments seems considerably lower in carnivore and primate hearts than is the case in rodent heart. In thin sections, intermediate filaments are seldom encountered in substantial quantities along the longitudinal axis of the main body of the myocardial cell, a finding confirmed by immunologic observations {34,35}. When found, small numbers of longitudinal intermediate filaments appear at the cell periphery and in myofibrillar interstices. The intercalated disc is a prominent site at which intermediate filaments are found, specifically associated with the intracellular plaques of desmosomes (figs. 1-16 and 1-29).

MITOCHONDRIA

These organelles are the second most populous constituent of ventricular myocardial cells (myofibrils forming the greatest portion {5}; Table 1-1). The typical locations for mitochondria are the myoplasmic spaces, where they form longitudinal columns among the myofibrils (figs. 1-1, 1-2, 1-7, 1-8, 1-19, 1-22, and 1-27), in the subsarcolemmal spaces, and in the myoplasm leading away from the nucleus (figs. 1-17 and 1-32). Speculation has been offered that the intermyofibrillar mitochondria constitute a population that in functional nature is different from the subsarcolemmal collection of mitochondria {34–36}. Subsarcolemmal mitochondria have the singular quality, in a variety of mammalian myocardial cells, of forming "tailored" appositions with gap junctions {39}. Such complexes frequently incorporate connecting strands that seem to form an adhesive bond between the juxtaposed structures; this apparently specific attachment may be related to regulation of ${Ca^{2+}}_i$ in the immediate vicinities of gap junctions, which in turn may affect the electrochemical functioning of such junctions {40,41}.

Mitochondria in conventionally preserved heart cells, even though they assume orthodox (metabolically inactive) configurations, nevertheless exhibit a number of variations in internal pattern, for example, the rather densely packed, shelflike cristae of mouse ventricle (figs. 1-14 and 1-27) and the elaborate scalloped cristae of cat {42}, dog (fig. 1-19), and monkey (figs. 1-7 and 1-13). Rarely are mitochondria of working myocardial cells small or poorly endowed with internal membranes. In fact, in apparently

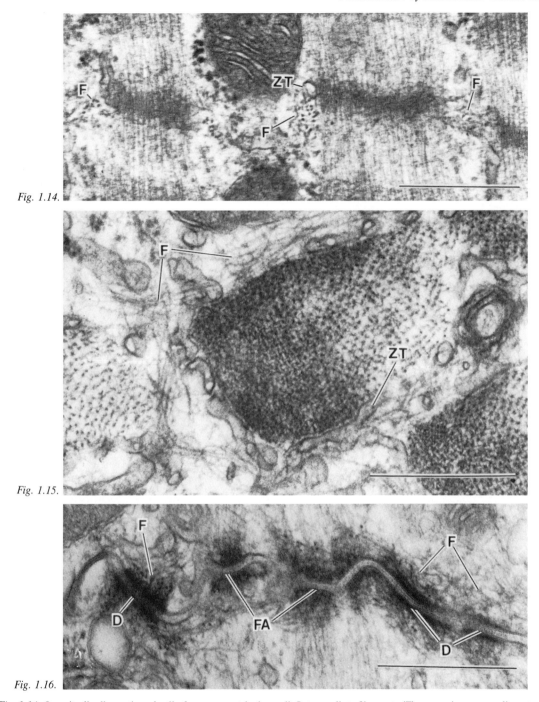

Fig. 1.14.

Fig. 1.15.

Fig. 1.16.

Fig. 1-14. Longitudinally sectioned cell of mouse ventricular wall. Intermediate filaments (F) appear in groups adjacent to the Z bands of the myofibrils. The transverse section of a *Z tubule* of sarcoplasmic reticulum (ZT) is also present in the Z-level myoplasm. Scale bar represents 0.5 μm.

Fig. 1-15. Transverse section of mouse ventricular myocardial cell. A Z disc is partially encircled by bundles of intermediate filaments (F). Z tubules (ZT) adhere closely to the surface of the myofibril. Scale bar represents 0.5 μm.

Fig. 1-16. Mouse ventricle. Intercalated disc formed between two apposed cell tips. Webworks of intermediate filaments (F) are closely associated with the intracellular plaques of desmosomes (D). Note the termination of actin filaments in the opaque substance of the *fascia adherens* junctions (FA). Scale bar represents 0.5 μm.

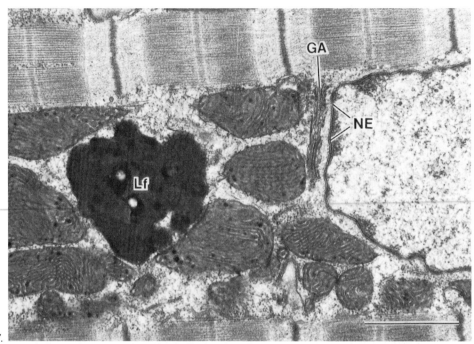

Fig. 1.17.

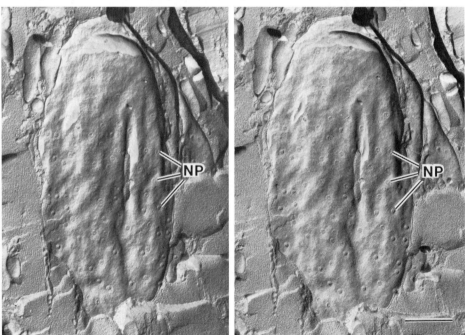

Fig. 1.18.

Fig. 1-17. Right ventricular wall of dog heart. This field, from a longitudinally sectioned myocardial cell, demonstrates typical contents of the "nuclear pole myoplasm," which extends longitudinally from the nuclear tips. A large lipofuscin body (Lf) dominates the field. Numerous mitochondria, which display dense granules and a variety of cristal configurations, also are packed into this myoplasmic compartment. The Golgi apparatus (GA) in this cell is a simple stack of saccules closely apposed to the nuclear envelope (NE). Scale bar represents 1 μm.

Fig. 1-18. Stereomicrographs that demonstrate the surface contours of a nucleus in mouse ventricular myocardium (stereo angle 20°). Numerous nuclear pores (NP) are distributed evenly in the nuclear membrane. Creases and folds also characterize the nuclear surface. Scale bar represents 1 μm.

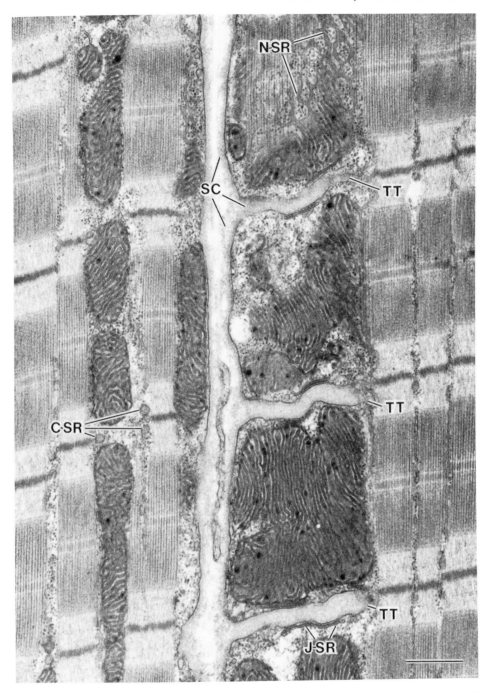

Fig. 1-19. Ventricular myocardial cells from dog right ventricular wall. The sarcolemma of the right-hand cell forms three T tubules (TT) oriented in register with Z bands of the nearest myofibrils. The substance of the myocardial surface coat (SC) can be seen both in association with the surface sarcolemma and within the T tubules' lumina. Three categories of sarcoplasmic reticulum can be discerned: network SR (N-SR) on the face of one myofibril; junctional SR (J-SR), flattened saccules apposed to the T tubules; and corbular SR (C-SR) (cf. figs. 1-7 and 1-26). Note mitochondria, either arranged in an intermyofibrillar row or located just beneath the surface sarcolemma. Scale bar represents 0.5 μm.

normal cells mitochondria may assume proportions that are truly gigantic, though giant mitochondria also may be symptomatic of pathology {43}.

Mitochondria in cells of the mammalian AVCS can vary widely in size, even within the same cells, and sometimes are small and poorly supplied with cristae (figs. 1-39, 1-42 to 1-44, and 1-46).

Nuclei

As mentioned in the section, *Cell shape and size*, multinucleate cells are the rule rather than the exception in mammalian ventricular cells. Binuclearity attains the majority (70%) by the end of the first postnatal week of life in the mouse {44}; approximately half of the right ventricular cells in human heart are binucleate by the end of the first year {45}; and in the rat 85% of muscle cells are binucleate in the adult {21}. Swine heart {46} and human heart {47} both achieve a high degree of polynuclearity, with as many as 22 nuclei observed in single myocardial cells of the pig {46}. The presence of multiple nuclei is likely the result of the persistence of karyokinesis, past the neonatal state, without the accompaniment of cytokinesis. This conclusion is supported by the discovery of single tetraploid nuclei in cells of neonatal mouse {44}. Complete mitosis ceases early in the postnatal life of the mammal {e.g., 48}, and in adults only atrial cells display any ability to divide {49}. It seems likely that the development of a stratified, oriented internal architecture is partly responsible for the inhibition of cytokinesis in ventricular muscle cells {e.g., 50}, though additional structural peculiarities of the myocardial cell may be involved (see *Centrioles*).

Myocardial nuclei generally are fusiform (figs. 1-1 and 1-18) and conform to the overall longitudinal arrangement of other major organelles (particularly myofibrils and mitochondria). Numerous infoldings and indentations may be present in nuclear envelopes (fig. 1-18). The elongate form of the nucleus may be controlled not only by the presence of surrounding myofibrils, but also by the microtubules that envelop them {29,30}. The lateral insertion and/or attachment of intermediate filaments {29} may be the agent responsible for the nuclear crenations that develop upon contraction of the myocardial cell {51}.

Myocardial nuclei may be located in peripheral or interior positions within the myoplasm (figs. 1-1, 1-7, 1-8, 1-13, and 1-19). Each nuclear pole has associated with it a conical myoplasmic region in which there appear Golgi saccules, centrioles (when present), mitochondria, rough and smooth endoplasmic (sarcoplasmic) reticulum, and a variety of lysosomes (including lipofuscin; fig. 1-17). Within individual cells examined in the same sample, the regions of "nuclear pole myoplasm" may range from being quite limited to occupying an extensive volume (fig. 1-32).

The surfaces of myocardial nuclei possess numerous rounded depressions ("pores"; fig. 1-18) at whose peripheries the outer and inner nuclear membranes fuse, and across which amorphous "diaphragms" extend.

Membrane systems

SURFACE SARCOLEMMA AND CAVEOLAE

The unit membrane that encloses the myocardial cell is usually referred to as the *sarcolemma*. The fact that there exist numerous folds, invaginations, and inpocketings of the sarcolemma has necessitated its terminological subdivision into (1) the *surface* or *peripheral sarcolemma*, that portion composing the large planar portions of the myocardial cell surface; (2) the *interior sarcolemma*, more commonly known as *transverse (T) tubules* or as the *transverse-axial tubular system* (TATS {8}; see the following section); and (3) *caveolae*, membrane-bounded vesicular structures that project inward from the cell surface, retaining luminal continuity with the extracellular fluid. The intercalated discs, which comprise sarcolemma regions containing specialized junctions and which are located at and near the cell ends, are considered separately (see *Intermembranous junctions*).

The majority of the surface sarcolemma is invested with a glycoproteinaceous covering, the least committal term for which is the *surface coat* (also referred to as *glycocalyx* and *basal lamina*). The surface coat is indistinct and largely amorphous in most electron-microscopic preparations (figs. 1-7, 1-19, 1-33, and 1-35). It is continuous over the mouths of caveolae, but does not appear to fill the caveolar lumina (fig. 1-35). In regions of close cell-to-cell apposition (e.g., the intercalated discs), the surface coat thins or disappears altogether. The surface coat has been thought to function in the trapping of certain ions, notably Ca^{2+} {52}, but the contribution of this particular external Ca^{2+} pool to the process of excitation-contraction coupling may not be especially significant {53}.

Caveolae bestow significant amounts of surface area to myocardial cells {54,55}, particularly to those cells that lack a TATS {56,57}. The evidence now available strongly suggests that proliferation of caveolae, from the surface of the muscle cell toward its interior, is the means whereby the TATS is formed in the course of myocardial development {8,26,58–60}.

TRANSVERSE-AXIAL TUBULAR SYSTEM (TATS)

The myocardial cells of mammals are essentially unique among vertebrates in their possession of extensive invaginations, conventionally refered to as transverse (T) tubules. Even in mammals, all cardiac muscle cells do not form T tubules; for example, certain atrial cells of the rat heart {56}, most atrial myocardial cells of guinea pig {61,62}, and many elements of the atrioventricular conducting system lack them. Where T tubules are found, they often are accompanied by longitudinally oriented (axial) tubules {8,60–62}. The interconnection in myocardial cells of transversely and axially oriented tubules has produced the concept of a *transverse-axial tubular system* or TATS {6,8,60–62}. The constituents of the TATS vary considerably among mammals. The tubules of mouse heart are characterized by small diameters and irregular profiles (fig. 1-20) {60}; on the other hand, the

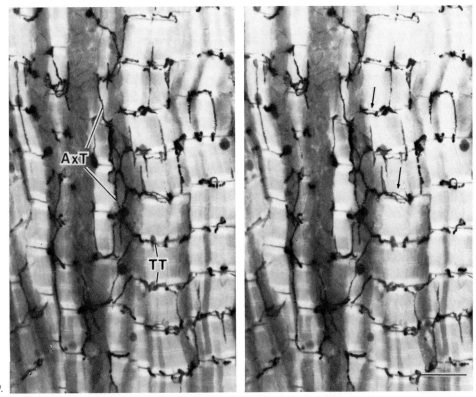

Fig. 1.20.

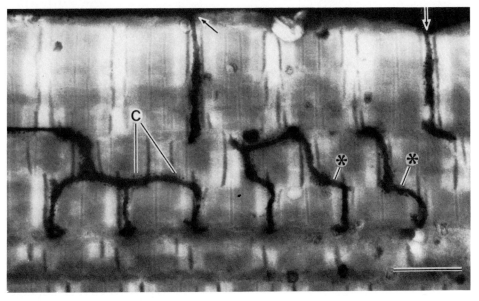

Fig. 1.21.

Fig. 1-20. Mouse ventricle. "Semithin" (ca. 1 μm thick) longitudinal section (stereo separation of 12°) of tissue whose system of extracellular spaces has been infiltrated with opaque material by means of postfixation in ferrocyanide-reduced osmium tetroxide (OsFeCN). Although many transversely oriented tubular structures are present (TT), numerous longitudinal and oblique tubules (collectively known as *axial* tubules: AxT) can be seen that frequently form connections between transverse tubules. "Beaded" segment profiles can be discerned (examples shown at arrows), the presence of which implies origin of the tubules from the proliferation of caveolar elements. The irregular contours, dilatations, and branching are typical of the mouse transverse-axial tubular system (TATS). Scale bar represents 2 μm.

Fig. 1-21. A 2 μm-thick section of OsFeCN-infiltrated TATS of rhesus monkey papillary muscle cell. The continuity of some T tubules with the surface sarcolemma is clearly shown (arrows). Deeper in the cell, transverse tubules are anastomosed with truly axial tubules (at the left), and toward the right half of the micrograph, obliquely oriented *axial* segments (*) connect T tubules oriented along Z lines of out-of-register myofibrils. The small opaque dots that decorate the TATS along much of its profiles are caveolae (C). Scale bar represents 2 μm.

TATS of guinea pig and monkey hearts (for example) is a collection of large-diameter tubules that often anastomose in rather regular latticeworks (fig. 1-21) that pervade the entire ventricular cell {6,8,61,62}.

The points of invagination of the transverse members of the TATS usually form at or near the successive sarcolemmal levels nearest the Z lines of the outermost myofibrils, and quite regular arrays of T-tubule openings are frequently apparent (figs. 1-19 to 1-21). Even if a T tubule does not originate squarely across from a Z line, it usually veers into a configuration so as to become aligned with the Z-line myoplasm {8,28,60} (figs. 1-20 and 1-21). As mentioned in the preceding section, the vectorial proliferation of caveolar elements from the sarcolemma, as well as from the caveolar chains themselves, is likely the mechanism, by which the TATS comes to exist. Profiles of the TATS in mouse heart very often reflect its caveolar origin (fig. 1-20; also see Forbes and Sperelakis {8,64} and Forbes et al. {60}), and in addition, caveolae are prominent along fully formed tubules (fig. 1-21). The significance of this latter finding is unclear, but it may indicate that the process of caveolation continues to a limited degree in the adult heart cell and can be called upon under conditions, such as cardiac hypertrophy, that necessitate additional growth of the TATS. In both neonatal and adult heart, the caveolae directly connected to the surface sarcolemma are seldom found as individual entities, but instead form alveolar collections of three to five fused caveolae; these have been found on occasion to form couplings with saccules of peripheral junctional SR {64}.

The larger examples of TATS elements are lined with surface-coat material (fig. 1-19), and it is likely that many of the smaller, more "primitive" transverse and axial tubules, such as those of mouse heart, are also coated {8}. A great deal of polymorphism is evident when the TATSs of various mammals are compared; average diameters of the tubules can range from ca. 50 to 500 nm (see the summary in Forbes and Sperelakis {8}), various cardiac muscle cells of mouse, rat, and shrew providing the lower values, and ventricular cells of guinea pig {61,62}, seal {65}, and golden hamster {66} achieving values at the upper end of the scale. The use of electron-opaque "tracer" materials, such as colloidal lanthanum hydroxide, horseradish peroxidase-diaminobenzidine-H_2O_2 reaction product, and the precipitate formed by postfixation in ferrocyanide-reduced osmium tetroxide (OsFeCN), has been vital in achieving appreciation of the form and extent of development of the TATS in mammalian heart {see 8 and 60 for further discussion}. Recently the combination of confocal scanning microscopy and membrane-specific fluorescent dyes has been used with some success to demonstrate the T system and SR of insect muscle {67}, and this approach is likely to be useful in mammalian cardiac muscle as well.

The contribution of the TATS to myocardial cells is considerably greater than that of the skeletal muscle T system. If the function of the cardiac TATS is primarily to bestow an optimum surface-to-volume ratio to each muscle cell, there would seem to be some physiologic disparity, since skeletal myocytes possess far greater

volumes (though the constitution of the TATS elements may be considerably different between the two types of muscle {5}). Substantial additional surface area is conferred to myocardial cells by caveolae, whether joined to the surface sarcolemma or to the TATS, or participating in extensive three-dimensional tubulovesicular arrays (*labyrinths*) found in mouse {8,58,59,63,68} and shrew hearts {8}. The development of a TATS is not directly attributable to the attainment of a certain cell diameter; it has been shown that large (30–50 mm diameter) conducting system muscle cells lack a TATS {e.g., 5} and that T-tubule development in the dog is initiated in cells of the left ventricle, which are of smaller average diameter than their counterparts in the right ventricle {69}. It has been suggested {5} that the TATS is an accommodative feature of those myocardial cells that can undergo hypertrophy, since cells of the AVCS lack a TATS and do not undergo enlargement. The fact remains that regions of excitable membrane and extracellular fluid are provided to all levels of the myocardial cells that contain the TATS {6}, and furthermore, that TATS distribution is reasonably even among different regions and depths of the ventricles {70}, thus potentially optimizing the conditions and processes that result in excitation-contraction coupling.

The TATS is the final system to develop in myocardial cells, and under culture conditions may not develop at all {71}, though some workers have now documented the reformation of T tubules in cultured adult myocytes {72,73} as well as the induction of T-tubule formation in cultures of neonatal cells {73}. The majority of mammalian hearts have not achieved TATS development by the time of birth, but the precocity of some species has been documented (e.g., the guinea pig {26,27}). It has been pointed out, however, that for different species the stages during which the TATS begins development are the same, that is, the heart of guinea pig and rat are equivalent in structural development when T tubules form, even though in the two species these stages occur, respectively, at the eight week of gestation and 1–2 weeks postnatally {27}.

SARCOPLASMIC RETICULUM

The equivalent of endoplasmic reticulum in muscle cells, *sarcoplasmic reticulum* (SR), exists in heart muscle in a variety of configurations that are structurally distinct yet contiguous. The bulk of the SR is made up of the *network SR* (N-SR), which appears in the form of meshworks that are closely applied to the myofibrillar surfaces (figs. 1-22 and 1-23). Specialization and segmentation of the N-SR according to the pattern of the underlying sarcomeres is commonly observed (figs. 1-22 and 1-23); in particular, closely packed tubules may anastomose over the central regions of the A bands to form fenestrated collars {74–76}, and *Z tubules* of SR encircle the myofibrils at their Z-line levels in the mouse and other mammals {e.g., 8,28} (figs. 1-14 and 1-15). Distended regions of N-SR have also been described {8,77,78}. Such *cisternal* SR is not limited in incidence to any particular level of the sarcomere, and can thus be readily distinguished from *extended junctional* SR (see below), which is formed primarily at the Z-line

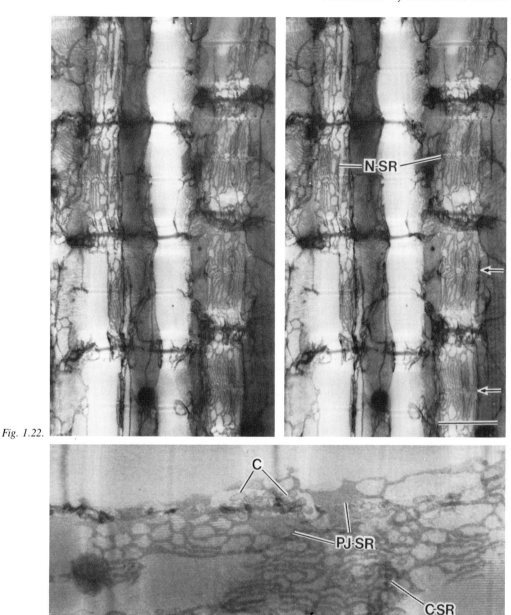

Fig. 1.22.

Fig. 1.23.

Fig. 1-22. Stereoscopic micrograph pair (12° stereo angle) of mouse ventricular tissue treated in such a manner that OsFeCN postfixation results in opacification of the sarcoplasmic reticulum (SR). In this semithin (ca. 0.3 µm) section, extensive arrays of SR are superimposed on the faces of myofibrils. Although the SR is continuous across the Z lines, it nevertheless forms a similar segmented pattern over each sarcomere. Over the A bands, most elements of network SR (N-SR) are found in the form of closely packed, parallel longitudinal tubules that mass in perforated retes (*fenestrated collars*: arrows) over the M-band level. Over the I bands, a looser meshwork of SR tubules appears. Such a pattern is typical of deep regions of the mouse myocardial cell (cf. fig. 1-23). Scale bar represents 1 µm.

Fig. 1-23. Tissue same as fig. 1-22. The section passes close to the surface of an SR-stained cell (note caveolae, C), where the loose-mesh N-SR configuration tends to dominate, the tubules anastomosing with expanded areas of junctional SR (in this case, peripheral J-SR, PJ-SR). Corbular SR (C-SR) also appears over a Z line. Scale bar represents 0.5 µm.

level. This complex three-dimensional arrangement of SR relative to sarcolemma, TATS, and myofibrils has recently been confirmed in elegant SEM studies of rat heart in which the *ground cytoplasm* has been extracted {79}. A substantial amount of rough endoplasmic reticulum (RER) also appears to be continuous with N-SR in adult heart, especially in association with Z tubules {80}.

The second major division of myocardial SR comprises the various categories of *junctional* SR (J-SR), the most noticeable examples of which form couplings (figs. 1-19 and 1-23 to 1-25). Myocardial couplings have often been called *triads* (two elements of J-SR complexed with a single T tubule), the term being derived from the study of skeletal muscle ultrastructure. Although the derivative *diad*, which describes the apposition of a single J-SR element with the sarcolemma (see fig. 1-25), seems adequate, the use of *triad* has been vitiated by the finding of numerous couplings (in the mouse, for example {8,60, 63}) that incorporate widely varying configurations, including circles of J-SR around TATS elements, *reversed triads* in which two TATS profiles flank a single J-SR saccule, S-shaped entwinements of J-SR and the TATS, and other formations.

Viewed en face, junctional SR saccules appear as roughly discoidal or oblong expansions into which N-SR tubules lead (figs. 1-23 and 1-24). In sagittal section (side view, so to speak), the J-SR is flattened in the vertical plane relative to the associated tubules of N-SR (in contrast to the situation in skeletal muscle, in which each example of the J-SR {*terminal cisterna*} is substantially distended). In the vertical plane of section, the two hallmarks of cardiac J-SR are apparent. These are (a) the intrasaccular *junctional granules*, which fall into a somewhat linear array along the length of the J-SR profile (fig. 1-25); and (b) the *junctional processes*, which are represented by a variety of amorphous and membranelike profiles (fig. 1-25). The subject of junctional process structure in muscle (skeletal, cardiac, and smooth muscle cells inclusive) has recently received intense attention, which has now led to the description in the junctional gap of *pillars* {64,81–83}, which are thin bodies that exist in apparent continuity with the unit membranes of the J-SR and sarcolemma (or, in addition, the T-axial tubules, in the case of skeletal and cardiac myocytes). The elucidation of pillars among the population of junctional processes has been fomented by such techniques as membrane intensification by tannic acid mordanting {81,84} or en bloc staining with uranyl acetate solution combined with stereoscopic analysis {64}. In the latter instance, it appears that even small degrees of tilt of the plane of section with respect to the incident electron beam are sufficient to resolve quasi-membranous bodies in spaces where before in the junctional gap there appeared only amorphous substance {64}.

The spatial configuration of myocardial junctional processes remains unresolved. Modifications of freeze-fracture technology that have demonstrated junctional processes of skeletal J-SR {85} have not yet been successfully applied to cardiac muscle. In addition, thin-section analysis is made difficult by the superposition of the various layers of the coupling (see discussions in Forbes and

Sperelakis {8,86}). Nevertheless, it has been deemed likely that junctional processes of cardiac muscle, like those of skeletal muscle, are disposed in rows {5,7}.

Additional forms of junctional SR have been described in heart, all of which anastomose with N-SR, contain electron-opaque granules, and bear external projections that resemble junctional processes, but do not come into apposition with the sarcolemma or TATS. The overall classification for these bodies is *extended junctional SR* (EJ-SR) {5,7,8,87}. A commonly encountered variety of EJ-SR is *corbular SR* (*coated SR* {4}), 80- to 120-nm spherules that appear to bud from the N-SR or exist in vesicular chains, usually near the Z lines (figs. 1-7, 1-26, 1-40). Corbular SR appears with widely varying frequency among different species and between different regions of the myocardium, and when found may exist singly, in small groups, or in clusters containing 5–10 vesicles. A peculiar form of EJ-SR has been described in mouse atrium {76}, in which circlets of SR bearing junctional processes and containing junctional granules appear in the myoplasm free of any connection of sarcolemma or TATS element, but are located where couplings with the TATS would be expected, i.e., at the Z-line levels.

Cisternal or saccular expansions of the SR have now been described in mouse heart {8}; these lie in deeper myoplasmic regions and are positioned over Z lines. They resemble nothing so much as J-SR components of interior couplings that have formed in the absence of contact with the TATS, a phenomenon first described in avian heart {87}. Additional variations of myocardial SR structure have been noted, including proliferations of J-SR {e.g., 88} and of N-SR {8}, as well as dense-cored segments of the N-SR {8}.

Enzymes and other proteins (e.g., Ca^{2+}, Mg^{2+}-ATPase, calsequestrin: {89–91}) associated with the cardiac SR are likely to be involved primarily in the sequestration and release of Ca^{2+} ion, and the pillarlike structures within couplings may be electromechanical devices whereby the action potential or other signals are relayed to the J-SR, thence to the rest of the internal SR membrane system that envelops the myofibrils {e.g., 64,83}.

During myocardial development, couplings first appear at the cell periphery, but as the TATS forms, increasing numbers of interior couplings arise, to the degree that the latter preponderate by far in adult heart {75,92,93}. In mouse ventricular cells, between 13% and 16% of the TATS surface is involved in couplings, and is thus equivalent in this respect to the situation for the surface sarcolemma {75,93}. The mechanism(s) by which couplings are formed may be related to an inductive effect derived from sarcolemma-SR contact; however, in consideration of the presence of EJ-SR, other influences, such as that of the Z lines and associated myoplasm {28}, should also be considered.

Intermembranous junctions: Intercalated discs

Myocardial cells are joined to one another by numerous intermembranous junctions, most of which are collected into adhesive complexes known as *intercalated discs*. These

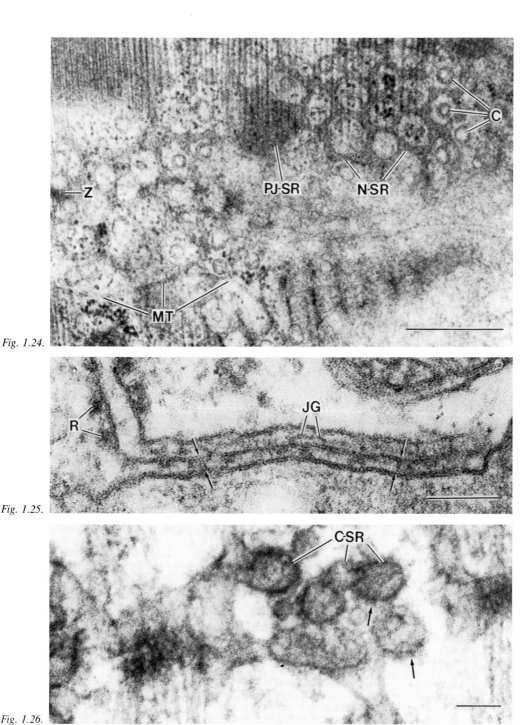

Fig. 1.24.

Fig. 1.25.

Fig. 1.26.

Fig. 1-24. Vervet monkey. Thin section, grazing surface of myocardial cell from right ventricular wall. Note caveolae (C) interspersed with meshes of network SR (N-SR) (cf. fig. 1-23). In this conventionally stained tissue, the greater opacity (relative to the N-SR) of the contents of the junctional SR saccule (PJ-SR) can be readily appreciated; this results in part from the presence of junctional granules and processes. The undulating profile of a microtubule (MT), oriented transversely across a myofibrillar face (Z, Z band), appears at the lower left. Scale bar represents 0.5 μm.

Fig. 1-25. Mouse ventricle. High magnification of peripheral J-SR saccule, showing its connection with N-SR tubule, here studded with ribosomes (R). Salient J-SR features are present, including the intrasaccular junctional granules (JG) and the junctional processes in the gap between the J-SR and surface sarcolemma. Some processes (*pillars*: between arrows) appear to join the apposed membranes and themselves appear membranelike. Scale bar represents 0.1 μm.

Fig. 1-26. Mouse ventricle. At the Z-line level, several examples of corbular SR (C-SR) are found, fused with N-SR tubules. Opaque contents and surface-connected projections, some membranelike (arrows), characterize these spherules of *extended junctional SR*. Scale bar represents 0.1 μm.

complexes incorporate the sarcolemma, that borders the ends of the cells, as well as additional, variable expanses of lateral sarcolemma near the cell ends (figs. 1-1 and 1-27). The sarcolemma of the intercalated disc is divided into four structural areas, those occupied by (a) *fasciae adherentes* ("intermediate" junctions), (b) *maculae adherentes* (desmosomes), (c) *maculae communicantes* (gap junctions, nexuses), and (d) unspecialized or "general" sarcolemma {94,95}.

For the most part, *fasciae adherentes* are regions in which the myofibrils terminate, the actin filaments apparently anchoring in the vague, opaque substance underneath the sarcolemma (figs. 1-16 and 1-27). Structured material is sometimes found in the intercellular gap of the *fascia adherens* {3,94}, but at best this extracellular material does not approach the complexity of the central lamella of desmosomes, a structure that may to a large degree be the basis of adhesion between adjacent myocardial cells {96}. Desmosomes are characterized additionally by discrete collections of opaque subsarcolemmal material (*plaques*), which face one another across the intercellular space and are matched in length in each of the apposed cells (fig. 1-29). The central lamella appears to receive filamentous projections from the sarcolemma; it has been proposed that different linking proteins are present between intermediate filaments and the intracellular portions of the desmosome {97}. The third junctional category, gap junctions, as well may be instrumental in cell-to-cell connection, both in mechanical and in electrical terms. In the mechanical sense, the integrity of the gap junction has been shown to be resistant both to pathologic conditions {98} and to processes that attempt by enzymatic and/or ionic means to separate the cells {99}; such findings necessarily ascribe to the gap junction some measure of adhesion. The more generally acclaimed function of gap junctions, particularly those of myocardium, is one of electrical communication via fluid-filled channels, which may exist in continuity with the myoplasm of both connected cells. The intercalated disc is a patchwork of the three types of junction, which are interspersed with areas of general sarcolemma that bear no intracellular or extracellular adornments (figs. 1-27 to 1-29 and 1-31). The contours of intercalated discs can be both species specific — and also region specific — within the same heart. Among mammalian ventricles, the discs in rodent heart exhibit a "wavy" pattern because of the presence of extensive, fingerlike longitudinal excursions and incursions (fig. 1-27). On the other hand, the tips of carnivore and primate ventricular cells are far more geometric in contour; wide expanses of the intercalated discs in such hearts are truly discoidal (figs. 1-1 and 1-28) {89}, and the longitudinal deviations are rectangular in profile, thus creating the classic "steplike" appearance of the intercalated disc (fig. 1-1). Intercalated discs of atrial and conductive cells incorporate a great deal of longitudinal sarcolemma (figs. 1-37, 1-39, and 1-42), and the disc segments are much less tightly corrugated than is usually the case in working ventricular muscle cells (fig. 1-28) {also see review in 94}.

The interdigitation of the various junctional categories is largely the product of the positions taken by the myofibrils, which specifically terminate in the *fasciae adherentes* (fig. 1-27). Therefore the majority of the transversely oriented sarcolemma — as well as some of the longitudinal component — of the disc is immutably occupied. Desmosomes and gap junctions therefore are relegated for the most part to the longitudinal folds, and only secondarily appear in the limited available sarcolemma in the intermyofibrillar spaces of the transverse component of the intercalated disc (figs. 1-27 to 1-30). Perhaps because of their intercalated discs' substantial investment in large expanses of longitudinally disposed sarcolemma, the ventricular cells of mouse and guinea pig exhibit gap junctions that are quite extensive {94,100}; this possible interspecies disparity in the total contribution of gap junction membrane is deserving of morphometric study, in view of both the controversy that remains concerning the electric properties of myocardial intercalated discs {e.g., 94,101} and the substantial underestimates that apparently result from measurements of tissue not specifically stained to reveal obliquely sectioned gap junctions {102}.

Freeze-fracture replication and extracellular tracer techniques have both led to a better understanding of gap junctions, collectively revealing the distribution of subunits (*connexons*) in hexagonally packed aggregates (at least in conventionally prepared tissue: see Raviola et al. {103}) and the central dot {104} within each connexon (figs. 1-30 and 1-31), the cavity of which may be the basis of cell-to-cell ionic communication. Gap junctions and desmosomes are recognizable in freeze-fracture replicas, which afford a two-dimensional view of the distribution and extent of such junctions (fig. 1-31), whereas *fasciae adherentes* are seldom clearly defined in replicas {94}.

As pointed out in the section, *Intermediate (10-nm) filaments*, myocardial desmosomes are frequently associated with intermediate filaments. As stated above, the specific intracellular associate of the *fascia adherens* junction is the myofibril. We have recently demonstrated {39}, furthermore, that there may be gravitation of subsarcolemmal mitochondria to myocardial gap junctions (see *Mitochondria*).

Other organelles

GOLGI APPARATUS AND ASSOCIATED STRUCTURES

Stacks of flattened, fenestrated sacs form the major portion of Golgi apparati. Each Golgi apparatus may be limited, in the heart, to a few saccules that lie against the tips of nuclei (fig. 1-17), which is often the case in ventricular fibers, or may comprise, in a single cell, numerous sets of lamellae throughout the nuclear pole myoplasm (fig. 1-32). This latter configuration is especially characteristic of atrial myocytes, in which the Golgi collections at the nuclear tips are connected by additional Golgi saccules that extend longitudinally about the nucleus {105}. An additional feature of the atrial Golgi apparati is their generation of *atrial specific granules*, opaque spheroidal bodies that have been extensively investigated and found to comprise several morphologic subcategories, to contain

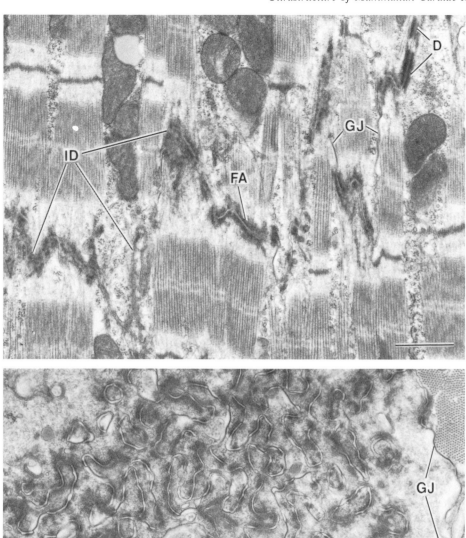

Fig. 1.27.

Fig. 1.28.

Fig. 1-27. Longitudinal thin section through intercalated disc (ID) of mouse ventricular wall. The actin filaments of the subjacent myofibrils terminate in the opaque intracellular material of the *fasciae adherentes* junctions (FA). The transverse portions of the intercalated disc thus substitute at these sarcomere levels for Z lines. Extensive, longitudinally aligned stretches of cell-to-cell appositions are common in hearts of rodents such as mouse and guinea pig, and these are the sarcolemmal sites at which desmosomes (D) and gap junctions (GJ) typically appear. Scale bar represents 1 µm.

Fig. 1-28. Transverse section of intercalated disc in dog ventricular myocardium. In working ventricular cells of carnivores and primates, the intercellular attachments form transverse planar arrays (cf. fig. 1-1), which in fact are disclike, and thus large expanses may be captured in a single transverse section (cf. fig. 1-4). As in the case of rodent heart (fig. 1-27), the longitudinal disc surfaces are the primary repository of desmosomes and gap junctions. An extensive gap junction (GJ) is present, in addition to a circular profile of gap junction membrane (C-GJ). Scale bar represents 1 µm.

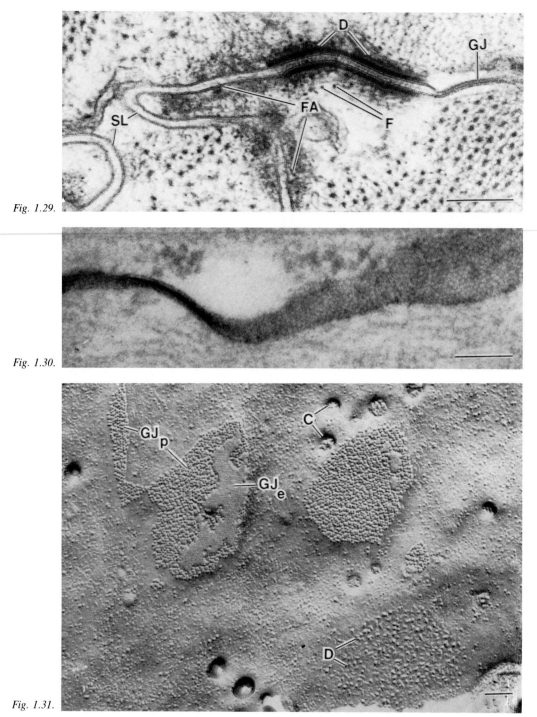

Fig. 1.29.

Fig. 1.30.

Fig. 1.31.

Fig. 1-29. Transverse section of mouse ventricular wall. Examples of the four sarcolemmal constituents of the intercalated disc are shown: the gap junction (GJ), septilaminar, and the most narrow region of the disc; the desmosome (D), characterized by a linear extracellular structure (the central lamella) and extremely opaque intracellular plaques, near which appear profiles of intermediate filaments (F); the *fascia adherens* (FA), which lacks the distinctly organized extracellular and intracellular components of the desmosome; and general sarcolemma (SL), the region in which caveolae and peripheral couplings are formed (see fig. 1-35). Scale bar represents 0.2 μm.

Fig. 1-30. Guinea pig papillary. Gap junction infiltrated with electron-opaque precipitate formed as a result of block staining with uranyl acetate. The thin section passes through a region in which the plane of the sarcolemma tilts, thus revealing the gap junction in side view at the left and en face at the right of the field. At the upper right the characteristic hexagonal packing of gap junction subunits (*connexons*), as well as the opaque central dot within each connexon, are made clear by the presence of the uranium precipitate. Scale bar represents 0.1 μm.

Fig. 1-31. Mouse ventricle. Freeze-fracture replica of lateral sarcolemmal region of intercalated disc (cf. fig. 1-27). In addition to the evenly distributed intramembranous particles on the P face of the general sarcolemma, there appear several groups of larger, tightly packed P-face particles of gap junctions (GJ$_p$); atop these aggregates appear small portions of the gap junction E face (GJ$_e$), which separated from the cell above in the fracturing process. The large particles distributed in a discoidal array at the lower right of the field are characteristic of a desmosome (D). C = caveolar openings. Scale bar represents 0.1 μm.

both carbohydrate and protein moieties, but not to consist of catecholamines {e.g., 106}. Specific granules are found throughout atrial cells (fig. 1-36) but are particularly concentrated in the nuclear pole myoplasm. The granules are apparently the source of peptides (e.g., *atrial natriuretic factor*, *atrial natriuretic peptide* {ANP}, *cardiodilatin*), which bring about vasodilatation and induce natriuresis and diuresis {107–109}.

Associated with Golgi apparatus in all cardiac cells are numerous vesicles of various sizes and appearances, including large and small pleiomorphic dense-cored bodies (fig. 1-32) and small clear-cored coated vesicles (fig. 1-32). Short segments of rough endoplasmic reticulum and of smooth-surfaced (sarcoplasmic) reticulum are frequent occupants of the nuclear pole cytoplasm, and thus can be found in apparent association with the Golgi region {80}; it is not yet clear, however, what confluency may exist between the membranes of the Golgi and the ER or SR {110}.

CENTRIOLES

When found, centrioles are located in the nuclear pole myoplasm, often in the vicinity of the Golgi apparatus. There are few published micrographs of centrioles in the ventricular cells of adult mammalian heart; however, centrioles are often discernible in atrial cells. It has been historically difficult to explain the exact function of centrioles, since they are not the intrinsic point from which microtubules become assembled to form the mitotic spindle. The paucity of centrioles in ventricular myocytes has been attributed to the low probability of encountering, in thin sections, these small, presumably paired, bodies within large volumes of myoplasm {42}. In view of the great frequency with which centrioles are encountered in developing ventricular myocytes of guinea pig and mouse (unpublished observations), an alternative, though speculative, explanation comes to mind, namely, that centrioles degenerate and disappear as a consequence of the completion of development of ventricular cells, which lose their cytokinetic competence in the adult heart (see *Nuclei*). It has been proposed that the loss of activity of DNA polymerase, leading to progressive DNA fragmentation and cessation of DNA replication, is responsible for terminal differentiation of the adult mammalian myocardial cell {111}. It was recently noted {112} that ventricular cells of transplanted human hearts are capable of regeneration of a sort, such that under conditions of transplant rejection, some myocytes appear to undergo dedifferentiation and redifferentiation. In ultrastructural aspect these cells resemble embryonic and neonatal cardiomyocytes from a variety of avian and mammalian species. No evidence of mitosis is seen in such hearts, however, and this supports the conclusion that cytokinesis is not normally within the purview of adult mammalian ventricular myocytes.

COATED VESICLES

A variety of different vesicular structures appears in heart cells. As noted above (*Golgi apparatus and associated structures*), small coated vesicles are characteristically associated with the Golgi apparatus, and may exist — in the static thin section — either free in the myoplasm or fused with a Golgi saccule (fig. 1-32), indicating the participation of such vesicles in a dynamic process. Larger coated vesicles are present in small numbers throughout myocardial cells (figs. 1-33 to 1-35); neither their origin nor function has yet been explained. The vesicles may be found fused with the sarcolemma (fig. 1-33) or TATS, or free in the myoplasm (figs. 1-34 and 1-35).

LYSOSOMES AND OTHER INCLUSIONS

The incidence of lysosomes per se is quite low in heart {5}, but membrane-bounded lipofuscin bodies (fig. 1-17; also known collectively as *aging pigment*) become increasingly common in the nuclear pole myoplasm as the animal grows older {113}. Lipofuscin is likely a form of residual body, the product of lysosomal engulfment and degradation of other organelles, most likely mitochondria {4,5}. Multivesicular bodies are found on occasion, and these have been likened to lysosomes {4}.

Lipid bodies and peroxisomes (microbodies) have been noted in myocardial intermyofibrillar and subsarcolemmal spaces, and can be distinguished cytochemically from one another. Peroxisomes, in addition to their reaction with diaminobenzidine and H_2O_2, also are characterized by their positions at the A-I levels of the sarcomeres {114,115}.

Glycogen particles occur with varying frequency in myocardial cells; individual *beta* particles are more prominent in slower beating hearts (such as those of cat and dog) than in fast-beating myocardia such as that of the mouse. Glycogen granules grouped together to form *alpha* particles appear in developing and neonatal hearts, and in some conductive cells {109}, but are not a common feature of mature working myocytes. McNutt and Fawcett {4} have noted the rather specific disposition of beta particles between the myofilaments in the I bands, and glycogen particles can be found in the various myoplasmic spaces, such as those adjacent to the nuclear poles, where they and ribosomes may easily be confused with one another (fig. 1-32).

CONDUCTIVE MYOCARDIAL CELLS: THE ATRIOVENTRICULAR CONDUCTING SYSTEM

Several relatively recent reviews are concerned with characterization of the conductive cells and pathways of the mammalian heart {e.g., 116–120}. These and other broader reviews of myocardial structure point out the great deal of anatomic variation that can exist between physiologically similar cells of different species. No attempt will be made here to summarize all these variations, but some of the more salient ultrastructural features of conductive cells will be considered, largely in the context of descriptions of working myocardial cells given in the preceding sections.

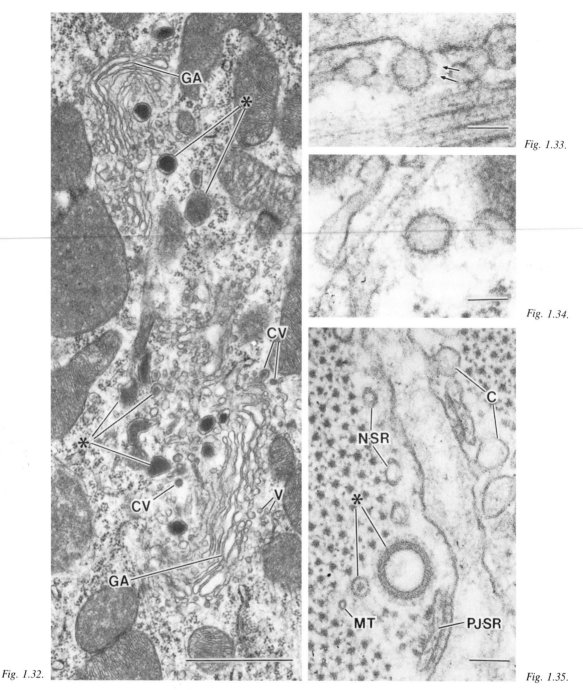

Fig. 1.33.

Fig. 1.34.

Fig. 1.32.

Fig. 1.35.

Fig. 1-32. Mouse ventricular myocardial cell; nuclear pole myoplasm, occupied in large part by Golgi apparati (GA). Although an extensive Golgi system is not a frequent constituent of ventricular cells, these profiles provide a composite view of the numerous aspects of the Golgi region. In addition to the dense-cored vesicles of varying sizes and shapes (*), which appear at the concave faces of the stacks of curved cisternae, there are numbers of small vesicles (V), largely associated with the forming convex Golgi saccules. Coated vesicles (CV) are present as well at both Golgi faces. Ribosomes, microtubules, and mitochondria coexist with the Golgi in nuclear pole myoplasm. Scale bar represents 1 μm.

Figs. 1-33 to 1-35. Coated vesicles of various configurations and locations in mouse ventricular myocardium.

Fig. 1-33. Coated vesicle fused with surface sarcolemma. Bristle-like projections (arrows) form part of the characteristic coating. Scale bar represents 0.1 μm.

Fig. 1-34. Coated vesicle deep in myoplasm. Note the similarity of its coating to that of the vesicle shown in fig. 1-33. Scale bar represents 0.1 μm.

Fig. 1-35. Transverse section of portions of two cells, demonstrating a variety of vesiclelike profiles, some of which are not truly spheroidal bodies, including cross sections of network SR (N-SR) at the myofibril periphery, and a microtubule (MT). Associated with the sarcolemma are surface-connected caveolae (C) and saccules of peripheral junctional SR (PJ-SR). Two atypical vesicles are present (*), one of which exhibits an opaque core. Scale bar represents 0.1 μm.

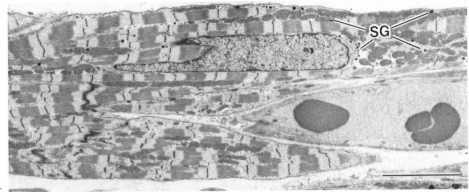

Fig. 1.36.

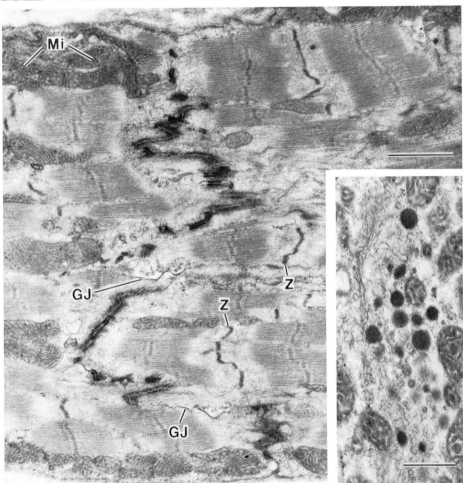

Fig. 1.37.

Fig. 1.38.

Figs. 1-36 to 1-38. Left atrial wall (longitudinal sections) from rhesus monkey heart.

Fig. 1-36. This section illustrates the thinness of the muscle cells of the atrium (cf. fig. 1-5). Atrial specific granules (SG) are scattered through the myoplasm of the upper cell. Scale bar represents 5 μm.

Fig. 1-37. The contours of this intercalated disc are irregular and largely involved in longitudinal folds, some of which contain gap junctions (GJ). Mitochondria (Mi) are smaller and less numerous than in working ventricular cells (cf. fig. 1-7). The lower degree of organization of these atrial cells also is denoted by their sarcomeric components (including Z bands: Z), which may be misaligned even in the same myofibril. Scale bar represents 1 μm.

Fig. 1-38. Golgi region, illustrating forming and mature atrial specific granules. Scale bar represents 0.5 μm.

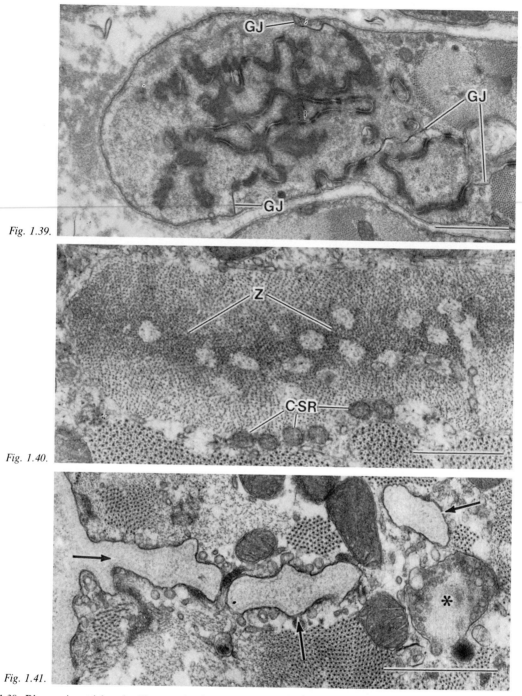

Fig. 1.39.

Fig. 1.40.

Fig. 1.41.

Fig. 1-39. Rhesus sinoatrial node. The complex interdigitations of apposed cells typifies nodal groupings (also see fig. 1-6). Gap junctions (GJ) are prominent in these intercalated disc profiles. Scale bar represents 1 μm.

Fig. 1-40. Rhesus SA nodal cell. Z discs (Z) in many of these cells exhibit numbers of circular defects (*perforations*). Numerous spherules of corbular SR (C-SR) also are characteristic of such cells. Scale bar represents 0.5 μm.

Fig. 1-41. Cat SA node. Certain nodal cells exhibit definite sarcolemmal infoldings (arrows), which are filled with surface-coat material. Granule-filled bodies (*) are common in these cells, and some of these can be traced to connection with the surface sarcolemma. Scale bar represents 1 μm.

Nodal cells

The major nodes of the AVCS, found in the right atrial region, are the sinoatrial (SA) and atrioventricular (AV) nodes. The two are connected by pathways often dismissed as being — in practical terms — more physiologic than anatomic; the AV node, in turn, gives rise to pathways that penetrate into the ventricles and ramify there in the form of the so-called Purkinje cell network. (Other pathways, from SA node to left atrium, apparently exist, however {117,120}). There often are described two major cell types in the nodes, those that are relatively myofibril rich and those that possess rather little contractile material; forms transitional between working atrial muscle cells and conductive cells have also been discerned {116}.

In thin sections, a reasonably dependable distinguishing characteristic of nodal cells is their tendency to group into clusters that contain several cells (figs. 1-6 and 1-39); this grouping appears to be the result of the involved interdigitation of cells via their *intercalated discs*, which in such cell groups are far less disclike than those of working myocardium, instead consisting largely of laterally placed junctional complexes (fig. 1-39). The interdigitation of cells within a nodal group typically is sufficiently involved that some cells may be wound about others, with tiny cell protrusions appearing in the midst of the intertwined members (fig. 1-39). The three main types of intermembranous junctions (see *Intermembranous junctions*) can usually be identified, but opinion has it that gap junctions do not occupy a major portion of nodal cell sarcolemma {5}.

The Z substance of myofibrils in SA and AV nodal cells often displays unusual morphologies. In some instances circular perforations appear in transversely cut Z discs (fig. 1-40). Longitudinal sections confirm the discontinuity of the Z bands across the widths of some myofibrils. An additional oddity of conductive cell myofibrils is the occasional presence of proliferated Z substance {121}, which forms intensely opaque myofibril segments (figs. 1-44 and 1-45) that resemble the nemaline rods of skeletal myopathy. Similar bodies are seen in working myocardium, particularly in older animals {122}. Such *Z rods* {22} are likely made up in large part (but not in their entirety) of tropomyosin. Their function in normal cells is not clear, but morphologically similar bodies have been proposed as the framework on which new sarcomeres are produced {123}. Their presence in pathologic skeletal muscle is thought to compromise myofibrillar contractility, but such an impediment is probably of minor consequence to cells of the AVCS, since their primary function is electrical rather than mechanical.

The sarcoplasmic reticulum of nodal cells consists of network SR, peripheral junctional SR, and numerous examples of corbular (extended junctional) SR (fig. 1-40; see *Sarcoplasmic reticulum*). In some cells, collections of N-SR are not specifically associated with the myofibrils, but instead occupy subsarcolemmal locations, intermingling there with filamentous material and glycogen particles {124}.

No clear-cut evidence has been presented to support the general presence of transverse tubules, much less a TATS (cf. *Transverse-axial tubular system*), in cells of the AVCS. Nevertheless a number of observations suggest that a variety of invaginations can form in such cells. For example, Osculati and Garibaldi {125,126}, Osculati et al. {127,128}, and Rybicka {124} have published micrographs that display indentations that emanate from the surface sarcolemma of Purkinje-type cells. In the SA node of cat myocardium, certain cells (fig. 1-41) contain large, membrane-bounded, granule-filled cavities that appear to be continuous with the sarcolemma, in view of occasional J-SR saccules that are attached to them. Some sarcolemmal intrusions, similar in form to T tubules, can be found as well (fig. 1-41). The above findings cast some doubt on the pat concept that AVCS cells can be distinguished de facto by their lack of a TATS. Whether or not the invaginations described are generated by a process similar to that which creates the TATS of working myocardial cells remains to be investigated. Such a determination will be significant in defining the parallels in construction that exist between contractile and conductive cells of the heart.

Purkinje cells

A great deal of controversy has developed over the conductive network of mammalian ventricle, beginning presumably with the work of Purkinje himself {129} (more properly spelled *Purkyně* {130}) and continuing with numerous other investigations that have questioned the singular identity and regional specificity of such cells (e.g., see Sherf and James {120}). The term continues to be readily recognized, however, even though exact definition seems yet forthcoming. Suffice it to say that the AVCS within the ventricle is largely composed of a highly ramified network of cells, subendocardial in location, which can be distinguished from the sometimes adjacent working fibers on the basis of one, or another, or more structural criteria. At this point the collection of qualified cells burgeons. Rodent Purkinje cells differ from working ventricular myocytes by little more than the lack of the TATS, it seems {131,132}. In shrew heart {133}, Purkinje cells are characterized by their small diameters and by relatively sparse complements of myofibrils and mitochondria. Purkinje-type cells of certain other species, however, display T-tubule-like structures (see the preceding section). Ungulates occupy an extreme of the spectrum, in having extraordinarily enlarged conductive fibers, often grossly discernible on ventricular surfaces, whose contractile apparati are virtually nil, which are devoid of T tubules, and whose volume is largely taken up by glycogen {e.g., 134,135}. Subdivision into categories of the Purkinje fibers of monkey heart has been attempted as well {116}.

Our own observations on rhesus monkey heart confirm the existence of at least two general types of cells in the subendocardial network. As in the case of nodal cells, the dichotomy is based on the greater and lesser incidence of myofibrillar material (figs. 1-42 and 1-43). The conductive cell having a prominent complement of myofibrils seems predominant; each example of this category, like nodal cells, is joined to its fellow cells by intercalated discs that

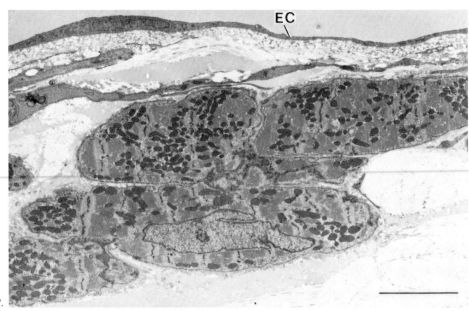

Fig. 1.42.

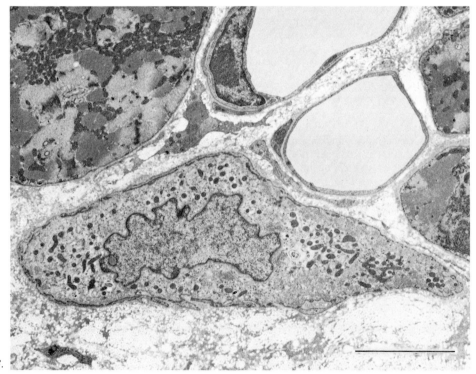

Fig. 1.43.

Figs. 1-42 and 1-43. "Purkinje" cells from ventricular subendocardial network of conductive cells in rhesus monkey heart.

Fig. 1-42. Small, myofibril-rich Purkinje cells, connected to one another by short, side-to-side appositions (see fig. 1-44) to form a thin network just beneath the endocardium (EC). Scale bar represents 5 μm.

Fig. 1-43. Transverse section of subendocardial "type I" {116} Purkinje fiber, identifiable by its overall lucent appearance relative to the adjacent working ventricular cells. Detail shown in fig. 1-46. Scale bar represents 5 μm.

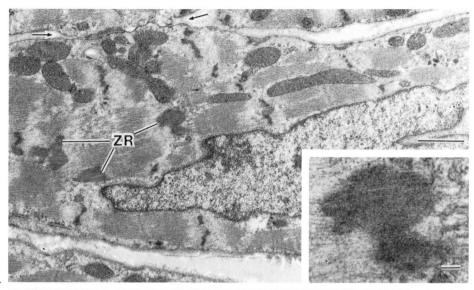

Fig. 1.44.

Fig. 1.45.

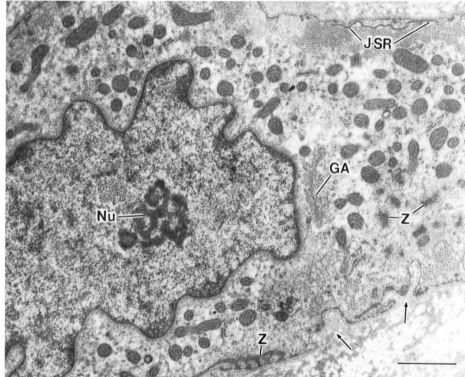

Fig. 1.46.

Fig. 1-44. Purkinje fibers in section alternate to that shown in fig. 1-42. Cell-to-cell adhesions are short (between arrows) and the substance of Z bands frequently proliferated to form *Z rods* (ZR). Scale bar represents 1 μm.

Fig. 1-45. Detail of Purkinje Z rod, illustrating its distinct substructure. Scale bar represents 0.1 μm.

Fig. 1-46. Detail of "clear" Purkinje cell. The nucleus exhibits a prominent nucleolus (Nu) and a crenated envelope. Myofibrillar material is sparse and tends to be located at the outer rim of the cell. Z-band material (Z) forms small dense profiles of various shapes. A limited Golgi apparatus (GA) is juxtaposed to the nucleus, and numerous small mitochondria are present in the electron-lucent myoplasm. Short sarcolemmal invaginations, lined with surface coat material, are seen (arrows). An elongate saccule of junctional SR (J-SR) undulates into and away from contact with the surface sarcolemma. Scale bar represents 1 μm.

are heavily invested in longitudinally oriented expanses of sarcolemma (fig. 1-42). There is also significant occurrence of nemalinelike aggregates of Z-disc substance (figs. 1-44 and 1-45), a phenomenon seen also in Purkinje cells of cow {136} and dog {137}. Myofibril-poor cells (probably equivalent to the type-I cells described by Virágh and Challice {116}) are spectacularly evident because of their "clear" appearance relative to other cells in their immediate vicinity (figs. 1-43 and 1-46). The contractile elements of such cells, like those of ungulate Purkinje fibers, are located primarily at the cell periphery. Their boundaries are convoluted, and the intermyofibrillar spaces (fig. 1-46) contain small mitochondria, microtubules, and some loosely arranged filamentous material (possibly composed in part of intermediate filaments {cf. 138}). Short sarcolemmal invaginations create undulated surfaces along stretches of cell border, and junctional SR of exceptional length — which becomes *extended J-SR* at some points (fig. 1-46) — is a notable characteristic of such cells.

CONCLUSIONS

Heart muscle, by dint of its essentiality to the survival of the body — particularly in regard to that of humans — has enjoyed commensurate interest in the form of scientific research. Understanding of the structure of heart muscle has been almost unbelievably expanded over the relatively short period during which cardiac ultrastructure has been studied {139}. Still the adjurations of Raymond Truex {119} come to mind as particularly apt. He has pointed out that the limitations imposed by light and electron microscopy are both significant and very different. By means of the first mode, light microscopy, the cell boundaries cannot be clearly identified; in the other (specifically transmission electron microscopy), the small sample size offered by thin sections is potentially deceptive, in terms of such tasks as measuring maximal cell diameters, even though resolution is increased as much as a thousandfold. In recent years the use of evolved techniques, for example, scanning electron microscopy in combination with single-cell isolation, freeze-fracture replication, stereoscopic thick-section examination of selectively opacified heart tissue, and computer-based reconstruction of cell shapes, has helped to close the information gap that existed in 1974 between 5-μm and 50-nm tissue sections. Nevertheless there remain additional problems, which are largely a product of the global Heisenberg principle: Nothing can be evaluated without being somehow altered. Isolation of myocardial cells can rupture their intercalated discs, procedures such as dehydration and critical-point drying may shrink cells severely, and so forth. Yet if the various limitations can be recognized and countered insofar as possible, in future reviews there will continue to be demonstrated the fact that the study of the heart has been well served by the broad technical field of ultrastructure research.

ACKNOWLEDGMENTS

This work was supported by grants from both the Public Health Service (HL-28329 to M.S.F., HL-18711 to N.S.) and the American Heart Association (grant-in-aid 78-753, and a grant-in-aid from the Virginia Affiliate of the A.H.A., both to M.S.F.). Dr. Forbes was also recipient from 1979–1984 of Research Career Development Award 5 KO4 HL-00550 from the National Institutes of Health.

REFERENCES

1. Sperelakis N, Rubio R: Ultrastructural changes produced by hypertonicity in cat cardiac muscle. *J Mol Cell Cardiol* 3:139–156, 1971.
2. Page E, McCallister LP: Quantitative electron microscopic description of heart muscle cells: Application to normal, hypertrophied and thyroxin-stimulated hearts. *Am J Cardiol* 31:172–181, 1973.
3. Simpson FO, Rayns DG, Ledingham JM: The ultrastructure of ventricular and atrial myocardium. In: Challice CE, Virágh S (eds) *Ultrastructure of the Mammalian Heart.* New York: Academic Press, 1973, pp 1–41.
4. McNutt NS, Fawcett DW: Myocardial ultrastructure. In: Langer GA, Brady AJ (eds) *The Mammalian Myocardium.* New York: John Wiley and Sons, 1974, pp 1–49.
5. Sommer JR, Johnson EA: Ultrastructure of cardiac muscle. In: Berne RM, Sperelakis N, Geiger SR (eds) *Handbook of Physiology,* Sect 2: The Cardiovascular System, Vol 1: The Heart. Bethesda, MD: American Physiological Society, 1979, pp 113–186.
6. Sperelakis N, Forbes MS, Rubio R: The tubular systems of myocardial cells: Ultrastructure and possible function. In: Dhalla NS (ed) *Recent Advances in Studies on Cardiac Structure and Metabolism,* Vol 4: Myocardial Biology. Baltimore, MD: University Park Press, 1974, pp 163–194.
7. Sommer JR, Waugh RA: The ultrastructure of the mammalian cardiac muscle cell — with special emphasis on the tubular membrane systems. *Am J Pathol* 82:191–232, 1976.
8. Forbes MS, Sperelakis N: The membrane systems and cytoskeletal elements of mammalian myocardial cells. In: Dowben RM, Shay JW (eds) *Cell and Muscle Motility,* Vol 3. New York: Plenum Press, 1983, pp 89–155.
9. Jordan HE, Banks JB: A study of the intercalated discs of the heart of the beef. *Am J Anat* 22:285–339, 1917.
10. Sjöstrand FS, Andersson-Cedergren E, Dewey MM: The ultrastructure of the intercalated disc of frog, mouse and guinea pig cardiac muscle. *J Ultrastruct Res* 1:271–287, 1958.
11. Rhodin JAG, del Missier P, Reid LC: The structure of the specialized impulse-conduction system of the steer heart. *Circulation* 24:349–367, 1961.
12. Hayashi K: An electron microscope study on the conduction system of the cow heart. *Jpn Circ J* 26:765–842, 1962.
13. Jacobson SL: Culture of spontaneously contracting myocardial cells from adult rats. *Cell Struct Funct* 2:1–9, 1977.
14. Vahouny GV, Wei RW, Tamboli A, Albert EN: Adult canine myocytes: Isolation, morphology and biochemical characterizations. *J Mol Cell Cardiol* 11:339–357, 1979.
15. Robinson TF, Hayward BS, Krueger JW, Sonnenblick EH, Wittenberg BA: Isolated heart myocytes: Ultrastructural case study technique. *J Microsc (Oxford)* 124:135–142, 1981.
16. Phillips SJ, Dacey DM: Mammalian ventricular heart cell shape, surface and fiber organization as seen with the

scanning electron microscope (SEM). *J Cell Biol* 70:85, 1976.

17. Phillips SJ, Dacey DM, Bove A, Conger AD: Quantitative data on the shape of the mammalian ventricular heart cell. *Fed Proc* 36:601, 1977.

18. Marino TA, Cook PN, Cook LT, Dwyer SJ III: The use of computer imaging techniques to visualize cardiac muscle cells in three dimensions. *Anat Rec* 198:537–546, 1980.

19. Janicki JS, Weber KT, Gochman RF, Shroff S, Geheb FJ: Three-dimensional myocardial and ventricular shape: A surface representation. *Am J Physiol* 241:H1–H11, 1981.

20. Nag AC, Fischman DA, Aumont MC, Zak R: Studies of isolated adult rat heart cells: The surface morphology and the influence of extracellular calcium ion concentration on cellular viability. *Tissue Cell* 9:419–436, 1977.

21. Bishop SP, Drummond JL: Surface morphology and cell size measurement of isolated rat cardiac myocytes. *J Mol Cell Cardiol* 11:423–433, 1979.

22. Goldstein MA, Shroeter JP, Sass RL: Optical diffraction of the Z lattice in canine cardiac muscle. *J Cell Biol* 75:818–836, 1977.

23. Goldstein MA, Schroeter JP, Sass RL: The Z lattice in canine cardiac muscle. *J Cell Biol* 83:187–204, 1979.

24. Landon DN: The influence of fixation upon the fine structure of the Z-disk of rat striated muscle. *J Cell Sci* 6:257–276, 1970.

25. Anversa P, Olivetti G, Bracchi P-G, Loud AV: Postnatal development of the M-band in rat cardiac myofibrils. *Circ Res* 48:561–568, 1981.

26. Forbes MS, Sperelakis N: The presence of transverse and axial tubules in the ventricular myocardium of embryonic and neonatal guinea pigs. *Cell Tissue Res* 166:83–90, 1976.

27. Hirakow R, Gotoh T: Quantitative studies on the ultrastructural differentiation and growth of mammalian cardiac muscle cells. II. The atria and ventricles of the guinea pig. *Acta Anat* 108:230–237, 1980.

28. Forbes MS, Sperelakis N: Structures located at the level of the Z bands in mouse ventricular myocardial cells. *Tissue Cell* 12:467–489, 1980.

29. Ferrans VJ, Roberts WC: Intermyofibrillar and nuclear-myofibrillar connections in human and canine myocardium: An ultrastructural study. *J Mol Cell Cardiol* 5:247–257, 1973.

30. Goldstein MA, Entman ML: Microtubules in mammalian heart muscle. *J Cell Biol* 80:183–195, 1979.

31. Cartwright J Jr, Goldstein MA: Microtubules in the heart muscle of the postnatal and adult rat. *J Mol Cell Cardiol* 17:1–7, 1985.

32. Park RS, Legier G, Cartwright J Jr, Goldstein MA: Perinuclear microtubules in postnatal rat heart. *J Morphol* 179:13–19, 1984.

33. Behrendt H: Effect of anabolic steroids on rat heart muscle cells. I. Intermediate filaments. *Cell Tissue Res* 180:303–315, 1977.

34. Fuseler JW, Shay JW, Feit H: The role of intermediate (10-nm) filaments in the development and integration of the myofibrillar contractile apparatus in the embryonic mammalian heart. In: Dowben RM, Shay JW (eds) *Cell and Muscle Motility*, Vol 1. New York: Plenum Press, 1981, pp 205–259.

35. Carlsson E, Kjörell U, Thornell L-E, Lambertsson A, Strehler E: Differentiation of the myofibrils and the intermediate filament system during postnatal development of the rat heart. *Eur J Cell Biol* 217:62–78, 1982.

36. Palmer JW, Tandler B, Hoppel CL: Biochemical properties of subsarcolemmal and interfibrillar mitochondria isolated from rat cardiac muscle. *J Biol Chem* 252:8731–8739, 1977.

37. Wolkowicz PE, McMillan-Wood J: Respiration-dependent calcium ion uptake by two preparations of cardiac mitochondria. *Biochem J* 186:257–266, 1980.

38. Matlib MA, Rebman D, Ashraf M, Rouslin W, Schwartz A: Differential activities of putative subsarcolemmal and interfibrillar mitochondria from cardiac muscle. *J Mol Cell Cardiol* 13:163–170, 1981.

39. Forbes MS, Sperelakis N: Association between gap junctions and mitochondria in mammalian myocardial cells. *Tissue Cell* 14:25–37, 1982.

40. Peracchia C: Calcium effects on gap junction structure and cell coupling. *Nature* 271:669–671, 1978.

41. Baldwin KM: Cardiac gap junction configuration after an uncoupling treatment as a function of time. *J Cell Biol* 82:66–75, 1979.

42. Fawcett DW, McNutt NS: The ultrastructure of the cat myocardium. I. Ventricular papillary muscle. *J Cell Biol* 42:1–45, 1969.

43. Kraus B, Cain H: Giant mitochondria in the human myocardium — morphogenesis and fate. *Virchows Arch {B}* 33:77–89, 1980.

44. Brodsky WK, Arefyeva AM, Uryvaeva IV: Mitotic polyploidization of the mouse heart myocytes during the first postnatal week. *Cell Tissue Res* 210:133–144, 1980.

45. Schmid G, Pfitzer P: Mitoses and binucleated cells in perinatal human hearts. *Virchows Arch {B}* 48:59–67, 1985.

46. Gräbner W, Pfitzer P: Number of nuclei in isolated myocardial cells of pigs. *Virchows Arch {B}* 15:279–294, 1974.

47. Schneider R, Pfitzer P: Die Zahl der Kerne in isolierten Zellen des menschlichen Myokards. *Virchows Arch {B}* 12:238–258, 1973.

48. Bugaisky L, Zak R: Cellular growth of cardiac muscle after birth. *Tex Rep Biol Med* 39:123–138, 1979.

49. Rumyantsev PP: Ultrastructural reorganization, DNA synthesis and mitotic division of myocytes in atria of rats with left ventricle infarction: An electron microscopic and autoradiographic study. *Virchows Arch {B}* 15:357–378, 1974.

50. Rumyantsev PP, Snigirevskaya ES: The ultrastructure of differentiating cells of the heart muscle in the state of mitotic division. *Acta Morphol Acad Sci Hung* 16:271–283, 1968.

51. Bloom S, Cancilla PA: Conformational changes in myocardial nuclei of rats. *Circ Res* 24:189–196, 1969.

52. Langer GA: Ionic movements and the control of contraction. In: Langer GA, Brady AJ (eds) *The Mammalian Myocardium*. New York: John Wiley and Sons, 1974, pp 193–217.

53. Isenberg G, Klöckner U: Glycocalyx is not required for slow inward calcium current in isolated rat heart myocytes. *Nature* 284:358–360, 1980.

54. Gabella G: Inpocketings of the cell membrane (caveolae) in the rat myocardium. *J Ultrastruct Res* 65:135–147, 1978.

55. Levin KR, Page E: Quantitative studies on plasmalemmal folds and caveolae of rabbit ventricular myocardial cells. *Circ Res* 467:244–255, 1980.

56. Forssmann WG, Girardier L: A study of the T system in rat heart. *J Cell Biol* 44:1–19, 1970.

57. Masson-Pévet M, Gros D, Besselsen E: The caveolae in rabbit sinus node and atrium. *Cell Tissue Res* 208:183–196, 1980.

58. Forbes MS, Sperelakis N: A labyrinthine structure formed from a transverse tubule of mouse ventricular myocardium. *J Cell Biol* 56:865–869, 1973.

59. Ishikawa H, Yamada E: Differentiation of the sarcoplasmic reticulum and T-system in developing mouse cardiac muscle. In: Lieberman M, Sano T (eds) *Developmental and Phy-*

siological Correlates of Cardiac Muscle. New York: Raven Press, 1976, pp 21–35.

60. Forbes MS, Hawkey LA, Sperelakis N: The transverse-axial tubular system (TATS) of mouse myocardium: Its morphology in the developing and adult animal. *Am J Anat* 170:143–162, 1984.

61. Sperelakis N, Rubio R: An orderly lattice of axial tubules which interconnect adjacent transverse tubules in guinea-pig ventricular myocardium. *J Mol Cell Cardiol* 2:211–220, 1971.

62. Forbes MS, Van Niel EE: Membrane systems of guinea pig myocardium: Ultrastructure and morphometric studies. *Anat Rec* 222:362–379, 1988.

63. Forbes MS, Sperelakis N: Myocardial couplings: Their structural variations in the mouse. *J Ultrastruct Res* 58:50–65, 1977.

64. Forbes MS, Sperelakis N: Bridging junctional processes in couplings of striated, cardiac, and smooth muscle cells. *Muscle Nerve* 5:674–681, 1982.

65. Ayettey AS, Navaratnam V: The fine structure of myocardial cells in the grey seal. *J Anat* 131:748, 1980.

66. Ayettey AS, Navaratnam V: The ultrastructure of myocardial cells in the golden hamster *Cricetus auratus*. *J Anat* 132:519–524, 1981.

67. Baumann O, Kitazawa T, Somlyo AP: Laser confocal scanning microscopy of the surface membrane/T-tubular system and the sarcoplasmic reticulum in insect striated muscle stained with DilC$_{18}$(3). *J Struct Biol* 105:154–161, 1990.

68. Forbes MS, Plantholt BA, Sperelakis N: Cytochemical staining procedures selective for sarcotubular systems of muscle: Applications and modifications. *J Ultrastruct Res* 60:306–327, 1977.

69. Legato MJ: Cellular mechanisms of normal growth in the mammalian heart. II. A quantitative and qualitative comparison between the right and left ventricular myocytes in the dog from birth to five months of age. *Circ Res* 44:263–279, 1979.

70. Tidball JG, Cederdahl JE, Bers DM: Quantitative analyses of regional variability in the distribution of transverse tubules in rabbit myocardium. *Cell Tissue Res* 264:293–298, 1991.

71. Legato MJ: Ultrastructural characteristics of the rat ventricular cell grown in tissue culture, with special reference to sarcomerogenesis. *J Mol Cell Cardiol* 4:299–317, 1972.

72. Moses RL, Claycomb WC: Disorganization and reestablishment of cardiac muscle cell ultrastructure in cultured adult rat ventricular muscle cells. *J Ultrastruct Res* 81:358–374, 1982.

73. Moses RL, Claycomb WC: Ultrastructure of the transverse tubular system in cultured cardiac muscle cells. *Dev Cardiol Med* 49:422–440, 1985.

74. Van Winkle WB: The fenestrated collar of mammalian cardiac sarcoplasmic reticulum: A freeze-fracture study. *Am J Anat* 149:277–282, 1977.

75. Forbes MS, Hawkey LA, Jirge SK, Sperelakis N: The sarcoplasmic reticulum of mouse heart: Its divisions, configurations, and distribution. *J Ultrastruct Res* 93:1–16, 1985.

76. Forbes MS, Van Niel EE, Purdy-Ramos SI: The atrial myocardial cells of mouse heart: A structural and stereological study. *J Structural Biol* 103:266–279, 1990.

77. Dolber PC, Sommer JR: Freeze-fracture appearance of rabbit cardiac sarcoplasmic reticulum: A freeze-fracture study. In: Bailey G (ed) *Thirty-Eighth Annual EMSA Meeting.* Baton Rouge, LA: Claitor's, 1980, pp 630–631.

78. Scales DJ: Aspects of the cardiac sarcotubular system revealed by freeze fracture electron microscopy. *J Mol Cell Cardiol* 13:373–380, 1981.

79. Ogata T, Yamasaki Y: High-resolution scanning electron microscopic studies on the three-dimensional structure of the transverse-axial tubular system, sarcoplasmic reticulum and intercalated disc of the rat myocardium. *Anat Rec* 228:277–287, 1990.

80. Slade AM, Severs NJ: Rough endoplasmic reticulum in the adult mammalian cardiac muscle cell. *J Submicrosc Cytol* 17:531–536, 1985.

81. Somlyo AV: Bridging structures spanning the junctional gap at the triad of skeletal muscle. *J Cell Biol* 80:743–750, 1979.

82. Eisenberg BR, Gilai A: Structural changes in single muscle fibers after stimulation at a low frequency. *J Gen Physiol* 74:1–16, 1979.

83. Eisenberg BR, Eisenberg RS: The T-SR junction in contracting single skeletal muscle fibers. *J Gen Physiol* 79:1–19, 1982.

84. Brunschwig JP, Brandt N, Caswell AH, Lukeman DS: Ultrastructural observations of isolated intact and fragmented junctions of skeletal muscle by use of tannic acid mordanting. *J Cell Biol* 93:533–542, 1982.

85. Kelly DE, Kuda AM: Subunits of the triadic junction in fast skeletal muscle as revealed by freeze-fracture. *J Ultrastruct Res* 68:220–233, 1979.

86. Forbes MS, Sperelakis N: Spheroidal bodies in the junctional sarcoplasmic reticulum of lizard myocardial cells. *J Cell Biol* 60:602–615, 1974.

87. Jewett PH, Sommer JR, Johnson EA: Cardiac muscle: Its ultrastructure in the finch and hummingbird with special reference to the sarcoplasmic reticulum. *J Cell Biol* 49:50–65, 1971.

88. Waugh RA, Sommer JR: Lamellar junctional sarcoplasmic reticulum: A specialization of cardiac sarcoplasmic reticulum. *J Cell Biol* 63:337–343, 1974.

89. Jorgensen AO, Shen A C-Y, Daly P, MacLennan DH: Localization of Ca^{2+} + Mg^{2+}-ATPase of the sarcoplasmic reticulum in adult rat papillary muscle. *J Cell Biol* 93:883–892, 1982.

90. Jorgensen AO, Campbell KP: Evidence for the presence of calsequestrin in two structurally different regions of myocardial sarcoplasmic reticulum. *J Cell Biol* 98:1597–1602, 1984.

91. Jorgensen AO, Shen A C-Y, Campbell KP: Ultrastructural localization of calsequestrin in adult rat atrial and ventricular muscle cells. *J Cell Biol* 101:257–268, 1985.

92. Bossen EH, Sommer JR, Waugh RA: Comparative stereology of the mouse and finch left ventricle. *Tissue Cell* 10:773–784, 1978.

93. Page E, Surdyk-Droske M: Distribution, surface density, and membrane area of diadic junctional contacts between plasma membrane and terminal cisterns in mammalian ventricle. *Circ Res* 45:260–267, 1979.

94. Forbes MS, Sperelakis N: Intercalated discs of mammalian heart: A review of structure and function. *Tissue Cell* 17:605–648, 1985.

95. McNutt NS: Ultrastructure of the myocardial sarcolemma. *Circ Res* 37:1–13, 1975.

96. Rayns DG, Simpson FO, Ledingham JM: Ultrastructure of desmosomes of mammalian intercalated disc: Appearances after lanthanum treatment. *J Cell Biol* 42:322–326, 1969.

97. Kelly DE, Kuda AM: Traversing filaments in desmosomal and hemidesmosomal attachments: Freeze-fracture approaches toward their characterization. *Anat Rec* 199:1014, 1981.

98. Kawamura K, James TN: Comparative ultrastructure of cellular junctions in working myocardium and the conduction system under normal and pathologic conditions. *J Mol Cell Cardiol* 3:31–60, 1971.

99. Berry MN, Friend DS, Scheuer J: Morphology and metabolism of intact muscle cells isolated from adult rat heart. *Circ Res* 26:679–687, 1970.

100. Kensler RW, Goodenough DA: Isolation of mouse myocardial gap junctions. *J Cell Biol* 86:755–764, 1980.

101. Sperelakis N: Propagation mechanisms in heart. *Annu Rev Physiol* 41:441–457, 1979.

102. Severs NJ: The cardiac gap junction and intercalated disc. *Int J Cardiol* 26:137–173, 1990.

103. Raviola E, Goodenough DA, Raviola G: Structure of rapidly frozen gap junctions. *J Cell Biol* 87:273–279, 1980.

104. McNutt NS, Weinstein RS: The ultrastructure of the nexus: A correlated thin-section and freeze-cleave study. *J Cell Biol* 47:666–688, 1970.

105. Rambourg A, Segretain D, Clermont Y: Tridimensional architecture of the Golgi apparatus in the atrial muscle cell of the rat. *Am J Anat* 170:163–179, 1984.

106. Cantin M, Benchimol S, Castonguay Y, Berlinguet J-C, Huet M: Ultrastructural cytochemistry of atrial muscle cells. V. Characterization of specific granules in the human left atrium. *J Ultrastruct Res* 52:179–192, 1975.

107. Cantin M, Gutkowska J, Thibault G, Milne RW, Ledoux S, MinLi S, Chapeau C, Garcia R, Hamet P, Genest J: Immunocytochemical localization of atrial natriuretic factor in the heart and salivary glands. *Histochemistry* 80:113–127, 1984.

108. Forssmann WG, Birr C, Carlquist M, Christmann M, Finke R, Henschen A, Hock D, Kirschheim H, Kreye V, Lottspeich F, Metz J, Mutt V, Reinecke M: The auricular myocardiocytes of the heart constitute an endocrine organ. Characterization of a porcine cardiac peptide hormone, cardiodilatin-126. *Cell Tissue Res* 238:425–430, 1984.

109. Chapeau C, Gutkowska J, Schiller PW, Milne RW, Thibaut G, Garcia R, Genest J, Cantin M: Localization of immunoreactive synthetic atrial natriuretic factor (ANF) in the heart of various animal species. *J Histochem Cytochem* 33:541–550, 1985.

110. Goldfischer S: The internal reticular apparatus of Camillo Golgi: A complex, heterogeneous organelle, enriched in acid, neutral and alkaline phosphatases, and involved in glycosylation, secretion, membrane flow, lysosome formation, and intracellular digestion. *J Histochem Cytochem* 30:717–733, 1982.

111. Claycomb WC: DNA fragmentation as a developmental program for cellular aging in cardiac muscle. *Dev Cardiol Med* 49:399–409, 1985.

112. McMahon JT, Ratliff NB: Regeneration of adult human myocardium after acute heart transplant rejection. *J Heart Transplant* 9:554–567, 1990.

113. Tomanek J, Karlsson UL: Myocardial ultrastructure of young and senescent rats. *J Ultrastruct Res* 42:201–220, 1973.

114. Herzog V, Fahimi HD: Identification of peroxisomes (microbodies) in mouse myocardium. *J Mol Cell Cardiol* 8:271–281, 1976.

115. Hicks L, Fahimi HD: Peroxisomes (microbodies) in the myocardium of rodents and primates. A comparative ultrastructural cytochemical study. *Cell Tissue Res* 175:467–481, 1977.

116. Viràgh S, Challice CE: The impulse generation and conduction system of the heart. In: Challice CE, Viràgh S (eds) *Ultrastructure of the Mammalian Heart.* New York: Academic Press, 1973, pp 43–90.

117. James TN, Sherf L: Specialized tissues and preferential conduction in the atria of the heart. *Am J Cardiol* 28:414–427, 1971.

118. James TN, Sherf L, Urthaler F: Fine structure of the bundle-branches. *Br Heart J* 36:1–18, 1974.

119. Truex RC: Structural basis of atrial and ventricular conduction. *Cardiovasc Clin* 6:2–24, 1974.

120. Sherf L, James TN: Fine structure of cells and their histological organization within internodal pathways of the heart: Clinical and electrocardiographic implications. *Am J Cardiol* 44:345–369, 1979.

121. Colborn GL, Carsey E Jr: Electron microscopy of the sinoatrial node of the squirrel monkey *Saimiri sciureus. J Mol Cell Cardiol* 4:525–536, 1972.

122. Fawcett DW: The sporadic occurrence in cardiac muscle of anomalous Z bands exhibiting a periodic structure suggestive of tropomyosin. *J Cell Biol* 36:266–270, 1968.

123. Legato MJ: Sarcomerogenesis in human myocardium. *J Mol Cell Cardiol* 1:425–437, 1970.

124. Rybicka K: Sarcoplasmic reticulum in the conducting fibers of the dog heart. *Anat Rec* 189:237–262, 1977.

125. Osculati F, Garibaldi E: Particolari strutturali delle fibre del Purkinje del cuore di ratto; osservazioni al microscopio elettronico effuttuate anche applicando la tecnica della perossidasei. *Boll Soc Med Chir (Pavia)* 88:403–437, 1974.

126. Osculati F, Garibaldi E: Fine structural aspects of the Purkinje fibres of the dog's heart. *J Submicr Cytol* 6:39–53, 1974.

127. Osculati F, Amati S, Petrini E, Francheschini F, Cinti S: Ultrastructural investigation of the Purkinje fibres of rabbit's and cat's heart. *J Submicrosc Cytol Pathol* 10:185–197, 1978.

128. Osculati F, Amati S, Petrini E, Marelli M, Gazzanelli G: A study on the organization of the tubular endoplasmic reticulum in the rat heart conduction fibres. *J Submicrosc Cytol Pathol* 10:371–380, 1978.

129. Robb JS: Comparative Basic Cardiology. New York: Grune and Stratton, 1965.

130. Moravec M, Moravec J: Intrinsic innervation of the atrioventricular junction of the rat heart. *Am J Anat* 171:307–319, 1984.

131. Sommer JR, Johnson EA: Cardiac muscle: A comparative study of Purkinje fibers and ventricular fibers. *J Cell Biol* 36:497–526, 1968.

132. Kim S, Baba N: Atrioventricular node and Purkinje fibers of the guinea pig heart. *Am J Anat* 132:339–354, 1971.

133. Forbes MS, Mock OB, Van Niel EE: Ultrastructure of the myocardium of the least shrew, *Cryptotis parva* Say. *Anat Rec* 226:57–70, 1990.

134. Thornell L-E: The fine structure of Purkinje fiber glycogen: A comparative study of negatively staining and cytochemically stained particles. *J Ultrastruct Res* 49:157–166, 1974.

135. Thornell LE: An ultrahistochemical study on glycogen in cow Purkinje fibers. *J Mol Cell Cardiol* 6:439–448, 1974.

136. Thornell LE: Ultrastructural variations of Z bands in cow Purkinje fibers. *J Mol Cell Cardiol* 5:409–417, 1973.

137. Martinez-Palomo A, Alanis J, Benitez D: Transitional cardiac cells of the conductive system of the dog heart: Distinguishing morphological and electrophysiological features. *J Cell Biol* 47:1–17, 1970.

138. Thornell L-E, Eriksson A: Filament systems in the Purkinje fibers of the heart. *Am J Physiol* 241:H291–H305, 1981.

139. Weinstein HJ: An electron microscope study of cardiac muscle. *Exp Cell Res* 7:130–146, 1954.

CHAPTER 2

Basic Pathological Processes of the Heart: Relationship to Cardiomyopathies

L. MAXIMILIAN BUJA

INTRODUCTION

Cardiomyopathy is broadly defined as heart muscle disease. The purpose of this chapter is to review certain basic pathological processes affecting the heart and to discuss the relationship of these processes to various cardiomyopathies. Additional information regarding several of these pathological processes is provided in other chapters of this book.

MYOCARDIAL ISCHEMIA

Myocardial ischemia is a state of relative deficiency of oxygen supply in relation to the global or regional oxygen demands of the heart {1,2}. The initial consequence of ischemia is altered excitation-contraction coupling, leading to a decrease or loss of contractile activity. Ischemic myocardium also develops abnormal electrical activity, which may lead to the generation of arrhythmias. The third consequence of ischemia, when it is of sufficient severity and duration, is the progression of cell injury to an irreversible phase of cell death (myocardial infarction).

Etiology and pathophysiology

Ischemic heart disease in humans usually develops as a consequence of coronary atherosclerosis, a disease that impairs coronary perfusion by the formation of atherosclerotic plaque and thrombus {2–4}. The coronary arteries also are subject to nonatheromatous diseases, including congenital anomalies, vasculitis, embolization, dissection, and aneurysms. Coronary diseases ordinarily affect the epicardial arteries, but involvement of intramural (small) arteries may be significant in some cases of ischemic heart disease.

The dynamic nature of ischemic heart disease is indicated by the imperfect relationship between the severity of anatomic lesions of the coronary vasculature and the variety and severity of clinical manifestations of ischemic heart disease {5–10}. A number of factors influence the interplay between the myocardium and the coronary vasculature. It is known that the primary determinants of myocardial oxygen demand are heart rate, blood pressure (myocardial wall stress), and myocardial contractile state. It is also known that ventricular hypertrophy and failure create a state of increased oxygen demand by their influence on these parameters. With a discrete area of coronary obstruction, 50% reduction in luminal diameter (75% reduction in area) is needed to reduce hyperemic blood flow, and 80% reduction in diameter is required to impair resting blood flow {2}. However, a number of factors can influence the functional significance of a coronary stenosis, including the presence of multiple stenoses, the extent of the coronary collateral circulation, and an excessive myocardial oxygen demand. Coronary perfusion is also influenced by coronary tone, blood pressure (particularly diastolic perfusion pressure), and hemic factors, including blood volume, hematocrit, viscosity, oxygen-hemoglobin dissociation properties, coagulation, and platelet function.

Increased myocardial oxygen demand in the presence of coronary atherosclerosis can induce myocardial ischemia, which usually is manifest by typical angina pectoris of effort. Other forms of ischemic heart disease, including acute myocardial infarction, usually are associated with localized alterations of the coronary arteries, including coronary spasm, platelet aggregation, and thrombosis (fig. 2-1) {2–15}. Occlusive coronary thrombi are frequently associated with evidence of plaque erosion, ulceration, rupture, and/or hemorrhage, suggesting that the initiating events leading to coronary thrombosis occur in the vessel wall {2–10}. These lesions typically involve soft plaques with prominent atheromatous cores and thin fibrous capsules (fig. 2-2). The key initiating factor appears to be endothelial injury caused by chronic hemodynamic trauma to the intimal surface, or inflammatory or chemical injury to endothelium and subendothelial tissue. Platelet aggregation and, to a variable extent, vasospasm are important in the evolution of the thrombotic lesion, as discussed below.

Coronary thrombosis plays an important role in the progression of coronary heart disease {2–10}. Thrombi are composed of granular aggregates of platelets, deposited at the site of thrombus initiation, as well as platelet-leukocyte lamellae and a fibrin-rich blood coagulum with trapped erythrocytes and leukocytes deposited proximal and distal to the initiation site. Repeated episodes of

N. Sperelakis (ed.), *Physiology and Pathophysiology of the Heart, Third Edition.*
© *1995 Kluwer Academic Publishers. ISBN 0-7923-2612-1. All rights reserved.*

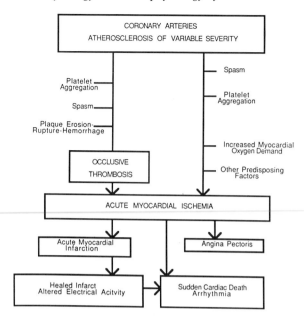

Fig. 2-1. Pathogenetic mechanisms operative in the major syndromes of acute ischemic heart disease. Modified from Buja et al. {6}, with permission.

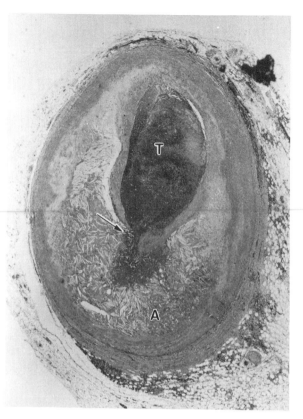

Fig. 2-2. Coronary artery from a patient with an acute myocardial infarct is occluded by a thrombus (T) superimposed on an atherosclerotic plaque (A) that exhibits a fissure in the capsule (arrow) and hemorrhage (dark material) at the fissure site. Hematoxylin and eosin stain, ×10. From Buja et al. {4}, with permission.

formation of small thrombi contribute to the growth of complicated atherosclerotic plaques. In addition, occlusive thrombi are involved in the pathogenesis of major episodes of ischemic heart disease. Occlusive coronary thrombi occur in over 90% of cases of transmural myocardial infarction, approximately a third of cases of subendocardial myocardial infarction, and a lower percentage of patients with unstable angina pectoris (without evidence of major infarction), and in those who die suddenly prior to hospitalization {5,16,17}. The available evidence indicates that occlusive coronary thrombosis is of major importance in the ultimate extent of an evolving myocardial infarction, although additional factors may be involved in the initiation of acute ischemic events that may or may not ultimately involve thrombus formation and further progression of the severity of the insult. In some cases, the important factor may be an excessive increase in myocardial oxygen demand. In other cases, the factors are vessel wall injury, platelet aggregation, and coronary vasospasm.

Coronary spasm is a localized, exaggerated increase in vascular tone leading to an acute narrowing or occlusion of an artery {6,7}. Spasm of a major coronary artery has been shown to be the cause of Prinzmetal's variant angina pectoris. Spasm of large and small coronary arteries also may play a role in other forms of ischemic heart disease. The etiology of coronary spasm is uncertain and may well differ from case to case. One possible mechanism is an alteration of the autonomic nervous system {6,7}. Although generalized autonomic dysfunction has not been found in patients with coronary spasm, an association of coronary spasm with other vasospastic disorders has been reported. In addition, activation of the alpha-adrenergic system by the cold pressor maneuver in patients with ischemic heart disease can result in coronary vasoconstriction and reduced coronary blood flow. Another possible mechanism is that spasm may be induced by primary alterations in medial smooth muscle, and these changes may involve alterations in calcium and/or magnesium homeostasis {6,7}. A third potential mechanism of spasm involves endothelial dysfunction in which endothelium-dependent relaxing factors, including nitric oxide, are deficient and/or the dysfunctional endothelial cells produce endothelin and related vasoconstrictive agents {6,7,18–21}. Finally, as a fourth mechanism, coronary spasm may develop secondary to platelet aggregation, activation, and release of vasoconstrictive agents {6,7,11–15}.

A complex interaction exists between vascular endothelium and platelets, since the former usually produces substances with vasodilator and antiplatelet aggregatory properties, including prostacyclin and nitric oxide, whereas the latter, when activated, produce thromboxane A_2 and other mediators, which promote vasoconstriction and platelet aggregation {6,7,11–15}. Recent studies have

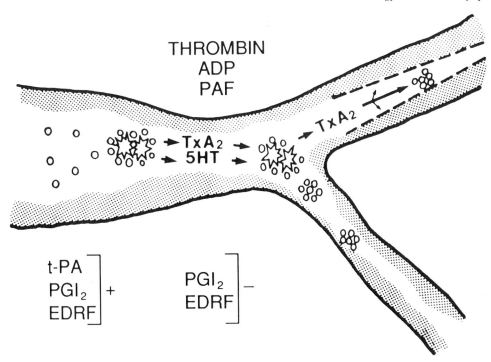

THROMBIN
ADP
PAF

TxA_2

TxA_2
5HT

$\begin{bmatrix} \text{t-PA} \\ \text{PGI}_2 \\ \text{EDRF} \end{bmatrix} +$ $\begin{bmatrix} \text{PGI}_2 \\ \text{EDRF} \end{bmatrix} -$

Fig. 2-3. Schematic diagram indicating the possible mechanisms by which thromboxane A_2 (TxA_2), serotonin (5HT), adenosine diphosphate (ADP), platelet activating factor (PAF), and thrombin promote platelet aggregation and decrease coronary blood flow in the patients with ischemic heart disease. Aggregating platelets (stars) release thromboxane A_2 (TxA_2) serotonin (5HT), ADP, PAF, and thrombin at sites of coronary artery stenosis and endothelial injury, which cause further platelet aggregation in the coronary artery, dynamic coronary vasoconstriction, and partial or total coronary artery thrombosis. Absence or reductions in endothelially derived relaxing factor (EDRF), prostacylin (PGI_2), and tissue plasminogen activating factor ($\pm$PA) at vascular sites with endothelial injury, and/or release of endothelins, probably contribute to the development of vasoconstriction and thrombosis. Modified from Hirsh et al. {11} and reproduced from Willerson et al. {14}, with permission.

demonstrated enhanced platelet aggregability and increased thromboxane levels in patients with active ischemic heart disease {11,12,22}. The clinical findings have been supported by experimental evidence that recurrent platelet aggregation at the site of a coronary stenosis with endothelial injury can produce episodes of coronary blood flow reduction {11–15}. In these models, a number of chemical mediators have been implicated in the platelet aggregation, including thromboxane, serotonin, adenosine diphosphate, and platelet activating factor. Thus platelet aggregation is associated with the release of chemical mediators that may, in turn, be involved in the initiation of spasm or the perpetuation of spasm initiated by other mechanisms. These findings indicate that platelet aggregation can induce myocardial ischemia by anatomic obstructive effects as well as the production of spasm (fig. 2-3). Furthermore, these platelet products, as well as platelet-derived growth factor (PDGF), can contribute to intimal proliferation, which leads to restenosis in significant numbers of patients treated with percutaneous coronary angioplasty (PTCA) {4,15}.

The interrelationship of coronary spasm and platelet aggregation varies in different clinical syndromes of ischemic heart disease. In patients with classical Prinzmetal's

angina pectoris, particularly those with minimal coronary artery disease, the primary event is coronary spasm, with platelet aggregation possibly contributing as a secondary phenomenon. In other patients with unstable angina pectoris, particularly those with significant atherosclerosis, available evidence suggests that platelet aggregation on atheromatous plaques is the primary event.

It is now clear that an important distinction exists between the pathophysiology of the common form of sudden cardiac death and acute myocardial infarction {16,17}. Most cases of sudden cardiac death are produced by a ventricular arrhythmia, usually ventricular fibrillation. This arrhythmia may be induced by an episode of acute ischemia, produced by platelet aggregation, vasospasm, or increased oxygen demand, or by an ectopic focus generated in an area of chronic myocardial damage with altered electrical activity (fig. 2-1). Most of the resuscitated survivors of sudden cardiac death do not evolve evidence of a major myocardial infarction. A minority of subjects with sudden cardiac death show evidence of an occlusive coronary thrombosis and/or an acute myocardial infarct. In these patients, the arrhythmia develops secondary to the coronary and myocardial lesions.

Survivors of one or more episodes of acute ischemic

TRANSMURAL MYOCARDIAL INFARCT

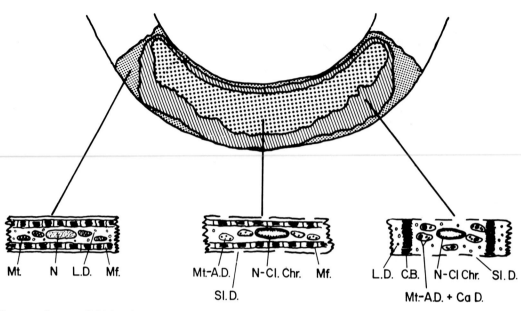

Fig. 2-4. Patterns of myocardial injury in acute myocardial infarction. C.B. = myofibrillar contraction band; L.D. = lipid droplet; Mf. = myofibril; Mt. = mitochondrion; Mt-A.D. = mitochondrion with amorphous matrix (flocculent) densities; Mt.A.D.+CaD. = mitochondrion with amorphous matrix densities and calcium phosphate deposits; N. = nucleus; N.-Cl. Chr. = nucleus with clumped chromatin; SI.D. = sarcolemmal defect.

damage may develop significant chronic ischemic heart disease. Manifestations include recurrent angina pectoris, arrhythmias, conduction abnormalities, cardiomegaly, and congestive heart failure. Pathologically, the heart shows coronary atherosclerosis, frequently with one or more occlusions; cardiac enlargement with left ventricular hypertrophy and dilatation; and extensive patchy myocardial fibrosis and/or one or more healed regional myocardial infarcts. Advanced cases with severe clinical and pathological changes have been termed *ischemic cardiomyopathy* {23–25}.

Experimental ischemic injury

Important information regarding mechanisms of myocardial cell injury has been obtained from studies of myocardial ischemia produced by coronary occlusion in experimental animals {26–29}. Myocardial infarction evolves within a risk region (bed-at-risk) supplied by the occluded vessel {26}. The ultimate basic lesion is coagulative necrosis. However, within the risk region topographical differences occur in the pattern of myocyte injury (fig. 2-4) {30,31}. In the central, mostly subendocardial region, the predominant cell type exhibits stretched myofibrils, clumped nuclear chromatin, mitochondria with flocculent (amorphous) matrix densities, and plasma membrane defects. The latter two features are indicative

of irreversible injury. An intermediate region contains necrotic muscle cells; with evidence of calcium overloading manifested by myofibrillar hypercontraction with contraction bands and, in some cells, mitochondria with calcium phosphate deposits. Necrotic cells in the intermediate region also exhibit amorphous matrix densities in the mitochondria, plasma membrane defects, clumped chromatin, and variable numbers of lipid droplets. In the outer region, the muscle cells exhibit marked accumulation of lipid droplets and other changes of cell injury, but they lack the changes of necrosis.

Many studies have addressed the question of progression of irreversible injury within the bed-at-risk {26–29}. The observations indicate that the rate of progression is a function of a severity-time index. The progression of necrosis is influenced by the size of the bed-at-risk and the severity of the ischemia, which, in turn, is influenced by the amount of collateral blood flow into the bed-at-risk shortly after the onset of coronary occlusion {26–29}. When ischemia is severe (less than 10–15% of normal blood flow), extensive irreversible injury occurs throughout the subendocardium after 40–60 minutes of coronary occlusion. The predisposition of the subendocardium is related to the more tenuous oxygen supply-demand relationship of this region with coronary occlusion; local metabolic differences in myocytes of the subendocardium also may be operative. After 3–6 hours of coronary

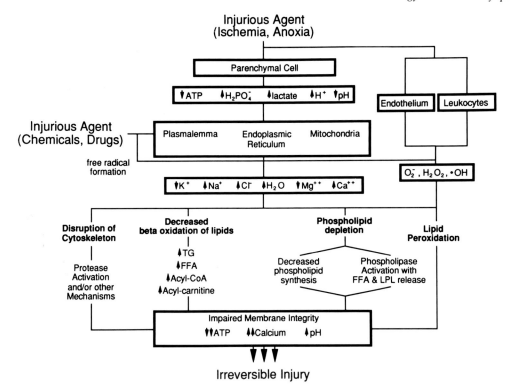

Fig. 2-5. Scheme of the pathogenesis of irreversible cell injury applicable to ischemic and toxic myocardial injury. ATP = adenosine triphosphate; FFA = free fatty acids; LPL = lysophospholipids; TG = triglycerides. Other abbreviations are standard chemical designations for ions and toxic oxygen species. From Buja et al. {39}, with permission.

occlusion, a wavefront of necrosis has progressed into the subepicardium. Little further progression of necrosis occurs thereafter.

The different patterns of myocardial injury observed in an established infarct are related to the rate of progression of damage in different regions of the bed-at-risk. In addition to coagulative necrosis, ischemia also may produce myocytolysis, when the ischemia is less rapid in onset, less severe, or chronic {32}. Myocytolysis is characterized by hydropic change and lysis of myofibrils with potential progression to complete cytolysis.

Mechanisms of irreversible injury

Following the onset of ischemia or hypoxia, numerous metabolic alterations occur in the oxygen-starved myoctyes {1}. Progressive dysfunction of the plasma membrane also occurs {33–39}. Extensive evidence indicates that progressive damage to the sarcolemma and organellar membranes is the key factor in the evolution of irreversible myocardial injury {39}. The functional consequences of altered membrane function involve (a) altered flux of sodium, potassium, chloride, and water, leading to cell swelling; and (b) net influx of calcium, leading to toxic effects of this cation {31,33,39–44}. Experimental evidence suggests that the onset of irreversibility correlates with the development of a severe permeability defect to

polyvalent ions {34,35,39–44}. However, injured myocytes may experience a reversible phase of calcium increase prior to irreversible calcium loading {39–44}. The magnitude of the cell swelling and calcium accumulation is determined by access to extracellular fluid. However, in severely ischemic areas subtle shifts in electrolytes and water between the intracellular and extracellular spaces likely have important consequences on progression of cell injury.

Several mechanisms are involved in the pathogenesis of myocardial membrane injury {38,39} (fig. 2-5). Progressive membrane phospholipid degradation occurs as a result of activation of phospholipase(s) and leads to accumulation of lysophospholipids and free fatty acids, including arachidonic acid {35–38}. Impaired mitochondrial beta oxidation also leads to accumulation of free fatty acids, which are partially reesterified into triglycerides, as well as long-chain acyl CoAs and acyl carnitines {35,38}. The various amphipathic lipid moieties accumulate in the membranes, altering their fluidity and permeability {35–38}. Peroxidation of membrane lipids is induced by free radicals and toxic oxygen products, which are produced by myocytes, endothelium, and invading leukocytes {45,46}. Damage to the cytoskeleton also occurs {47,48}. This further destabilizes the biochemically altered sarcolemma and predisposes to it rupture as a terminal event. The onset of irreversibility is associated with reversal of intracellular acidosis to a neutral pH {49,50}. Calcium-independent as well as calcium-dependent mechanisms of irreversible injury have been identified {51}.

Effects of adrenergic factors, reperfusion, preconditioning, and stunning

The progression of irreversible ischemic injury may be influenced by various pathophysiological factors, including alterations of the adrenergic nervous system. Coronary occlusion is followed by an increase in the population of membrane-associated beta- and alpha-adrenergic receptors in the ischemic myocardium {52,53}. Ischemia also results in a release of norepinephrine from nerve endings {54}. Thus, exposure of ischemic myocytes with altered receptor populations to increased amounts of catecholamines may contribute to the progression of ischemic injury and the genesis of ventricular arrhythmias {55,56}, as may the electrolyte alterations described above.

Reperfusion can profoundly influence the progression of myocardial ischemia. However, the effects of reperfusion are complex {57,58}. If instituted early enough after the onset of coronary occlusion, reperfusion clearly can limit the extent of myocardial necrosis and salvage significant amounts of jeopardized myocardium. However, reperfusion also changes the pattern of myocardial injury by causing hemorrhage within the severely damaged myocardium, by producing myofibrillar contraction bands and mitochondrial calcification in the injured myocytes, and by accelerating the release of intracellular enzymes from damaged myocardium. The latter effect leads to a marked elevation of serum levels of these enzymes without necessarily implying further myocardial necrosis. The timing of reperfusion is critical to the outcome, with the potential for myocardial salvage being greater the earlier the intervention. Although reperfusion can salvage myocardium, it may also induce additional injury. The concept of reperfusion injury implies the development of further damage, as a result of the reperfusion, to myocytes that were injured but that remained viable during a previous ischemic episode. Such injury may involve functional impairment, arrhythmia, and/or progression to cell death. The first two phenomena have been clearly documented, whereas reperfusion-induced cell death remains controversial.

Prior short intervals of coronary occlusion and reperfusion can influence the rate of progression of myocardial necrosis. Specifically, Murry and associates showed that the extent of myocardial necrosis following 60–90 minutes of coronary occlusion is significantly less in animals that had been pretreated with one or more 5-minute intervals of coronary occlusion prior to the induction of permanent occlusion {59,60}. However, after 120 minutes of coronary occlusion, the effect on infarct size is lost. This phenomenon is known as *preconditioning* {59,60}. Experimental evidence indicates that a reduced rate of ATP depletion correlates with the beneficial effects of preconditioning and that activation of adenosine receptors may mediate the process of preconditioning {61,62}. Other effects of intermittent ischemia are gene activation and induction of

synthesis of stress (heat shock) proteins, which may have a role in modulating the response of myocardium to subsequent injury {39}.

Myocardial *stunning* is the phenomenon of prolonged functional depression, requiring up to 24 hours or more for recovery, which develops on reperfusion, even after relatively brief periods of coronary occlusion, on the order of 15 minutes, which are insufficient to cause myocardial necrosis {57,58}. A related condition, termed *hibernation*, refers to chronic depression of myocardial function due to a chronic moderate reduction of perfusion. Preconditioning and stunning are independent phenomena, since the preconditioning effect is short term, transient, and not mediated through stunning. Free-radical effects and calcium loading have been implicated in the pathogenesis of stunning as well as other components of reperfusion injury {57,58,63,64}. After longer intervals of coronary occlusion on the order of 2–4 hours, necrosis of the subendocardium develops and even more severe and persistent functional depression occurs {65}. In experimental studies, after 2 hours of coronary occlusion, left ventricular regional sites of moderate dysfunction during ischemia recovered normal or near-normal regional contractile function after 1–4 weeks of reperfusion, whereas after 4 hours of coronary occlusion contractile dysfunction persisted after 4 weeks of reperfusion {65}. Thus, depending on the interval of coronary occlusion before reperfusion, variable degrees of either contractile dysfunction, necrosis, or both are seen with reperfusion. These observations emphasize the need for early intervention in order to salvage myocardium {9,66}.

CARDIAC CONDUCTION SYSTEM ABNORMALITIES

Abnormalities of the cardiac conduction system can lead to significant cardiac dysfunction and potentially fatal arrhythmias. Pathology can involve the sinoatrial (SAN) node, the atrioventricular (AVN) node, the atrioventricular bundle (AVB) (bundle of His), and the right and left bundle branches {67,68}. Most serious conduction system abnormalities are associated with anatomic alterations, but some, notably the prolonged Q-T syndrome, are not.

Ischemic injury and age-related degeneration of the SA node can lead to the sick sinus syndrome, which is characterized by a spectrum of arrhythmias. Altered atrioventricular conduction, including complete heart block, can result from damage to the AV node and bundle from acute or chronic coronary artery disease or age-related degenerative change unassociated with ischemia (Lev-Lenègre disease). Atrioventricular block also can occur on a congenital basis, as a consequence of primary tumor of the AV node and secondary to infective endocarditis. The presence of an aberrant AV conduction pathway, on a congenital basis, causes the Wolf-Parkinson-White and Lown-Ganong-Levine syndromes. Certain abnormalities of the conduction system are manifest by a prolonged Q-T interval on ECG, and this ECG change is strongly associated with sudden death. Recent evidence indicates an association of prolonged Q-T with mutations in the H-*ras*-1 gene {69,70}.

TOXIC MYOCARDIAL INJURY

It is known that a number of toxic insults produce myocardial injury independent of interruption in coronary blood flow {71–74}. The classical example of acute toxic myocardial injury is the damage produced by administration of excessive amounts of isoproterenol or other biogenic amines {75,76}. Catecholamine-induced cardiotoxicity is characterized by damaged muscle cells with myofibrillar hypercontraction, contraction bands, and mitochondrial calcium deposition. The pattern of injury is similar to that observed in peripheral regions of myocardial infarcts. This pattern of injury appears to be a general response of the myocardium when severe injury develops and some degree of coronary perfusion exists (either as occlusion-reperfusion, collateral perfusion, or toxic injury with normal perfusion). A similar pattern of acute myocardial injury has been observed with many other toxic insults to the heart {71,72}.

The progression of catecholamine-induced myocardial injury involves activation of adrenergic receptors, stimulation of myocardial metabolism, and increased oxygen consumption. A relatively severe mismatch in the oxygen-supply demand ratio may result and trigger phenomena operative in ischemic injury. There is evidence that direct stimulation of cardiac adrenergic receptors, either on myocardial cells, blood vessels, or both, can trigger norepinephrine-induced myocardial necrosis {77}. The irreversible phase of injury is associated with a marked defect in sarcolemmal permeability {75,76,78}.

Another pattern of toxic injury is characterized by the myocardial response to the anthracycline antibiotics, daunomycin and adriamycin {72,73,79,80}. In addition to acute effects, these agents produce chronic cardiotoxicity, which can lead to severe cardiac failure. Biologically, the phenomenon is characterized by a delayed response to the cumulative effects of the drug. Affected subjects exhibit cardiac dilatation and serous effusions. Microscopically, the characteristic lesion is a multifocal vacuolar change of the myocytes associated ultrastructurally with variable amounts of dilatation of the sarcoplasmic reticulum and T tubules, lysis of myofibrils, degeneration of mitochondria, and unusual nucleolar and nuclear changes {72,73,79}. Morphologically, these lesions represent a distinctive type of myocytolysis, which represents another general pattern of response to myocardial injury {2,32}.

The pathogenesis of adriamycin cardiotoxicity has been extensively investigated but has not been fully defined {80–82}. Potential mechanisms involve membrane damage, mediated in part by the generation of free radicals {83–86}, impaired protein synthesis mediated through effects on nucleic acids {87–89}, alterations in catecholamines and histamine {90}, and induction of heat shock proteins {91}. Toxic injury to the heart has been implicated in the etiology and pathogenesis of cardiomyopathy. However, progression from an acute to a chronic stage of

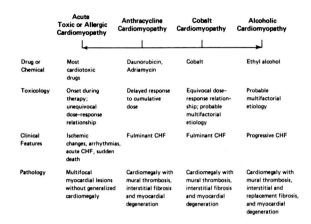

Fig. 2-6. The clinicopathological spectrum of drug-related cardiomyopathies. From Buja et al. {72}, with permission.

disease has not been proven for many agents. Anthracycline cardiotoxicity is conceptually important because this entity demonstrates that cardiomyopathy can result as a delayed response to the cumulative effects of an exogenous chemical (fig. 2-6).

INFECTION AND INFLAMMATION

A number of viruses, bacteria, and other microbes can produce acute myocarditis {92–95}. The end result may be death or complete resolution, but some cases can have a recurrent course, resulting in a picture resembling cases of idiopathic cardiomyopathy {92–95}. Studies of the pathogenesis of viral myocarditis suggest that, although the process is initiated by viral infection, the disease is perpetuated by the host response. One such mechanism is the proliferation of a specific population of cytotoxic lymphocytes that attack the myocytes altered by the initial viral infection {94}. Expression of stress (heat-shock) proteins on the surfaces of the altered myocytes may serve as an antigenic stimulus for the cytotoxic lymphocytes {91}.

Heart disease can result from autoimmune injury, as shown by the entities of acute rheumatic fever and chronic rheumatic heart disease. It is possible that less well-defined autoimmune phenomena contribute to the development or progression of certain cardiomyopathies {96–100}.

HYPERTROPHY AND FAILURE

Hypertrophy is a basic response of the heart in which one or both of the ventricles or atria increase in mass in response to an increased load {101–106}. This process is accomplished primarily by an increase in the mass of the cardiac myocytes without an increase in their number.

Normal growth and development of the mammalian heart is influenced by important changes occurring at the time of parturition. During early fetal development, growth of the heart involves multiplication and differentiation of myocytes. At or around the time of birth, myocytes lose the ability to undergo mitotic division. At this time a significant number of myocytes become binucleate, probably as a result of a final nuclear division without cytokinesis {107}. Subsequent normal growth of the heart is mediated by synthesis of myofibrils and other organelles in the existing myocytes.

Hypertrophy implies a further increase in cardiac mass above the normal value in response to an increased hemodynamic load, either an afterload (pressure load), preload (volume load), or both. Hypertrophy occurs in response to physiological stimuli, such as exercise, and in a variety of pathological states. There is debate as to whether or not the processes of physiological hypertrophy and pathological hypertrophy, at least in the early stages, represent the same or different patterns of response {108–111}. There is also uncertainty as to the basic stimulus for hypertrophy at the cellular level {106,112–118}. One view is that the physical forces of the increased stress directly stimulate a burst of protein synthesis, leading to increased cell mass. At the level of the whole ventricle, normalization of an increased wall stress by an appropriate hypertrophic response, according to the law of LaPlace, is an important predictor of the cardiac response to a variety of stimuli {108,111,116,117}. Alternative hypotheses emphasize the importance of other factors, such as transient ischemia, changes in high-energy phosphates, or other alterations in cellular metabolism {106,112–115,118}. These factors are postulated to function as couplers of the hemodynamic stimuli to enhanced gene expression, increased protein synthesis, and myocytes enlargement {106,118}. A schema for the potential interactions of these factors leading to myocardial hypertrophy in one disease state, namely, coronary heart disease, is shown in fig. 2-7 {119}. Addi-

tional insight into the molecular basis of hypertrophy is being derived from basic studies of the genetic regulation of nucleic acid and protein metabolism in the heart.

Cardiac failure is another important pathophysiological process affecting the heart {120,121}. This alteration is a pathophysiological state in which the heart looses its ability to provide an output sufficient for the metabolic demands of the peripheral tissues. Cardiac failure usually is the result of myocardial failure of the left, right, or both ventricles. However, cardiac failure also can result from pericardial disease, mitral stenosis, massive acute valvular insufficiency, or other causes. Cardiac failure may occur in a previously normal heart or one with hypertrophy. The usual response is chamber dilatation. However, the presence of chamber dilatation does not have a one-to-one relationship with overt failure, because a ventricle with a chronic volume load may exhibit dilatation when the subject does not show evidence of cardiac failure {127}.

Experimental studies have identified a number of biochemical alterations in the failing heart {122–126}. The critical lesion could involve defective energy production, defective energy utilization, or defective excitation-contraction coupling. Available evidence has implicated defective excitation-contraction coupling, due to defective calcium homeostasis, as the earliest alteration in certain models of myocardial failure. Specifically, these studies have identified defective uptake and release of Ca^{2+} from the sarcoplasmic reticulum with the potential result that less Ca^{2+} is available for activation of cardiac contraction {122–126}.

The above considerations imply a diffuse subcellular defect as the basis for myocardial failure. An alternative hypothesis for the pathogenesis of myocardial failure has been proposed by Sonnenblick, Factor, and associates {127}. According to their hypothesis, myocardial failure is initiated by factors that produce multifocal necrosis of myocardial fibers. Myocardial failure results when a critical mass of myocytes is lost such that the remaining myocytes, although functionally normal, are no longer able to maintain adequate ventricular function. Sonnenblick et al. have suggested that vasospasm may be the initiating cause of multifocal myocyte necrosis in several models of cardiomyopathy and cardiac failure {127}.

Alterations of the autonomic nervous system also contribute to the pathophysiology of congestive heart failure {126–128}. Progressive loss of catecholamines from failing myocardium and elevated circulating levels of catecholamines in subjects with cardiac failure have been documented. Recently cardiac failure has been shown to be associated with a decreased population of beta-adrenergic receptors and abnormalities of guanine nucleotide binding (G) proteins {126–129}. A depressed response of the heart to adrenergic stimulation appears to be important in the progression of cardiac dysfunction.

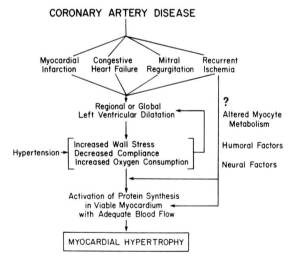

Fig. 2-7. Pathophysiological mechanisms leading to cardiac hypertrophy in chronic ischemic heart disease. From Buja et al. {119}, with permission.

PATTERNS OF CARDIOMEGALY

Patterns of cardiomegaly provide important information regarding the nature of the underlying pathologic process

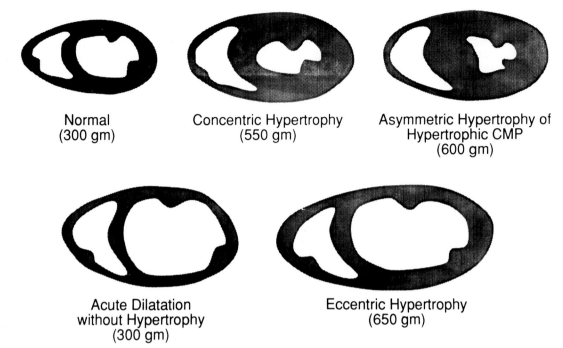

Normal
(300 gm)

Concentric Hypertrophy
(550 gm)

Asymmetric Hypertrophy of
Hypertrophic CMP
(600 gm)

Acute Dilatation
without Hypertrophy
(300 gm)

Eccentric Hypertrophy
(650 gm)

Fig. 2-8. Patterns of cardiomegaly shown in transverse sections through the cardiac ventricles. Values in parentheses represent corresponding heart weights. From Buja and Petty {130}, with permission.

(fig. 2-8) {102,103,130}. Cardiac dilatation without hypertrophy is indicative of acute cardiac failure involving a previously normal heart. The process is characterized by a normal heart weight, chamber enlargement, and reduced thickness of the wall. Ventricular dilation involves the Frank–Starling mechanism with progressive recruitment of myocytes, with an optimal diastolic sarcomere length of 2.2 μm (L max) {120,131}. Slippage and loss of registration of myofibrils also may contribute {120}. However, a major factor is geometric rearrangement of myocytes within the ventricular wall rather than progressive stretching of the myocytes. As a result of the rearrangement of myocytes, the wall of the dilated ventricle becomes thinner and exhibits fewer myocytes in a given transmural cross section {102,103}. Disease processes producing acute cardiac dilatation without hypertrophy include the acute phase of myocarditis, infective endocarditis, valvular insufficiency, and ischemia-induced cardiac decompensation.

Concentric hypertrophy is characterized by a relative or absolute increase in ventricular weight, a small chamber size, and a symmetrical, excessively thickened chamber wall {102,103,130}. This type of cardiomegaly is produced by a pressure load (afterload) on the involved ventricle. Common etiologies of concentric hypertrophy are valvular stenosis and systemic hypertension. Eccentric hypertrophy is characterized by increased ventricular weight and chamber dilatation {102,103,130}. The dilated ventricle has an eccentric configuration. Even though the weight is increased, the involved chamber wall is usually not thickened because of the increased chamber size. Eccentric

hypertrophy is the typical response of the heart to a chronic volume load (preload). This pattern of cardiomegaly can result from (a) acute chamber dilatation followed by compensatory hypertrophy, (b) progressive dilatation and hypertrophy developing in parallel, and (c) concentric hypertrophy followed by dilatation. Eccentric hypertrophy may be produced by chronic valvular insufficiency of any cause, cardiac failure superimposed on chronic coronary heart disease or hypertensive heart disease, or congestive (dilated) cardiomyopathy. The latter is distinguished by diffuse cardiac involvement producing symmetrical, four-chamber hypertrophy and dilatation.

The natural history of cardiac hypertrophy involves an early stage, characterized by stable cardiac function and the potential for regression of hypertrophy, and a late stage, characterized by progressive myocardial failure and progressive decrease in the potential for regression {101–106}. Linzbach has proposed that a critical cardiac mass in the range of 550 g occurs at the point of transition from the early to the late stage of hypertrophy {102}. After the critical cardiac mass is surpassed, important structural changes develop in the hypertrophied ventricle that predispose to myocardial failure and hinder regression. The greatly hypertrophied heart may develop an increase in myocyte number as a result of amitotic, longitudinal fission of enlarged myocytes {102}. Progressive degeneration of myocytes and fibrosis develops, and these changes tend to be more extensive in the subendocardium {132,133}. Degeneration and fibrosis occur in part because the oxygen demands of the greatly hypertrophied ventricle exceed the capability of the vasculature to supply blood {102,119,133}. Increasing wall stress is another factor {108,111,116}. The end result is a fixed structural dilatation of the involved chamber of the heart. Specific disease processes and mechanisms of hypertrophy undoubtedly influence the progression of hypertrophy and the potential for regression {134}.

CARDIOMYOPATHIES

The cardiomyopathies encompass a wide spectrum of disease processes {135–142}. They may be classified according to etiology and pathophysiology (clinicopathological features; table 2-1). Unfortunately the cause of many cases of cardiomyopathy in humans is unknown or uncertain. The typical idiopathic cardiomyopathy is characterized by heart muscle disease occurring in the absence of hypertension, coronary artery disease, valvular lesions, congenital cardiac defects, or other recognized forms of heart disease. These cardiomyopathies may have a congenital, familial, or genetic bases, or they may be acquired secondary to injury from some exogenous agent. Primary (idiopathic) cardiomyopathies arise from poorly understood causes, which exert major or exclusive effects on the myocardium. Secondary cardiomyopathies have a known cause or arise as part of a well-defined systemic or multiorgan disease {23–25,141}.

Secondary cardiomyopathy may occur with neuromuscular diseases, such as Friedriech's ataxia and various muscular dystrophies; with connective tissue diseases, including systemic lupus erythematosus; with neoplastic diseases when cardiac metastases occur; with metabolic diseases, including diabetes mellitus, thyrotoxicosis, myxedema, and glycogen storage disease; with nutritional diseases, notably beriberi and kwashiorkor; with hematologic diseases, including various hypereosinophilia syndromes; with viral, parasitic, protozoal, and bacterial infections; with granulomatous diseases, notably sarcoidosis; with infiltrative diseases, notably amyloidosis; and with drugs and other toxins {141}.

Table 2-1. General classification of cardiomyopathy (CMP)

A. Etiology
  1. Primary or idiopathic CMP — Isolated heart muscle
    disease due to
    a) Genetic, familial, or congenital defect
    b) Acquired cause
  2. Secondary CMP — Heart muscle disease secondary to
    a) Recognized etiology
    b) Systemic disease
    c) Other cardiovascular disease
B. Pathophysiology
  1. Congestive (dilated) CMP
  2. Hypertrophic CMP
    a) With obstruction (IHSS)
    b) Without obstruction
  3. Restrictive (constrictive) CMP
  4. Obliterative CMP

Heart muscle disease also may result from an initial cardiac or cardiovascular lesion, such as valvular disease, a congenital defect, hypertension, or coronary artery disease {23–25,141}. The heart muscle disease may come to dominate the clinical picture unless the underlying cardiac lesion is ameliorated. Examples of this phenomenon are the occasional progression of ischemic cardiomyopathy following coronary bypass surgery {2,119} and the persistence of cardiac disease following valve replacement {134}. The basis for this phenomenon relates to the general factors governing the natural history of cardiac hypertrophy discussed in the previous section.

Cardiomyopathies also are classified according to their pathophysiological manifestations with associated clinical and pathological features. The pathophysiological classification originally proposed by Goodwin is a practical and clinically useful approach {135}. It must be stressed, however, that this classification is not an etiological one per se. Nevertheless, the pathophysiological manifestations of the cardiomyopathy frequently provide useful information in assigning the case to a broad etiologic group.

Congestive (dilated) cardiomyopathy

Most primary cardiomyopathies are of the congestive (dilated) type {135–142}. Congestive cardiomyopathy is a subacute or chronic disorder characterized clinically by congestive cardiac failure, which is usually recurrent or progressive, and leads to progressive cardiac enlargement. Arrhythmias are another important clinical manifestation. They may occur as the presenting feature, and they may dominate the clinical picture at later stages of the disease. The prognosis is poor once chronic congestive heart failure develops, although relatively long-term survival occurs in a minority of cases {137}. The two leading categories of end-stage heart disease treated by cardiac transplantation are advanced coronary artery disease (ischemic cardiomyopathy) and idiopathic congestive cardiomyopathy {143}. Clinical episodes resulting from systemic emboli frequently occur. At necropsy, the heart is flabby, enlarged with a globular shape, and exhibits hypertrophy and dilatation (eccentric hypertrophy) of all four chambers {136,139,140}. Mural thrombi are frequently present, especially in the left ventricle, and explain the frequency of systemic embolization. Less advanced cases may exhibit mild hypertrophy with mild dilatation. Histologic changes are nonspecific and consist of variation in size, shape, and staining of muscle cells and their nuclei, and variable degrees of muscle cell degeneration and fibrosis. Congestive cardiomyopathy typically develops as an acquired condition. However, congestive cardiomyopathy also may be familial and/or genetic in origin {144}.

Circumstantial evidence has implicated viral myocarditis and chronic alcoholism as the most likely etiologic factors in many cases of primary congestive cardiomyopathy {74,92–94}. Many viruses, including those in the influenza, poliomyelitis, and Coxsackie B groups, have a known propensity for infecting the myocardium and producing acute cardiac failure (acute myocarditis). It has been documented that acute myocarditis may progress into a subacute or chronic disorder with features indistinguishable from those of idiopathic congestive cardiomyopathy. In most cases of congestive cardiomyopathy, however, proof of a preceding or active viral infection cannot be obtained. Recently, however, viral nucleic acid has been demonstrated by molecular techniques in significant numbers of cases of cardiomyopathy {145–148} and in related experimental models {149–151}, although the significance of these findings requires clarification {148}.

The incidence of congestive cardiomyopathy is higher in chronic alcoholics than in the general population. Only a small percentage of chronic alcoholics, however, develop congestive cardiomyopathy, and the heart disease tends to occur in those alcoholics without severe liver disease. Nevertheless, there is evidence that alcohol can induce progressive myocardial injury {74,152,153}. The terms *postpartum cardiomyopathy* and *peripartum cardiomyopathy* are applied to congestive cardiomyopathy that occurs within 3–5 months after childbirth or in the last trimester to 3–5 months after childbirth, respectively {141,154,155}. A predisposition exists for women over 30 with three or more pregnancies. Specific factors related to pregnancy, including autoimmune phenomena, have been implicated in the pathogenesis of peripartum cardiomyopathy, but there is no definitive evidence regarding pathogenetic factors.

Another form of congestive cardiomyopathy occurs in cancer patients treated with adriamycin. An increased incidence of congestive cardiomyopathy occurs in patients who have received a total cumulative dose of $550\,\mathrm{mg/m^2}$ of the drug {72,73,79–83}. Further study is needed regarding the roles of chemical agents, including drugs (fig. 2-4) and immunological phenomena {95–100,141}, in the genesis of congestive cardiomyopathy. Endomyocardial biopsy is a useful technique for evaluating the presence or absence of an inflammatory component {156,158}. Therapy with corticosteroids and immunosuppressive agents remains under investigation {159,160}.

Hypertrophic cardiomyopathy

Hypertrophic cardiomyopathy includes the entities hypertrophic obstructive cardiomyopathy (HOCM) and idiopathic hypertrophic subaortic stenosis (IHSS). Most patients with clinicopathologic features of hypertrophic cardiomyopathy have a genetically induced disease, which is inherited in an autosomal dominant pattern with incomplete penetrance {161–167}. Manifestations of typical hypertrophic cardiomyopathy include cardiac murmur, reduced arterial pulse, angina, dyspnea, and sudden death {135,163}. Laboratory evaluation may reveal evidence of asymmetric septal hypertrophy (ASH) and/or systolic anterior motion (SAM) of the mitral valve {141}. Characteristic pathological features include cardiac hypertrophy, without dilatation; left ventricular hypertrophy with excessive thickening of the ventricular septum (asymmetric septal hypertrophy); a widespread disorganized arrangement of muscle cells (muscle cell disarray), primarily in the ventricular septum; endocardial fibrous plaque in the

left ventricle outflow tract; focal thickening of the anterior leaflet of the mitral valve; and normal aortic valve {136,139–141,164}.

Patients with hypertrophic cardiomyopathy frequently develop left ventricular outflow tract obstruction, which simulates valvular aortic stenosis (hence the designation IHSS). Outflow tract obstruction probably results from an abnormal pattern of ventricular contraction, which produces abnormal systolic anterior movement of the anterior mitral leaflet toward the bulging ventricular septum. The abnormal movement of the mitral valve can also produce variable degrees of mitral insufficiency. Anatomic markers of the functional left ventricular outflow obstruction are the areas of fibrosis involving the anterior mitral leaflet and endocardium of the left ventricular outflow tract. The abnormally hypertrophied left ventricle also causes resistance to ventricular filling (inflow resistance), even when features of the outflow tract obstruction are not prominent {141}. Patients may develop progressive congestive cardiac failure and ventricular dilatation late in the course of the disease. Characteristic pathological features, including asymmetric septal hypertrophy and extensive muscle cell disarray, are still recognizable, even in the heart with end-stage hypertrophic cardiomyopathy and ventricular dilatation.

The genetic basis of typical hypertrophic cardiomyopathy is suggested by the high incidence of a positive family history with this disease. In addition, the noninvasive clinical technique of echocardiography has documented the familial occurrence of asymmetric septal hypertrophy in asymptomatic relatives of patients with clinical disease in over 90% of families studied {161}. Some features of inherited hypertrophic cardiomyopathy, including asymmetric septal hypertrophy, can rarely develop in patients with other forms of heart disease, including cardiac hypertrophy induced by severe hypertension {162}. An important distinguishing feature of inherited hypertrophic cardiomyopathy versus secondary hypertrophic cardiomyopathy is the presence of extensive muscle cell disarray, indicating an unusual pattern of myocardial hypertrophy {164}.

An inherited pattern of abnormal response of the myocardium to catecholamines beginning during cardiac development has been suggested as the basis for the development of asymmetric left ventricular hypertrophy and extensive muscle cell disarray in patients with hypertrophic cardiomyopathy {162}. Recently, mutations in the cardiac beta-myosin heavy chain gene (beta-MHC) located on the long arm of chromosome 14 have been identified in some families with hypertrophic cardiomyopathy {168–173}. However, the studies have demonstrated genetic heterogeneity in hypertrophic cardiomyopathy, and the absence of cardiac myosin heavy chain and actin gene involvement in some families with the disease {168–173}.

Restrictive (constrictive) cardiomyopathy

Restrictive (constrictive) cardiomyopathy is a rare form of cardiomyopathy that is characterized by impaired diastolic ventricular filling due to reduced compliance of the myocardium {135,141}. Restrictive cardiomyopathy frequently mimics constrictive pericarditis clinically {174}. Patients typically show signs of elevated central venous pressure without cardiomegaly. Causes of restrictive cardiomyopathy include amyloidosis {175}, hemochromatosis (although most cases of hemochromatosis have a congestive pattern) {176}, and idiopathic disease. An association with chronic renal disease, particularly in chronic dialysis patients, also has been noted {177}.

Obliterative cardiomyopathy

Some cases of cardiomyopathy are characterized by massive filling of the ventricular cavities by mural thrombi, necrosis, and/or fibrosis of the subendocardial myocardium, and variable degrees of mitral or tricuspid valvular insufficiency. These cases are sometimes designated as *obliterative cardiomyopathy* {135}. They occur with endomyocardial fibrosis of Africa and with Löffler's fibroplastic parietal endocarditis, which is associated with chronic hypereosinophilia syndromes {136}.

Myocardial biopsy

Myocardial biopsy can be safely used to obtain tissue from cardiomyopathy patients during life {156–158,178–180}. Biopsy has been useful in the separation of constrictive pericarditis from restrictive cardiomyopathy due to amyloidosis and other causes. Myocardial biopsy also is useful in the identification and staging of transplant rejection and adriamycin cardiotoxicity {158,178–180}. However, in most cases biopsy reveals nonspecific changes of hypertrophy and myocyte degeneration, and a specific etiological diagnosis cannot be made.

Specific diagnosis of hypertrophic cardiomyopathy on myocardial biopsy is not possible because of the questionable significance of small foci of apparent muscle fiber disarray, especially in small muscle samples with poorly preserved orientation. A recent area of interest is the identification of a subgroup of patients with active inflammation in myocardial tissue obtained at biopsy {156–158,180,181}. Current studies are aimed at evaluating the therapeutic efficacy of treatment of these patients with steroids or other antiinflammatory agents {156–160,180–182}.

Animal models

Most animal models of cardiac hypertrophy and failure have involved the imposition of a hemodynamic overload {183}. As previously mentioned, much information regarding acute toxic and viral injury has come from animal models. However, documentation that these acute insults lead to chronic cardiomyopathy is often not available. Two extensively studied models of chronic disease are the cardiomyopathic Syrian hamster and adriamycin cardiotoxicity {183}.

SUMMARY

This chapter has summarized important pathological responses of the heart to injury. These responses are involved in complex and often poorly understood ways in the development of cardiomyopathy. The goal of ongoing research is to more precisely define the causes and mechanisms of progression of the various types of cardiomyopathies.

REFERENCES

1. Hillis LD, Braunwald E: Myocardial ischemia. *N Engl J Med* 296:971–978, 1034–1041, 1093–1096, 1977.
2. Willerson JT, Hillis LD, Buja LM: Pathogenesis and pathology of ischemic heart disease. In: Willerson JT, Hillis JD, Buja LM (eds) *Ischemic Heart Disease: Clinical and Pathophysiological Aspects*. New York: Raven Press, 1982.
3. Buja LM, Clubb JF Jr, Bilheimer DW, Willerson JT: Pathobiology of human familial hypercholesterolemia and a related animal model, the Watanabe heritable hyperlipidemic rabbit. *Eur Heart J* 11(Suppl E):41–52, 1990.
4. Buja LM, Willerson JT, Murphree SS: Pathobiology of arterial wall injury, atherosclerosis, and coronary angioplasty. In: Black AJR, Anderson HV, Ellis SG (eds) *Complications of Coronary Angioplasty*. New York: Marcel Dekker, 1991, pp 11–33.
5. Buja LM, Willerson JT: Clinicopathologic findings in acute ischemic heart disease syndromes. *Am J Cardiol* 47:343–356, 1981.
6. Buja LM, Hillis LD, Petty SC, Willerson JT: The role of coronary arterial spasm in ischemic heart disease. *Arch Pathol Lab Med* 105:221–226, 1981.
7. Shepherd JT, Vanhoutte PM: Spasm of the coronary arteries: Causes and consequences (the scientist's viewpoint). *Mayo Clin Proc* 60:33–46, 1985.
8. Buja LM, Willerson JT: The role of coronary artery lesions in ischemic heart disease: Insights from recent clinicopathologic, coronary arteriographic, and experimental studies. *Hum Pathol* 18:451–461, 1987.
9. Buja LM, Willerson JT: Infarct size — can it be measured or modified in humans? *Prog Cardiovasc Dis* 29:271–289, 1987.
10. Fuster V, Badimon L, Badimon JJ, Chesebo JH: The pathogenesis of coronary artery disease and the acute coronary syndromes. *N Engl J Med* 326:242–250, 310–318, 1992.
11. Hirsh PD, Hillis LD, Campbell WB, Firth BG, Willerson JT: Release of prostaglandins and thromboxane into the coronary circulation in patients with ischemic heart disease. *N Engl J Med* 304:685–691, 1981.
12. Hirsh PD, Campbell WB, Willerson JT, Hillis LD: Prostaglandins and ischemic heart disease. *Am J Med* 71:1009–1026, 1981.
13. Willerson JT, Golino P, Eidt J, Campbell WB, Buja LM: Specific platelet mediators and unstable coronary artery lesions: Experimental evidence and potential clinical implications. *Circulation* 80:198–205, 1989.
14. Willerson JT, Yao S-K, Ferguson JJ, Anderson HV, Golino P, Buja LM: Unstable angina pectoris and the progression to acute myocardial infarction: Role of platelets and palteletderived mediators. *Texas Heart Inst J* 18:243–247, 1992.
15. Willerson JT, Yao S-K, McNatt J, et al.: Frequency and severity of cyclic flow alteration and platelet aggregation predict the severity of neointimal proliferation following

experimental coronary stenosis and endothelial injury. *Proc Natl Acad Sci USA* 88:10624–10628, 1991.

16. Cobb LA, Werner JA, Trobaugh GB: Sudden cardiac death. 1. A decade's experience with out-of-hospital resuscitation. *Mod Concepts Cardiovasc Dis* 49:31–36, 1980.

17. Buja LM, Willerson JT: Relationship of ischemic heart disease to sudden cardiac death. *J Forensic Sci* 36:25–33, 1991.

18. Furchgott RF: The role of endothelium in the responses of vascular smooth muscle to drugs. *Annu Rev Pharmacol Toxicol* 24:175–197, 1984.

19. Gryglewski RJ, Botting RM, Vane JR: Mediators produced by the endothelial cell. *Hypertension* 12:530–548, 1988.

20. de Gouville A-CL, Lippton HL, Cavero I, Summer WR, Hyman AL: Endothelin — a new family of endothelium-derived peptides with widespread biological peptides. *Life Sci* 45:1499–1513, 1989.

21. Egashira K, Inou T, Hirooka Y, Yamada A, Maruoka Y, Kai H, Sugimachi M, Suzuki S, Takeshita A: Impaired coronary blood flow response to acetylcholine in patients with coronary risk factors and proximal atherosclerotic lesions. *J Clin Invest* 91:29–37, 1993.

22. Fitzgerald DJ, Roy L, Catella F, Fitzgerald GA: Platelet activation in unstable coronary disease. *N Engl J Med* 315:983–989, 1986.

23. Burch GE, Tsui CY, Harb JM: Ischemic cardiomyopathy. *Am Heart J* 83:340–350, 1972.

24. Gould KL, Lipscomb K, Hamilton GW, Kennedy JW: Left ventricular hypertrophy in coronary artery disease: A cardiomyopathy syndrome following myocardial infarction. *Am J Med* 55:595–601, 1973.

25. Anversa P, Sonnenblick EH: Ischemic cardiomyopathy: Pathophysiological mechanisms. *Prog Cardiovasc Dis* 33:49–70, 1990.

26. Reimer KA, Jennings RB: The "wavefront phenomenon" of myocardial ischemic cell death. II. Transmural progression of necrosis within the framework of ischemic bed size (myocardium at risk) and collateral flow. *Lab Invest* 40:633–644, 1979.

27. Reimer KA, Ideker RE: Myocardial ischemia and infarction: Anatomic and biochemical substrates for ischemic cell death and ventricular arrhythmias. *Hum Pathol* 18:462–475, 1987.

28. Buja LM, Willerson JT: Experimental analysis of myocardial ischemia. In: Silver MD (ed) *Cardiovascular Pathology*, 2nd ed. New York: Churchill Livingstone, 1991, pp 621–642.

29. Buja LM: Pathobiology of myocardial ischemic injury. In: Acosta D Jr (ed) *Cardiovascular Toxicology*, 2nd ed. New York: Raven Press, 1992, pp 115–130.

30. Willerson JT, Parkey RW, Bonte FJ, Lewis SE, Corbett J, Buja LM: Pathophysiologic considerations and clinico-pathological correlates of technetium-99m stannous pyrophosphate myocardial scintigraphy. *Semin Nucl Med* 10:54–69, 1980.

31. Buja LM, Hagler HK, Willerson JT: Altered calcium homeostasis in the pathogenesis of myocardial ischemic and hypoxic injury. *Cell Calcium* 9:205–217, 1988.

32. Schlesinger MJ, Reiner L: Focal myocytolysis of the heart. *Am J Pathol* 31:443–459, 1955.

33. Buja LM, Willerson JT: Abnormalities of volume regulation and membrane integrity in myocardial tissue slices after early ischemic injury in the dog: Effects of mannitol, polyethylene glycol and propranolol. *Am J Pathol* 103:79–95, 1981.

34. Burton KP, Hagler HK, Willerson JT, Buja LM: Relationship of abnormal intracellular lanthanum accumulation to

progression of ischemic injury in isolated perfused myocardium: Effect of chlorpromazine. *Am J Physiol: Heart Circ Physiol* 241:H714–H723, 1981.

35. Chien KR, Reeves JP, Buja LM, Bonte F, Parkey RW, Willerson JT: Phospholipid alterations in canine ischemic myocardium. Temporal and topographical correlations with Tc-99m-PPI accumulation and an in vitro sarcolemmal Ca^{2+} permeability defect. *Circ Res* 48:711–719, 1981.

36. Chien KR, Han A, Sen A, Buja LM, Willerson JT: Accumulation of unesterified arachidonic acid in ischemic canine myocardium: Cycle and depletion of membrane phospholipids. *Circ Res* 54:313–322, 1984.

37. Chien KR, Sen A, Reynolds R, Chang A, Kim Y, Gunn MD, Buja LM, Willerson JT: Release of arachidonate from membrane phospholipids in cultured neonatal rat myocardial cells during adenosine triphosphate depletion: Correlation with the progression of cell injury. *J Clin Invest* 75:1770–1780, 1985.

38. Buja LM: Lipid abnormalities in myocardial cell injury. *Trends Cardiovasc Med* 1:40–45, 1991.

39. Buja LM, Eigenbrodt ML, Eigenbrodt EH: Apoptosis and coagulation necrosis: Basic types and mechanisms of cell death. *Arch Pathol Lab Med* 117:1208–1214, 1993.

40. Morris AC, Hagler HK, Willerson JT, Buja LM: Relationship between calcium loading and impaired energy metabolism during Na^+, K^+ pump inhibition and metabolic inhibition in cultured neonatal rat cardiac myocytes. *J Clin Invest* 83:1876–1887, 1989.

41. Buja LM, Fattor RA, Miler JC, Chien KR, Willerson JT. Effects of calcium loading and impaired energy production on metabolic and ultrastructural features of cell injury in cultured neonatal rat cardiac myocytes. *Lab Invest* 63:320–331, 1990.

42. Thandroyen FT, Morris AC, Hagler HK, et al.: Intracellular calcium transients and arrhythmia in isolated heart cells. *Circ Res* 69:810–819, 1991.

43. Thandroyen FT, Bellotto D, Katayama A, Hagler HK, Willerson JT, Buja LM: Subcellular electrolyte alterations during progressive hypoxia and following reoxygenation in isolated neonatal rat ventricular myocytes. *Circ Res* 71:106–119, 1992.

44. Lemasters J, Di Guiseppi J, Nieminen A, Hermann B: Blebbing, free Ca^{2+} and mitochondrial membrane potential preceding cell death in hepatocytes. *Nature* 325:78–81, 1987.

45. Farber JL, Kyle ME, Coleman JB: Biology of disease. The mechanisms of cell injury by activated oxygen species. *Lab Invest* 62:670–679, 1990.

46. Burton KP, Morris AC, Massey KD, Buja LM, Hagler HK: Free radicals alter ionic calcium levels and membrane phospholipids in cultured rat ventricular myocytes. *J Mol Cell Cardiol* 22:1035–1047, 1990.

47. Steenbergen C, Hill ML, Jennings RB: Cytoskeletal damage during myocardial ischemia: Changes in vinculin immunofluorescence staining during total in vitro ischemia in canine heart. *Circ Res* 60:478–486, 1987.

48. Armstrong SC, Ganote CE: Flow cytometric analysis of isolated adult cardiomyocytes: Vinculin and tubulin fluorescence during metabolic inhibition and ischemia. *J Mol Cell Cardiol* 24:149–162, 1992.

49. Gores GJ, Nieminen A-L, Wray BE, Herman B, Lemasters JJ: Intracellular pH during "chemical hypoxia" in cultured rat hepatocytes. Protection by intracellular acidosis against the onset of cell death. *J Clin Invest* 83:386–396, 1989.

50. Bond JM, Herman B, Lemasters JJ: Protection by acidotic pH against anoxia/reoxygenation injury to rat neonatal cardiac myocytes. *Biochem Biophys Res Commun* 179:798–803, 1991.

51. Starke PE, Hoek J, Farber JL: Calcium-dependent and calcium-independent mechanisms of irreversible cell injury in cultured rat hepatocytes. *J Biol Chem* 161:3006–3012, 1986.

52. Mukherjee A, Bush LR, McCoy KE, Duke RJ, Hagler H, Buja LM, Willerson JT: Relationship between β-adrenergic receptor numbers and physiological responses during experimental canine myocardial ischemia. *Circ Res* 50:735–741, 1982.

53. Corr PB, Shayman JA, Kramer JB, Kipnis RJ: Increased alpha adrenergic receptors in ischemic cat myocardium: A potential mediator of electrophysiological derangements. *J Clin Invest* 67:1232–1236, 1981.

54. Muntz KH, Hagler HK, Boulas HJ, Willerson JT, Buja LM: Redistribution of catecholamines in the ischemic zone of the dog heart. *Am J Pathol* 114:64–78, 1984.

55. Willerson JT, Buja LM: Short- and long-term influence of beta-adrenergic antagonists after acute myocardial infarction. *Am J Cardiol* 54(Suppl E):16E–20E, 1984.

56. Thandroyen FT, Muntz KH, Buja LM, Willerson JT: Alterations in beta-adrenergic receptors, adenylate cyclase, and cyclic AMP concentrations during acute myocardial ischemia and reperfusion. *Circulation* 82(Suppl II):II30–II37, 1990.

57. Hearse DJ, Bolli R: Reperfusion-induced injury: Manifestations, mechanisms and clinical relevance. *Trends Cardiovasc Med* 1:233–240, 1991.

58. Virmani R, Kolodgie FD, Forman MB, Farb A, Jones RM: Reperfusion injury in the ischemic myocardium. *Cardiovasc Pathol* 1:117–130, 1992.

59. Murry CE, Jennings RB, Reimer KA: Preconditioning with ischemia: A delay of lethal cell injury in ischemic myocardium. *Circulation* 74:1124–1136, 1986.

60. Murry CE, Richard VJ, Reimer KA, Jennings RB: Ischemic preconditioning slows energy metabolism and delays ultrastructural damage during a sustained ischemic episode. *Circ Res* 66:913–931, 1990.

61. Liu GS, Thronton J, Van Winkle DM, Stanley AWH, Olsson RA, Downey JM: Protection against infarction afforded by preconditioning is mediated by A_1 adenosine receptors in rabbit heart. *Circulation* 84:350–356, 1991.

62. Downey JM, Liu GS, Thornton JD: Adenosine and the anti-infarct effects of preconditioning. *Cardiovasc Res* 27:3–8, 1993.

63. Bolli R, Patel BS, Jeroudi MO, Lai EK, McCay PB: Demonstration of free radical generation in "stunned" myocardium of intact dogs with the use of the spin trap alpha-phenyl N-tert-butyl nitrons. *J Clin Invest* 82:476–485, 1988.

64. Kusuoka H, Porterfield JK, Weisman HF, Weisfeldt ML, Marban E: Pathophysiology and pathogenesis of stunned myocardium: Depressed Ca^{2+} activation of contraction as a consequence of reperfusion-induced cellular calcium overload in ferret hearts. *J Clin Invest* 79:950–961, 1987.

65. Bush LR, Buja LM, Tilton G, Wathen M, Apprill P, Ashton J, Willerson JT: Effects of propranolol and diltiazem alone and in combination on the recovery of left ventricular segmental function after temporary coronary occlusion and long term reperfusion in conscious dogs. *Circulation* 72:413–430, 1985.

66. Gunnar RM, Passamani ER, Bourdillon PD, et al.: Guidelines for the early management of patients with acute myocardial infarction. *J Am Coll Cardiol* 16:249–292, 1990.

67. Davies MJ, Anderson RH: The pathology of the conduction system. In: Pomerance A, Davies MJ (eds) *The Pathology of the Heart*. Oxford: Blackwell, 1975, pp 367–412.

68. Hudson REB: The conducting system: Anatomy, histology, and pathology in acquired heart disease. In: Silver MD (ed)

69. Keating M, Atkinson D, Dunn C, et al. Linkage of a cardiac arrhythmia, the long QT syndrome, and the Harvey *ras*-1 gene. *Science* 252:704–706, 1991.

70. Keating M: Linkage analysis and long QT syndrome. Using genetics to study cardiovascular disease. *Circulation* 85:1973–1986, 1992.

71. Reichenbach DD, Benditt EP: Catecholamines and cardiomyopathy: The pathogenesis and potential importance of myofibrillar degeneration. *Hum Pathol* 1:125–150, 1970.

72. Buja LM, Ferrans VJ, Roberts WC: Drug-induced cardiomyopathies. In: Hamburger F (ed) *Comparative Pathology of the Heart, Advances in Cardiology*, Vol 13. Basel: Karger, 1974, pp 330–348.

73. Buja LM, Ferrans VJ: Myocardial injury produced by antineoplastic drugs. In: Fleckenstein A, Rona G (eds) *Pathophysiology and Morphology of Myocardial Cell Alteration, Recent Advances in Studies on Cardiac Structure and Metabolism*, Vol 6. Baltimore, MD: University Park Press, 1975, pp 487–497.

74. Rubin E: Alcohol: Toxic or tonic? *Cardiovasc Rev Rep* 2:23–29, 1981.

75. Csapo Z, Dusek J, Rona G: Early alterations of the cardiac muscle cells in isoproterenol-induced necrosis. *Arch Pathol* 93:356–365, 1972.

76. Rona G, Boutet M, Huttner I, Peters H: Pathogenesis of isoproterenol-induced myocardial alterations: Functional and morphological correlates. In: Dhalla NS (ed) *Myocardial Metabolism, Recent Advances in Studies on Cardiac Structure and Metabolism*, Vol 3. Baltimore, MD: University Park Press, 1973, pp 507–525.

77. Downing SE, Lee JC: Contribution of alpha adrenoreceptor activation to the pathogenesis of norepinephrine cardiomyopathy. *Circ Res* 52:471–478, 1983.

78. Dhalla NS, Yates JC, Naimark B, Dhalla KS, Beamish RE, Ostadal B: Cardiotoxicity of catecholamines and related agents. In: Acosta D (ed) *Cardiovascular Toxicology*, 2nd ed. New York: Raven Press, 1992, pp 239–282.

79. Ferrans VJ: Overview of cardiac pathology in relation to anthracycline cardiotoxicity. *Cancer Treat Rep* 62:995–961, 1978.

80. Young RC, Ozols RF, Myers CE: The anthracycline antineoplastic drugs. *N Engl J Med* 305:139–153, 1981.

81. Havlin KA: Cardiotoxicity of anthracyclines and other antineoplastic agents. In: Acosta D (ed) *Cardiovascular Toxicology*, 2nd ed. New York: Raven Press, 1991, pp 143–164.

82. Jackson JA, Reeves JP, Muntz KH, Kruk D, Prough RA, Willerson JT, Buja LM: Evaluation of free-radical effects and catecholamine alterations in adriamycin cardiotoxicity. *Am J Pathol* 117:140–153, 1984.

83. Olson RD, Boerth RC, Gerber JG, Nies AS: Mechanism of adriamycin cardiotoxicity: Evidence for oxidative stress. *Life Sci* 29:1393–1401, 1981.

84. Steinherz LJ, Steinherz PG, Tan CTC, Heller G, Murphy ML: Cardiac toxicity 4 to 20 years after completing anthracycline therapy. *JAMA* 266:1672–1677, 1991.

85. Davies KJA, Doroshow JH: Redox cycling of anthracyclines by cardiac mitochondria: I. Anthracycline radical formation by NADH dehydrogenase. *J Biol Chem* 261:3060–3067, 1986.

86. Doroshow JH, Davies KJA: Redox cycling of anthracycline by cardiac mitochondria: II. Formation of superoxide anion, hydrogen peroxide, and hydroxyl radical. *J Biol Chem* 261:3068–3074, 1986.

87. Dalbow DG, Jaenke RS: In vivo RNA synthesis in the

hearts of adriamycin-treated rats. *Cancer Res* 42:79–83, 1982.

88. Ito H, Miller SC, Billingham ME, et al.: Doxorubicin selectively inhibits muscle gene expression in cardiac muscle cells in vivo and in vitro. *Proc Natl Acad Sci USA* 87:4275–4279, 1990.

89. Papoian T, Lewis W: Anthracyclines selectively decrease α cardiac actin mRNA abundance in the rat heart. *Am J Pathol* 141:1187–1195, 1992.

90. Bristow MR, Minobe WA, Billingham ME, Marmor JB, Johnson GA, Ishimoto BM, Sageman WS, Daniels JR: Anthracycline-associated cardiac and renal damage in rabbits: Evidence for mediation by vasoactive substances. *Lab Invest* 45:157–168, 1981.

91. Huber SA: Heat-shock protein induction in adriamycin and picornavirus-infected cardiomyocytes. *Lab Invest* 67:218–224, 1992.

92. Lerner AM, Wilson FM: Virus cardiomyopathy. *Prog Med Virol* 15:63–91, 1973.

93. Abelman WH: Viral myocarditis and its sequelae. *Ann Rev Med* 22:145–152, 1973.

94. Woodruff JF: Viral myocarditis: A review. *Am J Pathol* 101:425–484, 1980.

95. Cambridge G, MacArthur CGC, Waterson AP, Goodwin JF, Oakley CM: Antibodies to Coxsackie B viruses in congestive cardiomyopathy. *Br Heart J* 41:692–696, 1979.

96. Kirsner AB, Hess EV, Fowler NO: Immunologic findings in idiopathic cardiomyopathy: A prospective serial study. *Am Heart J* 86:625–630, 1973.

97. Bolte HD, Schultheiss P: Immunological results in myocardial diseases. *Postgrad Med J* 54:500–503, 1978.

98. Jacobs B, Matsuda Y, Deodhar S, Shirey E: Cell-mediated cytotoxicity to cardiac cells of lymphocytes from patients with primary myocardial disease. *Am J Clin Pathol* 72:1–4, 1979.

99. Fowles RE, Dieber CP, Stinson EB: Defective in vitro suppressor cell function in idiopathic congestive cardiomyopathy. *Circulation* 59:483–491, 1979.

100. Hang LM, Izui S, Dixon FJ: (NZW × BXSB) F₁ hybrid: A model of acute lupus and coronary, vascular disease with myocardial infarction. *J Exp Med* 154:216–221, 1981.

101. Meerson FZ: The myocardium in hyperfunction, hypertrophy and heart failure. *Circ Res* 24,25(Suppl II):II1–II63, 1969.

102. Linzbach AJ: Heart failure from the point of view of quantitative anatomy. *Am J Cardiol* 5:370–382, 1960.

103. Hort W: Quantitative morphology and structural dynamics of the myocardium. In: Bajusz E, Jasmin G (eds) *Methods and Achievements in Experimental Pathology*, Vol 5. Basel: Karger, 1971, pp 3–21.

104. Alpert NR (ed): *Myocardial Hypertrophy and Failure*, Vol 7. Perspectives in Cardiovascular Research. New York: Raven Press, 1983.

105. Swynghedauw B, Delcayre C: Biology of cardiac overload. In: Ioachim HL (ed) *Pathobiology Annual*, Vol 12. New York: Raven Press, 1982, pp 137–183.

106. Bugaisky LB, Gupta M, Gupta MP, Zak R: Cellular and molecular mechanism of cardiac hypertrophy. In: Fozzard HA, Haber E, Jennings RB, Katz AM, Morgan HE (eds) *The Heart and Cardiovascular System: Scientific Foundations*, 2nd ed. New York: Raven Press, 1992, pp 1621–1640.

107. Clubb FJ Jr, Bishop SP: Formation of binucleated myocardial cells in the neonatal rat: An index for growth hypertrophy. *Lab Invest* 50:571–577, 1984.

108. Grossman W: Cardiac hypertrophy: Useful adaptation or pathologic process? *Am J Med* 69:576–584, 1980.

109. Wikman-Coffelt J, Parmley WW, Mason DR: The cardiac hypertrophy process. Analysis of factors determining pathological vs. physilogical development. *Circ Res* 45:697–707, 1979.

110. Scheuer J, Malhotra A, Hirsch C, Capasso J, Schaible TF: Physiologic cardiac hypertrophy corrects contractile protein abnormalities associated with pathologic hypertrophy in rats. *J Clin Invest* 70:1300–1305, 1982.

111. Nguyen N, Buja LM: The role of ventricular wall stress in cardiac hypertrophy. *Cardiovasc Pathol*, in press, 1994.

112. Rabinowitz M, Zak R: Biochemical and cellular changes in cardiac hypertrophy. *Ann Rev Med* 23:245–262, 1972.

113. Morkin E: Activation of synthetic processes in cardiac hypertrophy. *Circ Res* 34,35(Suppl II):II37–II48, 1974.

114. Cohen J: Role of endocrine factors in the pathogenesis of cardiac hypertrophy. *Circ Res* 34,35(Suppl II):II49–II57, 1974.

115. Schreiber SS, Evans CD, Oratz M, Rothschild MA: Protein synthesis and degradation in cardiac stress. *Circ Res* 48:601–611, 1981.

116. Grossman W, Jones D, McLaurin LP: Wall stress and patterns of hypertrophy in the human left ventricle. *J Clin Invest* 56:56–64, 1975.

117. Cooper G IV, Kent RL, Uboh CE, Thompson EW, Mariano TA: Hemodynamic versus adrenergic control of cat right ventricular hypertrophy. *J Clin Invest* 75:1403–1414, 1985.

118. Chien KR, Knowlton KU, Chiens: Regulation of cardiac gene expression during myocardial growth and hypertrophy: Molecular studies of an adaptive physiologic response. *FASEB J* 5:3037–3046, 1991.

119. Buja LM, Muntz KH, Lipscomb K, Willerson JT: Cardiac hypertrophy in chronic ischemic heart disease. In: Tarazi R (ed) *Mechanisms of Left Ventricular Hypertrophy*. New York: Raven Press, 1983, pp 287–294.

120. Braunwald E, Ross J Jr, Sonnenblick EH: *Mechanisms of Contraction of the Normal and Failing Heart*, 2nd ed. Boston: Little, Brown, 1976.

121. Braunwald E: Historical overview and pathophysiologic considerations. In: Braunwald E, Mock MB, Watson J (eds) *Congestive Heart Failure: Current Research and Clinical Applications*. New York: Grune and Stratton, 1982, pp 3–9.

122. Schwartz A, Sordahl LA, Entman ML, Allen JC, Reddy YS, Goldstein MA, Luchi RJ, Wyborny LE: Abnormal biochemistry in myocardial failure. *Am J Cardiol* 32:407–422, 1973.

123. Dhalla NS, Das PK, Sharma GP: Subcellular basis of cardiac contractile failure. *J Mol Cell Cardiol* 10:363–385, 1978.

124. Chidsey CA: Calcium metabolism in the normal and failing heart. In: Braunwald, E (ed) *The Myocardium: Failure and Infarction*. New York: H.P. Publishing, 1975, pp 37–47.

125. Willerson JT: What is wrong with the failing heart? *N Engl J Med* 307:243–245, 1982.

126. Katz AM: Heart failure. In: Fozzard HA, Haber E, Jennings RB, Katz AM, Morgan HE (eds) *The Heart and Cardiovascular System: Scientific Foundations*, 2nd ed. New York: Raven Press, 1992, pp 333–353.

127. Sonnenblick EH, Factor S, Strobeck JE, Capasso JM, Fein F: The pathophysiology of heart failure: The primary role of microvascular hyperactivity and spasm in the development of congestive cardiomyopathies. In: Braunwald E, Mock MB, Watson J (eds) *Congestive Heart Failure: Current Research and Clinical Applications*. New York: Grune and Stratton, 1982, pp 87–97.

128. Sole MJ: Alterations in sympathetic and parasympathetic neurotransmitter activity. In: Braunwald E, Mock MB, Watson J (eds) *Congestive Heart Failure: Current Research*

and Clinical Applications. New York: Grune and Stratton, 1982, pp 101–113.

129. Bristow MR, Ginsbury R, Minobe W, Cubicciotti RS, Sageman WS, Lurie K, Billingham M, Harrison DC, Stinson EB: Decreased catecholamine sensitivity and β-adrenergic-receptor density in failing human hearts. *N Engl J Med* 307:205–211, 1982.

130. Buja LM, Petty CS: Heart disease, trauma, and death. In: Curran WJ, McGarry AL, Petty CS (eds) *Modern Legal Medicine, Psychiatry, and Forensic Science*. Philadelphia: FA Davis, 1980, pp 187–206.

131. Yoran C, Covell JW, Ross J Jr: Structural basis for the ascending limb of left ventricular function. *Circ Res* 32:297–303, 1973.

132. Maron BJ, Ferrans VJ: Ultrastructural features of hypertrophied human ventricular myocardium. *Prog Cardiovasc Dis* 11:207–238, 1978.

133. Dick MR, Unverferth DV, Baba N: The pattern of myocardial degeneration in nonischemic congestive cardiomyopathy. *Hum Pathol* 13:740–744, 1982.

134. Tarazi RC, Sen S, Fouad FM: Regression of myocardial hypertrophy. In: Braunwald E, Mock MB, Watson J (eds) *Congestive Heart Failure: Current Research and Clinical Applications*. New York: Grune and Stratton, 1982, pp 151–163.

135. Goodwin JF: Congestive and hypertrophic cardiomyopathies: A decade of study. *Lancet* 1:731–739, 1970.

136. Roberts WC, Ferrans VJ: Pathologic anatomy of the cardiomyopathies: Idiopathic dilated and hypertrophic types, infiltrative types, and endomyocardial disease with and without eosinophilia. *Hum Path* 6:287–342, 1975.

137. Fuster V, Gersh BJ, Giuliani ER, Tajik AJ, Brandenburg RO, Frye RL: The natural history of idiopathic dilated cardiomyopathy. *Am J Cardiol* 47:525–631, 1981.

138. Johnson RA, Palacios I: Dilated cardiomyopathies of the adult. *N Engl J Med* 307:1051–1058, 1119–1126, 1982.

139. Davies MJ: The cardiomyopathies: A review of terminology, pathology and pathogenesis. *Histopathology* 8:363–393, 1984.

140. Gravanis MB, Ansari AA: Idiopathic cardiomyopathies. A review of pathologic studies and mechanisms of pathogenesis. *Arch Pathol Lab Med* 111:915–929, 1987.

141. Wynne J, Braunwald E: The cardiomyopathies and myocarditises. In: Braunwald E (ed) *Heart Disease: A Textbook of Cardiovascular Medicine*, 2nd ed. Philadelphia: WB Saunders, 1984, pp 1399–1456.

142. Keren A, Popp RL: Assignment of patients into the classification of cardiomyopathies. *Circulation* 86:1622–1633, 1992.

143. Graham AR: Autopsy findings in cardiac transplant patients: A 10-year experience. *Am J Clin Pathol* 97:369–375, 1992.

144. Michels VV, Moll PP, Miller FA, et al.: The frequency of familial dilated cardiomyopathy in a series of patients with idiopathic dilated cardiomyopathy. *N Engl J Med* 326:77–82, 1992.

145. Bowles NE, Richards PJ, Olsen EGJ, Archard LC: Detection of coxsackie-B-virus-specific RNA sequences in myocardial biopsy samples from patients with myocarditis and dilated cardiomyopathy. *Lancet* 1:1120–1123, 1986.

146. Bowles NE, Rose ML, Taylor P, et al.: End-stage dilated cardiomyopathy: Persistence of enterovirus RNA in myocardium at cardiac transplantation and lack of immune response. *Circulation* 80:1128–1136, 1989.

147. Jin O, Sole MJ, Butany JW, et al.: Detection of enterovirus RNA in myocardial biopsies from patients with myocarditis and cardiomyopathy using gene amplification by polymerase chain reaction. *Circulation* 82:8–16, 1990.

148. Chang KL, Billingham ME, Weiss LM: Detection of enteroviral RNA in idiopathic dilated cardiomyopathy (IDCM). *Lab Invest* 66:20A, 1992.

149. Kandolf R, Ameis D, Kirschner P, Canu A, Hofschneider PH: In situ detection of enteroviral genomes in myocardial cells by nucleic acid hybridization: An approach to the diagnosis of viral heart disease. *Proc Natl Acad Sci USA* 84:6272–6276, 1987.

150. Kyu B-S, Matsumori A, Sato Y, et al.: Cardiac persistence of cardioviral RNA detected by polymerase chain reaction in a murine model of dilated cardiomyopathy. *Circulation* 86:522–530, 1992.

151. Wee L, Liu P, Penn L, et al.: Persistence of viral genome into late stages of murine myocarditis detected by polymerase chain reaction. *Circulation* 86:1605–1614, 1992.

152. Rubin E: Alcoholic myopathy in heart and skeletal muscle. *N Engl J Med* 301:28–33, 1979.

153. Ahmed SS, Regan TJ: Cardiotoxicity of acute and chronic ingestion of various alcohols. In: Acosta D Jr (ed) *Cardiovascular Toxicology*, 2nd ed. New York: Raven Press, 1992, pp 345–407.

154. O'Connell JB, Costanzo-Nordin MR, Subramanian R, et al.: Peripartum Cardiomyopathy: Clinical, Hemodynamic, Histologic and Prognostic Characteristics. *J Am Coll Cardiol* 8:52, 1986.

155. Melvin KR, Richardson PJ, Olsen EGJ, Daly K, Jackson G: Peripartum cardiomyopathy due to myocarditis. *N Engl J Med* 307:731–734, 1982.

156. Aretz HT, Billingham ME, Edwards WD, et al.: Myocarditis. A histopathologic definition and classification (The Dallas criteria). *Am J Cardiovasc Pathol* 1:3–14, 1987.

157. Popma JJ, Cigarroa RG, Buja LM: Diagnostic and prognostic utility of right-sided catheterization and endomyocardial biopsy in idiopathic dilated cardiomyopathy. *Am J Cardiol* 63:955–958, 1989.

158. Billingham ME: Role of endomyocardial biopsy in diagnosis and treatment of heart disease. In: Silver MD (ed) *Cardiovascular Pathology*, 2nd ed. New York: Churchill Livingstone, 1991, pp 1465–1486.

159. Parrillo JE, Cunnion RE, Epstein SE, et al.: A prospective, randomized, controlled trial of prednisone for dilated cardiomyopathy. *N Engl J Med* 321:1061–1068, 1989.

160. O'Connell JB: Immunosuppression for dilated cardiomyopathy. *N Engl J Med* 321:1119, 1989.

161. Clark CE, Henry WL, Epstein SE: Familial prevalence and genetic transmission of idiopathic hypertrophic subaortic stenosis. *N Engl J Med* 289:709–714, 1973.

162. Goodwin JF: ?IHSS. ?HOCM. ?ASH. A plea for unity. *Am Heart J* 89:269–277, 1975.

163. Maron BJ, Roberts WC, McAllister HA, Rosing DR, Epstein SE: Sudden death in young athletes. *Circulation* 62:218–229, 1980.

164. Maron BJ, Roberts WC: Quantitative analysis of cardiac muscle cell disorganization in the ventricular septum of patients with hypertrophic cardiomyopathy. *Circulation* 59:689–706, 1979.

165. Maron BJ, Bonow RO, Cannon III RO, et al.: Hypertrophic cardiomyopathy. Interrelations of clinical manifestations, pathophysiology, and therapy. *N Engl J Med* 316:780–789, 844–852, 1987.

166. Maron BJ, Roberts WC, McAllister HA, Rosing DR, Epstein SE: Sudden death in young athletes. *Circulation* 62:218–229, 1980.

167. Evans AT, Korndorffer W, Boor PJ: Sudden death of two brothers while playing basketball: Familial hypertrophic cardiomyopathy. *Tex Med* 76:48–51, 1980.

168. Jarco JA, McKenna W, Pare JAP, et al.: Mapping a gene

for familial hypertrophic cardiomyopathy to chromosome 14q1. *N Engl J Med* 321:1372–1378, 1989.

169. McKenna WJ, Stewart JT, Nihoyannopoulos P, et al.: Hypertrophic cardiomyopathy without hypertrophy: Two families with myocardial disarray in the absence of increased myocardial mass. *Br Heart J* 63:287–290, 1990.

170. Watkins H, Rosenzweig A, Hwang D-S, et al.: Characteristic and prognostic implications of myosin missense mutations in familial hypertrophic cardiomyopathy. *N Engl J Med* 326:1108–1114, 1992.

171. Epstein ND, Fananapazir L, Lin HJ, et al.: Evidence of genetic heterogeneity in five kindreds with familial hypertrophic cardiomyopathy. *Circulation* 85:635–647, 1992.

172. Schwartz K, Beckmann J, Dufour C, et al.: Exclusion on cardiac myosin heavy chain and actin gene involvement in hypertrophic cardiomyopathy of several French families. *Circ Res* 71:3–8, 1992.

173. Elstein E, Liew C-C, Sole MJ: The genetic basis of hypertrophic cardiomyopathy. *J Mol Cell Cardiol* 24:1471–1477, 1992.

174. Benotti JR, Grossman W: Restrictive cardiomyopathy. *Ann Rev Med* 35:113–125, 1984.

175. Buja LM, Khoi NB, Roberts WC: Clinically significant cardiac amyloidosis: Clinicopathologic findings in 15 patients. *Am J Cardiol* 26:394–405, 1970.

176. Cutler DJ, Isner JM, Bracey AW, Hufnagel CA, Conrad PW, Roberts WC, Kerwin DM, Weintraub AM: Hemochromatosis heart disease: An unemphasized cause of

potentially reversible restrictive cardiomyopathy. *Am J Med* 69:923–928, 1980.

177. Parfey PS, Harnett JD, Barre PE: The natural history of myocardial disease in dialysis patients. *J Am Soc Nephrol* 2:2–12, 1991.

178. Billingham ME, Bristow MR, Mason JW, Joseph LJ: Endomyocardial biopsy. In: Braunwald E, Mock MB, Watson J (eds) *Congestive Heart Failure: Current Research and Clinical Applications.* New York: Grune and Stratton, 1982, pp 237–251.

179. Nippoldt TB, Edwards WD, Holmes DR Jr, Reeder GS, Hartzler GO, Smith HC: Right ventricular endomyocardial biopsy: Clinicopathologic correlates in 100 consecutive patients. *Mayo Clin Proc* 57:407–418, 1982.

180. Mason JW: Endomyocardial biopsy: The balance of success and failure. *Circulation* 71:185–188, 1985.

181. Mason JW, Billingham ME, Ricci DR: Treatment of acute inflammatory myocarditis assisted by endomyocardial biopsy. *Am J Cardiol* 45:1037–1044, 1980.

182. O'Connell JB, Robinson JA, Henkin RE, Gunnar RM: Immunosuppressive therapy in patients with congestive cardiomyopathy and myocardial uptake of gallium-67. *Circulation* 64:780–786, 1981.

183. Bishop SP: Animal Models. In: Braunwald E, Mock MB, Watson J (eds) *Congestive Heart Failure: Current Research and Clinical Applications.* New York: Grune and Stratton, 1982, pp 125–149.

CHAPTER 3

Basis of the Cardiac Resting Potential

NICHOLAS SPERELAKIS

INTRODUCTION

Cardiac muscle is a unique excitable tissue. The peculiar electrical properties of heart muscle determine the special mechanical properties of the heart, enabling it to serve as an effective pump for circulating the blood. The entire ventricle is rapidly activated in an all-or-none manner, within several hundredths of a second, by virtue of the rapidly conducting (2–3 m/s) specialized Purkinje fiber system and by rapid propagation (0.3–0.5 m/s) through the myocardium. Cardiac muscle cannot normally be tetanized because of the long functional refractory period resulting from the long-duration action potential (AP). The long-duration plateau component of the AP allows the mechanical active state to be maximally developed and maintained for a sufficiently long period.

The pumping action of the heart can be increased when required or decreased when conditions permit by various mechanisms, including release of the neurotransmitters norepinephrine and acetylcholine at the autonomic nerve terminals and by action of circulating hormones or autacoids (e.g., angiotensin II, histamine). Cardiac output can be increased by increasing heart rate (by increasing automaticity of the normal pacemaker for the heart, the SA node) and by increasing the force of contraction of the ventricles. In addition to the Starling mechanism, one key mechanism for increasing force of contraction is an increase in the number of functional Ca^{2+} slow channels (L-type) in the cell membrane available for voltage activation, thereby increasing the Ca^{2+} ion influx per cardiac cycle.

The cell membrane exerts tight control over the contractile machinery during the process of excitation-contraction (electromechanical) coupling. Some drugs and toxins exert primary or secondary effects on the electrical properties of the cell membrane, and thereby exert effects on automaticity, arrhythmias, and force of contraction. Therefore, for an understanding of the mode of action of cardioactive and cardiotoxic agents, neurotransmitters, hormones, and plasma electrolytes on the electrical and mechanical activity of the heart, it is necessary to understand the electrical properties and behavior of the myocardial cell membrane at rest and during excitation. The first step in gaining such an understanding is to examine the electrical properties of myocardial cells at rest, including the origin of the resting membrane potential (resting E_m). The resting E_m and AP result from properties of the cell membrane. Some of the electrical characteristics of the cells of the various tissues of the heart are summarized in table 3-1.

PASSIVE ELECTRICAL PROPERTIES

Membrane structure and composition

The cell membrane is composed of a bimolecular leaflet of phospholipid molecules (e.g., phosphatidylcholine and phosphatidylethanolamine) with protein molecules floating in the lipid bilayer. The nonpolar hydrophobic ends of the phospholipid molecules project toward the middle of the membrane, and the polar hydrophilic ends project toward the edges of the membrane bordering on the water phases (fig. 3-1). This orientation is thermodynamically favorable. The lipid bilayer membrane is about 50–70 Å thick, and the phospholipid molecules are about the right length (30–40 Å) to stretch across half of the membrane thickness. Cholesterol molecules are in high concentration in the cell membrane (of animal cells), giving a phospholipid : cholesterol ratio of about 1.0; they are inserted between the phospholipid molecules. Some of the large protein molecules inserted in the lipid bilayer matrix protrude through the entire membrane thickness, e.g., the Na,K-ATPase, Ca-ATPase, and the various ion channel proteins, whereas other proteins are inserted into one leaflet (inner or outer) only, e.g., G proteins and adenylate cyclase enzyme. These proteins "float" in the lipid bilayer matrix, and the membrane has fluidity (reciprocal of microviscosity), such that the protein molecules can move around laterally in the plane of the membrane.

The outer surface of the cell membrane is lined with strands of mucopolysaccharides (the cell coat or glycocalyx), which endow the cell with immunochemical properties. The cell coat is highly negatively charged and therefore can bind cations, such as the Ca^{2+} ion. Treatment with neuraminidase, to remove sialic acid residues, destroys the cell coat.

N. Sperelakis (ed.), Physiology and Pathophysiology of the Heart, Third Edition.

Table 3-1. Comparison of the resting potentials and action potentials of cells in different regions of the mammalian heart

Parameter	Ventricular cell	Atrial cell	Sinoatrial nodal cell	Atrioventricular nodal cell	Purkinje fiber
Resting potential (mV)	−80 to 90	−80 to 90	−50 to 60	−60 to 70	−90 to 95
Action potential					
Magnitude (mV)	110–120	110–120	60–70	70–80	120
Overshoot (mV)	30	30	0–10	5–15	30
Duration (ms)	200–300	100–300	100–300	100–300	300–500
Maximal rate of rise (V/s)	100–200	100–200	1–10	5–15	500–700
Propagation velocity (m/s)	0.3–0.4	0.3–0.4	<0.05	0.1	2–3
Fiber diameter (μm)	10–16	10–15	5–10	5–10	100

The action potential duration is about 120 ms in avian heart and about 400–500 ms in amphibian heart. The duration is a function of heart rate and temperature. The propagation velocity at the atrial-atrioventricular nodel junction is considerably less than in the atrioventricular node proper. Cell length is about 100–200 μm for myocardial cells.

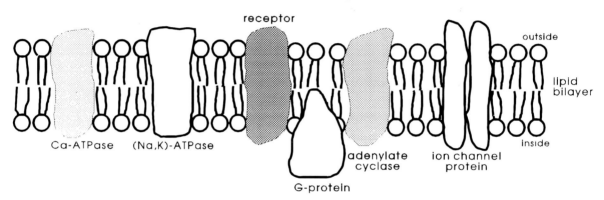

Fig. 3-1. Diagrammatic illustration of cell membrane substructure showing the lipid bilayer. Nonpolar hydrophobic tail ends of the phospholipid molecules project toward the middle of the membrane, and polar hydrophilic heads border on the water phase at each side of the membrane. The lipid bilayer is about 50–100 Å thick. For simplicity the cholesterol molecules are not shown. Large protein molecules protrude through the entire membrane thickness or are inserted into one leaflet only, as illustrated. These proteins include various enzymes associated with the cell membrane as well as membrane ionic channels. Membrane has fluidity so that the protein and lipid molecules can move around in the plane of the membrane and fluorescent probe molecules inserted into the hydrophobic region of the membrane have freedom to rotate.

Membrane capacitance and resistivity

Lipid bilayer membranes made artificially have a specific membrane capacitance (C_m) of 0.4–1.0 μF/cm², which is close to the value for biologic membranes. The capacitance of cell membranes is due to the lipid bilayer matrix. Calculation of membrane thickness (δ) from the following equation for capacitance, assuming a measured membrane capacitance (C_m) of 0.7 μF/cm² and a dielectric constant (ε) of 5, gives 63 Å:

$$C_m = \frac{\varepsilon A_m}{\delta} \frac{1}{4\pi k} \tag{3-1}$$

where A_m is the membrane area (in cm²) and k is a constant (9.0×10^{11} cm/F). Most oils have dielectric constants of 3–5. The more dipolar the material, the greater the dielectric constant (e.g., water, which is very dipolar, has a value of 81).

The artificial lipid bilayer membrane, on the other hand, has an exceedingly high specific resistance (R_m) of 10^6 to $10^9 \,\Omega$-cm², which is several orders of magnitude higher than the biologic cell membrane (about $10^3 \,\Omega$-cm²). R_m is greatly lowered, however, if the bilayer is doped with certain proteins or substances, such as macrocyclic-polypeptide antibiotics (ionophores). The added ionophores may be of the ion-carrier type, such as valinomycin, or of the channel-former type, such as gramicidin. Therefore, the presence of proteins that span across the thickness of the cell membrane must account for the relatively low resistance (high conductance) of the cell membrane. These proteins include those associated with the voltage-dependent gated ion channels of the excited membrane and the ion channels of the resting membrane. In summary, the *capacitance* is due to the *lipid bilayer matrix*, and the *conductance* is due to *proteins* inserted in the lipid bilayer.

The dielectric property of the cell membrane is very good. For a resting E_m of about 80 mV and a thickness of about 60 Å, the voltage gradient sustained across the membrane is about 133,000 V/cm. Thus the cell membrane tolerates an enormous voltage gradient.

Membrane fluidity

The electrical properties and the ion transport properties of the cell membrane are determined by the molecular composition of the membrane. The lipid bilayer matrix even influences the function of the membrane proteins, e.g., the Na,K-ATPase activity is affected by the surrounding lipid. A high cholesterol content lowers the fluidity of the membrane, and a high degree of unsaturation and branching of the tails of the phospholipid molecules raises the fluidity; chain length of the lipids also affects fluidity. The polar portion of cholesterol lodges in the hydrophilic part of the membrane, and the nonpolar part of the planar cholesterol molecule is wedged between the fatty acid tails, thus restricting their motion and lowering fluidity. Phospholipids with unsaturated and branched-chain fatty acids cannot be packed tightly because of steric hindrance due to their greater rigidity; hence such phospholipids increase membrane fluidity. Low temperature decreases membrane fluidity, as expected. Ca^{2+} and Mg^{2+} may diminish the charge repulsion between the phospholipid head groups; this allows the bilayer molecules to pack more tightly, thereby constraining the motion of the tails and reducing fluidity. Each phospholipid tail occupies about 20–30 Å^2, and each head group about 60 Å^2 {14}. Membrane fluidity changes occur in muscle development and in certain disease states such as cancer, muscular dystrophy (Duchenne type), and myotonic dystrophy.

The hydrophobic portion of local anesthetic molecules may interpose between the lipid molecules. This separates the acyl chain tails of the phospholipid molecules further, reducing the Van der Waals forces of interaction between adjacent tails, and so increasing the membrane fluidity. Local anesthetics depress the resting conductance of the membrane for K^+ and Na^+, and depress the voltage-dependent changes in g_{Na}, g_K, and g_{Ca}; that is, the local anesthetics produce a nonselective depression of most conductances of the resting and the excited membrane. At least part of this depression could come about indirectly by the anesthetics' effect on the fluidity of the lipid matrix. At the concentration of a local anesthetic required to completely block excitability, its estimated concentration in the lipid bilayer is more than 100,000/μm^2. Part of the depression of the Na,K-ATPase activity by local anesthetics {9} also could be explained by an effect on the fluidity, although a direct effect on the protein enzyme is also possible.

Potential profile across membrane

The cell membrane has *fixed negative charges* as its outer and inner surfaces. The charges are presumably due to acidic phospholipids in the bilayer and to protein mole-

cules, either embedded in the membrane (islands floating in the lipid bilayer matrix) or tightly adsorbed to the surface of the membrane. Most proteins have an acid isoelectric point, so that at a pH near 7.0 they possess a net negative charge. The charge at the outer surface of the cell membrane, with respect to the solution bathing the cell, is known as the *zeta potential*. This charge is responsible for the electrophoresis of cells in an electric field, the cells

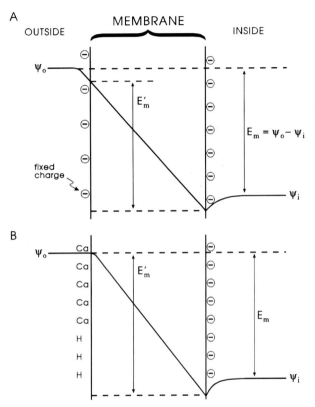

Fig. 3-2. Potential profile across the cell membrane. **A:** Because of fixed negative charges (at pH 7.4) at the outer and inner surfaces of the membrane, there is a negative potential that extends from the edge of the membrane into the bathing solution on both sides of the membrane. This surface potential falls off exponentially with distance into the solution. Magnitude of the surface potential is a function of the charge density. Ψ_o is the electrical potential of the outside solution, Ψ_i is that of the inside solution, and membrane potential (E_m) is the difference ($\Psi_o - \Psi_i$). E_m is determined by the equilibrium potentials and relative conductances. The profile of the potential through the membrane is shown as linear (the constant-field assumption), although this need not be true for the present purpose. If the outer surface potential is exactly equal to that in the inner surface, then the true transmembrane potential (E_m') is exactly equal to the (microelectrode) measured membrane potential (E_m). **B:** If the outer surface potential is different from the inner potential, for example, by elevating the extracellular Ca^{2+} concentration or lowering the pH to bind Ca^{2+} or H^+ to more of the negative charges, then the E_m' is greater than the measured E_m. Diminution of the inner surface charge decreases E_m'. The membrane ion changes are controlled E_m'.

58   *Physiology and Pathophysiology of the Heart*

moving toward the anode (positive electrode) because unlike charges attract. The surface charge affects the true potential difference (PD) across the membrane, as illustrated in fig. 3-2A. At each surface, the fixed charge produces an *electric field* that extends a short distance into the solution and causes each surface of the membrane to be slightly more negative (by a few millivolts) than the extracellular and intracellular solutions. The potential theoretically recorded by an ideal electrode, as the electrode is driven through the solution perpendicular to the membrane surface, should become negative as the electrode approaches within a few Angstrom units of the surface. The potential difference between the membrane surface and the solution declines exponentially as a function of distance from the surface. The *length constant* is a function of the ionic strength (or resistivity) of the solution: The lower the ionic strength, the greater the length constant is. The magnitude of the PD depends on the density of the charge sites (number per unit of membrane area); the number of charges is also affected by the ionic strength and pH.

In fig. 3-2A, the membrane potential measured by an intracellular microelectrode (E_m) is the potential of the outer solution (Ψ_o, the reference electrode) minus the potential of the inner solution (Ψ_i, the active microelectrode):

$$E_m = \Psi_o - \Psi_i. \tag{3-2}$$

The true PD across the membrane (E'_m), however, is really that PD directly across the membrane, as shown in the figure. If the surface charges at each surface of the membrane are equal, then $E'_m = E_m$. If the outer surface charge is decreased to zero by extra binding of protons or cations, such as Ca^{2+}, then the membrane becomes slightly hyperpolarized ($E'_m > E_m$), although this is not measurable by the intracellular microelectrode (fig. 3-2B). Conversely, if the outer surface charge were restored and if the inner surface charge were neutralized, then the membrane would become slightly depolarized ($E'_m < E_m$); again this change is not measurable by the microelectrode, which measures the PD between the two solutions.

Because the membrane ionic conductances are controlled by the PD directly across the membrane (i.e., by E'_m and not by E_m), changes in the surface charges (e.g., by drugs, ionic strength, or pH) can lead to apparent shifts in the threshold potential, activation curve, and inactivation curve. For example, elevated $[Ca]_o$ is known to raise the *threshold potential* (i.e., the *critical depolarization* required to reach electrical threshold), as expected from the small increase in E'_m that should occur. The apparent *mechanical threshold* (the E_m value at which contraction of muscle just begins) can also be shifted by a similar mechanism.

ION DISTRIBUTIONS AND THEIR MAINTENANCE

Resting potentials and ion distributions

The transmembrane potential in resting atrial and ventricular myocardial cells is about $-80\,mV$ (table 3-1). The resting E_m or maximum diastolic potential in Purkinje fibers is somewhat greater (about $-90\,mV$), whereas that in the nodal cells is lower (about $-60\,mV$).

The ionic composition of the extracellular fluid bathing the heart cells is similar to that of the blood plasma. It is high in Na^+ (about 145 mM) and Cl^- (about 100 mM), but low in K^+ (about 4.5 mM). The Ca^{2+} concentration is about 2 mM. In contrast, the intracellular fluid has a low concentration of Na^+ (about 15 mM or less) and Cl^- (about 6–8 mM), but a high concentration of K^+ (about 150–170 mM). The free intracellular Ca^{2+} concentration ($[Ca]_i$) is about $10^{-7}\,M$, but during contraction it may rise as high as $10^{-5}\,M$. The total intracellular Ca^{2+} is much higher (about 2 mM/kg), but most of this is bound to molecules such as proteins or is sequestered into compartments such as mitochondria and the sarcoplasmic reticulum (SR). Most of the intracellular K^+ is free, and it has a diffusion coefficient only slightly less than K^+ in free solution. Thus, under normal conditions the myocardial cell maintains an internal ion concentration markedly different from that in the medium bathing the cells, and it is these ion concentration differences that underlie the resting potential and excitability. The ion distributions and related pumps and exchange reactions are depicted in fig. 3-3.

Na-K pump

The intracellular ion concentrations are maintained differently from those in the extracellular fluid by active ion transport mechanisms that expend metabolic energy to push specific ions against their concentration or electrochemical gradients. These ion pumps are located in the cell membrane at the cell surface and probably also in the transverse tubular membrane. The major ion pump is the Na-K-linked pump, whch pumps Na^+ out of the cell against its electrochemical gradient, while simultaneously pumping K^+ in against its electrochemical gradient (fig. 3-3). The coupling of Na^+ and K^+ pumping is obligatory, since in zero $[K]_o$ the Na^+ can no longer be pumped out; that is, a coupling ratio of $3\,Na^+:0\,K^+$ is not possible. The coupling ratio of Na^+ pumped out to K^+ pumped is generally 3:2. If the ratio were 3:3, the pump would be electrically neutral or nonelectrogenic, because the pump would pull in three positive charges (K^+) for every three positive charges (Na^+) it pushed out. When the ratio is 3:2, the pump is electrogenic and directly produces a potential difference (PD) that causes the membrane potential (E_m) to be greater (more negative) than it would be otherwise, namely, on the basis of the ion concentration gradients and relative permeabilities or net diffusion potential (E_{diff}) alone. A coupling ratio of $3\,Na^+:1\,K^+$ would produce a greater electrogenic pump potential (V_p). Under normal steady-state conditions, the contribution of the Na^+-K^+ electrogenic pump potential to E_m (ΔV_{mp}) in myocardial cells is only a few millivolts (see section, *Electrogenic sodium pump potential*).

The driving mechanism for the Na-K pump is a membrane ATPase, the Na,K-ATPase, which spans across the membrane and requires both Na^+ and K^+ ions for acti-

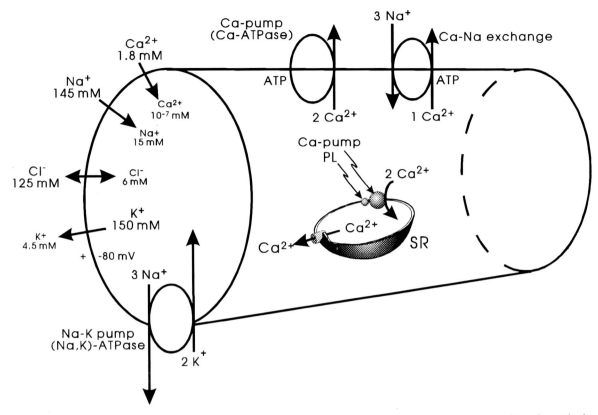

Fig. 3-3. Intracellular and extracellular ion distributions in a vertebrate myocardial cell. Also given are the polarity and magnitude of the resting potential. Arrows give direction of the net electrochemical gradient. Invagination transverse (T) tubules found in mammalian ventricular cells are continuations of the cell surface membrane into the cell interior. The Na^+-K^+ pump is located in the cell surface and the T-tubule membranes. A Ca-ATPase/Ca pump, similar to that in the SR, may be located in the cell membrane. A Ca-Na exchange carrier is located in the cell membrane.

vation. This enzyme requires Mg^{2+} for activity, and it is inhibited by Ca^{2+}. ATP, Mg^{2+}, and Na^+ are thus required at the inner surface of the membrane, and K^+ is required at the outer surface. A phosphorylated intermediate of the Na,K-ATPase occurs in the transport cycle, its phosphorylation being Na^+ dependent and its dephosphorylation being K^+ dependent (for references, see Sperelakis {42}). The pump enzyme usually drives three Na^+ ions in and two K^+ ions out for each ATP molecule hydrolyzed. The Na,K-ATPase is specifically inhibited by vanadate ion and by the cardiac glycosides (digitalis drugs) acting on the outer surface. The pump enzyme is also inhibited by vanadate ion and by sulfhydryl reagents (such as N-ethylmaleimide, mercurial diuretics, and ethacrynic acid), thus indicating that the SH groups are crucial for activity.

Blockade of the Na-K pump produces only a small immediate effect on the resting E_m: a small depolarization of about 2–6 mV, representing the contribution of V_p to E_m (ΔV_{mp}). Since excitability and generation of APs are almost unaffected at short times, excitability is independent of active ion transport. However, over a period of many minutes, depending on the ratio of surface area to volume of the cell, the resting E_m slowly declines because of gradual dissipation of the ionic gradients. The progressive depolarization depresses the rate of rise of the AP, and hence the propagation velocity, and eventually all excitability is lost. Thus, a large resting potential and excitability, although not immediately dependent on the Na-K pump, are ultimately dependent on it.

The rate of Na-K pumping in myocardial cells must change with the heart rate in order to maintain the intracellular ion concentrations relatively constant. A higher frequency of APs results in a greater overall movement of ions down their electrochemical gradients, and these ions must be repumped. For example, the cells tend to gain Na^+, Cl^-, and Ca^{2+} and to lose K^+. The factors that control the rate of Na-K pumping include $[Na]_i$ and $[K]_o$. In cells that have a large surface area to volume ratio (such as small-diameter nonmyelinated neurons), $[Na]_i$ may increase by a relatively large percentage during a train of APs, and this would stimulate the pumping rate. Likewise, an accumulation of K^+ externally occurs and also stimulates the pump (the K_m value for K^+, i.e., the concentration for half-maximal rate, is about 2 mM). It has been shown that $[K]_o$ is significantly increased during the AP in cardiac muscle.

Cl⁻ distribution

In many invertebrate and vertebrate nerve or muscle cells, Cl⁻ ion does not appear to be actively transported, that is, there is no Cl⁻ ion pump. In such cases, Cl⁻ distributes itself passively (no energy used) in accordance with E_m. In such a case, E_{Cl} is equal to E_m in a resting cell. In mammalian myocardial cells, Cl⁻ also seems to be close to passive distribution, because $[Cl]_i$ is at, or only slightly above, the value predicted by the Nernst equation from the resting E_m (for references, see Sperelakis {42}). When passively distributed, $[Cl]_i$ is low because the negative potential inside the cell (the resting potential) pushes out the negatively charged Cl⁻ ion (like charges repel) until the Cl⁻ distribution is at equilibrium with the resting E_m. Hence, for a resting E_m of $-80\,mV$, and taking $[Cl]_o$ to be $100\,mM$, $[Cl]_i$ calculated from the Nernst equation (see section on *Equilibrium potentials*) would be at $4.9\,mM$:

$$E_m = +61\,mV \log \frac{[Cl]_i}{[Cl]_o}$$

$$= -61\,mV \log \frac{[Cl]_o}{[Cl]_i}$$

$$\frac{-80\,mV}{-60\,mV} = \log \frac{100\,mM}{[Cl]_i}$$

$$\frac{100\,mM}{[Cl]_i} = \text{anti} \log \frac{-80\,mV}{-61\,mV} = \text{anti} \log 1.31 = 20.4$$

$$[Cl]_i = \frac{100\,mM}{20.4} = 4.90\,mM \qquad (3\text{-}3)$$

During the AP, the inside of the cell goes in a positive direction, and a net Cl⁻ influx (outward Cl⁻ current, I_{Cl}) will occur and thus increase $[Cl]_i$. The magnitude of the Cl⁻ influx depends on the Cl⁻ conductance (g_{Cl}) of the membrane:

$$I_{Cl} = g_{Cl}(E_m - E_{Cl}) \qquad (3\text{-}4)$$

This equation is discussed below in the section on *Electromechanical driving forces and membrane ionic currents*. Thus the average level of $[Cl]_i$ in myocardial cells of the beating heart should depend on the frequency and duration of the AP, that is, on the mean E_m averaged over many AP cycles.

Ca²⁺ distribution

NEED FOR CALCIUM PUMPS

For the positively charged Ca²⁺ ion, there must be some mechanism for removing Ca²⁺ from the myoplasm. Otherwise the myocardial cell would continue to gain Ca²⁺ until there was no electrochemical gradient for net influx of Ca²⁺. Ca²⁺ loading would occur until the free $[Ca]_i$ in the myoplasm was even greater than that outside (ca. 2 mM) because of the negative potential inside the cell. Therefore, there must be one or more Ca²⁺ pumps in operation. The SR membrane contains a Ca²⁺-activated ATPase (which also requires Mg²⁺) that actively pumps two Ca²⁺ ions from the myoplasm into the SR lumen at the expense of one ATP. This pump ATPase is capable of pumping down the Ca²⁺ to less than $10^{-7}\,M$. The Ca-ATPase of the SR is regulated by an associated low molecular weight protein, *phospholamban*. Phospholamban is phosphorylated by cyclic AMP-dependent protein kinase and, when phosphorylated, stimulates the Ca-ATPase and Ca²⁺ pumping. The sequestration of Ca²⁺ by the SR is essential for muscle relaxation. The mitochondria also can actively take up Ca²⁺ almost to the same degree as the SR, but this Ca²⁺ pool probably does not play an important role in normal excitation-contraction coupling processes.

However, the resting Ca²⁺ influx and the extra Ca²⁺ influx that enters with each AP must be returned to the interstitial fluid. Several mechanisms have been proposed for this (for references, see Sperelakis {42}): (a) A Ca-ATPase, similar to that in the SR, is present in the sarcolemma, and (b) a Ca-Na exchange occurs across the cell membrane. It has been reported that there is a Ca-ATPase in the sarcolemma of myocardial cells {5,15} and smooth muscle {4} that actively transports two Ca²⁺ outward against an electrochemical gradient, utilizing one ATP in the process. Phospholamban is not associated with the sarcolemmal Ca-ATPase. It has been speculated that some of the Ca²⁺ sequestered into the SR network may be transported across the junctional coupling formed between the junctional SR and the sarcolemma in cardiac muscle. If this were the case, this would allow a more direct reequilibration of the Ca²⁺ taken up by the SR with the ISF space.

Ca/Na EXCHANGE REACTION

The Ca_i/Na_o exchange reaction exchanges one internal Ca²⁺ ion for three external Na⁺ ions via a membrane carrier molecule (for references, see Sperelakis {42}; fig. 3-3). This reaction is facilitated by ATP, but ATP is not hydrolyzed (consumed) in this reaction. Instead, the energy for the pumping of Ca²⁺ against its large electrochemical gradient comes from the Na⁺ electrochemical gradient; that is, the uphill transport of Ca²⁺ is coupled to the downhill movement of Na⁺. Effectively, the energy required for this Ca²⁺ movement is derived from the Na,K-ATPase. Thus, the Na-K pump, which uses ATP to maintain the Na⁺ electrochemical gradient, indirectly helps to maintain the Ca²⁺ electrochemical gradient. Hence, the inward Na⁺ leak is greater than it would be otherwise. A complete discussion of the Ca/Na exchange is given in Chapter 15.

The energy cost (ΔG_{Ca}, in joules/mole) for pumping out Ca²⁺ ion is directly proportional to its electrochemical gradient. These energetic equations are as follows (where Δ_G is the change in free energy):

$$\Delta G_{Ca} = zF(E_m - E_{Ca}). \qquad (3\text{-}5)$$

The energy available from the Na⁺ distribution is directly proportional to its electrochemical gradient:

$$\Delta G_{Na} = zF(E_m - E_{Na}). \qquad (3\text{-}6)$$

Depending on the exact values of $[Na]_i$ and $[Ca]_i$ at rest in a cardiac cell, the energetics would be about adequate for

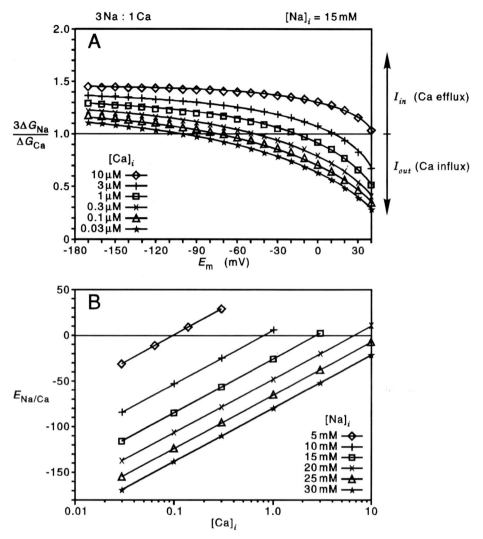

Fig. 3-4. Electrogenic Na/Ca exchange for $[Na]_i$ of 15 mM. Calculated ratio of the free energies for Na^+ versus Ca^{2+} ($3\,\Delta G_{Na}/\Delta G_{Ca}$) plotted as a function of membrane potentials (E_m) for coupling ratio of $3\,Na^+:1\,Ca^{2+}$ (**A**) for six different intracellular Ca^{2+} concentrations ($[Ca]_i$). At a ratio of 1.0, $3\,\Delta G_{Na} = -\Delta G_{Na}$ and the sum equals zero: $3\,\Delta G_{Na} + \Delta G_{Ca} = 0$. Therefore, the exchange would be at equilibrium at the E_m value at which each $[Ca]_i$ curve crosses the ratio of 1.0 line, i.e., this gives the value of the exchanger equilibrium potential, $E_{Na/Ca}$. At ΔG ratios >1.0, there is a net inward current carried by Na^+ ion, coupled with net Ca^{2+} efflux from the cell; that is, this represents the forward mode of operation of the exchanger. At ΔG ratios <1.0, there is a net outward current carried by Na^+ ion, coupled with net Ca^{2+} influx into the cell. This reflects the reverse mode of operation of the exchanger. Note that at the higher (more positive) E_m levels, the ΔG ratio is reduced. Also note that at the higher $[Ca]_i$ levels, there is a rightward shift of $E_{Na/Ca}$. **B:** The reversal potential ($E_{Na/Ca}$) for the Na/Ca exchanger, assuming a coupling ratio of $3\,Na^+:1\,Ca^{2+}$, is plotted on the ordinate as a function of $[Ca]_i$ on the abscissa. The family of curves is for six different $[Na]_i$ levels.

an exchange ratio of $3\,Na^+:1\,Ca^{2+}$. An exchange ratio of 3:1 would produce a small depolarization due to a net inward flow of current ($3\,Na^+$ in to $1\,Ca^{2+}$ out) via this electrogenic Ca_i/Na_o exchanger. This net exchanger current can be measured in whole-cell voltage-clamp studies when all ionic currents and Na/K pump current are blocked.

The exchange reaction depends on relative concentrations of Ca^{2+} and Na^+ on each side of the membrane and on relative affinities of the binding sites to Ca^{2+} and Na^+. Because of this Ca_i/Na_o exchange reaction, whenever the cell gains Na^+ it will also gain Ca^{2+}, because the Na^+ electrochemical gradient is reduced and the exchange reaction becomes slowed. The Ca/Na exchange process has been proposed as the mechanism of the positive inotropic action resulting from cardiac glycoside inhibition of the Na-K pump.

In addition, when the membrane is depolarized during

the AP plateau, the exchange carriers will exchange the ions in reverse, namely, internal Na^+ for external Ca^{2+}, and thus increase Ca^{2+} influx. The net effect of this mechanism is to elevate $[Ca]_i$. Such *reversed Ca_o/Na_i exchange* appears to be a significant source of Ca^{2+} for contraction in cardiac muscle of some species.

The ratio of free energy changes for Na^+ to Ca^{2+} were calculated for a coupling ratio of $3 Na^+ : 1 Ca^{2+}$ ($3 \Delta G_{Na}/\Delta G_{Ca}$) and a $[Na]_i$ of 15 mM, and plotted as a function of membrane potential, for different $[Ca]_i$ levels (fig. 3-4A). This plot allows a simple assessment of how the directionality of the exchanger is affected by E_m, i.e., *forward mode* versus *reverse mode* of operation, and how the *reversal potential* of the exchanger is shifted by $[Ca]_i$. When the ratio is 1.0, $3 \Delta G_{Na} = -\Delta G_{Ca}$, and the sum equals zero: $3 \Delta G_{Na} + -\Delta G_{Ca} = 0$. Therefore, the exchanger would be at equilibrium. For ΔG ratios >1.0, there is a net *inward current* carried by Na^+ ion, coupled with net Ca^{2+} *efflux* from the cell. This represents *forward mode* of operation of the exchanger. For ΔG ratios <1.0, there is a net *outward current* carried by Na^+ ion, coupled to a net Ca^{2+} *influx* into the cell. This represents *reverse mode* of operation of the exchanger.

The *equilibrium potential* or *reversal potential* for the Ca/Na exchanger ($E_{Na/Ca}$), for an exchange ratio of $3 Na^+ : 1 Ca^{2+}$, is

$$E_{Na/Ca} = 3 E_{Na} - 2 E_{Ca}, \tag{3-7}$$

where E_{Na} and E_{Ca} are the equilibrium potentials for Na^+ and Ca^{2+}, respectively, as calculated from the Nernst equation. Thus, the $E_{Na/Ca}$ varies with the $[Na]_i$ level and during changes in $[Ca]_i$ levels that occur with contraction. $E_{Na/Ca}$ is less negative (more positive) when $[Ca]_i$ is elevated, and shifts to more negative potentials when $[Na]_i$ is elevated (fig. 3-4B).

Therefore, when a myocardial cell changes from the resting potential (ca. -80 mV) to the AP plateau (ca. $+20$ mV), simultaneous with $[Ca]_i$ being elevated from about 0.1 μM to 3 μM, the exchanger switches to the reverse mode of operation, with Ca^{2+} influx. As stated previously, this Ca^{2+} influx can be a significant source of the total Ca^{2+} influx during excitation-contraction coupling. If the $[Na]_i$ level were 25 or 30 mM, the exchanger would always operate in the *reverse mode* at the physiological E_m levels.

EQUILIBRIUM POTENTIALS

For each ionic species distributed unequally across the cell membrane, an equilibrium potential (E_i) or battery can be calculated for that ion from the *Nernst equation* (for 37°C):

$$E_i = \frac{-61 \, mV}{z} \log \frac{C_i}{C_o}, \tag{3-8}$$

where C_i is the internal concentration of the ion, C_o is the extracellular concentration, and z is the valence (with sign). The -61 mV constant (2.303 RT/F) becomes -59 mV at 22°C (R is the gas constant of 8.3 joules/M·°K), T is the absolute temperature (°K = 273 + °C), F is the

Faraday constant (96,500 coul/equiv), zF = coul/M, and 2.303 is the conversion factor for natural log to $\log_{10}$. The Nernst equation gives the potential difference (PD; electrical force) that would *exactly oppose the concentration gradient* (diffusion force). Only very small charge separation (Q, in coulombs) is required to build up a very large PD:

$$E_m = \frac{Q}{C_m}, \tag{3-9}$$

where C_m is the membrane capacitance. For the ion distributions given previously, the approximate equilibrium potentials are

$$E_{Na} = +60 \, mV$$
$$E_{Ca} = +129 \, mV$$
$$E_K = -94 \, mV$$
$$E_{Cl} = -80 \, mV.$$

The sign of the equilibrium potential is for the inside with reference to the outside of the cell (fig. 3-5). In a concentration cell, the side of higher concentration becomes negative for positive ions (cations) and positive for negative ions (anions). Any ion whose equilibrium potential is different from the resting potential (e.g., -80 mV) is off equilibrium, and therefore must effectively be pumped at the expense of energy. In the myocardial cell, only Cl^- ion appears to be at or near equilibrium, whereas Na^+, Ca^{2+}, and K^+ are actively transported. Even H^+ ion is off equilibrium, E_H being close to zero potential. Extensive discussion of concentration cells and diffusion is given by Sperelakis {42}, and the mechanisms for development of the equilibrium potential are depicted in fig. 3-6 and discussed in its legend.

ELECTROCHEMICAL DRIVING FORCES AND MEMBRANE IONIC CURRENTS

The *electrochemical driving force* for each species of ion is the algebraic difference between its equilibrium potential, E_i, and the membrane potential, E_m. The total driving force is the sum of two forces: an *electrical force* (the negative potential in a cell at rest tends to pull in positively charged ions, because unlike charges attract) and a *diffusion force* (based on the concentration gradient; fig. 3-7). Thus in a resting cell the driving force for Na^+ is

$$(E_m - E_{Na}) = -80 \, mV - (-60 \, mV) = -140 \, mV. \tag{3-10}$$

The negative sign means that the driving force is directed to bring about net movement of Na^+ inward. The driving force for Ca^{2+} is

$$(E_m - E_{Ca}) = -80 \, mV - (+129 \, mV) = -209 \, mV. \tag{3-11}$$

The driving force for K^+ is

$$(E_m - E_K) = -80 \, mV - (-94 \, mV) = +14 \, mV. \tag{3-12}$$

Hence, the driving force for K^+ is small and directed outward. The driving force for Cl^- is nearly zero for a cell at rest:

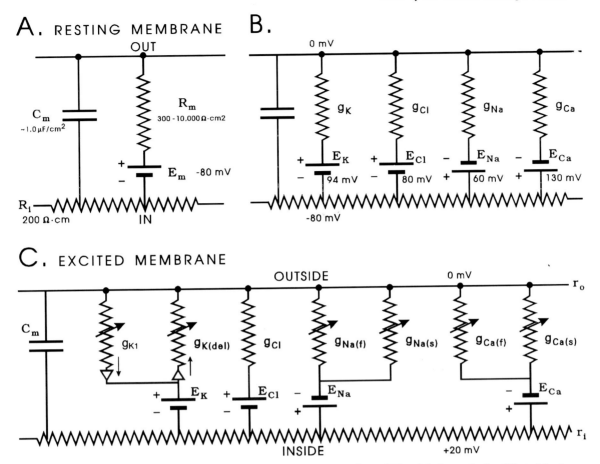

A. RESTING MEMBRANE   **B.**

C. EXCITED MEMBRANE

Fig. 3-5. Electrical equivalent circuits for a myocardial cell membrane at rest (A and B) and during excitation (C). **A:** Membrane as a parallel resistance-capacitance circuit, the membrane resistance (R_m) being in parallel with the membrane capacitance (C_m). Resting potential (E_m) is represented by an 80-mV battery in series with the membrane resistance, the negative pole facing inward. **B:** Membrane resistance is divided into its four component parts, one for each of the four major ions of importance: K$^+$, Cl$^-$, Na$^+$, and Ca^{2+}. Resistances for these ions (R_K, R_{Cl}, R_{Na}, and R_{Ca}) are parallel to one another and represent totally separate and independent pathways for permeation of each ion through the resting membrane. These ion resistances are depicted as their reciprocals, namely, ion conductances (g_K, g_{Cl}, g_{Na}, and g_{Ca}). Equilibrium potential for each ion (e.g., E_K), determined solely by the ion distribution in the steady state and calculated from the Nernst equation, is shown in series with the conductance path for that ion. Resting potential of -80 mV is determined by the equilibrium potentials and by the relative conductances. **C:** Equivalent circuit is further expanded to illustrate the voltage-dependent conductances that are activated during excitation. There are at least two separate K$^+$-conductance pathways [labelled here g_{K1} and $g_{K(del)}$]. Arrowheads in series with the K$^+$ conductances represent rectifiers, the arrowhead points giving the direction of least resistance to current flow. Thus $g_{K(o)}$ allows K$^+$ flux to occur more readily in the outward direction (outwardly directed rectification), whereas g_{K1} allows K$^+$ flux to occur more readily in the inward direction (inwardly directed rectification). There is a kinetically fast Na$^+$ conductance pathway (g_{Na}^f). In addition, there is a kinetically slow pathway that allows Ca2+ to pass through. Arrows drawn through the resistors represent that the conductances are variable, depending on membrane potential and time.

$$(E_m - E_{Cl}) = -80 \, mV - (-80 \, mV) = 0. \tag{3-13}$$

However, during the AP, when E_m is changing, the driving force for Cl$^-$ becomes large, and there is a net driving force for inward Cl$^-$ movement (*Cl$^-$ influx is an outward Cl$^-$ current*). Similarly, the driving force for K$^+$ outward movement increases during the AP, whereas those for Na$^+$ and Ca^{2+} decrease.

The *net current* for each ionic species (I_i) is equal to its *driving force times its conductance* (g_i, reciprocal of the resistance) through the membrane. This is essentially Ohm's Law:

$$I = V/R = g \cdot V, \tag{3-14}$$

modified for the fact that in an electrolytic system the total force tending to drive net movement of a charged particle must take into account both the electrical force and the concentration (or chemical) force. Thus, for the four ions, the net current can be expressed as

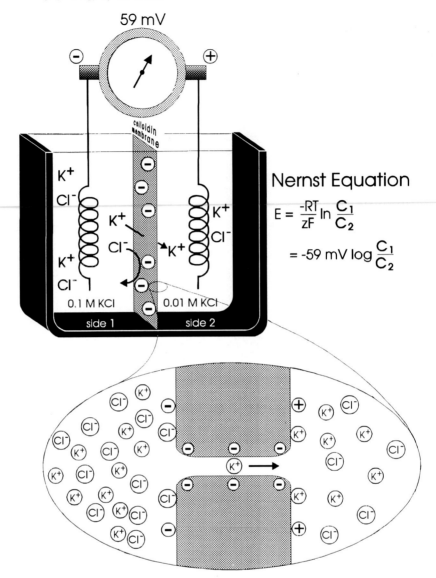

$$E = \frac{-RT}{zF} \ln \frac{C_1}{C_2}$$

$$= -59 \text{ mV} \log \frac{C_1}{C_2}$$

Fig. 3-6. **Upper diagram:** Concentration cell diffusion potential developed across an artificial membrane containing negatively charged pores. The membrane is impermeable to Cl$^-$ ions but permeable to cations such as Na$^+$. The concentration gradient for Na$^+$ causes a potential to be generated, the side of higher Na$^+$ concentration becoming negative. **Lower diagram:** Expanded diagram of a water-filled pore in the membrane, showing the permeability to Na$^+$ ions, but lack of penetration of Cl$^-$ ions. Potential difference is generated by charge separation, a slight excess of Na$^+$ ions being held close to the right-hand surface of the membrane; a slight excess of Cl$^-$ ions is plastered up close to the left surface.

$$I_{Na} = g_{Na}(E_m - E_{Na}) \tag{3-15}$$

$$I_{Ca} = g_{Ca}(E_m - E_{Ca}) \tag{3-16}$$

$$I_K = g_K(E_m - E_K) \tag{3-17}$$

$$I_{Cl} = g_{Cl}(E_m - E_{Cl}). \tag{3-18}$$

In a resting cell, Cl$^-$ and Ca^{2+} can be neglected, and the Na$^+$ current (inward) must be equal and opposite to the K$^+$ current (outward) in order to maintain a steady resting potential:

$$I_K = -I_{Na}. \tag{3-19}$$

Thus, although in the resting membrane the driving force for Na$^+$ is much greater than that for K$^+$, g_K is much larger than g_{Na}, so the currents are equal. Hence, there is a continual leak of Na$^+$ inward and K$^+$ outward, even in a resting cell, and the system would run down if active pumping were blocked. Since the ratio of the Na^+/K^+ driving forces ($-140\,mV/-14\,mV$) is 10, the ratio of conductances (g_{Na}/g_K) will be about $1:10$. The fact that g_K is much greater than g_{Na} accounts for the resting potential being close to E_K and far from E_{Na}.

The myocardial membrane has at least five separate voltage-dependent K^+ channels (fig. 3-5C). One of them, known as the I_{K1} channel, allows K^+ ion to pass more readily inward (against the usual net electrochemical gradient for K^+) than outward, the *inward-going rectifier* or *anomalous rectification*. This kinetically fast gated channel is responsible for the rapid decrease in K^+ conductance upon depolarization (and the increase in conductance with repolarization), and helps to set the resting potential and to bring about the terminal repolarization (phase 3) of the AP.

A second type of voltage-dependent K^+ channel is similar to the usual K^+ channel found in other excitable membranes, which slowly opens (increasing total g_K) upon depolarization, the *delayed rectifier* [I_K or $I_{K(del)}$]. This channel allows K^+ to pass more readily outward (down the usual electrochemical gradient for K^+) than inward, and so is also known as the *outward-going rectifier*. This delayed rectifier channel in myocardial cells turns on much more slowly than in nerve, skeletal muscle, or smooth muscle. The activation of this channel produces the increase in total g_K that terminates the cardiac AP plateau (phase 3 repolarization).

A third type of K^+ channel is activated by elevation of $[Ca]_i$, and is therefore known as the Ca^{2+}-activated K^+ channel or $I_{K(Ca)}$. With Ca^{2+} influx and internal release during the AP and contraction, the $I_{K(Ca)}$ channels are activated and help the $I_{K(del)}$ channels to repolarize the AP.

A fourth type of K^+ channel is kinetically fast [compared to $I_{K(del)}$] and provides a rapid outward K^+ current that produces a small amount of initial repolarization, known as phase 1 repolarization. This occurs immediately following the rapidly rising spike portion of the AP and is known as the *transient outward current* (I_{to}). There is some evidence that Cl^- current may contribute to I_{to} (Cl^- influx provides an outward I_{Cl}).

A fifth type of K^+ channel provides a current known as $I_{K(ATP)}$, and is regulated by ATP, such that in normal myocardial cells this K^+ channel is inhibited or masked or silent. However, in ischemic or hypoxic conditions, when the ATP level is lowered, the $I_{K(ATP)}$ channels become unmasked and provide a large outward I_K that prematurely shortens the cardiac AP. This channel provides a *protection mechanism* for the heart, namely, the ischemic region of the heart develops very abbreviated APs, and hence contraction is greatly depressed. This acts to *conserve ATP* in the afflicted cells, enabling full recovery if the blood flow returns to normal after a short time period.

DETERMINATION OF RESTING POTENTIAL AND NET DIFFUSION POTENTIAL (E_{diff})

For given ion distributions, which normally remain nearly constant under usual steady-state conditions, the resting

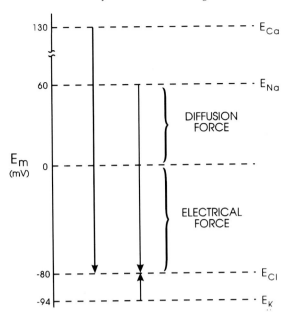

Fig. 3-7. Representation of the electrochemical driving forces for Na^+, Ca^{2+}, K^+, and Cl^-. Equilibrium potentials for each ion (e.g., E_{Na}) are positioned vertically according to their magnitude and sign; they were calculated from the Nernst equation for a given set of extracellular and intracellular ion concentrations. Measured resting potential is assumed to be $-80\,mV$. Electrochemical driving force for an ion is the difference between its equilibrium potential (E_i) and the membrane potential (E_m), that is, ($E_i - E_m$). Thus at rest the driving force for Na^+ is the difference between E_{Na} and the resting E_m; if E_{Na} is $+60\,mV$ and resting E_m is $-80\,mV$, the driving force is $140\,mV$; that is, the driving force is the algebraic sum of the diffusion force and the electrical force, and is represented by the length of the arrows in the diagram. Driving force for Ca^{2+} (about $210\,mV$) is even greater than that for Na^+, whereas that for K^+ is much less (about $14\,mV$). Direction of the arrows indicates the direction of the net electrochemical driving force, namely, the direction for K^+ is outward, whereas that for Na^+ and Ca^{2+} is inward. If Cl^- is passively distributed, then its distribution across the cell membrane can only be determined by the net membrane potential; for a cell sitting a long time at rest, $E_{Cl} = E_m$ and there is no net driving force.

potential is determined by the relative membrane conductances (g) or permeabilities (P) for Na^+ and K^+ ions; that is, the resting potential (of about $-80\,mV$) is close to E_K (about $-94\,mV$) because $g_K \gg g_{Na}$ or $P_K \gg P_{Na}$. There is a direct proportionality between P and g at constant E_m and concentrations. From simple circuit analysis (using Ohm's Law and Kirchhoff's Laws), one can prove that this should be true. Therefore, the membrane potential will always be closer to the battery (equilibrium potential) having the lowest resistance (highest conductance) in series with it (figs. 3-5 and 3-7). In the resting membrane, this battery is E_K, whereas in the excited membrane it will be E_{Na} (or E_{Ca}), because there is a large increase in g_{Na} (and g_{Ca}) during the AP. Any ion that is passively distributed cannot determine the resting potential; instead, the resting potential determines the distribution of that ion. Therefore, Cl⁻ drops out of consideration for myocardial cells because it seems to be passively distributed. However, transient net movements of Cl⁻ across the membrane do influence E_m; e.g., washout of Cl⁻ (in Cl⁻-free solution) produces a transient depolarization, and reintroduction of Cl⁻ produces a small hyperpolarization. Because of its relatively low concentration, coupled with its relatively low resting conductance, the Ca^{2+} distribution has only a relatively small effect on the resting E_m, and so it can be ignored. Therefore, a simplified version of the Goldman-Hodgkin-Katz constant-field equation can be given (for 37°C):

$$E_m = -61\,\text{mV}\log \frac{[K]_i + \frac{P_{Na}}{P_K}[Na]_i}{[K]_o + \frac{P_{Na}}{P_K}[Na]_o}. \qquad (3\text{-}20)$$

This equation shows that for a given ion distribution, the resting E_m is determined by the P_{Na}/P_K ratio, the relative permeability of the membrane to Na^+ and K^+. For myocardial cells, the P_{Na}/P_K ratio is about 0.04, whereas for nodal cells this ratio is closer to 0.10.

Inspection of the constant-field equation shows that the numerator of the log term will be dominated by the $[K]_i$ term [since the $(P_{Na}/P_k)[Na]_i$ term will be very small], whereas the denominator will be affected by both the $[K]_o$ and $(P_{Na}/P_K)[Na]_o$ terms. This relationship thus accounts for the deviation of the E_m versus log $[K]_o$ curve from a straight line (having a slope of 61 mV/decade) in normal Ringer solution (fig. 3-8). When $[K]_o$ is elevated ($[Na]_o$ reduced by an equimolar amount), the denominator becomes more and more dominated by the $[K]_o$ term, and less and less by the $(P_{Na}/P_K)[Na]_o$ term. Therefore, in bathing solutions containing high K^+, the constant-field equation approaches the simple Nernst equation for K^+, and E_m approaches E_K. As $[K]_o$ is raised stepwise, E_K becomes correspondingly reduced, since $[K]_i$ stays rela-

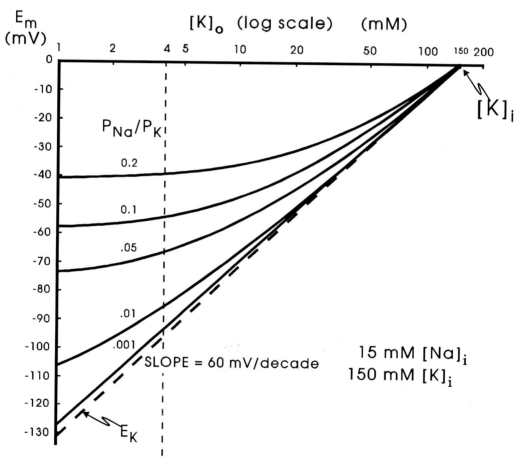

Fig. 3-8. Theoretical curves calculated from the Goldman constant-field equation for resting potential (E_m) as a function of $[K]_o$. The family of curves is given for various P_{Na}/P_K ratios (0.001, 0.01, 0.05, 0.1, and 0.2). The K^+ equilibrium potential (E_K) was calculated from the Nernst equation (broken straight line). Curves were calculated for a $[K]_i$ of 150 mM and a $[Na]_i$ of 15 mM. Calculations made holding $[K]_o + [Na]_o$ constant at 154 mM; i.e., as $[K]_o$ was elevated, $[Na]_o$ was lowered by an equimolar amount. Change in P_K as a function of $[K]_o$ was not taken into account for these calculations. The point at which E_m is zero gives $[K]_i$. The potential reverses in sign when $[K]_o$ exceeds $[K]_i$.

tively constant; therefore, the membrane becomes more and more depolarized (fig. 3-8).

An alternative method of approximating the resting potential is by the *chord-conductance equation*:

$$E_m = \frac{g_K}{g_K + g_{Na}} E_K + \frac{g_{Na}}{g_K + g_{Na}} E_{Na}. \qquad (3\text{-}21)$$

This equation can be derived simply from Ohm's Law and circuit analysis for the condition when net current is zero ($I_{Na} + I_K = 0$). The chord-conductance equation again illustrates the important fact that the g_K/g_{Na} ratio determines the resting potential. When $g_K \gg g_{Na}$, then E_m is close to E_K; conversely, when $g_{Na} \gg g_K$ (as during the spike part of the cardiac AP), E_m shifts to close to E_{Na}.

When $[K]_o$ is elevated (e.g., to 8 mM) in some cells, a hyperpolarization of up to about 10 mV may be produced. Such behavior is often observed in cells with a high P_{Na}/P_K ratio (due to low P_K) and therefore a low resting E_m, such as in young embryonic hearts. This hyperpolarization could be explained by several factors: (a) stimulation of the electrogenic Na^+ pump (V_p), (b) an increase in P_K (and therefore g_K) due to the $[K]_o$ effect on P_K, and (c) an increase in g_K (but not P_K) due to the concentration effect. A similar explanation may apply to the fallover in the E_m versus log $[K]_o$ curve, hence depolarizing the cells, when $[K]_o$ is lowered to 1 mM and less; this effect is prominent in rat skeletal muscle, for example.

Inhibition of the Na-K pump will gradually run down the ion concentration gradients. The cells lose K^+ and gain Na^+, and therefore E_K and E_{Na} become smaller. The cells thus become depolarized (even if the relative permeabilities are unaffected), which causes them to gain Cl^- (since $[Cl]_i$ was held low by the large resting potential) and therefore also water (cells swell). In summary, in the presence of ouabain (short-term exposure only) to inhibit the Na-K pump and V_p, the resting potential or *net diffusion potential E_{diff}* is determined by the ion concentration gradients for K^+ and Na^+, and by the relative permeability for K^+ and Na^+. When the Na-K pump is operating, there is normally a small additional contribution of V_{ep} to the resting E_m of about 2–8 mV in myocardial cells (discussed in following section).

ELECTROGENIC SODIUM PUMP POTENTIALS

A brief summary of the above principles is as follows. The Na-K pump is responsible for maintaining the cation concentration gradients. The diffusion potentials for K^+ (E_K) and Na^+ (E_{Na}) are about −94 mV and +60 mV, respectively. The resting potential value is usually near E_K, because the K^+ permeability (P_K) is much greater than P_{Na} in a resting membrane. The exact resting membrane potential (E_m) depends on the P_{Na}/P_K ratio, myocardial cells having P_{Na}/P_K ratios of 0.01–0.05, whereas smooth muscle or nodal cells of the heart have a ratio closer to 0.10–0.15. In the various types of heart cells, the resting E_m has a smaller magnitude (i.e., is less negative) than E_K by 10–40 mV. If there were no electrogenic pump poten-

tial contribution to the resting potential (that is, as though the Na-K pump was only indirectly responsible for the resting potential by its role in producing the ionic gradients), E_m would equal E_{diff}.

However, a direct contribution of the pump to the resting E_m can be demonstrated. For example, if the Na-K pump is blocked by the addition of ouabain, there usually is an immediate depolarization of 2–8 mV, depending on the type of heart cell; that is, the direct contribution of the electrogenic Na^+-K^+ pump to the measured resting E_m is small under physiologic conditions (but very important).

However, under conditions in which the pump is stimulated to pump at a high rate, e.g., when $[Na]_i$ or $[K]_o$ is abnormally high, the direct electrogenic contribution of the pump to the resting potential can be much greater, and E_m can actually exceed E_K by as much as 20 mV or more. For example, if the ionic concentration gradients are allowed to run down (e.g., by storing the tissues in zero $[K]_o$ and at low temperatures for several hours), then after allowing the tissues to restart pumping the measured E_m can exceed the calculated E_K (e.g., by 10–20 mV) for a period of time (fig. 3-9). The Na^+ loading of the cells is facilitated by placing them in cold low or zero $[K]_o$ solutions, since external K^+ is necessary for the Na-K-linked pump to operate; K_m of the Na,K-ATPase for K^+ is about 2 mM. After several hours in such a solution, the internal concentrations of Na^+, K^+, and Cl^- approach the concentrations in the bathing Ringer solution, and the resting potential is very low (< -20 mV). The tissue is then transferred to a pumping solution, which is the appropriate Ringer solution containing normal K^+ and at normal temperature. Under such conditions, the pump turns over at a maximal rate, because the major control over pump rate is $[Na]_i$ and $[K]_o$. The low initial E_m also stimulates the pump rate, because the energy required to pump out Na^+ is less. The measured E_m of such Na^+ preloaded cells increases rapidly and more rapidly than E_K, as shown in fig. 3-7. After this transient phase, however, a crossover of the two curves occurs, so that E_K again exceeds E_m, as in the physiologic condition. Cardiac glycosides prevent or reverse the transient hyperpolarization beyond E_K {8}. The possibility that ionic conductance changes (e.g., an increase in g_K or a decrease in g_{Na}) can account for the observed hyperpolarization can be ruled out whenever E_m exceeds (is more negative than) E_K.

Rewarming cardiac muscles that were previously cooled leads to the rapid restoration of the normal resting potential (within 10 minutes), whereas recovery of the intracellular Na^+ and K^+ concentrations is slower {28}. During prolonged hypoxia, the resting potential of cardiac muscle decreases much less than E_K decreases (a difference of about 25 mV) {20}. In such a situation, the electrogenic pump appears to act in an attempt to hold the resting potential constant, despite dissipating ionic gradients. It is not known whether the degree of electrogenicity of the pump (e.g., Na/K coupling ratio) might increase to compensate for a slowing pump rate.

Another method used to demonstrate that the pump is electrogenic is to inject Na^+ ions into the cell through a microelectrode. This procedure rapidly produces a

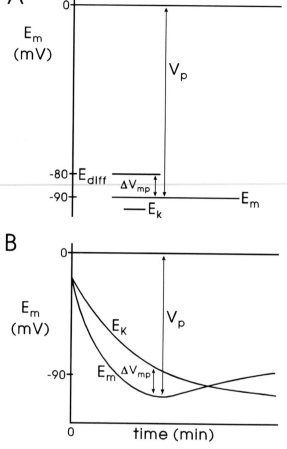

A

B

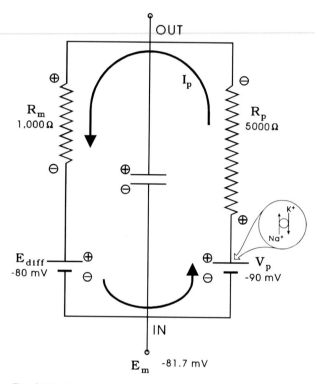

electrogenic, it must be demonstrated that the hyperpolarization produced upon Na^+ injection is not the result of enhanced pumping of an electroneutral pump. This could cause depletion of external K^+ in a restricted diffusion space just outside the cell membrane, the depletion thus leading to a larger E_K and thereby to hyperpolarization. Depletion could occur if the Na-K pump pumped in K^+ faster than it could be replenished by diffusion from the bulk interstitial fluid.

Fig. 3-9. Diagrammatic representation of an electrogenic sodium pump. **Upper graph:** Muscle cell in which the net ionic diffusion potential (E_{diff}, function of ion equilibrium potentials and relative conductances) is $-80\,mV$, yet exhibits a measured membrane resting potential (E_m) that is greater. Difference between E_m and E_{diff} represents the contribution of the electrogenic pump to the resting potential. The usual direct contribution of the pump is only a few millivolts and can be measured by the amount of depolarization produced immediately after complete inhibition of the Na,K-ATPase by cardiac glycosides. Because the pump pathway is separate from and parallel to the ionic conductance pathways, the electrogenic pump potential must be equal to V_{ep}. The contribution of the electrogenic pump potential to the resting potential ($E_m - E_{diff}$) is equal to ΔV_{ep}. **Lower graph:** Cell that was run down (Na loaded, K depleted) over several hours by inhibition of Na-K pumping, resulting in a low resting potential. Returning the muscle cell to a pumping solution allows the resting E_m to build back up as a function of time. Buildup in E_m occurs faster than buildup in E_K, as illustrated. Whenever E_m is greater (more negative) than the K^+ equilibrium potential (E_K), the difference (ΔV_{ep}) must reflect the contribution of the sodium pump potential.

small transient hyperpolarization, which is immediately abolished or prevented by ouabain. The pump current and the rate of Na^+ extrusion increase in proportion to the amount of Na^+ injected. To prove that the pump is

Fig. 3-10. Hypothetical electrical equivalent circuit for electrogenic sodium pump. The model consists of a pump pathway in parallel with the membrane resistance (R_m) pathway and the membrane capacitance (C_m) pathway. This model fits the evidence that the pump is independent of short-range membrane excitability and that the pump proteins and channel proteins are embedded in the lipid bilayer as parallel elements. Net diffusion potential (E_{diff}, determined by the ion equilibrium potentials and relative permeabilities) of $-80\,mV$ is depicted in series with R_m. The pump leg is assumed to consist of a battery in series with a fixed resistor (pump resistance, R_p) that does not change with changes in R_m and whose value is 5-fold higher than R_m. The pump battery is charged up to some voltage (V_{ep} of $-90\,mV$, for example) by a pump current generator. Net electrogenic pump current is developed by the pumping in of only 2 K^+ ions for every 3 Na^+ ions pumped out. For the values given in the figure (namely, R_m of $1000\,\Omega$, E_{diff} of $-80\,mV$, R_p of $5000\,\Omega$, and V_{ep} of $-90\,mV$), it may be calculated by circuit analysis that the measured membrane potential (E_m) is $-81.7\,mV$; that is, the direct electrogenic pump potential contribution to the resting potential is $-1.7\,mV$.

It has been suggested that the electrogenic Na^+ pump may be influenced by the membrane potential. From energetic considerations, depolarization should enhance the electrogenic Na^+ pump, whereas hyperpolarization should inhibit it. This is because depolarization reduces the electrochemical gradient (and hence the energy requirements) against which Na^+ must be extruded, whereas hyperpolarization increases the gradient. If the energetics are important, there should be a distinct potential, more negative than E_K, at which Na^+ pumping is prevented (e.g., a pump equilibrium potential). A value close to $-140 \, mV$ was reported for cardiac cells {7}.

Any method used to increase membrane resistance increases the contribution of the pump to the resting potential (fig. 3-10). That is, the electrogenic Na^+ pump contribution must be augmented under conditions that increase membrane resistance. The contribution of the pump potential to the measured E_m is the difference in E_m when the pump is operating versus immediately after the pump has been stopped by the addition of ouabain or zero $[K]_o$. Consequently, it appears as though the contribution from the electrogenic pump potential (ΔV_{mp}) were in series with the net cationic diffusion potential (E_{diff}).

$$E_m = E_{diff} + R_m I_p = E_{diff} + \Delta V_{mp}, \qquad (3\text{-}22)$$

where I_P is the electrogenic component of the pump current, and E_{diff} is the E_m that would exist solely on the basis of the ionic gradients and relative permeabilities in the absence of an electrogenic pump potential (as calculated from the constant-field equation). This equation states that E_m is the sum of E_{diff} and a voltage (IR) drop produced by the electrogenic pump. The electrogenic pump potential (V_p) can be considered to be in parallel with E_{diff} (fig. 3-10). Because the density of pump sites is more than 1000-fold greater than that of Na^+ and K^+ channels in resting membrane, there is no relation between the pump pathway (the active flux path) and R_m (the passive flux paths); that is, the pump path and the passive conductance paths are in parallel. The true potential is much greater than the ΔE_m measured in the absence and presence of ouabain; namely, the pump potential should be considered as the full potential between zero and the maximum negative pump potential (V_p) while the pump is pumping (fig. 3-7).

One possible equivalent circuit for an electrogenic Na^+ pump, which takes into account some of the known facts, is given in fig. 3-10. The pump pathway is in parallel with the resistance pathways, and the pump potential is the full potential (V_p) and not the ΔV_{mp}. The pump resistance (R_p) is estimated to be about 10-fold higher than R_m. If so, the pump resistance acts to minimize a short-circuit path to E_{diff} when the pump potential is low or zero (pump inhibited). The pump potential contribution to E_m (ΔV_{mp}) is a function of membrane resistance (R_m): The higher R_m is (R_p constant), the more nearly E_m approaches V_p. The pump battery is charged to some voltage by a *pump current generator*. If the pump is stopped by ouabain, V_p goes to zero. Using circuit analysis for the values of the parameters given in fig. 3-8, E_m would be $-81.8 \, mV$, moderately close to E_{diff} ($-80 \, mV$; table 3-2). If R_m is

Table 3-2. Summary of calculations of resting potential (E_m) for a model having an electrogenic pump potential (V_{ep}) in parallel with the net diffusion potential (E_{diff})

	E_{diff} (mV)	R_m (Ω-cm^2)	R_p (Ω-cm^2)	V_{ep} (mV)	Resting E_m (mV)	ΔV_{ep} ($E_m - E_{diff}$) (mV)
1.	-80	1000	10,000	-100	-81.8	-1.8
2.	-80	2000	10,000	-100	-83.3	-3.3
3.	-80	4000	10,000	-100	-85.7	-5.7
4.	-80	8000	10,000	-100	-88.9	-8.9
5.	-80	1000	10,000	0	-72.7	$+7.3$
6.	-80	1000	10,000	0	-79.2	$+0.8$
7.	-40	1000	10,000	-100	-45.5	-5.5
8.	-50	1000	10,000	-100	-54.5	-4.5
9.	-45	2000	10,000	-100	-54.2	-9.2
10.	-45	4000	10,000	-100	-60.7	-15.7

R_m = membrane resistivity; R_p = pump resistance; ΔV_{ep} = contribution of V_{ep} to the measured E_m. E_m was calculated from the following equation:

$$E_m = \frac{R_m}{R_m + R_p} V_p + \frac{R_p}{R_m + R_p}.$$

raised twofold (to $2000 \, \Omega$), E_m would be $-83.3 \, mV$. Thus this circuit clearly gives a pump potential contribution to E_m that is dependent on R_m. The higher R_m is relative to R_p, the more E_m reflects V_p. If E_{diff} is made smaller (e.g., in vascular smooth muscle cells with a higher P_{Na}/P_K ratio), then the relative contribution of the pump potential to E_m becomes greater (table 3-2).

In general, Cl^- ions are known to have a short-circuiting effect on the electrogenic Na^+ pump potential. For example, if the external Cl^- is replaced by less permeant anions, the magnitude of the hyperpolarization produced by the electrogenic Na^+ pump is substantially increased. This Cl^- effect could be caused by the lowering of membrane resistance in the presence of Cl^-. The greater R_m is, the greater is the contribution of the electrogenic pump potential to resting E_m (see fig. 3-10).

The density of Na-K pump sites, estimated by specific binding of [^3H] ouabain, is usually about $700–1000/\mu m^2$. The turnover rate of the pump is generally estimated to be $20–100/s$. The pump current (I_p) has been estimated as follows:

$$I_p = \Delta V_{mp}/R_m, \qquad (3\text{-}23)$$

where ΔV_{mp} is the pump potential contribution. Values of about $20 \, pM/cm^2$-s were obtained. A density of 1000 sites/mm^2 (10^{11} sites/cm^2) times a turnover rate of $40/s$ gives 4×10^{12} turnovers/cm^2-s. If $3 Na^+$ are pumped with each turnover, this gives 12×10^{12} Na^+ ions/cm^2-s; dividing by Avogadro's number (6.02×10^{23} ions/M) yields 20×10^{-12} M/cm^2-s, which is the same value as the $20 \, pM/cm^2$-s measured. The net pump current would be less, depending on the amount of K^+ pumped in the opposite direction, i.e., on the coupling ratio (e.g., $3 Na^+ : 2 K^+$). Whenever the Na-K pump is stimulated to turn over faster, e.g., by increasing $[Na]_i$ or $[K]_o$, the electrogenic pump potential contribution to $\dot{E}_m$ becomes larger. In skeletal muscle, insulin has been reported to increase the number of Na/K pump sites in the sarcolemma by increasing the rate of translocation from an internal pool {30}.

Ion flux (J) can be converted to current (I) by the following relationship:

$$I = J \cdot zF.$$

$$\frac{A}{cm^2} = \frac{M}{s\,cm^2}\frac{coul}{M}. \qquad (3\text{-}24)$$

Thus, a flux of $20\,pM/cm^2$-s is equal to approximately $2\,\mu A/cm^2$ $(20 \times 10^{-12}\,M/s\text{-}cm^2 \times 0.965 \times 10^5\,coul/M)$. Since $\Delta V_{mp} = i_p \cdot R_m$, if R_m were $1000\,\Omega\text{-}cm^2$ and i_p were $2\,\mu A/cm^2$, the electrogenic pump contribution to E_m would be $2\,mV$ $(E_m = E_{diff} + I_p R_m)$.

Because $3\,Na^+$ are known to be transported per molecule of ATP spent, it is assumed that the pump molecule has a net negative charge. The pump at the inner surface of the membrane may have a much higher affinity for Na^+ than for K^+, whereas the converse may be true at the outer surface. It is assumed that the pump cannot cycle unless fully loaded with $3\,Na^+$ ions. Two K^+ ions are usually carried in for every $3\,Na^+$ ions moved out. Since the pump is electrogenic, i.e., produces a net current (and hence potential) across the membrane, then the amount of K^+ pumped in must be less than the amount of Na^+ pumped out; e.g., the Na/K coupling ratio must be $3:2$ (or $3:1$). The coupling ratio cannot be $3:0$, because of the well-known fact that external K^+ must be present for the pump to operate. The coupling ratio might be increased under some conditions, e.g., when $[Na]_i$ is elevated. The pump potential contribution would become larger for a constant pumping rate if the coupling ratio were to increase (e.g., to $3:1$). The Na-K pump in several cell types can switch to a Na^+-Na^+ exchanging mode of operation, the mode change being governed by the $ATP/ADP/P_i$ ratios.

The electrogenic pump potential has physiologic importance in heart cells. Although small, the electrogenic pump potential contribution to the resting potential could have significant effects on the level of inactivation of the fast Na^+ channels, and hence on propagation velocity. Further, an electrogenic pump potential could act to delay depolarization under adverse conditions (e.g., ischemia and hypoxia) and would act to speed repolarization of the normal resting potential during recovery from the adverse conditions. It is crucial that the excitable cell maintain its normal resting potential as much as possible, because of the effect on the AP rate of rise and conduction velocity with small depolarizations, and complete loss of excitability with larger depolarizations. The rate of firing of pacemaker nodal cells is affected significantly by very small potential changes.

In cells in which there are lower resting potentials (e.g., vascular smooth muscle cells and cardiac nodal cell; table 3-1), the electrogenic pump potential contribution can be considerably larger (table 3-2). Sinusoidal oscillations in the Na-K pumping rate could produce oscillations in E_m, which could exert important control over the spontaneous

firing of the cell. The period of enhanced pumping hyperpolarizes the cell and suppresses automaticity, whereas slowing of the pump leads to depolarization and consequently to triggering of APs. Oscillation of the pump would be brought about by oscillating changes in $[Na]_i$. For example, the firing of several APs should raise $[Na]_i$ (nodal cells have a small volume/surface area ratio) and stimulate the electrogenic pump. The increased pumping rate, in turn, hyperpolarizes and suppresses firing, thus allowing $[Na]_i$ to become lower again and removing the stimulation of the pump; the latter depolarizes and triggers spikes, and the cycle could be repeated. Noma and Irisawa {26} concluded that in rabbit sinoatrial nodal cells the electrogenic Na^+ pump might be one factor that modulates the heart rate under physiologic conditions. When stimulated at a high rate, cardiac Purkinje fibers and nodal cells undergo a transient period of inhibition of automaticity after cessation of the stimulation, known as *overdrive suppression of automaticity*. Stimulation of the electrogenic pump due to elevation in $[Na]_i$ is the major cause of this phenomenon {29,45}.

PACEMAKER POTENTIALS AND AUTOMATICITY

In order to maintain a steady resting potential, the net outward current must equal the net inward current:

$$I_{out} = I_{in}. \qquad (3\text{-}25)$$

Assuming Cl^- is passively distributed, the outward K^+ current must be equal and opposite to the inward $Na^+ + Ca^{2+}$ current. If the inward current exceeds the outward current, then the membrane will depolarize along a certain time course (i.e., slope of the pacemaker potential or diastolic or phase-4 depolarization), depending on the excess (or net) inward current. The inward leak of Na^+ and Ca^{2+} currents is often called the *background inward current*. For the inward current to exceed the outward current (i.e., for a net inward current), either the inward current can be increased or the outward current I_K can be decreased. Both of these mechanisms are used for genesis of pacemaker potentials (automaticity). For example, if a time-dependent decrease (decay) in g_K occurs following an AP and hyperpolarizing afterpotential, then I_K decreases and the membrane depolarizes (g_{Na}/g_K progressively increases). Conversely, if an agent such as acetylcholine (ACh) were to increase the resting g_K, then the outward I_K is increased, the membrane hyperpolarizes, and the slope of the pacemaker potential decreases, thus reducing the frequency of firing. Some agents, such as norepinephrine, increase the background inward current, thereby increasing the slope of the pacemaker potential.

A prerequisite for automaticity is that the cells must have a relatively low Cl^- conductance (g_{Cl}). This condition holds true for all or most cell types in the heart. A high g_{Cl} acts to clamp E_m, making it difficult for a pacemaker potential to be developed. For example, addition of Ba^{2+} $(0.5\,mM)$ to frog sartorius muscle fibers, which have a high g_{Cl}/g_K ratio of about 4.0, has very little immediate effect. However, when the fibers are first equilibrated in Cl-free solution to reduce g_{Cl} to zero, Ba^{2+} produces a prompt depolarization, an increase in R_m, and automaticity {34}. Another way to view this effect of Cl^- is by Cole's {3} parallel capacitance-inductance (C_mL_m) circuit for an excitable membrane that tends to oscillate spontaneously when the R_{Cl} shunt resistance (and R_{Na}) is very high. The apparent inductance L_m arises because of the peculiar behavior of the K^+ resistance, namely, *anomalous rectification*. The rapid turnoff of this inwardly rectifying K^+ channel causes a very fast decrease in g_K with depolarization.

During the time course of the pacemaker potential, R_m increases progressively due to a decrease in g_K {35,43}. The progressive turnoff of the inwardly rectifying K^+ channels (I_{K1} current) causes R_m to increase progressively. In addition, there is a progressive turnoff of the g_K increase (delayed rectification) responsible for the rapid repolarizing phase of the AP and the subsequent *hyperpolarizing (positive) afterpotential* usually exhibited by pacemaker cells. The decreasing g_K helps to produce the depolarization. The *pacemaker depolarization* in heart cells is usually *linear* (or a ramp).

Myocardial cells can be made to exhibit abnormal automaticity of another type under pathophysiological conditions. A large depolarizing afterpotential arises from the hyperpolarizing afterpotential {34} and triggers the subsequent spike once the threshold potential (V_{th}) is reached. In this type of automaticity, each AP is triggered by the preceding one, and the abnormal automaticity of this type is known as *triggered automaticity*. Thus a train of spikes can be turned off by simply stopping one spike in the train from developing (e.g., by a brief hyperpolarizing current pulse) {34}. The depolarizing afterpotential is depressed by verapamil and is facilitated by cardiac glycosides and beta-adrenergic agonists {6,17}, the latter agents tending to produce *ectopic pacemaker activity*. They do so by increasing Ca^{2+} influx, and hence the degree of Ca^{2+} loading in the SR. Spontaneous release of Ca^{2+} from the overloaded SR activates a Ca^{2+}-regulated mixed Na^+-K^+ conductance ($g_{Na,K(Ca)}$) or *transient inward current (I_{ti})*. Turnon of these nonselective channels produces the observed depolarization: *delayed afterdepolarizations (DADs)* or *oscillatory afterpotentials (OAPs)* {19}. Calcium antagonist drugs block the DADs/OAPs by depressing Ca^{2+} influx, and thus preventing the Ca^{2+} overload of the SR.

All heart cells are capable of exhibiting automaticity under certain conditions. For example, ventricular cells placed into cell culture can develop automaticity {34}. Myocardial cells exposed to Ba^{2+} to decrease their g_K and depolarize them develop automaticity {10,35,39}. Ventricular muscle depolarized by the application of current also fires spontaneously during the current pulse {11,18,31,35}; that is, when E_m is brought into the voltage region that can develop pacemaker potentials, automaticity occurs.

In any cardiac pacemaker cell, if the membrane potential is hyperpolarized by a current pulse, the frequency of spontaneous firing is slowed and stopped; that is, automaticity is suppressed at high resting potentials {35}.

Conversely, application of depolarizing current increases the frequency of discharge. Thus, the slope of the pacemaker potential is exquisitely sensitive to small changes in E_m. The further E_m is above E_K (within limits), the greater the degree of automaticity. A low g_K, which also means a relatively lower resting E_m, facilitates automaticity. Elevations of $[K]_o$, which increases g_K, suppresses automaticity despite depolarizing {19,44}.

Under normal circumstances in the heart, the *hierarchy of automaticity* capability is SA nodal cells > AV nodal cells > Purkinje fibers. Ventricular or atrial myocardial cells develop automaticity only under pathologic conditions such as regional ischemia. The genesis of automaticity in Purkinje fibers is somewhat different from that in nodal cells {2,12,25}. Normally the automaticity of the cells lower in the hierarchy (e.g., the Purkinje cells) is latent (*latent pacemakers*), because the cells are driven at higher rates by the *primary pacemaker* (SA node). Because of the phenomenon of *overdrive suppression of automaticity* (fast drives of a pacemaker cell tend to hyperpolarize the cell and cause a pause in automaticity after the drive is terminated), the latent pacemakers normally may be *chronically in a state of overdrive suppression*. Thus a pacemaker potential may or may not be seen during diastole. One factor in the production of overdrive suppression is stimulation of the electrogenic Na^+ pump by the increase in $[Na]_i$ accompanying a high rate of driving {29,45}. In addition, K^+ tends to accumulate extracellularly during the fast drive.

One characteristic of a pacemaker cell is that *accommodation does not occur*; the cell fires no matter how slowly E_m is brought to the threshold potential V_{th}. This could reflect a homogeneous population of ionic channels with nearly identical voltage-sensitive gating, the low g_{Cl} (less clamping effect of Cl^-), and the decrease in g_K due to anomalous rectification. Little or no inactivation of slow Ca^{2+} channels occurs during the pacemaker depolarization because inactivation of slow channels occurs at more positive potentials (between about $-45\,mV$ and $-10\,mV$).

Automaticity of the heart (nodal cells) is normally under control of the autonomic nerves. The release of ACh from the *parasympathetic nerves* increases g_K, and thereby hyperpolarizes (toward E_K) and depresses automaticity. ACh also depresses the inward slow Ca^{2+} current, which also would tend to depress automaticity (for references, see Josephon and Sperelakis {16}). The release of norepinephrine from the sympathetic nerves tends to increase the inward slow Ca^{2+} current and to decrease g_K (kinetics of turnon), both of which tend to enhance automaticity. For a complete discussion of the electrogenesis of pacemaker potentials, the reader is referred to Chapter 9.

EFFECT OF RESTING POTENTIAL ON THE ACTION POTENTIAL

Any agent that affects the resting potential (e.g., depolarizes) will have important repercussions on the cardiac AP. Depolarization reduces the rate of rise of the AP and thereby also slows its velocity of propagation. A slow spread of excitation throughout the heart will interfere with the heart's ability to act as an efficient blood pump. This effect is progressive as a function of the degree of depolarization. If the myocardial cells and Purkinje fibers are depolarized to about −50 mV, then the rate of rise goes to zero and all excitability (and contraction) is lost, leading to cardiac arrest.

Hyperpolarizations usually produces only a small increase in the rate of rise, and large hyperpolarizations may actually slow the propagation velocity (because the critical depolarization required to bring the membrane to threshold is increased) or cause propagation block.

The explanation of the effect of resting E_m (or takeoff potential) on the maximum rate of rise (dV/dt max) of the AP is based on the sigmoidal h_∞ versus E_m curve. In Hodgkin–Huxley notation, h is the inactivation variable for the fast Na^+ conductance of the cell; it is a probability factor that deals with open (h = 1.0) versus closed (h = 0) positions of the inactivation (I) gate of each channel (figs.

3-11 and 3-12). The value of h is a function of E_m and time (t), and h_∞ is the h value at steady state or infinite time (practically, t > 20 ms). h_∞ is 0.9–1.0 at the normal resting potential (−80 mV) and diminishes with depolarization, becoming nearly zero at about −50 mV. The I gates are open in a resting membrane and close slowly (time constant of several milliseconds) upon depolarization, thus inactivating the fast Na^+ conductance (figs. 3-11 and 3-12).

The slow channels in myocardial cells are similar to the fast Na^+ channels, except that their A gates and I gates appear to operate much more slowly kinetically on a population basis; that is, the slow conductance turns on (activates) more slowly, turns off (inactivates) more slowly, and recovers more slowly (figs. 3-11 and 3-12). In addition, the voltage inactivation curve for the slow Ca^{2+} conductance is shifted to the right so that inactivation begins at about −45 mV and is not complete until about 0 mV {21,24}. The slow channels also have a lower activation (threshold) potential of about −35 mV (compared to about −60 mV for the fast Na^+ channels). When the fast

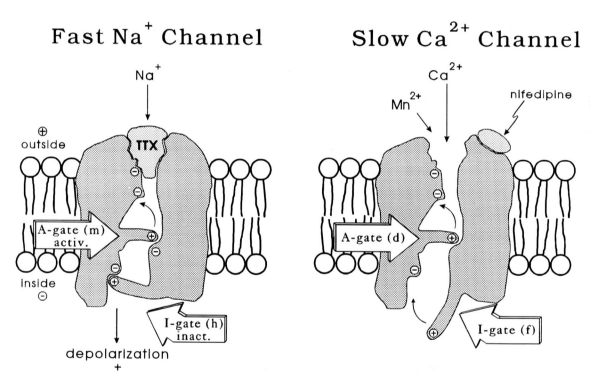

Fig. 3-11. Cartoon models for a fast Na^+ channel (left) and for a slow channel (right) in myocardial cell membrane. As depicted, two gates are associated with each type of channel: the activation (A) gate and inactivation (I) gate. Gates are presumably charged positively so that they can sense membrane potential. The I gate moves more slowly than the A gate. Gates of the slow channel are kinetically much slower than those of the fast Na^+ channel. The fast Na^+ channel is depicted in the resting state (A gate closed, I gate open) and just beginning the process of activation, whereas the slow channel is depicted in the active state (both gates open) and just beginning the process of inactivation. Depolarization causes the A gate to open quickly so that the channel becomes conducting (active state). However, the I gate slowly closes during depolarization and inactivates the channel (inactive state). During recovery upon repolarization, the A gate closes and the I gate opens (returns to resting state). Not depicted is the hypothesis that the protein constituent of the slow channel must be phosphorylated in order for the channel to be in a functional state available for voltage activation. Tetrodotoxin (TTX) blocks the fast Na^+ channel from the outside, presumably by binding in the channel mouth. Verapamil and Mn^{2+} block the slow channel.

resting state

active state

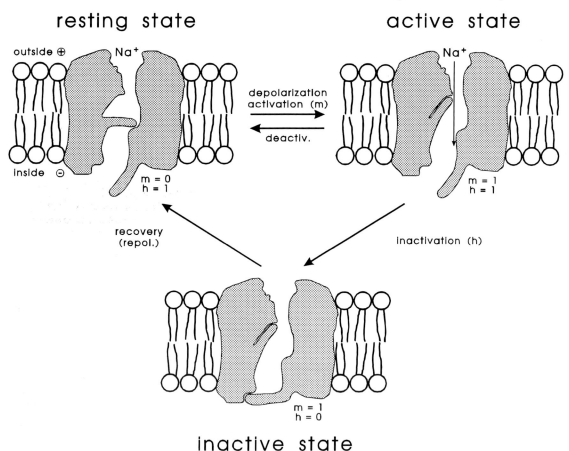

Fig. 3-12. Cartoon model of the three states of the fast Na^+ channel, patterned after Hodgkin–Huxley. In the resting state, the activation (m) gate is closed and the inactivation (h) gate is open. In the active state, the m gate is open while the h gate is still open. In the inactivated state, the m gate remains open, but the h gate was closed. During the recovery process, the inactivated channel is reverted back to the resting state by reclosing of the m gate and reopening of the h gate.

Na^+ channels are either blocked by tetrodotoxin (TTX) or voltage inactivated in elevated $[K]_o$ (25 mM; E_m of about -40 mV), positive inotropic agents, such as catecholamines or histamine, restore excitability in the form of slow-rising APs by increasing the number of Ca^{2+} slow channels available for voltage activation. The rate of rise of the slow AP is also dependent on the h_∞ variable (often termed the f_∞ *variable* for myocardial slow channels), with depression of dV/dt max beginning at -45 mV and going to zero at about -20 mV. These relationships are depicted in fig. 3-13.

The resting potential also affects the duration of the cardiac AP. With polarizing current, depolarization lengthens the AP, whereas hyperpolarization shortens it. In contrast, when elevated $[K]_o$ is used to depolarize the cells, the AP is usually shortened. (Under special conditions, such as Cl^--free solution, the AP may be prolonged with elevation of $[K]_o$ {2}.) One important determinant of the AP duration is the K^+ conduction (g_K). Agents or conditions that increase g_K, such as elevation of $]K]_o$, tend

to shorten the duration. In contrast, agents that decrease g_K or slow the activation of g_K, such as Ba^{2+} ion or tetraethylammonium ion (TEA^+), tend to lengthen the AP duration. Due to anomalous rectification (i.e., a decrease in g_K with depolarization), depolarization by current prolongs the AP and hyperpolarization shortens it.

Other factors are also important in determining the AP duration. For example, agents that slow the closing of the I gates of the fast Na^+ channels, such as veratridine, prolong the AP. Prolongation or stimulation of the inward slow current (I_{si}) tends to prolong the AP; conversely, agents that depress I_{si}, such as verapamil or Mn^{2+}, slightly shorten the AP. Conditions that depress metabolism of the heart and lower ATP, such as ischemia or hypoxia, greatly depress I_{si} and also act to turn on g_K earlier by removing ATP inhibition of an ATP-regulated K^+ channel [$g_{K(ATP)}$] {27} and so greatly abbreviate the cardiac AP {22,32, 38,46}. The cardiac AP shortens markedly at high heart rates. Three factors could contribute toward this effect: (a) the increase in $[Ca]_i$ (resulting from increase in $[Na]_i$)

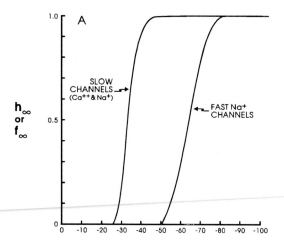

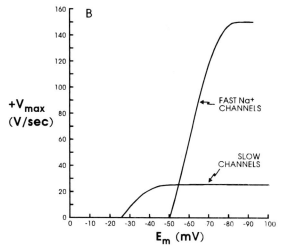

Fig. 3-13. Graphic representation of differences in behavior, with respect to voltage inactivation, of the fast Na^+ channels and slow (Na^+ and Ca^{2+}) channels. **A:** h_∞ inactivation factor of Hodgkin–Huxley ($g_{Na} = \bar{g}_{Na}m^3h$, where g_{Na} is the Na^+ conductance, m and h are probability variables, and overbar means maximal) for fast Na^+ channels or the comparable f_∞ factor for slow channels as a function of resting potential (E_m). The h_∞ or f_∞ represents h or f at t = infinity or steady state (practically, after 20 ms for h and after 1 s for f). This graph illustrates that fast Na^+ channels of myocardial cells begin to inactivate at about $-75\,mV$, and complete inactivation occurs at about $-50\,mV$ (h = 0). In contrast, slow channels inactivate between about $-45\,mV$ (f = about 1.0) and $-25\,mV$ ($f_\infty = 0$). **B:** Maximal rate of rise of the action potential (dV/dt max) as a function of resting E_m for the normal cardiac action potential (dependent on inward current through the fast Na^+ channels) and for the slow action potential (dependent on inward current through slow channels) elicited in cells whose fast Na^+ channels are blocked (by TTX or by depolarization to about $-45\,mV$). dV/dt max is a measure of the inward current intensity (everything else, such as membrane capacitance, held constant), which in turn is dependent on the number of channels available for activation.

produces an increase in resting g_K and enhances g_K activation kinetics by activation of a Ca^{2+}-regulated K^+ channel [$g_{K(Ca)}$; the Gardos-Meech effect] {1,13,23,33}; (b) K^+ accumulates outside the cell membrane, thereby increasing g_K; and (c) recovery of the slow channels is incomplete, thereby depressing I_{si}.

SUMMARY

Most of the factors that determine or influence the resting E_m of heart cells were discussed in this chapter. The structural and chemical composition of the cell membrane was briefly examined and correlated with the membrane's resistive and capacitative properties. The factors that determine the intracellular ion concentrations in myocardial cells were examined. These factors include the Na-K coupled pump, the Ca-Na exchange reaction, and a sarcolemmal Ca pump. The Na-K pump enzyme, the Na,K-ATPase, requires both Na^+ and K^+ for activity, and transports 3 Na^+ ions outward and usually 2 K^+ ions inward per ATP hydrolyzed. Cardiac glycosides are specific blockers of this transport ATPase. The Na-K pump is not directly related to excitability, but only indirectly related by its role in maintaining the Na^+ and K^+ concentration gradients.

The carrier-mediated Ca/Na exchange reaction may be driven by the Na^+ electrochemical gradient; i.e., the energy for transporting out internal Ca^{2+} by this mechanism comes from the Na,K-ATPase. The Ca/Na exchange reaction exchanges one internal Ca^{2+} ion for three external Na^+ ions when working in the *forward mode* in cells at rest. During the AP depolarization, the energetics cause the Ca/Na exchanger to operate in *reverse mode*, allowing Ca^{2+} influx.

The mechanism whereby the ionic distributions give rise to diffusion potentials was discussed, as were the factors that determine the magnitude and polarity of each ionic equilibrium potential. The equilibrium potential for any ion and the transmembrane potential determine the total electrochemical driving force for that ion, and the product of this driving force and membrane conductance for that ion determine the net ionic current or flux. The net ionic movement can be inward or outward across the membrane, depending on the direction of the electrochemical gradient.

The key factor that determines the resting E_m — in the absence of any electrogenic pump potential contributions and for fixed ionic distributions — is the relative permeability of the various ions, particularly of K^+ and Na^+, i.e., the P_{Na}/P_K ratio (or g_{Na}/g_K ratio), as calculated from the Goldman constant-field equation. The major physiologic ions that have some effect on the resting E_m or on the APs are K^+, Na^+, Ca^{2+}, and Cl^-. The Ca^{2+} electrochemical gradient has only a small direct effect on the resting E_m, although low external Ca^{2+} can affect the permeabilities and conductances for the other ions, such as Na^+ and K^+. Elevation of internal Ca^{2+} can increase the permeability to K^+ by activating Ca^{2+}-operated K^+-selective $I_{K(Ca)}$ channels.

Cl^- ion is passively distributed according to the membrane potential, i.e., not actively transported. However, there is some evidence indicating that $[Cl]_i$ may be about twice as high as that predicted from E_m in some cells; if so, this would give an E_{Cl} value of about $-66\,mV$ compared to a resting E_m of about $-80\,mV$. Before one can conclude that there is a Cl^- pump directed inward, however, the calculated E_{Cl} (concentrations corrected for activity coefficients) must be proven to be significantly more positive than the mean resting E_m of the cell averaged over a period of time; i.e., for example, any spontaneous APs must be taken into account. If Cl^- is passively distributed, it cannot determine the resting E_m. However, transient net movements of Cl^- ions, e.g., during the AP, can and do affect the E_m, particularly when g_{Cl} is high.

Elevation of $[K]_o$ to more than the normal concentration of about 4.5 mM decreases the K^+ equilibrium potential (E_K), as predicted from the Nernst equation ($[K]_i$ about constant), and depolarization is produced. Sometimes, however, some hyperpolarization is produced at a $[K]_o$ level between 5 and 9 mM. In addition, lowering $[K]_o$ to 0.1 mM often produces a prominent depolarization. These effects are usually explained on the basis that (a) P_K is lowered in low $[K]_o$ and elevated in higher $[K]_o$ and (b) an electrogenic Na-K pump potential is inhibited at a low $[K]_o$ (K_m of about 2 mM).

The resting E_m not only is the potential energy storehouse that is drawn upon for propagation of the APs, but because the membrane voltage-dependent cationic channels are inactivated with sustained depolarization, the rate of rise of the AP, and hence propagation velocity, are critically dependent on the level of the resting E_m. For example, a relatively small elevation of K^+ concentration in the blood has dire consequences for functioning of the heart.

The contribution of the Na-K pump to the resting E_m depends on (a) the coupling ratio of Na^+ pumped out to K^+ pumped in, (b) the turnover rate of the pump, (c) the number of pumps, and (d) the magnitude of the membrane resistance. The electrogenic pump potential is in parallel to the net ionic diffusion potential (E_{diff}), determined by the ionic equilibrium potentials and by the relative permeabilities. The contribution of the electrogenic pump potential to the measured resting E_m of myocardial cells is generally small (only a few millivolts), so that the immediate depolarization produced by complete Na-K pump stoppage with cardiac glycosides is only a few millivolts. Of course, long-term pump inhibition produces a larger and larger depolarization as the ionic gradients are dissipated. The rate of Na-K pumping, and hence the magnitude of the electrogenic pump contribution to E_m, is controlled primarily by $[Na]_i$ and by $[K]_o$. The electrogenic pump potential might be physiologically important to the heart under certain conditions that tend to depolarize the cells, such as transient ischemia or hypoxia. In such cases, the actual depolarization produced may be less because of a relatively constant pump potential in parallel with a diminishing E_{diff}. The electrogenic pump potential may also affect automaticity of the nodal cells.

REFERENCES

1. Bassingwaighte JB, Fry CH, McGuigan JAS: Relationship between internal calcium and outward current in mammalian ventricular muscle: A mechanism for the control of the action potential duration? *J Physiol* 262:15–37, 1976.
2. Carmeliet E, Vereecke J: Electrogenesis of the action potential and automaticity. In: Berne RM, Sperelakis N (eds) *Handbook of Physiology*. Bethesda, MD: American Physiological Society, 1979, pp 269–334.
3. Cole KS: *Membranes, Ions and Impulses: A Chapter of Classical Biophysics*. Berkeley: University of California, 1968.
4. Daniel EE, Kwan CY, Matlib MA, Crankshaw D, Kidwai A: Characterization and Ca^{2+}-accumulation by membrane fractions from myometrium and artery. In: Casteels R, Godfraind T, Ruegg JC (eds) *Excitation-Contraction Coupling in Smooth Muscle*. Amsterdam: Elsevier/North-Holland, 1977, pp 181–188.
5. Dhalla NS, Ziegelhoffer A, Hazzow JA: Regulatory role of membrane systems in heart function. *Can J Physiol Pharmacol* 55:1211–1234, 1977.
6. Ferrier GR, Moe GK: Effects of calcium on acetyl-strophanthidin-induced transient depolarizations in canine Purkinje tissue. *Circ Res* 33:508–515, 1973.
7. Gadsby DC, Nakao M: Steady-state current-voltage relationship of the Na/K pump in guinea pig ventricular myocytes. *J Gen Physiol* 94:511–537, 1989.
8. Glitsch HG: Activation of the electrogenic sodium pump in guinea-pig auricles by internal sodium ions. *J Physiol (Lond)* 220:565–582, 1972.
9. Henn FA, Sperelakis N: Stimulative and protective action of Sr^{2+} and Ba^{2+} on (Na^+,K^+)-ATPase from cultured heart cells. *Biochim Biophys Acta* 16 3:415–417, 1968.
10. Hermsmeyer K, Sperelakis N: Decrease in K^+ conductance and depolarization of frog cardiac muscle produced by Ba^{2+}. *Am J Physiol* 219:1108–1114, 1970.
11. Imanishi S, Surawicz B: Automatic activity in depolarized guinea pig ventricular myocardium. *Circ Res* 39:751–759, 1976.
12. Irisawa H: Comparative physiology of the cardiac pacemaker mechanism. *Physiol Rev* 58:461–498, 1978.
13. Isenberg G: Is potassium conductance of cardiac Purkinje fibres controlled by $[Ca^{2+}]_i$? *Nature* 253:273–274, 1975.
14. Jain MK: The Bimolecular Lipid Membrane: A System. New York: Van Nostrand, 1972.
15. Jones LR, Maddock SW, Besch HR Jr: Unmasking effect of alamethicin on the (Na^+,K^+)-ATPase, beta-adrenergic receptor-coupled adenylate cyclase, and cAMP-dependent protein kinase activities of cardiac sarcolemmal vesicles. *J Biol Chem* 255:9971–9980, 1980.
16. Josephson I, Sperelakis N: On the ionic mechanism underlying adrenergic-cholinergic antagonism in ventricular muscle. *J Gen Physiol* 79:69–86, 1982.
17. Kass RS, Tsien RS, Weingart R: Ionic basis of transient inward current induced by strophanthidin in cardiac Purkinje fibres. *J Physiol (Lond)* 281:209–226, 1978.
18. Katzung BG: Effects of extracellular calcium and sodium on depolarization-induced automaticity in guinea papillary muscle. *Circ Res* 37:118–127, 1975.
19. Kojima M, Sperelakis N: Properties of oscillatory afterpotentials in young embryonic chick hearts. *Circ Res* 55:497–503, 1984.
20. McDonald TF, MacLeod DP: Maintenance of resting potential in anoxic guinea pig ventricular muscle: Electrogenic sodium pumping. *Science* 172:570–572, 1971.

21. McDonald TF, Trautwein W: Membrane currents in cat myocardium: Separation of inward and outward components. *J Physiol* 274:193–216, 1978.
22. McDonald TF, MacLeod DP: Metabolism and the electrical activity of anoxic ventricular muscle. *J Physiol* 229:559–582, 1973.
23. Meech RW: Intracellular calcium injection causes increased potassium conductance in *Aplysia* nerve cells. *Comp Biochem Physiol* 42A:493–499, 1972.
24. New W, Trautwein W: Inward membrane currents in mammalian myocardium. *Pflügers Arch* 334:1–23, 1972.
25. Noble D: Initiation of the Heartbeat. Oxford: Clarendon, 1975.
26. Noma A, Irisawa H: Electrogenic sodium pump in rabbit sinoatrial node cell. *Pflügers Arch* 351:177–182, 1974.
27. Noma A, Matsuda H: Potassium channels identified with single channel recordings and their role in cardiac excitation. In: Dhalla NS, Pierce GN, Beamish RD (eds) *Heart Function and Metabolism.* Winnipeg, Canada: International Society for Heart Research, 1987, pp 67–78.
28. Page E, Storm SR: Cat heart muscle in vitro. VIII. Active transport of sodium in papillary muscles. *J Gen Physiol* 48:957–972, 1965.
29. Pelleg A, Vogel S, Belardinelli L, Sperelakis N: Overdrive suppression of automaticity in cultured chick myocardial cells. *Am J Physiol* 238:H24–H30, 1980.
30. Resh MD: Insulin activation of (Na^+,K^+)-adenosinetriphosphatase exhibits a temperature-dependent lag time. Comparison to activation of the glucose transporter. *Biochemistry* 22:2781–2784, 1983.
31. Reuter H, Scholz H: The regulation of the calcium conductance of cardiac muscle by adrenaline. *J Physiol (Lond)* 264:49–62, 1977.
32. Schneider JA, Sperelakis N: The demonstration of energy dependence of isoproterenol-induced transcellular Ca^{2+} current in isolated perfused guinea pig hearts — an explanation for mechanical failure of ischemic myocardium. *J Surg Res* 16:389–403, 1974.
33. Singer SJ, Nicolson GL: The fluid mosaic model of the structure of cell membranes. *Science* 175:720–731, 1972.
34. Sperelakis N, Schneider M, Harris EJ: Decreased K^+ conductance produced by Ba^{2+} in frog sartorius fibers. *J Gen Physiol* 50:1565–1583, 1967.
35. Sperelakis N, Lehmkuhl D: Effect of current on transmembrane potentials in cultured chick heart cells. *J Gen Physiol* 47:895–927, 1964.
36. Sperelakis N, Lehmkuhl D: Effects of temperature and metabolic poisons on membrane potentials of cultured heart cells. *Am J Physiol* 213:719–724, 1967.
37. Sperelakis N, Lehmkuhl D: Ionic interconversion of pacemaker and nonpacemaker cultured chick heart cells. *J Gen Physiol* 49:867–895, 1966.
38. Sperelakis N, Schneider JA: A metabolic control mechanism for calcium ion influxes that may protect the ventricular myocardial cell. *Am J Cardiol* 37:1079–1085, 1976.
39. Sperelakis N: (Na^+,K^+)-ATPase activity of embryonic chick heart and skeletal muscles as a function of age. *Biochim Biophys Acta* 266:230–237, 1972.
40. Sperelakis N: Changes in membrane electrical properties during development of the heart. In: Zipes DP, Bailey JC, Elharrar V (eds) *The Slow Inward Current and Cardiac Arrhythmias.* The Hague: Martinus Nijhoff, 1980, pp 221–262.
41. Sperelakis N: Electrophysiology of cultured chick heart cells. In: Sano T, Mizuhira V, Matsuda K (eds) *Electrophysiology and Ultrastructure of the Heart.* Bunkodo Co., Ltd., Tokyo, pp 81–108, 1967.
42. Tsien RW, Hess P, McCleskey EW, Rosenberg RL: Calcium channels: mechanisms of selectivity, permeation, and block. *Annual Review of Biophysics and Biophysical Chemistry* 16:265–290, 1987.
43. Trautwein W, Kassebaum DG: On the mechanism of spontaneous impulse generation in the pacemaker of the heart. *J Gen Physiol* 45:317–330, 1961.
44. Vassalle M: Cardiac pacemaker potentials at different extra- and intracellular K concentrations. *Am J Physiol* 208:770–775, 1965.
45. Vassalle M: Electrogenic suppression of automaticity in sheep and dog Purkinje fibers. *Circ Res* 27:361–377, 1970.
46. Vluegels A, Carmeliet E, Bosteels S, Zaman M: Differential effects of hypoxia with age on the chick embryonic heart. *Pflügers Arch* 365:159–166, 1976.

CHAPTER 4

Ionic Basis of Electrical Activity in the Heart

ROBERT S. KASS

INTRODUCTION

Cardiac muscle, like skeletal muscle and nerve, belongs to a class of tissues referred to as *excitable cells*. This classification reflects the ability of these cells to propagate impulses in a regenerative manner. The electrical activity of nerve and skeletal is rather uniform and is generated by similar ionic mechanisms. In contrast, the electrical activity in different regions of the heart consists of clearly distinguishable action potentials. This diversisty of action potential configuration reflects the multiple roles of electrical activity in the heart. But despite regional differences, these electrical impulses are generated by membrane permeability mechanisms that generally resemble those in other excitable cells.

This chapter presents a review of some of the major ionic currents in the heart and relates these currents both to the electrical activity of different regions and to some of the characteristic roles of this activity. The chapter emphasizes sodium, calcium, and potassium currents that have been studied in various mammalian cardiac cells. Where possible, structural information at the molecular level is integrated with the functional information about channel activity. This chapter is not intended to be a detailed review of each of these currents, but instead a source from which the reader may then pursue selected areas in more detail.

Excitation in the heart

NORMAL SPREAD OF THE IMPULSE: ROLES OF SPECIALIZED TISSUE

Electrical impulses in excitable cells are generated by local changes in the relative permeabilities of the surface membranes of these cells to various ions (see Chapter 3). These local permeability changes, in turn, regulate the electrical potential difference across the surface membrane through the electrochemical potential differences of the permeant ions. As a consequence of these local changes in membrane potential, voltage gradients are established both across the cell membrane and between local and distal longitudinal sites. These gradients force the movement of intracellular and extracellular ions. Ionic currents in combination with the cable properties (see Chapter 10) and morphology of different regions of the heart are responsible for the orderly pattern of cardiac excitation and contraction. This process depends on the unique electrical properties that have evolved for tissues that carry out specialized functions.

Electrical activity begins at the sinoatrial (SA) node, a strip of fine muscle fibers near the junction of the superior vena cava and the right atrium. The SA node generates electrical activity in a cyclic pattern, depolarizing and repolarizing spontaneously. The process of spontaneous depolarization is known as *pacemaker activity*. This region is not the only cardiac tissue that has this property (fig. 4-1), but it beats at the fastest rate and is thus the dominent pacemaker in the heart under normal conditions. In several pathological states, impulses from the SA node may not reach other regions of the heart. In such cases, cells that show slower (usually latent) pacemaker activity will drive the heart at a much lower than normal rate.

Under normal conditions, the impulse spreads rapidly from the SA node throughout the atrial muscle, where conduction is aided by special conducting tissue that resembles ventricular Purkinje fibers {1}. Electrical activity in the atrium is conducted into the ventricles through the atrioventricular node (AV node), a small strip of fine fibers that connects ventricular and atrial tissue. The small size of this tissue along with its electrical properties results in very slow impulse propagation through this node (typically on the order of 0.2 m/s). This slow AV node conduction ensures an adequate delay between atrial and ventricular contraction that is essential to proper filling and pumping of the ventricles.

From the AV node, the impulse is then conducted by specialized conducting tissue, the Purkinje fibers. In contrast to AV nodal tissue, Purkinje fibers consist of bundles of large cells that are well suited for rapid impulse conduction. Conduction velocity in the Purkinje network is on the order of 5 m/s (more than 10X the velocity in the AV node), and this ensures that the impulse spreads rapidly and uniformly throughout the ventricles. This rapid excitation of the ventricular muscle cells results in nearly synchronous contraction of these cells and a uniform pumping action on the blood in the ventricular chambers. When Purkinje fiber conduction is slowed in

N. Sperelakis (ed.), Physiology and Pathophysiology of the Heart, Third Edition.

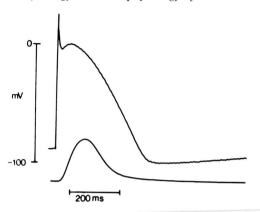

Fig. 4-1. Action potential and associated twitch tension in isolated Purkinje fiber. The upper trace is an intracellular recording of membrane potential obtained in an isolated Purkinje fiber that was driven by an external stimulus. Note the slow pacemaker activity following repolarization of the action potential. The lower trace, obtained using an optical monitor of contraction, shows the phasic tension developed by this fiber during the action potential. From R.S. Kass and D. Krafte, unpublished data.

diseased states, ventricular ejection is compromised due to the loss of synchrony in the contraction of individual muscle cells {1,2}.

Cardiac action potentials

As already suggested in the previous section, the distinct functional roles of electrical activity in each of these regions are closely related to the differences that have been found in the action potentials recorded in each area.

Nodal tissue

The duration of this action potential and all other cardiac action potentials is very long (on the order of 100 ms). The SA node shows spontaneous activity. The membrane potential changes from a negative value (near −65 mV) to a value greater than 0 mV and then returns to (repolarizes) the negative potential, where the cycle is repeated. Because the SA node determines heart rate, the slow change towards positive potentials (depolarization) occurring between beats is called the *pacemaker depolarization*. The most negative potential reached in this action potential is near −65 mV, a value much more positive than resting potentials of nerve or skeletal muscle. However, because the SA node is spontaneously active, it is not proper to refer to this as a resting potential. Instead the term *maximum diastolic potential* (MDP) is used to characterize this part of the nodal action potential. Another characteristic of this action potential is its maximum rate of polarization. This rate, on the order of 10 V/s, reflects the magnitude of the current that generates the voltage change (see eq. 4-4).

Electrical activity of cells in the AV node resemble that of the SA node, except that pacemaker activity is less

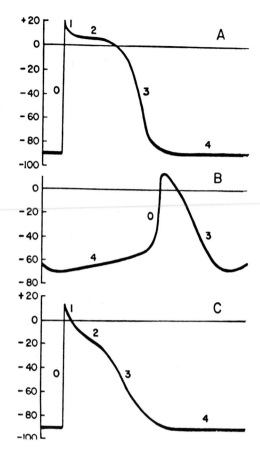

Fig. 4-2. Representative schematic records of transmembrane action potentials recorded from ventricular muscle (**A**), sinoatrial node (**B**), and atrial muscle (**C**). The vertical scale is in millivolts. The figure is from Hoffman and Cranefield {3}, with permission.

pronounced {3}. Thus, like SA node fibers, the maximum rate of rise of the action potential is on the order of 10 V/s and MDP is around −60 mV.

Purkinje fibers

Cells in Purkinje fiber bundles often also show some pacemaker activity (fig. 4-2), but this is much slower than pacing in the SA node. The Purkinje fiber MDP is much more negative (−90 mV) and the maximum rate of depolarization is much greater (500 V/s) than comparable parameters of the nodes. These differences are not entirely independent of each other and suggest the possibility that these action potentials are generated by two distinct mechanisms.

In the action potential shown, the membrane rapidly returns to approximately 0 mV following the initial depolarization. This rapid phase of repolarization seems to be most prominent in the Purkinje fiber (see *Calcium-activated currents*). After this rapid repolarization, there is a long-lasting phase of the action potential during which the membrane potential remains near $-20\,$mV to $0\,$mV with only a very slow repolarization evident. This is the plateau phase of the action potential. It is maintained by a delicate balance of small ionic currents and is easily altered by conditions such as drive rate or temperature.

Atrial and ventricular muscle

Like the Purkinje fiber, the most negative potentials reached in these cells is near $-90\,$mV, but under normal conditions these cells do not show pacemaker activity (fig. 4-2). The term *resting potential* is appropriate in describing these negative potentials. Neither atrial nor ventricular muscle cells have a rapid repolarization phase following the initial upstroke, but both have plateau phases of various shapes. Also, the maximum rate of rise of the rapid upstrokes of these cells resembles that of the Purkinje fiber.

Action potentials in the heart are the result of a complex interaction of several ionic currents. Regional differences in electrical activity often result from the varying contributions of different current. The next section discusses measurement of cardiac ionic currents and identification of some key current components that characterize electrical activity of the different anatomical regions.

Electrical analogs: Equivalent circuits

The mathematical description of impulse conduction based on local currents in nerve {4} is basically the same formalism originally developed by Kelvin to describe transmission of electrical signals along submerged telegraph cables and is thus referred to as *cable theory*. In addition to describing impulse conduction, cable theory provides the foundation upon which methods for measuring membrane currents in excitable cells are built. The cable properties of heart tissue are presented in more detail in Chapter 10, but some of the consequences of these properties will be briefly discussed here in the context of ionic current measurement.

One of the simplest and oldest biophysical representations of the permeability properties of cell membranes is the linear (ohmic) equivalent circuit. This circuit corresponds to the lumped electrical properties of local patches of membrane. It consists of membrane capacitance (C_m) and ionic conductances, which provide pathways for transmembrane movement of permeant ions. Although such a model does not provide insight into how ions actually move across membranes, it is extremely useful in studying both the cable properties and the electrical responses of excitable cells.

Membrane structure accounts for the membrane capacitance {2}, which is fairly constant in most biological membranes ($\mu F/cm^2$). Charge must be added to one side of the cell membrane and subtracted from the other in order to change the voltage across the membrane capacitance, as is the case for any two conducting surfaces that form a capacitor. This charge movement comprises a displacement, or capacity, current that is related to the rate of change in voltage across the membrane capacitance (C_m) as follows:

$$I_c = C_m dV_m/dt. \qquad (4\text{-}1)$$

According to this expression, membrane potential (V_m) will not change if there is no change in charge across the membrane capacitance. This equation also shows that when there is capacity current the rate of change of voltage is proportional to the magnitude of the current flowing into and out of the capacitor's conducting surfaces.

A region of membrane is referred to as *active* when the permeability to one or more ions suddenly increases in this region. Then positively charged ions move down their electrochemical gradients through open channels. This excitatory inward current adds positive charge to the inner surface of the cell membrane and thus leads to local depolarization. Intracellularly a longitudinal voltage difference is established between this depolarized region and more distant regions still at rest. This voltage drop forces ion movement (mostly K^+) from active to passive areas and sets up the local circuit currents that spread the depolarization.

At each patch of membrane, the total transmembrane current (I_m) divides between capacity current (which changes the voltage across the membrane) and ionic current (I_i), which flows through the conductive pathways, shunting the membrane capacitance. Total membrane current is thus the sum of these two components:

$$I_m = I_i + I_c \qquad (4\text{-}2)$$

or, using eq. (4-1) for I_c,

$$I_m = I_i + C_m dV_m/dt. \qquad (4\text{-}3)$$

Measurement of ionic current

Two important experimental conditions can be imposed to simplify eq. (4-3) and permit analysis of membrane current. In one case, longitudinal voltage gradients are considerably reduced, and that minimizes local circuit currents. In the squid axon this can be accomplished by short-circuiting the axon interior with an intracellular, low resistance, axial electrode. This condition has been termed *space-clamp*, and active electrical activity measured under space-clamp conditions is called a *membrane action potential*. In this case the net transmembrane current must be zero, and eq. (4-3) simplifies to

$$C_m dv/dt = -I_{ionic}. \qquad (4\text{-}4)$$

Although the multicellular nature of heart muscle precludes the experimental simplification used in nerve, eq. (4-4) can be applied to small isolated cardiac preparations. Then under conditions approximating zero longitudinal current, eq. (4-4) can be used to estimate net ionic current from time-dependent changes in membrane potential. However, this approach must be used with caution, as it is restricted by frequency-dependent changes in membrane capacity {5,6} as well as nonlinear characteristics of cardiac currents {7}.

Another simplification of eq. (4-3) occurs when membrane potential is measured and experimentally controlled by passing current from an intracellular current source. This technique is referred to as *voltage clamp*. Since voltage is controlled, capacity current (excluding brief transients) is eliminated, and the total applied current (which is measured) becomes transmembrane ionic current (I_i). Once again this requires uniform voltage control, a condition that can be attained in squid axon with axial wire arrangements, but only approximated in multicellular cardiac preparations. However, several recent advances have improved the reliability of cardiac voltage-clamp measurements. These include the computation of limiting properties of multicellular heart preparations {8} and the introduction of single isolated cardiac cells that can be voltage clamped {9}.

IONIC BASIS OF CARDIAC ELECTRICAL ACTIVITY

Some basic nomenclature

Before discussing the ionic basis of cardiac electrical activity, it will be useful to review some basic concepts that are used in descriptions of ionic currents. From the preceding section (eq. 4-4), it is clear that under experimental conditions that minimize impulse propagation (space clamp), the rate of change of membrane potential is given by the magnitude and direction of the total ionic current flowing across the membrane. By convention, negative current (inward movement of positive charge) depolarizes the membrane and thus produces a positive dV_m/dt. Total membrane current generally is the summation of several component ionic currents, and it is the experimenter's goal to characterize each current component. Each current is described as the product of a conductance (G_i) and a driving force ($E_m - E_i$):

$$I_i = G_i \times (E_m - E_i), \qquad (4\text{-}5)$$

where E_i is the equilibrium potential for a given channel (see Chapter 3) and E_m is membrane potential. In general, the conductance G_i may be a function of membrane potential and time.

Ions move across membranes through channels that can discriminate between possible charge carriers. The relative permeability of a channel to various ions, the channel selectivity, is reflected in the equilibrium potential. This is the potential of zero *net* current through the channel, and it is a function of the transmembrane concentration gradients of the permeant ions.

Two classes of inward currents in the heart

Action potentials in the heart may be divided into two general groups based on rate of depolarization. In one group (atrial and ventricular muscle, Purkinje fibers), the action potentials are characterized by very rapid (500 V/s) upstrokes, whereas in the second group (SA and AV nodal fibers) the action potential rises with a markedly slower upstroke (10 V/s). Using eq. (4-4) as a guide, this contrast

in upstroke velocity suggests that the regenerative inward current in the nodes might be much smaller than in other cardiac tissues. Another distinction between these groups is the voltage range from which these upstrokes emerge. The nodal tissues are activated over a considerably more positive voltage range than the other cardiac preparations.

These two observations provide clues to the existence of two inward currents in cardiac cells, which may be distinguished both by the voltage range over which they contribute to ionic current and by the differences in their sizes. Considerable experimental evidence now supports this view and provides several criteria for distinguishing these excitatory currents. One current, carried by sodium ions, resembles regenerative sodium current in nerve and skeletal muscle, and is responsible for the rapid upstroke and fast impulse conduction in atrial and ventricular muscle, as well as the special conducting tissue. A second current, carried principally by calcium ions, generates the nodal upstroke, underlies slow impulse conduction in the AV node, and maintains the plateau phase of the action potential in other parts of the heart.

SODIUM CURRENT

The upstroke of the action potential of working cardiac muscle and cells of the specialized conducting tracts, like action potentials in nerve and skeletal muscle, is due to a transient increase in membrane permeability to sodium ions. The very rapid rates of rise of the action potentials in these tissues predict [from eq. (4-4)] that the current responsible for these voltage changes is large (about $1\,\text{mA/cm}^2$).

Before the introduction of preparations that were suitable for voltage clamp analysis of large inward cardiac currents {8–10}, experiments on the upstroke and overshoot of the Purkinje fiber action potential demonstrated the sodium dependence of these parameters {11}. Later this same approach was used to probe the gating mechanisms of this channel {12} and to study interactions of calcium ions and some local anesthetics on them {13}.

Sodium currents have now been studied under voltage clamp in several multicellular cardiac preparations {9,10,14,15}. These currents appear similar to sodium currents in nerve and skeletal muscle. When the cell membrane is depolarized beyond $-65\,\text{mV}$, an inward current is initiated that rises to a peak and then declines within a few milliseconds (fig. 4-3A). As in other excitable cells, this current is described as current flow through channels regulated by time- and voltage-dependent activation and inactivation gates. At a particular time and voltage, the fraction of open sodium channels is determined by the product of the activation and inactivation gating parameters. Because of the unique anatomical properities, causing unusally wide intracellular clefts, the rabbit Purkinje fiber is particularly well suited for studies of large regenerative inward currents using microelectrodes to control membrane potential. The steady-state voltage dependence of these parameters obtained in the rabbit Purkinje fiber is given in fig. 4-3B.

As this product is zero at all potentials in fig. 4-3B,

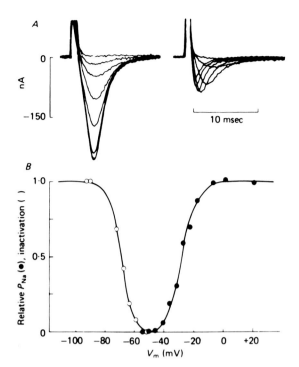

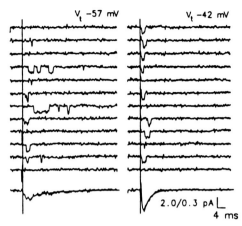

Fig. 4-4. Recordings of openings in the single-channel patch from canine cardiac Purkinje fiber cell membrane. Currents were recorded at the two voltages indicated in the figure. Each panel shows individual sweeps of current activity. Notice that some sweeps show no activity but that, when present, channel openings tend to occur near the beginning of each pulse. The averaged records are shown at the bottom of the figure, and these traces resemble "macrosopic" activity recorded in whole-cell mode or in multicellular preparations with microelectrodes (fig. 4-3). From Sconley et al. {25}, with permission.

Fig. 4-3. Sodium current in the rabbit Purkinje fiber. **A:** Families of total membrane current obtained using conventional protocols for inactivation (left) and permeability (right). The inactivation curve was measured at a constant test pulse voltage (-38 mV) following 500 ms prepulses. Permeability was measured from peak inward currents measured at various test pulses from a -58 mV holding potential. **B:** Voltage dependence of relative sodium current inactivation ($\bigcirc$) and permeability ($\bullet$). Data from Colatsky {14}.

these curves predict that the sodium conductance must also be zero in the steady state. These data were obtained at low temperatures. However at more physiological temperatures there appears to be a region of overlap of these two parameters that results in a "window" of steady-state sodium current over the plateau voltage range {16–18}. This current accounts for the effects of TTX and sodium removal on the cardiac action potential plateau {19,20}.

Membrane potential affects the fraction of sodium channels that are open, and thus determines the number of sodium channels available for impulse conduction. In the plateau potential range (fig. 4-3B) most of these channels are closed (inactivated). It is the time course of removal of sodium channel inactivation at diastolic potentials that determines the availability of these channels for impulse conduction, and consequently the periods in which the cells remain inexcitable (refractory). Sodium channels in the heart thus resemble sodium channels in other excitable cells in their voltage dependence and sensitivity to local anesthetic drugs. But some clues, such as a distinct low TTX sensitivity as well as voltage-dependent TTX block

{21}, suggest that cardiac sodium channels are structurally distinct from those of other cells.

Investigation of whole-cell cardiac sodium channel activity has been carried out in neonatal rat heart cells {22} and internally perfused canine cardiac Purkinje cells {23}. Measurements of single sodium-channel activity have been carried out in membranes of rat {24}, canine Purkinje {25} and guinea pig {26} hearts. Most of the kinetic and single-channel properties revealed in these studies resemble properties of sodium channel activity in multicellular cardiac and other cells. An example of single sodium channel activity as well as the averaged "macroscopic" activity of a patch of canine Purkinje cell membrane is shown in fig. 4-4.

The cloning and expression of a tetrodotoxin-resistant sodium channel from rat heart {27} have provided direct structural evidence for distinct channel proteins that form voltage-dependent sodium channels in heart, nerve, and other tissues. Studies are presently underway to determine further relationships between channel structure and function using the powerful tools of molecular genetics in combination with electrophysiological approaches {28,29}.

CALCIUM CHANNEL CURRENTS

In myocardial cells, Reuter {30} first showed that calcium entry can occur into the cytoplasm via calcium-sensitive inward current that is activiated by membrane potential. Calcium entry has since been shown to be key to maintainance of cardiac electrical and mechanical activity {31,32}. The discovery of calcium channel currents in the heart has led to extensive investigation of voltage- and agonist-modulated calcium channels in a wide variety of tissues. Some of the more important properties of cardiac calcium channels, as well as the experiments that led to their discovery, are outlined here.

Action potential experiments

The action potential of the Purkinje fiber or of working myocardial muscle can be made to resemble electrical activity of the SA or AV nodes by a variety of experimental conditions that depolarize the cells. Then the Purkinje fiber action potential is characterized by a very slow upstroke (about 10 V/s) and conduction velocity (0.1–0.01 m/s). Consequently, it is referred to as a *slow response action potential* {2,33}. Characteristics of the slow response are discussed in Chapter 12.

The current that generates the slow response was initially referred to as the *slow inward current* (I_{si}) in order to distinguish it from the fast and large regenerative inward sodium channel current (I_{Na}). It is carried principally by calcium ions and is as much as 100 times smaller than peak sodium currents. In addition to the slow response, it underlies impulse conduction in nodal tissue {34,35} and is crucial to maintenance of the plateau phase of action potentials of myocardial and special conducting tissues {36,37}.

Multiple types of calcium channels

Early voltage-clamp investigations in Purkinje fibers {30,38} and other preparations {39–41} demonstrated the existence of a calcium-sensitive inward current, which was then labeled the *slow inward current* (I_{si}). This current has many of the properties suggested by slow-response experiments: It is enhanced by catecholamines and blocked by Mn^{2+} and other metallic cations, and it has a voltage dependence distinct from I_{Na}.

In intact preparations, I_{si} was analyzed by Reuter, Trautwein, and others {42}. Subsequently, it has been investigated extensively in enzymatically isolated cell and membrane patches {43–46}. It is described analagously to the sodium current as current through a gated channel:

$$I_{Ca} = G_{Ca} \cdot d \cdot f \cdot (E_m - E_{si}). \tag{4-6}$$

G_{Ca} is the conductance when all I_{si} channels are fully open, d is the activation parameter, f the inactivation parameter, and E_{si} is the equilibrium potential. The voltage dependence and kinetics of these gating parameters differ from those of the sodium channel and account for the properties of calcium-dependent upstrokes. As suggested by the slow response data, the voltage range of I_{si} inactivation is so different from I_{Na} inactivation that calcium current can be activated from potentials at which the sodium current is almost completely inactivated.

It is now known that at least four calcium channel subtypes (P, T, N, and L) exist. Their identification and dissection is based on their pharmacological and/or biophysical properties {47,48}. Both T- and L-type channels have been studied in the heart {49}, but the physiological role of the T-type, or rapidly inactivating channel, remains

somewhat questionable, with evidence in favor of a link to calcium-induced calcium release and also a role in pacemaker activity of the sinoatrial node.

The L-type channel is the target of the most extensively developed calcium channel pharmacology. The drugs that have received the most attention belong to three distinct chemical classes: (a) phenylalkylamines (verapamil, D-600); (b) benzothiazepines [(+) cis-diltiazem]; and (c) the 1–4, dihydropyridines (PN 200-110, nitrendipine, nifedipine, nisoldipine). These drugs bind to distinct, but allosterically coupled, receptors on the channel protein {50}. Of all the chemical comounds that interact with calcium channels, the dihydropyridines (DHPs) have proven to be the most useful in molecular studies of the L-channel, because these drugs bind to the channel with highest affinity and specificity {51}.

CALCIUM CHANNEL AS A DIHYDROPYRIDINE RECEPTOR

Because of the high affinity of DHPs for calcium channels, the initial strategy for the isolation and purification of L-type calcium channels was to isolate and purify the protein component(s) as isolated DHP receptors with the chance that the purified components would constitute functional calcium channels {52}. This approach was applied to skeletal muscle t tubules, the richest source of L-type calcium channels, and yielded a purified DHP receptor that consisted of five subunits: α_1, α_2, β_2, γ, and δ {53–59}. Reconstitution experiments showed that the purified DHP receptor could function as a voltage-dependent calcium channel {54,60}.

The skeletal {61} and cardiac {62} DHP receptors were cloned using the purified rabbit skeletal muscle DHP receptor α_1 subunit as a probe. Both had marked structural resemblence to the voltage-gated sodium channel, providing indirect evidence that the α_1 subunit is the channel pore itself {59}. Functional channel activity could be measured after injection of the cardiac α_1 subunit mRNA into *Xenopus* oocytes {62}, and coexpression of the cardiac α, and skeletal β_2 subunits doubled the expressed currents, strongly suggesting the subunits other than α_1 were likely to have important functional roles in channel activity {62}. With this structural information in hand, it is now possible to begin to determine the molecular components that underlie important functional characteristics of the L-type channel in heart and other tissues.

Molecular pharmacology of calcium channels

Calcium channel antagonists, in general, and the dihydropyridine derivatives, in particular, regulate calcium influx by modulating channel gating {63–65}. Drug-induced gating changes resemble modes of gating that can occur under drug-free conditions {66,67}, supporting the view that molecular perturbations induced by these compounds promote indigenous conformational changes of the channel proteins. Since it has been shown that the α_1 subunit contains the specific binding sites for all three

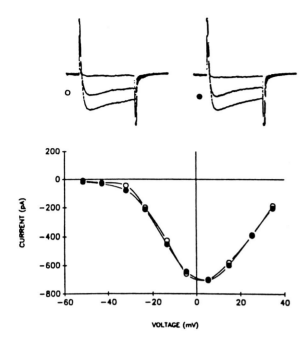

Fig. 4-5. L-type calcium channel currents recorded with whole-cell patch-clamp procedures from an isolated guinea-pig ventricular cell before (open symbols) and after (filled) exposure to the dihydropyridine calcium-channel blocker amlodipine (3 μM) at a −80 mV holding potential. At this voltage both the current traces and the corresponding current/voltage relationship (lower panel) are not affected by this voltage-dependent drug. From Kass and Arena {134}, with permission.

major classes of calcium channel blockers described above {50,52,59}, it is very likely that drug-induced conformational changes of the α_1 subunit underlie these gating changes.

Divalent ions inhibit the binding of radiolabeled phenlyalkylamines to membrane-bound L channels, but high-affinity dihydropyridine labeling of L-type channels in brain, cardiac, or smooth muscle membranes depends on the presence of divalent ions {50,55}, as does the binding of dihydropyridines to the purified DHP receptor {68}. Binding of calcium also has important regulatory roles in the permeability and gating properties of drug-free native L-type channels. Calcium influx and the high calcium selectivity of skeletal muscle and heart L-type channels is best explained by a multiple ion (at least two) binding model in which ion-ion repulsion is seen as the key to overcome strong intrapore cation binding {69}. Divalent ion binding has been shown to induce protein conformational changes, which, in turn, could affect the binding of other ions (notably H^+) {70}, and inactivation of cardiac L-channels has also been shown to be influenced by Ca^{2+} being enhanced with calcium entry {71,72}. Thus it is very likely that binding of calcium to at least one regulatory site changes the conformation of the α_1 subunit such that DHP-receptor interactions are modified, and possibly

permeation and/or gating are controlled in the absence of drug binding.

Examples of calcium channel current recorded using whole-cell conditions with the patch clamp are shown in fig. 4-5. The figure includes records taken in the absence and presence of the calcium channel blocker amlodipine at a negative holding potential (−80 mV). This drug, like other dihydropyridine calcium channel blockers, is very voltage dependent and does not block channels at this negative voltage.

Modulation by neurohormones

L-type calcium channel current in the heart is modulated by neurohormones. It is decreased by muscarinic agents {73,74} and increased by catecholamines {75}. Reuter and Scholz {76} suggested that the principal action of epinephrine on I_{si} is to increase the maximal conductance (G_{si}) of this channel. This can occur either by increasing the maximal conductance of each I_{si} channel or by creating more channels, each with a constant single-channel conductance.

Modulation of L-type channel activity by the beta-adrenergic pathway has been studied extensively using whole-cell and single-channel patch-clamp procedures. The reader is referred to one of many reviews for more details about the direct (G-protein limited) and indirect (cAMP-mediated) regulation of these channels {49}.

Potassium channel currents: Multiple roles in the heart

Heart K^+ channels include slowly activating voltage-dependent channels {77,78}; a background, relatively instaneous channel {79}; a channel regulated by cellular ATP concentrations {80–82}; a voltage- and calcium-activated transient channel {83–86}; and an acetylcholine-regulated potassium channel {87}. Still other, less well-characterized channels also exist in heart: a time-independent plateau channel {97} and a potassium channel activated by high intracellular sodium concentrations {88}.

REPOLARIZATION OF THE ACTION POTENTIAL: THE DELAYED RECTIFIER

The plateau phase of the cardiac action potential is maintained by a fine balance between small inward and outward currents. During the plateau phase, the membrane potential changes very slowly, indicating little net charge transfer across the membrane capacitance (see eq. 4-4). Then, as the balance tips in favor of outward current, the net movement of positive charge is from the inner surface to the outer surface of the membrane, and repolarization of the cell begins. The gradual transition to outward current is due both to the inactivation (decrease) in calcium channel currents and to the slow activation (increase) of a time-dependent outward current.

Noble and Tsien {77} investigated the repolarization process in the Purkinje fiber and found a time-dependent outward current that is activated over a potential range similar to the plateau of the action potential. Its time dependence consisted of two components: one relatively fast time constant ($\tau = 500\,\text{ms}$) and the other much slower ($\tau = 5\,\text{s}$). When they used voltage-clamp protocols to determine the equilibrium potential for this current, Noble and Tsien found the charge carrier of this current to be largely, but not exclusively, potassium ions. Because this channel is not completely selective for one charge carrier, it was labelled I_x, and expressed as the sum of its two components

$$I_x = I_{x1} + I_{x2}. \qquad (4\text{-}7)$$

I_{x1} is the faster component and I_{x2} is the slower component. This current is often also referred to as the *delayed rectifier* in order to relate it to repolarizing outward currents in nerve and skeletal muscle. Computer-generated reconstruction of the Purkinje fiber action potential confirmed that I_x is crucial to the repolarization process in these fibers {36}. Similar time-dependent outward currents have since been reported in SA nodal preparations, atrial preparations, and ventricular fibers {89,90}.

More recent pharmacological data {78,91} have confirmed the existence of multiple types of delayed rectifier channels in ventricular and atrial cells. The channel subtypes can be distinguished by their kinetics and pharmacology. A very rapidly activating component that is blocked by the benzenesulfonamide antiarrhythmic drug E-4031 and by lanthanum has been labeled I_{Kr} because, in addition to its delayed rectified characteristics, it also rectifies with depolarization. A second, approximately 10-fold larger component, which is lanthanum and E-4031-insensitive and does not inactivate, is labeled I_{Ks} because of its slow kinetics. Both channels contribute to the regulation of the action potential duration in atrial and ventricular cells, and thus their regulation by drugs or neurohormones is seen as key to control of the QT interval. Recent advances in drug development have, in fact, focused on drugs that specifically target these K^+ channels {92,93}.

SINGLE-CHANNEL RECORDINGS OF I_{kdr}

Little data are available reporting single-channel properties of mammalian ventricular delayed rectifier channels. Balser et al. {94} described single delayed rectifier channels in guinea pig ventricular myocytes with a mean chord conductance of $5.4\,\text{pS}$, but these channels appeared to inactivate. Walsh et al. {95} were unable to resolve single-channel events in excised patches of guinea pig myocytes, but described, instead, a macroscopic current consistent with a high-density, extremely low conductance K^+ channel. Regulation of isolated patch recordings of I_{Ks} has subsequently been reported {95}.

DELAYED RECTIFIER POTASSIUM CURRENT (I_{kdr}) IN NODAL CELLS

In mammalian sinoatrial and atrioventricular nodes, the repolarization phase of the action potential and, to a certain extent, pacemaking, are regulated by a delayed K^+ channel {96–98}. Shibasaki {99} measured single-channel activity of rabbit nodal delayed rectification and found a single-channel conductance much larger than that reported for I_{Ks} {100}. This channel may underlie I_r in ventricle and atria {34}. Delayed rectification of nodal tissue from other species can be comprised of both inactivating and non-inactivating components {101}, and the regulation of nodal delayed rectification may differ from that of the ventricle.

MODULATION OF DELAYED RECTIFICATION

It is well known that one component of delayed rectification in the heart is controlled by sympathetic stimulation: I_{Ks} is markedly enhanced by beta-adrenergic agonists. This has been demonstrated in multi-cell and single-cell preparations {75,102–105}. Studies of delayed rectification in single cells have provided evidence that beta-adrenergic enhancement of I_K is associated with phosphorylation of an intracellular protein by protein kinase A. Modulation of I_{Ks} by intracellular calcium {106} and protein kinase C {107,108} have also been demonstrated with evidence pointing towards distinct regulatory sites for different protein kinases {100}. Regulation of I_{Ks} occurs rapidly and probably contributes to control of action potential duration on a beat-by-beat basis. An example of the enhancement of I_{Ks} by protein kinase C is shown in fig. 4-6. The data in the figure illustrate the unique voltage-dependent effect of PKC on the channel activation curve. This effect distinguishes the actions of PKC from PKA, which shifts, but does not affect the slope of, I_{Ks} channel activation.

Background K^+ channel currents: The inward rectifier

The plateau phase of the cardiac action potential is characterized by high cellular input impedance {109}, and thus small changes in membrane current can cause dramatic changes in the duration of the action potential. One of the principal mechanisms underlying this unique property of heart action potentials is the rectification of the background (I_{k1}) K^+ channel conductance. This channel preferentially conducts K^+ in the outward direction across the cell membrane. As the membrane potential is made more positive than the K^+ equilibrium potential, this channel allows less and less current to flow and thus increases the background membrane impedance. The inward rectifier is important in determining the cellular resting potential and underlies changes in diastolic potentials during hyperkalemia and hypokalemia.

McAllister and Noble {110} were the first to measure the voltage-dependent properties of the current in a cardiac preparation (calf Purkinje fibers). They revealed a rectifying K^+-selective current. Sakmann and Trube {111} demonstrated inward rectification of this current at the single-channel level. Vandenberg {112} provided evidence that the basis for rectification is the occlusion of the K^+-channel pore by Mg^{2+}, which is driven into the channel as K^+ moves in the outward direction through the pore

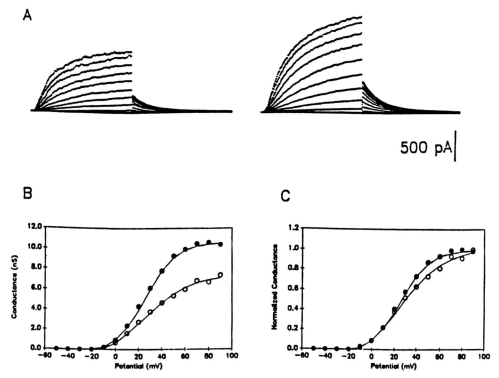

Fig. 4-6. Protein kinase C stimulation enhances I_{Ks} and changes the slope of its activation curve. Panel **A** shows traces of I_{Ks} recorded using whole-cell procedures in an isolated guinea-pig ventricular cell before (**left**) and after (**right**) exposure to 10 nM phorbol dibutyrate (PDB; a compound that stimulates protein kinase C activity). Notice the current enhancement, which is reflected in the un-normalized activation curve (**B**). Panel **C** (normalized activation curve) reveals an increase in the slope of the activation relationship caused by PDB. From Walsh and Kass {100}, with permission.

{113}. Matsuda et al. {114} confirmed the role of Mg^{2+} as the current-dependent plug that causes inward rectification in this channel, but they also detected a component of channel inhibition that was governed by membrane potential itself.

TRANSIENT OUTWARD CURRENT (I_{to})

The very rapid repolarization that follows the sodium-dependent upstroke of the Purkinje fiber action potential is also generated by a transition from inward to outward current. But in this case the transition is due to the inactivation of I_{Na} along with the activation and subsequent inactivation of a large outward current.

Early voltage-clamp studies showed a transient outward current component that dominated the early periods of currents recorded during strong depolarizing voltage pulses. These initial studies suggested that this was a chloride current, because it was greatly reduced by chloride removal {115,116}. But these effects of chloride substitution were later attributed to indirect effects on intracellular Ca activity {117}.

More recent studies have provided evidence that potassium ions are the most likely charge carrier for this transient outward current. This conclusion is based on pharmacological grounds: The transient outward current has been shown to be sensitive to compounds or procedures that block K channels in other excitable cells. It is sensitive to 4-aminopyridine and extracellular tetraethylammonium {92,117}, intracellular quaternary ammonium ion compounds {118}, and replacement of intracellular potassium by cesium {93,119}, although evidence has also been presented to implicate a role for a calcium-activated Cl^- channel as well {120}.

This current was initially labelled I_{qr} but now is referred to as I_{to} (for transient outward current). Its kinetic properties have not been completely analyzed, but it is clear that I_{to} activates quickly and inactivates, at least partially, with time constants near 50 ms. Recent studies have suggested that I_{to} may also consist of two components: one sensitive to intracellular calcium and a second component that is not calcium activated {121–123}. I_{to} is most prominent in the Purkinje fiber, where it contributes to the "notch" configuration of the action potential. It is also present in other cardiac cells, such as ventricular muscle, although it is not as important in these tissues {124}. Recently the possible contribution of a maintained component of I_{to} in the regulation of action potential duration has been explored. Dukes and Morad {125} have shown that tedisamil blocks I_{to} and shortens action potential duration in rat ventricular myoctyes. Furthermore, Litovsky and Antzelevitch {126} have reported regional differences in I_{to} channel density in the canine heart. They found I_{to} prominent in the ventricular epicardium but not in the endocardium. As a result, one would predict that if there were a maintained component of I_{to} in epicardial cells, differences between epicardial and endocardial action potential durations would, in part, be caused by the contrast in I_{to} channel density. If this were shown to be the case in other species, particularly in the human heart, then regional differences in I_{to} channel density could be the mechanism underlying the well-known phenomenon of T-wave inversion on the electrocardiogram.

Recently K^+ channel currents with rapid activation and slower inactivation components have been reported in both neonatal canine epicardium {13} and rat atrial myocytes {8}. Because of the activation kinetics, this type of channel would be expected to contribute to early phases of action potential repolarization, and, in addition, it has been suggested that it contributes to age-related changes in action potential duration {13}.

Calcium-activated currents

Calcium-activated K currents are known to exist in a wide variety of cells, and evidence has been presented that I_{to} is, at least in part, such a current. Siegelbaum et al. {127} first demonstrated a possible role of Ca_i in regulating the conductance of the I_{to} channel, and this work has been supported by further studies {83,121}. In this view the time-dependent changes in I_{to} are not entirely due to modulation of the I_{to} conductance by voltage-dependent gates. Instead, this conductance is enhanced by intracellular calcium ion concentration, which changes in a phasic manner during depolarizations.

Several properties of the delayed rectifier (I_K) have suggested that it too may be a calcium-activated current. Calcium influx (I_{si}) precedes the slower onset of I_K, and several compounds that block I_{Ca} also reduce I_x {128}. In addition, catecholamine-induced increases in I_{Ca} are accompanied by dramatic increases in I_K. However, recent experimental evidence has shown that I_x activation can be separated from I_{si} activation by a new calcium channel blocker, nisoldipine {129}. Nisoldipine, as well as D600, also prevents the increase of I_{Ca}, but not I_K, by norepinephrine {75}. Thus it is not likely that I_K is activated by intracellular calcium ions {130}, but it is clear that Ca^{2+} acts as a modulator of this channel {106}.

MOLECULAR BIOLOGY OF CARDIAC K CHANNELS

Based on homology with *Shaker* K^+ channels, several types of voltage-gated K^+ channels have now been cloned from rat and human heart {19–21,45}. All of these channels have *Shaker* like properties in that they are formed by four K^+ channel proteins, each with hydropathy profiles indicating six transmembrane spanning hydro-

phobic segments (S1, S2, S3, S4, S5, and S6), and they activate quickly and subsquently inactivate with continued depolarization. Thus it is not likely that these channel proteins underlie the very slowly activating delayed rectifier (I_{Ks}) channel, which does not inactivate, but they could be candidates for several important heart K^+ channels, including the transient outward current channel and the I_{Kr} channel.

The functional properties of I_{Ks} are not well correlated with any of reported for channels cloned from the *Shaker* family but instead resemble those of a unique channel, structurally very different from *Shaker*-type channels originally cloned from rat kidney {131} but later found in rat uterus {133}, human genomic DNA {134}, and also neonatal rat {131}, neonatal mouse {135,136} and human {132} hearts. The channel protein (minK because of its small size, or IsK) predicted by the cDNA contains 129–130 amino acids, only one *transmembrane-spanning domain*, and has no homology with other cloned channels {133}.

SUMMARY

This chapter has focused on the major ionic currents that contribute to cardiac electrical activity. It has not discussed pacemaker currents, electrogenic Na/K pump currents (see Chapter 3 and Noble and Tsien {77}); or possible roles of Na/Ca exchange in cardiac electrical activity (see Chapter 15). On the other hand, it has presented a review of sodium, potassium, and calcium channel currents that have been characterized in the heart as well as an introduction to the molecular biology of these channel types. In addition, it has provided references for more detailed study of each of them. Cardiac electrophysiology is an exciting area of study that is rapidly changing as newer and more quantitative experimental techniques are introduced. As this field of study expands, we are increasing our understanding of the mechanisms that underlie the complicated patterns of electrical activity in the normal heart, and we further our ability to correct electrical disturbances in diseased states.

REFERENCES

1. Noble D: The Initiation of the Heartbeat. Oxford: Clarendon Press, 1978.
2. Cranefield PF: The Conduction of the Cardiac Impulse. Mount Kisco, NY: Futura, 1975.
3. Hoffman BF, Cranefield PF: Electrophysiology of the Heart. Mount Kisco, NY: Futura, 1976.
4. Hodgkin AL, Rushton WAH: The electrical constants of a crustacean nerve fiber. *Proc R Soc Lon* B133:444–479, 1946.
5. Fozzard HA: Membrane capacity of the cardiac Purkinje fibre. *J Physiol* 182:255–267, 1966.
6. Carmeliet E, Willems J: The frequency dependent character of the membrane capacity in cardiac Purkinje fibres. *J Physiol* 213:85–84, 1971.
7. Strichartz GR, Cohen IS: V max as a measure of GNa in nerve and cardiac membranes. *Biophys J* 23:153–156, 1978.

8. Kass RS, Siegelbaum SA, Tsien RW: Three-microelectrode voltage clamp experiments in calf cardiac Purkinje fibers: Is slow inward current adequately measured? *J Physiol* 290:201–225, 1979.

9. Lee KS, Weeks TA, Kao RL, Akaike N, Brown AM: Sodium current in single heart muscle cells. *Nature* 278: 269–271, 1979.

10. Colatsky TJ, Tsien RW: Sodium channels in rabbit cardiac Purkinje fibres. *Nature* 278:265–268, 1979.

11. Draper MH, Weidmann S: Cardiac resting and action potentials recorded with an intracellular electrode. *J Physiol* 115:74–94, 1951.

12. Weidman S: The effect of the cardiac membrane potential on the rapid availability of the sodium carrying system. *J Physiol* 127:213, 1955.

13. Weidmann S: Effects of calcium ions and local anaesthetics on electrical properties of Purkinje fibres. *J Physiol* 129:568–582, 1955.

14. Colatsky TJ: Voltage clamp measurements of sodium channel properties in rabbit cardiac Purkinje fibres. *J Physiol* 305:215–234, 1980.

15. Ebihara L, Shigeto N, Lieberman M, Johnson EA: The initial inward current in spherical clusters of chick embryonic heart cells. *J Gen Physiol* 75:437–456, 1980.

16. Attwell D, Cohen I, Eisner D, Ohba M, Ojeda C: The steady state TTX-sensitive ("window") sodium current in cardiac Purkinje fibres. *Pflügers Arch* 379:137–142, 1979.

17. Colatsky TJ, Gadsby DC: Is tetrodotoxin block of background sodium channels voltage-dependent? *J Physiol* 306:20P, 1980.

18. Colatsky TJ: Mechanisms of action of lidocaine and quinidine on action potential duration in rabbit Purkinje fibers. An effect on steady state sodium currents? *Circ Res* 50:17–27, 1982.

19. Dudel J, Peper K, Rudel R, Trautwein W: Excitatory membrane current in heart muscle (Purkinje fibres). *Pflügers Arch* 292:255–273, 1966.

20. Coraboeuf E, Deroubaix E, Coulombe A: Effect of tetrodotoxin on action potentials of the conducting system in the dog heart. *Am J Physiol* 236:H561–H567, 1979.

21. Cohen CJ, Bean BP, Colatsky TJ, Tsien RW: Tetrodotoxin block of sodium channels in rabbit Purkinje fibers. *J Gen Physiol* 78:383–411, 1981.

22. Brown AM, Lee KS, Powell T: Sodium current in single rat heart muscle cells. *J Physiol* 318:479–500, 1981.

23. Makeilski MC, Sheets MF, Hanck DA, January CT, Fozzard HA: Sodium current in voltage clamped internally-perfused canine cardiac Purkinje cells. *Biophys J* 52:1–11, 1987.

24. Kunze DL, Lacerda AE, Wilson DL, Brown AM: Cardiac Na currents and the inactivity, reopening, and waiting properties of single cardiac Na channels. *J Gen Physiol* 86:697–719, 1985.

25. Scanley BE, Sheets MF, Fozzard HA: Kinetic analysis of single sodium channels from canine cardiac Purkinje cells. *J Gen Physiol* 95:411–438, 1990.

26. Lawrence JH, Yue DT, Rose WC, Marban E: Sodium channel inactivation from resting states in guinea-pig ventricular myocytes. *J Physiol* 443:629–650, 1991.

27. Rogart RB, Cribbs LL, Muglia LK, Kaiser MW, Kephart DD: Molecular cloning of a putative tetrodotoxin-resistant rat heart Na channel isoform. *Proc Natl Acad Sci USA* 86:8170–8174, 1989.

28. Backx PH, Yue DT, Lawrence JH, Marban E, Tamaselli GF: Molecular localization of an ion-binding site within the pore of mammalian sodium channels. *Science* 257:248–251, 1992.

29. O'Rourke B, Backx PH, Marban E: Phosphorylation-independent modulation of L-type calcium channels by magnesium-nucleotide complexes. *Science* 257:245–248, 1992.

30. Reuter H: The dependence of slow inward current in Purkinje fibres on the extracellular calcium-concentration. *J Physiol* 192:479–492, 1967.

31. Reuter H: Properties of two inward membrane currents in the heart. *Ann Rev Physiol* 41:413–424, 1979.

32. Kass RS, Krafte DS: Electrophysiology of Ca channels in excitable cells: Channel types, permeation, gating, and modulation. In: Structure and Physiology of the Slow Inward Calcium Channel. New York: Alan R. Liss, 1987.

33. Cranefield PF: Action potentials, afterpotentials, and arrhythmias. *Circ Res* 41:415–423, 1977.

34. Noma A, Yanagihara K, Irisawa H: Inward current of the rabbit sinoatrial node cell. *Pflügers Arch* 372:43–51, 1977.

35. Brown H, DiFrancesco D: Voltage-clamp investigations of membrane currents underlying pace-maker activity in rabbit sino-atrial node. *J Physiol* 308:331–351, 1980.

36. McAllister RE, Noble D, Tsien RW: Reconstruction of the electrical activity of cardiac Purkinje fibres. *J Physiol* 251:1–59, 1975.

37. Beeler GW, Reuter H: Reconstruction of the action potential of ventricular myocardial fibres. *J Physiol* 268: 177–210, 1977.

38. Vitek M, Trautwein W: Slow inward current and action potential in cardiac Purkinje fibres. The effect of Mn ions. *Pflügers Arch* 323:204, 1971.

39. Beeler GW Jr, Reuter H: Membrane calcium current in ventricular myocardial fibres. *J Physiol* 207:191–209, 1970.

40. Rougier O, Vassort G, Garnier D, Gargouil YM, Coraboeuf E: Existence and role of a slow inward current during the frog atrial action potential. *Pflügers Arch* 308:91–110, 1969.

41. New W, Trautwein W: Inward membrane currents in mammalian myocardium. *Pflügers Arch* 334:1–23, 1972.

42. Armstrong CM: Ionic pores, gates and gating currents. *Q Rev Biophys* 7:179–210, 1975.

43. Isenberg G, Klockner U: Glycocalyx is not required for slow inward calcium current in isolated rat heart myocytes. *Nature (Lond)* 284:358–360, 1980.

44. Hume JR, Giles W: Active and passive electrical properties of single bullfrog atrial cells. *J Gen Physiol* 78:19–42, 1981.

45. Lee KS, Lee EW, Tsien RW: Slow inward current carried by Ca^{2+} or Ba^{2+} in single isolated heart cells. *Biophys J* 33:143, 1981.

46. Lee KS, Tsien RW: Reversal of current through calcium channels in dialyzed single heart cells. *Nature (Lond)* 297:498–501, 1982.

47. Hess P: Calcium channels in vertebrate cells. *Ann Rev Neurosci* 13:337–356, 1990.

48. Bean BP: Classes of calcium channels in vertebrate cells. *Annu Rev Physiol* 51:367–384, 1989.

49. Pelzer D, Pelzer S, McDonald TF: Properties and regulation of calcium channels in muscle cells. *Rev Physiol Biochem Pharmacol* 114:108–207, 1990.

50. Glossmann H, Striessnig J: Molecular properties of calcium channels. *Rev Physiol Biochem Pharmacol* 114:1–105, 1990.

51. Janis RA, Triggle DJ: The Calcium Channel: Its Properties Function, Regulation and Clinical Relevance. CRC Press, Cleveland, 1990.

52. Hosey MM, Lazdunski M: Calcium channels: Molecular pharmacology, structure and regulation. *J Membr Biol* 104:81–105, 1988.

53. Borsotto M, Barhanin J, Norman RI, Lazdunski M: Purification of the dihydropyridine receptor of the voltage-

dependent calcium channel from skeletal muscle transverse tubule using (+)[^{3}H]PN200-110. *Biochem Biophys Res Commun* 122:1357–1366, 1984.

54. Curtis BM, Catterall WA: Purification of the calcium antagonist receptor of the voltage-sensitive calcium channel from skeletal muscle transverse tubules. *Biochemistry* 23:2113–2118, 1984.

55. Glossmann H, Striessnig J: Calcium channels. *Vitam Horm* 44:155–328, 1988.

56. Vaghy PL, Striessnig J, Miwa K, Knaus HG, Itagaki K, McKenna E, Glossmann H, Schwartz A: Identification of a novel 1,4-dihydropyridine and phenyl-alkylamine-binding polypeptide in calcium channel preparations. *J Biol Chem* 262:14337–14342, 1987.

57. Takahashi M, Seagar MJ, Jones JF, Reber BF, Catterall WA: Subunit structure of dihydropyridine-sensitive calcium channels from skeletal muscle. *Proceedings of the National Academy of Sciences of the United States of America* 84(15): 5478–5482, 1987.

58. Catterall WA, Seagar MJ, Takahashi M, Nunoki K: Molecular properties of voltage-sensitive calcium channels. *Advances in Experimental Medicine & Biology* 255:101–109, 1989.

59. Catterall WA: Structure and function of voltage-sensitive ion channels. *Science* 242:50–60, 1988.

60. Flockerzi V, Oeken HJ, Hofmann F, Pelzer D, Cavalie A, Trautwein W: Purified dihydropyridine-binding site from skeletal muscle T-tubules is a functional calcium channel. *Nature* 323:66–68, 1986.

61. Tanabe T, Takeshima H, Mikami A, Flockerzi V, Takahashi H, Kangawa K, Kojima M, Matsuo H, Hiose T, Numa S: Primary structure of the receptor for calcium channel blockers from skeletal muscle. *Nature* 328:313–318, 1987.

62. Mikami A, Imoto K, Tanabe T, Niidome T, Mori Y, Takeshima H, Narumiya S, Numa S: Primary structure and functional expression of the cardiac dihydropyridine-sensitive calcium channel. *Nature* 340:230–233, 1989.

63. Bean BP: Nitrendipine block of cardiac calcium channels: High-affinity binding to the inactivated state. *Proc Natl Acad Sci USA* 81:6388–6392, 1984.

64. Sanguinetti MC, Kass RS: Voltage-dependent block of calcium channel current in the calf cardiac Purkinje fiber by dihydropyridine calcium channel antagonists. *Circ Res* 55:336–348, 1984.

65. Hess, P, Lansman JB, Tsien RW: Different modes of gating behaviour favoured by dihydropyridine agonists and antagonists. *Nature* 311:538–544, 1984.

66. Pietrobon D, Hess P: Novel mechanism of voltage-dependent gating in L-type calcium channels. *Nature* 346:651, 1990.

67. Artalejo CR, Ariano MA, Perlman RL, Fox AP: Activation of facilitation calcium channels in chromaffin cells by D1 dopamine receptors through a cAMP/protein kinase A-dependent mechanism. *Nature* 348:239–242, 1990.

68. Flockerzi V, Oeken HJ, Hofmann F: Purification of a functional receptor for calcium channel blockers for rabbit skeletal muscle microsomes. *Eur J Biochem* 161:217–224, 1986.

69. Tsien RW, Hess P, McCleskey EW, Rosenberg RL: Calcium channels: Mechanisms of selectivity, permeation, and block. *Annu Rev Biophy Biophy Chem* 16:265–290, 1987.

70. Prod'hom B, Pietrobon P, Hess P: Direct measurement of proton transfer rates to a group controlling the dihydropyridine-sensitive Ca^{2+} channel. *Nature* 329:243–246, 1987.

71. Kass RS, Sanguinetti MC: Calcium channel inactivation in the cardiac Purkinje fiber. Evidence for voltage- and

72. Yue DT, Backx PH, Imredy JP: Calcium-sensitive inactivation in the gating of single calcium channels. *Science* 21:1735–1738, 1990.

73. Giles W, Noble SJ: Changes in membrane currents in bullfrog atrium produced by acetylcholine. *J Physiol* 261:103–123, 1976.

74. Ten Eick R, Nawrath H, McDonald TF, Trautwein W: On the mechanism of the negative inotropic effect of acetylcholine. *Pflügers Arch* 361:207–213, 1976.

75. Kass RS, Weigers SE: The ionic basis of concentration-related effects of noradrenaline on the action potential of calf cardiac Purkinje fibres. *J Physiol* 322:541–558, 1982.

76. Reuter H, Scholz H: The regulation of Ca conductance of cardiac muscle by adrenaline. *J Physiol* 264:49–62, 1977.

77. Noble D, Tsien RW: Outward membrane currents activated in the plateau range of potentials in cardiac Purkinje fibres. *J Physiol (Lond)* 200:205–231, 1969.

78. Sanguinetti MC, Jurkiewicz NK: Two components of cardiac delayed rectifier K$^+$ current. *J Gen Physiol* 96:195–215, 1990.

79. Hall AE, Hutter OF, Noble D: Current-voltage relations of Purkinje fibres in sodium deficient solutions. *J Physiol (Lond)* 166:225–240, 1963.

80. Noma A: ATP-regulated K$^+$ channels in cardiac muscle. *Nature* 305:147–148, 1983.

81. Noma A, Shibasaki T: Membrane current through adenosinetriphosphate-regulated potassium channels in guinea-pig ventricular cells. *J Physiol (Lond)* 363:463–480, 1985.

82. Trube G, Hescheler J: Inward-rectifying channels in isolated patches of the heart cell membrane: ATP-dependence and comparison with cell-attached patches. *Pflügers Arch* 401:178–184, 1984.

83. Siegelbaum SA, Tsien RW: Calcium-activated transient outward current in calf Purkinje fibers. *J Physiol (Lond)* 299:485–506, 1980.

84. Giles WR, Van Ginneken ACG: A transient outward current in isolated cells from the crista terminalis of rabbit heart. *J Physiol (Lond)* 368:243–264, 1985.

85. Kenyon JL, Sutko JL: Calcium and voltage-activated plateau currents of cardiac Purkinje fibers. *J Gen Physiol* 89:921–958, 1987.

86. Tseng G, Hoffman BF: Two components of transient outward current in canine ventricular myocytes. *Circ Res* 64:633–647, 1989.

87. Carmeliet E, Mubagwa K: Changes by acetylcholine of membrane currents in rabbit cardiac Purkinje fibres. *J Physiol* 371:201–217, 1986.

88. Kameyama M, Kakei M, Sato R, Shibasaki T, Matsuda H, Irisawa H: Intracellular Na$^+$ activates a K$^+$ channel in mammalian cardiac cells. *Nature* 309:354–356, 1984.

89. McDonald TF, Trautwein W: Membrane currents in cat myocardium: Separation of inward and outward components. *J Physiol (Lond)* 274:193–216, 1978.

90. Meier CF Jr, Katzung BG: Cesium blockade of delayed outward currents and electrically induced pacemaker activity in mammalian ventricular myocardium. *J Gen Physiol* 77:531–547, 1981.

91. Sanguinetti MC, Jurkiewicz NK: Delayed rectifier outward K current is composed of two currents in guinea pig atrial cells. *Am J Physiol* 260:H393–H399, 1991.

92. Kenyon JL, Gibbons WR: 4-aminopyridine and the early outward current of sheep cardiac Purkinje fibers. *J Gen Physiol* 73:139–157, 1979.

93. Marban E: Inhibition of transient outward current by intracellular ion substitution unmasks slow inward current in

cardiac Purkinje fibers. *Pflügers Arch* 390:102–106, 1981.

94. Balser JR, Bennett PB, Roden DM: Time-dependent outward current in guinea pig ventricular myocytes. Gating kinetics of the delayed rectifier. *J Gen Physiol* 96:835–863, 1990.

95. Walsh KB, Arena JP, Kwok WM, Freeman L, Kass RS: Delayed-rectifier potassium channel activity in isolated membrane patches of guinea pig ventricular myocytes. *Am J Physiol* 260:H1390–H1393, 1991.

96. Noma A, Irisawa H: A time and voltage-dependent potassium current in the rabbit sinoatrial node cell. *Pflügers Arch* 366:251–258, 1976.

97. DiFrancesco D, Noma A, Trautwein W: Kinetics and magnitude of the time-dependent potassiuim current in the rabbit sinoatrial node. *Pflügers Arch* 381:271–279, 1979.

98. Kokubun S, Nishimura M, Noma A, Irisawa H: Membrane currents in the rabbit atrioventricular node cell. *Pflügers Arch* 393:15–22, 1982.

99. Shibasaki T: Conductance and kinetics of delayed rectifier potassium channels in nodal cells of the rabbit heart. *J Physiol* 387:227–250, 1987.

100. Walsh KB, Kass RS: Distinct voltage-dependent regulation of a heart delayed IK by protein kinases A and C. *Am J Physiol (Cell)* 261:C1081–C1090, 1991.

101. Anumonwo JMB, Freeman LC, Kwok WM, Kass RS: Delayed rectification in single cells isolated from guinea pig sino-atrial node. *Am J Physiol (Heart Circ)* 262:H921–H925, 1992.

102. Tsien RW, Giles W, Greengard P: Cyclic AMP mediates the effects of adrenaline on cardiac Purkinje fibers. *Nature* 240:181–183, 1972.

103. Duchatelle-Gourdon I, Hartzell HC, Lagrutta AA: Modulation of the delayed rectifier potassium current in frog cardiomyocytes by β-adrenergic agonists and magnesium. *J Physiol (Lond)* 415:251–274, 1989

104. Harvey RD, Hume JR: Autonomic regulation of delayed rectifier K$^+$ current in mammalian heart involves G proteins. *Am J Physiol* 257 (Heart Circ Physiol 26):H818–H823, 1989.

105. Yazawa K, Kameyama M: Mechanism of receptor-mediated modulation of the delayed outward potassium current in guinea-pig ventricular myocytes. *J Physiol* 421:135–150, 1990.

106. Toshe N: Calcium-sensitive delayed rectifier potassium current in guinea pig ventricular cells. *Am J Physiol* 258: H1200–H1207, 1990.

107. Toshe N, Kameyama M, Irisawa H: Intracellular Ca and PKC modulate K current in guinea pig heart cells. *Am J Physiol* 253:H1321–H1324, 1987.

108. Walsh KB, Kass RS: Regulation of a heart potassium channel by protein kinase A and C. *Science* 242:67–69, 1988.

109. Weidmann S: Effect of current flow on the membrane potential of cardiac muscle. *J Physiol* 115:227–236, 1951.

110. McAllister RE, Noble D: The time and voltage dependence of the slow outward current in cardiac Purkinje fibres. *J Physiol* 186:632–662, 1966.

111. Sakmann B, Trube G: Conductance properties of single inwardly rectifying potassium channels in ventricular cells from guinea-pig heart. *J Physiol (Lond)* 347:641–657, 1984.

112. Vandenberg CA: Inward rectification of a potassium channel in cardiac ventricular cells depends on internal magnesium ions. *Proc Natl Acad Sci USA* 84:2560–2564, 1987.

113. Armstrong CM: Inactivation of the potassium conductance and related phenomena caused by quaternary ammonium

ion injection in squid axons. *J Gen Physiol* 54:553–575, 1969.

114. Matsuda H, Saigusa A, Irisawa H: Ohmic conductance through the inwardly rectifying K channel and blocking by internal Mg^{2+}. *Nature* 325:156–158, 1987.

115. Dudel J, Peper K, Rudel R, Trautwein W: The dynamic chloride component of membrane current in Purkinje fibers. *Pflügers Arch* 295:197–212, 1967.

116. Fozzard HA, Hiraoka M: The positive dynamic current and its inactivation properties in cardiac Purkinje fibers. *J Physiol (Lond)* 234:569–586, 1973.

117. Kenyon JL, Gibbons WR: Influence of chloride, potassium, and tetraethylammonium on the early outward current of sheep cardiac Purkinje fibers. *J Gen Physiol* 73:117–138, 1979.

118. Kass RS, Scheuer T, Malloy KJ: Block of outward current in cardiac Purkinje fibers by injection of quaternary ammonium ions. *J Gen Physiol* 79:1041–1063, 1982.

119. Marban E, Tsien RW: Effects of nystatin-mediated intracellular ion substitution on membrane currents in calf Purkinje fibres. *J Physiol*, 1982.

120. DiFrancesco D: A new interpretation of the pacemaker current IK2 in Purkinje fibers. *J Physiol* 314:359–376, 1981.

121. Coraboeuf E, Carmeliet E: Existence of two transient outward currents in sheep cardiac Purkinje fibers. *Pflügers Arch* 392:352–359, 1982.

122. Hiraoka M, Kawano S: Calcium-sensitive and insensitive transient outward current in rabbit ventricular myocytes. *J Physiol* 410:187–214, 1989.

123. Hiraoka M, Kawano S: Mechanism of increased amplitude and duration of the pateau with sudden shortening of diastolic intervals in rabbit ventricular cells. *Circ Res* 60:14–26, 1987.

124. McDonald TF, Pelzer D, Trautwein W: On the mechanism of slow calcium channel block in heart. *Pflügers Arch* 385:175–179, 1980.

125. Dukes ID, Morad M: Tedisamil inactivates transient outward K$^+$ current in rat ventricular myocytes. *Am J Physiol* H1746–H1749, 1989.

126. Litovsky SH, Antzelevitch C: Differences in the electrophysiological response of canine ventricular subendocardium and subepicardium to acetylcholine and isoprotererol. *Circulation Research* 67(3):615–627, 1990.

127. Siegelbaum SA, Tsien RW, Kass RS: Role of intracellular calcium in the transient outward current of calf Purkinje fibers. *Nature* 269:611–613, 1977.

128. Kass RS, Tsien RW: Multiple effects of calcium antagonists on plateau currents in cardiac Purkinje fibers. *J Gen Physiol* 66:169–192, 1975.

129. Kass RS: Nisoldipine: A new, more selective calcium current blocker in cardiac Purkinje fibers. *J Pharmacol Exp Ther* 223:446–456, 1982.

130. Kass RS: Delayed rectification in the cardiac Purkinje fiber is not activated by intracellular calcium. *Biophys J* 45:837–839, 1984.

131. Takumi T, Ohkubo H, Nakanishi S: Cloning of a membrane protein that induces a slow voltage-gated potassium current. *Science* 242:1042–1045, 1988.

132. Krafte DS, Dugrenier N, Dillon K, Volberg WA: Electrophysiological properties of a cloned, human potassium channel expressed in Xenopus oocytes. *Biophys J* 61:A378, 1992.

133. Pragnell M, Snay KJ, Trimmer JS, MacLusky NJ, Naftolin F, Kaczmarek LK, Boyle MB: Estrogen induction of a small, putative K channel mRNA in rat uterus. *Neuron* 4(5):807–812, 1990.

134. Murai T, Kakaizuka A, Takumi T, Ohkubo H, Nakanishi,

S: Molecular cloning and sequence analysis of human genomic DNA encoding a novel membrane protein which exhibits a slowly activating potassium channel activity. *Biochem Biophys Res Commun 161(1)*:176–181, 1989.

135. Folander K, Smith JS, Antanavage J, Bennett C, Stein RB, Swanson R: Cloning and expression of the delayed-rectifier IsK channel from neonatal rat heart and diethylstilbestrol-primed rat uterus. *PNAS 87(8)*:2975–2979, 1990

136. Honore E, Attali B, Romey G, Heurteaux C, Ricard P, Lesage F, Lazdunski M, Barhanin J: Cloning, expression, pharmacology, and regulation of a delayed rectifier K channel in mouse heart. *EMBO Journal 10(10)*:2805–2811, 1991

CHAPTER 5

Molecular Structure of the Cardiac Calcium Channel

VEIT FLOCKERZI & FRANZ HOFMANN

INTRODUCTION

Voltage-activated calcium channels are membrane-spanning proteins that allow the controlled entry of calcium ions into the cytoplasm of cells and thereby contribute to the genesis of the action potentials {54,62,73}. By raising $[Ca]_i$, calcium channels transduce electrical signals to chemical signals that command changes in secretion, metabolism, contraction, or excitability when decoded by appropriate calcium receptor proteins, such as synaptotagmin, calmodulin, troponin, and calcium-activated potassium channels {8,9,27}. Voltage-activated calcium channels are vital for several processes of the cardiovascular system. In the healthy heart they are essential for generation of normal cardiac rhythm, for induction of propagation through the atrioventricular node, and for contraction in atrial and ventricular muscle. In diseased myocardium, calcium channels can contribute to abnormal impulse generation and cardiac arrhythmias. In blood vessels they provide a direct supply of activating calcium, which controls smooth muscle contraction and vascular tone.

VOLTAGE-ACTIVATED CALCIUM CHANNELS IN MYOCARDIUM

In myocardium at least two types of voltage-activated calcium channels have been distinguished on the basis of their voltage and time dependence, conductance, and pharmacology; namely, slow or L-type (for long lasting) and fast or T-type channels (for tiny or transient; table 5-1) {3,24,44}.

T-type channels

T-type channels are predominantly localized within atrial cells. They contribute to the inward current only if cells are held at negative potentials, are opened at relatively small depolarization steps, and inactivate within tens of milliseconds. Atrial cells also contain L-type channels, which carry a substantial larger amount of ions than T channels, especially at the positive potentials that an atrial action potential quickly reaches. Therefore it is not clear whether the existence of the fast calcium channels has some special significance for the function of atrial cells. They would be useful in cells capable of spontaneous activity lacking functional sodium channels, like the cardiac pacemaker cells of the sinoatrial node, since they will be activated at relatively negative potentials and will help to depolarize the cell. The low threshold of the fast channels could also make them especially useful for the propagation of the atrioventricular calcium action potential. There are no specific blockers of T-type calcium channels available. Ni^{2+} has some selectivity for T channels compared with Cd^{2+}, whereas Cd^{2+} is more potent at L channels. Several agents may block T channels at micromolar concentrations (table 5-1) {1,37,67}. However, the selectivity of the effects of these drugs have still to be defined in regard to their similar actions on L-type calcium channels and sodium channels. The lack of high-affinity probes has hindered the pharmacological characterization and any structural definition of T-type calcium channels so far.

L-type calcium channels

L-type calcium channels are found in all excitable cells and are virtually ubiquitous within the myocardium {54,62,73}. They are the major pathways for voltage-gated calcium entry in heart. The L-type channel is high-voltage activated and has a high calcium conductance, contributing to a long-lasting current (table 5-1). It is highly sensitive to calcium channel blockers such as nifedipine, a dihydropyridine (dhp); verapamil, a phenyl-alkylamine (paa); and diltiazem. Dihydropyridines, for example, readily block the channel at concentrations below $10^{-6}\,M$.

SUBUNIT STRUCTURE OF THE L-TYPE CALCIUM CHANNEL

L-type voltage-activated calcium channels are present in high concentration in the transverse tubules of vertebrate skeletal muscle. Their high density has enabled purification of these calcium channels using high-affinity bound dhp calcium channel blockers as a specific label {12,20}. The purified channel complex has served as a model for

N. Sperelakis (ed.), Physiology and Pathophysiology of the Heart, Third Edition.

Table 5-1. Voltage-activated calcium channels in heart

	L	T
Properties		
Conductance	20–25 pS[1]	7–8 pS[1]
Activation	High voltage	Low voltage
Inactivation	Slow	Fast
Location	Atrial and ventricular cells	Atrial ≫ ventricular cells
Function	AP plateau ec coupling	(pacemaker)
Block	$Cd^{2+} > Ni^{2+}$ Phenylalkylamines Dihydropyridines Diltiazem	$Ni^{2+} > Cd^{2+}$ (flunarizine)[2] (niguldipine) (zonisamide) (tetrandine) (penfluridol)
Structure subunit (gene)	Hetero-oligomer α_1 (α_{1Ca}) α_2/δ (a_2/δ_a) β (B_2 and B_3)	Not determined

[1] 110 mM Ba^{2+} as charge carrier.
[2] None of these compounds is a high-affinity specific inhibitor of T-type channels.

structure-function studies. The L-type calcium channel from skeletal muscle is a complex of four proteins: the α_1 subunit (212,018 Da), which contains the binding sites for all known calcium channel blockers and the calcium conducting pore; the intracellularly located β subunit (57,868 Da); the transmembrane γ subunit (25,058 Da); and the α_2/δ subunit, a disulfide linked dimer of 125,018 Da {see 10,21,28 and references cited therein}. Reconstitution of the purified complex into phospholipid bilayers results in functional calcium channels that are reversibly blocked by calcium channel blockers and are modulated by cAMP-

dependent phosphorylation {19,30,41}. Complementary DNAs for the skeletal muscle calcium channel were isolated on the basis of peptide sequences derived from the purified proteins {6,18,31,57,68}. Using these cDNAs as probes, distinct gene products encoding α_1 and β subunits have been cloned from heart, smooth muscle, kidney, fibroblasts, endocrine, and neuronal cells. In contrast, the γ subunit appears to be expressed exclusively in skeletal muscle. The α_2/δ subunit is highly conserved in most tissues, including brain, and cardiac and smooth muscle, indicating that calcium channels in these tissues are heterooligomers formed from a common α_2/δ and different α_1 and β subunits (table 5-1).

ION-CONDUCTING PORE OF CALCIUM CHANNELS

The α_1 subunit is the ion-conducting pore of calcium channels, and complete cDNA clones of α_1 subunits have been isolated from a variety of tissues {22,38,40,43,49,58, 60,61,63,79,80,82}, including heart {5,17,39} and smooth muscle {4,35}, on the basis of sequence homology with their skeletal muscle counterpart. These cDNAs for α_1 subunits are derived from six different genes and encode polypeptides of predicted molecular masses of 212–273 kDa, which are structurally similar to voltage-activated sodium channels and are between 41% and 70% homologous. Hydropathicity analysis of all known α_1 subunits predicts four repeats, which are 45–60% homologous (fig. 5-1). Each repeat is composed of five transmembrane α-helices and one amphophilic segment, S4, which contains a positively charged residue at every third position and usually hydrophobic residues at the remaining positions. Two short amino acid sequences located between S5 and S6, called SS1 and SS2, may span part of the membrane. The positively charged S4 segment has been postulated to act as the voltage-sensing device

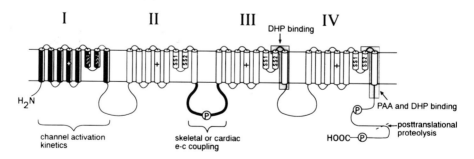

Fig. 5-1. Proposed transmembrane topology and structural features of the α_1 subunit of high-voltage activated calcium channels. The overall structure of all known calcium channel α_1 subunit cDNAs is taken from the hydropathicity analysis of the primary sequences and includes four homologous repeats (I, II, III, IV) containing six membrane-spanning regions. + = proposed transmembrane amphophilic segment (S)4, which is thought to be the voltage-sensing device of the channel. P = sites phosphorylated in vitro by cAMP kinase within the skeletal muscle α_1; the SS1–SS2 region suggested to be part of the channel pore is shown by the short barrels; DHP and PAA = dihydropyridine and phenylalkylamine binding sites; e-c coupling = excitation contraction coupling. The brackets indicate parts of the protein that are responsible for the skeletal (α_{1S}) or cardiac (α_{2C}) properties of the channel. The dash at the carboxy-terminal part indicates the area where the skeletal muscle α_1 subunit is processed post-translationally. The extracellular space is above the horizontal lines.

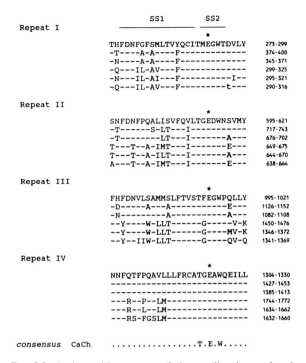

Fig. 5-2. Amino acid sequence of the predicted pore-forming region of the calcium channel. Alignment of the amino-acid sequences in the regions encompassing the SS1–SS2 segment of the four repeats of the different calcium channels. The glutamic acid residues (*) that occur at equivalent positions in the four repeats of all calcium channels but not in sodium or potassium channels are thought to be critical in determining the ion selectivity of the calcium channel and constitute part of the channel's selectivity filter. Replacing amino acid residues at equivalent positions in sodium channels by glutamic acid alters ion-selection properties of the sodium channel to resemble those of calcium channels {26}. The sequences are as follows: α_{1S}, skeletal muscle L type {68}; α_{1C}, cardiac and smooth muscle L-type {4,39}; α_{1D}, neuroendocrine L type {79}; α_{1A}, P type {40}; α_{1B}, N type {80}; α_{1E} {43}. Each of the six rows, in the four repeats, are respectively, from top to bottom: α_{1S}, α_{1C}, α_{1D}, α_{1A}, α_{1B}, and α_{1E}.

responsible for channel activation. It is thought that S4 responds to a change in the membrane potential with a slight shift of its positive charges and thereby induces a conformational change in the protein, which leads to channel opening {23}. This idea is supported by several mutagenesis experiments in sodium and potassium channels, where changing positively charged residues to noncharged residues alters the voltage dependency and/or shifts the voltage range of channel activation {47,66}. The SS1-SS2 region is predicted to form part of the channel pore {23}. The glutamic acid residues, which occur at equivalent positions in SS2 of the four repeats of all calcium channels (fig. 5-2) but not in sodium and potassium channels, seem to be critical in determining the ion selectivity of the calcium channel and constitute part of the channel's selectivity filter. Introducing glutamic acid residues at the respective positions in repeats III and IV of

a sodium channel alters ion-selection properties of the sodium channel to resemble those of calcium channels {26}.

By functional expression of chimeras of the skeletal and cardiac muscle, α_1-subunit-specific properties of the calcium channel were assigned to distinct parts of the ion conducting pore: Repeat I determines the activation time of the chimeric channel, i.e., slow activation upon membrane depolarization with the repeat from skeletal muscle and rapid activation with that from cardiac muscle {72} (fig. 5-1); the putative cytoplasmic loop between repeats II and III determines the type of excitation-contraction coupling (fig. 5-1). The loop from the skeletal muscle calcium channel α_1 subunit induces contraction in the absence of calcium influx, whereas the loop from the cardiac calcium channel α_1 subunit induces contraction only in the presence of calcium influx {70}.

Receptor sites for dihydropyridines and phenylalkylamines

The receptor sites for calcium channel blockers on the α_1 subunit of the skeletal muscle calcium channel can be covalently labeled with several dhps and the paa ludopamil. Proteolytic digestion of the skeletal muscle α_1 subunit photoaffinity labeled with dhp and ludopamil, and isolation of the labeled peptide fragments, either directly by reversed-phase hplc {53} or by mapping with antipeptide antibodies {42,64,65}, localizes portions of the dhp- and paa-binding sites to the sixth transmembrane helices of repeat III and IV, and their extracellular and intracellular ends (fig. 5-3) {42,64,65}. Another portion of the dhp side resides intracellularly adjacent to IVS6 (fig. 5-2) {53}. The photolabeling results suggest that transmembrane segments IIIS6 and IVS6 may be in close contact in the folded structure of the α_1 subunit and contribute to formation of the dhp receptor site. An allosteric interaction of the dhp and paa receptor sites has been infered from in vitro ligand binding studies and segment IVS6, which also forms part of the paa receptor site, might structurally link the two binding domains. Comparison of the amino acid sequences of different calcium channel α_1 subunits in the regions that are convalently labeled by dhp and paa indicates that especially IIIS6 and IVS6 and the following intracellular sequence is highly conserved among L-type calcium channels from skeletal muscle (CaCh1), cardiac and smooth muscle (CaCh2), and neural and endocrine tissues (CaCh3, fig. 5-3). Binding studies with radiolabelled DHPs demonstrate that the stably expressed α_1 subunits from skeletal, smooth, and cardiac muscle alone contain the allosterically coupled binding sites for the known calcium channel blockers {7,34}.

Various types of high-voltage activated calcium channels are formed from different α_1 subunits

L-type calcium channels contain α_1 subunits, which are encoded by the first, second, and third α_1 gene (CaCh1, CaCh2, and CaCh3). The product of the CaCh1 gene occurs in skeletal muscle in two isoforms: a minor form

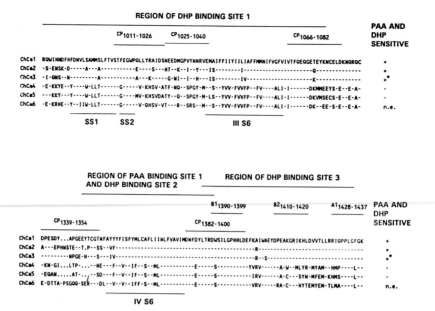

Fig. 5-3. Receptor sites for calcium channel blockers. Amino acid sequence comparisons in the dihydropyridine (DHP) and phenylalkylamine (PAA) binding regions of the α_1 subunit of voltage-activated calcium channels. Proteolytic digestion of the skeletal muscle α_1 subunit photoaffinity labeled with dihydropyridines and phenylalkylamines, and isolation of the labeled peptide fragments, either directly by reversed-phase hplc (peptides B1$_{1390-1399}$, B2$_{1410-1420}$, and A1$_{1428-1437}$) {53} or by mapping with antipeptide antibodies (directed against peptides CP1011–1026, CP1025–1040, CP1066–1082, CP1339–1354, CP1382–1400) {42,64,65} localizes portions of the dihydropyridine- and the phenylalkylamine-binding sites to the transmembrane helices IIIS6 (DHP 1) and IVS6 (PAA 1 and DHP 2), and their extracellular and intracellular ends. Another portion of the DHP site (DHP 3) resides intracellularly adjacent to the transmembrane helix IVS6. Sequence comparison in these regions reveal a high degree of homology among dihydropyridine-sensitive (L-type) Ca^{2+} channel clones from skeletal muscle (CaCh1) {68}, heart and smooth muscle (CaCh2) {4,39}, and neuroendocrine tissues (CaCh3) {79}. Dihydropyridine-insensitive channels, like P-(CaCh4) {40} and N-type (CaCh5) {80}, as well as B-type (CaCh6) {43} calcium channel clones, however, show significant sequence divergence in residues thought to be responsible for dihydropyridine or phenylalkylamine binding (e.g., peptide fragments B2 and A1). . . . , gap; — identical residues; *, PAA sensitivity has not been measured so far; n.e., not expressed so far.

(approx. 5%) of 212 kDa containing the complete amino acid sequence encoded by the α_1 mRNA, and a major form (approx. 95%) of 190 kDa, which is derived from the full-length product by post translational proteolysis close to amino acid residue 1690 {15} (fig. 5-1). The physiological function of this modification is not known because expression of the truncated form directs the synthesis of calcium channels, which are functionally indistinguishable from those synthesized from the full-length cDNA {2}. The short and long forms are phosphorylated rapidly in vitro by cAMP-dependent protein kinase at Ser$_{687}$ {55}, which is located at the cytosolic loop between repeat II and III, and Ser$_{1854}$ {56}, which is present only in the larger untruncated form.

The α_1 subunits from cardiac (CaCh2a) {39} and smooth muscle (CaCh2b) {5} are splice products of the second gene (CaCh2). A major difference between the two sequences are the different IVS3 segments, which result from alternative splicing of the primary transcript from the CaCh2 gene {49}. Complementary DNA or cRNA from CaCh2a and CaCh2b have been expressed transiently and stably {5,7,59}. No major differences have been observed

in basic electrophysiological and pharmacological properties of the two isoforms, including the amplitude of inward current, steady-state activation and inactivation, and DHP sensitivity {76}. However, Northern blots and PCR analysis shows that both splice variants are differentially expressed in heart and smooth muscle {5}, and during cardiac development {16}. The cDNA of a third gene (CaCh3) was isolated from neural and endocrine tissues, and represents a neuroendocrine-specific L-type calcium channel {58,79}.

The gene products of the fourth, fifth, and sixth gene (CaCh4, CaCh5, and CaCh6) have been found predominantly in brain but may also be expressed in other tissues {82}. Calcium channels transiently expressed from cRNA or cDNA of CaCh4 and CaCh5 induce high-voltage activated calcium currents that are insensitive to nifedipine, indicating that these channels are not of the L type. Channels directed by cRNA from CaCh4 are also insensitive towards ω-conotoxin but are inhibited by a mixture of toxins from the funnel web spider, characterizing this channel as a P-type calcium channel {40}. The gene product of CaCh5 binds and is irreversibly blocked by picomolar concentrations of ω-conotoxin, identifying the CaCh5 protein as a neural N-type calcium channel {17,80}. The CaCh6 gene product {43} encodes or low voltage activated T-type like channel, which is expressed in brain but not in heart.

AUXILIARY CALCIUM CHANNEL SUBUNITS

α_2/δ subunit

The skeletal muscle α_2/δ subunit (CaAl) is a glycosylated membrane protein of 125,018 Da {18} that is apparently highly conserved in most tissues. In the skeletal muscle the primary protein product of the α_2/δ gene is processed post-translationally by proteolysis, resulting in an α_2 protein containing amino acids 1–934 and a δ protein containing the amino acids 935–1080 {14}. The transmembrane δ subunit anchors the extracellularly located α_2 protein by disulfide bridges to the plasma membrane {32}. Immunoblots {45} and Northern blots {5,18} show that similar or identical α_2/δ subunits exist in skeletal muscle, heart, brain, vascular, airways, and intestinal smooth muscle. A splice variant of the skeletal muscle α_2/δ cDNA has been isolated from human and rat brain that encodes an identical δ but slightly different α_2 proteins {33,79}.

β subunit

The skeletal β subunit (CaB1) is an intracellularly located membrane protein consisting of 524 amino acids {57}. Its deduced amino acid sequence contains stretches of heptad repeat structure that are characteristic of cytoskeletal proteins. Differential splicing of the primary transcript of CaB1 results in at least three isoforms: CaB1a through CaB1c {51,52,57,79}. CaB1a is primarily expressed in skeletal muscle, whereas the two other isoforms are most abundant in brain. Transcripts of the CaB1 gene were detected in mRNA from heart and spleen {51}. Two other genes (CaB2 and CaB3) encoding β proteins different from the skeletal muscle β subunit have been isolated from a cardiac cDNA library {29}. Their deduced amino acid sequences show an overall homology to CaB1 of 71% (CaB2) and 66.6% (CaB3). Four different splice variants have been characterized for the CaB2 gene (CaB2a through CaB2d); CaB2a and CaB2b are primarily expressed in heart, whereas CaB2c and CaB2d have been cloned from rabbit and rat brain libraries {29,50}. Like the CaB1 gene, the CaB2 and CaB3 genes are tissue specifically expressed, with transcripts of CaB2 existing abundantly in heart, and to a lesser degree in aorta, trachea, and lung, whereas transcripts of CaB3 genes are expressed in brain and smooth muscle containing tissues such as aorta, trachea, and lung {29}. This suggests that the CaB3 gene product may be expressed predominantly in neuronal and smooth muscle cells.

γ subunit

The γ subunit (CaG1) consists of 222 amino acids and is an integral membrane protein {6,31}. Its deduced amino acid sequence contains four putative transmembrane domains and two glycosylation sites, which are located at the extracellular side. Northern and PCR analysis have not identified the presence of γ subunit in other tissues, suggesting that this protein may be specific for skeletal muscle.

FUNCTIONAL INTERACTION OF THE CALCIUM CHANNEL SUBUNITS

Although the calcium channel is an oligomeric structure, the α_1 subunits alone are able to function autonomously in some respect. Complementary DNAs or the corresponding messenger RNAs derived from CaCh1 and CaCh2 can direct expression of functional L-type calcium channels in *Xenopus* oocytes {4,39} or mammalian cell culture cells {7,38,48,76}. They can also restore both calcium currents and excitation-contraction coupling in myocytes from mice having the muscular dysgenesis mutation, which disrupts the endogenous α_1 gene {69,71}. Transient expression in *Xenopus* oocytes of CaCh2a {39,59,75} and CaCh2b cRNA {4} induced dhp-sensitive currents with electrophysiological properties similar to those reported from cardiac and smooth muscle. Heterologous coexpression of the cardiac α_1 subunit, together with the skeletal muscle β subunit and α_2/δ subunit, enhanced consistently the inward current to amplitudes greater than 1 μA/oocyte {59}. The α_2/δ or the β subunit alone or the combination of both decreased the activation time of the barium current twofold {59,75}. Oocytes containing all four subunits (α_1, α_2/δ, β, and γ subunits) had fast inactivating barium currents. The coexpression of the γ subunit shifted the steady-state inactivation of I_{Ba} by 40 mV to negative membrane potentials {59}. Under each condition inward currents were increased severalfold by the calcium channel agonist BayK8644. Homologous coexpression of the cardiac α_1 subunit with the cardiac β (CaB2) or the neuronal/smooth muscle β subunit (CaB3) with or without the α_2/δ subunit results in an increase in the amplitude of I_{Ba} as well as in an acceleration of channel activation {29}.

Similar effects of the subunits were obtained by stable coexpression of the skeletal muscle α_1 and β subunit in mouse fibroblasts (L cells), which do not contain endogenous calcium channels. The β subunit decreased the activation time of the expressed channel over 50-fold, and increased the number of DHP binding sites twofold {36}. In contrast to these results, it has been reported that coexpression of all four subunits in L cells resulted in a decreased amplitude of the barium current and in a diminished response toward the calcium channel agonist BayK 8644 {74}. This phenomenon has not been observed with other L-type calcium channels expressed in *Xenopus* oocytes or CHO cells.

The smooth muscle α_1 (CaCh2b) subunit induces barium currents in CHO cells, which are identical to those of native smooth muscle: The single channel conductance was 26 pS in the presence of 80 mM Ba^{2+}, the open probability increased with membrane depolarization, and the voltage dependence of activation and inactivation was similar to that of the native smooth muscle channel {7}.

Stable expression of the CaCh2b with the skeletal muscle β gene (CaB1) increased in parallel the number of DHP binding sites and the amplitude of whole-cell barium current, suggesting that the amplitude of the inward current is directly related to the number of expressed α_1 protein molecules {77}. In addition, the coexpression of the β subunit decreased the channel activation time twofold and shifted the voltage dependence of steady-state inactivation by 18 mV to −13 mV. The expression of the cardiac α_1 subunit (CaCh2a) in the same cells induces currents that are indistinguishable from that induced by the smooth muscle α_1 subunit. The only difference noted was a faster inactivation of the cardiac channel. This electrophysiological similarity is not surprising, since the primary sequence of both channels is 95% identical {4}. In contrast to the CaCh1 and CaC2 gene products, α_1 subunits derived from the neuroendocrine L-type CaCh3 gene, the neuronal P-type CaCh4 gene, and the neuronal N-Type CaCh5 gene induce barium currents only when coexpressed with the α_2/δ and β subunit {40,79,80}. The increase in current occurred always in the presence of the β subunit, most likely by an increased number of plasmalemmal calcium channel molecules. Overall these results show decisively that efficient expression of calcium channels with normal physiological properties is greatly enhanced by coexpression of α_2/δ and β subunits, and that each of these subunits can interact directly with the α_1 subunit to increase expression or restore some aspect of normal channel function. These findings imply that a three-subunit oligomer ($\alpha_1\alpha_2/\delta\beta$) is the physiologically functional calcium channel in most tissues (fig. 5-4). The only exception known so far is the calcium channel from skeletal muscle, where a fourth subunit, the γ subunit, might be necessary to shift the inactivation of the channel at the required membrane potential.

HORMONAL REGULATION OF THE CARDIAC CALCIUM CHANNEL

Activation of the L-type calcium channel is voltage dependent, yet the response to changes in the membrane potential is modulated by hormones. The beta-adrenergic receptor agonist isoproterenol increases the cardiac calcium current three- to sevenfold, either by cAMP-dependent phosphorylation of the channel {25,46}, or by the activated α subunits of the trimeric GTP binding protein G_s {81}, or a combination of the activated α subunits of the trimeric GTP binding protein G_s and the active cAMP kinase {11}. The L-type calcium current of isolated tracheal smooth muscle cells is also stimulated by activation of the beta-adrenergic receptor {78}. This beta-adrenergic receptor effect is mediated directly by a G protein and not by cAMP-kinase activation. These results suggest that the CaCh2 gene product may be regulated in vivo by the α subunit of a G protein and by cAMP-dependent phosphorylation. The primary sequences of cardiac and smooth muscle α_1 subunits are almost identical and contain identical phosphorylation sites. It is therefore conceivable that the cAMP-dependent stimulation of the cardiac cal-

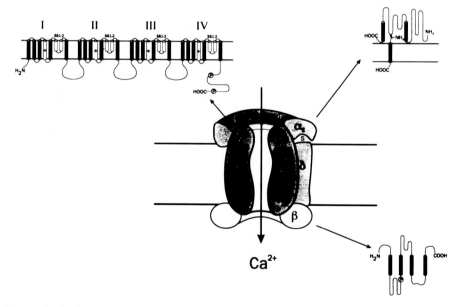

Fig. 5-4. Proposed subunit structure of the cardiac calcium channel. The cardiac L-type calcium channel is a three-subunit oligomer ($\alpha_1\alpha_2/\delta\beta$). The putative membrane configuration of individual subunits is taken from the hydropathicity analysis of the primary sequences. I, II, II, IV, repeats α_1 subunit; + = proposed transmembrane amphophilic segment (S)4; SS1-SS2 = predicted pore-forming region; (P) = predicted phosphorylation sites for cAMP kinase; s = disulfide bridge between the transmembrane δ and the extracellular located α_2 subunit. The extracellular space is above the horizontal lines.

cium channel depends not solely on the phosphorylation of the α_1 subunit but also on the tissue-specific coexpression of other proteins. The deduced amino acid sequence of the skeletal muscle β subunit (CaB1) contains several phosphorylation sites. Two of these sites, Ser_{182} and Thr_{205}, are phosphorylated in vitro by cAMP-dependent protein kinase {13,57}. The equivalent to Thr_{205} is conserved in the "cardiac" β subunit (Thr-165 in CaB2a and Thr-191 in CaB2b) but is not present in the "smooth muscle" β subunit CaB3. The sequence following this potential phosphorylation site is highly variable and determines several splice variants {29}. This variable region within β subunits may be responsible for the tissue-specific regulation of the L-type calcium currents by hormones and neurotransmitters.

VIEW IN PERSPECTIVE

High-voltage activated calcium channels are hetero-oligomers, and their tissue- and cell-specific functions depend on the α_2 subunit coexpressed with specific α_2/δ-, β-, and γ-like subunits. So far six distinct genes encoding α_1 subunits, three genes encoding β subunits, and one gene each for α_2/δ and γ have been identified and their cDNAs have been isolated from various tissues. Cardiac L-type calcium channels are oligomeric complexes of three subunits: α_1 (CaCh2a), α_2/δ (CaA1), and β (CaB2). In comparison, smooth muscle calcium channels have a similar composition but are made of different α_1 (CaCh2b) and β subunits (CaB3). L-type calcium currents in both tissues are sensitive towards dhp- and paa-type calcium channel blockers. The main pharmacological activities of these compounds are vasodilation and myocardial depression, and drugs of both classes may be distinguished with respect to the relative extend of these two major activities. Nifedipine, for example, a dhp, is more active at the smooth muscle calcium channel. At drug concentrations that relax smooth muscle the heart is unaffected. This might be due either to the different composition of the smooth and cardiac muscle calcium channels, or the cellular environment, for example, the resting potential, which influences dhp binding to its receptor site and is different in smooth and cardiac muscle cells. The current availability of the cDNAs for the expression of the various calcium channel subunits in cell culture cells, which do not contain endogenous calcium channels themselves and are a constant biological environment, allows further dissection of calcium channel pharmacology and offers a chance for a more refined drug therapy with more specific drugs than those on hand at present.

ACKNOWLEDGMENTS

The results obtained in the authors' laboratory were supported by grants from Deutsche Forschungsgemeinschaft, Thyssen Stiftung, and Fond der Chemie.

REFERENCES

1. Akaike N, Kostyuk PG, Osipchuk YV: Dihydropyridine-sensitive low-threshold calcium channels in isolated rat hypothalamic neurones. *J Physiol* 412:181–195, 1989.
2. Beam KG, Adams BA, Niidome T, Numa S, Tanabe T: Function of a truncated dihydropyridine receptor as both voltage sensor and calcium channel. *Nature* 360:169–171, 1992.
3. Bean BP: Two types of calcium channels in canine atrial cells. *J Gen Physiol* 86:1–30, 1985.
4. Biel M, Ruth P, Bosse E, Hullin R, Stühmer W, et al.: Primary structure and functional expression of a high voltage activated calcium channel from rabbit lung. *FEBS Lett* 269:409–412, 1990.
5. Biel M, Hullin R, Freundner S, Singer D, Dascal N, et al.: Tissue-specific expression of high-voltage-activated dihydropyridine-sensitive L-type calcium channels. *Eur J Biochem* 200:81–88, 1991.
6. Bosse E, Regulla S, Biel M, Ruth P, Meyer HE, et al.: The cDNA and deduced amino acid sequence of the γ subunit of the L-type calcium channel from rabbit skeletal muscle. *FEBS Lett* 267:153–156, 1990.
7. Bosse E, Bottlender R, Kleppisch T, Hescheler J, Welling A, et al.: Stable and functional expression of the calcium channel α_1 subunit from smooth muscle in somatic cell lines. *EMBO J* 11:2033–2038, 1992.
8. Brayden JE, Nelson MT: Regulation of aerterial tone by activation of calcium-dependent potassium channels. *Science* 256:1021–1024, 1992.
9. Brose N, Petrenko AG, Südhof TC, Jahn R: Synaptotagmin: A calcium sensor on the synaptic vesicle surface. *Science* 256:1021–1024, 1992.
10. Catterall WA, Seagar MJ, Takahashi M: Molecular properties of dihydropyridine-sensitive calcium channels in skeletal muscle. *J Biol Chem* 263:3533–3538, 1988.
11. Cavalié A, Allen TJA, Trautwein W: Role of the GTP-binding protein G_s in the β-adrenergic modulation of cardiac Ca channels. *Pflügers Arch* 419:433–443, 1991.
12. Curtis BM, Catterall WA: Purification of the calcium antagonist receptor of the voltage-sensitive calcium channel from skeletal muscle transverse tubules. *Biochemistry* 23:2113–2118, 1984.
13. De Jongh KS, Merrick DK, Catterall WA: Subunits of purified calcium channels: A 212-kDa form of α_1 and partial amino acid sequence of a phosphorylation site of an independent β subunit. *Proc Natl Acad Sci USA* 86:8585–8589, 1989.
14. De Jongh KS, Warner C, Catterall WA: Subunits of purified calcium channels; α_2 and δ are encoded by the same gene. *J Biol Chem* 265:14738–14741, 1990.
15. De Jongh KS, Warner C, Colvin AA, Catterall WA: Characterization of the two size forms of the α_1 subunit of skeletal muscle L-type calcium channels. *Proc Natl Acad Sci USA* 88:10778–10782, 1991.
16. Diebold RJ, Koch WJ, Ellinor PT, Wang J-J, Muthuchamy M, et al.: Mutually exclusive exon splicing of the cardiac calcium channel α_1 subunit gene generates developmentally regulated isoforms in the rat heart. *Proc Natl Acad Sci USA* 89:1497–1501, 1992.
17. Dubel SJ, Starr TVB, Hell J, Ahlijanian MA, Enyeart JJ, et al.: Molecular cloning of the α-1 subunit of an ω-conotoxin-sensitive calcium channel. *Proc Natl Acad Sci USA* 89:5058–5062, 1992.
18. Ellis SB, Williams ME, Ways NR, Brenner R, Sharp AH, et al.: Sequence and expression of mRNAs encoding the α_1 and α_2 subunits of a DHP-sensitive calcium channel. *Science* 241:1661–1664, 1988.

19. Flockerzi V, Oeken HJ, Hofmann F, Pelzer D, Cavalié A, et al.: Purified dihydropyridine-binding site from skeletal muscle t-tubules is a functional calcium channel. *Nature* 323:66–68, 1986.

20. Flockerzi V, Oeken HJ, Hofmann: Purification of a functional receptor for calcium-channel blockers from rabbit skeletal-muscle microsomes. *Eur J Biochem* 161:217–224, 1986.

21. Glossmann H, Striessnig J: Calcium channels. *Vitamin Horm* 44:155–328, 1988.

22. Grabner M, Friedrich K, Knaus HG, Striessnig J, Scheffauer F, et al.: Calcium channels from *Cyprinus carpio* skeletal muscle. *Proc Natl Acad Sci USA* 88:727–731, 1991.

23. Guy HR, Conti F: Pursuing the structure and function of voltage-gated channels. *Top NeuroSci* 13:201–206, 1990.

24. Hagiwara N, Irisawa H, Kameyama M: Contribution of two types of calcium currents to the pacemaker potentials of rabbit sino-atrial node cells. *J Physiol* 395:233–253, 1988.

25. Hartzell HC, Fischmeister R: Direct regulation of cardiac Ca^{2+} channels by G proteins: Neither proven nor necessary? *Top Pharm Sci* 13:380–385, 1992.

26. Heinemann SH, Terlau H, Stühmer W, Imoto K, Numa S: Calcium channel characteristics conferred on the sodium channel by single mutations. *Nature* 356:441–443, 1992.

27. Hille B: Calcium channels. In: *Ionic Channels of Excitable Membranes*, 2nd ed. Sunderland, MAss: Sinauer Associates, 1992, pp 83–114.

28. Hofmann F, Flockerzi V, Nastainczyk W, Ruth P, Schneider T: The molecular structure and regulation of muscular calcium channels. *Curr Top Cell Reg* 31:223–239, 1990.

29. Hullin R, Singer-Lahat D, Freichel M, Biel M, Dascal N, et al.: Calcium channel β subunit heterogeneity: Functional expression of cloned cDNA from heart, aorta and brain. *EMBO J* 11:885–890, 1992.

30. Hymel L, Striessnig J, Glossmann H, Schindler H: Purified skeletal muscle 1,4-dihydropyridine receptor forms phosphorylation-dependent oligomeric calcium channels in planar bilayers. *Proc Natl Acad Sci USA* 85:4290–4294, 1988.

31. Jay SD, Ellis SB, McCue AF, Williams ME, Vedvick TS, et al.: Primary structure of the c subunit of the DHP-sensitive calcium channel from skeletal muscle. *Science* 248:490–492, 1990.

32. Jay SD, Sharp AH, Kahl SD, Vedvick TS, Harpold MM, et al.: Structural characterization of the dihydropyridine-sensitive calcium channel α_2-subunit and the associated δ peptides. *J Biol Chem* 266:3287–3293, 1991.

33. Kim HL, Kim H, Lee P, King RG, Chin HR: Rat brain expresses an alternatively spliced form of the dihydropyridine-sensitive L-type calcium channel alpha-2 subunit. *Proc Natl Acad Sci USA* 89:3251–3255, 1992.

34. Kim HS, Wei X, Ruth P, Perez-Reyes E, Flockerzi V, et al.: Studies on the structural requirements for the activity of the skeletal muscle dihydropyridine receptor/slow Ca^{2+} channel. *J Biol Chem* 265:11858–11863, 1990.

35. Koch WJ, Ellinor PT, Schwartz A: cDNA cloning of a dihydropyridine-sensitive calcium channel from rat aorta. *J Biol Chem* 265:17786–17791, 1990.

36. Lacerda AE, Kim HS, Ruth P, Perez-Reyes E, Flockerzi V, et al.: Normalization of current kinetics by interaction between the α_1 and β subunits of the skeletal muscle dihydropyridine-sensitive Ca^{2+} channel. *Nature* 352:527–530, 1991.

37. Liu QY, Karpinski E, Rao M-R, Pang PKT: Tetrandine: A novel calcium channel antagonist inhibits type I calcium channels in neuroblastoma cells. *Neuropharmacology* 30:1325–1331, 1991.

38. Ma W-J, Holz RW, Uhler MD: Expression of a cDNA for a neuronal calcium channel α_1 subunit enhances secretion from adrenal chromaffin cells. *J Biol Chem* 267:22728–22732, 1992.

39. Mikami A, Imoto K, Tanabe T, Niidome T, Mori Y, et al.: Primary structure and functional expression of the cardiac dihydropyridine-sensitive calcium channel. *Nature* 340:230–233, 1989.

40. Mori Y, Friedrich T, Kim M-S, Mikami A, Nakai J, et al.: Primary structure and functional expression from complementary DNA of a brain calcium channel. *Nature* 350:398–402, 1991.

41. Mundiña-Weilenmann C, Chang CF, Gutierrez LM, Hosey MM: Demonstration of the phosphorylation of dihydropyridine-sensitive calcium channels in chick skeletal muscle and the resultant activation of the channels after reconstitution. *J Biol Chem* 266:4067–4073, 1991.

42. Nakayama H, Taki M, Striessnig J, Glossmann H, Catterall WA, et al.: Identification of 1,4-dihydropyridine binding regions within the α_1 subunit of skeletal muscle Ca^{2+} channels by photoaffinity labeling with diazipine. *Proc Natl Acad Sci USA* 88:9203–9207, 1991.

43. Niidome T, Kim MS, Friedrich T, Mori Y: Molecular cloning and characterization of a novel calcium channel from rabbit brain. *FEBS Lett* 308:7–13, 1992.

44. Nilius B, Hess P, Lansman JB, Tsien RW: A novel type of cardiac calcium channel in ventricular cells. *Nature* 316:443–446, 1985.

45. Norman RI, Burgess AJ, Allen E, Harrison TM: Monoclonal antibodies against the 1,4-dihydropyridine receptor associated with voltage-sensitive Ca^{2+} channels detect similar polypeptides from a variety of tissues and species. *FEBS Lett* 212:127–132, 1987.

46. Osterrieder W, Brum G, Hescheler J, Trautwein W, Flockerzi V, et al.: Injection of subunits of cyclic AMP-dependent protein kinase into cardiac myocytes modulates Ca^{2+} current. *Nature* 298:576–578, 1982.

47. Papazian DM, Timpe LC, Jan YN, Jan LY: Alteration of voltage-dependence of Shaker potassium channel by mutations in the S4 sequence. *Nature* 349:305–310, 1991.

48. Perez-Reyes E, Kim HS, Lacerda AE, Horne W, Wei X, Rampe D, Campbell KP, Brown AM, Birnbaumer L: Induction of calcium currents by the expression of the α_1-subunit of the dihydropyridine receptor from skeletal muscle. *Nature* 340:233–236, 1989.

49. Perez-Reyes E, Wei X, Castellano A, Birnbaumer L: Molecular diversity of L-type calcium channel. Evidence for alternative splicing of the transcripts of three nonallelic genes. *J Biol Chem* 265:20430–20436, 1990.

50. Perez-Reyes E, Castellano A, Kim HS, Bertrand P, Baggstrom E, et al.: Cloning and expression of cardiac/brain β subunit of the L-type calcium channel. *J Biol Chem* 267:1792–1797, 1992.

51. Powers PA, Liu S, Hogan K, Gregg RG: Skeletal muscle and brain isoforms of a β-subunit of human voltage-dependent calcium channels are encoded by a single gene. *J Biol Chem* 267:22967–22972, 1992.

52. Pragnell M, Sakamoto J, Jay SD, Campbell KP: Cloning and tissue-specific expression of the brain calcium channel β-subunit. *FEBS Lett* 291:253–258, 1991.

53. Regulla S, Schneider T, Nastainczyk W, Meyer HE, Hofmann F: Identification of the site of interaction of the dihydropyridine channel blockers nitrendipine and azidopine with the calcium channel α_1 subunit. *EMBO J* 10:45–49, 1991.

54. Reuter H: Calcium channel modulation by neurotransmitters, enzymes and drugs. *Nature* 301:569–574, 1983.

55. Röhrkasten A, Meyer HE, Nastainczyk W, Sieber M, Hofmann F: cAMP-dependent protein kinase rapidly phos-

phorylates serine-687 of the skeletal muscle receptor for calcium channel blockers. *J Biol Chem* 263:15325–15329, 1988.

56. Rotman EI, De Jongh KS, Florio V, Lai Y, Catterall WA: Specific phosphorylation of a COOH-terminal site on the full-length form of the α_1 subunit of the skeletal muscle calcium channel by cAMP-dependent protein kinase. *J Biol Chem* 267:16100–16105, 1992.

57. Ruth P, Röhrkasten A, Biel M, Bosse E, Regulla S, et al.: Primary structure of the β subunit of the DHP-sensitive calcium channel from skeletal muscle. *Science* 245:1115–1118, 1989.

58. Seino S, Chen L, Seino M, Blondel O, Takeda J, et al.: Cloning of the α_1 subunit of a voltage-dependent calcium channel expressed in pancreatic β cells. *Proc Natl Acad Sci USA* 89:584–588, 1992.

59. Singer D, Biel M, Lotan I, Flockerzi V, Hofmann F, et al.: The roles of the subunits in the function of the calcium channel. *Science* 253:1553–1557, 1991.

60. Snutch TP, Tomlinson WJ, Leonard JP, Gilbert MM: Distinct calcium channels are generated by alternative splicing and are differentially expressed in the mammalian CNS. *Neuron* 7:45–57, 1991.

61. Soldatov NM: Molecular diversity of L-type Ca^{2+} channel transcripts in human fibroblasts. *Proc Natl Acad Sci USA* 89:4628–4632, 1992.

62. Sperelakis N, Josephson I: The slow action potential and properties of the myocardial slow calcium channels. In: Sperelakis N (ed) *Physiology and Pathophysiology of the Heart*, 2nd ed. Boston: Kluwer Academic, 1989, pp 195–225.

63. Starr TVB, Prystay W, Snutch TP: Primary structure of a calcium channel that is highly expressed in the rat cerebellum. *Proc Natl Acad Sci USA* 88:5621–5625, 1991.

64. Striessnig J, Glossmann H, Catterall WA: Identification of a phenylalkylamine binding region within the α_1 subunit of skeletal muscle Ca^{2+} channels. *Proc Natl Acad Sci USA* 87:9108–9112, 1990.

65. Striessnig J, Murphy BJ, Catterall WA: Dihydropyridine receptor of L-type Ca^{2+} channels: Identification of binding domains for $[^3H](+)$-PN200-110 and $[^3H]$azidopine within the α_1 subunit. *Proc Natl Acad Sci USA* 88:10769–10773, 1991.

66. Stühmer W, Conti F, Suzuki H, Wang X, Noda M, Yahagi N, Kubo H, Numa S: Structural parts involved in activation and inactivation of the sodium channel. *Nature* 339:597–603, 1989.

67. Suzuki S, Rogawski MA: T-type calcium channels mediated the transition between tonic and phasic firing in thalamic neurons. *Proc Natl Acad Sci USA* 86:7228–7232, 1989.

68. Tanabe T, Takeshima H, Mikami A, Flockerzi V, Takahashi H, et al.: Primary structure of the receptor for calcium channel blockers from skeletal muscle. *Nature* 328:313–318, 1987.

69. Tanabe T, Beam KG, Powell JA, Numa S: Restoration of excitation-contraction coupling and slow calcium current in dysgenic muscle by dihydropyridine receptor complementary DNA. *Nature* 336:134–139, 1988.

70. Tanabe T, Beam KG, Adams BA, Niidome T, Numa S: Regions of the skeletal muscle dihydropyridine receptor critical for excitation-contraction coupling. *Nature* 346:567–569, 1990.

71. Tanabe T, Mikami A, Numa S, Beam KG: Cardiac-type excitation-contraction coupling in dysgenic skeletal muscle injected with cardiac dihydropyridine receptor. *Nature* 344:451–453, 1990.

72. Tanabe T, Adams BA, Numa S, Beam KG: Repeat I of the dihydropyridine receptor is critical in determining calcium channel activation kinetics. *Nature* 352:800–803, 1991.

73. Tsien RW, Ellinor PT, Horne WA: Molecular diversity of voltage-dependent Ca^{2+} channels. *Top Pharm Sci* 12:349–354, 1991.

74. Varadi G, Lory P, Schultz D, Varadi M, Schwartz A: Acceleration of activation and inactivation by the β subunit of the skeletal muscle calcium channel. *Nature* 352:159–162, 1991.

75. Wei X, Perez-Reyes E, Lacerda AE, Schuster G, Brown AM, et al.: Heterologous regulation of the cardiac Ca^{2+} channel α_1 subunit by skeletal muscle β and γ subunits. *J Biol Chem* 266:21943–21947, 1991.

76. Welling A, Bosse E, Ruth P, Bottlender R, Flockerzi V, et al.: Expression and regulation of cardiac and smooth muscle calcium channels. *J Pharmacol* 58(Suppl II):62–258, 1992.

77. Welling A, Bottlender R, Bosse E, Hofmann F: Stable expression of the calcium channel subunits in somatic cell lines. *Naunyn Schmiedebergs Arch Pharmacol* 345(Suppl):70, R18 (abstr), 1992.

78. Welling A, Felbel J, Peper K, Hofmann F: Hormonal regulation of calcium current in freshly isolated airway smooth muscle cells. *Am J Physiol* 262:L351–359, 1992.

79. Williams ME, Feldman DH, McCue AF, Brenner R, Velicelebi G, et al.: Structure and functional expression of α_1, α_2, and β subunits of a novel human neuronal calcium channel subtype. *Neuron* 8:71–84, 1992.

80. Williams ME, Brust PF, Feldman DH, Patti S, Simerson S, et al.: Structure and functional expression of an ω-conotoxin-sensitive human N-type calcium channel. *Science* 257:389–395, 1992.

81. Yatani A, Brown AM: Rapid β-adrenergic modulation of cardiac calcium channel currents by a fast G protein pathway. *Science* 245:71–74, 1989.

82. Yu ASL, Hebert SC, Brenner BM, Lytton J: Molecular characterization and nephron distribution of a family of transcripts encoding the pore-forming subunit of Ca^{2+} channels in the kidney. *Proc Natl Acad Sci USA* 89:10494–10498, 1992.

CHAPTER 6

Molecular Structure of Potassium and Sodium Channels and their Structure-Function Correlation

STEFAN H. HEINEMANN & WALTER STÜHMER

INTRODUCTION

The great improvements in genetic engineering and molecular biology have resulted in considerable progress in the development of biological sciences. This development has strongly affected cellular physiology, particularly in combination with the patch-clamp technique. The latter allows the indirect observation of conformational changes of a channel molecule in real time. The symbiosis of these techniques allows the identification of structural parts involved in the various functional properties of cloned ion channels. While Chapter 5 concentrated on the calcium channels, in this chapter we will summarize the actual knowledge on structure and function of voltage-dependent ion channels, in particular the ones selective for sodium and potassium.

Ion channels are proteins embedded in the membranes of cells. They consist of a linear sequence of amino acids, called the *primary sequence*. Using molecular biological techniques, it is possible to elucidate the primary sequence of these proteins. However, information on the folding of these chains of amino acids into functional proteins (secondary, tertiary, and quaternary structure) can only be obtained by additional methods such as x-ray crystallography or nuclear magnetic resonance spectroscopy. Membrane-bound proteins such as ion channels, however, are difficult to crystallize due to the simultaneous presence of hydrophobic and hydrophilic interfaces of the protein with its environment. In addition, in particular voltage-dependent ion channels tend to be very large structures with molecular weights in the range of some 100 kDa. Because of these reasons, only one class of membrane-bound proteins, the photoreaction center of *Rhodopseudomonas virids*, could be resolved at atomic resolution so far {1}. Structures with much lower spatial resolution of gap junction channels and the acetylcholine receptor channel could be obtained by electron microscopy of two-dimensional lattices {e.g., 2}.

SITE-DIRECTED MUTAGENESIS OF ION CHANNELS

Less rigorous methods can be applied in order to obtain more information on the role and structural aspects of protein domains or even of individual amino acid residues. The prerequisite for these methods is the deduction of the genetic information coding for the ion channel protein. There are several ways to obtain this information of the genetic code. If the protein of interest already exists in a purified form, microsequencing of a small part of the protein may be sufficient to identify the corresponding DNA in a cDNA library by DNA hybridization (e.g., sodium channel). A similar approach can be followed if genetic codes for proteins are searched that are closely related to sequences already known. In cases where the function of a protein is well characterized and where easy bioassays for channel function exist, expression cloning can be applied (e.g., glutamate receptor channel, chloride channel). In other cases, the localization of a genetic defect involving an ion channel protein on the chromosome can yield access to the primary sequence of the channel (e.g., *Shaker* potassium channel {3}, CFTR chloride channel (Cystic Fibrosis Transmembrane Conductance Regulator {4}).

The next step is to compare the deduced linear sequence of bases coding for a channel with other known protein sequences in order to identify homology and ancestral relationships among them. The linear sequence of amino acid residues can be analyzed in many ways with respect to the presence of secondary structural elements, such as potential α-helices, β-sheets, turns, and possible glycolysation and phosphorylation sites. Because the predictions of secondary structural elements are usually rather vague at this state, one mostly has to make do with a set of physical properties of the amino acids as a function of the position within the sequence. One of them is the hydrophobicity of the residues calculated in a sliding window of several residues. Such hydrophobicity plots are widely used for membrane-bound protein, because those are expected to possess several segments of the protein sequence that span the lipid bilayer, and that therefore are expected to have quite hydrophobic properties for energetic reasons. In fig. 6-1, such a plot is shown for a sodium channel (A) and a potassium channel (B). The regions that presumably form transmembrane segments, based on their length and their hydrophobicity, are marked with short horizontal bars.

For functional assay of the cloned channel proteins, the

N. Sperelakis (ed.), Physiology and Pathophysiology of the Heart, Third Edition.
© *1995 Kluwer Academic Publishers. ISBN 0-7923-2612-1. All rights reserved.*

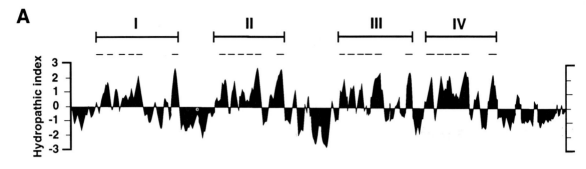

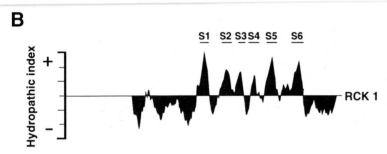

Fig. 6-1. Hydrophobicity plot of a Na (**A**) and a K (**B**) channel. The putative transmembrane segments are indicated by short bars above the hydrophobic segments. The S4 segments are not very hydrophobic due to the positive residues present. The longer bars above the Na channel indicate the four internal homologous repeats. Notice the two small peaks in the SS1–SS2 region between S5 and S6, thought to form part of the channel pore (particularly evident in the potassium channel sequence). Part **A** after Noda et al. {7}, part **B** after Stühmer et al. {57}.

message has to be expressed in a cell system. This is done in the following manner (fig. 6-2): cDNA-derived mRNA (cRNA) that corresponds to the channel being studied is injected into a cell that normally does not have these channels. A convenient expression system is the oocyte of the South African frog *Xenopus laevis* {5}. The cRNA will be processed in the same way as any other natural mRNA of the cell, that is, it will be translated, post-translationally modified, and inserted into the cell membrane. There the currents mediated by the expressed channels can be measured with electrophysiological techniques. The various steps involved in the preparation of *Xenopus* oocytes for electrophysiological recordings are shown in fig. 6-3. If channel proteins from mammalian sources are to be studied with respect to channel regulation, it is helpful to use mammalian cell lines for transfection with foreign plasmid DNA, yielding transient channel expression. With more involved methods, foreign DNA can be engineered into the genetic material of a host cell for stable channel expression.

The function of a specific amino acid can be studied by manipulating the residue in a site-specific manner (site-directed mutagenesis). Alternatively, entire domains of functionally different channels can be exchanged by formation of hybrid constructs (chimera). The topology of the channel, i.e., which parts of the channel protein face the extracellular side, which face the intracellular side, and which are not accessible at all, is often studied by antibody

binding to specific sites of the protein. The information obtained on the function of domains or single amino acids has to be interpreted with respect to a model of protein folding. Such models are obtained from hydrophobicity plots and secondary structure prediction plots. Although it should always be remembered that these are only models, they are essential in proposing testable hypotheses that will either be consistent with the model or will disprove it.

In addition, molecular cloning techniques allow the study of distribution and localization of mRNA in several tissues, indicating which cells possess these channels. Fractions of antisense mRNA of cloned channels that were labeled with radioactive markers can be hybridized *in situ* with the native mRNA of the tissue under consideration. Autoradiographs of these preparations then yield a spatial distribution of the channel. Recently, nonradioactive methods have been developed for *in situ* hybridization giving single-cell resolution {6}. Extensive studies were done with Na and K channels to localize their expression in the brain, as shown in fig. 6-4. However, other tissues, such as the heart, were also investigated in this respect (see below).

CHANNEL FAMILIES

The elucidation of the primary sequence of various channels made it clear that ion channels and receptors can be

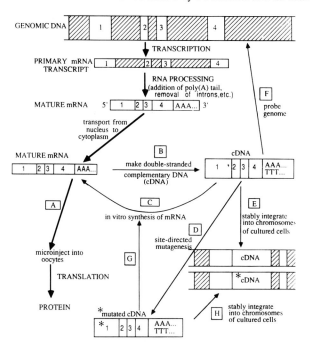

Fig. 6-2. Heterologous cRNA expression. The thick arrows on the left show the normal direction of flow for genomic information. Thin arrows indicate pathways used in recombinant DNA technology. **A:** Injection of mRNA coding for membrane channel protein into oocytes. **B:** Reverse transcriptase makes cDNA. **C:** cDNA can be used to synthesize mRNA directly. **D:** cDNA can be subjected to site-directed mutagenesis to produce mutations of a specific gene locus. **E:** cDNA can be integrated into chromosomes of cultured cells. **F:** cDNA can be used to probe DNA by means of hybridization screening. **G:** Mutated cDNA can be used to synthesize mRNA. **H:** mutated cDNA can be integrated into chromosomes of cultured cells. From Claudio {58}, with permission.

grouped into defined families of closely related proteins. This membership is not only based on similarity in function, but on sequence homology, probably arising from common ancestry early in evolution. For example, the nicotinic acetylcholine receptor belongs to the family of extracellular agonist-activated ion channels. Other members of this family include GABAa, glycine receptor, 5HT3, and ionotropic glutamate receptors. Interestingly, most of the agonists acting on the channels mentioned above also activate receptors of second messenger systems. These receptors are characterized as having seven putative membrane-spanning segments, such as the muscarinic acetylcholine receptor, GABAb, 5HT1, and metabotropic glutamate receptors. These receptors affect ion permeabilities indirectly through second messengers via G-protein-coupled systems.

There are several ways of assigning channels to certain groups. One of them is the distinction between the above-mentioned agonist-activated ion channels and those that are activated by depolarizing potentials. The latter group is classified according to their selectivity as potassium, sodium, and calcium channels. In addition, there are other members that are somewhere intermediate, such as the potassium channels activated by intracellular calcium, ATP-dependent channels, and the various chloride channels. These channels are only slightly voltage dependent and some are activated by an intracellular "agonist." Parts of the primary sequence of these channels are homologous to parts of the purely voltage-dependent channels. However, the classification of the latter channels is not clear at the moment and must await further sequence information from related channel types. The homologous regions between the various channel types probably arise because of the conservation of special motifs for specific functions, such as forming a potassium-selective ion pore in the case of the voltage-activated potassium channels, the ATP-sensitive potassium channels, and the calcium-activated potassium channels.

The voltage-dependent sodium and potassium channels are the main channels responsible for the propagation of action potentials. The properties of the sodium channels in the various excitable tissues in which they are found are quite homogeneous, although molecular biology has uncovered that this channel comes in many varieties. In contrast, potassium channels are quite variable with respect to properties in native tissue. This variety finds expression in the great number of variants found by cloning.

SUPERFAMILY OF VOLTAGE-GATED ION CHANNELS

The first sequence corresponding to a voltage-dependent sodium channel was described in 1984 {7}. This channel is the one found in the electric eel, *Electrophorus electricus*, and is involved in depolarizing one side of specialized muscle cells. These are arranged in series and form a battery stack. The synchronous depolarization gives rise to potentials of up to 800 V. During the discharge, each cell contributes on one side with the chloride equilibrium potential (−60 mV) and on the other, where the sodium channels are activated, with the sodium equilibrium potential (+50 mV). It is clear that in this tissue the density of voltage-dependent sodium channels is very high. This is a prerequisite to isolate the channel protein for microsequence analysis, a necessary first step in cloning this channel. The first sequence of a nicotinic acetylcholine receptor (n-AChR) was obtained from *Torpedo electroplax* tissue {8}. In this tissue the n-AChR has the equivalent function as the sodium channel in the specialized muscular tissue from the electric eel and is therefore of similar abundance.

Once a sequence of a certain protein is known, homologous sequences can be isolated by hybridization of a probe corresponding to the known protein with a genetic library of a novel tissue. In this manner, homologous sequences in the various tissues from different species are obtained. In the case of the voltage-gated sodium channel, different types have been found in rat brain {9–11}, human brain {12}, rat and human heart {13–15}, and two in skeletal muscle {16,17}. It consists of a main subunit of 260 kDa (α

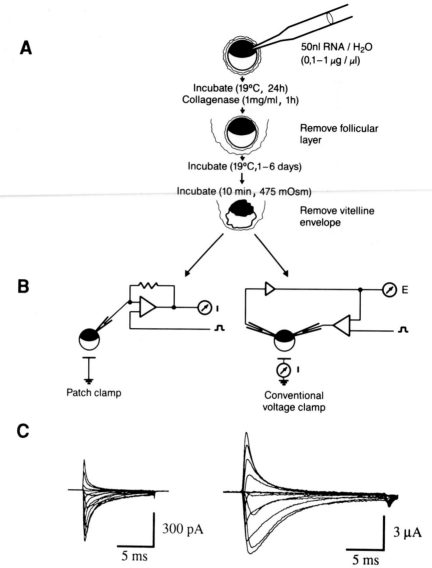

Fig. 6-3. **A:** Steps involved in preparation of oocytes for electrophysiological recording of exogenous ion channels. **B:** Schematic diagram of two recording techniques. **C:** Comparison of sodium currents recorded under patch-clamp (inside-out configuration) and under two-electrode voltage clamp. Responses to step depolarizations ranging from -50 to $+70$ mV in steps of 10 mV. The oocytes were injected with mRNA encoding a rat brain sodium channel. The traces were low-pass filtered prior to sampling with cutoff frequencies (-3 dB) of 10 kHz (left) and 3 kHz (right), respectively. Traces have been corrected for leakage and capacitive transients using a P/6 method. Note the differences in apparent channel kinetics obtained with these two methods. From Stühmer et al. {59}, with permission.

subunit) coding for some 2000 amino acids. In brain and muscle tissue, two additional subunits with molecular weights of 33 and 39 kDa have been found (β_1 and β_2 {18,19}), which are associated with the α subunit. The β_1 subunit increases the levels of expression and speeds up the inactivation when coexpressed with the α subunit {20}. However, the α subunit alone is capable of functionally expressing voltage-gated sodium channels in heterologous expression systems.

Detailed analysis of the primary sequence of the α subunit revealed that it contains four domains or repeats with a high degree of homology among them. Within each domain, six hydrophobic segments long enough to form a transmembrane α helix could be assigned (figs. 6-1 and

A

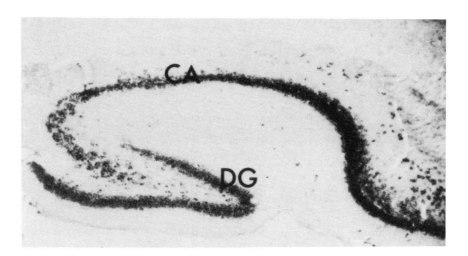

B

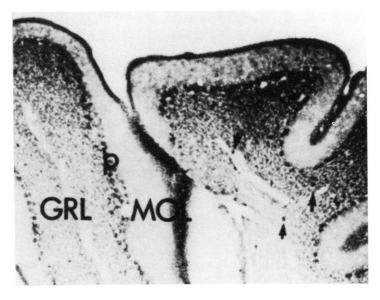

Fig. 6-4. In situ hybridization identifying a specific mRNA species at the single cell level. The RNA is hybridized in tissue sections to a specific probe labeled with radioactive or non-radioactive nucleotide analogs. The hybridization product is visualized either by film or emulsion autoradiography or by a colored enzymatic or fluorescent reaction product. The morphological conservation and cytological definition of the tissue cepends on the method employed. The figures shown identify single cells expressing Kv1.1 channels in rat hippocampus (**A**) and cerebellum (**B**). The 25 μm-thick parasagittal rat brain sections were hybridized with a digoxigenin-labeled riboprobe specific for Kv1.1. For visualization an alkaline phosphatase color reaction product was developed with nitroblue tetrazolium/5-bromo-4-chloro-3-indolyl-phosphate overnight {6}. CA = hippocampus; DG = dentate gyrus; GRL = granular layer; MOL = molecular layer; P = Purkinje cells. Arrows indicate Golgi cells. From S. Beckh and P. Wahle, unpublished data, with permission.

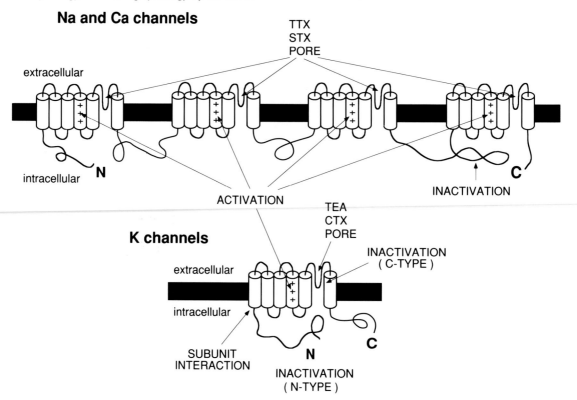

Fig. 6-5. Schematic diagram for the arrangement of the protein segments of Na, Ca, and K channels in the lipid membrane. The arrows point towards locations shown to be involved in the various functions indicated.

6-5). Therefore, the putative sodium channel α subunit would contain 24 transmembrane α helices. The amino terminal does not carry a leader sequence (which would be necessary for membrane crossing), and therefore this terminal is thought to be located intracellularly.

The first sequence corresponding to a voltage-gated potassium channel was obtained independently and simultaneously using reverse genetics on the *Shaker* mutant of *Drosophila melanogaster* {3,21,22}. The primary sequence corresponded to only 1 of the 4 repeats found in voltage-gated sodium channels. Therefore it was proposed that four of these subunits would assemble and form a functional channel. Elegant experiments combining wild-type channels and mutants that were made resistant to an open-channel blocker proved this to be correct {23}. Therefore, the assembled potassium channel structure would be similar to the one of the main α subunit of the voltage-gated sodium channel (see also figs. 6-1 and 6-5). In addition, there is a great sequence homology between the potassium channel and each repeat of the sodium channel. This means that equivalent structures in both channel families have equivalent function. This can be extended to voltage-gated calcium channels, which share sequence and structural homology to sodium channels.

CHANNEL ACTIVATION

A prominent feature found in all voltage-gated channels cloned so far is that the fourth segment of each repeat (or subunit), S4, carries a positive change every third residue. These charges have been proposed to form part of the voltage sensor required to respond to changes in the transmembrane potential {7,24}. This hypothesis was confirmed for both sodium and potassium channels by site-directed mutagenesis, in which the charged residues were replaced by neutral ones, giving a decrease in the voltage dependence of the mutant channels {25–27}. As expected, modification of the uncharged residues also resulted in modification of the voltage-dependent parameters, since this region is part of the voltage sensor. The steps involved, after sensing the electric field across the membrane, that lead to the actual opening of the ion channel are as yet unclear. For potassium channels, however, parts of the S5 segment and the intracellular linker between S4 and S5 were found to affect channel activation (e.g., {28}) and could therefore be playing a role in the final conformational transition leading to channel opening.

The activation of voltage-dependent ion channels is accompanied by so-called gating currents. They are expected to occur as a consequence of the displacement of the charges or dipoles that form part of the voltage sensor in the electric field. For ion channels in their native environment, the gating currents have been well characterized after blocking all of the ion currents by ionic substitution of permeant ions and/or ion current block using open-channel blockers. Gating current signals of other voltage-gated channel types that were also present in the preparation under investigation made the isolation of a current component specific for only one channel type difficult. The heterologous expression of voltage-gated ion channels provided an elegant way to study gating currents of a well-defined channel population, as shown for sodium and potassium channels. In addition, the activation mechanism assayed by gating current measurements can be studied on mutated channel variants. A dramatic example is the neutralization of the negative charge at position 384 (D384N) in rat brain sodium channel II. In this mutant, ionic currents are practically totally abolished, but the gating currents retain their normal properties {29}. These experiments gave evidence that the usual method of blocking ionic currents through sodium channels using TTX does not interfere with the gating mechanism, since gating currents measured using either TTX or a molecular ion conduction block give the same result in terms of gating currents.

INACTIVATION

A particular feature of nearly all voltage-dependent channels is their property to inactivate. This means that even though the stimulus, a depolarizing potential step, remains applied, the initially elicited current decreases (inactivates) with time. This property is important in shaping action potentials and is greatly responsible for the repolarization of the action potential. Using site-directed mutagenesis, regions involved in the inactivation process have been localized. Hoshi et al. {30} found that the amino-terminal region of potassium channels, localized intracellularly, forms a kind of plug that blocks the channel pore from the inside after the channel opens, causing inactivation (*N-type* inactivation). This *ball structure* is tied to the rest of the channel subunit by a sequence of amino acids acting as a *chain*, being the basis for the term *ball-and-chain model of inactivation*. Shortening of the chain results in faster inactivation, for the ball then has a higher probability of being close to the site where it binds to inactivate the channel.

For sodium channels, the linker region between repeats III and IV (also localized intracellularly) was found to be critical in inactivation. When the rat brain sodium channel II is expressed as two separate proteins, the first one from the N-terminal end through position 1504 in the linker between repeats III and IV, the second one from position 1506 to the C-terminal end, the fast inactivation is basically abolished {25}. Similar effects were obtained by antibody binding to this internal loop {31}. Site-directed mutagenesis in this linker revealed that hydrophobic amino acids are the major determinants for this linker to be an inactivation structure. A single point mutation in rat brain sodium channel IIA (F1489Q) was sufficient to abolish the fast component of the sodium channel inactivation to a great extent {32}.

The current molecular picture for this fast inactivation is that there are four inactivation "balls" in potassium channels (because there are four subunits, each having an N-terminal end), with only one being sufficient to inactivate the channel, and one inactivation "lid" for the sodium channel formed by the intracellular loop between repeats III and IV. These results are consistent with previous models and experiments on wild-type channels, in which proteolytic cleavage from the intracellular side removed inactivation. Moreover, intracellular perfusion with a peptide corresponding to the amino-terminal sequence of an inactivating potassium channel restored inactivation in potassium channels whose inactivation was removed by deleting the amino-terminal end of the protein {33}.

In addition to the main (and usually fast) inactivation, other slower and independent inactivation processes exist. For the potassium channels, these were termed *C-type* inactivation because mutations in the S6 segment, being the closest transmembrane segment to the C-terminal end of the protein sequence, showed strong effects on the time course of this inactivation process {34}. Mutations of amino acids in the pore region and in the end of the S5 segment were found to also affect this inactivation mechanism, leading to the hypothesis that C-type inactivation is basically determined by pore properties such as pore occupancy by ions.

PHARMACOLOGY

Another region of interest is the binding site of various toxins. Among these, sites affecting the action of small open-channel blockers are prominent, because these would pinpoint the location of the ion pore. For the sodium channel, tetrodotoxin (TTX) and saxitoxin (STX), and for the potassium channel tetraethylammonium (TEA) and charybdotoxin (CTX), are such specific open-channel blockers.

Here we would like to concentrate on that part of the channel molecule that forms the actual pore for the permeating ions. The first indication where the pore might be located in the channel molecule comes from experiments of Noda et al. {35}. They mutated residue E387 located in the linker between S5 and S6 of repeat I in the rat brain sodium channel II to a glutamine (Q) and found that the channel became basically insensitive to the specific blockers TTX and STX, which block the wild-type channel in nanomolar concentrations from the external side. TTX and STX are small, positively charged molecules, and the charge at E387 probably interacts directly with the toxins. In addition, the mutant had about a fivefold reduced single-channel conductance, indicating that the mutated site must be very close to the actual ion pore formed by the channel protein. These results obtained by mutating a D to Q in the pore region were consistent with earlier experiments by treating native channels with tetrame-

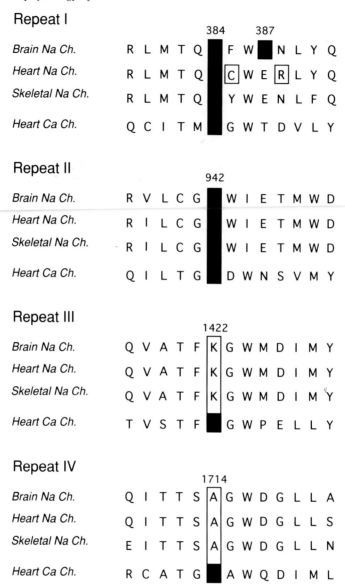

Fig. 6-6. Alignment of parts of the S5–S6 linker (called the *SS1–SS2 region* or also the *P region*) for various cloned sodium channels and a heart calcium channel. The boxes indicate residues discussed in detail in the text. The numbers refer to the residue numbers of the type II rat brain sodium channel. The standard single-letter amino acid code is used to designate the residues. Dark shading indicates negatively charged residues, light shading positive, and open boxes neutral residues.

thyloxonium, which acts by reducing negative charges {36}.

Figure 6-6 shows an alignment of sequences of this region for various channels. Pusch et al. {29} reported that the next negatively charged residue, D384, also seems to be important for toxin block. The mutant channel D384N was no longer blocked by TTX and STX, and it showed an extremely small single-channel conductance. With these experiments it was clearly shown that the ion channel pore must be directly at, or at least very close to, the above-mentioned amino acids. Similar to the first repeat, homologous residues of the other repeats proved also to be important for toxin block {37}. In addition, mutations of charged amino acids in this region resulted in reductions of the single-channel conductance (e.g., boxed residues in fig. 6-6). These two sets of results led to the conclusion that all four repeats contribute to the channel, thus forming a pore for the ions to travel through and a "pocket" for the toxins to bind. In these studies, special attention was paid to charged residues and, when mutated, they indeed showed the most pronounced effects with respect to toxin block and ion permeation. However, noncharged residues are also capable of determining differences between various sodium channels, as shown below.

These and other results on sodium channels were paralleled by studies of the TEA block of potassium channels. Within the S5–S6-linker, sites were identified that altered block by external TEA and CTX {e.g., 38,39}. Remarkably, one site even affected the channel block by internal TEA {40}, indicating that part of the S5–S6 linker has to be in contact with the intracellular side of the channel.

The results presented above confirmed the model put forward by Guy and collaborators {24,41} for the topological folding for the residues forming voltage-gated ion channels. This model assumes that the SS1–SS2 region, now termed the *P-region* (for pore region), dips into and out of the membrane, forming the narrow pore of the channel (see also fig. 6-5). This region can, in fact, be found in the hydrophobicity plot in fig. 6-1 between the fifth and sixth putative transmembrane region as two small hydrophobic peaks. Certainly, as proposed by Guy, other regions from the adjacent transmembrane segments will participate in pore formation.

Heart sodium channels are less sensitive to TTX and STX than neuronal sodium channels or sodium channels from innervated skeletal muscle. The contrary situation exists for the block by the external divalent cations Cd^{2+} and Zn^{2+}. Sequence comparison in the critical pore region of sodium channel II from rat brain and sodium channel I from heart muscle reveals only two salient modifications in repeat I; the other repeats are identical. In heart, arginine

is replaced for asparagine at position 388, and cysteine for phenylalanine at position 385 (for details see fig. 6-6). Site-directed mutagenesis experiments on both brain and cardiac sodium channels showed that it is the cysteine, and not arginine, that confers TTX and STX resistance to cardiac channels {42–44} (fig. 6-7A). Interestingly, the cysteine is also responsible for the increased blocking potency of Cd^{2+} and Zn^{2+} in the cardiac sodium channel (fig. 6-7B), while Co^{2+} and Ca^{2+} are less effective {42}. The cysteine residue in heart sodium channels, therefore, seems to undergo a specific interaction with Cd^{2+} and Zn^{2+}.

The binding of scorpion toxins was localized to external loops of the sodium channel between segments S5 and S6 in the first and fourth repeat by competition with antibodies raised against peptides having the same primary structure as the ion channel protein in these regions {45,46}.

CHANNEL PORE AND SELECTIVITY

After location of the channel pore, the most interesting question was what determines the selectivity of this pore. A clue to this problem is obtained by sequence alignment of various sodium channels with calcium channels that have a very similar overall structure (fig. 6-5). Concentrating on the pore region, it is striking that the inner columns of amino acids that were identified to be important for ion conduction and toxin block for the sodium channels are all glutamic acid residues (E) in the calcium channels (fig. 6-6). The sodium channel has negatively charged

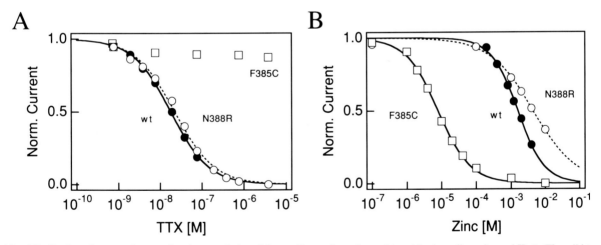

Fig. 6-7. Single point mutations confer characteristics of the cardiac sodium channel to rat brain sodium channel II. **A:** The wild-type rat brain sodium channel II (wt) is compared with two point mutants that introduce the amino acids into the pore region that are present at equivalent positions in the heart sodium channel. While N388R does not affect the channel block by external TTX, F385C reduces channel sensitivity for TTX by more than three orders of magnitude, as expected for cardiac sodium channels. **B:** While wt and F388R are blocked by external Zn^{2+} in the millimolar concentration range, the incorporation of a cysteine residue by F385C results in a specific channel block by external Zn^{2+} with a half-blocking concentration of 8 μM compared to a half-blocking concentration of 1.8 mM for wild-type brain channel. Part A after Heinemann et al. {42}, with permission.

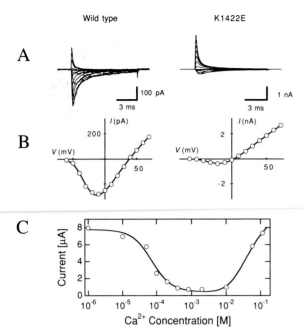

Fig. 6-8. Selectivity of the sodium channel. **A:** Inside-out macro patch recordings of the wild-type rat brain sodium channel II and point mutant K1422E as responses to voltage steps from −60 to +60 mV. Solutions in the pipette and bath were such that a sodium channel perfectly selective for Na⁺ over K⁺ should have a reversal potential of 46 mV. **B:** The plots of peak current versus test potential show that the current through the wild-type channels reverses at about 45 mV, whereas the reversal potential for the mutant K1422E is close to zero mV, indicating a complete loss of selectivity for Na⁺ over K⁺. **C:** As already apparent in A and B, the mutant K1422E carries much less inward current. This is due to channel block by external Ca²⁺. In this graph the peak inward current is shown for external solutions with increasing Ca²⁺ content compared to Na⁺. At the left side of this function, peak sodium inward current is progressively blocked by increasing amounts of Ca²⁺. On the right side of the minimum at about physiological Ca²⁺ concentrations the current increases again, because under these circumstances Ca²⁺ permeates through the channel, a phenomenon characteristic for Ca²⁺ channels. After Heinemann et al. {47}, with permission.

residues in the first two repeats but a positive amino acid in repeat III (K1422) and a neutral one in repeat IV (A1714). Measurements of reversal potentials in patch-clamp experiments revealed that the sodium channel mutant A1714E had a reduced selectivity for Na⁺ over K⁺ and mutant K1422E completely lost the selectivity {47} (fig. 6-8A,B). In addition, both mutants were blocked by external divalent cations such as Ca²⁺. Upon removal of external Ca²⁺, the mutant K1422E acted as a nonselective cation channel, and at higher Ca²⁺ concentrations Ca²⁺ itself became the charge carrier yielding large Ca²⁺ currents (fig. 6-8C). The combination mutant, K1422E·A1714E, was blocked by Ca²⁺ at even lower concentrations (IC₅₀ = 5.4 μM) and mainly conducted Ca²⁺ at physiological concentrations. This means that these two residues

are sufficient to confer the typical permeation characteristics of a calcium channel, namely, monovalent current block by divalent cations at low concentrations and divalent ion current at higher concentrations, onto a sodium channel. Hence a structure acting as a selectivity filter in the sodium channel, and presumably also in the calcium channel, was identified.

Potassium channels show a high homology to cyclic nucleotide-activated channels. These channels are strongly blocked by external Ca²⁺ and are not very selective for monovalent cations. In alignments of the pore region of potassium channels and the cGMP-activated channel, it becomes apparent that the high homology is spoiled by an extra GY motif, which is common to potassium channels. Deletion of these two amino acids indeed yielded ion channels with ion permeation properties reminiscent of cGMP-activated channels {48}.

Although the exact biophysical mechanisms of ion selectivity have as yet to be elucidated, site-directed mutagenesis of sodium and potassium channels clearly identified the linker between the transmembrane segments S5 and S6 to be at least part of the pore. By comparison with sequences of related channels with different selectivity properties (calcium-sodium channel, potassium-cGMP channel), amino acids within the P-region could be identified to play key roles in determining the selectivity of the channels for permeating ions.

HETEROGENEITY OF POTASSIUM CHANNELS

As mentioned, potassium channels exhibit a wide diversity of properties. How can such a variety be generated? In the case of channels cloned from the *Shaker* locus of *Drosophila melanogaster*, one way to generate variety is by alternative insertion of regions into the "original" sequence, a process called *alternative splicing*. For example, fast-inactivating and noninactivating channels can be generated just by alternative splicing of the amino-terminal end, leaving the transmembrane regions and the carboxy-terminal end unchanged. The slow-inactivating properties can in turn be modified by alternative splicing of the carboxy-terminal end. However, in rat there is no indication to date that alternative splicing plays a relevant role. The various divergent properties are rather encoded by different potassium channel genes. These different products differ in properties such as conductance, time course of fast and slow inactivation, and sensitivity to toxins and channel blockers.

Many homologous potassium channels have been identified using probes corresponding to the *Shaker* channel. The various channels found in *Drosophila* can be grouped into four subfamilies, which have been given the names of *Shaker*, *Shaw*, *Shal*, and *Shab*. The corresponding subfamilies are designated, in general, Kv1, Kv2, Kv3, and Kv4. The K stands for potassium, the v for voltage-gated, the number indicates the subfamily, and a second number after a period identifies each individual member. Another way to generate heterogeneity could thus be achieved by combining subunits from different subfamilies that assemble to form a functional channel. Potassium channels can indeed be formed by heteromultimers with properties in between those of the corresponding homomultimers.

The diversity of potassium channels is even increased by the specific assembly of α and small cytoplasmic β subunits. A β subunit cloned from rat brain (Mr 44.7 kD) was shown to provide an extra inactivating structure at the N-terminus with properties similar to the "ball" structures in α subunits of A-type potassium channels. Thus delayed rectifier channels can be converted into A-type channels by association of such a β subunit {49}.

CHANNEL REGULATION

Ion channels are regulated by various means. Phosphorylation is among the most important system for this modulation. Sites involved in phosphorylation of voltage-dependent ion channels have been localized using site-directed mutagenesis. In particular, cardiac calcium channels are strongly regulated by phosphorylation, and this modulation is essential for their physiological role. Chapter 5 focuses in more detail on this aspect.

Although apparently more important for calcium channels, effects of phosphorylation on Na and K channels were observed. Currents carried by rat brain sodium channel IIA, for example, are reduced in amplitude and slowed in inactivation kinetics by activation of protein kinase C {50}; they are increased in amplitude without effects on channel kinetics by protein kinase A {51,52}.

Another mechanism for regulation is the reduction-oxidation (redox) potential. The redox potential is tightly controlled in the cytoplasm and is subject to metabolic changes. Particular potassium channels, Kv1.4 and Raw3, are in fact regulated by the redox potential. In its reduced form, the currents mediated through Kv1.4 are fast inactivating, with a time constant of inactivation of about 50 ms. In the brain this current contributes to the so-called A current; in the heart it forms part of the transient potassium outward current (I_{TO}). This current component affects the shape of the action potential, since the transient outward currents speeds repolarization. During repetitive firing, this current will affect the firing rate. The normally fast inactivation of Kv1.4 is removed if the cytoplasmic side is oxidized. The site of this effect has been traced to a cysteine residue in the amino terminal of Kv1.4. This

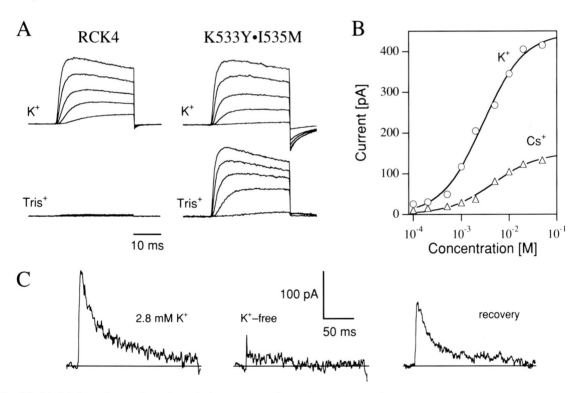

Fig. 6-9. Modulation of potassium channels by external K$^+$. **A:** Outward potassium currents through RCK4 channels and the RCK4-based mutant K533Y·I535M in presence of 10 mM external K$^+$ (upper panels), with all external K$^+$ replaced by the impermeable ion Tris$^+$ (lower panels), showing how RCK4-mediated currents are site-specifically modulated by external K$^+$. **B:** Dose-response curves for peak outward current through RCK4 channels as a function of external K$^+$ and Cs$^+$. The half-maximal current amplitude is obtained in 2.8 mM K$^+$, indicating that this channel is subject to K$^+$ regulation in the physiologically relevant concentration range. **C:** Transient outward potassium currents in acutely dissociated rat atrial cells in the presence (left and right) and in the absence of external K$^+$ (center trace). Parts A and B after Pardo et al. {55}, part C after Pardo et al. {56}.

cysteine is fixed by a disulfide bridge in the oxidized state, immobilizing the amino-terminal end responsible for inactivation. Reduction of the cytoplasmic milieu is capable of restoring fast inactivation to Kv1.4 {53}. Kv1.4 is abundant in brain tissue, but also has been found to be present in cardiac tissue {54}.

Another modulatory agent affecting Kv1.4 is the extracellular potassium concentration, $[K]_o$. The amount of current through Kv1.4 is proportional to $[K]_o$ in such a way that it overcomes the effect of changing the equilibrium potential for K^+ to more positive values {55}. Therefore, at higher $[K]_o$ more current flows through Kv1.4 channels, opposite to what is intuitively expected. Since $[K]_o$ depends on the previous activity of excitable tissue due to potassium accumulation in a restricted extracellular space, a component of I_{TO} will also depend on previous activity. In situations of low activity, K^+ will be cleared out of the extracellular space and reach a certain equilibrium concentration. At higher firing rates $[K]_o$ increases above this value. Therefore Kv1.4 might be an important regulator of pacemaking activity in cardiac tissue when action potentials are generated at a higher rate {56}. Under pathological conditions, especially cardiac ischemia, $[K]_o$ rises to very high values; this not only will alter the resting electrical properties of the cells, but also increase the fraction of I_{TO} flowing through Kv1.4 channels. Both effects combined would severely alter action potential shape and repolarization properties of the cardiac muscle, leading to severe rhythm disturbances. Figure 6-9 shows the effects of $[K]_o$ and $[Cs]_o$ on Kv1.4 channels, particularly in rat atrial cells (Fig. 6-9C).

SUMMARY AND CONCLUSIONS

In this chapter the molecular organization of voltage-gated ion channels has been presented. We concentrated on two members of this family, the sodium and potassium channels, since the calcium channels have been discussed in the previous chapter. This family shares common features such as consisting of four repeats (sodium and calcium) or four subunits (potassium), each of which has six putative transmembrane segments. In addition, two short segments form the pore region (P region), where determinants for open-channel blockers, conductance, and selectivity are located. A cysteine present in this region in cardiac sodium channels has been identified as the main factor responsible for the decreased sensitivity to TTX and STX, as well as the increased blocking ability of zinc in cardiac sodium channels. Parts of the voltage-sensing charges are located in the S4 segment, which carries several positively charged residues. Inactivation is associated with intracellular regions corresponding to the amino-terminal end in potassium channels and to the linker between repeats III and IV in sodium channels. Modulation of these channels by phosphorylation, redox potential, and extracellular potassium, have been discussed, in particular with respect to cardiac tissue.

REFERENCES

1. Deisenhofer J, Epp O, Miki K, Huber R, Michel H: X-ray structure analysis of a membrane protein complex. Electron density map at 3 Å resolution and a model of the chromophores of the photosynthetic reaction center from *Rhodopseudomonas viridis*. *J Mol Biol* 180:385–398, 1984.
2. Toyoshima C, Unwin N: Ion channel of acetylcholine receptor reconstructed from images of postsynaptic membranes. *Nature* 336:247–250, 1988.
3. Tempel BL, Papazian DM, Schwarz TL, Jan YN, Jan LY: Sequence of a probable potassium channel component encoded at *Shaker* locus of *Drosophila*. *Science* 237:770–775, 1987.
4. Rommens JM, Iannuzzi MC, Kerem B-S, Drumm ML, Melmer G, Dean M, Rozmahel R, Cole JL, Kennedy D, Hidaka M, Zsiga M, Buckwald M, Riordan JR, Tsui L-C, Collins FS: Identification of the cystic fibrosis gene: Chromosome walking and jumping. *Science* 245:1059–1065, 1989.
5. Gundersen CB, Miledi R, Parker I: Messenger RNA from human brain includes drug- and voltage-operated channels in *Xenopus* oocytes. *Nature* 308:421–424, 1984.
6. Wahle P, Beckh S: A method of in situ hybridization combined with immunocytochemistry, histochemistry, and tract tracing to characterize the mRNA expressing cell types of heterogeneous populations. *J Neurosci Methods* 41:153–166, 1992.
7. Noda M, Shimizu S, Tanabe T, Takai T, Kayano T, Ikeda T, Takahashi H, Nakayama H, Kanaoka Y, Minamino N, Kangawa K, Matuso H, Raftery MA, Hirose T, Inayama S, Hayashida H, Miyata T, Numa S: Primary structure of *Electrophorus electricus* sodium channel deduced from cDNA sequence. *Nature* 312:121–127, 1984.
8. Noda M, Takahashi H, Tanabe T, Toyosato M, Furutani Y, Hirose T, Asai M, Inayama S, Miyata T, Numa S: Primary structure of α-subunit precursor of *Torpedo californica* acetylcholine receptor deduced from cDNA sequence. *Nature* 299:793–797, 1982.
9. Noda M, Ikeda T, Kayano T, Suzuki H, Takeshima H, Kurasaki M, Takahashi H, Numa S: Existence of distinct sodium channel messenger RNAs in rat brain. *Nature* 320:188–192, 1986.
10. Suzuki H, Beckh S, Kubo H, Yahagi N, Ishida H, Kayano T, Noda M, Numa S: Functional expression of cloned cDNA encoding sodium channel III. *FEBS Lett* 228:195–200, 1988.
11. Auld VJ, Goldin AL, Krafte DS, Marshall J, Dunn JM, Catterall WA, Lester HA, Davidson N, Dunn RJ: A rat brain Na$^+$ channel α subunit with novel gating properties. *Neuron* 1:449–461, 1988.
12. Ahmed CMI, Ware DH, Lee SC, Patten CD, Ferrer-Montiel AV, Schinder AF, McPherson JD, Wagner-McPherson CB, Wasmuth JJ, Evans GA, Montal M: Primary structure, chromosomal localization, and functional expression of a voltage-gated sodium channel from human brain. *Proc Natl Acad Sci USA* 89:8220–8224, 1992.
13. Rogart RB, Cribbs LL, Muglia LK, Kephart DD, Kaiser MW: Molecular cloning of a putative tetrodotoxin-resistant rat heart Na$^+$ channel isoform. *Proc Natl Acad Sci USA* 86:8170–8174, 1989.
14. George AL, Knittle TJ, Tamkun MM: Molecular cloning of an atypical voltage-gated sodium channel expressed in human heart and uterus: Evidence for a distinct gene family. *Proc Natl Acad Sci USA* 89:4893–4897, 1992.
15. Gellens ME, George AL Jr, Chen L, Chahine M, Horn R, Barchi RL, Kallen RG: Primary structure and functional

expression of the human cardiac tetrodotoxin-insensitive voltage-dependent sodium channel. *Proc Natl Acad Sci USA* 89:554–558, 1992.

16. Trimmer JS, Cooperman SS, Tomiko SA, Zhou J, Crean SM, Boyle MB, Kallen RG, Sheng Z, Barchi RL, Sigworth FJ, Goodman RH, Agnew WS, Mandel G: Primary structure and functional expression of a mammalian skeletal muscle sodium channel. *Neuron* 3:33–49, 1989.

17. James WM, Emerick MC, Agnew WS: Affinity purification of the voltage-sensitive sodium channel from electroplax with resins selective for sialic acid. *Biochemistry* 28:6001–6009, 1989.

18. Harthorne RP, Catterall WA: Purification of the saxitoxin receptor of the sodium channel from rat brain. *Proc Natl Acad Sci USA* 78:4620–4624, 1981.

19. Barchi RL: Protein components of the purified sodium channel from rat skeletal muscle sarcolemma. *J Neurochem* 40:1377–1385, 1983.

20. Isom LL, De Jongh KS, Patton DE, Reber BFX, Offord J, Charbonneau H, Walsh K, Golding AL, Catterall WA: Primary structure and functional expression of the β_1 subunit of the rat brain sodium channel. *Science* 256:839–842, 1992.

21. Pongs O, Kecskemethy N, Muller R, Krah-Jentgens I, Baumann A, Kiltz HH, Canal I, Llamazares S, Ferrus A: *Shaker* encodes a family of putative potassium channel proteins in the nervous system of *Drosophila. EMBO J* 7:1087–1096, 1988.

22. Iverson LE, Tanouye MA, Lester HA, Davidson N, Rudy B: A-type potassium channels expressed from *Shaker* locus cDNA. *Proc Natl Acad Sci USA* 85:5723–5727, 1988.

23. MacKinnon R: Determination of the subunit stoichiometry of a voltage-activated potassium channel. *Nature* 350:232–235, 1991.

24. Guy HR, Seetharamulu P: Molecular model of the action potential sodium channel. *Proc Natl Acad Sci* USA 83:508–512, 1986.

25. Stühmer W, Conti F, Suzuki H, Wang X, Noda M, Yahagi N, Kubo H, Numa S: Structural parts involved in activation and inactivation of the sodium channel. *Nature* 339:597–603, 1989.

26. Papazian DM, Timpe LC, Jan YN, Jan LY: Alteration of voltage-dependence of *Shaker* potassium channel by mutations in the S4 sequence. *Nature* 349:305–310, 1991.

27. Liman ER, Hess P, Weaver F, Koren G: Voltage-sensing residues in the S4 region of a mammalian K^+ channel. *Nature* 353:752–756, 1991.

28. McCormack K, Tanouye MA, Iverson LE, Lin JW, Ramaswami M, McCormack T, Campanelli JT, Mathew MK, Rudy B: A role for hydrophobic residues in the voltage-dependent gating of *Shaker* K^+ channels. *Proc Natl Acad Sci USA* 88:2931–2935, 1991.

29. Pusch M, Noda M, Stühmer W, Numa S, Conti F: Single point mutations of the sodium channel drastically reduce the prore permeability without preventing its gating. *Eur Biophys J* 20:127–133, 1991.

30. Hoshi T, Zagotta WN, Aldrich RW: Biophysical and molecular mechanisms of *Shaker* potassium channel inactivation. *Science* 250:533–538, 1990.

31. Vassilev PM, Scheuer T, Catterall WA: Identification of an intracellular peptide segment involved in sodium channel inactivation. *Science* 241:1658–1661, 1988.

32. West JW, Patton DE, Scheuer T, Wang Y, Goldin AL, Catterall WA: A cluster of hydrophobic amino acid residues required for fast Na^+-channel inactivation. *Proc Natl Acad Sci USA* 89:10910–10914, 1992.

33. Zagotta WN, Hoshi T, Aldrich RW: Restoration of inactivation in mutants of *Shaker* potassium channels by a peptide derived from ShB.

34. Hoshi T, Zagotta WN, Aldrich RW: Two types of inactivation in *Shaker* K^+ channels: Effects of alteration in the carboxy-terminal region. *Neuron* 7:547–556, 1991.

35. Noda M, Suzuki H, Numa S, Stühmer W: A single point mutation confers tetrodotoxin and saxitoxin insensitivity on sodium channel II. *FEBS Lett* 259:213–216, 1989.

36. Sigworth FJ, Spalding BC: Chemical modification reduces the conductance of sodium channels in nerve. *Nature* 283:293–295, 1980.

37. Terlau H, Heinemann SH, Stühmer W, Pusch M, Conti F, Imoto K, Numa S: Mapping the site of block by tetrodotoxin and saxitoxin of sodium channel II. *FEBS Lett* 293:93–96, 1991.

38. MacKinnon R, Miller C: Mutant potassium channels with altered binding of charybdotoxin, a pore-binding peptide inhibitor. *Science* 245:1382–1385, 1989.

39. MacKinnon R, Yellen G: Mutations affecting TEA blockade and ion permeation in voltage-activated K^+ channels. *Science* 250:276–279, 1990.

40. Yellen G, Jurman ME, Abramson T, MacKinnon R: Mutations affecting internal TEA blockade identify the probable pore-forming region of a K^+ channel. *Science* 251:939–941, 1991.

41. Guy HR, Conti F: Pursuing the structure and function of voltage-gated channels. *Trends Neurosci* 13:201–206, 1990.

42. Heinemann SH, Terlau H, Imoto K: Molecular basis for pharmacological differences between brain and cardiac sodium channels. *Pflügers Arch* 422:90–92, 1992.

43. Satin J, Kyle JW, Chen M, Bell P, Cribbs LL, Fozzard HA, Rogart RB: A mutant of TTX-resistant cardiac sodium channels with TTX-sensitive properties. *Science* 256:1202–1205, 1992.

44. Backx PH, Yue DT, Lawrence JH, Marban E, Tomaselli GF: Molecular localization of an ion-binding site within the pore of mammalian sodium channels. *Science* 257:248–251, 1992.

45. Tejedor FJ, Catterall WA: Site of covalent attachment of α-scorpion toxin derivatives in domain I of the sodium channel α subunit. *Proc Natl Acad Sci USA* 85:8742–8746, 1988.

46. Thomsen WJ, Catterall WA: Localization of the receptor site for α-scorpion toxins by antibody mapping: Implications for sodium channel topology. *Proc Natl Acad Sci USA* 86:10161–10165, 1989.

47. Heinemann SH, Terlau H, Stühmer W, Imoto K, Numa S: Calcium channel characteristics conferred on the sodium channel by single mutations. *Nature* 356:441–443, 1992.

48. Heginbotham L, Abramson T, MacKinnon R: A functional connection between the pores of distantly related ion channels as revealed by mutant K^+ channels. *Science* 258:1152–1155, 1992.

49. Rettig J, Heinemann SH, Wunder F, Lorra C, Parcej DN, Dolly JO, Pongs O: Non-inactivating voltage-gated potassium channels are converted to A-type channels by association with a β subunit. Nature, in press, 1994.

50. Numann R, Catterall WA, Scheuer T: Functional modulation of brain sodium channels by protein kinase C phosphorylation. *Science* 254:115–118, 1991.

51. Smith RD, Golding AL: Protein kinase A phosphorylation enhances sodium channel currents in Xenopus oocytes. *Am J Physiol* 263:C660–C666, 1992.

52. Gershon E, Weigl L, Lotan I, Schreibmayer W, Dascal N: Protein kinase A reduces voltage-dependent Na^+ current in *Xenopus* oocytes. *J Neurosci* 12:3743–3752, 1992.

53. Ruppersberg JP, Stocker M, Pongs O, Heinemann SH, Frank R, Koenen M: Regulation of fast inactivation of cloned mammalian IK(A) channels by cysteine oxidation. *Nature* 352:711–714, 1991.

54. Tamkun MM, Knoth KM, Walbridge JA, Kroemer H, Roden DM, Glover DM: Molecular cloning and characterization of two voltage-gated K⁺ channel cDNAs from human venticle. *FASEB J* 5:331–337, 1991.

55. Pardo LA, Heinemann SH, Terlau H, Ludewig U, Lorra C, Pongs O, Stühmer W: Extracellular K⁺ specifically modulates a rat brain potassium channel. *Proc Natl Acad Sci USA* 89:2466–2470, 1992.

56. Pardo LA, Stühmer, W: Extracellular potassium modulates a transient current in rat atrial cells. 1994, in press.

57. Stühmer W, Ruppersberg JP, Schröter KH, Sakmann B, Stocker M, Giese KP, Perschke A, Baumann A, Pongs O: Molecular basis of functional diversity of voltage-gated potassium channels in mammalian brain. *EMBO J* 8:3235–3244, 1989.

58. Claudio T: Recombinant DNA technology in the study of ionic channels. *Trends Pharmacol Sci* 7:308–312, 1986.

59. Stühmer W, Terlau H, Heinemann SH: Xenopus oocytes for two-electrode and patch clamp recording. In: Kettenmann H, Grantyn R (eds) *Practical Electrophysiological Methods*, New York: Wiley-Liss, 1992, pp 121–125.

CHAPTER 7

Calcium Regulation of Ion Channels in Cardiomyocytes

NORITSUGU TOHSE & MORIO KANNO

INTRODUCTION

Excitation-contraction coupling is an indispensable process for heart contraction, and intracellular Ca^{2+} plays a central role in the coupling process. Since Irisawa {1} showed that rabbit sinoatrial nodal preparations ceased to contract when voltage clamped at the maximum diastolic potential, it is generally accepted that the electrical events in the sarcolemma primarily regulate an increase in cytoplasmic Ca^{2+} (Ca^{2+} transient) and thereby mechanical contraction. However, the introduction of the patch-clamp technique revealed that the Ca^{2+} transient also acts as one of the essential regulators of the membrane currents/channels in cardiac cells. The delayed rectifier K current (I_K), the transient outward current (I_{to}), and the hyperpolarization-activated inward current (I_f) were found to be increased by elevation of intracellular Ca^{2+} concentration ($[Ca]_i$). The Ca^{2+}-activated nonspecific cation current (I_{non}), which may contribute to the generation of cardiac arrhythmias in pathologic conditions, and the Na-Ca exchange current are also known to be Ca^{2+} sensitive. The Ca^{2+} sensitivity of these currents is important for understanding (a) the current systems underlying the action potentials and (b) changes in the action potentials enabled by hormonal regulations and produced by pathological interventions. In this chapter the new findings on Ca^{2+} regulation of I_K, I_{to}, I_f, and I_{non} channels obtained from use of the patch-clamp technique are described (Na-Ca exchange current is dealt with in another chapter).

Ca²⁺-ACTIVATED K⁺ CHANNEL (MEECH CHANNEL)

Meech {2,3} demonstrated in *Aplysia* neurons that K^+ conductance was markedly increased by intracellularly injected Ca^{2+}, and that EGTA injection abolished repetitive electrical activity. This phenomenon, sometimes called the *Meech effect*, provided evidence of an essential role of $[Ca]_i$ in modulating membrane currents. This Meech effect was thought to be generated by a class of K^+ channel different from the Hodgkin–Huxley K^+ channel, and these channels were called *the Ca^{2+}-activated K^+ channels*.

Cardiac electrophysiologists explored the Meech effect in cardiac muscles because of their dynamic change in $[Ca]_i$ (the Ca^{2+} transient) physiologically. The first such outstanding work was reported by Isenberg {4}. He demonstrated that intracellular injection of Ca^{2+} via a microelectrode produced a marked abbreviation of action potential duration and hyperpolarization of diastolic potential in sheep Purkinje fibers. This study implied that some Ca^{2+}-activated K^+ conductance produced the action potential shortening. In a subsequent paper {5}, he attributed these changes to Ca^{2+}-induced activation of steady-state K^+ current. However, single-channel activity of the Ca^{2+}-activated K^+ channel had not been detected in cardiac cells {6,7}.

In 1986, Callewaert et al. {8} demonstrated the existence of the Ca^{2+}-activated K^+ channels in cow cardiac Purkinje cells. This channel had a large conductance (120 pS) and did not exhibit activities in low $[Ca]_i$ (0.01 μM). These characteristics were very similar to the Meech channel reported by Pallotta et al. {9} in rat myotubule. However, the channel showed transient kinetics and seemed to carry a Ca^{2+}-dependent (caffeine-sensitive) transient outward current.

A steady-state Ca^{2+}-activated K^+ current, which is very similar to the Meech current, has been preliminarily reported by Baró and Escande {10}. In their reports a steady-state outward current blocked by Co^{2+} in guinea-pig atrial cells was observed as a mirror image of the Ca^{2+} current in use in the ramp pulse protocol. This finding in the atrial cells is very similar to that reported with the use of EGTA by Meech {3}. Recently Hagiwara et al. {11} reported that stretching of rabbit atrial cells produced a steady-state K^+ current. This current was abolished by removing the external Ca^{2+} and chelation of intracellular Ca^{2+}. Then an increase in $[Ca]_i$ up to a concentration of 0.3 μM activated the K^+ current without loading stretch stress. Therefore, stretch stress seems to activate the Meech channel through elevation of $[Ca]_i$.

The cardiac Meech channel requires a relatively higher $[Ca]_i$ for its activation than the physiological condition (1 μM for the transient type reported by Callewaert et al. {8}; 0.3 μM for the steady-state type reported by Hagiwara et al. {11}). Therefore, the cardiac Meech channel seems to be more important in the pathological condition than in

N. Sperelakis (ed.), Physiology and Pathophysiology of the Heart, Third Edition.

physiological condition. In the ischemic condition, $[Ca]_i$ is markedly elevated and then produces the muscle contracture. Therefore, it is likely that the cardiac Meech channel is related to the ischemia-induced abbreviation of the action potential, in addition to the ATP-sensitive K^+ channels {12}. Since only little information is available about the cardiac Meech channel, investigations of characteristics of this channel will be important for cardiac electrophysiologists.

DELAYED RECTIFIER K^+ CHANNELS

The delayed rectifier K^+ current (I_K) develops after the activation of the Ca^{2+} current. McGuigan {13} observed an increase in I_K with increasing frequency of applied voltage-clamp pulses, and suggested that the delayed rectification in calf and sheep ventricular muscles was modulated by intracellular Ca^{2+}. However, this study did not provide direct evidence for Ca^{2+} modulation of I_K. Brown and DiFrancesco {14} reported that I_K was de-

creased by D-600, a Ca^{2+} blocker, in rabbit sinoatrial node preparations, and its decrease was well correlated with the decrease in I_{Ca}. Goto et al. {15} showed that Co^{2+}, an inorganic Ca^{2+} channel blocker, reduced the delayed rectifier outward current $(I_{x(K)})$ of frog atrial muscle preparations and suggested the possible Ca^{2+} sensitivity of $I_{x(K)}$. However, other reports {16–18} disagreed on the Ca^{2+} sensitivity of I_K, claiming that the Ca^{2+} channel blockers used in these experiments had a nonselective interaction with other ionic channels. For example, Kass {17} showed that I_K of calf and dog Purkinje fibers was still activated in the presence of nisoldipine, a specific and potent Ca^{2+} channel blocker, though the drug abolished completely the Ca^{2+} current and contraction. In fact, Eisner and Vaughan-Jones {6} concluded in their 1983 review that there were no currents dependent upon $[Ca]_i$.

In the early 1980s, a great breakthrough occurred in the field of cardiac electrophysiology. Introduction of the patch-clamp method and single-cell preparations made possible estimation of the membrane current free from the influence of contraction and control of the intracellular

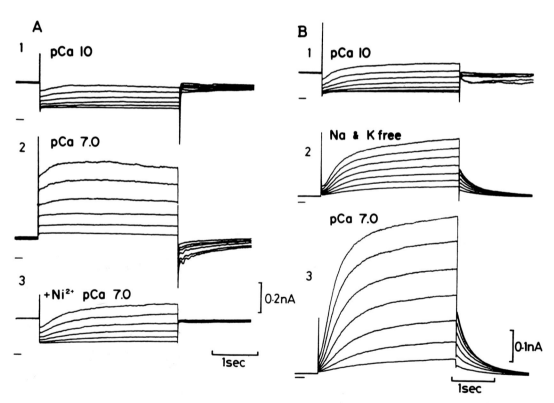

Fig. 7-1. **A:** Effects of Ni^{2+} on membrane currents in $[Ca]_i$ of pCa 7. Holding potential was $-37\,mV$ and test pulse duration was 3 seconds. **A-1** shows current traces at six different potentials by 10-mV steps between 13 and 63 mV in $[Ca]_i$ of pCa 10. **A-2** indicates a change of membrane current when $[Ca]_i$ was changed from pCa 10 to pCa 7. **A-3** indicates that Ni^{2+} (1 mM) blocked transient inward current and abolished the decline of the outward current at a depolarizing pulse in $[Ca]_i$ of pCa 7. The horizontal bar in each panel indicates 0 nA. **B:** Effects of external Na^+-free and K^+-free solution. **B-1** shows current traces at every 10-mV step from 3 to 63 mV in normal Tyrode's solution. The $[Ca]_i$ was pCa 10. **B-2** shows current traces in Na^+-free and K^+-free solution. **B-3** indicates that I_K markedly increased when $[Ca]_i$ changed from pCa 10 to pCa 7. The horizontal bar in each panel indicates 0 nA. Unpublished from Tohse, with permission.

environment. Thus, the Ca^{2+} sensitivity of I_K was re-examined by these new techniques. In single cells, Trautwein et al. {19} demonstrated that action potential duration was shortened by pressure injection of Ca^{2+}, consistent with Ca^{2+} activation of I_K. However, subsequent reports using voltage-clamp experiments revealed that the delayed rectifier K^+ current was not increased by elevation of $[Ca]_i$ {20–22}. Two drawbacks of these papers may be pointed out: the use of the two-microelectrode voltage-clamp method and not isolating I_K from other Ca^{2+}-activated currents.

In 1987, Tohse et al. succeeded in isolating I_K from other currents in guinea-pig ventricular cells. By combining the patch-clamp methods and the intracellular perfusion technique, we directly demonstrated the intracellular Ca^{2+} sensitivity of I_K {23,24}. Typical results are illustrated in fig. 7-1. Figure 7-1A-1 shows the delayed rectification in normal external solution and $[Ca]_i$ of 10^{-10}M (pCa 10). After elevation of $[Ca]_i$ to pCa 7, an oscillating inward tail current was evoked, in addition to a slowly declining outward current during the test pulse (fig. 7-1A-2). These current changes may be produced by the Na-Ca exchange system because Ni^{2+} (1 mM), a blocker of Na-Ca ex-

change {25}, abolished these changes (fig. 7-1A-3). In the presence of Ni^{2+} the delayed rectification was prominent, and its amplitude was increased in comparison with the control current shown in fig. 7-1A-1. These findings indicate that other Ca^{2+}-dependent currents mask the Ca^{2+}-induced increase in I_K if the isolation of I_K is not sufficient. Therefore, Na^+ was removed from the intracellular and extracellular solutions to inhibit the Na-Ca exchange system. In addition, K^+ was also removed from the extracellular solution to inhibit the inward rectifier K^+ current (I_{K1}). The current traces in the Na- and K-free external solution are shown in fig. 7-1B-2 (fig. 7-1B-1 shows the current traces in the normal external solution). The delayed rectification and outward tail currents were clearly observed, indicating that I_K was completely isolated from other currents. After $[Ca]_i$ was elevated from pCa 10 to 7 (using the intracellular perfusion technique), the isolated I_K was markedly increased (fig. 7-1B-3).

The concentration-response relation between $[Ca]_i$ and I_K is shown in fig. 7-2. I_K was sensitive to $[Ca]_i$ above 10 nM. $[Ca]_i$ in diastole in the heart is reported to be ~10 nM {26}. Therefore, this curve implies that the Ca^{2+}-induced increase in I_K takes place during physiological

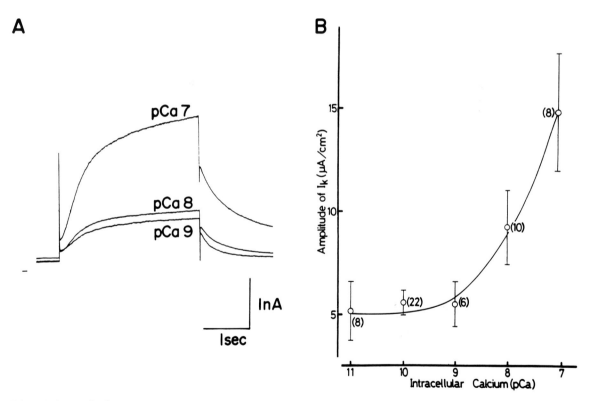

Fig. 7-2. **A:** Effect of $[Ca]_i$ elevation on the isolated I_K. Outward current traces were elicited by a 3-second test pulse from a holding potential of -30 mV to potentials of 50 mV in Na^+- and K^+-free solution at each $[Ca]_i$. The horizontal bar on the left, indicates the 0 current level. **B:** Concentration-response curve for I_K tail of $[Ca]_i$. The ordinate gives the current density of tail current of I_K elicited on return to a holding potential of -30 mV from a depolarizing pulse of 50 mV for 3 seconds. Numerals in parentheses are the number of different cells. Vertical bars indicate the standard error. Curves were fitted by eye. From Tohse {24}, with permission.

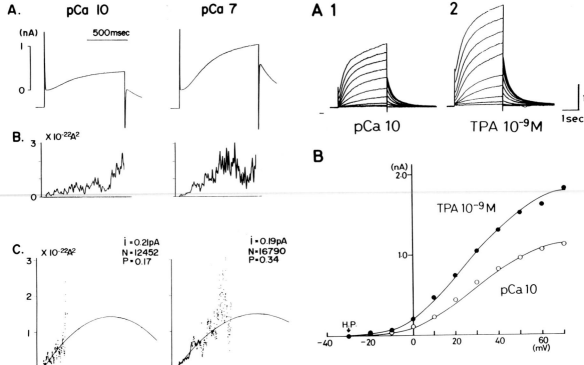

Fig. 7-3. Noise analysis of the isolated I_K. Ensembles of currents were elicited by a series of five identical pulses to 70 mV from −30 mV. **A:** Mean current corrected for leaked current. **B:** Variance (σ^2) of ion current as a function of time (t). **C:** σ^2 against mean current [I(t)]. Plots were fitted by parabolic curves given by the equation

$$\sigma^2 = iI(t) - I(t)^2/N,$$

where N is the number of functional channels per cell and i is unit amplitude of channel current. P is the probability of channels being in the open state. See Tohse {24} for details of the analysis. This illustration was taken from Tohse {24}, with permission.

Fig. 7-4. Effect of 10^{-9} M TPA on isolated I_K in Na$^+$- and K$^+$-free solution. **A:** Outward K$^+$ currents recorded by depolarizing pulses to 10 different potentials by 10-mV steps between −20 and 70 mV. The pulse duration was 3 seconds. The holding potential was −30 mV. **Left:** pCa 10 in pipette solution in the absence of TPA. **Right:** In the presence of 10^{-9} M TPA. Both the outward current on depolarization and its current tail on repolarization were increased by TPA. **B:** Current-voltage relations of tail current of I_K in the absence (open circles) and presence (closed circles) of TPA. It can be seen that TPA did not affect the voltage dependency of current activation. The zero current level is indicated by the horizontal bar at the lower left corner of A. From Tohse et al. {23}, with permission.

beating of the heart and plays an important role in repolarization of the action potential. The relation also indicates that I_K has a substantial basal activity, even at extremely low [Ca]$_i$ (pCa 11). Such basal activity was not observed in Ca^{2+}-activated K$^+$ channels (Meech channel) {27}.

Some studies reported on the single-channel activities of I_K {28–30}. However, there are no data about the relation between the I_K channel activity and [Ca]$_i$ because of difficulty with and the instability of continuous recording of the channel activity. Therefore, ensemble noise analysis was performed to investigate the effects of [Ca]$_i$ on properties of I_K channels (fig. 7-3) {24}. In the control condition (pCa 10), the unit amplitude, functional channel number per cell, and open probability of the I_K channel was 0.21 pA, 12,452, and 0.17, respectively. The elevation

of [Ca]$_i$ to pCa 7.0 increased the functional channel number and open probability of the I_K channel to 16,790 and 0.34, respectively, although there was no change in the unit amplitude.

Protein kinase C (PKC) is a Ca^{2+}-dependent protein kinase. When [Ca]$_i$ is elevated in the cardiac cytoplasm during physiological beating, it is possible that PKC is activated and modulates ion channels. Figure 7-4 shows the effects of a phorbol ester, and activator of PKC, on the isolated I_K in guinea-pig ventricular cells {23}. The phorbol ester TPA increased I_K and its tail current. Pretreatment with H-7, an inhibitor of PKC, abolished the effect of TPA.

Figure 7-5 provides more direct evidence for the PKC modulation {31}. Intracellular perfusion with purified PKC protein produced a marked increase in I_K. This observation indicates that PKC increases I_K by means of phosphorylation of the I_K channel protein. Therefore, it is quite important to examine the relation between the Ca^{2+}

A.

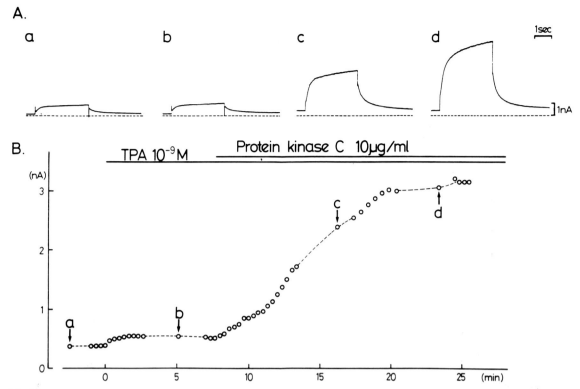

Fig. 7-5. Time course of the I_K increase produced by internal application of 10 µg/ml type III (α) protein kinase C. The amplitude of the I_K tail current was measured with a holding potential of -30 mV and a test potential of 50 mV. The $[Ca]_i$ was kept at pCa 9. At time 0, external perfusion of the cell with 10^{-9} M TPA was started. After 7 minutes, dialysis of the cell with protein kinase C was started. Examples of the current record are shown above the graph (**A–D**) for the time indicated on the graph. The broken lines indicate zero current level. From Tohse et al. {31}, with permission.

sensitivity of I_K and activation of PKC, since Ca^{2+} sensitivity appeared to be modulated by activated PKC. Figure 7-6 illustrates that the elevation of $[Ca]_i$ still increased I_K, even after inhibition of PKC by pretreatment with H-7. This result suggests that the I_K channel may possess an intracellular binding site for binding Ca^{2+}. On the other hand, the activation of PKC shifted the concentration-response curve for the I_K-increasing effects of $[Ca]_i$ leftward (fig. 7-7).

All these findings taken together suggest that the I_K channel possesses a phosphorylation site for PKC that is different from the site for protein kinase A {32,33}. The PKC-induced phosphorylation of the site may affect the affinity of the Ca^{2+}-binding site of the I_K channels (fig. 7-8). Recently we demonstrated {34} that stimulation of adrenergic α_1-receptors produced an increase in I_K through the activation of PKC in guinea-pig ventricular cells.

It is well known that I_K plays the most important role in the repolarization phase of the cardiac action potential. For example, sotalol and E-4031, which prolong action potential duration (APD), were found to specifically inhibit I_K {35,36}. Figure 7-9 illustrates the relationship between action potential, contraction time course, and I_K in guinea-pig ventricular muscles. This scheme suggests

that the Ca^{2+} transient occurring in advance of muscle contraction probably modulates the developing phase of I_K and, therefore, becomes one of the determinants of APD. In addition, the activation of PKC by stimulation of α_1-adrenoceptors may modulate a regulation of APD by $[Ca]_i$ through an enhancement of Ca^{2+} sensitivity of I_K. Irisawa and Hagiwara {37} reported that I_K in the rabbit sinoatrial cell was sensitive to $[Ca]_i$. It seems probable that regulation of APD by $[Ca]_i$ is also important for cardiac automaticity.

TRANSIENT OUTWARD CURRENT

In cardiac cell, two types of transient outward current (I_{to}) have been identified. One type showed slow inactivation and was blocked by 4-aminopyridine {38}. This current appeared to be insensitive to intracellular Ca^{2+} and appealed to be a K^+ current. Anther type of I_{to} showed rapid inactivation and was sensitive to intracellular Ca^{2+}. The first report about the Ca^{2+}-activated I_{to} appeared in 1980 {39}. In calf cardiac Purkinje fibers, removal of extracellular Ca^{2+} and intracellular injection of EGTA reduced I_{to}, which followed the Ca^{2+} current. Therefore Ca^{2+},

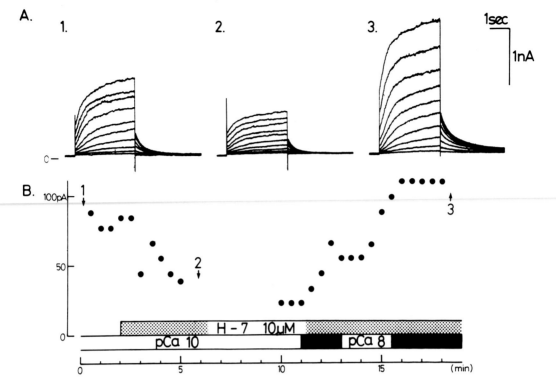

Fig. 7-6. Effect of the elevation of [Ca]$_i$ on I$_K$ in a PKC-inhibited cell. **A:** Panel 1 shows the isolated I$_K$ elicited by a 3-second test pulse between −20 and 70 mV, from a holding potential of −30 mV, at [Ca]$_i$ of pCa 10. The PKC inhibitor H-7 (10 μM) was treated with a cell to inhibit a basal activity of PKC (**panel 2**). The current was reduced by the treatment. **Panel 3** shows the I$_K$ increased by the elevation of [Ca]$_i$ from pCa 10 to 8, in the presence of H-7. **B:** Time course of I$_K$ tail current elicited by a 3-second pulse to 50 mV. Arrows indicate time points where the currents shown in panel A were recorded. Unpublished from Tohse, Kameyama, and Irisawa, with permission.

which enters intracellularly through Ca^{2+} channels, may activate the I$_{to}$. In 1982 Coraboeuf and Carmeliet {40} demonstrated the coexistence of two types of I$_{to}$ in sheep Purkinje fibers. They also showed that Ca^{2+}-activated I$_{to}$ was blocked by caffeine, which inhibits Ca^{2+} uptake of the sarcoplasmic reticulum.

After the introduction of the patch-clamp method, several studies {41–44} described Ca^{2+}-activated I$_{to}$ in various cardiac cells, including human atrial cells {41}. All these studies assumed that Ca^{2+}-activated I$_{to}$ was carried by K$^+$, although a reversal potential of the Ca^{2+}-activated I$_{to}$ was not demonstrated. Recently Zygmunt and Gibbons {45,46} examined the reversal potential of Ca^{2+}-activated I$_{to}$ in rabbit ventricular myocytes. Data indicated that Ca^{2+}-activated I$_{to}$ was carried by Cl$^-$. They also showed that Cl$^-$ channel blockers (SITS and DIDS) abolished the current. However, Ca^{2+}-activated K$^+$ channel activities, having a time course similar to I$_{to}$, were also directly recorded {8}. Therefore, at the present time the Ca^{2+}-activated I$_{to}$ is thought to consist of at least two types of current: the Ca^{2+}-activated Cl$^-$ current and the Ca^{2+}-activated K$^+$ current.

Although the Ca^{2+}-activated I$_{to}$ may contribute to developing phase 1 of the action potential (the notch) {42}, the precise kinetics and Ca^{2+} sensitivity is not clear. Because activity of the I$_{to}$ is exclusively dependent upon activation of the preceding Ca^{2+} current {45}, it is difficult to record I$_{to}$ isolated from the Ca^{2+} current. In addition, there is no report demonstrating a quantitative relation between I$_{to}$ and [Ca]$_i$. If these points are elucidated, the physiological significance of the Ca^{2+}-activated I$_{to}$ will be disclosed.

HYPERPOLARIZATION-ACTIVATED INWARD CURRENT

Hagiwara and Irisawa {47} reported that the hyperpolarization-activated inward current (I$_f$) was increased by intracellular Ca^{2+} in rabbit single sinoatrial node cells. The sensitivity of the intracellular Ca^{2+} of I$_f$ was independent of the cAMP-A-kinase system and PKC activities. They suggested that intracellular Ca^{2+} directly modulated the I$_f$ channels. However, Zaza et al. {48} did not observe Ca^{2+} sensitivity of I$_f$ in the isolated patch of rabbit sinoatrial cells and denied the direct action of Ca^{2+}. These are

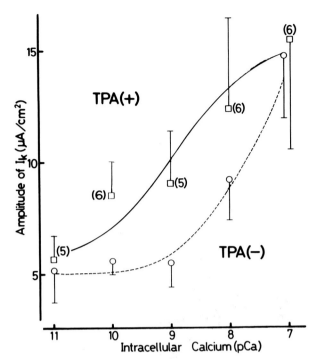

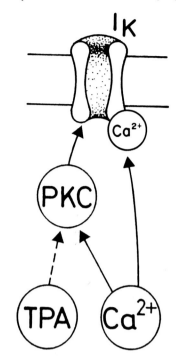

Fig. 7-7. Concentration-response curve for the increasing effect of $[Ca]_i$ on I_K in the presence of TPA. The ordinate gives the current density of the tail current of I_K elicited by a return to the holding potential of $-30\,mV$ from a depolarizing pulse of $50\,mV$ for 3 seconds. Squares indicate the mean values, and numerals in parentheses give the number of cells used in the presence of 1 nM TPA. Circles are the current density of the I_K tail obtained in the same condition, except in the absence of TPA, taken from fig. 7-2. Vertical bars give the standard error. Curves were fitted by eye. From Tohse et al. {31}, with permission.

Fig. 7-8. Cartoon of the interaction between PKC, $[Ca]_i$, and the I_K channel. $[Ca]_i$ directly binds to the I_K channel protein in addition to activating PKC. TPA enhances I_K channel activity through activation of PKC. PKC phosphorylates the I_K channel protein and then increases the sensitivity of I_K to $[Ca]_i$.

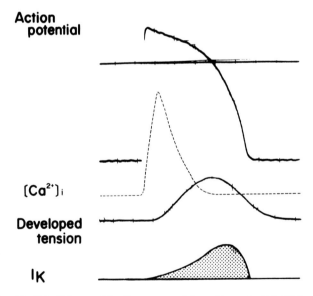

Fig. 7-9. Scheme of the time course of the action potential, $[Ca]_i$, developed tension, and I_K. The schematic time course of $[Ca]_i$, showed as a broken line, indicates the Ca^{2+} transient. The action potential and developed tension were recorded in guinea-pig papillary muscle preparations. The illustration shows the close relationship between the time courses of the Ca^{2+} transient and the activation of I_K.

the only two reports describing the Ca^{2+} sensitivity of I_f so far. More deep and broad-ranging investigation should be carried out to elucidate the effect of $[Ca]_i$ on this current.

Ca^{2+}-ACTIVATED NONSELECTIVE CATION CHANNELS

It was Colquhoun et al. {49} who firstly reported the single-channel activities of the Ca^{2+}-activated nonselective cation channels in cultured neonatal rat heart cells in 1981. Matsuda {22} depicted a nonselective current (I_{non}) in guinea-pig heart cells that was activated by the intracellular injection of Ca^{2+} and suggested that the current could be closely related to the nonselective cation channel described by Colquhoun et al. {49}. Later some reports {50–52} indicated that this channel produces the transient inward current that generates the arrhythmogenic delayed afterdepolarization in Ca^{2+}-loaded cells {53}. In adult heart cells, Ehara et al. {54} demonstrated the single-channel activities of the nonselective cation channel, and suggested that this activity of the channel might explain the Ca^{2+}-activated background current of single myocytes {22,55}. On the other hand, some reports {56–58} showed that the Na-Ca exchange current could also produce the transient inward current in the Ca^{2+}-loaded cells. Therefore, both currents may contribute to the generation of delayed afterdepolarization.

CONCLUSIONS

The patch-clamp method and its related techniques stimulated a remarkable accumulation of knowledge on ion channels activated by intracellular Ca^{2+}. Modification of ion channels by intracellular Ca^{2+} is very important for understanding the action potential configuration and automaticity, because the action potential is usually evoked with the Ca^{2+} transient. Ca^{2+} sensitivity of I_K and I_{to} may especially influence action potential duration. In fact, many previous experimental studies {4,19,21} showed that elevation of $[Ca]_i$ produced abbreviation of action potentials. However, there are only few studies {28–30} on single-channel activities of these currents. Therefore, study of single-channel activities should be done to obtain more precise data about the relation between these channels and $[Ca]_i$.

In the pathological condition, the nonselective cation channels are essential for the generation of delayed afterdepolarization. Because this channel requires very high $[Ca]_i$ (EC_{50} = 1.2 μM) {54}, it may open only in the pathological condition, i.e., in the ischemic condition and during intoxication of cardiac glycosides {20,21,55}. In addition, Ca^{2+} sensitivity of I_f may be arrhythmogenic. It is well known that I_f produces automaticity of the cardiac Purkinje cells {59,60}. This automaticity is often critical for the ectopic automaticity of the ischemic heart disease, although it is masked in the physiological condition. The ischemic damage produces elevation of $[Ca]_i$ in Purkinje cells and may enhance automaticity through a Ca^{2+}-induced increase in I_f.

The cardiac Meech channel may also be important in the ischemic condition because of its protective effect on diseased cells. In the ischemic condition, accumulated Ca^{2+} in the sarcoplasm may activate the Meech channel. Therefore, the Meech channel may produce ischemia-induced abbreviation of the action potential {12}. Ischemic-induced abbreviation of the action potential probably limits Ca^{2+} influx during the action potential, and then reduces Ca^{2+} accumulation during ischemia.

In summary, investigation of the Ca^{2+} sensitivity of the channels described in this chapter will disclose a new landscape to our understanding of the normal and pathological electroactivities of the heart.

REFERENCES

1. Irisawa H: Electrical activity of rabbit sino-atrial node as studied by double sucrose gap method. In: *Proceedings of the Satellite Symposium of the 25th International Congress of Europe 1972.* Brussels: Presses Académiques Européenes, 1972, pp 242–248.

2. Meech RW: Intracellular calcium injection causes increased potassium conductance in *Aplysia* nerve cells. *Comp Biochem Physiol* 42A:493–499, 1972.

3. Meech RW: The sensitivity of *Helix apersa* neurones to injected calcium ions. *J Physiol (Lond)* 237:259–277, 1974.

4. Isenberg G: Is potassium conductance of cardiac Purkinje fibres controlled by $[Ca^{2+}]_i$? *Nature* 253:273–274, 1975.

5. Isenberg G: Cardiac Purkinje fibres: $[Ca^{2+}]_i$ controls steady state potassium conductance. *Pflügers Arch* 371:71–76, 1977.

6. Eisner DA, Vaughan-Jones RD: Do calcium-activated potassium channels exist in the heart? *Cell Calcium* 4:371–386, 1983.

7. Kameyama M, Kakei M, Sato R, Shibasaki T, Mastuda H, Irisawa H: Intracellular Na^+ activates a K^+ channel in mammalian cardiac cells. *Nature* 309:354–356, 1984.

8. Callewaert G, Vereeke J, Carmeliet E: Existence of a calcium-dependent potassium channel in the membrane of cow cardiac Purkinje cells. *Pflügers Arch* 406:424–426, 1986.

9. Pallotta BS, Magleby KL, Barrett JN: Single channel recordings of Ca^{2+}-activated K^+ currents in rat muscle cell culture. *Nature* 293:471–474, 1981.

10. Baró I, Escande D: A Ca^{2+}-activated K^+ current in guinea-pig atrial myocytes. *Pflügers Arch* 414(Suppl 1):S168, 1989.

11. Hagiwara N, Matsuda N, Shoda M, Tamura K, Irisawa H: Calcium activated potassium current in single rabbit cardiac myocytes. *Jpn J Physiol* 42(Suppl):S266, 1992.

12. Nakaya H, Takeda Y, Tohse N, Kanno M: Effects of ATP-sensitive K^+ channel blockers on the action potential shortening in hypoxic and ischemic myocardium. *Br J Pharmacol* 103:1019–1026, 1991.

13. McGuigan JAS: Some limitations of the double sucrose gap, and its use in a study of the slow outward current in mammalian ventricular muscle. *J Physiol* 240:775–806, 1974.

14. Brown H, DiFrancesco D: Voltage-clamp investigations of membrane currents underlying pace-maker activity in rabbit sino-atrial node. *J Physiol* 308:331–351, 1980.

15. Goto M, Hyōdō T, Ikeda K: Ca-dependent outward currents in bullfrog myocardium. *Jpn J Physiol* 33:837–854, 1983.

16. Kass RS, Tsien RW: Control of action potential duration by calcium ions in cardiac Purkinje fibers. *J Gen Physiol* 67:599–617, 1976.

17. Kass RS: Delayed rectification in the cardiac Purkinje fiber is not activated by intracellular calcium. *Biophys J* 45:837–839, 1984.

18. Hume JR, Giles W, Robinson K, Shibata EF, Nathan RD, Kanai K, Rasmusson R: A time- and voltage-dependent K^+ current in single cardiac cells from bullfrog atrium. *J Gen Physiol* 88:777–798, 1986.

19. Trautwein W, Taniguchi J, Noma A: The effect of intracellular cyclic nucleotides and calcium on the action potential and acetylcholine response of isolated cardiac cells. *Pflügers Arch* 392:307–314, 1982.

20. Matsuda H, Noma A, Kurachi Y, Irisawa H: Transient depolarization and spontaneous voltage fluctuations in isolated single cells from guinea pig ventricles: Calcium-mediated membrane potential fluctuations. *Circ Res* 51:142–151, 1982.

21. Kurachi Y: The effects of intracellular protons on the electrical activity of single ventricular cells. *Pflügers Arch* 394:264–270, 1982.

22. Matsuda H: Effects of intracellular calcium injection on steady state membrane currents in isolated single ventricular cells. *Pflügers Arch* 397:81–83, 1983.

23. Tohse N, Kameyama M, Irisawa H: Intracellular Ca^{2+} and protein kinase C modulate K^+ current in guinea pig heart cells. *Am J Physiol* 253:H1321–H1324, 1987.

24. Tohse N: Calcium-sensitive delayed rectifier potassium current in guinea pig ventricular cells. *Am J Physiol* 258: H1200–H1207, 1990.

25. Kimura J, Miyamae S, Noma A: Identification of sodium-calcium exchange current in single ventricular cells of guinea-pig. *J Physiol (Lond)* 384:199–222, 1987.

26. Langer GA: Sodium-calcium exchange in the heart. *Annu Rev Physiol* 44:435–449, 1982.

27. Barrett JN, Magleby KL, Pallotta BS: Properties of single calcium-activated potassium channels in cultured rat muscle. *J Physiol (Lond)* 331:211–230, 1982.

28. Shibasaki T: Conductance and kinetics of delayed rectifier potassium channels in nodal cells of the rabbit heart. *J Physiol (Lond)* 387:227–250, 1987.

29. Clapham DE, Logothetis DE: Delayed rectifier K^+ current in embryonic chick heart ventricle. *Am J Physiol* 254: H192–H197, 1988.

30. Duchatelle-Gourdon I, Hartzell HC: Single delayed rectifier channels in frog atrial cells: Effects of β-adrenergic stimulation. *Biophys J* 57:903–909, 1990.

31. Tohse N, Kameyama M, Sekiguchi K, Shearman MS, Kanno M: Protein kinase C activation enhances the delayed rectifier potassium current in guinea-pig heart cells. *J Mol Cell Cardiol* 22:725–734, 1990.

32. Walsh KB, Kass RS: Regulation of a heart potassium channel by protein kinase A and C. *Science* 242:67–69, 1988.

33. Yazawa K, Kameyama M: Mechanism of receptor-mediated modulation of the delayed outward potassium current in guinea-pig ventricular myocytes. *J Physiol (Lond)* 421: 135–150, 1990.

34. Tohse N, Nakaya H, Kanno M: α_1-Adrenoceptor stimulation enhances the delayed rectifier K^+ current of guinea pig ventricular cells through the activation of protein kinase C. *Circ Res* 71:1441–1446, 1992.

35. Komeichi K, Tohse N, Nakaya H, Shimizu M, Zhu M-Y, Kanno M: Effects of N-acetylprocainamide and sotalol on ion currents in isolated guinea-pig ventricular myocytes. *Eur J Pharmacol* 187:313–322, 1990.

36. Sanguinetti MC, Jurkiewicz NK: Two components of cardiac delayed rectifier K^+ current: Differential sensitivity to block by class III antiarrhythmic agents. *J Gen Physiol* 96:195–215, 1990.

37. Irisawa H, Hagiwara N: Pacemaker mechanism of mammalian sinoatrial node cells. In: Mazgalev T, Dreifus LS, Michelson EL (eds) *Electrophysiology of the Sinoatrial and Atrioventricular Nodes*. New York: Alan R. Liss, 1988, pp 33–52.

38. Kenyon JL, Gibbons WR: 4-Aminopyridine and the early outward current of sheep cardiac Purkinje fibers. *J Gen Physiol* 73:139–157, 1979.

39. Siegelbum SA, Tsien RW: Calcium-activated transient outward current in calf cardiac Purkinje fibres. *J Physiol (Lond)* 299:485–506, 1980.

40. Coraboeuf E, Carmeliet E: Existence of two transient outward currents in sheep cardiac Purkinje fibers. *Pflügers Arch* 392:352–359, 1982.

41. Escande D, Coulombe A, Faivre J-F, Deroubaix E, Coraboeuf E: Two types of transient outward currents in adult human atrial cells. *Am J Physiol* 252:H142–H148, 1987.

42. Hiraoka M, Kawano S: Calcium-sensitive and insensitive transient outward current in rabbit ventricular myocytes. *J Physiol (Lond)* 410:187–212, 1989.

43. Tseng G-N, Hoffman BF: Two components of transient outward current in canine ventricular myocytes. *Circ Res* 64:633–647, 1989.

44. Dukes ID, Morad M: The transient K^+ current in rat ventricular myocytes: Evaluation of its Ca^{2+} and Na^+ dependence. *J Physiol (Lond)* 435:395–420, 1991.

45. Zygmunt AC, Gibbons WR: Calcium-activated chloride current in rabbit ventricular myocytes. *Circ Res* 68:424–437, 1991.

46. Zygmunt AC, Gibbons WR: Properties of the calcium-activated chloride current in heart. *J Gen Physiol* 99:391–414, 1992.

47. Hagiwara N, Irisawa H: Modulation by intracellular Ca^{2+} of the hyperpolarization-activated inward current in rabbit single sino-atrial node cells. *J Physiol (Lond)* 409:121–141, 1989.

48. Zaza A, Maccaferri G, Mangoni M, DiFrancesco D: Intracellular calcium does not directly modulate cardiac pacemaker (i_f) channels. *Pflügers Arch* 419:662–664, 1991.

49. Colquhoun D, Neher E, Reuter H, Stevens CF: Inward current channels activated by intracellular Ca in cultured cardiac cells. *Nature* 294:752–754, 1981.

50. Clusin WT: Caffeine induces a transient inward current in cultured cardiac cells. *Nature* 301:248–250, 1984.

51. Cannell MB, Lederer WJ: The arrhythmogenic current I_{TI} in the absence of electrogenic sodium-calcium exchange in sheep cardiac Purkinje fibres. *J Physiol (Lond)* 374:201–219, 1986.

52. Shimoni Y, Giles W: Separation of Na-Ca exchange and transient inward currents in heart cells. *Am J Physiol* 253: H1330–H1333, 1987.

53. Kass RS, Lederer WJ, Tsien RW, Weingart R: Role of calcium ions in transient inward currents and after-contractions induced by strophantidin in cardiac Purkinje fibres. *J Physiol (Lond)* 281:187–208, 1978.

54. Ehara T, Noma A, Ono K: Calcium-activated non-selective cation channel in ventricular cells isolated from adult guinea-pig hearts. *J Physiol (Lond)* 403:117–133, 1988.

55. Sato R, Noma A, Kurachi Y, Irisawa H: Effects of intracellular acidification on membrane currents in ventricular cells of the guinea pig. *Circ Res* 57:553–561, 1985.

56. Arlock P, Katzung BG: Effects of sodium substitutes on transient inward current and tension in guinea-pig and ferret papillary muscle. *J Physiol (Lond)* 360:105–120, 1985.

57. Fedida D, Noble D, Rankin AC, Spindler AJ: The arrhythmogenic transient inward current i_{TI} and related contraction in isolated guinea-pig ventricular myocytes. *J Physiol (Lond)* 392:523–542, 1987.

58. Lipp P, Pott L: Transient inward current in guinea-pig atrial myocytes reflects a change of sodium-calcium exchange current. *J Physiol (Lond)* 397:601–630, 1988.

59. DiFrancesco D: A new interpretation of the pace-maker current in calf Purkinje fibres. *J Physiol (Lond)* 314:359–376, 1981.

60. Callewaert G, Carmeliet E, Vereecke J: Single cardiac Purkinje cells: General electrophysiology and voltage-clamp analysis of the pace-maker current. *J Physiol (Lond)* 349: 643–661, 1984.

CHAPTER 8

ATP-Sensitive K Channels in the Cardiovascular System

W.J. LEDERER & COLIN G. NICHOLS

INTRODUCTION

The ATP-sensitive potassium channel was first "discovered" in heart muscle by Noma in 1983 {77}. Since that time it has been found in many cell types, including pancreatic betal cells {7,14}, skeletal muscle {90}, smooth muscle cells {24,55,108}, renal tubule cells {109,110}, and in other diverse cells, including cells in the central nervous system {14,15,71}. This channel appears to play an important and distinct role in the cellular physiology of the tissues involved. In the pancreatic beta cells, for example, the channels operate as sensors of the metabolic status of the cells and thus may indirectly act as glucose sensors. Thus [ATP] is an important factor in this signaling pathway. When intracellular ATP concentration rises, the cells depolarize because the ATP-sensitive K-channel activity declines. The depolarization activates calcium channels, and the influx of calcium causes the secretion of insulin. Increased insulin levels in the blood facilitate the transport of glucose into the cell, which, in turn, leads to an increase in intracellular [ATP]. The increase in intracellular [ATP] inhibits the K_{ATP} channels and consequently hyperpolarizes the pancreatic beta cells. In the cardiovascular system, the ATP-sensitive K channels also serve as metabolic sensors. The channels appear to be activated during ischemia and tend to "clamp" membrane potential in vascular smooth muscle and heart cells close to E_K. Depending on the degree of activation during ischemia or anoxia, the ATP-sensitive K channels may reduce the extent of contraction in vascular smooth or cardiac muscle, or may lead to decreased resting tone of the muscle (see below).

In this brief review we have focused on certain issues of particular interest. For more comprehensive discussion of other issues see several recent reviews {13,15,71}. It is important to note that many investigators have contributed significantly to our understanding of the ATP-sensitive K channel, much of which forms both the specifically cited and uncited background to this presentation, including Findlay {36–43}, Noma {48,52,53,77–80,83,84,94}, Weiss {27,45,105,106,111–114}, Ashcroft {6–11,13,15, 76}, Escande {31,32,99,100,115}, Standen {25,26,85,89–92}, Nelson {55,61,68,69,92}, Daut {24,108}, Carmeliet {21,22,54,82}, Hiraoka {33–35,46,67,107}, Kurachi

{122–123}, and Trube {12,18,81,88,103,117,118}. We apologize for not identifying all of the important contributors, but the scope of our presentation is limited.

WHAT IS THE ATP-SENSITIVE K CHANNEL?

There appear to be two characteristics of the the ATP-sensitive K channel (or K_{ATP} channel) that distinguish it from other potassium channels {13,15,71,77}. These two general features are functionally important in all tissues in which this channel type is found. (a) The channels are inhibited by intracellular ATP. Thus as intracellular ATP declines, the channels are activated further. In cells that have a resting potential positive to the equilibrium potential for the channel (E_{K-ATP}), the cells are hyperpolarized by the activation of the channel. In cells that have a resting potential very close to E_{K-ATP}, activation of the channels by low [ATP] tends to clamp the cell potential at E_{K-ATP}, thus opposing electrical depolarization by calcium and sodium channels. (b) The channels are blocked by sulfonylurea drugs (e.g., tolbutamide, glibenclamide). The exact sensitivity of the K_{ATP} channel to blockade by $[ATP]_i$ or the $k_{0.5}$ for inhibition by sulfonylureas such as glibenclamide varies from tissue to tissue. In the cardiovascular system, almost all of the detailed biophysical work has been done in heart muscle because of the abundance of expression found there. Nevertheless, the K_{ATP} channels in vascular smooth muscle, although sparsely distributed over the plasma membrane surface, appear to play an important regulatory role and have been hypothesized to be a central factor in the vascular response to metabolic stress {23,24,69}.

At normal intracellular [ATP] the K_{ATP} channel is almost always closed (see below). This raises the practical question, how is the channel modulated? Does intracellular [ATP] vary normally? When is [ATP] modulated by physiological events? When is it modulated by pathological events?

NORMAL [ATP]

Normal [ATP] has been reported to be between 5 and 15 mM {4,5,44}. During ischemia and anoxia, there ap-

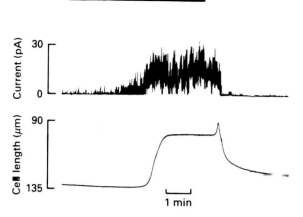

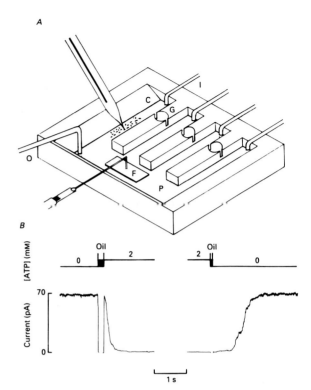

Fig. 8-1. Activation of K_{ATP} channels during chemical anoxia in a single rat heart muscle cell. Isolated rat ventricular myocytes were exposed to complete metabolic blockade by bathing the cells in a normal extracellular salt solution containing 10 mM 2-deoxyglucose and then adding 2 mM cyanide (at the time indicated by the bar in the figure). The **top panel** shows the single-channel records obtained from an on-cell patch-clamp electrode. The ***bottom trace*** shows a continuous measurement of cell length obtained optically. The very large shortening reveals the development of a "rigor contraction," which provides independent evidence that $[ATP]_i$ is very low. The activation of the K_{ATP} channels precedes the development of the rigor contraction and is rapidly reversed by the removal of cyanide. Parallel experiments show that as the K_{ATP} channel is activated, the cardiac action potential is shortened. The shortening of the cardiac action potential during anoxia is due in large part to the activation of the ATP-sensitive K channels. Other sarcolemmal channels in heart muscle are also affected by anoxia and ischemia, and contribute to the shortening of the action potential. Figure taken from Nichols and Lederer {70} and used with permission.

Fig. 8-2. The modified oil-gate bath is used to examine K_{ATP} channels in isolated sarcolemmal membrane patches. **A:** A schematic diagram of the modified oil-gate bath (derived from the chamber used by Qin and Noma {83}) is shown in panel A (top). The bath consists of four or more channels (C), each supplied by a separate solution supply line (I). The solution level within the chamber is controlled by an outflow pump that removes solution from the chamber via tube O under feedback control of a level indicator F {20}. Changing solutions is accomplished by moving the pipette from one channel into another through the oil-gate in partition G. **B:** Current records are shown for membrane patches containing about 40 active K_{ATP} channels in 0 mM ATP or in 2 mM ATP. As the electrode goes through the oil, a discontinuity in the current record is observed and on entering the 2 mM ATP solution, the current rapidly falls from about 70 pA to 0 pA. When the process is reversed the current rises from 0 pA to about 70 pA. The rapid change of extracellular solutions makes it possible to quickly measure the properties of the K_{ATP} channels in many solutions before channel rundown becomes unacceptably large. Figure taken from Lederer and Nichols {57} and used with permission.

pears to be only a moderate decline in intracellular [ATP], even when contraction is significantly affected by the experiment {4,5}. This fundamental observation, based on a whole-heart NMR spectroscopy analysis, raises an issue that has not been fully addressed even today: How important is [ATP] variation in controlling the function of the K_{ATP} channel? This is a research topic that is being actively investigated by many laboratories and it should also be stated that other factors play important roles in modulating K_{ATP} channels {71} (see below).

WHERE IS THE ATP-SENSITIVE K CHANNEL FOUND IN THE HEART? WHAT IS THE CHANNEL DENSITY?

The ATP-sensitive K channels have been identified by patch-clamp investigation in atrial and ventricular muscle cells, and by pharmacological implication in the coronary arteries and arterioles. A complete survey of the abundance of the K_{ATP} channels in the different myocardial cells is far

from complete, but ventricular muscle appears to have more channels per unit surface area than atrial muscle cells. In all myocardial cells examined to date, there are a very large number of channels when compared to other potassium channels or calcium channels. In rat ventricular muscle cells there may be more than 10 K_{ATP} channels per square micron. The large number of K_{ATP} channels per unit area combined with the presence of channels in virtually all myocardial cells suggests that the K_{ATP} channel is probably important in cardiac cellular physiology. This suggestion has led to widespread interest in the channel and a broad effort to elucidate its functional importance.

WHAT ARE THE PROPERTIES OF THE ATP-SENSITIVE K CHANNEL?

In heart muscle the channel can be described as an ATP-sensitive, inwardly rectifying potassium channel. The rectification appears to arise from blockade of outward current by intracellular magnesium, a feature found in other inwardly rectifying potassium channels. The single-channel conductance at around 0 mV in symmetrical KCl (140 mM) is about 70 pS in heart {53}. In physiological salt solutions, however, the conductance is less (approximately 25 pS over the voltage range −80 mV to +20 mV) {36,70}. The channels opening and closing probabilities are largely voltage independent. Thus, when the channel is opened at low [ATP], its opening and closing rates appear to be set largely by [ATP]. The channel appears to require phosphorylation in order to open (see fig. 8-4).

ATP sensitivity

Intracellular ATP blocks the K_{ATP} channel. In very low [ATP] the K_{ATP} channel has a high open probability, as shown in fig. 8-3. A graph of the relationship between [ATP] and P_o of the K_{ATP} channel shows that the P_o falls quite rapidly as [ATP] rises. The Hill coefficient of the relationship is around 2.0 with a $K_{0.5}$ of between 20 μM and 200 μM, depending on the conditions (see below). It has been suggested, because of the Hill coefficient and identified interactions between ATP and other nucleotide phosphates, that there are at least two ATP binding sites that regulate the opening and closing of the channel {71–73}. Significantly, ATP sensitivity is not the same for K_{ATP} channels from different tissues, nor is sulfonylurea sensitivity. Recent reports suggest that ATP sensitivity can be modified by brief treatment of the intracellular aspect of the sarcolemma with the proteolytic enzymes trypsin and chymotrypsin without altering conductance {74}. This result suggests that at least some of the regulation of the K_{ATP} channel is on a region of the channel protein (or on a channel subunit protein) that is distinct from the poreforming region of the channel {1,74}.

Sensitivity to other factors

Because there are many cellular factors that may change during anoxia or ischemia, it is important to determine if the sensitivity of the K_{ATP} channel changes as the possible modulators increase or decrease in concentration. While increasing ADP may reduce the sensitivity of the channel to ATP under normal conditions by a factor of 5 {70}, only smaller effects were observed with intracellular acidification (factor of 2), and no effect was found with increases in intracellular inorganic phosphate levels or lactate levels (see fig. 8-3). Other dinucleotide and trinucleotide phosphates can block and activate the K_{ATP} channel {57,123}.

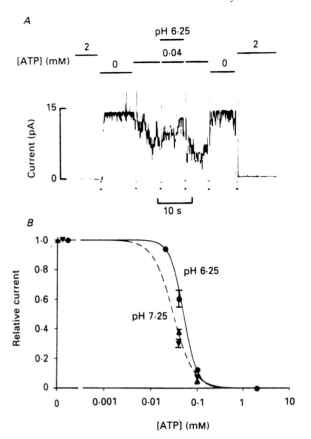

Fig. 8-3. Metabolic factors modulate the relationship between [ATP] and the probability that a K_{ATP} channel opens. The effect of [H$^+$], [lactate], and inorganic [phosphate] on the ATP dependence of the K_{ATP} channel activity. **A:** Record of current in a patch of membrane from a rat ventricular myocyte using the oil-gate bath described in fig. 8-2. The record shows how channel activity in 0.04 mM ATP changes when pH is changed from 7.25 to 6.25. **B:** The dose-response relationship for the [ATP]-dependent inhibition of K_{ATP} channels at two pH values: 7.25 (dashed line) and 6.26 (continuous line). The filled upside-down triangles (∇) show results obtained in the presence of 20 mM lactate, and the right-side-up filled triangles (Δ) show results obtained in the presence of 20 mM phosphate, both at pH 7.25. It is clear that intracellular acidification decreases the sensitivity of the K_{ATP} channels to [ATP], while there is virtually no effect of increases in intracellular lactate or phosphate. The fit curves are drawn according to the general equation:

$$I = \left[1 + \frac{ATP}{K}\right]^{-H},$$

where I is the relative current, ATP is the concentration of cytoplasmic ATP, K is the nucleotide concentration causing inhibition of the relative current to its half-maximal level, and H is the Hill coefficient. At pH 7.25, K = 25 μM and H = 2. At pH 6.25, K = 50 μM and H = 3. Figure taken from Lederer and Nichols {57} and used with permission.

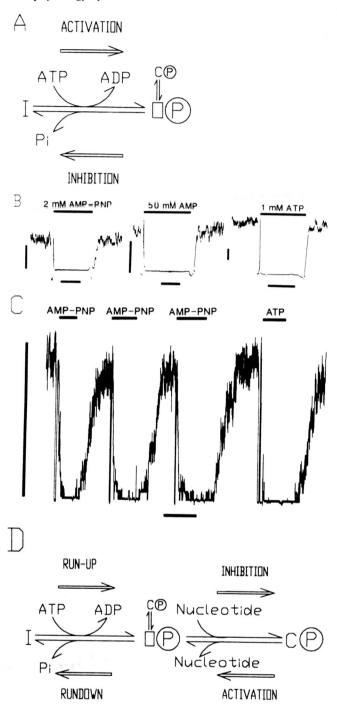

Fig. 8-4. Phosphorylation of the channel may be a necessary precondition for opening the K$_{ATP}$ channel, but the channel is "gated" without additional phosphorylation. **A:** Model of K$_{ATP}$ channel regulation according to Ribalet et al. {87}. Phosphorylation and dephosphorylation are responsible for the gating of the K$_{ATP}$ channel from the closed state to the open state, respectively. **B:** Reversible channel closure on exposure to nucleotides. From left to right the membrane patches were exposed to 2 mM AMP-PNP, 50 mM AMP, and 1 mM ATP. In each case reversible channel closure was the result. It does not matter whether or not the nucleotide can phosphorylate the K$_{ATP}$ channel. This result provides evidence that phosphorylation/dephosphorylation is the mechanism that controls the gating of the channel open and closed. It is widely recognized that phosphorylation of the K$_{ATP}$ channel appears to control, regulate, or significantly influence the "run-up" and "run-down" of the channel {36,43,63,81,87,102}. **C:** Evidence that the nonphosphorylating ATP analog, AMP-PNP (1 mM), can repeatedly inhibit K$_{ATP}$ channel activity and compares favorably to the response of ATP (0.5 mM). **D:** Model of the K$_{ATP}$ channel behavior describes how run-up requires phosphorylation but gating of the channel by ATP does not require further phosphorylation. Figure taken from Nichols and Lederer {72} and used with permission.

HOW DOES THE ATP-SENSITIVE K CHANNEL OPERATE IN FUNCTIONING MYOCARDIUM?

Our initial series of experiments began when we observed extremely large outward currents that were activated by chemical anoxia (exposure of cells to 5 mM 2-deoxy-glucose and 2 mM cyanide) {58}. Subsequent investigations showed similar effects with true anoxia {93,120}. Additional investigations demonstrated that the activation of these events and of single channels were due to the fall in intracellular [ATP] {57,70,93}. Such an experiment is shown in fig. 8-1. There is consequently primary support for Noma's initial speculation that the K_{ATP} channel may regulate or help to regulate contractile function during anoxia or ischemia {52,53,77}.

Given that the channels are plentiful but that their P_o (probability that the channels are open) is 0.5 at very low levels of [ATP], an important question is raised. Is there any way to investigate the possibility that the channels operate to affect cardiac behavior in normal or nearly normal heart muscle? The obstacle that is faced in any such investigation is the NMR spectroscopy results, which suggest that "global" intracellular [ATP] may fall by only 50%, possibly from around 5 mM to 2.5 mM {2-4,29,30}. The problem has been approached by trying to estimate by how much the intracellular [ATP] would have to decline in order for the activation of K_{ATP} channels to shorten the action potential by 50%. The result was that the [ATP] would have to fall to about 1.0 mM {75}. This result was very encouraging, but how was it possible?

The shortening of the action potential occurs at a relatively high level of intracellular [ATP] for at least two reasons. First, there are a large number of K_{ATP} channels compared with the number of other channels. Second, the single-channel conductance is larger than many channels (e.g., Na or Ca channels). The sum of these effects suggests that even if the channels are largely inhibited by millimolar [ATP], there are enough total K_{ATP} channels available so that some of the channels would be opened by the reduced [ATP] and those that did open would provide sufficient current to shorten the action potential significantly. The shorter action potential would be the more immediate cause of the negative inotropic effect of anoxia/ischemia because less calcium would enter the cell during the action potential.

Influence of spatial heterogeneity

The NMR data do not provide any spatial resolution. If the fall of intracellular [ATP] is not uniform within the heart during anoxia/ischemia, then that will have profound effects on the influence of the K_{ATP} channel in regulating the electrical activity of heart muscle. A simple calculation demonstrates this point. Assuming that the current produced by heart cells can freely affect all heart cells by conduction through gap junctions, then the following calculation can be completed. Assume that 1% of all heart cells consume all of their ATP so that [ATP] is zero. Assume that the remaining 99% of the heart cells have all of their ATP (i.e., no loss or change). Under these conditions, enough current would be activated in the 1% of cells to shorten the action potential by 50%, but essentially no change in [ATP] would be measured by the NMR spectroscopy analysis. Thus if spatial heterogeneity of [ATP] occurred within the myocardium, some regions may be metabolically unimpaired, while other regions may suffer metabolically and influence a much larger region because of the large amount of K_{ATP} channel current that can be activated from the very small region. At the present time the influence of spatial heterogeneity of [ATP] is appealing, makes physiological sense, but has not yet been proven.

HOW DOES THE ATP-SENSITIVE K CHANNEL OPERATE IN VASCULAR SMOOTH MUSCLE?

In coronary arteries Daut and coworkers have provided evidence that K_{ATP} channels are modulated under normal conditions by measuring changes in pressure and flow during the application of a sulphonylurea K_{ATP} channel blocker {24} Clapp and Gurney {23} showed that the resting membrane potential of pulmonary vascular smooth muscle cells was made more negative (from −55 mV) when a whole-cell patch-clamp pipette contained no ATP. The membrane potential of such a cell was made less negative when a step increase in intracellular [ATP] was produced by photorelease of caged ATP {23}. Thus one of the principal differences in the action of K_{ATP} channels in heart and smooth muscle is the effect of the channel opening on the resting potential. Because the resting potential of heart muscle is very close to E_{K-ATP}, there is little if any effect on the resting potential of heart muscle when the channels are activated by the fall in intracellular [ATP]. In smooth muscle, with a less negative resting potential, activation of the K_{ATP} channels leads to hyperpolarization. The hyperpolarization reduces the degree of activation of sarcolemmal calcium channels {69} and favors calcium efflux on the Na/Ca exchanger, and hence leads to relaxation. Thus, in vascular smooth muscle intracellular ATP appears to contribute significantly to the regulation of vascular tone by its influence on resting potential.

ADENOSINE HYPOTHESIS BECOMES THE "K CHANNEL HYPOTHESIS"

The adenosine hypothesis, formulated and well articulated by Berne and colleagues, states that blood flow to specific vascular beds is influenced by the metabolic state of the vascular bed. When blood flow is inadequate, [ATP] synthesis is not in balance with ATP consumption, and metabolites of ATP accumulate within the working cells of the vascular bed (e.g., skeletal muscle cells, brain cells, cardiac muscle cells). One of the metabolites of ATP, adenosine, can readily diffuse out of the working cells and diffuse to neighboring cells, including vascular smooth muscle cells. The action of adenosine on the smooth muscle leads to relaxation of the smooth muscle and hence increased blood flow {see, e.g., 62,101,116}. More recently specific potassium channels have been identified that are activated by the increase in adenosine {16,17}. A version of this hypothesis was recently presented that includes the role of the K_{ATP} channel {71}. In addition to the mechanisms described in the adenosine hypothesis, it is suggested that the same metabolic stress that leads to reduction in [ATP] in working cells in the vascular bed can affect the smooth muscle cells of the vascular bed. Thus when intracellular [ATP] falls, the vascular muscle relaxes and blood flow increases. This feedback control mechanism thus tends to respond to increased metabolic need by providing more blood flow to the needy region. Thus, in addition to any action of adenosine to cause relaxation of the vascular smooth muscle, there is also the action of the fall of the [ATP] within the vascular smooth muscle cell that leads to smooth muscle relaxation. As indicated in the previous paragraph, there is substantial evidence on the importance of intracellular [ATP] in the regulation of vascular smooth muscle cell tone. As intracellular [ATP] falls, the vascular flow increases. It should also be pointed out that adenosine has multiple actions in diverse cells and its role in smooth muscle relaxation may depend on additional factors, including which specific vascular bed is being considered.

ADDITIONAL RESULTS OF PARTICULAR INTEREST

Ischemic preconditioning and ischemic damage to the heart

Much recent work by Gross and others (e.g. ref 119,121) has provided evidence for a role of K_{ATP} channels in the

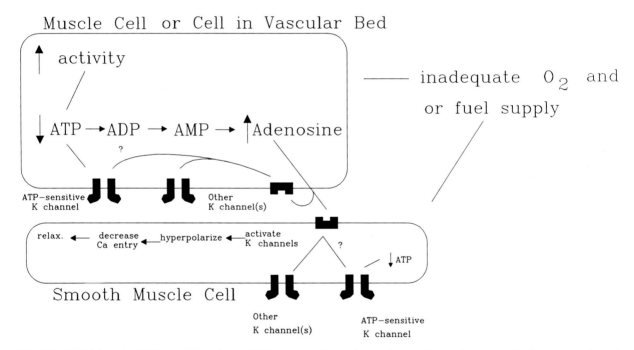

Fig. 8-5. ATP/Adenosine K-Channel Hypothesis. It is hypothesized that the regulation of more than one kind of potassium channel depends on intracellular [ATP] and/or on [adenosine]. Intracellular [ATP] falls during metabolic activity whenever synthesis of ATP lags behind consumption of ATP. The fall of intracellular [ATP] activates the K_{ATP} channels. The fall of intracellular [ATP] can activate K_{ATP} channels in many cells, including heart muscle cells and smooth muscle cells. In each case the activation of the potassium channels leads to either a hyperpolarization of the membrane potential towards E_{K-ATP} (the reversal potential for the K_{ATP} channel current) or tends to "clamp" the membrane potential near E_{K-ATP}. In either case the effect of the activation of the K_{ATP} channels is to decrease calcium entry and to lead to either relaxation or less contractile activation. In heart muscle the very large number of K_{ATP} channels means that even a small reduction of intracellular [ATP] can activate significant membrane current. Because the metabolic environment of a cell is influenced by its neighbors in its "nutrient field" (region of tissue in which cells share, to some extent, nutrient supply and waste product collection), cells consuming more ATP than they can resynthesize can influence the availability of nutrient substrate to their neighbors. Thus heart muscle cells may influence smooth muscle cells within their nutrient field. During the same metabolic activity, when consumption of ATP exceeds resynthesis of ATP, adenosine is produced within the active cells, and this adenosine, which can cross cell membranes, diffuses out of the active cells and can bind in increasing amounts to the sarcolemmal adenosine receptors on the active cell as well as on neighboring cells. Thus a heart muscle cell can influence a neighboring cell that may otherwise be in ATP balance. This binding of adenosine activates (by various pathways) potassium channels, which have largely the same effect on contraction as the activation of the K_{ATP} channels does. Additionally adenosine may have an indirect or direct action on the activity of the K_{ATP} channels. Figure modified from Nichols and Lederer {71}, with permission.

phenomenon of preconditioning, at least in certain animal models. *Ischemic preconditioning* is the term used to describe an experimental observation: The myocardium is made more resistant to a subsequent infarction when it is "preconditioned" by an earlier brief exposure to ischemia {19,28,49–51,59,60,64–66,86,95–98,104}. In other experiments {98} exposure to the K_{ATP} channel opener pinacidil led to no reduction in infarct size in the unpreconditioned hearts. However, such exposure to pinacidil did not prevent the preconditioning benefit otherwise observed. These observations led to the conclusion that ATP-sensitive K channels are not central to the "ischemia preconditioning" benefit. Nevertheless, pretreatment with glibenclamide, a K_{ATP} channel blocker, led to an increase in infarct size. From this it is concluded that ATP-sensitive K channels, when blocked, exacerbate the ultimate effects of ischemia. Importantly, adenosine receptor blockers do prevent the preconditioning benefit. Thus, consistent with the model shown in fig. 8-5, there are multiple pathways that link the effects of metabolic stress to cellular responses. There are adenosine-linked responses and also ATP-sensitive K-channel responses. Both sets of responses appear to significantly affect the impact of an ischemic insult on heart muscle.

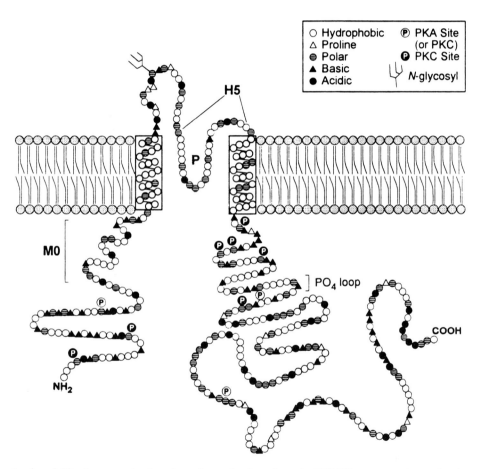

Fig. 8-6. Structural model for the new potassium channel superfamily — from the ROMK1 sequence. A pore-forming segment, labeled P, is located between two putative membrane-spanning segments of the ROMK1 sequence, M1 and M2. A region of sequence homology to Shaker K channels of the H5 region is shown. While the M0 region is assumed not to span the membrane, its hydrophobicity index indicates it could reside partly within the lipid bilayer. Both the amino and carboxy termini are thought to be cytoplasmic. On the C-terminus side is a possible ATP binding site, identified by the Walker type-A motif. A candidate for an N-linked glycosylation site is shown. Additionally, possible PKC and PKA (or PKC) phosphorylation sites are identified in the insert. Hydrophobic amino acid residues are A, G, M, I, L, V, F, W, C, P; uncharged polar residues are N, Q, S, T, Y; acidic residues are D, E; basic residues are K, R, H. Interestingly, while this member of the new superfamily appears to contain an ATP binding site, the other member, IRK1 {56}, has none. Nevertheless Northern blot analysis of ROMK1 indicates it is not found at significant levels within heart muscle but IRK1 is. Thus, it is not clear in what manner this new superfamily of potassium channels will help us in the quest for the gene(s) that code for the K_{ATP} channel. Figure taken from Ho et al. {47} and used with permission.

Stretch?

A somewhat more speculative report has been recently published, but the implications are nevertheless intriguing. Van Wagoner {124} has reported that the "sensitivity" of the ATP-sensitive K channels to [ATP] may be modulated by mechanical stretch in atrial muscle. More extensive investigations by independent groups should provide us with additional information on the role of sarcolemmal stretch in regulating the ATP-sensitive K channel. At the present time it is not clear how such modulation may affect normal physiological responses of heart or smooth muscle, or what role(s) this modulation may play in pathophysiological responses of the cardiovascular system.

MOLECULAR BIOLOGY OF THE ATP-SENSITIVE K-CHANNEL

Much effort has been expended to clone and express the K_{ATP} channel from diverse tissues. Early work by many laboratories, examining the possibility that the *Shaker* superfamily of potassium channels may include the K_{ATP} channel, has been unsuccessful to date. This recent effort is partly responsible for the identification of a new family of potassium channels obtained from kidney and mouse macrophage {47,56}. Both channels of this new family rectify inwardly and contain similar topology: two membrane-spanning regions and a poreforming or P region, which is illustrated in fig. 8-6. The kidney version, ROMK1 {47}, also contains a possible ATP-binding region. Nevertheless these channels are not in their present form blocked by ATP nor by sulfonylureas. Thus it is unclear whether this family, the *Shaker* family, or some new family of K^+ channels, yet to be discovered, will be linked to the K_{ATP} channel. It is also unclear whether a subunit (not yet identified) may modify or interact with a known or new channel subunit to provide it with the critical features, including inhibition by ATP and blockade by sulfonylureas.

SUMMARY

The ATP-sensitive K channel is found in cardiac and vascular smooth muscle cells, as well as in many other cells in the body. It is activated as intracellular [ATP] falls, tending to "clamp" membrane potential at a negative level or even to hyperpolarize it from its resting level. Given the properties of the channel, the channel's known abundance in heart and smooth muscle, and the established responses of cardiac and vascular smooth muscle to many metabolic factors (e.g., intracellular acidification, intracellular decline in [ATP], etc.), there is good evidence that the K_{ATP} channel plays a critical role in heart and vascular smooth muscle during anoxia and ischemia. Additionally, it is proposed that the K_{ATP} channels, along with other adenosine-activated potassium channels, play an important role in regulating the flow of blood to tissues during normal functioning. Thus it is suggested that the action

of the K_{ATP} channels in heart may be central to the regulation and limitation of metabolic load generated by the heart during its normal responses to activity (rest to maximum exercise). This final feature serves to limit the metabolic demands of heart muscle electrically under all conditions and thereby help to keep demand in balance with supply. Similarly the K_{ATP} channels in the smooth muscle, when activated by parallel events, help to keep supply at a level required by demand.

ACKNOWLEDGMENTS

This work has been supported by the NIH and the American Heart Association.

REFERENCES

1. Aguilar-Bryan L, Nichols CG, Rajan AS, Parker C, Bryan J: Coexpression of sulfonylurea receptors and K_{ATP} channels in hamster insulinoma tumor (HIT) cells. Evidence for direct association of the receptor with the channel. *J Biol Chem* 267:14934–14940, 1992.
2. Allen DG, Orchard CH: Myocardial contractile function during ischemia and hypoxia. *Circ Res* 60:153–160, 1987.
3. Allen DG, Lee JA, Smith GL: The consequences of simulated ischaemia on intracellular Ca^{2+} and tension in isolated ferret ventricular muscle. *J Physiol* 410:297–323, 1989.
4. Allen DG, Morris PG, Orchard CH, Pirolo JS: A nuclear magnetic resonance study of metabolism in the ferret heart during hypoxia and inhibition of glycolysis. *J Physiol* 361:185–204, 1985.
5. Allen DG, Orchard CH: Myocardial contractile function during ischemia and hypoxia. *Circ Res* 60:153–168, 1987.
6. Ashcroft FM: Adenosine 5-triphosphate-sensitive potassium channels. *Annu Rev Neurosci* 11:97–118, 1988.
7. Ashcroft FM, Harrison DE, Ashcroft SJH: Glucose induces closure of single potassium channels in isolated rat pancreatic β-cells. *Nature* 312:446–448, 1984.
8. Ashcroft FM, Kakei M: ATP-sensitive K^+ channels in rat pancreatic beta cells: Modulation by ATP and Mg^{2+} ions. *J Physiol* 416:349–367, 1989.
9. Ashcroft FM, Kakei M, Kelly RP: Rubidium and sodium permeability of the ATP-sensitive K^+ channel in single rat pancreatic beta-cells [published erratum appears in J Physiol (Lond) 412:557, 1989]. *J Physiol* 408:413–429, 1989.
10. Ashcroft FM, Rorsman P: ATP-sensitive K^+ channels: A link between β-cell metabolism and insulin secretion. *Biochem Soc Trans* 18:109–111, 1990.
11. Ashcroft FM, Rorsman P, Smith PA, Oosawa Y: The role of ion channels in stimulus secretion coupling in pancreatic β-cells. *Biophys J* 57:1990.
12. Ashcroft FM, Rorsman P, Trube G: Single calcium channel activity in mouse pancreatic β-cells. *Ann NY Acad Sci* 560:410–412, 1989.
13. Ashcroft SJ, Ashcroft FM: Properties and functions of ATP-sensitive K-channels. *Cell Signal* 2:197–214, 1990.
14. Ashcroft SJH, Ashcroft FM: Properties and functions of ATP-sensitive K-channels. *Cell Signal* 2:197–214, 1990.
15. Ashcroft SJH, Ashcroft FM: The sulfonylurea receptor. *Biochim Biophys Acta: Mol Cell Res* 1175:45–59, 1992.
16. Belardinelli L: Adenosine system in the heart. *Drug Dev Res* 28:263–267, 1993.

17. Belardinelli L, Shryock JC, Pelleg A: Cardiac electrophysiologic properties of adenosine. *Cor Art Dis* 3:1122–1126, 1992.

18. Belles B, Heschler J, Trube G: Changes of membrane currents in cardiac cells induced by long whole-cell recordings and tolbutamide. *Pflügers Arch* 409:582–588, 1987.

19. Bunch FT, Thornton J, Cohen MV, Downey JM: Adenosine is an endogenous protectant against stunning during repetitive ischemic episodes in the heart. *Am Heart J* 124. 1440–1446, 1992.

20. Cannell MB, Lederer WJ: A novel experimental chamber for single-cell voltage-clamp and patch-clamp applications with low electrical noise and excellent temperature and flow control. *Pflügers Arch* 406:536–539, 1986.

21. Carmeliet E: K$^+$ channels and control of ventricular repolarization in the heart. *Fund Clin Pharmacol* 7:19–28, 1993.

22. Carmeliet E, Biermans G, Callewaert G, Vereecke J: Potassium currents in cardiac cells. *Experientia* 43:1175–1184, 1987.

23. Clapp LH, Gurney AM: ATP-sensitive K$^+$ channels regulate resting potential of pulmonary arterial smooth muscle cells. *Am J Physiol: Heart Circ Physiol* 262:H916–H920, 1992.

24. Daut J, Maier Rudolph W, Von Beckerath N, Mehrke G, Gunther K, Goedel Meinen L: Hypoxic dilation of coronary arteries is mediated by ATP-sensitive potassium channels. *Science* 247:1341–1344, 1990.

25. Davies NW, Pettit AI, Agarwal R, Standen NB: The flickery block of ATP-dependent potassium channels of skeletal muscle by internal 4-aminopyridine. *Pflügers Arch* 419:25–31, 1991.

26. Davies NW, Spruce AE, Standen NB, Stanfield PR: Multiple blocking mechanisms of ATP-sensitive potassium channels of frog skeletal muscle by tetraethylammonium ions. *J Physiol* 413:31–48, 1989.

27. Deutsch N, Klitzner TS, Lamp ST, Weiss JN: Activation of cardiac ATP-sensitive K$^+$ current during hypoxia: Correlation with tissue ATP levels. *Am J Physiol: Heart Circ Physiol* 261:H671–H676, 1991.

28. Downey JM, Liu GS, Thornton JD: Adenosine and the anti-infarct effects of preconditioning. *Cardiovasc Res* 27:3–8, 1993.

29. Elliott AC, Smith GL, Allen DG: Simultaneous measurements of action potential duration and intracellular ATP in isolated ferret hearts exposed to cyanide. *Circ Res* 64:583–591, 1989.

30. Elliott AC, Smith GL, Eisner DA, Allen DG: Metabolic changes during ischaemia and their role in contractile failure in isolated ferret hearts. *J Physiol* 454:467–490, 1992.

31. Escande D, Cavero I: K$^+$ channel openers and "natural" cardioprotection. *Trends Pharm Sci* 13:269–272, 1992.

32. Escande D, Thuringer D, Le Guern S, Courteix J, Laville M, Cavero I: Potassium channel openers act through an activation of ATP-sensitive K$^+$ channels in guinea-pig cardiac myocytes. *Pflügers Arch* 414:669–675, 1989.

33. Fan Z, Nakayama K, Hiraoka M: Pinacidil activates the ATP-sensitive K$^+$ channel in inside-out and cell-attached patch membranes of guinea-pig ventricular myocytes. *Pflügers Arch* 415:387–394, 1990.

34. Fan Z, Nakayama K, Hiraoka M: Multiple action of pinacidil on adenosine-triphosphate-sensitive potassium channels in guinea-pig ventricular myocytes. *J Physiol* 430:273–295, 1990.

35. Fan Z, Nakayama K, Sawanobori T, Hiraoka M: Aromatic aldehydes and aromatic ketones open ATP-sensitive K$^+$ channels in guinea-pig ventricular myocytes. *Pflügers Arch* 421:409–415, 1992.

36. Findlay I: ATP-sensitive K$^+$ channels in rat ventricular myocytes are blocked and inactivated by internal divalent cations. *Pflügers Arch* 410:313–320, 1987.

37. Findlay I: Calcium-dependent inactivation of the ATP-sensitive K$^+$ channel of rat ventricular myocytes. *Biochim Biophys Acta* 943:297–304, 1988.

38. Findlay I: ATP4- and ATPMg inhibit the ATP sensitive K$^+$ channel of rat ventricular myocytes. *Pflügers Arch* 412:37–41, 1988.

39. Findlay I: Effects of ADP upon the ATP-sensitive K$^+$ channel in rat ventricular myocytes. *J Membr Biol* 101:83–92, 1988.

40. Findlay I: Effects of pH upon the inhibition by sulphonylurea drugs of ATP-sensitive K$^+$ channels in cardiac muscle. *J Pharmacol Exp Thera* 262:71–79, 1992.

41. Findlay I: Inhibition of ATP-sensitive K$^+$ channels in cardiac muscle by the sulphonylurea drug glibenclamide. *J Pharmacol Exp Ther* 261:540–545, 1992.

42. Findlay I, Deroubaix E, Guiraudou P, Coraboeuf E: Effects of activation of ATP-sensitive K$^+$ channels in mammalian ventricular myocytes. *Am J Physiol* 257:H1551–H1559, 1989.

43. Findlay I, Dunne MJ: ATP maintains ATP-inhibited K$^+$ channels in an operational state. *Pflügers Arch* 407:238–240, 1986.

44. Geisbuhler T, Altschuld RA, Trewyn RW, Ansel AZ, Lamka K, Brierley GP: Adenine nucleotide metabolism and compartmentalization in isolated adult rat heart cells. *Circ Res* 54:536–546, 1984.

45. Goldhaber JI, Parker JM, Weiss JN: Mechanisms of excitation-contraction coupling failure during metabolic inhibition in guinea-pig ventricular myocytes. *J Physiol* 443:371–386, 1991.

46. Hiraoka M, Fan Z: Activation of ATP-sensitive outward K$^+$ current by nicorandil (2-nicotinamidoethyl nitrate) in isolated ventricular myocytes. *J Pharmacol Exp Ther* 250:278–285, 1989.

47. HO K, Nichols CG, Lederer WJ, Lytton J, Vassilev PM, Kanazirska MV, Hebert SC: Cloning and expression of an inwardly rectifying ATP-regulated potassium channel. *Nature* 362:31–38, 1993.

48. Horie M, Irisawa H, Noma A: Voltage-dependent magnesium block of adenosine-triphosphate-sensitive potassium channel in guinea-pig ventricular cells. *J Physiol* 387:251–272, 1987.

49. Jennings RB, Murry C, Reimer KA: Myocardial effects of brief periods of ischemia followed by reperfusion. *Adv Cardiol* 37:7–31, 1990.

50. Jennings RB, Murry CE, Reimer KA: Energy metabolism in preconditioned and control myocardium: Effect of total ischemia. *J Mol Cell Cardiol* 23:1449–1458, 1991.

51. Jennings RB, Murry CE, Reimer KA: Preconditioning myocardium with ischemia. *Cardiovasc Drugs Ther* 5:933–938, 1991.

52. Kakei M, Noma A: Adenosine-5'-triphosphate-sensitive single potassium channel in the atrioventricular node cell of the rabbit heart. *J Physiol (Lond)* 352:265–284, 1984.

53. Kakei M, Noma A, Shibasaki T: Properties of adenosine-triphosphate-regulated potassium channels in guinea-pig ventricular cells. *J Physiol* 363:441–462, 1985.

54. Kantor PF, Coetzee WA, Carmeliet EE, Dennis SC, Opie LH: Reduction of ischemic K$^+$ loss and arrhythmias in rat hearts: Effect of glibenclamide, a sulfonylurea. *Circ Res* 66:478–485, 1990.

55. Kovacs RJ, Nelson MT: ATP-sensitive K^+ channels from aortic smooth muscle incorporated into planar lipid bilayers. *Am J Physiol: Heart Circ Physiol* 261:H604–H609, 1991.

56. Kubo Y, Baldwin TJ, Jan YN, Jan LY: Primary structure and functional expression of a mouse inward rectifier potassium channel. *Nature* 362:127–133, 1993.

57. Lederer WJ, Nichols CG: Nucleotide modulation of the activity of rat heart ATP-sensitive K^+ channels in isolated membrane patches. *J Physiol* 419:193–211, 1989.

58. Lederer WJ, Nichols CG, Smith GL: The mechanism of early contractile failure of isolated rat ventricular myocytes subjected to complete metabolic inhibition. *J Physiol* 413:329–349, 1989.

59. Li GC, Vasquez JA, Gallagher KP, Lucchesi BR: Myocardial protection with preconditioning. *Circulation* 82:609–619, 1990.

60. Liu GS, Thornton J, Van Winkle DM, Stanley AW, Olsson RA, Downey JM: Protection against infarction afforded by preconditioning is mediated by A1 adenosine receptors in rabbit heart. *Circulation* 84:350–356, 1991.

61. Mccarron JG, Quayle JM, Halpern W, Nelson MT: Cromakalim and pinacidil dilate small mesenteric arteries but not small cerebral arteries. *Am J Physiol: Heart Circ Physiol* 261:H287–H291, 1991.

62. Miller WL, Belardinelli L, Bacchus A, Foley DH, Rubio R, Berne RM: Canine myocardial adenosine and lactate production, oxygen consumption, and coronary blood flow during stellate ganglia stimulation. *Circ Res* 45:708–718, 1979.

63. Misler S, Falke LC, Gillis K, McDaniel ML: A metabolite-regulated potassium channel in rat pancreatic B cells. *Proc Natl Acad Sci USA* 83:7119–7123, 1986.

64. Murry CE, Jennings RB, Reimer KA: Preconditioning with ischemia: A delay of lethal cell injury in ischemic myocardium. *Circulation* 74:1124–1136, 1986.

65. Murry CE, Jennings RB, Reimer KA: New insights into potential mechanisms of ischemic preconditioning [editorial]. *Circulation* 84:442–445, 1991.

66. Murry CE, Richard VJ, Jennings RB, Reimer KA: Myocardial protection is lost before contractile function recovers from ischemic preconditioning. *Am J Physiol* 260:H796–H804, 1991.

67. Nakayama K, Fan Z, Marumo F, Sawanobori T, Hiraoka M: Action of nicorandil on ATP-sensitive K^+ channel in guinea-pig ventricular myocytes. *Br J Pharmacol* 103:1641–1648, 1991.

68. Nelson MT: Regulation of arterial tone by potassium channels. *Jpn J Pharmacol* 58(Suppl 2):238P–242P, 1992.

69. Nelson MT: Ca^{2+}-activated potassium channels and ATP-sensitive potassium channels as modulators of vascular tone. *Trends Cardiovasc Med* 3:54–60, 1993.

70. Nichols CG, Lederer WJ: The regulation of ATP-sensitive K^+ channel activity in intact and permeabilized rat ventricular myocytes. *J Physiol* 423:91–110, 1990.

71. Nichols CG, Lederer WJ: Adenosine triphosphate-sensitive potassium channels in the cardiovascular system. *Am J Physiol: Heart Circ Physiol* 261:H1675–H1686, 1991.

72. Nichols CG, Lederer WJ: The mechanism of K_{ATP} channel inhibition by ATP. *J Gen Physiol* 97:1095–1098, 1991.

73. Nichols CG, Lederer WJ, Cannell MB: ATP dependence of K_{ATP} channel kinetics in isolated membrane patches from rat ventricle. *Biophys J* 60:1164–1177, 1991.

74. Nichols CG, Lopatin AN: Trypsin and alpha-chymotrypsin treatment abolishes glibenclamide sensitivity of K_{ATP} channels in rat ventricular myocytes. *Pflügers Arch* 422:617–619, 1993.

75. Nichols CG, Ripoll C, Lederer WJ: ATP-sensitive potassium channel modulation of the guinea pig ventricular action potential and contraction. *Circ Res* 68:280–287, 1991.

76. Niki I, Kelly RP, Ashcroft SJ, Ashcroft FM: ATP-sensitive K-channels in HIT T15 beta-cells studied by patch-clamp methods, ^{86}Rb efflux and glibenclamide binding. *Pflügers Arch* 415:47–55, 1989.

77. Noma A: ATP-regulated K^+ channels in cardiac muscle. *Nature* 305:147–148, 1983.

78. Noma A, Shibasaki T: Membrane current through adenosine-triphosphate-regulated potassium channels in guinea-pig ventricular cells. *J Physiol (Lond)* 363:463–480, 1985.

79. Noma A, Takano M: The ATP-sensitive K^+ channel. *Jpn J Physiol* 41:177–187, 1991.

80. Notsu T, Tanaka I, Takano M, Noma A: Blockade of the ATP-sensitive K^+ channel by 5-hydroxydecanoate in guinea pig ventricular myocytes. *J Pharmacol Exp Ther* 260:702–708, 1992.

81. Ohno-Shosaku T, Zunkler BJ, Trube G: Dual effects of ATP on K^+ currents of mouse pancreatic β-cells. *Pflügers Arch* 408:133–138, 1987.

82. Opie LH, Carmeliet E: Introduction to the special issue on potassium channels. *Cardiovasc Res* 26:1010, 1992.

83. Qin D, Noma A: A new oil-gate concentration jump technique applied to inside-out patch clamp recording. *Am J Physiol* 255:H980–H984, 1988.

84. Qin D, Takano M, Noma A: Kinetics of ATP-sensitive K^+ channel revealed with oil-gate concentration jump method. *Am J Physiol* 26:H1624–H1633, 1989.

85. Quayle JM, Standen NB, Stanfield PR: The voltage-dependent block of ATP-sensitive potassium channels of frog skeletal muscle by caesium and barium ions. *J Physiol* 405:677–697, 1988.

86. Reimer KA, Murry CE, Yamasawa I, Hill ML, Jennings RB: Four brief periods of myocardial ischemia cause no cumulative ATP loss or necrosis. *Am J Physiol* 251:H1306–H1315, 1986.

87. Ribalet B, Ciani S, Eddlestone GT: ATP mediates both activation and inhibition of K(ATP) channel activity via cAMP dependent protein kinase in insulin secreting cell lines. *J Gen Physiol* 94:693–717, 1989.

88. Rorsman P, Trube G: Glucose dependent K^+ channels in pancreatic β-cells are regulated by intracellular ATP. *Pflügers Arch* 405:305–309, 1985.

89. Spruce AE, Standen NB, Stanfield PR: Studies of the unitary properties of adenosine-5'-triphosphate regulated potassium channels of frog skeletal muscle. *J Physiol* 382:213–236, 1987.

90. Spruce AE, Standen NB, Stanfield PR: Voltage-dependent ATP-sensitive potassium channels of skeletal muscle membranes. *Nature* 316:736–738, 1990.

91. Standen NB: Potassium channels, metabolism and muscle. *Exp Physiol* 77:1–25, 1992.

92. Standen NB, Quayle JM, Davies NW, Brayden JE, Huang Y, Nelson MT: Hyperpolarizing vasodilators activate ATP-sensitive K^+ channels in arterial smooth muscle. *Science* 245:177–180, 1989.

93. Stern MD, Silverman HS, Houser SR, Josephson RA, Capogrossi MC, Nichols CG, Lederer WJ, Lakatta EG: Anoxic contractile failure in rat heart myocytes is caused by failure of intracellular calcium release due to alteration of the action potential. *Proc Natl Acad Sci USA* 85:6954–6958, 1988.

94. Takano M, Qin DY, Noma A: ATP-dependent decay and recovery of K^+ channels in guinea pig cardiac myocytes. *Am J Physiol* 258:H45–H50, 1990.

95. Tanaka M, Earnhardt RC, Murry CE, Richard VJ, Jennings

RB, Reimer KA: Hypoxic reperfusion to remove ischaemic catabolites prior to arterial reperfusion does not limit the size of myocardial infarcts in dogs. *Cardiovasc Res* 25:7–16, 1991.

96. Thornton J, Striplin S, Liu GS, Swafford A, Stanley AW, Van Winkle DM, Downey JM: Inhibition of protein synthesis does not block myocardial protection afforded by preconditioning. *Am J Physiol* 259:H1822–H1825, 1990.

97. Thornton JD, Liu GS, Olsson RA, Downey JM: Intravenous pretreatment with A1-selective adenosine analogues protects the heart against infarction [see comments]. *Circulation* 85:659–665, 1992.

98. Thornton JD, Thornton CS, Sterling DL, Downey JM: Blockade of ATP-sensitive potassium channels increases infarct size but does not prevent preconditioning in rabbit hearts. *Circ Res* 72:44–49, 1993.

99. Thuringer D, Escande D: The potassium channel opener RP49356 modifies the ATP-sensitivity of K^+-ATP channels in cardiac myocytes. *Pflügers Arch* 414:S175, 1989.

100. Thuringer D, Escande D: Apparent competition between ATP and the potassium channel opener RP49356 on ATP-sensitive K^+ channels of cardiac myocytes. *Mol Pharmacol* 36:897–902, 1989.

101. Tominaga S, Curnish RR, Belardinelli L, Rubio R, Berne RM: Adenosine release during early and sustained exercise of canine skeletal muscle. *Am J Physiol* 238:H156–H163, 1980.

102. Trube G, Hescheler J: Inward-rectifying channels in isolated patches of the heart cell membrane: ATP-dependence and comparison with cell-attached patches. *Pflügers Arch Eur J Physiol* 401:178–184, 1984.

103. Trube G, Rorsman P, Ohno-Shosaku T: Opposite effects of tolbutamide and diazoxide on the ATP-dependent K^+ channel in mouse pancreatic β-cells. *Pflügers Arch* 407: 493–499, 1986.

104. Turrens JF, Thornton J, Barnard ML, Snyder S, Liu G, Downey JM: Protection from reperfusion injury by preconditioning hearts does not involve increased antioxidant defenses. *Am J Physiol* 262:H585–H589, 1992.

105. Venkatesh N, Lamp ST, Weiss JN: Sulfonylureas, ATP-sensitive K^+ channels, and cellular K^+ loss during hypoxia, ischemia, and metabolic inhibition in mammalian ventricle. *Circ Res* 69:623–637, 1991.

106. Venkatesh N, Stuart JS, Lamp ST, Alexander LD, Weiss JN: Activation of ATP-sensitive K^+ channels by cromakalim: Effects on cellular K^+ loss and cardiac function in ischemic and reperfused mammalian ventricle. *Circ Res* 71:1324–1333, 1992.

107. Virag L, Furukawa T, Hiraoka M: Modulation of the effect of glibenclamide on K_{APT} channels by ATP and ADP. *Mol Cell Biochem* 119:209–215, 1993.

108. Von Beckerath N, Cyrys S, Dischner A, Daut J: Hypoxic vasodilatation in isolated, perfused guinea-pig heart: An analysis of the underlying mechanisms. *J Physiol* 442: 297–319, 1991.

109. Wang W, Giebisch G: Dual modulation of renal ATP-sensitive K^+ channel by protein kinases A and C. *Proc Natl Acad Sci USA* 88:9722–9725, 1991.

110. Wang W, Sackin H, Giebisch G: Renal potassium channels and their regulation. *Annu Rev Physiol* 54:81–96, 1992.

111. Weiss JN, Lamp ST: Glycolysis preferentially inhibits ATP-sensitive K^+ channels in isolated guinea-pig cardiac myocytes. *Science* 238:67–69, 1987.

112. Weiss JN, Lamp ST: Cardiac ATP-sensitive K^+ channels. Evidence for preferential regulation by glycolysis. *J Gen Physiol* 94:911–935, 1989.

113. Weiss JN, Lamp ST, Shine KI: Cellular K^+ loss and anion efflux during myocardial ischemia and metabolic inhibition. *Am J Physiol* 256:H1165–H1175, 1989.

114. Weiss JN, Venkatesh N, Lamp ST: ATP-sensitive K^+ channels and cellular K^+ loss in hypoxic and ischaemic mammalian ventricle. *J Physiol* 447:649–673, 1992.

115. Wilde AAM, Escande D, Schumacher CA, Thuringer D, Mestre M, Flolet JWT: Glibenclamide inhibition of ATP-sensitive K^+ channels and ischemia-induced K^+ accumulation in the mammalian heart. *Pflügers Arch* 414:S176, 1989.

116. Winn HR, Rubio R, Berne RM: Brain adenosine production in the rat during 60 seconds of ischemia. *Circ Res* 45: 486–492, 1979.

117. Zunkler BJ, Lins S, Ohno-Shosaku T, Trube G, Panten U: Ctyosolic ADP enhances the sensitivity to tolbutamide of ATP-dependent K^+ channels from pancreatic β-cells. *FEBS Lett* 239:241–244, 1988.

118. Zünkler BJ, Trube G, Panten U: How do sulfonylureas approach their receptor in the β-cell plasma membrane. *Naunyn-Schmiedebergs Arch Pharmacol* 340:328–332, 1989.

119. Auchampach JA, Gross GJ: Adenosine A1 receptors, KATP channels, and ischemic preconditioning in dogs. *American Journal of Physiology: Heart and Circulatory Physiology* 264:H1327–H1336, 1993.

120. Benndorf K, Bollmann G, Friedrich M, Hirche H: Anoxia induces time-independent K^+ current through KATP channels in isolated heart cells of the guinea-pig. *Journal of Physiology* 454:339–357, 1992.

121. Gross, GJ, Auchampach JA: Blockade of ATP-sensitive potassium channels prevents myocardial preconditioning in dogs. *Circulation Research* 70:223–233, 1992.

122. Tung RT, Kurachi Y: G-protein activation of the cardiac ATP-sensitive K^+ channel. *Circulation* 82:III-462, 1990.

123. Tung RT, Kurachi Y: On the mechanism of nucleotide diphosphate activation of the ATP-sensitive K^+ channel in ventricular cell of guinea-pig. *Journal of Physiology* 437: 239–256, 1991.

124. Van Wagoner DR: Mechanosensitive gating of atrial ATP-sensitive potassium channels. *Circulation Research* 72: 973–983, 1993.

CHAPTER 9

Electrogenesis of The Pacemaker Potential as Revealed by Atrioventricular Nodal Experiments

H. IRISAWA[†], A. NOMA, & H. MATSUDA

INTRODUCTION

The atrioventricular (AV) node has two vitally important functions. One involves its role in the conduction through the atrium to the ventricle. The slow conduction of excitation within the node {1,2} provides an adequate time delay between contraction of the atria and that of the ventricles and enables the heart to function as an efficient pump. The other function of the AV node is its secondary pacemaker activity. When the sinoatrial (SA) node fails to control cardiac rhythm, as a result of either depressed automaticity or impaired conduction, the AV node functions as a pacemaker of the heart.

Following the discovery of the AV node {3}, major developments took place in the physiologic concept of the AV node in the late 1950s, when the membrane potentials of the AV node were recorded. Today, almost all features of the electrical activities of the intact AV node have been described. However, since the studies were limited to an analysis of the configuration of the action potentials and the maximum rate of depolarization, it remained unclear whether such measurements reflected the membrane properties of the AV nodal cell or the propagated action potential. Does the slurred upstroke with steps or notches frequently described in typical nodal cells (N cells {4}) represent an unknown characteristic of the inward current system or simply an artifact due to conduction block? Are there any regional differences in characteristics of the membrane current systems within the AV node? Does acetylcholine (ACh) increase the membrane potassium conductance? Is action potential generation independent of the membrane potentials? In order to answer these questions, direct measurements of the membrane current were awaited in the AV node.

Advances in the voltage-clamp technique made AV nodal or SA nodal experiments quite comparable to those involving other cardiac tissues, where membrane currents were examined. In 1976, Noma and Irisawa {5} developed small SA nodal preparations useful for voltage-clamp experiments. This method was introduced in several different laboratories for studying the SA and AV node (for review, see Irisawa {6} and Brown {7}). Single nodal cell

preparations have become available recently by treating the heart with collagenase {8,9}. Using the patch-clamp technique {10}, the single channel currents and also the whole cell currents can be recorded from single nodal cells {11,13; for review see 14}. Furthermore, the intracellular media can be replaced by switching the solution within the pipette {15}.

In this chapter, the results of our studies mainly on AV nodal cells are reviewed. The AV nodal cells exhibited very similar electrophysiologic characteristics to those observed in SA nodal cells. The membrane current systems of the nodal cells share essentially the same characteristics as those in other cardiac fibers.

SMALL AV NODE PREPARATIONS

The rabbit AV node lies between the ostium of the coronary sinus and the leaflet of the tricuspid valve {4}. Its size is approximately 5×3 mm. Before analyzing the membrane current in small dissected specimens, we examined the characteristics of the action potential in different regions of the intact AV node (fig. 9-1) {16}. An action potential similar to those of atrial cells was recorded from region I, but its maximum rate of rise was 28.6 V/s, which was smaller than the values usually obtained in atrial tissue. From region V, a pattern similar to that of the node-His cells (NH cells {4}) was recorded, but the maximum rate of rise was very small compared to that observed in the His bundle. In region III, the amplitude of the action potential was smallest, the resting potential being less negative than in the other two regions. All of these action potentials comprised the conducted action potential and were similar to those observed by Akiyama and Fozzard {17}, Ruiz-Ceretti and Ponce Zumino {18}, and Zipes and Mendez {19}, indicating that the region investigated by us was in fact the AV node defined by previous authors.

We then transected the AV nodal region perpendicularly to the AV ring into five 1-mm wide strands. Both sides of each strand were trimmed little by little to a width of 0.5 mm. The resultant strands were numbered from I to V (fig. 9-1A). We removed the epicardial side of these

[†] Deceased

N. Sperelakis (ed.), Physiology and Pathophysiology of the Heart, Third Edition.
© *1995 Kluwer Academic Publishers. ISBN 0-7923-2612-1. All rights reserved.*

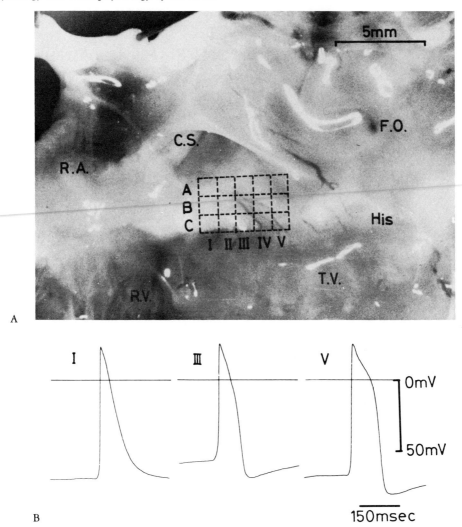

Fig. 9-1. **A:** Photography showing the AV node region of the rabbit heart: CS = coronary sinus; RA = right atrium; FO = foramen ovale; RV = right ventricle; TV = tricuspid valve; HIS = His bundle; A, B, and C, I-V, see text. B : I, III, and V correspond to the portion of I-B, III-B, and V-B in fig. 9-1A. From Kokubun et al. {16}, with permission.

thin-strand preparations, while the endocardial side remained intact. Each strand was then ligated with a silk suture into three equal portions, which were labelled A, B, and C. In the small AV nodal specimen, the action potentials recorded from different sites were almost superposable, indicating a synchronous excitation within the specimen. Thus, the action potential may faithfully reflect the membrane properties of the nodal cells.

Figure 9-2 shows one example of the action potentials recorded from a small specimen. Except for a few specimens from regions I-A, I-B, II-A, and V-C, the individual small preparations mostly showed spontaneous activity as seen by the slowly rising pacemaker depolarization (fig. 6-2). The action potential parameters from different AV nodal specimens revealed similar values in all 15 portions, suggesting that the AV nodal cells of different regions

share a common current system. The regional variation observed in the intact AV nodal specimens (fig. 9-1) is considered to be due to electrotonic influences from the atrial fibers or the His bundle. The amplitude of the action potential in the small specimens is slightly larger than that in N cells reported previously {17–19}, but the maximum rate of rise (8 ± 4 V/s) and the duration of the action potential are comparable to those given in many reports (fig. 6 in Mendez {20}). When the maximum rate of rise was smaller than 6 V/s, it was not affected by tetrodotoxin (TTX), while a larger maximum rate of rise was decreased to around 6 V/s with TTX, indicating a variable contribution of the sodium current.

Acetylcholine (ACh) consistently hyperpolarized the membrane in the same manner as in the SA nodal cell (fig. 9-3A) and depressed the spontaneous activity. Application

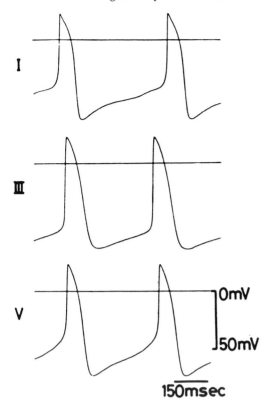

Fig. 9-2. Action potentials recorded in the small specimens of AV node: **I**, **III**, and **V** correspond to portions of I-B, III-B, and V-B in fig. 9-1A. From Kokubun et al. {16}, with permission.

Isolation of single AV nodal cells

A rabbit heart was mounted onto a Langendorff device and was perfused through the coronary artery with Ca-free Tyrode solution containing 0.04% w/vol collagenase (Sigma, type 1). After enzyme treatment for 30–40 minutes, the collagenase-treated heart was opened under a dissecting microscope and a small piece of tissue (1 × 1 mm) was dissected out from the same sites of the AV node as used for preparing the multicellular preparations described above. The small piece of tissue was teased in a recording chamber filled with control Tyrode solution to isolate single cells. After the isolated cells had settled to the floor of the chamber, they were perfused with Tyrode solution warmed at 35–36°C. In some experiments, we first dissected small preparations of the AV node from the intact heart and then treated them by incubation in the above collagenase-containing solution instead of perfusing the whole heart. No obvious difference was noted in the shape of the cells or in the electrical activities between these two isolation procedures.

Although the nodal cells are rod shaped in Ca-free solution (4–12 µm in width and 50–62 µm in length), they become round within an hour in normal Tyrode solution {12}. The viable single cells are clearly distinguishable from the dead cells, which show an irregular surface and are not transparent. The viable spherical or oval nodal cells, on the other hand, are revealed by phase-contrast microscopy to have a relatively smooth and shiny surface. The nodal cells display an oblate spheroidal shape along their major axes. The minor and major axes are 22 ± 4 µm and 31 ± 7 µm (n = 71), respectively. These values are quite similar to those for single SA nodal cells. About 10–30% of the cells contract spontaneously with a regular rhythm of 150–260/min and the contraction can be arrested by adding a small amount of ACh to the bath. Spontaneous contractions irregular in rhythm or insensitive to ACh were thought to be due to transient depolarizations and were regarded as a sign of Ca overload. Such cells were not used.

Voltage-clamp experiments on single cells were performed using patch electrodes {10}. The rhythmical contractions of the nodal cells were arrested by applying ACh, and the patch electrode was attached to the cell surface. Usually, ACh was washed out after establishing a giga seal. The membrane capacitance of the single nodal cells ranged from 15 to 60 pF and was corrected with the apparent size of the cell with a constant of about 1.3 µF/cm². The normalized membrane resistance was about 15 kohm·cm² at the resting membrane potential. The single cells revealed an action potential similar to that observed in the small nodal preparations. Figure 9-4 illustrates the action potentials recorded from single SA and AV nodal cells using the patch pipette. The amplitude of the action potentials was about 100 mV in the AV nodal cells and about 90 mV in the SA nodal cells. The duration at half repolarization was about 120 ms in the AV nodal cells and 100 ms in the SA nodal cells. The maximum diastolic potential was about −78 mV in the AV nodal cells, with a correction for the junctional potential of

of epinephrine increased both the maximum rate of rise and the spontaneous rate of the action potential.

The spontaneous action potentials were sensitive to current injections through a microelectrode in the small specimens, as has been observed using a suction electrode {21,22}. With depolarizing current pulses (fig. 9-3B), the maximum diastolic potential decreased and the frequency of the spontaneous discharge increased, whereas cessation of spontaneous activity occurred during application of a hyperpolarizing current (fig. 9-3C).

When we employed the voltage clamp method, the size was not sufficiently small to achieve spatial homogeneity of the membrane potential within the specimen. We had to trim the preparation further, stepwise, to 0.25 × 0.25 × 0.1 mm. The trimming procedure was deliberate, using a fragment of razor blade. The resting potential of the spontaneously active preparations is defined as the potential giving zero current with positive slope in the steady-state current voltage relationship {23}. The resting potential in the small AV nodal specimen was approximately −40 mV, and this value was clearly less negative than the resting potential of −62 mV, which was measured from the steady potential during diastole in the intact AV nodal specimen. The latter value is in good agreement with the data reported by other investigators {17–20}.

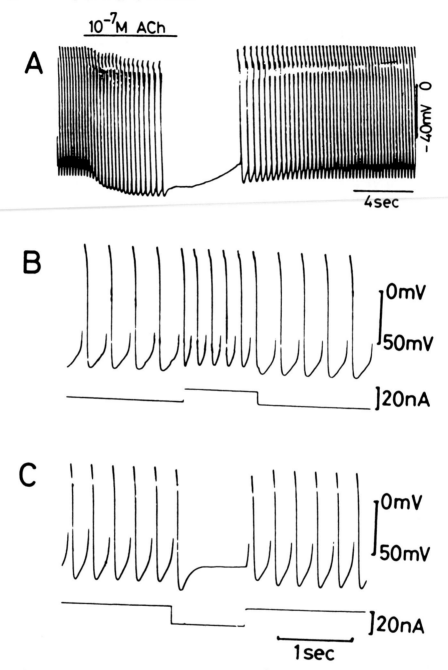

Fig. 9-3. **A:** Effect of acetylcholine on the small AV node specimen; 10^{-7} g/ml acetylcholine was superfused. Original trace by S. Kokubun. **B,C:** Effects of current injection on the spontaneous activity. In each panel the top trace represents the membrane potential, while the bottom represents the applied current. From Kukubun et al. {16}, with permission.

13 mV at the electrode tip. The characteristics of the action potential in the small specimens were thus reproduced in the single cells.

Membrane currents in the AV nodal cell

Voltage-clamp experiments are available both in small multicellular specimens and in single-cell preparations of the AV node. In the case of the small AV-node

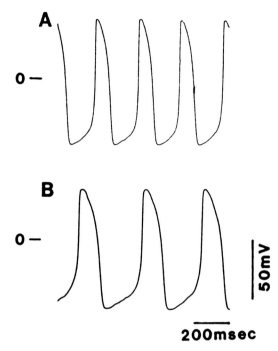

A

0 –

B

0 –

50 mV

200 msec

Fig. 9-4. Action potentials of single SA nodal (**A**) and AV nodal (**B**) cells. The patch electrode contained in mM; K-aspartate 130, KCl 10–20, EGTA 0.01–1, glucose 10, and 5 mM HEPES-KOH buffer (pH = 7.3). From Nakayama et al. {12}, with permission.

specimen, the conventional two-microelectrode voltage-clamp method was applied {24,25}, as has been done for the mammalian Purkinje fiber {26} and SA nodal preparations {5}. The membrane potentials of the single cells were clamped using the whole-cell clamp configuration of the patch-clamp technique. The experimental conditions for these two methods are different, but the results obtained were essentially similar. The following paragraphs summarize the data obtained by the two different methods.

Figure 9-5 compares the two families of voltage clamp traces obtained from a small AV nodal preparation (A) and those recorded from a single nodal cell (B). The clamp pulses were given in 10 mV steps from a holding potential of −40 mV. The sodium current is usually inactivated by employing such a low holding potential. A remarkable similarity was noted between these two specimens, except for the current amplitude. In the former specimen, the peak calcium current exceeded 50 nA, whereas in the latter cell it was about 0.3 nA. This suggests that the multicellular preparation contained about 200 cells, and that the cells within the preparation were clamped well spatially because of the electrical coupling between the cells through the gap junctions.

Depolarizing pulses that are more positive than −30 mV elicit an inward current through the Ca channels (I_{Ca}). This inward current is sensitive to various Ca blockers, such as verapamil, D 600, Cd^{2+}, etc. but is insensitive to TTX. The progressively activating outward current follows

the inactivation of the Ca current, and it decays gradually after the membrane is repolarized to the holding potential. This outward current (I_K) is carried by potassium ions as in the SA node. In general, the amplitude of the outward current tail was relatively smaller in the single-cell preparation than in the multicellular preparation; it appeared that washout of unknown substances or chelation of intracellular Ca^{2+} by EGTA, which is usually added to the pipette solution, reduced the amplitude of I_K.

On hyperpolarization from a holding potential of −40 mV at the first two or three steps (−50 to −60 mV), small gradual shifts in the current could be attributed to decaying I_K, but at a potential more negative than −70 mV the hyperpolarization-activated current (defined in different ways as I_h {27}, I_f {28,29}, and I_p {30} was activated (fig. 9-5A2). On return to the holding potential, transient activation of both the sodium current (I_{Na}) and the calcium current was observed. In about half of the specimens used, we could not register I_h while the specimen showed spontaneous activity.

In single-cell preparations, the current density can be obtained by assuming the cell shape to be a plane oblate spheroid. The amplitude of I_{Ca} peaked at 0 mV and its amplitude was about 18 μA/cm². I_K was activated in the voltage range positive to −50 mV and was saturated at about +20 mV. The amplitude of the fully activated I_K at −40 mV was about 3.3 μA/cm² and revealed an inward-going rectification. The amplitude of I_h varied from almost 0 μA/cm² to 3 μA/cm² at 002100 mV.

Ionic channels and their role in AV nodal excitation

Ten types of ionic channels have so far been identified in cardiac muscle as summarized in table 9-1. Most of them have been confirmed at the single-channel level. We consider that the ionic channel in the AV nodal cell poses precisely the same characteristics as those in other cardiac cells, since no evidence has yet been obtained to indicate any difference at the level of the single channel. However, the density of distribution of each channel may vary among different cardiac cells and characterizes the electrical excitability of the cardiac cells. The various characteristics are reviewed and the functions in AV nodal excitation are discussed in the following sections.

SODIUM CHANNEL

Ponce Zumino et al. {31} and De Ceretti et al. {32} have suggested that even in the midnodal region there is an Na channel. As shown in the SA nodal cell {33,34}, if the membrane was hyperpolarized more negatively than −70 mV, I_{Na} became activated. Figure 9-6 illustrates such an example in a small AV nodal specimen obtained from the midnodal region. Using the voltage-clamp method, we hyperpolarized the cell to −83 mV for 0.5 seconds to restore the availability of I_{Na}. On releasing the feedback circuit, a nodal break excitation was registered. The upstroke of this action potential contained two phases, fast (75 V/s) and slow (4.2 V/s). After superfusing TTX (10^{-7} g/ml), the fast-rising phase disappeared. The slow

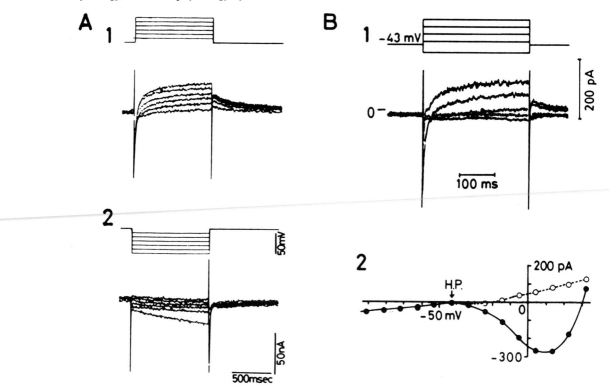

Fig. 9-5. Voltage-clamp records in the small AV nodal specimen (**A**) and from single AV nodel cell (**B**) of the rabbit. Current-voltage (I-V) relations in B-2 were measured from the same experiment shown in B-1 at the peak (filled circles) and near the end of the clamp pulse (open circles). The holding potential (H.P.) was about −40 mV, and various clamp pulses were applied (above each family of current traces). The records in A are modified from Kokubun et al. {24} and those in B from Nakayama and Irisawa {49}.

phase was activated after an initial foot, which reflects the time constant of the resting membrane. These findings clearly indicate that even in the midnodal region, I_{Na} contributes to the action potential.

When a holding potential negative to −50 mV was used in the voltage-clamp experiments, I_{Na} was activated on depolarization in almost every experiment. The sodium current, however, could not be controlled with the present voltage-clamp technique because of its limited frequency response and the series resistance within the cell.

CALCIUM CHANNEL

There has been some controversy about the ionic selectivity of the Ca channels in cardiac muscle or about the ionic basis of the slow inward current. The maximum rate of rise of the AV nodal action potential is increased with increasing Ca levels within a certain concentration range and the action potential is effectively suppressed by the application of Ca blockers. However, the action potential could be generated even in the absence of external Ca {24}. Recently, these paradoxical findings were finally explained by recording the single-channel current. The Ca channel acquires Na^+ conductance when the external free Ca^{2+} concentration is made to decrease below the micromolar level using EGTA in the ventricular cell (fig. 9-7) {35}. The amplitude of this Na current through the Ca channels is larger than that of the Ca current. However, Ca^{2+} of more than 10^{-5} M suppresses the Na conductance. Mg^{2+} also blocks the Na conductance of the Ca channel. Thus, under physiological conditions, the slow inward current is carried only by Ca^{2+}. Depression of the Ca current in the Na-depleted solution in the multicellular preparation is most probably explained by an increase in the intracellular Ca^{2+} level, which is caused by reversed operation of Na-Ca exchange.

The rising phase of the spontaneous action potential is generated by activation of the Ca channel. The contribution of the Ca channel to the later part of the pacemaker depolarization has also been assumed to explain the increase in the rate of diastolic depolarization induced by epinephrine. Application of epinephrine increases the amplitudes of I_{Ca}, I_K, and I_h. The increase of I_K on computer simulation decreased the spontaneous rate {36}. A positive chronotropic effect can be seen in a cell showing practically no I_h activation {37}. It seems likely, therefore, that an increase in the Ca channel conductance partially underlies the pacemaker depolarization.

Table 9-1.

Name of current		Ion selectivity	Single-channel conductance (pS)	Physiological significance	Voltage dependency	Traditional nomenclature	References
Voltage-gated channel current							
Sodium current	i_{Na}[a]	Na	15.1[c]	Excitation, conduction	+	I_{Na}[a]	4
Calcium current	i_{Ca}[b]	Ca, Ba, Sr	15–25	Excitation, secretion conduction, pacemaker	+	I_{Ca}, I_s, I_{si}	38
Inward rectifier	i_{Krec}	K	40–50	Resting potential plateau phase	+	I_{K1}	41,42
Delayed rectifier	i_K	K	1.6 (5.4 K)	Repolarization pacemaker	+	I_X, I_{X1}	47
Transient outward	i_{TO}, i_a	K, (Na & K) (Ca)	20	Early repolarization duration of action potential	+	Positive dynamic	49
Hyperpolarization activated current	I_h I_f	Na, K (Cl⁻)		Purkinje pacemaker depolarization of packmaker tissue	+	I_{K2}	53
Ligand-operated channel current							
ATP sensitive K current	i_{KATP}	K	90	Action potential duration	−		60
ACh sensitive K current	i_{KACh}	K	45–50	Vagal effect	+	Confused with I_{K1}	54,55
Na sensitive K current	i_{KNa}	K	200	Action potential duration	−		61
Ca sensitive K current	I_K, Ca	K	100				70,50
Carrier mediated current							
Na pump	I_{Na-K}			Electrogenic		—	64
Na-Ca exchange	I_{Na-Ca}			Electrogenic		—	65

[a] I is the net macroscopic current, i is the microscopic current.
[b] i_{Ca} is now subdivided into i_T and i_L, 8 and 15 pS in single-channel conductance, respectively.
[c] Single K channel conductances are with symmetric solutions unless mentioned (150 mM K/150 mM K).
[d] Cachelin et al. *J Physiol* 340, 389, 1983.

At least two different groups of Ca channel can be distinguished in the cardiac muscle. The usual and long-lasting type has a larger single-channel conductance ($I_{Ca,L}$) than the other ($I_{Ca,T}$) {38}. The threshold potential for activation of $I_{Ca,L}$ is around −30 mV, and that for $I_{Ca,T}$ is around −50 mV. The balance between the L and T currents is slightly different between different cardiac cells; $I_{Ca,L}$ exists more frequently than $I_{Ca,T}$ in ventricular cells as compared to atrial cells. The T-type channel exists in pacemaker cells {39}. Since no quantitative measurement of the channel is yet available, tests of the relationship between the pacemaker depolarization and the T-type Ca channel are awaited.

INWARD RECTIFIER K CHANNEL

This channel is predominant over other K channels in the ventricular and atrial cells. The inward rectifier K channel shows maximum open probability at around the resting membrane potential and provides the resting K conductance in these cell {40–43}. The open probability of the channel rapidly decrease on depolarization and ensures a low K conductance during the plateau potential. In SA and AV nodal cells, the K channel is scarcely found. This is easily tested by comparing the chance of recording the single-channel current in patch-clamp experiments. In the ventricular cell, most trials record one to three channels within a patch, but in the nodal cell about 95% of the trials fail to detect the channel (fig. 9-8).

In the whole-cell current recording, the amplitudes of the membrane currents were normalized with reference to the surface area of the single cells and are compared in fig. 9-9. In both the atrial and ventricular cells, the steady-state I-V relations revealed typical inward rectification. The large conductance in the hyperpolarizing potential range was due to the inward rectifier K channel. In contrast, the I-V curve of the SA nodal cell showed very shallow bending, which was due mostly to activation of the I_h current. It is interesting to note that the current density of the Ca current is not significantly different between these cells. It is concluded that the low resting potential of the pacemaker cells is due to a practical lack of the inward rectifier K channel.

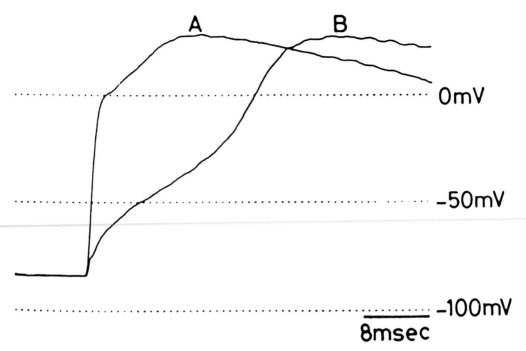

Fig. 9-6. Effect of TTX on the upstroke of the anodal break excitation in the small AV nodal specimen. The membrane potential was clamped to $-83\,mV$ to restore I_{Na}, and the clamp was switched off 0.5 seconds after the hyperpolarization. **A:** in Tyrode solution; **B:** $10^{-7}\,g/ml$ TTX was added to the control Tyrode solution. From Kokubun et al. {16}, with permission.

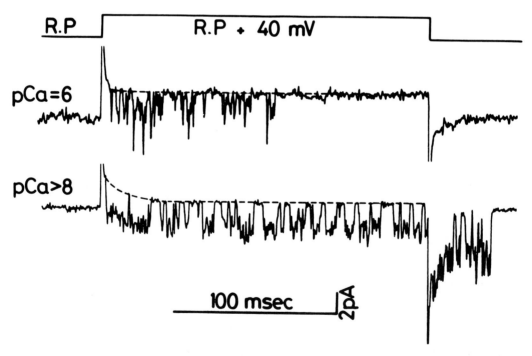

Fig. 9-7. Ca channel currents recorded from a guinea-pig ventricular cell with a patch pipette containing $144\,mM$ NaCl and TTX $31\,\mu M$ (cell-attached patch). The free Ca^{2+} concentration was adjusted to $P_{Ca} = 6.0$ (upper record) and 8.0 (lower record) using $2\,mM$ EGTA. Depolarizing clamp step of $40\,mV$ was applied from the resting membrane potential. The dotted line indicate the baseline with no channel opening. In the lower trace, the unit amplitude of the current was increased on repolarization because of the increased driving force. The cells were superfused with Tyrode solution containing $5\,\mu M$ BAY K 8664. Original recording by H. Matsuda.

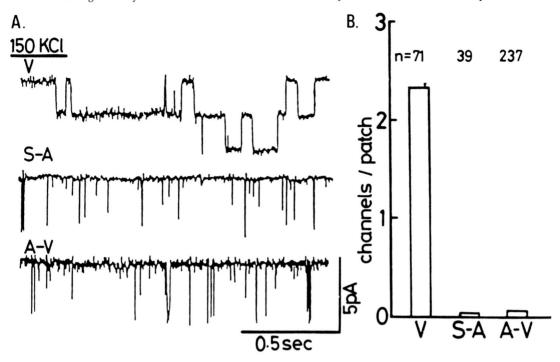

Fig. 9-8. Resting K conductances in the ventricular cells (V), SA nodal cells (S-A) and AV nodal cells (A-V). **A:** The cell-attached patch pipette contained 150 mM KCl and the pipette potential was set at 20 mV ± (resting potential). The single channel currents obtained from the ventricular cell is generated from the inward rectifier K channels and those from the nodal cells through the ACh-sensitive K channels. The pipette contained no ACh, and the activity is attributed to a basal activity of the K channel. If the pipette contained ACh, the open probability of the nodal-type channel is much increased. Note the unit amplitude of the inward rectifier K channel is smaller and the lifetime of the open state is longer than those of the ACh-sensitive K channels. **B:** The number of the inward rectifier K channels within a membrane patch was measured as the maximum number of overlapping open channels observed in a continuous recording for more than 5 minutes. This approximation was taken simply because it was easier than estimating the total number of channels by the leastsquares fit of the binominal distribution to the amplitude histogram. The average of channel number in the ventricular cell, SA nodal cell, and AV nodal cell are shown in the graph. n indicates the number of experiments. From Noma et al. {11}, with permission.

DELAYED RECTIFIER K CHANNEL

This current system contributes to the repolarizing process of the action potential. In the pacemaker tissue of the heart, the K current is thought to be responsible for diastolic depolarization. The outward current in the nodal cells, when examined in the absence of both I_{Ca} and I_{Na}, shows exponential activation during depolarization and deactivation on repolarization {12,44–46}. The time course fitted with the sum of at least two components. The early component was well described by a first-order Hodgkin–Huxley process for ion channel behaviour. The activation variable changed from 0 at about −50 mV to 1 at +10 mV. No significant effect of external K concentration on the channel kinetics was detected (cf. inward rectifier K channel). The fully activated current displayed anomalous rectification without any obvious negative slope.

Recently, Shibasaki {47} succeeded in recording the single-channel current (fig. 9-10). The ensemle average of the single-channel currents decayed with a time constant

of 40 ms on repolarization from 0 mV to −70 mV. The time course of activation of the channel on depolarization and deactivation of repolarization agreed well with the fast and major component of the whole-cell outward current. The channel behaved like a pure K channel, and its kinetics were voltage dependent, but were not dependent on the external K concentration. Due to the relatively small conductance of about 10 pS at 150 mV K_o, and also because of inward rectification, the outward-going current could not be detected.

TRANSIENT OUTWARD CURRENT

The presence of the transient outward current was documented as early as in 1964 by Deck and Trautwein {48}, and it is this current that is responsible for early repolarization of the action potential in the Purkinje fiber. In the AV nodal action potential, there is no rapid repolarization phase immediately after the rising phase of the action potential. Thus, the existence of this current system has long been overlooked. Recently, Nakayama and Irisawa

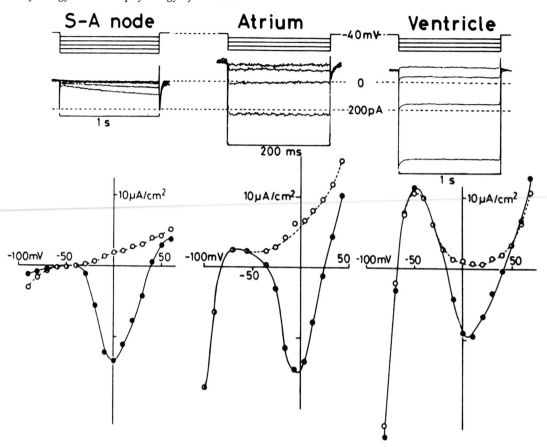

Fig. 9-9. Comparison of the I-V relations obtained from three different types of the cardiac cells. The amplitude of the whole cell current was normalized by referring to the surface area of the single cells to give the current density. In each family of voltage-clamp records the upper traces indicate the clamp program and the lower traces indicate the membrane currents. The I-V curves were measured at the peak of the inward current (filled circles) and near the end of the clamp steps (open circles). The larger resting conductances in the atrial and ventricular cells are due to the activity of the inward rectifier K channels. In the SA nodal cell, the time-dependent increase in the current during hyperpolarization is mainly due to the hyperpolarization-activated current.

{49} found a current in quiescent cells of the AV node of the rabbit that was very similar to the transient outward current (fig. 9-11A). When employing a low holding potential of about −40 mV, the current system is largely inactivated. The inactivation is removed with a time constant of 1–3 seconds by hyperpolarizing the membrane to more negative membrane potentials. When the membrane is depolarized from a holding potential of about −80 mV, the current is activated within several milliseconds and then inactivated. The time course of inactivation consisted of two exponential components: the fast time constants were in the range of 20–40 ms and the slower ones, 100–200 ms. The peak amplitude of the transient outward current in the AV nodal cells was very variable between different cells. In 13 out of 24 cells, the amplitude was negligible and in one case, giving the maximum amplitude, it was 21.4 μ/cm² at −17 mV, which is larger than that of the Ca current.

A voltage clamp protocol equivalent to the whole-cell clamp experiment induced a transient activation of a class of single channel (fig. 9-11B). When the patch pipette contained 5.4 mM K^+ and 134.6 mM Na^+, the single-channel current-voltage (I-V) relation was almost linear and showed a slope conductance of about 20 pS, and the reversal potential was around the resting membrane potential of the quiescent AV nodal cell. The channel was insensitive to variation of the external concentration of Cl^-. Nakayama and Irisawa {49} concluded that the P_{Na}/P_K ratio is around 0.2. It is suggested that the channel is not sensitive to the intracellular Ca^{2+}, since their pipette solution for the whole-cell clamp experiments always contained EGTA.

Single-channel currents that correspond to the transient outward current in the cow Purkinje fiber have recently been recorded by Callewaert et al. {50}. The I-V relation was linear in the voltage range between +10 mV and

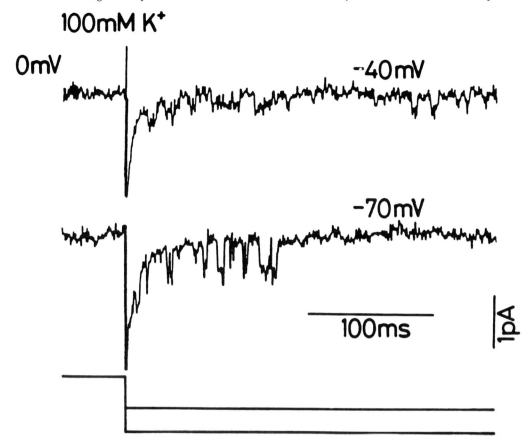

Fig. 9-10. The single-channel currents of the delayed rectifier K channel obtained in the rabbit nodal cell with the cell-attached patch recording. The pipette contained 100 mM KCl solution and the membrane potential was clamped back from 0 mV to −40 mV (**upper trace**) and to −70 mV (**lower trace**). The K channel was activated during the preceding depolarization, but no obvious single-channel current was observed because the potential was close to the reversal potential and also because of the inward-going rectification of the channel. On repolarization, an inward single channel current appeared. The channel is deactivated with time and the single-channel current disappeared. At −40 mV the activity lasted longer than at −70 mV, corresponding to the longer time constant of deactivation at −40 mV than at −70 mV in the whole cell current. Original traces from T. Shibasaki.

+110 mV, with a slope conductance of 120 pS at 10.8 mM external K^+. The channel was selective for K^+. Raising the internal Ca^{2+} activity from 0.01 μM to 1 μM markedly increased the frequency of opening of the K channel during depolarization. It seems that various channel types underlie the transient outward current in different cardiac cells.

HYPERPOLARIZATION-ACTIVATED CURRENT

In the SA node cell, hyperpolarization negative to −60 mV induced a gradual increase in the inward current {51}, and this current change was attributable to a current system I_h, which is activated by hyperpolarization {27}. The inward flow of I_h may accelerate the pacemaker depolarization and partially mediate the chronotropic effect of epinephrine {28,52}. In about one fifth of the small AV nodal preparations, activation of I_h became apparent at membrane

potentials negative to −80 mV, and in the remainder of the preparations the amplitude of I_h was negligibly small. Thus, no correlation between the amplitude of I_h and the pacemaker frequency was demonstrated in the AV nodal cells. This finding is consistent with the fact that the pacemaker activity was not markedly changed even when the I_h was nearly completely suppressed by application of Cs^+ in the SA node {37}. As has been suggested in the SA node, I_h does play a role in driving the membrane potential back to lower potential levels. Eventually, I_h may contribute to the action potential configuration of the AV nodal cell as an inward background current because of its slow time course compared to the cardiac cycle.

I_h is depressed by replacing the external Cl^- with organic anions and also by depleting the external Na^+. When the K concentration is increased, the amplitude is increased. Thus, the ionic selectivity of the channel is still undetermined. The relatively smooth current record

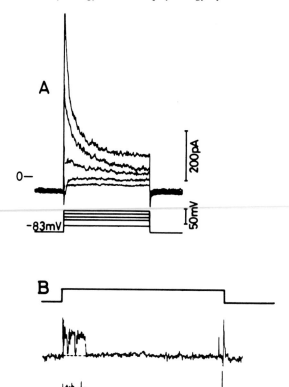

Fig. 9-11. **A:** Transient outward current observed in the quiescent AV nodal single cell of rabbit. The holding potential was −83 mV and depolarizing clamp pulses of 20, 40 50, 60, and 70 mV were applied. The transient outward current was activated at potentials positive to −40 mV. The peak of the current appeared within 10 ms after the onset of the pulse. The peak amplitude was 21 μA/cm². The current was completely inactivated when the holding potential was set at −43 mV. The patch pipette contained K aspartate 110, KCl 20, MgCl₂ 1, KH₂PO₄ 2, ATP 5, CrP 5, EGTA 1 mM and the pH was 7.2. **B:** Single channel recording of the transient outward current. The patch pipette was filled with solution containing 5.4 mM KCl and 134.6 mM NaCl. The membrane was first hyperpolarized by 34 mV from the resting potential to fully activate the channel and depolarized to a level positive by 66 mV from the resting potential. The channel inactivated with time during depolarization. Modified from Nakayama and Irisawa {49}, with permission.

during large activation of I_h suggests that the single channel conductance may be quite small. According to Brown et al. {53} the amplitude of single channel for this current was about 0.1 pA at −112 mV to about 0.05 pA at −72 mV with 70 mM external K.

MUSCARINIC RECEPTOR-OPERATED K CHANNEL

This channel mediates the increase in membrane K conductance induced by the application of ACh or during vagal stimulation. It had been a matter of debate whether ACh activates the inward rectifier K channel, which is responsible for the resting K conductance, or activates a discrete class of K channel. The question was definitely resolved, however, when a single-channel current different from the inward rectifier K channel was recorded {54}. The single-channel conductance of the ACh-sensitive channel is larger by about 50% and the lifetime is about 1/30 of that of the inward rectifier K channel (see fig. 9-8). The activity of the inward rectifier channel is not modulated by ACh. The outward current proved difficult to record by cell-attached patch recording. Thus, inward-going rectification was suggested. Recently, the effects of intracellular Mg²⁺ have been examined in inside-out patch recordings {Horie and Irisawa, personal communication}. It was found that in the absence of intracellular Mg²⁺, the channel conductance was almost ohmic.

Due to the characteristic delay before initiation of the muscarinic response, the involvement of an intracellular second messenger has been discussed. However, experiments injecting possible second messengers into single cell preparations failed to identify a second messenger {9}. Furthermore, the K channel responded to ACh applied in the patch pipette but did not respond to ACh applied in the bath {55}. In the latter case, almost the entire population of receptors, except for a few within the pipette tip, was stimulated by the bath application of ACh. It was concluded, therefore, that the regulation of the K channel by the muscarinic receptor is achieved within the membrane.

Recently, the involvement of GTP-binding protein in the activation of the K channel by the muscarinic receptor was demonstrated almost simultaneously in several laboratories {56–59}. The findings may be summarized as follows: (a) In the absence of GTP in the internal solution, the K current was not activated by agonists. (b) Pertussis toxin, which is a selective blocker of the inhibitory GTP-binding protein, blocked the muscarinic response. (c) In the presence of GTPγS, the agonist activated the K current irreversibly. The characteristic delay of the muscarinic ACh response may be explained by delayed interactions between the receptor, GTP-binding protein, and the channel on the plane of the surface membrane.

IONIC CHANNELS SENSITIVE TO INTRACELLULAR SUBTANCES

The ATP-regulated K channel opens when the intracellular ATP level decreases below 2 mM {13,60}. The channel is distributed at a high density (several channels per μm² surface membrane) in almost every cardiac tissue, including the nodal cells. The I-V relation is almost linear, with a slope of 80 pS in the presence of 150 mM external K. The intracellular Na⁺ and Mg²⁺ block the outward current of the channel in a voltage-dependent manner. The physiological significance of this ligand-gated channel has not yet been established, since the threshold of activation of the channel lies at a very low concentration of intracellular ATP. Recently, Ashcroft and Kakei (personal communication) found that the threshold for this current lies at the range of physiological concentration of ATP when ADP is coexisted within the cell. Activation of the channel may be responsible for the increased K permeability of the cell membrane under anoxic conditions. The pace-maker activity of the nodal cells may be depressed when the ATP-regulated K channels are activated.

A class of K channel having a very large single-channel conductance (200 pS at 150 mM K_o) was found in the ventricular cells when the intracellular Na^+ concentration was raised above 20 mM {61}. The activation of the channel by Na^+ was completely reversible. The physiological role of this channel in AV nodal excitation is entirely unknown.

Ca-activated K channels have been assumed in the nodal cells. However, no direct evidence is yet available for such channels.

ELECTROGENIC ION EXCHANGE SYSTEM

It has been shown that the pacemaker activity is depressed when the Na-K pump is enhanced by loading the nodal cells with Na^+ {62,63}. The activities of the Na-K pump and the Na-Ca exchange systems are assumed to change during the pacemaker cycle, since the influx of Na^+ and Ca^+ during excitation should be expelled during diastole. If the systems are electrogenic, the exchange systems may modulate the pacemaker activity. Employing the cell dialysis technique in single-cell preparations, both the Na-K pump and the Na-K pump and the Na-Ca exchange system have been demonstrated to generate a significant amplitude of membrane current in the ventricular cell {64,65}. The former system mostly generates outward current. The membrane current generated by the Na-Ca exchange system is largely dependent on the intracellular concentration of Ca^2 and Na^+. Thus, elucidation of the dynamic changes in the ion concentrations during activity of the AV is still awaited.

Most of the current systems are very sensitive to variations of the intracellular pH. The presence of the Na-H exchange system has been demonstrated in cardiac cells {66–68}. Although the system is electroneutral, it acts as buffer and so is very important in keeping the channel activities normal.

CONCLUSIONS

The above findings demonstrate that AV nodal cells possess dynamic current systems that are quite similar to those in the SA node. Thus, in the case of failure of the SA nodal rhythm and impaired atrial conduction, AV nodal cells can play the role of a pacemaker. The lack of the inward rectifier K channel in the nodal cells makes the membrane potential labile, and the cell can easily commence spontaneous activity through a small change in the membrane current. In the normal intact heart, however, AV nodal cells do not excite spontaneously. It is tempting

to assume that the membrane potential of the intact AV node cells is influenced by the high resting potential of the His fiber and the atrial fibers through the gap junctions. This is quite possible because the AV nodal cells possess a smaller I_h compared to SA nodal cells, where the I_h may counteract any kind of hyperpolarizing effects.

The Ca channel current makes a major contribution to the upstroke of the AV nodal action potential. The slow conduction of excitation through the AV node is attributable in part ot the fact that the action potential is generated by I_{Ca}, the maximum current density of which is only about 20 $\mu A/cm^2$. The amplitude of I_{Na} is of the order of mA/cm^2 in other myocardia and is involved in conducting the action potential. The weak electrical coupling resulting from a small number of gap junctions may also cause the slow conduction. The space constant of the AV node is 0.4–0.7 mm, which is approximately one half or one third of those for other myocardial fibers.

Through the experiments on the single-channel current and the whole-cell voltage clamp combined with internal dialysis, the membrane currents were shown to be very much dependent on intracellular factors. The activities of almost every channel are depressed when the intracellular ATP concentration is decreased. The ATP-regulated K channel detects a decrease in the ATP level and opens when the ATP level is decreased. Stimulation of cAMP-dependent protein kinase may increase the activity of both the Ca channel and the K channel {69}.

Intracellular Na^+ and Mg^+ ions block several types of K channels on strong depolarization and thereby ensure a low K conductance during the plateau of the action potential. If the intracellular Ca concentration is increased, both the nonselective cation channels {70} and the Na-Ca exchange mechanism are activated and generate an inward current at the resting membrane potential.

REFERENCES

1. Hoffman BF, Cranefield PF: Electrophysiology of the Heart, Mount Kisco, NY: Futura, 1960 (reprint 1976).
2. Matsuda K, Hoshi T, Kameyama S: Action potential of the atrioventricular node (Tawara). *Tohoku J Exp Med* 68:8, 1958.
3. Tawara S: Das Reizleitungssystem des Saugetierherzens. Jena: Gustav Fischer, 1906.
4. Paes De Carvalho A, Almeida DF: Spread of activity through the atrioventricular node. *Circ Res* 8:801–809, 1960.
5. Noma A, Irisawa H: Membrane current in the rabbit sinoatrial node cell as studied by the double microelectrode method. *Pflügers Arch* 364:45–52, 1976.
6. Irisawa H: Comparative physiology of the cardiac pacemaker mechanism. *Physiol Rev* 58:461–498, 1976.
7. Brown HF: Electrophysiology of the sinoatrial node *Physiol Rev* 62:505–530, 1982.
8. Taniguchi J, Kokubun S, Noma A, Irisawa H: Spontaneously active cells isolated from the sinoatrial and atrio-ventricular nodes of the rabbit heart. *Jpn J Physiol* 31:547–558, 1981.
9. Trautwein W, Taniguchi J, Noma A: The effects of intracellular cyclic nucleotides and calcium on the action potential and acetylcholine response of isolated cardiac cells. *Pflügers Arch* 392:307–314, 1982.

10. Hamill OP, Marty A, Neher E, Sakmann B, Sigworth FJ: Improved patch-clamp techniques for high-resolution current recording from cells and cell-free membrane patches. *Pflügers Arch* 391:85–100, 1981.

11. Noma A, Nakayama T, Kurachi Y, Irisawa H: Resting K conductances in pacemaker and non-pacemaker heart cells of the rabbit. *Jpn J Physiol* 34:245–254, 1984.

12. Nakayama N, Kurachi Y, Noma A, Irisawa H: Action potential and membrane currents of single pacemaker cells of the rabbit heart. *Pflügers Arch* 402:248–257, 1984.

13. Kakei M, Noma A: Adenosine-5'-triphosphate-sensitive single potassium channel in the atrioventricular node cell of the rabbit heart. *J Physiol* 352:265–284, 1984.

14. Irisawa H: Electrophysiology of single cardiac cells. *Jpn J Physiol* 34:375–388, 1984.

15. Matsuda H, Noma A: Isolation of calcium current and its sensitivity to monovalent cations in dialysed ventricular cells of guinea pig. *J Physiol* 357:553–573, 1984.

16. Kokubun S, Nishimura M, Noma A, Irisawa H: The spontaneous action potential of rabbit atrioventricular node cells. *Jpn J Physiol* 30:529–540, 1980.

17. Akiyama T, Fozzard HA: Ca and Na selectivity of the active membrane of rabbit AV node cells. *Am J Physiol* 236:C1–C8, 1979.

18. Ruiz-Ceretti E, Ponce Zumino A: Action potential changes under varied $[Na]_o$ and $[Ca]_o$ indicating the existence of two inward currents in cells of the rabbit atrioventricular node. *Circ Res* 39:326–336, 1976.

19. Zipes DP, Mendez C: Action of manganese ions and tetrodotoxin on atrioventricular nodal transmembrane potentials in isolated rabbit hearts. *Circ Res* 32:447–454, 1973.

20. Mendez C: The slow inward current and AV nodal propagation. In: Zipes DP, Bailey JC, Elharrar V (eds) *The Slow Inward Current and Cardiac Arrhythmias*. The Hague: Martinus Nijhoff, 1980, pp 285–294.

21. Shigeto N, Irisawa H: Slow conduction in the atrioventricular node of the cat; a possible explanation Experientia 28:1442–1443, 1972.

22. Shigeto N, Irisawa H: Effect of polarization on the action potentials of the rabbit AV node cells. *Jpn J Physiol* 24:605–616, 1974.

23. Noma A, Irisawa H: Effects of Na^+ and K^+ on the resting membrane potential of the rabbit sinoatrial node cell. *Jpn J Physiol* 25:287–302, 1975.

24. Kokubun S, Nishimura M, Noma A, Irisawa H: Membrane currents in the rabbit atrioventricular node cells. *Pflügers Arch* 393:15–22, 1982.

25. Noma A, Irisawa H, Kokubun S, Kotake H, Nishimura M, Watanabe Y: Slow current systems in the A-V node of the rabbit heart. *Nature* 285:228–229, 1980.

26. Deck KA, Kern R, Trautwein W: Voltage clamp technique in mammalian cardiac fibres. *Pflügers Arch* 280:50–62, 1964.

27. Yanagihara K, Irisawa H: Inward current activated during hyperpolarization in the rabbit sinoatrial node cell Pflügers Arch 385:11–19, 1980.

28. Brown HF, DiFrancesco D, Noble SJ: How does adrenaline accelerate the heart? *Nature* 280:235–236, 1979.

29. DiFrancesco D, Ferroni A, Mazzanti M, Tromba C: Properties of the hyperpolarizing-activated current (i_f) in cells isolated from the rabbit sino-atrial node. *J Physiol* 377:61–81, 1986.

30. Maylie J, Morad M, Weiss J: A study of pace-maker potential in rabbit sino-atrial node: Measurement of potassium activity under voltage-clamp conditions. *J Physiol (Lond)* 311:161–178, 1981.

31. Ponce Zumino AZ, Parisii IM, De Ceretti ERP: Effect of ischemia and low sodium medium on atrioventricular conduction. *Am J Physiol* 218:1489–1494, 1970.

32. De Ceretti E, Ruiz P, Ponce Zumino A, Parisii IM: Resolution of two components in the upstroke of the action potential in atrioventricular fibers of the rabbit heart. *Can J Physiol Pharmacol* 49:642–648, 1971.

33. Irisawa H: Ionic currents underlying spontaneous rhythm of the cardiac primary pacemaker cells. In: Bonke FIM (ed) *The Sinus Node*. The Hague: Martinus Nijoff, 1980, pp 368–375.

34. Kreitner D: Effects of polarization and inhibitors of ionic conductances on the action potentials of nodal and perinodal fibers in rabbit sinoatrial node. In: Bonke FIM (ed) *The Sinus Node*. The Hague: Martinus Nijhoff, 1980, pp 270–278.

35. Matsuda H: Sodium conductance in calcium channels of guinea-pig ventricular cells induced by removal of external calcium ions. *Pflügers Arch* 407:465–475, 1986.

36. Yanagihara K, Noma A, Irisawa H: Reconstruction of sinoatrial node pacemaker potential based on the voltage clamp experiments. *Jpn J Physiol* 30:841–857, 1980.

37. Noma A, Morad M, Irisawa H: Does the "pacemaker current" generate the diastolic depolarization in the rabbit SA node cells? *Pflügers Arch* 396:190–194, 1983.

38. Nilius B, Hess P, Lansman B, Tsien RW: A novel type of cardiac calcium channel in ventricular cells. *Nature* 316:443–446, 1985.

39. Hagiwara N, Irisawa H, Kameyama M: Transient type calcium current contributes to the pacemaker potential of rabbit sinoatrial node cells. *J Physiol* 395:233–253, 1988.

40. Sakmann B, Trube G: Conductance properties of single inwardly rectifying potassium channels in ventricular cells from guinea-pig heart. *J Physiol* 347:641–657, 1984.

41. Sakmann B, Trube G: Voltage-dependent inactivation of inward-rectifying single channel currents in the guinea-pig heart cells. *J Physiol* 347:659–683, 1984.

42. Kameyama M, Kiyosue T, Soejima M: Inward rectifier K channel in the rabbit ventricular cells. *Jpn J Physiol* 33:1039–1056, 1983.

43. Kurachi Y: Voltage-dependent activation of the inward-rectifier potassium channel in the ventricular cell membrane of guinea-pig heart. *J Physiol* 366:365–385, 1985.

44. Noma A, Irisawa H: A time- and voltage-dependent potassium current in the rabbit sinoatrial node cell. *Pflügers Arch* 366:251–258, 1976.

45. Yanagihara K, Irisawa H: Potassium current during the pacemaker depolarization in rabbit sinoatrial node cell. *Pflügers Arch* 388:255–260, 1980.

46. DiFrancesco D, Noma A, Trautwein W: Kinetics and magnitude of the time-dependent potassium current in the rabbit sinoatrial node: Effect of external potassium Pflügers Arch 381:271–279, 1979.

47. Shibasaki T: Single delayed rectifier K channels in pacemaker cells of rabbit heart. *J Physiol* 387:227–250, 1987.

48. Deck KA, Trautwein W: Ionic currents in cardiac excitation. *Pflügers Arch* 280:63–80, 1964.

49. Nakayama T, Irisawa H: Transient outward current carried by potassium and sodium in quiescent atrioventricular node cells of rabbits. *Circ Res* 57:65–73, 1985.

50. Callewaert G, Vereecke J, Carmeliet E: Existence of a calcium-dependent channel in the membrane of cow cardiac Purkinje cells. *Pflügers Arch* 406:424–426, 1986.

51. Seyama I: Characteristics of the rectifying properties of the sinoatrial node cell of the rabbit. *J Physiol* 255:379–397, 1976.

52. Noma A, Kotake H, Irisawa H: Slow inward current and its role mediating the chronotropic effect of epinephrine in the rabbit sinoatrial node. *Pflügers Arch* 388:1–9, 1980.

53. Brown HF, DiFrancesco D, Tromba C: Recording of single i_f channels in isolated rabbit sino-atrial node cells. *J Physiol* 377:111, 1986.
54. Sakmann B, Noma A, Trautwein W: Acetylcholine activation of single muscarinic K channels in isolated pacemaker cells of the mammalian heart. Nature 303:250–253, 1983.
55. Soejima M, Noma A: Mode of regulation of the Achsensitive K channel by the muscarinic receptor in rabbit atrial cells. *Pflügers Arch* 400:424–431, 1984.
56. Breitwieser GE, Szabo G: Uncoupling of cardiac β-adrenergic receptors from ion channels by a guanine nucleotide analogue. *Nature* 317:538–540, 1985.
57. Endoh M, Maruyama M, Iijima T: Attenuation of muscarinic cholinergic inhibition by islet-activating protein in the heart. *Am J Physiol* 249:H309–H320, 1985.
58. Pfaffinger PJ, Martin JM, Hunter DD, Nathanson NM, Hille B: CTP-binding proteins couple cardiac muscarinic receptors to a K channel. *Nature* 317:536–538, 1985.
59. Sorota S, Tsuji Y, Tajima T, Pappano AJ: Pertussis toxin treatment blocks hyperpolarization by muscarinic agonists in chick atrium. *Circ Rec* 57:748–758, 1985.
60. Kakei M, Noma A, Shibasaki T: Properties of adenosine-triphosphate-regulated potassium channels in guinea-pig ventricular cells. *J Physiol* 363:441–462, 1985.
61. Kameyama M, Kakei M, Sato R, Shibasaki T, Matsuda H, Irisawa H: Intracellular Na^+ activates a K channel in mammalian cardiac cells. *Nature* 309:354–356, 1984.
62. Noma A, Irisawa H: Contribution of an electrogenic sodium pump to the membrane potential in rabbit sinoatrial node cells. *Pflügers Arch* 358:289–301, 1975.
63. Kurachi Y, Noma A, Irisawa H: Electrogenic sodium pump in rabbit atrio-ventricular node cell. *Pflügers Arch* 391:261–266, 1981.
64. Gadsby DC, Kimura J, Noma A: Voltage dependence of Na/K pump current in isolated heart cells. *Nature* 315:63–65, 1985.
65. Kimura J, Noma A, Irisawa H: Na-Ca exchange current in mammalian heart cells. *Nature* 319:596–597, 1986.
66. Ellis D, Mac Leod KT: Sodium-dependent control of intracellular pH in Purkinje fibres of sheep heart. *J Physiol* 359:81–105, 1985.
67. Piwnica-Worms D, Jacob R, Horres R, Lieberman M: Na/H exchange in cultured chick heart cells: pH_i regulation. *J Gen Physiol* 85:43–64, 1985.
68. Sato R, Noma A, Kurachi Y, Irisawa H: Effects of intracellular acidification on membrane currents in ventricular cells of the guinea pig. *Circ Res* 57:553–561, 1985.
69. Kameyama M, Hofmann F, Trautwein W: On the mechanism of β-adrenergic regulation of the Ca channel in the guinea-pig heart. *Pflügers Arch* 405:285–293, 1985.
70. Colquhoun D, Neher E, Reuter H, Stevens CF: Inward current channels activated by intracellular Ca in cultured cardiac cells. *Nature* 294:752–753, 1981.

CHAPTER 10

Cardiac Excitability, Gap Junctions, Cable Properties, and Impulse Propagation

KENNETH S. GINSBURG & MORTON F. ARNSDORF

INTRODUCTION

Biophysical theory in the organization of knowledge

In this chapter we will review important concepts under-lying cardiac excitability. We will emphasize information that has appeared since the earlier editions of this chapter in 1984 {13} and 1986 {16} in the areas of cellular mechanisms of generation of excitation, communication between cells, spatial properties of conduction, and control of heart rhythm.

To a clinician cardiac excitability indicates the ability of cardiac cells regeneratively to depolarize and repolarize during the action potential, as well as the ease with which electrical activity propagates from cell to cell. To develop biophysical theories explaining excitability and other aspects of cardiac function has been a major challenge to the researcher, but such theories have become increasingly useful in organizing our knowledge. They form an intellectual framework within which one can assess critically what is known and what is unknown. For this reason we will review here, in a nonmathematical way, the logical basis for many of the biophysical results we will be summarizing. We will later introduce some biophysically based equations, along with qualitative discussion to help the reader assess their usefulness.

The practical use of a biophysical theory is to support predictions of how a system under study might respond to new contingencies. These predictions can be long term, for example, the risk of sudden cardiac death {134}, or short term, for example, the reconstruction of action potential waveforms from voltage-clamp currents {99}. They can be end results, but can also amount to new hypotheses for experimental testing.

Because of growth in computer and other technology, biophysical theories need no longer be rarefied or abstract; there is continued movement toward the testing and application of more refined theoretical models {197}. Nonetheless, in order to be useful, models need generality, parsimony, ease of application, and predictive power.

Biophysical system analysis

As shown in fig. 10-1A {45}, a biophysical theory is a model that describes a corresponding biophysical system

or process. Such a process normally has input(s) or stimuli, output(s) or responses, and possibly internal variables, all of which depend on time and are organized in space. The process may include intrinsic or artificially imposed feedback.

The process discussed most extensively in this chapter can be called *cardiac excitability*. In many cases, excitability is studied by measuring responses to stimuli that the experimenter controls. At the cellular level, either currents are injected into cells, in which case the responses are voltage changes, or voltages are imposed across cell membranes, in which case the responses are current flows. The former approach is called *current clamp* and is diagrammed in fig. 10-3A; the latter is called *voltage clamp*. In other cases, such as the study of the determinants of resting heart rate variability, there is no specific stimulus.

Because the action of a biophysical system or process involves storage and transfer of energy, the relationship between stimulus and response (the transfer characteristic), could in principle be expressed using the equations of dynamic system analysis, including linear and nonlinear differential equations. The physical properties of the system would be captured in the coefficients or parameters of these equations.

Key elements of the physical structure of a system under study are presumed initially to be unknown. Analysis consists of trying to infer this structure, using known physical laws as well as prior and new experimental (or clinical) observations. Many interesting analysis tasks involve showing how disturbances or perturbations, such as drugs or ischemic metabolism, change a system or process.

In many cases a graphical or numerical representation of the measured responses of a biophysical system will support inferences about its structure. In other cases we may need to find a specific set of equations to represent the system. Regardless of the representation, qualifying statements, quantitative constraints, and assumptions are required to define the conditions under which it was determined.

As seen in fig. 10-1B, when a system or process is to be represented by equations, analysis begins with choosing the equations and defining their known and unknown parameters. This part of the procedure is called *identification*. Ideally, the parameters should be related to actual

N. Sperelakis (ed.), Physiology and Pathophysiology of the Heart, Third Edition.
© *1995 Kluwer Academic Publishers. ISBN 0-7923-2612-1. All rights reserved.*

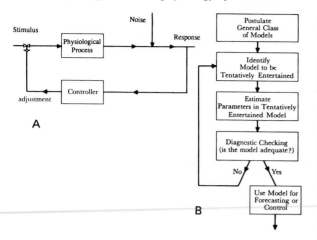

A

B

Fig. 10-1. **A:** A physiological process to which a stimulus is applied and from which a response is measured. Noise disturbances interfere with observation of the response. Feedback, if present, may occur naturally or may be imposed externally. **B:** The iterative procedure of building a model by identifying and estimating its parameters. Modified from Box and Jenkins {45}, with permission.

physical features. Analysis is completed by determinining the values of the identified parameters, a procedure called *estimation*. The responses described by these equations may be presented as mathematical solutions and/or graphically or numerically, and will normally be compared with experimentally measured responses.

Linear and nonlinear relationships between stimulus and response

Some phenomena of cardiac function, such as decremental conduction through cable-like tissues, can be described using linear differential equations. The requirement for a linear model is that all the system parameters can be taken as constant; they may, of course, change slowly over time and/or space, depending on factors such as developmental state, pathological conditions, and the type of tissue.

A key feature of a linear system is that many aspects of its responses can be predicted from the characteristics of the input(s). For instance, the strength of response is proportional to the strength of the stimulus, and multiple stimuli generate their respective responses independently. Analysis of linear systems from observations uses methods analogous with correlation, regression, and analysis of variance {45}. Powerful tools such as transform methods make these analyses more tractable {179}.

Whenever one or more parameters is not constant but rather depends on stimulus, internal, or response variables, nonlinear models are needed. Prior knowledge may indicate that nonlinear analysis is needed. For instance, nonlinear properties of the relationships between cellular transmembrane voltages and currents, such as thresholds, inactivation, and saturation, can be predicted

from the corresponding phenomena known to occur in individual ion channels.

Observation of a system's responses often clearly indicates that it is nonlinear. The response may have features inconsistent with the idea of proportional responses to stimuli {134}. These include, among others, bistability {201}, bifurcations {97}, and hysteresis {209}. In bistable systems, a given stimulus can lead to two or more kinds of response. In bifurcations, the character of the response evolves in time, or as a parameter is changed, in a specific sequence. In hysteresis, the response after a stimulus has reached some fixed amplitude differs, depending on how fast and/or in what direction the stimulus had been changed previously in the course of reaching that amplitude. When a periodic input is applied to a nonlinear system, the response can include harmonic and/or subharmonic frequencies, or can fall in arbitrary ratios (N:M) of integers, with respect to the input period. The response of a linear system to periodic inputs always has the same periodicities as the input.

Nonlinear behaviors may at first seem random or chaotic, making model identification and estimation seem formidably difficult. Indeed, there is no specific way to delimit what forms of models should be considered, and modeling is somewhat of an art. Usually a model is limited to somewhat specific conditions. Very large amounts of data may be needed to capture the considerable behavioral repertoire of many nonlinear systems.

Despite these problems, many nonlinear processes can behave according to specific and even simple rules {97,131,134}. Of note is the observation that a small change either in initial conditions (before a stimulus is applied) or system parameters can radically change the response of a system to a given stimulus {131,152}. Often a complex response can be made simple, or at least predictable, by a small change in conditions. One of us (MFA) has suggested that this phenomenon, which can be called an *assisted bifurcation*, is frequent in cardiac electrophysiology, and is useful as a therapeutic principle {19}.

A process under study is sometimes observable only at discrete time intervals. Approximating a linear continuous process with a discrete time model is often successful, because responses of a linear system have inherently limited rates of change. With a nonlinear system there is no such limit; that is, responses can be sudden or discontinuous. Although processes such as those governing heart rates have been modeled successfully using either nonlinear differential equation {131} or difference equation systems {324}, discrete approximations can lead to serious errors if discontinuities (in time or space) are present.

In most realistic cases, a system's responses to stimuli vary, as though either the system were responding to an unknown disturbance (fig. 10-1A) or the system parameters themselves varied. Thus identification and estimation are statistical and often iterative tasks (fig. 10-1B) {45}. Analysis then includes discrimination among alternative structures and sets of parameters, either to support one or another description of normal function, or to define and discriminate among health and disease states. For linear models, system properties can be expressed in terms of expectations or averages, and both the study of variance and discrimination among alternatives are relatively well formalized {65,154,179,264}.

The intrinsic variability of a system can change significantly in pathology. For instance, condution velocity {36} and refractoriness {3} develop specific patterns of variability in injured cardiac tissue, while heart rate is less variable during advanced heart failure {134}. Built in variability can be beneficial. For example, pacemaking cells synchronize optimally when they are not maximally coupled {183,271}. Discontinuities in the pattern of propagation through cardiac tissue may help to preserve function during injury {294}.

Variability can also be caused by technically imperfect (noisy) measurements. For instance, this source of variability affects the predictive power of signal-averaged electrocardiography {39,48}.

Techniques such as correlation {214} are applicable to some nonlinear systems, but can be difficult to use and interpret. To ease the difficulties of nonlinear analysis, advantage is sometimes taken of the fact that many nonlinear systems respond approximately linearly when the stimulus is a small disturbance of an idealized form, such as a step change. Often it is possible experimentally to reduce the order or complexity of a system. The voltage clamp is an elegant example of this approach {118}.

Electrophysiologists often distinguish cellular properties as being either active or passive. Properties that can be considered constant are passive. Under some conditions, intracellular and extracellular ionic activities, membrane capacitance, and intercellular coupling conductance are passive properties, or current sinks. Cellular properties such as the transmembrane ion conductances that are responsible for action potential generation and propagation, which are usually not constant, are referred to as *active properties* or *current sources*.

These and other properties will be described in some detail below. Whether a property should be thought of as passive or active depends on what stimulus is applied and what response is measured. When all cellular properties can be considered constant or passive, analysis using linear models is appropriate. As we noted, this condition can often be met when the stimulus is a relatively small perturbation. In general, however, one or more properties is active and nonlinear analysis must be used.

We will try to illustrate some biophysical ideas that have been applied to explain the ionic basis for excitation (generation of action potentials), communication between pairs of cells, and propagation of excitation over extensive areas. We will give some attention to disturbances of heart rhythm and their control, either by drugs or by pacing devices.

A complete biophysical consideration of cardiac function would include neurohumoral control, excitation-contraction coupling, analysis of the stress and strain relations of myocardial tissue during contraction, as well as the effects of contraction and mechanical loading on cellular electrophysiological properties {198,199}. These feedback phenomena must control cardiac excitability

closely under dynamic beat-to-beat conditions. As their study is beyond our scope, we will assume all of their influences remain constant. The appropriateness of this assumption should be considered carefully, especially in the study of pathological conditions.

Matrical concept of cardiac excitability

The matrical concept proposed previously by one of us {12,29} describes the essential nonlinear character of cardiac excitability and propagation in a way that is intuitive to the physiologist without requiring explicit mathematical equations. A matrix is drawn to show interrelationships among cellular properties. These properties are the system parameters we defined above, and therefore also have mathematical relationships.

Figure 10-2 {28} shows a sample matrix, which has a regular hexagonal shape, indicative of a normal state. To maintain a normal state, the bioelectrical events that allow the coordinated propagation of excitation, the contraction of the heart, and an efficient cardiac output must be controlled within very tight limits. Abnormalities in the regulatory mechanisms often accompany cardiac disease. As we will see in the examples below, abnormal states are represented by matrices of irregular polygonal shape.

In fig. 10-2, the bonds between the matrix elements show the interactions and mutual dependencies. This matrix includes the resting potential (V_r), threshold voltage (V_{th}), Na$^+$ conductance (g_{Na}), membrane resistance (R_m), length constant (λ), and, as a measure of overall excitability, the liminal length (LL), all of which will be defined below. The matrix has many more dimensions than are shown here, as each element is determined by underlying properties, such as ion channel conductances.

The active (source) and passive (sink) properties, which form the elements of the matrix, are not usually indepen-

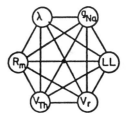

Fig. 10-2. A simplified normal matrix of active and passive cellular electrophysiologic properties that determine cardiac excitability. The elements include resting potential (V_r), threshold voltage (V_{th}), sodium conductance (g_{Na}), membrane resistance (R_m), length constant (λ), and liminal length (LL), all of which are defined in the text. Each element, in turn, depends on a set of more basic processes. The bonds connecting the elements indicate interactions and mutual dependencies. A normal state is indicated by the regular hexagonal shape. When quantities represented in the matrix change, the matrix changes shape; when a quantity decreases, the corresponding element shifts toward the center of the hexagon; when the quantity increases, the corresponding element shifts away from the center. From Arnsdorf and Wasserstrom {28}, with permission.

dent of each other. How any changes in the active and passive elements affect ongoing activity or responses to stimuli may be impossible to determine by experimentally changing just one element at a time. We will support this view with examples in analysis of propagation using cable theory {196,208}, description of conditions conducive to arrhythmias, and study of mechanisms and effects of anti-arrhythmic drugs {239,312}.

Recent valuable comprehensive reviews of cardiac electrophysiology include those edited by Fozzard et al. {121} and by Zipes and Jalife {352}. Reviews emphasizing non-linear analysis include Glass et àl. {129} and Jack et al. {171}. Specialized reviews will be mentioned as each topic area is introduced.

INDIVIDUAL MYOCARDIAL CELLS

Cell membrane components

The plasma membrane that separates the aqueous phases inside and outside the cells consists of a bilayer of phospholipids. These phospholipids are amphipathic, with their hydrophobic portions stably oriented toward the membrane interior and their charged hydrophilic portions oriented toward the internal and external aqueous phases. The phospholipids and other membrane constituents are subject to dielectric polarization, with the result that the membrane can store charge, as does an electrical capacitor.

The lipidic interior of the membrane bilayer should be a barrier to any flow of ions; however, the plasmalemma is significantly permeable to both ions and water. Transmembrane proteins, including ion channels and pumps or exchangers, mediate and impart specific properties to ion and water permeation. The ease or difficulty with which ions can pass through the membrane is determined by the physical properties of the transmembrane proteins and are measurable, respectively, as electrical conductance or resistance.

As fig. 10-3B shows, the arrangement, consisting of the lipid membrane, ion channels, and other membrane proteins, together behaves electrically as a parallel resistive and capacitive network with components R_m and C_m. Whenever a potential difference V_m exists across the membrane, a current I_m will flow, which consists of two components:

$$I_m = I_c + I_{ion}. \tag{10.1}$$

At any membrane potential V_m, the charge distribution held by membrane capacitance C_m represents stored energy. Whenever V_m changes, the physical work required to add or remove charge can only be done at a finite rate. This is described by

$$I_c = C_m \frac{dV_m}{dt}. \tag{10-2}$$

The relationship among I_{ion}, V_m, and R_m, is given by Ohm's Law:

$$I_{ion} = \frac{V_m}{R_m}. \tag{10-3}$$

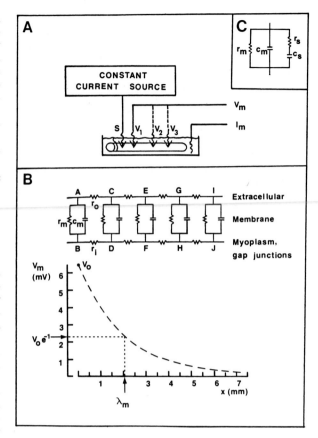

Fig. 10-3. **A:** Experimental arrangement for cable analysis. Stimulus is sudden application of a constant current, injected intracellularly through a microelectrode near the ligated end of a cardiac Purkinje fiber (S). Response is a change in transmembrane voltage (V_m), recorded by microelecrodes at several points along the preparation (VI, V2, V3, etc.). Stimulating current I_m is monitored via the bath ground. **B:** An electrical analog for a cable-like preparation, showing membrane resistance (r_m), membrane capacitance (c_m), internal longitudinal resistance (r_i) due to the myoplasm and gap junctions, and external resistance (r_o) due to the extracellular space. Below is plotted the transmembrane voltage as a function of distance in steady state after intracellular current application. Arrow marks length constant λ. **C:** An analog that represents membrane behavior more accurately by inclusion of series elements r_s and c_s, in addition to r_m and c_m.

Combining eqs. (10-1) through (10-3),

$$I_m = C_m \frac{dV_m}{dt} + \frac{V_m}{R_m}. \tag{10-4}$$

In studies on isolated cells, R_m, C_m, and I_m, expressed respectively as ohms (Ω), farads (F), and amperes (A), normally represent totals for the entire area of the cell membrane. In studies on isolated cable-like fibers or chains of cells end to end, with fixed geometry, the corresponding quantities, denoted in lower case as r_m, c_m, and i_m, can be expressed per unit length, and have the dimensions ohm-meter (resistivity; typical unit Ω-cm), farad/meter (typically μF/cm), and ampere/meter (typically μA/cm).

In reality, the electrical behavior of a cell membrane is more complex than is indicated by eq. (10-4). The membrane actually behaves as a capacitor, part of which is in series with a significant amount of resistance {109,115,171, 244} (fig. 10-3C). This property of C_m originates partly in details of the composition of the membrane, including the presence of proteins that can polarize without a conductance change {5}. However, it is due mainly to the T system, the transverse tubules that conduct action potentials into the interior of many types of cardiac cell and link the membrane of the sarcoplasmic reticulum (SR) with the extracellular membrane. Portions of the cell membrane (and thus of C_m) are accessible to the cell exterior only through T-system passages, which, although filled with extracellular medium, are narrow and resistive to ionic flow. As a consequence, the effective value of C_m is not truly constant, but rather depends on the frequency or rate of change of V_m.

Utrastructurally, the boundary of a cardiac muscle fiber (a cell) also includes extracellular matrix components such as glycocalyx, in addition to the cell membrane {288}. These features establish and maintain cell apposition and adhesion, but they also restrict the extracellular space, and can thereby affect excitation and propagation by restricting the flow and redistribution of ions.

Cellular excitability

As we noted above, cardiac excitability indicates the ability of cardiac cells regeneratively to depolarize and repolarize during the action potential, as well as the ease with which electrical activity propagates from cell to cell. These processes result from ionic flow through paths involving the cardiac cell membrane, the myoplasm, the gap junctions between cells, and the extracellular space.

In an individual cell, pumps driven by metabolic energy, particularly the Na/K-ATPase, along with electrochemical factors, establish a concentration gradient for each of the various ion species across the plasma membrane. If not opposed by the pumps, ionic currents would flow down these gradients through ion channels, the currents representing the rates at which the ions can permeate through the channels. At any instant, metabolically and electrochemically maintained nonequilibrium gradients of the permeable ions across the cell membrane represent stored energy, which is evident as a voltage difference, V_m. If V_m of a cell is constant, then there is no net inward or outward flux (current) of any ion species. The balance of current flowing through the ion channels of a cell is subject to disturbances, which can originate in the cell, in the activity of other cells, or in experimentally applied stimuli. Whenever any unopposed flux of ions occurs, V_m changes ($\Delta V_m = R_m \Delta I_m$). At the same time, the physical conformations of ion channel proteins, and hence their resistances to ionic flow, change whenever V_m changes. Because of this dependence on V_m, transmembrane resistance R_m, which is the net effect due to all of the ion channels present in the cell membrane, is a nonlinear active property, rather than a passive property.

Normally V_m is negative; positive charges would tend

to flow into a cell. If the net amount of positive charge flowing into the cell through some population of ion channels should increase transiently by a small amount, V_m will be reduced (made less negative). For a small change in V_m there is little or no change in R_m, and V_m will return to its original value when the transient disturbance is over, according to Ohm's Law. Such a disturbance in V_m is called an *electrotonic* or *decremental potential*.

However, the dependency of R_m on V_m is such that if a larger positive current disturbance occurs and V_m decreases (again, becomes less negative) beyond some point, R_m will decrease also. According to eq. (10-3), current I_m will then increase. The ion flux represented by I_m will further decrease V_m, leading to yet more I_m, and so on. This regenerative decrease in R_m (or increase in g_m) in response to a sufficient disturbance in I_m will result in an action potential (AP). It is sometimes called *negative slope conductance*.

The changes in V_m that occur during the generation of electrotonic and action potentials result in voltage differences among various points in a cell, and between any one cell and its neighbors. These potential differences will cause currents to flow through regions encompassing many cells. As we will describe, these currents, when properly regulated, lead to the coordinated propagation of excitation, which underlies normal contraction of the heart and an efficient cardiac output.

Ion currents and ion channel states

We noted above that the basis for generating electrotonic and action potentials is the dependence of R_m and resultant current I_m on V_m. Our current understanding of how transmembrane ion fluxes depend on voltage and time is based on voltage-clamp analysis. The voltage-clamp technique helps to clarify the complex nonlinear process relating I_m and V_m by allowing measurement of I_m while V_m is forced to change in a prescribed manner {118}.

When voltage clamping was combined with use of pharmacological and other chemical agents, it was confirmed that I_m has multiple components carried by different ions. The contribution to I_m from each ionic species is determined by both conductance for that species and the driving force behind that species. Conductance g is the reciprocal of resistance.

For a given ionic species, say y, the driving force is the difference between the instantaneous membrane voltage, V_m, and the equilibrium potential, E_y, so that

$$I_y = g_y(V_m - E_y). \tag{10-5}$$

E_y is the value of V_m that would have to exist at any instant to establish and maintain the existing transmembrane concentration gradient of ion species y. For any ion, when $V_m = E_y$, $I_y = 0$, regardless of g_y.

Recognizing that each ion species, say x, y, z, and so on, exists at a particular concentration inside and outside a cell and so has its own equilibrium potential E_x, E_y, or E_z, and that each ion conductance g_x, g_y, or g_z may depend on voltage, time, or both, in its own nonlinear way, we can write:

$$I_m \approx I_{ion} = \frac{V_m}{R_m} = V_m G_m$$

$$= g_x(V_m - E_x) + g_y(V_m - E_y)$$
$$+ g_z(V_m - E_z) + \cdots \qquad (10\text{-}6)$$

We have neglected capacitative current, I_c, and currents due to pump/exchange mechanisms, which determine intracellular ionic activities in a V_m-dependent manner {178, 203}, to show that I_m is mainly determined by ionic conductances. For modern examples of ion-selective voltage-clamp analysis see Hagiwara et al. {146} and Makielski et al. {213}.

The ion species of greatest interest are K^+ {60}, Na^+ {117}, and Ca^{2+} {247}. Usually, $V_m > E_K$, so that K^+ current will flow out of a cell whenever $g_K > 0$, tending to make V_m more negative. Usually, $V_m < E_{Na}$ and $V_m < E_{Ca}$, so whenever $g_{Na} > 0$ or $g_{Ca} > 0$, Na^+ or Ca^{2+}, respectively, will flow into a cell, tending to depolarize V_m.

The earliest formal model attempting to explain non-linearly voltage-dependent ion conductances was that of Hodgkin and Huxley {161}, which has subsequently been modified to better describe cardiac cells {107,238}. Taking as an example Na^+ conductance, g_{Na}, the Hodgkin–Huxley model can be explained as a modification of eq. (10-6):

$$I_{Na} = \overline{g_{Na}} \, m^3 h (V_m - E_{Na}). \qquad (10\text{-}7)$$

In this equation I_{Na} is the Na^+ current per unit area, E_{Na} is the equilibrium potential for Na^+, $\overline{g_{Na}}$ is the maximal value of g_{Na}, and m and h are dimensionless variable each of which weights $\overline{g_{Na}}$ in a voltage-dependent fashion.

At rest, when V_m has been quite negative for a long time, activation variable m, which can be thought of as a gate that permits g_{Na} to open, is 0, while inactivation variable h, which can be thought of a gate that forces g_{Na} into an inactive or nonresponsive state, is 1.

On depolarization to threshold V_{th}, the activation gate begins to open (m > 0), allowing Na^+ to rush into the cell. This further depolarizes the cell, leading to a further increase of m toward 1. In this way, variable m describes the regenerative activity (negative slope conductance) that produces the initial rapid upstroke (phase 0) of the AP. V_m can increase toward E_{Na} at a maximal rate in the range of 200–1000+ V/s.

During depolarization, the inactivation gate h begins to close (h < 1) slowly, stopping Na^+ flux and causing the AP to decay after reaching its peak. During the plateau phase, the inactivation gate will have closed completely (h = 0). In this inactivated state, g_{Na} is refractory to reactivation, even by repeated depolarizations, which would open the activation gate (m > 0). On repolarization, activation gate m quickly closes (m = 0) and inactivation gate h gradually opens (h = 1).

If a cell is gradually depolarized by a constant or slowly growing current, to a degree insufficient to trigger an AP, g_{Na} will become partially inactivated. This process is called *accommodation*. Such depolarization may be due to injury (especially hyperkalemia) or, in pacemaker tissue, the currents responsible for slow diastolic depolarization. Partial inactivation of g_{Na} may be an important feature of so-called slow response tissues, such as SA and AV nodes.

It is now of course known that the current of each ionic species is conducted by one or more types of ion-selective channel, which are conventionally named by the ion to which they are most permeable. Both macroscopic {49,70, 71,213} and unitary Na^+ channel currents {139} have been measured using patch-clamp techniques. Study of the probabilistic opening and closing of Na^+ and other channels has amply supported the inference of Hodgkin and Huxley that channels can be in one or more states of closure (at rest), opening (conductive), and inactivation (refractory).

The total conductance, say, g_y, of an ion species is well accounted for by contributions from an ensemble of individual channels carrying that species. As a reasonable approximation, an individual ion channel can be assumed to be either nonconductive or to have a fixed conductance. The time and voltage dependence of g_y then originates in the fact that channels can change between these conditions in binary probabilistic fashion, the probabilities depending on voltage and time.

Numerous cyclic or sequential state transition models have been offered that attempt to describe channel states explicitly {233}. In the Hodgkin–Huxley model, Na^+ channel activation and inactivation are both driven by changes in V_m but are otherwise independent. Some phenomena of Na^+ channel behavior can be explained more readily if it is assumed that inactivation does not depend on V_m, but rather follows as a normally obligatory consequence of activation {233}.

Action potentials of fast and slow response tissues

The problem of predicting or reconstructing electrotonic and action potentials from voltage dependences of ion conductances seen under the specialized condition of voltage clamp is formidable. The Hodgkin–Huxley model was actually the first attempt at reconstruction, but is often cited for its postulation of activation and inactivation states, and its inference of the existence of ion-selective channels. Modern comprehensive and quantitative action potential reconstructions have been proposed for Purkinje fibers {99,218}, for isolated atrial cells {106,253}, for ventricular cells {35}, and for SA node or pacemaker cells {254,349}.

An illustrative AP reconstruction appears in fig. 10-4 {254}. The composite AP waveform in this (panel A) and other reconstructions includes Na^+/Ca^{2+} and Na^+/K^+ exchange, and Ca^{2+} pump currents (fig. 10-4C), particularly affecting repolarization {64,116,218,239,313}, as well as ion channel currents (fig. 10-4E). A model and an experimental AP are compared in panel D. A few workers have simultaneously recorded ion channel activity and changes in V_m associated with APs {229}. We describe now the major features of the AP, considering mainly the contributions of ion channels (fig. 10-4B).

As we have noted, in cells not held under voltage clamp, transient depolarization of V_m beyond a threshold value V_{th} leads to regenerative growth of conductance

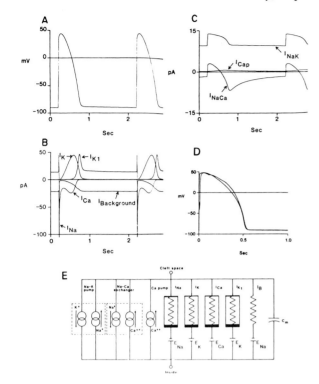

Fig. 10-4. Reconstruction of action potential (AP) from bullfrog atrial cell. **A:** Model AP waveform. **B:** Contributions of time- and voltage-dependent ion channel currents of Na⁺, K⁺, and Ca²⁺ to the AP. These currents are described in the text. Peak I_{Na} was $-6 \, nA$; therefore, the I_{Na} trace was scaled down to fit on the plot. **C:** Contributions of pump and exchanger currents to the AP. **D:** Comparison of experimental and model APs. Experimental AP has a slightly later peak and repolarization time course. **E:** Circuit analog showing membrane-bound ion channels and pumps/exchangers included in the AP reconstruction. The model also takes restricted extracellular space into account (not shown). From Rasmusson et al. {254}, with permission.

and consequent further rapid spontaneous depolarization, which initiates an AP. The maximal rate of depolarization at the start (phase 0) of the AP is related to the maximal conductance attained. The maximal depolarization rate is symbolized as dV_m/dt_{max} or V_{max}. It has long been recognized that cardiac tissues belong to either of two classes, those showing fast or slow phase 0 regenerative depolarizations {81,116,218,313}.

In so-called fast response tissues, namely, Purkinje fibers, atrial cells (fig. 10-4), and ventricular muscle cells, phase 0 depolarization is dominantly due to activation of Na⁺ channels, whose kinetics are fast. These fast response tissues show APs with faster V_{max} and have shorter refractory periods, faster conduction velocities, and other properties, which are listed in table 10-1.

In the so-called slow response tissues of the SA and AV nodes, the kinetically fast I_{Na} is not evident. This is so either because V_m rests at around $-60 \, mV$, at which

potential I_{Na} is completely inactivated and therefore eliminated functionally, or because fast Na⁺ channels are simply not expressed {232}. Instead, phase 0 depolarization is dominantly due to a current called I_{Ca}, carried by a Ca²⁺ channel (L-type), which can be blocked by phenylalkylamines (e.g., verapamil) and by dihydropyridines (e.g., nifedipine). I_{Ca} also contributes partly to rapid depolarization in fast tissues. The conductance of the L-type Ca²⁺ channel activates regeneratively, and then inactivates, analogous with that of fast Na⁺ channels, but with slower kinetics in both cases. The L-type Ca²⁺ channel imparts to slow response tissues many of the characteristics that are listed in table 10-1.

Fast response tissues can behave like slow response tissues if they are depolarized by injury or treated with drugs modifying the kinetics and states of the fast Na⁺ channel. In these cases, standing Na⁺ channel inactivation without recovery occurs. APs developed by fast tissues in these states depend on I_{Ca}.

Although both I_{Na} and I_{Ca} have been well characterized by direct measurement in cardiac tissue, phase 0 ionic conductance is often represented by the maximum rate of change of membrane voltage, V_{max}, especially in studying propagation in multicellular preparations {51} (see below).

The evolution of the AP after the peak depends on a balance among several ion channel phenomena. Inactivation of g_{Na} (in fast tissues) helps to form the initial decline after the peak (phase 1). In atrial and pacemaker tissues, an additional Ca²⁺ current, carried by T-type Ca²⁺ channels, activates on depolarization {239}. The T-Ca²⁺ channel also contributes to phase 1 decline of the AP, as it inactivates with faster kinetics than does the L-type Ca²⁺ current I_{Ca}. Part of phase 1 is also shaped by a transient outward current I_{to}, which, although not fully characterized, is in part carried by K⁺ in a Ca²⁺-dependent fashion.

The plateau (phase 2) of the AP is created and maintained largely by I_{Ca}, which continues or increases regeneratively once activated. At the same time, the plateau tends to be reduced by the Ca²⁺-dependent transient outward K⁺ current, I_{to}, which activates rapidly during depolarization {273}. The later part of the plateau is also profoundly influenced by Na⁺/Ca²⁺ exchange {239}.

The plateau of the AP is shortened {22,265,268}, cells are hyperpolarized {77,272}, intracellular Na⁺ activity is reduced, and, in slow tissues not expressing fast I_{Na}, phase 0 current is reduced, by tetrodotoxin (TTX). Before I_{Ca} had been identified specifically as due to Ca²⁺ flux through a highly selective channel {204}, inward current components not due to fast I_{Na}, being carried by both Ca²⁺ and Na⁺, and were called *slow inward current*, I_{si}. TTX sensitivity of inward currents may be due to complexities in the inactivation of a proportion of Na⁺ channels {120, 128}, or to the actions of electrogenic pump and transport processes, such as the Na⁺/K⁺-ATPase. Na⁺/Ca²⁺, or Na⁺/H⁺ exchange systems.

Phase 3 repolarization, the delayed but rapid return of V_m to the resting potential, is dominantly controlled by an outward K⁺ current that activates gradually during depolarization. The ion channel carrying this K⁺ current

Table 10-1. Comparision of electrophysiologic characteristics of so-called fast and slow response tissues

Properties	"Fast" response tissues	"Slow" response tissues (L-type calcium channel)
Geographic location	Atria; Purkinje fibers of the infranodal specialized conduction system; ventricles; AV bypass tracts (accessory pathways, Kent bundles, etc).	SA and AV nodes; perhaps valves and coronary sinus; depolarized fast respose tissues in which phase 0 dependence changes from I_{Na} to I_{Ca}.
"Passive" cellular properties		
Normal resting potential (V_r)	~ -80 to -95 mV	~ -40 to -65 mV
Subthreshold conductance	Primarily components of g_k, particularly g_{k_1}	Probably a component of g_k
"Active" cellular properties		
Curent responsible for phase 0	I_{Na}	I_{Ca} (I_{si})
Phase 0 channel kinetics of activation and inactivation	Fast	Slow. Activation multistep. Inactivation depends on V_m and $[Ca^{2+}]_i$
Maximal rate of rise of phase 0 (dV/dt_{max} or V_{max})	~ 300–1000 V/s	~ 1–50 V/s
Peak overshoot (V_{ov})	$\sim +20$ to $+40$ mV	~ -5 to $+20$ mV
Action potential amplitude	~ 90 to 135 mV	~ 30–70 mV
Properties importantly dependent on the interaction between active and passive properties		
"Threshold" voltage (V_{th})	~ -60 to -75 mV	~ -40 to -60 mV
Conduction	0.5–5 m/s	0.01–0.1 m/s
Safety factor	High	Low
Refractoriness and reactivation	Partial reactivation during phase 3 with complete reactivation in normal tissue 10–50 ms after return to normal V_r.	Partial and complete reactivation returns after attainment of V_r (>100 ms).
Relationship of rate to		
Action potential duration	Marked change	Slight change
Refractory period duration	Steep curve	"Flat" curve
Threshold	Independent	Varies directly with frequency
Conduction velocity	Independent	Decays with frequency
Characteristics conducive to reentry	Only with inactivation of sodium system with marked slowing of conduction velocity	Present even in normally I_{Ca}-dependent tissues (SA and AV nodes)
Automaticity	Yes. Depends in part or increasing I_k	Yes
Automaticity depressed by physiologic increases in $[K^+]_o$	Yes	No

is called the *delayed rectifier*, I_K. Repolarization is also associated with the gradual inactivation of I_{Ca} flowing through L-type Ca^{2+} channels. Finally, the repolarized state (phase 4) is promoted and stabilized by another outward K^+ current component, carried by a channel called the *inward* or *instantaneous rectifier*, I_{K1}, whose conductance increases with hyperpolarization {64}.

After initiation of an AP, tissues are refractory to further stimulation. In fast response tissues, I_{Na} normally inactivates rapidly, once activated by depolarization, but recovers partially as V_m repolarizes during the later part of the AP. Partial recovery of I_{Na}-dependent excitability is associated with properties such as accommodation. As soon as V_m returns to its maximal diastolic value (-80 to -95 mV) at the end of the AP, fast Na^+ channels recover fully and maximal excitability returns. In slow response tissues, by contrast, I_{Ca} recovers much more slowly, and reactivation cannot occur until well into electrical diastole, limiting the rate at which APs can be reinitiated. In the AV node, this property would limit the maximal impulse rate and thereby protect the ventricles in case of atrial fibrillation or flutter.

The ion channel complement of pacemaker cells is different in part from that of nonpacemakers {64,99}. In pacemakers, fast I_{Na} and instantaneous rectifier K^+ current I_{K1} are absent. Lacking these conductances, SA node cells have high input resistances, R_{in}. When R_{in}, which is the ratio $\Delta V_m / \Delta I_m$, is high, V_m is more sensitive to modulation and synchronization by extrinsic inputs or disturbances {9,312}, including neurohumoral ones (below), than when R_{in} is low. During diastole in SA node pacemakers, K^+ conductance does not dominate strongly in setting V_m. Nonselective currents designated I_b (background) {146} or I_f {100} flow. Presumably these currents destabilize V_m, so that it tends to depolarize more or less rapidly.

Neurohumoral control of the action potential

Two major neurohumoral pathways can sensitively modify AP properties. Stimulation of muscarinic acetylcholine receptors (especially in SA nodal tissues by vagal activation) potently activates a K^+ current, $I_{K(Ach)}$, found in SA and AV nodal as well as atrial cells. $I_{K(Ach)}$ shortens the AP and hyperpolarizes cells {64}. Acetylcholine also controls SA node pacing by affecting I_f {100}.

Beta-adrenergic stimulation is an important concomitant of acute ischemia. Through its action on numerous ion channels {151}, it shortens refractoriness and speeds conduction in the AV node, effects that are the targets of the beta-adrenergic blockers in common use clinically. Adrenergic stimulation greatly enhances an otherwise small chloride channel current, I_{Cl}, in ventricular cells {150}. This current would moderate and stabilize the effects of adrenergic stimuli {167}.

Action potentials in sequence

Having shown how nonlinearly V_m-dependent ion conductances can generate APs, we now consider some properties of the sequence of APs that drives normal cardiac contraction. We first observe qualitatively that the normal cardiac rhythm is at the same time regular and chaotically variable, a paradoxical behavior typical of nonlinear systems {15,19}.

We begin by asking why pacemaking behavior is not perfectly regular with constant intervals. One source of variability is the stochastic nature of ion channel currents {74}. Although ion channels behave to a first approximation independently, causing their variability to appear quite diluted in the ensemble behavior of a cell {65}, it should be remembered that in a nonlinear system, small variations can be amplified disproportionately. It is also known that ion channels can exhibit multiple quasistable modes of variability and sometimes act cooperatively.

A second source of variation lies in the extrinsic inputs received by each cell. Figure 10-5 shows that even isolated individual pacemakers can be driven to nonlinear behaviors, which could be related to cardiac rhythm disturbances {8}. A single depolarization during a diastolic interval (phase 4) shortened the time to the next AP, while a single depolarization during phase 3 of the AP lengthened the time to the next AP. Periodic driving entrained a pacemaker's AP sequence. Depending on the stimulation rate, the ratio (stimulation rate/AP rate) fell as integers, e.g., 1:1 (phase locking), 5:4, 3:2, 2:1 (subharmonic responses; fig. 10-5A–E), and so on. During periodic driving, each pulse changed the timing of the following AP as if it were a single pulse; that is, the effect of extrinsic driving was transient. By careful adjustment of the stimulus rate to intermediate values, chaotic patterns could be produced (not shown). It was also possible to terminate the spontaneous AP firing of a single cell by application of a single pulse of large amplitude (bistability) {142,201}.

In situ (aside from neurohumoral modulation), pacemakers are modulated mainly by neighboring cells via gap junction channels {63,89,224}, which are described further below. The high input resistances of SA node cells, which we mentioned above, would allow small electrotonic current flows and/or small variations of gap junctional conductance to modulate synchronization effectively. In spontaneously beating aggregates, cells determine a frequency of very near synchronous discharge by "mutual

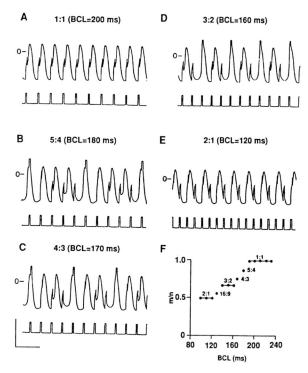

Fig. 10-5. Responses of an isolated rabbit sinus nodal cell to periodic depolarizations. **A:** At a basic cycle length (BCL) of 200 ms, 1:1 phaselocking was seen. **B–E:** When BCL was reduced to 120 ms, 1:2 subharmonic firing occurred. For 200 > BCL > 100 ms, synchronization had complex but stable patterns. **F:** Ratio of stimulus and response periods as dependent on stimulus period. Ticks below traces A–E mark stimulus times. From Anumonwo et al. {8}, with permission.

entrainment" on a "democratic" basis {224}. Modeling has suggested that the determination of a mutually acceptable beating frequency is optimized when the degree of coupling between cells is partial {182,271}.

Normally, cells within a certain region in the SA node have the fastest intrinsic rates and serve as primary pacemakers. These cells drive cells in closely adjacent regions, which also have pacemaker capability, but have lower intrinsic rates. The primary pacemakers reset those in subsidiary regions before they can generate APs spontaneously. Subsidiary cells do not then function as pacemakers unless the SA mode should fail.

Modeling has suggested that throughout the rest of the SA node and the atria, the degree of intercell coupling increases {64,182,183}. A corresponding shortening in AP duration has been noted {294}. Excitation propagates through the atria, AV node, and Purkinje fibers, at a rate that is normally locked to the SA node primary pacemaker rate. Cells of these regions do not normally demonstrate spontaneous activity. This activity is prevented by "overdrive suppression" {316}. In overdrive suppression, unlike transient entrainment to high frequency stimulation, humoral influences and redistribution of ion activities on repeated frequent use {67} persistenty change the balance of currents to one that does not support automaticity.

Pacemaker dominance and overdrive suppression appear under normal conditions to stabilize the heart rhythm and desensitize regions other than the SA node to adventitious extrinsic modulation.

The nonlinear phenomena that were described above for individual cells can also be evoked in aggregates of pacemaker cells {144,223}. In experiments on normal tissue, nonlinearities can be seen when the driving frequency is varied systematically. During ischemic injury, characteristics of the tissue, such as the time courses of repolarization and recovery from refractoriness, can change. These same nonlinearities might thus be evoked in injured tissue without requiring a change in the extrinsic driving frequency.

The nonlinear behaviors described above for active cells can also occur in cells that do not normally oscillate, including Purkinje fibers {62} and AV nodal tissue {277}. In contrast with the hierarchical view of rhythm control given above, it is also possible that atria and ventricles act as oscillators coupled and synchronized by a nonlinear mechanism {143}. Under pathological conditions (particularly reduced coupling), nonlinear behaviors, normally suppressed, may appear in other functional regions, including atrial or ventricular muscle.

INTERCELLULAR COMMUNICATION

Gap junctional structure

Our awareness of communication among cardiac cells dates back before the start of this century. The work of Heidenheim {156} and others led to the idea that the heart was an anatomical and electrical syncytium. Although Engelmann {111,112} had noted a sealing off of cells after injury in the frog heart, cells at a short distance from a cut surface remained excitable. In small myocardial segments connected by bridges of intact tissue, stimulation at any point caused contraction through the entire preparation, indicating that healthy cells were electrically connected with each other. In 1952 Weidmann {332} (see below) noted that the influence of stimulation extended over many cell lengths {see also 252}.

The electron microscopic studies of Sjöstrand and Anderson in 1954 {281}, however, described the intercalated disk and showed that cardiac cells were bound by membranes without any direct cytoplasmic connection between cells. The structure responsible for intercellular communication is the gap junction. The gap junction (hereafter GJ) is a specialized location where the membranes of neighboring cells meet within some 3 nm and are linked by hydrophilic channels that connect the interiors of the two cells and allow intercellular transport of small molecules and ions {38,195,210,243,248,305,319}.

The main (43-kDa) protein moiety of cardiac GJ channels, which differs from those of other tissues, is called a *connexin* {41}. As seen in fig. 10-9D {42}, it has four membrane-spanning regions and so terminates at both ends in the cytoplasm. Connexins group to form a hexameric structure containing a central pore. This structure is termed a *connexon* or *hemichannel*. A working GJ channel is formed when a connexon in one cell becomes localized in a cell membrane and matches sterically with a connexon from a neighboring cell {38}.

How this coupling of hemichannels is driven to occur is unknown {38}. At least an initial period of assembly into working channels can occur without de novo protein synthesis, as embryonic chick heart cells, reaggregating in culture, synchronize their rhythms within minutes after making physical contact {9,63,85,257,350}.

Electrically, a GJ channel connecting the interiors of two cells behaves as though it were shaped as a right cylinder. This functional geometry is distinctive from the locally narrowed (hourglass or funnel) shapes of other membrane channels {84}. Each type of nonjunctional channel has selectivity mainly for one species of ion, e.g., Na^+, Ca^{2+}, K^+, or Cl^-, attributable to the shape of its localized constriction. GJ channels are minimally ion selective; in fact, the pore is large enough to pass low molecular weight dyes or ATP. Because the long cylindrical path of a GJ channel slows permeation, the channel's conductance is comparable to those of nonjunctional channels.

The efficacy of intercellular communication is determined in large part by the conductance of GJs. Their importance in propagation will be considered in some detail below. Under some conditions, GJ conductance depends on transjunctional voltage, which can change rapidly (within milliseconds) during the normal generation and propagation of APs. Exogenous agents, such as alkanols {259,309}, strophanthidin {186}, or anesthetics {57,236}; changes in ionic milieu, including low ${Na^+}_i$ {186}; addition of Sr^{2+}, La^{3+}, or Mn^{2+} {91,92}; hypertonicity {108}; or Ca^{2+}-free EGTA solution {145}, as well as factors related to ischemia and injury, can also rapidly modify GJ conductance. The latter include transients in internal Ca^{2+} {82,191,207,307} and/or pH {53,307}, presence of lipophiles {54,55}, arachidonic acid pathway intermediates {114,215}, hypoxia {252,346}, and metabolic poisons {93,229,335}.

Rapid modulation could also occur via phosphaterelated phenomena. Cyclic nucleotides have diverse effects on GJ channel properties in different tissues {195,290}, but in pancreatic acinar cells {290} and in cardiac cells {200,305}, normal levels of cAMP and ATP together stabilize GJ channels in the open state, presumably by a protein kinase A-dependent phosphorylation {195}. In cardiac tissues, cAMP and cGMP have shown opposing effects {305}, respectively, increasing or decreasing coupling. Phosphorylation of single cardiac GJ channels has been seen to change unitary conductance, but not voltage dependence. These modulations notwithstanding, the phosphorylation site is not an absolute requirement for GJ channel activity {227}.

These rapid modulations indicate that GJ conductance is at some times an active physiological property. At the same time, GJ conductance can be considered a passive property, as indicated by the following considerations.

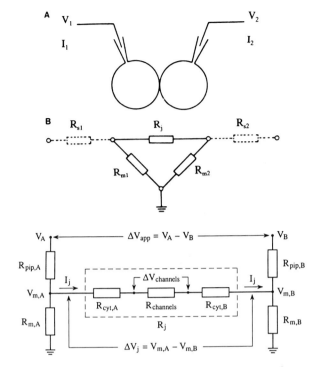

Fig. 10-6. Study of gap junctional channel conductance. **A:** Two coupled cells to which patch electrodes are sealed. When transmembrane voltages V_1 and V_2 are controlled (voltage clamp), currents I_1 and I_2 can be measured; when currents I_1 and I_2 are controlled (current clamp), voltages V_1 and V_2 can be measured. **B:** Idealized circuit analog for calculating junctional resistance (R_j) from current and voltage measurements. Effects of nonjunctional resistances (R_{m1} and R_{m2}) are considered. **C:** More realistic model for measuring R_j, which includes cytoplasmic resistances ($R_{cyt,A}$ and $R_{cyt,B}$), as well as nonjunctional ($R_{m,A}$ and $R_{m,B}$) and series or access resistances ($R_{pip,A}$ and $R_{pip,B}$). A,B: From Weingart {336}, with permission; C: from Wilders and Jongsma {341}, with permission.

GJ channels cluster together in plaques, driven to do so in part by interprotein forces and in part by forces originating in the tortuosity and other higher order properties of the cell membrane, the glycocalyx {1} and/or other cell surface components. Clustering profoundly affects electrical properties of GJ channels, as will be seen below.

The localization and distribution of GJ plaques in adult mammals {136}, including the dog {165}, are similar. The specific distribution depends on stage of development {137} and becomes less organized after injury {212,284}. In adult ventricular tissue, junctional placques appear to form exclusively and very densely within intercalated discs {137,165}, but at least in atria they also participate in lateral connections {136}. In SA node tissue, GJs are more sparse {216}, consistent with the total conductance between cell pairs {9}, which is much smaller than in ventricle {336}. Taken together, these features suggest

that the number of functioning junctional channels in a tissue is a point of physiological regulation.

Voltage-clamp analysis of gap junctional channels

In contrast with the V_m-dependent ion channels responsible for excitability, GJ channels are less accessible and have been more difficult to characterize under voltage clamp. We here summarize some properties of the GJ channel that are relevant to its crucial role in propagation.

Conductance of GJ channels has been studied by simultaneous voltage clamp of a pair of cells, mainly using the double whole-cell patch-clamp technique, which is shown in fig. 10-6A {234,319,341}. An idealized lumped electronic circuit analog for this type of experiment (fig. 10-6B) shows that current injected into either cell is conducted by both the sarcolemmal membrane (r_m) and the GJ (r_j) channels. The clamp currents in fig. 10.6B can be described by {336}

$$I_1 = \frac{V_1}{r_{m_1}} + \frac{(V_1 - V_2)}{r_j} = I_{m_1} + I_j. \tag{10-8}$$

$$I_2 = \frac{V_2}{r_{m_2}} + \frac{(V_2 - V_1)}{r_j} = I_{m_2} + I_j. \tag{10-9}$$

If experiments are designed so that V_1 is changed stepwise to various constant values while V_2 is held at zero, application of eqs. (10-8) and (10-9) are particularly simple. Substituting $V_2 = 0$, we have $I_1 = I_{m_1} + I_j$, $V_1 = V_j$, and $I_2 = I_j$, so that measurement of I_2 yields $g_j = I_2/V_1 = 1/r_j$ directly.

Voltage-clamp studies agree that cardiac GJ conductance is symmetric with respect to the direction of current flow {183,306,336}. As we will discuss below, a localized unidirectional disturbance of conduction is generally thought to be a substrate for reentrant cardiac arrhythmias. Unidirectional block could be explained by inhomogeneities in refractoriness and other tissue properties {207,220,322}. It is not known whether asymmetric GJ transmission, as occurs in invertebrate nervous systems {125}, could also be a contributing factor.

Dependence on transjunctional electric field (voltage gradient), a key issue in understanding how GJ conductance is regulated dynamically, has proven difficult to assess. In adult rat {217,222,336} and guinea pig {217, 259} ventricular preparations, g_j was high and was constant over the full range of variation of V_j expected during AP generation and propagation. In embryonic {318,321} and neonatal cardiac preparations, g_j showed transiency and voltage dependence {257,258}. Voltage-dependent conductance has also been found in GJs of adult rabbit SA node {9} and adult rat atria {200}, and in many noncardiac GJs {242,306}.

An example from our laboratory to illustrate how GJ conductance can depend on voltage appears in fig. 10-7 {200}. In panel A is shown current I_2, as defined in eq. (10-9), and measured with $V_2 = 0$ as described above. As V_1 was increased, the initial peak of I_2 grew proportionally, indicating a constant GJ conductance. For sufficiently large V_1, junctional current decayed to a lower steady value after the peak. It appears that junctional channels were initially open at rest ($V_j = 0$) and that some close or inactivate at large V_j, decreasing the observed conductance. The larger was the voltage, the more rapid was the decay. Initial (INST) and final values (SS) of I_j appear in panel B of fig. 10-7. As V_j was increased, GJ conductance, indicated by the slope of the corresponding line, was either constant (INST) or decreased (SS).

Figure 10-6C shows a model that represents the dual voltage-clamp whole-cell recording situation more accurately than does fig. 10-6B and can explain the disparate observations on V_j dependence {341}. Figure 10-6C shows that the voltage $\Delta V_{channels}$ that appears across the junctional channels can be smaller than the voltage ΔV_{app} that is applied to a cell pair because of voltage drops across $R_{pip,A}$ and $R_{pip,B}$ (which are exacerbated when current flows through $R_{m,A}$ and $R_{m,B}$), as well as $R_{cyt,A}$ and $R_{cyt,B}$. When the voltage loss due to these parasitic (unwanted) resistances is significant, the proportion of V_{app} that actually appears as $\Delta V_{channels}$ may be too little to cause the channel inactivation seen at higher values of V_{app}, such as that shown in fig. 10-7A {180,341}.

A feature that unifies many results on V_j dependence is that, regardless of the age or type of preparation, it only appears when the total g_j is relatively small {180,200,257, 258,309,341}. Many investigators have assumed junctional resistance ($R_{channels}$ in fig. 10-6C) to be much higher than the cytoplasmic resistances $R_{cyt,A}$ and $R_{cyt,B}$ {222,340}, owing to the very limited cross-sectional area represented by gap junctions. However, physical considerations predict that when many active GJ channels are clustered together in a plaque, enough current can flow through their large total conductance to drop significant voltage through the cytoplasmic resistance. Most of this loss will occur within submillimeter distance of the GJ channels {180}. The lack of voltage dependence in situations of large junctional conductance is consistent with this prediction {341}.

Although this clustering-related collapse of transjunctional electric fields is vexing experimentally, it may be functionally important. This question remains to be addressed. Junctional conductance per se is a critical parameter in the control of propagation {252}, as it is subject to many modulatory influences. However, many key issues in propagation, including differences between normal {181,184} and ischemic tissues {252}, can be discussed profitably in terms of the internal (also called axial or longitudinal) resistance r_i (fig. 10-3B), which includes both junctional resistance r_j (or $R_{channels}$) and cytoplasmic resistance (R_{cyt}).

Voltage loss across the series resistance of the recording electrodes ($R_{pip,A}$ and $R_{pip,B}$ in fig. 10-6C) has also been recognized {229,258,338,340}. Some workers have compensated series resistance electronically {229}. Although stable electronic compensation is readily attained with individual cells {278}, it is difficult to guarantee with two cells. Current shunting through nonjunctional conductances ($R_{m,A}$ and $R_{m,B}$), which increases voltage loss through $R_{pip,A}$ and $R_{pip,B}$ ($V_{m,A} \neq V_A$ and $V_{m,B} \neq V_B$ in fig. 10-6C), can often be measured approximately and corrected for in analysis, and/or partially suppressed.

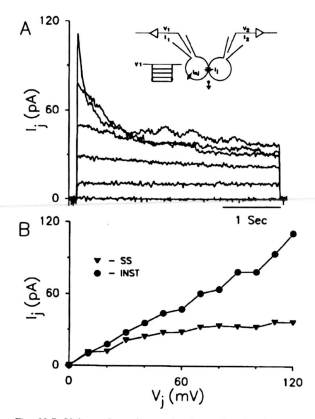

Fig. 10-7. Voltage dependence of cell gap junctional currents evoked by step stimulation in rat atrial cell pairs. **A:** Junctional current recorded from cell 2, which was held at $V_2 = 0\,mV$, while cell 1 was stepped to -120 (transient current with highest peak), -90, -60, -30, and $-10\,mV$ (lowest trace, not transient). See discussion of eqs. (10-8) and (10-9) in the text. **B:** Initial peak current (INST) was linearly proportional to step amplitude, indicating constant conductance. Steady current at the end of the step decreased relative to peak at larger step amplitudes, indicating voltage-dependent loss of conductance. From Lal and Arnsdorf {200}, with permission.

Most investigators have treated the network represented by a pair of coupled cells as purely resistive. Complexities of C_m that were attributed to extracellular resistivity (above) may also be influenced by junctional capacitances {37,61,124,157}. Cell and junctional membrane capacitances (not shown in fig. 10-6C) can reduce the temporal resolution of GJ channel records, especially when relatively few channels are active.

Figure 10-8 shows that the dual whose-cell patch voltage-clamp method can reveal the opening and closing of individual GJ channels. An example of such unitary events appears in fig. 10-8A {200}. Notice that the currents in each trace have one of two amplitudes, from whose difference ΔI_j the conductance of a single channel can be calculated as $\Delta I_j / \Delta V_j$. In practice, at each V_j many transitions are recorded and a suitable average value for ΔI_j is measured from amplitude histograms, such as that shown in the inset of panel A.

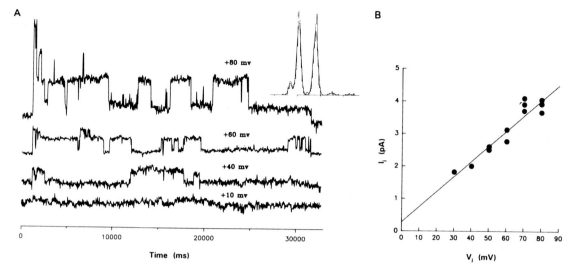

Fig. 10-8. Unitary conductance of gap junctional channel between members of a rat atrial cell pair. **A:** Examples of transitions between conducting and nonconducting states. Current I_2 was recorded after voltage V_1 was stepped to each stated value at time 0. **Inset:** Amplitude histogram of all points in a current record. The difference between currents represented by the two peaks provides a reliable estimate of the change in current between conducting and nonconducting states. **B:** Current-voltage relation calculated from histograms (such as that in the inset) at several voltages. Constant slope indicates that unitary conductance does not depend on voltage. From Lal and Arnsdorf {200}, with permission.

As shown in fig. 10-8B, at least in a given experimental situation, unitary conductance does not change with V_j, as the current-voltage relation has a constant slope. This means that the total junctional conductance between cells is determined mainly by the probabilities and durations of openings {56} and the number of functional channels {319}, analogously with macroscopic nonjunctional conductances.

Unitary conductance values as large as 165 pS have been measured {321}, but most workers have found values between 40 and 60 pS {9,56,57,305,309}. A portion of the dispersion in these values may originate with the measurement situation, as described above, and not as a true variance in the unitary conductance {341}.

Junctional channels can also demonstrate multiple conductive states {227,318,323}. The sizes and distributions of the conductive states depend on the relative expression of isoforms of the junctional channel proteins {187,323} and, for a given form, on phosphorylation state {227}. Further, unlike nonjunctional transmembrane ion channels, which show only abrupt transitions between conducting and nonconducting states, GJ channels appear able to make graded and/or slow conductance changes {234,258,290}. As seen in fig. 10-9A–C {38}, this behavior may represent constriction or relaxation of the GJ channel pore, which has been proposed to be formed as an array of helical screws {38,314}.

LINEAR CABLE THEORY AND DECREMENTAL CONDUCTION

Multiple cells: Regional specializations

Among the cells encountered along the pathway normally followed by cardiac excitation and propagation (SA node, atrial muscle, AV node, His-Purkinje fiber system, ventricular muscle) is found marked and purposeful heterogeneity. Differences exist not only in electrical properties of individual cells within each tissue type {294}, which depend on their complements of ion channels, but also in the spatial arrangement and types of gap junctions and connective tissues. Major phenomena that depend on these differences include not only AP waveform and automaticity, which we have described above, but also speed, safety, and directional properties of propagation, and finally, susceptibility to pathological disturbances.

Excitation normally spreads broadly in three dimensions through the masses of atrial and ventricular muscle. The pattern is not uniform; rather, it has specific anisotropy {295}. By contrast, the AV node and Purkinje fibers both form narrow pathways for the spread of excitation.

The Purkinje fiber system provides very rapid (0.5–5 m/s) and safe conduction of APs from the AV node to ventricular muscle, via the bundle of His, the bundle branches and fascicles, and the terminal branching system. In Purkinje fibers, cells are organized in many cases into essentially cylindrical columns, two to three cells in diameter, surrounded by connective tissue. End-to-end (as well as side-to-side) connections of cells allow the system to extend and transmit excitation over many cell

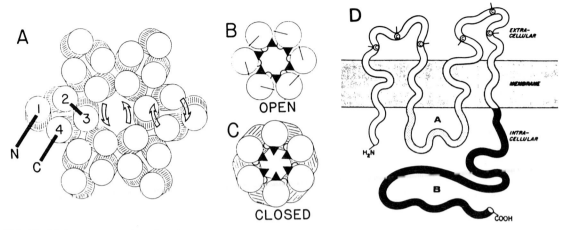

Fig. 10-9. Models for structure of gap junctional channels. **A:** Hexameric arrangement of connexins; end view of a hemichannel from cytoplasmic side. The four membrane-spanning regions of each connexin form a left-handed helix; the pore region is formed when membrane-spanning regions 3 of all six connexins associate as a right-handed helix. **B,C:** Open and closed states, respectively, of the pore. When connexins undergo torsion, possibly in response to a transjunctional voltage difference, phenylalanine residues, represented by dark triangles, move into the channel lumen and block permeation. **D:** Topological model showing situation of connexins in cell membrane. A,B,C: From Bennett et al. {38}, with permission; D: from Beyer et al. {42}, with permission.

lengths. Because of this structure, as well as their electrophysiology, long Purkinje fiber preparations resemble cables.

The AV node is not cable-like and supports much slower conduction than the His-Purkinje system. AV nodal conduction is relatively susceptible to failure, and many disturbances of heart rhythm originate there. In a recent computer simulation, several common modes of failure have been suggested to originate in one key nonlinear property, the recovery of excitability {141}.

One-dimensional cable theory

In 1952 Weidmann {332} studied the electrophysiological properties of cardiac Purkinje fibers. He applied subthreshold depolarizing and hyperpolarizing currents (i_m) intracellularly through a microelectrode and recorded V_m of the fiber at various points along its length (refer to fig. 10.3A). V_m decreased in graded fashion with increasing distance from the point of stimulation, but could be detected even several millimeters from the point of current application. The several cells that lay between the stimulating and recording microelectrodes must have been connected by a pathway with a low resistance to ionic flow. As the magnitude of the change in V_m was linearly related to the applied currents, electrical, rather than chemical, coupling appeared to be the mechanism of communication.

Weidmann {333} later also demonstrated long-range communication in ventricular muscle. He showed that ^{42}K diffused freely between cells, as would be predicted by cable theory. The upper limit for resistance between cells, $3\,\Omega$-cm, was almost 700-fold less than for the outer cell membrane.

The observations of Weidmann {332,333} were well described by uniform cable theory. This theory was used by Lord Kelvin in the mid-19th century to model the decrement in the signal carried by the trans-Atlantic telegraph cable. The model included terms corresponding with r_i, r_o, and r_m in fig. 10-3B. Hodgkin and Rushton in 1946 {162} showed that a modified cable equation rather well fit experimental observations in a nerve axon.

The passive membrane properties whose analogs appear in cable theory are of central importance for coordinated excitation and conduction under both normal and abnormal conditions. For this reason we will review this theory here. We will try to provide a reasoned approach to the cable equations. We will also examine how cablelike preparations can be assessed experimentally, including in our study the calculation of the variables r_m, C_m, and τ_m, which are relevant to the electrical analog in fig. 10-3B.

We will attribute the following properties to any preparation for which we want to claim a resemblance to the transmission line or one-dimensional cable of fig. 10-3B: The cells form a column in which the pathway through the cytoplasm and the connections between cells at their ends (R_i) has a low resistance. The outer membranes of the cells have a high resistance (R_m). Both R_i and R_m are assumed ohmic and linear; that is, they do not depend on V_m, at least for small changes in V_m.

The column of cells is assumed to be cylindrical. The surfaces of the cell membranes are uncomplicated by invaginations or other specializations, so that ions will not accumulate or become depleted in the intercellular space. The lipid component of the membrane will behave as an ideal capacitor. The volume of the solution outside the cells is assumed to be large, so that the resistance of the outside (r_o in fig. 10-3B) is negligible. Longitudinal current flow through the cable is considered uniform, and radial currents are considered negligible.

The basic cable equation is

$$i_m = \frac{1}{r_i} \frac{\partial^2 V_m}{\partial x} = \frac{V_m}{r_m} + c_m \frac{\partial V_m}{\partial t}, \quad (10\text{-}10)$$

where i_m is the current flow through any unit length of membrane (Am/cm), r_i is the longitudinal resistance of a unit length of the inside conductor or core of the cable (Ω/cm), V_m is the transmembrane voltage, and r_m and c_m, as previously defined, are the membrane resistance and capacitance for a unit length of cable (Ω/cm and F/cm, respectively).

To understand this partial differential equation, refer to fig. 10-3B. Any current i_i flowing to the right past a given point through the inside conductor must return to the same point by flowing leftward through the parallel segment of the outer conductor. The resistance for a given length (termed Δx) of the inside and outside conductors would be $r_i \Delta x$ and $r_o \Delta x$, respectively. According to Ohm's Law, the potential difference across any resistor spanning length Δx (say, resistor r_i between elements B and D in fig. 10-2B) is

$$\Delta V_i = i_i r_i \Delta x. \quad (10\text{-}11)$$

The length can be made smaller and smaller, so that Δx approaches zero. Mathematically, this is written

$$\frac{\partial V_i}{\partial x} = \lim \frac{\Delta V_i}{\Delta x} = -i_i r_i. \quad (10\text{-}12)$$

The negative sign indicates that the potential drops as the current passes through the amount of resistance corresponding with incremental length Δx.

Although r_o could be treated in the same manner as r_i, we consider r_o negligible because the outside solution is large. For this reason, the extracellular voltage will be constant. Conventionally, the extracellular voltage is taken as zero, so that $V_i = V_m$ at any point. Equation 10-9 can therefore be rewritten as

$$\frac{\partial V_m}{\partial x} = -i_i r_i. \quad (10\text{-}13)$$

The membrane of the cell is leaky; that is, a certain amount of current ($-i_m$) is lost through the membrane to the outside (via elements r_m and c_m) per unit length Δx of cable. This loss through the membrane {which can be described by eq. (10-4) with I_m substituted by i_m, R_m by r_m, and so on} reduces the current flowing longitudinally through the core. The loss in longitudinal current (Δi_i) in length Δx is

$$\Delta i_i = -i_m \Delta x. \quad (10\text{-}14)$$

Once again, we make the length of membrane smaller and smaller, letting Δx approach zero:

$$\frac{\partial i_i}{\partial x} = \lim \frac{\Delta i_i}{\Delta x} = i_m. \quad (10\text{-}15)$$

Differentiating eq. (10-13) and dividing through by r_i gives another expression for $\partial i_i / \partial x$:

$$\frac{\partial^2 V_m}{\partial x^2} = r_i \left(\frac{\partial i_i}{\partial x} \right), \quad (10\text{-}16)$$

and, substituting from eq. (10-13), the relationship becomes

$$\frac{\partial^2 V_m}{\partial x^2} = r_i i_m. \quad (10\text{-}17)$$

We obtain the cable equation, eq. (10-10), by substitution from eq. (10-4) (again with I_m substituted by i_m, R_m by r_m, and so on) and rearranging:

$$i_m = \frac{1}{r_i} \frac{\partial^2 V_m}{\partial x} = \frac{V_m}{r_m} + c_m \frac{\partial V_m}{\partial t}. \quad (10\text{-}10)$$

Experimental study of cable-like fibers

When a cable-like fiber is studied experimentally, it is normally stimulated by injection of a known current, and the relationship between the current and the ensuing voltage changes is sought. To describe this current-voltage relationship, the time and space constants, the input resistance, and the fiber's diameter and length are measured {252,332}. These experimentally observable electrical terms will now be defined using the quantities in fig. 10-3B.

Although the cable equation defines a relationship between i_m and V_m, this relationship cannot be known explicitly and used to compare with experimental results until the equation is solved for a particular pattern of i_m, such as a sudden step to a constant value. Solution of this equation requires transform methods and a consideration of error functions {see Hodgkin and Rushton 162}. Any solution also depends on boundary conditions that describe whether a fiber is long, or terminates by branching, with a short circuit, or with a cut end, the latter cases being relevant to injured tissues {87,122,332}. Here we illustrate instructive special cases.

After a sudden step change in i_m is forced (by current injection), V_m changes gradually, a reflection of the fact that work is required to add or remove charge from membrane capacitance C_m. After a time equal to the time constant τ_m, the change in V_m will have reached a fraction of its final value, which is characteristic of the structure. In a short fiber or cell, where $\tau_m = R_m C_m$,

$$V_m(t) = V_m(0)(1 - e^{t/\tau_m}) \quad (10\text{-}18a)$$

so that the fraction is 63%. In a long cablelike structure, in which $\tau_m = r_m c_m$,

$$V_m(t) = V_m(t = 0)\text{erf}(\sqrt{t/\tau_m}), \quad (10\text{-}18b)$$

so that, since erf(1) = 0.84, the fraction is 84%. τ_m also describes the rate at which I_m changes after a step change in V_m is forced.

When a constant current I_o has been injected into a long cable for a long duration, V_m at the point of stimulation $V_m(x = 0, t = \infty)$ is

$$V_o = \frac{r_i I o \lambda}{2}. \qquad (10\text{-}19)$$

The space constant, λ, will be defined next; the denominator 2 appears because half the current flows in one direction down the cable and the other half flows in the opposite direction. If current is introduced near a high-resistance barrier, such as the cut and ligated end of a Purkinje fiber, division by 2 is not required.

The distribution of V_m along the cable at a point x other than 0 along the cable (again, in steady state some time after starting the injection of a constant current) is approximated by

$$V_m(x) = V_m(x = 0) e^{-x/\lambda}. \qquad (10\text{-}20)$$

In eqs. (10-19) and (10-20), the length or space constant λ is the distance away from the point injection over which V_m falls to e^{-1} (about 37%) of its value at the point of injection. It is $\lambda = \sqrt{r_m/(r_i + r_o)}$ or, when r_o can be neglected, $\lambda = \sqrt{r_m/r_i}$.

Cable eq. 10-10 can be expressed using τ_m and λ by multiplying through by r_m, substituting, and rearranging:

$$-\lambda^2 \left(\frac{\partial^2 V_m}{\partial x^2} \right) + \tau_m \left(\frac{\partial_m}{\partial_t} + V_m \right) = 0. \qquad (10\text{-}21)$$

Equation (10-21) provides a relationship between V_m, x, and t that is amenable to experimental description.

Input resistance (R_{in}, measured in ohms) is the ratio of V_m to I_o at x = 0, the point of stimulation. It is normally measured with constat current in the steady state:

$$R_{in} = V_o/I_o. \qquad (10\text{-}22)$$

Realizing that $\lambda = \sqrt{r_m/r_i}$ and combining eq. (10-17) and eq. (10-20), the input resistance can be expressed as

$$R_{in} = \frac{\sqrt{r_m r_i}}{2}. \qquad (10\text{-}23)$$

When the diameter of a cable-like preparation, assumed to have a circular cross section, is known, we can define the specific resistance (the resistance of a unit area of membrane; in $\Omega\text{-cm}^2$),

$$R_m = 2\pi a r_m, \qquad (10\text{-}24)$$

as well as the internal or longitudinal resistivity (in $\Omega\text{-cm}$),

$$R_i = \pi a^2 r_i \qquad (10\text{-}25)$$

and the specific capacitance (in F/cm^2) of the membrane

$$C_m = \frac{c_m}{2\pi a}. \qquad (10\text{-}26)$$

Tissues that have been analyzed for cable properties include Purkinje fibers of sheep {20–23,25,27,87,103,115, 119,251,265,268,332}, dog {68,91,94}, and rabbit {71}; ventricular muscle of sheep {333,334}, dog {185,261}, calf and cow {335,346}, guinea pig {52,83,108}, and frog {61}; as well as bull frog atrium {145}, rabbit atrial trabeculae {44,47}, and rabbit SA node {43}. These studies have involved both pharmacological and physiological (e.g., hypoxia) manipulations. Considerations in comparing

experimental cable analyses with theory have been discussed by Walton and Fozzard {327,328}.

Figure 10-10 shows a representative experiment from our laboratory in which the above analyses were used to show how lysophosphatidylcholine (LPC) affected cable properties of Purkinje fibers {25}. LPC accumulates in ischemic, but not normal, myocardium. Its electrophysiological actions strongly suggest a role in arrhythmias that accompany acute myocardial ischemia {189,285,286, among others}. Our laboratory has also studied the effects of lidocaine on fibers previously altered by LPC {265}. This work will be described later.

Small hyperpolarizing constant current steps (I_o) were injected near the ligated end of a long unbranched Purkinje fiber. I_o was held at 45.5 nA for 100 ms (uppermost trace). This current produced changes of 5.44 mV and 4.05 mV in V_m, recorded, respectively, at 300 μm (middle trace) and 900 μm (lowest trace) from the stimulating site. V_m at these and other sites was plotted on a logarithmic scale as a function of the distance (x) from the stimulating site or was fit to a curve by linear regression. V_m at x = 0 was predicted by extrapolation back to x = 0 and was 6.30 mV. Using this datum and eq. (10-19), which holds for unidirectional current flow in this ligated fiber, $r_i = 1.36 \times 10^6$ Ω-cm was found. Putting V_m at x = 0 into eq. (10-22), $R_{in} = 139$ KΩ was found. λ, the value of x at which $V_m = e^{-1}V_o$, was 2.03 mm. τ_m, the time at which the change in V_m had reached 84% of its final value, was measured at x = 300 μm and was 26.8 ms (arrow in fig. 10-10). The fiber radius was 80 μm. Using this fact, specific resistance R_m was 1771 Ω-cm^2 {eq. (10-24)}, internal resistivity R_i was 215 Ω-cm {eq. (10-25)}, and specific capacitance C_m was 15.1 μF/cm^2 {eq. (10-26)}. After LPC, V_o increased to 8.4 mV and λ increased to 2.47 mm. R_{in} increased to 186 kΩ, R_m increased to 2883 Ω-cm^2, and R_i increased to 236 Ω-cm, but C_m was little changed at 12.0 μF/cm^2.

Limitations of linear cable analysis

The assumptions underlying one-dimensional cable analysis as described above are not strictly true and limit the method. Deviations originate in nonideal properties of each of c_m, r_m, and r_i {252}, as well as r_o, the latter being of special concern in tissues in situ and in injury {192}.

One source of discrepancy is the nonideal capacitive properties that result from the complexly infolded structure of the cell membrane (the T system). Not only does C_m behave as if part of it is in series with a resistance above {115, fig. 10-3C}, the narrow intercellular clefts {226,288} also radically enlarge the surface area and hence presumably the apparent magnitude of C_m.

In kid Purkinje fibers, Weidmann {332} found that R_i was about 100 Ω-cm, R_m was about 2000 Ω-cm^2, λ was about 2 mm, τ_m about 20 ms, and C_m was about 12 μF/cm^2. Although R_i was just somewhat lower than in nerve, C_m was 10 times higher. Assuming an average cell length of about 100 μM, λ would represent about 20 cells connected end to end. Weidmann recognized that his assumption that the fibers were smooth cylinders might be wrong. Indeed, Mobley and Page {226} later found that 80% of the total

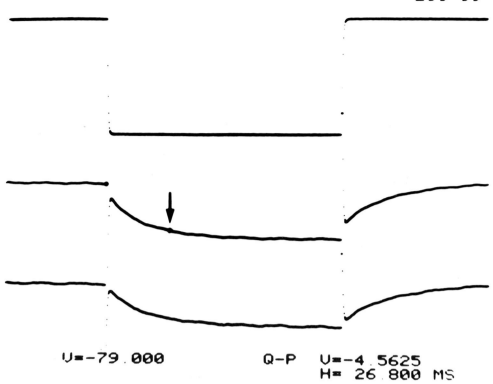

Fig. 10-10. Experimental measurement of cable properties in a long sheep Purkinje fiber. **Top trace:** Record of rectangular current step (I_m); amplitude during step was 45.5 nA. **Middle trace:** Record of transmembrane voltage response (V_m); final amplitude was 5.44 mV. **Bottom trace:** Record of V_m at a greater distance from the stimulating electrode than that of the middle trace; final amplitude was 4.05 mV. After the rectangular step change in I_m, V_m changes gradually as membrane capacitance c_m charges. In the middle trace, the arrow marks the time (26.8 ms) at which the change in V_m after current onset had reached 4.56 mV, 84% of its final value (arrow). The resting potential of this fiber was −79 mV. From Arnsdorf and Sawicki {25}, with permission.

membrane surface area was in the extracellular clefts, meaning that the total area was 10–12 times greater than assumed by Weidmann. This suggests that C_m should be about 1 μF/cm² {157,226} and R_m should be about 20,000 Ω-cm².

Charge injected at a given point on a passive Purkinje fiber will distribute nonhomogeneously over space due to the infoldings. Schoenberg et al. {268} modeled this effect using the geometrical ratios of Mobley and Page {226}. For charge injected at the surface of a 100-μM diameter fiber, the charging time constant for the clefts was 1–2 ms and the dc length constant for the clefts was of the order of 100 μM. These values are more than an order of magnitude smaller than τ_m and λ of an entire fiber. It can thus be expected that the clefts lead to only moderate deviation from cable theory, mainly affecting, for instance, the initial phase of response to a step current change. The role of K^+ accumulation or depletion in the clefts {33,34} in this nonideal behavior is unknown.

NONDECREMENTAL PROPAGATION OF ACTION POTENTIALS

Nonlinear behavior of cable-like fibers

In his classic study of Purkinje fibers, Weidmann {332} used small current steps that did not perturb V_m enough to induce APs regeneratively. Electrotonic transmission, which occurs in this range of V_m, where V_m and I_m are linearly related, is important, at least in regions where propagation has failed or been blocked (see below) {252}, and may influence propagation in normal tissues as well. Nonlinear V_m dependence of r_m is the basis for normal nondecremental propagation, just as it is the basis for normal cellular excitability. To account for the fact that r_m (or g_m) is voltage dependent, not constant, cable properties are studied with inputs that model APs.

Figure 10-11A shows the relationship between I_m and V_m in a Purkinje fiber into which constant currents were

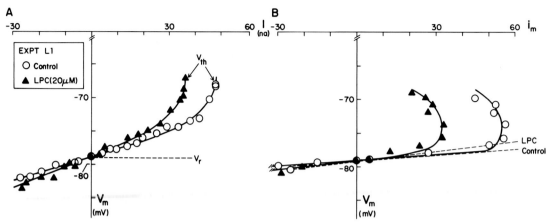

Fig. 10-11. Current-voltage relationships in a Purkinje fiber, showing nonlinear behavior in the subthreshold voltage range, before and after treatment with lysophosphatidyl choline (LPC), a toxic metabolite of ischemia. **A:** Total membrane current I versus V_m. **B:** Mathematically derived membrane current density i_m versus V_m. Tangents to the curves at $i_m = 0$ (dashed lines) show that LPC increased the membrane slope conductance (decreased R_m). LPC did not change the threshold voltage V_{th} nor the nonlinear shape of the current-voltage relation. From Arnsdorf and Sawicki {25}, with permission.

injected {25}. This relationship is linear for very small perturbations in I_m, when V_m is considerably negative of the threshold for regenerative depolarization (V_{th}), but not otherwise. The dependence of V_m on current density i_m may more accurately represent how a uniformly depolarized cable would behave than does dependence on total current I_m. As suggested by Cole and Curtis {72}, in a long cablelike fiber, i_m can be approximated by $i_m \propto I_m \cdot dI_m/dV_m$ {25,147}. dI_m/dV_m, also known as the membrane slope conductance (G_m), was measured by constructing tangents along the V_m versus I_m curve of fig. 10-11A. Then V_m was plotted as a function of i_m in fig. 10-11B. The nonlinearity of r_m is accentuated, and the negative slope conductance characteristic of excitable tissue for V_m near V_{th} is clearly revealed. LPC made V_m more steeply dependent on either I_m or i_m (slope conductance decreased) in the linear region, but changed neither resting potential (V_r) nor threshold voltage (V_{th}).

Study of cable properties becomes much more complex in the range of V_m where r_m is voltage dependent. For example, $\lambda = \sqrt{r_m/r_i}$ cannot be considered constant. It can fall by more than an order of magnitude when dV_m/dt is at maximum, as compared to its value during repolarization {196}. Voltage-dependent changes in r_m appeared similarly to reduce R_{in} and τ_m in sheep Purkinje fibers on repetitive pacing {251}. Longitudinal resistance r_i may also change. Pacing of Purkinje fibers does not change r_i or c_m {251}, but many modifiers of r_i, such as Ca^{2+} accumulation {217,252}, hypoxia {159}, or pH {51}, are themselves activity dependent.

Threshold and liminal length

An excitable cell has to be depolarized beyond a certain voltage to permit regenerative production of an AP, but this threshold voltage, V_{th}, cannot be defined as a scalar

quantity, because the ability of a stimulus to cause a regenerative response depends on many factors. Lapicque in 1907 {202} recognized that in nerve the current required to attain threshold was greater for stimuli of short duration than for stimuli of long duration. He found the following dependence of current strength on duration:

$$I_{th} = \frac{I_{rh}}{1 - e^{t/\tau}}, \qquad (10\text{-}27)$$

where I_{th} is the current required to provoke a regenerative response; I_{rh} is the rheobasic current, that is, the smallest current, regardless of length, that can cause a regenerative response; t is the duration of I_{th}; and τ approximates the membrane time constant. As an approximation, threshold was reached once a relatively constant amount of charge, $Q_{th} = I_{th} \cdot t$, had been transferred. However, threshold is complicated by the voltage- and time-dependent activation and inactivation properties of Na^+ conductance {161}. Noble and Stein {240} and Cooley and Dodge {76}, among others, concluded that threshold was crossed when the rapid depolarizing inward current equaled the slower repolarizing outward current.

In sheep Purkinje fibers, Dominguez and Fozzard {103} found that the time constant τ of the strength-duration curve was much shorter than the membrane time constant τ_m. Moreover, they observed that V_{th} depended on the duration of the stimulus. Fozzard and Schoenberg {122} interpreted these strength-duration relationships as resulting from the cable properties of the Purkinje fibers. They applied the concept of liminal length, first proposed by Hodgkin and Rushton {162} in nerve, to their results in short and long fiber preparations. In a unidimensional cable, a regenerative response will occur when the depolarizing current flowing into a certain length of tissue (the liminal length) exceeds the outward repolarizing current being sunk into adjacent segments of tissue. Near the tied end of a semi-infinite cable, the liminal length is very nearly

$$LL = \frac{\sqrt{2}\,e^{-1}\,Q_{th}}{\pi^3 a C_m \lambda V_{th}} \approx \frac{0.855\,Q_{th}}{2\pi^3 a C_m \lambda V_{th}}. \qquad (10\text{-}28)$$

This definition shows that the threshold for active regenerative depolarization depends greatly on passive cable properties {122}.

Since, according to the liminal length concept, threshold is space dependent, the question can be raised as to whether cable properties can be determined accurately from responses to current injected at a point. In fact, the space constant λ is poorly defined near a point of current stimulation {251,252}. Similarly, in a two- or three-dimensional array of cells, stimulation should ideally be applied over a finite area, rather than at a point, to avoid untoward effects due to excessive current density {190,196}.

Local circuit currents and traveling waves

When threshold is attained in some region within a cable-like fiber or other spatially extensive tissue, inward currents I_{Na} and I_{Ca} grow regeneratively, rendering the region positive as compared to neighboring regions. This locally positive V_m drives current, primarily of K^+, longitudinally through the myoplasm toward more negative regions, through longitudinal resistance r_i, which, as we have stated, is composed of both gap junctional resistance r_j and cytoplasmic resistance r_{cyt}. As is true under small signal (linear, subthreshold, electrotonic) conditions, a fraction of the longitudinal current charges c_m and flows out through conductances g_m. A complete circuit is formed as current flows back to the initially depolarized region via the extracellular space. As the initially depolarized region depolarizes further, beyond V_{th}, more longitudinal current will flow toward neighboring regions and may depolarize them enough to meet the liminal length requirement. Regenerative depolarization will ensue in these new regions, and as this occurs enough longitudinal current will soon flow to bring yet another region to threshold, and so on. In this way APs can be generated successively over extensive distances at a finite rate.

Normally, propagation can only occur in directions away from the region where suprathreshold depolarization first occurred. Once a given region has sustained an AP it will become refractory to stimulation by currents that may flow back longitudinally from newly excited regions along the exact same path. As we will see, backflow by alternative paths can be significant.

The one-dimensional cable model of eq. (10-10) can predict the nondecremental AP propagation {190} in response to suprathreshold stimuli that is actually observed in cable-like tissues. The solutions [eq. (10-18) through eq. (10-20)] of eq. (10-10) that we used in introducing cable theory were decremental responses that occurred after the current i_m was changed to a constant value in a sudden step. These solutions were found using linear system analysis. When nondecremental propagation occurs, V_m still changes in response to i_m as described by eq. (10-10);

however, i_m is not a constant or step, but rather must depend on V_m in a specified way. Describing the required form of dependence is somewhat involved {190}, but the essential feature is formally like the regenerative growth of current on depolarization (negative slope conductance), which was illustrated in fig. 10-8 and is a property of I_{Na} and I_{Ca}. Negative slope conductance is a key feature of all AP reconstruction models. Solutions of eq. (10-10) that support AP propagation through the dependence of i_m on V_m are called *traveling wave* or *nonlinear diffusion* solutions. Study of these solutions requires nonlinear computer approximation techniques.

Speed of propagation

We now consider how active and passive cellular properties affect speed of propagation. Considering first the active properties, in an isolated cell, $\dot{V}_{max}$ during phase 0 of the AP is expected to be proportional to the maximal ionic current of Na^+ or Ca^{2+} because most of the initial current flow recharges C_m and would be described by eq. (10-2). This is not always found experimentally {269}.

When APs propagate through a cable or extensive array of cells, ionic current flows longitudinally to neighboring regions, not just inward. Nonetheless, in a one-dimensional linear cable governed by eq. (10-10), $\dot{V}_{max}$ still measures the intensity of the maximal phase 0 ionic current, as we show here. When excitation propagates along the cable at a constant conduction velocity Θ (in m/s), the dependence of V_m (measured at a fixed instant of time) on distance along the cable should have the same form as its dependence on time (measured at a fixed point):

$$\frac{\partial^2 V_m}{\partial x^2} = \left(\frac{1}{\Theta^2}\right)\frac{\partial^2 V_m}{\partial t^2}. \qquad (10\text{-}29)$$

Combining the basic cable eq. (10-10) with eq. (10-29), and remembering that the ionic current is V_m/r_m, we have

$$\frac{1}{r_i \Theta^2}\frac{d^2 V_m}{dt^2} = c_m \frac{d V_m}{dt} + i_{ion}. \qquad (10\text{-}30)$$

At the moment when dV_m/dt is maximal, the second derivative, $d^2 V_m/dt$, becomes zero. Equation (10-30) then becomes

$$\dot{V}_{max} = \frac{i_{ion}}{c_m}. \qquad (10\text{-}31)$$

In practice, the relationship of $\dot{V}_{max}$ to the transmembrane current i_m is nonlinear in cable-like fibers {69}. Loading by neighboring cells' input impedances changes the shape of the AP waveform {90,196,205,260,292,320}. Distortion of $\dot{V}_{max}$ during phase 0 {173} is presumably somewhat mitigated by the fact that R_{in} is at its lowest then.

We can assume that maximal phase 0 I_{Na} or I_{Ca} is acceptably measured as $\dot{V}_{max}$ {328}. Intuitively, an increase of Θ with an increase of $\dot{V}_{max}$ should be expected. In fact, in slow response tissues where I_{Ca} generates phase 0, $\dot{V}_{max}$ and Θ are much slower than in fast tissues where I_{Na} generates phase 0. Cable theory predicts that Θ will depend approximately on the square root of $\dot{V}_{max}$ {168}. This was seen experimentally when $\dot{V}_{max}$ was modified using various Na^+ conductance modifiers {52}, although a linear relationship has also been seen {280}.

Pathological states are often associated with decreased Θ. Many of these conditions, such as those induced by injury or drugs, reduce maximal phase 0 currents. Evidently if passive properties are constant, Θ can be no faster than some limit set by $\dot{V}_{max}$, so these quantities can be expected to covary {51}. However, it should not be concluded when Θ decreases that reduced phase 0 current is always the cause {293}. Passive properties and the organization of propagation pathways require due consideration.

One measure of the relationship of passive properties and Θ is the duration of the subthreshold rising phase of the AP. During propagation along a given direction, the earliest effect of current spreading to a previously unexcited region is electrotonic depolarization. As C_m charges, V_m decreases exponentially until V_{th} is reached and rapid depolarization ensues. This early rise of V_m has been called the foot of the AP {310; see also 298}. It can be predicted approximately by solving eq. (10-30) for a step change in i_m. This solution is the sum of two exponentials, of which the dominant term is {196,310}

$$V_{m[foot]}(t) = A\ e^{r_i c_m t} = A\ e^{t/\tau_{foot}}, \qquad (10\text{-}32)$$

where A is an arbitrary constant. Recalling that $\lambda = \sqrt{r_m/r_i}$,

$$\tau_{foot} = \frac{1}{r_i c_m \Theta^2} = \left(\frac{\lambda_m}{\Theta}\right)^2 \frac{1}{\tau_m} = \frac{a}{2\ R_i C_m \Theta^2}. \qquad (10\text{-}33)$$

This relationship was found experimentally to hold in sheep Purkinje fibers {103}.

Analytical predictions of how passive cable properties affect Θ during active propagation of APs have been reviewed {208,327,328}. Θ decreases if c_m or r_i increase. This may be seen intuitively, as a larger c_m requires more charging current and a larger r_i leads to a steeper loss of V_m per unit fiber length at any instant. In either case, the length of fiber newly brought to V_{th} at each successive instant is correspondingly smaller. Active propagation has a specific speed, which is given by {190}

$$\Theta = \frac{k}{C_m \sqrt{R_m R_i}}, \qquad (10\text{-}34)$$

in which the constant k is a constant that depends on the diameter of the cable and on the specific function chosen to represent how i_m depends on V_m.

As we have noted, modulation of gap junctional resistance r_j can exert a large and possibly dominating effect on r_i, and so can partly control Θ. This has been predicted by modeling {32,73,86,98,181,208}, as well as in experiments in which exogenous uncoupling treatments such as alkanols {73,90,173} and ischemia {192} were shown to reduce Θ. Particularly to be noted is that increased r_i can lead to outright failure of impulse transmission {90,163,320,337}, a point that will be considered further below.

Larger fibers should conduct faster. Equation (10-34)

indicates that Θ of a fiber should increase in proportion to the square root of the radius {see also 160}. Θ has actually been found either to increase with diameter {105} or to be almost constant, independent of diameter {268}. In the latter case, internal resistivity R_i was larger in larger fibers, possibly opposing the expected effect of diameter a. In large Purkinje fibers the extracellular clefts are more prominent, contributing possibly significant r_o, which would also reduce Θ. Another possibility {251} is that large Purkinje fibers may consist of many parallel strands of small diameter cells, rather than few strands of large diameter cells. In situ, all strands would be largely independent, and so would retain r_i, r_m, and therefore Θ characteristic of the cell diameter, not the fiber diameter.

PROPAGATION IN SPATIALLY EXTENSIVE ARRAYS OF CELLS

Propagation through massive three-dimensional tissues such as ventricular myocardium is far more complex than one-dimensional propagation along cablelike fibers. Important earlier results are reviewed by Jack et al. {171}.

Anisotropic and discontinuous propagation patterns

Referring now to fig. 10-12 {295}, we first consider whether r_i, τ_m, and other factors determining the velocity Θ and safety of propagation are uniform in all dimensions (fig. 10-12A1) {295}. In a two-dimensional sheet of rat atrial cells, Woodbury and Crill, over 30 years ago {347}, observed that electrotonic potentials did not decay exponentially with distance from a point source of current [as in a one-dimensional cable, eq. (10-20)], but rather decayed as a Bessel function. Potential decay was much sharper with increasing distance transverse to the fiber axis than along the axis. It has also long been known that the velocity of nondecremental propagation is anisotropic; that is, Θ differs when measured at points that lie in different directions relative to the orientation of cells from a stimulation site {66,263}; see figs. 10-14 and 10.12A2.

Given that propagation velocity is different in two directions, say x and y, we can then ask if it is constant when measured in a given direction, say, y, regardless of the distance along the x direction, say, x_1 or x_2. Propagation meeting this condition can be called *uniformly anisotropic* {292,293,295}. In uniformly anisotropic propagation, how Θ depends on cable properties could be expressed mathematically as separate from how it depends on properties in the y direction {196}:

$$\Theta = f_{x,y}(x,y) = f_x(x)f_y(y). \qquad (10\text{-}35)$$

In this equation, $f_{xy}(x,y)$, $f_x(x)$, and $f_y(y)$ are all functions that describe the dependence of Θ on cable properties.

To describe anisotropic propagation empirically on a macroscopic scale, Spach et al. proposed measurement of the effective axial resistivity, $\overline{R_a}$ {300,301}. $\overline{R_a}$ is the value of internal resistivity that would account for the observed speed of propagation along any direction, not just along the long axis of muscle fibers. Unlike R_i in linear con-

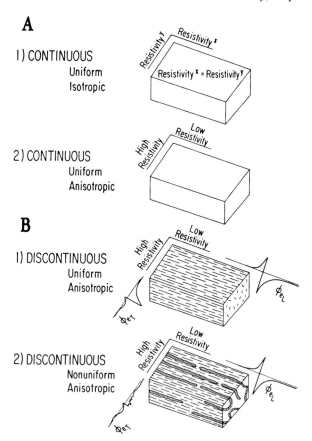

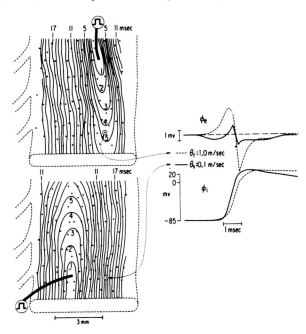

Fig. 10-13. Anisotropy of AP waveform and propagation velocity Θ in the crista terminalis. **Left:** Points of stimulation are indicated by square pulses; dots indicate sites of extracellular recording. **Right:** Extracellular (ϕ_e) and intracellular (ϕ_i) potentials at the right were recorded at points (circled and arrowed) longitudinal (dotted traces) and transverse (solid traces) to a point of stimulation. dV/dt_{max} was higher and τ_{foot} was longer in the transverse direction. Isochrone maps (left), constructed from the extracellular recordings, indicate uniform anisotropy; conduction velocity, calculated as the distance traveled normal to an isochrone per unit time, was lower transversely, despite higher dV_m/dt_{max}. From Spach et al. {300}, with permission.

Fig. 10-12. Characteristics of tissues viewed as conductive media supporting propagation. **A1:** Medium whose resistivity is constant and the same in all directions. **A2:** Medium whose resistivity is constant in a given direction but differs in different directions. **B1:** Medium with discrete impedances, such as high-resistance junctions, in the transverse direction. The resistivity is not constant, but the distribution of these impedances is similar throughout the medium. **B2:** Medium with irregularly arranged discrete transverse barriers. Transverse propagation can occur simultaneously via multiple paths. ϕ_e symbolizes extracellularly recorded potentials. From Spach et al. {295}, with permission.

tinuous cable theory, which incorporates only axial cytoplasmic resistivity and end-to-end GJ conductivity, $\overline{R_a}$ also includes implicitly the influences of cellular geometry and packing, extracellular resistivities, side-to-side couplings, and other features. Substituting $\overline{R_a}$ for R_i in the cable equation, we have

$$\frac{\pi a^2 \partial^2 V_m}{\overline{R_a} \partial x^2} = c_m \frac{\partial V_m}{\partial t} + i_{ion}. \qquad (10\text{-}36)$$

This equation has successfully predicted propagation on a macroscopic scale (several millimeters or more), even along pathways of complex or heterogeneous structure {300,301}.

On a microscopic scale (between a cell length and a few millimeters), eq. (10-36) is not applicable {292,293,295}. As fig. 10-14 {292} shows, recording extracellular potentials and their derivatives at multiple sites with high spatial resolution (separations of the order of 100 μm), Spach et al. {292,293,295} saw that excitation spread rapidly and along smooth contours in the axial direction. In young preparations (figs. 10-14A and 10.12B1), excitation also spread along smooth contours in directions off the long axis, indicating uniform anisotropy. However, in older preparations the fast longitudinal path was narrow and had abrupt borders. Off the long axis, excitation spread very slowly and in irregular or zigzag fashion (fig. 10-14B). Excitation often reached a transverse site multiphasically (see also fig. 10-12B2). This dissociation or fractionation indicates propagation by multiple paths, which could not occur in uniformly anisotropic tissue {293}. Propagation with these features has been called discontinuous {292}, dissociated microscopic {296}, or fractionated. Microscopically anisotropic propagation has also been confirmed using fast optical recording {230}.

Propagation velocity and other features of propagation

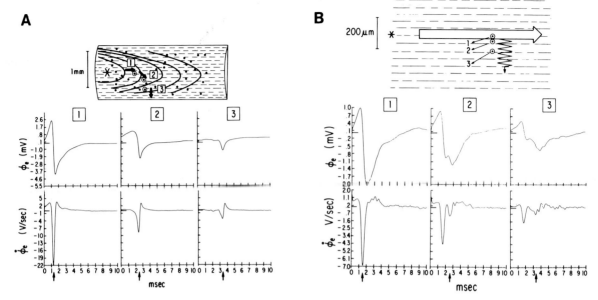

Fig. 10-14. Nonuniform anisotropic propagation in atrial tissue. **A:** Preparation from 2-year-old male. Excitation spread smoothly from site of initiation (*), as shown by the continuous isochrones (top). Smooth extracellular voltage waveforms (ϕ_e) and their time derivatives, recorded from circled points numbered (1,2,3), indicate monophasic excitation (bottom). The thin dashed lines show the orientation of the fibers. Arrows at the bottom of each panel mark the times of dV_m/dt_{max} of the underlying action potentials, which were used to construct the isochrones. Isochrones are separated by 1 ms. **B:** Preparation from 42-year-old male. The prominent open arrow on the preparation (top) indicates that in a narrow longitudinal region, propagation was fast and uniform, as shown in trace (1) at bottom. The sawtooth indicates that, in directions not collinear with the fiber axis, excitation spread along an irregular zigzag course. The corresponding extracellular waveforms and derivatives, seen in traces (2) and (3) at the bottom, are multiply peaked, indicating that excitation spread nonuniformly by multiple paths. From Spach and Dolber {292}, with permission.

are anisotropic in different ways. For example, as shown in fig. 10-13 {300}, despite faster propagation in the longitudinal direction, $\dot{V}_{max}$ was faster and τ_{foot} was shorter transversely {298,301}.

Anisotropic propagation must originate with structural features of cardiac muscle. Sperelakis and MacDonald {304} found that the bulk resistivity of ventricular muscle was much lower longitudinally than transversely. The fine structure of normal cardiac muscle is such that myocytes form "unit" bundles of 2–15 cells that have connections every 0.1–0.2 mm. These unit bundles are arranged into separate fascicles, connected with each other at longer distances, possibly related to diameter {287}. The fascicles, in turn, group into macroscopic bundles that have complex and varying interconnections {165}. The anisotropic distribution of gap junctions {136,137,165,289}, i.e., the localization (especially in adult tissue) of gap junctions dominantly or exclusively in end-to-end connections {136,137,165}, leaves transverse electrical coupling with a smaller magnitude and less uniformity than longitudinal coupling, consistent with slower and more indirect propagation off the long axis.

Nonuniform anisotropic propagation cannot be described using the cable equation, eq. (10-10), as this was derived using limiting arguments for infinitessimal distances. Another situation in which an infinitessimal

limit cannot apply is propagation through regions where conduction is decremental. If APs fail to propagate through a region, current transfer must have become electrotonic and have decremented to the point where the liminal length requirement at a downstream site is not met {9}. The converse of this is not true. As shown in fig. 10-15, Antzelevitch and Moe {7} have shown that electrotonic conduction through an inexcitable gap can support AP propagation. Purkinje fibers were put into a three-compartment bath in which the central (1.5 mm long) segment of tissue was rendered inexcitable by superfusing it with a solution that had $[K^+]_o$ of 15–20 mM. Enough current could be made to flow from the proximal compartment through the gap junctions in the inexcitable segment and into the distal compartment to evoke a regenerative AP.

Nonuniformly anisotropic propagation, involving indirect pathways and possibly regions of decremental conduction, is a feature of normal cardiac tissue. As we have noted, decremental coupling is the likely basis for optimal synchronization in pacemaker regions. Transverse propagation via relatively sparse lateral connections, possibly electrotonic, may help to stabilize the overall pattern of propagation through the myocardium.

Anisotropies are also relevant to pathology. As we will consider below, anisotropic structure changes in the

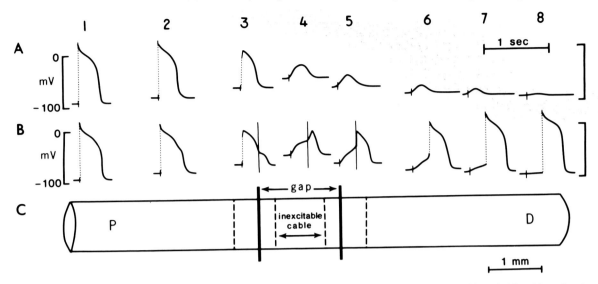

Fig. 10-15. An ischemic gap preparation that demonstrates electrotonic interaction can bridge an area of inexcitable cable and activate nondecremental conduction in a distal segment. **A:** Impulses were initiated by stimulating proximal segment P. They propagated as far as the border of the block and stopped there. Not enough electrotonic axial and local circuit current flowed in the inexcitable gap to bring the distal segment (D) to threshold. **B:** Same as A, but sufficient current did flow to trigger APs in the distal segment. **C:** Experimental arrangement. The middle compartment was rendered inexcitable by depolarization with a high $[K^+]_o$ solution, with inactivated both I_{Na} and I_{Ca}. From Antzelevitch and Moe {7}, with permission.

chronic phase after injury. Damaged longitudinal pathways can be supplanted by intact transverse-longitudinal-transverse alternates, which may be very long and have less than the normal strength of coupling {196,344}. Propagation through such restructured tissue could become very substantially slower and more variable than normal, and electrotonic coupling may become more prominent {212,284}. These features can support stable arrhythmic patterns of propagation {291,344}.

Considerations that limit the applicability of continuous cable theory differ in nerve and cardiac tissue. Propagation in myelinated nerve is spatially discrete in the sense that sparsely placed active nonlinear nodes are separated by long regions having only decremental conduction. In cardiac fibers each cell has extensive active membrane surface to support nondecremental conduction. Propagation is discrete because of the presence of high resistance gap junctions {196}.

Safety factor and propagation failure

Clinicians are well aware that propagation can fail more readily in certain tissues, such as the AV node, while propagation rarely fails in the His-Purkinje system or in atrial and ventricular muscle. The safety factor {328} is the excess of activating current or charge over that just required to produce a regenerative propagated response, the excess of source over sink.

Propagation should not fail in a continuous linear cable whose diameter and other properties are constant; nor should it fail in uniformly anisotropic multidimensional

tissues. Lower $\dot{V}_{max}$, higher R_i, longer τ_m, or lower R_m [see eqs. (10-29) and (10-30)] will slow propagation, but if R_i is finite and if the liminal length criterion is met anywhere in the cable, traveling waves should exist throughout.

Empirically, however, these expectations are not met. Both active and passive properties influence the safety of propagation. Regarding active properties, the tissues supporting safer propagation are those dependent on I_{Na} for phase 0 depolarization, while safety factor is poorer in tissues depending on I_{Ca}. Fast tissues depolarized during injury have a lower safety factor because of partial inactivation of I_{Na}.

Passive properties also critically affect the success of propagation. Failure can occur at points where passive properties change discontinuously, for example, at points of branching. If the cross-sectional area and length of a segment are constant, membrane surface area will increase and thus R_m will decrease at a branch point. As indicated by Goldstein and Rall {135}, Θ will change when fibers change their diameter or branch. In general, increased diameter or more branching led to smaller Θ as the sinking of current downstream was greater. Critically slowed conduction at times resulted in the failure of propagation and, at other times, in an echo beat, reflections, and other signs of mismatch {see also 207,220,322}. Extensive branching, as found in the AV node, is associated with lower safety.

Longitudinal propagation is faster {190}, but may or may not be safer, than transverse propagation. Heptanol uncoupling of gap junctions {31,88,90} and events generally associated with injury {191} blocked slow transverse propagation earlier than fast longitudinal propagation. Forcing normal tissue with increasingly premature extra stimuli blocked longitudinal propagation earlier than transverse {295,300,301}. Fast longitudinal propagation became first decremental and then ceased, while transverse propagation, though fractionated, continued.

When longitudinal propagation is less safe, one causal factor may be the loading effect of coupling on the AP waveform {196,205,320}. Referring to fig. 10-14, in the transverse direction higher coupling resistance leaves propagation speed slower, but leaves V_{max} higher {298,300}, contrary to expectation for a uniform linear continuous cable {160,293}. The underlying reason for disparate observations with respect to safety or failure of propagation is most likely differences in the microscopic non-uniform anisotropy of tissue structure {295}.

Spatially discrete cable theories

Spatially discrete cable theories have been discussed by Keener {190}. To provide a basis for a discrete cable theory, we return to the current balance equation, eq. (10-4), which applies to a single isolated cell, considered to be electrically homogeneous. We now modify this equation to describe a cell in contact with two neighbors (a segment of a one-dimensional cable). To the total capacitative current and the total ionic current of the cell, we add the total current flowing into or out of the cell from its neighbors {190}:

$$C_m A \frac{dV_m}{dt} = AI_{ion}(V_m,t) + I_{nbr}, \qquad (10\text{-}37a)$$

in which A is the total membrane surface area. We have written I_{ion} as dependent on V_m and t to remind the reader that a discrete cable, like a continuous one, must serve mainly to support nondecremental AP propagation. The currents (which total I_{nbr}) flowing in or out of a cell from its neighbors are driven by the potential differences between the cells and are controlled by the respective gap junctional resistances. Thus, for cell n having neighbors n − 1 and n + 1,

$$I_{nbr} = \frac{V_{n+1} - V_n}{r_j} - \frac{V_n - V_{n-1}}{r_j}$$
$$= \frac{V_{n+1} - 2V_n + V_{n-1}}{r_j}. \qquad (10\text{-}37b)$$

Combining and dividing through by A, we arrive at the discrete cable equation:

$$C_m \frac{dV_m}{dt} = I_{ion}(V_m,t) + \frac{V_{n+1} - 2V_n + V_{n-1}}{Ar_j}. \qquad (10\text{-}37c)$$

We assume that r_j is the same between all pairs of cells. More critically, we assume junctional resistance (r_j) to be large compared with cytoplasmic resistance. This may be the normal condition, the result of exogenous agents {73}, or of pathology. When r_j between cells is low {124}, in which case there is more intercellular current flow, or in long cells such as those of frog atria {166}, voltage loss in r_{cyt} becomes significant, and cells then cannot be considered homogeneous units {98,181,184}.

In highly coupled tissues such as ventricular muscle, macroscopic measures of resistivity [eq. (10-36)] or voltage distribution may show smooth variation. This smoothness does not preclude the existence of microscopic discontinuities of r_i, but may rather depend on the summed conductance of large numbers of parallel intercellular pathways {51,293} in both transverse and longitudinal directions.

The discrete eq. (10-37c) is the same as continuous eq. (10-10) with spatial derivative $\partial V_m/\partial x$ substituted by a finite difference, and internal longitudinal resistance r_i substituted by junctional resistance r_j. Because of this formal identity, eq. (10-37c) could be used to simulate numerically a continuous cable. However, eq. (10-37c) does not in general behave like eq. (10-10); the approximation is usefully close only when $\partial r_i/\partial x$ is constant; moreover, the spatial step size has no physical meaning and must be kept small. By contrast, in the discrete cable equation the step size represents a cell length {181,190}.

When using a discrete theory, it must be decided if quantities are to be measured relative to a unit of one cell (the step size) or along a continuous length scale. For instance, when measured on a continuous scale, longitudinal propagation is normally faster than transverse. However, if measured relative to numbers of cells, transverse propagation is normally faster {190}.

A key difference between continuous and discrete cable theories is in the relations governing propagation speed and safety. As we indicated above [eq. (10-30)], in continuous cable theory traveling waves will propagate when nonlinearly voltage-dependent excitation of an appropriate waveform is applied. If r_i should increase, propagation will slow, but traveling waves can be sustained as long as r_i is finite [eq. (10-30)]. On the other hand, in the discrete theory [as well as in numerical simulations of continuous theory using eq. (10-37c)], there is a maximum permissible value of r_j, dependent on the waveform of excitation, above which propagation will fail {190}.

Keener {190} has also considered the behavior of the continuous cable equation subject to constraints (boundary conditions), which are defined to describe conditions at the borders between cells. At each border a constraint states that $\partial V_m/\partial x$ is influenced by current flowing into or out of a cell via gap junctions. This current tends to change both V_m and, because of voltage dependence, i_m, in the vicinity of a border. When r_j is low, the constrained cable, driven by a transmembrane current i_m with regenerative nonlinear dependence on V_m, behaves like a continuous cable. When r_j is large, it behaves like a spatially discrete cable. An increase in r_j above some critical value causes propagation to fail {190}.

Continuous cable theory with boundary conditions takes into account that cytoplasmic resistance may be of greater or lesser significance to intercellular coupling. The theory predicts that larger cytoplasmic resistance reduces the ratio of longitudinal to transverse r_i. Thus a higher cytoplasmic resistance would make longitudinal propagation relatively more safe, while a lower r_{cyt} would make transverse propagation safer. This prediction may partly explain the disparate observations we noted above with respect to directional differences in safety. Apparent safety may also depend on the preparation used and the manipulation applied {190}.

Functional properties of gap junctions

Just as transmembrane ion currents, whose properties were revealed with the voltage clamp, determine the properties of APs, so also gap junctional conductances regulate the transfer of APs from cell to cell.

Metzger and Weingart {222} studied communication between paired adult rat ventricular cells by injecting current into one cell or the other. Current flowed through the nonjunctional membrane of the injected cell and also through r_j into the second or follower cell, where it perturbed the recorded V_m.

As with voltage-clamp studies of intercell communication (above), the responses were analyzed using the idealized lumped model of fig. 10-6A. From Kirchoff's laws, the input resistance (dV_i/dI_i) for either cell i (i = 1, 2) is given by

$$\frac{dV_1}{dI_1} = \frac{r_{m_1}(r_{m_2} + r_j)}{r_{m_1} + r_{m_2} + r_j},$$ (10-38)

which is the slope of the voltage-current relation for the injected cell, while the coupling coefficient (dV_{m_2}/dV_{m_1} or dV_{m_1}/dV_{m_2}) is given by

$$\frac{dV_{m_2}}{dV_{m_1}} = \frac{r_{m_2}}{r_{m_2} + r_j},$$ (10-39)

which is the ratio of the voltage change in the follower cell over the voltage change in the injected cell {37,221,330}. Measuring these quantities in both cells, in turn, generated four equations, which determined both nonjunctional membrane resistances (r_{m_1} and r_{m_2}) as well as junctional resistance r_j. As is true for voltage-clamp measurements of r_j [eqs. (10-8) and (10-9)], the accuracy of r_j measurements under current clamp is also limited. Both r_{m_1} and r_{m_2} are of course voltage dependent and are often much larger than r_j {338}.

Metzger and Weingart {222} found ventricular cells to be strongly coupled. Mean r_j was low and independent of voltage or direction of current flow, consistent with later voltage-clamp results. The value of r_j, 2.27 MΩ, corresponded to a specific R_j of 0.12 Ω-cm², which was low compared with the calculated specific R_m, 4.3 Ω-cm².

AP transfer requires an appropriate ratio of junctional and input resistances {319,337}. It has been suggested that unless $R_j/R_{in} < 12$, AP transfer or synchronization will not occur {63,320,337}. When $R_j/R_{in} < 5$, the delay in AP transfer should be very short compared to the AP duration. This is the normal situation in ventricular tissue (above). At intermediate ratios, $12 > R_j/R_{in} > 5$, delayed transfer occurs, which would slow propagation {208,337}. This may be the condition in pacemaker tissues.

Alternatively, the safety of transfer may be looked at in terms of numbers of open channels. The magnitudes of these resistances differ markedly among tissues. When input resistance is high, as in the SA node, junctional resistance can be low enough to allow partial synchroniza-

tion when there are only a few channels {9,337}. When input resistance is low, as in ventricular muscle, the rapid conduction needed for ventricular contraction requires several tens or hundreds of active channels {337,338}.

The spatial distribution and overall density of GJs are changed in injured tissue {212,284}. It may be predicted that injury, by reducing coupling, renders coupling-dependent properties, such as conduction velocity, more susceptible to modification by rate-dependent factors such as pH, $[Ca^{2+}]_i$ {51,159,217,252} or transjunctional voltage {180,341}, than normal tissue {299,319}. These influences may operate on a beat-to-beat time scale.

CARDIAC ARRHYTHMIAS, DRUG ACTIONS, AND CLINICAL IMPLICATIONS

Hypothesis of altered excitability and the electrophysiologic matrix

Any search for predictors of ventricular tachycardia (VT) or ventricular fibrillation (VF) will recognize that epidemiological and other data have clearly demonstrated that these potentially life-threatening arrhythmias rarely arise in normal hearts. This clinical observation led one of us (MFA) to suggest a number of years ago that excitability must be rendered abnormal for dangerous ventricular arrhythmias to arise, even in the presence of triggers such as PVCs. Restated in terms of the electrophysiologic matrix, the assumption is that the matrix of interacting active and passive cellular properties determines normal cardiac excitability. In the normal state, the heart is resistant to the development of cardiac arrhythmias, even in the presence of potential triggering beats. The normal matrical configuration must be altered by arrhythmogenic influences that affect one or several determinants of excitability. The result is a change in the matrical configuration that results in abnormal excitability and a proarrhythmic precursor state. In this state, PVCs and other triggers may give rise to reentrant or automatic arrhythmias.

As seen in fig. 10-16 {25}, our laboratory's measurements of the effects of lysophosphatidylcholine (LPC) on strength-duration relationships {25,265} show that arrhythmogenic disturbances affect both active and passive properties. As we noted previously, LPC is a metabolite that accumulates in ischemic myocardium {189,285,286}. In fig. 10-17A, strength duration curves measured on sheep Purkinje fibers are shown for control conditions (open circles) and application of 20 μM (closed triangles) and 45 μM LPC (closed squares). At 20 μM, the strength-duration curve was shifted downward, indicating that less current was required to attain threshold for any current duration; that is, the cells were more excitable in the classical sense. At 45 μM, the cells were less excitable, as indicated by the upward shift of the curve. As [LPC] was increased from 0 to 20 to 45 μM, V_{max} decreased monotonically. At 20 μM, increased excitability in the face of depressed Na$^+$ conductance indicates that passive mem-

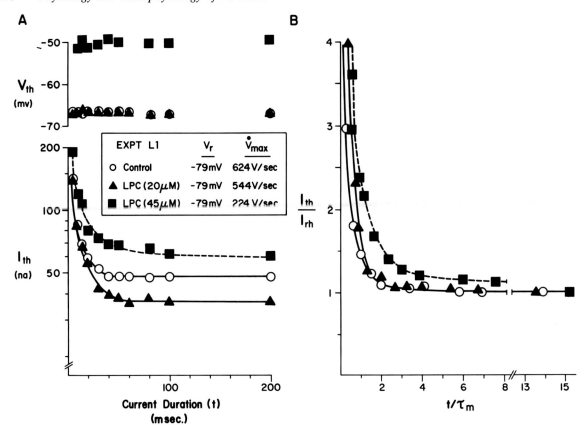

Fig. 10-16. Strength-duration (S-D) curves for a Purkinje fiber exposed to lysophosphatidylcholine (LPC) at 20 and 45 μM. **A:** At 20 μM, the S-D curve falls below control, indicating greater excitability. As dV_m/dt_{max} changed minimally, passive properties must have changed; indeed, λ was found to have increased. At 45 μM the curve lies above control, indicating lower excitability; g_{Na} was severely depressed. **B:** The S-D curves in A were normalized to minimize the influence of changes in passive properties. Control and 20 μM curves superimposed well. However, the 45 μM curve differed in shape, indicating a major change in active properties at this concentration. From Arnsdorf and Sawicki {25}, with permission.

brane properties must have been altered. In fact, R_m and λ were found to be larger than in control.

To minimize differences in the shapes of the strength-duration curves due to altered passive properties, threshold current was expressed relative to rheobasic current and duration was expressed relative to the membrane time constant, τ_m. As seen in fig. 10-16B, the normalized curves for control and 20 μM LPC were superimposible, indicating minimal change in active generator properties (compare fig. 10-12). By contrast, the normalized strength-duration curve at 45 μM was not superimposable on the control or 20 μM LPC curve, indicating that active properties had changed.

The transition from one equilibrium to another can be considered usefully with bifurcation diagrams. We can represent the outcome of this experiment in matrix form, as shown in fig. 10-22 {19}. The control condition representing the normal dynamic equilibrium is depicted by the regular hexagon (left edge). The accumulation of LPC by the tissue drives the equilibrium to the right along

the Y axis until point B is reached. At this point, normal homeostatic feedback mechanisms fail, resulting into a transition to a new dynamic equilibrium at points C or D. The conditions of the X axis, such as the anatomic substrate, the amount of LPC in the environment or in the membrane, the pH, and the $[K^+]_o$, cause one pathway (a or b, leading to equilibria C or D, respectively), to be preferred. This is termed an *assisted bifurcation*.

After 20 μM LPC (lower branch), the liminal length was shorter (shift in LL toward the center), and both R_m and λ were larger (lower matrix on lower branch). After 45 μM (upper branch) the liminal length was longer (shift in LL away from the center; lower figure on upper branch). Excitability had decreased despite increased R_m and λ, due to radical reduction in g_{Na}. In ischemia, other factors may contribute to the path chosen. Hyperkalemia, for example, will favor path a. We will return to some of the specific electrophysiologic changes in subsequent sections.

It follows that the proarrhythmic matrix at points C or D may be *fixed* or *transient*; fixed, as in the situation of an

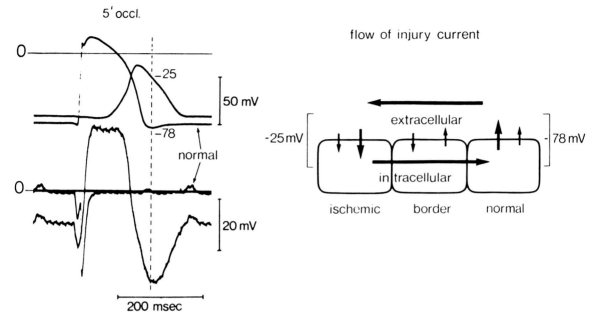

Fig. 10-17. Injury currents. **Left:** AP records (**top**) show depolarization, delay, loss of amplitude, and lower dV_m/dt_{max} at a site injured by ischemia of 5 minutes duration, compared with a normal site in the same tissue. Extracellular electrograms (**bottom**) show that injury current depended on the instantaneous difference between APs at the normal and injured sites. The preparation was canine heart in situ. **Right:** Schematic view of injury current circulation. From Janse and Kleber {175}, with permission.

anatomic substrate such as a ventricular aneurysm or a reentrant pathway around an anatomical obstacle, or transient, as with ischemia, drug toxicity, autonomic surges, and the like.

Antiarrhythmic and other drugs add another level of complexity and create yet another matrical configuration. The normal matrix or the matrix that has been reconfigured by arrhythmogenic influences interacts with the antiarrhythmic drug, creating yet another matrix that may be antiarrhythmic, antifibrillatory, or proarrhythmic. It follows that the predominant effect or effects of an antiarrhythmic drug depends on the type of matrix encountered. Returning again to fig. 10-22, note that a second bifurcation occurs after the tissue is exposed to lidocaine (C*,D*), which further alters the matrix. The final matrical configuration is also determined by the variables along the x axis for given points along the y axis. The arrhythmogenic matrix after LPC at point C is quite similar to the configuration after the interaction between LPC and lidocaine at point C*. Note the similarity between the presumed proarrhythmic and antiarrhythmic matrices This kite-shaped configuration is very similar to that we have observed for ethmozin, encainide, procainamide, and, at an elevated [K⁺]o, for quinidine, so it is not surprising that these drugs are proarrhythmic in a substantial number of patients.

A paradox and its resolution

One of us (MFA) has commented on an electrophysiologic paradox {18,19}. To restate {19}, the "paradox is that the

multiplicities, discontinuities, dynamic interactions and other complexities that exist in and among the active and passive properties underlying cardiac excitability should result in unpredictably complex behavior, yet electrophysiologic events usually are coordinated sufficiently to produce predictable outcomes. In other words, there is order in this seeming chaos."

The resolution to the paradox can be found in the bifurcation diagrams of fig. 10-22. The electrophysiologic universe in this experiment *moves as a system*, certain matrical configurations being favored by the variables along the X axis that assist bifurcation. *Self-organization, then, occurs through assisted bifurcations.* If some of these variables are known, then predictability is possible. In terms of arrhythmogenesis, for example, ischemia accompanied by the uptake of LPC and other metabolites, a decrease in pH and pO_2 and a rise in [K⁺]o almost invariably results in a matrix characterized by sodium channel inactivation and decreased excitability, such as appears at point C in fig. 10-22.

We reached our conclusions about the dynamics of arrhythmogenesis from clinical epidemiologic studies that led to the hypothesis of altered excitability and from our experiments in basic cellular electrophysiology that led to the concept of the electrophysiologic matrix. Others have reached similar conclusions from different vantages. Glass and Mackey {130} suggest that there are dynamical diseases that are characterized by abnormal temporal organization. They, and a number of other investigators, have been assessing normal and abnormal dynamical systems mathematically in terms of chaos, nonlinear dynamics, and fractal structure {132,172,342}. Glass and Mackey {130} theorize that spatial oscillations may produce abnormalities of conduction in one dimension, such as the Wenckebach phenomenon or reentry; spiral wave propagation in two dimensions, which may underly reentrant arrhythmias due to the leading circle mechanisms, which will be described later in this section; and scroll waves in three dimensions, which may be the basis for ventricular fibrillation.

Self-organization through assisted bifurcations is the probable reason that classifications of antiarrhythmic drugs, such as that of Vaughan–Williams, are empirically useful. Similarly, a drug that primarily decreases conductance through the sodium channel will predictably have this as its primary effect at point C in the ischemic matrix. In a situation filled with endless possibilities, ischemia favors certain bifurcations and a certain proarrhythmic matrix; and, as a result, drug action becomes predictable.

Origins, phenomena, and classification of arrhythmias

With the hypothesis of altered excitability and the concept of the electrophysiologic matrix in mind, we will turn to some of the mechanisms involved in creating the proarrhythmic matrical configurations of abnormal excitability. The underlying cause of cardiac rhythm disturbances often is tissue injury {10}, which may result from ischemia, reperfusion, and infarction {10,155,177}. Other influences, such as autonomic tone, drugs, and the like, may contribute to arrhythmogenesis and the proarrhythmic precursor matrix.

Traditionally clinicians and physiologists have related arrhythmogenesis to abnormalities of either impulse formation or impulse propagation {206,345}. We will discuss these sources of arrhythmia separately, although arrhythmogenesis may involve both mechanisms {199}. Any change in cellular mechanisms of AP generation must be localized, affecting some cells and not others {3,205,296}, and thereby creating spatial inhomogeneities of tissue properties that would not be present normally. Only by the juxtaposition of normal and injured tissues can the processes occur that define functionally arrhythmogenic pathways.

The classification of arrhythmias {345} presents difficulties typical of nonlinear systems. A given arrhythmic phenomenon can appear as a result of different mechanisms {312}. In some cases, the presumption is strong that a single "vulnerable parameter" has changed {312}, while in others, little or no information is available by which to decide the mechanism {351}. Conversely, one primary mechanism may generate varied arrhythmic behaviors, possibly in response to small changes in secondary factors.

Arrhythmogenesis during acute ischemia may differ from that during later phases of ischemia or when injured tissue has infarcted and healed over {177,188,191,344}. Taking the role of Ca^{2+} as an example, during acute ischemia, injury currents flow, as shown in fig. 10-17A {175}. These partially depolarize cells, and thereby may promote rhythm disturbances {138,175,177}. Injury currents are dynamic, flowing maximally at times when normal cells have repolarized and injured ones have not (vertical dotted line in fig. 10-17A) {175}. In infarcted tissue, injury currents do not flow because the cells are dead and uncoupled from the rest of the myocardial population, although actively ischemic areas may persist that may generate injury currents and remain coupled to neighboring cells. A rise in intracellular Ca^{2+} may isolate injured but potentially viable tissue by closing GJ channels. Often arrhythmias associated with acute ischemia are transient, while those associated with the healed infarct may be recurrent and often sustained {191}.

Arrhythmogenesis and changes in impulse generation

Abnormal excitability may occur when normally automatic tissues change their properties, when tissues that are not normally automatic become so {144,312}, or when normal tissues are stimulated from an ectopic location {297}. Ectopic activity may be induced by electrotonic coupling {176} and injury current flow. Excitability changes may be manifest as disturbances of the AP waveform, and can originate in altered ion channels, pumps, and/or exchangers {239}, or in changes in membrane resistance or cell-cell coupling.

Several phenomena related to excitability follow specifically as consequences of ATP depletion during ischemia {138}. AP duration shortens radically {239}, as seen in fig. 10-18 {175}. Initially a dominant cause of shortening is activation of ATP-inhibited K^+ channels {241}; this can occur as cells lose their charge of ATP, even within the physiological range {235,239}. As ATP depletion progresses further, over some minutes, Na^+/K^+ pumping begins to run down, leading to depolarization as $[K^+]_o$ increases {113}. Depolarization inactivates I_{Na} and slows V_{max} during phase 0 of the AP in fast tissues {206}, but it also promotes possible regenerative activation of I_{Ca}. Na^+/K^+ pump inhibition also increases $[Na^+]_i$ {113}, which stimulates Na^+/Ca^{2+} exchange, leading to modification of the late plateau of the AP {239}, increased internal Ca^{2+}, and likely Ca^{2+} overload, via amplified release from SR stores.

In cells that are partly depolarized and/or undergo unregulated changes in $[Ca^{2+}]_i$, such as overloads, APs often do not end with rapid repolarization, but rather with repetitive discharges {152}, or other aberrant time courses that are arrhythmogenic or represent ectopic automaticity {239}. Two common abnormal time courses are referred to as *early* or *delayed afterdepolarizations* (EADs and DADs, respectively) {239,312}. EADs and DADs are triggered activities in the sense that they are induced by a preceding AP.

Early afterdepolarizations (EADs) begin late in the plateau phase. They could represent activity of L-type Ca^{2+} channels. If V_m remains for an extended time at an intermediate level, many L-Ca^{2+} channels either remain open or recover from inactivation and subsequently reopen {276}. This behavior of L-Ca^{2+} channels could be promoted by beta-adrenergic stimulation {312}. Aside from quasi-stabilized Ca^{2+} currents, EADs could result

A. NORMAL

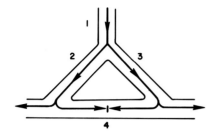

B. UNIDIRECTIONAL BLOCK WITH REENTRY

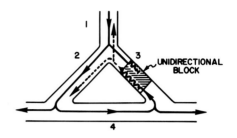

C. PRODUCTION OF BIDIRECTIONAL BLOCK

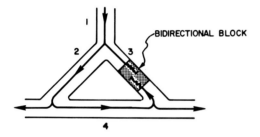

D. ABOLITION OF UNIDIRECTIONAL BLOCK

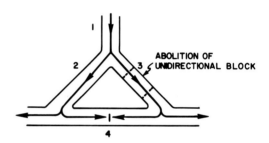

Fig. 10-18. Scheme of unidirectional block and reentrant propagation. **A:** Normally, impulses propagate from a central Purkinje fiber (1) down branches 2 and 3, and activate the ventricle (4), producing a QRS complex. **B:** Injury to branch 3 produces a depressed segment that unidirectionally blocks the impulse in that branch. The impulse travels normally down branch 2 and activates the ventricle, producing a normal QRS complex, but also conducts very slowly in the retrograde direction through the depressed segment in branch 3. If the tissue at the bifurcation has recovered its excitability by the time the impulse emerges from the depressed segment, this tissue will be reexcited. Excitation may travel down branch 2 to the ventricle, producing a premature depolarization (dashed arrow). Such reentrant excitation can occur repeatedly, leading to a sustained tachycardia. Excitation can also travel back up the central Purkinje fiber 1 (dashed arrow). **C:** A reentrant loop can be abolished by conversion of unidirectional to bidirectional block. If unidirectional block was induced by depression of I_{Na} and lowering of dV_m/dt_{max}, further depression of I_{Na} will lead to bidirectional block. **D:** The conditions for reentry are eliminated by abolishing the area of unidirectional block.

from prolonged Na^+ currents and/or loss of K^+ currents {312}, and can be induced {138} or suppressed {206} by drugs.

Late (delayed) afterdepolarizations (DADs) do not begin until after repolarization is largely complete. DADs are believed to represent currents of Na^+/Ca^{2+} exchange {312} or of a Ca^{2+}-dependent nonselective ion channel I_{ns} {75} and are initiated by Ca^{2+} overload, especially in ischemic hypoxia {51}. DADs are destabilizing positive feedback events, and are often highly rate dependent.

We reported a clinical case of an atrial tachyarrhythmia that might be ascribable to DADs, although the question remains as to the relationship between what is observed clinically and what is observed in the tissue bath {348}. EADs appear to be associated with known arrhythmias, particularly torsade de pointes {206}, possibly because cells generating them participate in loci where ectopic beats are generated {110,206}.

We have observed bistability as another manifestation of defective repolarization of an AP {24}. As seen in fig.

10-21, APs can end in either of two stable steady states, one at the resting potential and the other at the plateau potential. An AP evoked by a single triggering stimulus did not end normally, but rather with repeated depolarizations from the plateau voltage (fig. 10-17A,B). Such activity persisted for tens of minutes, until terminated by a hyperpolarizing pulse (panel B) or by the addition of lidocaine (panel C). This too can be considered in terms of a bifurcation diagram similar to that of fig. 10-22: The first bifurcation is from the steady state at the normal resting potential to a new steady state on the plateau. At the plateau, further bifurcation dependent on V_m on the x axis may result in afterdepolarizations if V_m in a critical range of plateau voltage that allows the opening and closing of L-type Ca^{2+} channels, or by quiescence if it is not.

When repolarization does occur, injury (as well as many drugs) can alter the time course of recovery of excitability afterward {177}. In normal fast I_{Na}-dependent tissues, refractoriness due to Na^+ channel inactivation does not limit response rates. Refractoriness lessens during phase 3 of the AP and is usually over by the time V_m has returned to V_r. Fast tissues can be driven at intervals as short as the AP duration. Recovery will be delayed whenever injury has prolonged the AP duration, e.g., in the case of EADs or DADs. However, recovery can be delayed beyond normal, even when injury has shortened the AP. Post repolarization refractoriness appears within minutes in acute ischemic injury {104}, and may be associated with slowed Na^+ channel inactivation.

Aside from leading to depolarization, increased $[K^+]_o$ due to loss of Na^+/K^+ pumping also modifies refractoriness {239,324}. Especially the relative refractory period is lengthened {194}. This may explain why localized increases of $[K^+]_o$ during acute ischemia {78,191} reduce conduction velocity Θ, and can even stop conduction altogether, at times when longitudinal resistance r_i will not have changed much.

Slow tissues, which depend normally on I_{Ca}, may be somewhat resistant to disturbances in refractoriness, since they are normally refractory beyond the recovery of the diastolic potential. To some extent, as we noted before, this property may be protective. Certainly, the average rate of transmission of impulses through the AV node is limited during atrial flutter and atrial fibrillation. Nonetheless, experiments suggest that rhythm disturbances can occur even if recovery in the AV node has the normal fixed monoexponential form, if the node is stimulated at rapid rates {141}. When recovery in the AV node follows a disturbed (nonmonotonic or supernormal) time course, abnormal or chaotic ventricular rhythms are likely {324}.

Arrhythmogenesis and changes in propagation

The situation most generally thought to lead to arrhythmias is reentry, which in a number of models has a basis in slow conduction and unidirectional block of propagation. Unidirectional block may originate with spatially inhomogeneous refractoriness {110,283}. In fast tissues, any localized influence reducing maximal Na^+ conductance could also slow conduction and/or cause partial block; so also could any inhomogeneity of conducting pathway geometry, or of ion distribution {207,220,322}. Excitation can propagate around an area of block by a long indirect path, or it can propagate slowly through it. In either case, it can ultimately reach back to and reenter an area of previously excited tissue that will have recovered. This reentrant mechanism, deduced originally by Mines in 1913 {225}, is illustrated in fig. 10-18. Normally (fig. 10-18A) excitation propagates along Purkinje fibers {2,3} to excite ventricular tissue {4}. Should injury produce unidirectional block of conduction (fig. 10-18B) in one fiber {3}, excitation would propagate down fiber {2} and possibly back along fiber (3). Owing to the length of the path and/or the condition of fiber (3) (compare fig. 10-15), excitation may propagate quite slowly back to site (1). Should site (1) have recovered excitability, path (1–2) will be reactivated, possibly in a sustained manner.

The duration of absolute refractoriness and the conduction velocity interact to determine a minimum path

length over which reentrant propagation (sometimes called *circus movement* {312}) could occur, as described approximately by {282}

$$L_c = \Theta RP, \qquad (10\text{-}40)$$

where L_c is the length of the reentrant path, Θ is the conduction velocity, and RP is the refractory period. In a normal Purkinje fiber, Θ is about $3\,m/s$ and RP is about 300 ms, so L_c would be $1\,m$, which is anatomically unlikely. However, if Θ is reduced to $0.01\,m/s$, then L_c is only $3\,mm$, a distance comparable to those over which discontinuities of propagation have been measured in normal tissue (above).

Both large- and small-scale reentrant circuits form commonly {110}. An example of a large circuit is bundle branch reentry. SA and AV nodes, because of their I_{Ca}-dependent APs and normally slow conduction, can readily participate in long reentrant circuits. Because of anisotropies in passive properties (especially r_i) related to the fine distribution of gap junctional connections, small or microscopic reentrant circuits may form within single Purkinje fibers or sections of ventricle.

Corrective strategies for reentry are directed toward eliminating triggering beats; changing path lengths (e.g., by stimulation, or surgical ablation, which can induce bidirectional blocks); decreasing propagation speeds (e.g., by drugs that influence $\dot{V}_{max}$ to nonpermissive values, or conversely, increasing conduction velocity in the area of slow conduction; and increasing the refractoriness of the tissue to be reexcited.

Arrhythmias could also occur when a previously excited region of tissue is reexcited electrotonically by way of a delayed reflected wave, or when propagating wavefronts collide. These events may cause waves of excitation to propagate off in a new direction that is not necessarily along, say, a defined reentrant loop {6}. Experimentally, reflection can also terminate arrhythmias. When drug interventions (heptanol, propafenone, and others) are effective in terminating reentrant arrhythmias, they may do so by changing the character of propagation in the involved circuit so that reflections occur. Reflected waves then collide with and annihilate those propagating orthodromically through the circuit {50}.

Reentrant excitation, as we have described it so far, is implied to follow circumscribed paths defined by anatomical changes such as infarcts; it is ordered {206}. However, this need not be the case. Inhomogeneous properties of conduction velocity {36} or refractoriness {3,283} in themselves are enough to support untoward propagation phenomena. A stable anatomical substrate, a fixed proarrhythmic matrix, may be a more likely concomitant of a chronic arrhythmia. Transient (or random) {206} modes of reentry, although usually associated with acute ischemia, may have no evident histological basis and can be induced in normal tissue. Transient arrhythmias reflect nonstationarity in time and/or space of the supporting properties (e.g., refractoriness, propagation velocity) {191}. A representative random reentry phenomenon is fibrillation, in which excitation progresses simultaneously along multiple wavefronts.

The reentrant circuit may be very short and functional, or, as Allessie put it, the head of the circulating waving front may be "biting on its own tail of relative refractoriness" {2,4}. Allessie has called this smallest possible circuit where the wave length equals the pathway length, the "leading circle" {3}. This type of reentrant movement does not require gross anatomical obstacles but creates its own refractory center. In two cases of Type II atrial flutter, Cosio and Arribas {79} have reported areas of localized continuous electrical activity consistent with the Allessie model. This suggests that the mechanism of Type II flutter is not intraatrial reentry around a gross anatomical obstacle but rather intraatrial reentry based on a leading circle.

Arrhythmogenesis, cable properties, anisotropy, and gap junctions

Historically, altered active properties have been thought more important than passive properties as the cause of arrhythmogenic conduction disturbances {25,55,148}. Inactivated sodium channel conductance, as reflected in an index such as a lowered $\dot{V}_{max}$, as we have noted, not only affects individual cells, but can abet the formation of reentrant pathways, as it is a sufficient cause of slowed conduction. However, conduction can be slowed in the presence of normal excitation {126,293,315}.

Type I or common atrial flutter is thought to be a reentrant arrhythmia {80,102,170,193,325,326,331, among others}. A single premature extrastimulus and rapid atrial pacing can initiate the arrhythmia. There is an excitable gap that allows the arrhythmia to be terminated by a single beat or by rapid pacing. The excitable gap is the portion of a reentrant circuit that has recovered its excitability and can again be reexcited. The excitable gap also allows entrainment with overdrive pacing during atrial flutter {325,326}. Recent experimental studies in the sterile pericarditis model suggest a role for anisotropic conduction in producing the functional area of slow conduction that is responsible for the reentrant phenomena {266,267, 274,275}.

Disturbances of conduction in acute ischemia have been thought mainly to be associated with AP generation {192,256,344}. For instance, as shown in fig. 10-19B {229}, metabolic inhibition via DNP or lowered [ATP]i led to radical decreases of R_{in} and loss of AP transfer in pairs of ventricular cells. Decreased R_{in} in injured cells creates

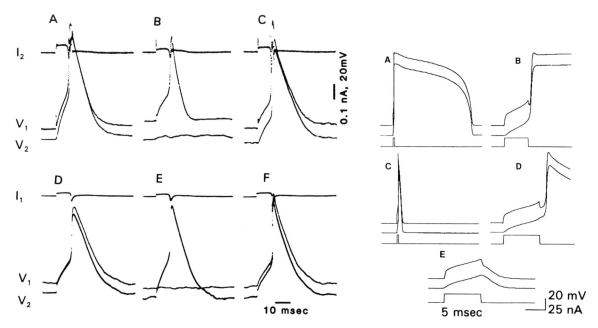

Fig. 10-19. Experimental demonstrations of loss of coupling (left) or cellular excitability (right) predicted for injured tissue in situ. **Left:** (**A–C**) APs were recorded from a pair of rat myocytes (V_1 and V_2) while cell 2 was stimulated (I_2). AP transfer (A) was eliminated when decanoic acid (1 mM) was applied (B), and restored on washout (C). (**D–F**) AP transfer was also eliminated reversibly by palmitoleic acid (50 μM). In this case cell 1 was stimulated (I_1). Decanoic and palmitoleic acids are representative of nonesterified fatty acids that accumulate in cells after many minutes of ischemia. The invariant shape of the APs indicate that neither of these fatty acids affected excitability. **Right:** (**A–E**) APs were recorded from paired guinea pig myocytes before (A) and during (C,E) treatment with the metabolic inhibitor dinitrophenol (DNP) at 80 μM. AP duration shortened (C) and ultimately failed (E). However, cell-to-cell current transfer remained robust and did not become delayed, as shown by traces (B) and (D), which expand in time the intial phases of (A) and (C), respectively, and by trace (E). Left from Burt et al. {55}, Right from Morley et al. {229}, with permission.

large sinks into which injury currents would flow, possibly causing arrhythmogenic heterogeneities in tissue properties, without anatomical barriers {229}. Junctional resistance r_j increased minimally, not enough to prevent electrotonic current transfer {229}.

After the initial phases of acute ischemia are past, longitudinal resistances increase in specific sequence. External longitudinal resistivity R_o begins to increase gradually within a few minutes, while internal resistivity R_i increases only after 10 minutes or more, but does so quite suddenly, completing its increase within 1 minute or so, following which conduction is blocked {192,256}.

In chronically infarcted myocardium, increased R_i enhances discontinuity of propagation above that normally predicted formally {181,260} and found experimentally {73,90,292,300}, as well as decreasing conduction velocity {237} and space constant {302}. Increased R_i is a consequence of derangement of gap junction organization after injury {30,87,95,96,212,237,284}. Associated with reduced GJ conductance is greater variance of conduction velocity {36} as well as predicted inhomogeneities in voltage distribution in response to injected current, which should be evident at a macroscopic scale {51}. These alterations may be destabilizing and lead to late potentials and arrhythmias, or may help to improve the stability of propagation in surviving tissue {297}. Tissues with structural heterogeneities, such as Purkinje-to-ventricular paths {220,322} or AV node {169}, may be more potently affected when R_i increases.

We assume that the influences that reduce GJ conductance during injury ultimately lead, in the healed-infarct period, to all-or-none loss of and redistribution in space of GJ channels that otherwise function normally. This assumption is based on the observed all-or-none modification of GJ conductance by injury-related influences, as we described in reviewing intercellular communication. Particularly to be noted is the synergism between increased $[Ca^{2+}]_i$ and cytoplasmic acidification {40,53,317}. Increasing $[Ca^{2+}]_i$ affected cable properties {191}. It decreased G_j, but not until $[Ca^{2+}]_i = 12\,\mu M$ was reached, high enough to induce contractures {82,307,338}. Normal transient increases in $[Ca^{2+}]_i$ due to I_{Ca} and Ca^{2+} release from the SR seem insufficient to affect G_j, which supports the earlier view of Weidman in 1970 {334}. Only changes in the phosphorylation state {227} and possible expression of the GJ channel isoforms in altered proportions {187,323} have been identified as factors likely to change the behavior of individual channels.

The view that a fraction of GJ channels remains intact is also supported by the fact that normal APs can be recorded within tissue areas infarcted after chronic ischemia, where propagation was delayed and fractionated {126,303,315}. One factor associated with closure of GJ channels in the face of intact or minimally disturbed excitability is the accumulation of nonesterified fatty acids in membranes. As fig. 10-19A {55} shows, at concentrations comparable to those found in ischemia, normal APs can be recorded in one member of a pair of cells, but do not transmit between cells. The mechanism of this disruption of GJs was proposed to be membrane disordering localized to channels, rather than gross membrane disruption or specific channel binding {55}.

Columns of cells with essentially normal action potentials may be physically separated from each other by collagen in a chronic infarction {126,315}. This may disrupt the GJ connections, resulting in loss of the integration of conduction velocities. Normally, rapidly conducting fibers would be slowed down by neighboring slowly conducting fibers, and vice versa, with the result being a uniform average conduction velocity. Disruption of the cell-cell communication would result in conduction at more disparate velocities. This, in part, may underly the fractionated electrograms and late potentials recorded by the epicardial electrogram. The microscopically heterogeneous properties that support arrhythmogenic pathways in infarcted tissue differ qualitatively from heterogeneities of normal tissue. Some cells must survive in an infarcted area if it participates in reentrant circuits; otherwise, the region would not support conduction at all {344}. In these cells, as mentioned, essentially normal APs can be recorded {126,315}, although there is evidence of electrotonic influences as well {303}. In thin strands of surviving tissue, propagation over very short distances may be almost normal. However, the borders of infarcted regions are not gradual but sharp and microscopically irregular {174}. Details of the border zone may correspond at least in scale with details of discontinuous propagation. Where arrhythmogenic circuits are sustained, they may be constrained to follow paths that are microscopically much longer than the apparent lengths that would be determined by interelectrode distances [refer to eq. (10-40)]. It is interesting to speculate that these may cause the fractionated potentials that are detected by the surface signal-averaged electrocardiogram.

These considerations have given rise to the hypothesis of anisotropic reentry, which is illustrated in fig. 10-20A, and in magnified form in fig. 10-20B {344}. Anisotropic reentry is proposed as a basis for sustained ventricular tachycardias, which can often be induced by a single stimulus in healed tissue {101}. During tachycardia, excitation was found to circulate through a narrow long strip of surviving ventricular tissue whose longer dimension was coaxial with the long axis of the cells {344}. It traveled longitudinally at about the normal rate, and transversely at a slow rate possibly not much different from that in normal anisotropic tissues. Wavefronts traveling mainly longitudinally propagated faster but followed longer paths, compared with those traveling mainly transversely, which moved slowly, but over short distances, and possibly electrotonically {303}. There was some dispersion or fractionation in the rearrival of these wavefronts at the start point, but regardless of the path, the transit time was long enough to allow the starting subarea to recover, so sustained reentry was supportable.

Teleologically the shutdown of GJs by increased $[Ca^{2+}]_i$ and/or lowered pH may serve mainly to isolate tissue elements that have undergone chronic ischemic/hypoxic injury from normal ones. This isolation means that normal cells will not lose their cytoplasmic contents or be depolarized by injured ones as a result of continued flow of

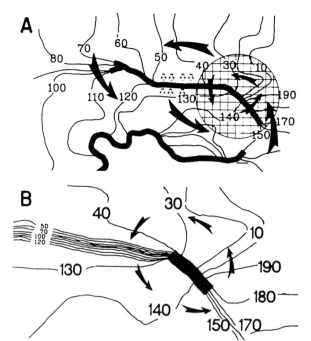

A

B

Fig. 10-20. The hypothesis of anisotropic reentry in infarct border zones. **A:** Heavy arrows and isochronal lines indicate excitation progressing around a long line where conduction appeared to be blocked (horizontal thick black lines). **B:** Expansion of area within gridwork from A, showing closely spaced isochrones. Slow transverse propagation is proposed to have occurred across the line of apparent block. From Wit {344}, with permission.

injury currents. In summary of observations on injured tissues, many observations support the idea that a decrease of cell membrane resistance R_m is the major initial acute effect of injury, while a decrease of R_j is the major late or chronic effect {175,191}.

Control of arrhythmias by drugs

PHENOMENOLOGY OF DRUG ACTION

We have already touched upon this topic. Traditionally, antiarrhythmic drugs have been classified according to some perceived predominant action {138,312}. The major classes are (I) those that reduce $\dot{V}_{max}$ and slow conduction (Na^+ conductance modifiers), (II) beta-adrenergic blockers, (III) those that extend AP durations (K^+ channel blockers), and (IV) those that shorten AP duration (Ca^{2+} channel conductance blockers) {312}. Within each class, drugs have been placed in a hierarchy. This scheme does not recognize drugs that modify ionic activities or metabolic processes, e.g., those that lower the activities of Mg^{2+}, K^+ {206}, or Cl^- {345}. Passive properties are not considered.

Antiarrhythmic drugs of Vaughan–Williams Class I (local anesthetic or membrane stabilizing), including

quinidine, procainamide, encainide, tocainide, and lidocaine, all seem similar if one simply looks at the "source" effect, reduction of $\dot{V}_{max}$. Indeed, all inhibit g_{Na}; Class I drugs bind specifically to and modify Na^+ channels directly, rather than acting indirectly, for instance, by modifying the cell membrane {270}. To some extent, the traditional classification has recognized differential effects. All Class I drugs reduce conduction velocity Θ, but those of Class IA (e.g., quinidine) prolong refractoriness, those of Class IB (e.g., mexilitine) shorten refractoriness, and those of Class IC (e.g., flecainide) leave refractoriness unaffected {206,312}. However, these drugs differ fundamentally in structure and physical properties, such as lipophilicity, and so must act at the Na^+ channel in measurably different ways.

Conversely, drugs that evoke phenomenologically similar responses can act by very different mechanisms. Experimentally, in ischemic isolated rat hearts the L and D isomers of verapamil are equally protective against induced ventricular fibrillation, but D-verapamil blocks fast Na^+ channels, while L-verapamil blocks Ca^{2+} channels {206}.

These complexities make the classification of antiarrhythmic drugs difficult. Any classification system must be considered a set of opinions, but the strength and usefulness of the system will improve as new knowledge validates or invalidates the underlying assumptions. Particularly important is new insight into the biophysical mechanisms of drug action at the cell membrane (pump, receptor, or ion channel) level {138}; a classification framework that extends the Vaughan–Williams scheme in this direction and is adaptable to new knowledge and newly developed drugs has been offered {312}.

SITES AND MECHANISMS OF DRUG ACTION

Regarding drugs active on ion channels, models including that of Hodgkin and Huxley {107,161,238} and linear or cyclic state transition schemes (reaction diagrams) {233} have been extended to account for the effects of drugs, in particular with the proposals of the modulated and guarded receptor theories {158,164,308}. Stated most generally, drugs interact with different affinities to a channel depending on the state (resting, activated, or inactivated) of the channel. When a drug molecule interacts with a channel in a certain state, it can change the likelihoods and rates with which the channel can enter other states. Finally, a drug molecule can modify or block ion permeation through a channel. These interactions can occur simultaneously or separately.

It is not possible to determine exhaustively how drugs and channels interact, because it is not possible to detect unambiguously the state of a channel. We cite here some common interactions that have been verified to occur at the unitary channel level.

Many drugs show use- or rate-dependent effects. Some drugs active on Na^+ channels modify phase 0 of the AP strongly only after one or more APs have occurred. This is consistent with the idea that these drugs affect Na^+ channels almost exclusively in the open state. Certain K^+

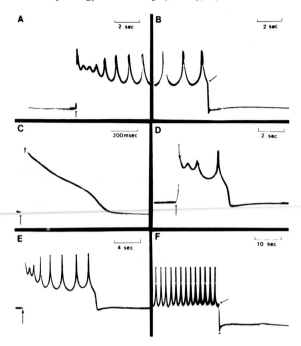

Fig. 10-21. Termination by lidocaine of triggered sustained rhythmic activity in a cardiac Purkinje fiber having an abnormality of repolarization. **A,B:** An electrically induced action potential triggered oscillatory activity, which increased in amplitude and persisted indefinitely, until terminated 45 minutes later by a hyperpolarizing intracellular current (arrow in panel B). **C:** After lidocaine treatment, this fiber repolarized and produced normal action potentials. **D–F:** During washout of lidocaine the action potential duration progressively prolonged, until a triggering stimulus was once again able to induce sustained rhythmic activity. From Arnsdorf and Mehlman {24}, with permission.

channel modifiers lengthen AP duration more when the heart rate is low, at which time the AP duration is normally longer in any case. This reverse use dependence is the opposite of what would be desired to better regulate the AP duration {138}. Certain drugs slow the rate at which channels inactivate after opening, or cause channels to open at a more negative V_m than normal, or prevent inactivation altogether.

Classification of drugs by the traditional scheme has been useful emprically, but has failed to recognize variations in mechanisms of action. It is paradoxical, for instance, that Class I antiarrhythmics, acting at Na^+ channels, should be efficacious when Ca^{2+} fluxes would appear to be a more sensitive point for regulation {206}, presumably because of their roles in triggered activity and in isolation of injured regions.

Research from our laboratory provides a plausible basis for explaining such unexpected behaviors. It has been shown that the effects of antiarrhythmics differ depending on the specific prior state of the tissue. Returning once again to fig. 10-22 {19}, we will review these data in greater detail in terms of the matrix. We showed above that the ischemic metabolite LPC has effects on active

and passive properties, the balance varying with concentration. As we saw in connection with fig. 10-16, $20\,\mu M$ LPC shifted the strength-duration curve downward, indicating increased excitability, despite some depression in Na^+ conductance. Increased excitability was due primarily to increased R_m in the subthreshold range (compare fig. 10-8). Lidocaine applied during LPC treatment decreased excitability, having further depressed Na^+ conductance, but also by decreasing R_m back toward the control value {265}.

Figure 10-22 shows how lidocaine's effects on active and passive properties depend on the prior state established by LPC. In the lower pathway, after LPC (say, at $20\,\mu M$) had increased excitability, the decrease in R_m (and concomitant increase in liminal length) occasioned by lidocaine tended to normalize the matrix. In the upper pathway, after LPC (say, at $45\,\mu M$; see fig. 10-16) had decreased excitability, additional lidocaine-mediated depression of g_{Na}-dependent excitability further deformed the matrix. This is a clear example of assisted bifurcation, which was first demonstrated in our laboratory with quinidine {26}.

We now cite several examples to support the state-dependent duality of drug effects. In normal sheep Purkinje fibers, it was found that procainamide {23}, encainide {25}, and quinidine {26} increase membrane resistance r_m, input resistance r_{in}, and length constant λ, while lidocaine {21,22} and the beta-adrenoreceptor blocker tolamolol {23} decrease the same parameters. Increased r_m and λ mean that excitation in a given region has a greater than normal effect on tissue regions at a distance, whether electrotonically or by nondecremental propagation. Such an increase in excitability may be arrhythmogenic, as seems to be the case after quinidine in normal tissue. On the other hand, it may be antiarrhythmic; drug-increased excitability may allow electrotonic conduction through an injured region that had been a site of unidirectional block that participated critically in a reentrant circuit.

Our laboratory has studied the effect of procainamide and lidocaine, in concentrations equivalent to clinically effective plasma levels, on excitability in normal Purkinje fibers {21,22}. Both drugs shifted the strength-duration curve upward, indicating less excitability; more current was required to attain threshold for any duration. However, procainamide decreased excitability by making V_{th} less negative, while lidocaine little affected V_{th} but decreased r_m in the subthreshold range. Procainamide increased and lidocaine decreased λ, indicating different effects on passive properties. Subsequently, studies have indicated that the effect of lidocaine on the Na^+ system depends greatly on the activation voltage, with the effect being much more intense in depolarized tissue. Other drugs for which we have found significant effects on passive properties include encainide {27} and quinidine {26}, both of which increase r_m.

State-dependent duality of drug action has demonstrated itself dramatically in the clinical situation. That antiarrhythmics could exacerbate rather than control arrhythmias has long been known {228}. Proarrhythmia

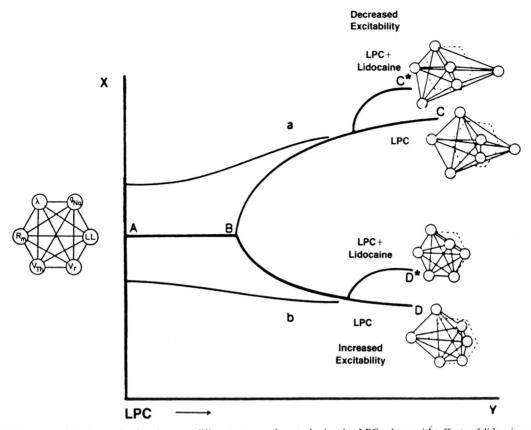

Fig. 10-22. Electrophysiologic matrix showing two different states of perturbation by LPC, along with effects of lidocaine, which depended on which state LPC had induced. At the left is a normal matrix (compare with fig. 10-2). When a quantity represented in the matrix decreases, the corresponding element shifts toward the center of the hexagon; a shift away indicates that the corresponding quantity has increased. LPC can increase excitability by increasing R_m and λ (lower pathway, A-B-D). To show this, R_m and λ have been moved further from the center in the lower matrix figure (D) on the lower pathway. In this LPC-induced state, lidocaine reduced R_m, LL (liminal length), and λ, renormalizing the matrix (upper matrix figure D* on lower pathway). LPC can also decrease excitability by depressing g_{Na} severely (upper pathway, lower matrix figure C). When LPC had decreased excitability, lidocaine reduced it further by depressing g_{Na} more and making V_{th} less negative (upper matrix figure C* on upper pathway). Bifurcations toward one state or the other, such as those induced by LPC and/or lidocaine, are proposed to be assisted; that is, they depend on the intial condition of the tissue. From Arnsdorf {19}, with permission.

was initially thought to be relatively uncommon, but awareness increased {228}. More recently, the Class IC drugs flecainide and encainide {58} proved in the Coronary Arrhythmia Suppression Trial (CAST) to have an unacceptably high association with fatal ventricular arrhthmias {206}. Patients in CAST had coronary artery disease and existing ventricular arrhythmias that had been well suppressed by these drugs {285}. These patients were randomized either to placebo or to treatment with the drug that had suppressed the ventricular arrythmia. An interesting observation was that the deaths were equally distributed throughout the period of drug treatment. As the Task Force of the working group on Arrhythmias of the European Society of Cardiology wrote about this aspect of the CAST trial {311}, this result suggested that "mechanisms other than early proarrhythmic effects must have been operative." The several possibilities discussed,

such as transient ischemia, would be the type of perturbations that would transiently alter the electrophysiologic matrix, changing a presumably antiarrhythmic matrix to a proarrhythmic matrix. Most likely, many patients with coronary and perhaps other types of heart disease have a fixed substrate and transient ischemia or autonomic surges that further deform the matrix and lead to potentially lethal arrhythmias. CAST suggested that antiarrhythmic drugs may also contribute. Subsequently, the moricizine arm of CAST was also discontinued {59}.

Proarrhythmia can be considered to represent either bifurcating chaotic or bistable system behavior. As discussed in the introductory portion of this section, the similarity of the arrhythmogenic and the allegedly antiarrhythmic matrices in fig. 10-22 is apparent, and it may be difficult or impossible to distinguish the inability of an antiarrhythmic drug to produce an antiarrhythmic matrical configuration from a drug-induced proarrhythmic matrix.

Effects of Class I and other drugs whose primary action is on "source" or active membrane properties on "sink" or passive properties need to be considered also. In fact, it is reasonable to ask how these primarily membrane-active agents work as antiarrhythmics when a reentrant pathway extends over a finite area. It has been suggested that depression of $\dot{V}_{max}$ by Class I agents may block reentry by turning a unidirectionally blocked or partly refractory area within a circuit into an area of total block {46}. The effectiveness of these drugs would then depend on both the degree of reduction of $\dot{V}_{max}$ and the geometry of the abnormal area {344}.

To date no clinical drugs have been proposed that would be effective on gap junctional properties {101,344}. In view of the complex anisotropic structures of circuits in healed tissues supporting reentry, the possibility of mechanisms relating to either modifying the electropharmacological properties of the existing GJs in surviving tissue elements or to changing the number and/or types of channels expressed merit consideration.

Electrical control of arrhythmias

Historically the development of electrical control (pacing, defibrillation) techniques has been driven by clinical and engineering considerations {262}. Empirical success has not depended on rigorous biophysical modeling. In electrical control, as in surgical ablation approaches {344}, success has not required microscopically accurate electrographic mapping of arrhythmic conduction pathways.

The mechanisms underlying current approaches to electrical control should not, however, be considered simple. Responses to extrinsic stimuli, such as pacing or defibrillation pulses, depend on the interactions between current flows forced by potential gradients over fairly extensive distances and the refractory state of the tissue {123}. The resulting three-dimensional patterns of excitation can be exceedingly complex {343}.

It can be predicted that strategies based more directly on system analysis will soon come into use. These strategies might take advantage of the extreme sensitivity of nonlinear systems to changes in initial state and/or parameters, particularly as manifest in bistability. The bistable (triggerable) behavior we described for Purkinje fibers (fig. 10-21) has long been observed in patients with sustained ventricular tachycardias; that is, such tachycardias can frequently be started or stopped by a single extra beat or stimulus {127,339}.

In the years after its initiation using fixed-rate stimulators, clinical pacing has grown steadily in capabilities {153}. We mention as highlights the development of demand pacing and similar adaptations related to heart rate changes, the ability to omit or delay a stimulating pulse, or to change automatically to an alternate pacing program, in response to a sensed event, and sequential pacing of the atrium then ventricle (with appropriate refractoriness). Recent trials have included a device that can sense two separate phenomena, such as activity and minute volume, and respond to both either according to

fixed weights or selectively according to a criterion on the sensed events {153}.

Despite all these advances, most pacing techniques applied to date clinically have relied on what can be called open-loop control. This means that all decisions as to what is the best corrective pacing algorithm to perform when any of various contingencies occurs are predetermined {329}.

One or more experimental devices use closed-loop or feedback control logic. In a closed-loop device, pacing is adjusted to minimize the difference between the value of a sensed variable and a criterion. Ideally the sensed variable would be an index of overall metabolic demand {329}. Closed-loop devices have the advantages of fast response to changes in demand (possibly within times as short as beat to beat) and robustness against unwanted sources of noise and variability.

Closed-loop control can be useful in preventing ventricular tachycardias (VT). Most attempts at interceding against VTs have relied on periodic overdrive pacing {219}; however, a recent experiment has shown that control based on chaotic system behavior might also be feasible {127}. As shown in fig. 10-23 {127}, ouabain was used to induce arrhythmia in a preparation of rabbit interventricular septum, during which interbeat intervals varied chaotically (panel B, left segment). Analysis of the intervals showed specific patterns of sequential dependence. These are shown in fig. 10-23A, in which the lengths of intervals are plotted as dependent on the lengths of previous intervals. At some times, the the lengths of the intervals tended toward stability; that is, a given interval tended to be similar in length to the immediately previous interval, and closer to the average length (intervals 163–165). At other times, the sequence tended to diverge; that is, a long interval tended to be followed by a short one, which was in turn followed by a yet longer interval, and so on (intervals 165–167). An approximate linear dynamic model for a stable rhythm was used to predict the expected length of each future interval. If a beat did not occur within this interval, it was concluded that a divergent sequence was beginning, and that correction was needed. Then an electrical stimulus was delivered. This stimulus was made strong enough to induce a beat, rather than merely producing electrotonically an advance or delay (phase resetting) {8}. Interrupting chaotically lengthened intervals in this way regularized the rhythm (fig. 10-23B, middle segment). The stimulus pattern that successfully controlled the rhythm was not overdrive or any similar form of periodic entrainment; in fact, during maintained control only about one third of intervals were found to diverge and needed to be terminated prematurely.

Long-term prediction of risk for sudden death

To draw causal connections between the experimental phenomena described in this chapter and the problems seen by the clinician has been persistently challenging. Clinically observable effects differ from those seen in acute electrophysiological experiments in both time scale and the complexity of the underlying systems {239}.

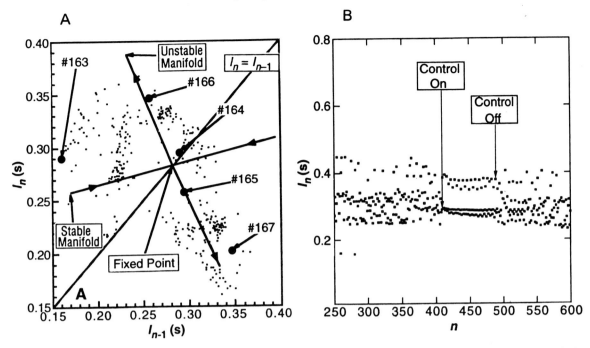

Fig. 10-23. Experimental closed-loop control of arrhythmia. Arrhythmia was induced by ouabain in a slice of rabbit interventricular septum. **A:** Chaotic arrhythmic sequence represented by a phase plot of the length of each interval as dependent on the length of the previous interval. In the sequence 163 . . . 167, intervals 163–165 appear to converge toward stability, while intervals 165–167 appear to diverge away from stability. **B:** In the left segment, interval length depended chaotically on time. In the middle segment, closed-loop control triggered a beat whenever the beat-to-beat interval was predicted to be divergently long. The rhythm regularized. Corrective stimuli were delivered occasionally. A periodic or overdrive correction was not effective. From Garfinkel et al. {127}, with permission.

Nonetheless it is at least intuitively true that similar information could be yielded by a large number of acute experiments as by a small number of long-term studies.

Clinicians would like to predict the risk of attempting to control ventricular tachycardia (VT) or fibrillation (VF) that lead to sudden death {177}. Until recently much work was based on what could be called the PVC hypothesis; namely, that PVCs are indicators of increased risk for sudden death {211}. In essence this was the basis of the CAST study {58,59}, and the PVC hypothesis has been largely discounted. Moreover, some protocols effective against VT or VF did not eliminate PVCs, and some patients at risk never demonstrated PVCs. Since a drug could be antifibrillatory independent of an antiarrhythmic effect {231}, it could be proposed that factors in the milieu, rather than a specific trigger, would lead to VT or VF.

This hypothesis of altered excitability has been expressed using the matrix concept {28,29}, and this has been discussed in some detail in the introductory portion of this section. As mentioned, the proarrhythmic matrix may be fixed or transient; fixed as with a ventricular aneurysm or an anatomical pathway; transient as with ischemia, drug toxicity, autonomic surges, and the like. Fixed matrical configurations may be studied acutely either pharmacologically or by electrophysiologic provo-

cative stimulation (EPS) using uniform pacing, with useful predictive accuracy. However, transient configurations that occur spontaneously in high risk patients may be difficult to simulate, even with highly complex EPS regimes {19}.

The value of long-term drug testing in at-risk patients has been pointed out {14}. To return to the CAST study, encainide, flecainide {58}, and moricizine {59} were seen to induce lethal proarrhythmic matrix configurations with unacceptably high probability, despite their suppression of PVCs. PVCs alone are poor predictors of proarrhythmic effects {250}; to identify additional predictors, studies such as CAST II {59} have relied on careful qualification of a homogeneous population {140}. Long-term control will be enhanced by automated drug delivery systems, and, complementing drug therapy, programmable pacemakers as well as implantable defibrillators.

It is reasonable to ask how biophysical system analysis could help in predicting sudden death {97,134,197}. One biophysical approach is the time-series analyses of heart rates. Heart rate can be presumed to be governed in large part by deterministic nonlinear laws. In the experimental example of electrical control we considered, normal behavior was almost periodic and pathological behavior was chaotic. Such a distinction is unlikely to hold generally {134}. Normal heart rhythm is not periodic but rather has a broad spectrum characteristic of random noise or a chaotic system, as does the rhythm in patients with congestive heart failure (CHF) {97,134}, but the rhythm that occurred shortly before death in CHF patients had a constant or periodically oscillating rate {133}.

We have cited examples of bistable behavior. Cellular responses to stimuli change, dependent on $[K^+]_o$, on stimulation rates, and other factors. Bistability is manifest at the tissue level in proarrhythmic effects of antiarrhythmic drugs and in responses to provocative electrical stimuli. The observation that these systems can be influenced toward desired or undesired responses by possibly minor changes in just one condition is expected to be the logical basis for new therapies {17,19}.

In the domain of clinical electrophysiology, averaging of surface ECG records, either in the time {48} or frequency {39} domain, is a strategy that gathers information at maximal rates in short periods, with the intention of detecting otherwise hidden long-term predictive factors. Effort has been made to contend with the statistical biases and inhomogeneities of signal averaging, which originate in the short recording periods and in nonstationarities (transiency) in the underlying physiological generators. Most frequently studied in signal-averaged ECG work are ventricular late potentials, namely, alterations in the amplitude and/or frequency content of the late portion of the QRS complex and ST segments {48}. Ventricular late potentials appear to originate in the same alterations, such as irregular infarct border zones, which can produce fractionation in invasively recorded electrograms {279}. Although these features have not been shown specifically to be associated with reentrant circuits, ventricular late potentials are rare in normal hearts and frequent in patients in whom VT has been demonstrated {48}, and thus may have considerable predictive value {46}.

CONCLUDING THOUGHTS

We began this chapter implying that biophysical theory was essential in the organization of knowledge. We have ranged widely in basic and clinical science. Our knowledge of the electrophysiologic events that determine normal and abnormal cardiac excitability has exploded in the decade since the first edition of this book, and important progress has been made in linking basic science to clinical realities. The maturation of the hypothesis of altered excitability, a hypothesis originally developed based on epidemiological reports, now comfortably includes subjects as diverse as the PVC hypothesis and the results of the CAST trial. Coupling the hypothesis of altered excitability with the new concept of the electrophysiologic matrix has indicated that electrophysiologic universes operate as systems resulting in predictible behavior, which, in turn, has led to understanding of our drug classification schemes; the similarity of electrophysiologic changes that may be antiarrhythmic or proarrhythmic, the importance of fixed and transient matrices in disease, arrhythmias, and sudden death; and other issues of immediate clinical relevance.

The practical use of a biophysical theory is to predict what might occur under a given set of circumstances. We are encouraged about the new types of information that have an important base in basic science, yet may be clinically very useful, such as the relationship between rate variability and sudden death, the positive and negative prognostic implications of the signal-averaged electrocardiogram, and other such meetings of the theoretical and the practical.

ACKNOWLEDGMENTS

This work was supported in part by NIH grant R37HL21778.

REFERENCES

1. Abney JR, Braun J, Owicki JC: Lateral interactions among membrane proteins. Implications for the organization of gap junctions. *Biophys J* 52:441–454, 1987.
2. Allessie MA, Bonke FIM, Kirchhof CJHJ: Atrial reentry. In: Rosen MR, Janse MJ, Wit AL (eds) *Cardiac Electrophysiology: A Textbook*. Mt Kisco, NY: Futura, 1990, pp 555–571.
3. Allessie MA, Bonke FI, Schopman FJ: Circus movement in rabbit atrial muscle as a mechanism of tachycardia. III. The leading circle concept: A new model of circus movement in cardiac tissue without the involvement of an anatomical obstacle. *Circ Res* 41:9–18, 1977.
4. Allessie MA, Lammers WJEP, Bonke FIM, Hollen J: Intra-atrial reentry as a mechanism for atrial flutter induced by acetylcholine and rapid pacing in the dog. *Circulation* 70:123–135, 1984.
5. Almers W: Gating currents and charge movements in excitable membranes. *Rev Physiol Biochem Pharmacol* 82:96–191, 1978.
6. Antzelevitch C: Electrotonus and reflection. In: Rosen MR, Janse MJ, Wit AI (eds) *Cardiac Electrophysiology: A Textbook*. Mt Kisco, NY: Futura, 1990, pp 491–516.
7. Antzelevitch C, Moe GK: Electrotonically mediated delayed conduction and reentry in relation to ventricular conducting tissue. *Circ Res* 49:1129–1139, 1981.
8. Anumonwo JMB, Delmar M, Vinet A, Michaels DC, Jalife J: Phase resetting and entrainment of pacemaker activity in single sinus nodal cells. *Circ Res* 68:1138–1153, 1991.
9. Anumonwo JMB, Wang H-Z, Trabka-Janik E, Dunham B, Veenstra BD, Delmar M, Jalife J: Gap junctional channels in adult mammalian sinus nodal cells. Immunolocalization and electrophysiology. *Circ Res* 71:229–239, 1992.
10. Arnsdorf MF: Membrane factors in arrhythmogenesis: Concepts and definitions. *Prog Cardiovasc Dis* 19:413–429, 1976.
11. Arnsdorf MF: The effect of antiarrhythmmic drugs on sustained rhythmic activity in cardiac Purkinje fibers. *J Pharmacol Exp Ther* 201:689–700, 1977.
12. Arnsdorf MF: Basic understanding of the electrophysiologic actions of antiarrhythmic drugs: Sources, sinks and matrices of information. *Med Clin North Am* 168:1247–1280, 1984.
13. Arnsdorf MF: Cable properties and conduction of the action potential: Excitability, sources, and sinks. In: Sperelakis N (ed) *Physiology and Pathology of the Heart*. Boston: Martinus Nijhoff, 1984, pp 109–140.
14. Arnsdorf MF: Discussion on intracardiac electrophysiologic

studies for drug selection in ventricular tachycardia: The need for new approaches based on perturbations of the electrophysiologic matrix. *Circulation* 75:137–139, 1987.

15. Arnsdorf MF: Cardiac excitability and antiarrhythmic drugs: A different perspective. *J Clin Pharmacol* 29:395–404 1989.

16. Arnsdorf MF: A matrical perspective of cardiac excitability, cable properties, and impulse propagation. In: Sperelakis N (ed) *Physiology and Pathophysiology of the Heart*, 2nd edi. Boston: Kluwer, 1989.

17. Arnsdorf MF: The cellular basis of cardiac arrhythmias. A matrical perspective. *Ann NY Acad Sci* 601:263–280, 1990.

18. Arnsdorf MF: Arnsdorf's paradox. *J Cardiovasc Electrophysiol* 1:42–52, 1990.

19. Arnsdorf MF: Cardiac excitability, the electrophysiologic matrix, and electrically induced ventricular arrhythmias: Order and reproducibility in seeming electrophysiologic chaos [editorial comment]. *J Am Coll Cardiol* 17:139–142, 1992.

20. Arnsdorf MF, Bigger JT Jr: Effect of lidocaine hydrochloride on membrane conductance in mammalian cardiac Purkinje fibers. *J Clin Invest* 51:2252–2263, 1972.

21. Arnsdorf MF, Bigger JT Jr: The effect of lidocaine on components of excitability in long mammalian cardiac Purkinje fibers. *J Pharmacol Exp Ther* 195:206–215, 1975.

22. Arnsdorf MF, Bigger JT Jr: The effect of procaine amide on components of excitability in long mammalian cardiac Purkinje fibers. *Circ Res* 38:115–122, 1976.

23. Arnsdorf MF, Friedlander I: The electrophysiologic effects of Tolamolol (UK-6558-01) on the passive membrane properties of mammalian cardiac Purkinje fibers. *J Pharmacol Exp Ther* 199:601–610, 1976.

24. Arnsdorf MF, Mehlman DJ: Observations on the effects of selected antiarrhythmic drugs on mammalian cardiac Purkinje fibers witgh two levels of steady-state potential: Influences of lidocaine, phenytoin, propranolol, disopyramide, and procainamide on repolarization, action potential shape and conduction. *J Pharmacol Exp Ther* 207:983–991, 1977.

25. Arnsdorf MF, Sawicki GJ: The effects of lysophosphatidylcholine, a toxic metabolite of ischemia, on the components of cardiac excitability in sheep Purkinje fibers. *Circ Res* 49:16–30, 1981.

26. Arnsdorf MF, Sawicki GJ: The effects of quinidine sulfate on the balance among active and passive cellular properties which comprise the electrophysiologic matrix and determine excitability in sheep Purkinje fibers. *Circ Res* 61:244–255, 1987.

27. Arnsdorf MF, Schmidt TA, Sawicki G: The effects of encainide on the determinants of cardiac excitability in sheep Purkinje fibers. *J Pharmacol Exp Ther* 223:40–48, 1985.

28. Arnsdorf MF, Wasserstrom JA: Mechanisms of action of antiarrhythmic drugs: A matrical approach. In: Fozzard HA, Haber E, Jennings RB, Katz AM, Morgan HE (eds) *The Heart and Cardiovascular System*. New York: Raven Press, 1986, pp 1259–1316.

29. Arnsdorf MF, Wasserstrom JA: A matrical approach to the basic and clinical pharmacology of antiarrhythmic drugs. *Rev Clin Basic Pharmacol* 6:131–188, 1987.

30. Baldwin KM: The fine structure of healing over in mammalian cardiac muscle. *J Mol Cell Cardiol* 9:959–966, 1977.

31. Balke CW, Lesh MD, Spear JF, Kadish A, Levine JH, Moore EN: Effects of cellular uncoupling on conduction in anisotropic canine ventricular myocardium. *Circ Res* 63:879–892, 1988.

32. Barr LM, Dewey M, Berger W: Propagation of action potentials and the structure of the nexus in cardiac muscle. *J Gen Physiol* 48:797–823, 1965.

33. Baumgarten CM, Isenberg G: Depletion and accumulation of potassium in the extracellular clefts of cardiac Purkinje fibers during voltage clamp hyperpolarization and depolarization. *Pflügers Arch* 368:19–31, 1977.

34. Baumgarten CM, Isenberg G, McDonald T, Ten Eick RE: Depletion and accumulation of potassium in the extracellular clefts of cardiac Purkinje fibers during voltage clamp hyperpolarization and depolarization. Experiments in sodium-free bathing media. *J Gen Physiol* 70:149–169, 1977.

35. Beeler GW, Reuter H: Reconstruction of the action potential of ventricular myocardial fibres. *J Physiol (Lond)* 268:177–210, 1977.

36. Ben-Haim SA, Palti Y: Intercellular conduction velocity variability as the basis for re-entrant arrhythmias in the ischemic myocardium. *J Theor Biol* 154:317–330, 1992.

37. Bennett MVL: Physiology of electrotonic junctions. *Ann NY Acad Sci* 137:509–539, 1966.

38. Bennett MVL, Barrio LC, Bargiello TA, Spray DC, Hertzberg E, Saez JC: Gap junctions: New tools, new answers, new questions. *Neuron* 6:305–320, 1991.

39. Berbari EJ, Albert DE, Lander P: Spectral estimation of the electrocardiogram. *Ann NY Acad Sci* 601:197–208, 1990.

40. Bers DM, Ellis D: Intracellular calcium and sodium activity in sheep heart Purkinje fibres. Effects of changes of external sodium and intracellular pH. *Pflügers Arch* 393:171–178, 1982.

41. Beyer EC, Paul DL, Goodenough DA: Connexin43: A protein from rat heart homologous to a gap junction protein from liver. *J Cell Biol* 105:2621–2629, 1987.

42. Beyer EC, Paul DL, Goodenough, DA: Connexin family of gap junction proteins. *J Membr Biol* 116:187–194, 1990.

43. Bonke FIM: Electrotonic spread in the sinoatrial node of the rabbit heart. *Pflügers Arch* 339:17–23, 1973.

44. Bonke FIM: Passive electrical properties of atrial fibers of the rabbit heart. *Pflügers Arch* 339:1–15, 1973.

45. Box GEP, Jenkins GM: Time Series Analysis: Forecasting and Control. San Fransisco: Holden-Day, 1976.

46. Boyden PA, Wit AL: Pharmacology of the antiarrhythmic drugs. In: Rosen MR, Hoffman BF (eds) *Cardiac Therapy*. The Hague, Netherlands: Martinus Nijhoff, 1983, pp 171–234.

47. Bredikis J, Bukauskas F, Veteikis R: Decreased intercellular coupling after prolonged rapid stimulation in rabbit atrial muscle. *Circ Res* 49:815–820, 1981.

48. Breithardt G, Borggrefe M, Martinez-Rubio A: Signal averaging. *Ann NY Acad Sci* 601:180–196, 1990.

49. Brown AM, Lee KA, Powell T: Sodium current in single rat heart muscle cells. *J Physiol (Lond)* 318:479–500, 1981.

50. Brugada J, Boersma L, Abdollah H, Kirchhof C, Allessie M: Echo-wave termination of ventricular tachycardia. *Circulation* 85:1879–1887, 1992.

51. Buchanan JW, Gettes LS: Ionic environment and propagation. In: Zipes DP, Jalife J (eds) *Cardiac Electrophysiology: From Cell to Bedside*. Philadelphia: WB Saunders, 1990, pp 149–156.

52. Buchanan JW Jr, Saito T, Gettes LS: The effects of antiarrhythmic drugs, stimulation frequency, and potassium-induced resting membrane potential changes on conduction velocity and dV/dtmax in guinea pig myocardium. *Circ Res* 56:696–703, 1985.

53. Burt JM: Block of intercellular communication: Interaction of intracellular H^+ and Ca^{2+}. *Am J Physiol* 253:C607–C612, 1987.

54. Burt JM: Uncoupling of cardiac cells by doxyl stearic acids: Specificity and mechanism of action. *Am J Physiol* 256:C913–C924, 1989.

55. Burt JM, Massey KD, Minnich BN: Uncoupling of cardiac

cells by fatty acids: Structure-activity relationships. *Am J Physiol* 260:C439–C448, 1991.

56. Burt JM, Spray DC: Single-channel events and gating behavior of the cardiac gap junction channel. *Proc Natl Acad Sci USA* 85:3431–3434, 1988.

57. Burt JM, Spray DC: Volatile anesthetics block intercellular communication between neonatal rat myocardial cells. *Circ Res* 65:829–837, 1989.

58. Cardiac Arrhythmia Suppression Trial (CAST) Investigators: Increased mortality due to encainide or flecainide in a randomized trial of arrhythmia suppression after myocardial infarction. *N Engl J Med* 321:406–412, 1989.

59. Cardiac Arrhythmia Suppression Trial II (CAST-II) Investigators: Effect of the antiarrhythmic agent moricizine on survival after myocardial infarction. *N Engl J Med* 327:227–233, 1992.

60. Carmeliet E: K^+ channels in cardiac cells: Mechanisms of activation, inactivation, rectification and $[K^+]e$ sensitivity. *Pflügers Arch* 414(Suppl 1):S88–S92, 1989.

61. Chapman RA, Fry CH: An analysis of the cable properties of frog ventricular myocardium. *J Physiol (Lond)* 283:263–282, 1978.

62. Chialvo DR, Jalife J: Non-linear dynamics of cardiac excitation and impulse propagation. *Nature* 330:749–752, 1987.

63. Clapham DE, Shrier A, DeHaan RL: Junctional resistance and action potential delay between embryonic heart cell aggregates. *J Gen Physiol* 75:633–654, 1980.

64. Clark JW, Shumaker JM, Murphey CR, Giles WR: Mathematical models of pacemaker tissue in the heart. In: Glass L, Hunter P, McCulloch A (eds) *Theory of Heart: Biomechanics, Biophysics, and Nonlinear Dynamics of Cardiac Function.* New York: Springer, 1991, pp 255–288.

65. Clay JR, DeHaan RL: Fluctuations in interbeat interval in rhythmic heart-cell clusters. Role of membrane voltage noise. *Biophys J* 28:377–389, 1979.

66. Clerc L: Directional differences of impulse spread in trabecular muscle from mammalian heart. *J Physiol (Lond)* 255:335–346, 1976.

67. Cohen IS, Falk RP, Kline RP: Membrane currents following activity in canine cardiac Purkinje fibers. *Biophys J* 33:281–288, 1981.

68. Cohen IS, Falk RT, Kline RP: Voltage-clamp studies on the canine Purkinje strand. *Proc R Soc Lond* B217:215–236, 1983.

69. Cohen CJ, Bean BP, Tsien RW: Maximal upstroke velocity as an index of available sodium conductance. Comparison of maximal upstroke velocity and voltage clamp measurements of sodium current in rabbit Purkinje fibers. *Circ Res* 54:636–651, 1984.

70. Colatsky TJ: Voltage clamp measurements of sodium channel properties in rabbit cardiac Purkinje fibres. *J Physiol (Lond)* 305:215–234, 1980.

71. Colatsky TJ, Tsien RW: Sodium channels in rabbit cardiac Purkinje fibers. *Nature* 278:265–268, 1979.

72. Cole KS, Curtis HJ: Membrane potential of the squid giant axon during current flow. *J Gen Physiol* 24:551–563, 1941.

73. Cole WC, Picone JB, Sperelakis N: Gap junction uncoupling and discontinuous propagation in the heart. A comparison of experimental data with computer simulations. *Biophys J* 53:809–818, 1988.

74. Colquhoun D, Hawkes AG: On the stochastic properties of single ion channels. *Proc R Soc Lond* B211:205–235, 1981.

75. Colquhoun D, Neher E, Reuter H, Stevens CF: Inward current channels activated by intracellular Ca in cultured cardiac cells. *Nature* 294:752–754, 1981.

76. Cooley JW, Dodge FA Jr: Digital computer solutions for excitation and propagation of the nerve impulse. *Biophys J* 6:583–599, 1966.

77. Coraboeuf E, Deroubaix E, Coulombe A: The effect of tetrodotoxin on action potentials of the conducting system in the dog heart. *Am J Physiol* 236:H561–H567, 1979.

78. Coronel R, Fiolet JW, Wilms-Schopman FJ, Schaapherder AF, Johnson TA, Gettes LS, Janse MJ: Distribution of extracellular potassium and its relation to electrophysiologic changes during acute myocardial ischemia in the isolated perfused porcine heart. *Circulation* 77:1125–1138, 1988.

79. Cosio FG, Arribas F: Role of conduction disturbances in atrial arrhythmias. In: Attuel P, Coumel P, Janse MJ (eds) *The Atrium in Health and Disease.* Mt Kisco, NY: Futura, 1989, pp 133–157.

80. Cosio FG, Arribas F, Barbero JM, et al.: Validation of double-spike electrograms as markers of conduction delay or block in atrial flutter. *Am J Cardiol* 61:775–780, 1988.

81. Cranefield PF: The Conduction of the Cardiac Impulse — The Slow Response and Cardiac Arrhythmias. Mt Kisco, NY: Futura, 1975.

82. Dahl G, Isenberg G: Decoupling of heart muscle cells: Correlation with increased cytoplasmic calcium activity and with changes of nexus ultrastructure. *J Member Biol* 53:63–75, 1980.

83. Daut J: The passive electrical properties of guinea pig ventricular muscle as examined with a voltage clamp technique. *J Physiol (Lond)* 330:221–242, 1982.

84. DeHaan RL: Dynamic behavior of cardiac gap junction channels. In: Hertzberg EL, Johnson RG (eds) *Gap Junctions: Proceedings of the International Conference on Gap Junctions, Pacific Grove, CA, July 6–10, 1987.* New York: Alan R. Liss, 1988.

85. DeHaan RL, Hirakowa R: Synchronization of pulsation rates in isolated cardiac myocytes. *Exp Cell Res* 70:214–222, 1972.

86. Del Castillo J, Moore JW: On increasing the velocity of a nerve impulse. *J Physiol (Lond)* 148:665–670, 1959.

87. Deleze J: The recovery of resting potential and input resistence in sheep heart injured by knife or laser. *J Physiol (Lond)* 208:547–562, 1970.

88. Delgado C, Steinhaus B, Delmar M, Chialvo DR, Jalife J: Directional differences in excitability and margin of safety for propagation in sheep ventricular epicardial muscle. *Circ Res* 67:97–110, 1990.

89. Delmar M, Jalife J, Michaels DC: Effects of changes in excitability and intercellular coupling on synchronization in the rabbit sino-atrial node. *J Physiol (Lond)* 370:127–150, 1986.

90. Delmar M, Michaels DC, Johnson T, Jalife J: Effects of increasing intercellular resistance on transverse and longitudinal propagation in sheep epicardial muscle. *Circ Res* 60:780–785, 1987.

91. DeMello WC: Effect of intracellular injection of calcium and strontium on cell communication in heart. *J Physiol (Lond)* 250:231–245, 1975.

92. DeMello WC: Effect of intracellular injection of La^{3+} and Mn^{2+} on electrical coupling of heart cells. *Cell Biol Int Rep* 3:133–149, 1979.

93. DeMello WC: Effect of 2,4 dinitrophenol on intercellular communication in mammalian cardiac fibres. *Pflügers Arch* 380:267–276, 1979.

94. DeMello WC: Effect of intracellular injection of cAMP on the electrical coupling of mammalian cardiac cells. *Biochem Biophys Res Commun* 119:1001–1007, 1984.

95. DeMello WC, Dexter D: Increased rate of sealing in beating heart muscle of the toad. *Circ Res* 26:481–489, 1970.

96. DeMello WC, Motta GE, Chapeau M: A study of the

healing-over of myocardial cells of toads. *Circ Res* 24: 475–487, 1969.

97. Denton TA, Diamond GA, Helfant RH, Khan S, Karagueuzian H: Fascinating rhythm: A primer on chaos theory and its application to cardiology. *Am Heart J* 120: 1419–1440, 1990.

98. Diaz PJ, Rudy Y, Plonsey R: The effects of the intercalated disc on the propagation of electrical activity in cardiac muscle. *Fed Proc* 40:393,1981.

99. DiFrancesco D, Noble D: A model of electrical activity incorporating ionic pumps and concentration changes. *Phil Trans R Soc Lond* B307:353–398, 1985.

100. DiFrancesco D, Zaza A: The cardiac pacemaker current I_f. *J Cardiovasc Electrophysiol* 3:334–344, 1992.

101. Dillon SM, Allessie MA, Ursell PC, Wit AL: Influences of anisotropic tissue structure on reentrant circuits in the epicardial border zone of subacute canine infarcts. *Circ Res* 63:182–206, 1988.

102. Disertori M, Inama G, Vergara G, Guarniero M, Del Favero A, Furlanello F: Evidence of a reentry circuit in the common type of atrial flutter in man. *Circulation* 67:434–440, 1983.

103. Dominguez G, Fozzard HA: Influence of extracellular K^+ concentration on cable properties and excitability of sheep cardiac Purkinje fibers. *Circ Res* 26:565–574, 1970.

104. Downar E, Janse MJ, Durrer D: The effect of acute coronary artery occlusion on subepicardial transmembrane potentials in the intact porcine heart. *Circulation* 56:217–224, 1977.

105. Draper MH, Mya-Tu M: A comparison of the conduction velocity in cardiac tissues of various mammals. *Q J Exp Physiol* 44:91–109, 1959.

106. Earm YE, Noble D: A model of the single atrial cell: Relation between calcium current and calcium release. *Proc R Soc Lond* B240:83–96, 1990.

107. Ebihara L, Johnson EA: Fast sodium current in cardiac muscle. A quantitative description. *Biophys J* 32:779–790, 1980.

108. Ehara T, Hasegawa J: Effects of hypertonic solution on action potential and input resistance in guinea pig ventricular muscle. *Jpn J Physiol* 33:151–167, 1983.

109. Eisenberg RS: Structural complexity, circuit models and ion accumulation. *Fed Proc* 39:1540–1543, 1980.

110. El-Sherif N: Electrophysiologic mechanisms of ventricular arrhythmias. *Int J Cardiac Imaging* 7:141–150, 1991.

111. Engelmann TW: Über die Leitung der Erregung im Herzmuskel. *Pflügers Arch* 11:465–480, 1875.

112. Engelmann TW: Vergleichende Untersuchungen zur Lehre von der Muskel-und Nervenelectricität. *Pflügers Arch* 15:116–148, 1877.

113. Fiolet JW, Baartscheer A, Schumacher CA, Coronel R, ter Welle HF: The change of the free energy of ATP hydrolysis during global ischemia and anoxia in the rat heart. Its possible role in the regulation of transsarcolemmal sodium and potassium gradients. *J Mol Cell Cardiol* 16:1023–1036, 1984.

114. Fluri GS, Rudisuli A, Willi M, Rohr S, Weingart R: Effects of arachidonic acid on the gap junctions of neonatal rat heart cells. *Pflügers Arch* 417:149–156, 1990.

115. Fozzard HA: Membrane capacity of the cardiac Purkinje fibre. *J Physiol (Lond)* 182:255–267, 1966.

116. Fozzard HA: Cardiac muscle. Excitability and passive electrical properties. *Progr Cardiovasc Dis* 19:343–359, 1977.

117. Fozzard HA: Sodium channels. In: Fozzard HA, Haber E, Jennings RB, Katz AM, Morgan HE (eds) *The Heart and Cardiovascular System*. New York: Raven Press, 1991, pp 1091–1120.

118. Fozzard HA, Beeler GW Jr: The voltage clamp and cardiac electrophysiology. *Circ Res* 37:403–413, 1975.

119. Fozzard HA, Dominguez G: Effect of formaldehyde and glutaraldehyde on electrical properties of cardiac Purkinje fibers. *J Gen Physiol* 53:530–540, 1969.

120. Fozzard HA, Friedlander I, January CT, Makielski JC, Sheets MF: Second order kinetics of Na^+ channel inactivation in internally dialysed canine cardiac Purkinje cells. *J Physiol (Lond)* 353:72P, 1984.

121. Fozzard HA, Haber E, Jennings RB, Katz AM, Morgan HE (eds): *The Heart and Cardiovascular System*. New York: Raven Press, 1991.

122. Fozzard HA, Schoenberg M: Strength-duration curves in cardiac Purkinje fibres: Effects of liminal length and charge distribution. *J Physiol (Lond)* 226:593–618, 1972.

123. Frazier DW, Wolf PD, Wharton JM, Tang AS, Smith WM, Ideker RE: Stimulus-induced critical point. Mechanism for electrical initiation of reentry in normal canine myocardium. *J Clin Invest* 83:1039–1052, 1989.

124. Freygang WH, Trautwein W: The structural implications of the linear electrical properties of cardiac Purkinje strands. *J Gen Physiol* 55:524–547, 1970.

125. Furshpan EJ, Porter DD: Transmission at the giant motor synapses of the crayfish. *J Physiol (Lond)* 145:289–325, 1959.

126. Gardner PI, Ursell PC, Fenoglio JJ Jr, Wit AL: Electro-physiologic and anatomic basis for fractionated electrograms recorded from healed myocardial infarcts. *Circulation* 72: 596–611, 1985.

127. Garfinkel A, Spano ML, Ditto WL, Weiss JN: Controlling cardiac chaos. *Science* 257:1230–1235, 1992.

128. Gintant GA, Datyner NB, Cohen IS: Slow inactivation of a tetrodotoxin-sensitive current in canine cardiac Purkinje fibers. *Biophys J* 45:509–512, 1984.

129. Glass L, Hunter P, McCulloch A (eds): *Theory of Heart: Biomechanics, Biophysics, and Nonlinear Dynamics of Cardiac Function*. New York: Springer, 1991.

130. Glass L, Mackey MC: From Clocks to Chaos. Princeton, NJ: Princeton University Press, 1988.

131. Glass L, Shrier A: Low dimensional dynamics in the heart. In: Glass L, Hunter P, McCulloch A (eds) *Theory of Heart: Biomechanics, Biophysics, and Nonlinear Dynamics of Cardiac Function*. New York: Springer, 1991, pp 290–312.

132. Gleick J. Chaos: Making a New Science. New York: Penguin, 1987.

133. Goldberger AL: Nonlinear dynamics, fractals and chaos: Applications to cardiac electrophysiology. *Ann Biomed Engr* 18:195–198, 1990.

134. Goldberger AL, Rigney DR: Nonlinear dynamics at the bedside. In: Glass L, Hunter P, McCulloch A (eds) *Theory of Heart: Biomechanics, Biophysics, and Nonlinear Dynamics of Cardiac Function*. New York: Springer, 1991, pp 584–605.

135. Goldstein SS, Rall W: Changes in action potential shape and velocity for changing core conductor geometry. *Biophys J* 14:731–757, 1974.

136. Gourdie RG, Green CR, Severs NJ: Gap junction distribution in adult mammalian myocardium revealed by an anti-peptide antibody and laser scanning confocal microscopy. *J Cell Sci* 99:41–55, 1991.

137. Gourdie RG, Green CR, Severs NJ, Thompson RP: Immunolabeling patterns of gap junction connexins in the developing and mature rat heart. *Anat Embryol (Berlin)* 185:363–378, 1992.

138. Grant AO Jr: On the mechanism of action of antiarrhythmic agents. *Am Heart J* 123:1130–1136, 1992.

139. Grant AO, Starmer CF, Strauss HC: Unitary sodium

channels in isolated cardiac myocytes of rabbit. *Circ Res* 53:823–829, 1983.

140. Greene HL, Roden DM, Katz RJ, Woosley RL, Salerno DM, Henthorn RW: The Cardiac Arrhythmia Suppression Trial: first CAST . . . then CAST-II. *J Am Coll Cardiol* 19:894–898, 1992.

141. Guevara MR: Iteration of the human atrioventricular (AV) nodal recovery curve predicts many rhythms of AV block. In: Glass L, Hunter P, McCulloch A (eds) *Theory of Heart: Biomechanics, Biophysics, and Nonlinear Dynamics of Cardiac Function.* New York: Springer, 1990, pp 313–358.

142. Guevara MR: Mathematical modeling of the electrical activity of cardiac cells. In: Glass L, Hunter P, McCulloch A (eds) *Theory of Heart: Biomechanics, Biophysics, and Nonlinear Dynamics of Cardiac Function.* New York: Springer, 1991, pp 239–253.

143. Guevara MR, Glass L: Phaselocking, period doubling bifurcations, and chaos in a mathematical model of a periodically driven oscillator. *J Math Biol* 14:1–23, 1982.

144. Guevara MR, Shrier A, Glass L: Phase-locked rhythms in periodically stimulated heart cell aggregates. *Am J Physiol* 254:H1–H10, 1988.

145. Haas HG, Meyer R, Einwachter HM, Stockem W: Intercellular coupling in frog heart muscle. Electrophysiological and morphological aspects. *Pflügers Arch* 399:321–335, 1983.

146. Hagiwara N, Irisawa H, Kasanuki H, Hosoda S: Background current in sino-atrial node cells of the rabbit heart. *J Physiol (Lond)* 448:53–72, 1992.

147. Hall AE, Hutter OF, Noble D: Current-voltage relations of Purkinje fibers in sodium deficient solutions. *J Physiol (Lond)* 166:255–240, 1963.

148. Harada H, Azuma J, Hasegawa H, Ohta H, et al.: Enhanced suppression of myocardial slow action potentials during hypoxia by free fatty acids. *J Mol Cell Cardiol* 16:261–276, 1984.

149. Harris AS, Bisteni A, Russell RA, Brigham JC, Firestone JE: Excitatory factors in ventricular tachycardia resulting from myocardial ischemia: Potassium a major excitant. *Science* 119:200–203, 1954.

150. Harvey RD, Hume JR: Autonomic regulation of a chloride current in heart. *Science* 244:983–985, 1989.

151. Harvey RD, Jurevicius JA, Hume JR: Intracellular Na$^+$ modulates the cAMP-dependent regulation of ion channels in the heart. *Proc Natl Acad Sci USA* 88:6946–6950, 1991.

152. Hauswirth O, Noble D, Tsien RW: The mechanism of oscillatory activity at low membrane potentials in cardiac Purkinje fibres. *J Physiol (Lond)* 200:255–265, 1969.

153. Hayes DL: The next 5 years in cardiac pacemakers: A preview. *Mayo Clin Proc* 67:379–384, 1992.

154. Hays WL: Statistics for the Social Sciences, 2nd ed. New York: Holt Rinehart Winston, 1973.

155. Hearse DJ, Bolli R: Reperfusion-induced injury: Manifestations, mechanisms, and clinical relevance. *Cardiovasc Res* 26:101–108, 1992.

156. Heidenheim M: Über die Structure des menschlichen Herzmuskels. *Anat Anz* 20:3–79, 1901.

157. Hellam DC, Studt JW: Linear analysis of membrane conductance and capacitance in cardiac Purkinje fibres. *J Physiol (Lond)* 243:661–694, 1974.

158. Hille B: Local anaesthetics: Hydrophilic and hydrophobic pathways for the drug-receptor reaction. *J Gen Physiol* 69:497–515.

159. Hiramatsu Y, Buchanan JW, Knisley SB, Gettes LS: Rate-dependent effects of hypoxia on internal longitudinal resis-

tance in guinea pig papillary muscles. *Circ Res* 63:923–929, 1988.

160. Hodgkin AL: A note on conduction velocity. *J Physiol* 125:221–224, 1954.

161. Hodgkin AL, Huxley AF: A quantitative description of membrane current and its application to conduction and excitation in nerve. *J Physiol (Lond)* 117:500–544, 1952.

162. Hodgkin AL, Rushton WAH: The electrical constants of a crustacean nerve fibre. *Proc R Soc Lond* B133:444–479, 1946.

163. Holland RP, Arnsdorf MF: Nonspatial determinants of electrograms in guinea pig ventricle. *Am J Physiol* 240:C148–C160, 1981.

164. Hondeghem LM, Katzung BG: Antiarrhythmic agents: The modulated receptor mechanism of action of sodium and calcium channel-blocking drugs. *Ann Rev Pharmacol Toxicol* 24:387–423, 1984.

165. Hoyt RH, Cohen ML, Saffitz JE: Distribution and three-dimensional structure of intercellular junctions in canine myocardium. *Circ Res* 64:563–574, 1989.

166. Hume JR, Giles WR: Active and passive electrical properties of single bullfrog atrial cells. *J Gen Physiol* 78:19–42, 1981.

167. Hume JR, Harvey RD: Chloride conductance pathways in heart. *Am J Physiol* 261:C399–412, 1991.

168. Hunter PJ, McNaughton PA, Noble D: Analytical models of propagation in excitable cells. *Prog Biophys Mol Biol* 30:99–144, 1975.

169. Ikeda N, Toyama J, Shimizu T, Kodama I, Yamada K: The role of electrical uncoupling in the genesis of atrioventricular conduction disturbance. *J Mol Cell Cardiol* 12:809–826, 1980.

170. Inoue H, Matsuo H, Takayanagi K, Murao S: Clinical and experimental studies of the effects of atrial extrastimulation and rapid pacing on the atrial flutter cycle. Evidence of macro-reentry with an excitable gap. *Am J Cardiol* 48:623–631, 1981.

171. Jack JJB, Noble D, Tsien RW: Electric Current Flow in Excitable Cells. Oxford: Clarendon Press, 1975.

172. Jalife J, Michaels DC: Phase-dependent interactions of cardiac pacemakers as mechanisms of control and synchronization in the heart. In: Zipes DP, Jalife J (eds) *Cardiac Electrophysiology and Arrhythmias.* Orlando, FL: Grune and Stratton, 1985, pp 109–119.

173. Jalife J, Sicouri S, Delmar M, Michaels DC: Electrical uncoupling and impulse propagation in isolated sheep Purkinje fibers. *Am J Physiol* 257:H179–189, 1989.

174. Janse MJ, Cinca J, Morena H, Fiolet JW, Kleber AG, de Vries P, Becker AE, Durrer D: The border zone in myocardial ischemia. An electrophysiological, metabolic, and histochemical correlation in the pig heart. *Circ Res* 44:576–588, 1979.

175. Janse MJ, Kleber AG: Electrophysiological changes and ventricular arrhythmias in the early phase of regional myocardial ischemia. *Circ Res* 49:1069–1081, 1981.

176. Janse MJ, van Capelle FJL: Electrotonic interactions across an inexcitable region as a cause of ectopic activity in acute regional myocardial ischemia: A study in intact porcine and canine hearts and computer models. *Circ Res* 50:527–537, 1982.

177. Janse MJ, Wit AL: Electrophysiological mechanisms of ventricular arrhythmias resulting from myocardial ischemia and infarction. *Physiol Rev* 69:1049–1169, 1989.

178. January CT, Fozzard HA: The effects of membrane potential, extracellular potassium, and tetrodotoxin on the intracellular sodium ion activity of sheep cardiac muscle. *Circ Res* 54:652–665, 1983.

179. Jenkins GM, Watts DG: Spectral Analysis and its Applications. San Fransisco: Holden-DAy, 1968.
180. Jongsma HJ, Wilders R, van Ginneken ACG, Rook MB: Modulatory effect of the transcellular electrical field on gap junction conductance. In: Peracchia C (ed) *Biophysics of Gap Junction Channels*. Boca Raton, FL: CRC Press, 1991, pp 163–172.
181. Joyner RW: Effects of the discrete pattern of electrical coupling on propagation through an electrical syncytium. *Circ Res* 50:192–200, 1982.
182. Joyner RW: Effects of spatial pattern of cell-cell coupling on cardiac action potential propagation. In: Sperelakis N, Cole WC (eds) *Cell Interactions and Gap Junctions*, Vol II. Boca Raton, FL: CRC Press, 1989, pp 155–164.
183. Joyner RW, VanCapelle FJL: Propagation through electrically coupled cells: How a small SA node drives a large atrium. *Biophys J* 50:1157–1164, 1986.
184. Joyner RW, Veenstra R, Rawling D, Chorro A: Propagation through electrically coupled cells. Effects of a resistive barrier. *Biophys J* 45:1017–1025, 1984.
185. Kameyama A, Matsuda K: Electrophysiological properties of the canine ventricular fiber. *Jpn J Physiol* 16:407–420, 1966.
186. Kameyama M: Electrical coupling between ventricular paired cells isolated from guinea pig heart. *J Physiol (Lond)* 336:345–357, 1983.
187. Kanter HL, Saffitz JE, Beyer EC: Cardiac myocytes express multiple gap junction proteins. *Circ Res* 70:438–444, 1991.
188. Kaplinsky E, Ogawa S, Balke CW, Dreifus LS: Two periods of early ventricular arrhythmia in the canine acute myocardial infarction model. *Circulation* 60:397–403, 1979.
189. Katz AM, Messineo FC: Lipid-membrane interactions and pathogenesis of ischemic damage in the myocardium. *Circ Res* 48:1–16, 1981.
190. Keener JP: Wave propagation in myocardium. In: Glass L, Hunter P, McCulloch A (eds) *Theory of Heart: Biomechanics, Biophysics, and Nonlinear Dynamics of Cardiac Function*. New York: Springer, 1991, pp 405–436.
191. Kleber AG, Janse MJ: Impulse propagation in myocardial ischemia. In: Zipes DP, Jalife J (eds) *Cardiac Electrophysiology: From Cell to Bedside*. Philadelphia: WB Saunders, 1990, pp 156–161.
192. Kleber AG, Riegger CB, Janse MJ: Electrical uncoupling and increase of extracellular resistance after induction of ischemia in isolated, arterially perfused rabbit papillary muscle. *Circ Res* 61:271–279, 1987.
193. Klein GJ, Guiraudon GM, Sharma AD, Milstein S: Demonstration of macroreentry and feasibility of operative therapy in the common type of atrial flutter. *Am J Cardiol* 57:587–591, 1986.
194. Kodama I, Wilde A, Janse MJ, Durrer D, Yamada K: Combined effects of hypoxia, hyperkalemia and acidosis on membrane action potential and excitability of guinea-pig ventricular muscle. *J Mol Cell Cardiol* 16:247–259, 1984.
195. Kolb H-A, Somogyi R: Biochemical and biophysical analysis of cell-to-cell channels and regulation of gap junctional permeability. *Rev Physiol Biochem Pharmacol* 118:1–47, 1991.
196. Kootsey JM: Electrical propagation in distributed cardiac tissue. In: Glass L, Hunter P, McCulloch A (eds) *Theory of Heart: Biomechanics, Biophysics, and Nonlinear Dynamics of Cardiac Function*. New York: Springer, 1991, pp 391–403.
197. Kovacs SJ: A clinical perspective on theory of heart. In: Glass L, Hunter P, McCulloch A (eds) *Theory of Heart: Biomechanics, Biophysics, and Nonlinear Dynamics of Cardiac Function*. New York: Springer, 1991, pp 608–611.

198. Lab MJ, Dean J: Myocardial mechanics and arrhythmia. *J Cardiovasc Pharmacol* 18(Suppl 2):S72–S79, 1991.
199. Lab MJ, Holden AV: Mechanically induced changes in electrophysiology: Implications for arrhythmia and therapy. In: Glass L, Hunter P, McCulloch A (eds) *Theory of Heart: Biomechanics, Biophysics, and Nonlinear Dynamics of Cardiac Function*. New York: Springer, 1991, pp 561–582.
200. Lal R, Arnsdorf MF: Voltage-dependent gating and single channel conductance of adult mammalian atrial gap junctions. *Circ Res* 71:737–743, 1992.
201. Landau M, Lorente P, Michaels D, Jalife J: Bistabilities and annihilation phenomena in electrophysiological cardiac models. *Circ Res* 66:1658–1672, 1990.
202. Lapicque L: Recherches quantitative sur l'excitation electriques des nerfs traitee comme un poplarisation. *J Physiol (Paris)* 9:620–635, 1907.
203. Lee CO: Ionic activities in cardiac muscle cells and application of ion-selective microelectrodes. *Am J Physiol* 241:H459–H478, 1981.
204. Lee KS, Tsien RW: High selectivity of calcium channels in single dialyzed heart cells of the guinea pig. *J Physiol (Lond)* 354:253–272, 1984.
205. Lesh MD, Pring M, Spear JF: Cellular uncoupling can unmask dispersion of action potential duration in ventricular myocardium. A computer modeling study. *Circ Res* 65:1426–1440, 1989.
206. Levy MN, Wiseman MN: Electrophysiologic mechanisms for ventricular arrhythmias in left ventricular dysfunction: Electrolytes, catecholamines, and drugs. *J Clin Pharmacol* 31:1053–1060, 1991.
207. Lewis MA, Grindrod P: One-way blocks in cardiac tissue: A mechanism for propagation failure in Purkinje fibers. *Bull Math Biol* 53:881–899, 1991.
208. Lieberman MM, Kootsey M, Johnson EA, Sawonobari T: Slow conduction in cardiac muscle. *Biophys J* 13:37–55, 1973.
209. Lorente P, Davidenko J: Hysteresis phenomena in excitable cardiac tissues. *Ann NY Acad Sci* 591:109–127, 1990.
210. Lowenstein WR: Junctional intercellular communication: The cell-to-cell membrane channel. *Physiol Rev* 61:829–913, 1981.
211. Lown B: Management of patients at high risk of sudden death. *Am Heart J* 103:689–695, 1982.
212. Luke RA, Safitz JE: Remodeling of ventricular conduction pathways in healed canine infarct border zones. *J Clin Invest* 87:1594–1602, 1991.
213. Makielski JC, Sheets MF, Hanck DA, January CT, Fozzard HA: Sodium current in voltage clamped internally perfused canine cardiac purkinje cells. *Biophys J* 52:1–11.
214. Marmarelis PZ, Marmarelis V: Analysis of Physiological Systems: The White-Noise Approach. New York: Plenum, 1978.
215. Massey KD, Minnich BN, Burt JM: Arachidonic acid and lipoxygenase metabolites uncouple neonatal rat cardiac myocyte pairs. *Am J Physiol* 263:C494–501, 1992.
216. Masson-Pevet M, Bleeker WK, Mackaay AJ, Bouman LN, Houtkooper JM: Sinus node and atrium cells from the rabbit heart: A quantitative electron microscopic description after electrophysiological localization. *J Mol Cell Cardiol* 11:555–568, 1979.
217. Maurer P, Weingart R: Cell pairs isolated from adult guinea pig and rat hearts: Effects of $[Ca^{2+}]i$ on nexal membrane resistance. *Pflügers Arch* 409:394–402, 1987.
218. McAllister RE, Noble D, Tsien RW: Reconstruction of the electrical activity of cardiac Purkinje fibres. *J Physiol (Lond)* 251:1–59, 1975.

219. Mehra R: Electrical stimulation techniques for prevention of ventricular arrhythmias. In: Saksena S, Goldschlager N (eds) *Electrical Therapy for Cardiac Arrhythmias.* Philadelphia: WB Saunders, 1990, pp 603–615.

220. Mendez C, Mueller WJ, Urquiaga X: Propagation of impulses across the Purkinje fiber-muscle junctions in the dog heart. *Circ Res* 26:135–150, 1970.

221. Metzger P, Weingart R: Electric current flow in a two-cell preparation from chironomus salivary glands. *J Physiol (Lond)* 346:599–619, 1984.

222. Metzger P, Weingart R: Electric current flow in cell pairs isolated from adult rat hearts. *J Physiol (Lond)* 366:177–195, 1985.

223. Michaels DC, Chialvo DR, Matyas EP, Jalife J: Chaotic activity in a mathematical model of the vagally driven sinoatrial node. *Circ Res* 65:1350–1360, 1989.

224. Michaels DC, Matyas EP, Jalife J: Mechanisms of sinoatrial pacemaker synchronization: A new hypothesis. *Circ Res* 61:704–714, 1987.

225. Mines GR: On the dynamic equilibrium of the heart. *J Physiol (Lond)* 46:349–383, 1913.

226. Mobley BA, Page E: The surface area of sheep cardiac Purkinje fibers. *J Physiol (Lond)* 220:547–563, 1972.

227. Moreno AP, Fishman GI, Spray DC: Phosphorylation shifts unitary conductance and modifies voltage dependent kinetics of human connexin43 gap junction channels. *Biophys J* 62:51–53, 1992.

228. Morganroth J: Proarrhythmic effects of antiarrhythmic drugs: Evolving concepts. *Am Heart J* 123:1137–1139, 1992.

229. Morley GE, Anumonwo JMB, Delmar M: Effects of 2,4-dinitrophenol or low [ATPi] on cell excitability and action potential propagation in guinea pig ventricular myocytes. *Circ Res* 71:821–830, 1992.

230. Müller W, Windisch H, Tritthart HA: Fast optical monitoring of microscopic excitation patterns in cardiac muscle. *Biophys J* 56:623–629, 1989.

231. Myerburg RJ, Zaman L, Kessler KM, Castellanos A: Evolving concepts of management of stable and potentially lethal arrhythmias. *Am Heart J* 103:615–622, 1982.

232. Nathan RD: Two electrophysiologically distinct types of cultured pacemaker cells from the rabbit sinoatrial node. *Am J Physiol* 250:H325–H329, 1986.

233. Neumcke B: Diversity of sodium channels in adult and cultured cells, in oocytes and in lipid bilayers. *Rev Physiol Biochem Pharmacol* 115:1–49, 1990.

234. Neyton J, Trautmann A: Single-channel currents of an intercellular junction. *Nature* 317:331–335, 1985.

235. Nichols CG, Lederer WJ: Adenosine triphosphate sensitive potassium channels in the cardiovascular system. *Am J Physiol* 261:H1675–H1686, 1991.

236. Niggli E, Rudisuli A, Maurer P, Weingart R: Effects of general anesthetics on current flow across membranes in guinea pig myocytes. *Am J Physiol* 256:C273–C281, 1989.

237. Nishiye H: The mechanism of Ca^{2+} action on the healing over process in mammalian cardiac muscles: A kinetic analysis. *Jpn J Physiol* 27:451–466, 1977.

238. Noble D: A modification of the Hodgkin–Huxley equations applicable to Purkinje fiber action and pacemaker potentials. *J Physiol (Lond)* 160:317–352, 1962.

239. Noble D: Ionic mechanisms determining the timing of ventricular repolarization: Significance for cardiac arrhythmias. *Ann NY Acad Sci* 644:1–22, 1992.

240. Noble D, Stein RB: The threshold conditions for initiation of action potentials by excitable cells. *J Physiol (Lond)* 187:129–162, 1966.

241. Noma A: ATP-regulated K^+ channels in cardiac muscle. *Nature* 305:147–148, 1983.

242. Obaid AL, Socolar SL, Rose B: Cell- co-cell channels with two independently regulated gates in series: Analysis of junctional conductance modulation by membrane potential calcium and pH. *J Membr Biol* 73:69–89, 1983.

243. Page E: Cardiac gap junctions. In: Fozzard HA, Haber E, Jennings RB, Katz AM, Morgan HE (eds) *The Heart and Cardiovascular System.* New York: Raven Press, 1991, pp 1003–1048.

244. Page E, Fozzard H: Capacitive, resistive, and syncytial properties of heart muscle — ultrastructural and physiological considerations. In: Bourne GH (ed) *The Structure and Function of Muscle,* Vol II, 2nd ed. Part 2: Structure. New York: Academic Press, 1973, pp 91–158.

245. Patlak J, Ortiz M: Slow currents through single sodium channels of the adult rat heart. *J Gen Physiol* 86:89–104, 1985.

246. Patlak J, Ortiz M: Two modes of gating during late Na^+ channel currents in frog sartorius muscle. *J Gen Physiol* 87:305–326, 1986.

247. Pelzer D, Pelzer S, McDonald TF: Calcium channels in heart. In: Fozzard HA, Haber E, Jennings RB, Katz AM, Morgan HE (eds) *The Heart and Cardiovascular System.* New York: Raven Press, 1991, pp 1049–1089.

248. Peracchia C (ed): *Biophysics of Gap Junction Channels.* Boca Raton, FL: CRC Press, 1991.

249. Peuch P, Gallay P, Grolleau R: Mechanism of atrial flutter in humans. In: Tourboul P, Waldo AL (eds) *Atrial Arrhythmias: Current Concepts and Management.* St. Louis, MO: Mosby-Year Book, 1990, pp 190–209.

250. Podrid PJ, Lampert S, Graboys TB, Blatt CM, Lown B: Aggravation of arrhythmia by antiarrhythmic drugs — incidence and predictors. *Am J Cardiol* 59:38E–44E, 1987.

251. Pressler ML: Cable analysis in quiescent and active sheep Purkinje fibres. *J Physiol (Lond)* 352:739–757, 1984.

252. Pressler ML: Passive electrical properties of cardiac tissue. In: Zipes DP, Jalife J (eds) *Cardiac Electrophysiology: From Cell to Bedside.* Philadelphia: WB Saunders, 1990, pp 108–122.

253. Rasmusson RL, Clark JW, Giles WR, Robinson K, Clark RB, Shibata EF, Campbell DL: A mathematical model of electrophysiological activity in a bullfrog atrial cell. *Am J Physiol* 259:H370–H389, 1990.

254. Rasmusson RL, Clark JW, Giles WR, Shibata EF, Campbell DL: A mathematical model of a bullfrog cardiac pacemaker cell. *Am J Physiol* 259:H352–H369, 1990.

255. Reber WR, Weingart R: Ungulate cardiac Purkinje fibres: The influence of intracellular pH on the electrical cell to cell coupling. *J Physiol (Lord)* 328:87–104, 1982.

256. Riegger CB, Alperovich G, Kleber AG: Effect of oxygen withdrawal on active and passive electrical properties of arterially perfused rabbit ventricular muscle. *Circ Res* 64:532–541, 1989.

257. Rook MB, de Jonge B, Jongsma HJ, Masson-Pevet MA: Gap junction formation and functional interaction between neonatal rat cardiocytes in culture: A correlative physiological and ultrastructural study. *J Membr Biol* 118:179–192, 1990.

258. Rook MB, Jongsma HJ, van Ginneken AC: Properties of single gap junctional channels between isolated neonatal rat heart cells. *Am J Physiol* 255:H770–H782, 1988.

259. Rüdisüli A, Weingart R: Electrical properties of gap junction channels in guinea-pig ventricular cell pairs revealed by exposure to heptanol. *Pflügers Arch* 415:12–21, 1989.

260. Rudy Y, Quan WL: A model study of the effects of the

discrete cellular structure on electrical propagation in cardiac tissue. *Circ Res* 61:815–823, 1987.

261. Sakamoto Y: Membrane characteristics of canine papillary muscle fiber. *J Gen Physiol* 54:765–781, 1965.

262. Saksena S, Goldschlager N (eds): *Electrical Therapy for Cardiac Arrhythmias*. Philadelphia: WB Saunders, 1990.

263. Sano TN, Takayama N, Shimamoto T: Directional difference of conduction velocity in cardiac ventricular syncytium studied by microelectrodes. *Circ Res* 7:262–267, 1959.

264. Saul JP, Berger RD, Albrecht P, Stein SP, Chen MH, Cohen RJ: Transfer function analysis of the circulation: Unique insights into cardiovascular regulation. *Am J Physiol* 261:H1231–1245, 1991.

265. Sawicki GJ, Arnsdorf MF: Electrophysiologic actions and interactions between lysophosphatidylcholine and lidocaine in the nonsteady state: The match between multiphasic arrhythmogenic mechanisms and multiple drug effects in cardiac Purkinje fibers. *J Pharm Exp Ther* 235:829–838, 1985.

266. Schoels W, Restivo M, Caref EB, Gough WB, el-Sherif N: Circus movement atrial flutter in canine sterile pericarditis model. Activation patterns during entrainment and termination of single-loop reentry in vivo. *Circulation* 83:1716–1730, 1991.

267. Schoels W, Yang H, Gough WB, el-Sherif N: Circus movement atrial flutter in the canine sterile pericarditis model. Differential effects of procainamide on the components of the reentrant pathway. *Circ Res* 68:1117–1126, 1991.

268. Schoenberg M, Dominguez G, Fozzard HA: Effect of diameter on membrane capacity and conductance of sheep cardiac Purkinje fibers. *J Gen Physiol* 65:441–458, 1975.

269. Sheets MF, Hanck DA, Fozzard HA: Nonlinear relation between V_{max} and I_{Na} in canine cardiac Purkinje cells. *Circ Res* 63:386–398, 1988.

270. Sheldon RS, Duff HJ, Hill RJ: *Clin Invest Med* 14:458–465, 1991.

271. Sherman A, Rinzel J: Model for synchronization of pancreatic β-cells by gap junction coupling. *Biophys J* 59:547–559, 1991.

272. Sheu S-S, Korth M, Lathrop DA, Fozzard HA: Intra and extracellular K^+ and Na^+ activities and resting membrane potential in sheep cardic Purkinje strands. *Circ Res* 47:692–700, 1980.

273. Shibata EF, Drury T, Refsum H, Aldrete V, Giles W: Contributions of a transient outward current to repolarization in human atrium. *Am J Physiol* 257:H1773–H1781, 1989.

274. Shimuzu A, Nozaki A, Rudy Y, Waldo AL: Multiplexing studies of effects of rapid atrial pacing on the area of slow conduction during atrial flutter in canine pericarditis model. *Circulation* 83:983–984, 1991.

275. Shimuzu A, Nozaki A, Rudy Y, Waldo AL: Onset of induced atrial flutter in the canine pericarditis model. *J Am Coll Cardiol* 17:1235–1236, 1991.

276. Shorofsky SR, January CT: L- and T-type Ca^{2+} channels in canine cardiac Purkinje cells. Single-channel demonstration of L-type Ca^{2+} window current. *Circ Res* 70:456–464, 1992.

277. Shrier A, Dubarsky H, Rosengarten M, Guevara MR, Nattel S, Glass L: Prediction of complex atrioventricular conduction rhythms in humans with use of the atrioventricular nodal recovery curve. *Circulation* 76:1196–1205, 1987.

278. Sigworth F: Electronic design of the patch clamp. In: Sakmann B, Neher E (eds) *Single Channel Recording*. New York: Plenum, 1983, pp 3–35.

279. Simson MB, Untereker WJ, Spielman SR, Horowitz LN, Marcus NH, Falcone RA, Harken AH, Josephson ME: Relation between late potentials on the body surface and directly recorded fragmented electrograms in patients with ventricular tachycardia. *Am J Cardiol* 51:105–112, 1983.

280. Singer DH, Lazzara R, Hoffman BF: Interrelationships between automaticity and conduction in Purkinje fibers. *Circ Res* 21:537–558, 1967.

281. Sjöstrand FS, Anderson E: Electron microscopy of the intercalated discs of cardiac muscle tissue. *Experientia* 10:369–372, 1954.

282. Smeets JL, Allessie MA, Lammers WJ, Bonke FI, Hollen J: The wavelength of the cardiac impulse and reentrant arrhythmias in isolated rabbit atrium. The role of heart rate, autonomic transmitters, temperature, and potassium. *Circ Res* 58:96–108, 1986.

283. Smith JM, Cohen RJ: Simple finite-element model accounts for wide range of cardiac dysrhythmias. *Proc Natl Acad Sci USA* 81:233–237, 1984.

284. Smith JH, Green CR, Peters NS, Rothery S, Severs NJ: Altered patterns of gap junction distribution in ischemic heart disease. *Am J Pathol* 139:801–821, 1991.

285. Sobel BE, Corr PB, Cain ME, Witkowski FX, Price DA: Potential arrhythmogenic electrophysiological derangements in canine Purkinje fibers induced by lysophosphoglycerides. *Circ Res* 44:822–832, 1979.

286. Sobel BE, Corr PB, Robinson AK, Goldstein RA, Witkowski FX, Klein MS: Accumulation of lysophosphoglycerides with arrhythmogenic properties in ischemic myocardium. *J Clin Invest* 62:546–553, 1978.

287. Sommer JR, Dolber PC: Cardiac muscle: The ultrastructure of its cells and bundles. In: Paes de Carvalho A, Hoffman BF, Lieberman M (eds) *Normal and Abnormal Conduction of the Heart Beat*. Mt Kisco, NY: Futura, 1981.

288. Sommer JR, Johnson EA: Ultrastructure of cardiac muscle. In: Berne RM (ed) *The Handbook of Physiology. I. The Cardiovascular System*. Baltimore, MD: The American Physiological Society, Williams and Wilkins, 1979, pp 113–186.

289. Sommer JR, Scherer B: The geometry of intercellular communication in cardiac muscle with emphasis on cell and bundle appositions. *Am J Physiol* 248:H792–H803, 1985.

290. Somogyi R, Kolb H-A: Cell-to-cell channel conductance during loss of gap junctional coupling in pairs of pancreatic acinar and Chinese hamster ovary cells. *Pflügers Arch* 412:54–65, 1988.

291. Spach MS: Anisotropic structural complexities in the genesis of reentrant arrhythmias [editorial comment]. *Circulation* 84:1447–1450, 1991.

292. Spach MS, Dolber PC: Relating extracellular potentials and their derivatives to anisotropic propagation at a microscopic level in human cardiac muscle: Evidence for electrical uncoupling of side-to-side fiber connections with increasing age. *Circ Res* 58:356–371, 1986.

293. Spach MS, Dolber PC: Discontinuous anisotropic propagation. In: Rosen MR, Janse MJ, Wit AL (eds) *Cardiac Electrophysiology: A Textbook*. Mt Kisco, NY: Futura, 1990.

294. Spach MS, Dolber PC, Anderson PA: Multiple regional differences in cellular properties that regulate repolarization and contraction in the right atrium of adult and newborn dogs. *Circ Res* 65:1594–1611, 1989.

295. Spach MS, Dolber PC, Heidlage JF: Properties of discontinuous anisotropic propagation at a microscopic level. *Ann NY Acad Sci* 591:62–74, 1990.

296. Spach MS, Dolber PC, Heidlage JF: Influence of the passive anisotropic properties on directional differences in propagation following modification of the sodium conductance in human atrial muscle. A model of reentry based on aniso-

tropic discontinuous propagation. *Circ Res* 62:811–832, 1988.

297. Spach MS, Dolber PC, Heidlage JF: Interaction of inhomogeneities of repolarization with anisotropic propagation in dog atria. A mechanism for both preventing and initiating reentry. *Circ Res* 65:1612–1631, 1989.

298. Spach MS, Dolber PC, Heidlage JF, Kootsey JM, Johnson EA: Propagating depolarization in anisotropic human and canine cardiac muscle: Apparent directional differences in membrane capacitance. A simplified model for selective directional effects of modifying the sodium conductance on V_{max}, τ_{foot}, and the propagation safety factor. *Circ Res* 60:206–219, 1987.

299. Spach MS, Kootsey JM, Sloan JD: Active modulation of electrical coupling between cardiac cells of the dog. A mechanism for transient and steady state variations in conduction velocity. *Circ Res* 51:347–362, 1982.

300. Spach MS, Miller WT, Dolber PC, Kootsey JM, Sommer JR, Mosher CE Jr: The functional role of structural complexities in the propagation of depolarization in the atrium of the dog. Cardiac conduction disturbances due to discontinuities of effective axial resistivity. *Circ Res* 50:175–191, 1982.

301. Spach MS, Miller WT, Geselowitz DB, Barr RC, Kootsey JM, Johnson EA: The discontinuous nature of propagation in normal canine cardiac muscle. Evidence for recurrent discontinuities of intracellular resistance that affect membrane currents. *Circ Res* 48:39–54, 1981.

302. Spear JR, Michelson EL, Moore EN: Reduced space constant in slowly conducting regions of chronically infarcted canine myocardium. *Circ Res* 53:176–185, 1983.

303. Spear JF, Michelson EL, Moore EN: Cellular electrophysiologic characteristics of chronically infarcted myocardium in dogs susceptible to sustained ventricular tachyarrhythmias. *J Am Coll Cardiol* 1:1099–1110, 1983.

304. Sperelakis N, MacDonald RL: Ratio of transverse to longitudinal resistivities of isolated cardiac muscle fiber bundles. *J Electrocardiol* 7:301–314, 1974.

305. Spray DC, Burt JM: Structure-activity relations of the cardiac gap junction channel. *Am J Physiol* 258:C195–205, 1990.

306. Spray DC, Harris AL, Bennett MVL: Equilibrium properties of a voltage-dependent junctional conductance. *J Gen Physiol* 77:77–93, 1981.

307. Spray DC, White RL, Mazet F, Bennett MVL: Regulation of gap junctional conductance. *Am J Physiol* 248:H753–H764, 1985.

308. Starmer CF, Grant AO, Strauss H: Mechanisms of use-dependent block of sodium channels in excitable membranes by local anesthetics. *Biophys J* 46:15–27, 1984.

309. Takens-Kwak BR, Jongsma HJ, Rook MB, Van Ginneken AC: Mechanism of heptanol-induced uncoupling of cardiac gap junctions: A perforated patch-clamp study. *Am J Physiol* 262:C1531–C1538, 1992.

310. Tasaki I, Hagiwara S: Capacity of muscle fiber membrane. *Am J Physiol* 188:423–429, 1957.

311. Task Force of the Working Group on Arrhythmias of the European Society of Cardiology (Akhtar M, Breithardt G, Camm AJ, Coumel P, Janse MJ, Lazara R, Myerburg RJ, Schwartz PJ, Waldo AL, Wellens HJJ, Zipes DP): CAST and beyond: Implications of the Cardiac Arrhythmia Suppression Trial. *Circulation* 91:1123–1127, 1990.

312. Task Force of the Working Group on Arrhythmias of the European Society of Cardiology: The Sicilian gambit. A new approach to the classification of antiarrhythmic drugs based on their actions on arrhythmogenic mechanisms. Circulation 84:1831–1851, 1991.

313. Trautwein W: Membrane currents in cardiac muscle fibers. *Physiol Rev* 53:793–835, 1973.

314. Unwin N: The structure of ion channels in membranes of excitable cells. *Neuron* 3:665–676, 1989.

315. Ursell PC, Gardner PI, Albala A, Fenoglio JJ Jr, Wit AL: Structural and electrophysiological changes in the epicardial border zone of canine myocardial infarcts during infarct healing. *Circ Res* 56:436–451, 1985.

316. Vassalle M: The relationship among cardiac pacemakers. Overdrive suppression. *Circ Res* 41:269–277, 1977.

317. Vaughan-Jones RD, Lederer WJ, Eisner DA: Ca^{2+} ions can affect intracellular pH in mammalian cardiac muscle. *Nature* 301:522–524, 1983.

318. Veenstra RD: Voltage-dependent gating of gap junctional conductance in embryonic chick heart. *Ann NY Acad Sci* 588:93–105, 1990.

319. Veenstra RD: Physiological modulation of cardiac gap junction channels. *J Cardiovasc Electrophysiol* 2:168–189, 1991.

320. Veenstra RD, DeHaan RL: Electrotonic interactions between aggregates of chick embryo cardiac pacemaker cells. *Am J Physiol* 250:H453–H463, 1986.

321. Veenstra RD, DeHaan RL: Measurement of single channel currents from cardiac gap junctions. *Science* 233:972–974, 1986.

322. Veenstra RD, Joyner RW, Rawling DA: Purkinje and ventricular activation sequences of canine papillary muscle. *Circ Res* 54:500–515, 1984.

323. Veenstra RD, Wang H-Z, Westphale EM, Beyer EC: Multiple connexins confer distinct regulatory and conductance properties of gap junctions in developing heart. *Circ Res* 71:1277–1283, 1992.

324. Vinet A, Chialvo DR, Jalife J: Irregular dynamics of excitation in biologic and mathematical models of cardiac cells. *Ann NY Acad Sci* 591:281–298, 1990.

325. Waldo AL, Carlson MD, Biblo LA, Henthorn RW: The role of transient entrainment in atrial flutter. in: Tourboul P, Waldo AL (eds) *Atrial Arrhythmias: Current Concepts and Management.* St. Louis, MO: Mosby-Year Book, 1990, pp 210–228.

326. Waldo AL, MacLean WAH, Karp RB, Kochoukos NT, James TN: Entrainment and interruption of atrial flutter with pacing. Studies in man following open heart surgery. *Circulation* 56:737–745, 1977.

327. Walton MK, Fozzard HA: The conducted action potential. Models and comparison to experiments. *Biophys J* 44:9–26, 1983.

328. Walton MK, Fozzard HA: Experimental study of the conducted action potential in cardiac Purkinje strands. *Biophys J* 44:1–8, 1983.

329. Ward D, Garratt C: Rate-responsive pacing and sensors. In: Saksena S, Goldschlager N (eds) *Electrical Therapy for Cardiac Arrhythmias.* Philadelphia: WB Saunders, 1990, pp 343–353.

330. Watanabe A, Grundfest H: Impulse propagation at the septal and commissural junctions of crayfish lateral giant axons. *J Gen Physiol* 45:267–308, 1961.

331. Watson RM, Josephson ME: Atrial flutter. I. Electrophysiologic substrates and modes of initiation and termination. *Am J Cardiol* 45:732–741, 1980.

332. Weidmann S: The electrical constants of Purkinje fibres. *J Physiol (Lond)* 118:348–360, 1952.

333. Weidmann S: The diffusion of radiopotassium across intercalated disks of mammalian cardiac muscle. *J Physiol (Lond)* 187:323–342, 1966.

334. Weidmann S: Electrical constants of trabecular muscle from

mammalian heart. *J Physiol (Lond)* 210:1041–1054, 1970.

335. Weingart R: The actions of ouabain on intercellular coupling and conduction velocity in mammalian ventricular muscle. *J Physiol (Lond)* 264:341–365, 1977.

336. Weingart R: Electrical properties of the nexal membrane studied in rat ventricular cell pairs. *J Physiol (Lond)* 370:267–284, 1986.

337. Weingart R, Maurer P: Action potential transfer in cell pairs isolated from adult rat and guinea pig ventricles. *Circ Res* 63:72–80, 1988.

338. Weingart R, Rüdisüli A, Maurer P: Cell to cell communication. In: Zipes DP, Jalife J (eds) *Cardiac Electrophysiology: From Cell to Bedside*. Philadelphia: WB Saunders, 1990, pp 122–127.

339. Wellens HJ, Duren DR, Lie KI: Observations on mechanisms of ventricular tachycardia in man. *Circulation* 54: 237–244, 1976.

340. White RL, Spray DC, Campos de Carvalho AC, Wittenberg BA, Bennett MVL: Some electrical and pharmacological properties of gap junctions between adult ventricular myocytes. *Am J Physiol* 249:C447–C455, 1985.

341. Wilders R, Jongsma HJ: Limitations of the dual voltage clamp method in assaying conductance and kinetics of gap junction channels. *Biophys J* 63:942–953, 1992.

342. Winfree AT: When Time Breaks Down: The Three-Dimensional Dynamics of Electrochemical Waves and Cardiac Arrhythmias. Princeton, NJ: Princeton University Press, 1987.

343. Winfree AT: Ventricular reentry in three dimensions. In: Zipes DP, Jalife J (eds) *Cardiac Electrophysiology: From Cell to Bedside*. Philadelphia: WB Saunders, 1990.

344. Wit AL: Anisotropic reentry: A model of arrhythmias that may necessitate a new approach to antiarrhythmic drug development. In: Rosen MR, Palti Y (eds) *Lethal Arrhythmias Resulting from Myocardial Ischemia and Infarction (Proceedings of the Second Rappaport Symposium)*. Norwell, MA: Kluwer Academic, 1989, pp 199–213.

345. Wit AL, Rosen MR: In: McFarlane PW, Lawrie-Veitch TD (eds) *Comprehensive Electrocardiology*. New York: Pergamon Press, 1989, pp 809–841.

346. Wojtczak J: Contractures and increases in internal longitudinal resistance of cow ventricular muscle induced by hypoxia. *Circ Res* 44:88–95, 1979.

347. Woodbury JW, Crill WE: On the problem of impulse conduction in the atrium. In: Florey L (ed) *Nervous Inhibition*. New York: Plenum Press, 1961, pp 24–35.

348. Wyndham RC, Arnsdorf MF, Levitsky S, Smith TM, Dhringra RC, Denes P, Rosen KM: Successful surgical excision of focal paroxysmal atrial tachycardia: Observations in vivo and in vitro. *Circulation* 62:1365–1372, 1980.

349. Yanagihara K, Noma A, Irisawa H: Reconstruction of sino-atrial node pacemaker potential based on the voltage clamp experiments. *Jpn J Physiol* 30:841–857, 1980.

350. Ypey DL, Clapham DE, DeHaan RL: Development of electrical coupling and action potential synchrony between paired aggregates of embryonic heart cells. *J Membr Biol* 51:76–96, 1979.

351. Zipes DP: Cardiac electrophysiology: Promises and contributions. *J Am Coll Cardiol* 13:1329–52, 1989.

352. Zipes DP, Jalife J (eds): *Cardiac Electrophysiology: From Cell to Bedside*. Philadelphia: WB Saunders, 1990.

CHAPTER 11

The Electrocardiogram and its Relationship to Excitation of the Heart

YORAM RUDY

INTRODUCTION

The electrical activity of cardiac muscle cells is projected to the surface of the torso by means of the intervening conducting medium. The surface potentials that are recorded as electrocardiograms reflect, therefore, both the heart generators as well as the surrounding volume conductor. The cardiac current sources are distributed throughout the myocardium and can be specified by giving the space-time distribution of dipole elements in the entire heart. A crude approximation is to represent the heart electrically by a single dipole, which is the vector sum of all these dipole elements. This is the basis of the *dipole hypothesis* introduced by Einthoven and associates as early as 1913 {1}. Interpretation of most clinical electrocardiograms (ECG) and vectorcardiograms (VCG) recorded today is still based on this simplified representation of the cardiac sources as a single *heart vector*. Moreover, almost all of the clinical ECG and VCG practiced today neglects the effects of the medium, i.e., the torso volume-conductor inhomogeneities, on the electrocardiogram. In spite of these simplifications, electrocardiography has been an extremely useful and reliable diagnostic tool for almost a century.

The last 40 years have seen major progress in several areas related to basic understanding of the electrocardiogram. In the 1950s the microelectrode was introduced, permitting direct recording of the membrane current-voltage relationships of cardiac cells. The recently developed patchclamp technique has allowed scientists to record the electrical activity of individual membrane ionic channels. Molecular biologists have started to determine the molecular structure of the channel proteins and to relate it to function. This activity at the cellular and subcellular level has provided important information on cellular processes that generate cardiac excitation and has helped us to characterized better the electrocardiographic sources on a microscopic (cellular) scale.

Advances in electronics and computers have made possible simultaneous recordings of electrical activity from many sites. These mapping techniques have been used to study the pattern of excitation and recovery in the myocardium, providing the basis for a macroscopic description of the cardiac sources as a function of time and space. Mapping techniques have also been used to record the potential distributions over the entire torso (the total surface ECG), extending the standard ECG approach that samples this potential distribution at only a small number of points. The advances in computers and digital computing have also lead to the development of detailed computer models and simulations of the electrocardiographic process, which have provided invaluable insights into the relationships between cardiac activity and the electrocardiographic fields. Considerable progress has also been made in attempts to solve the electrocardiographic inverse problem in which cardiac activity can be computed noninvasively from the body surface electrocardiographic data.

This chapter is an attempt to synthesize many of these concepts and to describe the genesis of the electrocardiographic potentials in terms of basic physiological processes and concepts from electromagnetic field theory. The discussion focuses on macroscopic phenomena (cellular and membrane processes are discussed extensively in other chapters of this volume) and relies on both quantitative and descriptive approaches. The emphasis is on basic principles rather than on specific questions, such as different designs of electrocardiographic lead systems. The two major determinants of the electrocardiographic potentials, namely, the cardiac sources and the torso volume conductor, are discussed first. Examples of electrocardiographic body surface potential maps (BSPMs) are provided. Finally, the principles introduced are used to describe an emerging electrocardiographic imaging modality (the "inverse problem") for noninvasive reconstruction of the electrical function of the heart.

ELECTRICAL SOURCES IN THE HEART

During the cardiac excitation process current sources arise in cell membranes throughout the heart. These sources can be characterized by a vector function $\vec{J}$, an impressed current density that depends on time and space. $\vec{J}$ is nonzero only in cellular membranes, where it can be identified with ionic currents that are carried mainly by sodium (Na), calcium (Ca), and potassium (K) ions. While this constitutes a rigorous formal description of the cardiac

N. Sperelakis (ed.), Physiology and Pathophysiology of the Heart, Third Edition.

sources, it is desirable to formulate alternative descriptions that lend themselves to quantitative evaluation, provide a basis for quantitative simulations of electric fields generated by the heart, and help relate the electrocardiographic potentials to the underlying cardiac activity. The goal of this section is to develop such representations of the electrocardiographic sources.

Single cardiac cell

Histologically the heart (cardiac tissue) is composed of many individual cells, each with a typical length of about 100 μm and a diameter of roughly 15 μm (fig. 11-1). Under normal conditions, these cells are electrically coupled through low resistance pathways (*gap junctions*) that permit current flow (carried by ions) between cells. This current provides the mechanism for conduction of the action potential and for the formation of an activation wave front that propagates through the heart and constitutes the locus of electrical sources during cardiac excitation. Since the single cardiac cell is the elementary unit of excitation, it is logical to begin the characterization of the cardiac electrical sources by first formulating the elementary source associated with a single cell.

The cellular action potential and the currents and membrane processes that are involved in its generation are discussed extensively in other chapters of this volume. We limit our discussion here to a brief summary of only the major ionic currents (many other currents also contribute to the action potential through ionic channels, ionic pumps, and ionic exchangers; they are omitted from this discussion

for the sake of simplicity and since the focus is on the cell as a source of extracellular potential rather than on membranee mechanisms of excitation). A simulated ventricular action potential, together with the major ionic currents, is shown in fig. 11-2 {3,4}. The action potential is characterized by a fast upstroke (phase 0), which is generated by voltage-dependent activation of a depolarizing sodium current (I_{Na}); a prolonged plateau (phase 2), which results from a balance between an inward current, carried mainly by calcium (I_{Ca}), and a time-dependent outward potassium current (I_K); and a fast repolarization phase (phase 3), which involves both time-dependent (I_K) and time-independent (I_{K1}) outward potassium currents.

The action potential is the transmembrane potential during excitation, defined as $V_m = \Phi_i - \Phi_o$ where Φ_i is the intracellular potential and Φ_o is the extracellular potential immediately adjacent to the cell membrane. Consider a single cell immersed in a uniform conducting medium (fig. 11-3). Since the plasma membrane is extremely thin (~75 Å), it can be treated as a mathematical surface of zero thickness that separates the intracellular and extracellular domains. Two conditions must hold across this surface:

$$\Phi_i - \Phi_o = V_m \neq 0. \tag{11-1}$$

(The potential difference is the transmembrane potential V_m, which is clearly not identically zero, and, in fact, varies with time during excitation, as shown in fig. 11-2A) and

$$\sigma_i \frac{\partial \Phi_i}{\partial n} = \sigma_o \frac{\partial \Phi_o}{\partial n} \tag{11-2}$$

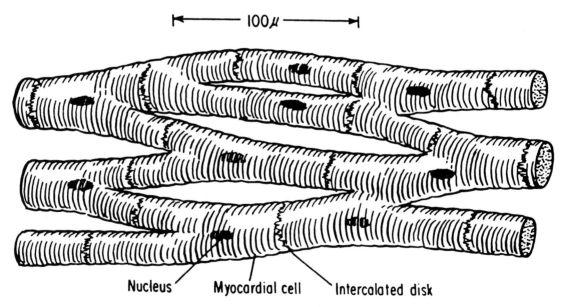

|← —— 100μ —— →|

Nucleus   Myocardial cell   Intercalated disk

Fig. 11-1. Cellular-level architecture of the myocardium. The tissue is composed of discrete cells that are interconnected at intercalated disks. The disks contain gap junctions that provide resistive pathways for current flow and electrical coupling between cells through cytoplasmic bridges (connexons). From Sonnenblick {2}, with permission.

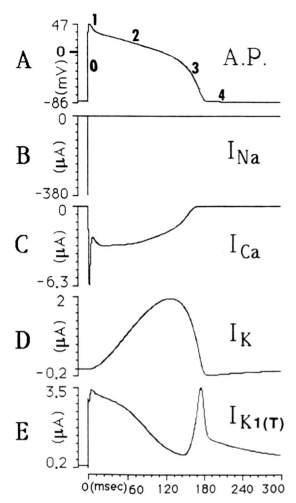

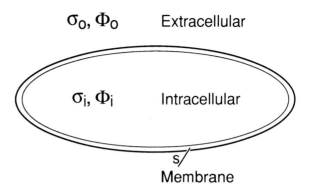

Fig. 11-3. A schematic representation of the single cell in a volume conductor. σ_i and σ_o are the intracellular and extracellular conductivities, respectively. Φ_i is the intracellular potential and Φ_o is the extracellular potential immediately adjacent to the cell membrane. The transmembrane potential V_m is given by $V_m = \Phi_i - \Phi_o$.

Fig. 11-2. A cardiac ventricular action potential (**A**) and major membrane ionic currents that determine its shape (**B–E**). Bold numbers in panel A indicate phase during the action potential. The fast kinetics and large amplitude of the sodium current, I_{Na} (panel **B**), result in the upstroke of the action potential (phase 0). The inward calcium current, I_{Ca} (panel **C**) supports the action potential plateau (phase 2) against the repolarizing potassium currents I_k (panel **D**) and $I_{k1(T)}$ (panel **E**). The large increase of I_k and the late peak of $I_{k1(T)}$ during phase 3 repolarize the membrane to the resting potential ($I_{k1(T)}$ is the total time-independent potassium current that includes a plateau current, I_{kp}; see Luo and Rudy {3}). Panel A depicts the action potential as a function of time. The action potential in space has a similar shape and is related to the temporal action potential through the velocity of propagation.

(The current density normal to the surface is continuous — no current is lost or gained in crossing the surface.)

We now define the scalar function Ψ {5}

$$\Psi = \sigma\Phi \tag{11-3}$$

where Φ is the desired potential and σ is the piecewise constant conductivity function, $\sigma = \sigma_i$ intracellularly and σ

$= \sigma_o$ extracellularly. Since Φ satisfies Laplace's equation in the source-free intracellular and extracellular domains, so does Ψ. Expressing eqs. (11-1) and (11-2) in terms of Ψ as defined in (11-3) gives

$$\Psi_i - \Psi_o = \sigma_i\Phi_i - \sigma_o\Phi_o \neq 0 \tag{11-4}$$

and

$$\frac{\partial\Psi_i}{\partial n} = \frac{\partial\Psi_o}{\partial n}. \tag{11-5}$$

In other words, Ψ is discontinuous across S while its normal derivative is continuous. This behavior identifies the surface S (the cell membrane) as the location of a double layer[1] of strength equal to the discontinuity in Ψ (that is, the strength of the double layer is given by $\vec{\tau} = (\Psi_i - \Psi_o)\hat{n})\{5\}$. The potential field, Ψ, generated by this dipole source distribution is {6}

$$\Psi = -\frac{1}{4\pi}\int_s (\Psi_i - \Psi_o)\nabla\left(\frac{1}{r}\right) \cdot \vec{ds} \tag{11-6}$$

where r is the distance from source to field point, ∇ is the gradient operator, and integration is performed over the entire cell surface, S.

Replacing Ψ by $\sigma\Phi$ according to (11-3) and restricting the field points to the extracellular domain (i.e., $\sigma = \sigma_o$ at the field points), we obtain the desired expression for the extracellular potential field, Φ_o, generated by an active cell:

$$\Phi_o = -\frac{1}{4\pi\sigma_o}\int_s (\sigma_i\Phi_i - \sigma_o\Phi_o)\nabla\left(\frac{1}{r}\right) \cdot \vec{ds} \tag{11-7}$$

In this expression $(\sigma_i\Phi_i - \sigma_o\Phi_o)\vec{ds}$ constitutes a dipole element in a small membrane area ds. Integration over the entire cell membrane, S, provides the potential generated by the entire cell.

Equation (11-7) identifies the source of the extracellular field arising from a single active cell to be a double layer located in the cell membrane. The strength of the double layer, $\sigma_i\Phi_i - \sigma_o\Phi_o$, is determined by the intracellular and extracellular conductivities and the transmembrane potential. This source is no longer identified with ionic currents within the membrane. It serves as an equivalent source that can be used to obtain [through eq. (11-7)] the potential field in the extracellular domain.

An alternative expression to (11-7) can be derived by noting that the quantity $-\nabla(1/r) \cdot \vec{ds}$ is an element of solid angle $d\Omega$ so that (11-7) can be written:

$$\Phi_o = \frac{1}{4\pi\sigma_o} \int_s (\sigma_i\Phi_i - \sigma_o\Phi_o)\, d\Omega. \qquad (11\text{-}8)$$

(The concept of a solid angle is defined at the end of this section.)

For a cell at rest, the transmembrane potential $V_m = \Phi_i - \Phi_o$ is constant over the entire cell membrane, which constitutes a closed surface. Since σ_i and σ_o are constants, the double-layer strength, $\sigma_i\Phi_i - \sigma_o\Phi_o$, is also constant (uniform) over the cell surface. Therefore, the double-layer strength term can be removed from under the integral sign to give

$$\Phi_o = \frac{1}{4\pi\sigma_o}(\sigma_i\Phi_i - \sigma_o\Phi_o)\int_s d\Omega = \frac{1}{4\pi\sigma_o}(\sigma_i\Phi_i - \sigma_o\Phi_o)\Omega = 0,$$

since, for exterior points the total solid angle subtended by a closed surface (the entire cell membrane in this case) is zero. Hence, a cell at rest does not contribute to the extracellular potential field, as expected. Similarly, when the cell is fully depolarized (at the plateau phase of V_m, see fig. 11-2), V_m is constant (to a good approximation) on the entire cell membrane and so is $\sigma_i\Phi_i - \sigma_o\Phi_o$. Therefore, a fully depolarized cell does not contribute significantly to the extracellular potential as well. It follows that a substantial contribution to the external potential field from a given cell occurs only during the rapid upstroke of the action potential (phase 0) and during the repolarization phase (phase 3). In the electrocardiogram, the QRS reflects the contribution of phase 0 (depolarization), while phase 3 (repolarization) is manifest in the T wave.

Comment — Definition of a Solid Angle. The solid angle, Ω, is proportional to the extent of opening of the cone that is formed by connecting all points on the boundary of the double layer, S, with the field point, P. Precisely, the solid angle is defined as the area intercepted on a unit sphere, centered at the field point, by this cone (fig. 11-4).

Sources associated with ventricular activation

The time course and pattern of normal activation of the human heart are depicted in fig. 11-5. Ventricular excitation is initiated at many subendocardial sites more or less simultaneously as a consequence of the anatomy (geometrical arrangement) and fast conduction velocity of the His-Purkinje system. Once excitation in the working myocardium is initiated, it spreads from cell to cell by means of current flow through gap junctions, which provide

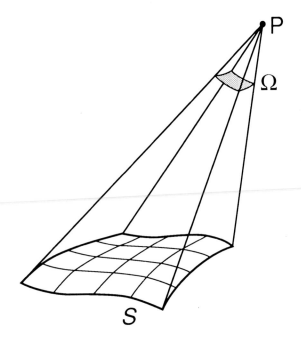

Fig. 11-4. A solid angle, Ω, associated with a surface, S, and an observation point, P. The area intercepted on a unit sphere is shown by the shaded area.

low resistance pathways between neighboring cells {7,8}. The distribution and properties of gap junctions {9} and the geometrical arrangement of the cardiac fibers in the myocardium {10} are such that the resistance to intracellular current flow is higher in the direction perpendicular to the fibers than along the fibers; a typical resistivity ratio is 9:1 {11,12} (cardiac fibers are elongated structures so that a longitudinal axis and a transverse axis can be defined; see fig. 11-1). As a result of this anisotropic property, excitation propagates at a higher velocity in the direction of the fibers than across fibers (a 3:1 velocity ratio is typical {12–14}).

The fibrous architecture of the heart is such that the cardiac fibers are parallel to the endocardial and epicardial surfaces {15,16}. The two factors discussed above (i.e., the Purkinje system and the anisotropic conduction velocity) lead to the formation of an activation front that is generally uniform and parallel to the endocardial surface. This activation front propagates (in both left and right ventricles) from endocardium to epicardium (fig. 11-5). An interesting (and somewhat parodoxical) observation is that propagation of the activation front proceeds across fibers, i.e., in the direction of slow conduction. Other observations regarding the sequence of normal excitation relate to the termination of activation; the latest parts to be activated are the posterobasal area or the posterolateral area of the left ventricle, and the pulmonary conus and the posterobasal area in the right ventricle (the reader is referred to {17} for a detailed description). As will be discussed below, the activation fronts are the loci of the

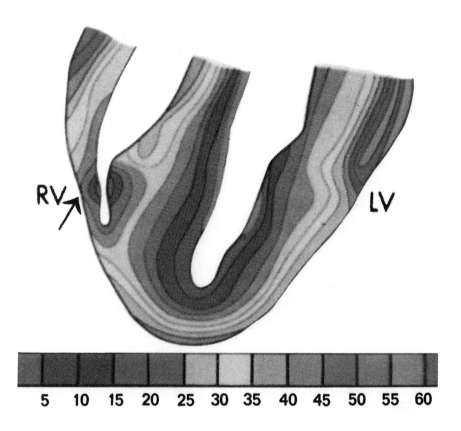

Fig. 11-5. Isochronic representation of normal activation of an isolated human heart displayed on a base-to-apex cross section. Each color represents a 5-ms interval (color scheme is shown at the bottom of the figure). RV = right ventricle; LV = left ventricle; arrow points to the site of right ventricular epicardial breakthrough. From Durrer et al. {17}, with permission.

electrocardiographic sources during the excitation process. Electrically these sources can be characterized as double layers.

For a typical propagation velocity of 50 cm/s and a rise time of 1 ms for the rising phase (phase 0) of the action potential, the spatial extent of the rising phase is (1 ms) * (50 cm/s) = 0.5 mm (a schematic description is provided in fig. 11-6). For each cell within this active region, the strength of the double-layer source in the membrane is not uniform (since V_m is not constant) and the integral expression (11-8) yields a finite (nonzero) contribution to the external potential. By superposition, the individual cellular double layers in this region of activation can be combined and replaced by an average dipole moment per unit volume. Since the extent of the rising phase is small compared with the wall thickness, it can be regarded as a two-dimensional surface of activation

(isochrone) that constitutes a double layer. A formal description of this averaging procedure can be obtained {18} by redefining the membrane discontinuity function, $\Delta\Psi = \Psi_i - \Psi_o$, to be an average of all values over the dimensions of a cell. With this definition, $\Delta\Psi$ becomes a volume function that exists at all points and is not restricted to the cell surfaces. As a result of this property, the divergence theorem {19} can be used to convert the surface integral [eq. (11-6)] to a volume integral:

$$\Psi = -\frac{1}{4\pi} \int_v \nabla \cdot \left[(\Psi_i - \Psi_o)\nabla\left(\frac{1}{r}\right) \right] dv \qquad (11\text{-}9)$$

Using the vector identity

$$\nabla \cdot (\Phi\vec{A}) = \vec{A} \cdot \nabla\Phi + \Phi\nabla \cdot \vec{A},$$

and noting that $r \neq 0$ for extracellular field points so that $\nabla^2(1/r) = 0$, we obtain

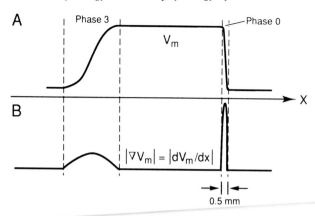

Fig. 11-6. Schematic representation of equivalent electrical sources associated with an action potential. **A:** Idealized spatial action potential, propagating in the positive × direction. **B:** Magnitude (absolute value) of the gradient of V_m, which is proportional to the volume dipole source density. Note that the source density is zero during the (idealized) plateau phase and that the source density is more confined in space and of much higher magnitude during depolarization (QRS) than during repolarization (T wave).

$$\Psi = -\frac{1}{4\pi} \int_v \nabla(\Psi_i - \Psi_o) \cdot \nabla\left(\frac{1}{r}\right) dv \qquad (11\text{-}10)$$

Using the definition of Ψ [eq. (11-3)]

$$\Phi_o = -\frac{1}{4\pi\sigma_o} \int_v \nabla(\sigma_i\Phi_i - \sigma_o\Phi_o) \cdot \nabla\left(\frac{1}{r}\right) dv \qquad (11\text{-}11)$$

where integration is over the volume of cardiac tissue. We can now define

$$\vec{j} = \nabla(\sigma_i\Phi_i - \sigma_o\Phi_o) \qquad (11\text{-}12)$$

which is identified as the (space-averaged) volume dipole moment source density. As stated above, during activation

this volume density can be approximated by a surface density (double layer) associated with the activation fronts in the heart.

Equation (11-12) relates the distribution and strength of the cardiac sources to the spatial behavior of the intracellular (Φ_i) and extracellular (Φ_o) potentials. With certain simplifications it could be related directly to the transmembrane action potential, V_m. If $\sigma_i = \sigma_o$ or if the extracellular space is extensive (i.e., $\Phi_o \ll \Phi_i$ and $V_m = \Phi_i - \Phi_o \approx \Phi_i$) then

$$\vec{j} = \sigma_i \nabla V_m$$

Note that $\nabla V_m = 0$ and the source density is zero in regions where V_m does not vary spatially (i.e., where cells are at rest or in an idealized plateau state). These regions do not contribute, therefore, to the extracellular potential field. In contrast, V_m is steep and ∇V_m is large, implying a large source density in regions that are being activated (rising phase of the action potential, phase 0) and that constitute the activation front (fig. 11-6). During the re-polarization phase (phase 3) V_m does vary spatially; however, ∇V_m during this phase is much smaller (~100 times smaller) than during the activation phase, since the change in V_m is much more gradual. Therefore, recovery is associated with a source density that is much smaller than the source density associated with the activation process. Note, however, that the activation sources are concentrated in a shell that is about 0.5 mm thick, while the recovery sources are distributed over the entire heart. As a result, the total source strength is roughly of the same order of magnitude for both processes.

A diagramatic illustration of double-layer activation fronts during ventricular excitation is provided in fig. 11-7. The double-layer strength is assumed uniform on the entire front, and its dipole components are perpendicular to the activation front, pointing toward the resting tissue (in the direction of the normal unit vector n̂). As will be discussed below, this uniform double-layer model is an

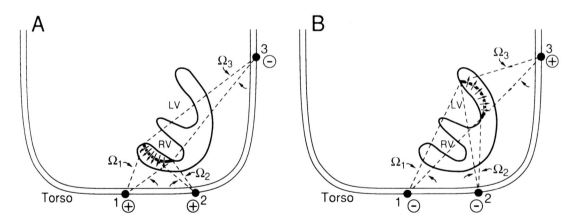

Fig. 11-7. Schematic description of broad double-layer fronts during normal activation of the right ventricle (RV, **A**) and of the left ventricle (LV, **B**). Polarity of potential and solid angles are shown for three torso sites ("ECG electrodes"). Note that polarity (+ or −) reflects orientation of the wavefront relative to the electrode (+ reflects an approaching front while − reflects a receding front). Potential magnitude is proportional to the solid angle.

adequate representation of the sources during normal activation. Solid angles associated with these activation fronts, as viewed from three selected field points ("electrodes") on the body surface, are also shown. Note that the potential magnitude at each "electrode" is proportional to the solid angle, which reflects the extent of the activation front, its orientation relative to the field point, and its proximity to the field point. Polarity of the body surface potentials is also indicated in the figure; the potential ahead of the advancing wave front is positive (+), while behind it the potential is negative (−). This principle, while extremely helpful to the interpretation of ECG potentials measured on the body surface, should be used cautiously. Realistic cardiac activation patterns may involve several simultaneous wave fronts. The potential is a superposition of contributions from all wave fronts and reflects their complex three-dimensional geometry. In addition, for certain activation patterns (e.g., point stimulation) the double layer can not be considered uniform (see below), and the potential ahead of some sections of the wave front may in fact be negative.

Equation (11-12) provides an expression for the cardiac sources in terms of intracellular and extracellular potentials and conductivities. This expression is general and does not require that the myocardium behaves isotropically on a macroscopic scale. During normal ventricular excitation, broad activation fronts are formed early in the process and propagate from endocardium to epicardium in a direction that is perpendicular to the orientation of the myocardial fibers. This implies that, on a macroscopic scale, all parts

of the activation fronts propagate in a direction of low conductivity and slow velocity; that is, in eq. (11-12) σ_i and σ_o in the direction of propagation are constant (or close to constant) everywhere on the wave front. For normal excitation, therefore, the source density $\bar{J}$ [eq. (11-12)] is approximately constant on a given wave front and the equivalent macroscopic cardiac sources can be represented, to a good approximation, as uniform double layers {20}.

The situation is entirely different when one considers the activation front produced by point stimulation (e.g., activation from an ectopic focus). For this condition the wave front is nearly ellipsoidal, with its major axis along the fiber direction (the direction of high conductivity and fast velocity) and its minor axes perpendicular to the fiber direction (the direction of low conductivity and slow velocity; fig. 11-8A). It is clear that different sections of the wave front "see" different conductivities in the direction of propagation, with the extremes being along (highest conductivity) and perpendicular (lowest conductivity) to the fiber direction. The conductivities in eq. (11-12) vary with the position on the wave front and the double-layer source density is no longer uniform. An analysis of the effects of myocardial anisotropy on the strength of the electrical sources can be found in Plonsey and Rudy {21}. An equivalent source representation that incorporates myocardial anisotropy is the oblique dipole-layer model {22,23}. This model consists of a double layer that is situated on the wave front and that can be viewed as the superposition of axial (along fiber direction) and

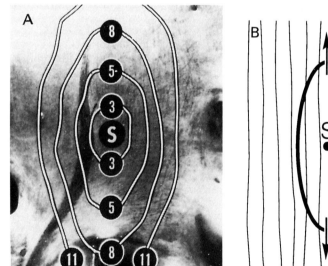
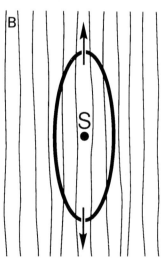
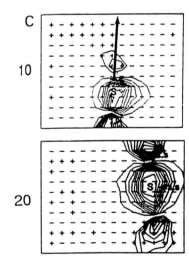

Fig. 11-8. Activation, equivalent sources, and potential patterns associated with point stimulation. **A:** Measured elliptical isochrones reflecting myocardial anisotropy (from Burger and Van Milaan {44}, by permission of the American Heart Association, Inc.). **B:** Hypothetical isochrone with the approximate source configuration of two opposite axial dipoles oriented along fibers. **C:** Measured potential patterns (isopotential maps) associated with point stimulation (top: 10 ms following stimulation; bottom: 20 ms following stimulation). Notice the central minimum with two maxima above and below it, all oriented in the direction of the fibers (indicated by the arrow in the 10 ms map). This pattern reflects the source configuration in panel B. In all panels S is the site of stimulation. (Panel C is from Watabe et al. {25}, by permission of the American Heart Association, Inc.)

transverse (perpendicular to fiber direction) component dipole densities, denoted as m_l and m_t, respectively. In general, the combination of the axial and transverse components results in a dipole layer whose dipoles are oblique to the activation front (unlike the uniform double layer where the dipoles are normal to the front). The potential is the superposition of the contributions from the axial and transverse components:

$$\Phi_o = \frac{1}{4\pi\sigma_o} \int_s [m_l(\hat{n} \cdot \hat{a}_l)\hat{a}_l + m_t(\hat{n} \cdot \hat{a}_t)\hat{a}_t] \cdot \nabla\left(\frac{1}{r}\right)ds. \quad (11\text{-}13)$$
$$\text{axial} \qquad \text{transverse}$$

In this expression, $\hat{n}$ is a unit vector normal to the wave front; $\hat{a}_l$ and $\hat{a}_t$ are unit vectors parallel and perpendicular to the local fiber direction, respectively (all unit vectors point toward the tissue at rest). Note that when the front is parallel to the fibers (propagation is across fibers) $\hat{n} \cdot \hat{a}_l = 0$, $\hat{a}_t = \hat{n}$, and the potential is due to a uniform double layer of density m_t that is normal to the front and to the fiber direction (this is the case during normal ventricular excitation). When the front is perpendicular to the fibers (propagation is along the fiber direction), $\hat{n} \cdot \hat{a}_t = 0$, $\hat{a}_l = \hat{n}$, and the potential is due to a uniform double layer of density m_l that is normal to the front and along the fiber direction. It is shown in Colli-Franzone et al. {22} that the ratio m_l/m_t equals the ratio of the intracellular axial and transverse conductivity coefficients, σ_l^i/σ_t^i, which is typically $9:1$ (in fact, $m_l/m_t \geq 15$ was required to reproduce the measured potential fields in Colli-Franzone et al. {22}). This implies that for point stimulation the maximum axial contribution (at the section of the ellipsoidal wave front that propagates along the fiber) is an order of magnitude greater than the maximum transverse contribution (at the sections of the wave front that propagate across fibers), suggesting that the source can be approximated (for the purpose of computing potentials sufficiently far from the activation front) by two equal and opposite axial dipoles, located on the long axis of the ellipsoidal wave front (fig. 11-8B).

An alternative (and equivalent) form of (11-13) is derived in Colli-Franzone et al. {22} by defining $m_a = m_l - m_t$ and $m_u = m_t$ (the subscripts a and u denote axial and uniform, respectively):

$$\Phi_o = \frac{1}{4\pi\sigma_o} \int_s [m_u\hat{n} + m_a(\hat{n} \cdot \hat{a}_l)\hat{a}_l] \cdot \nabla\left(\frac{1}{r}\right)ds \quad (11\text{-}14)$$
$$\text{uniform} \qquad \text{axial}$$
$$\text{normal}$$

This form represents the source as a superposition of a uniform double layer that is normal to the activation front and a non-uniform, axial double layer. From this perspective the oblique dipole layer model generalizes the classical, uniform double-layer model by adding to it a non-uniform, axial component. As discussed above, the uniform double-layer model provides the basis for the solid angle theory of electrocardiography. Note that the influence of the axial component decreases as the front surface becomes more parallel to the fiber direction since $\hat{n} \cdot \hat{a}_l$ decreases. This situation is realized by extensive

wave fronts, such as those during normal ventricular activation (figs. 11-5 and 11-7), and the use of the uniform double-layer model and of the solid angle theory is justified under these conditions. In contrast, during early ectopic activation the axial component dominates {22}, again suggesting that a simplified representation of the source by two axial dipoles may be used to provide a qualitative description of the potential field. (Note that for a closed wave front the contribution of the uniform component is zero since the solid angle subtended by a closed surface at any exterior point is equal to zero. For this situation, the entire contribution to the potential is from the axial component in eq. (11-14).) An example of the potential field generated by point stimulation is shown in fig. 11-8C. The pattern is characterized by a central negative area and two maxima that are positioned on a straight line that correlates well with the direction of the fibers near the pacing site. Such a pattern reflects the presence of a dominant axial source component in the fiber direction; in fact, similar potential patterns were generated experimentally by two dipoles oriented at $180°$ along a straight line {24}, validating the usefulness of the simple model in fig. 11-8B for a qualitative interpretation of the potentials associated with ectopic activation. A fascinating consequence of this source distribution is the counterclockwise rotation of the potential pattern (i.e., of the straight line connecting the potential maxima) with increasing intramural depth of stimulation relative to the epicardial surface {25}. This rotation reflects the intramural rotation of the fiber direction {16}, which implies a similar rotation of the axial component of the dipole layer source.[2]

We conclude the discussion of the electrocardiographic cardiac sources by reemphasizing that all dipole layer formulations assume the activation front to be a two-dimensional surface (i.e., the thickness of the front is small compared to its distance to the field point). This implies that such models are not suitable for studying the potential in the immediate vicinity of the front. An intracellular current model {13} that does not assume the sources to be restricted to the wave front surface may be more suitable for this purpose. Obviously, an accurate, quantitative description of the field in the vicinity of the front requires a realistic model of the membrane currents and of the anisotropic intracellular-extracellular ("bidomain") structure of the myocardium. However, for the purpose of relating cardiac activity to electrocardiographic potentials in regions that are sufficiently remote from the front, and in particular outside the myocardium and on the body surface, the dipole layer representations of the myocardial sources are extremely useful.

Example: Body surface potentials during normal ventricular activation

The principles and methods described in the previous sections provided the basis for many quantitative simulations of electrocardiographic potentials (the so-called forward problem, see Gulrajani et al. {27} for an extensive review). Notably, Miller and Geselowitz {28} used a stylized action potential along with isochrone data from the normal human heart {17} (some of these data are reproduced in fig. 11-5) to compute the potentials on the surface of a human torso model. The simulated isopotential surface maps were in good agreement with body surface potential distributions measured in normal subjects {29–32}. In the following example we will illustrate how these principles can be used to relate cardiac activity to body surface electrocardiographic potentials in a descriptive and qualitative (rather than quantitative) way. We will base our discussion on activation data of the human heart {17}, simultaneous recordings of body surface and epicardial potentials obtained in the chimpanzee {33} (whose chest geometry resembles the human), and the Miller–Geselowitz simulation mentioned above.

Figure 11-9 depicts body surface potential maps (BSPMs) generated by normal ventricular activation. Maps at selected time segments during the QRS are shown. BSPMs at the beginning of ventricular activation (fig. 11-9A) are characterized by a positive potential maximum in the upper sternal area and a negative potential region that is more inferior, to the left, and extends posteriorly. This pattern coincides in time with septal activation, which proceeds predominantly from left to right, and in an apical-basal direction (see fig. 11-5) {17}. The orientation of the heart in the torso (right ventricle more anterior than the left ventricle; see fig. 11-11) adds a posterior-anterior component relative to the torso. In terms of equivalent sources, a double-layer activation front is advancing from left to right, in an apical-basal direction, and is oriented somewhat posterior-anterior relative to the torso. As stated earlier (see fig. 11-7), potentials ahead of the front are positive and potentials behind it are negative. This explains the potential pattern on the body surface.

As activation progresses (fig. 11-9B) the maximum gradually moves inferiorly and to the left, while the minimum migrates posteriorly and then towards the right shoulder. This pattern coincides in time with endocardial to epicardial propagation of activation fronts in the walls of both ventricles (fig. 11-5); the gradual migration of the maximum downward and to the left probably reflects increasing dominance of the very extensive left ventricular fronts relative to the less extensive right ventricular fronts. A striking event is the sudden appearance of an intense and highly localized minimum in the upper sternal area (fig. 11-9B, 28 ms; in fact, this negative minimum is preceded by a decrease of positive potentials in the same location already at 26 ms and 24 ms). The appearance of this minimum is a reflection, on the body surface, of right ventricular epicardial breakthrough (fig. 11-5).

Double-layer activation fronts in the right ventricle just before breakthrough and immediately after breakthrough are shown diagramatically in fig. 11-10 (this diagram is based on the isochrones of fig. 11-5). Prior to breakthrough the surface potential in the sternal area is positive, due mostly to the proximity of the front advancing toward the breakthrough point (fig. 11-10A). The septal front contributes negative potential and acts to cancel part of the positive contribution from the free wall front, attenuating

the magnitude of the positive surface potential. However, its contribution is smaller since it is more remote from the surface field point (see fig. 11-11) and the potential (solid angle) decreases with the square of the distance. Note that the contribution from left ventricular activation to the surface potential in the sternal region is also relatively small due to the distance effect (fig. 11-11) and the large degree of cancellation between the free wall and septal fronts (fig. 11-5). Once breakthrough has occurred, a "window" is formed in the right ventricular free wall front (fig. 11-10B). The sternal region above the breakthrough point is now influenced mostly by the receding wave fronts in the free wall and in the septum, and a local minimum develops in this region.

Later during activation, the potential maximum shifts posteriorly (fig. 11-9C), reflecting activation of the posterior left ventricle. Finally, a new maximum appears in the upper sternal area and extends to the right shoulder (fig. 11-9D), reflecting the late activation of the pulmonary conus and of the posterobasal area of the right ventricle (fig. 11-5) {17}.

EFFECTS OF THE THORACIC VOLUME CONDUCTOR ON ELECTROCARDIOGRAPHIC BODY SURFACE POTENTIALS

The electrical activity of cardiac muscle cells is projected to the surface of the torso by means of the intervening conducting medium. The surface potentials that are recorded as electrocardiograms reflect, therefore, the properties of both the heart electrical generators (discussed in the previous section) and the surrounding passive volume conductor. Since the goal of electrocardiography is to reconstruct cardiac electrical events from body surface potential data, understanding the role played by the torso volume conductor in determining the surface potential distribution is essential. The major part of this section deals with the results of a theoretical simulation in which the electrocardiographic volume conductor is represented by a spherical "heart" eccentrically located in a spherical "torso." This idealized model permits a systematic study of the effects of the various torso compartments (inhomogeneities) on the electrocardiogram. Results of other theoretical and experimental studies, as well as electrocardiographic clinical observations, are discussed in relation to the findings of the eccentric spheres model. The section dealing with the model simulations is preceded by a discussion of the electrical properties of the various torso inhomogeneities and their representation in terms of equivalent sources. Similar presentation of this material can be found in Rudy {34}.

Electrical properties of the torso volume conductor

QUASI-STATIC APPROXIMATION

Although the bioelectric sources within the myocardium are time varying, most of the models that describe the potential fields generated by these sources in the sur-

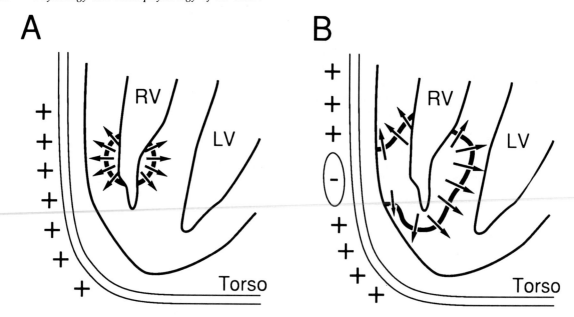

Fig. 11-10. Double-layer activation fronts in the right ventricle (schematic description based on fig. 11-5). **A:** Prior to break-through. **B:** Immediately after breakthrough. + and − indicate polarity of potential on the torso surface. The breakthrough "window" that is formed in the activation front is reflected as a local negative minimum (indicated by −) in the surface potential.

rounding volume conductor are static. In fact, they consider the spatial distribution of the sources at a certain instant of time, and solve for the potential distribution assuming steady-state conditions. The justification for this simplified representation of the electrophysiological system is considered in an article by Plonsey and Heppner {35} and will be reviewed here.

Since the emphasis in this chapter is on the volume conductor fields, we adopt an average macroscopic description of the cardiac sources by specifying an applied current density $\vec{J}$. For simplicity the time variation is assumed to be harmonic at an angular frequency ω. Under the assumption that the medium is linear, any arbitrary time variation can then be considered by using a Fourier series or integral representation.

For a linear, homogeneous, and isotropic medium the electric (scalar) and magnetic (vector) potentials are given by {6}

$$\Phi(x',y',z') = \frac{1}{4\pi(\sigma + j\omega\varepsilon)} \int_v \frac{-\nabla \cdot \vec{J}(x,y,z)e^{-jkR}}{R} dv \quad (11\text{-}15a)$$

$$\vec{A}(x',y',z') = \frac{\mu}{4\pi} \int_v \frac{\vec{J}(x,y,z)e^{-jkR}}{R} dv \quad (11\text{-}15b)$$

where $R^2 = (x - x')^2 + (y - y')^2 + (z - z')^2$. In the above (x,y,z) is the source point and (x',y',z') is the field point; ε (permitivity), μ (permeability), and σ (conductivity) are the physical parameters characterizing the medium; and

$$k^2 = \omega^2 \varepsilon \mu \left(1 + \frac{\sigma}{j\omega\varepsilon}\right).$$

The electric field is found from the scalar and vector potentials Φ and $\vec{A}$ by

$$\vec{E} = -j\omega\vec{A} - \nabla\Phi. \quad (11\text{-}15c)$$

Equations (11-15) can be simplified by making several assumptions using data relating to the electrical properties of biological materials. The assumptions involve the following phenomena: capacitive effects, propagation effects, inductive effects, and boundary conditions.

Capacitive effects

A conductive medium is characterized by its conductivity and permitivity. In eq. (11-15a), the coefficient $(\sigma + j\omega\varepsilon)$ can be written as $\sigma_c = \sigma(1 + j\omega\varepsilon/\sigma)$, where σ_c is a complex conductivity that includes displacement effects as well as pure conductivity. For quasi-static conditions to prevail, the medium must be purely resistive. Measurements by Schwan and Kay {36} show that $|j\omega\varepsilon/\sigma| < 0.15$ over the physiological range of frequencies. σ_c can therefore be approximated fairly well by σ and the medium can be considered purely resistive.

Propagation effects

Propagation effects are represented by the term e^{-jkR} in (11-15). Since

$$e^{-jkR} = 1 - jkR - \frac{(kR)^2}{2!} - j\frac{(kR)^3}{3!} + \dots,$$

these effects can be neglected if $|kR| \ll 1$. Setting the magnitude of $(1 + j\omega\varepsilon/\sigma)$ equal to the conservative value $\sqrt{2}$, and taking the highest component frequency of significance as 10^3 Hz; R_{max} as 1 m (an overall dimension of the human body); σ as 0.2 mho/m (a representative mean

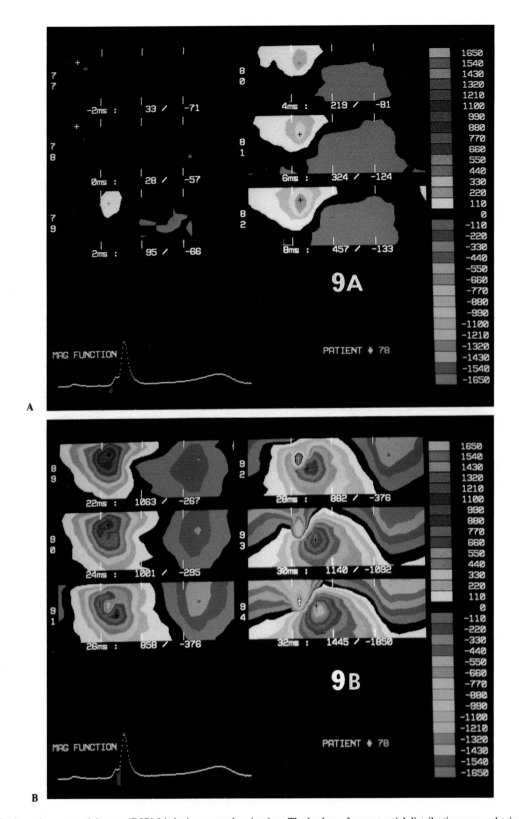

Fig. 11-9. Body surface potential maps (BSPMs) during normal activation. The body surface potential distributions were obtained with our 180-electrode mapping system. Potential levels are displayed as different colors (yellow to red are increasing positive potentials; green to blue are increasing negative potentials; the color scale on the right of each panel is in microvolts). Each panel displays six maps that are 2 ms apart (starting from the left top map and ending with the right, bottom map). The interval during the QRS covered by the six maps is indicated by the red segment on the MAG FUNCTION ECG trace. The times from the beginning of the QRS (in milliseconds) and the maximum and minimum potential values (in microvolts) are displayed below each map. Each map is divided into four segments, from left to right: right chest, left chest, left back, right back. **A:** Beginning of ventricular activation. The positive

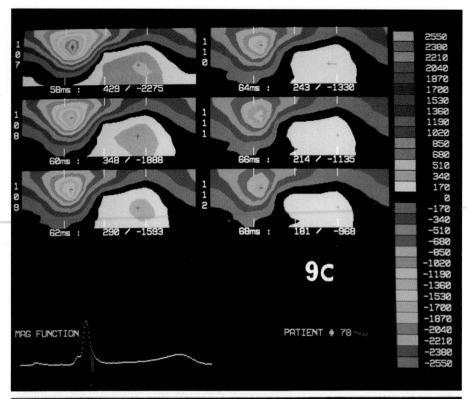

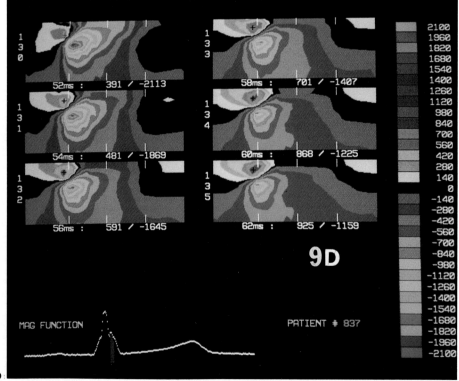

potential maximum in the upper sternal area and the negative region that is left inferior and extends posteriorly reflect early septal activation. **B:** Right ventricular epicardial breakthrough. The appearance of a "notch" in the anterior positive potential (26 ms, left, bottom map) and its development into a very localized anterior minimum (green "window" at 28 ms, right, top map) reflect right ventricular epicardial breakthrough. This minimum becomes more extensive and of higher amplitude as breakthrough progresses (30 ms and 32 ms, middle and bottom maps on right). **C:** Late ventricular activation. The posterior maximum and anterior minimum reflect activation of the posterior left ventricle. **D:** Late ventricular activation. The maximum in the upper sternal-right shoulder area reflects late activation of the pulmonary conus and of the posterobasal area of the right ventricle.

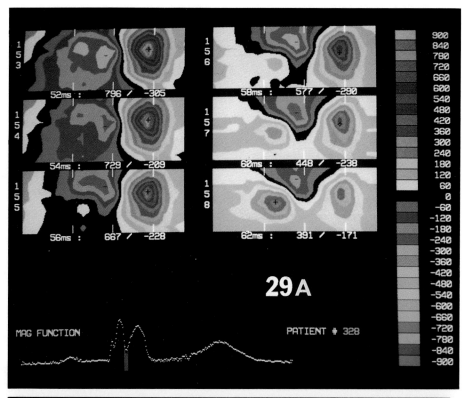

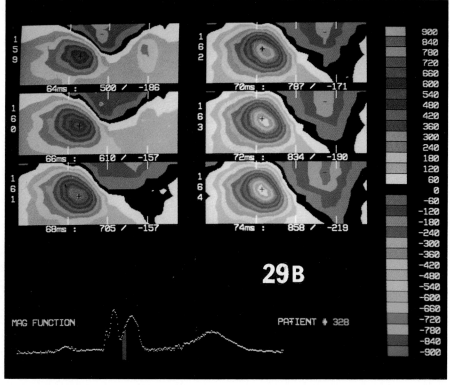

Fig. 11-29. Examples of regional cardiac events that are reflected in the body surface potential distribution. Format is the same as that in fig. 11-9. **A,B:** Right bundle branch block (RBBB). The posterior maximum (A, left column) reflects late stage of left ventricular activation. This maximum diminishes in amplitude, while a second anterior maximum develops (A, right column), reflecting the beginning of activation in the right ventricle. At 62 ms (A, right, bottom map) two distinct (posterior and anterior) potential maxima are present, reflecting activation in the left ventricle and right ventricle, respectively. While the posterior maximum diminishes in amplitude and finally disappears (reflecting completion of left ventricular activation), the anterior maximum increases in amplitude,

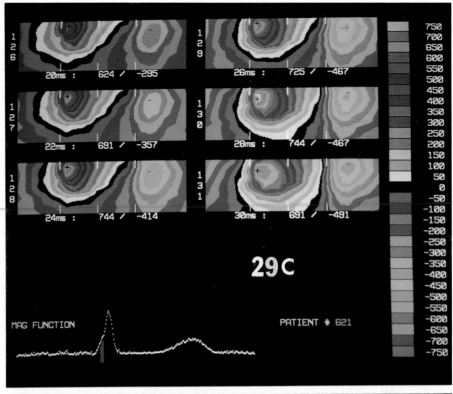

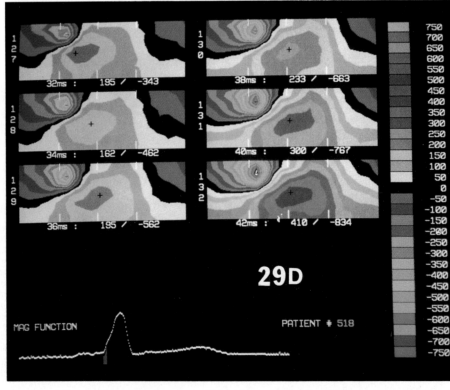

reflecting the late onset of right ventricular activation and the sequential nature of cardiac excitation (right ventricle after left ventricle) in RBBB. **C,D:** Wolff-Parkinson-White Syndrome. In C, the potential distribution (posterior minimum and anterior maximum) reflects an activation front traveling from posterior to anterior. The posterior location of the potential minimum corresponds to a preexcitation site along the atrioventricular groove in the posterior left ventricle. In D, the potential distribution reflects activation from right-superior to left-inferior and a preexcitation site at the anteroseptal right ventricle. The predicted locations of the preexcitation sites were confirmed during surgery. See Liebman et al. {104} for detail.

value of biological tissues); and μ as the permeability of free space, i.e., $\mu = \mu_o = 4\pi \times 10^{-7}$ Henry/m (noting the absence of magnetic materials in the body), we obtain

$$kR_{max} = (1 - j) \cdot \sqrt{2000\pi \cdot 4\pi \cdot 10^{-7} \cdot 0.2} = 0.0397(1 - j).$$

Thus, as an upper bound e^{-jkR} is unity to within 4%, and the phase-angle error of 0.0397 rad. (2.3°) is negligible. We can state, therefore, that propagation effects can be neglected and that changes at the source can be considered to be instantaneously detected at a field point.

Inductive effects

The component of electric field that arises from magnetic induction is given in (11-15c) by the term $j\omega \vec{A}$. By considering a differential current source element, Plonsey and Heppner {35} have shown that

$$\left| \frac{\omega A}{\nabla \Phi} \right| = |kR|^2,$$

and hence the inductive component in (11-15c) is negligible relative to $\nabla\Phi$ if $|kR|^2 \ll 1$. The criterion for ignoring propagation effects was that $|kR| \ll 1$. Since this criterion was shown to be satisfied by the physiological system under consideration, conditions for neglecting inductive effects are automatically met.

Boundary conditions

The conclusions obtained so far are readily generalized to an inhomogeneous medium. Thus the approximations that were shown to be valid in a homogeneous system can also be used in a region composed of several subregions, each of which is homogeneous but has a conductivity value different from the others. In electrocadiography, the medium actually consists of such subregions (lungs, muscle, blood, fat, etc.) that are approximately homogeneous, and hence the criteria described above are met in the real electrocardiographic system. Since boundaries between subregions are included in the system, boundary conditions at these interfaces must be examined.

At each interface between regions of different conductivity the potential and normal component of total current (conduction plus displacement) must be continuous (since the total current is solenoidal, i.e., $\nabla.\vec{J}_T = 0$). The rigorous condition involving the current can be written

$$\sigma_1\left(1 + \frac{j\omega\varepsilon_1}{\sigma_1}\right)E_{1_n} = \sigma_2\left(1 + \frac{j\omega\varepsilon_2}{\sigma_2}\right)E_{2_n} \qquad (11\text{-}16)$$

where σ_i is the conductivity of region i, and E_{i_n} is the normal electric field in region i, at the interface.

Since the displacement current can be ignored, as discussed in the section on capacitive effects, this condition reduces to

$$\sigma_1 E_{1_n} = \sigma_2 E_{2_n} \qquad (11\text{-}17)$$

which is the same expression as that obtained for stationary conditions. If one region has zero conductivity (i.e., the air

in which the body is embedded), we can use $\sigma_2 = 0$ in (11-16) to obtain

$$\sigma_1\left(1 + \frac{j\omega\varepsilon_1}{\sigma_1}\right)E_{1_n} = j\omega\varepsilon_2 E_{2_n} \qquad (11\text{-}18)$$

Since ε_2 is a free space dielectric constant, we utilize $\varepsilon_2 = \varepsilon_0 = 9 \times 10^{-12}$ farad/m, and with $\omega = 2000\pi$ and $\sigma_1 = 0.2$ mho/m, $\omega\varepsilon_2/\sigma_1 = 3 \times 10^{-7}$, which is clearly negligible. Thus it seems reasonable to assume that $E_{1_n} \sim 0$, which follows directly from the "static" form of the boundary condition (11-17) for $\sigma_2 = 0$.

In view of the above discussion, we can conclude that the electrocardiographic problem can be treated at any instant of time as if steady-state conditions were in effect; that is, at each instant of time the potential field satisfies Poisson's equation, and the boundary conditions are those that would exist if the source were stationary.

ELECTRICAL RESISTIVITY OF THORACIC TISSUES

The validity of the quasi-static approximation in the electrocardiographic problem implies that the (inhomogeneous) thoracic medium can be characterized as purely resistive. Quantitative knowledge of the resistivities of the various tissues within the thorax is therefore necessary to analyze the effects of internal inhomogeneities on surface potentials. A large amount of data on the resistivities of body tissues are available in the literature (see the Geddes and Baker compendium {37}), but the resistivity values are not always consistent, and the results reported by different investigators may spread over a wide range.

Two sets of exhaustive resistivity measurements in living animals were performed by Rush and associates {38} and by Schwan and Kay {36,39}. Both utilized techniques that minimize the nonlinear effect of electrode polarization {40} on the results. Schwan and Kay made theoretical corrections for the effect of polarization impedance. Rush and colleagues, on the other hand, used the "four-electrode" technique, which overcomes the polarization effect by using a constant-current source at the current electrodes, and a very high input impedance voltmeter at the potential measuring electrodes. Furthermore, both experiments were made under similar and well-controlled conditions. The following discussion concentrates on these two studies and is based, for the most part, on an excellent review of the subject by Rush and Nelson {41}.

Blood

The resistivity of blood is dependent on the percentage of blood volume occupied by the red cells (hematocrit). With fewer red blood cells, the resistivity is lower, confirming the view that the cells, because of their high-resistivity membranes, act as insulating bodies at low frequencies.

The effect of red blood cells on the resistivity of whole blood has been evaluated both theoretically and experimentally. Maxwell {42} derived an equation for a suspension of homogeneous insulating spheres in a conducting medium relating the combined resistivity of the suspension to the percentage of volume occupied by the spheres (hematocrit in the case of blood). The theoretical expression was modified later to account for various shapes of cells (see {43} for review), and the general relation is given by

$$\rho = \frac{\rho_o(f + H)}{f(1 - H)},$$

where ρ_o is the resistivity of serum, f is a form factor (for spheres f = 2, for cylinders f = 1, and for the shape of normal red cells f = 1.35), and H is the hematocrit. Experimentally the effect of red cell concentration on blood conductivity was measured in a series of dilution experiments {44}. The correspondence between the aforementioned theory and the experimental results is excellent.

In neither of the studies by Schwan and Kay, and Rush and associates, was blood resistivity measured. Rush and associates found it to be unnecessary in view of the good agreement between the results obtained in several different measurements {44,46}. The result obtained in these three studies for the resistivity of normal hematocrit blood at 37°C was 160 Ω-cm. Other studies {47,48}, not mentioned in the work by Rush and associates, all agree with this result.

Cardiac muscle

The results of the four-electrode measurements performed by Rush and associates show an anisotropy of about 2:1, with a high resistivity value of 563 Ω-cm and a low resistivity value of 252 Ω-cm. These results are considerably lower than the value of 965 Ω-cm obtained by Schwan and Kay using their catheterlike two-electrode system. According to a theoretical analysis by Rush {49}, the effective "random" value (referring to the random orientation of cell fibers in relation to the electric field) measured by Schwan and Kay should be somewhere around the geometric mean of the high and low resistivity values, i.e., ~430 Ω-cm arising from the four-electrode measurements. In order to investigate the origin of the remaining discrepancy, Rush and associates {38} employed a catheter electrode similar to that used by Schwan and Kay, and determined the resistivity value to be 516 Ω-cm before correcting for polarization effects (a procedure that will reduce the measured resistivity even further). Thus there is actually only a fairly small discrepancy between the results obtained by Rush using the four-electrode technique and the two-electrode system. Moreover, when the dog was killed by injection of nembutal, a rapid rise in resistivity (25% increase in 15 minutes) was observed toward the 800–1000 Ω-cm range measured by Schwan and Kay. Since the heart muscle measurements were taken by Schwan and Kay following poisoning of the experimental animal and cessation of all cardiac electrical activity, the high values obtained could be explained in this way. The last observation, together with the fact that both two- and four-electrode techniques gave essentially the same result in the living animal, seems to be a convincing proof of the validity of the lower resistivity values obtained by Rush and associates.

Lung

The resistivity measurements of lung tissue were performed by Rush and associates in an open-chested dog with the lungs under forced ventilation (duplicating breathing pressures during normal respiration). The electrodes were placed on the outside surface of the lung. In Schwan and Kay's experiment, on the other hand, the electrode holder was inserted through the trachea in the intact dog and placed in one of the smaller bronchi. The results obtained were 2170 Ω-cm (the Rush group) and 1120 Ω-cm (Schwan and Kay; mean values over the breathing cycle), i.e., a 2:1 difference in values. The low values of the latter measurements may be attributed to the uncertain conditions around the electrodes (location, collection of fluid, proximity to major blood vessels, and possible collapse of the lung about the plugged airway) and/or to the fact that the interior of the lung around the bronchi actually may have a lower mean resistivity than the regions nearer the outer lung surfaces.

Skeletal muscle

The skeletal muscle layer is highly anisotropic and the results obtained by the Rush group are 2300 and 150 Ω-cm in direction transverse and parallel, respectively, to the muscle fibers. Using the analysis of Rush {49}, the "random" value predicted for the Schwan and Kay measurement is in fairly good agreement with their actual result of 965 Ω-cm.

Fat

The results obtained by the Rush group show a value of 2500 Ω-cm, which is representative of the values obtained by several other groups, including Schwan and Kay.

After considering the effects of anisotropy on skeletal muscle, and the effects of death on the cardiac muscle resistivity, the two sets of measurements discussed above are in close agreement, except for lung tissue, where the difference may be attributed to the different locations of the electrodes in these two studies. The Rush and associates data, which will be used for typical resistivity values in the eccentric spheres model simulations, are given in table 11-1.

INHOMOGENEITIES — EQUIVALENT
SOURCES FORMULATION[3]

The final conclusion of the first section was that although the cardiac sources are time varying, the problem is a quasi-static one in a homogeneous system as well as in the more realistic system composed of several subregions, each of which is of a different (constant) conductivity value. A consequence of the above is that

$$\vec{E} = -\nabla\Phi \qquad (11\text{-}19)$$

Table 11-1. Thoracic tissue resistivities

Tissue		Resistivity (Ω cm)
Blood		162
Heart[a]	High	563
	Low	252
Lung		2150
Skeletal muscle[a]	High	2300
	Low	150
Fat		2500

[a] High and low refer to high and low resistivities of anisotropic tissue.
From Rush et al. {38,41}.

[the inductive component in eq. (11-15c) can be neglected]. In an infinite, homogeneous volume conductor we have

$$\Phi = \frac{1}{4\pi\sigma} \int_v \frac{-\nabla \cdot \vec{J}}{R} \, dv \qquad (11\text{-}20)$$

[since $|e^{-jkR}| \sim 1$, and $|j\omega\varepsilon| \ll \sigma$ in (11-15a)]. Taking the Laplacian of eq. (11-20) yields

$$\nabla^2 \Phi = \frac{\nabla \cdot \vec{J}}{\sigma} \qquad (11\text{-}21)$$

which is Poisson's equation with a source term $(\nabla \cdot \vec{J})/\sigma$. Under the same quasi-static conditions, the boundary conditions at each interface between regions of different conductivity are

$$\Phi_1 = \Phi_2 \qquad (11\text{-}22)$$

(continuity of potential),

$$\sigma_1 E_{1_n} = \sigma_2 E_{2_n} \qquad (11\text{-}23)$$

(continuity of normal component of current).
Using (11-19), (11-23) can be written as

$$-\sigma_1 \frac{\partial \Phi_1}{\partial n} = -\sigma_2 \frac{\partial \Phi_2}{\partial n}. \qquad (11\text{-}24)$$

Equations (11-22) and (11-24) can be expressed in terms of the scalar function $\Psi = \sigma\Phi$ that was introduced earlier [eq. (11-3)]. Since σ is constant in each subregion, it follows from (11-21) that

$$\nabla^2 \Psi = \sigma \nabla^2 \Phi = \nabla \cdot \vec{J}$$

and Ψ is solution to Poisson's equation. The boundary conditions of eqs. (11-22) and (11-24) when considered with respect to Ψ become

$$\Psi_2 - \Psi_1 = \sigma_2 \Phi_2 - \sigma_1 \Phi_1 = (\sigma_2 - \sigma_1)\Phi_1 \qquad (11\text{-}25)$$

$$\frac{\partial \Psi_1}{\partial n} = \frac{\partial \Psi_2}{\partial n} \qquad (11\text{-}26)$$

Thus, at each interface Ψ is discontinuous, while its normal derivative is continuous. This type of behavior characterizes a double layer of strength equal to the discontinuity in Ψ, placed at the interface location in an equivalent homogeneous medium. The potential field due to such a double layer is given by [see eqs. (11-6) and (11-7)]

$$\Psi_i = \frac{1}{4\pi} \int_{s_i} \Phi_i (\sigma_{i_2} - \sigma_{i_1}) \nabla \left(\frac{1}{R}\right) \cdot d\vec{s_i}. \qquad (11\text{-}27)$$

Replacing Ψ by $\sigma\Phi$, and including all the interfaces as well as the primary source field, we have

$$\Phi(p) = \frac{1}{4\pi\sigma_p} \left(\int_v \frac{-\nabla \cdot \vec{J}}{R} dv \right. \qquad (11\text{-}28)$$
$$\left. + \sum_i \int_{s_i} \Phi_i (\sigma_{i_2} - \sigma_{i_1}) \nabla \left(\frac{1}{R}\right) \cdot d\vec{s_i} \right)$$

where $\Phi(p)$ is the potential at an arbitrary point p, and σ_p is the conductivity at that point. The first integral represents the contribution of the primary cardiac sources, while the second integral represents the (double-layer) secondary sources that arise at the interfaces between regions of different conductivities in the torso.

Effects of torso inhomogeneities on body surface potentials (results of the eccentric spheres model simulations)

The torso volume conductor consists of several compartments of different conductivity (fig. 11-11). The heart consists of the blood cavities bounded by the myocardium and the very thin pericardium. The intracavitary blood has the highest conductivity of any tissue within the thorax — its value[4] (at normal hematocrit) is $\sigma_1 = 0.006$ mho/cm. It is surrounded by the myocardium, whose conductivity is one-third that of blood, i.e., $\sigma_2 = 0.002$ mho/cm (an average value of the "high" and "low" conductivities of this anisotropic tissue). The pericardium[5] is a very thin resistive layer and can be considered as two-dimensional membrane of resistance $1000 \Omega\text{-cm}^2$. The entire heart structure is enveloped by the very extensive lung region, which is a poor conductor, having a conductivity of $\sigma_3 = 0.0005$ mho/cm (an average over a respiratory cycle). Surrounding the lung region is the high-conductivity skeletal muscle shell. This tissue is highly anisotropic, having a "high" resistivity value $\rho_h = 2300 \Omega\text{-cm}$, and a "low" resistivity value $\rho_l = 150 \Omega\text{-cm}$. It can be shown {52} that 1-cm anisotropic muscle layer with resistivities as described becomes equivalent, under a scale transformation, to a 3-cm thick isotropic layer with resistivity of $800 \Omega\text{-cm}$ (conductivity $\sigma_4 = 0.00125$ mho/cm). Finally, the outermost layer is the subcutaneous fat. Its electrical characteristics are similar to those of the lung; it is a poor conductor, having a conductivity $\sigma_5 = 0.0004$ mho/cm.

In addition to the electrical characteristics described above, the geometry is another important factor in determining the current flow in the volume conductor and the surface potential distribution. In particular, the location of the heart, in which the sources are contained, must have a significant effect. A very prominent geometrical characteristic is the eccentricity of the heart within the torso and its proximity to the anterior chest wall.

The eccentric spheres model of the heart-torso system shown in fig. 11-12 was used in our simulation studies. This model is simple enough so that analytic solutions for the potentials can be obtained. Nevertheless, the model is reasonably sophisticated with respect to the conductivity

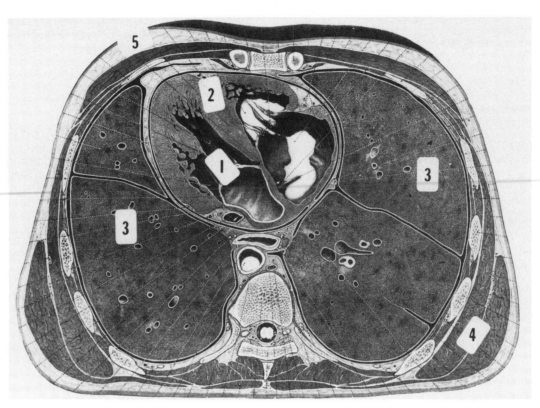

Fig. 11-11. A cross section of the human torso: 1, blood cavity; 2, myocardium; 3, lung; 4, skeletal muscle; 5, subcutaneous fat. From Eycleshymer HC, Schoemaker DM: *A Cross Section Anatomy.* New York: Appleton Century Crofts, 1911, with permission.

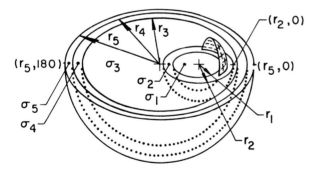

Fig. 11-12. The eccentric spherical model of the inhomogeneous torso. The double layer source is marked by + and − signs on its positive and negative surfaces, respectively. For normal values of conductivity (σ) see text. The eccentricity (distance between heart center and torso center) is typically 5 cm. From Rudy and Plonsey {60}, by permission of the American Heart Association, Inc.

and geometrical factors described above. The model consists of two eccentric systems of concentric spheres. The heart is represented as a sphere consisting of a central blood volume bounded by a spherical heart-muscle shell and pericardium; the heart, in turn, is placed eccentrically within a spherical torso, which includes a lung region bounded by spherical muscle and fat layers. The source of the field is a double-layer spherical cap lying concentrically within the myocardium, representing an activation wave. The direction of the double layer is radial, and since the spread of activation in the left ventricular wall during normal excitation is mainly from endocardium to epicardium, this is a realistic representation of the source during most of the QRS. The idealized spherical geometry is necessary for obtaining an analytic solution to the problem. Such a solution makes possible the inclusion of many inhomogeneous compartments in the model, and the easy manipulation of conductivities and geometrical parameters (such as the size of the heart, its location within the torso, the dimensions of the various torso compartments, etc.). The method of obtaining the analytic expressions for the potential field has been described in detail {53}.

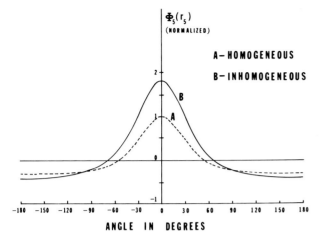

Fig. 11-13. Combined effect of torso inhomogeneities on the surface potential distribution generated by a double layer located endocardially. The potential is plotted as a function of the polar angle Θ. $\Theta = 0°$ corresponds to the midsternal line; $\Theta = 180°$ and $\Theta = -180°$ is the same point, representing the center of the posterior surface of the thorax. The potential is normalized so that the peak potential in the homogeneous case is unity. From Rudy and Plonsey {53}, with permission.

COMBINED EFFECTS OF THE TORSO INHOMOGENEITIES

The intergrated effect of all the inhomogeneities on the surface potential distribution is sown in fig. 11-13. Two different cases are described: A is the homogeneous case with conductivity everywhere equal to that of the myocardium. Only the body-air interface is included. B describes the complete inhomogeneous case, where all torso compartments are present with their typical values of conductivity. The eccentricity of the spherical heart was $d = 5$ cm. The central angle of the double-layer source was 120°. For this angle the surface area of the double layer is sufficiently extensive so that the source is a reasonable representation of a wave of activation located in the anterior wall of the ventricle.

Several important observations can be made by comparing the homogeneous (A) and the inhomogeneous (B) cases. First, it is apparent that the inhomogeneities do not change the general characteristics of the potential distribution. There is one maximum (at $\Theta = 0°$) and one minimum (at $\Theta = 180°$) in each case; in other words, a "dipolar" surface potential is obtained in the inhomogeneous as well as in the homogeneous case. This result conforms to other studies of this question by other investigators. The conclusion of a theoretical study by Rush {54} is that the appearance of extra peaks in the surface potential caused by the presence of inhomogeneities is possible, in principle, in a three-dimensional model of the torso, but is highly unlikely to result from the inhomogeneities that actually exist. A similar negative conclusion about the possibility that inhomogeneities can cause

the appearance of extra peaks in the surface potential was reached by Taccardi and d'Alche {55}, who considered the effect of the lung inhomogeneity, and by Geselowitz and Ishiwatari {56}, and Okada {57}, who studied the isolated effect of the intracavitary blood mass. A single dipole placed in a dog myocardium by Horan and associates {58} did not generate multiple potential peaks on the torso surface, leading to the same conclusion. A simulation study by Gulrajani and Milloux {59}, utilizing a realistically shaped human torso model, also confirms that the inhomogeneities do not change the general pattern of the potential distribution. We can conclude, therefore, that multipeaked surface potentials reflect nondipolarity in the cardiac electrical source itself rather than influences of the inhomogeneous torso volume conductor.

Another integrated effect of the inhomogeneities is the augmentation of body surface potential magnitudes. For an endocardial location of the double layer (fig. 11-13), with all inhomogeneities included in the model, the peak potential value is almost twice the value obtained for the homogeneous case. The augmentation is caused by the intracavitary blood and (for anterior points on the torso) by the lungs.

An important property of the volume conductor is the *smoothing effect*, illustrated in fig. 11-14 {60}. In this simulation, body surface (A) and epicardial potentials (B) are computed for three different configurations of activation wavefronts. In I the two activation waves are separated by 40°, in II by 80°, and in III by 120°. While the epicardial potential distribution reflects accurately the multi-wavefront nature of the underlying sources, the surface potentials do not. In the simulation, when two activation waves in the anterior part of the spherical myocardium are separated by less than 100° (I and II in fig. 11-14), two discrete maxima arise on the epicardium, whereas only a single broad maximum appears on the body surface. Only when the separation is greater than 100° (III in fig. 11-14) are two discrete maxima apparent on the body surface as well, reflecting the true nature of the myocardial sources. These results clearly demonstrate that surface potential distributions are smoothed out greatly by the torso volume conductor, and provide only a low resolution picture of regional cardiac events. In contrast, epicardial potentials accurately reflect details of the underlying activation pattern. In particular, discrete activation wavefronts are reflected as separate potential maxima on the epicardium. Moreover, the location of these maxima corresponds to the location of the underlying wavefronts.

The smoothing effect of the volume conductor was observed experimentally by King and associates {61} in the intact dog, and by Spach and associates {62,63} in the intact chimpanzee. Simultaneous recordings of body surface and epicardial potentials in the aforementioned studies, as well as a comparison of measured torso potentials with those simulated from epicardial recordings {64}, show that (at many instances) the body surface potential maps are simpler and less detailed than the epicardial maps. It is noted in these studies that potential maps on the anterior torso surface are capable of resolving those

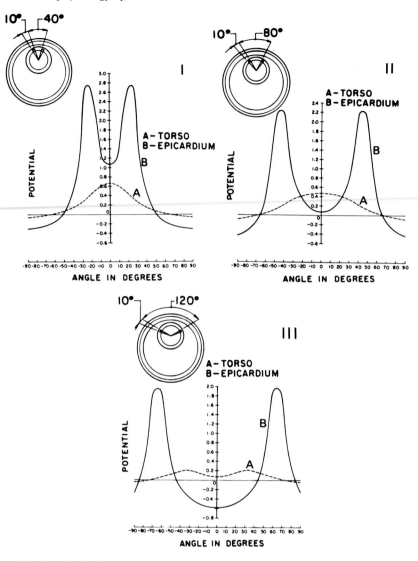

Fig. 11-14. Comparison of body surface (**A**) and epicardial (**B**) potentials originating from two discrete activation wavefronts located in the myocardium. The central angles of the two activation wave fronts are I = 40°, II = 80°, III = 120°. The geometry is illustrated by the cross section of the model in the left upper corner of each graph. From Rudy and Plonsey {60}, by permission of the American Heart Association, Inc.

epicardial extrema whose separation equals or exceeds their distance to the torso. When separation is less than the heart-torso distance, distinct details of epicardial events disappear from the surface potential distribution, in agreement with the theoretical results shown in fig. 11-14. Such conclusions also are supported by the work of Abildskov and colleagues {65}, who studied surface potential distributions arising from stimulated ectopic beats at different sites in the closed-chest dog. The smoothing effect was also demonstrated by Taccardi and associates {66–68} in tank studies of the potential distribution surrounding isolated turtle and dog hearts, as well as in a study of the potential field generated experi-

mentally by two dipoles in a circular homogeneous conducting medium {24}. An isolated, perfused rabbit heart technique was used by Mirvis and associates {69} to assess the ability to detect and localize multiple discrete epicardial events from body surface potential distributions. These researchers conclude that surface potentials accurately depict single and dual generators only if the two sources are sufficiently separated.

The eccentric spheres model simulations, and the experimental results described above, all demonstrate that details of the electrical activity of the heart are smoothed out by the torso volume conductor and do not appear in the body surface potential distribution. In contrast (fig. 11-

14B), epidardial potentials provide a high-resolution, accurate reflection of the underlying myocardial sources. Epicardial potentials permit, therefore, a direct interpretation of electrical events within the heart in a fashion that is not possible from surface distributions, and epicardial potential mapping constitutes a very important research and diagnostic tool.

CONDUCTIVITY EFFECTS

Blood cavity

Unlike the eccentric spheres model and the realistic-geometry model of Gulrajani and Mailloux {59}, most theoretical studies of the inhomogeneities have considered only single compartments of the torso volume conductor. Of these, the high conductivity (three times that of the surrounding myocardium) intracavitary blood is considered to be most influential, and its effect is best understood. This effect was first studied by Brody {70} and is known as the Brody Effect. The principle behind this effect can be readily understood by considering a dipole in a semiinfinite slab of finite conductivity (representing the myocardium) in front of a perfectly conducting slab (representing the high conductivity blood mass) (fig. 11-15a). The boundary conditions at the interface are satisfied by the image system shown in fig. 11-15b. For a dipole oriented normal to the interface ("radial" dipole P_n), the image dipole is of the same strength and in the same direction. In contrast, for the tangential dipole P_t the image is oppositely directed. The effect of the blood is, therefore, to enhance potentials due to radial excitation and to attenuate those due to excitation tangential to the blood cavity. It should be noted that for a more geometrically realistic blood cavity of infinite conductivity (a sphere rather than a semiinfinite

slab), the system of images consists of a dipole and two point sources {71}. The augmentation factor for radial dipoles in this case is 2.4, rather than the factor of 2.0 obtained from the planar geometry of fig. 11-15.

The effects of variations in blood conductivity on body surface potentials, as obtained from the eccentric spheres model, are shown in fig. 11-16 {72}. In this simulation, the conductivity of the intracavitary blood was varied, while all other inhomogeneities were present in the model with their typical (normal) conductivity values. The potential at the mid-anterior point (r_5, 0; see fig. 11-12) is plotted as a function of blood conductivity and hematocrit. Normal refers to the value of conductivity at normal hematocrit. Two different locations of the double-layer activation source are considered, namely, at the endocardium and the epicardium. The condition $\sigma_1 = 0.002$ mho/cm describes the case in which the blood region is homogeneous with the surrounding myocardium. (Under this condition no secondary sources are present at the blood-myocardium interface.) It is clear from fig. 11-16 that the surface potential increases monotonically with increasing blood conductivity (decreasing hematocrit); the effect is more pronounced for an endocardial double-layer source. The enhancement of surface potentials by the intracavitary blood is consistent with the prediction of the idealized system of images of fig. 11-15. As mentioned above, radial dipoles are augmented by the blood cavity. Since the source in the eccentric spheres model is a radial double layer respresenting the normal sequence of activation from endocardium to epicardium, augmentation of surface potentials by the intracavitary blood is to be expected.

The effect of the intracavitary blood mass can be appreciated by comparing the potential obtained for normal blood conductivity ($\sigma_1 = 0.006$ mho/cm) to the potential obtained when the blood conductivity is set equal to that of the surrounding myocardium ($\sigma_1 = \sigma_2 = 0.002$ mho/cm). The latter condition corresponds to the situation where the blood inhomogeneity is not included in the model (and, therefore, no secondary sources at the

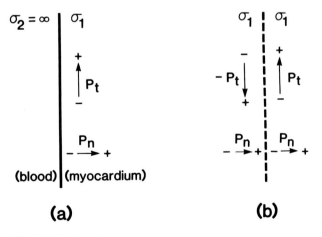

(a)

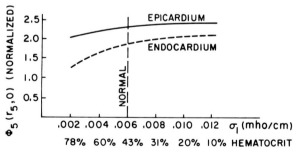

(b)

Fig. 11-15. The effects of a perfectly conducting region on a normal (P_n) and tangential (P_t) dipoles (**a**) The original system; (**b**) the image system that satisfies the correct boundary conditions at the interface and gives the correct field to the right of the boundary. From Rudy {34}, with permission.

Fig. 11-16. The effect of variations in intracavitary blood conductivity (hematocrit) on the surface potential. The potential is adjusted so that it attains a value of unity in the homogeneous case (conductivity everywhere is 0.002 mho/cm). ENDOCARDIUM and EPICARDIUM refer to endocardial and epicardial location of the source, respectively. From Rudy et al. {72}, by permission of the American Heart Association, Inc.

blood-myocardium interface are present). For a double-layer source located endocardially, the potential increases by 46.4% when the intracavitary blood is added. An interesting observation is that when the blood is added to an otherwise homogeneous model (conductivity of 0.002 mho/cm everywhere), the enhancement of the surface potential is 71.96%. This result shows that the net effect of the remaining torso compartments (lungs, skeletal muscle, fat, pericardium) is to diminish the augmentation effect of the blood. The Brody Effect is consequently less important than predicted by models that considered the isolated effect of the blood in an otherwise homogeneous medium {70}. Similar increases in magnitude of surface potentials were observed by Gulrajani and Mailloux {59} during simulated normal excitation.

Clinically, fig. 11-16 simulates the effect of variations in hematocrit on the ECG. Hence, patients with anemia (low hematocrit) are expected to have high surface potentials, whereas potentials lower than normal are expected in patients with polycythemia (high hematocrit). This type of behavior is in agreement with the experiments of Nelson and associates {73}, who studied the effect of variation in hematocrit on the surface potential in the dog. The same behavior was observed by Rosenthal and colleagues {74} in patients with polycythemia or anemia. Reduction of hematocrit in the polycythemic group resulted in increases in magnitude of the left maximal and anterior maximal spatial vectors. Raising the hematocrit in the anemic group decreased the magnitude of these vectors.

Pericardium

The dependence of the body surface potential at the mid-anterior point $(r_5, 0)$ on the conductivity of the pericardium is shown in fig. 11-17 {72}. Two different cases are considered: In A the pericardium is treated as an infinitely thin resistive membrane, whereas in B it is a layer of finite thickness (a thickness of 0.5 cm was chosen). The abscissa is a logarithmic scale of pericardial conductivity values normalized by σ_{pN}, the typical value of pericardial con-

ductivity [σ_{pN} = 0.001 mho/cm^2 for the thin membrane (A) and σ_{pN} = 0.0005 mho/cm for the finite layer (B)]. The potential is adjusted so that a value of unity is obtained for the typical conductivity ($\sigma = \sigma_{pN}$).

In the case of the infinitely thin resistive membrane (A), the potential increases monotonically with increasing conductivity. The behavior of the potential in the finite thickness pericardium case (B) is quite different. The potential attains a maximum at about twice the normal conductivity, and for higher conductivities voltages lower than normal are obtained. The similarity in behavior of both the resistive membrane and the finite layer for low conductivities is not surprising. In the infinitely thin membrane case, all current flow is normal to the pericardium and no tangential component is possible. The current flow in the finite layer of high resistivity behaves in a similar way, since most of the current has to flow radially (normal to the layer), and a tangential flow in this layer is greatly impeded by the high resistivity medium. For high conductivities the current flow through the membrane still is radial, whereas in the finite layer case a significant tangential current flow is possible. This difference accounts for the contrasting behavior of the potentials in A and B over the range of high pericardial conductivities.

The behavior predicted in B was observed experimentally by Manoach and associates {75}. In their experiments, the pericardial sac was filled with either saline (a high conductivity fluid) or olive oil (a poor conductor of electrical current). Since in both cases they measured low QRS voltages (relative to normal values), they concluded that the attenuation of potentials is independent of the conductivity but results from the compression of the heart by the fluid. The results obtained here (B) show that low voltages are to be expected for high as well as low conductivity, and can be explained on the basis of conductivity variations alone. This conclusion was confirmed by Kramer {76} in a set of well-controlled experiments. Similar to Manoach and colleagues, different conductivity fluids were added to the pericardial sac. However, three (rather than two) fluids were used, permitting actual examination of the nonmonotonic behavior of fig. 11-17B. Since all three fluids used (mineral oil, whole blood, and physiological saline) are of approximately the same density, their "compression" effects on the heart should be approximately equal when they are injected into the pericardium in the same volume quantities. In contrast, the conductivities of the three fluids are substantially different ($\sigma_{oil} = 50 \times 10^{-6}$ mho/cm, $\sigma_{blood} = 6 \times 10^{-3}$ mho/cm, and $\sigma_{saline} = 15 \times 10^{-3}$ mho/cm). These density and conductivity properties permit the study of conductivity variation independent of compression changes. The results show the same nonmonotonic behavior predicted by curve B of fig. 11-17, and support the eccentric-spheres model conclusion that this behavior results from conductivity changes rather than "compression" of the heart by the excess fluid. Moreover, the percentage change in body-surface potentials observed experimentally were in excellent quantitative agreement with those predicted by the eccentric-spheres model based on conductivity variations alone.

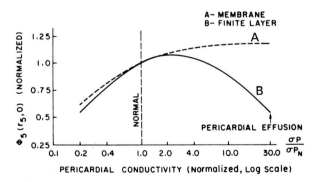

Fig. 11-17. The effect of variations in pericardial conductivity on the surface potential. In **A**, the pericardium is represented by an infinitely thin resistive membrane. In **B**, it is of finite thickness. From Rudy et al. {72}, by permission of the American Heart Association, Inc.

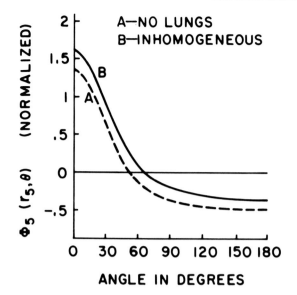

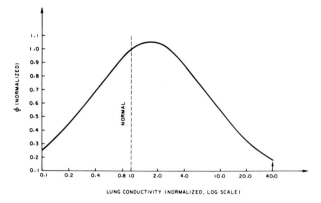

Fig. 11-19. The effect of variations in lung conductivity on the surface potential. The potential is normalized to a value of unity at the typical lung conductivity (NORMAL). The conductivity of physiological saline is indicated by the arrow. From Rudy et al. {86}, by permission of the American Heart Association, Inc.

Fig. 11-18. Effect of the lungs on the surface potential distribution: In **A** the conductivity of the lung region is made equal to that of the cardiac muscle layer. **B** is the complete inhomogeneous case, with the lung region represented in the model. From Rudy and Plonsey {53}, with permission.

In the clinical condition of pericardial effusion, the pericardial space is filled with high-conductivity fluid and constitutes a layer of finite thickness. Under this condition, which is similar to the experimental situation described above, the dependence of the surface potential on the conductivity of the pericardial sac is described by curve B in fig. 11-17. The voltages are low for high as well as low conductivities. The case of pericardial effusion is emphasized by the arrow in the figure, and is for fluid having a conductivity equal to that of plasma. A reduction of ECG potentials is therefore to be expected in patients with pericardial effusion.

Lungs

The low conductivity lung region is the most extensive inhomogeneity in the torso (see fig. 11-11). Together with the posterior mediastinum (also a poor conductor), the lungs envelope the heart, except for an anterior region, where the heart is in contact with the anterior chest wall. This asymmetry is introduced in the model (fig. 11-12) through the eccentric location of the spherical heart in the torso. For an eccentricity of 6 cm the spherical heart actually touches the anterior wall of the spherical torso. Figure 11-18 describes the effect of the lungs on the surface potential distribution. When the lungs are included in the model (B), the potentials at anterior chest points are enchanced (by about 16%), while the magnitude of posterior potentials is slightly reduced. This nonuniform behavior reflects the asymmetry of the lung compartment, which results in channeling of the electrical current in the

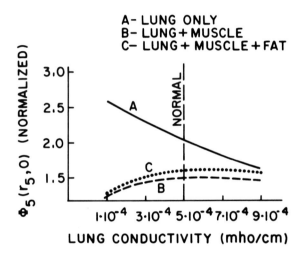

Fig. 11-20. The effect of variations in the conductivity of the lungs on the surface potential. In **A** the surface muscle and fat layers are excluded from the model and the conductivity of these regions is made equal to that of the lung. In **B** the surface muscle layer is included, having its typical conductivity value; whereas in **C** both muscle and fat layers (with their associated typical conductivities) are represented. From Rudy et al. {72}, by permission of the American Heart Association, Inc.

direction of smaller resistance (the anterior direction in this case). Slight magnitude increases in the anterior chest potentials were observed by Gulrajani and Mailloux {59} as well.

The simulated effect of variations in the conductivity of the lungs on the surface potential magnitude is shown in fig. 11-19. The behavior is bell-shaped with low potentials obtained for high as well as low conductivity values[6]. The potential attains a maximum at a conductivity that is very close to normal physiologic values. This nonmonotonic behavior is determined by the lung interaction with the surrounding muscle layer (i.e., by the effect of the secondary sources at the lung-muscle interface), as demonstrated by fig. 11-20 {72}. Three cases are considered: In A, the skeletal muscle and subcutaneous fat layer are made homogeneous with the underlying lung region (i.e., $\sigma_5 = \sigma_4 = \sigma_3 = 0.0005$ mho/cm). Under these conditions the surface potential increases monotonically as lung conductivity decrease. In B, the surface muscle layer is included in the model with its typical conductivity value ($\sigma_4 = 0.00125$ mho/cm), as a result of which the functional dependence of the potential on the conductivity of the lungs changes completely, so that low voltages are obtained for abnormally low lung conductivities. The effect of adding the subcutaneous fat layer to the model is very small (C in fig. 11-20), and the behavior is essentially the same as in B.

The model prediction of low surface potentials in cases of low lung conductivity is consistent with the clinical findings of low ECG voltages in patients with obstructive lung disease {78–83} (pulmonary emphysema, cystic fibrosis). In this condition, air — a nonconductor of electrical current — is trapped in the lungs, and as a result the average lung conductivity decreases. The same behavior was observed during experimentally induced overinflation of the lungs in the dog {84}. On the other end of the spectrum, abnormally high lung conductivity occurs clinically in cases of edema, pulmonary congestion, or infiltration {85}. To study experimentally the effect of increased lung conductivity on ECG potentials, we obtained scalar orthogonal ECG recordings and vectorcardiograms from human subjects undergoing pulmonary lavage of a whole lung {86}. In this procedure the air in the lung is replaced by physiologic saline solution (a high conductivity fluid). The ECG changes caused by filling the left lung are shown in fig. 11-21. The most obvious change is an overall decrease in the potential magnitude with maximal decrease in the posterior direction, clearly seen in the transverse and sagittal plane vectorcardiograms, as well as in the scalar Z-lead amplitude. That the largest effect is on the Z-lead voltages is consistent with the fact that most of the lung volume lies posterior to the heart. The decrease in potentials caused by the increased lung conductivity is consistent with the model prediction. Similar to the experiment, the model predicts the largest decrease in the Z-lead voltage.

We can conclude that low surface potentials result from high as well as low lung conductivities, and that an

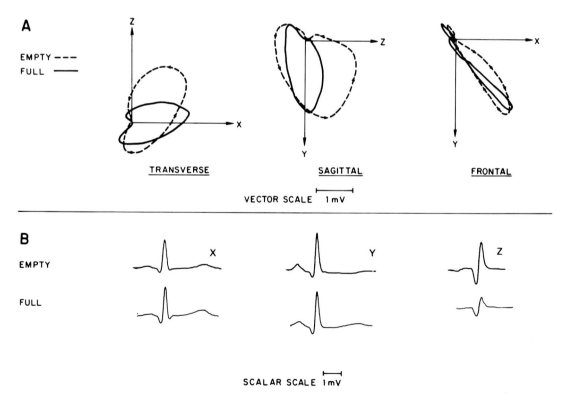

Fig. 11-21. ECG effects caused by filling the left lung with (high conductivity) saline. **A:** Transverse, sagittal, and frontal vectorcardiograms before (broken line) and after (solid line) the lung was filled with saline. **B:** Scalar recordings of leads X, Y, and Z obtained before (top) and after (bottom) the lung was filled with saline. From Rudy et al. {86}, by permission of the American Heart Association, Inc.

important role is played by the muscle layer in determining this behavior. This last observation adds to our understanding of the process. Under the condition of high lung conductivity, most of the current flow is confined to the lung region. When the lung conductivity is decreased, an alternative low-resistance pathway is available through the surface muscle layer. As a result, low potentials are generated at high as well as low lung conductivities, giving rise to the bell-shaped curve of fig. 11-19.

It should be mentioned that intuitive explanations that have been given in the literature consider the lungs to be the only cause for the *low* potentials detected in patients with obstructive lung disease. This conclusion is reached by arguing that the high-resistance lungs impede current flow to the surface and, as a result, low voltages are obtained. In fact, were the surface muscle layer absent, an abnormally *high* ECG potential field would result from low values of lung conductivity (A in fig. 11-20).

Surface muscle layer

The high-conductivity surface muscle layer plays an important role in determining the behavior of the body surface potential distribution. As described above, the functional dependence of the surface potential on the conductivity of the lungs is controlled by the effect of the skeletal muscle, and this surface layer is responsible for the abnormally low voltages obtained in cases of abnormally low lung conductivities.

The high-conductivity surface muscle layer attenuates the potentials at the surface of the torso (fig. 11-22). The decrease in the potential at the mid-anterior point $(r_5, 0)$

caused by the muscle layer is 22.56% (relative to the case in which the surface muscle layer is made homogeneous with the underlying lung region, i.e., $\sigma_4 = \sigma_3 = 0.0005$ mho/cm). This layer also acts to reduce potential differences between points on the torso. (The potential difference between $(r_5, 0)$ and $(r_5, 180)$ is reduced from 2.75 to 1.95 when the surface muscle is included; see fig. 11-22.) This implies that the muscle layer is an important contributor to the smoothing effect of the volume conductor discussed previously. It also explains the low voltages detected in cases of abnormally low lung conductivity, since under this condition most of the tangential current is confined to the high conductivity surface muscle layer, and the "short-circuiting" effect of this layer is reflected in the surface potential distribution. Similar smoothing and scaling down of potentials were observed by Gulrajani and Mailloux {59}. However, they question the importance of the muscle in determining the torso surface potential distribution. The apparent discrepancy arises from the fact that in the Gulrajani–Mailloux simulations a high conductivity surface layer way always present, even prior to inclusion of the muscle layer with its typical (fixed) conductivity value. This implies that in their study the effect of the muscle layer was determined by comparison with a situation in which a "muscle layer," with lower than normal conductivity, was already present. In contrast, in the eccentric spheres model the muscle layer can be completely eliminated (by making its conductivity equal to the conductivity of the underlying lung region). Under these conditions, no secondary sources arise at the lung-muscle interface so that a natural baseline is established for the study of the effects of such sources. As mentioned above, the presence of these secondary sources completely changes the behavior of surface potentials as a function of lung conductivity, demonstrating their importance in determining the potential distribution.

The effect of variations in skeletal muscle conductivity is shown in fig. 11-23. The potential decreases with in-

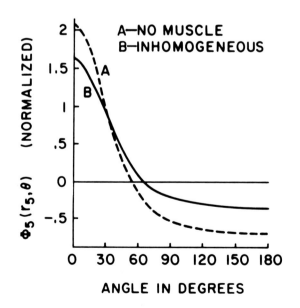

Fig. 11-22. Effect of the skeletal muscle layer on the surface potential distribution. In **A** the surface muscle layer region is made homogeneous with the underlying lung compartment. **B** is the complete inhomogeneous case, with the muscle layer included. From Rudy and Plonsey {53}, with permission.

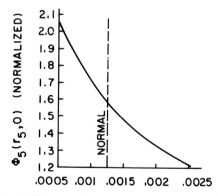

Fig. 11-23. The effect of variations in the conductivity of the skeletal muscle layer on the surface potential. From Rudy et al. {72}, by permission of the American Heart Association, Inc.

creasing muscle conductivity, and a fivefold increase in the conductivity (from 0.0005 mho/cm to 0.0025 mho/cm) causes the potential to drop from 2.05 to 1.22 (a 40.5% decrease).

A clinical condition that results in an abnormally low skeletal muscle conductivity is Pompe's disease. In this disease, large quantities of glycogen (a poor conductor) accumulate in skeletal muscle tissues, causing a decrease in the tissue conductivity. According to the behavior described in fig. 11-23, abnormally high surface potentials are to be expected with this abnormality. The clinical findings conform to this prediction: R voltages of 66 mm in V_5, 84 mm in V_6, and 88 mm in V_7 are observed (J.L. Potter, J.D. Kramer, The Children's Hospital Medical Center of Akron, Ohio, personal communication). Since a high degree of cardiomegaly is observed in patients with Pompe's disease, and since the effect of a dilated heart, according to the eccentric spheres model, is to augment surface potentials (the effect of heart size is discussed below), it is likely that the high ECG voltages result from a combination of two effects: a dilated heart and an abnormally low skeletal muscle conductivity.

Subcutaneous fat layer

The outermost compartment of the eccentric sphere model, namely, the subcutaneous fat layer, does not influence the surface potential distribution significantly. Its inclusion in the model causes the potential at the mid-anterior point to increase by only 6.8%, whereas the potentials at other locations on the torso are affected hardly at all.

An attempt to simulate the effect of obesity on the surface potential is shown in fig. 11-24. The potential at $(r_5,0)$ decreases with increasing fat layer thickness so that low potentials are expected in cases of obesity. The effect is not very significant, and an increase in fat thickness of 1 cm (from 0.5 to 1.5 cm) causes the potential to decrease by only 9.2%.

GEOMETRICAL EFFECTS

Heart position

The torso potential at the mid-anterior point $(r_5,0)$ and the potential magnitude at the corresponding point $(r_2,0)$ on the epicardium are shown in fig. 11-25 (A and B, respectively) as a function of the eccentricity (the displacement of the "heart" center from the "torso" center). Anatomical significance can be appreciated by noting that, in the model, for an eccentricity of 1 cm the anterior wall of the ventricle is 5 cm from the inner boundary of the anterior chest wall, whereas for an eccentricity of 5 cm the distance between the heart and the anterior chest wall is 1 cm. The behavior of the potential magnitude at other sites on the torso surface and on the epicardium is qualitatively the same as that plotted.

Figure 11-25A demonstrates that surface potentials are greatly affected by the heart position, in contrast to the epicardial potential behavior (fig. 11-25B). When the eccentricity is increased from 1 to 5 cm, the torso potential is almost doubled (the increase in potential is 97%). When the eccentricity is increased by 1 cm, from 4 to 5 cm (this could represent a normal variation in heart position), the potential is increased by 24.2%. In contrast, the epicardial potential (fig. 11-25B) is almost completely independent of the location of the heart within the torso. For an increase of eccentricity from 1 to 5 cm, the change in epicardial potential magnitude is less than 4%. This result implies that the entire epicardial potential distribution is not sensitive to variations in the location of the heart (as might be caused by changes in posture), and is essentially free from effects of body shape and size. This result is obtained because of all extracardiac secondary sources only the sources at the heart-lung interface are normally of sig-

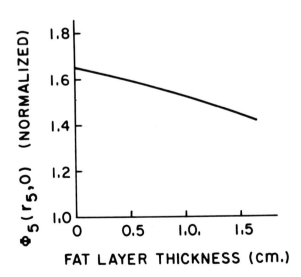

Fig. 11-24. The effect of variations in the thickness of the subcutaneous fat layer on the surface potential. From Rudy et al. {72}, by permission of the American Heart Association, Inc.

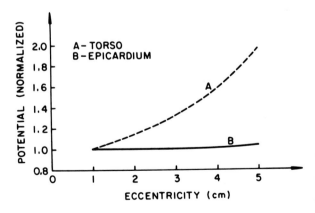

Fig. 11-25. The effects of variations in the eccentricity of the heart on body surface (**A**) and epicardial (**B**) potentials. The potentials are normalized to unity at an eccentricity of 1.0 cm. From Rudy and Plonsey {60}, by permission of the American Heart Association, Inc.

nificance in determining epicardial potentials {60}. Since this interface moves with the heart, the effect is independent of the heart position in the torso. It should be emphasized that, in principle, the epicardial potentials are affected by other extracardiac secondary sources (i.e., those at the lung-surface muscle interface, the surface muscle-fat interface, and the torso-air boundary). This phenomenon contradicts the intuitive view that the epicardium, being part of the heart, reflects the primary cardiac sources alone, independent of any torso effects. It should be recognized, however, that the potential field generated by the primary sources gives rise to secondary sources at the torso interfaces mentioned above. These secondary sources, in turn, affect the potential field everywhere, and in particular on the epicardial surface. As stated above, these effects are small and do not alter significantly the epicardial potential distribution.

These properties of epicardial potentials, together with the high resolution with which they reflect the myocardial source configuration (see earlier discussion on the smoothing effect) imply that epicardial potential distributions allow detailed examination of regional electrical events within the heart, are free from effects of body shape and size, and are only affected to a minimal degree by torso inhomogeneities. Epicardial potential maps provide, therefore, a detailed, high-resolution picture of the underlying cardiac electrical activity. They truly reflect the primary cardiac sources, with only minimal influences from secondary sources at the torso boundary and at boundaries between areas of different conductivities within the torso. It is as a result of these characteristics that epicardial potential mapping has become an important research and diagnostic tool. In addition, these properties identify the noninvasive reconstruction of epicardial potentials from body surface potential distributions as a very attractive goal of inverse electrocardiography {87,88}. This will be discussed further.

Size of the heart

The effect of variations in the size of the heart on the magnitude of body surface potentials is shown in fig. 11-26 {89}. The surface potential at the mid-anterior point on the spherical "torso" is plotted as a function of the radius of the heart. Two cases are considered: In A the size of the heart is varied while the area of the double-layer source is kept constant. This simulates the effect on the surface potential of an increased blood cavity due to its volume conductor properties alone. In B the enlargement of the blood cavity is accompanied by a proportional increase in the area of the source (the geometry is illustrated in fig. 11-27A and 11-27B, respectively). Although no information is available on the source distribution in the dilated heart, an increase in the area occupied by the activation wave is possible, assuming normal action potentials in the distended myocardial fibers and normal spread of activation (i.e., a normal Purkinje system).

The results in both cases show that the effect of dilation is to augment the magnitude of surface potentials. For an increase of 3 cm (from 5 to 8 cm) in the radius of the heart,

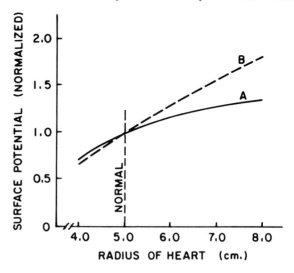

Fig. 11-26. The effect of variations in the size of the heart on the magnitude of surface potential. **A:** Area of the double-layer source is kept constant. **B:** Area of the source increases with increasing heart size. NORMAL refers to a typical heart size (radius of 5 cm in a torso of radius 12.5 cm). The potential is normalized so that a value of unity is obtained for the typical case. From Rudy and Plonsey {89}, by permission.

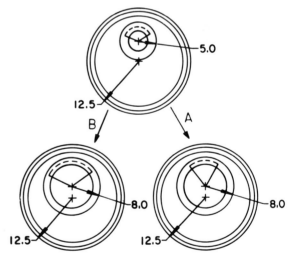

Fig. 11-27. Geometry of the changes in heart size simulated in fig. 11-26. **A:** No change in double-layer area. **B:** Area of the double layer increases with increasing heart size. From Rudy {34}, with permission.

the surface potential is increased by 35.3% in A and by 82.3% in B. In A, the augmentation is caused by the increase in the volume of the blood compartment alone, while in B the additional possible enhancement in the size of the source causes a further significant increase in potential.

The model prediction of an increase in the magnitude

of surface potentials due to an increase in heart volume is in keeping with experimental results. In a set of experiments, Manoach and coworkers {75,90,91} found that in normal cats a decrease in the intracavitary blood volume, produced by bleeding or by clamping of the abdominal inferior vena cava, caused a reduction in the QRS amplitude. Conversely, an increase in the amplitude of the QRS occurred when the blood volume was increased by clamping of the aorta or by overfilling of the left ventricle. Similar results were obtained by Angelakos and Gokhan {92}, who studied the influence of altering venous inflow on the magnitude of the ECG potentials in the dog. In their experiment, QRS potentials decreased in magnitude following occlusion of the superior and/or inferior vena cava. Reduction of ECG potentials was observed during bleeding in intact anesthetized dogs as well. Reinfusion of blood produced a prompt recovery of the magnitude of the potentials. A recent study by Kramer et al. {76}, in which the intracavitary blood volume was reduced by obstructing both the superior and inferior vena cava (with a ballon-tipped catheter), and increased by obstructing the aortic outflow tract, also confirms the theoretical results of fig. 11-26.

In contrast to the experimental results described above, a clinical study conducted by Ishikawa and coworkers {93} demonstrates a decrease in surface potentials in patients with an enlarged heart due to congestive heart failure. Clinical improvement and decrease in the cardiothoracic ratio (estimated from chest x-rays) were accompanied by an increase in magnitude of the spatial and transverse maximal QRS vectors. Since the volume conductor pro-

perties of a large blood cavity result in the augmentation of the surface potentials (fig. 11-26, and experimental results described above), other factors must be operative in congestive heart failure to account for the net attenuation of ECG potentials. It is possible that the excitation pattern and the source configuration and/or strength are modified in this abnormality in such a way that low potentials result in spite of the large blood cavity. Another possibility is increased lung conductivity due to edema caused by the congestive heart failure. As discussed earlier, the increased lung conductivity will cause an attenuation of the surface potentials. This effect is opposite to that produced by dilatation. It is possible, and in fact seems likely, that in patients with congestive heart failure the attenuation of the surface potential is cause by the increased lung conductivity, an effect that predominates over the augmentation due to dilatation, so that low potentials result in spite of the large blood cavity.

Thickness of the ventricular wall

The effect of increased myocardial thickness during hypertrophy is simulated in the eccentric spheres model by increasing the thickness of the spherical heart wall, keeping all other parameters (including the area of the double-layer source) constant. Three situations are illustrated in fig. 11-28. A is the typical case, with normal thickness of the ventricular wall (a thickness of 1 cm). When the thickness of the wall is doubled at the expense of the lung region (this situation is described in B), the potential at the mid-anterior point of the torso increases by 13.6% relative

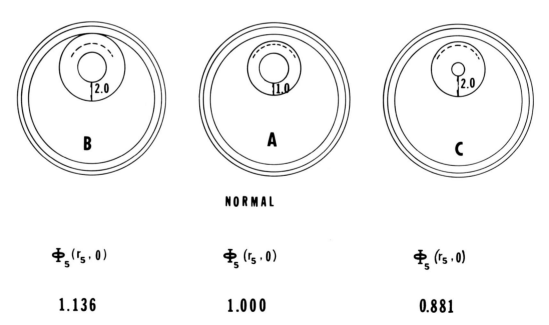

NORMAL

$\Phi_s(r_s, 0)$ $\Phi_s(r_s, 0)$ $\Phi_s(r_s, 0)$

1.136   **1.000**   **0.881**

Fig. 11-28. The effect of a thick ventricular wall on the surface potential. **A:** defines the typical case. The increase in myocardial thickness described in **B** is compensated for by a reduction in the lung region, and in **C** it is compensated for by a reduction in the intracavitary blood compartment. From Rudy {34}, with permission.

to the typical case. On the other hand, when the thickness of the wall is doubled at the expense of the blood chamber (C in the figure), the potential decreases by 12%.

The increase of 13.6% described in B is small and cannot account by itself for the high ECG voltages measured in cases of hypertrophy. (In these cases, an increase of 100% in potential values, relative to the normal, is common.) It seems, therefore, that factors other than the volume conductor effect considered here are influenced by hypertrophy. These factors might include the strength of the source and/or the area it occupies. The above simulation demonstrates the difficulty of predicting the effect of hypertrophy on the potential distribution without considerable information on both gemetrical effects, as well as modifications of the activation sources. Such details are, at present, poorly understood.

EMERGING NEW APPROACHES TO ELECTROCARDIOGRAPHY: BODY SURFACE POTENTIAL MAPPING AND ELECTROCARDIOGRAPHIC IMAGING

Introduction

The goal of electrocardiography is to noninvasively characterize the electrical function of the heart from potentials measured on the body surface. The limitations of standard electrocardiographic techniques (i.e., ECG and VCG) were mentioned in the introduction to this chapter. These techniques sample the body surface potentials at a small subset of points. As discussed earlier, cardiac electrical activity is a process that is spatially distributed throughout the myocardium. However, the standard techniques are very limited in their ability to provide information on regional electical activity and to locate bioelectric events (e.g., foci of arrhythmogenic activity) in the heart. In fact, VCG lumps all cardiac sources in a single dipole, located at the "center" of the heart (the so-called heart vector). Recent advances in electronics and computers simplify and reduce the cost of simultaneous potential recordings from many (100–250) torso sites {94}. This development has resulted in an ongoing extensive acquisition and study of body surface potential distributions both experimentally and clinically {95–99}. A result of this activity is the accumulating evidence that the potential distribution over the entire torso permits the detection and identification of regional electrical events in the heart in a fashion that is not possible from ECG and VCG. A study during cardiac pacing demonstrated that the body surface potential maps (BSPMs) reflect the different locations of endocardial pacing sites {100}. This ability to noninvasively relate surface potential patterns to regional cardiac events is of great physiological and clinical importance. An example of a clinical application already in use is the approximate localization of the accessory atrioventricular pathway in Wolff-Parkinson-White (WPW) syndrome prior to surgery or catheter ablation {101–104}.

Earlier we presented BSPMs during normal ventricular

activation (fig. 11-9) and demonstrated that they can reflect regional activity in the heart (e.g., right ventricular epicardial breakthrough; late activation of the pulmonary conus). Additional examples, for abnormal activation patterns, are provided in fig. 11-29.

The examples demonstrate that BSPMs provide information on regional electrical activity in the heart. However, they do so with very low resolution {60,105–108}. This property is a result of the smoothing effect of the torso volume conductor that was discussed earlier. Therefore, specific locations of cardiac events and accurate details of regional activity, such as the number and location of activation fronts in the heart, cannot be determined from visual inspection of the BSPMs. Obviously, a mathematical method for noninvasive, quantitative reconstruction of cardiac electrical events from body surface potential data is highly desirable. Such a method will constitute an electrocardiographic imaging modality for reconstructing function (i.e., the electrical activity of the heart), similar to other functional imaging modalities (e.g., positron emission tomography, PET) that provide information on regional myocardial function, such as blood flow and metabolic activity.

The availability of the potential distribution over the entire torso through body surface potential mapping makes such computations possible (the problem of computing events in the heart from data measured away from the heart constitutes an "inverse problem," while computing potentials away from the heart starting from the cardiac electrical activity constitutes a "forward problem"). Unfortunately, the actual three-dimensional distribution of activation fronts in the myocardium cannot be uniquely determined from the body surface potential distribution. Solutions to the inverse problem have been constructed in terms of equivalent cardiac-source representations (for review see {109}) or of epicardial isochrones {110}. The equivalent-generator approach does not have a unique solution, since there exist different source configurations that generate the same potential distribution on the body surface. To overcome this difficulty, constraints are introduced on the equivalent source configuration (e.g., a fixed or a moving single dipole, multiple fixed dipoles, etc.). The nature of the cardiac sources must be known a priori for a meaningful solution to be constructed (for example, a single moving dipole solution may provide useful information about a single well-localized activation front in the myocardium but cannot account for the general pattern of cardiac activity that is characterized by a complex, multifront configuration). As a result, this approach often fails and provides nonphysiological solutions when the actual, distributed nature of the cardiac sources does not conform to the constraints (e.g., number and/or location of dipoles) that are imposed on the equivalent-source representation. Because the solution is in terms of *equivalent* (rather than true) cardiac sources, the results cannot be validated directly by experimental measurements, and it is difficult to interpret the solution in terms of underlying physiological processes. The epicardial isochrones approach also suffers from serious limitations: (a) Isochrones provide the sequence of activation but do not maintain the entire information content of the potentials. (b) Epicardial isochrones are not defined for intramural activity prior to epicardial breakthrough. (c) The inverse solution in terms of epicardial isochrones {110} assumes that the myocardium is isotropic and that the source can be represented by a uniform-strength double layer. Realistically, however, the fibrous structure of the myocardium is highly anisotropic and, consequently, isochronal dipole-layer source models are nonuniform in general (importantly, ectopic activation from an arrhythmogenic focus gives rise to highly nonuniform sources).

Another possibility is to define the epicardial potential distribution (rather than the cardiac sources) as the solution to the electrocardiographic inverse problem, an approach that was pioneered by Barr and Spach {111} and by Colli Franzone et al. {112} (an extensive review of this approach is provided in Rudy and Messinger-Rapport {113}). Earlier we demonstrated that epicardial potentials mirror details of the electrical events within the myocardium with much higher resolution than the body surface potentials (see fig. 11-14 and related discussion). In addition, epicardial potentials are not sensitive to variations in heart position, (e.g., due to respiration or change of posture) and to body shape and size (fig. 11-25). Also, in contrast to body surface potentials, epicardial potential patterns are only minimally affected by the torso inhomogeneities {60}. All of these properties imply that epicardial potentials permit a direct interpretation of electrical events within the heart in a fashion that is not possible from body surface potential data. As a result, epicardial potential mapping has become an important experimental tool in the study of excitation (normal activation and activation during ventricular pacing have been studied using an array of 1124 electrodes distributed over the epicardial surface {114,115}), of various conduction abnormalities {116–118}, of myocardial ischemia and infarction {119}, and of mechanisms of arrhythmias {120, 121}. The development of multiplexing systems for simultaneous recordings from many epicardial sites permits the detailed study of arrhythmias on a beat-by-beat basis. Several laboratories utilize such systems for the study of reentrant arrhythmias associated with myocardial infarction {122,123} and with atrial flutter {124,125,126}. Clinically, epicardial potential mapping has become an essential intraoperative clinical tool {127,128}. It has been used to establish the site of reentry so that surgical interruption of the reentry pathway could be performed {129}. The site of origin of ventricular arrhythmias associated with myocardial ischemia and infarction was identified so that surgical excision of the site of earliest activation could be performed {130,131}. Clinical epicardial mapping has also been used to determine the location of the accessory pathway in WPW syndrome prior to surgical ablation {132–134}. A recent intraoperative epicardial mapping study has demonstrated that in a significant number of patients (25–30% of all cases mapped in the operating room) postinfarction ventricular tachycardia involves subepicardial reentry {135}. In these cases, epicardial laser photocoagulation interrupted the tachycardia by blocking conduction within critical elements of the reentrant pathway (in the slow-conducting segment of the pathway).

The above discussion clearly demonstrates the great importance of epicardial potentials for both experimental and clinical (diagnostic and treatment) purposes. A noninvasive method of reconstructing epicardial potentials from measured body surface potentials (a procedure termed *the inverse problem in terms of potentials*) is therefore highly desirable. Experimentally it can be used to characterize patterns of activation during arrhythmias and to study the effects of antiarrhythmic drugs and of neural activity on the cardiac activation sequence in an intact animal. It can also be used to study the onset and development of ventricular fibrillation and the effects of defibrillation. Clinically, it can be used to determine the site of origin of ventricular arrhythmias and their underlying mechanism, and to locate accessory pathways in WPW patients prior to surgical or catheter ablation. It can also be used to determine the nature of conduction abnormalities, to evaluate the efficacy of antiarrhythmic drug therapy, and to characterize ischemic and infarcted regions in the myocardium.

Formulation of the inverse problem in terms of potentials has several advantages over the equivalent generator approach. The solution is unique and can be more directly related to underlying physiological processes than the equivalent sources, which do not necessarily represent actual activation fronts. There is no need to make restrictive assumptions regarding the nature of the cardiac sources (e.g., number of activation fronts). The myocardial anisotropy and intracavitary blood inhomogeneity are taken into account implicitly in the potential formulation. Epicardial potentials reflect three-dimensional activity in the myocardium prior to epicardial breakthrough. Recent work by Taccardi and coworkers {25,136} has substantially advanced the ability to relate epicardial potentials to intracardiac events and to the myocardial structure. Finally (and importantly), inverse solutions in terms of potentials can be evaluated by direct comparison with measured epicardial potentials, such as those obtained simultaneously with surface potentials in the dog {111}, or in an electrolytic tank model of the human torso that contains a beating dog heart {112}. We have adopted this approach to the inverse problem of electrocardiography. A brief summary of the methodology and selected examples of inverse-computed epicardial potentials are provided in the following sections.

Methods

A detailed descripton of the mathematical methods, as applied to the inverse problem, can be found in {113, 137,138}. Briefly, Green's second theorem, together with the boundary element method {139}, was applied to the discretization of Laplace's equation in the volume between the epicardial surface and body surface to result in the following matrix equation:

$$AV_E = V_T \qquad (11-29)$$

where V_E is the vector of epicardial potentials, V_T is the vector of torso potentials, and A is a transfer matrix between the heart and torso that depends on the geometry. Equation (11-29) constitutes the forward problem, i.e., given V_E, V_T is computed. Solution to the inverse problem requires an inversion of A to give V_E in terms of V_T. Although a solution to the inverse problem is unique, it is ill posed in the sense that even small errors (noise) in the data can cause unbounded errors in the solution. Therefore, one cannot simply invert equation (11-29) to compute V_E. To overcome this difficulty, we utilized a Tikhonov regularization technique {140}, in which V_E is obtained by minimizing, with respect to V_E, the following objective function:

$$\| V_T - AV_E \|^2 + t \| V_E \|^2 \qquad (11\text{-}30)$$

where t is a regularization parameter. The first term in eq. (11-30) represents the least-square solution of eq. (11-29), while the second term is a regularization term that imposes bounds on the amplitude of the solution. The regularization parameter, t, controls the degree of regularization. For a small value of t, the first term in eq. (11-30) dominates, driving the solution towards the unstable least-squares solution. Large values of t make the solution more constrained because the second term in eq. (11-30) dominates. The optimal choice of t provides a balance between the accuracy and stability of the solution, resulting in a close estimate of the epicardial potential distribution that is also stable. The epicardial potential solution, V_E, obtained by minimizing the functional in (11-30) is given by

$$V_E = (A^*A + tI)^{-1}A^*V_T. \qquad (11\text{-}31)$$

Using this approach, we computed epicardial potentials throughout the cardiac cycle in normal sinus rhythm {141}. The experimental data were obtained at the University of Parma, Italy using an isolated dog heart placed in the proper human anatomical position inside a torso-shaped electrolytic tank, which was molded in the form of a 9-year-old male child (fig. 11-30). There were 216 epicardial electrodes and 400 body surface electrodes. The set of body surface potentials provided the data for our computations. Simultaneous recording of body surface and epicardial potentials provided a unique opportunity to evaluate the accuracy of the inverse procedure, with the measured epicardial potentials serving as the "gold standard" for comparison.

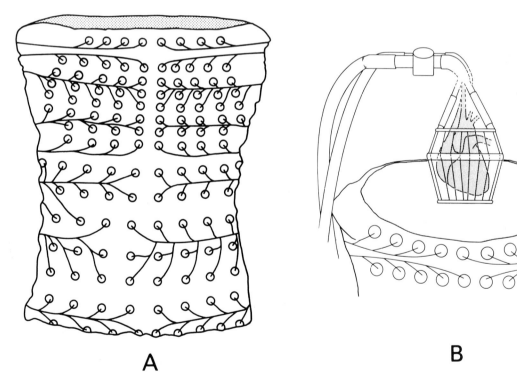

A   B

Fig. 11-30. The heart-torso preparation. **A:** Anterior view of the human-shaped torso tank. **B:** View of the canine heart within its epicardial cage as it is lowered into the tank. The tank was molded about a 9-year-old boy. During the experiment it was filled with a modified Ringer's solution with resistivity of $50\,\Omega$-cm. The heart, maintained by Langendorff perfusion by a donor dog, beat in sinus rhythm and was suspended in its cage in the correct anatomical position for the child as determined by x-rays. There were 408 measurement electrodes on the tank and 216 electrodes on the epicardial cage. From Messinger-Rapport and Rudy {141}, by permission of the American Heart Association, Inc.

Measured Body Surface Potentials

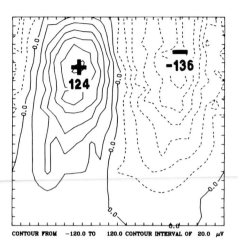

CONTOUR FROM −120.0 TO 120.0 CONTOUR INTERVAL OF 20.0 μV

Measured Epicardial Surface Potentials   ## Tikhonov Inversion, RE = .35

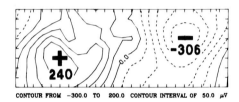

CONTOUR FROM −350.0 TO 250.0 CONTOUR INTERVAL OF 50.0 μV   CONTOUR FROM −300.0 TO 200.0 CONTOUR INTERVAL OF 50.0 μV

Fig. 11-31. Inverse reconstruction, early QRS. **Top:** Measured body surface potentials. **Lower left:** Measured epicardial optentials. **Lower right:** Inverse-recovered epicardial potentials using Tikhonov regularization. Relative inversion error, RE = 0.35. Maxima (+) and minima (−) values, as well as contour lines and intervals, are given in microvolts. Solid contour lines represent positive potentials. Broken contour lines indicate negative potentials. In each map anterior potentials are on the left and posterior potentials are on the right. The same is true for all succeeding maps. From Messinger-Rapport and Rudy {141}, by permission of the American Heart Association, Inc.

Examples of reconstructed epicardial potentials

The following maps of inverse-reconstructed epicardial potentials are selected examples of inverse computations throughout the cardiac cycle in normal sinus rhythm. The inverse-computed epicardial maps were evaluated by comparison with the actual, measured potential distribution. The relative error of inversion ranged from a minimum of 0.35 during the QRS to a maximum of 1.0 that occurred during the T-P interval. The average relative error during the entire QRS was 0.51. One particular example of inverse-recovered epicardial potentials during early QRS is shown in fig. 11-31. The computed epicardial potentials (bottom right) are displayed on a rectangular grid and are shown together with the measured body surface (top) and epicardial (bottom left) potentials. The relative inversion error for this particular map is 0.35. Note that the positions of the inverse-computed potential maximum (+) on the anterior and the potential minimum (−) on the posterior are each within 1 cm from the actual

measured ones. The amplitudes are somewhat diminished relative to the actual measured potentials.

A more rigorous test of the ability of the inverse procedure to reconstruct details of the epicardial potential distribution is shown in fig. 11-32 (same format as fig. 11-31). The maps are obtained during mid-QRS. Note that the epicardial pattern (bottom left) is complicated, displaying multiple maxima and minima. The body surface map (top) does not reflect this complexity and is relatively smooth (an example of the smoothing effect of the torso volume conductor discussed earlier). In spite of this smoothing, the inverse procedure is able to reconstruct all epicardial maxima and minima to within approximately 1 cm of their actual positions (bottom right).

An example of the ability to reconstruct cardiac electrophysiological events is provided in fig. 11-33 (examples of other events can be found in Messinger-Rapport and Rudy {141}). The anterior minimum (arrow) indicates right ventricular breakthrough and increases progressively in extent and in amplitude (from −3 μV to −429 μV to

Measured Body Surface Potentials

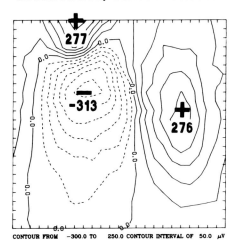

Measured Epicardial Surface Potentials   Tikhonov Inversion, RE = .42

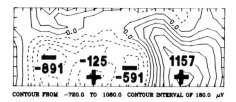

Fig. 11-32. Inverse reconstruction, mid-QRS. Same format as in fig. 11-31. Relative inversion error, RE = 0.42. From Messinger-Rapport and Rudy {141}, by permission of the American Heart Association, Inc.

−1057 µV, left column), reflecting the progression of the breakthrough process. This breakthrough minimum is reconstructed at the correct breakthrough position by the inverse procedure (right column), and the temporal progression is also captured. However, the inverse procedure fails to reconstruct this minimum at the first instant when breakthrough actually occurs, since its amplitude and extent are very small (top row). This limitation can be overcome by introducing temporal information on the progression of the activation process into the regularization procedure (*temporal regularization* {142}). By doing so (fig. 11-34), we were able to reconstruct the break-through minimum (arrow) even at 6 ms from the onset of QRS (compare to top row of fig. 11-33), the time of onset of right ventricular breakthrough as judged from the measured epicardial potentials. It should be stated that the ability to reconstruct local potential patterns and local cardiac events is very encouraging and of important clinical significance, since it is indicative of the capability of the inverse approach to detect and localize cardiac abnormalities (e.g., an ectopic arrhythmogenic focus) for the purposes of diagnosis and treatment. Direct evaluation of this capability is currently in progress in our laboratory.

The above discussion focused on the reconstruction of epicardial potentials from body surface potential data, reflecting efforts toward this goal (by us and others) in recent years. While these efforts continue and enter the phase of clinical implementation, an additional and more recent goal of inverse electrocardiography is the reconstruction of potentials on the "other surface" of the heart, namely, the endocardium. The endocardial surface of the heart is accessible through catheterization procedures. Electrode catheters have been used extensively during electrophysiology studies (EPS) for diagnosis and, more recently, for catheter-ablation treatment of arrhythmias {143}. Current electrode-catheter mapping is very limited, since it records information from a limited number of sites (typically 15 sites in the left ventricle) and the procedure is very time consuming (up to 45 minutes). Moreover, mapping from multiple sites is carried out over several cardiac cycles and cannot provide information on beat-to-beat changes in the activation pattern. To overcome these difficulties, a multi-electrode endocardial balloon was developed {144,145} and used to obtain detailed endocardial potential maps that were extremely helpful for the diagnosis and study of arrhythmogenic mechanisms {145} and for the localization of the arrhythmogenic site prior to surgical ablation {144}. However, this approach is

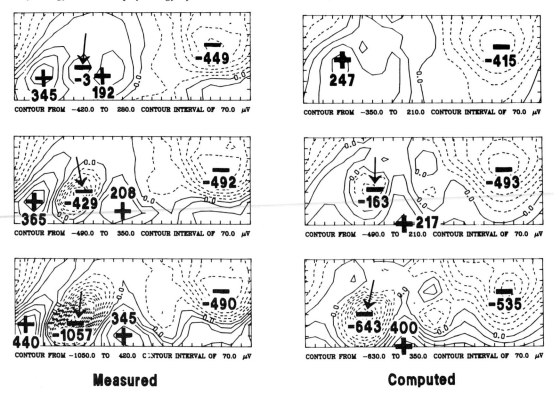

Measured   Computed

Fig. 11-33. Right ventricular epicardial breakthrough. Measured epicardial potential distributions are in the left column, and corresponding inverse-computed epicardial potential distributions are in the right column. Time in QRS (top to bottom): 6, 8, and 10 ms. Arrows in the maps identify the anterior minimum that reflects right ventricular epicardial breakthrough. From Messinger-Rapport and Rudy {141}, by permission of the American Heart Association, Inc.

extremely invasive and requires open heart surgery with a cardiopulmonary bypass.

The principles that govern the relationships between cardiac activation, myocardial sources, and the resulting potential fields were discussed earlier in this chapter. The same principles that we have applied to relate epicardial potentials and body surface potentials can be applied to relate endocardial potentials to potentials measured by a catheter in the blood cavity {146}. Recently, a multi-electrode probe was developed by Taccardi et al. {147} that contains 41 evenly distributed electrodes on its surface and that does not occlude the ventricular cavity. Our recent simulation studies {146} have demonstrated that, similar to the smoothing effect of the torso volume conductor on body surface potentials, the intracavitary probe potentials are smoothed out by the high conductivity of the intracavitary blood and can only provide a low-resolution reflection of the endocardial potentials. Since the endocardial potentials do reflect the complexities of the myocardial source configurations with higher resolution {146}, it is highly desirable to solve a second type of inverse problem, defined as the reconstruction of endocardial potential distribution from intracavitary potentials

measured by a multi-electrode catheter probe. Since the potential over a closed surface (the probe surface) is available, this constitutes a similar problem to the inverse computation of epicardial potentials from body surface potentials discussed above and has a unique solution. We have modified the methods used in solving the inverse-epicardial problem (discussed above) and applied them to the inverse-endocardial problem {148}. Results in an idealized model are encouraging, demonstrating that endocardial potentials can be computed with good accuracy and stability in the presence of simulated measurement noise and errors in probe position. Results from a first set of experiments in an isolated canine heart-intracavitary probe preparation also demonstrate the feasibility of the approach. With this procedure, detailed endocardial maps could be obtained in the catheterization laboratory on a beat-by-beat basis, permitting studies of arrhythmogenic mechanisms (e.g., determining the reentry pathway and the dynamic changes leading to initiation and termination) and of the effects of drugs, and allowing for an accurate determination of the arrhythmogenic site prior to catheter ablation. By applying this approach in combination with the inverse-epicardial procedure, potentials on both sur-

EARLY QRS
(110 msec)

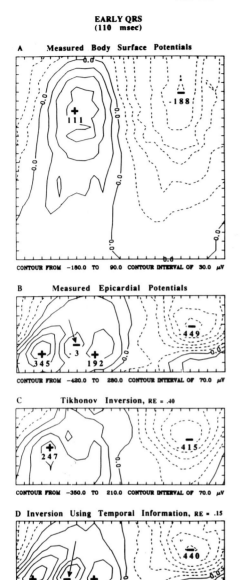

A   Measured Body Surface Potentials

CONTOUR FROM −180.0 TO 90.0 CONTOUR INTERVAL OF 30.0 μV

B   Measured Epicardial Potentials

CONTOUR FROM −420.0 TO 280.0 CONTOUR INTERVAL OF 70.0 μV

C   Tikhonov Inversion, RE = .40

CONTOUR FROM −350.0 TO 210.0 CONTOUR INTERVAL OF 70.0 μV

D   Inversion Using Temporal Information, RE = .15

CONTOUR FROM −420.0 TO 280.0 CONTOUR INTERVAL OF 70.0 μV

Fig. 11-34. Example of the advantage of temporal methods; right ventricular epicardial breakthrough (6 ms in QRS; 110 ms from onset of P). **A:** Measured torso potential distribution. **B:** Measured epicardial potential distribution. **C:** Inverse-recovered epicardial potentials obtained by Tikhonov quasistatic inversion. **D:** Inverse-recovered epicardial potentials obtained by temporal inversion. Arrows in the maps identify the anterior minimum that reflects right ventricular epicardial break-through. Note that details of the anterior potential distribution (the breakthrough minimum with its two flanking maxima) are reconstructed by the temporal method (D) but not by the quasistatic Tikhonov method (C). From Oster and Rudy {142}, with permission.

faces of the heart could be obtained nonsurgically, providing detailed information on the electrical function of the heart.

CONCLUDING REMARKS

It is interesting (and surprising) to note that the electrocardiogram has been used extensively and successfully as a clinical diagnostic tool before the principles of its genesis have been understood. Many of the principles that relate the electrocardiographic potentials to cardiac electrical events have been elucidated in recent years. However, the complete relationship between the ECG and the cardiac electrical excitation process is not yet fully established. Active research is conducted in many laboratories toward this goal. Very significant progress is being made in elucidating cellular mechanisms at the level of channel function and molecular structure. This will undoubtedly enhance our understanding of the basic biophysical processes underlying the ECG. Mapping studies of activation patterns and potentials are being conducted with increasing resolution and better signal quality. Combined with sophisticated visualization and graphics tools that are now available on computers, this activity will provide a more accurate description of the macroscopic distribution of sources in the heart in relation to the myocardial structure (e.g., anisotropy). A parallel effort involves theoretical, computer models of cellular processes and of macroscopic phenomena. As our understanding of the basic processes that generate the electrocardiographic potentials improves, our ability to interpret these potentials and to relate them to cardiac function will be significantly enhanced. This knowledge, if put into practice, is likely to completely change the way that electrocardiography is practiced as a research and clinical tool.

ACKNOWLEDGMENTS

Supported in part by the National Institutes of Health grant HL-33343 and by Grant-in-Aid from the American Heart Association. Computer time for inverse computations was provided by Pittsburgh Supercomputing Center grant PSCA 21. I wish to thank my graduate students Howard Oster and Dirar Khoury for reading the manuscript and Doris Fink for carefully typing it.

NOTES

1. A double layer is a surface distribution of dipole sources. A dipole is a source-sink pair separated by a short distance. The reader is referred to Jackson {6} for a review of these concepts.
2. Actually the rotation of the isochrones with increasing depth lags somewhat behind the rotation of fiber direction {26}.
3. A somewhat different representation of the equivalent sources was given by Plonsey {50}, and was also derived by Geselowitz {51} utilizing Green's theorem.
4. The conductivity values are based on the data of Rush and associates given in table 11-1.
5. The value $\rho_p = 1000\,\Omega\text{-cm}^2$ was provided by Dr. J. Clark from measurements on the pericardium of a dog.
6. Similar bell-shaped behavior was obtained by Arthur and

Geselowitz for the magnitude of an equivalent dipole source
{77}.

REFERENCES

1. Einthoven W, Fahr G, de Waart A: Uber die richtung und die manifesse grosse der potential — schwankungen im menschlichen herzen und uber die einfluss der herzlage auf die form des elektrokardiogramms. *Pflügers Arch* 150:275, 1913 (Translation: *Am Heart J* 40:163, 1950).
2. Sonnenblick EH: Myocardial ultrastructure in the normal and failing heart. In: Braunwald E (ed) *The Myocardium: Failure and Infarction.* New York: H.P. Publishing, 1974, pp 3–13.
3. Luo C, Rudy Y: A model of the ventricular cardiac action potential: Depolarization, repolarization, and their interaction. *Circ Res* 68:1501, 1991.
4. Luo C, Rudy Y: A dynamic model of the cardiac ventricular action potential: Ionic currents and concentration changes. AHA 65th Scientific Sessions, New Orleans, November 16–19, 1992. *Circulation* 86:I563, 1992 (abstr).
5. Plonsey R: The formulation of bioelectric source-field relationships in terms of surface discontinuities. *J Franklin Inst* 297:317, 1974.
6. Jackson WD: Classical Electrodynamics. New York: John Wiley, 1962.
7. Weingart R: Electrical properties of the nexal membrane studied in rat ventricular cell pairs. *J Physiol (Lond)* 370:267, 1986.
8. Rook MB, Jongsma HJ, Van Ginneken ACG: Properties of single gap junctional channels between isolated neonatal rat heart cells. *Am J Physiol* 255:H770, 1988.
9. Hoyt RH, Cohen ML, Saffitz JE: Distribution and three-dimensional structure of intercellular junctions in canine myocardium. *Circ Res* 64:563, 1989.
10. Sommer JR, Jennings RB: Ultrastructure of cardiac muscle. In: Fozzard HA, Jennings RB, Haber E, Katz AM, Morgan HE (eds) *The heart and Cardiovascular System: Scientific Foundations,* Vol 1. New York: Raven Press, 1986, pp 61–100.
11. Clerc L: Directional differences of impulse spread in trabecular muscle from mammalian heart. *J Physiol (Lond)* 255: 335, 1976.
12. Roberts D, Hersh LT, Scher AM: Influence of cardiac fiber orientation on wavefront voltage, conduction velocity, and tissue resistivity in the dog. *Circ Res* 44:701, 1979.
13. Spach MS, Miller WT 3rd, Miller-Jones E, Warren RB, Barr RC: Extracellular potentials related to intracellular action potentials during impulse conduction in anisotropic canine cardiac muscle. *Circ Res* 45:188, 1979.
14. Myerburg RJ, Gelband H, Nilsson K, Castellanos A, Morales AR, Bassett AL: The role of canine superficial ventricular muscle fibers in endocardial impulse distribution. *Circ Res* 42:27, 1978.
15. Streeter DD, Henry SM, Spotnitz HM, Patel DP, Ross J, Sonnenblick EH: Fiber orientation in the canine left ventricle during diastole and systole. *Circ Res* 24:339, 1969.
16. Hunter PJ, Nielsen PMF, Smaill BH, LeGrice IJ, Hunter IW: An anatomical heart model with applications to myocardial activation and ventricular mechanics. In: Pilkington TC, Loftis B, Thompson JF, Woo SL-Y, Palmer TC, Budinger TF (eds) *High-Performance Computing in Biomedical Research.* Boca Raton, FL: CRC Press, 1993, pp 3–26.
17. Durrer D, van Dam RT, Freud GE, Janse MJ, Meijer FL,
Arzbaecher RC: Total excitation of the isolated human heart. *Circ Res* 41:899, 1970.
18. Plonsey R: Introductory physics and mathematics. In: Macfarlane PW, Lawrie TDV (eds) *Comprehensive Electrocardiology,* Vol 1. Oxford: Pergamon Press, 1989, pp 41–76.
19. Smythe WR: Static and Dynamic Electricity. New York: McGraw-Hill, 1968.
20. van Oosterom A: Cell models — macroscopic source descriptions. In: Macfarlane PW, Lawrie TDV (eds) *Comprehensive Electrocardiology,* Vol 1. Oxford: Pergamon Press, 1989, pp 155–179.
21. Plonsey R, Rudy Y: Electrocardiogram sources in a 2-dimensional anisotropic activation model. *Med Biol Eng Comput* 18:82, 1980.
22. Colli-Franzone P, Guerri L, Viganotti C, Macchi E, Baruffi S, Spaggiari S, Taccardi B: Potential fields generated by oblique dipole layers modeling excitation wavefronts in the anisotropic myocardium. *Circ Res* 51:330, 1982.
23. Colli-Franzone P, Guerri L, Viganotti C: Oblique dipole layer potentials applied to electrocardiology. *Math Biol* 17:93, 1983.
24. DeAmbroggi L, Taccardi B: Current and potential fields generated by two dipoles. *Circ Res* 27:901, 1970.
25. Watabe S, Taccardi B, Lux RL, Ershler PR: Effect of nontransmural necrosis on epicardial potential fields — correlation with fiber direction. *Circulation* 82:2115, 1990.
26. Frazier DW, Krassowska W, Chen P, Wolf PD, Danieley ND, Smith WM, Ideker RE: Transmural activation and stimulus potentials in three-dimensional anisotropic canine myocardium. *Circ Res* 63:135, 1988.
27. Gulrajani RM, Roberge FA, Mailloux GE: The forward problem of electrocardiography. In: Macfarlane PW, Lawrie TDV (eds) *Comprehensive Electrocardiology,* Vol 1. Oxford: Pergamon Press, 1989, pp 197–236.
28. Miller WT 3rd, Geselowitz DB: Simulation studies of the electrocardiogram I. The normal heart. *Circ Res* 43:301, 1978.
29. Taccardi B: Distribution of heart potentials on the thoracic surface of normal human subjects. *Circ Res* 12:341, 1963.
30. Spach MS, Silverberg WP, Boineau JP, Barr RC, Long EC, Gallie TM, Gabor JB, Wallace AG: Body surface isopotential maps in normal children, ages 4 to 14 years. *Am Heart J* 72:640, 1966.
31. Liebman J, Thomas CW, Rudy Y, Plonsey R: Electrocardiographic body surface potential maps of the QRS of normal children. *J Electrocardiol* 14:249, 1981.
32. Widman L, Liebman J, Thomas CW, Fraenkel R, Rudy Y: Electrocardiographic body surface potential maps of the QRS and T of normal young adults — qualitative description and selected quantifications. *J Electrocardiol* 21:121, 1988.
33. Spach MS, Barr RC, Lanning CF, Tucek PC: Origin of body surface QRS and T wave potentials from epicardial potential distribution in the intact chimpanzee. *Circulation* 55:268, 1977.
34. Rudy Y: The effects of the thoracic volume conductor (inhomogeneities) on the electrocardiogram. In: Liebman J, Plonsey R, Rudy Y (eds) *Pediatric and Fundamental Electrocardiography.* Dordrecht: Martinus Nijhoff, 1987, p 49.
35. Plonsey R, Heppner D: Considerations of quasi-stationarity in electrophysiological systems. *Bull Math Biophys* 29:657, 1967.
36. Schwan HP, Kay CF: The conductivity of living tissues. *Ann NY Acad Sci* 65:1007, 1957.
37. Geddes LA, Baker LE: The specific resistance of biological material. A compendium of data for the biomedical engineer and physiologist. *Med Biol Eng* 5:271, 1967.

38. Rush S, Abildskov JA, McFee R: Resistivity of body tissues at low frequencies. *Circ Res* 12:40, 1963.
39. Schwan HP, Kay CF: Specific resistance of body tissues. *Circ Res* 4:664, 1956.
40. Cobbold RSC: Transducers for Biomedical Measurements. New York: John Wiley, 1974.
41. Rush S, Nelson CV: The effects of electrical inhomogeneity and anisotropy of thoracic tissues on the field of the heart. In: Nelson CV, Geselowitz DB (eds) *The Theoretical Basis of Electrocardiology*. Oxford: Clarendon Press, 1976, pp 323–354.
42. Maxwell JC: *A Treatise on Electricity and Magnetism*, Vol 1. Oxford: Clarendon Press, 1904.
43. Cole KS, Curtis HJ: Bioelectricity, electric physiology. In: Glasser O (ed) *Medical Physics*, Vol II. Chicago: Year Book Publishers, 1944.
44. Burger HC, Van Milaan JB: Measurement of the specific resistance of the human body to direct current. *Acta Med Scand* 114:584, 1943.
45. Burger HC, Van Dongen R: Specific electric resistance of body tissues. *Phys Med Biol* 5:431, 1961.
46. Hirsch FG, Texter EC, Wood LA, Ballard WC, Horan FC, Wright MD: The electrical conductivity of blood. 1. Relationship to erythrocyte concentration. *Blood* 5:1017, 1950.
47. Rosenthal RL, Tobias CW: Measurement of the electrical resistance of human blood; use in coagulation studies and cell volume determinations. *J Lab Clin Med* 33:1110, 1948.
48. Molnar GW, Nyboer J, Levine RK: The effect of temperature and flow on the specific resistance of human venous blood. Fort Knox, KY: U.S. Army Medical Research Laboratory Report, Rep. 127. Project 6-64-12-028, 1953, pp 1–118.
49. Rush S: Methods of measuring the resistivities of anisotropic conducting media in situ. *J Res Natl Bur Stand* 66c:217, 1962.
50. Plonsey R: Laws governing current flow in the volume conductor. In: Nelson CV, Geselowitz DB (eds) *The Theoretical Basis of Electrocardiology*. Oxford: Clarendon Press, 1976.
51. Geselowitz DB: On bioelectric potentials in an inhomogeneous volume conductor. *Biophy J* 7:1, 1967.
52. McFee R, Rush S: Qualitative effects of thoracic resistivity variations on the interpretation of electrocardiograms: The low-resistance surface layer. *Am Heart J* 76:48, 1968.
53. Rudy Y, Plonsey R: The eccentric spheres model as the basis for a study of the role of geometry and inhomogeneities in electrocardiography. *IEEE Trans Biomed Eng* 26:392, 1979.
54. Rush S: Inhomogeneities as a cause of multiple peaks of heart potential on the body surface: Theoretical studies. *IEEE Trans Biomed Eng* 18:115, 1971.
55. Taccardi B, D'Alche P: Verification of experimentale d'une method mathematique pour le calcul de la distribution des potentiels engendres par un dipole dans un milieu conducteur non homogene. *J Physiol (Paris)* 57:281, 1965.
56. Geselowitz DB, Ishiwatari H: A theoretic study of the effect of the intracavitary blood mass on the dipolarity of an equivalent heart generator. In: Hoffman I (ed) *Vectorcardiology 1965*. Amsterdam: North-Holland, 1966, pp 393–402.
57. Okada RH: An experimental study of multiple dipole potentials and the effects of inhomogeneities in volume conductors. *Am Heart J* 54:567, 1957.
58. Horan L, Flowers N, Brody D: Body surface potential distribution; comparison of naturally and artificially produced signals as analyzed by digital computer. *Circ Res* 13:373, 1963.
59. Gulrajani RM, Mailloux GE: A simulation study of the effects of torso inhomogeneities on electrocardiographic potentials, using realistic heart and torso models. *Circ Res* 52:45, 1983.
60. Rudy Y, Plonsey R: A comparison of volume conductor and source geometry effects on body surface and epicardial potentials. *Circ Res* 46:283, 1980.
61. King TD, Barr RC, Herman-Giddens GS, Boaz DE, Spach MS: Isopotential body surface maps and their relationship to atrial potentials in the dog. *Circ Res* 20:393, 1972.
62. Spach MS, Barr RC, Lanning CF, Tucek PC: Origin of body surface QRS and T wave potentials distributions in the intact chimpanzee. *Circulation* 55:268, 1977.
63. Spach MS, Barr RC, Lanning CF: Experimental basis for QRS and T wave potential distributions in the intact chimpanzee. *Circ Res* 42:103, 1978.
64. Ramsey III M, Barr RC, Spach MS: Comparison of measured torso potentials with those simulated from epicardial potentials for ventricular depolarization and repolarization in the intact dog. *Circ Res* 41:660, 1977.
65. Abildskov JA, Burgess MJ, Lux RL, Wyatt RF: Experimental evidence for regional cardiac influence in body surface isopotential maps of dogs. *Circ Res* 38:386, 1976.
66. Taccardi B: Contribution à la détermination quantitative des erreurs de la vectorcardiographie. *Arch Int Physiol* 59:63, 1951.
67. Taccardi B: La distribution spatiale des potentiels cardiaques. *Acta Cardiol* 13:173, 1958.
68. Taccardi B, Musso E, DeAmbroggi L: Current and potential distribution around an isolated dog heart. In: Rijlant P (ed) *Proceedings of the Satellite Symposium of the 25th International Congress on Physiological Science (The Electrical Field of the Heart) and the 12th Colloquium Vectorcardiographicum*. Brussels: Presses Academiques Europenees, 1972, pp 566–512.
69. Mirvis DM, Keller FW, Ideker RE, Cox JW, Zettergren DG, Dowdie RF: Values and limitations of surface isopotential mapping techniques in the detection and localization of multiple discrete epicardial events. *J Electrocardiol* 10:347, 1977.
70. Brody DA: A theoretical analysis of intracavitary blood mass influence on the heart lead relationship. *Circ Res* 4:731, 1956.
71. Rudy Y, Plonsey R: A note on the "Brody-Effect." *J Electrocardiol* 11:87, 1978.
72. Rudy Y, Plonsey R, Liebman J: The effects of variations in conductivity and geometrical parameters on the electrocardiogram, using an eccentric spheres model. *Circ Res* 44:104, 1979.
73. Nelson CV, Rand PW, Angelakos ET, Hugenholtz PG: Effect of intracardiac blood on the spatial vectorcardiogram. I. Results in the dog. *Circ Res* 31:95, 1972.
74. Rosenthal A, Restieaux NJ, Feig SA: Influence of acute variations in hematocrit on the QRS complex of the Frank electrocardiogram. *Circulation* 44:456, 1971.
75. Manoach M, Gitter S, Grossman E, Varon D: The relation between the conductivity of the blood and the body tissue and the amplitude of the QRS during heart filling and pericardial compression in the cat. *Am Heart J* 84:72, 1972.
76. Kramer DA, Hamlin RL, Weed HR: Effects of pericardial effusates of various conductivities on body surface potentials in dogs - documentation of the eccentric spheres model. *Circ Res* 55:788, 1984.
77. Arthur RM, Geselowitz DB: Effect of inhomogeneities on

the apparent location and magnitude of a cardiac current dipole source. *IEEE Trans Biomed Eng* 17:141, 1970.

78. Burch GE, DePasquale NP: Electrocardiographic diagnosis of pulmonary heart disease. *Am J Cardiol* 2:622, 1963.

79. Wasserburger RH, Kelle JR, Rasmaussen BS, Juhl JH: The electrocardiographic pentalogy of pulmonary emphysema. *Circulation* 20:831, 1959.

80. Selvester RH, Rubin HB: New criteria for the electrocardiographic diagnosis of emphysema and cor pulmonale. *Am Heart J* 69:437, 1965.

81. Littman D: The electrocardiographic findings in pulmonary emphysema. *Am J Cardiol* 5:339, 1960.

82. Kerr A, Adicoff A, Klingeman JD, Pipberger HV: Computer analysis of the orthogonal electrocardiogram in pulmonary emphysema. *Am J Cardiol* 25:34, 1970.

83. Flaherty JT, Blumenschein SD, Spock A, Canent RV, Gallie TM, Boineau JP, Spach MS: Cardiac potentials in pulmonary disease: Over-distension of the lung versus cor pulmonale (right ventricular hypertrophy). *Am J Cardiol* 20:29, 1967.

84. Toyama J, Okada A, Nagata Y, Okajima M, Yamada K: Electrocardiographic changes in pulmonary emphysema: Effects of experimentally induced over-inflation of the lungs on QRS complexes. *Am Heart J* 87:606, 1974.

85. Van De Water JM, Mount BE, Barela JR, Schuster R, Leacock FS: Monitoring the chest impedance. *Chest* 64:597, 1973.

86. Rudy Y, Wood R, Plonsey R, Liebman J: The effect of high lung conductivity on electrocardiographic potentials — results from human subjects undergoing bronchopulmonary lavage. *Circulation* 65:440, 1982.

87. Barr RC, Spach MS: Inverse solutions directly in terms of potentials. In: Nelson CV, Geselowitz DB (ed) *The Theoretical Basis of Electrocardiology*. Oxford: Clarendon Press, 1976, pp 294–304.

88. Rudy Y: Critical aspects of the forward and inverse problems in electrocardiography. In: Sideman S, Beyar R (eds) *Simulation and Imaging of the Cardiac System*. Dordrecht: Martinus Nijhoff, 1985, pp 279–298.

89. Rudy Y, Plonsey R: Comments on the effect of variations in the size of the heart on the magnitude of ECG potentials. *J Electrocardiol* 13:79, 1980.

90. Manoach M, Gitter S, Grossman E, Varon D, Gassner S: Influence of hemorrhage on the QRS complex of the electrocardiogram. *Am Heart J* 82:55, 1971.

91. Manoach M, Gassner S, Grossman E, Varon D, Gitter S: Influence of cardiac filling on the amplitude of the QRS complex in normal cats. *Isr J Med Sci* 8:566, 1972.

92. Angelakos ET, Gokhan N: Influence of venous inflow volume on the magnitude of the QRS potentials in-vivo. *Cardiologia* 43:337, 1963.

93. Ishikawa K, Berson AS, Pipberger HW: Electrocardiographic changes due to cardiac enlargement. *Am Heart J* 81:635, 1971.

94. Kavuru MS, Vesselle H, Thomas CW: Advances in body surface potential mapping (BSPM) instrumentation. In: Liebman J, Plonsey R, Rudy Y (eds) *Pediatric and Fundamental Electrocardiography*. Dordrecht: Martinus Nijhoff Publishing, 1987, pp 315–327.

95. Benson DW: Role of body surface maps in cardiac arrhythmias. In: Liebman J, Plonsey R, Rudy Y (eds) *Pediatric and Fundamental Electrocardiography*. Dordrecht: Martinus Nijhoff, 1987, p 361.

96. Van Dam R: Present state of the art of body surface mapping. In: Liebman J, Plonsey R, Rudy Y (eds) *Pediatric and Fundamental Electrocardiography*. Dordrecht: Martinus Nijhoff, 1987, p 347.

97. Yamada K, Harumi K, Musha T (eds): *Advances in Body Surface Potential Mapping*. Nagoya, Japan: University of Nagoya Press, 1983.

98. Mirvis DM: Body surface electrocardiographic mapping. Boston: Kluwer Academic, 1988.

99. Liebman J, Rudy Y, Diaz P, Thomas CW, Plonsey R: The spectrum of right bundle branch block as manifested in electrocardiographic body surface potential maps. *J Electrocardiol* 17:329, 1984.

100. Sippens Groenewegen A, Spekhorst H, Van Hamel NM, Kingma JH, Hauer RNW, Janse MJ, Dunning AJ: Body surface maping of ectopic left and right ventricular activation. *Circulation* 82:879–896, 1990.

101. Benson DW, Gallagher JJ, Spach MS, Barr RC, Edwards SB, Olkham HN: Accessory atrioventricular pathway in an infant: Prediction of location with body surface maps and ablation with cryosurgery. *J Pediatr* 96:41, 1980.

102. DeAmbroggi L, Taccardi B, Macchi E: Body surface maps of heart potentials: Tentative localization of preexcited area of forty-two Wolff-Parkinson-White patients. *Circulation* 54:251, 1976.

103. Yamada K, Toyama J, Walda M, Sugiyama S, Sugenoya J, Toyoshima H, Mizumo Y, Sotohata I, Kibayshi M: Body surface isopotential mapping in Wolff-Parkinson-White syndrome: Noninvasive methods to determine the localization of accessory atrioventricular pathway. *Am Heart J* 192:721, 1975.

104. Liebman J, Olshansky B, Zeno JA, Geha A, Rudy Y, Henthorn RW, Cohen M, Waldo AL: Electrocardiographic body surface potential mapping in the Wolff-Parkinson-White syndrome: Non-invasive determination of the ventricular insertion sites of AV connections. *Circulation* 83: 886–901, 1991.

105. King TD, Barr RC, Herman-Giddens GS, Boaz DE, Spach MS: Isopotential body surface maps and their relationship to atrial potentials in the dog. *Circ Res* 20:393, 1972.

106. Ramsey M, Barr RC, Spach MS: Comparison of measured torso potentials with those simulated from epicardial potentials for ventricular depolarization and repolarization in the intact dog. *Circ Res* 41:660, 1977.

107. Spach MS, Barr RC, Lanning CF, Tucek PC: Origin of body surface QRS and T wave potentials from epicardial potential distributions in the intact chimpanzee. *Circulation* 55:268, 1977.

108. Spach MS, Barr RC, Lanning CF: Experimental basis for QRS and T wave potential distributions in the intact chimpanzee. *Circ Res* 42:103, 1978.

109. Gulrajani RM, Savard P, Roberge FA: The inverse problem in electrocardiography: Solutions in terms of equivalent sources. *CRC Crit Rev Biomed Eng* 16:171–214, 1988.

110. Cuppen JJM, Van Oosterom A: Model studies with the inversely calculated isochrones of ventricular depolarization. *IEEE Trans Biomed Eng* 31:652–659, 1984.

111. Barr RC, Spach MS: Inverse calculation of QRS-T epicardial potentials from body surface potential distributions for normal and ectopic beats in the intact dog. *Circ Res* 42:661–675, 1978.

112. Colli-Franzone P, Guerri L, Tentoni S, Viganotti C, Baruffi S, Spaggiari S, Taccardi B: A mathematical procedure for solving the inverse problem of electrocardiography. *Math Biosci* 77:353–396, 1985.

113. Rudy Y, Messinger-Rapport BJ: The inverse problem in electrocardiography: Solutions in terms of epicardial potentials. *CRC Crit Rev Biomed Eng* 16:215, 1988.

114. Arisi G, Macchi E, Baruffi S, Spaggiari S, Taccardi B: Potential fields on the ventricular surface of the exposed dog heart during normal excitation. *Circ Res* 52:706, 1983.

115. Arisi G, Macchi E, Corradi C, Lux RL, Taccardi B: Epicardial excitation during ventricular pacing. *Circ Res* 71:840, 1992.

116. Christopher RC, Wyndham MB, Smith T, Mooideen KM, Mammana R, Levitsky S, Rosen KM: Epicardial activation in patients with left bundle branch block. *Circulation* 61:696, 1980.

117. Ohno M, Toyama J, Kohbe T, Isomura S, Kudama I, Yamada K: Effects of injury to the right ventricular conducting tissue on canine hearts on epicardial activation sequence and electrocardiogram. *Jpn Circ J* 46:1056, 1981.

118. Van Dam R: Ventricular activation in human and canine bundle branch block. In: Wellens, Lie, Janse (eds) *The Conduction System of the Heart.* Philadelphia: Lea and Febiger, 1976, p 377.

119. Holland RB, Brook H: Precordial and epicardial surface potentials during myocardial ischemia in the pig. *Circ Res* 37:471, 1975.

120. Allessie M, Bonke FIM, Schopman FL: Circus movement in rabbit atrial muscle as a mechanism of tachycardia. *Circ Res* 33:54, 1973.

121. Hayden WGE, Juirley EJ, Tyland DA: The mechanism of canine atrial flutter. *Circ Res* 20:496, 1967.

122. El-Sherif N, Mehra R, Gough WB, Zeiler RH: Reentrant ventricular arrhythmias in the late myocardial infarction period: Interruption of reentrant circuits by cryothermal techniques. *Circulation* 68:644, 1983.

123. Wit AL, Allessie M, Bonke FIM, Lammers W, Smeets J, Fenoglio JJ: Electrophysiologic mapping to determine the mechanism of experimental ventricular tachycardia initiated by premature impulses. Experimental approach and initial results demonstrating reentrant excitation. *Am J Cardiol* 49:166, 1982.

124. Shimizu A, Nozaki A, Rudy Y, Waldo AL: Onset of induced atrial flutter in the canine pericarditis model. *J Am Coll Cardiol* 17:1223–1234, 1991.

125. Shimizu A, Nozaki A, Rudy Y, Waldo AL: Multiplexing studies of the effects of rapid atrial pacing on the area of slow conduction during atrial flutter in the canine pericarditis model. *Circulation* 83:983–994, 1991.

126. Ortiz J, Igarashi M, Gonzalez X, Laurita K, Rudy Y, Waldo AL: Mechanism of spontaneous termination of atrial flutter in the canine pericarditis model. *PACE* 14:627, 1991.

127. Downar E, Parson ID, Mickleborough LL, Cameron DA, Yao KC, Waxman MB: On-line epicardial mapping of intraoperative ventricular arrhythmias: Initial clinical experience. *J Am Coll Cardiol* 4:703, 1984.

128. Gallagher JJ, Kasell JH, Cox JL, Smith WM, Ideker RE: Techniques of intraoperative electrophysiologic mapping. *Am J Cardiol* 49:211, 1982.

129. Spurrel RAJ, Yates SK, Thornburn CW, Sowton GE, Deuchar C: Surgical treatment of ventricular tachycardia after epicardial mapping studies. *Br Heart J* 27:115, 1975.

130. Fontaine G, Guiraudon G, Frank R: Stimulation studies and epicardial mapping in ventricular tachycardia: Study of mechanisms and selection for surgery. In: Kulbertus HE (ed) *Reentrant Arrhythmias.* Lancaster, England: MTP Press, 1977, pp 334–350.

131. Wittig JH, Boineau JP: Surgical treatment of ventricular arrhythmias using epicardial, transmural, and endocardial mapping. *Ann Thoracic Surg* 20:117, 1975.

132. Gallagher JJ, Kasell J, Sealy WC, Pritchett ELC, Wallace AG: Epicardial mapping in the Wolff-Parkinson-White syndrome. *Circulation* 57:854–866, 1978.

133. Josephson ME, Harken AH: Surgical therapy of arrhythmias. In: Rosen MR, Hoffman BF (eds) *Cardiac Therapy.* Boston: Martinus Nijhoff, 1983, pp 377–385.

134. Cox JL: Intraoperative computerized mapping techniques: Do they help us to treat our patients better surgically? In: Brugada P, Wellens HJJ (eds) *Cardiac Arrhythmias: Where to Go from Here?* Mount Kisco, NY: Futura, 1987, pp 613–637.

135. Littmann L, Svenson RH, Gallagher JJ, Selle JG, Zimmern SH, Fedor JM, Colavita PG: Functional role of the epicardium in post infarction ventricular tachycardia. *Circulation* 83:1577–1591, 1991.

136. Spaggiari S, Baruffi S, Arisi G, Macchi E, Taccardi B: Effect of intramural fiber direction on epicardial isochrone and potential maps (abstr). *Circulation* 76(Suppl IV):241, 1987.

137. Messinnger-Rapport BJ, Rudy Y: Computational issues of importance to the inverse recovery of epicardial potential in a realistic heart-torso geometry. *Math Biosci* 97:85, 1989.

138. Rudy Y, Oster HS: The electocardiographic inverse problem. In: Pilkington TC, Loftis B, Thompson JF, Woo SL-Y, Palmer TC, Budinger TF (eds) *High-Performance Computing in Biomedical Research.* Boca Raton, FL: CRC Press, 1993, pp 135–155.

139. Brebbia CA, Telles JCF, Wrobel LC: Boundary element techniques: Theory and applications in engineering. Berlin: Springer-Verlag, 1984.

140. Tikhonov AN, Arsenin VY: *Solutions of Ill-Posed Problems* (translated from Russian). New York: Wiley, 1977.

141. Messinger-Rapport BJ, Rudy Y: Non-invasive recovery of epicardial potentials in a realistic heart-torso geometry: Normal sinus rhythm. *Circ Res* 66:1023, 1990.

142. Oster HS, Rudy Y: The use of temporal information in the regularization of the inverse problem of electrocardiography. *IEEE Trans Biomed Eng* 39:65, 1992.

143. Fontaine G, Scheinman MM (eds): *Ablation in Cardiac Arrhythmias.* Mount Kisco, NY: Futura, 1987.

144. De Bakker JMT, Janse MJ, Van Cappelle FJL, Durrer D: Endocardial mapping by simultaneous recording of endocardial electrograms during cardiac surgery for ventricular aneurysm. *J Am Coll Cardiol* 2:947–953, 1983.

145. Downar E, Harris L, Mickleborough LL, Shaikh N, Parson ID: Endocardial mapping of ventricular tachycardia in the intact human ventricle: Evidence for reentrant mechanisms. *J Am Coll Cardiol* 11:783–791, 1988.

146. Khoury DS, Rudy Y: A model study of volume conductor effects on endocardial and intracavitary potentials. *Circ Res* 71:511, 1992.

147. Taccardi B, Arisi G, Macchi E, Baruffi S, Spaggiari S: A new intracavitary probe for detecting the site of origin of ectopic ventricular beats during one cardiac cycle. *Circulation* 75:272–281, 1987.

148. Khoury DS, Rudy Y: Reconstruction of endocardial potentials from intracavitary probe potentials: A model study. Computers in Cardiology, Durham, NC, October 11–14, 1992, IEEE Computer Society Press, pp 9–12.

CHAPTER 12

Slow Action Potential and Properties of the Myocardial Slow Ca Channels

NICHOLAS SPERELAKIS & IRA JOSEPHSON

SLOW Ca CHANNELS AND THEIR ROLE IN Ca^{2+} ENTRY

Hormones and neurotransmitters play an important role in regulating the force of contraction of the heart. The force of contraction of the heart is controlled by the Ca^{2+} influx across the cell membrane during the action potential (AP) in the process of excitation-contraction coupling (fig. 12-1). This Ca^{2+} influx occurs through the voltage-dependent and time-dependent gated slow channels of the cell membrane.[1] This chapter briefly reviews and summarizes some of the important properties of the myocardial slow Ca channels, particularly their dependence on metabolism and their regulation by cyclic AMP. In addition, the slow action potentials and their possible role in cardiac arrhythmias will be briefly discussed.

Besides the slow Ca channels, there are other types of voltage-dependent channels in heart cells, including fast Na^+ channels and several types of K^+ channels. In addition, there are at least two types of Ca^{2+}-dependent channels, one selective for K^+ [$g_{K(Ca)}$] and one mixed Na/K [$g_{Na,K(Ca)}$]. Each type of ionic channel is a specific protein that floats in the lipid bilayer matrix of the cell membrane (fig. 12-2). Each channel has a water-filled central pore for ion passage. A cation passing through its ion-selective channel probably binds to two or more negatively charged sites on its journey through the channel down its electrochemical (electrical plus concentration) gradient. The voltage-dependent fast Na^+ channels and slow channels may be modeled with a central activation (A, m, or d) gate and an inactivation (I, h, or f) gate at the inner surface of the membrane (fig. 12-3).

Compared to the fast Na^+ conductance, the slow Ca^{2+} conductance is kinetically slower, that is, the channels behave as if their gates open, close, and recover more slowly. In addition, the slow-channel gates operate over a less-negative (more-depolarized) voltage range, i.e., their threshold potential and the inactivation voltage range are higher (less negative, fig. 12-4). These two types of channels for carrying inward (depolarizing) current also are blocked by different drugs: tetrodotoxin (TTX) blocks fast Na^+ channels (by binding to the outer mouth of the channel and acting as a physical plug) but does not affect the slow channels; in contrast, calcium-antagonistic drugs,

such as verapamil, nifedipine, and diltiazem, block the slow channels with relatively little or no effect on the fast Na^+ channels.

There are three types of slow channels with respect to ion selectivity: Ca^{2+}, Na^+, and Ca-Na (fig. 12-5). The Ca-Na type allows both Ca^{2+} ions and Na^+ ions to pass through, perhaps with competition between them. An example of a pure Ca-selective slow channel is found in arterial vascular smooth muscle (VSM) cells {100} or in guinea-pig atrial and ventricular cells {77}. An example of a nearly pure Na-selective slow channel is found in young (2- to 3-day-old) embryonic chick hearts {104}. Since verapamil and D-600 (methoxy derivative of verapamil) block all three types of slow channels, such calcium-antagonistic drugs are more appropriately called *slow channel blockers*. Because Ca^{2+} ion entry into the cardiac cell during excitation is through the Ca or Ca-Na slow channels, the Ca antagonists are often called *calcium-entry blockers*. Since Ca^{2+} influx into the cell controls the force of contraction, the calcium antagonistic drugs partly or completely uncouple contraction from excitation. Slow channels are also found in nodal cells (SA and AV) and Purkinje fibers, as well as in working myocardial cells.

It was shown by Lee and Tsien {54}, in voltage-clamp experiments on internally dialyzed isolated single adult heart cells (from guinea-pig ventricle), that a reversal of the Ca slow-channel current occurs at large depolarizing clamps and that the outward current is carried by K^+ ion through the slow channel. (An outward movement of Cs^+ can also occur through the slow channels). D-600 blocked the current flow in either direction. This latter point must be remembered when considering all the actions of the calcium-antagonistic drugs.

ACTION OF NEUROTRANSMITTERS, HORMONES, AND POSITIVE INOTROPIC AGENTS

A number of positive inotropic agents exert an effect to increase the number of available slow channels in the myocardial cell membrane. This action may be the predominant explanation for their increase in cardiac contractility, since the amount of Ca^{2+} ion entering the cell

N. Sperelakis (ed.), Physiology and Pathophysiology of the Heart, Third Edition.
© 1995 Kluwer Academic Publishers. *ISBN 0-7923-2612-1. All rights reserved.*

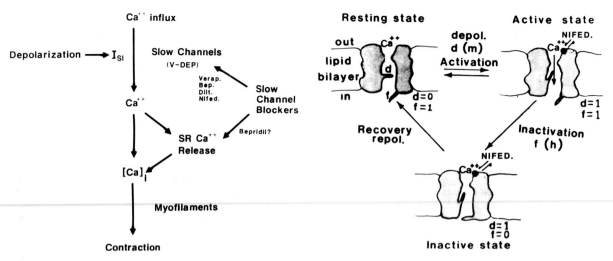

Fig. 12-1. Summary diagram for excitation-contraction coupling in myocardial cells. Ca^{2+} influx during excitation occurs through the voltage-dependent and time-dependent gated slow channels. This entering Ca^{2+} helps to raise the myoplasmic Ca^{2+} concentration $[(Ca)_i]$ to the level necessary to activate the contractile proteins (e.g., 10^{-5} M) and acts to bring about the release of additional Ca^{2+} from the SR by the mechanism of Fabiato and Fabiato {25}.

Fig. 12-3. Cartoon model for the three hypothetical states of a slow channel, patterned after the Hodgkin–Huxley states for the fast Na^+ channel. In the resting state, the d(m) gate is closed and the f(h) gate is open (d = 0; f = 1). Depolarization to the threshold activates the slow channel to the active state, the d gate opening rapidly and the f gate still being open (d = 1; f = 1). The activated channel spontaneously inactivates to the inactive state due to closure of the f gate (d = 1; f = 0). The recovery process upon repolarization returns the channel from the inactive state back to the resting state, which is again available for reactivation. Ca^{2+} ion is depicted as being bound to the outer mouth of the channel and poised for entry down its electrochemical gradient when both gates are in the open position (activated state of channel). Also depicted is the possible binding of nifedipine to the outer mouth of the slow channel (solid circle) in the active state or inactive state, and thereby either blocking the activated channel or slowing the recovery process for converting from the inactive state back to the resting state. Modified from Sperelakis {100}, with permission.

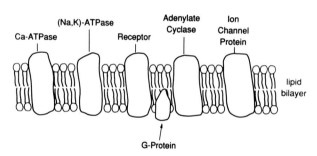

Fig. 12-2. Diagram of the Singer-Nicolson model for the cell membrane as a lipid bilayer with proteins floating in the bilayer. Some protein molecules are inserted in only one leaflet of the bilayer, such as the autonomic receptors on the external surface and the adenylate cyclase complex on the inner surface. Some large protein molecules protrude through the entire thickness of the membrane, such as the ion channel proteins. Redrawn from Sperelakis {101}, with permission.

through the slow channels controls the force of contraction. The Ca^{2+} entering directly elevates $[Ca]_i$ (which activates the myofilaments) and indirectly elevates [Ca], further by releasing Ca^{2+} from the intracellular sarcoplasmic reticulum (SR) stores. For example, the Ca^{2+} that entered the cell could bring about the release of more Ca^{2+} by the Ca trigger-Ca release hypothesis of Fabiato and Fabiato {25}. Blockade of the slow channels, and hence Ca^{2+} influx, by Ca^{2+}-antagonists agents (such as verapamil, nifedipine, diltiazem, Mn^{2+}, Co^{2+}, and La^{3+})

depresses or abolishes the contractions without greatly affecting the normal fast AP, i.e., contraction is uncoupled from excitation.

The positive inotropic agents that affect the number of available slow channels include beta-adrenergic receptor agonists (such as isoproterenol and norepinephrine), histamine (H_2 receptor), and methylxanthines (such as caffeine, theophylline, and methylisobutylxanthine). The action of these agents is very rapid, the peak effect often occurring within 1–3 minutes. The effect of the catecholamines is blocked by beta-adrenergic blocking agents, and the effect of histamine is blocked by H_2-receptor blocking agents (but not by H_1-receptor antagonists {41}). The addition of exogenous dibutyryl cyclic AMP exerts a similar effect, but relatively slowly, the peak effect occuring in 15–30 minutes {91}. Angiotensin II also stimulates the myocardial slow channels {27}.

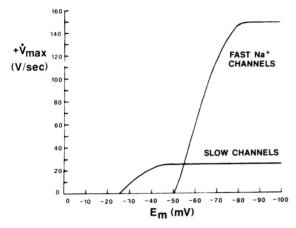

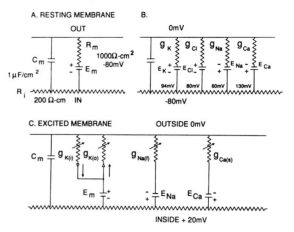

Fig. 12-4. Graphic representation of differences in behavior, with respect to voltage inactivation, of the fast Na^+ channels and slow (Na^+ and Ca^{2+}) channels. Maximal rates of rise of the action potential (+max dV/dt) as a function of resting E_m for the normal cardiac action potential (dependent on inward current through the fast Na^+ channels) and for the slow action potential (dependent on inward current through the slow channels) elicited in cells whose fast Na^+ channels are blocked (by TTX or by depolarization to about −45 mV). +max dV/dt is a measure of the inward current intensity (everything else, such as membrane capacitance, held constant), which in turn is dependent on the number of channels available for activation. From Sperelakis {101}, with permission.

ASSESSMENT OF SLOW CHANNEL FUNCTION

Slow action potential

One method of detecting the effect of agents on the slow channels is to first block the fast Na^+ channels and excitability by tetrodotoxin (TTX) or to voltage inactivate them by partially depolarizing the cells (e.g., to −40 mV) in elevated $[K]_o$ (e.g., 25 mM). Then, addition of agents, such as catecholamines, which rapidly increase the number of slow channels available for activation upon stimulation, causes the appearance of slowly rising overshooting APs (the slow responses), which resemble the plateau component of the normal fast AP {3,8} (fig. 12-6). The slow APs are accompanied by contractions that are nearly as large as the normal contractions {87}. The slow APs are blocked by agents that block inward slow current, including Mn^{2+}, La^{3+}, verapamil, D-600, nifedipine, and diltiazem {87,90}.

Changes in the maximum rate of rise (max dV/dt) of the slow AP may be used as an index of the changes in the slow inward current (I_{si}), since max $dV/dt \propto I_{si}/C_m$. The intensity of the slow inward current is a product of the conductance (g_{si}) times the electrochemical driving force. For example, if all of I_{si} is carried by Ca^{2+} ions, $I_{Ca} = g_{Ca}$ ($E_m - E_{Ca}$). Thus, for a constant driving force, I_{si} is directly proportional to g_{si}. The conductance, g_{si}, is proportional to the number of Ca^{2+} slow channels open at any

Fig. 12-5. A–B: Electrical equivalent circuits for a myocardial cell membrane at rest. C: Electrical equivalent circuit for a myocardial cell membrane during excitation. **A:** Membrane as a parallel resistance-capacitance network, the membrane resistance (R_m) being in parallel with the membrane capacitance (C_m). Resting potential (E_m) is represented by an 80-mV battery in series with the membrane resistance. **B:** Membrane resistance is divided into its four component parts, one for each of the four major ions of importance: K^+, Cl^-, Na^+, and Ca^{2+}. These represent totally separate and independent pathways for permeation of each ion through the resting membrane. Equilibrium potential for each ion (e.g., E_K), determined solely by the ion distribution in the steady state and calculated from the Nernst equation, is shown in series with the conductance path for that ion. Resting potential of −80 mV is determined by the equilibrium potentials and by the relative conductances. **C:** Equivalent circuit is further expanded to illustrate that for the voltage-dependent conductances there are at least two separate K^+-conductance pathways (labelled here g_k^o and g_k^i). Arrowheads in series with the K^+ conductances represent rectifiers, the arrowheads pointing in the direction of least resistance to current flow. There are two separate Na^+ conductances (g_{Na}^s). In addition, there is a nonspecific kinetically slow pathway that allows both Na^+ and Ca^{2+} to pass through, perhaps by competition with each other. The Ca^{2+}-selective pathway (g_{Ca}^s) is also kinetically slow. Arrows drawn through the resistors represent that the conductances are variable, depending on membrane potential (and time). From Sperelakis {101}, with permission.

instant in time. Thus the effect of a drug on depressing max dV/dt can be translated into an effect on the number of available (unblocked) slow channels, assuming that a channel can either be drug blocked or unblocked. Although the relationship between max dV/dt and number of open channels may be somewhat nonlinear, for our purposes we will assume that this relationship is a simple direct linear relationship.

Whole-cell and membrane patch-voltage clamp

A second method of detecting the effect of agents on the Ca^{2+} slow channels is by use of voltage-clamp analysis. Voltage clamp has been done on small cardiac muscle and Purkinje fiber strands (bundles) by various methods. In

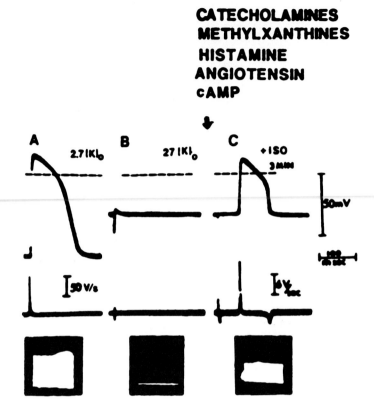

Fig. 12-6. Characterization of the slow AP responses induced by catecholamines, methylxanthines, histamine, angiotensin II, or cyclic adenosine monophosphate (cAMP) in isolated perfused guinea pig hearts. The fast Na^+ channels were inactivated in elevated K^+. **Upper tracings:** Intracellular potentials (V vs. t) recorded from myocardial cells of the ventricular wall. **Lower tracings:** The first time derivative of the action potential (dV/dt); the peak upward deflection of dV/dt gives the maximal rate of rise of the action potential (max dV/dt). The lower records in each panel are the contractions recorded on a penwriter at a slow speed. **A:** The normal fast action potential (2.7 mM K^+ Ringer perfusate). **B:** Perfusion with 27 mM K^+-Ringer solution depolarized the cells to -40 mV and inactivated the fast Na^+ channels; the heart was unresponsive to stimulation 10-fold greater than the normal threshold. **C:** Isoproterenol (10^{-7} M), caffeine (3 mM), histamine (10^{-6} M), and angiotensin II (10^{-7} M) rapidly restored electrical activity in the form of a slow AP response (max dV/dt of 15 V/s), the peak effect being attained within 1–3 minutes. Dibutyryl cAMP (10^{-4} M) slowly induced the slow APs with accompanying contractions, the peak effect occurring with 15–30 minutes. Contractions were always associated with these slow APs. Modified from Schneider and Sperelakis {85}, with permission.

the past few years, the voltage-clamp method has been applied to isolated single adult heart cells using single microelectrode (switching current and voltage), double microelectrode, suction pipette, and patch pipette methods. This preparation and techniques have yielded reliable and quantitative data for I_{si}. Voltage clamp of the entire single cell gives the macroscopic currents. In voltage clamp, the membrane potential is stepchanged from an initial steady-state holding potential (V_h), which is often near the natural resting potential (E_m), to the desired test potential (V_c) and held (clamped) there for a desired time period (e.g., 20–200 ms), and the current (inward and outward) required to hold E_m at V_c is measured. The conductance for the ion carrying the current is calculated from $g_i = I_i/(V_c - E_i)$. By clamping to different voltages, the complete relationship between g_i and E_m (V_c) can be obtained. If V_h is about -80 mV, then two inward currents are recorded: an initial fast inward Na^+ current and a second slow inward current, carried primarily by Ca^{2+} ions. The two inward currents overlap and are followed by an outward K^+ current, the delayed rectifier K^+ current. If TTX is added to block the fast Na^+ channels, or a V_h of about -50 mV is used to voltage inactivate the fast Na^+ channels, then the fast inward Na^+ current is abolished and the only inward current is I_{si} (fig. 12-7).

The technique of patch clamping of small cell membrane areas (e.g., $1-2 \mu^2$), either left attached to the intact cell (cell-attached patch) or cell-free isolated in the tip of the patch micropipette, has been used to study the Ca^{2+} slow channels and the effects of drugs on these channels {12,14,33,79,81,82}. In the isolated patch method, the patches can be made inside-out or outside-out, and very

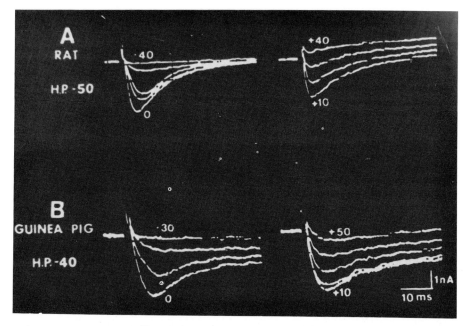

Fig. 12-7. Macroscopic I_{si}. The slow inward Ca^{2+} currents obtained from single rat (**A**) and guinea pig (**B**) ventricular cells. The holding current in A was -50 mV; in B it was -40 mV. Voltage steps were applied in 10-mV increments from the holding potential. The numbers next to the current traces indicate the step potentials. From Josephson et al. {46}, with permission.

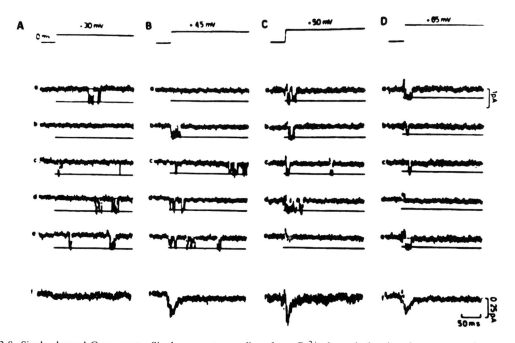

Fig. 12-8. Single-channel Ca currents. Single current recordings from Ca^{2+} channels (a–e) and reconstructed mean currents (f) in response to depolarizations (duration 300 ms) of various amplitudes (**A–D**). Cell-attached recordings were obtained with a 50-mM Ba^{2+}-filled pipette in Tyrode solution. Linear components of leakage and capacitance have been subtracted. In each panel (A–D, a–e), the average unitary current amplitude and the baseline level are indicated by the solid lines. Reconstructed mean currents (A–D, f) were obtained by averaging the individual current responses of 50–80 depolarizations of a given amplitude. The signals were low-pass filtered at 1 kHz. From Cavalie et al. {14}, with permission.

tight gigaohm ($10-100\,G\Omega$) seals are formed with the glass tip of the patch pipette to minimize short-circuiting of the patch. The small patch often contains only a single functional ion channel. For example, it is estimated that there may be only one Ca^{2+} slow channel per $1-10\,\mu m^2$ of cell membrane. The density of fast Na^+ channels is about $10-100$ times greater.

The openings and closings of the channels can be examined at different clamp potentials and in the presence of drugs. The probability (p) of the slow channel being open increases at greater depolarizing clamp steps and decreases at hyperpolarizing clamp voltages. The current that flows through the opened channel is usually about one picoampere (pA) and varies with the voltage step, and hence the electrochemical driving force. The values for the conductance of the Ca^{2+} slow channel usually range between 5 and 25 pS (pico-Siemens). The Ca^{2+} slow channel typically opens in bursts, and the length of the bursts increases at more depolarized voltages. The mean (or ensemble) current I(t) found by averaging over repetitive trials is: $I(t) = i_s \cdot N \cdot p(t)$, where i_s the current through the single channel (for a given driving force), N is the number of channels in the patch (e.g., one), and p is the average probability of the channel being in the open state during a depolarizing clamp step (as a function of time, fig. 12-8).

A three-state sequential model, with two closed states (C_1 and C_2) and one open state (0), has been proposed for the Ca^{2+} slow channel {33}:

$$C_1 \underset{k_{-1}}{\overset{k_1}{\rightleftharpoons}} C_2 \underset{k_{-2}}{\overset{k_2}{\rightleftharpoons}} O,$$

where k_1 and k_2 are the forward (opening) rate constants, and k_{-1} and k_{-2} are the backward (closing) rate constants.

The calcium antagonistic drugs were found to decrease the probability of the channel being opened with time and to increase the number of trials with no channel openings (mode 0 of Hess et al. {33}). This can account for the effect of these drugs on decreasing the macroscopic currents (I_{si}) measured from whole cells, and giving rise to a negative inotropic effect in cardiac muscle and vasodilation in vascular smooth muscle. In contrast, the calcium slow-channel agonistic drugs, e.g., the dihydropyridine derivative Bay-K-8644, increase the probability of channel opening and the mean open time (mode 2 of Hess et al. {33}). This can account for the effect of this class of drug on increasing the macroscopic currents (I_{si}) measured from whole cells, and giving rise to a positive inotropic effect in cardiac muscle and vasoconstriction in vascular smooth muscle.

TYPES OF CALCIUM CHANNELS

Recent work employing the patch-clamp method has demonstrated that multiple types of Ca channel activity can be recorded in a variety of excitable cells, including cardiac myocytes {2}. The channel types can be differentiated on the basis of voltage dependence, kinetics, permeability, and pharmacology (summarized in table 12-1). The following two main classes[2] of Ca channels have been described in myocardial cells:

1. (Long-lasting) L Type: Activation occurs at less negative potentials; the current has a slow time-dependent inactivation; Ba ions display a larger conductance than Ca ions; the probability of opening is increased by beta-adrenergic stimulation, cyclic AMP, etc.; the currents are dihydropyridine (DHP) sensitive (i.e., agonists and antagonists).
2. (Transient) T Type: Activation is at more negative potentials; the current shows a rapid time-dependent inactivation and equal conductances for Ba and Ca ions; and the current is insensitive to DHPs.

In the presence of external Ca ions the selectivity of the L-type Ca channel is Ca > Sr > Ba $\ggg$ Li $\gg$ Na > K > Cs; (Ca is about 1000-fold more permeable than Na). However, if external Ca ions are removed (i.e., by chelation with EGTA), then the Ca channel permits large

Table 12-1. Summary of major differences between the slow (L-type) and fast (T-type) Ca^{2+} channels

Properties	Ca^{2+} channels	
	Slow (L-type)	Fast (T-type)
Duration of current	Long lasting (sustained)	Transient
Inactivation kinetics	Slower	Faster
Activation kinetics	Slower	Faster
Threshold	High (ca. $-30\,mV$)	Low (ca. $-50\,mV$)
Half-activation potential	ca. $-20\,mV$	ca. $-50\,mV$
Single-channel conductance	High ($18-26\,pS$)	Low ($8-10\,pS$)
Regulated by cAMP and cGMP	Yes	No
Regulated by phosphorylation	Yes	No
Blocked by Ca^{2+} antagonist drugs	Yes	No (slight)
Opened by Ca^{2+} agonist drugs	Yes	No
Permeation by Me^{2+}	Ba > Ca	Ba $\approx$ Ca
Inactivation by $[Ca]_i$	Yes	Slight (?)
Recordings in isolated patches	Runs down	Rel. stable

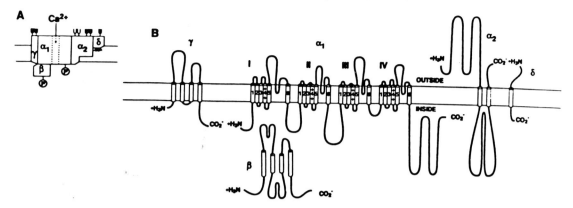

Fig. 12-9. Ca channel structure. The subunit structure of a calcium channel. **A:** Diagram of the five subunits that comprise the calcium channel, with phosphorylation sites indicated on the α_1 and β subunits. **B:** Transmembrane model of Ca^{2+} channel subunits derived from primary sequence determinations. Note the four repeated domains of the α_1 subunit. From W.A. Catterall, *Science* 253:1499–1500, 1991, with permission.

fluxes of monovalent cations. Under these conditions, the addition of micromolar amounts of external Ca^{2+} ions produces a block of the channel, which can be observed in single-channel recordings as a shortening in the mean open time {117}.

In addition, a new type of Ca^{2+} channel was discovered in 8-day-old fetal rat ventricular cells {108}. A residual I_{Ca} remaining in the presence of a high concentration (3 µM) of nifedipine (nifedipine-resistant I_{Ca}) was not blocked by diltiazem, tetramethrine (T-type channel blocker), or ω-conotoxin (N-type channel blocker), and had a half-inactivation potential about 20 mV more negative than the nifedipine-sensitive (L-type channel) I_{Ca}.

Structure of the cardiac L-type Ca^{2+} channel

Recently, great advances have been achieved in defining the structure of cardiac slow Ca^{2+} channels using molecular biological techniques {65}. A 185-kDa peptide subunit of the Ca^{2+} channel complex was found to contain the dihydropyridine binding site, and it was sufficient to produce Ca currents in reconstituted bilayer experiments; that is, the α_1 subunit contained the water-filled (gated) conducting pore of the channel. The primary amion acid structure of the α_1 subunit deduced from cloned cDNA suggests that there are four repeated units of homology, with each repeat containing five hydrophobic and one hydrophilic (membrane-spanning) α helices (fig. 12-9). The hydrophilic segment (S4) is positively charged and is thought to act as the voltage-sensing gate of the channel.

There are also four other subunits (α_2, β, γ, δ), which constitute the oligomeric structure of the Ca channel complex. The role of these other subunits is not as clear as for the α_1 subunit, and they may serve in a structural or modulatory capacity. In this regard, both the α_1 and β subunits contain phoshorylation sites, which may be involved in channel regulation, as described below.

SPECIAL PROPERTIES OF THE MYOCARDIAL SLOW CHANNELS

Cyclic-AMP dependence

Cyclic AMP is directly involved with the functioning of the slow channels (table 12-2) {80,87,91,98,129}. The first evidence for this was provided in 1972 by Shigenobu and

Table 12-2. Summary of mechanisms for the control of Ca^{2+} influx by myocardial cells, and hence force of contraction of the heart; control is exerted by altering the fraction of the slow channels in the phosphorylated state, the dephosphorylated channel being electrically silent

I. Extrinsic control
    Usually mediated by sarcolemmal receptors and adenylate cyclase activity
    A. Autonomic nerves
       1. Sympathetic nerves
          Neurotransmitter: norepinephrine
       2. Parasympathetic nerves
    B. Circulating hormones and autacoids
       1. Epinephrine and norepinephrine
       2. Histamine
       3. Angiotensin II
    C. Drugs
       1. Calcium antagonists (slow-channel blockers)
       2. Beta-adrenergic receptor blockers
       3. Histamine H_2-receptor blockers
       4. Methylxanthines
       5. Cardiac glycosides
II. Intrinsic control
    Usually activated by ischemia
    A. pH dependence of slow channels
    B. Metabolic (ATP) dependence of slow channels
    C. Cyclic-AMP dependence of slow channels
    D. Protection hypothesis

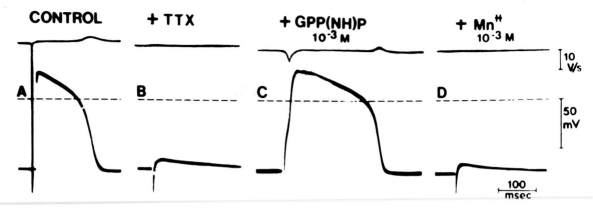

Fig. 12-10. GPP(NH)P induction of a slow AP response in cultured chick heart cell reaggregates in the presence of propranolol. The preparation was paced at a rate of 1/s. All recordings are from one cell. **A:** Control fast action potential recorded in normal Tyrode solution. **B:** The addition of TTX (3.1×10^{-6} M) completely blocked excitability. Propranolol (10^{-6} M) was then added to ensure that any effect observed was not due to activation of the beta-adrenergic receptor. **C:** Addition of GPP(NH)P (10^{-3} M) induced the slow APs in 15 minutes. **D:** Addition of Mn^{2+} (1 mM) abolished the slow APs within 1 minute. The upper traces give dV/dt. Modified from Josephson and Sperelakis {42}, with permission.

Sperelakis {91} and by Tsien et al. {116}. Histamine and beta-adrenergic agonists, subsequent to binding to their specific receptors, lead to rapid stimulation of adenylate cyclase with resultant elevation of cyclic-AMP levels. The methylxanthines enter into the myocardial cells and inhibit phosphodiesterase, the enzyme that destroys cyclic AMP, thus causing an elevation of cyclic AMP. These positive inotropic agents also rapidly induce the slow APs, along a parallel time course, presumably by making more slow channels available in the membrane and/or by increasing their mean open time. Dibutyryl cyclic AMP also induces the slow APs after a long lag period of 15–30 minutes, as expected from either slow penetration through the membrane or from slow elevation of intracellular cyclic AMP (fig. 12-6).

Several tests of the cyclic-AMP hypothesis were done. Josephson and Sperelakis {42} showed that a GTP analog (5'-guanylimidodiphosphate [GPP(NH)P], 10^{-5} to 10^{-3} M) that directly activates adenylate cyclase induced the slow APs in cultured reaggregates of chick heart cells within 5–20 minutes (fig. 12-10). GPP(NH)P binds to the GTP site on the regulatory component of the adenylate cyclase complex, but cannot be hydrolyzed by the GTPase activity of the enzyme, and so causes an irreversible activation of adenylate cyclase and elevation of cyclic AMP. Forskolin, a highly potent activator of adenylate cyclase activity, was shown to be a strong positive inotropic agent in isolated guinea-pig atrial muscle {18}, and induces slow action potentials and contractions in guinea-pig ventricle {95,125}.

Vogel and Sperelakis {121} demonstrated that cyclic AMP iontophoretically microinjected intracellularly into dog Purkinje fibers and guinea-pig ventricular muscle induced the slow APs in the injected cell for a transient period of 1–2 minutes (fig. 12-11). A second injection of cyclic AMP again induced a slow AP, which again decayed within 1–2 minutes. The effect of the injected cyclic AMP

was immediate, i.e., within seconds after the injection was stopped. The amplitude and duration of the induced slow APs were a function of the amount of cyclic AMP injected. Cyclic-AMP injections potentiated (increased their rate to rise and amplitude) slow APs induced by theophylline.

Li and Sperelakis {58} demonstrated that pressure injection of cyclic AMP, GPP(NH)P, and cholera toxin into single ventricular myocardial cells within guinea-pig papillary muscles rapidly induced and potentiated slow APs (figs. 12-12 and 12-13). As illustrated in fig. 12-12, pressure injection of cyclic AMP induced large, slow APs within 15–25 seconds after injection was started. The effect persisted as long as the pressure was applied, and the slow APs decayed within 25 seconds after the injecting pressure was discontinued. Thus, these results confirm the data obtained by electrophoretic injection of cyclic AMP. Intracellular injection of GPP(NH)P (for 5 seconds only) produced a very rapid effect, i.e., large slow APs were induced within 40–50 seconds, in contrast to the relatively slow effect (5–20 minutes) of GPP(NH)P added to the bathing medium. The induced slow APs persisted for over 3 minutes after the injecting pressure was stopped, indicating the relatively long-acting effect of GPP(NH)P. Figure 12-13 illustrates that injection of cholera toxin rapidly potentiates an ongoing slow AP, the effect beginning within 30 seconds and reaching maximum within 3 minutes (during a 3-minute injection period). The induced slow APs persisted for over 4 minutes after the injecting pressure was stopped, indicating the relatively long-acting effect of cholera toxin. (Cholera toxin has an effect on the adenylate cyclase complex that is similar to that of GPP(NH)P, namely, there is an irreversible activation of the regulatory component of the enzyme by inhibiting the hydrolysis of the GTP.)

Intracellular perfusion with cyclic AMP via a suction pipette enhanced I_{si} in isolated single adult cells {35}. Similarly, a photochemical activation method for suddenly

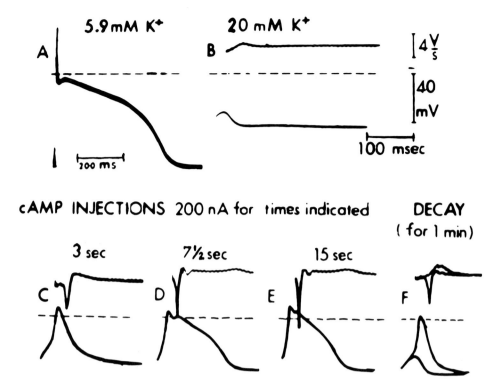

Fig. 12-11. Cyclic-AMP induction of slow action potentials in short canine Purkinje fibers. **A:** Normal fast action potential recorded from a fiber bathed in Krebs–Henseleit solution ($[K]_o = 5.9$ mM). **B:** Elevation of $[K]_o$ to 20 mM depolarized the fiber to about -40 mV and abolished excitability (field stimuli of 10-fold the normal threshold intensity applied). **C–E:** Induction of slow action potentials in a single fiber by cyclic-AMP injections of 200 nA for 3 seconds (C), 7.5 seconds (D), and 15 seconds (E), the induced responses were allowed to decay completely between injections (not illustrated for C and D). **F:** Decay (for 1 minute). At 1 minute after the injection in E, the slow action potential had decreased markedly in max dV/dt and duration (first sweep), and then disappeared nearly completely (second sweep). Note graded effects of the cyclic-AMP injections on the maximal upstroke velocity (+max dV/dt, upper traces). Horizontal dashed lines give the zero potential level. Different time calibrations in A and B–F. The preparation was paced at 0.3 Hz throughout. dV/dt trace arbitrarily shifted to the right, so as to not be obscured in the upstroke of the action potential. From Vogel and Sperelakis. {121}, with permission.

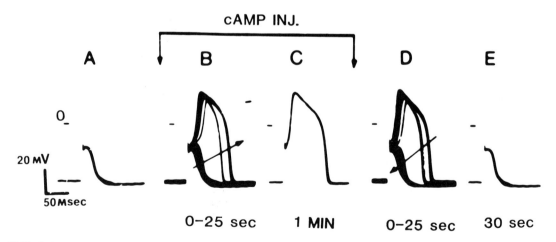

Fig. 12-12. Induction of slow action potentials in guinea-pig papillary muscle by intracellular pressure injection of cyclic AMP. The muscle was depolarized in 22 mM $[K]_o$ to voltage inactivate fast Na^+ channels. A microelectrode filled with 0.2 M Na^+-cAMP was used for both pressure injection and intracellular recording. **A:** Small graded response (stimulation rate 30/min). **B:** Superimposed records showing the gradual appearance of slow action potentials upon cyclic-AMP injection over a 25-second. **C:** Presence of stable slow action potential after injection for 1 minute. **D:** Gradual decrease of slow action potentials over a period of 25 seconds after stopping injection. **E:** Complete decay of slow action potentials 30 seconds after cessation of cyclic-AMP injection. All records were obtained from one impaled cell. From Li and Sperelakis {58}, with permission.

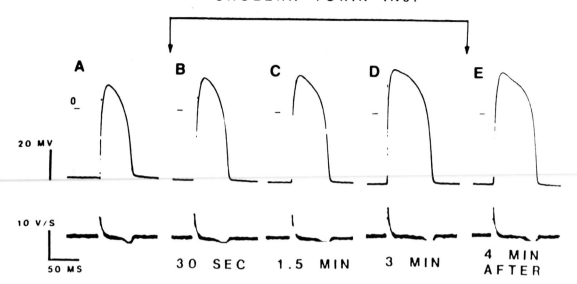

Fig. 12-13. Stimulation of slow action potentials by intracellular injection of cholera toxin. **A:** Slow action potential induced by electrical stimulation (30/min) in 22 mM $[K]_o$. **B–D:** Effect of intracellular pressure injection of cholera toxin. A microelectrode filled with reconstituted cholera toxin (1 mg/ml) solution containing 0.2 M NaCl was used both for intracellular injections and membrane potential recordings. An enhancement of the slow action potential occurred within 30 seconds (B) of the commencement of the injection period. The amplitude and duration of the slow action potential continued to increase during the injection, as seen at 1.5 minutes (C), until about 3 minutes (D), when an apparent steady state was reached. **E:** Persistent effect of cholera toxin after cessation of injection. The slow action potential remained enhanced 4 minutes after the injection had stopped. All records were obtained from one impaled cell. From Li and Sperelakis {58}, with permission.

increasing the intracellular cyclic AMP level enhanced I_{si} in bullfrog atrial cells {68}.

Results from patch-clamp analysis {1,12,112}, suggest that cyclic AMP increases the number of functional slow channels available in the myocardial sarcolemma and/or the probability of opening of a given channel. The net effect would be the same, i.e., an increase in the number of slow channels open at any instant of time. Reuter et al. {81} demonstrated that isoproterenol lengthened the mean open time of the channel and decreased the intervals between bursts (clustering of channel open states). Since the conductance of the single channel was not increased by isoproterenol, the increase in the total maximal slow conductance (g_{si}) produced by isoproterenol could be produced by the observed increase in the mean open time of each channel, as well as by an increase in the number of channels participating in the conductance on a stochastic basis.

These results support the hypothesis that the intracellular level of cyclic AMP controls the availability of the slow channels in the myocardial sarcolemma (table 12-2).

Metabolic dependence

It was shown by Schneider and Sperelakis {86,87,98} that the induced slow APs are blocked by hypoxia, ischemia, and metabolic poisons (including cyanide, dinitrophenol,

and valinomycin) within 5–15 minutes, accompanied by a lowering of the cellular ATP level. Only one example of the effect of metabolic interference will be given. Figure 12–14 shows that cyanide completely blocks the slow APs and contractions (figs. 12-14A–C) at a time when the fast APs (figs. 12-14D and 12-14E) are hardly affected; however, the contractions are nearly completely abolished, i.e., there is uncoupling of contraction from the fast AP. These data suggest that interference with metabolism leads to blockade of the slow channels. The fast APs are unaffected under these conditions, indicating that the fast Na^+ channels are essentially unaffected. However, the contractions accompanying the normal fast APs are depressed or abolished, indicating that contraction is uncoupled from excitation, as expected if the slow channels were blocked. The slow APs blocked by valinomycin or by hypoxia are restored by elevation of the glucose concentration {122}, indicating that the effect of metabolic poisons or hypoxia is indeed mediated by metabolic interference. Thus, there is a specific dependence of the slow channels on metabolic energy. The ATP dependence of I_{si} in isolated myocytes has been demonstrated by several groups {35,69,105,112}.

With prolonged metabolic interference, e.g., 60–120 minutes of hypoxia or cyanide, there is a gradual shortening of the duration of the normal fast AP, until a relatively brief spikelike component only remains, but which is still

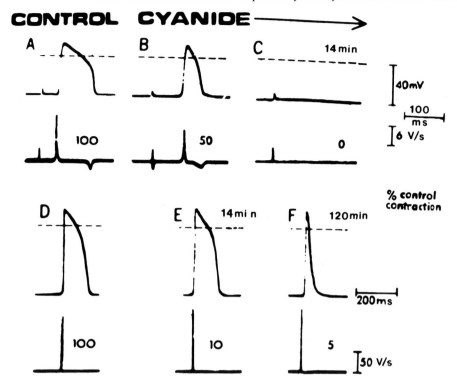

Fig. 12-14. Inhibition by cyanide (10^{-3} M) of the inward Ca^{2+} current induced by catecholamines in hearts partially depolarized by 27 mM K^+ (fast Na^+ channels inactivated). Intracellular recordings shown in upper traces; first derivatives of the action potentials are shown in the lower traces. Percent of control contractile force is numerically indicated in each panel. **A:** Control slow AP response induced by isoproterenol (10^{-7} M). **B,C:** The slow AP was depressed at 13 minutes (B) and abolished by 16 minutes (C) following addition of KCN to the perfusate. Depression and loss of contractions followed a parallel time course. **D:** Normal fast action potential in normal Ringer (2.7 mM K^+). **E:** At 14 minutes after KCN addition. There was almost no effect on the fast AP (max dV/dt, amplitude or duration) at a time when the slow channels were blocked (C). However, the contractions were greatly depressed. **F:** After 120 minutes in cyanide, the fast APs became greatly shortened in duration but retained fast rates of rise. Modified from Schneider and Sperelakis {86}, with permission.

rapidly rising (fig. 12-14F). Thus, metabolic interference exerts a second, but much slower, effect on the membrane. This effect is due to a K^+ conductance that is turned on by the reduction in the intracellular ATP concentration {70}.

Several K^+ channel currents are dependent on ATP levels in cardiac cells {69,70,115}. In isolated single ventricular cells from adult guinea-pig heart, the marked shortening of the APD_{50} produced by 0.1 mM DNP was accompanied by a pronounced increase of time-independent K^+ current {38}. When the patch pipette contained only 0.5 mM ATP, the Ca^{2+} slow current was decreased to less than 10% of the control value, and the time-dependent delayed-rectifier outward K^+ current was depressed {69}. At normal ATP levels, the inwardly rectifying K^+ channels have a slope conductance of approximately 25 pS {115}. In the presence of metabolic inhibitors (cell-attached patch) or in the absence of ATP in the solution bathing the cytoplasmic side (inside-out patch), this type of single-channel current disappears and a new type appears. The new current is also an inwardly rectifying K^+ current, but the slope conductance is approximately 80 pS; that is, the 80-pS channel appeared only after inhibition of cellular metabolism to lower the ATP level. Thus the type and conductance of K^+ channel current depends on the ATP level. ATP stimulates the normal low-conductance (25 pS) inwardly rectifying K^+ channel and inhibits the high-conductance (80 pS) inwardly rectifying K^+ channel. The ATP channel is also blocked by other intracellular triphosphates (GTP and UTP), as well as a nonhydrolyzable ATP analog, AMP-PNP. ADP is less effective than ATP in blocking the channel. Inward rectification is caused by a voltage-dependent blockade of the channel by intracellular Na^+ and Mg^{2+} ions at positive potentials. The channels display no time dependence of the kinetics of opening and closing; therefore, the macroscopic current is essentially time invariant. It was suggested {70} that this ATP-sensitive K^+ channel underlies the increased outward K^+ current that occurs in conditions of hypoxia or metabolic poisons, and that the ATP-inhibited K^+ channel may serve as a link between cellular energy metabolism and regulation of membrane excitability. ATP depletion produces shortening of the APD_{50}, and this

Phosphorylation Hypothesis for Slow Channel

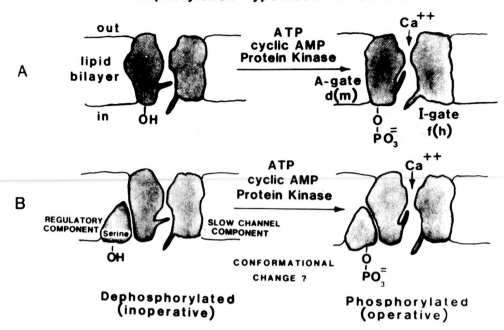

Fig. 12-15. Cartoon model for a slow channel in myocardial cell membrane in two hypothetical forms: dephosphorylated (or electrically silent) form (left diagrams) and phosphorylated form (right diagrams). The two gates associated with the channel, an activation (A, d, or m) gate and an inactivation (I, f, or h) gate, are kinetically much slower than those of the fast Na^+ channel. The hypothesis states that a protein constituent of the slow channel itself (**A**) or a regulatory protein associated with the slow channel (**B**) must be phosphorylated in order for the channel to be in a functional state available for voltage activation. Phosphorylation occurs by a cyclic-AMP-dependent protein kinase in the presence of ATP. Presumably a serine or threonine residue in the protein becomes phosphorylated. Phosphorylation of the slow channel protein or of an associated regulatory protein may produce a conformation change that effectively allows the channel gates to operate so that Ca^{2+} can pass through. Modified from Sperelakis and Schneider {85}, with permission.

results in a negative inotropic effect, thus sparing ATP. Hence, when ATP is lowered by hypoxia and ischemia, activation of the ATP-inhibited K^+ channel prevents further depletion of ATP and thus would help to protect the ischemic cells from irreversible damage.

It has also been shown that both the unstimulated (native) and the stimulated (induced) myocardial slow channels are similar with respect to their blockade by metabolic poisons {127}.

Phosphorylation hypothesis

Because of the relationship between cyclic AMP and the number of available slow channels, and because of the dependence of the functioning of the slow channels on metabolic energy, Shigenobu and Sperelakis {91} and Sperelakis and Schneider {98} postulated that a membrane protein must be phosphorylated in order for the slow channel to become available for voltage activation (fig. 12-15). A similar hypothesis has been proposed by Tsien and colleagues {116}, Watanabe and colleagues {129}, and Rinaldi and colleagues {83} for myocardial slow channels and by Kandel et al. for the serotonin-sensitive K^+ channel in *Aplysia* {13,92,93}. Elevation of cyclic AMP by a

positive inotropic agent activates a cyclic-AMP-dependent protein kinase (dimer split into two monomers), which phosphorylates a variety of proteins in the presence of ATP. Several myocardial membrane proteins become phosphorylated under these conditions.

To test whether the regulatory effect of cAMP is exerted by means of cA-PK and phosphorylation, intracellular injection of the catalytic subunit of the cA-PK was done. Such injections induced and enhanced the slow APs {9} and potentiated I_{Ca} {73,112,113}. Another test of the phosphorylation hypothesis was done by liposome injection of an inhibitor (protein) of the cA-PK into heart cells and showing that it inhibited the spontaneous slow APs {9}. This protein kinase inhibitor also was shown to inhibit I_{Ca} of cardiac cells {47}.

Based on the rapid decay of the response to injected cAMP, the mean life span of a phosphorylated channel is likely to be only a few seconds at most, and it is possible that the channels are phosphorylated and dephosphorylated with every cardiac cycle {58}. Hence, agents that affect or regulate the phosphatase would affect the life span of the phosphorylated channel. Thus, channel stimulation can be produced either by increasing the rate of phosphorylation (by cA-PK) or by decreasing the rate of dephosphorylation (inhibition of the phosphatase) {119}. For example, the Ca^{2+}-dependent phosphatase, calcineurin, inhibits the slow APs in 3-day-old embryonic chick hearts. Phosphatases have been shown to decrease the Ca^{2+} current in neurons {117} and ventricular myocardial cells {29}. The catalytic subunit of the protein phosphatases 1 and 2A inhibited the Ca^{2+} channel, and okadaic acid, a protein inhibitor, enhanced the amplitude of the I_{Ca}, prestimulated by beta-adrenergic agents {31}.

The protein that is phosphorylated might be a protein constituent of the slow channel itself (fig. 12-16A). The phosphorylation required to make the slow channel functional need not be of the channel protein itself, but of a contiguous regulatory type (e.g., phospholambanlike) of protein associated with the myocardial slow channel. For example, Rinaldi et al. {83} suggested that the function of

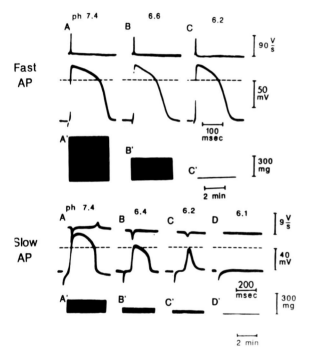

Fig. 12-16. Selective blockade of the slow channels by acid pH; bicarbonate-CO_2 buffer. A 20-day-old chick embryo heart was perfused with normal Ringer solution and paced at a rate of 0.5/s. **Upper row**: Normal fast APs. **A**: Normal fast action potential and contractions at pH 7.4. **B**: At pH 6.6, the force of contraction was greatly reduced, whereas the action potentials were almost unaffected. **C**: At pH 6.2, contractions were completely abolished, with almost no effect on the fast APs, i.e., excitation-contraction uncoupling was produced. **Lower row**: Blockade of isoproterenol (10^{-6} M)-induced slow AP responses at low pH (bicarbonate-CO_2 buffer system; 25 mM $[K]_o$). **A**: Control slow AP response and mechanical record at pH 7.4. **B–C**: Progressive blockade of slow AP responses and accompanying contractions as pH of perfusing solution was lowered. **D**: At pH 6.1, complete blockade of slow APs and contractions occurred. Upper traces gives dV/dt, from which the maximal rate rise of action potentials was obtained. Modified from Vogel and Sperelakis {120}, with permission.

cardiac slow Ca^{2+} channels in isolated sarcolemmal vesicles is modulated by a cyclic-AMP-dependent phosphorylation of a 23,000 Mw sarcolemmal protein (calciductin).

Phosphorylation could make the slow channel available for activation by a conformational change that either allowed the activation gate to be opened upon depolarization or effectively increased the diameter of the water-filled pore (the selectivity filter portion) so that Ca^{2+} and Na^+ could pass through. The phosphorylated form of the slow channel would be the active (operational) form, and the dephosphorylated form would be the inactive (inoperative) form; that is, only the phosphorylated form would be available to become activated upon depolarization to threshold. The dephosphorylated channels would be electrically silent. An equilibrium would probably exist between the phosphorylated and dephosphorylated forms of the slow channels for a given set of conditions, including the level of cyclic AMP. Thus, agents that act to elevate the cyclic-AMP level would increase the fraction of the slow channels that are in the phosphorylated form, and hence available for voltage activation. Such agents would increase the force of contraction of the myocardium.

There are some positive inotropic agents that induce the slow channels, but do not elevate cyclic AMP, e.g., angiotensin II {32} and fluoride ion (<1 mM) {39,119}. Fluoride ion may act by inhibiting the phosphoprotein phosphatase that dephosphorylates the slow-channel protein, thereby resulting in a larger fraction of phosphorylated channels; that is, inhibition of the rate of dephosphorylation should have the same effect as stimulation of the rate of phosphorylation. Angiotensin may activate a non-cyclic-AMP-dependent protein kinase. Thus, the results with angiotensin and fluoride can be fitted within the framework of the phosphorylation hypothesis.

G protein regulation of slow Ca channels

The guanine nucleotide binding proteins (G proteins) are interposed between membrane receptors and their effectors (e.g., enzymes and ion channels). Upon receptor activation, the G protein involved (G_s or G_i) becomes dissociated into its component subunits, namely, the α subunit and the βδ subunit. It is the α subunit that is possibly involved in activating certain membrane enzymes (such as adenylate cyclase) and Ca^{2+} and K^+ ion channels. The βδ subunit has been shown to activate certain membrane enzymes, such as phospholipase C.

As mentioned previously, β-receptor stimulation leads to the activated GTP-associated form of the regulatory protein (G_s^*). The active subunit ($α_s^*$) associates with the catalytic subunit of adenylate cyclase and increases the production of cAMP. The increase in cAMP levels stimulates the catalytic subunit of protein kinase A (PKA), which leads to phosphorylation of the Ca channel protein. This well-known pathway is an example of indirect regulation of Ca channels via guanine nucleotide binding (G) proteins {78}.

Recently, it has been discovered that G_s^* can directly activate Ca^{2+} channels in myocytes in which the cAMP-phosphorylation pathway has been blocked {132}. This direct, or membrane-delimited, pathway may allow for a more rapid response in Ca channel activity following β-receptor activation, in comparison with the more indirect pathway utilizing phosphorylation.

CYCLIC GMP ANTAGONISM OF CYCLIC AMP

Superfusion of isolated guinea pig papillary muscles with 8-Br-cGMP (10^{-5} to 10^{-3} M) abolished the Ca^{2+}-dependent slow APs and accompanying contractions within 7–20 minutes {126}. Intracellular pressure injection of cyclic GMP into cells of guinea-pig papillary muscle transiently depressed or abolished slow APs much more quickly (e.g., 1–2 minutes) {126}. Injection of cyclic GMP into cultured chick heart cells by the liposome method also abolished the slow APs {8}.

Therefore, cyclic GMP regulates the functioning of the myocardial Ca^{2+} slow channels in a manner that is antagonistic to that of cyclic AMP. The effect of cyclic GMP may be mediated through phosphorylation of a protein that regulates the functioning of the slow channel. It is possible that the slow-channel protein, or an associated regulatory protein, has a second site that can be phosphorylated and that, when phosphorylated, inhibits the slow channel. Another possibility is that there is a second type of regulatory protein that is inhibitory when phosphorylated. Another mechanism proposed for frog ventricular muscle, in which db-cAMP potentiates the twitch and 8-Br-cGMP depresses it, is based on the fact that cGMP depressed the cAMP level (i.e., there was a reciprocal relationship between cGMP and cAMP), namely, that cGMP may serve to regulate cAMP level {94}. Consistent with this, cyclic GMP was reported to have negligible effects on basal I_{Ca} in voltage-clamped single frog ventricular cells, but greatly decreased the potentiated I_{Ca} produced by beta-adrenergic agonists or intracellular perfusion with cyclic AMP {28}. They suggested that the decrease in I_{Ca} was mediated by cyclic-AMP hydrolysis via a cyclic-GMP-stimulated phosphodiesterase.

It was recently demonstrated cGMP inhibition of Ca^{2+} slow channel activity at both the whole-cell and the single-channel levels {110}. Cyclic GMP did not change unit amplitude and slope conductance of the Ca^{2+} channel, but prolonged the closed time and shortened the open times. Because 8-Br-cGMP is a potent activator of G-kinase and does not stimulate cAMP hydrolysis, cGMP inhibition of the basal activity of the Ca^{2+} channels may be mediated by G kinase.

In 3-day-old embryonic chick heart cells, the Ca^{2+} slow channels often exhibited long-lasting openings (e.g., for 300 ms) under normal conditions, especially at the more positive command potentials {110}; that is, the Ca^{2+} slow channels naturally possessed mode 2 behavior, in the absence of any added Ca^{2+} channel agonist such as the dihydropyridine, Bay-K-8644. Addition of Bay-K-8644 did not further prolong the open times, but appeared to recruit silent Ca^{2+} channels {106}. Long-lasting openings were much less frequently observed in 17-day-old embryonic

cells {110}. Addition of 8-Br-cGMP to the bath of 3-day cells exhibiting long openings completely inhibited Ca^{2+} slow channel activity.

Calmodulin-protein kinase and protein kinase C

Inhibitors of calmodulin (trifluoperazine and calmidazolium) inhibit the slow APs of heart cells {6,7,40}. Subsequent injection of calmodulin reverses the inhibition produced by calmidazolium. It appears that maximal activation of the slow channels requires two separate phosphorylation steps (calmodulin dependent and cAMP-dependent). These may be on the same protein or on two separate proteins.

A high concentration of the alpha-adrenergic agonist, phenylephrine, causes a positive inotropic effect in cardiac muscle {10}. The alpha-adrenoceptor agonists stimulate the phosphatidyl inositol cycle and generation of inositol trisphosphate (IP_3) and diacyl glycerol (DAG). IP_3 acts as a second messenger to release stored Ca^{2+} from the sarcoplasmic reticulum (SR). DAG and Ca^{2+} activate PK-C, which phosphorylates a number of proteins. It is presently controversial whether PK-C is involved in regulation of the myocardial slow Ca^{2+} channels. One group reported that phorbol ester and ang-II stimulated I_{Ca} {24}, whereas another group did not observe such stimulation {107}. There have been variable findings with respect to the effect of activation of alpha-adrenoceptor agonists on elevation of cAMP.

Selective blockade by acidosis

The myocardial slow channels are selectively blocked by acidosis {18,120}. Vogel and Sperelakis {120} showed that the slow APs induced by isoproterenol, for example, are depressed in rate of rise, amplitude, and duration as the pH of the perfusing solution is lowered below 7.0 (fig. 12-16). The slow AP is 50% inhibited at pH 6.6 and is completely abolished at pH 6.1. (The slow APs should be abolished before all the slow channels are blocked because of the requirement of a minimum density of slow channels for regenerative and propagating responses.) The contractions are depressed in parallel with the slow APs. Similar findings were recently reported using internally perfused and voltage-clamped guinea-pig ventricular myocytes {36}. When the Na-H exchange mechanism is blocked, a 50% reduction in I_{Ca} was found at pH_i 6.5, and I_{Ca} was blocked by pH_i 6.0. It was found that a lower external pH (5.5) was necessary for 50% reduction of I_{Ca}. Thus the Ca channel is more sensitive to internal, than to external, protons.

Acidosis has little or no effect on the normal fast AP, i.e., the rate of rise remains fast and the overshoot and duration are only slightly affected. However, the contractions become depressed and abolished as a function of the degree of acidosis; that is, excitation-contraction uncoupling occurs, as expected from a selective blockade of the slow channels.

Since the myocardium becomes acidotic during hypoxia and ischemia (glycolysis is increased and lactic acid diffuses into the interstitial fluid space), it is likely that part of the effect of these metabolic interventions on the slow channels is mediated by the accompanying acidosis and not solely by a decrease in ATP level. Consistent with this, the effects of hypoxia on the slow AP were almost immediately reversed, but only partially and transiently, by changing the pH of the perfusing solution to 8.0; the responses gradually diminished further during hypoxia at the alkaline pH {5}.

Intrinsic control over Ca^{2+} influx: Protection hypothesis

The Ca^{2+} influx of the myocardial cell is controlled by extrinsic factors (table 12-2). For example, stimulation of the sympathetic nerves to the heart or circulating catecholamines or other hormones can have a positive inotropic action, whereas stimulation of the parasympathetic neurons has a negative inotropic effect. The mechanism for some of these effects is mediated by changes in the levels of the cyclic nucleotides. This extrinsic control of the Ca^{2+} influx is enabled by the peculiar properties of the slow channels, as, for example, the postulated requirement for phosphorylation.

However, in addition, there is intrinsic control by the myocardial cell itself over its Ca^{2+} influx (table 12-2). For example, under conditions of transient regional ischemia, many of the slow channels become unavailable (or silent). This effect may be mediated by lowering the ATP level of the affected cells and by the accompanying acidosis (since slow-channel blockade during hypoxia occurs faster at acid pH than at alkaline pH). Acidosis presumably blocks the slow channels directly, and metabolic interference causes indirect inactivation of the slow channels. Both effects are relatively selective for the slow channels.

Thus the myocardial cell can partially or completely suppress its Ca^{2+} influx (which is part of the inward slow current, I_{si}) under adverse conditions. This causes the affected cells to contract weakly or not at all, and since most of the work done by the cell is mechanical, this conserves ATP. Such a mechanism may serve to protect the myocardial cells under adverse conditions, such as transient regional ischemia during coronary vasospasm. If the myocardial cell could not control its Ca^{2+} influx, then the ATP level might drop so low under such conditions that irreversible damage would be done, i.e., the cells would become necrotic. Because of the peculiar properties of the slow channels, they become inactivated, thus uncoupling contraction from excitation and conserving ATP. The cells could then recover fully when the blood flow returns to normal.

The almost normal resting potential and retention of fast APs in the ischemic zone would allow propagation through this area to be normal, thus minimizing the chances for the induction of arrhythmias. The effect of metabolic interference on shortening the AP after 30–120 minutes (due to enhanced g_K, which terminates the AP) would also help to shut off I_{si} more quickly, thereby reducing the total Ca^{2+} influx per impulse and so helping to conserve ATP.

The AP in the ischemic region may be either a slow-channel AP or a depressed fast-channel AP. The depression of the rate or rise is caused by the partial depolarization of the cells due to K^+ accumulation in the interstitial space and perhaps to depression of electrogenic Na^+ pumping. (Progressive depolarization voltage inactivates a progressively larger fraction of the fast Na^+ channels due to closing of their inactivation [I] gates.) Many of the slow channels also would be expected to be blocked because of the acidosis and lowered ATP level.

BLOCKADE OF THE SLOW CHANNELS BY ACETYLCHOLINE AND ADENOSINE

The parasympathetic neurotransmitter, acetylcholine (ACh), exerts a negative inotropic effect on the heart, as well as a negative chronotropic effect by action on the SA nodal cells. Because of the positive treppe (staircase) phenomenon of cardiac muscle, the latter effect also produces a negative inotropic effect. ACh is well known to increase g_K and thereby can hyperpolarize SA nodal cells (therefore depressing automaticity) and shorten the duration of the AP in atrial myocardial cells {20}. This would also tend to suppress slow APs in atrial cells by increasing the overlapping outward K^+ current and so diminishing the net inward (slow) current.

In ventricular myocardial cells, activation of the muscarinic receptor by ACh reverses the stimulation of the adenylate cyclase complex produced by the beta-adrenergic agonists. Activation of the beta-adrenergic receptor activates the (stimulatory) regulatory component of the adenylate cyclase complex, whereas activation of the muscarinic receptor activates an inhibitory regulatory component of the enzyme (see fig. 12-18).

Activation of the muscarinic receptor by ACh exerts an inhibitory effect on adenylate cyclase and cyclic AMP level, via the G_i (inhibitory) coupling protein, to reverse the stimulation of adenylate cyclase produced by means of the G_s coupling protein due to, for example, activation of the beta-adrenoceptor or H_2 receptor; that is, the muscarinic receptor antagonizes or opposes the stimulation of adenylate cyclase produced by other receptors, such as the beta-adrenoceptor or H_2 receptor. Thus ACh depresses Ca^{2+} influx and contraction not only by elevation of cyclic GMP, but also by reversing cyclic AMP elevation produced by beta-adrenergic agonists and H_2 agonists.

Josephson and Sperelakis {44}, in voltage-clamp experiments on cultured chick ventricular cells stimulated by isoproterenol, demonstrated that ACh depresses the inward slow current, I_{si} (fig. 12-17). It is possible that the depression of the ISO-potentiated I_{is} is mediated by a lowering of the cyclic-AMP level, which was elevated by activation of the beta-adrenergic receptor. It is not known whether part of this effect of ACh is also mediated through elevation of the intracellular cyclic-GMP level, which would act to antagonize the effects of cyclic AMP. ACh did not increase the outward K^+ current (I_K) in these ventricular cells. This suggests that the ACh-activated K^+ channel may be absent from ventricular cells.

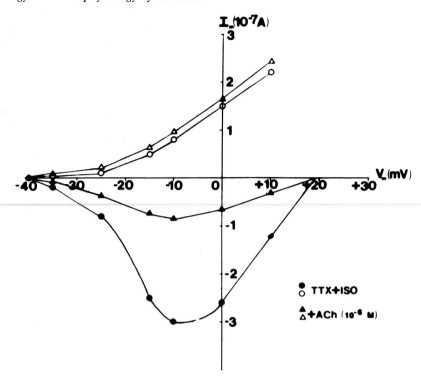

Fig. 12-17. Acetylcholine (ACh) depression of the inward slow current (I_{si} or I_{Ca}) that was potentiated by isoproterenol (ISO) in a cultured reaggregate of embryonic chick ventricular cells. Current/voltage (I/V) curves obtained by a two-microelectrode voltage clamp. The fast Na^+ current was suppressed by use of tetrodotoxin (TTX, 10^{-6} M) and by using a holding potential of -40 mV). Filled circles represent I_{si} potentiated by 10^{-6} M ISO; unfilled circles give the steady-state outward K^+ current. Addition of 10^{-6} M ACh depressed I_{si} (filled triangles, 3 minutes), whereas there was little or no effect on outward I_K (unfilled triangles). Note that ACh depressed the ISO-stimulated I_{Ca} but did not potentiate I_K in these ventricular cells. Taken from Josephson and Sperelakis {44}, with permission.

ACh not only depressed the slow APs induced by isoproterenol, but also the slow APs that were induced by forskolin {124,131}. If forskolin's action resulted from a direct stimulation of the catalytic subunit of the adenylate cyclase complex, then activation of the muscarinic receptor may somehow reverse this stimulation.

Adenosine (ADO) has effects on the heart that are virtually identical to those of ACh. For example, in isolated rabbit SA node, both ADO and ACh depress automaticity and hyperpolarize {130}. In atrial cells, both ADO and ACh markedly shorten the action potential and produce a small hyperpolarization and depression of automaticity {3}. In contrast, in ventricular muscle of birds {91} and mammals {84}, ACh and ADO do not shorten the APD_{50} and do not hyperpolarize. Consistent with this, Belardinelli and Isenberg {3} showed that ADO did not shorten the APD in isolated ventricular myocytes (bovine and guinea pig). However, if the APD_{50} is first prolonged by isoproterenol (ISO), then ADO counteracted the effects of ISO, including on the plateau overshoot {3}.

The Ca^{2+}-dependent slow APs of atrial muscle of guinea pig {88} are blocked by ADO. In guinea-pig ventricular cells, however, ADO had little or no effect on the ISO-induced slow APs {84}. This was confirmed in voltage-clamp measurements of I_{si} (I_{Ca}) in isolated guinea-pig ventricular myocytes (in 25 mM $[K]_o$ to suppress the fast I_{Na}) {37}. The stimulation of I_{Ca} by ISO (10^{-8} M) was not counteracted by ADO (2×10^{-4} M). However, if these experiments were repeated in normal low $[K]_o$ (5.4 mM), ADO was able to counteract the stimulatory effect of ISO {37}. Hence, for some unknown reason, in high $[K]_o$ ADO cannot antagonize the potentiating effect of ISO on I_{Ca}.

Consistent with the ability of ADO to counteract the stimulatory effect of ISO on I_{Ca} in ventricular muscle, ADO (10^{-5} M) was shown to reverse the elevation of cyclic AMP produced by ISO (3×10^{-8} and 10^{-7} M) to nearly the control (basal) level in embryonic chick (12-day-old) ventricular muscle {4}. Further support for the view that the anti-adrenergic effect of ADO in ventricular muscle is due to inhibition of adenylate cyclase was provided by West et al. {131}, who showed that the increased APD in response to forskolin was antagonized by ADO.

The mechanism whereby ADO and ACh shorten the normal AP and hyperpolarize in atrial muscle, in addition

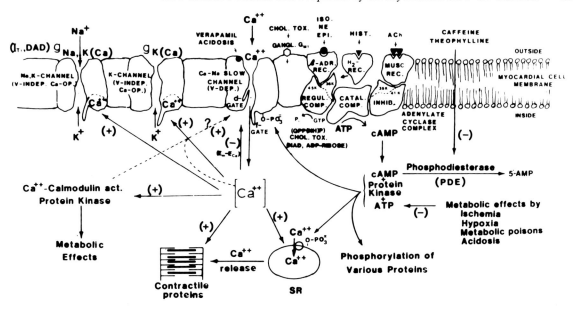

Fig. 12-18. Model for actions of adenosine (ADO) in various heart tissues. As depicted, in all cardiac tissues, specifically ventricular, atrial, SA nodal, and AV nodal, ADO activates an ADO receptor (A_1), which inhibits the catalytic subunit of adenylate cyclase via the G_s (N_s) coupling protein. This action antagonizes or reverses the stimulatory effects of activation of the beta-adrenergic receptor or histaminic H_2 receptor on the adenylate cyclase exerted via the G_s (N_s) coupling protein, thereby returning the cyclic AMP level back towards the basal level. Also depicted is the fact that ACh exerts a similar effect via activation of the muscarinic receptor. As illustrated, muscarinic receptor activation also stimulates the guanylate cyclase and thereby elevates the cyclic GMP level. Cyclic AMP stimulates the Ca^{2+} slow channels via phosphorylation by a cyclic AMP-dependent protein kinase (cA-PK). Cyclic GMP inhibits the Ca^{2+} slow channels. In all cardiac tissues except ventricular, ADO and ACh act, via their respective receptors, to activate a special K^+ channel via a G_x (G_o or N_o) type of coupling protein, as depicted at the right side of the diagram. This effect increases a K^+ conductance [$g_{K(ACh)}$ and $g_{K(ADO)}$], and therefore gives rise to ADO-induced and ACh-induced K^+ current.

to inhibition of I_{Ca}, is an increase in K^+ conductance (g_K). For example, in measurements of the steady-state outward I_K (using voltage clamp of isolated guinea-pig atrial myocytes), Belardinelli and Isenberg {3} found that ADO and ACh increased outward I_K; that is, there was similarity between the ADO-induced current and ACh-induced current. The increased outward K^+ current would shorten the APD and hyperpolarize (towards E_K).

The effects of ADO and ACh in various cardiac tissues are summarized diagrammatically in fig. 12-18. As depicted, the ventricular cell does not possess the ADO- or ACh-activated K^+ conductance channel, whereas the atrial and nodal cells do. This would explain why the normal AP is not shortened in ventricular muscle, whereas it is shortened in atrial muscle and nodal cells, and hyperpolarization is produced. As depicted, all cardiac tissues possess ADO and ACh receptors, which when connected to the G_i coupling protein antagonize the stimulatory effects of the beta-adrenergic and histaminic H_2 receptors exerted on the catalytic subunit of adenylate cyclase via the G_s coupling protein. This would explain the lowering of the cyclic AMP level by ADO or ACh that was elevated by ISO and the reversal of the increase in I_{Ca} produced by ISO. Stimulation of the guanylate cyclase by muscarinic

receptor activation, with consequent elevation of cyclic GMP, would also act to depress I_{Ca}.

BLOCKADE OF SLOW CHANNELS BY DRUGS AND ANESTHETIC AGENTS

The calcium-antagonistic drugs, such as verapamil, D-600, nifedipine, diltiazem, and bepridil, block the voltage-dependent slow channels (Ca^{2+} and Ca-Na types) found in myocardial cells (fig. 12-20), Purkinje fibers, nodal cells, and VSM cells. Some Ca antagonists, such as verapamil, D-600, and nifedipine (but not diltiazem, bepridil, and mesudipine), also block the slow Na^+ channels found in young (3-day-old) embryonic chick hearts {52,90}.

Figure 12-18 illustrates the effect of verapamil on blocking the slow APs in guinea-pig papillary muscle and of nifedipine on blocking the isoproterenol-induced slow APs in guinea-pig papillary muscle (fig. 12-19A–D) and guinea-pig Purkinje fibers (fig. 12-19E–H) driven at a constant rate of 0.5 Hz. As indicated, nifedipine is more potent than verapamil in blocking the slow channels {66,67}. The general order of potency of the calcium antagonistic drugs in blocking the slow channels of various

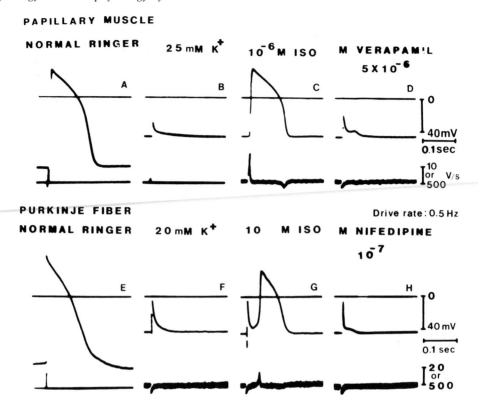

PAPILLARY MUSCLE

NORMAL RINGER   25 mM K⁺   10⁻⁶ M ISO   M VERAPAMIL
5 X 10⁻⁶

PURKINJE FIBER   Drive rate: 0.5 Hz

NORMAL RINGER   20 mM K⁺   10   M ISO   M NIFEDIPINE
10⁻⁷

Fig. 12-19. Induction of the slow action potentials (APs) and their block by calcium-antagonistic drugs. **A–D:** Papillary muscle (guinea pig). **E–H:** Purkinje fiber (guinea pig). A and E: Normal fast APs. B and F: Elevation of $[K_o]$ to 25 mM (B) or 20 mM (F) depolarized to about −45 mV and blocked excitability (shock artifacts only visible). C and G: Addition of isoproterenol (10^{-6} M) rapidly induced slowly rising APs and slow APs. D and H: Addition of verapamil (5×10^{-6} M; D) or nifedipine (10^{-7} M; H) rapidly depressed and blocked the slow APs. The driving rate for the slow APs was 0.5 Hz. The upper straight line in each panel is the zero potential level, and the lower trace is dV/dt, the peak excursion of which gives max dV/dt. The voltage and time calibrations are the same throughout; the dV/dt calibration bars represent 500 V/s for A and E, and 10 V/s for B–D or 20 V/s for F–H. Modified from Molyvdas and Sperelakis {66,67}, with permission.

heart tissues is nifedipine > diltiazem ≥ verapamil > bepridil {57}.

By definition, to be a member of this class of compounds a drug must block the slow channel by direct action on the cell membrane channel itself (and not indirectly via metabolic depression or acidosis, for example), and this action must be relatively specific for the slow channel, in contrast to the other types of voltage-dependent ion channels (e.g., fast Na⁺ channel or delayed rectifier K⁺ channel). Thus, this definition would distinguish Ca antagonists from local anesthetics or metabolic poisons, for example.

Some Ca antagonists, such as bepridil, may exert, in addition, a second action, e.g., intracellularly to depress Ca^{2+} uptake into or release from the SR {118}. The evidence for a second effect of bepridil was the fact that this drug depressed cardiac contractile force more than could be accounted for by the depression of the inward slow Ca^{2+} current. Consistent with the possibility of a second intracellular effect, bepridil and verapamil were shown to enter the myocardial cells, the order of uptake

being bepridil > verapamil ≥ nitrendipine ≫ nifedipine > diltiazem {75,76}. This order of uptake followed the order of lipid solubilities {76}. In addition, those Ca antagonists that readily enter the cells have the possibility of exerting their effect on the slow channels from the inner surface of the cell membrane. For example, it was shown that a charged quaternary ammonium derivative of D-600 had no effect on the inward slow current of myocardial cells when added to the bathing solution, but did depress I_{si} when injected intracellularly {39}.

Ca^{2+} binding to isolated sarcolemmal membranes (vesicles) was inhibited by verapamil and bepridil in a dose-dependent manner, verapamil being the more potent of the two, as it is in inhibition of slow APs {75}. Since Ca^{2+} binding to the outer mouth of the slow channel (as depicted in fig. 12-1) is probably the first step in ion permeation through the channel, Ca^{2+} displacement could be one possible mechanism for blockade of Ca^{2+} entry by verapamil and bepridil, although this would not readily account for the frequency dependency of the effect of

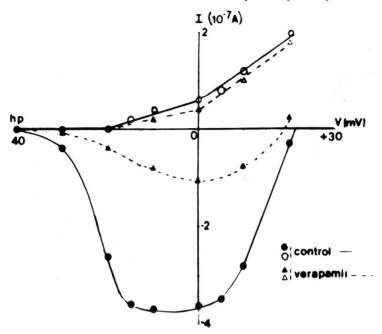

Fig. 12-20. Effect of verapamil (10^{-6} M) on membrane currents recorded from a reaggregate cell culture. Solid circles are peak I_{si} recorded with TTX (10^{-6} M) and isoproterenol (10^{-6} M) present; open circles represent outward currents (at 300 ms). The triangles are values after 3-minute exposure to verapamil (10^{-6} M); open triangles show outward currents and filled triangles the values for I_{si}. These data show that verapamil depresses I_{si} and has almost no effect on the outward I_K. From Josephson and Sperelakis {44}, with permission.

these two drugs. On the other hand, the frequency-independent block of Ca^{2+} entry by Mn^{2+}, Co^{2+}, or La^{3+} ions could be by such a mechanism. Nifedipine and diltiazem did not inhibit Ca^{2+} binding {74}. Thus there are great differences in properties of the calcium-antagonistic drugs, and they may block the slow channels by different molecular mechanisms, as might be predicted from their widely different chemical structures.

Apparent reversal of the block of the slow APs and contractions by the Ca antagonists by elevation of $[Ca]_o$ may result from either of two mechanisms: (a) competition between Ca^{2+} and drug for binding to the outer mouth of the channel, or (b) the increased electrochemical driving force for Ca^{2+} influx through the fraction of slow channels not blocked by the drug. The latter mechanism probably operates in all cases, whereas the former mechanism may be involved with some of the drugs, such as verapmil and bepridil.

The effect of most of the calcium-antagonistic drugs on depression of the slow APs and inward slow Ca^{2+} current (I_{si}) is frequency dependent; that is, the higher the frequency of stimulation, the greater the blocking effect on the slow channels. For example, a dose of drug that completely blocks the slow APs at a drive rate of 1 Hz may exhibit no effect at 0.1 Hz. This effect is prominent in the action of all of this class of drugs, although nifedipine seems to have a lesser frequency dependence than the other drugs. In contrast, Ca^{2+}-entry blockers, such as

Mn^{2+}, Co^{2+}, and La^{3+}, do not exhibit a frequency dependency; that is, the effect of Mn^{2+}, for example, is present even to the first stimulation after equilibration of the Mn^{2+} under resting conditions.

This frequency dependency of effect suggests that the calcium-antagonistic drugs do not act as simple blockers for the Ca^{2+} slow channels, as perhaps Mn^{2+} or La^{3+} might act. Rather, this property suggests that the drug might act to slow the recovery process of the slow channel from the inactive state back to the resting state (see fig. 12-3). If so, then a slow drive rate of a long quiescent period (e.g., 20–60 seconds) would allow complete recovery of the drugged slow channel before the next excitation occurred. To exert such an effect on the gate recovery kinetics, the drugs could bind anywhere on the channel protein. An alternative possibility is that the drug binds to the channel only in the active state or inactive state (membrane also depolarized) to block it, and then dissociates before conversion of the channel to the resting state. There is substantial evidence that binding of the drug is voltage dependent, depolarization favoring binding and hyperpolarization favoring unbinding.

Another possibility to be considered is that any drug that affected the phosphorylation of the slow channels by some direct means would also effectively block the slow channels selectively and could account for the drug's frequency dependence. Consistent with this possibility, it was recently found that several of the calcium-antagonistic drugs, such as verapamil, inhibited the cyclic-AMP-dependent phosphorylation in vitro of three membrane proteins (Carry, Sperelakis, and Villar-Palasi, unpublished observations).

A number of other agents and drugs also block the myocardial slow channels, including high concentrations of ouabain {45}, local anesthetics {43}, and volatile general anesthetics {59}. The local anesthetics, lidocaine and procainamide, however, blocked the slow channels nonspecifically; that is, the dose-response curve for the slow APs were similar to that for the fast APs. In contrast, depressed fast APs, produced in 10 mM $[K]_o$, were about 10-fold more sensitive to lidocaine {96}. Halothane and enflurane are more selective in inhibiting the slow channels of the heart than the fast Na^+ channels {21}.

EXCITATION AND CONDUCTION OF THE SLOW ACTION POTENTIALS

The slow APs have a stimulation threshold nearly 10-fold higher than that for the fast APs, i.e., slow APs have a lower excitability. The threshold potential (V_{th}) for the slow APs is at an E_m of about -35 mV, whereas that for the fast APs is about -55 mV, i.e., the critical depolarization required to excite is large for the slow APs (assuming an unchanged resting potential of -80 mV). Chronaxie of the slow AP (0.9 ms) is about 10-fold higher than that for the fast AP {21}.

The slow APs propagate at a velocity of about 4–10 cm/s {61}. In a simple cable, conduction velocity (θ) should vary directly with the max dV/dt {97}; that is, the faster the rate of rise of the AP, the faster the propagation. (There are exceptions to this in cardiac muscle when comparing transverse propagation versus longitudinal propagation, because the tissue is not a simple cable). Thus, if the fast AP in cardiac muscle propagates at 0.40 m/s for a max dV/dt of 150 V/s, then if max dV/dt is reduced to 15 V/s for the slow AP, θ should be reduced by 10 times or to 0.127 m/s. However, propagation velocity is decreased more than the predicted amount in both myocardium (12.7 m/s predicted vs. <4–10 cm/s actual) and Purkinje fibers (0.2 m/s predicted vs. <0.1 cm/s actual) {23}. The latter authors attributed the discrepancy to the slow AP, seeing a higher effective membrane capacitance (C_m), i.e., a higher capacitive reactance (X_o). It is not known to what degree decremental conduction may occur, i.e., decreasing propagation velocity and response amplitude as a function of the distance along the muscle.

Some studies have focused on the ability of propagating fast APs to trigger slow APs. In rabbit left atrial strips (composed of homogenous parallel bundles of fibers) compartmentalized into three functional segments, the left (test) segment being exposed to 12.7 mM $[K]_o$ and 1 mM $[Ba]_o$ to depolarize sufficiently to block the fast APs, Masuda et al. {61} found that high-frequency (0.63–2.5 Hz) stimulation caused 2:1 block due to fatigue of the slow AP (slowness of recovery of excitability). However, low-frequency (0.13–0.4 Hz) stimulation also produced complete block. Therefore, there was a limited frequency range in which a normal fast AP could stimulate slow APs at a sustained 1:1 ratio. The low-frequency block was attributed to the observed reduced amplitude and duration of the atrial fast AP, since ACh, which shortens the plateau of the atrial AP, also blocked the development of the slow AP in the test compartment when it was added to the middle compartment. Hence, the amplitude, duration, and frequency of the fast APs determined whether they served as effective stimuli for the slow APs in the depolarized region.

Cukierman and Paes de Carvalho {21} studied the properties of membrane (nonpropagated) slow APs induced (stimulated with a suction electrode) in short (2–3 mm) atrial trabeculae from rabbit left atrium by 1 mM $[Ba]_o$ and 10 mM $[K]_o$. The resting potential in the high K^+-Ba^{2+} solution was -55 mV, the amplitude of the slow APs was 60 mV, and the APD_{50} was 84 ms. The slow AP upstroke was always initiated from a small subthreshold-depolarizing step. The slow AP was all or none. The slow AP fatigued at high pacing rates (>1 Hz), and a fully developed slow AP could only be obtained within a certain frequency range, as found in the long-strip preparation of Masuda et al. {61}.

POSSIBLE ROLE OF SLOW ACTION POTENTIALS IN ARRHYTHMIAS

Slow APs have been implicated in the genesis of arrhythmias {19–21}. Propagating fast APs can trigger slow APs in depolarized regions {23}. Slow conduction in a pathway allows circus movement of excitation around that pathway and may lead to reentrant type of arrhythmias. There is a requirement of one-way conduction through the depressed area, and the length of the reentry loop is critical, depending on velocity. In an ischemic or infarcted zone, and the surrounding border zone, there is a depressed area with slowed conduction. Partial depolarization of the cells in this area occurs because of a high $[K]_o$ due to the hypoxia/ischemia and consequent impaired metabolism. In addition, there is norepinephrine (NE) release for the sympathetic nerve terminals.

NE release should elevate cyclic AMP and increase the number of available slow channels, tending to increase I_{si} in the cells in the ischemic zone. However, the hypoxia/ischemia should tend to depress I_{si} because of the accompanying lowered ATP level and the metabolic dependence of the slow-channel functioning. Therefore, the ischemic AP can be either (a) a depressed fast AP (i.e., an AP whose inward current is carried through fewer fast Na^+ channels) due to the partial depolarization (and the h_∞ vs. E_m relationship) or (b) a pure slow AP (i.e., an AP whose inward current is carried only through slow channels) if the K^+ depolarization is great enough such that complete voltage inactivation of all (or most) fast Na^+ channels has occurred (at about -55 mV). There is some evidence for both possibilities {20}.

Evidence that the ischemic AP is a depressed fast AP includes the fact that TTX blocks the AP, whereas verapamil does not {53,133}. Additional points supporting the view the ischemic AP is a depressed fast AP and not a slow AP are (a) the metabolic dependence of the functioning of the slow channels and (b) the dyskinesis or akinesis of the ischemic area. It is likely that the degree of K^+ accumulation, and hence depolarization, is one factor determining the nature of the AP in the ischemic zone; other factors may be the amount of catecholamines released that persist in the interstitial fluid and the degree of ATP depletion and acidosis in the afflicted cells.

Although local anesthetics depress and block slow APs at concentrations similar to those that depress the normal fast APs {43}, the depressed fast APs are nearly 10-fold more sensitive to these drugs {96}. Thus lidocaine and procainamide, and related antiarrhythmic agents, can relatively selectively suppress fast APs in ischemic/infarcted regions and thereby suppress dysrhythmias.

The APs in the ischemic area have slow upstroke velocities (max dV/dt), are conducted slowly (ca. 0.05 m/s), and about 35% of the APs have notched upstrokes or two peaks {19}. There are delays and possibly decremental conduction. The depressed area exhibits one-way block, frequency-dependent block, and the Wenckebach phenomenon. There is a low safety factor for conduction, causing the impulse to be prone to block at impediments. Structural inhomogeneities/asymmetries and pathologic changes can act as impediments to conduction {19}. In addition, premature excitation can unmask asymmetries, and so a premature impulse may travel more readily in one direction than the other. Such undirectional block of a premature implulse sets up one condition necessary for circus movement, namely, one-way conduction. Increase in resistance of the cell-to-cell junctions (or in juctional cleft width) during hypoxia/ischemia were suggested as a cause of conduction impediment {19}.

EFFECT OF [Ca]$_i$ ON MEMBRANE CHANNELS

[Ca]$_i$ has profound effects on membrane electrical properties (fig. 12-20). A depolarizing afterpotential following a conventional hyperpolarizing afterpotential was first described in cultured embryonic chick heart cells by Lehmkuhl and Sperelakis {55}, who turned trains of spontaneous APs on and off by applying hyperpolarizing current pulses of various intensities. They thereby demonstrated that each AP in a train was triggered by the preceding AP by means of the delayed depolarizing afterpotential. Ferrier and Moe {26} subsequently described this phenomenon in mammalian heart and called it a *delayed afterdepolarization* (DAD). They showed that cardiac glycosides and elevated [Ca]$_o$ potentiate the DAD, and that calcium-antagonistic drugs depress and abolish the DAD, and pointed out its possible importance in arrhythogenesis.

Kass et al. {49} showed that the DAD is not directly produced by an inward Ca^{2+} current, but rather indirectly by release of Ca^{2+} from the SR, which, in turn, produces an increase in a nonspecific leakage-type conductance for a net inward depolarizing current, the transient inward current (I_{Ti}). The reversal potential (E_{rev}) for I_{Ti} is about

$-5 \, mV$ and is sensitive to [Na]$_o$ but not to [Ca]$_o$. The increase in APs opens a nonspecific voltage-independent postsynaptic type of ion channel that allows both Na^+ and K^+ to pass through. This type of channel would be somewhat analogous to the Ca^{2+}-activated K^+ channels [$g_{K(Ca)}$] {39}.

I_{Ti} and concomitant aftercontractions are enhanced by digitalis, K^+-free solution, catecholamine, and elevated [Ca]$_o$. The effects of digitalis and K-free solution can be explained by inhibition of the Na-K pump. For example, ouabain potentiates I_{Ti} by inhibiting the Na-K pump, thereby increasing [Na]$_i$, which increase [Ca]$_i$ via the Ca-Na exchange system. The elevated [Ca]$_i$, in turn, triggers Ca^{2+} release from the SR by the Ca-trigger-Ca mechanism of Fabiato and Fabiato {25}. An oscillatory release of Ca^{2+} can account for the damped oscillations in I_{Ti} (and in DADs and aftercontractions) sometimes observed. I_{Ti} is abolished by pretreatment with caffeine (10 mM) to deplete the SR stores of Ca^{2+}. The progressive potentiation of the DAD or I_{Ti} during a train of impulses can be explained by progressive loading of the SR with Ca^{2+}.

Thus, elevation in [Ca]$_i$ activates at least two different types of ion channel: (a) the nonspecific channel conductance [$g_{Na,K(Ca)}$], which underlies I_{Ti} and DAD, and which may be important in genesis of dysrhthmias and even in cardiac plateau formation; and (b) the Ca^{2+}-activated transient outward K^+ channel conductance, which may be important in shortening of the cardiac AP. In addition, Marban and Tsien {60} provided evidence that elevation of [Ca]$_i$ (but not Sr^{2+}) increases the voltage-dependent I_{Ti} in Purkinje fibers, and that this might mediate some of the effects of cardiac glycosides. The mechanism for this effect of [Ca]$_i$ could involve the Ca-calmodulin-activated protein kinase and phosphorylation of the slow channels {see also 15,16}. This positive feedback effect of [Ca]$_i$ may not continue because higher [Ca]$_i$ could inhibit Ca^{2+} entry (negative feedback), either by somehow blocking the channels and/or decreasing the electrochemical gradient for Ca^{2+} entry.

INACTIVATION OF I$_{Ca}$ BY Ca

Evidence favoring the former mechanism has been collected from voltage-clamp experiments using a variety of excitable cells, including isolated ventricular myocytes from rat and guinea pig {46} and from Purkinje fibers {48}. The results suggest that the rate of inactivation or time-dependent decay of I_{Ca} during a depolarization may depend not only on the voltage, but also on the Ca^{2+} influx through the Ca channels. Double-pulse voltage-clamp experiments have demonstrated that the amount of Ca ions entering the myocyte during a prepulse affects the magnitude of a subsequent Ca current {46}. In addition, substitution of external Ba^{2+} ions for Ca^{2+} ions slows the rate of inactivation, thereby demonstrating that an ion-specific interaction with the channel contributes to this process. The rate of inactivation is also slowed by intracellular injection of EGTA, which lowers the intracellular free Ca^{2+} concentration {46}. It has also been shown that an elevation in external Ca produces a larger Ca current, which decays more rapidly {34}. Thus, the Ca^{2+} ion itslef plays an important role in providing negative feedback in order to help regulate the Ca current.

SUMMARY AND CONCLUSIONS

Ca^{2+} ion influx through voltage-dependent and time-dependent slow channels during the cardiac action potential is the key step in excitation-contraction coupling and determines the force of contraction of the heart. The model for slow Ca channels is similar to that for fast Na^+ channels, except that the slow Ca channels (a) have gates that open and close more slowly, (b) have gates that operate over a different voltage range (less negative activation and inactivation voltages), and (c) are blocked by different agents (e.g., by calcium-antagonistic drugs such as verapamil and nifedipine). In addition, the slow channels have some special properties (in comparison with fast Na^+ channels and various types of K^+ channels) that enable the myocardial cells to exercise control over its Ca^{2+} influx in response to intrinsic and extrinsic factors and hormones/neurotransmitters. These unusual properties include (a) energy dependence, (b) pH dependence, (c) cyclic-AMP dependence, and (d) Ca-dependent inactivation.

The sympathetic neurotransmitter, norepinephrine, catecholamine hormones, angiotensin II, histamine, and methylxanthines rapidly induce slow Ca channels in myocardial cells. Following blockade of the fast Na^+ channels with TTX or by voltage inactivating them in 25 mM $[K]_o$, these agents rapidly allow the production of slowly rising APs by increasing the number of slow channels available for voltage activation and/or their mean open time. Concomitantly, these compounds rapidly elevate intracellular cyclic-AMP levels, suggesting that cylic AMP is somehow related to the functioning of the slow channels. Exogenous cyclic AMP produces the same effect, but much more slowly.

Exposure of intact myocardial cells to the GTP analog, GPP(NH)P, also induces slow APs within 10–20 minutes. This effect is presumably by activation of the adenylate cyclase complex. Intracellular injection of cyclic AMP, GPP(NH)P, and cholera toxin (also an activator of the adenylate cyclase complex) rapidly induces or potentiates ongoing slow APs in the injected cell. Thus the time delay between exposure to the agent and an observed effect is greatly reduced by intracellular application of the agent. These results clearly indicate the key role played by cyclic AMP in regulation of the Ca^{2+} slow channel and hence Ca^{2+} influx and force of contraction.

The induced slow channels are very sensitive to blockade by metabolic poisons, hypoxia, and ischemia (fig.

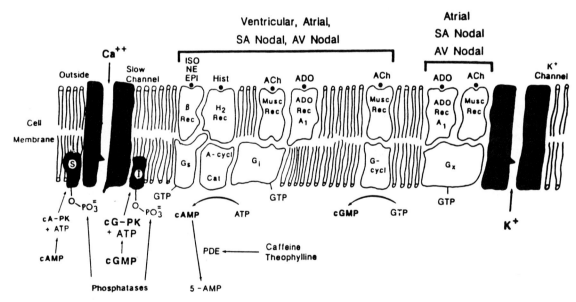

Fig. 12-21. Diagrammatic summary of some of the properties of the ion channels in myocardial cell membrane. Included are the mechanism of action of some positive inotropic agents, such as beta-adrenergic agonists, histaminic H_2 agonists, and methylxanthines (phosphodiesterase inhibitors). The beta agonists and H_2 agonists act on the regulatory component (guanine nucleotide binding protein) of the adenylate cyclase complex to stimulate cyclic-AMP production. The voltage-dependent myocardial slow channels are dependent on cyclic AMP and on metabolism, presumably because a protein constituent (or regulatory component) of the slow channel must be phosphorylated in order for it to be in a form that is available for voltage activation. The sites of action of GPP(NH)P and cholera toxin on the regulatory component of adenylate cyclase are shown. Also depicted are the facts that the slow channels are selectively blocked by acidosis and by calcium-antagonistic drugs (slow-channel blockers). Also schematized are two types of ion channels that are activated by internal Ca^{2+} ion: a K^+-selective channel [$g_{K(Ca)}$] and a non-selective Na-K channel ($g_{Na,K(Ca)}$). From Sperelakis {103}, with permission.

12-21). The slow AP is blocked at a time when the rate of rise and duration of the normal fast AP is essentially unaffected. However, the contraction accompanying the fast AP is depressed or abolished, i.e., contraction is uncoupled from excitation, as expected from slow-channel blockade. The ATP level is greatly reduced by the metabolic poisons, e.g., by valinomycin and DNP, at the same time that the slow channels are blocked {85}. Therefore, the slow channels are metabolically dependent, presumably on ATP, whereas the fast Na^+ channels are not.

The dependence of the myocardial slow channels on cyclic-AMP level and on metabolism suggests that phosphorylation of a membrane protein constituent of the slow channel, or of an associated regulatory protein, by a cyclic-AMP-dependent protein kinase and ATP, may make it available for voltage activation {see Sperelakis 99,102}. The dephosphorylated slow channel would be electrically silent, i.e., nonfunctional. Phosphorylation may produce a conformational change that allows the gates of the slow channel to operate in response to membrane potential.

The slow channels are also selectively sensitive to blockade by acid pH; that is, at pH 6.8–6.1, the slow AP is depressed or blocked. In contrast, the fast AP is not much affected, but excitation-contraction uncoupling occurs. Part of the rapid effect of ischemia in blocking the slow channels appears to be mediated by the concomitant acidosis.

By these special properties of the slow channels, Ca^{2+} influx into the myocardial cell can be controlled by extrinsic factors, such as by autonomic nerve stimulation or circulating hormones, and by intrinsic factors, such as cellular pH or ATP level. During transient regional ischemia, the selective blockade of the slow channels, which results in depression of the contraction and work of the afflicted cells, might serve to protect the cells against irreversible damage by helping to conserve their ATP content.

The parasympathetic neurotransmitter, ACh, depresses the inward slow current (I_{si}) stimulated by beta-adrenergic agonists in ventricular cells, without potentiating the outward K^+ current. Similar results are produced by adenosine.

The majority of the slow channels have a threshold potential at about -35 mV (compared to about -65 mV for the fast Na^+ channels). The max dV/dt of the slow AP is about 10 V/s, and the propagation velocity (0.04–0.10 m/s) is about one-sixth to one-third that of the fast AP. The slow APs fatigue at frequencies above 1 Hz. Fast APs can trigger slow APs in K^+ depolarized regions. Slow APs have been implicated in the genesis of reentrant types of arrhythmias in ischemic zones, but there is also evidence that some ischemic APs are depressed fast APs rather than true slow APs; regardless, propagation velocity will be slow and there will be conduction disturbances that can predispose to dysrhythmias. Although local anesthetics depress and block slow APs and fast APs over a similar range of concentrations, depressed fast APs are more sensitive to these drugs.

Delayed depolarizing afterpotentials have also been implicated in the genesis of arrhythmias of the triggered automaticity type. These afterpotentials are due to an increase in $[Ca]_i$ opening up a voltage-independent nonspecific postsynaptic type of ion channel having an equilibrium (reversal) potential at about -5 mV. Any condition, such as hypoxia/ischemia, digitalis, or catecholamines, that elevates $[Ca]_i$ potentiates the depolarizing afterpotential, and hence the possible triggering of AP trains from these ectopic foci and producing dysrhythmias. Calcium-antagonistic drugs, by their action to block the slow channels and thereby suppress Ca^{2+} influx and loading of the SR, suppress these afterpotentials and prevent such arrhythmogenesis.

The myocardial Ca^{2+} slow channels are also regulated by cyclic GMP in a manner that is opposite to that of cyclic AMP. The effect of cyclic GMP is presumably mediated by means of phosphorylation of a protein, for example, a regulatory protein (inhibitory-type) associated with the slow channel.

Preliminary data suggest that calmodulin also may play a role in regulation of the myocardial slow Ca^{2+} channels, possibly mediated by the Ca^{2+}-calmodulin protein kinase {6,7} and phosphorylation of some regulatory-type protein.

Thus it appears that the Ca^{2+} slow channel is a complex structure, perhaps consisting of several proteins, including perhaps two associated regulatory proteins, one stimulatory and one inhibitory, both of which may require phosphorylation in order to express their regulatory function. Some cardioactive drugs could conceivably affect the phosphorylation-dephosphorylation steps. The mean life span of a phosphorylated channel is likely to be of the order of 1 second or less.

NOTES

1. The terms *slow channel*, *slow Ca channel*, and *Ca channel* are used interchangably in this chapter. In addition, the term *slow inward current (I_{si})* is used interchangably with *calcium current (I_{Ca})*.
2. A third class of Ca channels, termed *N-type*, has also been reported and displays the following characteristics: Activation and steady-state inactivation occur with relatively strong depolarization, the current displays a moderately rapid inactivation, and the current is insensitive to DHPs {117}.

REFERENCES

1. Bean BP, Nowysky MC, Tsien RW: β-adrenergic modulation of calcium channels in frog ventricular heart cells. *Nature* 307:371–375, 1984.
2. Bean BP: Two kinds of calcium channels in canine atrial cells. *J Gen Physiol* 86:1–30, 1985.
3. Belardinelli L, Isenberg G: Actions of adenosine and isoproterenol on isolated mammalian ventricular myocytes. *Circ Res* 53:287–297, 1983.
4. Belardinelli L, Vogel S, Linden J, Berne RM: Antiadrenergic action of adenosine on ventricular myocardium in embryonic chick hearts. *J Mol Cell Cardiol* 14:291–294, 1982.

5. Belardinelli L, Vogel SM, Sperelakis N, Rubio R, Berne RM: Restoration of inward slow current in hypoxic heart muscle by alkaline pH. *J Mol Cell Cardiol* 11:877–892, 1979.

6. Bkaily G, Sperelakis N, Eldefrawi M: Effects of the calmodulin inhibitor, trifluoperazine, on membrane potentials and slow actions potentials of cultured heart cells. *Eur J Pharm* 105:23–31, 1984.

7. Bkaily G, Sperelakis N: Calmodulin is required for a full activation of the calcium slow channels in heart cells. *J Cyclic Nucleotide Prot Phosphy Res* 11:25–34, 1986.

8. Bkaily G, Sperelakis N: Injection of cyclic GMP into heart cells blocks the slow action potentials. *Am J Physiol (Heart Circ Physiol)* 248:H745–H749, 1985.

9. Bkaily G, Sperelakis N: Injection of protein kinase inhibitor into cultured heart cells blocks the calcium slow channels. *Am J Physiol (Heart Circ Physiol)* 246:H630–H634, 1984.

10. Bruckner R, Scholz H: Effects of alpha-adrenoceptor stimulation with phenylephrine in the presence of propranolol on force of contraction, slow inward current and cyclic AMP content in the bovine heart. *Br J Pharmacol* 82:223–232, 1984.

11. Brum G, Flockerzi V, Hofmann F, Osterreider W, Trautwein W: Injection of catalytic subunit of cAMP-dependent protein kinase into isolated cardiac myocytes. *Pflügers Arch* 398:147–154, 1983.

12. Cachelin AB, dePeyer JE, Kokubun S, Reuter H: Ca^{2+} channel modulation by 8-bromocyclic AMP in cultured heart cells. *Nature* 304:462–464, 1983.

13. Camardo JS, Shuster MJ, Siegelebaum SA, Kandel ER: Modulation of a specific potassium channel in sensory neurons of Aplysia by serotonin and cAMP-dependent protein phosphorylation. *Cold Spring Harbor Symp Quant Biol* 48:213–220, 1983.

14. Cavalie A, Ochi R, Pelzer D, Trautwein W: Elementary currents through Ca^{2+} channels in guinea pig myocytes. *Pflügers Arch* 398:284–297, 1983.

15. Chad J, Eckert R: Calcineurin, a calcium-dependent phosphatase, enhances Ca-mediated inactivation of Ca current in perfused snail neurons (abstr). *Biophys J* 47:266, 1985.

16. Chad J, Eckert R: Leupeptin, an inhibitor of Ca-dependent proteases, retards the kinase-irreversible, Ca-dependent loss of calcium current in perfused snail neurons (abstr). *Biophys J* 47:266, 1985.

17. Chad JE, Eckert RJ: An enzymatic mechanism for calcium current inactivation in dialysed Helix neurones. *J Physiol* 378:31–51, 1986.

18. Chesnais JM, Coraboeuf E, Sauvain MP, Vasses JM: Sensitivity to H, Li and Mg ions of the slow inward sodium current in frog atrial fibres. *J Mol Cell Cardiol* 7:627–642, 1975.

19. Cranefield PF, Dodge FA: Slow conduction in the heart. In: Zipes DP, Bailey JC, Elharrar V (eds) *The Slow Inward Current and Cardiac Arryhthmias.* The Hague: Martinus Nijhoff, 1980, pp 149–171.

20. Cranefield PF: *The Conduction of the Cardiac Impulse.* Mt Kisco, NY: Futura, 1975.

21. Cukierman S, Paes de Carvalho A: Slow response excitation: Dependence on rate and rhythm. In: Paes de Carvalho A, Hoffman BF, Lieberman M (eds) *Normal and Abnormal Conduction in the Heart.* Mt Kisco, NY: Futura, 1982, pp 413–428.

22. Cuppoletti J, Thakkar J, Sperelakis N, Wahler G: Cardiac sarcolemmal substrate of the cGMP-dependent protein kinase. *Membr Biochem* 7:135–142, 1988.

23. Dodge FA, Cranefield PF: Nonuniform conduction in cardiac Purkinje fibers. In: Paes de Carvalho A, Hoffman BF, Lieberman M (eds) *Normal and Abnormal Conduction in the Heart.* Mt Kisco, NY: Futura, 1982, pp 379–396.

24. Dosemeci A, Dhalla RS, Cohen NM, Lederer WJ, Rogers TB: Phorbol ester increases calcium current and stimulates the effects of angiotensin II on cultured neonatal rat heart myocytes. *Circ Res* 62:347, 1988.

25. Fabiato A, Fabiato F: Calcium and cardiac excitation-contraction coupling. *Ann Rev Physiol* 41:473–484, 1979.

26. Ferrier GR, Moe GK: Effect of calcium on acetyl-strophanthidin-induced transient depolarizations in canine Purkinje tissue. *Circ Res* 33:508–515, 1973.

27. Freer RJ, Pappano AJ, Reach MJ, Bing KT, McLean MJ, Vogel SM, Sperelakis N: Mechanism of the positive inotropic effect of angiotenisn II on isolated cardiac muscle. *Circ Res* 39:178–183, 1976.

28. Hartzell HC, Fischmeister R: Opposite effects of cyclic GMP and cyclic AMP on Ca^{2+} current in single heart cells. *Nature* 323:273–275, 1986.

29. Hescheler J, Kameyama M, Trautwein W, Mieskes G, Soling HD: Regulation of the cardiac calcium channel by protein phosphatases. *Eur J Biochem* 165:261–266, 1987.

30. Hescheler J, Kameyama M, Trautwein W: On the mechanism of muscarinic inhibition of the cardiac Ca current. *Pflügers Arch* 407:182–1989, 1986.

31. Hescheler J, Mieskes G, Ruegg JC, Takai A, Trautwein W: Effects of a protein phosphatase inhibitor, okadaic acid, on membrane currents of isolated guinea-pig cardiac myocytes. *Pflügers Arch* 412:248–252, 1988.

32. Hescheler J, Pelzer D, Trube G, Trautwein W: Does the organic calcium channel blocker D-600 act from inside or outside on the cardiac cell membrane? *Pflügers Arch* 393:287–291, 1982.

33. Hess P, Lansman JB, Tsien RW: Modulation of single calcium channels by the calcium agonist Bay K 8644 (abstr). *Biophys J* 45:394, 1984.

34. Irisawa H, Kokubun S: Effects of various intracellular Ca ion concentrations on the Ca current of guinea pig single ventricle cells. *Jpn J Physiol* 34:599–611, 1984.

35. Irisawa H, Kokubun S: Modulation by intracellular ATP and cyclic AMP of the slow inward current in isolated single ventricular cells of the guinea pig. *J Physiol* 338:321–327, 1983.

36. Irisawa H, Sato R: Intra- and extracellular actions of protons on the calcium current of isolated guinea-pig ventricular cells. *Circ Res* 59:348–355, 1987.

37. Isenberg G, Belardinelli L: Ionic basis for the antagonism between adenosine and isoproterenol on isolated mammalian ventricular myocytes. *Circ Res* 55:309–325, 1984.

38. Isenberg G, Vereecke J, van der Heyden G, Carmeliet E: The shortening of the action potential by DNP in guinea pig ventricular myocytes is mediated by an increase of a time-independent K conductance. *Pflügers Arch* 397:251–259, 1983.

39. Isenberg G: Cardiac Purkinje fibers: $[Ca^{2+}]_i$ controls the potassium permeability via the conductance components g_{k1} and g_{k2}. *Pflügers Arch* 371:77–85, 1977.

40. Johnson JC, Wittenauer LA, Nathan RD: Calmodulin Ca^{2+}-antagonists and Ca^{2+}-transporter in nerve and muscle. *J Neural Trans Suppl* 18:97–111, 1983.

41. Josephson I, Renaud JF, Vogel S, McLean M, Sperelakis N: Mechanism of the histamine-induced positive inotropic action in cardiac muscle. *Eur J Pharmacol* 35:393–398, 1976.

42. Josephson I, Sperelakis N: 5'-guanylimidodiphosphate stimulation of slow Ca^{2+} current in myocardial cells. *J Mol Cell Cardiol* 10:1157–1166, 1978.

43. Josephson I, Sperelakis N: Local anesthetic blockade of Ca^{2+}-mediated action potentials in cardiac muscle. *Eur J Pharmacol* 40:201–208, 1976.

44. Josephson I, Sperelakis N: On the ionic mechanism underlying adrenergic-cholinergic antagonism in ventricular muscle. *J Gen Physiol* 79:69–86, 1982.

45. Josephson I, Sperelakis N: Ouabain blockade of inward slow current in cardiac muscle. *J Mol Cell Cardiol* 9:409–418, 1977.

46. Josephson IR, Sanchey-Chapula J, Brown AM: A comparison of calcium currents in rat and guinea pig single ventricular cells. *Circ Res* 54:144–156, 1984.

47. Kameyama M, Hofmann F, Trautwein W: On the mechanism of β-adrenergic regulation of the Ca^{2+} channel in the guinea-pig heart. *Pflügers Arch* 405:285–293, 1986.

48. Kass RS, Sanguinetti M: Inactivation of Ca channel current in the calf cardiac Purkinje fiber. *J Gen Physiol* 84:705–726, 1984.

49. Kass RS, Tsien RS, Weingart R: Ionic basis of transient inward current induced by strophanthidin in cardiac Purkinje fibres. *J Physiol (Lond)* 281:209–226, 1978.

50. Kohlhardt M, Bauer B, Krause H, Fleckenstein A: Differentiation of the transmembrane Na and Ca channels in mammalian cardiac fibres by the use of specific inhibitors. *Pflügers Arch* 335:309–322, 1972.

51. Kohlhardt M, Fleckenstein A: Inhibition of the slow inward current by nifedipine in mammalian ventricular myocardium. *Naunyn-Schmiedebergs Arch Pharmacol* 298:267–272, 1977.

52. Kojima M, Sperelakis N: Calcium antagonistic drugs differ in blockade of slow Na^+ channels in young embryonic chick hearts. *Eur J Pharmacol* 94:9–18, 1983.

53. Lazzara R, Sherlag B: Role of the slow current in the generation of arrhythmias in ischemic myocardium. In: Zipes DP, Bailey JC, Elharrar V (eds) *The Slow Inward Current and Cardiac Arrhythmias*. The Hague: Martinus Nijhoff, 1980, pp 399–416.

54. Lee KS, Tsien RW: Reversal of current through calcium channels in dialysed single heart cells. *Nature* 297:498–501, 1982.

55. Lehmkuhl D, Sperelakis N: Electrical activity of cultured heart cells. In: Tanz RD, Kavaler F, Roberts J (eds) *Factors Influencing Myocardial Contractility*. New York: Academic Press, 1967, pp 245–278.

56. Levi RC, Alloatti G, Fischmeister R: Cyclic GMP regulates the Ca-channels current in guinea pig ventricular myocytes. *Pflügers Arch* 413:685–687, 1989.

57. Li T, Sperelakis N: Calcium antagonist blockade of slow action potentials in cultured chick heart cells. *Can J Physiol Pharmacol* 61:957–966, 1983.

58. Li T, Sperelakis N: Stimulation of slow action potentials in guinea-pig papillary muscle cells by intracellular injection of cAMP, Gpp(NH)p, and cholera toxin. *Circ Res* 52:111–117, 1983.

59. Lynch C, Vogel S, Sperelakis N: Halothane depression of myocardial slow action potentials. *Anesthesiology* 55:360–368, 1976.

60. Marban E, Tsien RW: Enhancement of calcium current during digitalis inotropy in mammalian heart: Positive feedback regulation by intracellular calcium? *J Physiol* 329:589–614, 1982.

61. Masuda MO, Paula-Carvalho M, Paes de Carvalho A: Excitability and propagation of slow responses in rabbit atrium partially depolarized by added K^+ and Ba^{2+}. In: Paes de Carvalho A, Hoffman BJ, Lieberman M (eds) *Normal and Abnormal Conduction in the Heart*. Mt Kisco, NY: Futura, 1982, pp 397–412.

62. Mehegan JP, Muir WW, Unverferth DV, Fertel RH, McGiurk SM: Electrophysiological effects of cylic GMP on canine cardiac Purkinje fibers. *J Cardiovasc Pharmacol* 7:30–35, 1985.

63. Mery PF, Lohmann SM, Walter U, Fischmeister R: Ca^{2+} current is regulated by cylic GMP-dependent protein kinase in mammalian cardiac myocytes. *Proc Natl Acad Sci USA* 88:1197–1201, 1991.

64. Metzer H, Lindner E: The positive inotropic-acting forskolin, a potent adenylate cyclase activator. *Arzneim Forsch* 31:1248–1250, 1981.

65. Mikami A, Imoto K, Tanabe T, Niidome Y, Mori H, Takeshima, Narumiya M, Numa S: Primary structure and functional expression of the cardiac dihydropyridine sensitive calcium channel. *Nature* 340:230–233, 1989.

66. Molyvdas P-A, Sperelakis N: Comparison of the effects of several calcium antagonistic drugs (slow-channel blockers) on the electrical and mechanical activities of guinea pig papillary muscle. *J Cardiovasc Pharmacol* 5:162–169, 1983.

67. Molyvdas P-A, Sperelakis N: Comparison of the effects of several calcium antagonistic drugs on the electrical activity of guinea pig Purkinje fibers. *Eur J Pharmacol* 88:205–214, 1983.

68. Nargeot J, Nerbonne JM, Engels J, Lester HA: Time course of the increase in the myocardial slow inward current after a photochemically generated concentration jump of intracellular cAMP. *Proc Natl Acad Sci USA* 80:2395–2399, 1983.

69. Noma A, Shibasaki T: Membrane current through adenosine-triphosphate-regulated potassium channels in guinea pig ventricular cells. *J Physiol* 363:463–480, 1985.

70. Noma A: ATP-regulated K channels in cardiac muscle. *Nature* 305:147–148, 1983.

71. Nowycky MC, Fox AP, Tsien RW: Three types of calcium channels in chick dorsal root ganglion cells (abstr). *Biophys J* 47:67, 1985.

72. Ono K, Trautwein W: Potentiation by cyclic GMP of β-adrenergic effect on Ca^{2+} current in guinea-pig ventricular cells. *J Physiol* 443:387–404, 1991.

73. Osterrieder W, Brum G, Hescheler J, Trautwein W, Flockerzi V, Hoffman F: Injection of subunits of cyclic AMP-dependent protein kinase into cardiac myocytes modulates Ca^{2+} current. *Nature* 298:576–578, 1982.

74. Pang DC, Sperelakis N: Differential actions of calcium antagonists on calcium binding to cardiac sarcolemma. *Eur J Pharmacol* 81:403–409, 1982.

75. Pang DC, Sperelakis N: Nifedipine, diltiazem, verapamil and bepridil uptake into cardiac and smooth muscles. *Eur J Pharmacol* 87:199–207, 1983.

76. Pang DC, Sperelakis N: Uptakes of calcium antagonists into muscles as related to their lipid solubilities. *Biochem Pharmacol* 33:821–826, 1984.

77. Pappano AJ: Calcium-dependent action potentials produced by catecholamines in guinea pig atrial muscle fibers depolarized by potassium. *Circ Res* 27:379–390, 1970.

78. Pelzer D, Pelzer S, McDonald TF: Properties and regulation of calcium channels in muscle cells. *Rev Physiol Biochem Pharmacol* 114:107–207, 1990.

79. Reuter H, Cachlin AB, DePeyer JE, Kokubun S: Modulation of calcium channels in cultured cardiac cells by isoproterenol and 8-bromo-cAMP. *Cold Spring Harbor Sym Quant Biol* 48:193–200, 1983.

80. Reuter H, Scholz H: The regulation of the calcium conductance of cardiac muscle by adrenaline. *J Physiol* 264:49–62, 1977.

81. Reuter H, Stevens CF, Tsien RW, Yellen G: Properties of

single calcium channels in cardiac cell culture. *Nature* 297: 501–504, 1982.

82. Reuter H: Calcium channel modulation by neurotransmitters, enzymes and drugs. *Nature* 301:569–574, 1983.

83. Rinaldi ME, Capony J-P, Demaille JG: The cyclic AMP-dependent modulation of cardiac sarcolemmal slow calcium channels. *J Mol Cell Cardiol* 14:279–289, 1982.

84. Schneider JA, Shigenobu K, Sperelakis N: Valinomycin inhibition of the inward slow current of cardiac muscle. In Roy PE, Dhalla NS (eds) *Recent Advances in Studies on Cardiac Structure and Metabolism*, Vol 9. Baltimore, MD: University Park Press, 1976, pp 33–52.

85. Schneider JA, Sperelakis N: Slow Ca^{2+} and Na^+ responses induced by isoproterenol and methylxanthines in isolated perfused guinea pig hearts exposed to elevated K^+. *J Mol Cell Cardiol* 7:249–273, 1975.

86. Schneider JA, Sperelakis N: The demonstration of energy dependence of the isoproterenol-induced transcellular Ca^{2+} current in isolated perfused guinea pig hearts: An explanation for mechanical failure in ischemic myocardium. *J Surg Res* 16:389–403, 1974.

87. Schneider JA, Sperelakis N: Valinomycin blockade of slow channels in guinea pig hearts perfused with elevated K^+ and isoproterenol. *Eur J Pharmacol* 27:349–354, 1974.

88. Schrader J, Rubio R, Berne RM: Inhibition of slow action potentials of guinea pig atrial muscle by adenosine: A possible effect on Ca^{2+} influx. *J Mol Cell Cardiol* 7:427–433, 1975.

89. Schramm M, Thomas G, Towart R, Franckowiak G: Activation of calcium channels by novel 1,4-dihydropyridines. *Arzneim Forsch/Drug Res* 33:1268–1272, 1983.

90. Shigenobu K, Schneider JA, Sperelakis N: Verapamil blockade of slow Na^+ and Ca^{2+} responses in myocardial cells. *J Pharmacol Exp Ther* 190:280–288, 1974.

91. Shigenobu K, Sperelakis N: Ca^{2+} current channels induced by catecholamines in chick embryonic hearts whose fast Na^+ channels are blocked by tetrodotoxin or elevated K^+. *Circ Res* 31:932–952, 1972.

92. Shuster MJ, Camardo JS, Siegelbaum SA, Kandel ER: Cyclic AMP-dependent protein kinase closes the serotonin-sensitive K^+ channels of Aplysia sensory neurones in cell-free membrane patches. *Nature* 313:392–395, 1985.

93. Siegelbaum SA, Camardo JS, Kandel ER: Serotonin and cyclic AMP close single K^+ channels in Aplysia sensory neurones. *Nature* 299:413–417, 1982.

94. Singh J, Flitney FW: Inotropic responses of the frog ventricle to dibutyryl cyclic AMP and 8-bromo cyclic GMP and related changes in endogenous cyclic nucleotide levels. *Biochem Pharmacol* 30:1475–1481, 1981.

95. Spah F: Forskolin, a new positive inotropic agent, and its influence on myocardial electrogenic cation movements. *J Cardiovasc Pharmacol* 6:99–106, 1984.

96. Sperelakis N, Belardinelli L, Vogel SM: Electrophysiological aspects during myocardial ischemia. In: Hayase S, Murao S (eds) *Proceedings of 8th World Congress of Cardiology*. Amsterdam: Excerpta Medica, 1979, pp 229–236.

97. Sperelakis N, Mayer G, MacDonald R: Velocity of propagation in vertebrate cardiac muscles as functions of tonicity and $[K^+]_o$. *Am J Physiol* 219:952–963, 1970.

98. Sperelakis N, Schneider JA: A metabolic control mechanism for calcium ion influx that may protect the ventricular myocardial cell. *Am J Cardiol* 37:1079–1085, 1976.

99. Sperelakis N: Cyclic AMP and phosphorylation in regulation of Ca^{2+} influx into myocardial cells, and blockade by calcium-antagonistic drugs. *Am Heart J* 107:347–357, 1984.

100. Sperelakis N: Electrophysiology of vascular smooth muscle of coronary artery. In: Kalsner S (ed) *The Coronary Artery*. Croom Helm, London 1982, pp 118–167.

101. Sperelakis N: Origin of the cardiac resting potential. In: Berne RM, Sperelakis N (eds) *Handbook of Physiology. The Cardiovascular System*, Vol 1: *The Heart*. Bethesda, MD: American Physiological Society, 1979; pp 187–267.

102. Sperelakis N: Properties of calcium-dependent slow action potentials and their possible role in arrhythmias. In: Opie LH, Krebs R (eds) *Calcium Antagonists and Cardiovascular Disease*. New York: Raven Press, 1983.

103. Sperelakis N: Regulation of calcium slow channels of cardiac muscle by cyclic nucleotides and phosphorylation. *J Mol Cell Cardiol* 20:75–105, 1988.

104. Sperelakis N: Changes in membrane electrical properties during development of the heart. In: Zipes DP, Bailey JC, Elharrar V (eds) *The Slow Inward Current and Cardiac Arryhythmias*. The Hague: Martinus Nijhoff, 1980, pp 221–262.

105. Taniguchi J, Noma A, Irisawa H: Modification of the cardiac action potential by intracellular injection of adenosine triphosphate and related substances in guinea pig single ventricular cells. *Circ Res* 53:131–139, 1983.

106. Tohse N, Conforti L, Sperelakis N: Bay K 8644 enhances Ca^{2+} channel activities in embryonic chick heart cells without prolongation of open times. *Eur J Pharmacol* 203:307–310, 1991.

107. Tohse N, Kameyama M, Sakiguchi K, Shearman MS, Kanno M: Protein kinase C activation enchances the delayed recifier K^+ current in guniea-pig heart cells. *J Mol Cell Cardiol* 22:725–734, 1990.

108. Tohse N, Masuda H, Sperelakis N: Novel isoform of Ca^{2+} channel in rat fetal cardiomyocytes. *J Physiol (Lond)*, 451: 295–306, 1992.

109. Tohse N, Nakaya H, Takeda Y, Kanno M: Inhibitory Effect of Human Atrial Natriuretic Peptide on cardiac L-type CA channels. *Jpn J Pharmacol* 58:184p, 1992.

110. Tohse N, Sperelakis N: Cyclic GMP inhibits the activity of single calcium channels in embryonic chick heart cells. *Circ Res* 69:325–331, 1991.

111. Tohse N, Sperelakis N: Long-lasting openings of the single slow (L-type) Ca^{2+} channels in chick embryonic heart cells. *Am J Physiol* 259:H639–H642, 1990.

112. Trautwein W, Hoffmann F: Activation of calcium current by injection of cAMP and catalytic subunit of cAMP-dependent protein kinase. *Proc Int Union Physiol Sci* 15:75–83, 1983.

113. Trautwin W, Taniguchi J, Noma A: The effect of intracellular cyclic nucleotides and calcium on the action potentials and acetycholine response of isolated cardiac cells. *Pflügers Arch* 392:307–314, 1982.

114. Tripathi O, Sperelakis N: Effect of 8-bromo cyclic GMP on slow channel mediated action potentials of 3-day-old embryonic chick ventricle. *J Dev Physiol* 16:309–316, 1991.

115. Trube G, Heschler T: Inwardly rectifying channels in isolated patches of the heart cell membrane. *Pflügers Arch* 401: 178–184, 1984.

116. Tsien RW, Giles W, Greengard P: Cyclic AMP mediates the effects of adrenaline on cardiac Purkinje fibers. *Nature (New Biol)* 240:181–183, 1972.

117. Tsien RW, Hess P, McClesky EW, Rosenberg RL: Calcium channels: Mechanisms of selectivity, permeation and block. *Ann Rev Biophys Biophys Chem* 16:265–290, 1987.

118. Vogel S, Crampton R, Sperelakis N: Blockade of myocardial slow channels by Bepridil (CERM-1978), *J Pharmacol Exp Ther* 210:378–385, 1979.

119. Vogel S, Sperelakis N, Josephson I, Brooker G: Fluoride

stimulation of slow Ca^{2+} current in cardiac muscle. *J Mol Cell Cardiol* 9:461–475, 1977.

120. Vogel S, Sperelakis N: Blockade of myocardial slow inward current at low pH. *Am J Physiol* 233:C99–C103, 1977.

121. Vogel S, Sperelakis N: Induction of slow action potentials by microiontophoresis of cyclic AMP into heart cells. *J Mol Cell Cardiol* 13:51–64, 1981.

122. Vogel S, Sperelakis N: Valinomycin blockade of myocardial slow channels is reversed by high glucose. *Am J Physiol* 235:H46–H51, 1978.

123. Wahler GM, Rusch NJ, Sperelakis N: 8-bromo-cyclic GMP inhibits the calcium channel current in embryonic chick ventricular myocytes. *Can J Physiol Pharm* 68:531–534, 1990.

124. Wahler GM, Sperelakis N: Cholinergic attenuation of the electrophysiological effects of forskolin. *J Cyclic Nucleotide Prot Phosphoryl Res* 11:1–10, 1986.

125. Wahler GM, Sperelakis N: Induction and enhancement of cardiac slow action potentials (APs) by forskolin (abstr). *Biophys J* 47:515, 1985.

126. Wahler GM, Sperelakis N: Intracellular injection of cyclic GMP depresses cardiac slow action potentials. *J Cyclic Nucleotide Prot Phosphoryl Res* 10:83–95, 1985.

127. Wahler GM, Sperelakis N: Similar metabolic dependence of stimulated and unstimulated myocardial slow channels. *Can J Physiol Pharmacol* 62:569–574, 1983.

128. Wahler GM, Sperelakis N: The new Ca^{2+} agonist (Bay K 8644) potentiates and induces slow action potentials. *Am J Physiol (Heart Circ Physiol)* 247:H337–H340, 1984.

129. Watanabe AM, Besch HR Jr: Cyclic adenosine monophosphate modulation of slow calcium influx channels in guinea pig hearts. *Circ Res* 35:316–324, 1974.

130. West GA, Belardinelli L: Correlation of sinus slowing and hyperpolarization caused by adenosine in sinus node. *Pflügers Arch* 403:75–81, 1985.

131. West GA, Isenberg G, Belardinelli L: Antagonism of forskolin effects by adenosine in isolated hearts and ventricular myocytes. *Am J Physiol* 250:H769–H777, 1986.

132. Yatani A, Brown AM: Rapid β-adrenergic modulation of cardiac calcium channel currents by a fast G protein pathway. *Science* 245:71–74, 1989.

133. Zipes DP, Rinkenberger RL, Heger JJ, Prystowski EN: The role of the slow inward current in the genesis and maintenance of supraventricular tachyarrhythmias in man. In: Zipes DP, Bailey JC, Elharrar V (eds) *The Slow Inward Current and Cardiac Arrhythmias*. The Hague: Martinus Nijhoff, 1980, pp 481–506.

CHAPTER 13

Excitation-Contraction Coupling: Relationship of Calcium Currents to Contraction

LESYA M. SHUBA & TERENCE F. MCDONALD

INTRODUCTION

Physiological contractions of striated muscle cells are triggered by action potentials that elicit transient increases in calcium (Ca) concentration at the myofilaments. The immediate source of the myofilament-activating Ca depends on cell type. In frog heart it primarily flows from extracellular locations, in mammalian heart it mainly comes from intracellular sarcoplasmic reticulum (SR) stores, and in skeletal muscle it is almost exclusively from these stores.

Despite the fact that activator Ca released from SR powers contraction in mammalian cardiac and skeletal muscle, and that both muscle types utilize the action potential to trigger the release, they differ in the way that the electrical signal is coupled to release. In skeletal muscle, depolarization per se suffices for the task {124, 131}, whereas the evidence from studies on excitation-contraction coupling in heart muscle {e.g., 18,43,45–47} strongly suggests that Ca release is contingent on the electrical impulse *and* a rapid influx of extracellular Ca. This influx is thought to move through depolarization-activated Ca channels, to control the release of activator Ca from the SR stores, and then to replenish them, with little direct influence on myofilament activation.

In the sections below we expand on this core concept of cardiac excitation-contraction coupling. The concept owes much to pioneering studies on cardiac action potentials and contraction {4,102,155}, but here we place particular emphasis on the role of channel-carried Ca movements (currents) as deduced from voltage-clamp experiments on ventricular tissues and myocytes. The next section sets the stage for the main topic by providing brief overviews of methodologies, cellular mechanisms, and concepts related to Ca movement and contraction. The subsequent sections present experimental results that not only justify designation of L-type Ca current ($I_{Ca,L}$) as the primary trigger for internal Ca release and contraction, but also demonstrate that the early phase of $I_{Ca,L}$ modulates the amount of Ca released, and that inward Ca-channel flux replenishes SR Ca stores.

Needless to say, there are many important aspects of excitation-contraction coupling that cannot be covered in any detail here. The reader should consult both older

{e.g., 10,36,50,53,76,101} and newer {e.g., 18,31,55,59, 78,79,100,110,151,152} reviews for a comprehensive view of the subject.

OVERVIEW OF CALCIUM MOVEMENTS DURING CONTRACTION AND RELAXATION

We use this section to serve a potpourri that provides brief notes on methods, mechanisms, and concepts that are central to the major topic. It is organized into subsections on methods and measurements, properties of L-type and T-type Ca channel currents, sodium-calcium (Na-Ca) exchange, Ca storage and release, types of contraction, and relaxation.

Methods and measurements

The development of methods to inject current and voltage-clamp thin bundles of mammalian cardiac tissue was a major step forward in the study of excitation-contraction coupling. When these were combined with simultaneous measurement of contractile force, the nature of membrane potential control of contraction began to take shape {e.g., 54,56,97,102,148,155}. The addition of Ca current measurements brought further insight {13,57,58,107,119,146}. Although this current was labelled I_{Ca} between 1970 and 1976, an incorrect consensus that Na might be contributing up to one half of the current led to general use of the *slow inward current* (I_{si}) tag. The latter fell into disuse during the 1980s when voltage-clamp experiments on isolated myocytes indicated that Ca channels were highly selective for Ca over monovalent cations {70,82,88,90}. With the discovery of a second species of Ca channels (T-type) in cardiac cells {11,99,109} (see next subsection), the predominant component historically measured from depolarized holding potentials became known as *L-type* Ca current or $I_{Ca,L}$ With this hindsight, we refer to earlier I_{Ca} and I_{si} as $I_{Ca,L}$ when appropriate.

One large advantage of myocytes over multicellular preparations in studying the relations between Ca current and contraction is that the smaller membrane area and low access resistance to the cytoplasm in myocytes permit quicker, more faithful control of the membrane potential.

N. Sperelakis (ed.), Physiology and Pathophysiology of the Heart, Third Edition.

This quality of control is rarely, if ever, achieved in voltage-clamp studies on multicellular preparations, which generally also suffer from ion accumulation/depletion in restricted extracellular spaces and overlap of non-Ca currents {e.g., 12}. Despite these limitations, the results obtained on both types of preparations are surprisingly coherent.

The other side of the coin is that multicellular preparations are closer to the true physiological state of heart cells in vivo than myocytes that have weathered enzymatic dissociation procedures. Therefore, there are grounds for believing that Ca movement, Ca handling, and contractile activity in myocytes may be somewhat distorted and different than in the donor tissue. However, as the material below unfolds, it will be apparent that divergent responses are more the exception than the rule. This is good news because in addition to improved clamp fidelity and the possibility of cell dialysis with pipette-filling solutions, myocytes are extremely convenient experimental models for measurements of Ca_i transients and responses to photorelease of caged Ca_i {e.g., 105}. The Ca_i measurements are made after loading of myocytes with Ca-sensing fluorescent probes such as indo-1 and fura 2 {61}. They provide an extremely useful correlate to myocyte contraction/shortening measurements, which is in part verified by important studies on multicellular preparations that indicate a near-linear relation between imaged Ca_i and the rate/degree of force development {156,157}. Furthermore, Ca light measurements help distinguish between changes in Ca_i related to Ca channel activity, Na-Ca exchange, and release of Ca from the SR, especially when they are used in conjunction with specific blockers such as the Ca antagonists for Ca channels and ryanodine for SR Ca-release channels. A drawback is that these indicators are Ca buffers that can affect the rate and degree of myocyte shortening {e.g., 40}. A recent in-depth review of the methodology by Wier {152} also points out that these measurements reflect average Ca_i in the cytoplasm, and average Ca_i may be markedly different than regional Ca_i at short times after powerful dynamic events such as Ca channel influx and SR Ca release.

Properties of L-type and T-type calcium channel currents

Ca ions flow through highly specific channels in cardiac cell membranes. There are two types of Ca channels, L-type and T-type, which are similar in some respects but very different in others {see 92 for review}. Both channels are three to four orders more selective for Ca than Na or K ions, and can transfer on the order of one million Ca ions per second. Both currents ($I_{Ca,L}$, $I_{Ca,T}$) are activated by cell membrane depolarization and are inactivated in a time- and voltage-dependent manner when the depolarization is maintained. One major difference is that the $I_{Ca,T}$ threshold is around -60 mV and peak amplitude -30 mV, compared to ca. -40 mV and $+5$ mV for much larger $I_{Ca,L}$ (see fig. 13-3). The amplitude of both currents declines at more positive potentials, and is zero at the respective reversal potentials of ca. $+40$ mV for $I_{Ca}T$ {e.g., 2,6} and ca. $+70$ mV for $I_{Ca,L}$ {70,81,90,115}. $I_{Ca,T}$ and $I_{Ca,L}$

activate at about the same rate (7–10 ms (22°C) and 2–4 ms (35°C) near 0 mV), but $I_{Ca,T}$ inactivates much more quickly and completely, especially at potentials positive to -30 mV {6,11,115,126}. Although both current types are fully available on depolarizations from -90 mV, $I_{Ca,T}$ is fully inactivated when cells are steadily depolarized to -50 mV, whereas $I_{Ca,L}$ remains nearly fully available {6,116}. Further major differences between the two currents are that (a) classical cardiac stimulants such as isoproterenol and Bay K8644 have pronounced effects on $I_{Ca,L}$ but not on $I_{Ca,T}$; and (b) classical organic blockers such as D600 and nifedipine are much more potent blockers of $I_{Ca,L}$ than $I_{Ca,T}$ {6,11,115,126}.

Sodium-calcium exchange

The electrogenic Na-Ca transporter in the sarcolemma exchanges three Na ions for each Ca ion {e.g., 37,65, 74,117}. Building on earlier work on cardiac {122} and nerve {24} preparations, Mullins {103} proposed that the exchanger extrudes Ca at negative potentials but imports it at positive potentials. The three Na ions move down an electrochemical gradient, and the single Ca ion moves uphill, with the equilibrium potential (E) given by E_{Na-Ca} $= 3 E_{Na} - 2E_{Ca}$. Thus an inward-directed exchange current I_{Na-Ca} (and Ca extrusion) will occur at potentials negative to E_{Na-Ca}, and an outward-directed current (and Ca influx) at potentials positive to E_{Na-Ca}. E_{Na-Ca} may be near -40 mV in most cardiac cells at rest, ensuring Ca extrusion during exchanger operation. (However, unusually high Na_i combined with $Ca_i \leq 100$ nM can position E_{Na-Ca} slightly negative to resting potential in rat ventricular cells {135}.)

Although negative E_{Na-Ca}, and Ca extrusion, is the usual situation during diastole, the action potential upstroke carries the membrane potential above E_{Na-Ca} and shifts the exchanger into the Ca influx mode. However, the rapid opening of Ca channels during/after the action potential upstroke triggers the release of Ca from the SR (see below), and this can elevate free Ca_i by 10-fold or more within tens of milliseconds. The result is a shift in E_{Na-Ca} to potentials above the plateau, and conversion of the exchanger back to the Ca efflux mode. It may stay in this mode for the remainder of the action potential (and subsequent diastole) because even though Ca_i gradually falls from its peak and pushes E_{Na-Ca} to more negative values, the membrane is also repolarizing. Substantive support for this view of dynamic changes in E_{Na-Ca} during the action potential comes from studies of extracellular Ca concentration changes in ventricular tissue during the action potential {16,64}. Modeling studies {66} and measurements of I_{Na-Ca} currents during the AP {41} are also consistent with this view.

The situation during a maintained voltage-clamp depolarization is different. If the step is to 0 mV, there will be a short period of Ca influx immediately after depolarization but the driving force for the current ($0-E_{Na-Ca}$) will be significantly smaller than that achieved by an action potential overshoot. The Ca_i transient upon release of Ca from the SR will switch the exchanger to the Ca efflux mode within tens of milliseconds. However, unlike the action potential situation, the fall in Ca_i and relaxation due to subsequent SR pumping may drive E_{Na-Ca} below $0\,mV$ and switch the exchanger to the Ca influx mode. These dynamic changes will be attenuated during depolarizations to clamp potentials below $0\,mV$, and accentuated during clamps to more positive potentials.

Calcium storage and release

As reviewed by Fabiato and Baumgarten {48}, evidence from experiments on isolated SR vesicles and skinned cardiac cells indicate that the site of the internal Ca store is almost certainly the SR. A recent computer model of cardiac SR structure and function {154} incorporates (a) a main Ca store in which Ca is predominantly bound, (b) a "releasable" terminal in which mainly free Ca is available for triggered release and myofilament activation, and (c) the longitudinal SR, which sequesters cytoplasmic Ca and promotes relaxation (although other SR probably participates as well).

The dominant hypothesis of Ca release from cardiac SR is that a rapid increase in cytoplasmic Ca near the SR triggers the release of a large quantity of Ca from the SR; release is terminated by time- and Ca-dependent inactivation {45–47,154}. The incorporation of isolated SR vesicles into planar lipid bilayers has permitted studies on single SR Ca-release channels. They indicate that the high conductance Ca-selective channels are activated by Ca, ATP, and caffeine, and inhibited by magnesium, ruthenium red, and calmodulin {3,75,127,128,141,142}. These agents modify channels by altering their open time probability without affecting the unit conductance. The single-channel studies have led to kinetic models that suggest two open states and two or three closed states {127,141}. The plant alkaloid ryanodine binds with high affinity to the SR Ca-release channels and disrupts excitation-contraction coupling by 'locking' the channel protein into an open but very low conductance state {3,128}.

Types of contraction

There are three "types" of contraction discussed in this chapter. The relatively fast isometric contraction triggered by an action potential in mammalian atrial or ventricular tissue at ca. 36°C is the normal phasic (twitch) event. Its time course and amplitude are reproduced by 100–300 ms voltage-clamp pulses to potentials around $0\,mV$. The fast phasic shortening of unloaded myocytes appears to have similar features. Phasic contractions/shortenings are almost abolished by Ca channel blockade, as well as by ryanodine, indicating that they are activated by Ca released from the SR (see below). Prolonged action potentials and prolonged clamp pulses can produce a post-twitch maintained tension in cardiac tissue. These "tonic tension" responses are also seen in myocytes, are intensified at positive potentials, last as long as the plateau/pulse, and are possibly due to the Na-Ca exchanger operating in the Ca-influx mode {55} (see fig. 13-2).

Two other contractile events are most often observed under unphysiological conditions. Repolarization-activated contractions are generally smaller versions of normal phasic events. They have most often been recorded after pulses to high positive potentials and are covered later. The final type, delayed aftercontractions, is noted here but not discussed in further sections. These events are seen after action potentials or specific clamp pulses when tissues or myocytes are suffering from Ca overload, arising, for example, from digitalis poisoning {e.g., 72} or reoxygenation {63}. They are due to random spontaneous releases of Ca from overloaded SR that are transiently synchronized into a significant coordinated release by a preceding triggered release {15,34,45–47,63}.

Relaxation

A number of processes are involved in producing the relaxation phase of the twitch. The combination of Ca uptake by the SR and Ca extrusion via the Na-Ca exchanger is quite capable of restoring Ca concentration to resting levels within the appropriate timeframe {e.g., 19,21,23, 27,28,40,41}. Contributions by sarcolemmal Ca-ATPase pumping and mitochondrial uptake are negligible under physiological conditions; in the absence of the primary mechanisms, however, the latter two can effect slow relaxation. Bers et al. {21} and Bassani et al. {9} have highlighted this situation by demonstrating that inhibition of both Na-Ca exchange and SR Ca pumping dramatically slows relaxation. Separate inhibition of the two pathways indicates that they probably compete against each other, with the SR Ca pump usually having the upper hand {21}. The voltage dependence of the electrogenic Na-Ca exchanger {7,21,28} is responsible for the enhanced rate of relaxation at more negative potentials.

L-TYPE CALCIUM CURRENT IS THE PHYSIOLOGICAL TRIGGER FOR CALCIUM RELEASE AND CONTRACTION

Bell-shaped voltage dependencies of $I_{Ca,L}$, Ca_i, and phasic contraction

Since $I_{Ca,L}$ flows through channels whose gating is dependent on voltage and time, its amplitude can be varied over a wide range by the application of selected voltage-clamp sequences. A standard approach in investigating the relation between cardiac $I_{Ca,L}$ amplitude and the force of contraction is to clamp the membrane potential to a negative holding potential and impose a series of voltage-clamp pulses to more positive potentials. The pulses usually have a duration approximating that of the action potential, and an amplitude that is incremented in small steps to explore the voltage range from -60 to $+60\,mV$ or beyond. Figure 13-1 shows the voltage dependencies of $I_{Ca,L}$ amplitude and force of contraction (developed tension) in a cat papillary muscle pulsed with 300-ms pulses from $-50\,mV$. The schematic above the plots indicates that the preparation was maintained in a steady state with 0.33 Hz pulsing

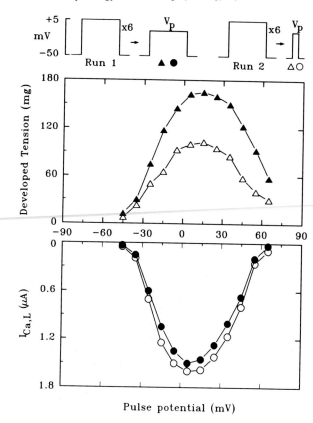

Fig. 13-1. Bell-shaped dependence of developed tension (**top**) and $I_{Ca,L}$ (**bottom**) in a cat papillary muscle stimulated at 0.33 Hz. The preparation was kept in a steady state with 300-ms pulses from −50 to +5 mV except for every seventh pulse. The latter were to pulse potentials V_p between −45 and +65 mV, and were 300 ms long in run 1 and 25 ms long in run 2. Temperature was 36°C and Ca_o was 1.8 mM.

to +5 mV, except for interposed 300-ms test pulses. The threshold for both $I_{Ca,L}$ and phasic contraction was around −40 mV, both peaked in the range 0 to +20 mV, and both declined at more positive potentials. The curves for $I_{Ca,L}$ and contraction/shortening are bell shaped, and this is a hallmark of cardiac tissue {57,58,101,119,144,145} and myocyte {18,38,69,71,86,98} function in all mammalian species tested. Several regions of these typical $I_{Ca,L}$ and contraction relations deserve further scrutiny.

1. *Threshold potential.* Threshold potentials for the activation of $I_{Ca,L}$ and the activation of phasic contraction are very similar, if not identical, in ventricular muscle from dog {13}, cat {107}, sheep {119} (fig. 13-2), and bull (McDonald and Trautwein, unpublished), as well as in sheep atrial {144} and Purkinje {57,58} fibers. In fact, New and Trautwein {107} went so far as to state that they never saw $I_{Ca,L}$ without phasic tension, nor phasic tension without $I_{Ca,L}$, in cat papillary muscles under satisfactory voltage-clamp control. London and Krueger {86} made a similar observation on guinea pig ventricular myocytes.

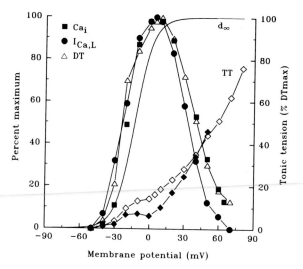

Fig. 13-2. Bell-shaped dependence of twitch contraction and $I_{Ca,L}$ in a sheep ventricular bundle stimulated with trains of six 300-ms pulse at 0.33 Hz from −50 mV to successively higher potentials. Values were measured on the sixth pulse of each train. Tonic tension (right-hand Y-axis) was measured at the end of 2-second pulses in the same preparation, and at 10-mV intervals from a cat papillary muscle clamped by a 3 mV/s voltage ramp (temperature 35°C; Ca_o 1.8 mM). Shown for comparison are the changes in Ca_i measured by Cleemann and Morad {38} in a rat ventricular myocyte (temperature 23°C, Ca_o 2 mM), a generic steady-state $I_{Ca,L}$ activation curve (d_∞) (Boltzmann distribution with $V_{0.5}$ at −13 mV and slope 8 mV) that fits data from a variety of ventricular tissues and myocytes {see 114}.

2. *Ascending limb.* There is generally a good correspondence between $I_{Ca,L}$ amplitude and developed tension at potentials between threshold and maximum magnitude. This correspondence is adequately illustrated by the data in figs. 13-1–13-3.

3. *Descending limb.* The curves in fig. 13-1 indicate that the decline in $I_{Ca,L}$ amplitude is much steeper than the decline in peak tension at test potentials more positive than +10 mV. This is a common finding in ventricular tissues {e.g., 13,91,145} (see fig. 13-2) and myocytes {18,38,69,71} (see fig. 13-3), and leads to the question of how a relatively large contraction can be triggered by very small inward (or even outward) $I_{Ca,L}$ at potentials near E_{rev}.

There are several plausible explanations for the divergence at positive potentials, and we begin with one that still allows a role for $I_{Ca,L}$ as trigger. The central thesis is that $I_{Ca,L}$ is a mixed ionic current at positive potentials. Whereas *net* $I_{Ca,L}$ approaches zero at the reversal potential of ca. +70 mV {70,81,82,107,115}, an inward-directed Ca component should be present at voltages up to the estimated Ca equilibrium potential (E_{Ca}) of ca. +120 mV (Ca_o about 10,000 times Ca_i). This inward Ca component is undetected in $I_{Ca,L}$ because it is offset by the outward movement of monovalent cations (mainly K) through the channels. Even though the latter have very limited perme-

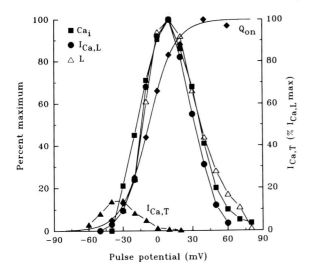

Fig. 13-3. Bell-shaped relations for $I_{Ca,L}$, shortening (ΔL), and Ca_i transient from data on guinea pig ventricular myocytes obtained by Rose et al. {125}, Isenberg and Wendt-Gallitelli (71), and Bueckelmann and Wier {22}, respectively. T-type current from Balke et al. {6} is expressed as a percent of maximum $I_{Ca,L}$ (right-hand Y-axis) reported by the same group {125}. Charge movement associated with L-type Ca channel activation (Q_{on}) is from Hadley and Lederer {62}. The myocytes were pulsed with 200–500 ms pulses and superfused with ca. 2 mM Ca solution (except Q_{on} 4 mM Cd) at room temperature (except $I_{Ca,L}$ 36°C).

The discussion to this point is based on the concept that the predominant factor in shaping the bell-shaped contraction relation is $I_{Ca,L}$-mediated release of Ca from the SR. Fabiato's studies {43,45–47,49} clearly demonstrated that $I_{Ca,L}$-shaped pulses of Ca triggered the release of Ca from the SR of skinned cardiac cells. Complementary investigations by Wier {150} and Wier and Isenberg {153} on cardiac Purkinje fibers injected with the Ca indicator aequorin suggested that Ca_i transients related to SR Ca release were related to voltage in the same manner as $I_{Ca,L}$. Subsequent experiments on voltage-clamped myocytes loaded with Ca indicator dyes such as indo-1 or fura-2 indicate that the magnitude of SR-engendered Ca_i transients is voltage dependent {e.g., 18,22,32,38, 104,137}. Examples of the bell-shaped dependence of the Ca_i transient on voltage are shown in figs. 13-2 and 13-3; they are in very good agreement with $I_{Ca,L}$ and phasic contraction/shortening relations shown in the same figures.

Calcium channel activation is an insufficient condition for triggering of phasic cardiac contraction

The activation of contraction in skeletal muscle is linked to voltage-dependent intramembrane charge movement that is sensitive to organic Ca channel blockers {124,131}. Charge movement and contractile force activation have sigmoidal dependencies on voltage that are quite similar to those of the steady-state activation of $I_{Ca,L}$ (d_∞, fig. 13-2) and L-type Ca channel gating charge movement (Q_{on}, fig. 13-3) in cardiac preparations, and quite different from bell-shaped $I_{Ca,L}$ relations in both skeletal {129} and cardiac (fig. 13-1) muscle. The coupling of skeletal muscle SR Ca release to voltage sensors rather than Ca influx explains the well-known indifference of skeletal muscle contraction to the presence of external Ca. By contrast, cardiac muscle cells do not contract in the absence of external Ca, even when they are depolarized by pulses that move maximal charge and fully activate Ca channels (see Q_{on} curve). The missing link in the latter case is not simply a requirement for L-type current flow per se; large L-type currents carried by Ba or Na fail to trigger contractions in cardiomyocytes {104}.

Robust phasic contraction requires more than calcium current

Both $I_{Ca,T}$ and $I_{Ca,L}$ are possible suppliers of Ca to the myofilaments during an action potential or voltage-clamp pulse. However, any $I_{Ca,T}$ contribution is likely to be miniscule, since it is very small at plateau potentials and inactivates quickly and completely {6} (also see fig. 13-3). Although $I_{Ca,L}$ is far larger than $I_{Ca,T}$ (see fig. 13-3), and inactivates more slowly, it also seems to make little impression on Ca_i compared to the contribution of Ca released from the SR. A recent estimate by Sipido and Wier {140} is that the increment in Ca_i due to peak $I_{Ca,L}$ is about 5% of that produced by the accompanying release of Ca from well-filled SR. There are several other observations reinforcing the view that $I_{Ca,L}$ makes only a minor direct contribution to myofilament activation. (a) Con-

ability compared to Ca {82,90,121}, they are at relatively high concentration in the cell and experience a large electrochemical gradient at high positive potentials. Thus the amplitude of $I_{Ca,L}$ becomes a poorer and poorer estimator of inward Ca flux as the potential approaches E_{rev}.

The second possibility is that Ca entry via the Na-Ca exchange mechanism enhances contraction at positive potentials. As noted earlier, the exchanger may operate in the Ca-influx mode at positive potentials and increase Ca_i {7,39}. Recent studies {30,111,134,137} suggest that this elevation can induce release of Ca from the SR and/or modulate contraction. These releases are far slower and smaller than those elicited by $I_{Ca,L}$. As a result, the contractions are small and slow in onset. Although exchanger Ca entry could contribute to reloading of the SR stores, and to slowly rising maintained tonic tension (see *Tonic tension*), it is doubtful that it has any impact on a given Ca release and contraction triggered by an action potential under physiological conditions due to the relatively short duration of the action potential overshoot (see *Sodium-calcium exchange*). However, contractions elicited by clamp pulses to positive potentials may be influenced by exchanger Ca entry because step pulses (unlike the action potential) hold the membrane at the positive potential for a prolonged period of time. When these pulses are short (e.g., 30 ms in fig. 13-1, run 2), exchanger Ca entry will be minimal; even when the pulses are 300 ms long (fig. 13-1, run 1), entry may be insufficient to elicit Ca release.

tractions are very small after SR Ca depletion manipulations such as long rests {e.g., 1,71}, subthreshold pulsing {13}, slow pulsing (see fig. 13-9), and shortened pulses (see fig. 13-10), despite large $I_{Ca,L}$ {13,71} (figs. 13-9 and 13-10). (b) Ryanodine block of SR Ca release can reduce phasic contraction and the Ca_i transient by up to 90% in rat ventricular preparations {8,143} without reducing the influx of L-type Ca {32}. (c) Ca carried by a large $I_{Ca,L}$ of 3 nA peak flowing for 25 ms (estimated time to peak of Ca_i transient) at 37°C into a restricted space of 10 pL in a 30-pl guinea pig ventricular cell would change Ca_i by roughly 25 µM (without buffering); this translates to an increment of 0.1–0.2 µM in free Ca_i {44} and minimal contractile activation.

Phasic contraction triggered by $I_{Ca,L}$ tails

Contractions with time courses resembling those elicited by depolarizing pulses can also be triggered by repolarizations from large positive potentials. These were originally reported by McGuigan {97} and Beeler and Reuter {13} in clamp experiments on mammalian ventricular tissue, and have since been noted in many other studies on tissues and myocytes. Unlike the situation with aftercontractions (see *Types of contraction*), there is no requirement for a preceding triggered event. As demonstrated by London and Krueger {86} on guinea pig ventricular myocytes, depolarizations to +100 mV failed to trigger detectable phasic contractions, but repolarizations from this potential were always effective stimuli. In similar cells, Sipido and Wier {140} found that repolarization from +60 mV provoked a large increase in Ca_i. The latter must be due to release from the SR for the following reasons: (a) Even if one assumes that Ca channels are fully activated after several hundred milliseconds at high positive potentials, a straightforward calculation indicates that the fast deactivation of a large $I_{Ca,L}$ at negative repolarizing potentials (ca. 0.4 ms at 22°C) {92} would only result in a ca. 1-µM change in an unbuffered cytoplasmic space of 10 pL. This is only 1/25th of the charge that would be carried by a 25-ms flow of $I_{Ca,L}$ at 0 mV (see previous subsection). Taking buffering into account {cf. 44}, this influx is too small to have any activating effect on the contractile machinery. Indeed, it is even difficult to make a case for SR Ca release by such a small Ca influx. However, it seems to do precisely that since repolarization contraction and Ca_i transient are blocked by ryanodine {8,23,32}. Perhaps the extremely rapid influx on the $I_{Ca,L}$ tail has a salutary effect on Ca release that can only be duplicated by a much larger influx during the much slower $I_{Ca,L}$ transient elicited by depolarization. In this regard, Fabiato {46} has shown that rapid increases of Ca_i near the SR are more effective release triggers than slow, large increases.

The case against a trigger role for I_{Ca},T

Although there have been suggestions that "fast" I_{Ca-T} might be the trigger, or one of the triggers, for contraction in heart muscle cells {5,99,100}, there are a number of strong arguments against this suggestion. (a) There is no correlation between the location of the bell-shaped I_{Ca-T} voltage relation and the phasic contraction and Ca_i transient relations (fig. 13-3). (b) Contraction is essentially unaffected when depolarizing pulses are applied from strongly negative potentials (where $I_{Ca,T}$ and $I_{Ca,L}$ are available) compared to −50 mV (where only $I_{Ca,L}$ is available) in both ventricular tissue (fig. 13-5A) and myocytes {69}. (c) Preferential block of L-type channels with nisoldipine completely abolished the Ca_i transient {5}. Finally, (d) there is the question of just how much Ca is likely to flow through T-type channels during an action potential. The upstroke of a ventricular action potential is so fast over the voltage range (say, −50 to −10 mV: fig. 13-3) pertinent for $I_{Ca,T}$ that the time available (≪1 ms) is simply too short for significant $I_{Ca,T}$ activation. Assuming relatively equal degrees of T-type and L-type channel activation as the upstroke slows towards its peak, current through T-type channels will only be a few percent of that through L-type channels (fig. 13-3). In summary, a triggering role for $I_{Ca,T}$ seems highly improbable in adult mammalian ventricular cells.

Tonic tension

Tonic tension is a maintained tension that is readily apparent when cardiac muscle preparations have been depolarized to positive potentials for > ca. 300 ms. It can emerge as a sustained contraction after partial relaxation of a twitch {e.g., 136}, slowly develop over several hundred milliseconds after relaxation of a twitch {e.g., 144}, or slowly develop to a quasi-steady state without a preceding twitch {e.g., 86,146}, depending on the preparation and experimental conditions. These contractile events were first observed when action potentials were prolonged at positive potentials by current injection {102, 155}. They were also observed when long voltage-clamp pulses were applied to cardiac tissue preparations {e.g., 29,112} and have been likened to the tonic tension in frog heart tissue {cf. 101} that has been attributed to Ca influx via the Na-Ca exchanger {67}.

The open diamonds in fig. 13-2 illustrate the voltage dependence of the tonic tension in sheep ventricular muscle. In this experiment it was measured as the steady post-twitch tension developed in response to 2-second depolarizations. It was small at potentials below 0 mV but waxed in exponential fashion at positive potentials. With the exception of being a causative factor in the small bump that can sometimes be detected in the L-type window-current region centred near −20 mV {cf., 92,146}, $I_{Ca,L}$ appears to play no role in this type of force development. For example, depolarizing ramp-clamps that are slow enough (e.g., 3 mV/s) to ensure full L-type channel inactivation at plateau voltages also produce exponential increases in tonic tension in cat (filled diamonds, fig. 13-2) and dog {101} ventricular muscle. Additional evidence against $I_{Ca,L}$ involvement is that tonic tension in ventricular myocytes is not blocked by Ca-channel blocking concentrations of Cd {86} and verapamil {8}.

Proof that long clamps to positive potentials can increase Ca_i was provided by Wier and colleagues {8,23}.

The small slow increase in Ca_i was attributed to Ca influx through the Na-Ca exchanger since it was unaffected by high concentrations of ryanodine and verapamil. There are two other indications of exchanger involvement: (a) The exponential-like rise in tension with positive potential is paralleled by the voltage-dependent behavior of exchanger current {e.g., 23,74}, and (b) reduction of E_{Na-Ca} by increasing Na_i enhances tonic tension in sheep Purkinje fibers {42}. A final remark is that a slow ryanodine-insensitive SR Ca release that is activated at positive potentials has not yet been ruled out.

Results contrary to the party line

A consistent picture of $I_{Ca,L}$ as the physiological trigger for phasic contraction has been built up in this section. There is a voluminous literature that contributes to this picture, only some of which has been cited. Even so, we would be remiss in not pointing out a few of the studies that suggest that other mechanisms may also deserve consideration. Since it would take a further chapter to discuss the strengths and weaknesses of the experimental evidence, it is more prudent to point the reader to representative papers where the evidence and background can be appreciated first hand. One of these, authored by Leblanc and Hume {77}, makes the case in favor of a Na current-induced SR Ca release. They explained such coupling by a Ca-induced Ca release mechanism, with Na-Ca exchange causing influx of Ca in response to a rise of intracellular Na (Ca-influx mode). Other studies have also addressed the possible roles of I_{Na-Ca} {30,111, but see 20} and membrane voltage {14} as triggers for SR Ca release. In the latter study {14}, the preparations were in a Ca-overloaded state, and it is worth noting that breakdown of the relation between $I_{Ca,L}$ and force of contraction when muscle cells are in this state has often been reported since the initial observation by Beeler and Reuter {13}. One way to look at the situation is that the SR is an undisciplined organelle when it is overloaded with Ca and surrounded by unusually high Ca_i. The normally tight rein on Ca-release channel opening becomes progressively weaker with cell Ca accumulation until almost any (secondary?) signal can cause a large spillage. A delayed aftercontraction (see *Types of contraction*) is a particular example of unfettered release.

$I_{Ca,L}$ GRADES CONTRACTILE FORCE

The close correspondence between the bell-shaped voltage dependencies of $I_{Ca,L}$ amplitude, Ca_i transient, and contraction in ventricular tissues and myocytes (figs. 13-1–13-3) strongly suggests that there is more than a passing relationship between them. However, the data are all based on a single protocol, i.e., depolarizing pulses from a constant negative holding potential to more positive potentials. This raises the possibility that the results are fortuitous. A firming up of the hypothesis that $I_{Ca,L}$ amplitude grades Ca release and force requires that (a) the relation hold under other pulsing patterns, (b) the bell-shaped Ca release relation not be due to an unknown

influence of voltage, and (c) the grading of $I_{Ca,L}$ by altering external ionic conditions or pharmacological treatment results in a complementary grading of contractile strength. These aspects are covered in the three subsections below.

$I_{Ca,L}$ and contraction graded by degree of channel availability

The purpose of the experiments described below was to examine how the force of contraction responds to changes in $I_{Ca,L}$ amplitude produced by voltage sequences that alter the availability of L-type Ca channels. Figure 13-4 compares a control response in cat papillary muscle with responses obtained when channels were either completely or partially inactivated. The control depolarization from -50 to $+10\,mV$ for 300 ms elicited large $I_{Ca,L}$ and contraction (left-hand panel). The Ca channels were then inactivated by moving the holding potential to $0\,mV$. A subsequent test pulse to the same potential as before ($+10\,mV$) produced negligible $I_{Ca,L}$ and barely detectable contraction (middle panel). Repolarization of the preparation from $0\,mV$ to more negative potentials results in a time- and voltage-dependent recovery from inactivation. When inactivation was partially removed with a 200-ms repolarization to $-50\,mV$, the subsequent test activation to $+10\,mV$ elicited $I_{Ca,L}$ and contraction whose respective amplitudes were about 60% of control values (right-hand panel).

The protocol shown in the right-hand panel of fig. 13-4 was expanded to investigate the proportionality between $I_{Ca,L}$ and contraction over the entire range of channel availability. Figure 13-5A indicates that long repolarizations from the holding potential of $+10\,mV$ to potentials between 0 and $-80\,mV$ produced a recovery of both parameters along a sigmoidal course. This proportionality was also observed when the time course of $I_{Ca,L}$ restoration was probed with repolarizing pulses of varying duration (fig. 13-5B). As inactivation was removed, $I_{Ca,L}$ and peak contraction recovered along similar exponential time courses. The time courses are not always as well correlated as in this example {e.g., 55}, which is not surprising considering that species-dependent restitution of contraction {e.g., 59} and dynamic feedback on $I_{Ca,L}$ (see *Replenishment of SR calcium stores by $I_{Ca,L}$*) can be quite complex.

Bell-shaped Ca_i release is not due to an unknown influence of voltage

The results shown in figs. 13-4 and 13-5 were obtained with clamp protocols that incorporated test pulses to a constant potential. This helps remove the insecurities related to fortuitous bell-shaped relations mentioned earlier. A recent study by Niggli and Lederer {108} on guinea pig ventricular myocytes has produced a strong additional argument against an unknown bell-shaped Ca-release dependence on voltage per se. They found that the time course and degree of ryanodine-sensitive shortening following photorelease of caged Ca_i to trigger Ca release was

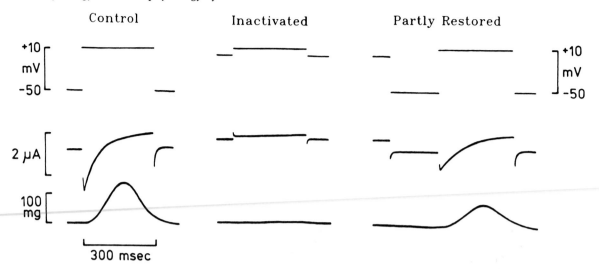

Fig. 13-4. $I_{Ca,L}$ and contraction after inactivation and partial restoration of Ca channels in cat ventricular muscle. After the control response (left-hand panel), channels were inactivated by moving the holding potential from −50 mV to 0 mV. Pulses to +10 mV now produced negligible $I_{Ca,L}$ and tension (middle panel). A 200-ms repolarization to −50 mV resulted in partial restoration of both $I_{Ca,L}$ and tension on the subsequent test pulse to +10 mV (right-hand panel). Temperature 35°C, Ca$_o$ 1.8 mM.

independent of clamp pulse potentials (−100, −40, 0, +100 mV) and time (0–2 seconds) after pulse application. The records from these critical experiments are reproduced in fig. 13-6.

Grading of $I_{Ca,L}$ and contraction by other physiological and pharmacological interventions

Varying the ionic composition of the external solution, or application of pharmacological agents such as beta-adrenergic agonists, Ca channel activators, and Ca channel blockers, may well have effects on contraction that are unrelated to effects on $I_{Ca,L}$. In the first instance, however, and in the absence of hard evidence on "side effects," one expects that directional changes in the current will elicit complementary changes in contractile force. Examples of this congruence are given in the subsections below.

EXTRACELLULAR Ca

Early experiments on the modulation of $I_{Ca,L}$ and developed tension by Ca$_o$ in mammalian ventricular muscle established that changes in one parameter closely paralleled changes in the other {13,107}. New and Trautwein {107} reported that a reduction in Ca$_o$ from 3.6 to 0.9 mM reduced both maximum $I_{Ca,L}$ and accompanying contractile force by 55–60% in cat papillary muscles. Using a fast perfusion method, Lipp et al. {85} reported that switching from 2 to 0 mM Ca immediately abolished $I_{Ca,L}$ and the Ca$_i$ transient in guinea pig atrial myocytes.

INORGANIC BLOCKERS

Divalent cations such as Cd, Co, and Mn depress both $I_{Ca,L}$ and contraction. In cat and bovine ventricular trabe-

culae there was a close correspondence between the concentration-dependent attenuation of $I_{Ca,L}$ by Co and the accompanying depression of contractile force {94}. Similarly, a concomitant reduction in the two parameters has been reported for frog {149}, sheep, and pig {73} myocardial preparations treated with Mn and La, respectively.

ORGANIC BLOCKERS

The phenylalkylamine Ca-channel blockers D600 and AQA39 have been shown to have concentration-dependent effects on $I_{Ca,L}$ that are paralleled by depressions of developed tension in cat papillary muscle {106,147}. In more recent experiments on guinea pig ventricular myocytes, Arreola et al. {5} observed that block of $I_{Ca,L}$ by the dihydropyridine nisoldipine abolished Ca release by the SR in guinea pig ventricular myocytes. A well-characterized feature of organic Ca channel blockers is that the degree of block is "use dependent" {e.g., 92,93,95}. This feature can be used to explore the grading of contraction by $I_{Ca,L}$. For example, nearly full block of $I_{Ca,L}$ by steady pulsing from −50 to 0 mV can be largely relieved by long rest periods at potentials negative to −50 mV. Since the unblocking effectiveness of shorter (e.g., 3 minutes) rests is minimal at −50 mV, but improves to about 80% at −110 mV, rests at different potentials can be used to grade $I_{Ca,L}$ amplitude and to measure tension development on subsequent test pulses to 0 mV. The results of an experiment of this type on a cat papillary muscle treated with 2 μM D600 for 90 minutes are shown in fig. 13-7. The grading of force by test $I_{Ca,L}$ was quite remarkable; for example, very small $I_{Ca,L}$ and contraction after rest at −40 mV were augmented 5.7-fold and 5.5-fold,

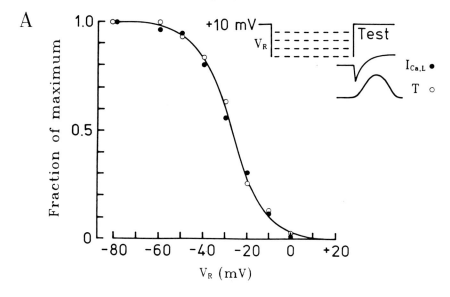

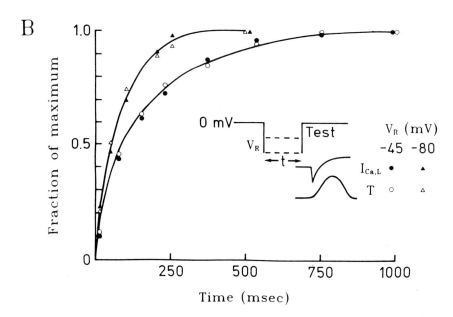

Fig. 13-5. The correspondence between $I_{Ca,L}$ and the force of contraction when $I_{Ca,L}$ amplitude is varied by varying channel availability. **A:** From the holding potential of $+10\,mV$ (complete inactivation of $I_{Ca,L}$), the membrane potential of a cat papillary muscle was repolarized to potentials V_R for 1500 ms. $I_{Ca,L}$ (filled circles) and contraction (open circles) were triggered by the subsequent test pulse to $+10\,mV$. Pulses to V_R were applied at a rate of 0.1 Hz **B:** Time-dependent restoration of $I_{Ca,L}$ and contraction. The $-45\,mV$ data were extracted from the results of Reuter {119} on sheep ventricular muscle (Ca_o 1.8 mM); the $-80\,mV$ data were obtained from cat ventricular muscle (McDonald and Trautwein, unpublished; Ca_o 3.6 mM). Temperature was 35–37°C.

respectively, after unblock by a rest at $-110\,mV$. A further relevant finding is that early transient stimulation of $I_{Ca,L}$ by D600 is accompanied by similar-sized transient stimulation of contraction {96}.

CTAECHOLAMINES AND CYCLIC AMP ELEVATION

An important study by Grossman and Furchgott {60} first established that catecholamines increase Ca exchange in

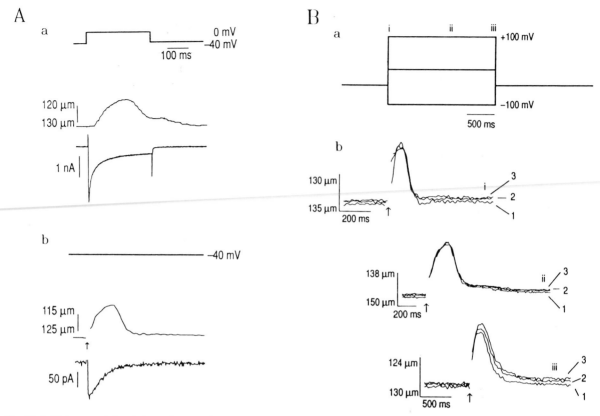

Fig. 13-6. Voltage and time independence of Ca release in guinea pig ventricular myocytes. **A:** (a) Contraction and $I_{Ca,L}$ triggered by a voltage-clamp depolarization from -40 to $0\,mV$. (b) Contraction and associated largely I_{Na-Ca} inward transient current induced by photolysis of caged Ca^{2+} (arrow) at a fixed potential of $-40\,mV$. Temperature 31°C, Ca_o 1 mM. **B:** (a) Protocol: The membrane potential was changed from the holding potential of $-40\,mV$ to $-100\,mV$, $0\,mV$, or $+100\,mV$ for 2 seconds. Flashes were applied at (i), (ii), or (iii). (b) Twitch contractions induced by photolysis of caged Ca^{2+} at different membrane potentials. Flashes were applied at (i) the same time as the voltage change, (ii) 500 ms into the voltage step, or (iii) upon returning to the holding potential. Superimposed contractions are shown for each series. Traces 1–3 were at -100, 0, and $+100\,mV$, respectfully. Series (ii) and (iii) were performed at 22°C, and series (i) at 31°C; Ca_o 1 mM. The figure was composed (with permission) from records in Niggli and Lederer {108}.

beating but not in quiescent cardiac preparations. The link between the extra Ca influx and excitation was then determined by Reuter {118}, who found that beta-adrenergic agonists augment $I_{Ca,L}$ in cardiac Purkinje fibers. Reuter {120} also established that increased force of contraction in ventricular muscle treated with catecholamines was commensurate with an increase in $I_{Ca,L}$, and that these effects were duplicated by a membrane-permeable cyclic AMP analogue. Photorelease of caged cyclic AMP injected into frog atrial fibers also increased $I_{Ca,L}$ and contraction in tandem {123}. In agreement with these earlier results, Callewaert et al. {32} concluded that enhanced Ca release from the SR in myocytes treated with epinephrine was directly related to enhanced $I_{Ca,L}$.

BAY K8644

The dihydropyridine Ca channel agonist Bay K8644 increases Ca influx and the force of contraction in heart muscle {133}. Sanguinetti and Kass {130} investigated $I_{Ca,L}$ and contraction in calf Purkinje fibers treated with the agonist. They found that when the cell membrane holding potential was more negative than $-50\,mV$, Bay K8644 increased both $I_{Ca,L}$ and twitch contraction. Bay K8644 became a partial blocker of Ca channels when the holding potential was moved to more positive potentials than -50 {cf. 115}, and pulsing from the latter holding potentials produced a parallel inhibition of $I_{Ca,L}$ and contraction.

CARDIAC GLYCOSIDES

The effects of cardiac glycosides on $I_{Ca,L}$, and whether these affect glycoside-induced positive inotropy, are still contentious. A voltage-clamp study on cat ventricular muscle by McDonald et al. {91} suggested that the increase in contractility was independent of an effect on $I_{Ca,L}$; there was no change in $I_{Ca,L}$ during the onset of

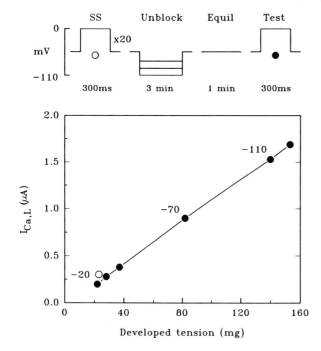

Fig. 13-7. Grading of developed tension by $I_{Ca,L}$ in a cat papillary muscle treated with 2 μM D600 for 90–120 minutes. The preparation was kept in a steady state with 300-ms pulses from −50 to 0 mV at 0.33 Hz (open circle, lower left). After 20 pulses, the muscle was rested (unblock) for 3 minutes at a potential between −110 and −30 mV. A further 1 minute equilibration at −50 mV was followed by a test pulse to 0 mV, and restimulation to steady state. $I_{Ca,L}$ and contraction recovered, in tandem, the more negative the unblocking voltage (bottom left to top right). From McDonald and Pelzer (unpublished). Ca_o was 3.6 mM and temperature was 36°C.

inotropy, and a moderate depression when inotropy was fully developed. A later study by Marban and Tsien {87} on cardiac Purkinje fibers indicated that in these tissues there can be an enhancement of $I_{Ca,L}$, with a time course similar to the development of the positive inotropic effect. Recent investigations of cardiac glycoside action on isolated myocytes have also produced disparate results. Fischmeister et al. {52} reported inhibitory, stimulatory, and transient stimulatory effects on $I_{Ca,L}$ in frog myocytes. Similarly, ouabain produced short transient $I_{Ca,L}$ increases in frog atrial myocytes {2} and guinea pig ventricular myocytes {83} prior to moderate or marked inhibition. On the other hand, Levi {84} did not detect any change in $I_{Ca,L}$ during inotropy onset in guinea pig ventricular myocytes treated with strophanthidin, but did observe inhibition as inotropy progressed. Possible mechanistic reasons for the divergent results {cf. 87,89} and the "dual" effect {52} have not yet been rigorously examined, but it is likely that delayed inhibition of $I_{Ca,L}$ is related to increased Ca_i following inhibition of Na pumping. In this regard, Levi {84} found that delayed inhibition of Ca channel

current during glycoside treatment was absent when Ba was the charge carrier.

REPLENISHMENT OF SR CALCIUM STORES BY $I_{Ca,L}$

Relaxation in heart muscle cells is primarily due to sequestration of Ca by the SR and extrusion of Ca by the Na-Ca exchanger, with a minor contribution from extrusion by the sarcolemmal Ca-ATPase pump. The fraction of SR-released Ca that is extruded from the cell during each relaxation must be replenished if steady-state contractile activity is to be maintained. In this section, we key on experimental results suggesting that replenishment is mainly due to the Ca charge carried through L-type channels, although likely contributions of Ca influx via the Na-Ca exchanger {e.g., 111} should be kept in mind in assessing these results.

Postrest recovery of contractile force

The first contraction after long rest periods is generally a slowly rising weak event in cardiac tissue and myocytes {e.g., 1,26,71,94}. Continued stimulation produces a marked increase in twitch rate of rise and amplitude during the first 5–8 beats, followed by slower recovery to steady state. Measurements of postrest Ca influx {17}, Ca_i release {40}, and SR Ca concentration {71}, are consistent with SR store depletion during rest and refilling during subsequent activity.

Whereas pulsing to relatively positive potentials likely leads to SR reloading with Ca carried into the cell by both $I_{Ca,L}$ and Na-Ca exchange in the Ca-influx mode, pulsing to around 0 mV enhances the possible contribution of the former and restricts that of the latter (see *Sodium-calcium exchange*). Voltage-clamp stimulation to ca. 0 mV after a rest period has been shown to produce marked positive staircases over 6–8 pulses in the contraction of ventricular bundles from dog {13}, sheep {119}, and cat {107,138}, as well as of ventricular myocytes from guinea pig {71} and cat {40}. Two examples are shown in fig. 13-8. The most straightforward explanation for this type of inotropy is that (a) a pulse-to-pulse buildup of SR stores is fuelled by an avid SR uptake of L-type channel influx of Ca that temporarily exceeds sarcolemmal Ca extrusion, and (b) graded release of a near-constant fraction of the SR stores by a near-constant $I_{Ca,L}$ produces larger and larger absolute release, and contraction, until steady state is reached. In fact, in all of the examples cited above (but see next subsection), $I_{Ca,L}$ actually *declined* by ca. 10–30% during the positive tension staircase, lending additional emphasis to the interpretation that the positive staircase in force is due to enhanced filling rather than enhanced fractional release by $I_{Ca,L}$.

Effects of stimulus frequency on $I_{Ca,L}$ and contraction

The effects of stimulus frequency on the action potential configuration and force of contraction are exceedingly

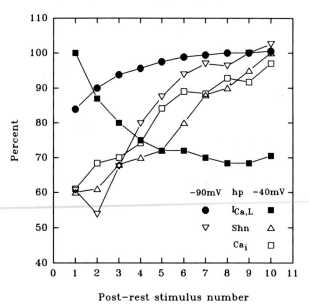

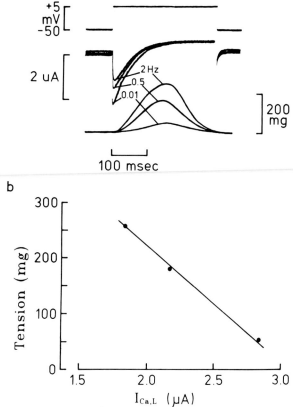

Fig. 13-8. Postrest changes in myocyte $I_{Ca,L}$ and shortening during stimulation from −40 or −90 mV holding potential. The positive staircase in contractile strength (open triangles) was not greatly affected by the holding potential during restimulation at 0.5 Hz to 0 or +10 mV. However, $I_{Ca,L}$ was facilitated when the holding potential was −90 mV (filled circles) and depressed when it was −40 mV (filled squares). The −90 mV data were taken from the Hryshko and Bers {68} study on rabbit ventricular myocytes (30°C, 2 mM Ca_o), and the −40 mV data (including indo-1-monitored Ca_i) from that of DuBell and Houser {40} on cat ventricular myocytes (22°C, 2 mM Ca_o).

Fig. 13-9. Effect of stimulus frequency on $I_{Ca,L}$ and tension in cat ventricular muscle. Stimulation with trains of eight 300-ms pulses from −50 mV to +5 mV was at 0.01, 0.5, and 2 Hz. **A:** Superimposed records from the eighth pulse at each frequency. **B:** A plot of the data in A. Temperature was 36°C and Ca_o was 1.8 mM.

complex, and are dependent on both tissue type and species {25,26,35,132}. Therefore, there is little ground for believing that frequency will have simple effects on $I_{Ca,L}$ and contraction. In most species (rat is one exception), contractile force is much weaker at low frequencies (i.e., 0.1 Hz) than at higher ones (e.g., 2 Hz). The concomitant changes in $I_{Ca,L}$ generally fall into one of two categories: a decline (inverse relation) or an increase (facilitation) in amplitude with higher frequency. These categories are discussed further below.

A synopsis of the frequency-dependent changes in $I_{Ca,L}$ and contraction of cat papillary muscle is shown in fig. 13-9. In this experiment trains of eight voltage-clamp 300-ms pulses from −50 to +5 mV were applied at frequencies of 0.01, 0.5, and then 2 Hz. The superimposed records of the membrane currents and contractions on the eighth pulse at each frequency indicate that $I_{Ca,L}$ was largest, and force of contraction smallest, at the 0.01-Hz pulsing rate (fig. 13-9A). A plot of $I_{Ca,L}$ amplitude versus contractile force depicts the extent of the inverse relation (fig. 13-9B).

Similar inverse relations have also been noted in studies on dog and cat ventricular bundles {138,139}, as well as on bovine ventricular {69} and guinea pig atrial {85} myocytes. These observations are consistent with the results on

postrest stimulation covered in the previous subsection. Stores are nearly empty after long rests {71}, and infrequent pulsing has much the same effect. Conversely, the more frequent the pulsing, the larger the influx per unit time of Ca through L-type channels (even if there is a moderate decline in per-pulse influx at higher frequency). In addition, it seems likely that shorter diastolic intervals during higher frequency stimulation will help fill SR stores by curtailing the time available for optimal Ca extrusion by sarcolemmal transporters.

An important aspect of the foregoing studies is that the negative frequency staircase in $I_{Ca,L}$ occurred during pulsing from holding potentials of −60 to −40 mV. In a number of other studies on myocytes pulsed from about −90 mV, a change in stimulation from a low rate (e.g., 0.1 Hz) to a higher one (e.g., 1–3 Hz) resulted in a positive frequency staircase in $I_{Ca,L}$, which has been termed *potentiation* or *facilitation* {e.g., 51,80,99,113,158}. The question of facilitation versus negative frequency staircase of $I_{Ca,L}$ is discussed below.

Modulation by short-duration pulses

INTERPOSED SINGLE SHORT PULSES

The open symbols in fig. 13-1 show the effects of interposing a single 25-ms pulse to various potentials during otherwise steady pulsing with 300-ms depolarizations from -50 to 5 mV. Since the duration of the 25-ms pulses still allowed $I_{Ca,L}$ to reach a peak at each potential, the $I_{Ca,L}$-voltage relation for the interposed short pulses was similar to that for interposed 300-ms pulses (bottom graph, fig. 13-1). However, the contractions triggered by the short pulses were roughly one-third smaller (top graph, fig. 13-1). Although the contractions on the short pulses developed with the same latencies and initial rates of activation as those on the 300-ms pulses, relaxation began earlier than on contractions elicited by regular pulses. Similar abbreviation of activation in cat ventricular muscle was observed when the action potential was prematurely terminated by current injection {102} or when short depolarizations were applied {148}. Short depolarizing steps also abbreviated contraction in sheep Purkinje fibers {56} and guinea pig ventricular myocytes {71}. In agreement with these observations, Ca_i transients relaxed more quickly when depolarization was shortened in guinea .pig {22} and rat {33} ventricular myocytes. Since large $I_{Ca,L}$ tail currents on repolarization from quite positive potentials can trigger phasic contractions in ventricular tissue preparations (see *Robust phasic contraction . . .*), the shortened contractions probably reflect a premature shutting-off of "late" $I_{Ca,L}$-mediated release during depolarization, and/or the early onset of Ca_i extrusion by the Na-Ca exchanger, rather than lamed Ca release at negative potentials (cf. fig. 13-6).

INTERPOSED TRAINS OF SHORT PULSES

When a train of short pulses is interposed during regular stimulation with longer pulses, the depressant effects observed with a single short pulse are accentuated until a new steady state is reached after 6–8 pulses of the train. The filled symbols in fig. 13-10 depict the time courses of these negative tension staircases in cat and bovine ventricular tissues, and in rat and guinea pig ventricular myocytes. A notable feature is that the first curtailed pulse in tissues cost the tissues a far greater fraction (40–60%) of long (300-ms) pulse contractile force than was the case in myocytes ($\pm10\%$), suggesting tighter control of release in the tissues. Otherwise, the patterns of weakening with short pulses and recovery with subsequent long pulses were similar. The open symbols on the graph indicate that Ca_i transients in ventricular myocytes decline and increase in agreement with the force data. Thus these results support the concept that $I_{Ca,L}$ flowing at post-peak-current times makes an important contribution to the replenishment of SR Ca stores {cf. 47}.

STEADY STATE AT DIFFERENT PULSE DURATIONS

The results in fig. 13-10 indicate that a change in pulse duration produces a new steady-state contractile response

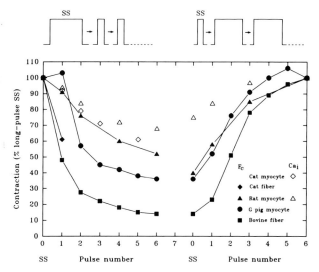

Fig. 13-10. Dependence of contractile force and Ca_i on the duration of the depolarizing clamp pulse. The protocols are shown in the schematic on top, and the experimental conditions (preparation, long pulse, short pulse, temperature, Ca_o) were as follows: cat papillary muscle (300 ms, 25 ms, 36°C, 1.8 mM Ca_o), bovine ventricular strand (300 ms, 25 ms, 36°C, 1.8 mM Ca_o), guinea pig ventricular myocyte (500 ms, 100 ms, 35°C, 1.8 mM Ca_o; data from Isenberg and Wendt-Gallitelli {71}), rat ventricular myocyte (220 ms, 20 ms, 23°C, 2 mM Ca_o; data from Cleemann and Morad {38}), and cat ventricular myocyte (500 ms, 25 ms, 22°C, 2 mM Ca_o; data from DuBell and Houser {40}).

after 6–8 pulses. Steady-state responses in sheep atrial and cat ventricular fibers stimulated with pulses ranging from 8 to 300 ms duration are plotted in fig. 13-11. Shortening of pulse duration from 300 to 200 ms had little effect on contraction (filled symbols). Further shortening caused depression, with the precipitating duration being shorter in the atrial fiber. The steady-state contractile force with 10–15 ms pulses was only about 20% of the 200/300-ms values, despite a 25–30% increase in $I_{Ca,L}$ amplitude. The depression of contraction provides a rough indication of SR refilling reliance on L-type Ca flux flowing between 10- and 15 ms and ca. 200 ms for steady-state long-pulse responses. It is only a rough indication because short pulses probably ensure that a greater fraction of the Ca released by the SR is pumped out of the cell on each cycle. In other words, early repolarization will boost the Na-Ca exchanger's ability to compete with the SR pump for a share of the released Ca.

Positive versus inverse relations

Both postrest stimulation {80} and an increase from low to moderately high stimulation frequency {e.g., 99,158} can produce pulse-to-pulse facilitation of $I_{Ca,L}$ and contractile force when resting/holding potential is around -90 mV. In addition to the increase in amplitude, the inactivation of $I_{Ca,L}$ is slowed down. A full discussion of $I_{Ca,L}$ facilitation

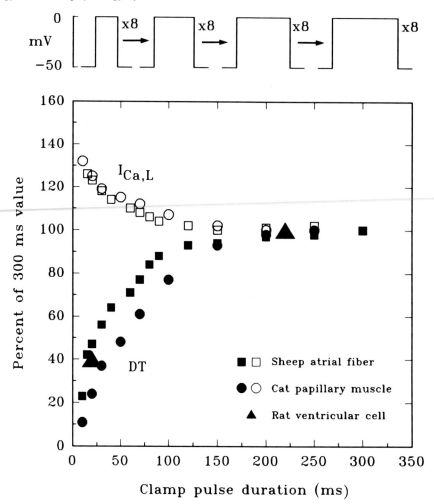

Fig. 13-11. $I_{Ca,L}$ and force of contraction in a sheep atrial fiber and a cat papillary muscle stimulated with trains of eight pulses from −50 to 0 mV at 0.4 Hz. The duration of the pulses was progressively increased, and the data are from the last pulse in each train. Temperature was 36°C and Ca_o was 1.8 mM. Shown for comparison are two measurements of shortening in rat ventricular myocytes (22°C, 2 mM Ca_o). Reported by Cleeman and Morad {38}, with permission.

is beyond the scope of this chapter {see 92 for review}, but brief comments on the contrast with negative $I_{Ca,L}$ staircases are merited.

Facilitation of $I_{Ca,L}$ has obvious benefits for force development: since release should be enhanced by the larger amplitude, and SR filling enhanced by both the larger amplitude and slower inactivation of the current. However, pulse-to-pulse negative staircases in $I_{Ca,L}$ also generate robust positive inotropic staircases, and while one might expect the latter to develop more slowly and less fully than those generated by facilitated $I_{Ca,L}$, it is by no means a given since there will be less Ca extrusion at a holding potential of −50 mV than at −90 mV. That matter aside, why would a change in holding potential from −90 to −50 mV convert a positive $I_{Ca,L}$ staircase into a negative one? Some authors have suggested that slower potential-

dependent recovery from inactivation at the less negative potential could be the culprit. However, this seems unlikely (except at high frequency) because the inverse relation is seen even at quite slow pulsing rates (fig. 13-9) and with short minimally inactivating pulses (fig. 13-11). Nor can an unknown feedback of SR Ca concentration on a future or currently activating $I_{Ca,L}$ be considered a likely answer, since the SR seems to fill and empty in much the same manner during staircases from the two holding potentials. One factor may be that Ca_i close to L-type channels is likely to be higher at the end of diastole at −50 mV than at −90 mV due to less effective extrusion by voltage-dependent Na-Ca exchange {cf. 74}. A buildup of this Ca_i with repetitive pulsing could lead to a progressive partial Ca-induced inactivation of L-type Ca channels. On the other hand, since facilitation is generally not seen when Ba rather than Ca is the charge carrier, one of the most attractive explanations for facilitation is that an increase in Ca_i with repetitive pulsing is due to a Ca_i-potentiating effect on channels {cf. 87,89,92}.

SUMMARY OF THE ROLE OF $I_{Ca,L}$ IN CONTRACTION

The evidence presented in this chapter points to $I_{Ca,L}$ having three major functions in heart excitation-contraction. First, it serves as the trigger for the release of activator Ca from the internal SR stores. The supporting evidence is that phasic contraction and $I_{Ca,L}$ share a common threshold, and block of $I_{Ca,L}$ blocks contraction and Ca release from the SR. Conversely, $I_{Ca,L}$ cannot trigger meaningful contraction when Ca release channels are blocked, or when the SR stores are depleted. The mechanism by which Ca is released from the SR is likely to involve the Ca-activated Ca release process detailed by Fabiato. The second role of $I_{Ca,L}$ is the grading of the fraction of Ca released from the SR. The supporting evidence is that when the amount of Ca available for release is held constant, grading of $I_{Ca,L}$ amplitude by a variety of protocols results in a closely correlated grading of the force of contraction. Of importance here is that Ca-activated Ca release in skinned cardiac cells can be graded by grading the concentration of the trigger Ca solution; the range of trigger Ca concentrations required is not out of line with that expected from Ca influx associated with the early phases of $I_{Ca,L}$. A third identified role for $I_{Ca,L}$ is that it replenishes SR stores. The supporting evidence is that an alteration in the charge carried by $I_{Ca,L}$, whether by modification of current amplitude, duration, or frequency of activation, has a predictable effect on Ca_i transients and contractility triggered by subsequent depolarizations.

The material covered in this chapter indicates that a firm foundation has been laid. However, there is undoubtedly much more to be learned about the properties of the individual elements involved in excitation-contraction coupling, and especially the dynamic interplay between them.

ACKNOWLEDGMENTS

Lesya Shuba was supported by a Killan Trust Scholarship. Support to Terence F. McDonald from the Medical Research Council (Canada) and the Heart and Stroke Foundation of Nova Scotia is gratefully acknowledged.

REFERENCES

1. Allen DG, Jewell BR, Wood EH: Studies of the contractility of mammalian myocardium at low rates of stimulation. *J Physiol* 254:1–17, 1976.
2. Alvarez JL, Vassort G: Properties of the low threshold Ca current in single frog atrial cardiomyocytes: A comparison with the high threshold Ca current. *J Gen Physiol* 100:519–545, 1992.
3. Anderson K, Lai FA, Liu Q-Y, Rousseau E, Erickson HP, Meissner G: Structural and functional characterization of the purified cardiac ryanodine receptor-Ca^{2+} release channel complex. *J Biol Chem* 264:1329–1335, 1989.
4. Antoni H, Jacob R, Kaufmann R: Mechanical response of the frog and mammalian myocardium to changes in the action potential duration by constant current pulses. *Pflügers Arch* 306:33–57, 1969.
5. Arreola J, Dirksen RT, Shieh R-C, Williford DJ, Sheu S-S: Ca^{2+} current and Ca^{2+} transients under action potential clamp in guinea pig ventricular myocytes. *Am J Physiol* 261:C393–C397, 1991.
6. Balke CW, Rose WC, Marban E, Wier WG: Macroscopic and unitary properties of physiological ion flux through T-type Ca^{2+} channels in guinea-pig heart cells. *J Physiol* 456:247–265, 1992.
7. Barcenas-Ruiz L, Beuckelmann DJ, Wier WG: Sodium-calcium exchange in heart: Membrane currents and changes in $[Ca^{2+}]_i$. *Science* 238:1720–1722, 1987.
8. Barcenas-Ruiz L, Wier WG: Voltage dependence of intracellular $[Ca^{2+}]_i$ transients in guinea pig ventricular myocytes. *Circ Res* 61:148–154, 1987.
9. Bassani RA, Bassani JWM, Bers DM: Mitochondrial and sarcolemmal Ca^{2+} transport reduce $[Ca^{2+}]_i$ during caffeine contractures in rabbit cardiac myocytes. *J Physiol* 453:591–608, 1992.
10. Bassingthwaighte JB, Reuter H: Calcium movements and excitation-contraction coupling in cardiac cells. In: de Mello WC (ed) *Electrical Phenomena in the Heart*. New York: Academic Press, 1972, pp 353–393.
11. Bean BP: Two kinds of calcium channels in canine atrial cells. Differences in kinetics, selectivity, and pharmacology. *J Gen Physiol* 86:1–30, 1985.
12. Beeler GW Jr, McGuigan JAS: Voltage clamping of multicellular preparations: Capabilities and limitations of existing methods. *Prog Biophys Mol Biol* 34:219–254, 1978.
13. Beeler GW Jr, Reuter H: The relation between membrane potential, membrane currents and activation of contraction in ventricular myocardial fibres. *J Physiol* 207:211–229, 1970.
14. Berlin JR, Cannell MB, Lederer WJ: Regulation of twitch tension in sheep cardiac Purkinje fibers during calcium overload. *Am J Physiol* 253:H1540–H1547, 1987.
15. Berlin JR, Cannell MB, Lederer WJ: Cellular origins of the transient inward current in cardiac myocytes. *Circ Res* 65:115–126, 1989.
16. Bers DM: Early transient depletion of extracellular Ca during individual cardiac muscle contractions. *Am J Physiol* 244:H462–H468, 1983.
17. Bers DM: Ca influx and sarcoplasmic reticulum Ca release in cardiac muscle activation during post-rest recovery. *Am J Physiol* 248:H366–H381, 1985.
18. Bers DM: *Excitation-Contraction Coupling and Cardiac Contractile Force*. Boston: Kluwer Academic, 1991, pp 93–118.
19. Bers DM, Bridge JHB: Relaxation of rabbit ventricular muscle by Na-Ca exchange and sarcoplasmic reticulum calcium pump: Ryanodine and voltage sensitivity. *Circ Res* 65:334–342, 1989.
20. Bers DM, Christensen DM, Nguyen TX: Can Ca entry via Na-Ca exchange directly activate cardiac muscle contraction? *Mol Cell Cardiol* 20:405–414, 1988.
21. Bers DM, Lederer WJ, Berlin JR: Intracellular Ca transients in rat cardiac myocytes: Role of Na-Ca exchange in excitation-contraction coupling. *Am J Physiol* 258:C944–C954, 1990.
22. Beuckelmann DJ, Wier WG: Mechanism of release of cal-

cium from sarcoplasmic reticulum of guinea pig cardiac cells. *J Physiol* 405:233–255, 1988.

23. Beuckelmann DJ, Wier WG: Sodium-calcium exchange in guinea-pig cardiac cells: Exchange current and changes in intracellular Ca^{2+}. *J Physiol* 414:499–520, 1989.

24. Blaustein MP, Hodgkin AL: The effect of cyanide on the efflux of calcium from squid axons. *J Physiol* 200:497–527, 1969.

25. Bouchard RA, Bose D: Analysis of the interval-force relationship in rat and canine ventricular myocardium. *Am J Physiol* 257:H2036–H2047, 1989.

26. Boyett MR, Jewell BR: Analysis of the effects of changes in rate and rhythm upon electrical activity in the heart. *Prog Biophys Mol Biol* 36:1–52, 1980.

27. Bridge JHB, Smolley JR, Spitzer KW: The relationship between charge movements associated with I_{Ca} and I_{Na-Ca} in cardiac myocytes. *Science* 248:376–378, 1990.

28. Bridge JHB, Spitzer KW, Ershler PR: Relaxation of isolated ventricular cardiomyocytes by a voltage-dependent process. *Science* 241:823–825, 1988.

29. Brill DM, Fozzard HA, Makielski JC, Wasserstrom JA: Effect of prolonged depolarizations on twitch tension and intracellular sodium activity in sheep cardiac Purkinje fibres. *J Physiol* 384:355–375, 1987.

30. Brooksby P, Levi AJ: Does Ca influx via Na-Ca exchange trigger intracellular Ca release and contraction in isolated rat ventricular myocytes? *J Physiol* 452:227P, 1992.

31. Callewaert G: Excitation-contraction coupling in mammalian cardiac cells. *Cardiovasc Res* 26:923–932, 1992.

32. Callewaert G, Cleemann L, Morad M: Epinephrine enhances Ca^{2+} current-regulated Ca^{2+} release and Ca^{2+} reuptake in rat ventricular myocytes. *Proc Natl Acad Sci USA* 85:2009–2013, 1988.

33. Cannell MB, Berlin JR, Lederer WJ: Effect of membrane potential changes on the calcium transient in single rat cardiac muscle cells. *Science* 238:1419–1423, 1987.

34. Capogrossi MC, Stern MD, Spurgeon HA, Lakatta EG: Spontaneous Ca^{2+} release from the sarcoplasmic reticulum limits Ca^{2+}-dependent twitch potentiation in individual cardiac myocytes. *J Gen Physiol* 91:133–155, 1988.

35. Carmeliet E: Repolarisation and frequency in cardiac cells. *J Physiol (Paris)* 73:903–923, 1977.

36. Chapman RA: Control of cardiac contractility at the cellular level. *Am J Physiol* 245:H535–H552, 1983.

37. Chapman RA: Sodium/calcium exchange and intracellular calcium buffering in ferret myocardium: An ion-sensitive micro-electrode study. *J Physiol* 373:163–179, 1986.

38. Cleemann L, Morad M: Role of Ca^{2+} channel in cardiac excitation-contraction coupling in the rat: Evidence from Ca^{2+} transients and contraction. *J Physiol* 432:283–312, 1991.

39. Crespo LM, Grantham CJ, Cannell MB: Kinetics, stoichiometry and role of the Na-Ca exchange mechanism in isolated cardiac myocytes. *Nature* 345:618–621, 1990.

40. DuBell WH, Houser SR: Voltage and beat dependence of Ca^{2+} transient in feline ventricular myocytes. *Am J Physiol* 257:H746–H759, 1989.

41. Egan TM, Noble D, Noble SJ, Powell T, Spindler AJ, Twist VW: Sodium-calcium exchange during the action potential in guinea-pig ventricular cells. *J Physiol* 411:639–661, 1989.

42. Eisner DA, Lederer WJ, Vaughan-Jones RD: The control of tonic tension by membrane potential and intracellular sodium activity in the sheep cardiac Purkinje fibre. *J Physiol* 335:723–743, 1983.

43. Fabiato A: Myoplasmic free calcium concentration reached during the twitch of an intact isolated cardiac cell and during

calcium-induced release of calcium from the sarcoplasmic reticulum of a skinned cardiac cell from the adult rat or rabbit ventricle. *J Gen Physiol* 78:457–497, 1981.

44. Fabiato A: Calcium-induced release of calcium from the cardiac sarcoplasmic reticulum. *Am J Physiol* 245:C1–C14, 1983.

45. Fabiato A: Rapid ionic modifications during the aequorin-detected calcium transient in a skinned canine cardiac Purkinje cell. *J Gen Physiol* 85:189–246, 1985.

46. Fabiato A: Time and calcium dependence of activation and inactivation of calcium-induced release of calcium from the sarcoplasmic reticulum of a skinned canine cardiac Purkinje cell. *J Gen Physiol* 85:247–289, 1985.

47. Fabiato A: Simulated calcium current can both cause calcium loading in and trigger calcium release from the sarcoplasmic reticulum of a skinned canine cardiac Purkinje cell. *J Gen Physiol* 85:291–320, 1985.

48. Fabiato A, Baumgarten CM: Methods for detecting calcium release from the sarcoplasmic reticulum of skinned cardiac cells and the relationship between calculated transsarcolemmal calcium movements and calcium release. In: Sperelakis N (ed) *Function of the Heart in Normal and Pathological States*. The Hague: Martinus Nijhoff, 1987.

49. Fabiato A, Fabiato F: Calcium-induced release of calcium from the sarcoplasmic reticulum of skinned cells from adult human, dog, cat, rabbit, rat and frog hearts and from fetal and new-born rat ventricles. *Ann NY Acad Sci* 307:491–522, 1978.

50. Fabiato A, Fabiato F: Calcium and cardiac excitation-contraction coupling. *Ann Rev Physiol* 41:473–484, 1979.

51. Fedida D, Noble D, Spindler AJ: Use-dependent reduction and facilitation of Ca^{2+} current in guinea-pig myocytes. *J Physiol* 405:439–460, 1988.

52. Fischmeister R, Brocas-Randolph M, Lechêne P, Argibay JA, Vassort G: A dual effect of cardiac glycosides on Ca current in single cells of frog heart. *Pflügers Arch* 406:340–342, 1986.

53. Fozzard HA: Slow inward current and contraction. In: Zipes DP, Bailey JC, Elharrar V (eds) *The Slow Inward Current and Cardiac Arrhythmias*. The Hague: Martinus Nijhoff, 1980, pp 173–203.

54. Fozzard HA, Hellam DC: Relationship between membrane voltage and tension in voltage clamped cardiac Purkinje fibres. *Nature* 218:588–589, 1968.

55. Gibbons WR: Cellular control of cardiac contraction. In: Fozzard et al. (eds) *The Heart and Cardiovascular System*, 2nd ed. New York: Raven Press, 1986, pp 747–778.

56. Gibbons WR, Fozzard HA: Voltage dependence and time dependence of contraction in sheep cardiac Purkinje fibers. *Circ Res* 28:446–460, 1971.

57. Gibbons WR, Fozzard HA: Relationships between voltage and tension in sheep cardiac Purkinje fibers. *J Gen Physiol* 65:345–365, 1975.

58. Gibbons WR, Fozzard HA: Slow inward current and contraction in sheep cardiac Purkinje fibers. *J Gen Physiol* 65:367–384, 1975.

59. Gibbons WR, Zygmunt AC: Excitation-contraction coupling in heart. In: Fozzard HA et al. (eds) *The Heart and Cardiovascular System*, 2nd ed. New York: Raven Press, 1992, pp 1249–1279.

60. Grossman A, Furchgott RF: The effects of various drugs on calcium exchange in the isolated guinea-pig left auricle. *J Pharmacol Exp Ther* 145:162–172, 1964.

61. Grynkiewicz G, Poenie M, Tsien RY: A new generation of Ca^{2+} indicators with greatly improved fluorescence properties. *J Biol Chem* 260:3440–3450, 1985.

62. Hadley RW, Lederer WJ: Comparison of the effects of Bay K 8644 Ca^{2+} current and Ca^{2+} channel gating current. *Am J Physiol* 262:H472–H477, 1992.
63. Hayashi H, Ponnambalam C, McDonald TF: Arrhythmic activity in reoxygenated guinea pig papillary muscles and ventricular cells. *Circ Res* 61:124–133, 1987.
64. Hilgemann DW: Extracellular calcium transients at single excitations in rabbit atrium. Measured with tetramethylmurexide. *J Gen Physiol* 87:707–735, 1986.
65. Hilgemann DW: Numerical approximations of sodium-calcium exchange. *Prog Biophys Mol Biol* 51:1–45, 1988.
66. Hilgemann DW, Noble D: Excitation-contraction coupling and extracellular calcium transients in rabbit atrium: Reconstruction of basic cellular mechanisms. *Proc R Soc Lond* [Biol] 230:163–205, 1987.
67. Horackova M, Vassort G: Sodium-calcium exchange in regulation of cardiac contractility: Evidence for an electrogenic, voltage-dependent mechanism. *J Gen Physiol* 73: 403–424, 1979.
68. Hryshko LV, Bers DM: Ca current facilitation during postrest recovery depends on Ca entry. *Am J Physiol* 259: H951–H961, 1990.
69. Isenberg G: Ca entry and contraction as studied in isolated bovine ventricular myocytes. *Z Naturforsch* 37:502–512, 1982.
70. Isenberg G, Klöckner U: Calcim currents of isolated bovine ventricular myocytes are fast and of large amplitude. *Pflügers Arch* 395:30–41, 1982.
71. Isenberg G, Wendt-Gallitelli MF: Cellular mechanisms of excitation contraction coupling. In: Piper HM, Isenberg G (eds) *Isolated Adult Cardiomyocytes: Electrophysiology and Contractile Function*. Boca Raton, FL: CRC Press, 1989, pp 213–248.
72. Kass RS, Tsien RW, Weingart R: Ionic basis of transient inward current induced by strophanthidin in cardiac Purkinje fibres. *J Physiol* 281:209–226, 1978.
73. Katzung BG, Reuter H, Porzig H: Lanthanum inhibits Ca inward current but not Na-Ca exchange in cardiac muscle. *Experientia* 29:1073–1075, 1973.
74. Kimura J, Miyamae S, Noma A: Identification of sodium-calcium exchange current in single ventricular cells of guinea-pig. *J Physiol* 384:199–222, 1987.
75. Lai FA, Anderson K, Rousseau E, Liu Q-Y, Meissner G: Evidence for a Ca^{2+} channel within the ryanodine receptor complex from cardiac sarcoplasmic reticulum. *Biochem Biophys Res Comm* 151:441–449, 1988.
76. Langer GA: Sodium-calcium exchange in the heart. *Ann Rev Physiol* 44:435–449, 1982.
77. Leblanc N, Hume JR: Sodium current-induced release of calcium from cardiac sarcoplasmic reticulum. *Science* 248: 372–376, 1990.
78. Lederer WJ, Berlin JR, Cohen NM, Hadley RW, Bers DM, Cannell MB: Excitation-contraction coupling in heart cells: Roles of the sodium-calcium exchange, the calcium current, and the sarcoplasmic reticulum. *Ann NY Acad Sci* 588:190–206, 1990.
79. Lederer WJ, Vaughan-Jones RD, Eisner DA, Sheu SS, Cannell MB: The regulation of tension in heart muscle by intracellular sodium. In: Nathan RD (ed) *Cardiac Muscle: The Regulation of Excitation and Contraction*. Orlando, FL: Academic Press, 1986, pp 217–235.
80. Lee KS: Potentiation of the calcium-channel currents of internally perfused mammalian heart cells by repetitive depolarization. *Proc Natl Acad Sci USA* 84:3941–3945, 1987.
81. Lee KS, Tsien RW: Reversal of current through calcium channels in dialysed single heart cells. *Nature* 297:498–501, 1982.
82. Lee KS, Tsien RW: High selectivity of calcium channels in single dialysed heart cells of the guinea-pig. *J Physiol* 354: 253–272, 1984.
83. Le Grand B, Deroubaix E, Coulombe A, Coraboeuf E: Stimulatory effect of ouabain on T- and L-type calcium currents in guinea pig cardiac myocytes. *Am J Physiol* 258:H1620–H1623, 1990.
84. Levi AJ: The effect of strophanthidin on action potential, calcium current and contraction in isolated guinea-pig ventricular myocytes. *J Physiol* 443:1–23, 1991.
85. Lipp P, Pott L, Callewaert G, Carmeliet E: Calcium transients caused by calcium entry are influenced by the sarcoplasmic reticulum in guinea-pig atrial myocytes. *J Physiol* 454:321–338, 1992.
86. London B, Krueger JW: Contraction in voltage-clamped internally perfused single heart cells. *J Gen Physiol* 88:475–505, 1986.
87. Marban E, Tsien RW: Enhancement of calcium current during digitalis inotropy in mammalian heart: Positive feedback regulation by intracellular calcium? *J Physiol* 329:589–614, 1982.
88. Matsuda H, Noma A: Isolation of calcium current and its sensitivity to monovalent cations in dialysed ventricular cells of guinea-pig. *J Physiol* 357:553–573, 1984.
89. McDonald TF: The slow inward calcium current in the heart. *Ann Rev Physiol* 44:425–434, 1982.
90. McDonald TF, Cavalié A, Trautwein W, Pelzer D: Voltage-dependent properties of macroscopic and elementary calcium channel currents in guinea pig ventricular myocytes. *Pflügers Arch* 406:437–448, 1986.
91. McDonald TF, Nawrath H, Trautwein W: Membrane currents and tension in cat ventricular muscle treated with cardiac glycosides. *Circ Res* 37:674–682, 1975.
92. McDonald TF, Pelzer S, Trautwein W, Pelzer D: Regulation and modulation of calcium channels in cardiac, skeletal and smooth muscle cells. *Physiol Rev*, 74:365–507, 1994.
93. McDonald TF, Pelzer D, Trautwein W: On the mechanism of slow calcium channel block in heart. *Pflügers Arch* 385: 175–179, 1980.
94. McDonald TF, Pelzer D, Trautwein W: Does the calcium current modulate the contraction of the accompanying beat? A study of E-C coupling in mammalian ventricular muscle using cobalt ions. *Circ Res* 49:576–583, 1981.
95. McDonald TF, Pelzer D, Trautwein W: Cat ventricular muscle treated with D600: Characteristics of calcium channel block and unblock. *J Physiol* 352:217–241, 1984.
96. McDonald TF, Pelzer D, Trautwein W: Dual action (stimulation, inhibition) of D600 on contractility and calcium channels in guinea-pig and cat heart cells. *J Physiol* 414: 569–586, 1989.
97. McGuigan J: Tension in ventricular fibres during a voltage clamp. *Helv Physiol Acta* 26:CR362–CR363, 1968.
98. Mitchell MR, Powell T, Terrar DA, Twist VW: Influence of a change in stimulation rate on action potentials, currents and contractions in rat ventricular cells. *J Physiol* 364:113–130, 1985.
99. Mitra R, Morad M: Two types of calcium channels in guinea pig ventricular myocytes. *Proc Natl Acad Sci USA* 83:5340–5344, 1986.
100. Morad M, Cleemann L: Role of Ca^{2+} channel in development of tension in heart muscle. *J Mol Cell Cardiol* 19:527–553, 1987.
101. Morad M, Goldman Y: Excitation-contraction coupling in heart muscle: Membrane control of development of tension.

Prog Biophys Mol Biol 27:257–313, 1973.

102. Morad M, Trautwein W: The effect of the duration of the action potential on contraction in the mammalian heart muscle. *Pflügers Arch* 299:66–82, 1968.

103. Mullins LJ: The generation of electric currents in cardiac fibers by Na/Ca exchange. *Am J Physiol* 263:C103–C110, 1979.

104. Näbauer M, Callewaert G, Cleemann L, Morad M: Regulation of calcium release is gated by calcium current, not gating charge, in cardiac myocytes. *Science* 244:800–803, 1989.

105. Näbauer M, Morad M: Ca^{2+}-induced Ca^{2+}-release as examined by photolysis of caged Ca^{2+} in single ventricular myocytes. *Am J Physiol* 258:C189–C193, 1990.

106. Nawrath H, Ten Eick RE, McDonald TF, Trautwein W: On the mechanism underlying the action of D-600 on slow inward current and tension in mammalian myocardium. *Circ Res* 40:408–414, 1977.

107. New W, Trautwein W: The ionic nature of slow inward current and its relation to contraction. *Pflügers Arch* 334:24–38, 1972.

108. Niggli E, Lederer WJ: Voltage-independent calcium release in heart muscle. *Science* 250:565–568, 1990.

109. Nilius B, Hess P, Lansman JB, Tsien RW: A novel type of cardiac calcium channel in ventricular cells. *Nature* 316:443–446, 1985.

110. Noble D: Sodium-calcium exchange and its role in generating electric current. In: Nathan RD (ed) *Cardiac Muscle: The Regulation of Excitation and Contraction.* Orlando, FL: Academic Press, 1986, pp 171–200.

111. Nuss HB, Houser SR: Sodium-calcium exchange-mediated contractions in feline ventricular myocytes. *Am J Physiol* 263:H1161–H1169, 1992.

112. Ochi R, Trautwein W: The dependence of cardiac contraction on depolarization and slow inward current. *Pflügers Arch* 323:187–203, 1971.

113. Peineau N, Argibay JA: Transient changes in action potential duration and calcium current after an increase in stimulation frequency in isolated guinea-pig ventricular cardiocytes. *J Physiol* 446:338P, 1992.

114. Pelzer D, Cavalié A, McDonald TF, Trautwein W: Macroscopic and elementary currents through cardiac calcium channels. *Prog Zool* 33:83–98, 1986.

115. Pelzer D, Pelzer S, McDonald TF: Properties and regulation of calcium channels in muscle cells. *Rev Physiol Biochem Pharmacol* 114:108–207, 1990.

116. Pelzer D, Pelzer S, McDonald TF: Calcium channels in heart. In: Fozzard HA (ed) *The Heart and Cardiovascular System,* 2nd ed. New York: Raven Press, 1991, pp 1049–1089.

117. Reeves JP, Hale CC: The stoichiometry of the cardiac sodium-calcium exchange system. *J Biol Chem* 259:7733–7739, 1984.

118. Reuter H: The dependence of slow inward current in Purkinje fibres on the extracellular calcium-concentration. *J Physiol* 192:479–492, 1967.

119. Reuter H: Time and voltage-dependent contractile responses in mammalian cardiac muscle. *Eur J Cardiol* 1:177–181, 1973.

120. Reuter H: Localization of beta adrenergic receptors and effects of noradrenaline and cyclic nucleotides on action potentials, ionic currents and tension in mammalian cardiac muscle. *J Physiol* 242:429–451, 1974.

121. Reuter H, Scholz H: A study of the ion selectivity and the kinetic properties of the calcium dependent slow inward current in mammalian cardiac muscle. *J Physiol* 264:17–47, 1977.

122. Reuter H, Seitz N: The dependence of calcium efflux from cardiac muscle on temperature and external ion composition. *J Physiol* 195:451–470, 1968.

123. Richard S, Nerbonne JM, Nargeot J, Lester HA, Garnier D: Photochemically produced intracellular concentration jumps of cAMP mimic the effects of catecholamines on excitation-contraction coupling in frog atrial fibers. *Pflügers Arch* 403:312–317, 1985.

124. Ríos E, Pizarro G: Voltage sensor of excitation-contraction coupling in skeletal muscle. *Physiol Rev* 71:849–908, 1991.

125. Rose WC, Balke CW, Wier WG, Marban E: Macroscopic and unitary properties of physiological ion flux through L-type Ca^{2+} channels in guinea-pig heart cells. *J Physiol* 456:267–284, 1992.

126. Rose WC, Marban E, Wier WG, Balke CW: Densities of T- and L-type calcium channels estimated from comparison of macroscopic and unitary currents in cardiac ventricular myocytes (abstr). *Circ* 84(Suppl):II, 181, 1991.

127. Rousseau E, Meissner G: Single cardiac sarcoplasmic reticulum Ca^{2+}-release channel: Activation by caffeine. *Am J Physiol* 256:H328–H333, 1989.

128. Rousseau E, Smith JS, Henderson JS, Meissner G: Single channel and $^{45}Ca^{2+}$ flux measurements of the cardiac sarcoplasmic reticulum calcium channel. *Biophys J* 50:1009–1014, 1986.

129. Sánchez JA, Stefani E: Kinetic properties of calcium channels of twitch muscle fibres of the frog. *J Physiol* 337:1–17, 1983.

130. Sanguinetti MC, Kass RS: Regulation of cardiac calcium channel current and contractile activity by the dihydropyridine Bay K 8644 is voltage-dependent. *J Mol Cell Cardiol* 16:667–670, 1984.

131. Schneider MF, Chandler WK: Voltage dependent charge movement in skeletal muscle: A possible step in excitation-contraction coupling. *Nature* 242:244–246, 1973.

132. Schouten VJA, ter Keurs HEDJ: Role of I_{Ca} and Na^+/Ca^{2+} exchange in the force-frequency relationship of rat heart muscle. *J Mol Cell Cardiol* 23:1039–1050, 1991.

133. Schramm M, Thomas G, Towart R, Frankowiak G: Novel dihydropyridines with positive inotropic action through activation of Ca^{2+} channels. *Nature* 303:535–537, 1983.

134. Sham JSK, Cleemann L, Morad M: Gating of the cardiac Ca^{2+} release channel: The role of Na^+ current and Na^+-Ca^{2+} exchange. *Science* 255:850–853, 1992.

135. Shattock MJ, Bers DM: Rat vs. rabbit ventricle: Ca flux and intracellular Na assessed by ion-selective microelectrodes. *Am J Physiol* 256:C813–C822, 1989.

136. Shepherd N, Vornanen M, Isenberg G: Force measurements from voltage-clamped guinea pig ventricular myocytes. *Am J Physiol* 258:H452–H459, 1990.

137. Shieh RC, Williford DJ: Na-Ca exchange current during physiological excitation-contraction coupling in guinea-pig ventricular myocytes (abstr). *FASEB J* 6:A443, 1992.

138. Šimurda J, Šimurdová M, Bravený P, Šumbera J: Slow inward current and action potentials of papillary muscles under non-steady state conditions. *Pflügers Arch* 362:209–218, 1976.

139. Šimurda J, Šimurdová M, Bravený P, Šumbera J: Activity-dependent changes of slow inward current in ventricular heart muscle. *Pflügers Arch* 391:277–283, 1981.

140. Sipido KR, Wier WG: Flux of Ca^{2+} across the sarcoplasmic reticulum of guinea-pig cardiac cells during excitation-contraction coupling. *J Physiol* 435:605–630, 1991.

141. Sitsapesan R, Williams AJ: Mechanisms of caffeine activation of single calcium-release channels of sheep cardiac sarcoplasmic reticulum. *J Physiol* 423:425–439, 1990.

142. Stern MD, Lakatta EG: Excitation-contraction coupling in

the heart: The state of the question. *FASEB J* 6:3092–3100, 1992.

143. Sutko JL, Willerson JT: Ryanodine alteration of the contractile state of rat ventricular myocardium: Comparison with dog, cat, and rabbit ventricular tissues. *Circ Res* 46: 332–343, 1980.

144. Ten Eick R, Nawrath H, McDonald TF, Trautwein W: On the mechanism of the negative inotropic effect of acetylcholine. *Pflügers Arch* 361:207–213, 1976.

145. Trautwein W: The slow inward current in mammalian myocardium: Its relation to contraction *Europ J Cardiol* 1/2: 169–175, 1973.

146. Trautwein W, McDonald TF, Tripathi O: Calcium conductance and tension in mammalian ventricular muscle. *Pflügers Arch* 354:55–74, 1975.

147. Trautwein W, Pelzer D, McDonald TF, Osterrieder W: AQA 39, a new bradycardiac agent which blocks myocardial calcium channels in a frequency- and voltage-dependent manner. *Naunyn Schmiedeberg's Arch Pharmacol* 317:228–232, 1981.

148. Tritthart H, Kaufmann R, Volkmer H-P, Bayer R, Krause H: Ca-movement controlling myocardial contractility I. Voltage-, current- and time-dependence of mechanical activity under voltage clamp conditions (cat papillary muscles and trabeculae). *Pflügers Arch* 338:207–231, 1973.

149. Vassort G, Rougier O: Membrane potential and slow inward current dependence of frog cardiac mechanical activity. *Pflügers Arch* 331:191–203, 1972.

150. Wier WG: Calcium transients during excitation-contraction coupling in mammalian heart: Aequorin signals of canine Purkinje fibers. *Science* 207:1085–1087, 1980.

151. Wier WG: Cytoplasmic [Ca^{2+}] in mammalian ventricle: Dynamic control by cellular processes. *Annu Rev Physiol* 52:467–485, 1990.

152. Wier WG: [Ca^{2+}]$_i$ transients during excitation-contraction coupling of mammalian heart. In: Fozzard et al. (eds) *The Heart and Cardiovascular System*, 2nd ed. New York: Raven Press, 1992, pp 1223–1248.

153. Wier WG, Isenberg G: Intracellular [Ca^{2+}] transients in voltage clamped cardiac Purkinje fibers. *Pflügers Arch* 392: 284–290, 1982.

154. Wong AY, Fabiato A, Bassingthwaigthe JB: Model of calcium-induced calcium release mechanism in cardiac cells. *Bull Math Biol* 54:95–116, 1992.

155. Wood EH, Heppner RL, Weidmann S: Inotropic effects of electric currents. *Circ Res* 24:409–445, 1969.

156. Yue DG: Intracellular [Ca^{2+}] related to rate of force development in twitch contraction of heart. *Am J Physiol* 252: H760–H770, 1987.

157. Yue DT, Wier WG: Estimation of intracellular [Ca^{2+}] by nonlinear indicators. A quantitative analysis. *Biophys J* 48: 533–537, 1985.

158. Zygmunt AC, Maylie J: Stimulation-dependent facilitation of the high threshold calcium current in guinea-pig ventricular myocytes. *J Physiol* 428:653–671, 1990.

CHAPTER 14

Cardiac Excitation-Contraction Coupling: From Global to Microscopic Models

GERRIT ISENBERG

INTRODUCTION

Excitation couples to contraction through an increase in the concentration of calcium ions in the myofibrillar space (or cytosol). Most of this activator Ca^{2+} is released from the intracellular stores of the sarcoplasmic reticulum (SR). The mechanisms by which the depolarization of the surface membrane leads to SR Ca^{2+} release, however, are not yet fully understood. This article describes the related problems in three sections. The first section considers excitation-contraction (E-C) coupling in the framework of "global" models that approximate the concentration of calcium ions in the cytosol ($[Ca^{2+}]_c$) as a homogeneous pool. This approximation will be used for describing recent results on transient changes in $[Ca^{2+}]_c$ as they are monitored by Ca^{2+}-sensitive fluorescent dyes fura-2 or indo-1 {13,106,127,128}. Special attention will be paid to a comparison between $[Ca^{2+}]_c$ and the concentration of total calcium (ΣCa_c, i.e., the sum of ionized and bound calcium) as it is measured by electron probe microanalysis {121,122}.

$[Ca^{2+}]_c$ and ΣCa_c change with time due to Ca^{2+} fluxes that are driven by electrochemical gradients. There is a first Ca^{2+} gradient between the extracellular space and the cytosol, which is provided by the diffusional barrier of the plasma surface membrane (sarcolemma) in combination with the Ca^{2+} extrusion by the Na-Ca exchanger and the plasmalemmal Ca^{2+} ATPase. A second Ca^{2+} gradient exists between the SR and the cytosol, which is maintained by the SR Ca^{2+} ATPase (SERCa). Detailed information on the Ca^{2+} ATPases and the Na-Ca exchanger are given in other chapters of this book {10,80,110}. Hence, the second section of this chapter will concentrate on the new literature about those proteins that channel the Ca^{2+} fluxes into the cytosol, namely, the dihydropyridine- (DHP-) sensitive L-type Ca^{2+} channels of the sarcolemma (DHP-R) and the ryanodine-sensitive Ca^{2+}-release channel (RyR) of the SR.

The third section will demonstrate that some fundamental properties of cardiac E-C coupling are difficult to understand without taking into consideration the spatial arrangement of the Ca^{2+} channels in sarcolemma and SR, and the correspondent Ca^{2+} heterogeneities. A speculative outlook on those "microscopic models" of cardiac E-C coupling {22,54,107,199} will be presented.

METHODS

Microfluometry

Since the invention of fluorescent Ca^{2+} indicators like fura-2 or indo-1 {45}, a whole series of new experiments on cardiac E-C coupling has started. Usually the membrane-impermeable indicator is dialyzed from the patch electrode into the cytosol of the single myocyte {128}. In case of indo-1, fluorescence is excited by UV light of 310 nm, and the emitted fluorescence is measured at both 410 nm (Ca^{2+}-indo-1) and 470 nm (indo-1). $[Ca^{2+}]_c$ can be calculated from the ratio of the 410/470 nm fluorescence, independent of the dye concentration and of possible movement artifacts. The fluorescence signals have also been analyzed with imaging techniques. The ratiometric methods with indo-1 used a pair of charge-coupled device cameras. With the spatial resolution of light microscopy and a time resolution of 16.7 ms, the images indicated that $[Ca^{2+}]_c$ changed homogeneously during a twitch {128}.

Voltage clamp

The $[Ca^{2+}]_c$ transients can be measured under the condition of the voltage clamp, thereby controlling the trans-sarcolemmal Ca^{2+} fluxes through DHP-R and the Na-Ca exchanger {17,18,44,57,58,113,114}. Since a large fraction of the Ca^{2+} influx loads the SR with releasable Ca^{2+}, voltage-clamp programs are suitable for modulating the SR Ca^{2+} load {44,52,55,58,119,120}. To the recorded current wave, the Ca^{2+} influx through DHP-sensitive Ca^{2+} channels contributes as a negative current surge (I_{Ca}), and the Ca^{2+} efflux through Na-Ca exchange as a negative tail current component (I_{ex} in fig. 14-1). Dissection of the individual current components from the net current is not feasible if the block of a Ca^{2+} flux interferes with the Ca^{2+} homeostasis of the cell.

Voltage-clamp experiments using wide-opened patch pipettes go along with "cell dialysis." One should bear in

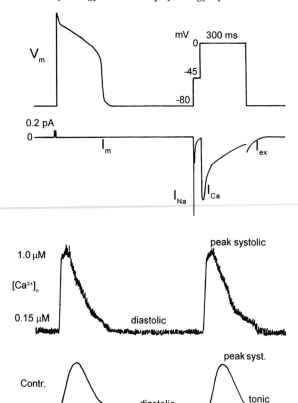

after a 15-ms delay and peaks within ca. 30-ms to 1 μM. *Contractions* of mechanically unloaded myocytes are usually measured as isotonic shortening. At diastole, sarcomere length is ca. 1.85 μm. During systole, it shortens within 130-ms to ca. 1.65 μm. Relaxation may remain incomplete as long as the membrane is not repolarized (tonic component of contraction).

Fig. 14-1. Schematic of the basic events during cardiac E-C coupling (guinea-pig ventricular cell). From top to bottom: V_m action potential or voltage-clamp depolarization, I_m stimulus current or ionic membrane currents, $[Ca^{2+}]_c$ transients, and contraction. *Action potentials during current clamp* are triggered by stimulus current or in vivo by conduction. Action potentials start from a diastolic membrane potential of ca. −80 mV. The fast upstroke changes the potential within less than 1-ms to an overshoot of ca. +40 mV. After an initial fast phase, repolarization is retarded, which causes the ca. 250-ms plateau phase. Finally, the membrane rapidly repolarizes to the diastolic potential. *Membrane currents during voltage clamp.* The membrane is integrated into an electronic feedback system (voltage clamp) that "clamps" the potential to the wanted value by feeding current into the cell. For this schematic, potassium currents were blocked. The 20-ms prepulse from −80 to −45 mV activates and inactivates I_{Na}, the inward sodium current through TTX-sensitive channels; I_{Na} is largely out of scale and would peak to ca. −100 nA per cell. The step to 0 mV activates and inactivates an inward calcium current (I_{Ca}) through dihydropyridine (DHP)-sensitive Ca^{2+} channels. Approximately 5% of I_{Ca} does not inactivate. Repolarization to −80 mV switches off non-inactivated I_{Ca} and recovers the Ca^{2+} channels from the inactivated to the resting available state. I_{Ca} is discussed (a) to trigger Ca^{2+} release from the SR, (b) to load the SR with Ca^{2+}, and (c) to contribute to the Ca^{2+} that activates the myofilaments. The current I_{ex} is generated by the electrogenic Na-Ca exchange, i.e., it represents Ca^{2+} efflux from the cell. *$[Ca^{2+}]_c$, the concentration of cytosolic Ca^{2+} ions*, can be measured with fluorescent Ca^{2+}-indicators such as fura-2 or indo-1. The diastolic $[Ca^{2+}]_c$ of 0.15 μM is typical for myocytes that are stimulated at 1 or 2 Hz. During the depolarization, $[Ca^{2+}]_c$ rises

mind that cell dialysis not only loads the cell with the dye but also washes out essential cytosolic constituents, such as protein kinases, calmodulin, ATP, etc., and perhaps other unknown soluble "factors." Presumably due to this washout, the recordings are stable only for a limited period of time (e.g., 15 minutes at 36°C), and usually there is a subsequent rundown of Ca^{2+} channel current {88} and contractility {53,100}.

Electron probe microanalysis

Electron probe microanalysis (EPMA) measures the total calcium concentration, ΣCa, with approximately 16-nm resolution {121,122}. The ΣCa distribution of a given functional state can be preserved by shock-freezing the cell. After cryosectioning and freeze-drying, the 25-nm thin section is analyzed in the electron microscope. EPMA attributes the spatial distribution of Σ Ca to morphological compartments {119}. EPMA analyzes a volume of $16 \cdot 16 \cdot 25$ nm^3 in which the number of Ca atoms is extremely small; that is, precise measurements (low standard deviation) require long analysis times, e.g., of 1000 seconds per point. For elemental imaging, e.g., of $128 \cdot 128$ pixels, a 1-second analysis time and 2-second computer time per point results in an on-line analysis of approximately 13-hours per image. As a consequence, the spatial information is contaminated with a relatively high statistical error. Since shock-freezing ends the experiment, EPMA can give only a snapshot view of the ΣCa. The evaluation of the entire time course {123} requires tremendous experimental effort, because due to cell-to-cell variability more than six cells have to be shock-frozen and analyzed for each time point (see fig. 14-3).

Skinned preparations

Skinning means the destruction of the plasmalemmal membrane as a permeation barrier without impairment of the intracellular membranes. Skinning can be done chemically (e.g., by saponin or α-toxin) or mechanically. The mechanical skinning procedure described by Fabiato {34–39} uses 4–7 μm thick and 20–60 μm long bundles of myofibrils, which are surrounded by SR. In such skinned bundles, externally applied solutions have direct access to the outer surface of the SR. Thus slow diffusion of Ca^{2+} takes place only through each myofibril once Ca^{2+} has been released from the SR. In the myofibrillar space of skinned bundles, $[Ca^{2+}]_c$ has been measured by aequorin fluorescence.

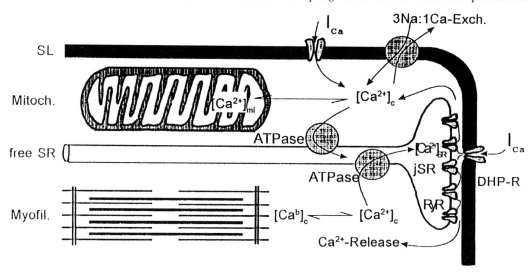

Fig. 14-2. Simplified schema of the possible Ca^{2+} compartments in a ventricular cell. Extracellular Ca^{2+} enters primarily as calcium current (I_{Ca}) through dihydropyridine-sensitive Ca^{2+} channels (DHP-R) of the sarcolemma (SL). In the narrow space between SL and junctional SR (jSR), I_{Ca} may increase $[Ca^{2+}]_c$ sufficiently for activation of Ca^{2+} release channels of the SR (ryanodine receptors or RyR). SR Ca^{2+} release is driven by the high intra-SR Ca^{2+} concentration $[Ca^{2+}]_{SR}$. SR Ca^{2+} release is the main source for the fast rise in $[Ca^{2+}]_c$. Ca^{2+} ions bind to endogenous Ca^{2+} ligands, thereby increasing the concentration of bound Ca^{2+} $[Ca^b]_c$. $[Ca^b]_c$ exceeds $[Ca^{2+}]_c$ by a factor of 1000. Binding of Ca^{2+} to troponin C activates contraction. The systolic rise in $[Ca^{2+}]_c$ increases $[Ca^{2+}]$ of other cell compartments, e.g., of mitochondria. Sequestration of Ca^{2+} by SR Ca^{2+}-ATPase starts during systole. Ca^{2+} efflux from the cell is mostly due to electrogenic Na-Ca exchange. The less important Ca^{2+} efflux through plasma membrane Ca^{2+}-ATPase is not shown.

Ca^{2+} measurements in cell organelles and microsomes

Microfluometry and EPMA analyze the calcium concentration "in vivo," that is, in myocytes in which the integrity of the intracellular organization has not been disturbed. The calcium concentration of cell compartments can also be measured by means of disruptive techniques: The ventricular muscle is homogenized and the organelle under investigation, e.g., mitochondria {29}, is separated by centrifugation through a density gradient. The method applies also to SR vesicles {40,75}. Vesicle studies have revealed many of the basic properties of the SR Ca^{2+} transport, i.e., the Ca^{2+}-ATPase (SERCa) {71,110}. For the studies of SR Ca^{2+} release through the RyR, the vesicles are loaded with $^{45}Ca^{2+}$, the release is activated by exposing the vesicles to a high $[Ca^{2+}]$ in a stop-flow apparatus, followed by rapid filtration and quenching {74, 75}. The time resolution of this method is on the order of 1 second.

Protein purification and expression

From vesicle preparations proteins can be solubilized by detergents. Purification of the proteins is done with columns equipped with ligands that bind the proteins specifically. Accordingly, the purified protein is called a *ryanodine receptor* (RyR) {40,74,86} or a *dihydropyridine receptor* (DHP-R) {41,62}. The physiological function of the purified proteins, for example, to produce ionic currents through Ca^{2+} release channels (RyR), can be monitored after reconstitution of the protein into a lipid bilayer. However, the specific function may be lost when one of the purification steps has unfolded the protein and an incorrect tertiary conformation has been reconstituted. The channel proteins can also be expressed from mRNA in an oocyte or another expression system. In the case of a channel protein, the function can be studied by measuring the membrane current through the expressed protein. Knowledge of primary protein structure has been gained from molecular biology, which has succeeded in screening genomic libraries and in expressing complementary DNA {76,112}.

Single-channel analysis

Currents through single channels {26,50,85,88,93–96} have amplitudes up to several picoamperes. The currents flow discontinuously, suggesting that the channel protein fluctuates between conducting and nonconducting conformations. Statistical analysis provides insight into the molecular mechanism of gating from "closed" to "open" (how many transitions, rate constants, etc.). Single-channel activity can be analyzed in patches attached to the native cells or to oocytes with the expressed channels. Channel activity can also be analyzed from cell-free isolated patches: Either the patch is excised from the cell or the channel protein is reconstituted into a patch with a lipid bilayer {93–96}.

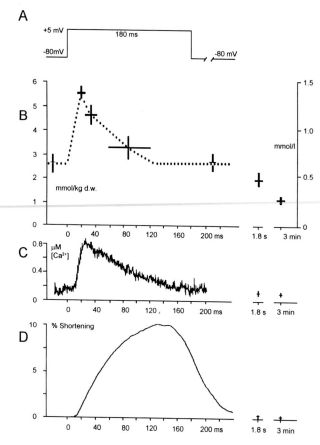

Fig. 14-3. Time course of total myofibrillar ΣCa_c (**B**) in comparison with $[Ca^{2+}]_C$ (**C**) and cell shortening (**D**) induced by a 180-ms voltage-clamp step to 0 mV (**A**) (prepulse to −4.5 mV not shown for clarity). In B, vertical bars indicate SEM and horizontal bars indicate the period from which measurements were grouped together. C and D are averages of 10 sweeps. $[Ca^{2+}]_c$ was calculated from the 410/470-nm indo-1 fluorescence ratio by computer. Note: The points at 1.8 seconds and 3 minutes show that ΣCa_c recovers along a slower time course than $[Ca^{2+}]_c$. Modified after Wendt-Gallitelli and Isenberg, with permission {22}. *Method.* Ventricular myocytes were potentiated with a train of paired voltage-clamp pulses. Potentiation was monitored by the extent of cell shortening and the inward tail current I_{ex}. Movement of ions within the cell was arrested by shock-freezing with propane (−196°C). Frozen myocytes were cut at −150°C, and the 80-nm thick sections were freeze-dried at 10^{-6} Torr and analyzed at −100°C in an electron microscope equipped with an energy-dispersive detector. For analysis the beam diameter of 16 nm was focused on the myofilaments, i.e., SR or mitochondria were excluded.

GLOBAL CONCEPTS OF CARDIAC E-C COUPLING {13,28,29,49,77}

Requirement for $[Ca^{2+}]_o$

In contrast to skeletal or smooth muscles, cardiac muscle has an absolute requirement for extracellular Ca^{2+} to contract: At zero $[Ca^{2+}]_o$ the heart stops beating, although excitability is retained. In the absence of $[Ca^{2+}]_o$ contraction can be elicited by inducing Ca^{2+} release from the SR with caffeine. Hence, it has been concluded that influx of extracellular Ca^{2+} is the necessary link between the electrical events (action potential) and the SR Ca^{2+} release. This phenomenon of *Ca^{2+}-induced Ca^{2+} release (CICR)* {34–39} is the key event in cardiac E-C coupling.

Gradation of contraction

In fast vertebrate skeletal muscle, gradation of contraction is achieved by the recruitment of more muscle fibers whose individual responses are not graded but are all or none {6}. In the heart each excitation activates the whole muscle, but at yet nearly identical excitations the strength of the heart-beat can change markedly. This must mean that the gradation of cardiac contraction is a property inside the individual muscle cell. How excitations grade the activation of CICR in the single cell is another key question about cardiac E-C coupling.

Schema of Ca^{2+} movements

Activation of contraction occurs by binding of Ca^{2+} to troponin C (TnC) {103,104}. During the cardiac action potential extracellular Ca^{2+} enters the cell through DHP-R, and to some extent through the Na-Ca exchanger. Some of this Ca^{2+} may bind to the myofilaments and directly activate contraction. Most of this Ca^{2+} binds to the SERCa protein and is sequestered into the SR. A fraction of the entering Ca^{2+} may bind to RyR and activate CICR. Most experimental results support the hypothesis that most of the activator Ca^{2+} stems from SR Ca^{2+} release.

For relaxation Ca^{2+} is removed from the cytoplasm so that Ca^{2+} will dissociate from TnC. At least three processes are involved, the Ca^{2+} ATPase of the SR (SERCa) {71,110}, the Ca^{2+} ATPase of the plasmalemma (PMCa) {24}, and the Na-Ca exchanger {32,78,79}. A small leak of Ca^{2+} out of the SR into the cytoplasm may be important for the loss of cellular Ca^{2+} in unstimulated cells. Presumably this loss is the basis for the rest decay of contractility {3,19,20,90}.

Ca^{2+} compartments

Functionally, a Ca^{2+} compartment is a space in which the Ca^{2+} concentration differs from the Ca^{2+} concentration in the surrounding space {58,97}. In a morphological sense, compartments are surrounded by lipid membranes that act as permeability barriers. The permeability barrier between the extracellular and intracellular spaces is the *sarcolemma* of the cell surface and the T tubules {42,105}. The Ca^{2+} flux through the sarcolemma is localized at those relevant molecules, such as Ca^{2+} channels (DHP-R), the Na-Ca exchanger, and Ca^{2+}-ATPases (PMCa). A major structural specialization of the sarcolemma is the formation of junctions with the SR. Those junctions can occur either at the surface sarcolemma or at the T-tubular membrane.

SARCOPLASMIC RETICULUM

The sarcoplasmic reticulum {42,105} is an entirely intracellular, membrane-bound Ca^{2+} compartment. The main function of the SR is the sequestration and release of Ca^{2+}. Among different species, and also between different regions of the heart, the volume fraction of the SR varies between 5% and 8%, which may reflect the differing importance of the SR. In the *junctional SR*, the T-tubular membrane is separated from the SR membrane by a 12-nm *junctional gap* {43}. The gap is bridged by *foot proteins*, which have been identified as the SR Ca^{2+} release channel or RyR {40}. The RyR appear with a periodic spacing of approximately 30-nm {43}, and there is a match of approximately 7 RyR to one DHP-sensitive Ca^{2+} channel of the sarcolemma {16,126}. The potential implication of this arrangement for cardiac E-C coupling will be considered later. *Corbular SR* (also called *extended junctional SR*) bears foot proteins that do not come into contact with the sarcolemma; e.g., corbular SR occurs along the Z-disk {42}. The *free SR* is a network of tubules 25–60-nm wide that is continuous with the junctional SR, but free of the foot proteins. Fenestrated collars (at the M lines) enlarge the surface-to-volume ratio and, presumably, provide a high rate of Ca^{2+} sequestration.

LUMINAL PROTEINS

Luminal proteins inside the SR {71} bind Ca^{2+} with low affinity and high capacity. Most abundant is calsequestrin, a protein present in the junctional SR as a matrix. Cardiac calsequestrin has a mass of 45,269 kDa; each molecule can bind 20–40 Ca^{2+} ions with millimolar affinity. The amount of calsequestrin suggests that the majority of the intraluminal Ca^{2+} is bound to calsequestrin. During CICR, the rapid dissociation of Ca^{2+} from the Ca^{2+}-calsequestrin complex permits a far more extensive Ca^{2+} release to the cytoplasm than would be the case in the absence of such a Ca^{2+} buffer. Also, the sequestration of luminal free Ca^{2+} reduces the gradient against which the Ca^{2+} must be pumped {13,71}. Due to calsequestrin, the SR Ca^{2+} load can improve by an increase in ΣCa_{SR} at an almost constant $[Ca^{2+}]_{SR}$.

MITOCHONDRIA

Twenty to 35% of the ventricular cell volume is occupied by mitochondria {13,29,42,55,105}. The mitochondria are the sites of oxidative phosphorylation; hence, the large mitochondrial content reflects the high demands of cardiac tissue for ATP. Cardiac mitochondria are usually cylindrical. Layers of mitochondria are found just under the sarcolemma and between adjacent myofibrils. Frequently the mitochondria are surrounded by a network of free SR {42,123,125}.

MYOFIBRILS

The myofibrils occupy 45–50 vol% of ventricular cells {13,42,105,124,125}. The myofibrils are composed of myosin, actin, and associated components. The myofilaments run in bundles or fibrils. The z lines anchor the actin filaments with intermediate filaments of the cytoskeleton. From the z lines the actin filaments project approximately 1 μm toward the center of the sarcomere. The 1.6-μm long myosin filaments center on the m line, where they are connected to each other in a hexagonal array by radial crosslinks.

Ca^{2+} binding in the myofibrillar space

Contraction of cardiac muscle is activated if Ca^{2+} binds to the Ca^{2+}-specific or *activator site* of troponin C {103,104}. Usually the concentration of the Ca-TnC complex is extrapolated from $[Ca^{2+}]_c$ and the binding constants of Ca-TnC {34,87,91}. With TnC as the only Ca^{2+} ligand, one can calculate the amount of calcium bound to TnC from measured $[Ca^{2+}]_c$. However, the presence of multiple Ca^{2+} ligands with different Ca^{2+} affinities makes the calculations more difficult; that is, for Ca^{2+} binding TnC competes with other Ca^{2+} binding sites as calmodulin, SERCa, lipids, etc. Taking into account all the ligands known until 1983, Fabiato {34} suggested that activation of contraction to 50% of the maximum (3 μM $[Ca^{2+}]_c$) requires ΣCa_c to increment by approximately 125 μmol/l cell water.

Ca^{2+} BUFFER VALUES

The ratio of total ΣCa to ionized $[Ca^{2+}]$ defines the buffer value {13,122,123}; the buffer value is 1000, for example, if from 1000 parts only one part is ionized. The relation between ΣCa and $[Ca^{2+}]$ was measured in ventricular homogenates after equilibration {89}. The buffer value decreased with increasing $[Ca^{2+}]_c$, it was approximately 800 at 0.3 μM $[Ca^{2+}]_c$, 250 at 0.5 μM $[Ca^{2+}]_c$, and only 20 for $[Ca^{2+}]_c$ higher than 1 μM, indicating that the Ca^{2+} buffer became exhausted with increasing $[Ca^{2+}]_c$.

For the myofibrillar space, ΣCa_c has been measured by EPMA and compared with $[Ca^{2+}]_c$ {120,123}. For $[Ca^{2+}]_c$ between 0.09 and 0.18 μM, the buffer value was 5500, and between 0.18 and 0.9 μM $[Ca^{2+}]_c$ it was approximately 1000, i.e., again exhaustion was observed. There are two consequences of these results. (a) A forceful contraction requires that ΣCa_c increments in the myofibrillar space by ca. 700 μM {123}. In cardiac muscle only part of this calcium binds to TnC. Other cytoplasmic Ca^{2+} binding sites remain to be identified; possible candidates are the E-F hands on such proteins as S100α, CACY, and CAPL {33}. (b) A change in Ca^{2+} buffer saturation can interfere with quantitative evaluation of $[Ca^{2+}]_c$ transients. For example, ryanodine treatment does not only suppress systolic $[Ca^{2+}]_c$ transients, but it also increases diastolic $[Ca^{2+}]_c$ {47}; since the Ca^{2+} buffers are saturated to a different extent, one cannot subtract the ryanodine-insensitive from the ryanodine-sensitive $[Ca^{2+}]_c$ signal and identify the difference signal with SR Ca^{2+} release.

CONTRIBUTION OF MITOCHONDRIA
TO SYSTOLIC Ca^{2+} BUFFERING

Experiments on isolated mitochondria have suggested that the mitochondrial Ca^{2+} transport is a slow and low affinity system, i.e., not suited to interfere with the myofibrillar $[Ca^{2+}]_c$ transients {29}. Hence, most models do not include mitochondria in the space in which Ca^{2+} ions equilibrate {13,34,49}. However, the isolation procedure may have washed out cytosolic factors that activate mitochondrial Ca^{2+} transport {72}. In situ measurements by EPMA indicated that intramitochondrial ΣCa does increase during the initial systole. As expected from a Ca^{2+} buffer, the ΣCa_{mito} peak occurred 20-ms later and reached only 80% of the peak of ΣCa_c {55, 123}. During later systole and during diastole the mitochondria released the calcium again. The beat-to-beat changes as well as the slow changes in mitochondrial calcium control the activity of dehydrogenase, a rate limiting step in ATP formation. Hence, mitochondrial calcium has been suggested to couple the production of ATP to the demands of the cell {29,48,72}.

Time course of $[Ca^{2+}]_c$ and ΣCa_c during systole

During a voltage-clamp step to 0 mV, $[Ca^{2+}]_c$ and ΣCa_c peak within 20–40-ms and decay within the following 80–120-ms {123}. The similar time course of ΣCa_c and $[Ca^{2+}]_c$ (fig. 14-3) suggests that the endogenous Ca^{2+} ligands bind and unbind Ca^{2+} at rates that are equal to or larger than the rate of Ca^{2+} binding to the Ca^{2+} indicator indo-1. From the 700 µM increment in ΣCa_c, up to 40% may bind to the "fast" Ca^{2+}-specific sites of TnC; additional sites with similar affinities and rate constants have been postulated (see above). The time course of ΣCa and $[Ca^{2+}]_c$ is much faster than the time course of force development {100} or of unloaded shortening (fig. 14-3). When the extent of shortening peaks after 130-ms, ΣCa_c has almost returned to the diastolic value. This discrepancy may suggest that the time course of contraction is rate limited not by the lifetime of Ca-TnC complex but by the slow kinetics of the crossbridges {123}.

Ca^{2+} influx alone is insufficient for activation of contraction

In ventricular muscle, it is the "DHP-sensitive Ca^{2+} channel" that delivers the vast majority of Ca^{2+} entry {13,22,80,127,128}. The question of whether Ca^{2+} carried by I_{Ca} through DHP-sensitive channels is sufficient for activation of contraction has been addressed repetitively {10,34,52}. For a rhythmically beating mammalian heart, the answer is that less than 10% of the activator is derived from influx of extracellular Ca^{2+}, whereas the remaining part is released from the SR {13,17,18,23,47,101}. For the experimental separation of the two Ca^{2+} sources, one cannot just block I_{Ca} (e.g., by adding a Ca^{2+} channel blocker like nifedipine) and evaluate the difference signal in the force or $[Ca^{2+}]_c$ transient because block of I_{Ca} simultaneously removes the SR Ca^{2+} release trigger. Hence, the separation has been performed more indirectly.

ESTIMATED AMOUNT OF Ca^{2+} INFLUX

It is the initial 20-ms period that determines the amplitude of the fast rise in $[Ca^{2+}]_c$ and the fast force twitch (see below). The 20-ms time integral of I_{Ca} (fig. 14-5B) indicates that ca. 20 pA · s or $1 \cdot 10^{-16}$ mol Ca^{2+} are added to the cell {10,52,54}. Distributed over the volume of the myofilament space (50 vol% · 12 pL), this Ca^{2+} influx would increase the concentration of total calcium (ΣCa_c) by 17 µM, which is only 2.4% of the measured rise in ΣCa_c; that is, the amount of Ca^{2+} influx is insufficient for any

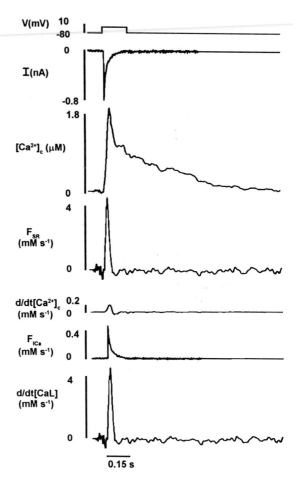

Fig. 14-4. Evaluation of net SR Ca^{2+} flux (F_{SR}) from the $[Ca^{2+}]_c$ transients in the absence of Na-Ca exchange during a 150-ms pulse from −80 to 10 mV. Current I was measured as a verapamil-sensitive current, $[Ca^{2+}]_c$ was evaluated from fura-2 fluorescence. F_{SR} was calculated from the time derivative $d/dt[Ca^{2+}]$. F_{ICa} is the Ca^{2+} influx through DHP-sensitive Ca^{2+} channels and $d[CaL]/dt$, the rate of change in total concentration of ligands complexed with Ca^{2+}. Ca^{2+} efflux through Na-Ca exchange was suppressed by sodium-free extracellular medium. Ca^{2+} efflux through SL Ca^{2+}-ATPase and mitochondrial Ca^{2+} uptake were thought to be negligible. Hence, the net SR Ca^{2+} flux F_{SR} could be calculated according to $F_{SR} = d/dt[Ca^{2+}]_c − I_{Ca} + d/dt[CaL]$. From Sipido and Wier {101}, with permission.

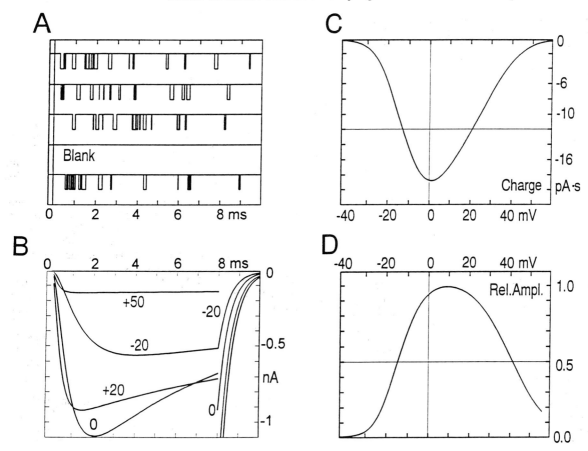

Fig. 14-5. Basic properties of the DHP-sensitive L-type Ca^{2+} channel. **A:** Idealized single channel currents during 10-ms depolarizations from −80 to 0 mV. The contribution of records without channel activity ("blank") has been artificially reduced. Note: There is always a waiting time until the first opening. Simulation after results measured at 37°C, and with 2 mM $[Ca^{2+}]_o$ and 1 µM of the Ca^{2+} channel opener BAYK 8644 in the patch pipette {61}. **B:** Time course of I_{Ca} during an 8-ms depolarization to the indicated potential. Note: At more positive potentials, I_{Ca} activates faster and the peak is reached at a shorter time. Repolarization to −80 mV (at 8-ms) increases the Ca^{2+} driving force, and therefore the current I_{Ca} rapidly decays because repolarization closes (deactivates) the Ca^{2+} channels. (For illustration purposes, the amplitude of the resulting Ca^{2+} tail current is reduced to 50%). **C:** Bell-shaped voltage dependence of the 20-ms time integral of I_{Ca}. **D:** Bell-shaped voltage dependence of the peak $[Ca^{2+}]_c$ transients recorded from myocytes with moderate SR Ca^{2+} load.

direct activation of contraction if the high concentration of intracellular Ca^{2+} buffers is considered.

If the membrane remains depolarized, ventricular cells can develop *tonic contractions*, which amount to ca. 10% of the peak contraction (fig. 14-1). Tonic tension is probably caused by sustained Ca^{2+} influx, either through non-inactivated L-type Ca^{2+} channels or through the Na-Ca exchanger {13,28,77,100,115}. Although the amplitude of sustained Ca^{2+} influx is small, it can have a pronounced effect because (a) amount of Ca^{2+} influx increases with the duration of the clamp step, (b) Ca^{2+} efflux through the Na-Ca exchanger is absent or low at 0 mV, and (c) the Ca^{2+} buffer value may be lower than during complete relaxation. For potentials between −40 mV and +20 mV the tonic component was related to the L-type Ca^{2+} channels because it followed the expected voltage depen-

dence {115} and was increased by Ca^{2+} channel openers like BAYK8644. At more positive potentials, the tonic component of contraction or of $[Ca^{2+}]_c$ seemed to be caused by Ca^{2+} influx through the Na-Ca exchanger, i.e., it increased when the potentials were set more positive or when the sodium gradient was reduced {15,18,57}. At low frequencies of stimulation, myocytes from guinea pig or rabbit show a "slow" or second component of contraction that slowly increases with time until the membrane is repolarized {68,90}. Again, the slow component increases when influx of extracellular Ca^{2+} is augmented.

PHARMACOLOGICAL BLOCK OF THE SR FUNCTION

The SR can be functionally removed {13} by blocking the Ca^{2+}-ATPase, e.g., by thapsigargin {9,67}, or one can prevent the SR Ca^{2+} release channels from closure with application of ryanodine or caffeine {9,67,94,101}. The functional removal of the SR has been used to dissect the effects of Ca^{2+} influx and Ca^{2+} release on the $[Ca^{2+}]_c$ signal (see below). Often the functional removal of the SR increases the diastolic $[Ca^{2+}]_c$; then a quantitative evaluation is difficult. For example, if the intervention has reduced the diastolic buffer value from 2000 to 1000, a similar Ca^{2+} flux will cause a larger increment in $[Ca^{2+}]_c$ {59}. Qualitatively, however, there is general agreement that functional removal of the SR does not only reduce the peak of contraction but also changes the time course from a fast to a slow contraction {13,53,59,67}.

Ca^{2+} induced Ca^{2+} release from the SR

SKINNED CARDIAC PREPARATIONS

Experiments in skinned cardiac preparations have shown that a small elevation of $[Ca^{2+}]_c$ leads to a larger Ca^{2+} release from the SR (Ca^{2+}-induced Ca^{2+} release or CICR) {34–39}. It has been questioned if CICR is of physiological relevance because at physiological millimolar Mg^{2+} concentration Ca^{2+} release channels (Ry-R) open only when the concentration of "trigger Ca^{2+}" is $10\,\mu M$ or higher (see *Ryanodine receptor*, below). Fabiato {34–39}, however, demonstrated that CICR does operate under physiological conditions, provided the trigger $[Ca^{2+}]_c$ is raised sufficiently quickly, e.g., from $0.1\,\mu M$ to $0.6\,\mu M$ within 1 ms. Since CICR implies a positive feedback, one might suppose that it ends only if all Ca^{2+} is released. However, gradation of CICR could be attributed to a Ca^{2+}-dependent inactivation mechanism of the Ca^{2+} release channel {36,38}. On the basis of these findings, a four-state model with two Ca^{2+} binding sites was proposed long before any of the single-channel recordings from reconstituted Ry-R had been done. The states are open (O), closed (C), refractory or inactivated (R, also closed), and available (A, also closed):

In this scheme, the solid circle represents the Ca^{2+} binding site that causes activation and the open circle represents the Ca^{2+} binding causing inactivation. According to the model, Ca^{2+} binds with modest affinity and at a high rate to the activation site but with high affinity and at a low rate to the inactivation site. A rapid increase in trigger $[Ca^{2+}]_c$ primarily occupies the activation site and opens the channel. The inactivation site binds Ca^{2+} more slowly, thereby turning off Ca^{2+} release. The inactivation of the Ca^{2+} release channel explains how the SR Ca^{2+} release can be graded by the amount of trigger Ca^{2+} and the rate of its rise. The model fitted not only the results from skinned cells but also provided a working hypothesis for a long period of time.

Ca^{2+} induced Ca^{2+} release: support from $[Ca^{2+}]_c$ transients

WHAT IS EXPECTED?

In the cytoplasm, the spatial distribution of Ca^{2+} ions changes with time. The spatial pattern will be determined by the activity and spatial location of the various cellular processes, such as Ca^{2+} influx and Ca^{2+} release or Ca^{2+} efflux and Ca^{2+} reuptake. Some important morphological structures may cause inhomogeneities in Ca^{2+} distribution {13,22,54,107,109,128}. It is thought that most of the Ca^{2+} is released into the 12-nm junctional gap and that longitudinal Ca^{2+} gradients drive the Ca^{2+} ions from the z to the m line of the sarcomere. Theoretical considerations suggested that Ca^{2+} is distributed with inhomogeneities for the initial 20-ms of the rise in $[Ca^{2+}]_c$, while Ca^{2+} homogeneity for later periods, was justified {129}. However, it seems to be impossible that one can experimentally verify the expected spatial cytosolic $[Ca^{2+}]$ inhomogeneities {128}. Therefore, modeling has been tried. In a recent review Wier {128} has defined spatial-temporal Ca^{2+} movements by a set of simultaneous differential equations. Essentially, in an element of the cytosol the rate of a change in $[Ca^{2+}]_c$ was described as the linear superimposition of fluxes due to diffusion, binding, and Ca^{2+} fluxes through membranes. A general solution was not obtained because too many border values were unknown.

Assuming spatial uniformity, the equations simplify to ordinary differential equations {49,101,128}. The solutions of these equations have been used to describe the spatial average of the Ca^{2+} distribution or the "global" $[Ca^{2+}]_c$ transient, as it is measured by fluorescent indicators. The equation

$$d/dt\{[Ca^{2+}]_c\} = d/dt\{[Ca^{2+}]_c, \text{binding}\} + d/dt\{[Ca^{2+}]_c, \text{membrane flux}\}$$

considers the entire cell as one homogenous volume, bounded by the sarcolemma, and containing organelles and Ca^{2+}-binding ligands that have no spatial properties. Ca^{2+} fluxes across organelles are represented simply as cellular processes distributed uniformly within the volume. According to Stern {107,109}, models that simplify the spatial heterogeneities of Ca^{2+} distribution to a "common pool" of homogeneous $[Ca^{2+}]_c$ are called *global models* of cardiac E-C coupling.

Ca^{2+} influx through channels triggers CICR

Excitation is thought to trigger SR Ca^{2+} release in skeletal muscle through an electrical charge movement in the sarcolemma {6,25}, in smooth muscle through the release of the second messenger IP_3, and in cardiac muscle through the influx of extracellular Ca^{2+}. Numerous studies that compared the influence of membrane potential on $[Ca^{2+}]_c$ transients with that on I_{Ca} support the view that Ca^{2+} influx through DHP-sensitive L-type Ca^{2+} channels triggers cardiac SR Ca^{2+} release, at least under physiological circumstances {13,17,18,22,36,38,58,77,81,99–101,114, 127,128}.

For example, small depolarizations that did not activate I_{Ca} did not elicit $[Ca^{2+}]_c$ transients {22,80,128}. Positive to the threshold of I_{Ca}, the peak $[Ca^{2+}]_c$ transients (or peak contractions) followed a similar bell-shaped voltage dependence as the time integral of I_{Ca} (see fig. 14-5D; compare {13,17,22,99}). Depolarizations close to the Ca^{2+} equilibrium potential ($+120$ mV) maximally activated the Ca^{2+} channels but did not induce Ca^{2+} influx, and the Ca^{2+} release signals were missing. However, SR Ca^{2+} release was triggered by the Ca^{2+} tail current upon repolarization from $+120$ to -80 mV {17,18,23}, a result that nearly excluded that the charge-movement hypothesis applies to cardiac SR Ca^{2+} release. This conclusion has gained further support from the different molecular biology of skeletal and cardiac Ca^{2+} channels (see Chapter 5).

There is agreement that the membrane potential controls cardiac E-C coupling, primarily through Ca^{2+} mediated by Ca^{2+} channels {13,22,128}. At a high SR Ca^{2+} load, stimulated Ca^{2+} influx through Na-Ca exchange could trigger SR Ca^{2+} release as well {15,57}. Block of DHP-sensitive Ca^{2+} channels with Ca^{2+} abolished the $[Ca^{2+}]_c$ transients due to short (4 ms) depolarizations but not those during long depolarizations, although the latter rose at a slower rate {54}. Since the efficacy of I_{Ca} in triggering $[Ca^{2+}]_c$ transients was much higher than the efficacy of Ca^{2+} influx through Na-Ca exchange, it was speculated that Ca^{2+} influx through DHP-sensitive Ca^{2+} channels has preferential access to Ca^{2+} release channels {99} (see also *Microscopic models*).

Estimation of the Ca^{2+} release flux

Whereas the sarcolemmal Ca^{2+} fluxes are easily measured, the SR Ca^{2+} release flux is not. Direct electrical measurements are not possible because the intracellular membrane system has no access to the patch electrodes, and the SR membrane cannot be voltage clamped. Hence SR Ca^{2+} release is evaluated from $[Ca^{2+}]_c$ transients {101,128}. However, the $[Ca^{2+}]_c$ transient is caused by superimposition of several Ca^{2+} fluxes. Sipido and Wier {101} tried to dissect individual components. They suppressed Ca^{2+} influx through DHP-sensitive Ca^{2+} channels by verapamil, Ca^{2+} efflux through Na-Ca exchange by sodium-free extracellular solutions, and Ca^{2+} fluxes in and out of the SR with 10 mM caffeine. Assuming independence, the individual components were subtracted and the net rate of movement of Ca^{2+} into or out of the SR was estimated. The results indicated an early peak of net release of Ca^{2+} (between 3 and 9 mM/s) for SR Ca^{2+} flux, followed by a prolonged and slow phase of net uptake of Ca^{2+} (fig. 14-4). Presumably, these values are underestimates, since spatial Ca^{2+} gradients could not be considered.

Assessment of the SR Ca^{2+} content

INDIRECT METHODS {13,14,21}

During an individual twitch, the SR releases only part of the stored Ca^{2+} {13}. Nearly complete SR Ca^{2+} release can be induced by rapid application of caffeine or of cold solutions (1°C). For these experiments the amplitude of the corresponding $[Ca^{2+}]_c$ transient has been demonstrated to vary with the SR Ca^{2+} load. Quantitative evaluation of these indirect results has been hampered by the fact that released Ca^{2+} quickly binds to an unknown number of intracellular ligands. However, the ability to use these approaches, which are reproducible in the same myocyte, makes them very sensitive means of assessing the relative changes in SR Ca^{2+} content. *Caffeine* {9,74} keeps Ca^{2+} release channels in the open state, i.e., although released Ca^{2+} is sequestered back by SERCa it cannot reaccumulate due to SR leakiness. In the constant presence of caffeine, $[Ca^{2+}]_c$ transients slowly decay from a peak of ca. 1.4 μM {9}, suggesting that the released Ca^{2+} was extruded by the Na-Ca exchanger. Also *rapid cooling* increases the open probability of the SR Ca^{2+} release channels {130}; in addition, it inhibits Ca^{2+} redistribution by SERCa and Na-Ca exchange. Rapid cooling raised $[Ca^{2+}]_c$ to values that were close to the level given by Ca^{2+} saturation of indo-1 {14}. This high level was steady for at least 1 minute, suggesting that Ca^{2+} redistribution by SERCa and Na-Ca exchange worked at a very low rate. $[Ca^{2+}]_c$ transients due to rapid cooling suggested that the SR contains releasable Ca^{2+} at a concentration of 3.5 mnol/per liter SR volume {13,14}.

EPMA

Assessment by EPMA is a more direct method for measuring total calcium concentration in the SR and its compartments. During diastole ΣCa was 2.4 mM in the junctional SR and 0.6 mM in the cytosol. During the initial 20 ms of the systole, this concentration gradient disappeared (fig. 14-3). A similar disappearance of the diastolic calcium gradients at the peak of contraction or during poisoning with ryanodine has been reported for the junctional and corbular SR of multicellular preparations {78,119}. In cardiac muscle, the dimensions of junctional SR are much smaller than the dimensions of the terminal cisternae in skeletal muscle; hence, these concentrations are presumably underestimates. More recent results from 80-nm thin cryosections yielded calcium concentrations as high as 20 mM inside junctional, corbular, and free SR mM {124,125}. Presumably most of this calcium is bound to calsequestrin.

IS THE JUNCTIONAL SR THE RELEASE COMPARTMENT?

The junctional SR has been considered as the Ca^{2+} release compartment because its RyR face the DHP-R of the sarcolemmal membrane ({13,22,54,99} and section "microscopic models of E-C coupling"). However, the junctional SR comprises only 0.3% of the cell volume {42,104,106}. Since the SR Ca^{2+} release should end when ΣCa in the junctional SR and $ΣCa_c$ are equal (1.4 mM), the amount of calcium released from junctional SR could increase $ΣCa_c$ in the water space between the myofilaments (50 vol%) by

$$\Delta\Sigma Ca_c = \{(20\,mM - 1.4\,mM) \cdot 0.3\,vol\%\}/50\,vol\%$$
$$= 0.11\,mM.$$

This increase is insufficient to account for the measured $\Delta\Sigma Ca_c$ of 0.75 mM. If one assumes that Ca^{2+} ions can rapidly diffuse from the other parts of the SR to the junctional SR, then the balance is

$$\Delta\Sigma Ca_c = \{(20\,mM - 1.4\,mM) \cdot 5\,vol\%\}/50\,vol\%$$
$$= 1.9\,mM.$$

The comparison of this value with the measured $\Delta\Sigma Ca_c$ of 0.75 mM suggests not only that SR calcium content is sufficient for the activation of the systole, but also that the entire SR calcium content is not released during a normal twitch.

Modulation of SR Ca^{2+} load, inotropy

BETA-ADRENERGIC INOTROPY {13,69}

Adrenalin or isoproterenol largely increase the peak I_{Ca}, $[Ca^{2+}]_c$ transients, and contractions. Beta-stimulation increases the total intra-SR calcium concentration {120}. This "filling effect" can be attributed to both higher Ca^{2+} influx through DHP-sensitive Ca^{2+} channels {106,116,117} and enhanced Ca^{2+} sequestration by SERCa (phosphorylation of phospholamban {71}). Details are described in another chapter of this book {69}.

POST REST POTENTIATION {13,67,68,90}

The level of SR Ca^{2+} load varies with the Ca^{2+} fluxes through the sarcolemma. During a rest period there is no Ca^{2+} influx. However, Ca^{2+} "leaks" out of the SR and is extruded {12,13}. After a 5-min rest period, the SR of guinea-pig ventricular cells is almost Ca^{2+} depleted {12, 13,119,120}. The first few postrest excitations cannot release much Ca^{2+}; hence, the contractions are small and slow {52,90}. During the initial postrest contractions, there is little Ca^{2+} efflux {12}, i.e., the Ca^{2+} influx (time integral of I_{Ca}) increments the total cellular calcium concentration by 50–100 µM per excitation {52,58,90}. The Ca^{2+} influx is thought to fill the SR with releasable Ca^{2+} to a higher extent, an idea that has been used to explain why the amplitude of the $[Ca^{2+}]_c$ transients or contractions increases in a beat-to-beat fashion (positive staircase). Within ca. 10 beats a new steady state is achieved, at which the SR Ca^{2+} load has been regained and Ca^{2+} influx is compensated by Ca^{2+} efflux. The refilling of junctional SR with Ca^{2+} after a rest period has been proven by EPMA {123} as well as by indirect tests using caffeine or rapid cooling {13,14}.

FREQUENCY INOTROPY {5,13,19,20,67,68,90,97}

Increasing the Ca^{2+} influx per unit time, i.e., increasing the frequency of stimulation from 1 to 3 Hz (or application

of paired pulses) increases the SR Ca^{2+} load, and the better Ca^{2+}-filled SR can release more activator Ca^{2+}. The increase in Ca^{2+} influx is mostly through the higher open probability of DHP-sensitive Ca^{2+} channels per unit time. Also, the membrane potential lasts for a longer period of unit time at positive values when the Na-Ca exchanger is in the Ca^{2+} influx rather than in the Ca^{2+} efflux mode. High frequencies of stimulation increase the *intracellular* Na^+ activity a_{Na}^i {20}, thereby reducing the Na^+ gradient and the Ca^{2+} efflux across the sarcolemma {64}. Hence, part of the frequency inotropy should be attributed to the Na-Ca exchanger. Improved Ca^{2+} filling has been assessed with caffeine {20}, rapid cooling {13}, and EPMA {123}. The frequency inotropy has a frequency upper limit: If the interval between the beats is too short, Ca^{2+} influx falls because part of the DHP-sensitive channels does not recover from inactivation. In case SR Ca^{2+} release channels would inactivate, they may be refractory as well {36}.

DIASTOLIC $[Ca^{2+}]_c$ STAIRCASE

A change in stimulation frequency from less than 0.1 to 2 Hz increases the cellular calcium content {64,65,90}. This increase is reflected in better Ca^{2+} filling of the SR (see above); in addition, there is a moderate rise of diastolic $[Ca^{2+}]_c$ {20,59,65} and diastolic ΣCa_c {123}. After the end of stimulation, the elevated ΣCa_c and $[Ca^{2+}]_c$ return to resting levels within several seconds {123}. The diastolic tension or sarcomere length do not change severely, suggesting that Ca^{2+} ions are bound not to troponin C but to other cytosolic Ca^{2+} ligands that have a high affinity and a slow off rate. The increase in diastolic ΣCa_c (of $[Ca^{2+}]_c$) reduces the cellular Ca^{2+} buffer value; hence, from a given amount of SR Ca^{2+} release, a larger fraction can bind to troponin C {59}. Assuming that part of the slow high-affinity sites are the Ca^{2+},Mg^{2+} sites on troponin C, a cooperative interaction could Ca^{2+}-sensitize the fast Ca^{2+}-specific sits on troponin C and contribute to the inotropy as well {59,127}.

GLYCOSIDE INOTROPY {2}

Since the recognition of digitalis glycosides as specific inhibitors of the plasma membrane K^+,Na^+-ATPase {102}, it has been suggested that this action is primarily responsible for the positive inotropic effects. Even partial inhibition of the K^+,Na^+-ATPase and small increases in intracellular sodium concentration can have a large impact on the balance of Ca^{2+} fluxes through the Na-Ca exchanger {20,32}, with the effect that the SR is loaded with Ca^{2+} more heavily. Also, the concomitant rise in diastolic $[Ca^{2+}]_c$ may contribute to the inotropy. The digitalis inotropy still occurs after SR has been functionally removed with ryanodine {13}. In these experiments the contractions are no longer very sensitive to dihydropyridines, indicating that in the case of elevated a_{Na}^i Ca^{2+} influx through the stimulated Na-Ca exchanger can activate the contraction directly {13,15}.

Cardiac Excitation-Contraction Coupling: From Global to Microscopic Models 299

Ca^{2+} OVERLOAD AND SPONTANEOUS Ca^{2+} RELEASE {13,108}

High concentrations of cardioactive glycosides decrease the amplitude of $[Ca^{2+}]_c$ transients and systolic contraction. This toxic effect is caused by oscillatory aftercontractions that occur as a consequence of SR Ca^{2+} overload. Spontaneous SR Ca^{2+} release is blocked by caffeine or ryanodine. The result suggests that spontaneous SR Ca^{2+} release occurs through SR Ca^{2+} release channels. One hypothesis suggests that the same channels (RyR) that release Ca^{2+} during the normal twitch are activated by leakiness highly amplified by the positive feedback of the CICR {107}. Another hypothesis attributes spontaneous Ca^{2+} release through RyR to an activation mechanism that is completely different than the one considered for CICR {38}. When spontaneous Ca^{2+} release precedes stimulated SR Ca^{2+} release, the stimulated $[Ca^{2+}]_c$ transient and corresponding contraction are depressed. This attenuation may result from reduced Ca^{2+} filling of the SR, from refractoriness of the SR Ca^{2+} release channels, or from net loss of Ca^{2+} from the cell. In intact single cells, spontaneous Ca^{2+} release spreads out within $\approx 100\,\mu m/s$ as a propagating wave {128}.

Ca^{2+} CHANNEL PROTEINS

Ca^{2+} release channel or ryanodine-receptor (RyR)

The SR Ca^{2+} release channel has been purified {4,40,71, 130} and cloned {86}. The cardiac RyR is a homotetramere, with monomers of 4969 amino acids and a molecular weight of about 565,000 kDa. The hydrophobic sequences near the COOH terminus suggest that the SR membrane is spanned by six segments; accordingly, the protein has been classified in superfamily III of ligand-gated channels. Image reconstruction from negatively stained RyR molecules {4,40} suggests a 3.7-nm Ca^{2+} channel that originates in the SR lumen and forms a 3.7-nm pore in the small baseplate between the six segments. A far larger part of the RyR protrudes into the cytosol, where the channel is surrounded by structures of fourfold symmetry with the dimensions $27 \times 27 \times 14\,nm$. Here the channel branches into four radial channels that empty into the cytosol. Up to now, no Ca^{2+} binding domain has been distinguished in the protein; however, some evidence suggests that ATP, Ca^{2+}, calmodulin may bind near residues 3600–4500. Cardiac RyR also contains a potential site for phosphorylation by cAMP-dependent protein kinase {111,131}.

MODULATION OF $^{45}Ca^{2+}$ RELEASE BY LIGANDS

Purified SR vesicles were the first preparation in which the function of RyR was analyzed {74,75}. Usually the vesicles are preloaded with $^{45}Ca^{2+}$. $^{45}Ca^{2+}$ efflux was started by rapid exposure to a medium containing $10\,\mu M$ Ca^{2+}, and half of the preloaded $^{45}Ca^{2+}$ was released within 30 seconds . The results suggested that cardiac SR contains a ligand-gated Ca^{2+} channel that is activated by

Ca^{2+}. In the absence of Mg^{2+}, dependence of $^{45}Ca^{2+}$ efflux on the concentration of cytosolic Ca^{2+} was bell shaped {75}, i.e., it increased for $[Ca^{2+}]_c > 0.5\,\mu M$, had a maximum at $10\,\mu M$ $[Ca^{2+}]_c$, and fell when $[Ca^{2+}]_c$ was higher. $^{45}Ca^{2+}$ efflux was also activated by adenine nucleotides, and ATP increased Ca^{2+} release up to 200-fold. A similar stimulating effect was measured for caffeine; however, caffeine acted on a site different from the adenine site. $^{45}Ca^{2+}$ efflux was inhibited by Mg^{2+}, H^+, and calmodulin. In the presence of $5\,mM$ ATP (activating the Ca^{2+} release) and $3\,mM$ free Mg^{2+}, activation of $^{45}Ca^{2+}$ efflux required $[Ca^{2+}]_c$ higher than $3\,\mu M$, and a maximum was not achieved up to $1\,mM$. Presumably, the physiological conditions of $5\,mM$ ATP and $0.5\,mM$ free Mg^{2+} require more than $20\,\mu M$ $[Ca^{2+}]$ for full activation {74,75}. There was no evidence that $^{45}Ca^{2+}$ efflux inactivates with time.

SINGLE CHANNEL ANALYSIS {6,10,95,130}

Purified cardiac RyR were incorporated into planar phospholipid bilayers, and the single-channel currents were measured under voltage-clamp conditions. The analysis indicated that the RyR functions as a ligand-gated, cation-selective ion channel. Opening of the Ca^{2+} release channel was not influenced by membrane potential; however, the open probability P_o increased by micromolar concentrations of Ca^{2+}. With Ca^{2+} as the only activator, P_o was usually below 0.4, and a higher degree of activation was achieved when Ca^{2+} activation was combined with millimolar concentrations of ATP. P_o was reduced by millimolar concentrations of Mg^{2+}. In summary, the modifications of single-channel gating and conductance are consistent with flux experiments on vesicles. Based on this evidence, it would appear that the RyR-channel of cardiac muscle can be purified and reconstituted without loosing the functional sites for interaction with the regulatory ligands. The question of whether RyR channels inactivate and become refractory has recently been tested with rapid solution changes; the result was negative: A sudden rise in $[Ca^{2+}]$ from $<10^{-8}$ to 10^{-4} increased P_o with a time constant of $4\,ms$; however, P_o remained at the high level for at least 1 second. Application of rapid concentrations jumps at 1 or $5\,Hz$ resulted in very similar mean currents, i.e., there was no evidence of inactivation and refractoriness {96}.

ION SELECTIVITY

The single-channel current increased with the free Ca^{2+} concentration to the luminal side along a saturation curve, and the half-maximal conductance was achieved at a free Ca^{2+} concentration of $4\,mM$ {70}. When $50\,mM$ Ca^{2+} was the permeant ion, the single-channel slope conductance was $70\,pS$ {130}. The RyR were somewhat more permeable to divalent cations than monovalent cations ($P_{Ca^{2+}}/P_{K^+} = 6.6$) but showed relatively little discrimination between divalent cations $P_{Ca^{2+}}/P_{Mg^{2+}} = 2.3$). From the permeation of ions of known ionic radius, a "selectivity filter" has been deduced, and its minimum cross-sectional area is similar to that of the acetylcholine-gated channel of the endplate {130}. The properties of the RyR-channel are consistent with the idea that the channel functions as a single ion channel (i.e., no multiple-ion occupancy) and that the length of the pore with restricted diffusion is short {130}.

Although the ligand-operated RyR seems to have the properties required to explain Ca^{2+}-induced SR Ca^{2+} release and cardiac E-C coupling, fundamental problems remain. Since CICR constitutes a positive feedback, Ca^{2+} release should be regenerative: A small amount of Ca^{2+} can trigger the release of more Ca^{2+} from the SR, which in turn releases more Ca^{2+} in a regenerative process; the release will not terminate until the Ca^{2+} driving force is abolished.

L-type Ca^{2+} channel or dihydropyridine-receptor (DHP-R)

The DHP-sensitive channels of cardiac tissue have been purified {41} and cloned from both human and rabbit cDNA {1,30,62,76}. The Ca^{2+} channel is a pentameric complex: α_1, α_2/δ, β, and γ. α_1 is the pore-forming subunit with four membrane-spanning repeats. Dihydropyridines presumably bind to the extracellular site of α_1. The side for cAMP-dependent phosphorylation has not been clarified up to now. The isoforms of skeletal and cardiac α_1 subunits have large homologies. However, expression of the skeletal α_1 isoform into myotubes from dysgenic mice without endogenous DHP-sensitive channels restored the musclelike, $[Ca^{2+}]_o$-independent type of contractile activation {1,112}. Expression of the cardiac α_1 isoform induced a type of coupling that was suppressed by $[Ca^{2+}]_o$ removal or by block of Ca^{2+} permeation with Ca^{2+} channel blockers {112}. These differences correspond to differences in the cytosolic loop between repeat II and III of the α_1 subunits, which is thought to determine the specific ways of skeletal versus cardiac ECC.

In cardiac cells, two types of Ca^{2+} channels, L and T, have been distinguished on the basis of differences in gating, pharmacological sensitivity, and unitary conductance {8,11,82}. L-type Ca^{2+} channels {46,56,115,116} predominate during strong depolarizations, remain available at weakly negative holding potentials, and exhibit a clear-cut sensitivity to dihydropyridines (therefore, the name *DHP-sensitive channels*). In contrast, T-type channels operate over a more negative voltage range, are generally not very sensitive to DHPs, and exhibit a small single-channel conductance. The density of functional channels ($N_T \cdot P_f$, see below) is ca. 2 L-type and 0.1 T-type Ca^{2+} channels per μm^2 {8,88}. The low density of T-type Ca^{2+} channels, as well as the fact that they are not found in the cardiac muscle of several species {11}, suggests that L-type but not T-type Ca^{2+} channels are necessary for cardiac E-C coupling.

Ca^{2+} INFLUX

The open L-type Ca^{2+} channel allows passage of Ca^{2+} ions from the extracellular space into the cytoplasm. The channel is permeable for divalent cations such as Ca^{2+},

Sr^{2+}, or Ba^{2+} but nor for Mg^{2+} {93}. Extracellular Ca^{2+} ions are more than 2000-fold more permeable than extracellular Na^+ or intracellular K^+ ions {52,66,116}. The absence of external divalent cations removes the channel's selectivity, and external monovalent cations can carry large inward-going currents {50,66}. At 2 mM $[Ca^{2+}]_o$, intrachannel Ca^{2+} ions block Na^+ movement; therefore, under physiological conditions Na^+ ions make a negligible contribution to the Ca^{2+} current {88}. The results were modeled with a pore through which the ions permeate in single file, interacting with multiple binding sites along the way, suggesting that ion binding rather than filtering determines selectivity {50,116}.

In cell-attached patches, Ca^{2+} flux from a pipette containing 2 mM Ca^{2+} generates an open-channel current of -0.4 pA (36°C, 0 mV) {61}, which translates to a Ca^{2+} influx of 1.2 million Ca^{2+} ions per second. Presumably Ca^{2+} ions that permeate through the channel accumulate to submillimolar concentrations near the cytosolic channel exit {107,132}. Ca^{2+} influx through single channels increases with $[Ca^{2+}]_o$ along a curve that achieves half-saturation at 2 mM $[Ca^{2+}]_o$ {61}. The whole-cell current I_{Ca} and the single-channel current i_{Ca} are related by

$$I_{Ca}(t,V) = N_T \cdot P_f(V) \cdot P_o(t,V) \cdot i_{Ca}.$$

N_T is the total number of L-type Ca^{2+} channels per cell. $P_f(V)$ is the probability that the channel will open upon depolarization to the potential V. $P_o(V,t)$ is the probability of finding the channel open at a given time {88}. According to fig. 14-5B, depolarizations to 0 mV let I_{Ca} peak to -1.1 nA within 4 ms. At this time, $P_o(0 mV, 4 ms)$ may approximate 0.5. The ratio peak of $I_{Ca}/i_{Ca} = -1.1$ nA/-0.4 pA/0.5 suggests $N_T \cdot P_f = 5500$ functional DHP-sensitive Ca^{2+} channels per ventricular myocyte or 1 Ca^{2+} channel/μm^2. Beta-adrenergic stimulation and cAMP-dependent channel phosphorylation can increase peak I_{Ca} approximately three-fold. The result suggests that N_T is at least 16,500, or that phosphorylation increases P_f from basal 0.3 towards 1 {85,116,117}. However, only 30% ($P_o = 0.3$) of the total number of channels (N_T) are available at basal phosphorylation.

As in other voltage-gated channels, the open probability of the L-type Ca^{2+} channel is controlled by membrane potential. Close to threshold (i.e., -30 mV), P_f is low, that is, most depolarizations fail to induce openings [$P_f = 0.01$ is equivalent to $(1 - P_f) = 99\%$ blank records]. More positive potentials increase P_f along a sigmoidal Boltzmann curve up to a maximum at $+10$ mV {26}. When a membrane is depolarized by a voltage-clamp pulse, macroscopic I_{Ca} activates along a sigmoidal time course (fig. 14-5B). At 36°C, the *activation* time constants vary between 5 ms at -20 mV to 0.5 ms at $+20$ mV. Macroscopic activation is reflected by transitions in the channel conformation that are summarized by $P_o(V,t)$. Depolarization favors the transition from the available resting state (C_1) through another closed state (C_2), from which the channel can pass to the open state (O)

$$C_1 \leftrightarrow C_2 \leftrightarrow O.$$

The sigmoidal macroscopic activation time course is attributed to passage through the state C_2, which generates the "waiting time" between the start of depolarization and the first channel opening (fig. 14-5A). At more positive potentials, the rate for the transition $C_1 \rightarrow C_2$ increases and the waiting time becomes shorter. The life time of the open state O is short (0.1 to 0.4 ms at 0 mV, fig. 14-5A); however, the channel frequently reopens (transition $0 \leftrightarrow C_2 \leftrightarrow O \leftrightarrow C_2$, etc.).

The decay of macroscopic I_{Ca} is called *inactivation* {88}. Macroscopic inactivation is not reflected in the lifetime of the singe-channel openings {8,92}, and the time constants of leaving and reentering the open state (sub-milliseconds) are much shorter than the time constants of macroscopic I_{Ca} inactivation (10 and 50 ms). A simple model adds a single transition to an inactivated state ($C_1 \leftrightarrow C_2 \leftrightarrow O \rightarrow I$); however, this model can account only for some properties of $P_o(t,V)$. For example, channel openings are found not only early but also late during depolarization, which is described by a change between different "modes" of channel activity {117}. This complex behavior may be attributed to spontaneous phosphorylation and binding of Ca^{2+} {92}.

At the resting potential of -80 mV, the channels are closed (mostly C_1). Channel openings become prominent for potentials positive to -30 mV ("threshold"). More positive potentials reduce the number of blanks, i.e., increase P_f, and let P_o peak at earlier time to higher values. At 0 mV, the amount of Ca^{2+} influx through L-type Ca^{2+} channels is maximal. For a given potential, a Ca^{2+} influx of approximately. $1 \cdot 10^{-16}$ mol can be calculated from the time integral over I_{Ca}

$$Ca^{2+} \text{ influx} = \{z \cdot F\}^{-1} \int_{0\,ms}^{20\,ms} I_{Ca}(0\,mV)dt = \{z \cdot F\}^{-7} \cdot 18_p As$$
$$= \{z \cdot F\}^{-1} \cdot N_T \cdot i_{Ca} \cdot P_f(0\,mV) \int_{0\,ms}^{20\,ms} P_o(0\,mV,t)dt,$$

where z is the equivalence charge (2 for Ca^{2+}) and F the Faraday constant (96,500 As/mol). Figure 14-5C illustrates that Ca^{2+} influx follows "bell-shaped" voltage dependence {26,72}, i.e., it increases with less negative potentials, reaches a maximum at 0 mV, and decreases again when the potentials are more and more positive (fig. 14-5C). Ca^{2+} influx decreases at positive potentials because the potential V approximates the Ca^{2+} equilibrium potential $E_{Ca}(+120\,mV)$ where the driving force $(V - E_{Ca})$ for Ca^{2+} influx disappears. Repolarization to negative potentials (i.e., from 0 to -80 mV) increases the driving force $(V - E_{Ca})$, resulting in a large tail current (fig. 14-5B). The amplitude of the tail current is proportional to the degree of preceding activation $(P_o \cdot P_f)$, and its fast decay represents channel "deactivation" from state O to C_2.

MICROSCOPIC MODELS OF CARDIAC E-C COUPLING

Graded versus regenerative $[Ca^{2+}]_c$ transients

The influx of Ca^{2+} through L-type channels can be graded by both the amplitude and duration of the depolarizing

voltage-clamp steps. How the gradation of Ca^{2+} influx translates into a gradation of SR Ca^{2+} release or a gradation of contraction has been a key question in cardiac E-C coupling for years. As can be expected from the positive feedback due to CICR, the gradation of Ca^{2+} release depends on the SR Ca^{2+} load. The SR Ca^{2+} load can be modulated by repetitive stimulation or by trains of voltage-clamp pulses. For the example of guinea-pig ventricular myocytes, 0.1-Hz stimulation provides a low Ca^{2+} load and 1-Hz stimulation a moderate Ca^{2+} load {20,47}. At low Ca^{2+} load, the amplitude of the peak $[Ca^{2+}]_c$ transients follows the amount of trigger Ca^{2+} (time integral of I_{Ca}) over a wide range. When the influx of trigger Ca^{2+} was graded by the amplitude of 20-ms voltage-clamp steps, the peak of the $[Ca^{2+}]_c$ transients followed a similar bell-shaped voltage dependence as the amount of Ca^{2+} influx (fig. 14-5B,D; compare {13,22,80,113,115}). When the influx of trigger Ca^{2+} was graded by the duration of clamp steps to 0 mV, the $[Ca^{2+}]_c$ transients gradually increased with the time integral of I_{Ca} (fig. 14-6C, dashed line, compare {13,15,17,47}).

The SR Ca^{2+} load of guinea-pig ventricular cells can be increased to an optimum by 3-Hz stimulation {20}, the frequency at which the heart beats in vivo. A similar potentiation is achieved by trains of paired voltage-clamp pulses {20,123}. The high SR Ca^{2+} load increased the amplitude of the $[Ca^{2+}]_c$ transients, indicating that indeed better-filled SR can release more Ca^{2+}. In addition, potentiation to a high SR Ca^{2+} load changed the relation between the peak $[Ca^{2+}]_c$ transients and the amount of trigger Ca^{2+}. For example, the gradation of peak $[Ca^{2+}]_c$ by positive potentials was almost absent (fig. 14-6C, solid curve, compare {57}). When the amount of trigger Ca^{2+} was graded by the duration of the test step, repolarization after 4-ms did not curtail the $[Ca^{2+}]_c$ transient. Whether Ca^{2+} entry was turned off by repolarization or continued for 120-ms, the $[Ca^{2+}]_c$ transient started after the same 5-ms delay, rose at a nearly identical rate, and reached a similar peak 36-ms after the start of depolarization (fig. 14-6A). The result that $[Ca^{2+}]_c$ transients, once triggered, continue independently of the trigger suggests that the underlying mechanism is regenerative. Presumably CICR achieves saturation if the high SR Ca^{2+} load provides a high positive feedback amplification.

The results that SR Ca^{2+} release is both graded and regenerative seem to be incompatible. The dilemma is re-solved by leaving the concepts of *global models* of cardiac E-C coupling that summarize all cytosolic $[Ca^{2+}]$ concentrations in a *common Ca^{2+} pool*. Here we introduce the *microscopic models* {107}, which pay special attention to the microheterogeneities of $[Ca^{2+}]$ in the cytosol. It is postulated that the local $[Ca^{2+}]$ concentration that activates SR Ca^{2+} release through RyR differs from the $[Ca^{2+}]_c$ that is measured around the myofilaments. The spatial $[Ca^{2+}]$ heterogeneities were already discussed earlier with the remark that they cannot be resolved by the available optical methods. This remark is true also in the present context; hence, the following paragraphs are highly speculative.

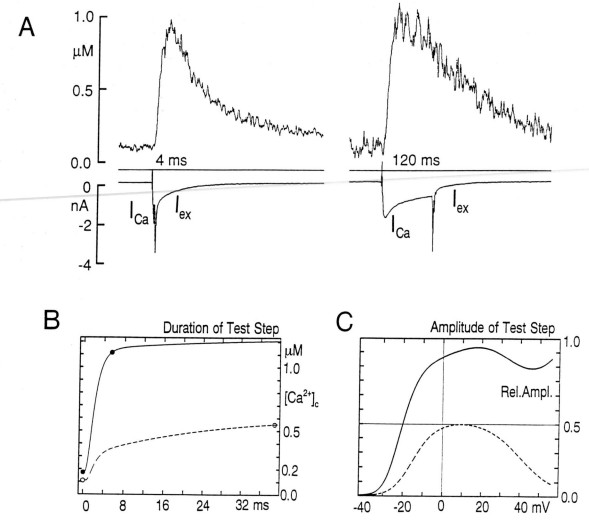

Fig. 14.6. Graded versus regenerative $[Ca^{2+}]_c$ transients from cells at high SR Ca^{2+} load. **A:** $[Ca^{2+}]_c$ transients evoked by 4-ms or 120-ms pulses to $0\,mV$. Labels for I_{Ca} and I_{ex}, the current due to Ca^{2+} efflux through Na-Ca exchange. **B,C:** Gradation of peak $[Ca^{2+}]_c$ transients recorded from cells at low (dashed lines) or high SR Ca^{2+} load (solid lines). Method: To test the trigger effect at a comparable Ca^{2+} load, the cells were conditioned with pulse trains. Every seventh of the conditioning pulses was substituted by a test pulse that was varied in either duration (A,B) or amplitude (C). Trains of paired pulses were used for high, and trains of single pulses for low Ca^{2+} load. **B:** The amount of trigger Ca^{2+} was graded by the duration of the test step to $0\,mV$. Dots for highly Ca^{2+} loaded cells mark diastolic $[Ca^{2+}]_c$ and peak $[Ca^{2+}]_c$ induced by 5-ms pulses achieving 90% of peak $[Ca^{2+}]_c$ induced by 160-ms pulses. Circles for cells with low Ca^{2+} load mark diastolic $[Ca^{2+}]_c$ and peak $[Ca^{2+}]_c$ induced by 40-ms pulses approximating 90% of peak $[Ca^{2+}]_c$ induced by 160-ms pulses. C: The amount of trigger Ca^{2+} was graded by amplitude of 160-ms test steps. The peak $[Ca^{2+}]_c$ transients have been normalized by the response to $+20\,mV$. Note: In cells with low Ca^{2+} load, the curve follows a bell (dashed). In cells with high Ca^{2+} load cells, gradation is nearly lost for positive potentials.

Macroscopic $[Ca^{2+}]_c$ transients are graded by recruitment of active release clusters

RELEASE CLUSTER: POSSIBLE RELATION
TO ULTRASTRUCTURE

The 12-nm junctional gap between the sarcolemma with the SR L-type Ca^{2+} channels (DHP-R) and the SR release channels (RyR) is considered as the functional unit of a *release cluster* {99,107,109}. In a simple approximation, a model cluster would comprise a gap that extends over an area of 300×300-nm^2 together with 36 Ry-R, spaced at $30\,nm$ lateral distance, and 4 DHP-R, each them surrounded by 9 RyR {16,126}. The membranes on both sides of the gap restrict the Ca^{2+} diffusion; hence, Ca^{2+} fluxes through DHP-R or RyR can increase local $[Ca^{2+}]$

inside the gap ($[Ca^{2+}]_{jG}$) to values far beyond $[Ca^{2+}]_c$. The current through a single Ca^{2+} channel can raise $[Ca^{2+}]_{jG}$ to more than $20\,\mu M$, sufficiently high to induce openings of RyR with high probability. Once the DHP-R and Ry-R close, diffusion will dissipate $[Ca^{2+}]_{jG}$. The rise and fall of $[Ca^{2+}]_{jG}$ should occur within less than a millisecond; however, the time course may be retarded by Ca^{2+} binding site within the gap. The following postulates consider primarily the situation in which SR Ca^{2+} load is potentiated to its optimum.

1. Postulate: Ca^{2+} influx through single DHP-R is sufficient for activation of RyR in the local neighborhood. During a 0.3-ms single opening, L-type channel Ca^{2+} currents of $-0.4\,pA$ transport ca. 300 Ca^{2+} ions. Despite the small number, at the cytosolic exit of the channel $[Ca^{2+}]_{jG}$ rises by ca. $100\,\mu M$ {51,107,132}. Due to diffusion, this high concentration falls steeply with distance. Hence, only RyR in the closest neighborhood (distance 15 nm?) can become Ca^{2+} activated.

2. Postulate: Within one cluster CICR is regenerative (high SR Ca^{2+} load). The current through a single Ca^{2+} release channel (RyR) is ca. $2\,pA$ {7,94–96,130}. This current rises $[Ca^{2+}]_{jG}$ over larger distances, i.e., it activates the next RyR. Hence, once Ca^{2+} activation of one RyR has started, CICR spreads out within the junctional gap until all RyR are activated. All RyR that activate as a unit constitute the *release cluster*. Since regenerative CICR is activated by Ca^{2+} influx during the first opening of DHP-R, later reopening of the DHP-R can be neglected.

3. Postulate: RyR close without inactivation. At 20 ms after excitation, the calcium gradient between the inside of the junctional SR and the gap space is abolished {123}; hence, CICR is ended. Ca^{2+} diffuses from the gap rapidly into the myofibrillar space. Refilling of the junctional SR with releasable Ca^{2+} occurs with a delay of 20 ms or more {123}, which could be a property of the SERCa {97}. Hence, within 20–40 ms $[Ca^{2+}]_{jG}$ can fall to the myofibrillar $[Ca^{2+}]_c$ of $\approx 1\,\mu M$ {129} and RyR can close.

4. Postulate: CICR does not spread out between individual clusters. Outside the junctional gap diffusional barriers are missing, and the high $[Ca^{2+}]$ is dissipated by diffusion; over a distance of 20 nm it may have fallen to less than 30% of $[Ca^{2+}]_{jG}$. We thus postulate that Ca^{2+} activation of RyR does not spread out over the entire cell. Recent studies of CICR activated by photorelease from caged precursors are in line with this postulate {81,84}.

5. Activation of Ca^{2+} release from corbular SR is not well understood. The corbular SR bears RyR {98} that are localized 50–500 nm away from DHP-R. Ca^{2+} influx through DHP-R is unlikely to activate RyR over such a distance. However, the individual sacs of corbular SR are only 50 nm apart. Presumably Ca^{2+} activation can spread out like a wave jumping from one sac to the next of corbular SR.

6. Postulate: Macroscopic CICR is graded by recruitment of individual clusters through the number of open L-type Ca^{2+} channels DHP-R (Synon. DHP-R).

7. At low SR Ca^{2+} load, Ca^{2+} release within one cluster might be graded. This is because low Ca^{2+} release flux increases the open probability of neighboring RyR only moderately, i.e., due to statistical properties RyR will close if $[Ca^{2+}]_{jG}$ is only moderately increased {107}. Hence, when the SR Ca^{2+} load is low, there is no or only little positive feedback (low amplification) in the cluster and CICR does not become regenerative. The net effect is that the probability of open RyR within one cluster (and the amount of Ca^{2+} release) follows more directly the influx of trigger Ca^{2+}. Consecutive opening of the same DHP-R or simultaneous opening of the 4 DHP-R channels within the cluster may superimpose in their effects on CICR. The activation of RyR on corbular SR may require summation of several $[Ca^{2+}]$ waves converging from several active release clusters.

Examples of gradation

Some examples shall illustrate how the model attributes the gradation of macroscopic signals to the recruitment of the release cluster.

GRADATION BY PULSE DURATION (PULSES TO 0 MV)

On average, 25% of the DHP-R respond to steps of $0\,mV$ with channel openings $[P_f(0\,mV) = 0.25]$ and 75% with blanks (see Chapter ●●). Since a cluster has four independent DHP-R, the cluster remains inactive with the probability that all four DHP-R are closed, which is $(1 - P_f)^4$ or 0.32; that is, 68% of the clusters will open if the duration of the step is much longer than the time to the first opening. Pulses shorter than 4 ms will reduce the macroscopic response according to the probability $P_o(t)$ (fig. 14-6B, solid line), i.e., the duration dependence of macroscopic CICR will follow the steep activation time course of the DHP-sensitive Ca^{2+} channels {54}.

RECRUITMENT OF ACTIVE CLUSTERS BETWEEN THRESHOLD AND 0 MV

Pulses to $-25\,mV$, close to threshold of I_{Ca}, produce mostly (97%) blanks; i.e., openings occur at $P_o(-25\,mV) = 0.03$. The probability that a cluster does not become active during long steps is $(1 - P_o)^4$ or 89%; that is, the steps to $-25\,mV$ activate 11% of all clusters or 15% of the CICR obtained with pulses to $0\,mV$ (see fig. 14-5D). For pulses to $-10\,mV$, a similar calculation with $P_o(-10\,mV) = 0.15$ results in 48% of all clusters being active, or the global response being 70% of the maximum. In summary, gradation by pulse amplitude is a consequence of the voltage dependence of the open probability of the DHP-R, as the higher open probability recruits a larger number of active clusters. However, due to the assumption that one cluster has four DHP-R, the two bell-shaped curves resemble each other only in a qualitative way.

GRADATION AT POSITIVE POTENTIALS

At the Ca^{2+} equilibrium potential ($+120\,mV$) Ca^{2+} influx through DHP-R is zero, and without influx of trigger Ca^{2+} the release cluster should remain inactive. At intermediate potentials, however, the situation is more complex. For example, steps to $+40\,mV$ induce macroscopic $[Ca^{2+}]_c$ transients that peak to 50% of the maximal response (fig. 14-5D) whereas the macroscopic Ca^{2+} influx achieves only 10% of the maximum (fig. 14-5B). At $+40\,mV$, the small microscopic current through single DHP-R is ca. $-0.1\,pA$ and cannot achieve the $20\,\mu M\,[Ca^{2+}]_{iG}$ needed for maximal activation of RyR, i.e., RyR are activated at a low probability. In such a situation, RyR have a high chance of closing spontaneously, and $[Ca^{2+}]_{iG}$ dissipates by diffusion before regenerative activation of the release cluster has occurred.

At $+40\,mV$, a P_f of 0.3 gives a definite high probability that two or more of the four DHP-R of the cluster will activate simultaneously. Hence there is a chance that the effects of two nonregenerative processes superimpose, thereby increasing $[Ca^{2+}]_{iG}$ beyond the $20\,\mu M$ at which the regenerative release in the cluster was postulated to start. The net effect of this superimposition depends on the SR Ca^{2+} load. *At low SR Ca^{2+} load*, Ca^{2+} flux through RyR is low, and the rise in $[Ca^{2+}]_{iG}$ remains local. The net effect is that the probability of the RyR releasing Ca^{2+} is more or less proportionate to the local $[Ca^{2+}]_{iG}$ provided by Ca^{2+} influx through DHPR. Thus the global $[Ca^{2+}]_c$ response will fall at potentials more positive than the Ca^{2+} influx (fig. 14-5B,D).

At high SR Ca^{2+} load, the Ca^{2+} flux through RyR is large and amplifies local $[Ca^{2+}]_{iG}$ to a high degree, and eventually the positive feedback rises $[Ca^{2+}]_{iG}$ beyond the threshold at which CICR within the cluster becomes regenerative. Thus the macroscopic $[Ca^{2+}]_c$ signals will fall less steeply with positive potentials at high than at low SR Ca^{2+} load (fig. 14-6C: solid vs. dashed line). Also at high SR Ca^{2+} load, the macroscopic $[Ca^{2+}]_c$ should fall with strongly positive potentials, and it should be zero at $+120\,mV$, when Ca^{2+} influx through DHP-R is zero. Experimentally, however, cells with high SR Ca^{2+} load respond to steps to $+120\,mV$ with a macroscopic CICR. The result can partially be attributed to an artifact, i.e., the voltage clamp needs ca. $1\,ms$ to change the potential form $-80\,mV$ to $+120\,mV$, and during this time sufficient Ca^{2+} could enter through DHP-R. In addition, the strongly positive potentials augment Ca^{2+} influx through the Na-Ca exchanger to such an extent that it can trigger regenerative CICR {15,55,114}, provided the amplification of the positive feedback is high.

CONCLUSIONS

Despite overwhelming information on molecules, structure, and function, general understanding of cardiac E-C coupling has not yet been achieved. Although recent microscopic models try to synthesize the details, they are highly speculative because many of the assumptions are unproven at present. The microscopic models indicate that deeper understanding of cardiac E-C coupling depends not only on further insight into molecular biology, but also on information about how the molecules interact with their neighbors within the spatial architecture of the cell. Analysis of Ca^{2+} distribution as a function of space and time will hopefully help us to understand how these interactions control cardiac E-C coupling on the cellular level.

REFERENCES

1. Adams BA, Tanabe T, Mikami A, Numa S, Beam KG: Intramembrane charge movement restored in dysgenic skeletal muscle by injection of dihydropyridine receptor cDNAs. *Nature* 346:569–572, 1990.
2. Akera, T, Brody TM: Pharmacology of cardiac glycosides. In: Sperelakis N (ed) *Physiology and Pathophysiology of the Heart.* Dordrecht, The Netherlands: Kluwer Academic, Publishers 1989, pp 453–469.
3. Allen DG, Jewell BR, Wood EH: Studies of the contractility of mammalian myocardium at low rates of stimulation. *J Physiol (Lond)* 254:1–17, 1976.
4. Anderson K, Lai FA, Liu Q-Y, Rousseau E, Erickson HP, Meissner G: Structural and functional characterization of the purified cardiac ryanodine receptor-Ca^{2+} release channel complex. *J Biol Chem* 264,2:1329–1335, 1989.
5. Antoni H, Jacob R, Kaufmann R: Mechanische Reaktionen des Frosch- und Säugetiermyokards bei Veränderung der Aktionspotentialdauer durch konstante Gleichstromimpulse. *Pflügers Arch* 306:33–57, 1969.
6. Ashley CC, Mulligan IP, Lea TJ: Ca^{2+} and activation mechanisms in skeletal muscle. *Q Rev Biophys* 24:1–73, 1991.
7. Ashley RH, Williams AJ: Divalent cation activation and inhibition of single calcium release channels from sheep cardiac sarcoplasmic reticulum. *J Gen Physiol* 95:981–1005, 1990.
8. Balke CW, Rose WC, Marban E, Wier WG: Macroscopic and unitary properties of physiological ion flux through T-type Ca^{2+} channels in guinea-pig heart cells. *J Physiol (Lond)*, 456:247–265, 1992.
9. Baró I, O'Neill SC, Eisner DA: Changes of $[Ca^{2+}]_i$ during refinlling of the sarcoplasmic reticulum in rat ventricular and vascular smooth muscle. *J Physiol (Lond)*, 1993, in press.
10. Baumgarten CM, Fabiato A: Calculated transsarcolemmal calcium movements in cardiac muscle. In: Sperelakis N (ed) *Physiology and Pathophysiology of the Heart.* Dordrecht, The Netherlands: Kluwer Academic, 1989, pp 253–265.
11. Bean BP: Two kinds of calcium channels in canine atrial cells. Differences in kinetics, selectivity, and pharmacology. *J Gen Physiol* 86:1–30, 1985.
12. Bers DM: Ca influx and sarcoplasmic reticulum Ca release in cardiac muscle activation during postrest recovery. *Am J Physiol (Heart Circ Physiol)* 248:H366–H381, 1985.
13. Bers DM: *Excitation-Contraction Coupling and Cardiac Contractile Force.* Dordrecht, The Netherlands: Kluwer Academic, 1991.
14. Bers DM, Bridge JHB, Spitzer KW: Intracellular Ca^{2+} transients during rapid cooling contractures in guinea-pig ventricular myocytes. *J Physiol (Lond)* 417:537–553, 1989.
15. Bers DM, Lederer WJ, Berlin JR: Intracellular Ca transients in rat cardiac myocytes: Role of Na-Ca exchange in excitation-contraction coupling. *Am J Physiol Cell Physiol* 258:C944–C954, 1990.

16. Bers DM, Stiffel VM: The ratio of ryanodine:dihydropyridine receptors (RYR:DHPR) in cardiac and skeletal muscle and implications for E-C coupling. *J Mol Cell Cardiol* 24 (Suppl IV):P39, 1992.

17. Beuckelmann DJ, Wier WG: Mechanism of release of calcium from sarcoplasmic reticulum of guinea-pig cardiac cells. *J Physiol (Lond)* 405:233–255, 1988.

18. Beuckelmann DJ, Wier WG: Sodium-calcium exchange in guinea-pig cardiac cells: Exchange current and changes in intracellular Ca^{2+}. *J Physiol (Lond)* 414:499–520, 1989.

19. Blinks JR, Koch-Weser J: Physical factors in the analysis of the actions of drugs on myocardial contractility. *Pharmacol Rev* 15:531–599, 1963.

20. Boyett MR, Frampton JE, Harrison SM, Kirby MS, Levi AJ, McCall E, Milner DR, Orchard CH: The role of intracellular calcium, sodium and pH in rate-dependent changes of cardiac contractile force. In: Noble MIM Seed WA (eds) *The Interval-Force Relationship of the Heart.* Cambridge, UK: Cambridge University Press, 1992, pp 111–172.

21. Bridge JHB: Relationships between the sarcoplasmic reticulum and transarcolemmal Ca transport revealed by rapidly cooling rabbit ventricular muscle. *J Gen Physiol* 88:437–473, 1986.

22. Callewaert G: Excitation-contraction coupling in mammalian cardiac cells. *Cardiovasc Res* 26:923–932, 1992.

23. Cannell MB, Berlin JR, Lederer WJ: Effect of membrane potential changes on the calcium transient in single rat cardiac muscle cells. *Science* 238:1419–1423, 1987.

24. Carafoli E: The plasma membrane calcium pump. Structure, function, regulation. *Biochim Biophys Acta Bio-Energetics* 1101:266–267, 1992.

25. Caswell AH, Brandt NR: Does muscle activation occur by direct mechanical coupling of transverse tubules to sarcoplasmic reticulum? *Trends Biochem Sci* 14:161–165, 1989.

26. Cavalié A, Ochi R, Pelzer D, Trautwein W: Elementary currents through Ca^{2+} channels in guinea pig myocytes. *Pflügers Arch* 398:284–297, 1983.

27. Chapman RA: Excitation-contraction coupling in cardiac muscle. *Prog Biophys Mol Biol* 35:1–52, 1979.

28. Chapmann RA: Control of cardiac contractility at the cellular level. *Am Heart J* 245:H535–H552, 1983.

29. Crompton M: The role of Ca^{2+} in the function and dysfunction of heart mitochondria. In: Langer GA (ed) *Calcium and the Heart.* New York: Raven Press, 1990, pp 167–198.

30. Diebold RJ, Koch WJ, Ellinor PT, Wang J-J, Muthuchamy M, Wieczorek DF, Schwartz A: Mutually exclusive exon splicing of the cardiac calcium channel α_1 subunit gene generates developmentally regulated isoforms in the rat heart. *Proc Natl Acad Sci USA* 89:1497–1501, 1992.

31. Egan TM, Noble D, Noble SJ, Powell T, Spindler AJ, Twist VW: Sodium-calcium exchange during the action potential in guinea-pig ventricular cells. *J Physiol (Lond)* 411:639–611, 1989.

32. Eisner DA, Smith TW: The Na-K pump and its effectors in cardiac muscle. In: Fozzard HA (ed) *The Heart and Cardiovascular System.* New York: Raven Press, 1992, pp 863–902.

33. Engelkamp D, Schäfer BW, Erne P, Heizmann CW: S100α, CAPL, and CACY: Molecular cloning and expression analysis of three calcium-binding proteins from human heart. *Biochemistry* 31:10258–10264, 1992.

34. Fabiato A: Calcium-induced release of calcium from the cardiac sarcoplasmic reticulum. *Am J Physiol* 245:C1–C14, 1983.

35. Fabiato A: Rapid ionic modifications during the aequorin-detected calcium transient in a skinned canine cardiac Purkinje cell. *J Gen Physiol* 85:189–246, 1985.

36. Fabiato A: Time and calcium dependence of activation and inactivation of calcium-induced release of calcium from the sarcoplasmic reticulum of a skinned canine cardiac Purkinje Cell. *J Gen Physiol* 85:247–290, 1985.

37. Fabiato A: Simulated calcium current can both cause calcium loading in and trigger calcium release from the sarcoplasmic reticulum of a skinned canine cardiac Purkinje cell. *J Gen Physiol* 85:291–320, 1985.

38. Fabiato A: Two kinds of calcium-induced release of calcium from the sarcoplasmic reticulum of skinned cardiac cells. *Adv Exp Med Biol* 311:245–262, 1992.

39. Fabiato A, Fabiato F: Contractions induced by a calcium-triggered release of calcium from the sarcoplasmic reticulum of single skinned cardiac cells. *J Physiol (Lond)* 249:469–495, 1975.

40. Fleischer S, Inui M: Biochemistry and biophysics of excitation-contraction coupling. *Annu Rev Biophys Chem* 18:333–364, 1989.

41. Flockerzi V, Oeken H-J, Hofmann F, Pelzer D, Cavalié A, Trautwein W: Purified dihydropyridine-binding site from skeletal muscle t-tubules is a functional calcium channel. *Nature* 323:66–68, 1986.

42. Forbes MS, Sperelakis N: Ultrastructure of mammalian cardiac muscle. In: Sperelakis N (ed) *Physiology and Pathophysiology of the Heart.* Dordrecht. The Netherlands: Kluwer Academic, 1989, pp 3–41.

43. Frank JS: Ultrastructure of the unfixed myocardial sarcolemma and cell surface. In: Langer GA (ed) *Calcium and the Heart.* New York: Raven Press, 1990, pp 1–25.

44. Gibbons WR, Fozzard HA: Slow inward current and contraction of sheep cardiac Purkinje fibers. *J Gen Physiol* 65:367–384, 1975.

45. Grynkiewicz G, Poenie M, Tsien RY: A new generation of Ca^{2+} indicators with greatly improved fluorescence properties. *J Biol Chem* 260:3440–3450, 1985.

46. Hadley RW, Lederer WJ: Properties of L-type calcium channel gating current in isolated guinea pig ventricular myocytes. *J Gen Physiol* 98:265–285, 1991.

47. Han S, Schiefer A, Isenberg G: The efficacy of brief Ca^{2+} currents as a trigger for Ca^{2+} release increases with SR Ca^{2+} load (guinea-pig ventricular myocytes). *J Physiol (Lond)*, in press, 1993.

48. Hansford RG: Dehydrogenase activation by Ca^{2+} in cells and tissues. *J Bioenerg Biomembr* 23:823–854, 1991.

49. Hilgemann DW, Noble D: Excitation-contraction coupling and extracellular calcium transients in rabbit atrium: Reconstruction of basic cellular mechanisms. *Phil Trans R Soc Lond* 230:163–205, 1986.

50. Hille B: *Ionic Channels of Excitable Membranes*, 2nd ed. Sunderland, MA: Sinauer Associates, 1992.

51. Imredy JP, Yue DT: Submicroscopic Ca^{2+} diffusion mediates inhibitory coupling between individual Ca^{2+} channels. *Neuron* 9:197–207, 1992.

52. Isenberg G: Ca^{2+} entry and contraction as studied in isolated bovine ventricular myocytes. *Z Naturforsch Teil C* 37:502–512, 1982.

53. Isenberg G, Beresewicz A, Mascher D, Valenzuela F: The two components in the shortening of unloaded ventricular myocytes: Their voltage dependence. *Basic Res Cardiol* 80:117–122, 1985.

54. Isenberg G, Han S: Gradation of Ca^{2+} induced Ca^{2+} release by depolarizing clamp steps in potentiated guinea-pig ventricular myocytes. *J Physiol (Lond)*, in press, 1993.

55. Isenberg G, Han S, Schiefer A, Wendt-Gallitelli M-F: Changes in mitochondrial calcium concentration during the cardiac contraction cycle. *Cardiovasc Res*, in press, 1993.

56. Isenberg G, Klöckner U: Calcium currents of isolated bovine ventricular myocytes are fast and of large amplitude. *Pflügers Arch* 395:30–41, 1982.

57. Isenberg G, Spurgeon H, Talo A, Stern M, Capogrossi M, Lakatta E: The voltage dependence of the myoplasmic calcium transient in guinea pig ventricular myocytes is modulated by sodium loading. In: Clark WA, Decker RS Borg TK (eds) *Biology of Isolated Adult Cardiac Myocytes.* New York: Elsevier Science, 1988, pp 354–357.

58. Isenberg G, Wendt-Gallitelli M-F: Cellular mechanisms of excitation contraction coupling. In: Piper HM, Isenberg G (eds) *Isolated Adult Cardiomyocytes.* Boca Raton, FL: CRC Press, 1989, pp 213–248.

59. Isenberg G, Wendt-Gallitelli M-F: Binding of calcium to myoplasmic buffers contributes to the frequency-dependent inotropy in heart ventricular cells. *Basic Res Cardiol* 87: 411–417, 1992.

60. Kentish JC, Barsotti RJ, Lea TJ, Mulligan IP, Patel JR, Ferenczi MA: Calcium release from cardiac sarcoplasmic reticulum induced by photorelease of calcium or Ins(1,4,5)P$_3$. *Am J Physiol* 258:H610–H615, 1990.

61. Klöckner U, Isenberg G: Currents through single L-type Ca^{2+} channels studied at 2 mM [Ca^{2+}]$_o$ and 36°C in myocytes from the urinary bladder of the guinea-pig. *J Physiol (Lond)* 438:P228, 1991.

62. Kuniyasu A, Oka K, Ide-Yamada T, Hatanaka Y, Abe T, Nakayama H, Kanaoka Y: Structural characterization of the dihydropyridine receptor-linked calcium channel from porcine heart. *J Biochem (Tokyo)* 112:235–242, 1992.

63. Lakatta EG: Aging of the adult heart. In: Sperelakis N (ed) *Physiology and Pathophysiology of the Heart.* Dordrecht, The Netherlands: Kluwer Academic, 1989, pp 625–641.

64. Langer GA: Calcium exchange in dog ventricular muscle. Relation to frequency of contraction and maintenance of contractility. *Circ Res* 361:361–378, 1965.

65. Lee HC, Clusin WT: Cytosolic calcium staircase in cultured myocardial cells. *Circ Res* 61:934–939, 1987.

66. Lee KS, Tsien RW: High selectivity of calcium channels in single dialyzed heart cells of the guinea-pig. *J Physiol (Lond)* 354:253–272, 1984.

67. Lewartowski B, Hansford RG, Langer GA, Lakatta EG: Contraction and sarcoplasmic reticulum Ca^{2+} content in single myocytes of guinea pig heart: Effect of ryanodine. *Am J Physiol Heart Circ Physiol* 259:H1222–H1229, 1990.

68. Lewartowski B, Pytkowski B, Janczewski A: Calcium fraction correlating with contractile force of ventricular muscle of guinea-pig heart. *Pflügers Arch* 401:198–203, 1984.

69. Lindemann JP, Watanabe AM: Mechanisms of adrenergic and cholinergic regulation of myocardial contractility. In: Sperelakis N (ed) *Physiology and Pathophysiology of the Heart.* Dordrecht, The Netherlands: Kluwer Academic, 1989, pp 423–452.

70. Lindsay ARG, Williams AJ: Functional characterization of the ryanodine receptor purified from sheep cardiac muscle sarcoplasmic reticulum. *Biochim Biophys Acta Bio-Membr* 1064:89–102, 1991.

71. Lytton J, MacLennan DH: Sarcoplasmic reticulum. In: Fozzard HA (ed) *The Heart and Cardiovascular System.* New York: Raven Press, 1992, pp 1203–1222.

72. McCormack JG, Crompton M: The role and study of mammalian mitochondrial Ca^{2+} transport and matrix Ca^{2+}. In: McCormack JG, Cobbold PH (ed) *Cellular Calcium, a Practical Approach.* Oxford: IRL Press, 1991, pp 345–382.

73. McDonald TF, Cavalié A, Trautwein W, Pelzer D: Voltage-dependent properties of macroscopic and elementary calcium channel currents in guinea pig ventricular myocytes. *Pflügers Arch* 406:437–448, 1986.

74. Meissner G, Darling E, Eveleth J: Kinetics of rapid Ca^{2+} release by sarcoplasmic reticulum. Effects of Ca^{2+}, Mg^{2+} and adenine nucleotides. *Biochemistry* 25:236–244, 1986.

75. Meissner G, Henderson JS: Rapid calcium release from cardiac sarcoplasmic reticulum vesicles is dependent on Ca^{2+} and is modulated by Mg^{2+}, adenine nucleotide, and calmodulin. *J Biol Chem* 262:3065–3073, 1987.

76. Mikami A, Imoto K, Tanabe T, Niidome T, Mori Y, Takeshima H, Narumiya S, Numa S: Primary structure and functional expression of the cardiac dihydropyridine-sensitive calcium channel. *Nature* 340:230–233, 1989.

77. Morad M, Goldman Y: Excitation-contraction coupling in heart muscle: Membrane control of development of tension. *Prog Biophys Mol Biol* 27:259313, 1973.

78. Moravec CS, Bond M: Calcium is released from the junctional sarcoplasmic reticulum during cardiac muscle contraction. *Am J Physiol* 260:H989–H997.

79. Mullins LJ: Role of Na-Ca exchange in heart. In: Sperelakis N (ed) *Physiology and Pathophysiology of the Heart.* Dordrecht, The Netherlands: Kluwer Academic, 1989, pp 241–265.

80. Näbauer M, Callewaert G, Cleemann L, Morad M: Regulation of calcium release is gated by calcium current, not gating charge, in cardiac myocytes. *Science* 244:800–803, 1989.

81. Näbauer M, Morad M: Ca^{2+}-induced Ca^{2+} release as examined by photolysis of caged Ca^{2+} in single ventricular myocytes. *Am J Physiol* 258:C189–C193, 1990.

82. Nilius B, Hess P, Lansman JB, Tsien RW: A novel type of cardiac calcium channel in ventricular cells. *Nature* 316: 443–446, 1985.

83. Noble D, Powell T: The slowing of Ca^{2+} signals by Ca^{2+} indicators in cardiac muscle. *Proc Natl Acad Sci USA* 246: 167–172, 1991.

84. O'Neill SC, Mill JG, Eisner DA: Local activation of contraction in isolated rat ventricular myocytes. *Am J Physiol* 258:C1165–C1168, 1990.

85. Ochi R, Kawashima Y: Modulation of slow gating process of calcium channels by isoprenaline in guinea-pig ventricular cells. *J Physiol (Lond)* 424:187–204, 1990.

86. Otsu K, Willard HF, Khanna VK, Zorzato F, Green NM, MacLennan DH: Molecular cloning of cDNA encoding the Ca^{2+} release channel (ryanodine receptor) of rabbit cardiac muscle sarcoplasmic reticulum. *J Biol Chem* 265:13472–13483, 1990.

87. Pan BS, Solaro J: Calcium-binding properties of troponin C in detergent-skinned heart muscle fibers. *J Biol Chem* 262: 7839–7849, 1987.

88. Pelzer D, Pelzer S, McDonald TF: Calcium channels in heart. In: Fozzard HA (ed) *The Heart and Cardiovascular System.* New York: Raven Press, 1992, pp 1049–1089.

89. Pierce GN, Philipson KD, Langer GA: Passive calcium-buffering capacity of a rabbit ventricular homogenate preparation. *Am J Physiol Cell Physiol* 249:C248–C255, 1985.

90. Pytkowski B, Lewartowski B, Prokopczuk A, Zdanowski K, Lewandowska K: Excitation- and rate-dependent shifts of Ca in guinea-pig ventricular myocardium. *Pflügers Arch* 398:103–113, 1983.

91. Robertson SP, Johnson JD, Potter JD: The time-course of Ca^{2+} exchange with calmodulin, troponin, parvalbumin, and myosin in response to transient increases in Ca^{2+}. *Biophys J* 34:559–569, 1981.

92. Rose WC, Balke CW, Wier WG, Marban E: Macroscopic and unitary properties of physiological ion flux through L-

type Ca^{2+} channels in guinea-pig heart cells. *J Physiol (Lond)* 456:267–284, 1992.

93. Rosenberg RL, Hess P, Reeves JP, Smilowitz H, Tsien RW: Calcium channels in plannar lipid bilayers: Insights into mechanisms of ion permeation and gating. *Science* 231:1564–1566, 1986.

94. Rousseau E, Meissner G: Single cardiac sarcoplasmic reticulum Ca^{2+}-release channel: Activation by caffeine. *Am J Physiol (Heart Circ Physiol)* 256:H328–H333, 1989.

95. Rousseau E, Smith JS, Henderson JS, Meissner G: Single channel and $^{45}Ca^{2+}$ flux measurements of the cardiac sarcoplasmic reticulum calcium channel. *Biophys J* 50:1009–1014, 1986.

96. Schiefer A, Meissner G, Isenberg G: Activation of reconstituted cardiac SR Ca^{2+} release channels by fast Ca^{2+} concentration jumps: No evidence for Ca^{2+} inactivation. *Pflügers Arch*, in press, 1993.

97. Schouten VJA, Van Deen JK, De Tombe P, Verveen AA: Force-interval relationship in heart muscle of mammals: A calcium compartment model. *Biophys J* 51:13–26, 1987.

98. Schwarz H, Meissner G, Wendt-Gallitelli MF: Immuno-gold labeling of ryanodine receptors in ventricle of the guinea-pig. *Proc 32nd IUPS* (abstr).

99. Sham JSK, Cleemann L, Morad M: Gating of the cardiac Ca^{2+} release channel: The role of Na^+ current and Na^+-Ca^{2+} exchange. *Science* 255:850–853, 1992.

100. Shepherd N, Vornanen M, Isenberg G: Force measurements from voltage-clamped guinea pig ventricular myocytes. *Am J Physiol* 258:H452–H459, 1990.

101. Sipido KR, Wier WG: Flux of Ca^{2+} across the sarcoplasmic reticulum of guinea-pig cardiac cells during excitation-contraction coupling. *J Physiol (Lond)* 435:605–630, 1991.

102. Skou JC: Enzymatic basis for active transport of Na^+ and K^+ across cell membrane. *Physiol Rev* 45:596–617, 1965.

103. Solaro RJ, Pan B-S: Control and modulation of contractile activity of cardiac myofilaments. In: Sperelakis N (ed) *Physiology and Pathophysiology of the Heart*. Dordrecht, The Netherlands: Kluwer Academic, 1989, pp 291–303

104. Solaro RJ, Wise RM, Shiner JS, Briggs FN: Calcium requirements for cardiac myofibrillar activation. *Circ Res* 34:525–530, 1974.

105. Sommer JR, Jennings RB: Ultrastructure of cardiac muscle. In: *Handbook of Physiology*. The Cardiovascular System 1, 1979, pp 113–185.

106. Spurgeon HA, Stewrn MD, Baarts G, Raffaeli S, Hansford RG, Talo A, Lakatta EG, Capogrossi MC: Simultaneous measurement of Ca^{2+}, contraction, and potential in cardiac myocytes.

107. Stern MD: Theory of excitation-contraction coupling in cardiac muscle. *Biophys J* 63:497–517, 1992.

108. Stern MD, Capogrossi MC, Lakatta EG: Spontaneous calcium release from the sarcoplasmic reticulum in myocardial cells: Mechanisms and consequences. *Cell Calcium* 9:247–256, 1988.

109. Stern MD, Lakatta EG: Excitation-contraction coupling in the heart: The state of the question. *FASEB J* 6:3092–3100, 1992.

110. Tada M, Shigekawa M, Kadoma M, Nimura Y: Uptake of calcium by sarcoplasmic reticulum and its regulation and functional consequences. In: Sperelakis N (ed) *Physiology and Pathophysiology of the Heart*. Dordrecht, The Netherlands: Kluwer Academic, 1989, pp 267–290.

111. Takasago T, Imagawa T, Shigekawa M: Phosphorylation of the cardiac ryanodine receptor by cAMP-dependent protein kinase. *J Biochem (Tokyo)* 106:872–877, 1989.

112. Tanabe T, Beam KG, Adams BA, Niidome T, Numa S:

Regions of the skeletal muscle dihydropyridine receptor critical for excitation-contraction coupling. *Nature* 346:567–569, 1990.

113. Terrar DA, White E: Changes in cytosolic calcium monitored by inward currents during action potentials in guinea-pig ventricular cells. *Proc R Soc Lond B* 238:171–188, 1989.

114. Terrar DA, White E: Mechanisms and significance of calcium entry at positive membrane potentials in guinea-pig ventricular muscle cells. *Q J Exp Physiol* 74:121–139, 1989.

115. Trautwein W, McDonald TF, Tripathi O: Calcium conductance and tension in mammalian ventricular muscle. *Pflügers Arch* 354:55–74, 1975.

116. Tsien RW: Calcium channels in excitable cell membranes. *Annu Rev Physiol* 45:341–358, 1983.

117. Tsien RW, Bean BP, Hess P, Lansman JB, Nilius B, Nowycky MC: Mechanisms of calcium channel modulation by β-adrenergic agents and dihydropyridine calcium agonists. *J Mol Cell Cardiol* 18:691–710, 1986.

118. Tsien RW, Tsien RY: Calcium channels, stores, and oscillations. *Annu Rev Cell Biol* 6:715–760, 1990.

119. Wendt-Gallitelli M-F: Ca pools involved in the regulation of cardiac contraction under positive inotropy. X-ray microanalysis of rapidly frozen ventricular muscles of the guinea-pig. *Basic Res Cardiol* 81:25–32, 1986.

120. Wendt-Gallitelli MF, Isenberg G: X-ray microanalysis of single cardiac myocytes frozen under voltage-clamp conditions. *Am J Physiol* 256:H574–H583, 1989.

121. Wendt-Gallitelli MF, Isenberg G: X-ray microprobe analysis of voltage-clamped single heart ventricular myocytes. In: Conn M (ed) *Methods is Neurosciences*. London: Academic Press, 1991, pp 103–126.

122. Wendt-Gallitelli MF, Isenberg G: X-ray microanalysis. In: McCormack JG Cobbold PH (eds) *Cellular Calcium: A Practical Approach*. New York: Oxford University Press, 1991, pp 133–157.

123. Wendt-Gallitelli MF, Isenberg G: Total and free myoplasmic calcium during a contraction cycle: X-ray microanalysis in guinea-pig ventricular myocytes. *J Physiol (Lond)* 435:349–372, 1991.

124. Wendt-Gallitelli M-F, Isenberg G, Voigt T: Calcium imaging of free sarcoplasmic reticulum. X-ray microanalysis of voltage-clamped guinea-pig ventricular myocytes. *Pflügers Arch* 420:R78, 1992.

125. Wendt-Gallitelli M-F, Voigt T, Isenberg G: Contribution of free SR to the release of activator calcium. Quantitative calcium imaging by X-ray microanalysis of voltage-clamped guinea-pig ventricular myocytes. *J Physiol (Lond)* 459:222, 1992.

126. Wibo M, Godfraind T: Stoichiometric ratio of dihydropyridine and ryanodine receptors in junctional areas of rat ventricle. J Mol Cell Cardiol 24(Suppl IV):P23, 1992.

127. Wier WG: Cytoplasmic $[Ca^{2+}]$ in mammalian ventricle: Dynamic control by cellular processes. *Annu Rev Physiol* 52:467–485, 1990.

128. Wier WG: $[Ca^{2+}]_i$ transients during excitation-contraction coupling of mammalian heart. In: Fozzard HA et al. (eds) *The Heart and Cardiovascular System*, 1992.

129. Wier WG, Yue DT: Intracellular calcium transients underlying the short-term force interval relationship in ferret ventricular myocardium. *J Physiol (Lond)* 376:507–530, 1986.

130. Williams AJ: Ion conduction and discrimination in the sarcoplasmic reticulum ryanodine receptor/calcium-release channel. *J Muscle Res Cell Motility* 13:7–26, 1992.

131. Witcher DR, Kovacs RJ, Schulman H, Cefali DC, Jones LR: Unique phosphorylation site on the cardiac ryanodine receptor regulates calcium channel activity. *J Biol Chem* 266:11144–11152, 1991.

132. Zucker RS, Fogelson AL: Relationship between transmitter release and presynaptic calcium influx when calcium enters through discrete channels. *Proc Natl Acad Sci USA* 83: 3032–3036, 1986.

CHAPTER 15

Cardiac Sodium-Calcium Exchange System

JOHN P. REEVES

INTRODUCTION

The Na/Ca exchange system is a carrier-mediated transport process that is found in the plasma membrane of cardiac myocytes. It couples the movement of three Na ions across the membrane in exchange for a single Ca ion moving in the opposite direction. Hence, it establishes a connection between the transmemembrane gradient of Na and the intracellular Ca concentration ($[Ca]_i$). It is a bidirectional transport process, capable of moving Ca in either direction across the plasma membrane. However, because of the inwardly directed concentration gradient of Na, established by the action of the Na,K-ATPase, its principal mode of operation is in the direction of Ca efflux. In cardiac myocytes, the exchanger is the predominant Ca efflux process in the cell and competes with the sarcoplasmic reticulum (SR) Ca-ATPase for cytosolic Ca (fig. 15-1). Approximately 20% of the Ca released by the SR is transported out of the cell via the Na/Ca exchanger with each beat. Changes in the driving force for Na/Ca exchange therefore exert a profound influence on the amount of Ca taken up by the SR and on the force of contraction of subsequent beats (fig. 15-1).

The exchanger is especially abundant in cardiac cells, but it is also found in other cell types, such as smooth and skeletal muscle, kidney, and intestinal epithelia, and in many other tissues as well. It is not ubiquitous, however, and there are cell types such as the human erythrocyte that do not exhibit Na/Ca exchange. There is another type of Na/Ca exchanger in retinal rods; it has a stoichiometry of 4 Na/(1 Ca + 1 K) and is a different molecular entity than the cardiac exchanger. Most of the discussion of this chapter will focus on the cardiac exchanger, although references will be made to the retinal rod exchanger from time to time. This chapter will discuss the fundamental properties of Na/Ca exchange as a transport process and describe the essential elements of its role in cardiac physiology. The interested reader may consult one of several recent reviews {1–4} for more detailed information on Na/Ca exchange.

FUNDAMENTAL PROPERTIES OF Na/Ca EXCHANGE

Stoichiometry

There is now abundant evidence that the stoichiometry of the cardiac Na/Ca exchanger is 3 Na/Ca {1–4}. This value was established experimentally by a thermodynamic approach in which the membrane potential and the magnitudes of the ion gradients for Na and Ca are measured under conditions where the exchange system is in equilibrium. This condition can be defined as follows: For an exchange process in which the movement of the n Na ions is obligatorily coupled to the movement of a single Ca ion, the thermodynamic driving force ($\Delta\mu_{Na\text{-}Ca}$) can be written as

$$\Delta\mu_{Na\text{-}Ca} = n\Delta\mu_{Ca} - \Delta\mu_{Ca}$$
$$= (n - 2)E_m - nE_{Na} + 2 E_{Ca}, \qquad (15\text{-}1)$$

where $\Delta\mu_i = n_i(E_m - E_i)$ is the electrochemical potential of the ionic species i, n_i is the valence of i, E_m is the membrane potential, and E_i is the equilibrium potential for i, defined for Na and Ca as

$$E_{Na} = -RTF^{-1}\ln\{[Na]_i/[Na]_o\}, \qquad (15\text{-}2)$$
$$E_{Ca} = -(1/2)RTF^{-1}\ln\{[Ca]_i/[Ca]_o\}, \qquad (15\text{-}3)$$

where intracellular and extracellular concentrations have been substituted for the respective ionic activities, R is the gas constant, T is the absolute temperature, and F is the value of the Faraday. It can be seen that when n = 2 the process is electroneutral and the term involving the membrane potential drops out. For any other stoichiometry, however (and n need not be an interger), the membrane potential will constitute a part of the thermodynamic driving force for Na/Ca exchange. The relation in eq. (15-1) is formulated such that Ca moves out of the cell if $\Delta\mu_{Na\text{-}Ca}$ is negative and moves into the cell if it is positive. At equilibrium ($\Delta\mu_{Na\text{-}Ca} = 0$), there is no net Ca movement in either direction. The condition of equilibrium provides a means for determining the stoichiometry if E_{Na}, E_{Ca}, and E_m are known, i.e.,

$$n = 2(E_m - E_{Ca})/(E_m - E_{Na}) \quad [\Delta\mu_{Na\text{-}Ca} = 0]. \qquad (15\text{-}4)$$

309

N. Sperelakis (ed.), Physiology and Pathophysiology of the Heart, Third Edition.

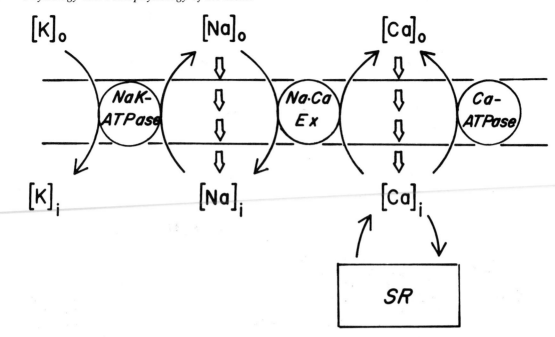

Fig. 15-1. Ionic homeostasis in myocardial cells. The transmembrane [Na] and [K] gradients are maintained by the operation of the Na,K-ATPase. The open arrows represent Na and Ca entry through voltage-gated channels. Note that both the Na/Ca exchanger and the plasma membrane Ca-ATPase compete for cytosolic Ca with the sarcoplasmic reticulum (SR) Ca-ATPase; the plasma membrane Ca-ATPase appears to be less important than the Na/Ca exchanger as a Ca efflux mechanism in myocardial cells. Reproduced from Reeves {33}, with permission.

Using this approach, radioactive Ca flux studies in cardiac membrane vesicles and electrophysiological measurements in whole cardiac cells established the stoichiometry of the exchange process as 3 Na per Ca {5, 6}.

Because the stoichiometry of the exchange system involves a net imbalance of charge, one positive charge moves out of the cell for every Ca ion moving into the cell via the exchanger and vice versa. Thus, the exchange system generates a current across the cardiac cell membrane {6}. By convention, the direction of a current is specified as the direction of movement of positive charge. Thus, Ca entry into the cell via Na/Ca exchange is associated with an outward current, whereas the exchanger generates an inward current when Ca moves out of the cell. Much of our present knowledge of the kinetics and regulatory properties of Na/Ca exchange comes from electrophysiological measurements of exchange currents using either internally perfused whole myocytes {6} or giant sarcolemmal membrane patches {7}. The latter is a particularly versatile system since it allows easy access to the cytoplasmic surface of the membrane.

It is useful to discuss the thermodynamics of Na/Ca exchange in terms of its reversal potential $E_{Na\text{-}Ca}$. This is the membrane potential at which the exchange system is in equilibrium i.e., when the net ion flux mediated by the exchanger is zero. From the relations given above in eqs. (15-1) to (15-4), we can see that the reversal potential (with n = 3) is defined as

$$E_{Na\text{-}Ca} = 3\,E_{Na} - 2\,E_{Ca}$$
$$= -RTF^{-1}\ln\{([Ca]_o/[Ca]_i)([Na]_i/[Na]_o)^3\}. \tag{15-5}$$

At membrane potentials that are more negative than $E_{Na\text{-}Ca}$, positive current will flow into the cell and the exchange system will operate in the direction of Ca efflux. At membrane potentials that are more positive than the reversal potential, the exchange current will be outward and Ca will move into the cell. For typical values of the intracellular and extracellular concentrations of Na and Ca ($[Na]_o = 140\,mM$, $[Ca]_o = 2\,mM$, $[Na]_i = 6\,mM$, and $[Ca]_i = 0.1\,\mu M$), $E_{Na\text{-}Ca}$ is approximately $-12\,mV$. Thus, for this example the driving force for Na/Ca exchange at a resting potential of $-80\,mV$ will be in the direction of net Ca efflux. The reversal potential is obviously highly sensitive to changes in the intracellular concentrations of Na and Ca. It will be important to keep this relationship in mind when the roles of Na/Ca exchange in Ca homeostasis are discussed in later sections of this chapter.

As mentioned above, the retinal rod exchanger has a different stoichiometry than the cardiac exchanger {8,9}. In the case of the rod exchanger, K is cotransported with Ca and the stoichiometry is 4 Na/(1 Ca + 1 K). With this stoichiometry, the reversal potential for Na/Ca+K exchange in retinal rods is

$$E_{Na\text{-}(Ca+K)} = 4\,E_{Na} - 2\,E_{Ca} - E_K$$
$$= RTF^{-1}\ln\{([Ca]_o/[Ca]_i)([K]_o/[K]_i)([Na]_i/[Na]_o)^4\}.$$

For the ionic concentrations given in the example in the previous paragraph, with $[K]_o = 4 \, mM$ and $[K]_i = 140 \, mM$, the reversal potential becomes $+163 \, mV$. Thus, there is a much larger driving force in favor of Ca efflux for the retinal rod exchanger compared to the cardiac exchanger. In retinal rods, however, it is likely that the steady-state concentration of intracellular Na in retinal rods is higher than the value of 6 mM assumed in the above example; this is because there is a continual entry of Na through the light-sensitive, cGMP-gated cation conducting channel, which elevates $[Na]_i$. Indeed, it is thought that one of the benefits of a K-coupled exchanger in retinal rods is that the driving force of Ca efflux is maintained in the face of relatively high concentrations of intracellular Na.

Kinetics of Na/Ca exchange

Although the thermodynamic considerations discussed above and the concept of the reversal potential for Na/Ca exchange can tell us the direction of Na/Ca exchange, it tells us nothing about the efficiency of this process. There are several factors to consider in discussing the rate of movement of ions by Na/Ca exchange. The first is the maximal rate of turnover of the exchanger, i.e., the rate of ion movement when the exchanger is fully saturated with Na and Ca. Recent measurements suggest that each exchange carrier can generate a maximal flux of 1000–5000 Ca ions per second. Maximal exchange current densities in cardiac ventricular cells correspond to the movement of 4 $\times \, 10^{10}$ Ca ions per cell per second {10}. Comparison of these two numbers suggest that each ventricular cell contains 8–40 million Na/Ca exchange carriers. Thus, the exchanger has the capacity to generate large Ca fluxes in myocardial cells.

The second factor determining the rate of Na/Ca exchange is the concentration of the transported ions needed to activate the exchange system. Since the external concentrations of Na and Ca under phsiological conditions are constant and are at nearly saturating levels with respect to exchanger activation, exchange activity is controlled mainly by the intracellular concentrations of these ions. Activation of exchange activity by Na involves the co-operative interaction of three Na ions, and therefore activity increases with the second or third power of the Na concentration. As a consequence, exchange activity increases from 10% to 90% of maximal with only a 5- to 10-fold increase in the Na concentration. Half-maximal activation of exchange activity by Na occurs at approximately 15 mM at the cytoplasmic surface. Half-maximal activation of exchange activity by cytosolic Ca occurs at approximately 4 μM at $[Na]_o = 150 \, mM$. Activation by Ca does not involve the cooperative interaction of more than 1 Ca ion and so exchange activity is less sensitive to variations in $[Ca]_i$, requiring an 80-fold increase to go from 10% to 90% of maximal activity.

In cardiac cells, the cytoplasmic concentrations of Na (4–8 mM) and Ca (40–100 nM) are substantially below their respective K_ms for Na/Ca exchange. This means that the exchanger is operating at only a small percentage of its maximal capacity under resting conditions. Even during

contraction, the cytoplasmic concentration of Ca does not rise much above 1 μm in normal cardiac cells; with a K_m for Ca of 4 μm this would be sufficient to activate Na/Ca exchange to 20% of its maximal capacity. In considering this figure, however, it should be borne in mind that transient local concentrations of Ca immediately adjacent to the cytoplasmic surface of the sarcolemma may be substantially higher than the bulk concentration in the cytoplasm. Moreover, the capacity of the exchanger is so large that even when it is operating at only a fraction of its maximal rate, it is still capable of exerting a profound influence on intracellular $[Ca^{2+}]$.

The third factor that determines the efficiency of the exchanger in mediating Ca fluxes is the influence of various intracellular regulators of exchange activity. These will be discussed in the next section.

Regulation of Na/Ca exchange

There are two well-defined modes of regulation of the cardiac Na/Ca exchanger: (a) secondary activation by intracellular Ca and (b) regulation by intracellular ATP {reviewed in 2 and 11}. Secondary activation by intracellular Ca was first observed in squid axons in experiments where the injection of intracellular EGTA, a Ca chelator, was found to block Na_i-dependent Ca influx. It should be noted that Na was the cytoplasmic transport substrate in this instance so that chelation of intracellular Ca should have had no effect on exchange activity unless Ca was necessary to activate the exchanger at an additional, non-transport site. In cardiac cells, some studies have suggested that secondary activation occurs at very low concentrations of Ca ($5 \times 10^{-8} \, M$), whereas others have indicated that Ca activation occurs within the low micromolar range. It is uncertain whether secondary activation by Ca is required for the operation of the exchanger in the Ca efflux mode; the reason for the uncertainty is that it is difficult experimentally to distinguish between the actions of cytosolic Ca as an activating cation and its actions as a transport substrate. If Ca efflux is regulated in the same way as Ca influx, secondary activation by Ca would provide a mechanism for switching the exchanger "off" at low concentrations of intracellular Ca. Turning "off" the exchanger in this way might be important for maintaining sufficient amounts of Ca within the sarcoplasmic reticulum and the mitochondria for normal cardiac function. This appears to be a feature of the retinal rod exchanger, which ceases to transport Ca out of the rod when $[Ca]_i$ declines to approximately 100 nM despite the large thermodynamic driving force in favor of Ca efflux under these conditions {12}.

Many independent studies have indicated that Na/Ca exchange is regulated by intracellular ATP, despite the fact that exchange activity is not associated with or dependent upon ATP hydrolysis. Studies with squid axons, cardiac myocytes, and smooth muscle cells have indicated that removal or depletion of intracellular ATP produces a profound depression in Na/Ca exchange activity, and this is associated with changes in the kinetics of the exchanger. Specifically, the K_m for intracellular Ca is shifted to higher

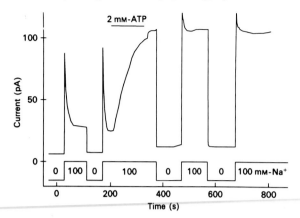

Fig. 15-2. Na-dependent inactivation of the Na/Ca exchanger. Currents are shown for giant sarcolemmal patches {7} from cardiac myocytes. The Na-free patch pipette buffer (extracellular membrane surface) contained 5 mM $CaCl_2$ {13}. Repetitive applications of a solution containing 100 mM Na were made at the cytoplasmic membrane surface. Mg-ATP was also applied for 110 seconds, as indicated by the bar. Data taken from Collins et al. {13}, with permission.

concentrations by a factor of approximately 10 in the absence of ATP. A shift to higher concentrations is also observed for the interaction of Ca at the secondary activation site.

In giant membrane patches, ATP has been shown to counteract what has been called *Na-dependent inactivation* {13}. This process is depicted in fig. 15-2. As shown, upon the addition of Na there is a nearly instantaneous rise in exchange current, which then declines over a period of several seconds to a fraction (30% in fig. 15-2) of its initial value. When Mg-ATP is added following the period of decline, there is a profound increase in exchange current. Subsequent cycles of Na addition reveal a much smaller degree of Na-dependent inactivation. As shown in fig. 15-2, the effect of ATP persists after its removal. It has been suggested that Na-dependent inactivation represents the time-dependent entry of the exchanger into an inactive state, a process that is associated with the binding of Na at the cytoplasmic surface of the exchanger. Apparently, this inactivation is specific for the Na-bound configuration, since no such inactivation is associated with the binding of Ca at the cytoplasmic surface. Na-dependent inactivation may be an important mechanism for protecting the cell against Ca overload under conditions (e.g., ischemia) when ATP levels decline and intracellular Na levels rise.

The mechanism underlying the regulatory effects of ATP is unknown. Experiments with squid axons suggest that phosphorylation is involved {11}, although it is uncertain whether it is the exchanger itself that is phosphorylated or an associated intracellular protein. In contrast, studies with giant membrane patches from cardiac myocytes suggest that ATP exerts its effects by activating ATP-dependent aminophospholipid translocase, an

enzyme that transports negatively charged phospholipids from the external membrane surface to the cytoplasmic surface {14}. Most cells maintain an asymmetric distribution of phospholipid species between the two surfaces of the bilayer, with negatively charged phospholipid species such as phosphatidylserine located almost exclusively in the cytoplasmic half of the bilayer leaflet. This distribution is maintained in part by the activity of the phospholipid translocase and in part by interaction of phosphatidylserine with cytoskeletal constitutents. Experiments with reconstituted phospolipid vesicles indicate that Na/Ca exchange activity is markedly stimulated by negatively charged amphiphilic species, including phosphatidylserine {15}. An attractive hypothesis for the effects of ATP depletion on exchange activity is that the disruption of the cytoskeleton and inhibition of translocase activity leads to a loss of phosphatidylserine at the cytoplasmic membrane surface and a consequent inhibition of Na/Ca exchange activity. This hypothesis, which is currently being tested experimentally, does not preclude the involvement of phosphorylation in the regulation of exchange activity, since phosphorylation of cytoskeletal elements could be important in maintaining the asymmetric distribution of phosphatidylserine.

Reaction mechanism

One can imagine two basic mechanisms by which Na/Ca exchange takes place: Either the Na and Ca ions are translocated in separate steps during the exchange process (fig. 15-3) or else the carrier binds Na and Ca simultaneously on opposite sides of the membrane, and both ions are translocated at the same time. The consecutive and simultaneous models, as they are called, have different

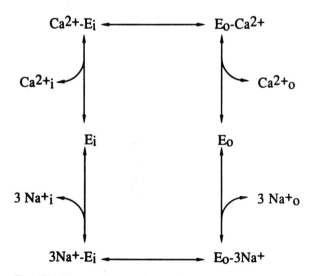

Fig. 15-3. Consecutive reaction mechanism for Na/Ca exchange. In this model, the Na (lower) and Ca (upper) translocation steps are separate. Reproduced from Durkin et al. {34}, with permission.

kinetic characteristics and, at present, the bulk of the kinetic evidence favors the consecutive mechanism (fig. 15-3). Experiments with membrane patches indicate the K_m for the transported ion decreases toward zero as the concentration of the exchange partner on the opposite side of the membrane decreases. This behavior is characteristic of the consecutive mechanism and reflects the fact that the concentration of unloaded carriers on one side of the membrane depends (in part) upon the rate at which the carrier is translocated from the opposite side. The most direct evidence in favor of the consecutive model comes from experiments indicating that the translocation of Na (in the absence of Ca) is associated with a transient current in membrane patches, which reflects a redistribution of exchange carriers. These results suggest that the Na-loaded form of the carrier is positively charged. However, some investigators have also reported transient currents associated with the Ca translocation step, suggesting that both branches of the exchange process may involve charge movement. Further details regarding the reaction mechanism of Na/Ca exchange have been presented in recent reviews {1,4}.

Na/Ca EXCHANGE AND CARDIAC PHYSIOLOGY

Figure 15-4 depicts the changes in membrane potential and reversal potential for Na/Ca exchange (cf. above) during a typical cardiac action potential of a ventricular myocyte. The figure indicates that $E_{Na\text{-}Ca}$ changes markedly during the course of the cardiac action potential; this reflects the increase in intracellular [Ca] due to Ca entry from the exterior and Ca release from internal stores. It can be seen

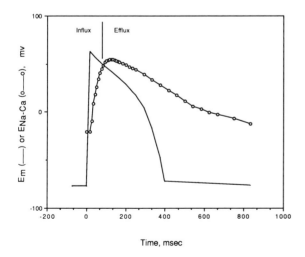

Fig. 15-4. Membrane potential (E_m) and Na-Ca exchange reversal potential ($E_{Na\text{-}Ca}$) during a ventricular myocyte action potential. $E_{Na\text{-}Ca}$ was calculated assuming $[Na]_o = 140\,mM$, $[Na]_i = 6\,mM$, $[Ca]_o = 2\,mM$, and values of $[Ca]_i$ taken from Wier and Beuckelmann {16}.

that for most of the cardiac action potential, and during the period of rest between action potentials, the membrane potential is more negative than the $E_{Na\text{-}Ca}$. This indicates that the exchanger will mediate Ca efflux during these periods. At the begining of the action potential, however, there is a brief period during which the action potential is more positive than $E_{Na\text{-}Ca}$. During this period the exchanger could theoretically mediate Ca influx and contribute to the activation of cardiac contraction. It should be stressed that this is a hypothetical diagram and that the precise concentrations of intracellular Ca and Na during the cardiac action potential are not known with great certainty. The figures used here for $[Ca]_i$ are based primarily on studies with intracellular Ca-sensitive dyes {16} and reflect bulk concentrations in cytoplasmic Ca. However, there may be cellular compartments in which the local concentrations of Na and or Ca deviate significantly from those in the bulk cytoplasm. Despite the limitations of this approach, we will use fig. 15-4 as a point of departure for our discussion of ion fluxes mediated by the exchanger.

Ca efflux

Several experimental studies have demonstrated that the Na/Ca exchanger is the primary Ca efflux mechanism of cardiac myocytes; two experiments will be cited to illustrate this conclusion. In the first study, extracellular Ca-indicating dyes were used to monitor $[Ca]_o$ in functioning myocardium {17}. The results revealed that $[Ca]_o$ rapidly decreased during the early portions of the cardiac action potential and then gradually regained its initial level prior to the next beat. The early decline in $[Ca]_o$ is due to entry of Ca into the cells through voltage-dependent Ca channels. The gradual restoration of $[Ca]_o$ was apparently mediated by the cardiac Na/Ca exchanger, since the return of $[Ca]_o$ to its initial value was abolished in the absence of Na.

The second study {18} employed a cold-shock procedure to release Ca from the SR and to produce a contracture in rabbit ventricular muscle. Subsequent warming of the tissue produced a relaxation of tension that is due to a combination of Ca reuptake into the SR and Ca transport to the exterior. The decline in tension upon rewarming is shown in fig. 15-5. In the presence of caffiene, which maintains the SR Ca release channel in an open state, relaxation is due solely to Ca transport out of the cell. Relaxation under these conditions was greatly slowed by the removal of Na from the medium, indicating that Ca transport occurs primarily by Na/Ca exchange. Note that in the absence of caffeine, removal of external Na had only a marginal effect on relaxation of tension (fig. 15-5); relaxation under these conditions is due solely to Ca uptake into the SR. The results indicate that there is a strong competition between the SR Ca ATPase and the plasma membrane Na/Ca exchanger for reuptake of Ca into the SR and transport of Ca to the cell exterior, respectively (cf. fig. 15-1). Recent results suggest that the exchanger extrudes approximately 20% of the Ca released from the SR during each beat {19}. It will be important to

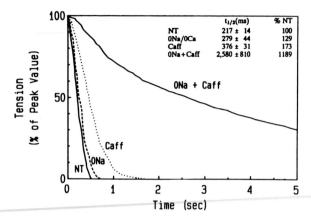

Fig. 15-5. Relaxation of cooling contractures upon rapid re-warming in media containing normal or Na-free Tyrode's solution, with or without 10 mM caffeine as indicated. Reproduced from Bers and Bridge {18}, with permission.

keep this competition in mind when considering the effects of Na/Ca exchange in mediating the inotropic effects of agents (e.g., cardiac glycosides) that affect intracellular Na levels (cf. below).

Other experiments have shown that the Na/Ca exchanger is an important Ca efflux mechanism, even during periods of rest, when [Ca]$_i$ is 100 nM or less {20}. This conclusion is based on studies with rabbit ventricular tissue which indicate that the amount of Ca remaining in the SR declines during a prolonged period of rest and the rate of decline is dependent upon [Na]$_o$ and the ratio of [Na]$_o$ to [Ca]$_o$. Thus, the exchanger can effect a transfer of Ca from internal stores to the cell exterior during rest; this probably reflects the activity of the exchanger in removing Ca from the cytosol and should not be taken to indicate that there is a direct transfer of Ca from the SR to the exterior. There is an interesting species specificity to this effect {21}. In contrast to the data with rabbit ventricular tissue, the SR Ca content in the rat actually *increases* during a prolonged rest. Measurements with ion-selective microelectrodes have shown that rabbit cells exhibit a net loss of Ca during rest while the rat cells exhibit a net gain. The difference between the two species was correlated with a difference in resting [Na]$_i$, which in the rabbit was 9–10 mM and in the rat was 16–17 mM. The increased [Na]$_i$ in the rat decreased the calculated E$_{Na-Ca}$ to a value below that of the resting potential (so that the driving force is in favor of net Ca influx), whereas E$_{Na-Ca}$ > E$_m$ in the rabbit and the driving force favors Ca efflux. These results underscore the sensitivity of the exchange system to changes in [Na]$_i$ and the versatility of its physiological activity.

Ca influx

As indicated in fig. 15-4 there is a brief period of time during which the membrane potential is more positive than the reversal potential for Na/Ca exchange. This

represents the period during which the exchanger could theoretically mediate net Ca influx. What fig. 15-4 does not take into consideration is the possibility that local Na concentrations might be significantly elevated in a restricted space immediately beneath the cardiac sarcolemma. This could result from Na influx through Na channels during the initial phases of the cardiac action potential. Such an elevation in the local Na concentration would further increase the driving force for Ca influx by the Na/Ca exchanger. Experiments have recently been described that support this possibility {22,23}. When Ca channels are blocked, Ca release from the SR can be initiated by a process that is sensitive to the Na channel blocker tetrodotoxin (TTX). This Ca release is dependent upon the presence of extracellular Ca and was not observed if Li was used as a substitute for Na. (Li can be conducted by the Na channel but cannot replace Na in mediating Ca fluxes by Na/Ca exchange.) The results suggested that Ca influx mediated by Na/Ca exchange can initiate Ca release from the SR by a "Ca-induced Ca release process." A TTX-sensitive component of the Ca transient was also observed under more physiological conditions (i.e., in the absence of Ca channel blockers), suggesting that this might be a physiological mechanism that contributes to release of Ca from intracellular stores. At present the importance of this process in cardiac physiology is uncertain. Nevertheless, it is important to recognize the possibility that the exchanger may play multiple roles in mediating Ca fluxes during cardiac function.

Immunohistochemical results conducted with antibodies to the cardiac exchanger indicate that the exchanger is located in the T tubules of the cardiac cell {24,25}. (There is currently disagreement as to whether its distribution is *restricted* to the T-tubules or if it also abundant within the bulk sarcolemma.) In smooth muscle cells, microscopic studies with fluorescently labeled antibodies suggest that the exchanger, the Na, K-ATPase, and underlying SR are distributed within similar domains over the membrane surface {26}. These results with different types of muscle cells raise the possibility that the exchanger is distributed topographically in such a manner as to maximize its influence on the SR. This could be an important factor in the exchanger's ability to regulate the amount of releasable Ca in the SR, as discussed above under *Ca efflux*, or in contributing to the events that trigger Ca release from the SR, as discussed in the preceding paragraph. It should be emphasized, however, that the distribution of the exchanger over the membrane surface and its contribution to initiating Ca release are unsettled issues and that the present evidence is not sufficiently precise to delineate the intimacy of the exchanger's relationship with the SR.

Na/Ca exchange currents and the cardiac action potential

As mentioned previously, the Na/Ca exchanger generates a current during activity due to the charge imbalance inherent in its stoichiometry. One might therefore expect that the current generated by exchanger during Ca efflux would make a contribution to the plateau phase of the action potential. Mathematical models based on the ionic

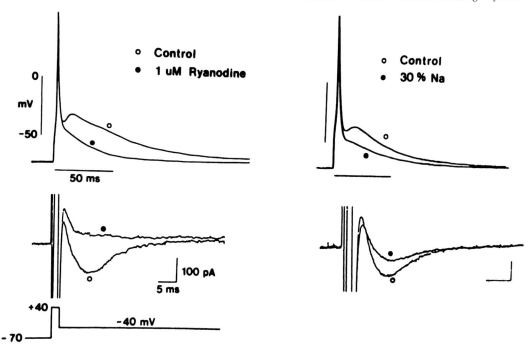

Fig. 15-6. Effect of ryanodine (left) and low Na (right) on action potential (top) and slow inward current (bottom) in rabbit atrial cells. From Noble et al. {27}, with permission.

changes occurring during the cardiac action potential suggest that this is so. In atrial cells, a current has been demonstrated that is dependent on release of intracellular Ca and the presence of extracellular Na (fig. 15-6), and is presumably due to Na/Ca exchange. Abolishing this current by treatment of rabbit atrial cells with ryanodine (which blocks SR Ca release), or by substitution of Na_o with Li_o, dramatically reduces the late plateau phase of the atrial action potential (fig. 15-6) {27}. Thus, in atrial cells the Na/Ca exchange current exerts a profound influence on the shape of the action potential. In ventricular cells, currents due to Na-Ca exchange during an action potential have also been demonstrated {27}, although the prolonged duration of the Ca current and elevated potential of the plateau phase in some species has made its influence on the shape of the action potential more difficult to discern.

Inotropism and Na/Ca exchange

There are a number of agents and conditions, such as digitalis administration or an increase in stimulation frequency, which tend to increase the cytoplasmic concentration of Na. This is associated with an increase in the force of cardiac contraction. As discussed previously, the activation of exchange activity by intracellular Na is dependent upon the second or third power of $[Na]_i$. Moreover, the competitive effect of cytoplasmic Na in blocking Ca efflux increases with $[Na]^2$. Thus, the ability of the exchanger to promote Ca influx, or to inhibit Ca efflux, is highly sensitive to small changes in $[Na]_i$. Remembering that the exchanger and the SR Ca-ATPase compete for cytosolic Ca during relaxation, the sigmoidal dependence of the SR Ca-ATPase on [Ca] will result in a further amplication of the exchanger's effects on the amount of Ca stored in the SR. Finally, the strength of contraction is itself a steeply rising function of the Ca concentration. The overall result is that the amount of Ca stored in the cardiac SR and the strength of contraction that results from its release are exquisitely sensitive to small changes in the intracellular Na ion concentration. Measurements of $[Na]_i$ with ion-selective microelectrodes have indicated that developed tension is proportional to the sixth or seventh power of the intracellular Na ion concentration {28}. Thus, it is no surprise that inotropic interventions that exert only a small effect on $[Na]_i$ can have a disproportionately large effect on the strength of cardiac contraction. The Na/Ca exchanger obviously plays a central role in mediating these effects.

MOLECULAR NATURE OF THE Na/Ca EXCHANGER

The cardiac Na/Ca exchanger has been purified, cloned, and sequenced by Philipson and his colleagues {29}. The deduced amino acid sequence of the protein predicts an M_r of 105 kDa, and it appears in SDS polyacrylamide gels as two bands at approximately 120 and 160 kDa. The

Cardiac Na/Ca Exchanger

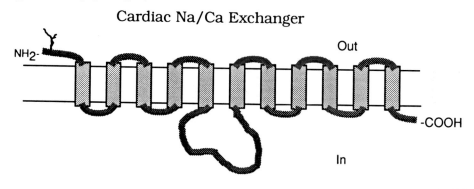

Retinal Rod Na/Ca,K Exchanger

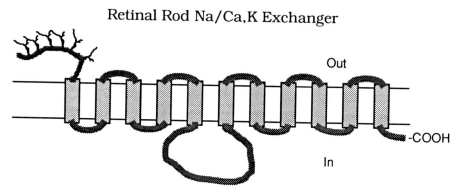

Fig. 15-7. Membrane topology of the cardiac (top) and retinal rod (bottom) exchangers. Transmembrane segments are depicted as shaded recangles within the membrane. Modified from Reeves {4}, with permission.

increase in molecular size over that predicted by the amino acid sequence is probably due to glycosylation of the exchanger. However, the reason for the presence of two bands in SDS gels, as opposed to only a single band, is unknown. COS cells transfected with a clone for the bovine cardiac exchanger exhibit only a single band at approximately 115 kDa, whereas CHO cells transfected with the same clone exhibit two bands, at 130 and 150 kDa. Perhaps the difference between the two types of transfected cells reflects differences in processing or glycosylation of the exchanger during synthesis.

The exchanger is unique among transport carrier proteins in possessing a cleaved, NH$_2$-terminal signal sequence. The signal sequence is a 32 amino acid stretch at the NH$_2$-terminal end of the protein and is a recognition element for the molecular machinery involved in translocating the initial portion of the exchanger to the extracellular surface of the membrane during biosynthesis. The signal sequence is removed from the mature protein by a specific peptidase in the endoplasmic reticulum during synthesis of the protein. The mature protein consists of 938 amino acids and contains 11 hydrophobic stretches that appear to constitute transmembrane segments. A large 520 amino acid cytoplasmic loop is found between

the fifth and sixth putative transmembrane segment. The suggested orientation of the exchanger in the membrane is depicted in fig. 15-7.

The amino acid sequence of the exchanger is highly conserved between mammalian species. The sequences of the cardiac exchangers from dog, cow, cat, and human hearts are more than 95% identical. A substantial fraction of the differences between the species occurs within the 32 amino acid signal sequence. The rabbit renal exchanger has also been cloned and sequenced {30}, and it is nearly identical to the cardiac sequence, although a cluster of amino acid differences, including a 28-residue deletion, is found within a portion of the central hydrophilic domain.

The function of the central hydrophilic domain of the exchanger is unknown. Mutants in which 440 of the 520 amino acids of this region have been deleted carry out Na/Ca exchange with no obvious change in the [Na] or [Ca] dependence of the exchange process, although the overall exchange rate in these mutants is reduced compared to the wild type {31}. Thus, the hydrophilic domain does not appear to be involved in binding or translocation of the transported ions. However, the mutant exchanger does not display secondary activation by cytoplasmic Ca, suggesting that the hydrophilic domain is responsible for

```
NaCa Exchanger....  Y T W L  Y I I L S V S S P G  V V E V W E G L L  T F F F

Na,K-ATPase.......  Y T W L  E A V I F L I G I I  V A N V P E G L L  A T V T
SR Ca-ATPase.......  R G A I  Y Y F K I A V A L A  V A A I P E*G L P  A V I T
PM Ca-ATPase.......  Q Y F V  K F F I I G V T V L  V V A V P E G L P  L A V T
H,K-ATPase........  Y T F I  R A M V F F M A I V  V A Y V P E G L L  A T V T
```

Fig. 15-8. Homology between cardiac Na/Ca exchanger and cation-transporting ATPases. The area within the shaded box shows an average 61% identity between the exchanger and the ATPases in pairwise comparisons. The asterisk indicates the essential glutamate residue in the SR Ca-ATPase, as discussed in the text. Modified from Reeves {4}, with permission.

mediating this mode of regulation of exchange activity. Whether the hydrophilic domain is involved in ATP-dependent regulation is currently under investigation.

The cardiac exchanger is not homologous to any other known protein, although a small region of the exchanger exibits a limited degree of homology to the Na,K-ATPase. This region occurs in the fourth and fifth transmembrane segments immediately prior to the central hydrophilic domain (fig. 15-8). A portion of this sequence is highly conserved among various ATP-dependent cation transporting ATPases; in the sarcoplasmic reticulum (SR) Ca-ATPase, this region contains a glutamate residue (asterisk in fig. 15-8), which has been shown to be essential for Ca transport {32}. Recent experiments have shown that this glutamate residue is also essential for Na/Ca exchange activity (K.D. Philipson, personal communcation). Thus, it seems likely, by analogy to the Ca-ATPase, that the interaction of the exchanger with transported cations involves specific polar residues within the hydrophobic membrane-spanning regions of the exchanger. This conclusion is consistent with the properties of the deletion mutant discussed above, which shows essentially normal K_m values for Na/Ca exchange despite the removal of most of the central hydrophilic domain.

The retinal rod Na/(Ca+K) exchanger has also been cloned and sequenced {33}. The rod exchanger is 1134 amino acids long and, like the cardiac exchanger, contains 11 putative transmembrane domains with a large hydrophilic domain (445 amino acids) between the fifth and sixth transmembrane segment (fig. 15-8). The rod exchanger also appears to exhibit an NH_2-terminal signal sequence. The region of the retinal rod exchanger from the NH_2 terminus to the first transmembrane segment is 380 amino acids long and is much more extensive than the corresponding regions of the cardiac exchanger (40 amino acids); these regions are presumably extracellular due to the presence of the signal sequence. Despite the similarities in membrane topology and in functional activity, there is remarkably little amino acid homology between the two proteins. There are only two regions of these exchangers that show a significant degree of similarity, and these occur within two pairs of membrane-spanning regions on either side of the central hydrophilic domain {33}. It is clear from these results that the two types of exchangers have evolved independently.

CONCLUSIONS

Na/Ca exchange is an important participant in the complex process that regulates the intracellular Ca content and the force of contraction of cardiac muscle. Its role as the predominant Ca efflux mechanism in myocardial cells is now clear, and this activity has a major influence in regulating the amount of Ca stored within the SR through an exquisite sensitivity of the exchange process to $[Na]_i$. Other functions for Na/Ca exchange have been suggested, such as its possible contribution to promoting Ca release in the SR through Na_i-dependent Ca influx and the effects of the exchange current on the shape of the action potential. The cloning of the cardiac exchanger and the application of molecular biological techniques may uncover still other roles for Na/Ca exchange in cardiac physiology.

REFERENCES

1. Blaustein MP, DiPolo R, Reeves JP (eds): Sodium-calcium exchange. *Ann NY Acad Sci* 639, 1991.
2. Reeves JP: Sodium-calcium exchange. In: Bronner F (ed) *Intracellular Calcium Regulation*. New York: Wiley-Liss, 1990, pp 305–347.
3. Philipson KD: The cardiac Na-Ca exchanger. In: Langer GA (ed) *Calcium and the Heart*. New York: Raven Press, 1990, pp 85–108.
4. Reeves JP: Molecular aspects of sodium-calcium exchange. *Arch Biochem Biophys* 292:329–334, 1992.
5. Reeves JP, Hale CC: The stoichiometry of the cardiac sodium-calcium exchange system. *J Biol Chem* 259:7733–7739, 1984.
6. Kimura J, Miyamae S, Noma A: Identification of sodium-calcium exchange current in single ventricular cells of guinea pig. *J Physiol* 384:199–222, 1987.
7. Hilgemann DW: Giant excised cardiac sarcolemmal membrane patches: Sodium and sodium-calcium exchange currents. *Pflügers Arch* 415:247–249, 1989.
8. Schnetkamp PPM, Basu DK, Szerencsei RT: Na-Ca exchange in bovine rod outer segments requires and transports K. *Am J Physiol* 257:C153–C157, 1989.
9. Cervetto L, Lagnado L, Perry RJ, Robinson DW, McNaughton PA: Extrusion of calcium from rod outer segments is driven by both sodium and potassium gradients. *Nature* 337:740–743, 1989.
10. Li J, Kimura J: Translocation mechanism of cardiac Na-Ca exchange. *Ann NY Acad Sci* 639:48–60, 1991.

11. DiPolo R, Beaugé: Regulation of Na-Ca exchange. An overview. *Ann NY Acad Sci* 639:100–111, 1991.
12. Schnetkamp PPM, Basu DK, Li X-B, Szerencsei RT: Regulation of intracellular free Ca concentration in the outer segments of bovine retinal rods by Na-Ca-K exchange measured with fluro-3. II. Thermodynamic competence of transmembrane Na and K gradients and inactivation of Na-dependent Ca extrusion. *J Biol Chem* 266:22983–22990, 1991.
13. Collins A, Somlyo AV, Hilgemann DW: The giant cardiac membrane patch method: Stimulation of outward Na-Ca exchange current by MgATP. *J Physiol* 454:27–57, 1992.
14. Hilgemann DW, Collins A: Mechanism of cadiac Na-Ca exchange current stimulation by MgATP: Possible involvement of aminophospholipid translocase. *J Physiol* 454:59–82, 1992.
15. Vemuri R, Philipson KD: Phospholipid composition modulates the Na-Ca exchange activity of cardiac sarcolemma in reconstituted vesicles. *Biochim Biophys Acta* 937:258–268, 1987.
16. Wier WG, Beuckelmann DJ: Sodium-calcium exchange in mammalian heart: Current-voltage relation and intracellular calcium concentration. *Mol Cell Biochem* 89:97–102, 1989.
17. Hilgemann DW: Extracellular calcium transients and action potential configuration changes related to post-stimulatory potentiation in rabbit atrium. *J Gen Physiol* 87:675–706, 1986.
18. Bers DM, Bridge JHB: Relaxation of rabbit ventricular muscle by Na-Ca exchange and sarcoplasmic reticulum calcium pump. Ryanodine and voltage sensitivity. *Circ Res* 65:334–342, 1989.
19. Bers DM, Lederer WJ, Berlin JR: Intracellular Ca transients in rat cardiac myocytes: Role of Na-Ca exchange in excitation-contraction coupling. *Am J Physiol* 258:C944–C954, 1990.
20. Sutko JL, Bers DM, Reeves JP: Postrest inotropy in rabbit ventricle: Na-Ca exchange determines sarcoplasmic reticulum Ca content. *Am J Physiol* 250:H654–H661, 1986.
21. Shattock MJ, Bers DM: Rat vs. rabbit ventricle: Ca flux and intracellular Na assessed by ion-selective microelectrodes. *Am J Physiol* 256:C813–C822, 1989.
22. Leblanc N, Hume JR: Sodium current-induced release of calcium from cardiac sarcoplasmic reticulum. *Science* 248:372–375, 1990.
23. Levesque PV, LeBlanc N, Hume JR: Role of reverse Na-Ca exchange in excitation-contraction coupling in the heart. *Ann NY Acad Sci* 639:386–397, 1991.
24. Frank JS, Mottino G, Reid D, Molday RS, Philipson KD: Distribution of the Na-Ca exchange protein in mammalian cardiac myocytes: An immunofluorescence and immunocolloidal gold-labelling study. *J Cell Biol* 117:337–345, 1992.
25. Kieval RS, Bloch RJ, Lindenmayer GE, Ambesi A, Lederer WJ: Immunogluorescence localization of the Na-Ca exchanger in heart cells. *Am J Physiol* 263:C545–C550, 1992.
26. Moore EDW, Fogarty KE, Fay FS: Role of Na-Ca exchanger in β-adrenergic relaxation of single smooth muscle cells. *Ann NY Acad Sci* 639:543–549, 1991.
27. Noble D, Noble SJ, Bett GCL, Earm YE, Ho WK, So IK: The role of sodium-calcium exchange during the cardiac action potential. *Ann NY Acad Sci* 639:334–353, 1991.
28. Lee CO: 200 years of digitalis: The merging central role of the sodium in the control of cardiac force. *Am J Physiol* 249:C367–C378, 1985.
29. Nicoll DA, Longoni S, Philipson KD: Molecular cloning and functional expression of the cardiac sarcolemmal Na-Ca exchanger. *Science* 250:562–565, 1990.
30. Reilly RF, Shugrue CA: cDNA cloning of a renal Na-Ca exchanger. *Am J Physiol* 262:F1105–F1109, 1992.
31. Matsuiko S, Nicoll DA, Reilly RF, Hilgemann DW, Philipson KD: Identification of regulatory regions of the cardiac sarcolemmal Na-Ca exchanger. *Proc Natl Acad Sci USA* 90:3870–3874, 1991.
32. Clarke DM, Loo TW, Inesi G, MacLennan DH: Location of high affinity Ca-binding sites within the predicted transmembrane domain of the sarcoplasmic reticulum Ca-ATPase. *Nature* 339:476–478, 1989.
33. Reiländer H, Achilles A, Friendel U, Maul G, Lottspeich F, Cook NJ: Primary structure and functional expression of the Na/Ca, K exchanger from bovine rod photoreceptors. *EMBO J* 11:1689–1695, 1992.
34. Reeves JP: Na-Ca exchange, [Ca]$_i$ and myocardial contractility. In: Stone HL, Weglicki SB (eds) *Pathobiology of Cardiovascular Injury*. Boston: Martinus Nijhoff, 1985, pp 232–243.
35. Durkin JT, Ahrens DC, Aceto JF, Condrescu M, Reeves JP: Molecular and functional studies of the cardiac sodium-calcium exchanger. *Ann NY Acad Sci* 639:189–201, 1991.

CHAPTER 16

Basic Calculations of Transsarcolemmal Calcium Movements in Cardiac Excitation-Contraction Coupling

CLIVE MARC BAUMGARTEN & ALEXANDRE FABIATO

INTRODUCTION

The mechanism of excitation-contraction coupling is not established for any type of muscle {1}. In cardiac muscle there is not even universal agreement on whether Ca^{2+} is released from the sarcoplasmic reticulum (SR) during excitation-contraction coupling. This will be this question addressed in this chapter. In the discussion of the question, emphasis will be placed on estimation of the Ca^{2+} fluxes across the sarcolemma and their possible relationships with the Ca^{2+} movements in and out of the SR. A detailed description of the simple calculations that permit this correlation will provide a tool for a critical analysis of the literature.

Since previous editions of this book appeared {2,3} there have been important advances in studies of sodium-calcium exchange and of the calcium channel in the heart sarcolemma. Quantitative models of sodium-calcium exchange have been developed to estimate calcium entry and efflux by this mechanism {4–11}, direct measurements of the sodium-calcium exchange current have been made {12–24}, and the cardiac exchanger protein has been cloned and expressed {25}.

New results have also changed the views on calcium channels {26–28}. First, two types of channels have been identified in heart {29–32}. The L Ca^{2+} channel inactivates more slowly, is affected by catecholamines and dihydropyridine calcium blockers, corresponds to the calcium current most often studied previously, and is thought to have a role in excitation-contraction coupling. It is now clear that L calcium channels undergo both a voltage-dependent and a calcium-dependent inactivation {33,34}. The second type of Ca^{2+} channel, the T channel, activates transiently with both a negative threshold and a rapid voltage-dependent inactivation, requires a negative holding potential to be observed, and is insensitive to catecholamines and dihydropyridines. Under physiologic conditions the T channel probably comprises less than 10% of the total calcium current {26,27,29,30}. Some have suggested that the T Ca^{2+} channel may be involved in triggering the release of Ca^{2+} from the SR {35}. The low T-channel density, small current at the plateau voltage, and apparent absence of T Ca^{2+} channels in some ventricular muscle studies argue its role in excitationcontraction

coupling is likely to be minor, however. Finally, the L Ca^{2+} channel α_1 subunit, the pore-containing portion of the molecule, has been cloned and expressed {36,37}.

Despite these new pieces of information about calcium channels and sodium-calcium exchange, it is not certain that we are more able to estimate the transmembrane calcium fluxes during the action potential than 6 years ago {3} because of the following difficulties. Studies of single calcium channels often use high concentrations of unphysiologic divalent cations, such as barium, as charge carriers instead of calcium. These high concentrations of divalent cations shield surface charge and may have direct effects on the channels, altering their conductances, voltage dependence, and kinetics. Intracellular ions are also substituted. Often ethyleneglycol-bis(β-aminoethyl ether)-N,N'-tetraacetic acid (EGTA) is added to the intracellular solution. Consequently, the calcium-dependent inactivation that is seen under physiologic conditions may be reduced. Thus one cannot simply take the calcium current observed under nonphysiologic experimental conditions for computations of the physiologic transsarcolemmal calcium influx {38}. Similar arguments can be made regarding Ca^{2+} fluxes mediated by Na^+-Ca^{2+} exchange. In order to isolate this exchange current from other membrane currents, investigators are forced to modify ionic conditions and to utilize a variety of blockers with imperfect selectivity. Although we know more about the mechanism of calcium entry and efflux, we still cannot be certain of the amplitude of the fluxes under physiologic conditions. The principles relating transmembrane calcium fluxes to the calcium transient in the cell remain the same as in previous versions of this chapter {2,3}, and the present chapter reviews some of these principles.

EVIDENCE FOR A CALCIUM RELEASE FROM THE CARDIAC SARCOPLASMIC RETICULUM

Detailed analyses of the force-frequency relationships of the adult mammalian heart have generally been interpreted as evidence that the Ca^{2+} influx across the sarcolemma during one action potential is not entirely used for activating the myofilaments during the corresponding contraction, but rather, fills a store with Ca^{2+} that can be

N. Sperelakis (ed.), Physiology and Pathophysiology of the Heart, Third Edition.

released during subsequent contractions {39–41}. These experiments do not, however, provide clues to the ultrastructural location of the Ca^{2+} store.

Pharmacologic tools acting specifically on the SR would help in locating the Ca^{2+} store in the SR {42}. Caffeine often has been used for this purpose because it is well established that it specifically releases Ca^{2+} from the skeletal muscle SR. Unfortunately, the situation is more complex in cardiac muscle, where caffeine has multiple sites of action, including the sarcolemma {43}. Ryanodine modulates the SR Ca^{2+} release channel with relatively high selectivity but presents the disadvantage of an irreversibility of action {44}. Nevertheless, recent experiments with ryanodine favor the SR as the primary Ca^{2+} storage site in mammalian cardiac muscle, as discussed below.

Until recently, the evidence suggesting that the Ca^{2+} store is located in the SR came mostly from experiments in preparations permitting direct access to the SR, including isolated SR vesicles and skinned cardiac cells. These studies demonstrate that the SR has the capacity to store the amount of Ca^{2+} necessary to activate the myofilaments sufficiently to produce the physiologic contraction {45–47}. In skinned cardiac cells it is possible to ascertain that the Ca^{2+} release by caffeine comes from the SR since the sarcolemma has been removed {48}. It is also possible to destroy the ability of the SR to actively accumulate and release Ca^{2+} by detergent treatment; then the Ca^{2+} store disappears {48}. Some skinned cardiac cells, such as those from mammalian atrium {48}, dog Purkinje tissue {49}, and pigeon ventricle {49}, do not contain transverse tubules. The observation of a Ca^{2+} release in these preparations demonstrates that the transverse tubules are not the Ca^{2+} storage site {48,49}. Finally, the mitochondria do not appear to be able to accumulate Ca^{2+} when the myoplasmic [free Ca^{2+}] is in the physiologically relevant range, whereas they do accumulate Ca^{2+}, but extremely slowly, at unphysiologically high myoplasmic [free Ca^{2+}] {48}. In addition, inhibitors and uncouplers of the mitochondrial respiration do not modify the Ca^{2+} release from the internal store at physiologically relevant myoplasmic [free Ca^{2+}] {48}. These findings demonstrate that the mitochondria cannot be the intracellular storage site. Therefore, the data from skinned cardiac cells permit the firm conclusion that Ca^{2+} can be released from the SR, at least in these preparations.

More recently evidence favoring the SR as the Ca^{2+} storage site has been obtained from intact cardiac cells treated with ryanodine. It has been found that ryanodine depresses the Ca^{2+} transient by up to 90% in isolated intact guinea pig {50,51} and rat {52,53} ventricular myocytes. At low concentrations, ryanodine causes a depletion of the SR Ca^{2+} stores by forcing the SR Ca^{2+} release channels to open nearly continuously to a subconductance level but, at higher concentrations, it closes the release channel {22,53–56}. In either case, ryanodine limits the contribution of the SR. The depression of the Ca^{2+} transient by ryanodine does not appear to result from any effects on I_{Ca}. For example, at a concentration sufficient to depress fura-2 fluorescence during the Ca^{2+}

transient by a factor of four, ryanodine had no effect on peak I_{Ca} or its voltage dependence, although the rate of I_{Ca} decay was slowed {52}. If anything, slowing the decay of I_{Ca} should enhance the Ca^{2+} transient rather than depress it.

ARGUMENTS AGAINST A CALCIUM RELEASE FROM THE SARCOPLASMIC RETICULUM

Although the subcellular preparations permit a direct access to the SR, the techniques used to obtain them may damage this organelle and give it unphysiologic properties {1,48}. This criticism is very difficult to answer in a definitive manner. Effort has been made to evaluate and correct some of the unphysiologic conditions of the skinned cardiac cells: unphysiologic level of myoplasmic [free Mg^{2+}], excessive Ca^{2+} loading of the SR, and swelling of the SR {48}. Nevertheless, it is obviously not possible to identify and correct all of the potentially unphysiologic conditions created by skinning of the membrane and substitution of computed solutions for the intracellular milieu. Therefore the conclusion that Ca^{2+} can be released from the SR is still widely open to alternative hypotheses. These hypotheses are of two types: (a) those admitting the presence of an intracellular Ca^{2+} store, but suggesting that its location is in structures other than the SR; and (b) those assuming that activation is possible by direct transsarcolemmal influx without the help of Ca^{2+} release from an internal store.

Among the first type of hypotheses suggesting an intracellular Ca^{2+} store different from the SR, it has been proposed that the mitochondria could be the storage site {57}. But this hypothesis has been almost completely abandoned because the affinity of the mitochondria for Ca^{2+} and their rate of Ca^{2+} accumulation and release are much too low to account for the physiologic changes of myoplasmic [free Ca^{2+}] known to take place inside the cardiac cell {48,58,59}.

Another hypothesis locates the store in high-affinity, *polarization-dependent* binding sites at the inner face of the sarcolemma {41,60}. It has been proposed that these sites could be acidic lipids such as phosphatidylserine {60}, which is observed at a high concentration in the isolated sarcolemmal preparation {61}. It is not possible to eliminate such a possibility, although it is not supported by any direct evidence. If this hypothesis were supported by data, the presence of binding sites inside the sarcolemma would not eliminate the possibility of additional Ca^{2+} storage in the SR {62}. The concept of *polarization dependence* renders the hypothesis difficult to exclude. Otherwise, the Ca^{2+} binding sites studied in isolated sarcolemmal vesicles have a very low affinity (in the range of $10^4 M^{-1}$ at most) in the presence of the physiologic myoplasmic concentrations of K^+ and Mg^{2+} {63,64}. Evidence from Ca^{2+} indicator studies in voltage-clamped guinea pig {50,51} and rat {52,65} myocytes indicates, however, that depolarization without Ca^{2+} entry cannot induce the rapid rise in [Ca^{2+}]$_i$ associated with a normal contraction. Upon strong depolarizations to potentials positive to the Ca^{2+} equilibrium potential, $[Ca^{2+}]_i$ increased only slowly and was attributable to Na^+-Ca^{2+} exchange. A rapid Ca^{2+} transient was observed in these experiments on *repolarization*, however. It appears to be initiated by the small transsarcolemmal influx of Ca^{2+} during the brief Ca^{2+} tail current {66} that occurs on repolarization. These data are quite different from those in skeletal muscle, where neither Ca^{2+} transients nor Ca^{2+} tail currents are observed on repolarization {68}. Furthermore, neither the Ca^{2+} transient nor cell shortening occurs in rat ventricular myocytes when depolarizations result in entry of Na^+ or Ba^{2+} rather than Ca^{2+} through Ca^{2+} channels {68}. These observations on Ca^{2+} transients build on earlier studies comparing the voltage dependence of the Ca^{2+} current and tension and argue against both depolarization per se {69–71} and a depolarization-dependent release of Ca^{2+} from sarcolemmal binding sites (this article) as the mechanism of excitation-contraction coupling.

The second type of hypotheses negates any intracellular release of Ca^{2+} {72,73}. To raise this possibility appears legitimate in view of the following findings: (a) the removal of Ca^{2+} from the bathing fluid results in the disappearance of cardiac contraction within a few tens of seconds {74} while the action potential remains present {75}[1]; and (b) the peak of the Ca^{2+} transient has a bell-shaped voltage dependence that matches the voltage dependence of I_{Ca} {50–52,65}. These observations support the conclusion that transsarcolemmal influx of Ca^{2+} is an essential step in excitation-contraction coupling of cardiac muscle, but they by no means exclude the possiblitiy of an additional release of Ca^{2+} from an intracellular store {2,63,76}. The argument most often used to exclude the release of Ca^{2+} from the SR is a quantitative one: there is enough Ca^{2+} bound outside the sarcolemma to activate the myofilaments directly {72}. This argument can be challenged at two levels. First, even if it were demonstrated that there is enough Ca^{2+} influx across the sarcolemma to activate the myofilaments directly, this would not eliminate the possibility that an intracellular store of Ca^{2+}, such as the SR, could modify the transsarcolemmal Ca^{2+} before it reaches the myofilaments {48}. Thus, for instance, most of the transsarcolemmal Ca^{2+} influx could be accumulated into the SR, while an approximately equal amount would be released from the SR. Secondly, this quantitative argument is not yet supported by data. Neither the transsarcolemmal Ca^{2+} influx necessary to activate the myofilaments directly nor the actual value of the systolic transsarcolemmal Ca^{2+} influx has yet been established with certainty.

The amount of transsarcolemmal Ca^{2+} influx that would be necessary for activating the myofilaments directly is discussed in detail by Fabiato {77}, taking into account what was known in 1982 of the intracellular calcium buffering in the cardiac cell. More recent analyses by Sipido and Wier {66} and Bers {78} modify the calcium buffering parameters used by Fabiato {77} only slightly. The computer program used to generate the relation between any increase of myoplasmic total calcium resulting from

transsarcolemmal calcium influx and the resulting increase of myoplasmic [free Ca^{2+}] is available {79}.[2]

The systolic transsarcolemmal Ca^{2+} influx is not known either. Displacement of Ca^{2+} by lanthanum {72}, an ion that does not cross the sarcolemma, only establishes the presence of a pool of Ca^{2+} superficial to the surface membrane; this is, at least qualitatively, consistent with the large binding capacity of the isolated sarcolemmal vesicles {61–64,80}. Compartmental analysis of the ionic flux data with ^{45}Ca {72} is difficult in the presence of multiple potential compartments {81}. This analysis confirms that the lanthanum-displaceable Ca^{2+} is superficially located {72}; but since it is done through the integration of many beats, the compartmental analysis does not indicate at what time during the cardiac cycle the superficial Ca^{2+} enters the cell and does not permit a quantification of what fraction of superficial Ca^{2+} enters the cell. The very interesting measurements of systolic Ca^{2+} influx with Ca^{2+} ion-selective electrodes {82–86} or antipyrylazo III or tetramethylmurexide {87–90} are still open to many potential technical problems, and hence, will not be analyzed here. Therefore, the only data for quantifying the systolic transsarcolemmal influx of Ca^{2+} discussed here are those derived from voltage-clamp studies. The rationale for the calculation of the transsarcolemmal influx from these voltage-clamp studies is explained in the next section.

ESTIMATE OF THE TRANSSARCOLEMMAL CALCIUM INFLUX THROUGH THE CALCIUM CURRENT

Voltage-clamp studies demonstrate a slow inward current (I_{si}), which is distinguished from the fast Na^+ inward current by the fact that it is not inhibited by tetrodotoxin {91}. This current is largely attributable to Ca^{2+} influx {92,93, cf. 94} and more recently has been referred to as the Ca^{2+} current (I_{Ca}). In the past, the amplitude of the Ca^{2+} current has been difficult to estimate, in part because of the superimposition of outward K^+ currents. If I_{Ca} can be isolated from other currents, it is possible to calculate the transsarcolemmal Ca^{2+} influx caused by the Ca^{2+} current and to consider whether the Ca^{2+} influx is of sufficient magnitude to directly activate the myofilaments. Measurements of the Ca^{2+} current using the whole-cell variant of the patch-clamp technique provide superior voltage control and excellent separation of currents by dialyzing the cell's interior with impermeant K^+ substitutes. We have chosen not to use such studies for the present calculation, however, in part because of the uncertain effects on I_{Ca} of dialysis with EGTA and of the loss of soluble intracellular modulators of Ca^{2+} channels and soluble intracellular Ca^{2+} buffers. Instead, we will illustrate the principles involved using data from Marban and Tsien {91}, who measured I_{Ca} with a two-microelectrode voltage clamp in a multicellular strand of Purkinje fibers from the calf after blocking the superimposed currents. The experiments were done in the presence of

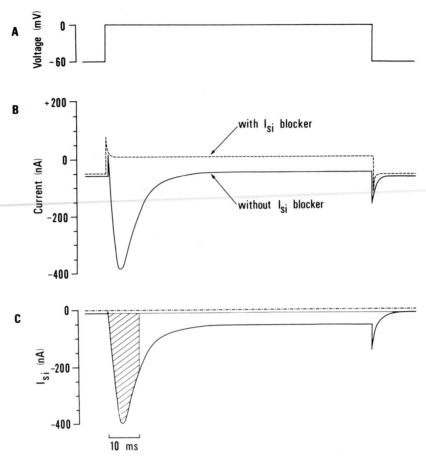

Fig. 16-1. Schematic representation of the fast and slow components of the slow inward current derived from experiments by Marban and Tsien {91} and others (as referenced in the text). The fiber was treated with tetrodotoxin to block the fast sodium current and cesium loaded to block the outward K$^+$ current. **A:** Voltage-clamp step. **B:** Current with D-600 treatment (dotted curve) and without D-600 (solid curve). Note that the capacitance currents at the onset of the end of the clamp step have been modified to avoid superimposition. **C:** Difference between solid and dotted curve, which represents the time course of the Ca^{2+} current (I$_{Ca}$). The area used for integrating the initial fast component of Ca^{2+} current is hatched. This integration over 10 ms yields an average value of 70% of peak I$_{Ca}$.

tetrodotoxin to block the Na$^+$ current and after cesium loading to block the outward K$^+$ currents.

The following equation can be derived to calculate the Ca^{2+} influx by the slow inward current:

$$\frac{d[\text{total Ca}]}{dt} = \int_0^t \frac{J}{zF} \times \frac{S}{V} \times \frac{f_i}{f_v}, \qquad (16\text{-}1)$$

where d[total Ca] = change in myoplasmic total calcium concentration in mol/l (M) (no ionic charge is shown to emphasize that total rather than free calcium is meant); dt = change in time, from 0 to t (s); J = current density (current/surface area) (coul/s·cm^2); z = valence, for Ca^{2+} = 2 (dimensionless); F = Faraday's constant, 9.65×10^4 (coul/mol); S/V = surface/volume ratio (cm^2/l); f$_i$ = fraction of I$_{si}$ carried by Ca^{2+} (dimensionless); and f$_v$ = fraction of cell volume Ca^{2+} enters (dimensionless).

The calcium current per surface area [variable J in eq. (16-1)] can be calculated as follows: Upon depolarization from −60 to 0 mV (fig. 16-1A), an inward current rapidly turns on and reaches a peak (fig. 16-1B, solid curve) in about 5 ms. Then the current largely inactivates in about 20 ms to reach a plateau of remaining inward current while the depolarization is maintained. Upon repolarization the current returns to its original value. Exposure to a calcium channel blocker (such as D-600) abolishes the transient inward current and shifts the current in an outward direction to a given level (fig. 16-1B, dotted curve). The difference between this level of current obtained with D-600 and the time-dependent current obtained without D-600 permits an inference {95} of the time course and magnitude to the calcium current (fig. 16-1C). In the schematic drawing of fig. 16-1C, the amplitude of the peak current was $5 \times 10^{-6} \text{A/cm}^2$ (from Marban and Tsien {91}). D-600 experiments revealed a noninactivating component of the calcium current that was about 20% of peak current at 0 mV, whereas some noninactivating Ca^{2+} current remained after repolarization to -60 mV.

The level of noninactivating Ca^{2+} current shown in fig. 16-1 was not directly derived from the data of Marban and Tsien {91}, but was an average estimate derived from a critical review of the literature on the experiments with Ca^{2+} channel blockers. Accurate measurements of noninactivating Ca^{2+} current require a highly selective blockage, which is unlikely {96} unless all K^+ currents are blocked. Estimates vary widely in different preparations {26,97} and also vary in the same preparation when different blocking agents are applied. For example, studies with D-600 in calf Purkinje fibers {95,98} suggest that up to 50% of calcium channels do not inactivate during depolarizatin to 0 mV. After calf Purkinje fibers have been loaded with cesium to block the outward current, however, the shift of the late current in an outward direction by D-600 suggests that only about 20% of the current does not inactivate at -10 mV (fig. 7C in Marban and Tsien {91}). Yet, exposure to manganese shifts that late current in an inward direction, a result that cannot be explained simply by a blockade of noninactivating calcium channels (fig. 7B in Marban and Tsien {91}). In isolated cardiac cells, estimates also range from 15% in cow ventricular cells {99} to 50% in guinea pig ventricular cells {100}. On the other hand, there is no evidence for noninactivating calcium current channels in guinea pig or cat ventricular muscle, rabbit sinoatrial node, and rat ventricular muscle treated with cobalt {101,102}, D-600 {99,103,104}, or verapamil {105}.

The percentage of calcium channels that remain noninactivated near the resting potential is even more controversial. No steady-state calcium current was found at -40 mV in one study {98}, while 20–25% of the peak current was found at -60 mV in another study {100}.

Although the selectivity of the channel is quite high {92,93}, all of the current measured as I_{Ca} is not carried by Ca^{2+}. Recent studies on single-cell preparations under relative physiologic conditions find a reversal potential of near +50 mV {92}, and some Na^+ and K^+ must also pass through the channel. The fraction of I_{Ca} carried by Ca^{2+} in Marban and Tsien's experiments {91} can be estimated by using the approach of Reuter and Scholz {94, cf. 92,93}. Assuming that the constant-field equation applies, permeability ratios can be calculated from the reversal potential for the slow inward current at different extracellular $[Ca^{2+}]$ and from the intracellular and extracellular ion activities. The data of Marban and Tsien {91} are reasonably fitted by a ratio of permeabilities to Ca^{2+} and Na^+, respectively, P_{Ca}/P_{Na} of about 100, and a ratio P_{Ca}/P_K of about 200. These ratios are independent of voltage, although the current carried by Ca^{2+} is dependent on voltage. Then, at 0 mV the fraction of slow inward current carried by Ca^{2+} is estimated as 0.9 [variable f_i in eq. (16-1)]. Different assumptions regarding surface potential could raise this estimate, and higher permeability ratios, e.g., $P_{Ca}/P_{Na} \sim 1000$ and $P_{Ca}/P_K \sim 10,000$, have

been estimated in isolated myocytes {92}. On the other hand, the constant-field calculations of the current carried by each permeant ion can be criticized, especially when applied to the Ca^{2+} channel. In several instances, ions with higher permeabilities as judged by E_{rev} have lower single-channel conductances {93}. For this analysis, which is intended to determine whether Ca^{2+} entry via sarcolemmal calcium channels is sufficient to activate the myofilaments directly, using 0.9 or 1.0 as the fraction of the calcium current carried by Ca^{2+} does not alter the conclusion, and much larger variations in the magnitude of the peak calcium current have been reported.

We were unable to find values for the surface-volume ratio for the calf Purkinje tissue. For Purkinje tissue of sheep another ungulate, a value of $0.39 \times 10^7 \text{cm}^2/\text{l}$ has been reported {106}. This value will be used for the ratio, S/V, in eq. (16-1). Data on the fraction of the cell volume that Ca^{2+} enters are also lacking. As a first approximation, we will assume that Ca^{2+} is excluded from the volume of the mitochondria. The mitochondrial volume fraction, again from the sheep Purkinje tissue data, is 0.103 {106}. Thus, the variable f_v in eq. (16-1) is 0.897.

This simple approach implicitly assumes that calcium entry from discrete channels gives rise to a spatially homogenous increase in myoplasmic [free Ca^{2+}]. Ca^{2+} gradients certainly may occur close to the sarcolemmal Ca^{2+} channels but are thought to decay in <1 μm {107}. During a normal contraction, Ca^{2+} determined with digital imaging fluorescence microscopy appears to be uniform {108}. This method is, however, unlikely to have sufficient spatial resolution to detect critical gradients, which may occur over distances much smaller than one sarcomere. Finite-element analysis has been used to estimate the spatial and temporal gradients of Ca^{2+} based on estimates of transmembrane and SR Ca^{2+} fluxes and Ca^{2+} binding to intracellular buffer {109}. This analysis suggests that Ca^{2+} release from junctional SR is likely to result in up to a twofold Ca^{2+} gradient over a distance <1 μm during the rising phase of the intracellular Ca^{2+} transient. The gradient is expected to reach its peak at 40 ms, to be greater longitudinally than radially, and to dissipate within 70 ms. During the rising phase of the Ca^{2+} transient detected by indo-1 in atrial myocytes, the simultaneously measured Na^+-Ca^{2+} exchange current is greater than at the same $[Ca^{2+}]_i$ during the failing phase {110}. These data are consistent with the idea that Ca^{2+} higher immediately under the membrane than on average. A subsarcolemmal accumulation of Ca^{2+} was first proposed on the basis of shifts in the E_{rev} for the Ca^{2+} current a number of years ago, along with a quantitative model of Ca^{2+} movements, diffusion, and binding {111}.

There is also uncertainty about how much of the Ca^{2+} current might be used for activating the corresponding contraction. Obviously, the late slow component of the Ca^{2+} influx, corresponding to noninactivated slow inward channels, cannot be responsible for the level of peak tension, since this current continues after the tension has already reached its peak. Yet it is difficult to decide how much of the initial peak of relatively fast Ca^{2+} current is used for generating the peak tension. If one decides, as shown in fig. 16-1 (hatched area), that the initial 10 ms of the Ca^{2+} current are responsible for the peak tension, then the integration of the current during this initial 10 ms gives an average current amplitude equal to 70% of the peak Ca^{2+} current. Since in the experiments of Marban and Tsien {91} the peak Ca^{2+} current was 5×10^{-6} A, the parameter $\int_t^0 J$ in eq. (16-1) is $0.70 \times 5 \times 10^{-6}$.

Substituting these values in eq. (16-1) gives a rate of Ca^{2+} influx of

$$\frac{d[\text{total Ca}]}{dt} = \frac{0.70 \times 5 \times 10^{-6}}{2 \times 9.6 \times 10^4} \times 0.39 \times 10^7 \times \frac{0.90}{0.897}$$

$$= 71 \times 10^{-6} \text{ M/s},$$

which gives an increase of [total Ca] in the myoplasm of 0.71 µM during the initial 10 ms.

If one decides instead that the initial 20 ms are responsible for generating the peak tension, then the integration from 0 to 20 ms gives an average current amplitude of 50% of the peak current. It is just necessary to replace 0.70 by 0.50 to obtain

$$\frac{d[\text{total Ca}]}{dt} = 51 \times 10^{-6} \text{ M/s},$$

which gives an increase of [total Ca] in the myoplasm of 1.0 µM during the initial 20 ms. Considering what is known of the intracellular Ca^{2+} buffers {66,77,79}, this increase of [total Ca] would produce an increase of [free Ca^{2+}] that would be unquestionably insufficient to induce any direct activation of the myofilaments.[2]

Some recent experiments in single cardiac cells permit the calculations of higher values of increase of [total Ca] during an action potential. The reason for these higher values is uncertain, although a partial explanation may be that series resistance in a multicellular preparation causes an underestimate of the slow inward current {99}. We have calculated the increase of [total Ca] during the peak slow inward current measured by Isenberg and Klöckner {99} in isolated adult rat ventricular cells. These investigators found a peak current of 2.8×10^{-9} A during voltage clamp at 0 mV, but they did not relate the current to membrane surface area. The current density can be obtained as follows. An isolated adult rat cardiac cell has an average length of 93 µm, width of 19 µm, and thickness of 11 µm {46}, which gives a volume of 19.4×10^{-12} l. The surface-volume ratio of the rat ventricular cell is 0.44×10^7 cm²/l {112}. Then,

$$S = S/V \times V = 0.44 \times 10^7 \times 19.4 \times 10^{-12} = 8.54 \times 10^{-5} \text{ cm}^2$$

Thus, the peak current is

$$I/S = 2.8 \times 10^{-9}/8.54 \times 10^{-5} = 32.8 \times 10^{-6} \text{ A/cm}^2.$$

The fraction of cell volume occupied by the mitochondria in rat ventricular cells is 0.34 {112}. Thus variable f_v in eq. (16-1) is 0.66. One can estimate the fraction of slow inward current carried by Ca^{2+} (variable f_i) to be 0.90 as previously. Finally, we have assumed that the Ca^{2+} current in the study by Isenberg and Klöckner {99} has the same time course as that observed in the study by Marban and Tsien {91}. On the one hand, the time course of the slow

inward current in single cells might be expected to be faster than in multicellular preparations because the series resistance is lower. On the other, the time course observed by Marban and Tsien {91} is already much more rapid than found in other multicellular preparations.

Substituting these values in eq. (16-1) and integrating the current during the initial 10 ms gives a rate of increase of [total Ca] of 714×10^{-6} M/s, thus an increase of [total Ca] of 7.14 µM during the initial 10 ms. If the integration is done during the initial 20 ms, then the increase of myoplasmic [total Ca] is 10.2 µM. With such a change in [total Ca], precise calculations of the amount of Ca^{2+} buffering inside a cardiac cell are required to decide whether this Ca^{2+} influx is sufficient to partially activate the myofilaments. These computations are reported elsewhere with the conclusion that this Ca^{2+} influx would be insufficient to activate the myofilaments directly {77,79}.[1] Although there is considerable variation in the magnitude of I_{Ca} reported, the 2.8 nA peak current considered here {99} is larger than average for ventricular cells; I_{Ca} often is in the range of ~1–1.5 nA {51,52}.

The preceding computations and discussion of Isenberg and Klöckner {99} were those of earlier versions of this chapter {2,3}, and they are maintained here to explain the rationale for such calculations. The increase of [total Ca] caused by the Ca^{2+} current in isolated bovine cardiac myocytes now has been computed by Isenberg {113}. A detailed discussion of these highly pertinent data can be found in Fabiato {77}.

COMPUTATION OF THE SODIUM-CALCIUM EXCHANGE

To infer the direction of the net flux of calcium across the sarcolemma during rest and during Ca^{2+} release from the SR shown in fig. 16-2, the information relative to the intracellular [free Ca^{2+}] and [free Na^+] and on the coupling ratio of the Na^+-Ca^{2+} exchange were critically reviewed previously {2}. The free ion values have been expressed in terms of activity. Translation to free concentrations can be obtained by dividing the values by the activity coefficients at 37°C: 0.74 for Na^+ and 0.32 for Ca^{2+} {115}. The ion activities are identified by the symbol a followed by a subscript indicating the ion and a superscript o for the external activity or i for the myoplasmic activity. The following values were selected: $a_{Na}^o = 115 \times 10^{-3}$ M; $a_{Na}^i = 6.4 \times 10^{-3}$ M {115}; $a_{Ca}^o = 0.58 \times 10^{-3}$ M; resting $a_{Ca}^i = 2.56 \times 10^{-8}$ M (from skinned cardiac cell experiments {46}; a critical review {2} of the data from Ca^{2+} ion-selective electrodes {115–117} gave somewhat higher values, but potential errors in this method tend to cause overestimation of a_{Ca}^i; a typical fura-2 estimate for resting a_{Ca}^i is 3.2×10^{-8} M {51}. In the hypothesis of a Ca^{2+} release from the SR, the Ca^{2+} influx across the sarcolemma would result in an a_{Ca}^i of at least 6.4×10^{-8} M {46,77}. The maximum Ca^{2+} activity reached during Ca^{2+} release would be 1.28×10^{-6} M {46,77}. In the hypothesis of a direct activation of the myofilaments by the trans-sarcolemmal Ca^{2+} influx, the influx would cause a_{Ca}^i to increase to no more than 1.28×10^{-6} M. This myoplasmic activity would generate the maximum level of tension that an intact cardiac cell is able to develop {46}. This remains far from a full activation of the myofilaments, which is never obtained in an intact cell {46}.

The electrochemical gradient for Na^+ ($\bar{\mu}_{Na}$) is calculated according to eq. (16-2):

$$\bar{\mu}_{Na} = zFE_m - RT \ln \frac{a^o_{Na}}{a^i_{Na}}, \tag{16-2}$$

where $\bar{\mu}_{Na}$ = electrochemical gradient for Na, in $V \times F$; R = gas constant, 8.3151 J/mol $\times$ °K; T = temperature in Kelvin degrees (°K); z = valence; F = Faraday's constant, 9.65×10^4 coul/mol; E_m = membrane potential in V.

The Nernst equation permits the calculation of the Nernst equilibrium potential for Na^+ (E_{Na}):

$$E_{Na} = +\frac{RT}{zF} \ln \frac{a^o_{Na}}{a^i_{Na}}, \tag{16-3}$$

which gives a value of $+77$ mV for E_{Na}. Then,

$$\bar{\mu}_{Na} = zF(E_m - E_{Na}), \tag{16-4}$$

where a negative value of $\bar{\mu}_{Na}$ implies that the gradient favors an inward movement of Na^+. Assuming $E_m = -85$ mV at rest and 0 during depolarization, one can calculate $\bar{\mu}_{Na}$ at the relevant times in the cardiac cycle.

Similar equations permit the calculation of E_{Ca}, which is found to be $+134$ mV at rest and $+85$ mV during Ca^{2+} release, and the computation of $\bar{\mu}_{Ca}$ at rest, during the Ca^{2+} influx across the sarcolemma, and during Ca^{2+} release from the SR.

The energy available for ion transport by Na^+-Ca^{2+} exchange depends upon the electrochemical gradients ($\bar{\mu}_{Na}$ and $\bar{\mu}_{Ca}$) and the Na^+-Ca^{2+} coupling ratio (n) of the transport. There is now general agreement that the coupling ratio is 3 {118,119}, and accordingly, the computation has been done for this value (fig. 16-2).

At equilibrium, the energy available in the Na^+ and Ca^{2+} electrochemical gradients is equal, and no net transport occurs:

$$nzF(E_m - E_{Na}) = zF(E_m - E_{Ca}). \tag{16-5}$$

This is equivalent to

$$3(E_m - E_{Na}) = 2(E_m - E_{Ca}). \tag{16-6}$$

If the Na^+ gradient multiplied by three is larger in magnitude than the Ca^{2+} gradient, Na^+ enters the cell via Na^+-Ca^{2+} exchange, causing Ca^{2+} efflux. If the magnitude of the Ca^{2+} gradient is the larger one, then there is Ca^{2+} influx coupled with Na^+ efflux. Based on a coupling ratio of three, this computation shows that during diastole the Na^+-Ca^{2+} exchange would cause Na^+ efflux.

To describe the systolic Ca^{2+} movements via Na^+-Ca^{2+} exchange, we shall consider first the hypothesis of a Ca^{2+} release from the SR and, secondly, the hypothesis of a direct activation of the myofilaments by the transsarcolemmal Ca^{2+} influx. In the first case, depolarization of the membrane reverses the net gradient for Na^+-Ca^{2+} exchange [eq. (16-6)], and the Na^+-Ca^{2+} exchanger would cause an additional Ca^{2+} influx (sometimes referred to as

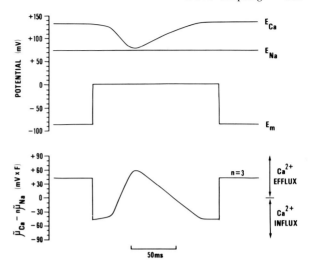

Fig. 16-2. Direction of the net Ca^{2+} flux by Na^+-Ca^{2+} exchange during a voltage-clamp depolarization to the systolic potential and at resting potential in the mammalian myocardium. The computations are based on a critical review of the literature relative to the intracellular and extracellular Ca^{2+} and Na^+ activity and a coupling ratio, n, of three for the Na^+-Ca^{2+} exchanger. E_m = membrane potential; E_{Na} = Nernst potential for Na^+; E_{Ca} = Nernst potential for Ca^{2+}; $\bar{\mu}_{Na}$ = the electrochemical gradient for Na^+; $\bar{\mu}_{Ca}$ = the electrochemical gradient for Ca^{2+}. The arrows on the right of the lowest panel indicate the direction of net Ca^{2+} movement by Na^+-Ca^{2+} exchange; the horizontal bar corresponds to equilibrium, at which there is no net movement of Ca^{2+} or Na^+.

reverse Na^+-Ca^{2+} exchange) during the initial part of the transsarcolemmal Ca^{2+} influx caused by the Ca^{2+} current. The velocity of the Na^+-Ca^{2+} exchange derived from experiments in isolated sarcolemmal vesicles {120,121} seems to be sufficient to permit it to cause Ca^{2+} influx during the approximately 20 ms between the transsarcolemmal influx and the time when the Ca^{2+} release from the SR would cause the Na^+-Ca^{2+} exchange to reverse its direction. The amount of Ca^{2+} influx via Na^+-Ca^{2+} exchange during this time can be assumed to be small compared to that brought by the Ca^{2+} current in the view of the high K_m of the Na^+-Ca^{2+} exchange {120}. If a significant Ca^{2+} influx occurs during this time, the resulting outward movement of Na^+ might somewhat complicate the measurement of the Ca^{2+} current. When Ca^{2+} release from the SR reaches its peak, permitting the activation of the myofilaments, the Na^+-Ca^{2+} exchange functions in the Ca^{2+} extrusion mode. The Na^+-Ca^{2+} exchanger has a high capacity, yet this system will work efficiently only when the myoplasmic [free Ca^{2+}] is still high, because its K_m is relatively high, $0.6-1.5 \times 10^{-6}$ M, with a Hill coefficient of 1 {9,120}. At the lower myoplasmic [free Ca^{2+}] during diastole, the Ca^{2+} extrusion by the sarcolemmal Ca^{2+} pump is relatively more important than during the Ca^{2+} transient (see below).

With the hypothesis that the activation of the myofilaments results directly from transsarcolemmal Ca^{2+} influx {72}, the Na^+-Ca^{2+} exchange would still be biphasic during systole. Initially it would transport Ca^{2+} inward at the beginning of the transsarcolemmal Ca^{2+} influx while the [free Ca^{2+}] is low, then Ca^{2+} would be transported outward when the transsarcolemmal Ca^{2+} influx has reached a level sufficient to activate the myofilaments. Thus, even in this case the Na^+-Ca^{2+} exchange would not function monophasically in the direction of a pure Ca^{2+} influx during the action potential, as was proposed by Mullins {122}.

Recent studies have considered the possibility that the Ca^{2+} entry initially resulting from Na^+-Ca^{2+} exchange on depolarization may contribute to excitation-contraction coupling. This might occur in two ways: (a) Ca^{2+} influx might be sufficient to directly elevate myoplasmic [free Ca^{2+}] to a level sufficient to activate the myofilaments; and (b) Ca^{2+} influx via Na^+-Ca^{2+} exchange might act as the trigger for Ca^{2+}-induced Ca^{2+} release. Based on immunohistology, the density of the Na^+-Ca^{2+} exchanger appears to be highest in the transverse tubular system {123}, near the Ca^{2+} release channel of the SR. As for the first hypothesis, several groups agree that Ca^{2+} influx by this route is sufficient to directly contribute to the Ca^{2+} transient during strong depolarizations, e.g., to +80 mV, but the kinetics of the rise in Ca^{2+} are much slower than those during a normal twitch {51,66,124–126}. The amount of Ca^{2+} entry by Na^+-Ca^{2+} exchange is dependent on $[Na^+]_i$, and increasing intracellular Na^+ by application of cardiac glycosides, for example, stimulates Ca^{2+} influx under these conditions {16,127}. The second hypothesis has also received some support. Leblanc and Hume {128} found that 5 μM TTX reduced the Ca^{2+} transient in indo-1 dialyzed guinea-pig ventricular myocytes without altering action potential duration or plateau configuration. This effect was abolished by ryanodine, required external Ca^{2+}, but was insensitive to block of L Ca^{2+} channels with nisoldipine and D-600. These data suggested to the authors that I_{Na} increases subsarcolemmal Na^+ sufficiently to augment Ca^{2+} influx by Na^+-Ca^{2+} exchange and that exchanger-mediated Ca^{2+} entry induces Ca^{2+} release from the SR. Accumulation of Na^+ could result from diffusional delays {111} or from a postulated {129} partial diffusion barrier ("fuzzy space") under the membrane. Although trains of five stimuli were used to load the SR with Ca^{2+} {128}, it is uncertain whether the Ca^{2+} stores were the same before and after TTX; TTX reduces a_{Na}^i and increases the gradient for Ca^{2+} efflux by Na^+-Ca^{2+} exchange {130}. Another study failed to find a Ca^{2+} release induced by I_{Na} over the voltage range of the action potential, under somewhat different experimental conditions, however {126}. Despite these issues, the hypothesis of Leblanc and Hume {128} remains an interesting conjecture and will certainly be tested further.

SARCOLEMMAL CALCIUM PUMP

Initial descriptions of a Ca^{2+}-ATPase in the sarcolemma sensitive to free Ca^{2+} in the micromolar range were by Sulakhe and St. Louis {131}. There was some question, however, as to whether this sarcolemmal ATPase was in fact due to contamination of the preparation by SR vesicles {132}. However, Caroni and Carafoli {133,134} have provided compelling evidence that this ATPase activity indeed takes place in the sarcolemma and that its affinity for Ca^{2+} is higher ($K_m = 0.3 \times 10^{-6}$ M) than that of the Na^+-Ca^{2+} exchanger. The sarcolemmal Ca^{2+} pump has a lower capacity than the Na^+-Ca^{2+} exchanger, and the rate of transport is also lower. Thus, the sarcolemmal Ca^{2+} pump is likely to function at concentrations near or at the diastolic level. It is not unreasonable to suspect that there is redundancy built into the mechanisms for Ca^{2+} extrusion from the cell whereby the sarcolemmal Ca^{2+} pump would back up the Na^+-Ca^{2+} exchanger. Under normal conditions, the Na^+-Ca^{2+} exchanger may be sufficient to maintain $[Ca^{2+}]_i$ at resting levels. With Na^+ loading and partial depolarization, however, the lowest [free Ca^{2+}] at which Na^+-Ca^{2+} exchange can extrude Ca^{2+} is elevated, and the sarcolemmal Ca^{2+} pump would be necessary to lower Ca^{2+} to resting levels.

The amount of total calcium that can be extruded from the cardiac cell by the sarcolemmal Ca^{2+} pump during a beat and between two beats could theoretically be calculated from the affinity of the pump for Ca^{2+}, its maximum rate of transport per milligram sarcolemmal protein as derived from experiments in isolated sarcolemma, and the concentration of sarcolemmal protein per milligram wet weight of tissue. The resulting change of myoplasmic [free Ca^{2+}] could then be derived by dividing the result of this calculation by the product of the tissue water, expressed as percentage of wet weight, multiplied by the intracellular water, expressed as a percentage of the total water. There are still too many uncertainties about the degree of purity of the isolated sarcolemmal preparation and the percentage of vesicles inside-out versus right-side-out for such calculations to be meaningful at the present time. Nevertheless, several studies that directly assessed the contributions of various Ca^{2+} transport mechanisms to the Ca^{2+} transient argue that the role of the sarcolemmal Ca^{2+} pump in Ca^{2+} efflux during a normal Ca^{2+} transient is quite small and can be ignored {15,66,135}.

SOME LIMITATIONS OF THE ANALYSIS

A fully satisfactory analysis of the questions addressed here require detailed consideration of not only transsarcolemmal Ca^{2+} fluxes, but also the kinetics of binding of Ca^{2+} to intracellular ligands, the diffusion constant for Ca^{2+}, which may vary in different parts of the myoplasm, and the complex geometrical arrangement of each of the Ca^{2+} transport proteins and binding sites. The extreme heterogeneity of the cell and our lack of knowledge of these details preclude a rigorous theoretical reconstruction of the Ca^{2+} transient at this time. Nevertheless, an important advance has come from the application of finite-element analysis to calculation of the temporal and spatial distribution of Ca^{2+} within a ventricular myocyte {66,109}.

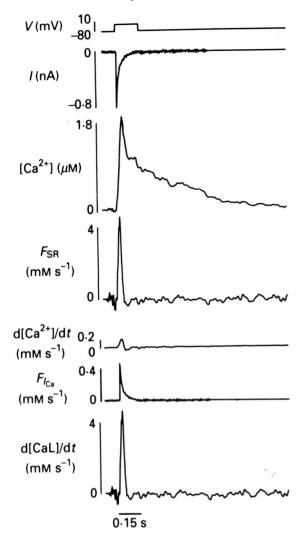

Fig. 16-3. Measured verapamil-sensitive Ca^{2+} current (I) and Ca^{2+} transient ($[Ca^{2+}]$), calculated spatially averaged Ca^{2+} flux from the SR (F_{sr}) and I_{Ca} (F_{ICa}), and derivatives of [free Ca^{2+}] ($d[Ca^{2+}]/dt$) and [bound Ca^{2+}] ($d[CaL]/dt$) in a guinea-pig ventricular myocyte in response to a 150-ms depolarization from -80 to $10\,mV$ (V). Na^+-Ca^{2+} exchange was inhibited by omitting both internal and external Na^+. Under these conditions, the Ca^{2+} flux from the SR was about 20 times greater than the Ca^{2+} flux through L Ca^{2+} channels. From Sipido and Wier {66}, with permission of the authors and Cambridge University Press.

For example, fig. 16-3, taken from the work of Sipido and Wier {66}, shows I_{Ca} and the intracellular Ca^{2+} transient recorded in a guinea-pig ventricular myocyte during a 150-ms depolarizing pulse from -80 to $10\,mV$ along with the calculated SR and Ca^{2+} channel fluxes and the calculated rate of Ca^{2+} binding to intracellular ligands. The experi-

ment was done in the total absence of Na^+, so Na^+-Ca^{2+} exchange was blocked. Under these conditions the Ca^{2+} flux from the SR was about 20 times greater than the Ca^{2+} flux through L Ca^{2+} channels. But a complexity introduced by Ca^{2+} binding is also apparent. Both the flux of Ca^{2+} from the SR and the rate of binding to ligands were much greater than the transmembrane Ca^{2+} flux through Ca^{2+} channels and the rate of change of cytoplasmic Ca^{2+}. Determining the fraction of Ca^{2+} from the SR and the fraction that enters as I_{Ca} that remain free is not yet possible with any certainty. Such calculations would require detailed knowledge of local conditions and the geometry of Ca^{2+} transport and binding sites, which are not presently available.

DIFFICULTIES WITH THE HYPOTHESIS OF A DIRECT ACTIVATION OF THE MYOFILAMENTS BY TRANSSARCOLEMMAL CALCIUM INFLUX

In conclusion, the currently available information with respect to the quantification of the Ca^{2+} influx and efflux during a cardiac beat does not provide any compelling reason to infer or eliminate a role of the SR in cardiac excitation-contraction coupling. Irrespective of the amplitude of these Ca^{2+} movements whenever they are established, and even if they were sufficient to activate or inactivate the myofilaments, this would not permit the elimination of a role for the SR. As previously emphasized, the Ca^{2+} accumulation in a release from the SR could modify the changes of myoplasmic [free Ca^{2+}] resulting from Ca^{2+} movements across the sarcolemma before and after the activation of the myofilaments.

If one were to accept the hypothesis that the transsarcolemmal Ca^{2+} influx could activate the myofilaments directly without Ca^{2+} release from the SR, then it would be necessary to deal with the role of the SR in Ca^{2+} accumulation. One suggestion {72,73} is that the SR is involved in Ca^{2+} reaccumulation, but not in Ca^{2+} release. Consequently one has to assume a unidirectional net flux of Ca^{2+} across the SR {72,73}. If such a route were to exist, then the total calcium influx per beat should be larger than the total calcium efflux throught the Ca^{2+} pump and the Na^+-Ca^{2+} exchange by an amount equal to the calcium efflux through this specific route involving the SR. At the present time, however, the calcium efflux through Na^+-Ca^{2+} exchange and the sarcolemmal Ca^{2+} pump is not known. The total calcium influx during a beat is not known quantitatively either; there are uncertainties about the amount of total calcium carried by the Ca^{2+} current, no reliable information on the amount of total calcium entering by Na^+-Ca^{2+} exchange, and, in addition, no knowledge about the passive Ca^{2+} leak through the membrane following the concentration gradient, which is likely to bring additional Ca^{2+} into the cell during the rest between beats. Although this hypothesis cannot be eliminated and can indeed explain some data in an internally consistent manner {72,73}, it poses a difficult kinetics problem to explain how Ca^{2+} returns to the surface membrane to be reused during a subsequent beat {136}.

In addition, this hypothesis is not compatible with some known properties of the cardiac SR {137}.

An alternative hypothesis for direct activation of the myofilaments by the transsarcolemmal Ca^{2+} influx is conceptually simpler. This hypothesis assumes that the SR plays no role at all in the beat-to-beat Ca^{2+} regulation. The Ca^{2+} efflux would then be entirely accomplished by the surface membrane through Na^+-Ca^{2+} exchange and the Ca^{2+} pump of the sarcolemma.

A direct activation of the myofilaments by transsarcolemmal Ca^{2+} influx and a Ca^{2+} extrusion entirely supported by Na^+-Ca^{2+} exchange and the sarcolemmal Ca^{2+} pump has been suggested for the cardiac cells that have the smallest diameter, paricularly for the ventricular cell of the adult frog, as first proposed in great detail by Morad and Goldman {138} and subsequently by others {e.g., 139,140}. In the skinned single cardiac cells from the adult frog ventricle and in the fetal ventricular cells of mammalian species, there is no evidence of rapid Ca^{2+} release induced by Ca^{2+} or by caffeine {48,49}. This lack of rapid release is also observed in pluricellular preparations, from the same tissues, in which the sarcolemma remains present but is disrupted, so that the superficial cisternae of the SR are preserved {48}. Yet even in frog heart, and especially in frog atrium {77}, it is not possible to exclude completely a participation of a Ca^{2+} release from the SR in excitation-contraction coupling {42,141}.

For the adult mammalian ventricle, a similar mechanism of direct activation and inactivation of the myofilaments by transsarcolemmal Ca^{2+} influx {72} and efflux is quantitatively neither supported nor excluded by any of the data on transsarcolemmal influx and efflux that have been discussed in this chapter. The hypotheses suggesting a direct activation of the myofilaments in adult mammalian myocardium are challenged by experiments in skinned cardiac cells, however. These experiments indicate that the SR has the capability to accumulate Ca^{2+} and to modify, by a release, the transsarcolemmal Ca^{2+} influx irrespective of its magnitude {1,46,48}. Thus the hypothesis of the direct activation of the myofilaments by the transsarcolemmal influx of Ca^{2+} must disregard the results obtained from skinned cardiac cells on the grounds that these preparations may be in an unphysiologic condition {72}, which is certainly a legitimate concern. In contrast, it does not seem possible to attribute the properties of the SR of skinned cardiac cells to transverse tubules {60}, which do not exist in several of the tissues used for preparing skinned cardiac cells {48,49}.

NOTES

1. In fact, Ringer's observations were made on frog ventricle and to apply them to mammalian ventricle is unwarranted {142}. Repeating Ringer's experiments on small trabeculae from the frog ventricle, but with observation under the high-power microscope, confirmed Ringer's findings. Not only was contraction abolished within 2–3 minutes by Ca^{2+} removal, but microscopic examination found the preparation to be completely quiescent {142}. In contrast, when the experiments were done in a mammalian (e.g., adult rat) ventricular tissue, Ca^{2+} removal resulted in an almost complete abolition of the contraction detected from the ends of the trabecula with a highly sensitive transducer but observation under the microscope showed localized cyclic contractions. This very prominent but desynchronized contractile behavior persisted for many hours in a Ca^{2+}-free solution {142}. Therefore, this observation is, in fact, one of many pieces of evidence suggesting that, in addition to the transsarcolemmal Ca^{2+} influx, an intracellular Ca^{2+} store participates in the excitation-contraction coupling of the adult mammalian cardiac tissue. Other experiments have demonstrated that the Ca^{2+} store is located in the sarcoplasmic reticulum {142}.

2. It suffices to run example no. 4, which is included in diskette no. 2, which is freely distributed with this article, to generate a table of total calcium concentration versus free calcium concentration, taking into account what was known in 1982 of the steady-state calcium buffering within the mammalian cardiac cells.

REFERENCES

1. Fabiato A, Fabiato F: Calcium release from the sarcoplasmic reticulum. *Circ Res* 40:119–129, 1977.
2. Fabiato A, Baumgarten CM: Methods for detecting calcium release from the sarcoplasmic reticulum of skinned cardiac cells and the relationships between calculated transsarcolemmal calcium movements and calcium release. In: Sperelakis N (ed) *Physiology and Pathophysiology of the Heart*. Boston: Martinus Nijhoff, 1984, pp 215–254.
3. Baumgarten CM, Fabiato A: Calculated transsarcolemmal calcium movements in cardiac muscle. In: Sperelakis N (ed) *Physiology and Pathophysiology of the Heart*, 2nd ed. Boston: Kluwer Academic Publishers, 1988, pp 253–265.
4. Eisner DA, Lederer WJ: Na-Ca exchange: Stoichiometry and electrogenicity. *Am J Physiol* 248:C189–C202, 1985.
5. Johnson EA, Kootsey JM: A minimum mechanism for Na^+-Ca^{2+} exchange: Net and unidirectional Ca^{2+} fluxes as a function of ion composition and membrane potential. *J Memb Biol* 86:167–187, 1985.
6. Läuger P: Voltage dependence of sodium-calcium exchange: Predictions from kinetic models. *J Memb Biol* 99:1–11, 1987.
7. Hilgemann DW, Noble D: Excitation-contraction coupling and extracellular calcium transients in rabbit atrium: Reconstruction of basic cellular mechanisms. *Proc R Soc Lond B* 230:163–205, 1987.
8. Hilgemann DW: Numerical approximations of sodium-calcium exchange. *Prog Biophys Mol Biol* 51:1–45, 1988.
9. Miura Y, Kimura J: Sodium-calcium exchange current: Dependence on internal Ca and Na and competitive binding of external Na and Ca. *J Gen Physiol* 93:1129–1145, 1989.
10. Li J, Kimura J: Translocation mechanism of Na-Ca exchange in single cardiac cells of guinea pig. *J Gen Physiol* 96:777–788, 1990.
11. Matsuoka S, Hilgemann DW: Steady-state and dynamic properties of cardiac sodium-calcium exchange. Ion and voltage dependencies of the transport cycle. *J Gen Physiol* 100:963–1001, 1992.
12. Mentard D, Vassort G, Fischmeister R: Changes in external Na induce a membrane current related to the Na-Ca exchange in cesium-loaded frog heart cells. *J Physiol* 84:201–220, 1984.
13. Hume JR, Uehara A: "Creep currents" in single frog atrial cells may be generated by electrogenic Na/Ca exchange. *J Gen Physiol* 87:857–884, 1986.

14. Hume JR, Uehara A: Properties of "creep currents" in single frog atrial cells. *J Gen Physiol* 87:833–855, 1986.

15. Barry WH, Rasmussen CAF Jr, Ishida H, Bridge JHB: External Na-independent calcium extrusion in cultured ventricular cells. *J Gen Physiol* 88:393–411, 1986.

16. Kimura J, Noma A, Irisawa H: Na-Ca exchange current in mammalian heart cells. *Nature* 319:569–597, 1986.

17. Kimura J, Miyamae S, Noma A: Identification of sodium-calcium exchange current in single ventricular cells of guinea-pig. *J Physiol* 384:199–222, 1987.

18. Fedida D, Noble D, Shimoni Y, Spindler AJ: Inward current related to contraction in guinea-pig ventricular myocytes. *J Physiol* 385:565–589, 1987.

19. Lipp P, Pott L: Transient inward current in guinea-pig atrial myocytes reflects a change of sodium-calcium exchange current. *J Physiol* 397:601–630, 1988.

20. Egan T, Noble D, Powell T, Spindler AJ, Twist VW: Sodium-calcium exchange during the action potential in guinea-pig ventricular cells. *J Physiol* 411:630–661, 1989.

21. Hilgemann DW: Giant excised cardiac sarcolemmal membrane patches: Sodium and sodium-calcium exchange currents. *Pflügers Arch* 415:247–249, 1989.

22. Bers DM, Bridge JHB: Relaxation of rabbit ventricular muscle by Na-Ca exchange and the sarcoplasmic reticulum. *Circ Res* 65:334–342, 1989.

23. Bridge JHB, Smolley J, Spitzer KW, Chin TK: Voltage dependence of sodium-calcium exchange and the control of calcium extrusion in the heart. *Ann NY Acad Sci* 639:34–47, 1991.

24. Horackova M, Vassort G: Sodium-calcium exchange in regulation of cardiac contractility. *J Gen Physiol* 73:403–424, 1979.

25. Nicoll DA, Longoni S, Philipson KD: Molecular cloning and functional expression of the cardiac sarcolemmal Na^+-Ca^{2+} exchanger. *Science* 250:562–565, 1990.

26. Pelzer D, Pelzer S, McDonald TF: Calcium channels in heart. In: Fozzard HA, Haber E, Jennings RB, Katz AM, Morgan HE (eds) *The Heart and Cardiovascular System. Scientific Foundations*, 2nd ed. New York: Raven Press, 1992, pp 1049–1089.

27. Bean BP: Classes of calcium channels in vertebrate cells. *Annu Rev Physiol* 51:367–384, 1989.

28. Porzig H: Pharmacological modulation of voltage-dependent Ca channels in intact cells. *Rev Physiol Biochem Pharmacol* 114:209–262, 1990.

29. Bean BP: Two kinds of calcium channels in canine atrial cells. Differences in kinetics, selectivity, and pharmacology. *J Gen Physiol* 86:1–30, 1985.

30. Nilius B, Hess P, Lansman JB, Tsien RW: A novel type of cardiac calcium channel in ventricular cells. *Nature* 316:443–446, 1985.

31. Mitra R, Morad M: Two types of calcium channels in guinea pig ventricular myocytes. *Proc Natl Acad Sci USA* 83:5340–5344, 1986.

32. Hirano Y, Fozzard HA, January CT: Characteristics of L- and T-type Ca^{2+} currents in canine cardiac Purkinje cells. *Am J Physiol* 256:H1478–H1492, 1989.

33. Lee KS, Marban E, Tsien RW: Inactivation of calcium channels in mammalian heart cells: Joint dependence on membrane potential and intracellular calcium. *J Physiol* 364:395–411, 1985.

34. Bechem M, Pott L: Removal of Ca current inactivation in dialyzed guinea-pig atrial cardioballs by Ca chelators. *Pflügers Arch* 404:10–20, 1985.

35. Morad M, Cleemann L: Role of Ca^{2+} channels in development of tension in heart muscle. *J Mol Cell Cardiol* 19:527–553, 1987.

36. Mikami A, Imoto K, Tanabe T, Niidome T, Mori Y, Takeshima H, Narumiya S, Numa S. Primary structure and functional expression of the cardiac dihydropyridine-sensitive calcium channel. *Nature* 340:231–233, 1989.

37. Catterall WA: Molecular properties of voltage-gated ion channels in the heart. In: Fozzard HA, Haber E, Jennings RB, Katz AM, Morgan HE (eds) *The Heart and Cardiovascular System. Scientific Foundations*, 2nd ed. New York: Raven Press, 1992, pp 945–962.

38. McDonald TF, Cavalie A, Trautwein W, Pelzer D: Voltage-dependent properties of macroscopic and elementary calcium channel currents in guinea pig ventricular myocytes. *Pflügers Arch* 406:437–448, 1986.

39. Antoni H, Jacob R, Kaufmann R: Mechanische Reaktionen des Frosch- und Saugetiermyokards bei Veranderung der Aktionspotential-Dauer durch konstante Gleichstromimpulse. *Pflügers Arch* 306:33–57, 1969.

40. Boyett MR, Jewell BR: Analysis of the effects of changes in rate and rhythm upon electrical activity in the heart. *Prog Biophys Mol Biol* 36:1–52, 1980.

41. Wohlfart B, Noble MIM: The cardiac excitation-contraction cycle. *Pharmacol Ther* 16:1–43, 1982.

42. Chapman RA: Control of cardiac contractility at the cellular level. *Am J Physiol* 245:H535–H552, 1983.

43. Blinks JR, Olson CB, Jewell BR, Braveny P: Influence of caffeine and other methylxanthenes on mechanical properties of isolated mammalian heart muscle: Evidence for a dual mechanism of action. *Circ Res* 30:367–392, 1972.

44. Fabiato A: Effects of ryanodine in skinned cardiac cells. *Fed Proc* 44:2970–2976, 1985.

45. Solaro RJ, Briggs FN: Estimating the functional capabilities of the sarcoplasmic reticulum in cardiac muscle: Calcium binding. *Circ Res* 34:531–540, 1974.

46. Fabiato A: Myoplasmic free calcium concentration reached during the twitch of an intact isolated cardiac cell and during calcium-induced release of calcium from the sarcoplasmic reticulum of skinned cardiac cell from the adult rat or rabbit ventricle. *J Gen Physiol* 78:457–497, 1981.

47. Levitsky DO, Benevolensky DS, Levchenki TS, Smirnov VN, Chazzov EI: Calcium-binding rate and capacity of cardiac sarcoplasmic reticulum. *J Mol Cell Cardiol* 13:785–796, 1981.

48. Fabiato A, Fabiato F: Calcium-induced release of calcium from the sarcoplasmic reticulum of skinned cells from adult human, dog, cat, rabbit, rat, and frog hearts and from fetal and newborn rat ventricles. *Ann NY Acad Sci* 307:491–522, 1978.

49. Fabiato A: Calcium release in skinned cardiac cells: Variations with species, tissues, and development. *Fed Proc* 41:2238–2244, 1982.

50. Barcenas-Ruiz L, Wier WG: Voltage dependence of $[Ca^{2+}]_i$ transients in guinea pig ventricular myocytes. *Circ Res* 61:148–154, 1987.

51. Beuckelmann DJ, Wier WG: Mechanism of release of calcium from s.r. of guinea-pig cardiac cells. *J Physiol* 405:233–255, 1988.

52. Callewaert B, Cleemann L, Morad M: Epinephrine enhances Ca^{2+} current-regulated Ca^{2+} release and Ca^{2+} reuptake in rat ventricular myocytes. *Proc Natl Acad Sci USA* 85:2009–2013, 1988.

53. Hansford RG, Lakatta EG: Ryanodine releases calcium from sarcoplasmic reticulum in calcium-tolerant rat cardiac myocytes. *J Physiol* 390:453–467, 1987.

54. Meissner G: Ryanodine activation and inhibition of the Ca^{2+}-release channel of sarcoplasmic reticulum. *J Biol Chem* 261:6300–6306, 1986.

55. Nagaski K, Fleischer S: Ryanodine sensitivity of the calcium

release channel of sarcoplasmic reticulum. *Cell Calcium* 9:1–7, 1988.

56. Sutko JL, Kenyon JL: Ryanodine modification of cardiac muscle responses to potassium-free solutions. Evidence for inhibition of sarcoplasmic reticulum calcium release. *J Gen Physiol* 82:385–404, 1983.

57. Affolter H, Chiesi M, Dabrowska R, Carafoli E: Calcium regulation in heart cells: The interaction of mitochondrial and sarcoplasmic reticulum with troponin-bound calcium. *Eur J Biochem* 67:389–396, 1976.

58. Scarpa A, Graziotti P: Mechanisms for intracellular calcium regulation in heart. I. Stopped-flow measurements of Ca^{2+} uptake by cardiac mitochondria. *J Gen Physiol* 62:756–772, 1973.

59. Somlyo AP, Somlyo AV, Shuman H, Scarpa A, Endo M, Inesi G: Mitochondria do not accumulate significant Ca concentrations in normal cells. In: Bronner F, Peterlik M (eds) *Calcium and Phosphate Transport Across Biomembranes*. New York: Academic Press, 1981, pp 87–93.

60. Lullman H, Peters T, Preuner J: Role of the plasmalemma in calcium-homeostasis and for excitation-contraction coupling in cardiac muscle. In: Noble MIM, Drake A (eds) *Cardiac Metabolism*. London: Wiley and Sons, 1983, pp 1–18.

61. Philipson KD, Bers DM, Nishimoto AY: The role of phospholipids in the Ca^{2+} binding of isolated cardiac sarcolemma. *J Mol Cell Cardiol* 12:1159–1173, 1980.

62. Fabiato A: Appraisal of the hypothesis of the "depolarization-induced" release of calcium from the sarcoplasmic reticulum in skinned cardiac cells from the rat or pigeon ventricle. In: Fleischer S, Tonomura Y (eds) *Structure and Function of the Sarcoplasmic Reticulum*. New York: Academic Press, 1985, pp 479–519.

63. Bers DM, Philipson KD, Langer GA: Cardiac contractility and sarcolemmal calcium binding in several cardiac muscle preparations. *Am J Physiol* 240:H576–H583, 1981.

64. Bers DM: A Correlation of the Effects of Cationic Uncouplers on Intact Cardiac Muscle and on Ca^{2+} Bound to Isolated Cardiac Muscle Plasma Membranes. UCLA PhD thesis, 1978. Ann Arbor, MI: University Microfilms.

65. Cannell MB, Berlin JR, Lederer WJ: Effects of membrane potential changes on the calcium transient in single rat cardiac muscle cells. *Science* 238:1419–1423, 1987.

66. Sipido KR, Wier WG: Flux of Ca^{2+} across the sarcoplasmic reticulum of guinea-pig cardiac ventricular cells during excitation-contraction coupling. *J Physiol* 435:605–630, 1991.

67. Brum G, Stefani E, Rios E: Simultaneous measurements of Ca^{2+}-currents and intracellular Ca^{2+}-concentrations in single skeletal muscle fibers of the frog. *Can J Physiol Pharm* 65:681–685, 1986.

68. Näbauer M, Callewaert G, Cleemann L, Morad M: Regulation of calcium release is gated by calcium current, not gating charge, in cardiac myocytes. *Science* 244:800–803, 1989.

69. New W, Trautwein W: The ionic nature of the slow inward current and its relationship to contraction. *Pflügers Arch* 334:24–38, 1972.

70. Gibbons WR, Fozzard HA: Slow inward current and contraction of sheep cardiac Purkinje fibers. *J Gen Physiol* 65:367–384, 1975.

71. London B, Kruger JW: Contraction in voltage clamped internally perfused single heart cells. *J Gen Physiol* 88:475–505, 1986.

72. Langer GA: Events at the cardiac sarcolemma: Localization and movement of contractile-dependent calcium. *Fed Proc* 35:1274–1278, 1976.

73. Mensing HJ, Hilgemann DW: Inotropic effects of activation and pharmacological mechanisms in cardiac muscle. *Trends Pharmacol Sci* 2:303–307, 1981.

74. Ringer S: A further contribution regarding the influence of the different constituents of the blood on the contraction of the heart. *J Physiol* 4:29–42, 1883.

75. Mines GR: On functional analysis by the action of electrolytes. *J Physiol* 46:188–235, 1913.

76. Langer GA: The role of calcium in the control of myocardial contractility: An update. *J Mol Cell Cardiol* 12:231–239, 1980.

77. Fabiato A: Calcium-induced release of calcium from the cardiac sarcoplasmic reticulum. *Am J Physiol* 245:C1–C14, 1983.

78. Bers DM: Excitation-Contraction Coupling and Cardiac Contractile Force. Boston: Kluwer Academic Publishers, 1991.

79. Fabiato A: Computer programs for calculating total from specified free or free from specified total ionic concentrations in aqueous solutions containing multiple metals and ligands. In: Fleischer S, Fleischer B (eds) *Methods in Enzymology, Biomembranes*, Vol 157: *ATP-Driven Pumps and Related Transport*. Orlando, FL: Academic Press, 1988, pp 378–417.

80. Philipson KD, Bers DM, Nishimoto AY, Langer GA: Binding of Ca^{2+} and Na^{+} to sarcolemmal membranes: Relation to control of myocardial contractility. *Am J Physiol* 238:H373–H378, 1980.

81. Solomon AK: Compartmental methods of kinetic analysis. In: Comar CL, Bronner F (eds) *Mineral Metabolism: An Advanced Treatise*. Vol 1: *Principles, Processes, and Systems*, Part A. New York: Academic Press, 1960, pp 119–167.

82. Bers DM: Early transient depletion of extracellular Ca during individual cardiac muscle contractions. *Am J Physiol* 244:H462–H468, 1983.

83. Bers DM, MacLeod KT: Cumulative depletions of extracellular calcium in rabbit ventricular muscle monitored with calcium-selective microelectrodes. *Circ Res* 58:769–782, 1986.

84. Bers DM, Bridge JHB, MacLeod KT: The mechanism of ryanodine action in rabbit ventricular muscle evaluated with Ca-selective microelectrodes and rapid cooling contractures. *Can J Physiol Pharmacol* 65:610–618, 1987.

85. MacLeod KT, Bers DM: The effects of rest duration and ryanodine on changes of extracellular calcium concentration in cardiac muscle from rabbits. *Am J Physiol* 253:C398–C407, 1987.

86. Bers DM: Ca influx and sarcoplasmic reticulum Ca release in cardiac muscle activation during postrest recovery. *Am J Physiol* 248:H366–H381, 1985.

87. Hilgemann DW, Delay MJ, Langer GA: Activation-dependent cumulative depletions of extracellular free calcium in guinea pig atrium measured with antipyrylazo III and tetramethylmurexide. *Circ Res* 53:779–793, 1983.

88. Hilgemann DW: Extracellular calcium transients and action potential configuration changes related to post-stimulatory potentiation in rabbit atrium. *J Gen Physiol* 87:675–706, 1986.

89. Hilgemann DW: Extracellular calcium transients at single excitations in rabbit atrium measured with tetramethylmurexide. *J Gen Physiol* 87:707–735, 1986.

90. Pizarro G, Cleemann L, Morad M: Optical measurement of voltage-dependent Ca^{2+} influx in frog heart. *Proc Natl Acad Sci USA* 82:1864–1868, 1985.

91. Marban E, Tsien RW: Effects of nystatin-mediated intracellular ion substitution on membrane currents in calf Purkinje fibres. *J Physiol* 329:569–587, 1982.

92. Campbell DL, Giles WR, Hume JR, Noble D, Shibata EF:

Reversal potential of the calcium current in bull-frog atrial myocytes. *J Physiol* 403:267–286, 1988.

93. Hess P, Lansman JB, Tsien RW: Calcium channel selectivity for divalent and monovalent cations: Voltage and concentration dependence of single channel current in ventricular heart cells. *J Gen Physiol* 88:293–319, 1986.

94. Reuter H, Scholz H: A study of the ion selectivity and the kinetic properties of the calcium dependent slow inward current in mammalian cardiac muscle. *J Physiol* 264:17–47, 1977.

95. Siegelbaum SA, Tsien RW: Calcium-activated transient outward current in calf cardiac Purkinje fibres. *J Physiol* 299:485–506, 1980.

96. Kass RS, Tsien RW: Multiple effects of calcium antagonists on plateau currents in cardiac Purkinje fibers. *J Gen Physiol* 66:169–192, 1975.

97. McDonald TF: The slow inward calcium current in the heart. *Annu Rev Physiol* 44:425–434, 1982.

98. Kass RS, Siegelbaum S, Tsien RW: Incomplete inactivation of the slow inward current in cardiac Purkinje fibres. *J Physiol* 263:127P–128P, 1976.

99. Isenberg G, Klockner U: Glycocalyx is not required for slow inward calcium current in isolated rat heart myocytes. *Nature* 284:358–360, 1980.

100. Lee KS, Tsien RW: Reversal of current through calcium channels in dialyzed single heart cells. *Nature* 297:498–501, 1982.

101. Hino N, Orchi R: Effect of acetylcholine on membrane currents in guinea-pig papillary muscle. *J Physiol* 307:183–197, 1980.

102. McDonald TF, Pelzer D, Trautwein W: Does the calcium current modulate the contraction of the accompanying beat? A study of E-C coupling in mammalian ventricular muscle using cobalt ions. *Circ Res* 49:576–583, 1981.

103. Nawrath H, Ten Eick RE, McDonald TF, Trautwein W: On the mechanism underlying the action of D-600 on slow inward current and tension in mammalian myocardium. *Circ Res* 40:408–414, 1977.

104. Noma A, Kotake H, Irisawa H: Slow inward current and its role mediating the chronotropic effect of epinephrine in the rabbit sinoatrial node. *Pflügers Arch* 388:1–9, 1980.

105. Ehra T, Kaufman R: The voltage- and time-dependent effects of (−)-verapamil on the slow inward current in isolated cat ventricular myocardium. *J Pharmacol Exp Ther* 207:49–55, 1987.

106. Mobley BA, Page E: The surface area of sheep cardiac Purkinje fibres. *J Physiol* 220:547–563, 1972.

107. Smith SJ, Augustine GJ: Calcium ions, active zones, and synaptic transmitter release. *Topics Neurosci* 11: 458–464, 1988.

108. Takamatsu T, Wier WG: High temporal resolution video imaging of intracellular calcium. *Cell Calcium* 11:111–120, 1990.

109. Wier WG, Yue DT: Intracellular calcium transients underlying the short-term force-interval relationship in ferret ventricular myocardium. *J Physiol* 376:507–530, 1986.

110. Lipp P, Pott L, Callewaert G, Carmeliet E: Simultaneous recording of Indo-1 florescence and Na^+-Ca^{2+} exchange current reveals two components of Ca^{2+} release from the sarcoplasmic reticulum of cardiac atrial myocytes. *FEBS Lett* 275:181–184, 1990.

111. Bassingthwaighte JB, Reuter H: Calcium movements and excitation-contraction coupling in cardiac cells. In: DeMello WC (ed) *Electrical Phenomena in the Heart*. New York: Academic Press, 1972, pp 353–395.

112. Stewart JM, Page E: Improved stereological techniques for studying myocardial cell growth: Application to external

sarcolemma, T system, and intercalated disks of rabbit and rat hearts. *J Ultrastruct Res* 65:119–134, 1978.

113. Isenberg G: Ca entry and contraction as studied in isolated bovine ventricular myocytes. *Z Naturforsch* 37c:502–512, 1982.

114. Baumgarten CM: A program for calculation of activity coefficients at selected concentrations and temperatures. *Comput Biol Med* 11:189–196, 1981.

115. Sheu S-S, Fozzard HA: Transmembrane Na^+ and Ca^{2+} electrochemical gradients in cardiac muscle and their relationship to force development. *J Gen Physiol* 80:325–351, 1982.

116. Marban E, Rink TJ, Tsien RW, Tsien RY: Free calcium in heart muscle at rest and during contraction measured with Ca^{2+}-sensitive microelectrodes. *Nature* 286:845–850, 1980.

117. Lee CO: Ionic activities in cardiac muscle cells and application of ion-selective microelectrodes. *Am J Physiol* 241:H459–H478, 1981.

118. Reves JP, Hale CC: The stoichiometry of the cardiac sodium-calcium exchange system. *J Biol Chem* 259:7733–7739, 1984.

119. Sheu S-S, Blaustein MP: Sodium/calcium exchange and regulation of cell calcium and contractility in cardiac muscle, with a note about vascular smooth muscle. In: HA Fozzard, E Haber, RB Jennings, AM Katz, HE Morgan (eds) *The Heart and Cardiovascular System: Scientific Foundations*, 2nd ed. New York: Raven Press, 1992, pp 903–943.

120. Caroni P, Reinlib L, Carafoli E: Charge movements during the Na^+-Ca^{2+} exchange in heart sarcolemmal vesicles. *Proc Natl Acad Sci USA* 77:6354–6358, 1980.

121. Kadoma M, Froehilich J, Reeves J, Sutko J: Kinetics of sodium ion induced calcium ion release in calcium ion loaded cardiac sarcolemmal vesicles: Determination of initial velocities by stopped-flow spectrophotometry. *Biochemistry* 21:1914–1918, 1982.

122. Mullins LJ: Interactions between Na/K and Na/Ca pumps. In: *Ion Transport in Heart*, New York: Raven Press, 1981, pp 61–74.

123. Frank JS, Mottino G, Reid D, Molday RS, Philipson KD: Distribution of the Na^+-Ca^{2+} exchange protein in mammalian cardiac myocytes: An immunofluorescence and immunocolloidal gold-labeling study. *J Cell Biol* 117:337–345, 1992.

124. Barcenas-Ruiz L, Beuckelmann DJ, Wier WG: Sodium-calcium exchange in heart: Currents and changes in $[Ca^{2+}]_i$. *Science* 238:1720–1722, 1987.

125. Crespo LM, Grantham CJ, Cannell MB: Kinetics, stoichiometry and role of the Na-Ca exchange mechanism in isolated cardiac myocytes. *Nature* 345:618–621, 1990.

126. Sham JS, Cleemann L, Morad M: Gating of the cardiac Ca^{2+} release channel: The role of Na^+ current and Na^+-Ca^{2+} exchange. *Science* 255:850–853, 1992.

127. Bers DM, Christensen DM, Nguyen TX: Can Ca entry via Na-Ca exchange directly activate cardiac muscle contraction? *J Mol Cell Cardiol* 20:405–414, 1988.

128. Leblanc N, Hume JR: Sodium current-induced release of calcium from cardiac sarcoplasmic reticulum. *Science* 248:372–376, 1990.

129. Lederer WJ, Niggli E, Hadley W: Sodium-calcium exchange in excitable cells: Fuzzy space. *Science* 248:283, 1990.

130. January CT, Fozzard HA: The effects of membrane potential, extracellular potassium and tetrodotoxin on intracellular sodium ion activity in sheep cardiac muscle. *Circ Res* 54:652–665, 1984.

131. Sulakhe PV, St Louis PJ: Passive and active calcium fluxes across plasma membranes. *Prog Biophys Mol Biol* 35: 135–195, 1980.

132. Jones LR, Besch HR Jr, Flemins JW, McConnaughey MM,

Watanabe AM: Separation of vesicles of cardiac sarcolemma from vesicles of sarcoplasmic reticulum: Comparative biochemical analysis of component activities. *J Biol Chem* 254:530–539, 1979.

133. Caroni P, Carafoli E: An ATP-dependent Ca^{2+}-pumping system in dog heart sarcolemma. *Nature* 283:765–767, 1980.

134. Caroni P, Carafoli E: The Ca^{2+}-pumping ATPase of heart sarcolemma. *J Biol Chem* 256:3263–3270, 1981.

135. Carafoli W: Membrane transport of calcium: An overview. *Methods Enzymol* 157:3–11, 1988.

136. Solaro RJ, Briggs FN: Calcium conservation and the regulation of myocardial contraction. In: Dhalla NS (ed) *Recent Advances in Studies on Cardiac Structure and Metabolism. Myocardial Biology*, Vol 4. Baltimore, MD: University Park Press, 1974, pp 359–374.

137. Van Winkle WB, Schwartz A: Ions and inotropy. *Annu Rev Physiol* 38:247–272, 1976.

138. Morad M, Goldman Y: Excitation-contraction coupling in heart muscle: Membrane control of development of tension. *Prog Biophys Mol Biol* 27:257–313, 1973.

139. Kavaler F, Anderson TW: Indirect evidence that calcium extrusion causes relaxation of frog ventricular muscle. *Fed Proc* 37:300, 1978.

140. Kavaler F, Anderson TW, Fisher VJ: Sarcolemmal site of caffeine's inotropic action on ventricular muscle of the frog. *Circ Res* 42:285–290, 1978.

141. Niedergerke R, Page S: Analysis of caffeine action in single trabeculae of the frog heart. *Proc R Soc Lond B* 213:303–324, 1981.

142. Fabiato A: Calcium both activates and inactivates calcium release from cardiac sarcoplasmic reticulum. In: Rubin RP, Weiss GB, Putney JW Jr (eds) *Calcium in Biological Systems*. New York: Plenum, 1985, pp 269–375.

CHAPTER 17

Uptake of Calcium by Sarcoplasmic Reticulum and its Regulation and Functional Consequences

MICHIHIKO TADA & MASAAKI KADOMA

INTRODUCTION

The contraction-relaxation cycle of the myocardium is physiologically regulated by a change in the intracellular Ca^{2+} concentration {1–3}. The cardiac contractile system, like that of skeletal muscle, is activated maximally when the ionized Ca^{2+} concentration reaches the value of $\sim 10^{-5}$ M, while the active state can be converted to the resting one when the ionized Ca^{2+} falls below 10^{-7} M. In the fast skeletal muscle, this change in the intracellular Ca^{2+} is regulated solely by the sarcoplasmic reticulum (SR). Release and subsequent accumulation of Ca^{2+} by this organelle induce contraction and relaxation of the contractile system. In the cardiac muscle, however, the intracellular Ca^{2+} concentration during the contraction relaxation cycle is controlled not only by the SR but also by other cellular organelles such as the sarcolemma {4–8}. The extent to which the SR participates in the regulation of the beat-to-beat Ca^{2+} movement varies among different animal species {5,6}. In the mammalian ventricle, the SR is fairly well developed {9}, and there is evidence that the SR plays a major role in initiating contraction and relaxation {5–7}. In contrast, in the cardiac muscle of lower vertebrates, such as frog ventricle, the SR appears to be less developed, and available data indicate that the sarcolemma plays a more important role {5,6}. Although mitochondria have long been implicated in the control of cardiac relaxation, recent experiments indicate that they do not play a significant role both in amphibian and mammalian cardiac muscle under physiologic conditions {5,7}.

Accumulation by and release of Ca^{2+} from the SR have been studied using various experimental systems ranging from the preparations of isolated SR vesicles to the intact fiber, obtained mainly from the mammalian cardiac muscle. The mechanism by which the SR accumulates Ca^{2+} to induce relaxation, and its regulation, which is physiologically and pharmacologically important, have been elucidated fairly well {10}. Of particular interest is the notion that cardiac SR exhibits a unique mechanism by which Ca pumping function is controlled by phosphorylation of its regulatory protein phospholamban {11}. More extensive studies are leading us to the understanding of Ca pump ATPase and phospholamban at the molecular level. The

mechanism by which the SR releases Ca^{2+} to initiate contraction is another issue of importance {12}. Although the chemical and structural bases for this process have been obscure, great progress has evolved quite recently, and has led to the new notion that the molecular machinery of Ca release exists in a specified portion of the SR {13}. As the molecular structure and function of the SR Ca release channel have been intensively elucidated, this protein has proven to be responsible for the release of Ca^{2+} from SR. As the latter subject is discussed elsewhere in this book (Chapter 12), this chapter summarizes the present knowledge of Ca transport across the SR membranes and its regulation, with an emphasis on the molecular mode by which Ca^{2+} is accumulated by the Ca pump of the cardiac SR.

STRUCTURE AND COMPOSITION OF SARCOPLASMIC RETICULUM MEMBRANES

The SR of the mammalian myocardium consists of a membrane-limited structure that forms a network surrounding the bundles of myofilaments {9}. The lumen of the SR forms a closed intracellular system that is not continuous with the extracellular space. The transverse tubular system (T system), another tubular structure running mainly perpendicular to the long axis of the myocardial cell and thus segmenting the SR at the Z lines, is continuous with the surface membrane, its lumen communicating with the extracellular space. The SR can be divided into two components: the free SR and the junctional SR {9,14}. The former does not participate in the formation of any junction with other membranes, but surrounds the myofilaments mainly in the center of the sarcomere. The latter is located beneath the cell surface membrane to form a peripheral coupling with the sarcolemma or situated alongside the T system to form an interior coupling with the membranes of the T system. The interior couplings occur in the forms of the dyads or triads in which one or two elements of junctional SR form coupling on one or either side of the T tubules, respectively. The junctional SR that forms peripheral and interior couplings is often referred to as the *subsarcolemmal cisternae* and the *terminal cisternae*, respectively. The

N. Sperelakis (ed.), Physiology and Pathophysiology of the Heart, Third Edition.

junction between the junctional SR and either the cell surface membrane or the membrane of the T system is characterized by the presence of "feet," regular periodic projections extended from the membrane of the junctional SR {9,14}. These structures may provide the basis for transmission of a signal from the sarcolemma to the SR. In addition to feet, the junctional SR is further characterized by the presence of dense granular material inside its lumen. These dense materials are negatively charged and are considered to represent a Ca-binding protein, calsequestrin (see below) {15}. In addition to these portions of SR, specialized forms of junctional SR called corbular SR, which differ from ordinary junctional SR in geometry and in topographic aspect, can be identified in the cardiac muscle {9}. In contrast, the free SR is devoid of these features of the junctional SR. Therefore, different portions of the SR have special structural features, suggesting that different functions may be assigned to these portions of the SR. In accord with this notion, storage and release of Ca^{2+} occur primarily at the terminal cisternae {16,17}, while Ca uptake appears to occur alongside the entire surface of the SR membrane.

The ionic composition of the SR in situ has been studied with electron-probe analysis of skeletal muscle {17}. The contents of K^+, Na^+, and Cl^- in the SR in the resting muscle are not very different from those in the cytoplasm, but are quite different from those of the extracellular space. Such observations indicate that the SR is an intracellular compartment and argue against the existence of a resting potential across the SR membranes if the in-situ SR membranes are permeable to K^+, Na^+, and Cl^-, as in the isolated SR vesicles. When a short tetanus is induced in frog muscle, it has been shown that the terminal cisternae release more than half of their Ca^{2+} content into the cytoplasm {17}. This Ca^{2+} release is associated, with a significant uptake of Mg^{2+} and K^+ into the terminal cisternae. As Ca^{2+} released significantly exceeds the total measured cation accumulation, it was suggested that protons and/or organic ions are also taken up by the terminal cisternae to compensate for a large charge deficit. These results thus indicate that various ions are moving into or out of the SR, coupled to the Ca movement during activation and relaxation of the muscle fiber.

Preparation of fragmented sarcoplasmic reticulum

When cardiac muscle is homogenized, the SR membranes are fragmented and then reseal spontaneously into small vesicles. These vesicles can be isolated in microsomal fractions by differential centrifugation of homogenized cardiac muscle {18–22}. The microsomes sedimented between 8000–10,000 and 37,000–40,000 g are usually further treated with 0.6 M KCl to remove contaminating contractile proteins. The resultant preparations, which are used commonly in most laboratories, are highly enriched in the SR membranes, as judged on the basis of the marker enzyme activities (Ca uptake and Ca^{2+}-dependent ATPase activities, and Ca^{2+}-dependent acylphosphoenzyme formation; see below). The yield of this preparation from dog heart is about 0.63 mg/g wet muscle, which is approxi-

mately 10% of the SR membranes present in the muscle homogenate {21}. These preparations are contaminated with mitochondrial fragments so that their ATPase activity is inhibited significantly by sodium azide, a mitochondrial inhibitor {18,23–25}. Their Ca-uptake activity, however, is not affected by this reagent {18,21}. These preparations are also significantly contaminated with the sarcolemmal membranes, the latter content being estimated to be up to 15% {26}. Recently a more elaborate procedure has been developed for isolation of cardiac SR membranes {27}. Although the new procedure takes a long time (16–18 hours), the preparation has considerably improved Ca transport properties, stability, and purity. The isolated cardiac SR membrane vesicles are largely spherical, with a diameter of about 0.1–0.2 µ when examined in an electron microscope {27}. These vesicles are considered to be sealed and retain the original right-side-out orientation, Ca^{2+} thus being transported into their lumen.

As can be predicted from the finding that the SR in situ is composed of different regions, the isolated fragmented SR membranes are not homogenous. Meissner {28} separated the fragmented SR membranes isolated from fast skeletal muscle into subfractions of different density by centrifugation through sucrose gradient. Subsequent biochemical and morphologic data have indicated that light and heavy fractions are derived from the longitudinal SR (free SR) and the terminal cisternae (junctional SR), respectively {28,29}. Jones and his coworkers {30,31} have shown that cardiac SR membranes also consist of heterogeneous subpopulations. They differentiated the fraction derived from the juncional SR from that from the free SR by their protein composition and Ca transport properties. The junctional SR fraction contains high contents of calsequestrin and high molecular weight proteins, and its Ca-uptake activity is selectively stimulated by both ryanodine and ruthenium red. This subfraction also contains a high content of the specific binding site for calcium antagonist [^{3}H] nitrendipine {32}.

Protein and lipid composition

When cardiac SR vesicles are subjected to polyacrylamide gel electrophoresis in the presence of sodium dodecylsulfate, a considerable number of protein bands can be observed. Cardiac SR membranes appear to have more complex protein composition than the skeletal SR membranes {27}. The major component is a polypeptide with a molecular weight of approximately 100,000 Da. This polypeptide represents the ATPase protein of the SR, which plays a central role in the Ca transport by the SR. The ATPase protein has recently been partially purified from pigeon-heart {22} and dog-heart {33,34} SR membranes after solubilizing the membrane proteins by deoxycholate or Triton X-100. The ATPase protein accounts for 35–40% of the total SR protein in the highly purified cardiac SR preparation {27}. Electrophoresis of cardiac SR membranes also demonstrates other protein bands corresponding to calsequestrin (Mw 44,000–55,000 Da), the intrinsic glycoproteins (Mw 53,000 and 160,000 Da), and the high molecular weight proteins (Mw 290,000–350,000 Da) {31,

35,36}. In addition to these proteins, which are also components of skeletal-muscle SR membranes, cardiac SR membranes contain phospholamban, a specific low molecular weight protein that serves as the substrate for protein kinases and controls the function of the Ca pump of the SR (see below and Tada and Katz {11}).

MOLECULAR STRUCTURE OF Ca PUMP ATPase

The ATPase protein is an amphipathic single chain polypeptide. One mole of the ATPase protein contains approximately 2 moles of high-affinity Ca-binding sites (K_d, ~0.3 μM) and 1 mole each of high-affinity (K_d, 0.5–3.0 μM) and low-affinity ATP-binding sites (K_d, ~1 mM) {22,37–40}. Its molecular weight determined by sedimentation equilibrium in the analytic ultracentrifuge in the presence of detergents is 115,000–119,000 {41}. The hydrophobic region of the ATPase polypeptide is intimately associated with the membrane lipid phse, while its hydrophilic portion appears to be exposed on the cytoplasmic side of the SR membrane. Limited trypsin digestion of the intact closed SR vesicles cleaves the ATPase polypeptide first into two fragments (at T1, see fig. 17-1): fragment A (Mr ~ 55,000) and fragment B (Mr ~ 45,000). By further trypsin digestion, fragment A is cleaved into two fragments (at T2): fragment A_1 (Mr ~ 33,000) and fragment A^2 (Mr ~ 22,000) {42,44}. These tryptic fragments contain both the hydrophilic and hydrophobic portions, each of which is independently anchored in the membrane. The active site of the ATPase, which is phosphorylated by the terminal phosphate of ATP during the enzyme catalysis (see below), is located on the tryptic fragment A_1, a specific aspartate residue being phosphorylated. In contrast, the nucleotide-binding site, which also constitutes the active site, is located on fragment B and can be labelled with fluorescein isothiocyanate {45}. The Ca-transporting site may be associated with the tryptic fragment A_2 since this fragment appears to posses Ca ionophore activity when incorporated into lipid bilayer {44} and is covalently labelled with dicyclohexylcarbodimide (DCCD) under conditions in which high-affinity Ca binding to the ATPase is inhibited by this reagent {46}.

The complete amino acid sequence of the rabbit SR ATPase polypeptide has been deduced by MacLennan and his cowokers from its cDNA sequence {47,48}. They demonstrated the existence of two closely crosshybridizing genes that encode ATPase proteins of fast-skeletal and of slow-skeletal/cardiac SR, respectively. With the advent of recombinant DNA technology, their approaches have led to a rather thorough understanding of the composition of the sarco(endo)plasmic reticulum in different tissues. Table 17-1 shows that there are at least three kinds of Ca

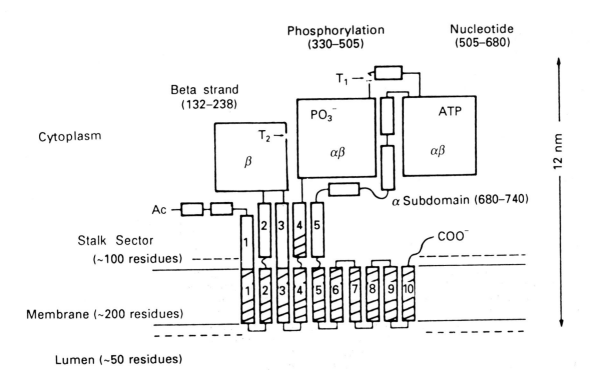

Fig. 17-1. Assembly of ATPase domains. The predicted arrays of helices and the three major domains are laid out in a planar diagram. In the ATPase molecule the helices would form tight clusters. The ATP-binding domain would be folded beside the other two major domains, permitting interaction among all three and accounting for the approximately triangular molecular profile derived from electron micrographs of ordered arrays by optical diffraction and for the molecular shape deduced from hydrodynamic measurements and electron microscopy. Modified from MacLennan et al. {47}.

Table 17-1. Expression and chromosomal localization in human genes encoding sarco(endo)plasmic reticulum proteins {49–55}

Gene	Tissue					Chromosome
	Fast	Slow	Cardiac	Smooth	Non-muscle	
Ca-ATPase[a]						
SERCA1	+[b,c]	–	–	–	–	16
SERCA2	–	+[b]	+[b]	+[c]	+[c]	12
SERCA3	–	+	+	+	+	
Phospholamban	–	+	+	+	–	6

[a] Nomenclature based upon Burk et al. {55}.
[b,c] Expression of alternatively spliced forms.

ATPase genes expressed in sarco(endo)plasmic reticulum (SERCA) {49–55}. The type gene, SERCA 1, expressed in fast skeletal muscle, gives rise to two alternatively spliced transcripts, thus producing an adult pump, SERCA 1a, and a neonatal pump, SERCA 1b. The type 2 gene, SERCA 2, encodes two alternatively spliced products. SERCA 2a is expressed in slow skeletal muscle and cardiac muscle, while SERCA 2b is expressed in smooth muscle and nonmuscle tissues. The type 3 gene, SERCA 3, was found to be expressed in a broad variety of both muscle and nonmuscle tissues. As shown below, the ATPase enzyme expressed by type 2 gene (SERCA 2a) exhibits a unique molecular interaction with phospholamban. The slow/cardiac muscle ATPase protein contains 997 amino acid residues with a calculated molecular weight of 109,529 Da, while the fast skeletal ATPase contains 1001 amino acid residues with a molecular weight of 110,331 Da {47,48}. Although there are 164 differences in amino acid sequence between the two ATPases, overall topographical maps based on the predicted secondary structure were found to be similar. Figure 17-1 shows a diagram of the submolecular structure of the ATPase protein deduced from its primary structure and other chemical and morphologic data (see below) {47}. In this diagram each functional site of the ATPase protein is considered to form a functional domain in the tertiary structure: It is made up of a cytoplasmic headpiece, creating a tripartite structure. The headpiece, made up of three globular domains, lies on top of the pentahelical stalk, and the 10 transmembrane helices form the intramembrane structure. Based on mutational analyses, the high-affinity Ca binding sites are proposed to be located near the center of the transmembrane domain {56,57}. Therefore, the Ca-binding and the ATP-processing domains are considered to be physically separated, which is consistent with a report that the distance between nucleotide and Ca sites, as estimated in the luminescence energy-transfer experiments, was 35–47 Å {58}. In this diagram it is postulated that the gross conformational change of the ATPase protein provides the link between the events occurring within the Ca-binding and the ATP-processing domains. It should be mentioned, however, that the model shown in the diagram is still speculative, although it is plausible. It remains to be examined how these functional sites interact mutually within the three-dimensional structure of the ATPase protein.

IDENTIFICATION OF OTHER SR COMPONENTS

Calsequestrin is loosely bound to the membrane and is easily extracted by treatment with detergents or alkaline solutions {35,36}. Cardiac calsequestrin is a protein of strong negative charge, its molecular weight varying between 44,000 and 55,000 Da, depending on the conditions used for gel electrophoresis. Based on cDNA-deduced amino acid sequence, its molecular weight is calculated to be 45,269 {59}. This protein, presumably localized inside the SR vesicles, has a low affinity but a large binding capacity for Ca^{2-}. It binds an appreciable amount of Ca^{2+} when intravesicular Ca^{2+} concentration exceeds millimolar ranges. This protein varies greatly in its content, being practically absent in the ryanodine-insensitive fraction and greatly enriched in the ryanodine-sensitive fraction (see above) {30,31}. It is suggested that this protein primarily serves as a storage site of the accumulated Ca.

The 53,000-Da and 160,000-Da glycoproteins are, like the ATPase protein, intrinsic membrane proteins of the cardiac SR {35,36}. These are alternatively spliced products of the same gene: The larger molecular weight isoform is termed *sarcalumenin* {60}. It is exposed on both the outside and inside surfaces of the SR vesicles. However, their physiologic role is not known at present.

In addition to these major proteins, SR membranes contain many other proteins. In fast skeletal SR, two of these proteins were characterized {42,44}. One is the 12,000-Da proteolipid that is an intrinsic membrane protein and often copurifies with the ATPase protein in detergents. The other is the high-affinity Ca-binding protein (Mr ~ 55,000, termed *calreticulin*), which is a water-soluble extrinsic protein. This protein has recently been reported to be present in cardiac and smooth muscle tissues as well as in nonmuscle cells {61}. Functions of these proteins are not known.

LIPID COMPOSITION

In the SR preparations isolated from fast skeletal muscle, phospholipids make up about 80% of the total lipids on a molar basis, choline glycerophospholipids being the most prominent molecular species (65–73%) {10}. The low cholesterol content and the relatively high degree of unsaturation of the fatty acid component of the major phospholipids are characteristics of the SR membranes of rabbit fast skeletal muscle. The phospholipid composition of cardiac SR is generally similar to that of fast skeletal muscle, except that it contains a significantly high level of ethanolamine glycerophospholipids {27}. A recent report {62} has demonstrated that the major phospholipid in cardiac SR membrane is plasmalogen and that choline glycerophospholipid in the cardiac SR contains over five times the amount of plasmalogen compared to that in fast skeletal SR. The purified ATPase protein contains phospholipid, the composition of which is similar to that of the intact SR membrane {42}. Phospholipid molecules intimately associated with the ATPase protein are required for its enzymic activity. Thus, phospholipase treatment of the purified ATPase protein or the native SR membranes results in inhibition of ATP hydrolysis and/or Ca transport by the membranes {63}.

Structural organization of sarcoplasmic reticulum membranes

The structural organization of the SR membranes of skeletal and cardiac muscles, either isolated or in situ, has been studied using various electron-microscopic preparations {9,14,20,27,35,42,64}. Electron-microscopic pictures of freeze-fractured SR membranes indicate that the hydrophobic interior of the membranes is filled with globular particles 80–90 Å in diameter. The majority of these particles are concentrated in the outer leaflet of the membrane bilayer. Negative staining of the SR membrane vesicles reveals the presence of smaller particles (about 40 Å in diameter) with stalks projecting from the surface of the membranes. These surface and intramembranous particles have been shown to represent the structural features of the ATPase protein. It is thus suggested that a large part of the ATPase protein is localized in the cytoplasmic leaflet of the bilayer membrane of the SR and that this protein extends into the cytoplasm to form 40-Å particles. The structure of isolated SR membranes of skeletal muscle have also been investigated using the x-ray and neutron diffraction techniques {65}. The use of these techniques reveals that the ATPase protein spans the entire SR membrane with its major portion (about 50% of its total mass) localized externally to the membrane lipid bilayer, thus confirming the asymmetric distribution of the ATPase protein visualized by electron microscope.

The density of the ATPase protein in the membrane may be less in the cardiac SR than in the fast skeletal SR. The densit of 90-Å intramembraneous particles in the cardiac SR as seen by freeze-fracture electron microscopy {9,27} was reported to be about half that in fast skeletal SR. The lower density of the small surface particles was also suggested for the cardiac SR using thin-section and negative-staining electron microscopy {27}.

There is uncertainty as to the state of aggregation of the ATPase polypeptide in the native SR membranes.

Because the density of the smaller surface particles was found to be three to four times more than that of the intramembraneous particles and because there has been some experimental evidence for occurrence of functional interactions between the ATPase polypeptides {41,64,66}, the ATPase has been considered to form oligomers within the SR membrane. Franzini-Armstrong and Ferguson {67}, however, have recently shown that the disposition of ATPase in the SR membrane is primarily disorderly and that the ATPase does not form oligomers of uniform size. They also reported that counting the intramembraneous particles on the fractured membrane is not a reliable means of obtaining the ATPase density. There is also uncertainty as to the size of the functional unit for the Ca pump in the membrane. Although the monomeric form of the ATPase obtained in the presence of detergents has been shown to be catalytically active {41}, some recent kinetic, spectroscopic, and radiation inactivation experiments suggest that the minimum functional unit of the Ca pump may be a oligomer (possibly a dimer) of the ATPase polypeptide {41,66,68}. When the SR membranes are treated with vanadate, extensive two-dimensional crystalline arrays of the ATPase are formed {69}. The ATPase crystals contains dimers as structural units. On the other hand, when the crystals were formed in the presence of Ca^{2+} or lanthanide ions, the crystallographic unit is a monomer {70}. At present, however, the functional significance of these forms of the ATPase-ATPase interaction are not clear.

Ca UPTAKE BY THE FRAGMENTED SARCOPLASMIC RETICULUM

Ca uptake and ATP hydrolysis

Isolated cardiac SR vesicles can take up Ca^{2+} in the presence of Mg^{2+} and ATP, thereby reducing markedly Ca^{2+} concentration in the reaction medium {1,63}. At relatively low ionized Ca^{2+} (3–50 μM) and in the absnce of Ca^{2+}-precipitating anions such as oxalate or phosphate, SR vesicles rapidly accumulate up to 70 nM Ca^{2+}/mg protein {19–21, 71–73}. This Ca^{2+} flows out of the vesicles at a slow rate in the presence of EGTA, a membrane-impermeable Ca-chelating agent. This Ca^{2+}, however, is rapidly and completely released when the SR membrane is made leaky with detergents or Ca ionophores {74}. These observations indicate that Ca^{2+} is transported across the SR membranes and stored within their lumen. If the internal space of the cardiac SR vesicles is assumed to be 4–5 μl/mg protein, which is the value reported for the skeletal SR vesicles {63}, the intravesicular Ca^{2+} concentration could be as high as 17 mM. Although a significant portion of this Ca^{2+} may be bound to the intravesicular structures, such as Ca-binding proteins and membrane phospholipids, the intravesicular ionized Ca^{2+} would still be at the millimolar range, indicating that Ca^{2+} is transported against the concentration gradient under these conditions.

After a steady-state level of up to 70 nM Ca^{2+}/mg

protein is reached, further Ca accumulation is not observed even when the Ca^{2+} and ATP concentrations in the medium are sufficient to activate the Ca pump. The constant level of Ca accumulation indicates that both the rates of active Ca influx by the pump and passive Ca efflux are equal. The influx depends on the degree of activation of the Ca pump and the concentration of intravesicular Ca^{2+}, while the efflux depends on the intravesicular Ca^{2+} concentration and the Ca permeability of the SR membranes. As noted below, intravesicular Ca^{2+} at millimolar ranges inhibits the Ca pump by interfering with an intermediary step of ATP hydrolysis. The passive permeability of Ca^{2+} is relatively low, about 50–100 times slower than the maximal initial rate of Ca uptake in skeletal muscle SR [63]. This low permeability to Ca^{2+} primarily reflects the intrinsic property of the lipid bilayer matrix on which SR membranes are built. It was found, however, that the SR permeability to Ca^{2+} increases markedly during ATP-supported Ca uptake when Ca^{2+} concentrations outside the SR vesicles increase [75,76].

When oxalate is included in the reaction medium, cardiac SR vesicles take up as much as 6–10 μM Ca^{2+}/mg protein [21,22]. An equimolar amount of Ca^{2+} and oxalate is taken up under these conditions and Ca oxalate crystal is formed inside the SR vesicles [1,18,77], indicating that the intravesicular concentrations of Ca oxalate is higher than its solubility product. Ca uptake observed under these conditions proceeds linearly over a considerable period of time until Ca^{2+} concentrations in the medium become too low to activate the Ca pump or until Ca uptake is limited by the Ca oxalate storing capacity of the vesicles. Therefore, oxalate, which is freely permeable to the SR membranes and forms crystal with Ca^{2+}, appears to sustain Ca uptake by maintaining the intravesicular Ca^{2+} concentrations at a low level, thereby removing an inhibitory effect of intravesicular high Ca^{2+} on Ca transport [78].

Ca uptake by SR vesicles is usually measured using radioactive $^{45}Ca^{2+}$ by the membrane filtration method, which allows rapid separation of $^{45}Ca^{2+}$-loaded vesicles from the reaction medium. This technique is appropriate for following the time course of Ca uptake in a time scale of minutes. The reported maximal rates of Ca uptake by cardiac SR vesicles measured with this technique in the presence of oxalate range from 0.2 μM/mg protein/min at 25°C [79] to 1.5 μM/mg protein/min at 37°C [21]. In the absence of Ca-precipitating anion, this technique does not allow accurate determination of the rate of Ca uptake because Ca uptake proceeds linearly only for a short time. Ca uptake in time scales of milliseconds to seconds can be followed with stopped-flow techniques or the quench-flow method. In the former, a rapid time-dependent spectral change of Ca indicator dyes such as murexide or arsenazo III, which reflects variation of the Ca^{2+} concentration in the medium, is monitored spectrophotometrically; while, in the latter, fast ^{45}Ca uptake by the vesicles is measured after quenching the uptake reaction with EGTA or La^{3+} using a rapid-quenching apparatus. The initial rate of ATP-supported Ca uptake by cardiac SR vesicles measured with murexide through the stopped-flow technique was

reported to be 16–21 nM Ca^{2+}/mg protein/150 ms at 25°C [71]. In contrast, an initial uptake rate of 33.4 nM Ca^{2+}/mg protein/s was measured at 22°C in the presence of 18.9 μM Ca^{2+} with a rapid-quenching apparatus and EGTA [80]. It should be noted that these values of Ca-uptake rate are much greater than those obtained at the steady state in the presence of oxalate (see above).

Ca transport across cardiac SR membranes is an energy-requiring process [1,77]. SR vesicles exhibit Ca^{2+}-dependent and Ca^{2+}-independent ATP hydrolysis. In the usual preparations of cardiac SR membranes, a large portion of Ca^{2+}-independent ATPase activity appears to be derived from the activity associated with the contaminating mitochondrial cragments [18,23–25]. In contrast, the Ca^{2+}-dependent portion of ATP hydrolysis is catalyzed by the ATPase protein of the SR. In fast skeletal muscle SR, the Ca^{2+}-dependent ATP hydrolysis and Ca uptake parallel each other under a variety of conditions [1,77], indicating that the former represents an energy source for the latter. Ca^{2+}-dependent ATP hydrolysis and Ca uptake are tightly coupled, two moles Ca^{2+} being transported for one mole ATP hydrolyzed both in the presence and absence of oxalate [1,64,77]. In accord with this coupling ratio, one mole of ATPase protein was shown to contain two moles of high-affinity Ca-binding sites and one mole of high-affinity ATP-binding site (see above). A coupling ratio of two moles Ca^{2+} taken up per mole ATP hydrolyzed is also observed in the intact cardiac SR vesicles [24]. The coupling ratio, however, decreases when the passive permeability of SR membranes to Ca^{2+} is increased by various means. Treatment of SR vesicles with detergents or ionophores, for example, renders the SR membranes leaky and prevents net uptake of Ca^{2+} while a high rate of ATP hydrolysis is maintained for a prolonged period of time. Low coupling ratios have often been reported even in intact SR vesicles [27,30,31]. This may indicate that a significant fraction of the SR vesicles in these preparations is open membrane fragments or that some mechanisms may be operating to maintain increased permeability of the SR membranes to Ca^{2+} [75,76]. The latter possibility is consistant with the recent finding that ryanodine and ruthenium red improve this coupling ratio significantly [30,31].

Ca uptake and Ca^{2+}-dependent ATP hydrolysis by cardiac SR vesicles are activated by very low Ca^{2+} concentrations in the medium outside SR vesicles [1,63]. The rates of both activities rise with increasing Ca^{2+} concentrations, reaching a maximum' at 3–10 μM Ca^{2+}. Half-maximal activation is seen at 0.3–4.7 μM Ca^{2+} (K_{Ca}) at pH 6.8–7.0 [19–21,25,72,73,79,81]. This rather large variation of the optimal range of Ca^{2+} for activation arises partly from the different binding constants for the Ca-EGTA complex employed by different investigators. It should be noted that the optimal range of Ca^{2+} (K_{Ca}) for Ca uptake and ATP hydrolysis measured in the presence of oxalate is approximately fivefold greater than that for the steady-state Ca accumulation obtained in the absence of Ca-precipitating anions [21]. The former, being in agreement with that for formation of a phosphoenzymes intermediate of ATP hydrolysis (see below), appears likely to reflect Ca^{2+} dependence of Ca influx effected by the Ca pump. The latter, however, may not give true Ca^{2+} dependence of the pump activity because a steady-state Ca accumulation is determined by the dynamic equilibrium between Ca influx into and Ca efflux from the SR vesicles. Because the permeability of the SR membrane to Ca^{2+} increases with increasing Ca^{2+} outside the SR vesicles {75,76}, the high intravesicular Ca^{2+}, which is the result of the pump activity, would increase Ca efflux significantly at higher Ca^{2+} in the medium. This, together with the decreased turnover of the Ca pump caused by high intravesicular Ca^{2+} (see below), could lower Ca^{2+} concentrations at which Ca^{2+} dependence of the steady-state accumulation exhibits a saturation. The activating effect of Ca^{2+} can be mimicked by Sr^{2+} or Mn^{2+} {1,82}. La^{3+} at relatively high concentrations inhibits both Ca uptake and ATP hydrolysis {10}. Both activities are inhibited by high Ca^{2+} inside SR vesicles, as mentioned above.

In cardiac SR, like in skeletal SR {10}, an equimolar complex of Mg^{2+} and ATP appears to serve as the physiologic substrate for Ca uptake and Ca^{2+}-dependent ATP hydrolysis. The complex of Ca^{2+} and ATP also serves as a substrate for these activities, but the activities are much less when CaATP serves as a substrate than when MgATP is used as a substrate {83,84}. The Ca^{2+}-dependent ATP hydrolysis exhibits a complex MgATP dependence: in the presence of an ATP-regenerating system, the ATPase activity shows saturation at about $10\,\mu M$ MgATP (K_m, $1-2\,\mu M$), while a further increase in activity is observed at higher MgATP concentrations ($K_m \sim 0.18\,mM$) {25,85}. The K_m value obtained at low ATP is similar to that for formation of phosphoenzyme intermediate of the ATPase (see below), indicating that this low K_m site corresponds to a high-affinity catalytic site. The stimulatory effect of high ATP is considered to arise from the regulatory action of the nucleotide on the turnover of the Ca pump, because high concentrations of ATP exert an activating effect on the intermediary steps of ATP hydrolysis (see below). In addition, the analogues of ATP, which are not hydrolyzed or are hydrolyzed little by the enzyme, mimic the effect of high ATP {39,40,86}. Besides ATP, the Ca pump of SR utilizes other natural nucleotide triphosphates {1,10,87}. The rates of utilization at 5 mM by the cardiac Ca pump are in the following order; ATP > CTP > ITP > GTP > UTP {18}. Van Winkle et al. {85}, however, have recently reported that GTP does not support the calcium translocation and that the mechanism of GTP hydrolysis is different from that for ATP. Other phosphate compounds such as acetylphosphate and *p*-nitrophenylphosphate also serve as substrates, although the rates of utilization are very slow {89}.

Mg^{2+}, in addition to serving as the component of the physiologic substate MgATP, accelerates an intermediary step of ATP hydrolysis (see below). The possibility that Ca uptake is obligatorily coupled to countertransport of Mg^{2+} has been excluded by recent experiments with skeletal SR vesicles {82,90}.

Monovalent cations such as K^+ are required for the full activation of the Ca-pump activity {91–93}. Removal of monovalent salts from reaction medium reduces the rates of Ca uptake and Ca^{2+}-dependent ATP hydrolysis to approximately one fourth of those observed in the presence of optimal concentrations of these salts. The effectiveness of these salts at 100 mM is graded in the following order: $K^+ > Na^+ > NH^{3+} > Rb^+ > Cs^+ > Li^+$ {91–93}. A recent study {94} showed that K^+ activates the Ca pump activity on the cytoplasmic surface of the SR membrane and that K^+ does not serve as a counterion for Ca transport. As discussed later, these monovalent salts also accelerate one of the intermediary steps of ATP hydrolysis.

pH dependence of the rates of Ca uptake and Ca^{2+}-dependent ATP hydrolysis by the cardiac SR vesicles exhibits a bell-shaped profile with the optimum at pH 6.2–6.5 for Ca uptake and at pH 7.5–8.0 for ATP hydrolysis {25,95}.

Effects of ion fluxes and the membrane potential on Ca uptake have been studied using native fastskeletal SR vesicels {96,97} or purified skeletal SR ATPase protein incorporated into phospholipid bilayer vesicles {98}. The rate of ATP-dependent Ca uptake is stimulated when a membrane potential, negative inside, is imposed across the reconstituted SR membrane with a K^+-concentration gradient and valinomycin. This observation suggests that the Ca pump of the SR is electrogenic. pH gradient (inside acidic) was also shown to increase the initial rate of Ca uptake {96,99}. H^+ was found to be ejected from the SR vesicles during the initial phase of Ca uptake {82,100}. This H^+ ejection and Ca uptake may be tightly coupled in such a way that H^+ is obligatorily exchanged for Ca^{2+} in an antiport system. On the other hand, the native SR membranes have been shown to be highly permeable to ions such as K^+, Na^+, H^+, and Cl^-, although they are relatively impermeable to Ca^{2+}, Mg^{2+}, and larger ions such as $Tris^+$, $choline^+$, or $gluconate^-$ {97,101}. A specific K^+ channel has been identified and extensively characterized in the skeletal SR membranes {102,103}. An anion channel that is blocked by aniontransport inhibitors was also identified in the skeletal SR membranes {104}. It is, therefore, also possible that charge displacement caused by the activity of the electrogenic Ca pump may be counterbalanced by fluxes of these highly permeable ions that are not directly coupled to the Ca-pump activity.

Mechanism of ATP hydrolysis

As mentioned earlier, Ca uptake by cardiac SR is an energy-requiring process and is stoichiometrically linked to ATP hydrolysis. As Ca uptake can be reconstituted from the ATPase protein purified from skeletal SR and phospholipids {44,105}, the ATPase protein is considered to serve not only as a Can transporter but also as a transducer of chemical energy into the osmotic energy. To elucidate the mechanism by which Ca^{2+} is transported across SR membranes, analysis of the elementary steps of Ca^{2+}-dependent ATP hydrolysis and comparison of these with those of Ca transport must be carried out. A current view of the mechanism of ATP hydrolysis by the Ca-pump ATPase is summarized below.

During Ca^{2+}-dependent ATP hydrolysis by cardiac SR

vesicles, the terminal phosphate of ATP is incorporated into the ATPase protein {23,25,81,106–109}. The phosphoenzyme formation requires micromolar ranges of Ca^{2+} and ATP, indicating that high-affinity sites for Ca^{2+} and ATP, which are responsible for activation of ATP hydrolysis (see above), are involved in phosphorylation of the ATPase {25,81,107}. When concentrations of Ca^{2+} and ATP are varied at a relatively low concentration range, complete parallelism can be observed between the steady-state level of phosphoenzyme and the rate of ATP hydrolysis {25}, supporting the view that the phosphoenzyme is an intermediate of ATP hydrolysis. The chemical characteristics of the phosphoenzyme isolated by the addition of acid are those of an acylphosphoprotein {25,107}. In skeletal SR, the phosphoryl group was shown to be covalently bound to the carboxyl group of aspartic acid residue {110}. The maximum amount of phosphoenzyme formed in the oridinary preparations of cardiac SR, which could reflect the amount of the ATPase protein in the preparations, varies significantly from one animal species to the other, the SR preparation from dog heart giving the highest value of up to 1.3 nM/mg protein {23,25,107}. When the SR preparations from pigeon heart are further purified by sucrose density gradient after Ca oxalate loading, a phosphoenzyme level as high as 2.45 mM/mg protein can be obtained {22}.

Steady-state and transient kinetic studies of ATP hydrolysis by cardiac and skeletal SR membranes and the extensive use of various conformational probes revealed that the ATPase enzyme undergoes successive conformational transitions during catalysis {10,64,66,87,108, 111–113}. The results may be summarized as shown in the following scheme (scheme 1):

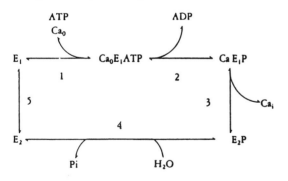

where Ca_o and Ca_i refer to Ca^{2+} located outside and inside the SR vesicles, respectively. The ATPase is considered to assume two major conformations E_1 and E_2, the former (E_1 or E_1P) having high Ca affinity and the latter (E_2 or E_2P) having low Ca affinity. The micromolar range of Ca^{2+} stabilized the E_1 conformation of the free enzyme, whereas removal of Ca^{2+} from the medium at low pH and high temperature, or addition of vanadate, stabilized the E_2 type of the free enzyme {112–114}. Under physiologic conditions, two moles of Ca^{2+} and one mole of MgATP react with one mole of the ATPase (E_1) on the outside surface of the SR membranes to form a Michaelis complex (step 1). Formation of the E_1-type phosphoenzyme (E_1P)

(step 2) is accompanied by the transient occlusion of Ca bound to the Ca-transport site {115}. Metal-free ADP is released on the outside surface of the membranes {84}. Mg^{2+} thus remains bound to the enzyme at this stage {116}. Ca^{2+} is then released into the vesicular lumen when E_1P is converted to the E_2 type of phosphoenzyme (E_2P) (step 3). E_1P is a high-energy type of phosphoenzyme, as it donates its phosphate group to added ADP to form ATP, while E_2P is a low-energy type because it does not react with added ADP. Therefore, a change in orientation of the Ca site with respect to the membrane and decrease of the affinity of the Ca site for Ca^{2+} appear to be coupled to the conversion of the high-energy to low-energy states of the phosphoenzyme. In step 4, E_2P decomposes to yield inorganic phosphate (P_i) on the outside surface of the SR vesicles. Mg^{2+} appears to be released from the ATPase at this step. Then, E_2 is transformed to E_1, with the resultant change in orientation of the Ca site, the enzyme thus completing a catalytic cycle.

Enzyme phosphorylation in cardiac SR vesicles is very rapid (fig. 17-2) {108,117,118}. It reaches a maximum level at 30 ms at 20–22°C when ATP (10 μM) is added to cardiac SR vesicles in a Ca^{2+}-containing medium. After reaching a maximum level, phosphoenzyme decreases slightly to the steady-state level (overshoot). In contrast, P_i liberation exhibits a distinct lag phase during accumulation of phosphoenzyme, indicating that P_i is derived from the turnover of phosphoenzyme. When enzyme phosphorylation is started by the addition of ATP and Ca^{2+} to the reaction medium containing the enzyme and EGTA, phosphorylation proceeds at a much slower rate and the overshoot cannot be observed (fig. 17-2). These observations are taken to indicate that the E_2 to E_1 transition (step 5), which is induced by Ca^{2+} addition, is slow and controls the rate of enzyme phosphorylation. The slow transition of E_2 to E_1 (step 5) can also be followed by monitoring changes of intrinsic fluorescence of the enzyme or the fluorescence of fluorescein bound to the enzyme {113,114,119}.

Ca^{2+} release from E_1P appears to be tightly coupled to the conformational transition of the enzyme from E_1P to E_2P, which can be monitored by measuring the increase in the fluorescence of 2′,3′-0-(2,4,6-trinitrocyclohexadienylidene)-ATP (TNPATP), a structural analogue of ATP, bound at the active site of the enzyme {120,121}. The Ca release from E_1P is accelerated by high pH, high ATP, and the insidenegative membrane protential {121}.

Phosphoenzyme decomposition is accelerated by Mg^{2+} or K^+, but inhibited by high Ca^{2+} {23,25,10,64,91,109}. At high Ca^{2+} (>1.0 mM), the E_1P to E_2P conversion is inhibited because Ca binding to the low-affinit Ca-binding site on E_2P accelerates reversal of this reaction step, thereby decreasing the concentration of E_2P. Mg^{2+} accelerates the phosphoenzyme hydrolysis by increasing the rate of the E_1P to E_2P conversion {111}. Recent reports {83,116} have shown that Mg^{2+}, which is derived from the metal component of the physiologic substrate MgATP and remains bound to the enzyme during catalysis, is responsible for this fast turnover of the phosphoenzyme intermediate.

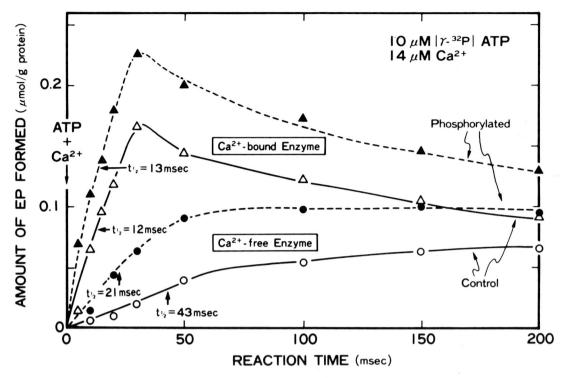

Fig. 17-2. Time courses of formation of phosophoenzyme intermediate before (○, △) or after (●, ▲) the treatment with cyclic AMP-dependent protein kinase: △, ▲, ATPase reaction started with SR plus Ca^{2+}; ○, ●, ATPase reaction started with Ca^{2+}-free SR. The final reaction medium contained $10 \mu M$ [γ-^{32}P]ATP and $14 \mu M$ ionized Ca^{2+}. Temperature was 22°C and pH was 6.8. From Tada et al. {117}, with permission.

Monovalent cations such as K^+ accelerate E_2P hydrolysis {122,123}, thus shifting the equilibrium of step 4 markedly to E_2 plus P_i. In the absence of K^+, E_2P hydrolysis is slow and limits the overall rate of ATP hydrolysis. In the presence of 100 mM KCl, which is usually included in the reaction medium for the measurement of Ca uptake and ATP hydrolysis by the SR, E_2P hydrolysis is much faster than the rate of the E_1P to E_2P conversion {122,123}. High concentrations of ATP also exert stimulatory effects on the intermediary steps of ATP hydrolysis {124,125}. Almost all the reaction steps (steps 2, 3, 4, and 5) have been shown to be accelerated by ATP, but apparently at different concentrations {10,112,121,122,125, 126}.

It was shown in skeletal SR vesicles that the reaction sequence outlined above is completely reversible {10,87, 112}. Lowering Ca^{2+} in the medium outside the Ca-loaded intact SR vesicles by a Cachelating agent leads to ATP synthesis from ADP and P_i, which is coupled with Ca efflux, Synthesis of one mole of ATP is coupled to the outflow of two moles of Ca^{2+} {127}. Reversal of Ca transport requires that ADP, P_i, and Mg^{2+} are present in the medium outside the SR vesicles. The free enzyme should be in the E_2 conformation for the reversal of the Ca pump to occur. Therefore, high ATP or the micromolar range of Ca^{2+}, which stabilizes the E_1 conformation, inhibits the pump reversal. During the pump reversal, the

ATPase is phosphorylated by P_i. The resultant phosphoenzyme reacts with added ADP to form ATP, which is coupled to Ca efflux. Phosphorylation of the ATPase by Pi also occurs even when the SR vesicles are rendered leaky or solubilized so that Ca gradient across the SR membranes cannot be developed {87,112}. The resultant phosphoenzyme, however, does not react with added ADP to form ATP. Under these conditions, simultaneous addition of high Ca^{2+} and ADP to the phosphoenzyme leads to the net synthesis of ATP {112,128}. The Ca^{2+} concentration required for the synthesis of ATP is in the millimolar range, which presumably reacts with the low-affinity Ca-binding site on the enzyme. Therefore, reversal of ATP hydrolysis can be achieved without using the osmotic energy that might be derived from the concentration gradient of Ca^{2+} across the SR membrane. For the synthesis of ATP in the intact SR vesicles, therefore, the concentration gradient of Ca^{2+} appears to be required only to provide high intravesicular Ca^{2+} concentrations and to saturate the internal low-affinity Ca-binding site {112}.

Comparison of Ca pumps of cardiac and skeletal muscle sarcoplasmic reticulum

As described in the preceding section, the mechanism of Ca uptake and ATP hydrolysis by cardiac SR vesicles is generally similar to that by skeletal SR vesicles. However, significant differences are noted in the two types of SR preparations: (a) Ca uptake and ATP hydrolysis are considerably slower in cardiac than in skeletal SR preparations {1,63}. (b) In the cardiac SR membranes, a specific regulatory mechanism, which is physiologically and pharmacologically important, controls Ca transport and ATP hydrolysis (see below) {11}. (c) The cardiac and fast skeletal SR ATPases are products of different genes, and there are some differences in the primary structure of these ATPases (see above).

To define the basis for the slower Ca uptake by the cardiac SR preparations, the steady-state ATPase reactions by dog-cardiac and rabbit fast-skeletal SR preparations were compared under the identical experimental conditions {25}. ATP hydrolysis by cardiac preparations at saturating Ca^{2+} is three to six times slower than that by skeletal preparations, whereas, at low Ca^{2+} (1–2 μM), the former is more than 10 times slower than the latter. A study on ATP dependence of the rate of ATP hydrolysis revealed that the K_m value for ATP is similar in both types of SR preparation while the maximum rate of ATP hydrolysis is about fourfold less in cardiac preparations. The maximum level of enzyme phosphorylation, which reflects the density of the ATPase protein in each SR preparation, was also found to be about fourfold less in dog cardiac preparations. In addition, the concentration of ionized Ca^{2+} that elicits half-maximal activation of the ATPase of dog cardiac preparation (K_{Ca}) is three to four times higher than that of the corresponding value for K_{Ca} in rabbit skeletal preparations. These results therefore indicate that the relatively slow rate of Ca uptake by dog cardiac preparations primarily reflects a low content of the ATPase and lower Ca affinity of the enzyme, rather than a low enzyme turnover rate. It may be added that the pH optimum for ATP hydrolysis is at a slightly more alkaline level in cardiac SR preparations.

In addition to these results obtained in the steady-state analysis of ATP hydrolysis, the transient-state kinetic data indicate that there are quantitative differences in the rate constants of some of the partial reactions of the ATPase of both types of SR {108,129}. When the ATPase reaction is started by the addition of ATP and Ca^{2+} to the reaction medium containing EGTA and enzyme, enzyme phosphorylation is slow, reflecting the slow conformational transition of E_2 to E_1 (step 5 of scheme 1). In dog cardiac preparations, the estimated rate constant of the E_2 to E_1 transition in the presence of 10 μM ATP is approximately five times smaller than that in rabbit skeletal preparations. The rate of phosphorylation, however, is the same for both types of SR preparation when the reaction is started by the addition of ATP (10–50 μM) to SR vesicles in a Ca^{2+}-containing medium, indicating that steps 1 and 2 of scheme 1 occur at similar rates in the two types of SR preparation.

It was shown that dissociation of Ca^{2+}, which is bound to the ATPase protein during the initial phase of enzyme activation, is 1.5-fold slower in the dog cardiac preparations. Phosphoenzyme decomposition, as measured after the new formation of phosphoenzyme is prevented by

chelation of Ca^{2+} by EGTA in the presence of 3 mM $MgCl_2$ and 100 mM KCl, exhibits complex time courses but appears to be slightly slower in the dog cardiac SR preparations. These transient-state kinetic data collectively indicate that the slower conformational transition of the E_2 to E_1 (step 5) in the dog cardiac preparations is the most prominent difference observed. The difference in the rate of this reaction step could be responsible for the lower rates of ATP hydrolysis and Ca uptake by cardiac SR preparations at low ATP. At high ATP concentrations, however, the E_2 to E_1 transition may not control the overall rate of reaction because high ATP enhances this reaction step {112}. It should be added that enzyme phosphorylation (steps 1 and 2), when started by the addition of ATP to the enzyme in a Ca^{2+}-containing medium, is significantly slower in the absence of added KCl than in the presence of this salt at 100 mM in the dog cardiac SR preparations {118}. This effect of KCl was not observed in the rabbit fast-skeletal preparations {84,130}.

REGULATION OF Ca UPTAKE BY FRAGMENTED SARCOPLASMIC RETICULUM

In cardiac SR membrane, a regulatory mechanism exists in which a specific protein component of the SR membranes (phospholamban) serves as a regulator controlling the Ca-pump ATPase activity. Such a mechanism is responsible for altering Ca transients within the cell and is considered to play a key role in mediating the actions of hormones and drugs on heart muscle. Phospholamban was first found in the membrane of SR to serve as a substrate for cyclic-AMP-dependent protein kinase. Upon phosphorylation of its serine residue, Ca pump ATPase was greatly enhanced, indicating the possibility that phospholamban fnctions as a regulator of Ca pump. In this sense, phospholamban serves to link the two important intracellular messengers Ca^{2+} and cyclic AMP. Phospholamban polypeptide was sequenced quite recently, indicating the existence of a unique molecular structure.

Cyclic-AMP regulation of Ca uptake

PHOSPHOLAMBAN PHOSPHORYLATION

A membrane protein of cardiac SR was found to be phosphorylated by cyclic-AMP-dependent protein kinase. The phosphoprotein, unlike the phosphorylated intermediate of the ATPase of the SR, exhibits stability characteristics of a phosphoester in which the phosphate is largely incorporated into serine residue {131–133}. On the SDS-polyacrylamide gel electrophoresis, this phosphorylatable peptide exhibits the apparent molecular weight of 22,000. Since this 22,000-Dal protein is specifically associated with functional alterations in the SR (see below), it was termed *phospholamban* in view of its ability to receive phosphate from ATP {134,135}. The molecular weight of phospholamban is found to be higher when estimated from its amino acid sequence (see below). Phospholamban was also found to serve as a substrate for calmodulin-dependent protein kinase {136}, which phosphorylates a site different from that for cyclic-AMP-dependent protein kinase. Protein kinase C was reported to catalyze phosphorylation of phospholamban {137}, although the site for the phosphorylation was not defined.

STIMULATION OF Ca UPTAKE

The rate of Ca uptake by cardiac SR vesicles in the presence of oxalate is more than doubled when the SR vesicles are previously phosphorylated by incubation with an optimum concentration of cyclic AMP and cyclic-AMP-dependent protein kinase {24}. This stimulation was also found in the absence of oxalate, when the rapid initial phase of Ca uptake (up to 300 ms) was determined by a special device {80,117}. In contrast, Ca uptake by the SR vesicles isolated from fast skeletal muscle does not exhibit such stimulation, nor is there any significant phosphorylation of similar protein {138}. The extent to which Ca uptake by cardiac SR vesicles is stimulated is correlated well with the increase in phospholamban phosphorylation, but not with other phosphoproteins {139}. Protein kinase obtained from cardiac muscle (type-II kinase) produces such stimulation, while that obtained from skeletal muscle (type-I kinase) is also functional, but to a much lesser extent {131}. When the rate of Ca uptake by cardiac SR vesicles is examined at different Ca^{2+} concentrations, cyclic-AMP-dependent phosphorylation of phospholamban reduces by approximately threefold the Ca^{2+} concentration at which a half-maximal activation of Ca uptake is observed {24,140}. When the phosphorylated SR membranes are incubated with phosphoprotein phosphatase obtained from bovine heart, most of the phosphorylated phospholamban is dephosphorylated {141,142}. Dephosphorylation leads to a complete reversal of the effect produced by protein kinase. When Ca uptake and phospholamban phosphorylation are compared in the presence of a fixed amount of protein kinase and different amounts of protein kinase inhibitor (modulator), a linear relationship is observed between the decrease in Ca uptake and the inhibition of phosphorylation of the SR membranes {143}.

Calmodulin-dependent phosphorylation of phospholamban is also associated with the stimulation of oxalate-facilitated Ca uptake by cardiac SR {144–147}. Such stimulation, which occurs in the absence of cyclic-AMP-dependent phosphorylation, is apparently indistinguishable from that induced by cyclic-AMP {146,147}. Like cyclic-AMP-dependent stimulation, calmodulin-dependent stimulation of Ca uptake is produced by the enhancement of Ca pump ATPase {146,147}.

EFFECT OF PHOSPHOLAMBAN ON PARTIAL REACTIONS OF ATP HYDROLYSIS

Ca uptake by SR vesicles is coupled with Ca^{2+}-dependent ATP hydrolysis. The observed stimulation of Ca uptake by phospholamban phosphorylation could be derived either from the enhanced turnover of the ATPase or from the increased efficiency of the Ca pump, namely, the increased

coupling ratio between Ca uptake and ATP hydrolysis. In fact, acceleration of Ca uptake is accompanied by the enhanced rate of concomitant ATP hydrolysis, the stoichiometry between Ca^{2+} taken up and ATP hydrolyzed being maintained at about 2 after phospholamban is phosphorylated {24}. The observed alteration in kinetic proterties of Ca^{2+}-dependent ATPase induced by phospholamban phosphorylation can be interpreted using the reaction sequence described in scheme 1. When phospholamban is phosphorylated, the ATPase activity in the presence of saturating concentrations of Ca^{2+} and ATP increases without alteration of a phosphoenzyme intermediate level {81}, suggesting that the increased rate of ATP hydrolysis may be due to the enhanced turnover of the phosphoenzyme intermediate. Studies on partial reaction of ATPase, employing steady-state and pre-steady-state kinetic measurements, are consistent with a view that the two rate-limiting steps of ATPase (steps 3 and 5 in scheme 1) are greatly enhanced when phospholamban is at phosphorylated state. The enhanced rate of decay in EP by phospholamban phosphorylation {81, 148,149} probably represents that step 3 is accelerated, since it is the rate-limiting step during phosphoenzyme decomposition under conditions where saturating concentrations of Ca^{2+}, Mg^{2+}, and K^+ are present (see above). It is important to note that step 3, where E_1P is converted to E_2P, is characterized by the reaction state at which the affinity for Ca^{2+} is greatly altered.

The acceleration of step 5 is the other feature of ATPase enzyme when phospholamban is phosphorylated. This is evidenced by an experiment shown in fig. 17-2, in which the reaction is initiated by the addition of ATP and Ca^{2+} to the reaction medium containing EGTA and the enzyme {117}. However, the rate of phosphoenzyme formation is not affected significantly when ATP is added to cardiac SR vesicles in a Ca^{2+}-containing medium. These studies indicate that the effect of phospholamban phosphorylation is manifest when the ATPase reaction is initiated at E_2 state but not at E_1 state, suggesting that phospholamban phosphorylation enhances step 5, the rate-limiting step during the formation of EP. Like step 3, step 5 is characterized by a great change in the affinity for Ca^{2+}, when E_2 is converted to E_1.

It is of interest to note that phospholamban phosphorylation enhances two rate-limiting steps (steps 3 and 5) in the reaction sequence of ATP hydrolysis {11,148}. These are the steps at which a significant conformational change of the ATPase enzyme occurs and the affinity of enzyme for Ca^{2+} is greatly altered. The mechanism by which phospholamban affects the key elementary steps of ATPase is not known at the present time. However, it is intriguing to assume that phospholamban could exert a critical action on ATPase by a protein-protein interaction. The possible mode of molecular contacts between these two proteins remains to be elucidated.

Molecular structure of phospholamban

Early observations indicated that phospholamban, either in native or purified form, exists as an oligomer.

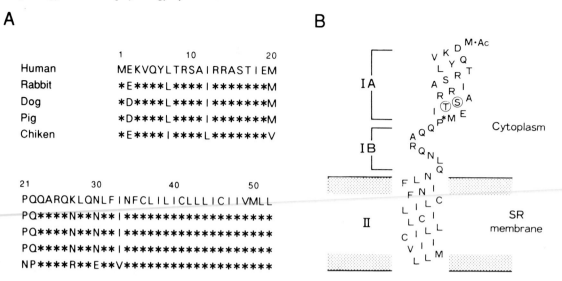

Fig. 17-3. **A:** Comparison of amino acid sequences of phospholamban monomer among human, dog, rabbit, pig, and chicken {49,50,156–158}. Residues are represented by the one-letter code. Identical residues among these five species are shown as asterisks, except the human sequence. **B:** Secondary structure of canine phospholamban monomer {159}. The two alpha-helices, domain IA and domain II, are connected by domain IB, which forms a random structure. Domain I is exposed at the cytoplasmic surface, while domain II is anchored in the SR membrane. The circled residues, S and T, represent Ser 16 and Thr 17, which are phosphorylated by cAMP-dependent and Ca/calmodulin-dependent protein kinase, respectively. The asterisk indicates the helix-braking Pro 21.

Temperature-dependent stepwise conversion between the oligomer and monomer has actually been demonstrated {136}. The molecular weight of phospholamban oligomer is 27,000 and that of monomer is 6000 based on their mobility in an SDS-polyacrylamide gel of Laemmli's system. Upon phosphorylation, the mobility of phospholamban is decreased on SDS polyacrylamide gels. The pattern of temperature-dependent and phosphorylation-dependent mobility shift suggested that phospholamban is a pentamer comprised of five identical monomers {150}. The application of the low-angle laser light scattering technique indicated that the molecular weight of phospholamban oligomer is 30,400, so phospholamban is a pentamer {151}. Mutation analyses indicated that Cys residues, particularly Cys 41, are important for stabilizing the oligomeric structure. It is unlikely, however, that these Cys residues in the neighboring monomers could form disulfide bonds for oligomer formation, because these Cys residues exist as free SH groups {152}. Instead, formation of hydrogen bonds between neighboring Cys residues is likely to be responsible for pentamer formation. The fact that the mutant in which Cys was replaced with Ala does exist as an oligomer at ambient temperature supports this idea. Probably the size, hydrophobicity, and polarity of the side chain of Cys residues exactly matches the micro-environment, thus allowing the hydrophobic residues in neighboring helices to create optimal stabilizing forces.

Purification of canine phospholamban {153,154} and its cDNA sequencing {152,155,156} revealed its molecular structure. The amino acid sequence of phospholamban deduced from the nucleotide sequence is 52 amino acids long, which corresponds to the calculated molecular weight of 6080 {155,156}. Figure 17-3 shows that the amino acid sequences of phospholamban deduced from cDNA nucleotide sequence are well conserved among several species, including human {49,50,156–158}. Phospholamban is encoded by only one gene, which is located on human chromosome 6 {50}. Thus phospholamban is a homo-pentamer. Hydropathy plots suggested that this peptide is an amphipathic peptide; the N-terminal half (Met 1 to Asn 30, named *domain I*) is hydrophilic, whereas the C-terminal half (Leu 31 to Leu 52, named *domain II*) is extremely hydrophobic. As shown in fig. 17-3, domain I is exposed at the cytoplasmic surface, while domain II is embedded within the SR membrane {159}. Analysis of predicted secondary structure indicated that this molecule is rich in alpha-helices; two helices (domains IA and II) are connected by the less structured domain IB. Secondary structure analysis using circular dichroism supports this prediction {160}. Domain I was demonstrated to contain the specific phosphorylation sites. cAMP-dependent protein kinase phosphorylates Ser 16, and Ca/calmodulin-dependent protein kinase phosphorylates Thr 17 {152, 161}. Two Arg residues (Arg 13 and 14) adjacent to the two phosphorylatable residues were proven to be essential for phosphorylation {161}, in accord with the consensus sequence for protein kinase substrate. The same phospholamban sequence is expressed in slow skeletal, cardiac, and smooth muscle SR (table 17-1).

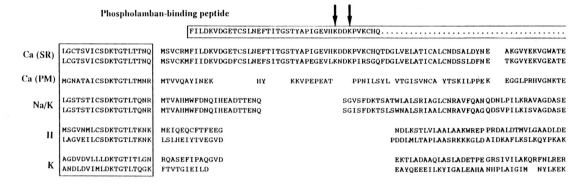

Fig. 17-4. The amino-acid sequence of the crosslinked peptides obtained from rabbit cardiac SR ATPase and from canine fast skeletal muscle SR ATPase is shown aligned with homologous regions in other sequences {162}. Phospholamban was conjugated with ^{125}I labeled Denny–Jaffe reagent. Light activation of conjugated phospholamban incubated with purified ATPase resulted in the formation of a complex. The phospholamban-ATPase complex was cleaved at the azo linkage using sodium dithionite. This cleavage leaves ^{125}I label attached to the domain that interacts with phospholamban. The ATPase was then digested with CNBr and fractionated using reverse-phase HPLC followed by ion-exchange column chromatography. The ^{125}I-labeled peptides were sequenced. Two arrows indicate the lysine residues where the crosslinking reagent bound. Each line represents the following ATPase sequences from top to bottom: rabbit slow-twitch/cardiac muscle SR Ca-ATPase, rabbit fast-twitch muscle SR Ca-ATPase, human plasma membrane Ca-ATPase, sheep plasma membrane Na/K ATPase, torpedo plasma membrane Na/K ATPase, *Saccharomyces cervisiae* H-ATPase, *Neurospora crassa* H-ATPase, *Escherichia coli* K-ATPase, and *Streptococcus faecalis* K-ATPase.

Intermolecular interaction between SR Ca pump ATPase and phospholamban

A line of indirect evidence suggested that phospholamban exerts critical action on ATPase by a protein-protein interaction {11,162}. The experiment using a crosslinking agent demonstrated the direct interaction between the two SR proteins, Ca pump ATPase and phospholamban {163}. The Lys residue of purified phospholamban (Lys 3) was conjugated with Denny–Jaffe crosslinking reagent. Light activation of conjugated phospholamban incubated with purified Ca pump ATPase from cardiac muscle resulted in the formation of a complex only when phospholamban was in the unphosphorylated state and the Ca ATPase was in the Ca-free state (E2 conformation). The domain of the ATPase that interacts with phospholamban was identified by sequencing the photoaffinity labeled peptide. This peptide, whose two Lys residues (Lys 397 and Lys 400) were labeled, was found to originate from a region that is just six amino acids from the C-terminal side of the phosphorylation domain (fig. 17-4). The Asp residue (Asp 351) in this phosphorylation domain is phosphorylated to form EP during the transport cycle of ATPase. It remains to be examined which particular residue(s) is essential for binding. Interestingly, ATPase from fast-twitch skeletal muscle was also shown to contain a putative phospholamban binding domain, although phospholamban was not found to exist in SR of this type of muscle {49,138}. Our preliminary data showed that phospholamban can interact with coexpressed SERCAl Ca ATPase in COS-1 cells. The amino acid sequence in the phosphorylation site among cation-transporting ATPase shares a high degree of homology, whereas the putative phospholamban-binding domain is present only in SR-type ATPase, but not in other plasma membrane ATPases (fig. 17-4). The finding that the phospholamban-binding domain exists in close proximity to the active phosphorylation site of Ca ATPase (Asp 351) indicates that binding of phospholamban to this site could cause significant effects on steps involving phosphorylation of Ca ATPase.

Assuming that phospholamban exhibits its function by binding to a specific region in the ATPase enzyme, it is not yet clear how such a protein-protein interaction could result in significant alterations in the enzymatic activity of Ca pump ATPase, depending upon phosphorylated and unphosphorylated states of phospholamban. It is feasible to propose the following mechanism, based upon our data on enzyme kinetics and chemical observations. The unphosphorylated phospholamban serves to suppress the ATPase activity by binding to the region very close to the phosphorylation site in Ca ATPase {11,140}. Such suppression is relieved when phosphate incorporation into phospholamban dissociates this protein from ATPase, resulting in augmentation of the ATPase activity. Experiments using reconstitution techniques {164,165} or controlled tryptic digestion {166} of phospholamban support this hypothesis.

There are several new observations concerning the mode by which phospholamban interacts with ATPase. These data also lead to the notion that phospholamban would operate to suppress ATPase. Anti-phospholamban monoclonal antibody A1, the epitope that was identified to be a region involving Arg 9 {161}, was reported to enhance Ca uptake of cardiac SR vesicles {167}. The antibody activated Ca uptake and ATPase activity by increasing its affinity for Ca^{2+} {168}. These effects were comparable to those of dual phosphorylation of phospholamban by cAMP-dependent and Ca/calmodulin-dependent protein kinases. The effects of the antibody and phosphorylation by cAMP-dependent protein kinase were not additive. The stoichiometry between Ca and ATP was not altered in these procedures. These results suggested that the monoclonal antibody A1 and phosphorylation of phospholamban activated Ca uptake via a common mechanism, increase in the turnover of ATPase enzyme. Phospholamban coexpressed with slow/cardiac Ca ATPase in COS cells diminished the affinity of ATPase for Ca^{2+} {169}.

Recent work using synthesized phospholamban peptides reconstituted into liposomes with purified Ca pump ATPase clearly demonstrated the interaction between the two SR proteins. The peptide corresponding to 25 amino acid residues from the N-terminus (Met 1 to Arg 25) inhibited Ca uptake, and its inhibition was diminished by phosphorylation of the peptide {165}. Our recent experiments have shown that the synthetic peptide corresponding to domain I of phospholamban (Met 1 to Asn 31) inhibited purified cardiac SR Ca pump ATPase activity in a dose-dependent manner; the inhibition was reduced by phosphorylation of the peptide. However, the affinity of the ATPase activity for Ca^{2+} was not changed by these maneuvers {170}, i.e., this peptide has effects only on V_{max} of Ca ATPase activity. On the other hand, peptides containing domain II, the intramembrane portion of phospholamban, decreased the Ca affinity of ATPase with phosphorylation of the peptide, reducing this inhibitory effect {170}.

These results are consistent with our hypothesis that unphosphorylated phospholamban acts as a suppressor of Ca pump ATPase and that phosphorylation of phospholamban de-suppresses its inhibitory effect. Our results also indicate that, in terms of phospholamban-mediated regulation of Ca pump ATPase, not only the cytoplasmic domain but also the intramembrane portion of phospholamban are required. Since the peptides devoid of N-terminal 7 residues had no effects on Vmax, the residues responsible for the Vmax effect could reside in this N-terminal portion. The C-terminal intramembrane domain could contribute to the effects on Ca affinity. A conformational change of domain I caused by the change in electrostatic forces by incorporation of phosphate into phospholamban or steric hindrance brought by the antibody would be transmitted to the transmembrane domain of phospholamban, which leads to functional dissociation of phospholamban with Ca pump ATPase.

Taking these kinetic and chemical properties into consideration, we might predict the mechanism of regulation of the SR Ca pump ATPase by phospholamban. Domain I of unphosphorylated phospholamban may interact directly with the E_2 form of the ATPase to inhibit conversion between E_2 and E_1. The interaction is diminished by phosphorylation of phospholamban. Changes in electrostatic properties of the SR membrane on phospholamban phosphorylation may also contribute to the increased Ca affinity of the ATPase {171,172}. Domain II of phospholamban may not be a mere anchor, but should also play an important role in the interaction between the two proteins in addition to domain I for the two reasons: (a) the domain is well conserved among mammalian and avian species, (b) synthetic peptide corresponding to domain I of phospholamban did not mimic phospholamban function completely; domain II was necessary for the shift in Ca affinity, as mentioned above. It remains to be examined how transmembrane helices of Ca pump ATPase and domain II of phospholamban interact and how the signal of phosphorylation and dephosphorylation of domain I is transduced into the changes in the interaction between domain II of phospholamban and the intramembrane helices of Ca pump ATPase. It is also intriguing to know how the oligomeric structure of phospholamban contributes to the intermolecular interaction between the two molecules. The studies using synthetic phospholamban variants corresponding to the intramembrane portion or biologically synthesized mutants could give us more clues. Furthermore, mutations on key domain and other related regions of the two proteins may give us the ultimate answers.

PHYSIOLOGIC RELEVANCE

In the mammalian myocardium, the SR is considered to be the major system involved in bringing about relaxation {5–8}. The SR is also implicated as the major source of Ca^{2+} for activation of contraction (see Chapter 12). The molecular mechanism of the Ca pump of the SR, which affects cardiac relaxation, is fairly well understood, as described in the preceding sections. In the following section, the physiologic relevance of the Ca-pump activity of the isolated cardiac SR membranes is discussed briefly.

Ca uptake by the sarcoplasmic reticulum and cardiac relaxation

In the isolated cardiac contractile system, full activity occurs when $50–100 nM$ Ca^{2+}/g wet muscle are available for binding to the contractile proteins {3,173}. In the intact mammalian heart cells, however, the myoplasmic free Ca^{2+} reached during the physiologic contraction appears to be significantly lower than that necessary for the full activation of the contractile system {174,175}. In heart cells from adult rat or rabbit, the tension developed during the maximum twitch was estimated to be about 70% of the maximum tension {175}. In addition, in intact rabbit ventricular cells the tension developed during regular single-pulse stimulation at 12/min was only 20% of the maximum {175}. According to the estimate by Solaro et al. {173}, 70% and 20% maximal force development require that 25.8 and 17.1 nM Ca^{2+}/g wet muscle are delivered to the dog cardiac myofibrils, respectively, suggesting that this range of Ca^{2+} must bind to and be removed from the contractile system in vivo during each cardiac cycle under physiologic conditions.

ATP-supported Ca accumulation by the isolated cardiac

SR vesicles has been studied in the presence and absence of Ca-precipitating anions. Ca accumulation in the absence of Ca-precipitating anions is clearly the one that is more physiologically relevant because a Ca^{2+}-trapping mechanism like that provided by oxalate has not been defined in vivo. The steady-state levels of Ca accumulation by the isolated cardiac vesicles, obtained at the physiologic ranges of Ca^{2+} in the absence of Ca-precipitating anions, and the maximum yield of the SR vesicles isolated from the heart muscle, can give an estimate of the maximum capacity of the SR in vivo to accumulate Ca^{2+} at corresponding Ca^{2+} concentrations. The estimate given by Solaro and Briggs {21} indicates that the SR in dog heart can accumulate Ca^{2+} in amounts well in excess of those necessary to activate the contractile proteins under the comparable conditions. Therefore, the Ca-accumulating capacity of the isolated SR vesicles can adequately explain the relaxed state of cardiac muscle at the steady state.

There have been some uncertainties, however, regarding the relationship between the quantitative aspects of the rate of Ca uptake by the isolated SR vesicles and of relaxation in the intact heart. The rate of Ca uptake by cardiac SR vesicles in vitro, as measured in the presence of oxalate over a time scale of minutes, is about 5–20 times less than the physiologic requirement {63}. Recent experiments in which fast Ca accumulation by the SR vesicles is followed with stopped-flow or quench-flow techniques, however, provide different results. One group reported that the amount of Ca^{2+} taken up by the cardiac SR vesicles during an interval of 0–150 ms, when measured with stopped-flow techniques in the presence of murexide, was 37 nM/mg protein at 37°C {71}. If adjustment is made for the SR content in the heart muscle (~6.3 mg/g wet muscle {21}), the SR vesicles could remove as much as 250 nM/g wet muscle during times required for heart relaxation (~200 ms). This amount of Ca^{2+} is significantly greater than that which must be removed from the fully activated contractile system to effect complete relaxation. In contrast to this report, one to two orders of magnitude smaller rate of Ca uptake was measured by another group using a similar experimental method {176}. It should be pointed out, however, that the experimental conditions employed by the latter group are likely to be the reason for the very low rate of Ca uptake observed. The reaction mixture used as described in the figure legends does not contain Mg^{2+}, which is essential for the optimum activity of the Ca pump of the SR (see above).

The fast rate of uptake by the cardiac SR vesicles was also measured with a rapid-quenching apparatus using Ca^{2+} chelator as a quencher of the uptake reaction {80}. The amount of Ca^{2+} accumulated by the cardiac SR vesicles at 0.2–18.9 μM Ca^{2+} during the first 200 ms of the uptake reaction was found to be comparable to that which is necessary to activate the isolated contractile system at corresponding Ca^{2+} concentrations. Although the data described above do not provide an adequate quantitative description of Ca uptake by the SR in vivo during cardiac relaxation, they are consistent with the view that the SR plays the major role in the relaxation of the mammalian myocardium, especially since it is known that mitochondria do not take up Ca^{2+} significantly under physiologic conditions {5,7,73}.

Physiologic relevance of phospholamban phosphorylation

Tada et al. {24,134,135} first proposed that cyclic-AMP-mediated acceleration of Ca uptake by cardiac SR may explain the two principal mechanical effects of catecholamines on heart muscle: abbreviation of systole and increased contractility. Cyclic-AMP-mediated stimulation of the rate of Ca uptake by the SR could explain abbreviation of systole, because Ca^{2+} would be removed from troponin at an increased rate. The increased rate of Ca uptake following phospholamban phosphorylation could increase the amount of Ca^{2+} stored inside the SR membranes, allowing the cell to retain some of the Ca^{2+} that would otherwise be lost during diastole. This Ca^{2+} could add to the amount of Ca^{2+} available for delivery to the contractile proteins in subsequent contractions, thus promoting augmentation of myocardial contractility {177}.

The proposed sequence of events appears to find support from experiments in skinned and intact heart cells. Catecholamines produce relaxation at the very early phase, followed by augmentation of contraction {178}. The onset of increased tension development after exposure of the heart to catecholamines is gradual, reaching the steady state after about 20 beats {179}. A recent experiment in which the Ca transient in the intact heart cell is studied with the use of aequorin, a Ca-sensitive bioluminescent protein, indicates that catecholamines augment the initial rate of Ca release into the cytoplasm during the early phase of contraction as well as the rate of reduction of Ca^{2+} during relaxation {180}. Employing a skinned cardiac cell, which exhibits cycles of phasic contractions upon addition of an appropriate amount of Ca^{2+}, Fabiato and Fabiato {181} demonstrated that a brief preincubation with cyclic AMP results in an increased amplitude of contraction and faster rates of tension development and relaxation.

The intracellular level of cyclic AMP appears to increase prior to the development of increased contractility after exposure of the heart cell to catecholamines {182,183}. Others found, however, that there is no detectable increase in cyclic AMP when catecholamines covalently attached to glass beads augment contraction {184,185}. It is not known at present whether a subtle increase in cyclic AMP, which might have been too low to detect, could have given rise to significant mechanical changes. Alternatively, dissociation of inotropic responses from cyclic-AMP formation may reflect some other effect of catecholamines on sarcolemmal systems such as calcium channels.

Phospholamban phosphorylation was demonstrated to occur in the intact heart. The addition of the isoproterenol to the heart perfused with $^{32}P_i$ results in increased ^{32}P incorporation into the microsomal protein (phospholamban) with simultaneous increase in the rates of tension development and relaxation {186,187}. It is of interest to note that the extent of phospholamban phosphorylation and the rate of Ca uptake are significantly increased in the cardiac SR preparations of the hyperthyroid rat {188}. Aging does not affect the extent to which Ca uptake by the SR is accelerated by the cyclic-AMP-phospholamban system {189}.

In addition to cyclic-AMP-mediated phosphorylation of phospholamban, phosphorylation of this protein is also catalyzed by Ca^{2+} and calmodulin-dependent protein kinase. Phospholamban phosphorylation by the calmodulin system appears to function in the intact heart cell because calmodulin inhibitor (fluphenazine) significantly reduced phospholamban phosphorylation in vivo {186}. As Ca uptake by the isolated cardiac SR vesicles is enhanced when either of the cyclic-AMP-dependent or calmodulin-dependent systems is operational, Ca uptake by the SR in vivo may be regulated by these two systems in separate manners. Such an assumption may find support from the molecular structure of phospholamban, which exhibits a specific site (Thr 17) for calmodulin-dependent kinase, occurring adjacent to the site for cyclic-AMP-dependent protein kinase (Ser 16). It is premature to speculate on the physiologic relevance of calmodulin-dependent phosphorylation of phospholamban. Possibly, however, this system may be activated when the myocardial cell is overloaded with Ca^{2+}.

Acknowledgments

This work was supported by research grants from the ministries of Education, Science and Culture, and of Health and Welfare of Japan and a Grant-in-Aid from the Muscular Dystrophy Association of America.

REFERENCES

1. Weber A: Energized calcium transport and relaxing factors. *Curr Top Bioenerg* 1:203–254, 1966.
2. Ebashi S, Endo M: Calcium ion and muscle contraction. *Prog Biophys Mol Biol* 18:123–183, 1968.
3. Katz AM: Contractile proteins of the heart. *Physiol Rev* 50:63–158, 1970.
4. Langer GA: Heart: Excitation-contraction coupling. *Ann Rev Physiol* 35:55–86, 1973.
5. Chapman RA: Excitation-contraction coupling in cardiac muscle. *Prog Biophys Mol Biol* 35:1–52, 1979.
6. Fabiato A, Fabiato F: Calcium and cardiac excitation-contraction coupling. *Ann Rev Physiol* 41:473–484, 1979.
7. Winegrad S: Electromechanical coupling in heart muscle. In: Berne RM, Speralakis N, Geiger SR (eds) *Handbook of Physiology*, Sect 2: *The Cardiovascular System*, Vol 1: *The Heart*. Bethesda: American Physiological Society, 1979, pp 393–428.
8. Katz AM: Congestive heart failure: Role of altered myocardial cellular control. *N Engl J Med* 293:1184–1191, 1975.
9. Sommer JR, Johnson EA: Ultrastructure of cardiac muscle. In: Berne RM, Sperelakis N, Geiger SR (eds) *Handbook of Physiology*, Sect 2: *The Cardiovascular System*, Vol 1: *The Heart*. Bethesda: American Physiological Society, 1979, pp 113–186.
10. Tada M, Yamamoto T, Tonomura Y: Molecular mechanism of active calcium transport by sarcoplasmic reticulum. *Physiol Rev* 58:1–79, 1978.
11. Tada M, Katz AM: Phosphorylation of the sarcoplasmic reticulum and sarcolemma. *Ann Rev Physiol* 44:401–423, 1982.
12. Endo M: Calcium release from the sarcoplasmic reticulum. *Physiol Rev* 57:71–108, 1977.
13. Fleischer S, Inui M: Biochemistry and biophysics of excitation-contraction coupling. *Annu Rev Biophys Chem* 18:333–364, 1989.
14. Franzini-Armstrong C: Structure of sarcoplasmic reticulum. *Fed Proc* 39:2403–2409, 1980.
15. Jorgensen AO, Campbell KP: Evidence for the presence of calsequenstrin in two structurally different regions of myocardial sarcoplasmic reticulum. *J Cell Biol* 98:1597–1602, 1984.
16. Winegrad S: Intracellular calcium movements of frog skeletal muscle during recovery from tetanus. *J Gen Physiol* 51:65–83, 1968.
17. Somlyo AV, Gonzalez-Serratos H, Shuman H, McClellan G, Somlyo AP: Calcium release and ionic changes in the sarcoplasmic reticulum of tetanized muscle: An electron-probe study. *J Cell Biol* 90:577–594, 1981.
18. Fanburg B, Gergely J: Studies on adenosine triphosphate-supported calcium accumulation by cardiac subcellular particles. *J Biol Chem* 240:2721–2728, 1965.
19. Harigaya S, Schwartz A: Rate of calcium binding and uptake in normal animal and failing human cardiac muscle. *Circ Res* 25:781–794, 1969.
20. Pretorius PJ, Pohl WG, Smithen CS, Inesi G: Structural and functional characterization of dog heart microsomes. *Circ Res* 25:487–499, 1969.
21. Solaro RJ, Briggs FN: Estimating the functional capabilities of sarcoplasmic reticulum in cardiac muscle: Calcium binding. *Circ Res* 34:531–540, 1974.
22. Levitsky DO, Aliev MK, Kuzmin AV, Levchenko TS, Smirnov VN, Chazov EI: Isolation of calcium pump system and purification of calcium ion-dependent ATPase from heart muscle. *Biochim Biophys Acta* 443:468–484, 1976.
23. Pang DC, Briggs FN: Reaction mechanism of the cardiac sarcotubule calcium (II) dependent adenosine triphosphatase. *Biochemistry* 12:4905–4911, 1973.
24. Tada M, Kirchberger MA, Repke DI, Katz AM: The stimulation of calcium transport in cardiac sarcoplasmic reticulum by adenosine 3′: 5′-monophosphate-dependent protein kinase. *J Biol Chem* 249:6174–6180, 1974.
25. Shigekawa M, Finegan JM, Katz AM: Calcium transport ATPase of canine cardiac sarcoplasmic reticulum. *J Biol chem* 251:6894–6900, 1976.
26. Jones LR, Besch HR Jr, Fleming JW, McConnaughey MM, Watanabe AM: Separation of vesicles of cardiac sarcolemma from vesicles of cardiac sarcoplasmic reticulum: Comparative biochemical analysis of component activities. *J Biol Chem* 254:530–539, 1979.
27. Chamberlain BK, Levitsky DO, Fleischer S: Isolation and characterization of canine cardiac sarcoplasmic reticulum with improved Ca^{2+} transport properties. *J Biol Chem* 258:6602–6609, 1983.
28. Meissner G: Isolation and characterization of two types of sarcoplasmic reticulum vesicles. *Biochim Biophys Acta* 389:51–68, 1975.
29. Campbell KP, Franzini-Armstrong C, Shamoo AE: Further characterization of light and heavy sarcoplasmic reticulum vesicles: Identification of the "sarcoplasmic reticulum feet" associated with heavy sarcoplasmic reticulum vesicles. *Biochim Biophys Acta* 602:97–116, 1980.
30. Jones LR, Cala SE: Biochemical evidence for functional heterogeneity of cardiac sarcoplasmic reticulum vesicles. *J Biol Chem* 256:11809–11818, 1981.

31. Seiler S, Wegener AD, Whang DD, Hathaway DR, Jones LR: High molecular weight proteins in cardiac and skeletal muscle junctional sarcoplasmic reticulum vesicles bind calmodulin, are phosphorylated, and are degraded by Ca^{2+}-activated protease. *J Biol Chem* 259:8550–8557, 1984.

32. Williams LT, Jones LR: Specific binding of the calcium antagonist [^{3}H]nitrendipine to subcellular fractions isolated from canine myocardium: Evidence for high affinity binding to ryanodine-sensitive sarcoplasmic reticulum vesicles. *J Biol Chem* 258:5344–5347, 1983.

33. Van Winkle WB, Pitts BJR, Entman ML: Rapid purification of canine cardiac sarcoplasmic reticulum Ca^{2+}-ATPase. *J Biol Chem* 253:8671–8673, 1978.

34. Nakamura J, Wang T, Tsai L-I, Schwartz A: Properties and characterization of a highly purified sarcoplasmic reticulum Ca^{2+}-ATPase from dog cardiac and rabbit skeletal muscle. *J Biol Chem* 258:5079–5083, 1983.

35. Campbell KP, MacLennan DH, Jorgensen AO, Mintzer MC: Purification and characterization of calsequestrin from canine cardiac sarcoplasmic reticulum and identification of the 53,000 dalton glycoprotein. *J Biol Chem* 258:1197–1204, 1983.

36. Cala SE, Jones LR: Rapid purification of calsequestrin from cardiac and skeletal muscle sarcoplasmic reticulum vesicles by Ca^{2+}-dependent elution from phenyl-Sepharose. *J Biol Chem* 258:11932–11936, 1983.

37. Meissner G: ATP and Ca^{2+} binding by the Ca^{2+} pump protein of sarcoplasmic reticulum. *Biochim Biophys Acta* 298:906–926, 1973.

38. Ikemoto N: The calcium binding sites involved in the regulation of the purified adenosine triphosphatase of the sarcoplasmic reticulum. *J Biol Chem* 249:649–651, 1974.

39. Dupont Y: Kinetics and regulation of sarcoplasmic reticulum ATPase. *Eur J Biochem* 72:185–190, 1977.

40. Dupont Y, Pougeois R, Ronjat M, Verjovsky-Almeida S: Two distinct classes of nucleotide binding sites in sarcoplasmic reticulum Ca-ATPase revealed by 2′,3′-0-(2,4,6-Trinitrocyclohexadienylidene)-ATP. *J Biol Chem* 260:7241–7249, 1985.

41. Møller JV, Andersen JP, Le Marie M: The sarcoplasmic reticulum Ca^{2+}-ATPase. *Mol Cell Biochem* 42:83–107, 1982.

42. MacLennan DH, Holland PC: Calcium transport in sarcoplasmic reticulum. *Ann Rev Biophys Bioeng* 4:377–404, 1975.

43. Green NM, Allen G, Hebdon GM: Structural relationship between the calcium-v and magnesium-transporting ATPase of sarcoplasmic reticulum and the membrane. *Ann NY Acad Sci* 358:149–158, 1980.

44. MacLennan DH, Reithmeier RAF, Shoshan V, Campbell KP, Le Bel D, Herrmann TR, Shamoo AE: Ion pathways in proteins of the sarcoplasmic reticulum. *Ann NY Acad Sci* 358:138–148, 1980.

45. Pick U, Karlish SJD: Indications for an oligomeric structure and for conformational changes in sarcoplasmic reticulum Ca^{2+}-ATPase labelled selectively with fluorescein. *Biochim Biophys Acta* 626:255–261, 1980.

46. Pick U, Racker E: Inhibition of the (Ca^{2+}) ATPase from sarcoplasmic reticulum by dicyclohexycarbodiimide: Evidence for location of the Ca^{2+} binding site in a hydrophobic region. *Biochemistry* 18:108–113, 1979.

47. MacLennan DH, Brandl CJ, Korczak B, Green NM: Aminoacid sequence of a Ca^{2+} + Mg^{2+}-dependent ATPase from rabbit muscle sarcopasmic reticulum, deduced from its complementary DNA sequence. *Nature* 316:696–700, 1985.

48. Brandl CJ, Green NM, Korczak B, MacLennan DH: Two Ca^{2+} ATPase genes: Homologies and mechanistic implications of deduced amino acid sequences. *Cell* 44:597–607, 1986.

49. Fujii J, Lytton J, Tada M, MacLennan DH: Rabbit cardiac and slow-twitch muscle express the same phospholamban gene. *FEBS Lett* 227:51–55, 1988.

50. Fujii J, Zarain-Herzberg A, Willard HF, Tada M, MacLennan DH: Structure of the rabbit phospholamban gene, cloning of the human cDNA, and assignment of the gene to human chromosome 6. *J Biol Chem* 266:11669–11675, 1991.

51. Brandl CJ, deLeon S, Martin DR, MacLennan DH: Adult forms of the Ca^{2+}ATPase of sarcoplasmic reticulum. Expression in developing skeletal muscle. *J Biol Chem* 262:3768–3774, 1987.

52. Lytton J, MacLennan DH: Molecular cloning of cDNAs from human kidney coding for two alternatively spliced products of the cardiac Ca^{2+}-ATPase gene. *J Biol Chem* 263:15024–15031, 1988.

53. Gunteski-Hamblin A-M, Greeb J, Shull GE: A novel Ca^{2+} pump expressed in brain, kidney, and stomach is encoded by an alternative transcript of the slow-twitch muscle sarcoplasmic reticulum Ca-ATPase gene. *J Biol Chem* 263:15032–15040, 1988.

54. Lytton J, Zarain-Herzberg A, Periasamy M, MacLennan DH: Molecular cloning of the mammalian smooth muscle sarco(endo)plasmic reticulum Ca^{2+}-ATPase. *J Biol Chem* 264:7059–7065, 1989.

55. Burk SE, Lytton J, MacLennan DH, Shull GE: cDNA cloning, functional expression, and mRNA tissue distribution of a third organellar Ca^{2+} pump. *J Biol Chem* 264:18561–18568, 1989.

56. Clarke DM, Loo TW, Inesi G, MacLennan DH: Location of high affinity Ca^{2+}-binding sites within the predicted transmembrane domain of the sarcoplasmic reticulum Ca^{2+}-ATPase. *Nature* 339:476–478, 1989.

57. MacLennan DH: Molecular tools to elucidate problems in excitation-contraction coupling. *Biophys J* 58:1355–1365, 1990.

58. Scott TL: Distances between the functional sites of the (Ca^{2+} + Mg^{2+})-ATPase of sarcoplasmic reticulum. *J Biol Chem* 260:14421–14423, 1985.

59. Scott BT, Simmerman HKB, Collins JH, Nadal-Ginard B, Jones LR: Complete amino acid sequence of canine cardiac calequestrin deduced by cDNA cloning. *J Biol Chem* 263:8958–8964, 1988.

60. Leberer E, Charuk JH, Green NM, MacLennan DH: Molecular cloning and expression of cDNA encoding a lumenal calcium binding glycoprotein from sarcoplasmic reticulum. *Proc Natl Acad Sci USA* 86:6047–6051, 1989.

61. Fliegel L, Burns K, MacLennan DH, Reithmeier RA, Michalak M: Molecular cloning of the high affinity calcium-binding protein (calreticulin) of sekeletal muscle sarcoplasmic reticulum. *J Biol Chem* 264:21522–21528, 1989.

62. Gross RW: Identification of plasmalogen as the major phospholipid constituent of cardiac sarcoplasmic reticulum. *Biochemistry* 24:1662–1668, 1985.

63. Martonosi A: Biochemical and clinical aspects of sarcoplasmic reticulum function. *Curr Top Membr Transp* 3:83–197, 1972.

64. Inesi G: Transport across sarcoplasmic reticulum in skeletal and cardiac muscle. In: Giebish G, Tosteson DC, Ussing HH (eds) *Membrane Transport in Biology*. Berlin: Springer, 1979, pp 357–393.

65. Herbette L, DeFoor P, Fleischer S, Pascolini D, Scarpa A, Blasie JK: The separate profile structures of the functional calcium pump protein and the phospholipid bilayer within isolated sarcoplasmic reticulum membranes determined by

X-ray and neutron diffraction. *Biochim Biophys Acta* 817:103–122, 1985.

66. Ikemoto N: Structure and function of the calcium pump protein of sarcoplasmic reticulum. *Ann Rev Physiol* 44: 297–317, 1982.

67. Franzini-Armstrong C, Ferguson DG: Density and disposition of Ca^{2+}-ATPase in sarcoplasmic reticulum membrane as determined by shadowing techniques. *Biophys J* 48:607–615, 1985.

68. Chamberlain BK, Berenski CJ, Jung CY, Fleischer S: Determination of the oligomeric structure of the Ca^{2+} pump protein in canine cardiac sarcoplasmic reticulum membranes using radiation inactivation analysis. *J Biol Chem* 258: 11997–12001, 1983.

69. Taylor K, Dux L, Martonosi A: Structure of the vanadate-induced crystals of sarcoplasmic reticulum Ca^{2+}-ATPase. *J Mol Biol* 174:193–204, 1984.

70. Dux L, Taylor KA, Ting-Beall HP, Martonosi A: Crystallization of the Ca^{2+}-ATPase of sarcoplasmic reticulum by calcium and lanthanide ions. *J Biol Chem* 260:11730–11743, 1985.

71. Besch HR Jr, Schwartz A: Initial calcium binding rates of canine cardiac relaxing system (sarcoplasmic reticulum fragments) determined by stopped-flow spectrophotometry. *Biochem Biophys Res Commun* 45:286–292, 1971.

72. Repke DI, Katz AM: Calcium-binding and calcium-uptake by cardiac microsomes: A kinetic analysis. *J Mol Cell Cardiol* 4:401–416, 1972.

73. Kitazawa T: Physiological significance of Ca uptake by mitochondria in the heart in comparison with that by cardiac sarcoplasmic reticulum. *J Biochem* 80:1129–1147, 1976.

74. Entman ML, Gillette PC, Wallick ET, Pressman BC, Schwartz A: A study of calcium binding and uptake by isolated cardiac sarcoplasmic reticulum: The use of a new ionophore (X537A). *Biochem Biophys Res Commun* 48: 847–853, 1972.

75. Katz AM, Repke DI, Fudyma G, Shigekawa M: Control of calcium efflux from sarcoplasmic reticulum vesicles by external calcium. *J Biol Chem* 252:4210–4214, 1977.

76. Chamberlain BK, Volpe P, Fleischer S: Calcium-induced calcium release from purified cardiac sarcoplasmic reticulum vesicles. General characteristics. *J Biol Chem* 259:7540–7546, 1984.

77. Hasselbach W: Relaxing factor and the relaxation of muscle. *Prog Biophys Mol Biol* 14:167–222, 1964.

78. Weber A: Regulatory mechanisms of the calcium transport system of fragmented rabbit sarcoplasmic reticulum. I. The effect of accumulated calcium on transport and adenosine triphosphate hydrolysis. *J Gen Physiol* 57:50–70, 1971.

79. Suko J: The calcium pump of cardiac sarcoplasmic reticulum: Functional alterations at different levels of thyroid state in rabbits. *J Physiol* 228:563–582, 1973.

80. Will H, Blanck J, Smettan G, Wollenberger A: A quench-flow kinetic investigation of calcium ion accumulation by isolated cardiac sarcoplasmic reticulum: Dependence of initial velocity on free calcium ion concentration and influence of preincubation with a protein kinase, MgATP, and cyclic AMP, *Biochim Biophys Acta* 449:295–303, 1976.

81. Tada M, Ohmori F, Yamada M, Abe H: Mechanism of the stimulation of Ca^{2+}-dependent ATPase of cardiac sarcoplasmic reticulum by adenosine 3':5'-monophosphate-dependent protein kinase: Role of the 22,000-dalton protein. *J Biol Chem* 254:319–326, 1979.

82. Chiesi M, Inesi G: Adenosine 5'-triphosphate dependent fluxes of manganese and hydrogen ions in sarcoplasmic reticulum vesicles. *Biochemistry* 19:2912–2918, 1980.

83. Shigekawa M, Wakabayashi S, Nakamura H: Reaction mechanism of Ca^{2+}-dependent adenosine triphosphatase of sarcoplasmic reticulum: ATP hydrolysis with CaATP as a substrate and role of divalent cation. *J Biol Chem* 258: 8698–8707, 1983.

84. Yamada S, Ikemoto N: Reaction mechanism of calcium-ATPase of sarcoplasmic reticulum: Substrates for phosphorylation reaction and back reaction, and further resolution of phosphorylated intermediates. *J Biol Chem* 255: 3108–3119, 1980.

85. Van Winkle WB, Tate CA, Bick RJ, Entman ML: Nucleotide triphosphate utilization by cardiac and skeletal muscle sarcoplasmic reticulum: Evidence for a hydrolysis cycle not coupled to intermediate acylphosphate formation and calcium translocation. *J Biol Chem* 256:2268–2274, 1981.

86. Shigekawa M, Akowitz AA, Katz AM: Stimulation of adenosine triphosphatase activity of sarcoplasmic reticulum by adenylyl methylene diphosphate. *Biochim Biophys Acta* 526:591–596, 1978.

87. Hasselbach W: The reversibility of the sarcoplasmic calcium pump. *Biochim Biophys Acta* 515:23–53, 1978.

88. Van Winkle WB, Tate CA, Bick RJ, Entman ML: Nucleotide triphosphate utilization by cardiac and skeletal muscle sarcoplasmic reticulum: Evidence for a hydrolysis cycle not coupled to intermediate acylphosphate formation and calcium translocation. *J Biol Chem* 256:2268–2274, 1981.

89. Trumble WR, Sutko JL, Reeves JP: ATP-dependent calcium transport in cardiac sarcolemmal membrane vesicles. *Life Sci* 27:207–214, 1980.

90. Salama G, Scarpa A: Magnesium permeability of sarcoplasmic reticulum. Mg^{2+} is not countertransported during ATP-dependent Ca^{2+} uptake by sarcoplasmic reticulum. *J Biol Chem* 260:11697–11705, 1985.

91. Shigekawa M, Pearl LJ: Activation of calcium transport in skeletal muscle sarcoplasmic reticulum by monovalent cations. *J Biol Chem* 251:6947–6952, 1976.

92. Jones LR, Besch HR Jr, Watanabe AM: Monovalent cation stimulation of Ca^{2+} uptake by cardiac membrane vesicles: Correlation with stimulation of Ca^{2+}-ATPase activity. *J Biol Chem* 252:3315–3323, 1977.

93. Duggan PF: Calcium uptake and associated adenosine triphosphatase activity in fragmented sarcoplasmic reticulum: Requirement for potassium ions. *J Biol Chem* 252:1620–1627, 1977.

94. Shigekawa M, Wakabayashi S: Sidedness of K^+ activation of calcium transport in the reconstituted sarcoplasmic reticulum calcium pump. *J Biol Chem* 260:11679–11687, 1985.

95. Tate CA, Van Winkle WB, Entman ML: Time-dependent resistance to alkaline pH of oxalate-supported calcium uptake by sarcoplasmic reticulum. *Life Sci* 27:1453–1464, 1980.

96. Meissner G: Calcium transport and monovalent cation and proton fluxes in sarcoplasmic reticulum vesicles. *J Biol Chem* 256:636–643, 1981.

97. Meissner G: Monovalent ion and calcium ion fluxes in sarcoplasmic reticulum. *Mol Cell Biochem* 55:65–82, 1983.

98. Zimniak P, Racker E: Electrogenicity of Ca^{2+} transport catalyzed by the Ca^{2+}-ATPase from sarcoplasmic reticulum. *J Biol Chem* 253:4631–4637, 1978.

99. Ueno T, Sekine T: A role of H^+ flux in active Ca^{2+} transport into sarcoplasmic reticulum vesicles. I. Effect of an artificially imposed H^+ gradient on Ca^{2+} uptake. *J Biochem* 89:1239–1246, 1981.

100. Madeira VMC: Proton movements across the membranes of sarcoplasmic reticulum during the uptake of calcium ions. *Arch Biochem Biophys* 200:319–325, 1980.

101. Meissner G, McKinley D: Permeability of canine cardiac sarcoplasmic reticulum vesicles to K^+, Na^+, H^+, and Cl^-. *J Biol Chem* 257:7704–7711, 1982.

102. McKinley D, Meissner G: Evidence for a K^+, Na^+ permeable channel in sarcoplasmic reticulum. *J Membr Biol* 44:159–186, 1978.

103. Miller C: Voltage-gated cation conductance channel from fragmented sarcoplasmic reticulum: Steady-state electrical properties. *J Membr Biol* 40:1–23, 1978.

104. Kasai M, Kometani T: Inhibition of anion permeability of sarcoplasmic reticulum vesicles by 4-aceto-amido-4′-isothiocyano-stilbene-2,2′-disulfonate. *Biochim Biophys Acta* 557:243–247, 1979.

105. Racker E: Reconstitution of a calcium pump with phospholipids and a purified Ca^{2+}-adenosine triphosphatase from sarcoplasmic reticulum. *J Biol Chem* 247:8198–8200, 1972.

106. Fanburg BL, Matsushita S: Phosphorylated intermediate of ATPase of isolated cardiac sarcoplasmic reticulum. *J Mol Cell Cardiol* 5:111–115, 1973.

107. Suko J, Hasselbach W: Characterization of cardiac sarcoplasmic reticulum ATP-ADP phosphate exchange and phosphorylation of the calcium transport adenosine triphosphatase. *Eur J Biochem* 64:123–130, 1976.

108. Sumida M, Wang T, Mandel F, Froehlich JP, Schwartz A: Transient kinetics of Ca^{2+} transport of sarcoplasmic reticulum: A comparison of cardiac and skeletal muscle. *J Biol Chem* 253:8772–8777, 1978.

109. Jones LR, Besch HR Jr, Watanabe AM: Regulation of the calcium pump of cardiac sarcoplasmic reticulum: Interactive roles of potassium and ATP on the phosphoprotein intermediate of the (K^+, Ca^{2+})-ATPase. *J Biol Chem* 253:1643–1653, 1978.

110. Degani C, Boyer PD: A borohydride reduction method for characterization of the acyl phosphate linkage in proteins and its application to sarcoplasmic reticulum adenosine triphosphatase. *J Biol Chem* 248:8222–8226, 1973.

111. Shigekawa M, Dougherty JP: Reaction mechanism of Ca^{2+}-dependent ATP hydrolysis by skeletal muscle sarcoplasmic reticulum in the absence of added alkali metal salts. III. Sequential occurrence of ADP-sensitive and ADP-insensitive phosphoenzymes. *J Biol Chem* 253:1458–1464, 1978.

112. De Meis L, Vianna AL: Energy interconversion by the Ca^{2+}-dependent ATPase of the sarcoplasmic reticulum. *Ann Rev Biochem* 48:275–292, 1979.

113. Pick U, Karlish SJD: Regulation of the conformational transition in the Ca-ATPase from sarcoplasmic reticulum by pH, temperature, and calcium ions. *J Biol Chem* 257:6120–6126, 1982.

114. Pick U: The interaction of vanadate ions with the Ca-ATPase from sarcoplasmic reticulum. *J Biol Chem* 257:6111–61119, 1982.

115. Dupont Y: Occlusion of divalent cations in the phosphorylated calcium pump of sarcoplasmic reticulum. *Eur J Biochem* 109:231–238, 1980.

116. Shigekawa M, Wakabayashi S, Nakamura H: Effect of divalent cation bound to the ATPase of sarcoplasmic reticulum: Activation of phosphoenzyme hydrolysis by Mg^{2+}. *J Biol Chem* 258:14157–14161, 1983.

117. Tada M, Yamada M, Ohmori F, Kuzuya T, Inui M, Abe H: Transient state kinetic studies of Ca^{2+}-dependent ATPase and calcium transport by cardiac sarcoplasmic reticulum: Effect of cyclic AMP-dependent protein kinase–catalyzed phosphorylation of phospholamban. *J Biol Chem* 255:1985–1992, 1980.

118. Briggs FN, Wise RM, Hearn JA: The effect of lithium and potassium on the transient state kinetics of the $(Ca + Mg)$-ATPase of cardiac sarcoplasmic reticulum. *J Biol Chem* 253:5884–5885, 1978.

119. Dupont Y: Fluorescence studies of the sarcoplasmic reticulum calcium pump. *Biochem Biophys Res Commun* 71:544–550, 1976.

120. Dupont Y, Pougeois R, Evaluation of H_2O activity in the free or phosphorylated catalytic site of Ca^{2+}-ATPase. *FEBS Lett* 156:93–98, 1983.

121. Wakabayashi S, Shigekawa M: Factor influencing calcium release from the ADP-sensitive phosphoenzyme intermediate of the sarcoplasmic reticulum ATPase. *J Biol Chem* 261:9762–9769, 1986.

122. Shigekawa M, Dougherty JP: Reaction mechanism of Ca^{2+}-dependent ATP hydrolysis by skeletal muscle sarcoplasmic reticulum in the absence of added alkali metal salts. II. Kinetic properties of the phosphoenzyme formed at the steady state in high Mg^{1+} and low Ca^{2+} concentrations. *J Biol Chem* 253:1451–1457, 1978.

123. Shigekawa M, Akowitz AA: On the mechanism of Ca^{2+}-dependent adenosine triphosphatase of sarcoplasmic reticulum: Occurrence of two types of phosphoenzyme intermediates in the presence of KCl. *J Biol Chem* 254:4726–4730, 1979.

124. Froehlich JP, Taylor EW: Transient state kinetic studies of sarcoplasmic reticulum adenosine triphosphatase. *J Biol Chem* 250:2013–2021, 1975.

125. McIntosh DB, Boyer PD: Adenosine 5′-triphosphate modulation of catalytic intermediates of calcium ion activated adenosinetriphosphatase of sarcoplasmic reticulum subsequent to enzyme phosphorylation. *Biochemistry* 22:2867–2875, 1983.

126. Scofano HM, Vieyra A, De Meis L: Substrate regulation of the sarcoplasmic reticulum ATPase: Transient kinetic studies. *J Biol Chem* 254:10227–10231, 1979.

127. Makinose M, Hasselbach W: ATP synthesis by the reverse of the sarcoplasmic calcium pump. *FEBS Lett* 12:271–272, 1971.

128. Knowles AF, Racker E: Formation of adenosine triphosphate from Pi and adenosine diphosphate by purified Ca^{2+}-adenosine triphosphatase. *J Biol Chem* 250:1949–1951, 1975.

129. Sumida M, Wang T, Schwartz A, Younkin C, Froehlich JP: The Ca^{2+}-ATPase partial reactions in cardiac and skeletal sarcoplasmic reticulum: A comparison of transient state kinetic data. *J Biol Chem* 255:1497–1503, 1980.

130. Shigekawa M, Kanazawa T: Phosphoenzyme formation from ATP in the ATPase of sarcoplasmic reticulum: Effect of KCl or ATP and slow dissociation of ATP from precursor enzyme-ATP complex. *J Biol Chem* 257:7657–7665, 1982.

131. Kirchberger MA, Tada M, Katz AM: Adenosine 3′,5′-monophosphate-dependent protein kinase-catalyzed phosphorylation reaction and its relationship to calcium transport in cardiac sarcoplasmic reticulum. *J Biol Chem* 249:6166–6173, 1974.

132. La Raia RJ, Morkin E: Adenosine 3′5′-monophosphate-dependent membrane phosphorylation: A possible mechanism for the control of microsomal calcium transport in heart muscle. *Circ Res* 35:298–306, 1974.

133. Will H, Levchenko TS, Levitsky DO, Smirnov VN, Wollenberger A: Partial characterization of protein kinase-catalyzed phosphorylation of low molecular weight proteins in purified preparations of pigeon heart sarcolemma and sarcoplasmic reticulum. *Biochim Biophys Acta* 543:175–193, 1978.

134. Tada M, Kirchberger MA, Katz AM: Phosphorylation of a 22,000-dalton component of the cardiac sarcoplasmic reticulum by adenosine 3′:5′-monophosphate-dependent

protein kinase. *J Biol Chem* 250:2640–2647, 1975.

135. Katz AM, Tada M, Kirchberger MA: Control of calcium transport in the myocardium by the cyclic AMP-protein kinase system. *Adv Cyclic Nucleotide Res* 5:453–472, 1975.

136. Le Peuch CJ, Haiech J, Demaille JG: Concerted regulation of cardiac sarcoplasmic reticulum calcium transport by cyclic adenosine monophosphate dependent and calcium-calmodulin-dependent phosphorylations. *Biochemistry* 18:5150–5157, 1979.

137. Movsesian MA, Nishikawa M, Adelstein RS: Phosphorylation of phospholamban by calcium-activated, phospholipid-dependent protein kinase. *J Biol Chem* 259:8029–8032, 1984.

138. Kirchberger MA, Tada M: Effects of adenosine 3′:5′-monophosphate-dependent protein kinase on sarcoplasmic reticulum isolated from cardiac and slow and fast contracting skeletal muscles. *J Biol Chem* 251:725–729, 1976.

139. Kirchberger MA, Chu G: Correlation between protein kinase-mediated stimulation of calcium transport by cardiac sarcoplasmic reticulum and phosphorylation of a 22,000 dalton protein. *Biochim Biophys Acta* 419:559–562, 1976.

140. Hicks MJ, Shigekawa M, Katz AM: Mechanism by which cyclic adenosine 3′:5′-monophosphate-dependent protein kinase stimulates calcium transport in cardiac sarcoplasmic reticulum. *Circ Res* 44:384–391, 1979.

141. Tada M, Kirchberger MA, Li HC: Phosphoprotein phosphatase-catalyzed dephosphorylation of the 22,000 dalton phosphoprotein of cardiac sarcoplasmic reticulum. *J Cyclic Nucleotide Res* 1:329–338, 1975.

142. Kirchberger MA, Raffo A: Decrease in calcium transport associated with phosphoprotein phosphatase-catalyzed dephosphorylation of cardiac sarcoplasmic reticulum. *J Cyclic Nucleotide Res* 3:34–53, 1977.

143. Tada M, Ohmori F, Nimura Y, Abe H: Effect of myocardial protein kinase modulator on adenosine 3′:5′-monophosphate-dependent protein kinase-induced stimulation of calcium transport by cardiac sarcoplasmic reticulum. *J Biochem (Tokyo)* 82:885–892, 1977.

144. Katz S, Remtulla MA: Phosphodiesterase protein activator stimulates calcium transport in cardiac microsomal preparations enriched in sarcoplasmic reticulum. *Biochem Biophys Res Commun* 83:1373–1379, 1978.

145. Kranias EG, Bilezikjian LM, Potter JD, Piascik MT, Schwartz A: The role of calmodulin in regulation of cardiac sarcoplasmic reticulum phosphorylation. *Ann NY Acad Sci* 356:279–291, 1980.

146. Tada M, Inui M, Yamada M, Kadoma M, Kuzuya T, Abe H, Kakiuchi S: Effects of phospholamban phosphorylation catalyzed by adenosine 3′:5′-monophosphate- and calmodulin-dependent protein kinases on calcium transport ATPase of cardiac sarcoplasmic reticulum. *J Mol Cell Cardiol* 15:335–346, 1983.

147. Kirchberger MA, Antonetz T: Calmodulin-mediated regulation of calcium transport and (Ca^{2+} + Mg^{2+})-activated ATPase activity in isolated cardiac sarcoplasmic reticulum. *J Biol Chem* 257:5685–5691, 1982.

148. Tada M, Yamada M, Kadoma M, Inui M, Ohmori F: Calcium transport by cardiac sarcoplasmic reticulum and phosphorylation of phospholamban. *Mol Cell Biochem* 46:73–95, 1982.

149. Kranias EG, Mandel F, Wang T, Schwartz A: Mechanism of the stimulation of calcium ion dependent adenosine triphosphatase of cardiac sarcoplasmic reticulum by adenosine 3′,5′-monophosphate dependent protein kinase. *Biochemistry* 19:5434–5439, 1980.

150. Wegener AD, Jones LR: Phosphorylation-induced mobility shift in phospholamban in sodium dodecyl sulfate-polyacrylamide gels. Evidence for a protein structure consisting of multiple identical phosphorylatable subunits. *J Biol Chem* 259:1834–1841, 1984.

151. Watanabe Y, Kijima Y, Kadoma M, Tada M, Takagi T: Molecular weight determination of phospholamban oligomer in the presence of sodium dodecyl sulfate: Application of low-angle laser light scattering photometry. *J Biochem (Tokyo)* 110:40–45, 1991.

152. Simmerman HK, Collins JH, Theibert JL, Wegener AD, Jones LR: Sequence analysis of phospholamban. Identification of phosphorylation sites and two major structural domains. *J Biol Chem* 261:13333–13341, 1986.

153. Inui M, Kadoma M, Tada M: Purification and characterization of phospholamban from canine cardiac sarcoplasmic reticulum. *J Biol Chem* 260:3708–3715, 1985.

154. Jones LR, Simmerman HK, Wilson WW, Gurd FR, Wegener AD: Purification and characterization of phospholamban from canine cardiac sarcoplasmic reticulum. *J Biol Chem* 260:7721–7730, 1985.

155. Fujii J, Kadoma M, Tada M, Toda H, Sakiyama F: Characterization of structural unit of phospholamban by amino acid sequencing and electrophoretic analysis. *Biochem Biophys Res Commun* 138:1044–1050, 1986.

156. Fujii J, Ueno A, Kitano K, Tanaka S, Kadoma M, Tada M: Complete complementary DNA-derived amino acid sequence of canine cardiac phospholamban. *J Clin Invest* 79:301–304, 1987.

157. Verboomen H, Wuytack F, Eggermont JA, De Jaegere S, Missiaen L, Raeymaekers L, Casteels R: cDNA cloning and sequencing of phospholamban from pig stomach smooth muscle. *Biochem J* 262:353–356, 1989.

158. Toyofuku T, Zak R: Characterization of cDNA and genomic sequences encoding a chicken phospholamban. *J Biol Chem* 266:5375–5383, 1991.

159. Tada M, Kadoma M: Regulation of the Ca^{2+} pump ATPase by cAMP-dependent phosphorylation of phospholamban. *Bioessays* 10:157–163, 1989.

160. Simmerman HK, Lovelace DE, Jones LR: Secondary structure of detergent-solubilized phospholamban, a phosphorylatable, oligomeric protein of cardiac sarcoplasmic reticulum. *Biochim Biophys Acta* 997:322–329, 1989.

161. Fujii J, Maruyama K, Tada M, MacLennan DH: Expression and site-specific mutagenesis of phospholamban. Studies of residues involved in phosphorylation and pentamer formation. *J Biol Chem* 264:12950–12955, 1989.

162. Tada M, Kadoma M, Inui M, Fujii J: Regulation of Ca^{2+}-pump from cardiac sarcoplasmic reticulum. *Methods Enzymol* 157:107–154, 1988.

163. James P, Inui M, Tada M, Chiesi M, Carafoli E: Nature and site of phospholamban regulation of the Ca^{2+} pump of sarcoplasmic reticulum. *Nature* 342:90–92, 1989.

164. Inui M, Chamberlain BK, Saito A, Fleischer S: The nature of the modulation of Ca^{2+} transport as studied by reconstitution of cardiac sarcoplasmic reticulum. *J Biol Chem* 261:1794–1800, 1986.

165. Kim HW, Steenaart NA, Ferguson DG, Kranias EG: Functional reconstitution of the cardiac sarcoplasmic reticulum Ca$^{2(+)}$-ATPase with phospholamban in phospholipid vesicles. *J Biol Chem* 265:1702–1709, 1990.

166. Kirchberger MA, Borchman D, Kasinathan C: Proteolytic activation of the canine cardiac sarcoplasmic reticulum calcium pump. *Biochemistry* 25:5484–5492, 1986.

167. Suzuki T, Wang JH: Stimulation of bovine cardiac sarcoplasmic reticulum Ca^{2+} pump and blocking of phospholamban phosphorylation and dephosphorylation by a

phospholamban monoclonal antibody. *J Biol Chem* 261: 7018–7023, 1986.

168. Kimura Y, Inui M, Kadoma M, Kijima Y, Sasaki T, Tada M: Effects of monoclonal antibody against phospholamban on calcium pump ATPase of cardiac sarcoplasmic reticulum. *J Mol Cell Cardiol* 23:1223–1230, 1991.

169. Fujii J, Maruyama K, Tada M, MacLennan DH: Co-expression of slow-twitch/cardiac muscle Ca^{2+}-ATPase (SERCA2) and phospholamban. *FEBS Lett* 273:232–234, 1990.

170. Sasaki T, Inui M, Kimura K, Kuzuya T, Tada M: Molecular mechanism of regulation of Ca^{2+} pump ATPase by phospholamban in cardiac sarcoplasmic reticulum. Effects of synthetic phospholamban peptides on Ca^{2+} pump ATPase. *J Biol Chem* 267:1674–1679, 1992.

171. Xu ZC, Kirchberger MA: Modulation by polyelectrolytes of canine cardiac microsomal calcium uptake and the possible relationship to phospholamban. *J Biol Chem* 264:16644–16651, 1989.

172. Chiesi M, Schwaller R: Involvement of electrostatic phenomena in phospholamban-induced stimulation of Ca uptake into cardiac sarcoplasmic reticulum. *FEBS Lett* 244:241–244, 1989.

173. Solaro RJ, Wise RM, Shiner JS, Briggs FN: Calcium Requirements for cardiac myofibrillar activation. *Circ Res* 34:525–530, 1974.

174. Winegrad S: Studies of cardiac muscle with a high permeability to calcium produced by treatment with ethylenediaminetetraacetic acid. *J Gen Physiol* 58:71–93, 1971.

175. Fabiato A: Myoplasmic free calcium concentration reached during the twitch of an intact isolated cardiac cell and during calcium-induced release of calcium from the sarcoplasmic reticulum of a skinned cardiac cell from the adult rat or rabbit ventricle. *J Gen Physiol* 78:457–497, 1981.

176. Scarpa A, Williamson JR: Calcium binding and calcium transport by subcellular fractions of heart. In: Drabikowski W, Strzelecka-Gotaszewska H, Carafoli E (eds) *Calcium Binding Proteins*. Amsterdam: Elsevier, 1974, pp 547–585.

177. Tada M, Inui M: Regulation of calcium transport by the ATPase-phospholamban system. *J Mol Cell Cardiol* 15:565–575, 1983.

178. Morad M, Rolett EL: Relaxing effects of catecholamines on

mammalian heart. *J Physiol (Lond)* 224:537–558, 1972.

179. Reuter H: Localization of beta adrenergic receptors, and effects of noradrenaline and cyclic numleotides on action potentials, ionic currents and tension in mammalian cardiac muscle. *J Physiol (Lond)* 242:429–451, 1974.

180. Allen DG, Blinks JR: Calcium transients in aequorin-injected frog cardiac muscle. *Nature* 273:509–513, 1978.

181. Fabiato A, Fabiato F: Relaxing and inotropic effects of cyclic AMP on skinned cardiac cells. *Nature* 253:556–558, 1975.

182. Tsien RW: Cyclic AMP and contractile activity in heart. *Adv Cyclic Nucleotides Res* 8:363–420, 1977.

183. Schümann HJ, Endoh M, Brodde OE: The time course of the effects of β- and α-adrenoceptor stimulation by isoprenaline and methoxamine on the contractile force and cAMP level of the isolated rabbit papillary muscle. *Naunyn-Schmiedebergs Arch Pharmacol* 289:291–302, 1975.

184. Ingebretsen WR Jr, Becker E, Friedman WF, Mayer SE: Contractile and biochemical responses of cardiac and skeletal muscle to isoproterenol covalently linked to glass beads. *Circ Res* 40:474–484, 1977.

185. Venter JC, Ross J Jr, Kaplan NO: Lack of detectable change in cyclic AMP during the cardiac inotropic response to isoproterenol immobilized on glass beads. *Proc Natl Acad Sci USA* 72:824–828, 1975.

186. Le Peuch CJ, Guilleux J-C, Demaille JG: Phospholamban phosphorylation in the perfused rat heart is not solely dependent on β-adrenergic stimulation. *FEBS Lett* 114:165–168, 1980.

187. Lindemann JP, Jones LR, Hathaway DR, Henry BG, Watanabe AM: β-adrenergic stimulation of phospholamban phosphorylation and Ca^{2+}-ATPase activity in guinea pig ventricles. *J Biol Chem* 258:464–471, 1983.

188. Limas CJ: Enhanced phosphorylation of myocaridal sarcoplasmic reticulum in experimental hyperthyroidism. *Am J Physiol* 234:H426–H431, 1978.

189. Kadoma M, Sacktor B, Froehlich JP: Stimulation by cAMP and protein kinase of calcium transport in sarcoplasmic reticulum from senescent rat myocardium (abstr). *Fed Proc* 39:2040, 1980.

CHAPTER 18

Control Mechanisms Regulating Contractile Activity of Cardiac Myofilaments

R. JOHN SOLARO

INTRODUCTION

In this chapter we focus on the molecular machine responsible for the ability of cardiac muscle cells to shorten and develop force. This machine, which is housed in the sarcomeres, consists of bundles of thin and thick filaments. Active mechanical changes in the sarcomere are due to interactions between the thin and thick myofilaments, which are triggered by release of Ca^{2+} into the myofilament space and powered by hydrolysis of ATP {1}. The result of these interactions is a translation of the thin filaments toward the center of the sarcomere. This sliding process is the fundamental mechanism by which the cardiac chambers develop pressure and eject blood. In this chapter we consider (a) the elements of thin and thick filaments responsible for the transduction of chemical energy into mechanical activity, (b) the regulation of this process by Ca^{2+} ions and by feedback mechanisms involving the interactions themselves, and (c) modulation of the regulation by short-term processes involving second messenger cascades and protein phosphorylation.

STRUCTURE AND FUNCTION OF CARDIAC MYOFILAMENT PROTEINS

Coupling of ATP hydrolysis to the relative motion of thick and thin filaments has been intensively studied at various levels of organization, and there is enough information to present a plausible and detailed concept of the chemomechanical transduction process. The molecular structure of thin and thick filaments is shown in fig. 18-1.

The thick filament of mammalian cardiac muscle is composed mainly of myosin, which itself is an enzyme capable of splitting ATP. Myosin is an elongated hexameric protein consisting of two heavy chains and four light chains. Each of the two heavy chains consists of a long α-helical tail and a globular head. The two tails are intertwined, forming a two-headed structure. The head contains the ATPase and an actin-binding site. Attached noncovalently to each head are two different light chains. One light chain is releasable in alkali and is called *alkali-light chain* or *LCI* and the other, which is phosphorylatable, is called the *P-light chain* or *LCII*. The

backbone of the thick filament is formed by an assembly of a large portion of the myosin tail, with the head and a short segment of the tail, the so-called crossbridge, projecting from the thick filament. The globular head region of the myosin molecule can be cleaved from the tail portion by proteolysis to yield a two-headed fragment called *heavy meromyosin* (HMM) or a single-headed fragment called *subfragment* (S-1). Both HMM and S-1, which retain the actin-binding and ATPase sites, are often used in biochemical studies because they are soluble at physiological ionic strength.

The major component of the thin filament is actin. Actin monomer (G-actin) is a single polypeptide (MW 43,000). In the presence of physiological ionic strength ATP and Mg^{2+}, G-actin spontaneously assembles into F-actin, which constitutes the backbone of the thin filament. F-actin is commonly represented as two strands of monomers coiled around each other. In addition, the thin filament contains tropomyosin (Tm) and troponin (Tn). Tm is a fibrous molecule consisting of two subunits. There are two subunit isoforms, which are very similar in amino acid sequence. The subunits, which are at least 90% α-helix, are arranged in a Tm molecule as a two-stranded coiled coil. In thin filaments, Tm exists as a linear polymer, a rigid molecule in which the monomers are bound head to tail with an eight to nine amino acid residue overlap between the C and N termini. There is a Tm filament in each of the two major grooves formed by the twisted actin filaments, with each Tm monomer spanning seven actin monomers.

Tn, which is a complex of three functionally distinctive peptides, is distributed periodically along the thin filament with an interval of about 40 nm. The three units of Tn are designated on the basis of three major functional characteristics reflected in their names: troponin C (TnC) for Ca-binding subunit, troponin I (TnI) for the inhibitory subunit, and troponin T (TnT) for Tm-binding subunit. The Tn complex interacts with both Tm at multiple interaction sites and at a limited number of actin monomers in the thin filament. Before considering how alterations in the interactions among Tn units, and Tm and actin, are related to activation of the thin filament, we consider how the actin-myosin reaction is related to force and shortening.

N. Sperelakis (ed.), Physiology and Pathophysiology of the Heart, Third Edition.

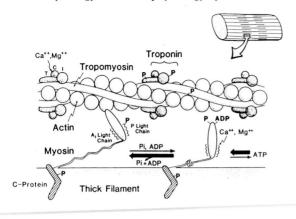

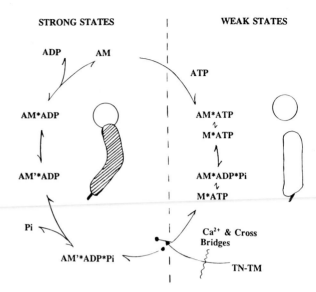

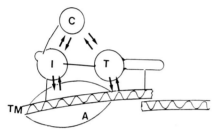

Fig. 18-1. **Top:** Cartoon depicting the array of proteins in cardiac myofilaments. The symbol P indicates a site of potential covalent phosphorylation. **Bottom:** Schematic representation of interaction among troponin components (C, I, and T), tropomyosin (TM), and actin (A). Arrows indicate reactions that are reversibly altered during activation and relaxation by Ca^{2+} binding to troponin C and removal. Straight lines indicate Ca^{2+}-insensitive interactions presumed to maintain structural integrity. See text for details.

Fig. 18-2. Schematic representation of the crossbridge cycle showing intermediates in the kinetic cycle. The crossbridge on the right denotes a "weak" crossbridge predominating in relaxation. The crosshatched crossbridge on the left denotes a strong, force-generating state. The vertical dashed line separates weak from strong states and, as indicated, redistribution of the population of crossbridges occurs with release of the block by troponin-tropomyosin (Tn-Tm). The wavy line denotes that the inhibition by Tn-Tm may be released by the action of Ca^{2+} and strong crossbridges themselves. See text for details.

CHEMOMECHANICAL TRANSDUCTION

It is the reaction between the myosin crossbridges and actin that couples ATP hydrolysis to a motion of the filaments. Although the exact molecular events for chemomechanical transduction are not certain, it is clear that motion and force are related to states of the crossbridge in a reaction cycle {2}. The nature of these states is shown schematically in fig. 18-2, which depicts intermediates in the reaction cycle of actin with the myosin heads.

The scheme is a composite of those used by Millar and Homsher {3} and Walker et al. {4} to analyze kinetic experiments aimed at determining rate processes in the cycle. As indicated in fig. 18-2, during diastole crossbridges are in a 'weak' binding state in rapid equilibrium with actin. With systole and Ca^{2+} release into the myofilament space, the crossbridges redistribute to a population containing strongly attached and force-generating states. A key feature is the change in orientation of the crossbridge state during hydrolysis of ATP and product release. This change, depicted schematically as the strong force-generating crossbridge in fig. 18-2, is believed to impel the thin filaments toward the center of the sarcomere, to

generate force, and to cause shortening depending on the loading conditions. It is apparent that the number of force-generating crossbridges reacting with the thin filament is related to the force-generating capability of the myofilaments, and that the rate of crossbridge cycling is related to the shortening velocity. Ultimately it is this redistribution that establishes the diastolic and systolic states of cardiac myofilaments. In diastole, weak states predominate because of inhibition of the redistribution to the strong state by the action of Tn-Tm. As indicated in the scheme in fig. 18-2, redistribution of crossbridge states is associated with release from inhibition by two mechanisms. One involves the action of Ca^{2+} on the functional unit of the thin filament (7 mol actin to 1 mol TnC, TnI, TnT, and Tm); the other involves feedback effects of the crossbridge on TnC and interactions among functional units that spread activation along the thin filament to near-neighbor functional units.

REGULATION OF THE ACTIN–CROSSBRIDGE REACTION

The key reaction in the diastolic/systolic transition is the delivery of Ca^{2+} to the myofilaments. Ca^{2+} binds to TnC, the main Ca receptor of the myofibrils. Ca-TnC triggers the actin-myosin reaction, by promoting disinhibition of functional units in thin filament. Under normal conditions, regulation of the release of Ca^{2+} into the myofibrillar space and the control of flows of Ca^{2+} to and from Tn sites are mediated by the sarcolemma and sarcoplasmic reticulum. The roles of these membrane systems in excitation-contraction coupling, in regulation of relaxation, and as determinants of the frequency of Ca^{2+} triggering are treated in detail elsewhere in this book and will not be considered here.

In diastole, the intracellular Ca^{2+} ion concentration is about $0.1\,\mu M$ and during systole it rises to about $1.0\,\mu M$, depending on the activity of the various membrane channels and transport systems. Diastolic levels of free Ca^{2+} are associated with little or no Ca binding to regulatory sites on TnC and, as described in detail below, the force-generating actin-myosin reaction is blocked and myosin ATPase activity is essentially arrested. Associated with electrical depolarization of the cells is an increase in free Ca^{2+}, which under normal, resting inotropic states appears to deliver enough Ca^{2+} to the myofilaments to bring them to 10–25% of full activation {5}. Thus, there is the possibility for recruitment of crossbridges into the actin-myosin reaction by alterations in the Ca^{2+} delivered to the myofilaments during systole. This, of course, is an important mechanism for altering cardiac contractile state by the autonomic nervous system and by various pharmacological interventions.

The steady-state relation between free Ca^{2+} ion concentration and myofilament force and/or ATPase activity can be demonstrated in so-called skinned fiber preparations in which the sarcolemma and other membranes have been dissolved away using nonionic detergents such as Triton X-100 {6}. Developed tension is measured by soaking the preparation held isometric in a force-measuring setup in solutions similar to the intracellular environment and containing free Ca^{2+} buffered to various concentrations using EGTA. With the aid of ^{45}Ca, Ca^{2+} binding to myofilament TnC can also be measured in these preparations. The steady-state relation between force developed by skinned fibers and Ca^{2+} binding to sites on TnC is depicted in fig. 18-3. The figure shows results of experiments in which we measured TnC-Ca^{2+} binding measured with the aid of ^{45}Ca in the same isometric skinned fibers in which force was measured {5}. The higher affinity sites (2 mol/mol myofilament TnC) are nearly saturated with Ca^{2+} at pCa values at which force has yet to increase. On the other hand, the single lower affinity site titrates Ca^{2+} over the range of activating pCa values. Kinetic studies showed that the high-affinity sites exchange Ca^{2+} very slowly with a half-time of the order of minutes {7}, whereas the lower affinity site exchanges Ca^{2+} with a half-time within the contraction/relaxation cycle {8}. It is apparent, therefore, that contraction/relaxation is associated with exchange of Ca^{2+} with this single regulatory site. Inasmuch as removal of Ca^{2+} and Mg^{2+} from higher affinity sites causes dissociation of TnC from myofibrils, these sites have been assigned a structural role in maintaining the integrity of the troponin molecule {9}.

An intriguing aspect of the relations among myofilament force, TnC bound Ca^{2+}, and pCa is that whereas force is a steep function of pCa, indicative of a cooperative response to Ca^{2+}, binding of Ca^{2+} to myofilament TnC

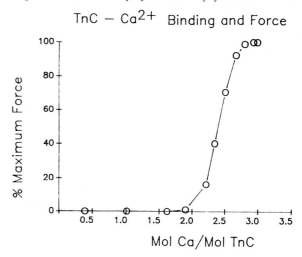

Fig. 18-3. Relation between force developed by skinned fiber preparations and stoichiometry of Ca^{2+} binding to myofilament TnC. Both measurement were made in the preparation held isometric at a sarcomere length of $2.0\,\mu m$ at pH 7.0 and room temperature. Conditions in mM were 5 $MgATP^{2-}$, 2 Mg^{2+}, and 150 ionic strength. Various levels of force were achieved by varying the free Ca^{2+} over a broad range with the aid of EGTA buffers. Data are recalculated from those reported by Pan and Solaro {5}.

can be fit with a noncooperative model with independent sites or with some small cooperativity. The implication of this is illustrated in the data plotted in fig. 18-3. They show that full activation of the myofilaments may occur with only a fraction of the TnC regulatory sites filled with Ca^{2+}. Thus, full activation of the myofilament may be associated with processes other than binding of Ca^{2+} to TnC. Moreover, the cooperative response of force to pCa may lie in features of the regulatory process other than Ca^{2+} binding to TnC. Ideas on the mechanism of the cooperative response are presented following a more complete description of mechanisms for myofilament activation by Ca^{2+}.

Thin-filament related Ca regulation

As depicted in fig. 18-2, one mode of redistribution of weak crossbridges to strong crossbridges involves Ca^{2+} release and myofilament Ca^{2+} binding, which releases the functional unit from a prevailing inhibition resulting from the action of Tm. Interactions among thin filament proteins that signal release of the myofilaments from the inhibitory activity of Tn-Tm are illustrated in the lower panel of fig. 18-1. In diastole, tight binding of TnI to actin and interactions of TnT with TnI, actin, and Tm promote a population of crossbridges that are in the weak binding state {10}. Reversible disinhibition of the inhibitory activity of TnT-TnI-Tm on actin-myosin reactions requires the presence of TnC. A key reaction is tight binding of TnC to TnI triggered by Ca^{2+} binding to the regulatory site {5,8}. This tight binding weakens the TnI-actin interaction and alters the TnT-TnI-actin-Tm interactions in such a way that Tm moves into the groove of the thin filament {11}.

The reaction of TnI with TnC occurs in two regions of the molecule at a near-amino-terminal domain and in an inhibitory domain, which, as shown in fig. 18-1, shuttles between binding to TnC and to actin. TnI also reacts with a carboxy-terminal half of TnT, as does actin and Tm. These interactions are Ca^{2+} sensitive. On other hand, the reaction of the amino-terminal half of TnT with Tm is not sensitive to Ca^{2+} and occurs in the region of overlap between adjacent Tm molecules. This has led to the idea that the tadpole-shaped Tn complex is anchored to Tm at its tail and during Ca^{2+} activation actually lifts off the thin filament {12}.

How Ca binding to TnC ultimately switches the interaction between myosin and actin on and off is not fully understood, although it is generally believed that tropomyosin plays a pivotal role in the transmission of the on/off signal to actin. There are two hypotheses for the mode of regulation of actin-myosin interactions leading to force and shortening of striated muscle. One line of experiments supports the idea that the regulation of the transitions is "all or none," i.e., that activation involves increases in the number of myosin heads reacting with actin as strongly bound force-generating crossbridges, but with little or no gradation of the reaction in the form of regulation of a kinetic transition in the overall cycle {4}. The other hypothesis holds that Ca^{2+} controls one or more rate constants in the transition among crossbridge states, resulting in graded activation {13}. Evidence in favor of the "all or none" mechanism comes from studies that determined the Ca^{2+} dependence of rate constants from pre-steady-state measurements. In these experiments, photolysis of caged Pi was used to rapidly release Pi into the myofilament space, resulting in a transient fall of force due to product inhibition and transition of the crossbridges from strong to weak states. These studies showed that Ca^{2+} had no {3} or little {4} effect on the rate constant associated with the fall in force with release of caged Pi.

Role of metal binding to myosin light chain II in activation

Although it has been shown that removal of the Tn-Tm complex from cardiac myofibrillar preparations results in a loss of the Ca^{2+} dependence of acto-myosin ATPase activity {19}, in the presence of Ca^{2+} binding sites on myosin of vertebrate striated muscle, there has been persistent interest in the possibility that there is an additional Ca^{2+} switch at the level of thick filaments. The idea of a myosin-linked regulatory mechanism was also inspired by observations showing Ca^{2+}-binding-induced conformation changes in isolated thick filaments {14}, and early X-ray diffraction studies of frog muscle stretched beyond overlap showing activation-related changes in the intensity of equatorial reflections, suggesting crossbridge movement independent of thin filaments {15}.

The divalent ion binding sites of myosin of vertebrate striated muscle have been studied extensively. Myosin molecules contain a relatively high-affinity nonspecific ion binding site on each of the two light chains. The sites bind Ca^{2+} and Mg^{2+} competitively, with the affinity for Ca^{2+} being higher than that for Mg^{2+}. The Mg^{2+} reported affinities for Ca^{2+} and Mg^{2+} of the site vary greatly, but it is likely that the affinities are significantly lower than Ca^{2+} binding to TnC {16}. Studies of the primary structure of the LCII, also known as PLC, suggest there are four domains in the sequence that are analogous to the Ca^{2+} binding domains of parvalbumin, whereas only one domain is complete. Bagshaw and Reed {17} have demonstrated the nonspecific high-affinity site is indeed located in domain 1. Equilibrium binding studies show that purified myosin can bind some Ca^{2+} at pCa 5 in the presence of physiological level of Mg^{2+} (1 mM). However, since the rate constant for dissociation of Mg is low (0.05–0.06 s), the exchange of Ca^{2+} and Mg^{2+} at the site is expected to take tens of seconds to complete and is apparently too slow to contribute to rapid initiation of contraction of striated muscle. The data are, therefore, against a mechanism involving direct Ca^{2+} interaction with myosin as a switch for activation of cardiac myofilaments. There may, however, be effects of PLC that modify the response of myofilaments to Ca^{2+} that occur on a relatively long time scale with sustained changes in the rate or level of contractility. In this case one might expect a change in the level of metal bound to PLC.

Cooperative response to Ca^{2+}

The mechanisms underlying the steep dependence of steady-state force/ATPase on pCa are not well understood. An early explanation for the phenomenon was that the activation of a functional unit requires simultaneous occupancy of two or all four independent binding sites of TnC {18,19}. However, the Hill coefficient of the pCa/response curves computed based on these models is only slightly higher than one unit and therefore are far from sufficient to account for the steep response of actomyosin ATPase to increasing Ca {19}. Recently, much attention has been given to possible involvement of cooperative protein-protein interactions. Cooperative interactions likely to play a role in determining the characteristics of the pCa-force/ATPase relation may be loosely classified into two categories: (a) cooperativity in Ca binding to TnC and (b) interactions among Tn-Tm in different functional units along the thin filament.

The evidence that regulation of force and ATPase activity involves a single Ca^{2+} binding site on cardiac TnC rules out the possibility that the Ca^{2+} switch is a two- or three-power switch. There is, however, evidence that the affinity of cardiac TnC for Ca^{2+} may be affected by a cooperative mechanism involving crossbridge interactions with the thin filament. Such an effect is expected on theoretical grounds {20}, since energies of interaction from Ca-TnC to myosin sites on actin would also be expected to occur in the reverse direction when actin sites bind myosin. Bremel and Weber {21} were the first to demonstrate that crossbridges attached to actin in the absence of ATP (rigor links) induced an increased affinity of skeletal TnC for Ca^{2+}. This effect of rigor crossbridges on TnC was supported by experiments using skinned fibers that showed reductions in the level of MgATP result in an increase in Ca sensitivity of force development {22}.

Similar results have been obtained in the case of cardiac muscle {5}.

It has been suggested that the attachment of force-generating crossbridges may have a similar effect on TnC. There are conflicting data relevant to the idea. Ridgway et al. {23} found that in aequorin-injected, voltage-clamped barnacle single muscle fibers, the level of steady-state force associated with a particular Ca^{2+} concentration depends on the immediate history of the fiber; the same Ca^{2+} level can produce more force if the fiber previously experienced a high force. The results were confirmed by the observation that the pCa/force relation of skinned fibers exhibited hysteresis. To explain these findings, the authors suggest that crossbridge interactions modulate Ca affinity of TnC, and thereby, Ca sensitivity of the contractile system. Direct support for this idea comes from observations showing that a quick release of intact heart muscle produces a burst of extra Ca^{2+} in the myoplasm, as detected using the luminescent protein aequorin {24}. This effect is presumed to reflect changes in the Ca affinity of myofilaments due to crossbridge detachment. On the other hand, Wnuk et al. {25} found that during steady-state ATP hydrolysis, TnC in regulated crayfish actomyosin displays Ca-binding properties essentially the same as those of regulated actin without myosin. Fuchs {26} showed that under conditions of steady-state force development, there is no enhancement of Ca binding to myofilaments of skinned psoas fibers, as compared to the relaxed state produced by vanadate. One explanation for the discrepancy is that because the predominant steady-state crossbridge intermediates, $M \cdot ADP \cdot Pi$ and $M \cdot ADP$, have much lower affinities for actin than rigor state, AM {13}, the alteration in the Ca affinity of TnC due to interaction of the crossbridges with actin would be too small to measure by direct binding assays used by Wnuk et al. {25} and Fuchs {26}.

Interactions between different functional units along a thin filament

The idea that the steep dependence of force/ATPase rate of regulated actomyosin on free Ca^{2+} concentration could arise from an interaction between adjacent tropomyosin molecules was first suggested explicitly by Tawada and Tawada {27}. Tawada et al. {28} found that the relation between pCa and the rate of superprecipitation of actomyosin regulated by nonpolymerizable Tm, from which several C-terminal residues were removed enzymatically, was much less steep that found with actomyosin-containing untreated Tm. To account for the finding, a theoretical model {28} was proposed that assumed the transition of the tropomyosin-troponin unit from the inhibitory to the noninhibitory position primarily occurs as a result of saturation of the Ca binding sites of TnC in the same unit; however, because of end-to-end interactions of tropomyosin molecules along the thin filament, the transition of a particular unit can also occur before saturation of the Ca binding sites of a TnC. The cooperativity was introduced by means of postulating that the equilibrium constant for transition of a Ca-free troponin-tropomyosin

from an inhibitory to a noninhibitory position increases with the increase in the fraction of tropomyosin molecules to the noninhibitory position.

Another interesting feature of the model was that the Ca-affinity constants of TnC were assumed to be independent of the state of tropomyosin and crossbridge interaction. The theoretical analysis based on the model demonstrated that a steep dependence of the activation of actomyosin interaction could be obtained without any cooperativity in Ca binding {28}. More recent work provides further support for these ideas. For example, at low ATP, which favors a population of strongly attached (rigor) crossbridges (fig. 18-2), force and ATPase activity can be activated in the absence of Ca^{2+}, and the pCa force curve is shifted to the left {22}. One hypothesis {19,20,28,29} for these effects is that the movement of Tm promoted by strong crossbridges acts to spread activation along the thin filament to neighboring functional units that are not activated by Ca^{2+}-TnC. This idea has been supported by studies showing that removal of the Tm overlap by proteolytic digestion leads to less cooperativity in Ca^{2+} regulation of myofilament activity {28}. Cooperativity in the reaction of the crossbridges with thin filaments has been described formally by the model of Hill et al. {29}, in which functional units are viewed as being in an on state or off state with binding constants of crossbridges for the "on" and "off" state of actin monomers. The free energy of interaction, Y, between these two states is also included, and, for example, when Tm is clipped at its C-terminal end to removal overlap, Y fell to about 10% of its value in the intact system {30}.

Studies {31,32} on skinned muscle fibers in which either TnC or Tn was partially removed provided important evidence for a role of nearest neighbor interaction in Ca regulation of force production. TnC can be extracted from skinned fast skeletal muscle fibers by brief treatment with EDTA without significant loss of other myofibrillar proteins {31}. Partial removal of TnC from rabbit psoas fibers resulted in a reduction in active tension during maximum Ca activation. This is presumably due to permanent inhibition of the functional units devoid of TnC. Brandt et al. {32} reported that extraction of slightly less than half of the total TnC resulted in a dramatic decrease in the Hill coefficient (from 5.8 to 2) of the pCa-force relation of skinned rabbit psoas fibers. They suggested that the decrease in apparent cooperativity in the activation process was caused by tropomyosin-troponin units without TnC, which constitute inactive gaps preventing cooperative propagation of activation along a thin filament. Based on the observation that extraction of as little as one TnC per tropomyosin-troponin strand brought about a detectable decrease in the Hill coefficient, these investigators suggested that an intact thin filament activates as a cooperative unit {32}.

Moss et al. {33} reported that proteolytic removal of a small portion of Tn complexes from skinned rabbit psoas fibers resulted in development of Ca-insensitive active tension and increased Ca sensitivity of tension development. It was argued that the development of Ca-insensitive active tension was most likely due to disinhibition of all or some actin monomers of those functional units in which troponin had been removed. Thus the results strongly suggest that activation of some of the functional units along a thin filament enhanced Ca sensitivity of tension development involving functional units with troponin still bound. Another very interesting finding in the study was that, in the absence of Ca^{2+}, only one third or one half of the functional groups along a thin filament needed to be activated by removal of troponin in order to activate the entire thin filament. By analogy, one may speculate that in an intact contractile filament assembly, only a portion of the troponins need to be saturated by Ca to achieve full activation of the thin filament. This possibility is very attractive because it offers a mechanism whereby the contractile machinery can respond to changes in Ca concentration in a highly cooperative manner without significant cooperativity in Ca binding to TnC.

MODULATION OF CA ACTIVATION OF CARDIAC MYOFILAMENTS

The regulation of cardiac function can be designated as arising from three main mechanisms. The first, known as Starling's Law of the Heart, is intrinsic to the cells and involves changes in end-diastolic volume with no change in end-systolic volume. The second mechanism involves extrinsic control involving mainly influences of the autonomic nerves and neurohumors on the end-systolic length of cells. Here we consider these two mechanisms as short term in that they occur over several beats. A third mechanism, which we consider to be long term, involves altered gene expression. All of these major physiological mechanisms for control of cardiac function involve modulation of the activity and regulation of the cardiac myofilaments.

Length-dependent activation

The Starling relation, i.e., the relation between end-diastolic volume and stroke volume, is a reflection of the rising limb of the length-tension curve of cardiac muscle. There is convincing evidence that the shape of the rising limb of the sarcomere length twitch tension relation of mammalian cardiac muscle is determined by a length-dependent alteration in myofilament Ca activation. The hypothesis is that the myofilaments are relatively inactive at short lengths due to a reduced sensitivity to free Ca^{2+}. It has been known for some time {34} that the overall muscle length-tension relation of isolated mammalian papillary muscle or ventricular trabeculae is quite different from that of tetanized skeletal muscle, in that the active tension of cardiac muscle decreases much more steeply with reduction of muscle length from the length at which maximum active tension occurs. A good example of the steep dependence of active force on sarcomere length can be found in a study by Ter Keurs et al. {35}. Within the range of sarcomere length from 1.55 to 2.35 μm, the active tension of trabeculae rose continuously with sarcomere length. There was not a plateau, nor a descending limb, and active

tension approached zero at a sarcomere length of about 1.6 μm. At an external Ca concentration 0.5 mM, tension decreased linearly with decreasing sarcomere length; a reduction in sarcomere length from 2.3 μm (at which the maximum active tension occurs) to 2.0 μm resulted in a near-50% drop in active tension; at a sarcomere length 1.7 μm, the tension was reduced to 5%–10% of maximum tension. At higher Ca, the dependence of tension on sarcomere length became nonlinear; nevertheless, it was still quite steep. The steep decline of force with decreasing sarcomere length differs dramatically from the behavior of skeletal muscle fibers undergoing tetanic contractions. The sarcomere-length tension relation for tetanic of skeletal muscle fibers {36} has a plateau of maximum tension development between sarcomere lengths of about 2 and 2.2 μm; in the range of sarcomere length between 2 and 1.7 μm, the tension does not decrease steeply with decreasing sarcomere length; thus at a sarcomere length of 1.7 μm, a skeletal muscle fiber develops about 70–80% maximum tension.

The possibility that a mechanical restoring force underlies the steep ascending limb of cardiac muscle has been considered by Jewell {37}. It is known that when a papillary muscle is actively shortened to a sarcomere length below 1.9 μm, it will, upon removal of stimulations, recoil back to a resting length of about 1.9 μm. The observation suggests the presence of restoring forces at sarcomere lengths below 1.9 μm. As pointed out by Jewel {37}, since the restoring force is absent above 1.9 μm, the sharp decline of tension with a decrease of sarcomere length from 2.3 to 1.9 μm cannot be accounted for by the restoring forces. Jewell {37} analyzed the length-force relations of papillary muscle at various external Ca^{2+} concentrations and found a Ca-sensitive elastic restoring force is required to account for the data if one assumes that the steep drop of force at short sarcomere lengths was solely due to length-dependent restoring forces. Since a Ca-sensitive internal load is not likely, the analysis suggests that restoring force alone cannot account for the shape of the length-force relation of cardiac muscle. However, a partial contribution of restoring force cannot be excluded.

Jewell {37} proposed that a decrease in activation of the contractile system with decreasing sarcomere length is the most likely explanation for the steep length-force relation of cardiac muscle in the range of sarcomere length between 2.2 and 1.9 μm. The hypothesis has been strongly supported by experimental evidence. For example, when the degree of activation of the muscle is varied by raising extracellular Ca^{2+} {34,35}, increasing stimulus frequency {37}, and paired pulse stimulation {37}, the shape of the length-tension relation of cardiac muscle changes in a manner suggesting that inotropic interventions are more effective in potentiating force production at short sarcomere lengths than at long ones. The observations are interpreted as suggesting the activation of the contractile system is less complete at short sarcomere lengths. Further support for the hypothesis has come from experiments demonstrating that the Ca^{2+} sensitivity of contractile machinery decreases with sarcomere length, as detailed below.

Research to date has established that the length dependence of activation of mammalian striated muscle is, at least partly, due to variation of Ca sensitivity of the myofilament with sarcomere length. In addition, there is less conclusive evidence suggesting the sarcomere length may also affect other steps of the excitation-contraction coupling. Only the evidence bearing on the dependence of Ca sensitivity of the contractile system is considered here. Summaries of the data relevant to possible effects of muscle length on processes in sarcolemma and sarcoplasmic reticulum can be found in a review by Allen and Kentish {38}. Use of skinned muscle preparations has made possible the direct investigation of the effect of sarcomere length on the sensitivity of the contractile machinery to Ca^{2+}.

Endo {39} reported the first evidence that Ca sensitivity of myofilaments is dependent on sarcomere length. An increase in Ca sensitivity of the contractile machinery with increasing sarcomere length has since been demonstrated for virtually all skinned fiber preparations of vertebrate skeletal and cardiac muscles studied {38}. However, for a comparable change in sarcomere length, the effect is much more pronounced in mammalian slow-twitch and cardiac muscle than in fast-twitch mammalian or amphibian muscles. Most recent reports {38} found that in skinned fast-twitch or cardiac-muscle fibers, variation of sarcomere length resulted in a parallel shift of the pCa-force relation without marked effects on the steepness of the relation, in contrast to early observations by Endo {39} that the effect was only detected at Ca^{2+} concentrations at which the active force was low.

The most straightforward hypothesis proposed to explain the dependence of Ca sensitivity on muscle length is that the affinity of TnC for Ca^{2+} increases with sarcomere length {38}. Several reports have provided data that can be accounted for by a length dependence of Ca binding to TnC. There is evidence from direct Ca^{2+}-binding determinations for an increase in myofilament-bound Ca^{2+} with increases in sarcomere length in heart muscle {40}. Moreover, at relatively long sarcomere lengths, the declining phase of the Ca transient of papillary muscle is faster than at shorter lengths, while the duration of the contraction is prolonged {42}. These data are most easily explained by an increase in the affinity of TnC and are not likely to be a result of enhanced Ca uptake by SR, which would cause an abbreviated duration of contraction. A reduction in Ca binding to TnC at short sarcomere lengths was also inferred from the observation that over the ascending limb of the cardiac muscle length-tension relation, shortening caused an immediate increase in the amplitude of the Ca transient {24}. The data were compatible with a reduction in Ca binding to TnC at shorter lengths. However, the results can also be explained by rapid changes in Ca release or Ca entry as a function of muscle length. In addition, step releases of cardiac muscle in its ascending limb and barnacle muscle near slack length during the later stage of a twitch produces a bump on the Ca transient. The bump has been attributed to a release of Ca from the myofilaments as a consequence of reduced Ca affinity during or after the release of the muscle {41}.

Several mechanisms by which length changes could affect the Ca-binding constant of TnC have been postulated. Based on assumption that crossbridges in active muscle increase the affinity of TnC for Ca as rigor linkages do in the suspension of myofibrils, Allen and Kurihara {41} proposed that the Ca affinity of TnC depends on the number of crossbridges attached and therefore will vary with the magnitude of tension production. Such a mechanism cannot explain the increase in the sensitivity of the contractile system to Ca^{2+} when the muscle is stretched beyond optimum overlap {33}. Sarcomere length per se may determine the Ca sensitivity of the contractile machinery. It is also possible that changes in filament spacing and/or accompanying changes in crossbridge kinetics may be responsible for the length dependence of the Ca sensitivity of myofilaments. Whatever the mechanism, it is interesting that the special features of cardiac myofilaments with respect to length-dependent activation may not be associated with TnC itself but other proteins. Complete substitution of cTnC for fsTnc did not alter the length dependence of activation in skinned fiber preparations {31,43}, indicating that the variant of TnC present in the myofilaments is not important. It has been hypothesized that the difference between fast and cardiac myofilaments in the effect of crossbridges on TnC Ca^{2+} binding may be due to the slower cycle time (longer duty cycle) of the actin–crossbridge reaction in cardiac myofilaments {31,44}. In any case, a detailed molecular mechanism as to how changes in muscle length could directly affect the Ca affinity of TnC awaits further investigation.

Modulation by protein phosphoryation

It is now clear that many of the myofilament proteins are substrates for kinases and phosphatases that covalently attach and remove phosphate largely from serine and threonine residues in the various proteins (see Solaro {45} for review). In the thin filament, these proteins include TnI, TnT, and Tm. In thick filaments, the phosphorylatable proteins are C protein, a myosin-associated protein attached at intervals along the thick filament (fig. 18-1), and LCII or the P-light chain (PLC). In vitro, TnI and C-protein are substrates for PKA (cAMP-dependent protein kinase); PLC, C-protein for Ca-calmodulin dependent kinase; and C-protein, PLC, TnI, and TnT for protein kinase C (PKC). There are also more or less specific kinases (TnT-kinase and Tm-kinase) for TnT and Tm. Which of these proteins is phosphorylated in intact preparations subjected to various inotropic mechanisms has been studied by perfusion of hearts or superfusion of myocytes with ^{32}P-ortho-phosphate added to physiological buffers such as Krebs Henseleit {46,47}.

There is good agreement among various investigators that interventions, such as perfusion with isoproterenol, that activate PKA, phosphorylate only TnI and C protein. The phosphorylation site is unique to the cardiac variant of TnI {46}, and this provides evidence that the phosphorylation may be of functional significance in heart function per se. In vitro phosphorylation of TnI reduces the affinity of TnC for Ca^{2+} by enhancing the "off-rate" for Ca binding to the single regulatory site on cardiac TnC {8}. As expected from this observation, pCa-force and pCa-ATPase activity relations of the myofilaments shift to the right following phosphorylation of TnI {45}. In situ, there is also clear evidence that beta-adrenergic stimulation of heart preparations is associated with a desensitization of the myofilaments to Ca^{2+}.

Although it has been proposed that this reduced Ca sensitivity of the myofilaments in hearts beating under the influence of beta-adrenergic stimulation may be a negative feedback mechanism or may play a role in the enhanced relaxation rate {45–47}, how these mechanical changes are associated with TnI or C-protein phosphorylation remains uncertain. The uncertainly comes from evidence showing that phosphorylation of TnI and C-protein does not correlate well with the inotropic state, especially following the decay of activity with pulse perfusion with isoproterenol {45–47}. This may be related to the existence of multiple sites of phosphorylation on these proteins. For example, in the case of TnI there are serial serines in the unique amino-terminal extension of the cardiac variant {48}. Which of these sites is actually phosphorylated in situ and which is functionally significant has yet to be determined. As discussed below, there are also multiple sites of phosphorylation on C-protein and TnI involving other kinases that may be activated during adrenergic stimulation of the heart.

Apart from the effect of beta-adrenergic stimulation of the heart on the response of the myofilaments to Ca^{2+}, there is evidence that there is also an associated crossbridge kinetics. Yet there are conflicting data regarding whether catecholamines increase crossbridge kinetics, and the idea that myosin might be directly affected by beta-adrenergic related signals is controversial and not yet accepted. Earlier results indicating that adrenergic agonists might affect crossbridge kinetics have not been confirmed, and most recent evidence indicates that catecholamines do not affect crossbridge cycling, as determined from measurements of unloaded shortening velocity.

Winegrad and Weisberg {49} and colleagues reported evidence using EGTA-extracted heart muscle preparations that beta-adrenergic stimulation is associated with an increase in the maximum force-generating capability depending on the myosin isoform population. Preparations predominant in the fast ATPase isoform of myosin heavy chain (V1) showed the effect, whereas those with the slow ATPase isoform (V3) did not. This intriguing and potentially significant result has not been confirmed in skinned fiber preparations {50,51}. Moreover, investigation of the effects of catecholamines in intact hearts containing either mostly V1 and mostly V3 myosin have also not confirmed this result {52}. One explanation for the differences in results is that the specific conditions (phosphodiesterase inhibition; detergent treatment and EGTA skinning) required to show these effects may not be relevant to the intact situation.

The measurements may also depend on the particular experimental situation. Various measurements of crossbridge kinetics may not all reflect the same rate-limiting step in the cycle and may also depend on the state of thin and thick filament activation reflecting relative phosphorylation of various sites at the time the measurement was made. In any case, whether or not catecholamines affect the crossbridge cycling rate and unloaded shortening velocity is important to our understanding of the regulation of contractions of the heart. The lack of an effect of catecholamine stimulation on unloaded shortening velocity in the heart has several important implications. First, it is certain that at least some sites on C-protein and TnI were phosphorylated in these preparations. This then would indicate that phosphorylation of these sites does not affect crossbridge kinetics. The result also indicates that the increased rate of force generation present when heart preparations are stimulated with beta-adrenergic agonists is due to a separate mechanism, most likely the availability of Ca^{2+}, and not regulation of the reaction of crossbridges with actin.

Protein kinase C and TnT and TnI

An important and unresolved question is the relation between phosphorylation at PKC-dependent sites on the myofilaments and their activity and regulation. Both TnI and TnT become phosphorylated in situ {53,54} with activation of the PKC cascade by alpha-adrenergic stimulation {54}. In the case of TnI, one site is at Ser-43 in the N-terminus in cTnI that binds to TnC and TnT; the other is located at Thr-143, a unique residue in the inhibitory region of cTnI {55}. The position at Thr-143 corresponds to a proline in the slow skeletal TnI and fast skeletal TnI sequence. The location of this substitution lends support to the hypothesis that this may be a functionally significant difference between cTnI and skeletal TnI. In the case of TnT, there is evidence that phosphorylation of the PKC sites, which are all located in the C-terminal portion of the molecule, inhibit binding of TnT to Tm {53}. Thus, phosphorylation of TnI and TnT may alter myofilament activation by different routes — one involving the level of activation of the thin filament by altered interactions of the TnI-inhibitory region with TnC and actin and TnI with TnT; and the other by altering thin filament activation by altered activity of TnT.

In view of all of these complexities, it may not be surprising that studies on the effects of PKC-dependent phosphorylations of myofilaments have led to conflicting results. Noland and Kuo {53} reported that phosphorylation of Thr-143 was associated with a decrease in actomyosin Mg ATPase activity in reconstituted preparations with no change in pCa_{50} for activation. In contrast, there are reports {56} that PKC-dependent phosphorylation of TnI in single cells is associated with a change in the Hill n of the pCa-force relation with no effect on force or the pCa_{50}. These results suggest that the effect of PKC is most prominent when LC2 has been first phosphorylated by MLCK. Yet treatment of isolated heart preparations with phorbol esters results in a negative inotropic effect {57} and agonists thought to work through PKC-dependent mechanisms show negative inotropic effects. Moreover, results of work reported by Endoh and Blinks {59} indicate that alpha-adrenergic stimulation is associated with an increase in the responsiveness of the myofilaments to Ca^{2+}.

Work from Noland and Kuo {57} and Venema and Kuo {54} indicates that PKC-dependent phosphorylation of TnT inhibits its binding to Tm and thus results in inhibition of acto-S1 and myofibrillar ATPase activity. An important aspect of all of these results with phosphorylation by the PKC-dependent pathways is the notion that thin filament activation may be regulated by phosphorylation in a way that may regulate the level of thin filament activation. A reasonable hypothesis for this regulation is that the phosphorylation of the regulatory proteins such as TnI and TnT provides a mechanism for grading the energies of interaction among functional units of the thin filament and thus the level of thin filament activation at a particular fractional occupancy with strong crossbridges.

C-protein phosphorylation and activation of cardiac myofilaments

C-protein is a thick filament associated protein present in the myofilaments of cardiac muscle {60}. It is arranged in seven to eight transverse stripes 10 nm wide at 43-nm intervals along the thick filament in two 300-nm zones on either side of the M-line; the zones are separated by 400 nm. As shown in fig. 18-1, C protein binds to the subfragment-2 region of the myosin molecule and to light meromyosin (LMM). The stoichiometry of C protein in the thick filament indicates that three C-protein molecules wrap around the thick filament. There is also evidence that C protein can bind to actin. The rod-shaped molecule is also apparently able to span the gap between thick and thin filaments. Evidence from in vitro reconstitution experiments indicated that C protein affects the ATPase rate of myosin, yet these experiments are difficult to put in a physiological context due to the dependence of the results on the ratio of C protein to myosin and to the conditions of pH and ionic strength {60}.

More recently, though, clearer evidence has been presented on the role of C-protein in the regulation of striated muscle contraction. Hoffman et al. {61} measured the force-pCa relation before and after partial extraction of C protein from ventricular myocytes and after reconstitution with exogenous C protein. Maximum tension was about the same in all these preparations; however, the active tension at submaximally activating levels of free Ca^{2+} was increased in the preparations missing 60–70% of their C protein. This effect of C protein was similar in preparations in which there was partial extraction of TNC, indicating that the C-protein removal did not alter cooperative nearest neighbor interactions among functional units in the thin filament. Hoffman et al. {61} proposed from the results of these experiments that at least one effect of C protein is to modify the range of movement of crossbridges in such a way that its removal from the thick filament increases the probability of binding of the myosin head with actin at submaximally activating free Ca^{2+}. At maximally activating levels of free Ca^{2+}, this effect of C

protein is of less significance, presumably because the probability of myosin crossbridge reaction with actin is relatively high.

Cardiac muscle C protein is phosphorylated in vitro by protein kinase A and in vivo by adrenergic stimulation of the heart. In vitro, C protein is also a substrate for Ca/calmodulin-dependent protein kinase II (CaM-kinase II), as well as phosphorylase kinase and protein kinase C {45,62}. A new aspect of our understanding of the potential role of C-protein phosphorylation in the regulation of cardiac contractility is identification of peptides on the protein that are substrates for the various kinases {62}. Moreover, recent evidence indicates that a kinase known to copurify with C protein is most likely CaM-kinase II. The phosphorylation of C-protein peptides in the experiments of Schlender and Bean {62} show that phosphorylation by protein kinase A and CaM-kinase II at one domain are not additive and involve the same site. In addition to the common sites of phosphorylation, they show evidence for unique CaM-kinase II sites. The presence of phosphatase activity in partially purified preparations of C protein indicates that the phosphorylation/dephosphorylation of these sites may be rapid.

The functional significance of C-protein phosphorylation as a modulator of the activity or Ca^{2+} sensitivity of the myofilaments is not clear. C-protein phosphorylation does not appear to affect the pCa_{50} for activation of myofibrillar MgATPase activity {27}. However, there is evidence that the phosphorylation state of C protein can stimulate or inhibit myosin ATPase activity depending on the ratio of C protein to myosin in the reaction mixture {60}. The successful extraction and reconstitution of C protein in skinned fiber preparations indicates that it should not be too long before we know more precisely the role of C-protein phosphorylation in terms of the mechanical activity of the myofilaments. It will be of interest to do site-directed phosphorylation of C protein and reconstitution in such preparations.

Role of P light chain phosphorylation

Considerable efforts have been made to explore the possible roles of light chain II phosphorylation in the regulation of actomyosin ATPase of striated muscles. Early studies in Perry's (see Solaro {45} for review) laboratory found little or no effect of phosphorylation of myosin on myosin ATPase or actomyosin ATPase. On the other hand, Cooke et al. {63} have reported that thiophosphorylation of LC-2 in skinned psoas fibers held at constant length, and in myofibrils crosslinked with glutaraldehyde to prevent shortening, decreased the ATPase activity by a factor of two. They suggest that the expression of such inhibitory effect requires an intact filament structure. In agreement with this finding, Crow and Kushmerick {64} reported that in intact fast skeletal muscle, there is good correlation between the increased phosphorylation of PLC and a decrease in the rate of high-energy phosphate usage and a parallel decrease in the maximum velocity of shortening. It was suggested that

PLC phosphorylation may be capable of downmodulation of the rate of crossbridge turnover in tetanized muscle.

However, Barsotti et al. {65} demonstrated convincingly that in tetanized fast skeletal muscles there is no consistent relationship between the degree of PLC phosphorylation and the rate of chemical energy usage, a finding arguing against a role of phosphorylation of PLC as a modulator of the rate of crossbridge cycling. Moreover, a more recent study employing permeabilized skeletal muscles has indicated quite clearly that in the presence of an ATP-regenerating system, creatine phosphate, and creatine kinase, phosphorylation of PLC has no effect on the maximum shortening velocity and force-velocity curves at maximally activating Ca^{2+}. According to the hypothesis that the maximum velocity of shortening is proportional to the intrinsic rate of actin-activated ATPase activity of myosin, the data can thus be interpreted as indicating a lack of effect of phosphorylation of PLC on crossbridge cycling. One effect of phosphorylation of PLC that appears to be well supported has been demonstrated in permeabilized skeletal and cardiac muscle fibers. These studies show that increases in PLC phosphorylation correlate with an increase in the force level at submaximum Ca and an associated leftward shift of the initial portion of the P_{Ca}-force relation {64}. Although long-term changes in heart rate are known to alter the level of PLC phosphorylation in the heart, the implication of this phenomenon is not yet clear {67}.

SUMMARY AND CONCLUSIONS

The regulation of cardiac myofilament chemomechanical transduction is, in general, similar to that of other striated muscles, but there are clear differences that appear to be related to the specialized functional activity and physiological properties of the heart. Recruitment of crossbridges appears to occur by means of alterations in the amounts of Ca^{2+} delivered to the myofilaments. This does not appear to be the case in skeletal striated muscle. In addition, the modulation of Ca binding appears to be more prominent in heart versus other striated muscle. The length dependence of activation, the apparent basis of Starling's Law of the Heart, is most prominent in heart. Moreover, modulation of Ca activation by protein phosphorylation also appears to be a unique feature of regulation of cardiac myofilaments. Thus, intrinsic and extrinsic regulation of cardiac muscle appears to involve alterations in the response of the myofilaments to Ca^{2+}. This mechanism appears to be an important part of the overall regulation of cardiac activity, which clearly also involves alterations in Ca^{2+} delivery to the myofilaments by mechanisms involving membrane pumps and channels.

REFERENCES

1. Woledge RC, Curtin NA, Holmsher E: Energetic Aspects of Muscle Contraction. Monographs of the Physiological Society No 41. New York: Academic Press, 1985, pp 39–46.
2. Lymn RW, Taylor EW: Mechanism of adenosine triphosphate hydrolysis by actomyosin. *Biochemistry* 10:4617–4624, 1971.
3. Millar NC, Homsher E: The effect of phosphate and calcium on force generation in glycerinated rabbit skeletal muscle fibers. *J Biol Chem* 265:20234–20240, 1990.
4. Walker JW, Lu Z, Moss RL: Effects of Ca^{2+} on the kinetics of phosphate release in skeletal muscle. *J Biol Chem* 267:2459–2456, 1992.
5. Pan BS, Solaro RJ: Calcium-binding properties of troponin C in detergent-skinned heart muscle fibers. *J Biol Chem* 262:7839–7849, 1987.
6. Solaro RJ, Pang DC, Briggs N: The purification of cardiac myofibrils with Triton X-100. *Biochim Biophys Acta* 245:259–262, 1971.
7. Pan BS, Palmiter KA, Plonczynski M, Solaro RJ: Slowly exchanging calcium binding sites unique to cardiac/slow muscle troponin C. *J Mol Cell Cardiol* 22:1117–1124, 1990.
8. Robertson SP, Johnson JD, Holroyde MJ, Kranias EG, Potter JD, Solaro RJ: The effect of troponin I phosphorylation on the Ca^{2+}-regulatory site of bovine cardiac troponin. *J Biol Chem* 257:260–263, 1982.
9. Zot HG, Potter JD: A structural role for the Ca^{2+}-Mg^{2+} sites on troponin C in the regulation of muscle contraction. *J Biol Chem* 257:7678–7683, 1982.
10. Leavis PC, Gergely J: Thin filament proteins and thin-filament-linked regulation of vertebrate muscle contraction. *CRC Crit Rev Biochem* 16:233–305, 1984.
11. Huxley HE: Structural changes in the actin- and myosin-containing filaments during contraction. *Cold Spring Harbor Symp Quant Biol* 37:361–376, 1972.
12. Zot AS, Potter JD: Structural aspects of troponin-tropomyosin regulation of skeletal muscle contraction. *Ann Rev Biophys Chem* 16:535–559, 1987.
13. Chalovich JM, Eisenberg E: Inhibition of actomyosin ATPase activity by troponin-tropomyosin without blocking the binding of myosin to actin. *J Biol Chem* 257:24342–2437, 1982.
14. Morimoto K, Harrington WF: Evidence for structural changes in vertebrate thick filament induced by calcium. *J Mol Biol* 88:693–709, 1974.
15. Kress M, Huxley HE, Faruqi AR, Koch MHJ, Hendrix J: Thin filament x-ray diffraction in contracting frog muscle. In: *The Eighth International Biophysics Congress Abstracts.* Bristol, England, 1984, p 119.
16. Holroyde MJ, Potter JD, Solaro RJ: The calcium binding properties of phosphorylated and unphosphorylated cardiac skeletal myosins. *J Biol Chem* 254:6478–6482, 1979.
17. Bagshaw CR, Reed GH: The significance of the slow dissociation of divalent metal ions from myosin regulatory light chains. *FEBS Lett* 81:386–390, 1977.
18. Potter JD, Gergely J: The calcium and magnesium binding sites on troponin and their role in the regulation of myofibrillar adenosine triphosphatase. *J Biol Chem* 250:4628–4633, 1975.
19. Weber A, Murray JM: Molecular control mechanisms on muscle contraction. *J Biol Chem* 254:6470–6477, 1973.
20. Shiner JS, Solaro RJ: Activation of thin filament-regulated muscle by calcium ion: Considerations based on nearest-neighbor lattice statistics. *Proc Natl Acad Sci USA* 79:4637–4641, 1982.
21. Bremel RD, Weber A: Cooperation within actin filament in vertebrate skeletal muscle. *Nature (New Biol)* 238:97–101, 1972.
22. Godt RE: Calcium-activated tension of skinned muscle fibers of the frog: Dependence on magnesium adenosine triphosphate concentration. *J Gen Physiol* 63:722–739, 1974.
23. Ridgway EB, Gordon AM, Martyn DM: Hysteresis in the

force-calcium relation in muscle. *Science* 219:1075–1077, 1983.

24. Housmans PR, Lee NKM, Blinks JR: Active shortening retards the decline of the intracellular calcium transient in mammalian heart muscle. *Science* 221:159–161, 1983.

25. Wnuk W, Schoechlin M, Stein EA: Regulation of actomyosin ATPase by a single Ca-binding site on troponin C from crayfish. *J Biol Chem* 259:9017–9623, 1984.

26. Fuchs F: The binding of calcium to detergent-extracted rabbit psoas muscle fibers during relaxation and force generation. *J Muscle Res Cell Motil* 6:477–486, 1985.

27. Tawada Y, Tawada T: Co-operative regulation mechanism of muscle contraction: Inter-tropomyosin co-operation model. *J Theor Biol* 50:269–283, 1975.

28. Tawada Y, Ohara H, Ooi T, Tawada K: Nonpolymerizable tropomyosin and control of the superprecipitation of actomyosin. *J Biochem* 78:65–72, 1975.

29. Hill TL, Eisenberg E, Greene LE: Theoretical model for the cooperative equilibrium binding of myosin subfragment 1 to actin-troponin-tropomyosin. *Proc Natl Acad Sci USA* 77:3186–3190, 1983.

30. Pan B-S, Gordon AM, Luo Z: Removal of tropomyosin overlap modifies cooperative binding of myosin S-1 to reconstituted thin filaments of rabbit striated muscle. *J Biol Chem* 264:8495–8598, 1989.

31. Moss RL: Ca^{2+} regulation of mechanical properties of striated muscle: Mechanistic studies using extraction and replacement of regulatory proteins. *Circ Res* 70:865–884, 1992.

32. Brandt PW, Diamond MS, Schachat FH: The thin filament of vertebrate skeletal muscle cooperatively activates as a unit. *J Mol Biol* 180:379–384, 1984.

33. Moss RL, Swinford AE, Greaser ML: Alteration in the Ca^{2+} sensitivity of tension development by single skeletal muscle fibers as stretched lengths. *Biophys J* 43:115–119, 1983.

34. Allen DG, Jewell BR, Murray JW: The contribution of activation processes to the length-tension relation of cardiac muscle. *Nature (Lond)* 248:606–607, 1974.

35. Ter Keurs HEDJ, Rijinsburger WH, van Heuningen R, Nagelsmit MJ: Tension development and sarcomere length in rat cardiac trabeculae. Evidence of length-dependent activation. *Circ Res* 46:703–714, 1980.

36. Gordon AM, Huxley AF, Julian FJ: The variation in isometric tension with sarcomere length in vertebrate muscle fibres. *J Physiol* 184:170–192, 1966.

37. Jewell BR: A re-examination of the influence of muscle length on myocardial performance. *Circ Res* 40:321–330, 1977.

38. Allen DG, Kentish JC: The cellular basis of the length-tension relation in cardiac muscle. *J Mol Cell Cardiol* 17:821–840, 1985.

39. Endo M: Length dependence of activation of skinned muscle fibers by calcium. *Cold Spring Harb Symp Quant Biol* 37:505–510, 1973.

40. Hoffman PA, Fuchs F: Bound calcium and force development in skinned cardiac muscle bundles: Effect of sarcomere length. *J Mol Cell Cardiol* 20:667–677, 1988.

41. Allen DG, Kurihara S: The effects of muscle length on intracellular calcium transients in mammalian cardiac muscle. *J Physiol* 327:79–94, 1982.

42. Allen DG, Smith GL: The first calcium transient following shortening in skinned ferret ventricular muscle. *J Physiol (Lond)* 366:83P, 1985.

43. Moss RL, Nwoye LO, Greaser ML: Substitution of cardiac troponin C into rabbit muscle does not alter the length dependence of Ca^{2+}-sensitivity of tension. *J Physiol (Lond)* 440:273–289, 1991.

44. Hannon JD, Martyn DA, Gordon AM: Effects of cycling and rigor crossbridges on the conformation of cardiac troponin C. *Circ Res* 71:984–991, 1992.

45. Solaro RJ: Protein phosphorylation and the cardiac myofilaments. In: Solario RJ (ed) *Protein Phosphorylation in Heart.* Boca Raton, FL: CRC Press, 1986, pp 129–156.

46. Solaro RJ, Moir AJG, Perry SV: Phosphorylation of TnI and the inotropic effect of adrenaline in the perfused rabbit heart. *Nature (Lond)* 262:615–616, 1976.

47. England PJ: Cardiac function and phosphorylation of contractile proteins. *Phil Trans R Soc Lond* B302:83–90, 1983.

48. Leszyk J, Dumaswala R, Potter JD, Collins JH: Amino acid sequence of bovine cardiac troponin I. *Biochemistry* 27:2821–2827, 1988.

49. Winegrad S, Weisberg A: Isozyme specific modification of myosin ATPase by cAMP in rat heart. *Circ Res* 60:384–392, 1987.

50. Miller DJ, Smith GL: The contractile behaviour of EGTA and detergent-treated muscle. *J Muscle Res Cell Motil* 6:541–567, 1985.

51. Kentish JC, Jewell BR: Some characteristics of Ca^{2+}-regulated force production in EGTA treated muscles from rat heart. *J Gen Physiol* 84:83–99, 1984.

52. de Tombe PP, ter Keurs EDJ: Lack of effect of isoproterenol on unloaded velocity of sarcomere shortening in rat cardiac trabeculae. *Circ Res* 68:382–391, 1991.

53. Noland TA, Kuo JF: Protein kinase C phosphorylation of cardiac troponin T decreases Ca-dependent actomyosin MgATPase and troponin T binding to tropomyosin-F-actin complex. *Biochem J* 288:123–129, 1992.

54. Venema RC, Kuo JF: Protein kinase C-mediated phosphorylation of troponin I and C-protein in isolated myocardial cells is associated with inhibition of myofibrillar actomyosin ATPase. *J Biol Chem* 268:2705–2711, 1993.

55. Noland TA Jr, Raynor RL, Kuo JF: Identification of sites phosphorylated in bovine cardiac troponin I and troponin T by protein kinase C and comparative substrate activity of synthetic peptides containing the phosphorylation sites. *J Biol Chem* 264:20778–20785, 1989.

56. Clement O, Puceat M, Walsh MP, Vassort G: Protein kinase C enhances myosin light-chain kinase effects on force development and ATPase activity in rat single skinned cardiac cells. *Biochem J* 285:311–317, 1992.

57. Noland TA Jr, Kuo JF: Protein kinase C phosphorylation of cardiac troponin I or troponin T inhibits Ca^{2+}-stimulated actomyosin MgATPase activity. *J Biol Chem* 266:4974–4978, 1991.

58. Gwathmey JK, Hajar RJ: Effect of protein kinase C activation on sarcoplasmic reticulum function and apparent myofibrillar Ca^{2+} sensitivity in intact and skinned muscles from normal and diseased human myocardium. *Circ Res* 67:744–652, 1990.

59. Endoh M, Blinks JR: Action of sympathomimetic amines on the Ca^{2+}-transients and contractions of rabbit myocardium: Reciprocal changes in myofibrillar responsiveness to Ca^{2+} mediated through alpha and beta-adrenoceptors. *Circ Res* 62:247–265, 1988.

60. Hartzell HC: Effects of phosphorylated and unphosphorylated C-protein on cardiac actomyosin ATPase. *J Mol Biol* 186:185–195, 1985.

61. Hoffman PA, Hartzell HC, Moss RL: Alterations in Ca^{2+} sensitive tension due to partial extraction of C-protein from rat skinned cardiac myocytes and rabbit skeletal muscle fibers. *J Gen Physiol*, in press, 1991.

62. Schlender KK, Bean LJ: Phosphorylation of chicken cardiac

C-protein by calcium/calmodulin-dependent protein kinase II. *J Biol Chem* 266:2811–2817, 1991.

63. Cooke R, Franks K, Stull JT: Myosin phosphorylation regulates the ATPase activity of permeable skeletal muscle fibers. *FEBS Lett* 144:33–37, 1982.

64. Crow MT, Kushmerick MJ: Myosin light chain phosphorylation is associated with a decrease in the energy cost for contraction in fast twitch mouse muscle. *J Biol Chem* 257:2121–2124, 1982.

65. Barsotti R, Butler T: Chemical energy usage and myosin light chain phosphorylation in mammalian skeletal muscle. *J Muscle Res Cell Motil* 5:45–64, 1984.

66. Persechini A, Stull JT, Cooke R: The effect of myosin phosphorylation on the contractile properties of skinned rabbit skeletal muscle fibers. *J Biol Chem* 260:7951–7954, 1985.

67. Stull JT, Sanford CJ, Manning DR, Blumenthal DK, High CW: Phosphorylation of myofibrillar proteins in striated muscle. *Cold Spring Harb Conf Cell Prolif* 8:823–891, 1981.

CHAPTER 19

Contractile and Mechanical Properties of the Myocardium

ALLAN J. BRADY

INTRODUCTION

One of the principal concerns of cardiac muscle mechanics is the understanding of the relation between the contractile properties of the whole heart and the myofilaments. In its most superficial sense this relation is one of geometry. Dimensionally, a measure of whole-heart performance should be understandable from studies of the mechanical properties of long thin papillary muscles or trabeculae. From such one-dimensional analyses one could surmise that the three-dimensional complexity of the whole heart could be approximated. Indeed, there have been numerous attempts to formulate ventricular performance in terms of constitutive parameters, i.e., in terms of parameters that are independent of external influences but that are based on the mechanical characteristics of papillary muscles. These approaches, however, generally prove inadequate where functional differences in organ contractility are of interest. These deficiencies, in the large part, arise from the geometrical approximations required to describe the thick-walled asymmetrical ventricle and from an inappropriate characterization of the one-dimensional mechanical properties of papillry muscle or trabecular preparations. This chapter will discuss the characterization of the functional relations between force and length that have been used as the basis for the formulation of constitutive relations.

Specifically, force-length relations will be discussed relating sarcomere length and muscle length to force development. Particular emphasis will be given to those parameters that add to the complexity of force development, such as nonuniform sarcomere length, length-dependent activation, restoring forces, and shortening deactivation. Also, the status of the force-velocity relation in heart muscle will be discussed as it relates to earlier concepts of its use as an index of contractility. Finally, stepwise and cyclic perturbation analysis will be mentioned, as this approach promises insight into muscle contractile properties of crossbridge kinetics and their relation to known biochemical steps of the cardiac contractile process.

FORCE DEVELOPMENT

The sliding filament mechanism of contraction originally proposed in 1954 by Huxley and Hansen {58} and by Huxley and Niedergerke {57}, and elaborated in 1971 by Huxley and Simmons {59}, has gained wide acceptance for striated muscle. Indeed, while some of the kinetics of myofilament interaction of skeletal and cardiac muscle are obviously different, the myofilament structures are similar, calcium is an essential element in the initiation of contraction, and many of the contractile properties of force generation and of shortening are related. Based on these common factors it is prudent to look for similarities in myofilament interaction processes in these two systems.

Briefly, as summarized in various accounts in Ingels {60}, the sliding filament crossbridge attachment concept of force development is the following: Calcium released from the sarcoplasmic reticulum (SR) by sarcolemmal excitation binds to troponin-C on the tropomyosin (summarized in Murray and Weber {84}). Tropomyosin then translates deeper into the thin filament groove, exposing binding sites on the actin to which a bead (or heads) of the myosin thick filament cross-bridge (CB) can attach (fig. 19-1). This attachment is manifested as an increase in muscle stiffness (resistance to stretch), although not necessarily as an increase in active force development (see Julian {65} for a resume of the steps of the CB mechanical cycle). Presumably, force development occurs following CB attachment as the head undergoes a rotation about a flexible "joint" between the S-1 and S-2 segments of the CB (fig. 19-1). During the process of this rotation two events are hypothesized to occur as force is developed and longitudinal translation begins to occur: (a) A spatial sequence of interactions of a CB head with actin sites occurs {60}, and (b) the rotation results in an elongation of the S-2 segment of the CB. [For the present, a highly extensible S-2 segment (composed of a coiled-coil, alpha-helix element) should be considered more hypothetical than real, as discussed by Julian {65}.] In this manner, the CB head rotation and consequent S-2 elongation are presumed to create a translational force between the two sets of filaments.

For the sake of analytical simplicity in some considerations {71} (and as also depicted in fig. 19-1), this

N. Sperelakis (ed.), Physiology and Pathophysiology of the Heart, Third Edition.
© 1995 Kluwer Academic Publishers. ISBN 0-7923-2612-1. All rights reserved.

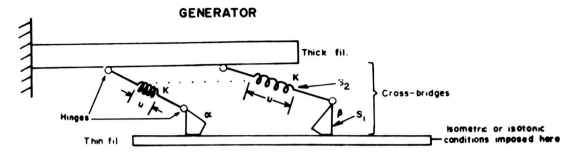

Fig. 19-1. Sketch of crossbridge (CB) attachment mechanism showing two attached states: **(a)** before head rotation and **(b)** after head rotation. SI and S2 denote CB head and extensible connecting element, respectively. K is the elastic constant of S2 and u is the extension of S2 from its zero force position. From Julian {65}, with permission.

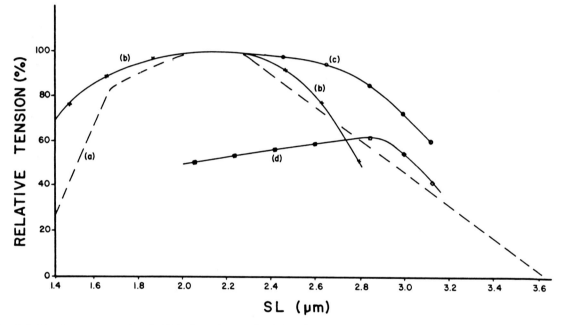

Fig. 19-2. Tension-sarcomere length (SL) plots of normalized data from various muscle preparations. Dashed curve **(a)**: Skeletal muscle {43}. Curve **(b)**: Tonically activated mechanically skinned rat ventricular fiber. Data at short SL from Fabiato and Fabiato {34}; data at long SL from Fabiato and Fabiato {36}. Curve **(c)**: Similar data for dog mechanically skinned ventricular fiber. Curve **(d)**: Partially activated mechanically skinned rat ventricular fiber. Tensions are relative to peak active tension (P_o) in the respective muscle preparations.

rotational event is assumed to be a two-step process for each CB, i.e., attachment and rotation; however, from energetic considerations {53,54} the rotation needs to be continuous, perhaps with many steps, but is limited, nevertheless, to a specific maximum rotational angle.

These concepts of CB attachment and rotation lead to the prediction that total active force and stiffness in a muscle should be directly proportional to the number of attached CBs. It must be kept in mind, however, that an attached CB may not be in a force-developing mode (i.e., the CB head may not have rotated to a force-developing position but, if attached to actin, would still contribute to a resistance to stretch or compression. In any case, the current most widely accepted operating hypothesis of muscle force development relates active force development directly to the number of attached crossbridges.

FORCE-LENGTH RELATIONS

Intermediate and long sarcomere lengths

At the next level of structural organization, i.e., the sarcomere, force development should be directly related to sarcomere length if force development is assumed to be directly related to the number of attached crossbridges.

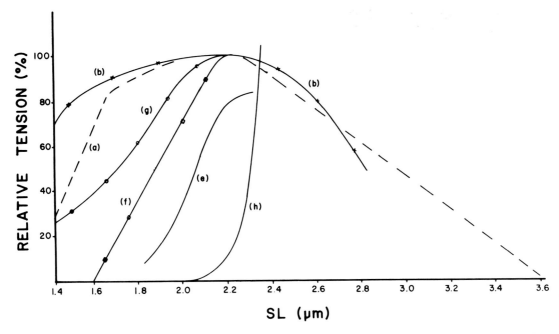

Fig. 19-3. Tension-SL plots of normalized data from various muscle preparations. Dashed curve **(a)**: Skeletal muscle {43}. Curve **(b)**: Mechanically skinned rat ventricular fiber, as in fig. 19-2. Curve **(e)**: Data from thin intact papillary muscle with SL measured at peak of isometric muscle contraction {99}. Curve **(f)**: Same reference as (e) but SL maintained constant by controlled stretch during contraction. Curve **(g)**: Phasic contractions of mechanically skinned rat ventricular fiber induced by Ca^{2+}-induced Ca^{2+} release {34}. Tensions are relative to peak active tension (P_o) in respective muscle preparations.

More specifically, force development should be related to the volume of overlap or interfilament surface between the sets of thick and thin filaments. In fully activated fibers this expectation appears to be realized [fig. 19-2, dashed curve (a)] in skeletal muscle {43,70} over the range of sarcomere lengths (SL) 2.2–3.6 µm, and in cardiac muscle as well {36}, to the extent that long sarcomere lengths can be obtained without undue constraints from other structural elements [fig. 19-2, curves (b) and (c)]. Measurement of active force in intact cardiac fibers is severely limited by the rapid rise in rest tension above SL = 2.2 µm [fig. 19-3, curve (h)], and no plateau in total tension appears. The plateau of active tension, however, can be very broad in tonically activated skinned cardiac fibers [fig. 19-2, curve (b)].

A simple relation between myofilament overlap and force development is challenged by some investigators {61}, who, using laser diffraction to measure SL, found a positive slope for the length-tension relation of conditioned skinned rabbit soleus fibers at all sarcomere lengths up to 3.0 µm [similar to curve (d)]. In contrast, Julian and Moss {67}, noting sarcomere uniformity by direct photomicrography of skinned frog anterior tibial fibers, found a linear decline in force from SL = 2.2 to 3.6 µm, similar to previous studies in intact frog semitendinosus [curve (a)] {43}.

Deviations from a simple relation between overlap and tension in this range of SL are apparent in partially

activated cardiac muscle [fig. 19-2, curve (d)] {67,131}, in papillary muscle during controlled stretch {69}, and in skeletal muscle {19,31,61,101}. In these responses active force development continues to increase with extension of SL up to 3.0 µm (2.3 µm in Julian et al. {69}) before beginning to decline. This observation that peak active force development in partially activated fibers occurs at less than optimum overlap challenges the simplicity of the overlap model and comples us to be concerned about other parameters of CB attachment or force development. Fabiato and Fabiato {36} discuss the possibility that myofilament sensitivity to Ca may be increased at longer sarcomere lengths. Some indication of this possibility is found in recent observations in intact skeletal muscle {78} that maximum Ca^{2+} activation in skeletal muscle does indeed occur on the descending limb of the force-length relation.

In fully activated muscle, including heart muscle [fig. 19-2, curves (b) and (c)], a plateau of active force development occurs over the range of sarcomere lengths of 1.8–2.2 µm (or −2.4 µm in mechanically skinned skeletal and cardiac fibers {36,67}). In fact, the force-SL relation in mechanically skinned muscle appears to lie above that of intact fibers at SL >2.2 µm (fig. 19-2).

Maximum tension (stress) is about 120 kN/m^2 (1.2 kg/cm^2) for papillary muscle {99} compared to 300–400 kN/m^2 in single skeletal muscle fibers {43}. However, if allowance is made for the lower fractional cross-sectional area of myofilaments in heart muscle {87}, the maximal force-generating capabilities of the two types of muscle myofilaments are similar.

Force-length relations at short sarcomere length (Frank–Starling Relation)

A remarkable variation in the force-length relations occurs in heart muscle below $SL = 2.2\,\mu m$ (fig. 19-3), depending on the mode of activation and the amount of shortening that occurs during contraction. Comparison of curve (e) (force plotted versus initial muscle length in an intact papillary muscle) with (f) (the same muscle force developed at constant controlled SL) shows the reduction in force development that can occur in a so-called isometric contraction [curve (e)] {99}. Curve (g) is a plot of the same parameters in a mechanically skinned rat ventricular fiber activated by phasic Ca^{2+}-induced Ca^{2+} release, and curve (b) shows the response of a similar preparation with tonic Ca^{2+} activation. Curve (a), as in fig. 19-2, gives the force-length relation of a tetanized single skeletal muscle fiber preparation. Comparison of the curves for rat cardiac muscle emphasizes the fact that the full contractile potential of a fiber at a shortened length far excels the performance seen in an isometric muscle contraction [curve (e)].

At least four factors are presumed to be responsible for this disparity of force-length relations at sarcomere lengths below $2.0\,\mu m$: (a) a mechanical interference of the ends of the thin filaments from adjacent halves of the sarcomere as they meet and overlap in the mid-A-band region {43}, (b) the possible limitation of force development by external and internal elastic structures that are distorted by muscle shortening, (c) shortening deactivation in which active shortening per se tends to reduce the ability of muscle to develop tension {28}, and (d) length-dependent activation in which Ca^{2+}-induced Ca^{2+} release is reduced at short sarcomere lengths {35} or the activation of thin filament sites by Ca^{2+} is limited at short sarcomere lengths {124}.

All four factors would be expected to significantly influence the shape of the ascending limb of the Frank–Starling force-length relation. Allen and Kentish {1} have discussed these factors at some length in their review of the cardiac length-tension relation. Their arguments, along with others, will be summarized in the next four sections.

FILAMENT INTERFERENCE

A distinct change occurs in the slope of the ascending limb of the tension-length relation in skeletal muscle at a sarcomere length at which the thin filaments would begin to overlap ($SL = 2.0\,\mu m$). In the range of sarcomere lengths of $2.0{-}1.6\,\mu m$, the decline in force development has been attributed to either a physical interaction (resistance) of the overlapping thin filaments or to an interference of crossbridge attachment in the overlapping regions {43}. The thin filaments of cardiac muscle are reported to be slightly longer than in skeletal muscle {102} so that, on the basis of thin filament interference, the beginning of the decline might be expected to occur at a

somewhat longer sarcomere length in cardiac muscle. While a sharp angle in the ascending limb of the tension-length relation of heart muscle is not evident, the plateau of the tension-length relation is less broad than in skeletal muscle and suggests that, as in skeletal muscle, thin-filament overlap may contribute to the decline in tension at a somewhat longer sarcomere length.

However, the broader plateau obtainable in tonic contractions of skinned cardiac cells (fig. 19-3B) indicates that cardiac cells are capable of substantial force generation at sarcomere lengths at which considerable thin filament overlap would be expected to occur. Hence, additional factors must be involved to account for the steep decline of the cardiac tension-length relation.

RESTORING FORCES (EXTRACELLULAR)

Actively shortened muscle fibers (even single mechanically skinned fibers) will not remain at short sarcomere lengths ($>1.85{-}1.90\,\mu m$) during relaxation. Hence some restoring force must exist in the structural network of the muscle or within the cells themselves. In this regard it might be expected that as the muscle fibers increase in diameter with active shortening at constant volume, the extracellular structures would offer some elastic resistance and this constraint would limit the amount of force that the fibers could develop in the longitudinal direction. Additionally, compression of the extracellular collagen in the longitudinal direction with fiber shortening might also tend to reduce active force development external to the cells. In fact, Robinson and Winegrad {103} described a network of microfibrils and microthreads, as well as collagen fibrils, that link cells of the rat myocardium together. They suggested that this network might influence fiber motion.

It is apparent, though, that if contraction against restoring forces were solely responsible for the decline in tension at short sarcomere lengths, the difference between peak tension at L_{max} and isometric tension at shorter SL should be a measure of the restoring force (assuming that the same number of CBs attach between $SL = 1.6\,\mu m$ and $2.2\,\mu m$). Since the restoring force, then, should be strictly length dependent, the same restoring force-length correction should apply at all sarcomere lengths along the ascending limb of the Frank–Starling curve. Jewell {62} and Bodem et al. {6} tested this hypothesis (fig. 19-4) by noting, in varied external Ca^{2+}, the difference between peak tension at L_{max} and peak tension along the ascending limb. They found that the difference factor (i.e., the restoring force component) must also be Ca^{2+} dependent.

With respect to shortening capabilities in rat papillary muscle and frog atrial cells, a comparison of the minimum sarcomere length to which unloaded multicellular and isolated single cell preparations can shorten indicates little difference in their minimal sarcomere lengths. For example, rat papillary muscle {44,47,99,124} and mechanically skinned single rat ventricular fibers {35} will contract to a minimum sarcomere length of about $1.6\,\mu m$ in unloaded shortening. In intact frog atrial trabeculae, Winegrad {130} reported a minimum sarcomere length of $1.5{-}1.6\,\mu m$ in freely shortening preparations, while Tarr

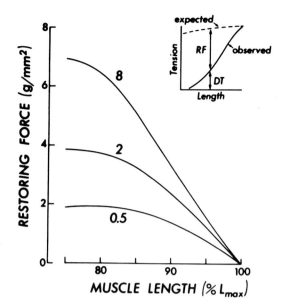

Fig. 19-4. Plot of restoring force (RF, see **inset**) necessary to account for the decline in developed tension (DT) at short lengths. Curves show the Ca^{2+} dependence of this restoring force factor. Numbers on curves give $[Ca^{2+}]$ in millimoles. From Jewell {62} and by permission of the American Heart Association.

et al. {119} showed shortening to about 1.45 μm in very lightly loaded single atrial fibers. Contrasting the single-fiber and multifiber preparations, these observations would suggest that the limitation to shortening probably lies within the cells rather than in external constraints to diameter change or longitudinal resistance to shortening. Similar conclusions were reached by Parsons and Porter {90}. They observed, in cultured chick heart cells, some kinked fibrils at rest that straightened during contraction, indicating that an internal restoring force exists that re-established the kinked state during relaxation.

In skeletal muscle, Brown et al. {15} and Gonzales-Serratos {42} observed that the myofibrils of contracted fibers embedded in gelatin became wavy during relaxation but straightened again during activation. Similar responses occurred in skinned cardiac cells {33,35}. Thus restoring forces do appear to exist in contacted muscle, but the major component must lie within the cell at short sarcomere lengths.

These conclusions are not surprising when considering the fact that while the collagen fiber direction appears to be predominantly parallel to the fiber direction, an absence of elastic constraints oriented radially to the muscle fibers {103} indicates that the collagen probably is not rigidly linked in the transverse direction.

RESTORING FORCES (INTRACELLULAR)

One consideration for a restoring force in intact heart muscle is a compression of the sarcolemma, the SR, or mitochondria during muscle shortening. This seems unlikely, however, in view of the observation that relaxation to initial rest length still occurs in skinned preparations after Brij 58 treatment to remove all membrane structures {35}.

Fabiato and Fabiato {35} reported that relaxation in highly activated (pCa = 6) mechanically skinned rat ventricular fibers occurred in two phases, i.e., a fast component of relaxation from SL = 1.10 μm to 1.57 μm occurring in about 0.6 second and a slow component of further relaxation to 1.91 μm occurring in about 43 seconds. Since there were no external forces on these fibers, the restoring forces must all lie within the skinned fiber. Fabiato and Fabiato {124} attempted to measure this restoring force by letting a contracted cell relax against the force transducer. The restoring force amounted to only 4% maximum contractile force (P_o).

Krueger et al. {75} considered internal elastic restoring forces as the basis for the spontaneous and rapid relaxation that occurs in intact cardiac myocyte twitches. However, they concluded from these studies that since the velocity of shortening in highly activated fibers was constant over the range SL = 2.0–1.7 μm, no simple or appreciable elastic restoring force could be responsible for the constant shortening velocity.

Ter Keurs et al. {124} studied these shortening responses in more detail by deactivating isotonically contracting rat trabeculae late in the contractile cycle with small-amplitude high-frequency (150-Hz) sinusoidal length perturbations. These responses were compared with similar contractions in which the muscle was linearly unloaded during the perturbation-induced premature deactivated relaxation phase. They found that the force reduction necessary to prevent the premature relaxation only amounted to less than 2% P_o. Similarly, a force of 1% P_o was sufficient to produce a rapid elongation to control length when applied following the early unloading of an isotonic contraction. From these observations they conclude that the restorng force producing of maximum contractile force and thus could not explain the reduction of active force development at short sarcomere lengths.

Collectively, these data indicate that the restoring force in these preparations seems insufficient to account for the major portion of the slope of the ascending limb of the Frank–Starling relation.

SHORTENING DEACTIVATION

One of the proposed factors that may influence the shape of the length-tension relation is the observation that shortening tends to reduce the ability of muscle to develop tension (in skeletal muscle {24,26,64} and heart muscle {5,7,28,77}). Figure 19-5 shows several possible manifestations of the influence of shortening on the ability of a muscle to develop force. In these responses, releases to a light load are given at various times during contraction. These responses show that shortening following early releases reduces the later force-generation capacity of the muscle relative to its capability, when it remains isometric until the later period. This deactivation is apparent im-

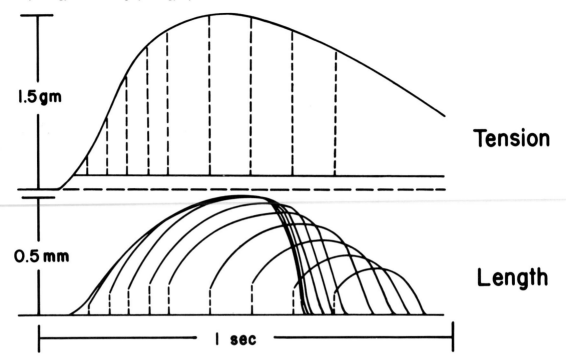

Fig. 19-5. Tension **(upper curves)** and length change **(lower curves)** showing releases of a rabbit papillary muscle to a small load at various times during contraction. Note the reduced ability of the muscle to shorten or bear the load (deactivation) following the releases, i.e., early releases reduce the period of shortening or force-generating capability. Modified from Brady {8}, with permission.

mediately upon the onset of shortening, since only brief transient shortening intervals (<20 ms) initiate deactivation and the effect can last beyond a given contraction. Shortening deactivation is more prominent the later in a contraction the perturbation occurs.

Shortening during the first 25–30% of a twitch has little effect on subsequent tension generation or shortening capacity, but shorteing during the relaxing phase of contraction may abruptly terminate the contraction (see also Ter Keurs {124}) and also reduce the force-generation or shortening capacity of a subsequent contraction. The magnitude and time of occurrence of shortening during a contraction seem to be the primary factors that influence this negative inotropic effect. Ekelund and Edman {29} found similar shortening deactivation effects in skinned frog and mouse skeletal muscle, which could be reduced with elevated Ca^{2+} and with increased ionic strength and could be enhanced by elevated Mg^{2+}. They suggest that shortening may lead to a decrease in troponin-calcium binding or that with shortening the number of crossbridges in a braking position (attached but compressed) is increased so that the net shortening force is reduced.

Shortening deactivation may thus play a significant role in the determination of the shape of the force-length relation, particularly in heart muscle. Considerable series compliance is evident in most cardiac multicellular preparations, and sarcomeric nonuniformity is evident in both

multicellular and loaded single-cell preparations. Thus even during an isometric contraction, some degree of sarcomere shortening (and/or lengthening) probably occurs, so that it is likely that the sarcomeric shortening that occurs during these isometric muscle contractions reduces the peak developed force. Resting sarcomere length in most multicellular preparations (i.e., slack length) is between 1.9 and 2.2 μm. Therefore, the force developed at a mean sarcomere length of, say, 1.6 μm requires extensive sarcomere shortening, and probably deactivation, before the contraction becomes isometric at 1.6 μm. The magnitude of this deactivation is difficult to evaluate because of the above-mentioned factors of internal loading with shortening and length-dependent activation (next section).

Some evidence for the magnitude of shortening deactivation was obtained by Pollack and Krueger {99}, who measured force development at short sarcomere lengths using an exponential controlled stretch to compensate for SL shortening (similar to the method proposed by Brady {9}). They found that this method reduces series compliance to 1–2% (from about 5%) but that peak tension still fell at reduced SL, even with this minimal shortening; hence, they concluded that while shortening deactivation may be significant, the steep ascending limb of the length-tension relation is not primarily due to shortening deactivation.

LENGTH-DEPENDENT ACTIVATION

In the operational range for heart muscle, i.e., 1.6–2.2 μm, our concept of the relation between myofilament overlap and active force development is extremely unclear in both cardiac and skeletal muscle. It is readily apparent that in all kinds of preparations (from intact multicellular preparations to length-clamped glycerinated myofibrils), active force development declines at sarcomere lengths below 2.0 μm. In the early proposals of the sliding-filament hypothesis {43}, and as proposed still by Julian and Moss {67}, the fall in developed tension at short sarcomere lengths (1.6–2.0 μm) was related to a resistive elastic interaction between overlapping thin filaments and to a distortion of thick filaments abutting against the Z bands at less than 1.6 μm SL. In this scheme total CB force would decline very little, but sarcomere force would be reduced by the magnitude of the elastic interaction between thin-filament regions of the sarcomere.

This interpretation was called into question when it was observed that the deeper sarcomeres of myofibrils in a whole muscle fiber at short SL became wavy during the twitch responses and that this waviness disappeared with tetanic stimulation or in the presence of caffeine {121,122}. These observations suggested that perhaps activation was graded at short SL and that a reduction in CB force development (i.e., a reduction in the number of CB attachments) might be responsible for the decline in active force development at short SL.

In support of the length-dependent activation concept, Kentish et al. {73} found a striking shift to the right of the force-pCa relation at reduced sarcomere length in chemically skinned rat trabeculae. They conclude that the steep force-Pca relation at short sarcomere length cannot be explained by a positive cooperativity of calcium binding on troponin sites but that the steepness may be due to an increase in the number of available force-generating crossbridges, as length is increased over the range 1.65–2.15 μm. In mechanically skinned cardiac cells, Fabiato {32} found an increasing relation between Ca^{2+} induced Ca^{2+} release (determined with Arsenazo III) and SL over the range of 1.8–2.3 μm. These two observations suggest both a reduction in released Ca^{2+} and a reduction in Ca^{2+} sensitivity at short sarcomere lengths.

Again, the picture is not yet clear. Moss {83} found a similar shape of the ascending limb in unskinned (tetanized) and skinned skeletal muscle fibers in fixed Ca^{2+} concentrations and concluded that length-dependent variation in activator Ca^{2+} did not play a major role in determining the shape o the ascending limb. In support of this interpretation, he cites the observation of Blinks et al. {4} that peak light responses of aequorin declined only gradually with sarcomere length from SL = 2.4–1.4 μm. However, Lopez et al. {78} indicate that Ca^{2+}-induced activation (measured by aequorin fluorescence) in skeletal muscle is in fact decreased at short lengths and reaches its maximum on the descending limb of the length-tension relation (SL = 3.0–3.2 μm).

A novel concept suggesting a basis for an apparent dependence of contractile activation on length, rather than a length dependence of Ca^{2+} release, comes from the reevaluation of some earlier data in a recent report of Allen and Kurihara {2}. Rather than taking the average of the calcium (aequorin) transients immediately following a length change {2}, they find that the first calcium transient following a reduction in length is increased while the force is reduced. They interpret this to mean that less calcium is bound by the myofilaments at the short length so that cytosol calcium is elevated (given that the release of calcium from the SR is unchanged). Further, they showed a reduced duration of aequorin fluorescence in twitches at increasing length (80% to 100% L_{max}) {2}, consistent with a greater binding of Ca^{2+} to troponin at increased length and increased force development.

Also, they point out that a force-dependent increase in the binding constant of troponin for Ca^{2+} would predict a steepening relation between pCa and tension {17} and also would account for the shift in P_{Ca}-tension relation noted by Kentish et al. {73}. This mechanism offers an alternative to the concept of a length dependence of Ca^{2+}-induced Ca^{2+} release {35}, which does not explain well either the relative constancy of the peak aequorin signal with muscle length noted by Allen and Kurihara {2} in the above report or the shallow slope of the tension-length relation in tonically activated skinned heart cells [curve (b), fig. 19-3]. An increase in Ca^{2+} release from SR has also been questioned by Chuck and Parmley {18} as a basis for the slow caffeine-reversible increase in tension following a length change in cat papillary muscle.

Ter Keurs {123} has combined many of these observations into a working hypothesis in which the principal factor responsible for the steep ascending limb of the Frank–Starling relation is attributed to a length dependence of myofilament activation. He suggests that the length dependence arises from a limitation of calcium binding to the myofilaments in the double-overlapping regions of the thin filaments.

Obviously, the data are incomplete, and furthermore, a detailed mechanism for the length dependence of activation has not been substantiated so that we have little direct insight into the details of this phenomenon. At this point we can only recognize that a length dependence of contractile activation is readily demonstrable and must be considered in any evaluation of cardiac performance.

Unfortunately, the relative contribution of these four factors (mechanical interference of overlapping thin filaments, elastic restoring forces, shortening deactivation, and length-dependent activation) to the ascending limb of the Frank–Starling relation is not well quantified, but each may be significant under particular contractile conditions. The data from sarcomere-length-controlled multicellular preparations are helpful, but these data still reflect the mean response of many cells in which the uniformity of sarcomere response has not been clearly evaluated. More definitive data will need to come from studies on single myocytes in which sarcomere length can be accurately monitored.

Relation between sarcomeric and muscle force-length relations

As an example of the problem of relating muscle length to sarcomere length, consider the following data. Julian and Sollins {68} measured sarcomere lengths in thin rat papillary muscles by direct photomicrography of the sarcomeres. Resting sarcomere length averaged 2.23 μm at L_{max}. Although the muscle was restrained at L_{max}, sarcomere shortening occurred in the body of the muscle to a mean length of 1.98 μm (i.e., about 11%) during isometric contraction. At 0.75 L_{max}, 3–6% sarcomere shortening occurred with isometric muscle contraction. At some points between these two muscle lengths, sarcomere shortening up to 15% was noted at constant muscle length. Similar results were obtained by Pollack and Huntsman {98}, who found that about 40% of this length change could be attributed to end compliance, but the rest occurred as nonuniformity within the body of the muscle.

Thus it is evident that an isometric muscle contraction cannot be assumed to occur at constant sarcomere length or constant myofilament overlap. Furthermore, whether we attempt to deduce myofilament interactions from measurements in multifiber preparations or whether we try to predict papillary muscle or whole-heart function from myofilament properties, we must contend with the complex structural organization and variability of this tissue.

SARCOMERIC AND SEGMENTAL NONUNIFORMITY

Since nearly all force measurements in heart muscle have been made in multicellular preparations, it has generally been presumed that muscle length was synonymous with sarcomere length. Only in the last few years have investigators become concerned with the now-established observation that, particularly in heart muscle, sarcomere lengths can vary considerably from segment to segment and even from cell to cell within the preparation. Thus measured force-length relations in these preparations give only force-mean sarcomere length relations and cannot be interpreted in terms of myofilament overlap directly. The degree to which sarcomere nonuniformity exists in both resting and active heart muscle has been documented in a number of studies {56,68,74,91,94,98}. In these studies sarcomere uniformity existed only in segments of varied length. A compliance of as much as 7% occurred in the end regions of these preparations, but significant nonuniformity also existed within the body of the muscle.

Several techniques have been introduced to reduce the nonuniformity problem so that a relation between contractile force and myofilament overlap could be determined. As a measure of segment length, Pollack and Krueger {99} and van Heuningen et al. {126} used the first-order laser diffraction line generated by the sarcomeres in a selected uniformly responding segment of a thin papillary muscles of the rat. This diffraction line served as the sensing element for segment control in a servo system. Donald et al. {22} inserted transverse pins

through a papillary muscle and used the image of these pins projected onto a light-sensing device (CCD) to control segment length.

Brady {9} attempted to determine the series elastic component (SE) of papillary muscles (including end compliance) by quick-stretch techniques and then used the force-extension relation of this SE to control a linear motor device attached to the muscle. All these approaches led to a large reduction in SE (to about 1.5–2%) and a broader plateau of the active force-length relation. However, while these techniques offer better control of sarcomere length during force-length evaluations, they still do not assure sarcomere uniformity in contractile responses. Similar approaches applied to single cardiac myocytes are needed where sarcomere uniformity can be more clearly determined.

The advantage of the single cardiac myocyte for these studies is indicated by the fact that sarcomere lengths in unrestrained single isolated cardiac cells display a remarkable uniformity, even during contraction {13,21,35, 75,104}. These observations indicate that either the collagen matrix within which the cells exist in multicellular preparations, or the application of mechanical constraints (i.e., ties, clamps), or both, lead to a nonuniform distribution of stress during contraction. However, attachment to single cardiac myocytes for twitch measurements remains a challenge.

VISCOELASTIC PROPERTIES OF HEART MUSCLE

The interpretation of the contractile properties of heart muscle, including its many inotropic states, requires an appreciation of the viscoelastic character of both resting and active muscle. Resting muscle length presages the subsequent contractile response, but resting length in multicellular and whole-heart preparations is determined by both internal and external viscoelastic properties.

The passive time and velocity-dependent stress components of heart muscle responses are complex and play a significant role in the dertermination of sarcomere length and in the manifestation of muscle force. The more dramatic viscoelastic component active muscle is stress relaxation, which is multiexponential in its decay. It is most pertinent to rapid perturbation studies and will be discussed in that section. In resting muscle stress relaxation is less dramatic, since the forces involved are usually of lower magnitude; however, stress relaxation is present and usually displays different decay factors than that of active muscle {104}. Creep is another long-term phenomenon that must be dealt with when sarcomere length over an extended time period is of interest. These phenomena have been quantified in intact heart muscle {92} and in isolated cardiac cells {37}, but we have little information regarding their structural or molecular basis. Consequently, we can do little more than describe their appearance and discuss how they relate to contractile responses. In the case of viscoelasticity and creep of passive heart muscle, this will be mentioned in the section *resting tension*.

Mechanical analogs

When considering the relation between passive resting tension and active force development, it is not clear that resting tension can be simply subtracted from total tension in order to obtain active tension. Such an operation presumes that these two forces are arranged in parallel. In general we do not know that this is the case. Indeed, if compliance at the ends of the muscle preparation is appreciable, as is apparent in the work of Pollack and Huntsman {98} and Julian and Sollins {68}, the simple additive relation of resting and active tension is invalid, because passive parallel elastic elements in the body of the muscle will be unloaded during active contraction while their counterparts at the ends of the muscle become more loaded. For a meaningful measurement of active force, the mechanical relation between these two passive components must be known. Similarly, since it is well established that active force development is highly dependent upon sarcomere length over much of the operating length of the sarcomeres, sarcomere length must be known in order to establish the relation between active force and sarcomere length. However, with the presence of end compliance and with the possibility of nonuniformity of stress distribution in the muscle during contraction, sarcomere length variations within the preparation are likely to occur. Additonally, as mentioned above, there is evidence that shortening or extension of the sarcomere during active contraction alters its subsequent contractility. All these factors will influence the transform (or constitutive relation) that must develop in order to relate myofilament mechanics to, say, papillary muscle behavior or whole heart performance.

A good deal of information has been obtained in the past two decades in regard to these problems. While we cannot say that the ideal and unique transform has been derived for heart muscle, many previous simplifying assumptions in model analysis are now invalidated and the types of experiments that must be done are more clearly defined.

In recent years a large number of mechanical analogs have been evaluated in an attempt to define a unique analytical relation that would make possible an interpretation of myofilament force and length interactions in terms of mechanical parameters measurable at the ends of the muscle. These models generally have tended to ignore viscous properties and have mostly dealt with the undamped elastic response of the preparation. To this extent, these models only relate to instantaneous elastic properties of the muscle. Some more complex models include dampers, but the inclusion of these additional elements result in a model with so many parameters that unique characterization of a preparation is beyond experimental verification. While muscle viscosity cannot be ignored, there is little advantage in phenomenological attempts to model it until the structures with which it is associated can be identified. In any case the following models are based on rapid perturbation data (quick stretch and releases) and do not include viscous components.

The models in question include first a discussion of the classical three-element model of A.V. Hill {50} (i.e., the so-called Maxwell model), in which resting tension was assumed to be attributable to passive elastic elements (PE) that solely bore rest tension and thus determined initial sarcomere length. Additional passive elastic elements (SE) that became evident in an active muscle were presumed to be in series with the force-generating elements of the muscle. This series elastic component was most vividly demonstrated by releasing an active muscle to zero load during a contraction {63}. In multicellular heart preparations, SE compliance thus defined is of the order of 5% L_o) (muscle length at maximum active force development) {82,99}. PE varies widely with species from a relatively small stiffness at sarcomere lengths of $3.0-3.6\,\mu m$ in frog heart {61} to an exceedingly stiff PE in rat ventricle such that rest tension at $SL = 2.8\,\mu m$ can be as large as active tension {36}.

The Hill model has been popular because resting tension-length relations could be algebraically subtracted from total length-tension relations in order to calculate active tension. It is obvious, however, that this simple analog has serious limitations, particularly in preparations in which considerable compliance exists at the ends of, or in the attachments to, the muscle.

Recognition of this end compliance suggests an alternate three-element model, i.e., the so-called Voigt arrangement, in which the series elasticity (SE) bears both resting and active contractile force. The interpretation of myofilament force-length relations in terms of this analog gives different characteristics for myofilament interactions than the Maxwell arrangement if short-term myofilament interactions is assumed to be stiff, i.e., if the contractile element is assumed to be rigid to short, fast perturbations {9,48, 97}. Fung {39} did not accept this assumption and claimed that the two models were indistinguishable. The issue is more complex, however, because neither of these two analogs includes the additional elastic component of the crossbridges.

Brady et al. {14} considered a large number of mechanical analogs and attempted to describe a unique arrangement of elastic elements, including parallel, series, and CB elasticity, which would be applicable to a given cardiac preparation. He used the stiffness-force relation at varied initial muscle lengths to describe elastic responses of rabbit papillary muscle (see also Fung {38}). Perturbations of $1-2\,ms$ duration were employed in order to obtain some limited measure of CB elasticity as well as to characterize passive elasticity of the muscle. In some preparations a three-elastic element lumped parameter model appeared to be adequate to fully describe the elastic properties of papillary muscle over the functional range of muscle lengths ($0.75-1.05\ L_o$). It was recongnized, however, that considerable segmental inhomogeneity existed in these preparations, as indicated by the movement of opaque microspheres placed in the vasculature of the papillary muscle prior to excision of the muscle.

Furthermore, consideration of these stiffness-force data as a two-segment distributed system made up of two

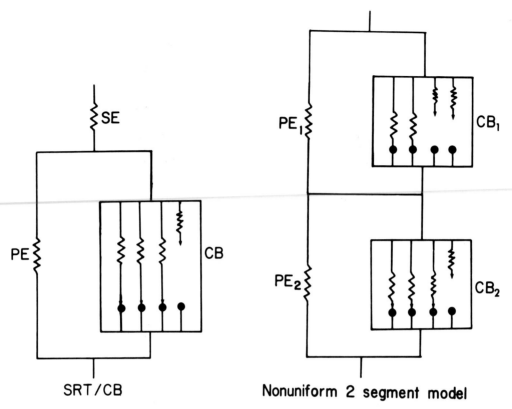

Fig. 19-6. Lumped three-element mechanical analog **(left)** and two-segment, four-element distrivuted analog **(right)** of papillary muscle. PE = parallel elastic element; SE = series elastic element; CB = crossbridge elastic and force-generating element. Numerical subscripts on distributed analog denote the two populations, which may have different characteristics. Modified from Brady et al. {14}, with permission.

populations of sarcomeres with different stiffness-force characteristics (right diagram, fig. 19-6) led to an analog analytically indistinguishable from the lumped three-element system (SRT/CB model, fig. 19-6). In other words, the elastic constants for the PE, SE, and crossbridges for either model (lumped or distributed parameters) could be derived from the stiffness-force data. Thus, without an independent measurement of segmental motion during contraction, it was impossible to determine which analog applied to a given preparation. It is clear, then, that this ambiguity makes it impossible to interpret myofilament interactions from measurements of whole-muscle preparations where sarcomere nonuniformity is present.

Resting tension

EXTRACELLULAR ORIGINS

Since the collagen matrix in which heart cells are embedded form a three-dimensional system around the cells, these elastic structures may contribute to resting tension by resisting longitudinal extension of the muscle fibers. As with restoring forces that may occur with muscle

shortening, other candidates for elements bearing resting tension with muscle extension are the membrane structures [sarcolemma (SR) and mitochondria] and intermediate filaments. The availability of single intact myocytes of several species and procedures for partial extraction of cellular components makes possible a comparison of length-tension relations in single, multicellular, and partially extracted preparations of the same species. These components are discussed below.

The contribution of extracellular elastic structures to muscle force has received considerable attention in the past two decades (see Brady {10}). Cardiac muscle exhibits substantial rest tension at much shorter lengths than skeletal muscle so that the meshowork of collagen around the cells is a prime candidate for the higher rest tension. For example, Winegrad {130} concluded that connective tissue must limit the extension of frog atrial trabeculae, because locally contracting cells could stretch the sarcomeres of quiescent cells that were in series with the active cells more effectively than did a simple extension of the whole trabecular preparation. Adjacent cells were not influenced by these local contractions.

The contribution of extracellular structures to rest

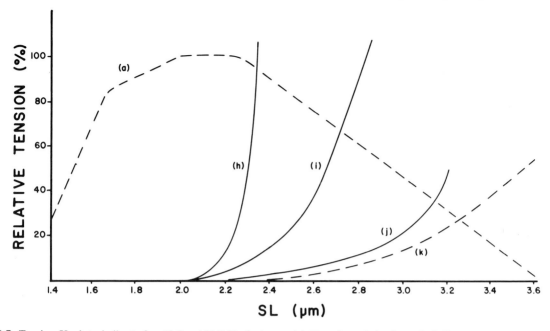

Fig. 19-7. Tension-SL plots similar to figs. 19-2 and 19-3. Dashed curve **(a)**: Data from skeletal muscle {70}. Curve **(h)**: Resting tension data from thin rat papillary muscle {98}. Curve **(i)**: Resting tension data from mechanically skinned rat ventricular fiber {36}. Curve **(j)**: Resting tension data from mechanically skinned dog ventricular fiber {36}. Curve **(k)**: Resting tension data from chemically or mechanically skinned frog anterior tibial muscle {67}. Tensions are relative to peak active tension (P_o) in respective muscle preparations.

tension at long sarcomere lengths was more clearly shown in this preparation by Tarr et al. {120}, who found that resting stress in the range of SL = 2.35–3.45 μm was 8- to 30-fold greater in intact frog atrial trabeculae than in the same isolated single cells.

In contrast, several studies show that in the operating range of heart, muscle extracellular structures may not be the major components of resting tension {11}. A particularly definitive study was conducted by Grimm and Whitehorn {46}, which showed that the extraction of the myofilaments of a rat papillary muscle with high salt (0.6 M KCl) destroyed the high rest tension of this muscle, while the collagen and other cellular structures were left intact. On the other hand, enzymatic disruption of the cellular integrity (presumably the intercalated discs) reduced both active and passive rest tension, again suggesting that some structure within the cells, as well as cell-to-cell contact, was responsible for rest tension.

CELLULAR COMPONENTS OF RESTING TENSION

As indicated above, cellular components that might be sources of resting tension are the sarcolemma, intracellular membrane structures, and intermediate filaments {76}. Studies in mechanically skinned skeletal muscle by Natori {85} and Podolsky {95}, however, all show that the sarcolemma does not contribute to rest tension until SL = 3.0 μm.

On the other hand, there is evidence in mammalian heart tissue that some detergent-soluble structures may be involved, at least to a limited extent, in the development of resting tension. For example, Fabiato and Fabiato {36} found that in dog mechanically skinned ventricular fibers had a high resting tension until detergent treatment, whereupon they exhibited resting tension less than one-quarter P_o at SL = 3.0 μm [fig. 19-7, curve (j)]. In contrast, skinned frog ventricular cells had a low resting tension (10% P at S = 3.0 μm), which was not significantly affected by the detergent Brij 58, and these fibers could be extended to SL = 8 μm. They also noted that these ventricular cells had a higher resting tension than similarly prepared frog semitendinosus fibers.

In mechanically skinned rat ventricular fiber {36}, detergent treatment reduced resting tension in the range of sarcomere lengths of 2.1–2.4 μm, but not at longer sarcomere lengths [fig. 19-7, curve (i)]. Only treatment of the preparation with elastase reduced resting tension at the longer sarcomere lengths. This treatment also tended to disrupt lateral connections between myofibrils.

Collectively, these findings indicate that the structural source of resting tension in heart muscle at SL below 3.0 μm probably is not related to extracellular collagen but must be a property of the muscle fibers themselves. In the range of SL = 2.0–2.4 μm, the sarcolemma or other detergent-soluble structures probably bear a substantial portion of resting tension (depending on species), but in preparations such as the rat ventricle, other intracellular elastic structures must bear a major portion of the rest tension.

Other candidates for bearing rest tension are the longitudinal distributions of intermediate filaments of heart cells, e.g., titin {127} or connectin {80,81}, desmin {125}, and tubulin {3,107,108}. The mechanical properties of these elements are not yet established, but preliminary studies indicate that little stiffness remains in the observable residue of single rat heart myocytes after detergent (0.5% Triton X-100) and high-salt (0.6 M KI) treatment {12}. The data of Brady and Farnsworth {12} and those of Grimm and Whitehorn {46} cited above indicate that the contractile filaments must be intact in order for heart cells to bear appreciable resting tension. Therefore, it seems unlikely that the principal resting-stress-bearing elements run simply from Z line to Z line without intermediate attachments to the contractile filaments. Armstrong and Ganote {3} and Samuel et al. {107,108} have shown that microtubules proliferate and reorganize during sarcomerogenesis but that tubulin is present only in low concentration (0.01% total protein) in adult cardiac myocytes. Thus the microtubules would appear to play only a minor role in resting tension development in normal adult heart cells.

On the other hand, titin filaments appear to be present in considerable quantities in myofibrils (~10% total cell protein), and immunofluorescence analyses {12,129} suggest that these filaments are in a position to transfer stress between the A- and I-band filaments. In this regard, Wang et al. {128} have shown that labelled epitopes of titin in the I-band regions of skeletal muscle are extensible with changes in sarcomere length but labelled regions of A-band titin are not. Titin is abundant in cardiac muscle {81}, but its extensibility has not been studied.

Horowits et al. {55} have shown that resting tension in skeletal muscle can be reduced with intense x-ray irradiation, which presumably selectively destroyed the large molecular-weight titin filaments. However, less severe methods of high molecular weight protein disruption have not been reported; such measurements are critical, obviously, in order to specifically define the elements of muscle that are responsible for resting tension.

It is also interesting to consider whether the presence of titin in the crossbridge environment might influence active force development. No specific data have been reported in this regard but titin can be phosphorylated {109}, which suggests some possible regulatory role for this strategically located set of giant molecules.

Viscosity and creep

It has long been appreciated that muscle, particularly cardiac muscle, undergoes a slow continuous increase in length when subjected to a constant load. Similarly, at constant length force may decline continuously. These phenomena have been described as creep (distinct from stress relation) and are characteristic of many long-chain highly crosslinked substances. In papillary muscle, creep has been characterized phenomenologically by Pinto and

Patitucci {93}. It has also been briefly described in hamster single cardiac myocytes {37}. Pinto and Patitucci showed that at a load corresponding to the peak stress-strain ratio (0.2–1.0 g/mm^2, depending on species) an extension of 2–3% occurred (logarithmically in time) over a period of 100 seconds. Large initial extensions (>15%) resulted in less creep in this interval. Creep was not strongly dependent on temperature.

A most critical observation in these studies was that in conditioned preparations (i.e., following cyclic perturbations for a given period of time), creep deformation was symmetrically reversible in time. The initial creep rate was about 1%/s following an applied stress equal to the peak stress-strain ratio. Based on these observations, we would expect creep extensions less than 1% during the normal cardiac cycle (70 beats/min). Also, since creep is symmetrically reversible, in the normal heart cycle creep occurring during systole should be reversed during diastole. Only with sustained changes in diastolic tension (or pressure) would the creep phenomenon affect successive contractions differently.

In the study by Pinto and Patitucci {93}, some attention was given to the tied ends of the preparation but no consistent relation between creep and end effects was noted. They concluded that the creep effect was not specifically related to the end regions, although the distribution of the creep deformation between the ends and the body of the muscle was not clear in their study. They noted that the relative creep rate in a 14-mm cat ventricular strip was almost identical to that in a 4-mm cat papillary muscle, so that these creep rate values are probably indicative of the changes in mean sarcomere length under these loading conditions. In the worst case, it appears that changes in force development, expected from SL changes of 1%, should be anticipated during short-term changes in resting tension. Long-term changes (>100 seconds) may correspond to SL changes of 2–3%.

FORCE-VELOCITY-LENGTH RELATIONS

In cardiac muscle the interest in the force-velocity (P-V) relation has been twofold. First, there is the common interest with skeletal muscle that the P-V relation might provide a relation between the mechanical and energetic relations of the contracting muscle. Second, the fact that heart muscle functions on the ascending limb of the force-length relation makes difficult the separation of inotropic contractile changes from length-dependent change. Previous work with mammalian papillary muscle indicated that shortening velocity reached its maximum early in contraction {16} and also suggested that V_{max} (maximum shortening velocity) might be independent of initial muscle length so that V_{max} could serve as an index of contractility that relates only to changes in the nongeometrical aspects of the muscle {16,110}. More detailed studies show, however, that problems with the extrapolation of force velocity curves, the complicated interactions of contractile parameters, such as length-dependent force changes, nonlinear elastic elements, shortening inactivation, nonuniformity of sarcomeres, and the time dependence of force generation {23,28,86,88,89,96,99,132}, leave serious doubts as to the utility of finding such a simple index of contractility in multicellular preparations.

Parmley et al. {88} surveyed a number of possible indices of contractility and found that indices that were sensitive to the contractile state were also sensitive to preload (initial length), while indices that were less preload sensitive were also less reflective of contractile state changes. In their analysis, the maximum rate of isometric tension development (dP/dt) seemed most sensitive to the state of contractility.

Edman and Hwang {27} and Edman {25} introduced a measure of unloaded shortening velocity (V_o) whereby velocity is measured as the length change of a quick release to zero force divided by the time interval to take up the slack of the release. He showed that in skeletal muscle V_o compared favorably with V_o in single fibers. Each has a similar Q10 (2.67) between 2C and 12C, V_o was independent of sarcomere length from 1.65 to 2.7 μm, and V_o was similar for both twitch and tetanus. Tarr et al. {119} also found shortening velocity in single intact frog atrial fibers to be constant down to SL = 1.6 μm. In contrast, Pollack and Krueger {99} and Daniels et al. {20} used this technique, along with a measurement of sarcomere length with laser diffraction in a servo loop, and showed that in thin rat papillary muscles P_o and V_o varied in parallel with changes in sarcomere length in the range SL = 1.6–2.1 μm (1.6–1.85 μm in Daniels et al. {20}) but was constant only between SL = 2.1–2.3 μm (1.85–2.3 μm in Daniels et al. {20}). Furthermore, Daniels et al. {20} found that V_o reached a maximum early in contraction when force development was only 50% P_o. At SL = 1.85 μm, where V_o became constant, contractile force was still only 60% P_o. In view of the these observations in heart muscle, the possibility of obtaining a length-independent measure of contractility in terms of shortening velocity seems to be ruled out at the sarcomere level also.

By way of comparison of shortening velocities in intact and isolated cells, Pollack and Krueger {99} measured V_o at 10 μs at 26°C at SL = 2.0 μm. Daniels et al. {20} give a value of 13.6 μm/s. At the next level of structural simplicity, Fabiato and Fabiato {36} calculated a maximum shortening velocity of 20 μm/s in maximally activated mechanically skinned rat myocytes.

These values compare with an extrapolated V_{max} in cat papillary muscle in the range of 0.5–2.0 muscle lengths/s at comparable temperatures {23,86,111}. Obviously, the shortening velocity in isolated cells can be much higher than in the larger multicellular preparations and can be dramatically increased with full activation. These comparisons suggest that intercellular interactions considerably impede shortening-rate capabilities of the fibers; although if force generation is sustained, the same ultimate sarcomere length may be achieved.

Velocity-length relations have been considered in cardiac muscle {16} and show an early maximum shortening rate followed by a constancy in the velocity-length profile of contraction that is independent of initial muscle length and time. These results were interpreted to indicate

that during the twitch the effects of shortening inactivation exactly balance the rising activation from Ca^{2+} release. While this balance of interactions seems rather fortuitous, it demonstrates the complexity and reinforces the reservations that must be considered in the interpretation of the measured parameters of cardiac contraction.

The conclusions to be drawn from two decades of study of P-V relations in heart muscle are (a) shortening velocity, because of the many contractile parameters that influence its measurement, cannot serve as a useful index of cardiac contractility independent of length factors; but (b) the high constant velocity of shortening in isolated cardiac cell systems, perhaps only minimally complicated by internal loading, may indicate more directly the shortening kinetics of CB turnover. This shortening rate may reflect the net effect of length-dependent activation and shortening deactivation, but these processes now seem more amenable to experimental control, particularly if force measurements and SL can be simultaneously determined in intact isolated cells.

PERTURBATION ANALYSIS

As mentioned in the introduction, a primary objective of the study of muscle function is to understand the mechanism whereby metabolic energy is transformed into mechanical work. Considerable advances have been made in muscle physiology at the biochemical level that relate the splitting of ATP to actomyosin interactions. Understandably, the most detailed information on this energy transduction process comes from the most isolated or more completely extracted muscle systems. From these structurally and chemically simplified systems, we now have a large number of rate constants of reaction kinetics that pertain to the CB cycle. However, the effect of structural order and mechanical stress on these reaction kinetics is more difficult to obtain.

In an attempt to derive this information from structured and mechanically stressed muscle preparations, a number of laboratories have introduced perturbation techniques (both stepwise and sinusoidal) to analyze the force or length response of intact muscle preparations to changes in applied strain or stress. The rationale for this approach in terms of stepwise perturbations is that when an actively contracting muscle in a steady state of activation is subjected to an abrupt change in stress or strain, the time course of the subsequent response should reveal kinetic properties of myofilament interactions.

In the case of sinusoidal perturbations, this approach is prompted by observations in asynchronous muscle systems (e.g., insect fibrillar flight muscle) that an optimal range of frequencies exist over which an oscillatory perturbation leads to a phase shift between muscle force and length such that the muscle does work against the system rather than simply dissipating the applied energy, as would a viscoelastic body. The frequency and amplitude characteristics of these critical oscillations should also reflect the interaction of chemical and mechanical kinetics of the active contractile system and, in resting muscle, possibly

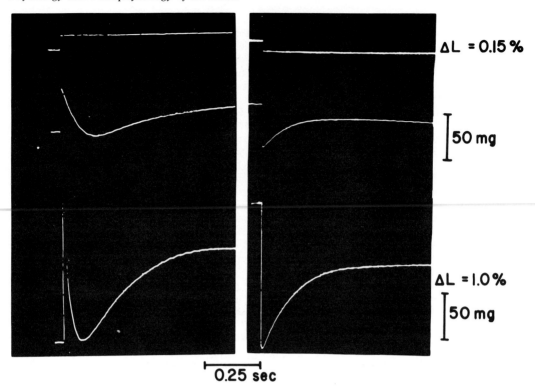

Fig. 19-8. Delayed tension responses of glycerol extracted rabbit papillary muscle to quick stretch **(left panel)** and quick release **(right panel)**. **a:** Imposed length change (stretch or release). **b:** Tension responses following 0.15% length step. **c:** Tension responses following 1.0% length step. Active tension (T_o) prior to each step is about 250 mg. From Steiger {114}, with permission.

weak crossbridge interaction at higher frequencies as in asynchronous flight muscle (~2 kHz) {45}.

Steiger {113,114} and Herzig and Ruegg {49} found that, as in insect fibrillar flight muscle {41,79} and glycerinated rabbit psoas muscle {72,105}, glycerol-extracted rabbit ventricular muscle activated with Ca^{2+} responded to a quick stretch or release with a delayed tension change (at constant length). Figure 19-8 shows typical tension responses of glycerol extracted heart muscle to two levels of step length perturbations [curves (b) and (c)]. The first phase of the response following the step (stretch or release) is a rapid, temperature-insensitive return of tension towards T. Phase 2 is an order of magnitude slower, and in fig. 19-8 appears as the slow tail on the first phase before reversing direction (stretch response) to redevelop delayed tension (phase 3). Delayed tension with releases is not as dramatic as with stretches. Phase 2 is Ca^{2+} sensitive and reflects inotropic states of the muscle. Phase 3 rate constants correspond with the normal heart rate of a wide variety of animals from frog and pig (30–50 beats/min) to hummingbird (2000 beats/min) {115}. While the responses in heart muscle are an order of magnitude slower than in insect and skeletal muscle preparations, they display the same mechanical features that are responsible for the oscillatory behavior of

asynchronous insect fibrillar flight muscle. Superimposed high-frequency length perturbations (100 Hz) also show that muscle stiffness parallels the force changes during delayed tension responses, indicating that these induced force changes involve CB attachments {118}.

Further studies in living cardiac muscle {118} in which steady-state activation was achieved by short period of caffeine or Ba^{2+} contracture also showed the delayed tension effect in response to step perturbations and further identified a range of oscillatory frequencies (0.05–1.2 Hz) in which muscle force lagged the imposed length change so as to to work on the system.

A further elaboration of these studies {116,117} suggests that the rate constants fitted to the transient mechanical responses should correspond to the following chemical rate constants: k1, the fast temperature-insensitive phase, may correspond to acto-myosin dissociation; k2, which is strongly temperature and perturbation amplitude dependent, to recombination and dissociation of the (myosin-products) component of the CB with actin; and k3, which characterizes the delayed tension, to V_{max}, i.e., the maximum ATPase and attachment of new cross-bridges. In a four-state CB cycle model, Steiger and Abbott {117} have matched these rate constants obtained in several muscle types to known biochemical rate constants.

Rate constants for some of these processes have also been derived by Kawai and Brandt {72} from Nyquist plots of complex stiffness of the skeletal muscle of several species using sinusoidal perturbation analysis. Although the correspondences of the mechanical and biochemical rate constants are somewhat arbitrary, and they give only a measure of net reaction rates rather than specific forward and backward rate constants; nevertheless, they look promising in terms of developing useful relations between mechanical and chemical muscle contractile processes.

At this stage these correspondences can only be considered speculative because (a) the data were not obtained in muscle systems with controlled sarcomere lengths, i.e., series compliance and sarcomere uniformity are not controlled, and (b) the identification of specific mechanical rate constants with certain biochemical reaction processes is presumptive. In any case, some correlations between perturbation-related mechanical and chemical events are now plausible. Indeed, it will be interesting to consider the possible role of stress-dependent weak crossbridge attachments {45} as a step in the delayed tension response of cardiac muscle.

ACTIVE STATE

The concept of the active state was originally defined as the ability of a muscle to develop force at constant length {51}. In this respect the onset of the active state is slow, particularly in heart muscle, since force development requires considerable time to reach its maximum. In contrast, in terms of shortening capability, the maximum velocity of shortening occurs very early (in skeletal muscle {151}; in heart muscle {25,93}). The question then arises as to which parameter should be the measure of activation.

The active-state concept has been critically evaluated in several discussions {63,66,97,100}, with the recommendation in the latter review that the concept be abandoned. For example, Pollack and coworkers {97} could not determine a unique elastic modulus for series elasticity in heart muscle. Julian and Moss {66} considered force development and shortening in terms of a crossbridge model and series elasticity, and concluded that such a model predicted both a slow development of force and an early maximum shortening capability, as observed experimentally. However, since muscle activation is now recognized to be regulated by myoplasmic Ca^{2+}, and both shortening velocity and force development are strongly dependence on myoplasmic Ca^{2+}, the uniqueness of the classical active-state concept in terms of force development alone is lost. Indeed, the concept has little definitive value and should be abandoned.

IMPLICATIONS FOR WHOLE-HEART FUNCTION

From this discussion it is apparent that the formulation of a fundamental constitutive relation that would describe heart muscle contractility in an effective manner is still premature. The complex dependence of contractile force on such factors as shortening deactivation, restoring forces, length-dependent activation, and sarcomere nonuniformity, and in addition, our inability to quantitatively represent these factors makes anything but an empirical formulation of little use. Also, even empirical relations will have to be prescribed for very specific functional situations and would likely only apply to a narrow range of cardiac function.

Similar concerns are expressed by Elzinga and Westerhof {30}, who have considered the merits of isolated myocardium variables as they might serve as a means to quantify the pump function of the heart. Their conclusion is that force-length relations of isolated heart tissue are not necessarily related to the shape of the left ventricular function curve. For example, end-systolic volume can be larger when stroke volume is increased by an increase in end-diastolic volume, as might be predicted from the above discussion of shortening deactivation. Their suggestion is that an understanding of the basis of the cardiac pump function curve should come from the consideration of muscle fibers as they operate in the wall of the heart rather than in terms of parameters that are under rigidly controlled length and force conditions.

The complexity and ambiguity of the cardiac contractile process at short muscle lengths emphasizes these recommendations insofar as the search goes for a unique index of cardiac contractility. Thus it seems unlikely that a simple constitutive relation {40} will be found that can be related to pump function with only a three-dimensional geometrical transfer function. It is possible that empirical constitutive relations may be determined that may be useful clinically {106}, but these relations will give little insight into molecular mechanisms of contractile function.

Therefore, it becomes critical to understand the functional basis of the ascending limb of the Frank–Starling relation so that the relative contributions of more of the underlying factors, i.e., external and internal loading, shortening deactivation, nonuniformity, and length-dependent activation, can be included in the constitutive relation. Additionally, there must also be a consideration of the contribution of the three-dimensional geometry of the heart to these intrinsic factors. Certainly, the shape, structure, and strain and stress distribution of the wall, as well as complex pressure loading, will have an effect on these interactions between contractile parameters.

From these considerations we must conclude that mechanical studies at the level of the myocyte and new insight into myocyte integration into whole-heart structure and function are high priorities for future investigation.

REFERENCES

1. Allen DG, Kentish JC: The cellular basis of the length-tension relation in cardiac muscle. *J Mol Cell Cardiol* 17: 821–840, 1985.
2. Allen DG, Kurihara S: The effects of muscle length on intracellular calcium transients in mammalian cardiac muscle. *J Physiol* 327:79–94, 1982.
3. Armstrong SC, Ganote CE: Flow cytometric analysis of

isolated adult cardiomyocytes — vinculin and tubulin fluorescence during metabolic inhibition and ischemia. *J Mol Cell Cardiol* 24:149–162, 1992.

4. Blinks JR, Rudel R, Taylor SR: Calcium transients in isolated amphibian skeletal muscle fibres: Detection with aequorin. *J Physiol* 277:291–323, 1978.

5. Bodem R, Sonnenblick EH: Deactivation of contraction by quick releases in the isolated papillary muscle of the cat. Effects of lever damping, caffeine, and tetanization. *Circ Res* 34:214–225, 1974.

6. Bodem R, Skelton CL, Sonnenblick EH: Inactivation of contraction as a determinant of the length-active tension relation in heart muscle of the cat. *Res Exp Med* 168:1–13, 1976.

7. Brady AJ: Onset of contractility in cardiac muscle. *J Physiol* 184:560–580, 1966.

8. Brady AJ: Length-tension relations in cardiac muscle. *Am Zool* 7:603–610, 1967.

9. Brady AJ: Active state in cardiac muscle. *Physiol Rev* 48:570–600, 1968.

10. Brady AJ: Mechanical properties of isolated cardiac myocytes. *Physiol Rev* 71:413–428, 1991.

11. Brady AJ: Length dependence of passive stiffness in single cardiac myocytes. *Am J Physiol* 260:H1062–H1071, 1991.

12. Brady AJ, Farnsworth SP: Cardiac myocyte stiffness following extraction with detergent and high salt solutions. *Am J Physiol* 250:H932–H943, 1986.

13. Brady AJ, Tan ST, Ricchiuti NV: Contractile force measured in unskinned isolated adult rat heart fibers. *Nature* 282:728–729, 1979.

14. Brady AJ, Tan ST, Ricchiuti NV: Perturbation measurements of papillary muscle elasticity. *Am J Physiol* 241:H155–H173, 1981.

15. Brown LM, Gonzales-Serratos H, Huxley AF: Electron microscopy of frog muscle fibers in extreme passive shortening. *J Physiol (Lond)* 208:86P, 1970.

16. Brutsaert DL: The force-velocity-length-time interaction of cardiac muscle. In: *The Physiologic Basis of Starling's Law of the Heart*. London: Ciba Foundation, 1974.

17. Chapman RA: Excitation-contraction coupling in cardiac muscle. *Prog Biophys Mol Biol* 35:1–52, 1979.

18. Chuck LHS, Parmley WW: Caffeine reversal of length-dependent changes in myocardial contractile state in the cat. *Circ Res* 47:592–598, 1980.

19. Close RI: The relations between sarcomere length and characteristics of isometric twitch contraction of frog sartorius muscle. *J Physiol* 220:745–762, 1972.

20. Daniels M, Noble MIM, Ter Keurs HEDJ, Wohlfart B: Velocity of sarcomere shortening in rat cardiac muscle: Relationship to force, sarcomere length, calcium and time. *J Physiol* 355:367–381, 1984.

21. De Clerck NM, Claes VA, Van Ocken ER, Brutsaert DL: Sarcomere distribution patterns in single cardiac cells. *Biophys J* 35:237–242, 1981.

22. Donald TC, Reeves DNS, Reeves RC, Walker AA, Hefner LL: Effects of damaged ends in papillary muscle preparations. *Am J Physiol* 238:H14–H23, 1980.

23. Donald TC, Unnoppetchara K, Peterson D, Hefner LL: Effect of initial muscle length on V_{max} in isotonic contraction of cardiac muscle. *Am J Physiol* 223:262–267, 1972.

24. Edman KAP: Mechanical deactivation induced by active shortening in isolated fibres of the frog. *J Physiol* 246:255–275, 1975.

25. Edman KAP: The velocity of unloaded shortening and its relation to sarcomere length and isometric force in vertebrate muscle fibers. *J Physiol* 291:143–159, 1979.

26. Edman KAP: Depression of mechanical performance by

active shortening during twitch and tetanus of vertebrate muscle fibers. *Acta Physiol Scand* 109:15–26, 1980.

27. Edman KAP, Hwang JC: The force-velocity relationship in vertebrate muscle fibers at varied tonicity of the extracellular medium. *J Physiol* 269:255–272, 1977.

28. Edman KAP, Nilsson E: Time course of the active state in relation to muscle length and movement: Comparative study on skeletal muscle and myocardium. *Cardiovasc Res* 1(Suppl):3–10, 1971.

29. Ekelund MC, Edman KAP: Shortening-induced deactivation of skinned fibres of frog and mouse striated muscle. *Acta Physiol Scand* 116:189–199, 1982.

30. Elzinga G, Westerhof N: How to quantify pump function of the heart: The value of variables derived from measurements on isolated muscle. *Circ Res* 44:303–308, 1979.

31. Endo M: Stretch-induced increase in activation of skinned fibers by calcium. *Nature* 237:211–213, 1972.

32. Fabiato A: Sarcomere length dependence of calcium release from the sarcoplasmic reticulum of skinned cardiac cell demonstrated by differential microspectrophotometry with Arsenazo III. *J Gen Physiol* 76:15, 1980.

33. Fabiato A, Fabiato F: Activation of skinned cardiac cells. Subcellular effects of cardioactive drugs. *Eur J Cardiol* 1:143–155, 1973.

34. Fabiato A, Fabiato F: Dependence of the contractile activation of skinned cardiac cells on the sarcomere length. *Nature* 256:54–56, 1975.

35. Fabiato A, Fabiato F: Dependence of the calcium release tension generation and restoring forces on sarcomere length in skinned cardiac cells. *Eur J Cardiol* 4(Suppl):13–27, 1976.

36. Fabiato A, Fabiato F: Myofilament-generated tension oscillations during partial calcium activation and activation dependence of the sarcomere length-tension relation of skinned cardiac muscle. *J Gen Physiol* 72:667–699, 1978.

37. Fish D, Orenstein J, Bloom S: Passive stiffness of isolated cardiac and skeletal myocytes in the hamster. *Circ Res* 54:267–276, 1984.

38. Fung YC: Elasticity of soft tissues in simple elongation. *Am J Physiol* 213:1532–1544, 1967.

39. Fung YC: Comparison of different models of the heart muscle. *J Biomechan* 4:289–295, 1971.

40. Ghista DN, Brady AJ, Radhakrishnan S: A three-dimensional analytical (rheological) model of the human left ventricle in passive-active states: Non-traumatic determination of the in vivo values of the rheological parameters. *Biophys J* 13:832–854, 1973.

41. Goodall MC: Autooscillations of extracted muscle fibers. *Nature* 177:1238–1239, 1956.

42. Gonzales-Serratos H: Inward spread of activation in vertebrate muscle fibers. *J Physiol (Lond)* 211:777–799, 1971.

43. Gordon AM, Huxley AF, Julian FJ: The variation in isometric tension with sarcomere length in vertebrate muscle fibers. *J Physiol* 184:170–192, 1966.

44. Gordon AM, Pollack GH: Effects of calcium on the sarcomere length-tension relation in rat cardiac muscle. Implications for the Frank-Starling mechanism. *Circ Res* 47:610–619, 1980.

45. Granzier HLM, Wang K: Interplay between passive tension and strong and weak crossbridges in insect asynchronous flight muscle: A functional dissection by gelsolin mediated thin filament removal. *J Gen Physiol* 101:235–270.

46. Grimm AF, Whitehorn WV: Characteristics of resting tension of myocardium and localization of its elements. *Am J Physiol* 210:1362–1368, 1966.

47. Grimm AF, Whitehorn WV: Myocardial length-tension

sarcomere relationships. *Am J Physiol* 214:1378–1387, 1968.

48. Hefner LL, Bowen TE Jr: Elastic components of cat papillary muscle. *Am J Physiol* 212:1221–1227, 1967.

49. Herzig JW, Ruegg JC: Myocardial cross-bridge activity and its regulation by Ca^{2+}, phosphate and stretch. In: Riecher G, Weber A, Goodwin J (eds) *Myocardial Failure*. New York: Springer-Verlag, 1977.

50. Hill AV: The heat of shortening and the dynamic constants of muscle. *Proc R Soc Lond B* 126:136–195, 1938.

51. Hill AV: The onset of contraction. *Proc R Soc Lond B* 136:242–254, 1949.

52. Hill AV: The transition from rest to full activity in muscle: The velocity of shortening. *Proc R Soc Lond B* 138:329–338, 1951.

53. Hill TL: Theoretical formalism for the sliding filament model of contraction of striated muscle. Part I. *Prog Biophys Mol Biol* 28:267–340, 1974.

54. Hill TL: Theoretical formalism for the sliding filament model of contraction of striated muscle. Part II. *Prog Biophys Mol Biol* 29:105–159, 1975.

55. Howorits R, Kempner ES, Bisher ME; Podolsky RJ: Evidence for a physiological role of titin and nebulin in skeletal muscle. *Biophys J* 49:421, 1986.

56. Huntsman LL, Joseph DS, Oiye MY, Nichols GL: Auxotonic contractions in cardiac muscle segments. *Am J Physiol* 237:H131–H138, 1979.

57. Huxley AF, Niedergerke R: Interference microscopy of living muscle fibers. *Nature* 173:971–973, 1954.

58. Huxley HE, Hanson J: Changes in the cross-striations of muscle during contraction and stretch and their structural interpretation. *Nature* 173:973–976, 1954.

59. Huxley AF, Simmons RM: Proposed mechanism of force generation in striated muscle. *Nature* 233:533–538, 1971.

60. Ingels NB Jr (ed): *The Molecular Basis of Force Development*. Palo Alto, CA: Palo Alto Medical Research Foundation, 1979.

61. Iwazumi T, Pollack GH: The effect of sarcomere non-uniformity on the sarcomere length-tension relationship of skinned fibers. *J Cell Physiol* 10:321–337, 1981.

62. Jewell BR: A reexamination of the influence of muscle length on myocardial performance. *Circ Res* 40:221–226, 1977.

63. Jewell BR, Wilkie DR: An analysis of the mechanical components in muscle. *J Physiol (Lond)* 143:515–540, 1958.

64. Jewell BR, Wilkie DR: The mechanical properties of relaxing muscle. *J Physiol* 152:30–47, 1960.

65. Julian FJ: Some theories for muscle contraction based on cyclic, short-range interactions between actin and myosin. In: Ingels NB Jr (ed) *The Molecular Basis of Force Development*. Palo Alto, CA: Palo Alto Medical Research Foundation, 1979.

66. Julian FJ, Moss RL: The concept of active state in striated muscle. *Circ Res* 38:53–59, 1976.

67. Julian FJ, Moss RL: Sarcomere length-tension relations of frog skinned muscle fibers at lengths above the optimum. *J Physiol* 304:529–539, 1980.

68. Julian FJ, Sollins MR: Sarcomere length-tension relations in living rat papillary muscle. *Circ Res* 37:299–308, 1975.

69. Julian FJ, Sollins MR, Moss RL: Absence of a plateau in length-tension relationship of rabbit papillary muscle when internal shortening is prevented. *Nature* 260:340–342, 1976.

70. Julian FJ, Sollins MR, Moss RL: Sarcomere length non-uniformity in relation to tetanic responses of stretched skeletal muscle fibers. *Proc R Soc Lond B* 200:109–116, 1978.

71. Julian FJ, Sollins KR, Sollins MR: A model for the transient and steady-state mechanical behavior of contracting muscle. *Biophys J* 14:546–562, 1974.

72. Kawai M, Brandt PW: Sinusoidal analysis: A high resolution method of correlating biochemical reactions with physiological processes in activated skeletal muscles of rabbit, frog and crayfish. *J Muscle Res Cell Motil* 1:279–303, 1980.

73. Kentish JC, Ter Deurs HEDJ, Ricciardi L, Bucx JJJ, Noble MIM: Comparison between the sarcomere length-force relations of intact and skinned trabeculae from rat right ventricle. Influence of calcium concentrations on these relations. *Circ Res* 58:755–768, 1986.

74. Krueger JW, Farber S: Sarcomere length "orders" relaxation in cardiac muscle. *Eur Heart J* 1(Suppl A):37–47, 1980.

75. Krueger JW, Forletti D, Wittenberg BA: Uniform sarcomere shortening behavior in isolated cardiac muscle cells. *J Gen Physiol* 76:587–607, 1980.

76. Lazarides E: Intermediate filaments as mechanical integrators of cellular space. *Nature* 283:249–256, 1980.

77. Leach JK, Brady AJ, Skipper BJ, Millis DL: Effects of active shortening on tension development of rabbit papillary muscle. *Am J Physiol* 238:H8–H13, 1980.

78. Lopez JR, Wanek LA, Taylor SR: Skeletal muscle length-dependent effects of potentiating agents. *Science* 214:79–82, 1981.

79. Lorand L, Moos C: Autooscillations of extracted muscle fibers. *Nature* 177;1239–1240, 1956.

80. Magid A, Ting-Beal HP, Carvell M, Kontis T, Lucaveche C: Connecting filaments, core filamen and side-struts: A proposal to add three new load-bearing structures to the sliding filament model. In: Pollack GH, Sugi H (eds) *Contractile Mechanisms of Muscle*. New York: Plenum Press, 170:397–328, 1984.

81. Maryama K, Kimura S, Kuroda M, Handa K: Connectin, an elastic protein of muscle: Its abundance in cardiac myofibrils. *J Biochem* 82:347–350, 1977.

82. McLaughlin RJ, Sonnenblick EH: Time behavior of series elasticity in cardiac muscle. Real-time measurements by controlled-length techniques. *Circ Res* 34:798–811, 1974.

83. Moss RL: Sarcomere length-tension relations of frog skinned muscle fibers during calcium activation at short lengths. *J Physiol* 292:177–192, 1979.

84. Murray JM, Weber A: A cooperative action of muscle proteins. *Science* 230:58–71, 1974.

85. Natori R: The property and contractile process of isolated myofibrils. *Jikeikai Med J* 1:119–126, 1954.

86. Noble MTM, Bowen TE, Hefner LL: Force-velocity relationship of cat cardiac muscle, studied by isotonic and quick-release techniques. *Circ Res* 24:821–833, 1969.

87. Page E, McCallister LP, Power B: Stereological measurements of cardiac ultrastructure implicated in excitation-contraction coupling. *Proc Natl Acad Sci USA* 68:1465–1466, 1971.

88. Parmley WW, Chuck L, Yeatman L: Comparative evaluation of the specificity and sensitivity of isometric indices of contractility. *Am J Physiol* 228:506–510, 1975.

89. Parmley WW, Yeatman L, Sonnenblick E: Differences between isotonic and isometric force velocity relations in cardiac and skeletal muscle. *Am J Physiol* 219:546–550, 1970.

90. Parsons C, Porter KR: Muscle relaxation: Evidence for an intrafibrillar restoring force in vertebrate striated muscle. *Science* 153:426–427, 1966.

91. Pinto JG: Macroscopic inhomogeneities in the mechanical response of papillary muscles. *Biorheology* 15:511–522, 1978.

92. Pinto JG, Fung YC: Mechanical properties of the heart muscle in the passive state. *J Biomech* 6:597–616, 1973.

93. Pinto JG, Patitucci PJ: Creep in cardiac muscle. *Am J Physiol* 232:H553–H563, 1977.
94. Pinto JG, Win R: Non-uniform strain distribution in papillary muscle. *Am J Physiol* 233:H410–H416, 1977.
95. Podolsky RJ: The maximum sarcomere length for contraction of isolated myofibrils. *J Physiol (Lond)* 170:110–123, 1964.
96. Pollack GH: Maximum velocity as an index of contractility in cardiac muscle. *Circ Res* 26:111–127, 1970.
97. Pollack GH, Huntsman LL, Verdugo P: Cardiac muscle models. An overextension of series elasticity? *Circ Res* 31:569–579, 1972.
98. Pollack GH, Huntsman LL: Sarcomere length-active force relations in living mammalian cardiac muscle. *Am J Physiol* 227:383–389, 1974.
99. Pollack GH, Krueger JW: Sarcomere dynamics in intact cardiac muscle. *Eur J Cardiol* 4(Suppl):53–75, 1976.
100. Pringle JWS: Models of muscle. *Symp Soc Exp Biol* 14:41–68, 1960.
101. Rack PMH, Westbury DR: The effects of length and stimulus rate on tension in isometric cat soleus muscle. *J Physiol* 204:443–460, 1969.
102. Robinson TF, Winegrad S: The measurement and dynamic implications of thin filament lengths in heart muscle. *J Physiol* 286:607–619, 1979.
103. Robinson TF, Winegrad S: A variety of intercellular connections in heart muscle. *J Mol Cell Cardiol* 13:185–195, 1981.
104. Roos KP, Brady AJ, Tan ST: Direct measurement of sarcomere length from isolated cardiac cells. *Am J Physiol* 242:H68–H78, 1982.
105. Ruegg JC, Steiger GJ, Schadler M: Mechanical activation of the contractile system. *Pflügers Arch* 319:139–145, 1970.
106. Sagawa K: The ventricular pressure-volume diagram revisited. *Circ Res* 43:677–687, 1978.
107. Samuel J-L, Marotte F, Delcayre C, Rappaport L: Microtubule reorganization is related to rate of heart myocyte hypertrophy in rat. *Am J Physiol* 251:H1118–H1125, 1986.
108. Samuel J-L, Schwartz K, Lompre AM, Delcayre C, Marotte R, Swynghedauw B, Rapppaport L: Immunological quantitation and localization of tubulin in adult rat heart isolated myocytes. *Eur J Cell Biol* 31:99–106, 1983.
109. Somerville LL, Wang K: In vivo phosphorylation of titin and nebulin in frog skeletal muscle. *Biochem Biophys Res Comm* 147:986–992, 1987.
110. Sonnenblick EH: Implications of muscle mechanics in the heart. *Fed Proc* 21:975–990, 1962.
111. Sonnenblick EH: Determinants of active state in heart muscle; force, velocity, instantaneous muscle length, time. *Fed Proc* 24:1396–1409, 1965.
112. Sonnenblick EH, Parmley WW, Parmley CW: The contractile state of the heart as expressed by force velocity relations. *Am J Cardiol* 23:488–503, 1969.
113. Steiger GJ: Stretch activation and myogenic oscillation of isolated contractile structures of heart muscle. *Pflügers Arch* 330:347–361, 1971.
114. Steiger GJ: Tension transients in extracted rabbit heart muscle preparations. *J Mol Cell Cardiol* 9:671–685, 1977.
115. Steiger GJ: Stretch activation and tension transients in cardiac, skeletal and insect flight muscle. In: Tregear RT (ed) *Insect Flight Muscle*. Amsterdam: Elsevier/North-Holland Biomedical, 1977.
116. Steiger GJ: Kinetic analysis of isometric tension transients in cardiac muscle. In: Sugi H, Pollack GH (eds) *Cross-Bridge Mechanism in Muscle Contraction*. Tokyo: University of Tokyo, 1979.
117. Steiger GJ, Abbott RH: Biochemical interpretation of tension transients produced by a four-state mechanical model. *J Muscle Res Cell Motil* 2:245–260, 1981.
118. Steiger GJ, Brady AJ, Tan ST: Intrinsic regulatory properties of contractility in the myocardium. *Circ Res* 42:339–350, 1978.
119. Tarr M, Trank JW, Goertz KK, Leiffer P: Effect of initial sarcomere length on sarcomere kinetics and force development in single frog atrial cardiac cells. *Circ Res* 49:767–774, 1981.
120. Tarr M, Trank JW, Leiffer P, Shepherd N: Sarcomere length-resting tension relation in single frog atrial cardiac cells. *Circ Res* 45:554–559, 1979.
121. Taylor SR: Decreased activation in skeletal muscle fibres at short lengths. In: *The Physiological Basis of Starling's Law of the Heart*. London: Ciba Foundation Symposium, 24, 1974.
122. Taylor SR, Rudel R: Striated muscle fibers; inactivation of contraction induced by shortening. *Science* 167:882–884, 1970.
123. Ter Keurs HEDJ: Calcium and contractility. In: Drake-Holland AJ, Noble MIM (eds) *Cardiac Metabolism*. New York: Wiley & Sons, 1983.
124. Ter Keurs HEDJ, Rijnsburger WH, van Heunigen, R: Restoring forces and relaxation of rat cardiac muscle. *Eur Heart J* 1(Suppl A):67–80, 1980.
125. Tokuyasu KT: Visualization of longitudinally oriented intermediate filaments in frozen section of chick cardiac muscle by a new staining method. *J Cell Biol* 97:562–565, 1983.
126. Van Heuningen R, Rijnsburger WH, Ter Keurs HEDJ: Sarcomere length control in striated muscle. *Am J Physiol* 242:H411–H420, 1982.
127. Wang K: Cytoskeletal matrix in striated muscle: The role of titin, nebulin and intermediate filaments. In: Pollack GH, Sugi H (eds) *Contractile Mechanisms in Muscle*. New York: Plenum Press, 170: 1984, pp 285–305.
128. Wang K, McCarter R, Wright J, Beverly J, Ramirez-Mitchell R: Viscoelasticity of the sarcomere matrix of skeletal muscles. The titin-myosin composite filament is a dual-stage molecular spring. *Biophys J* 64, 1993, pp 1161–1177.
129. Wang S-M, Greaser NL: Immunocytochemical studies using a monoclonal antibody to bovine cardiac titin on intact and extracted myofibrils. *J Muscle Res Cell Motil* 6:293–312, 1985.
130. Winegrad S: Resting sarcomere length-tension relation in living frog heart. *J Gen Physiol* 64:343–355, 1974.
131. Winegrad S, McClellan G, Robinson T, Lai N-P: Variable diastolic compliance and variable Ca^{2+} sensitivity of the contractile system in cardiac muscle. *Eur J Cardiol* 4(Suppl): 41–46, 1976.
132. Yeatman LA Jr, Parmley WW, Sonnenblick E: Effects of temperature on series elasticity and contractile element motion in heart muscle. *Am Physiol* 217:1030–1034, 1969.

CHAPTER 20

Substrate and Energy Metabolism of the Heart

L.H. OPIE

INTRODUCTION

Metabolism comes from the Greek word meaning "change". Our knowledge of metabolism of the heart is evolving and also changing, partially in response to renewed interest by clinical cardiologists, so that the field of cardiac metabolism is now going through a period of resurgence and emerging from earlier neglect {1}.

When glucose or fatty acids are changed into simple two- or three-carbon units, which can enter the Krebs citrate cycle, then metabolic pathways are in operation. Breakdown of ATP and its resynthesis is likewise part of the process of cardiac metabolism, as is the regulation of the oxygen requirement for these processes, and hence the myocardial oxygen uptake.

Because of the very high turnover rate of ATP in the myocardium, a correspondingly high rate of mitochondrial production of ATP is required. Within the mitochondria, the citrate cycle of Krebs breaks down the critical compound acetyl CoA to CO_2 and hydrogen atoms; the latter, in turn, yield electrons that are pumped out of the mitochondria to form a proton gradient across the mitochondrial membrane, a gradient that is required for the synthesis of ATP by oxidative phosphorylation. During this process the protons reenter the mitochondria, finally to combine with oxygen to form water.

Acetyl CoA is an activated two-carbon fragment, eventually derived from one of the three major substrates of the myocardium: glucose, lactate, or free fatty acids. Strictly speaking, a substrate is a chemical compound that an enzyme catalytically converts to the product of that reaction. As each energy source needs a series of catalytic reactions before it can be converted to acetyl CoA, the term *substrate* simply means a fuel for the myocardium.

This chapter discusses the pathways whereby each of the major substrates is broken down to acetyl CoA, the role of each substrate in myocardial energy production, and the metabolic reactions to myocardial ischemia and reperfusion.

GLUCOSE

Importance of glucose for metabolism of the heart

Glucose is a myocardial fuel of special historical and evolutionary interest, although the major fuel only after a carbohydrate meal (table 20-1). Historically, interest in glucose metabolism dates back to at least 1907, when Locke and Rosenheim {2} found glucose uptake by the isolated heart. Evans {3} in 1914 suggested that only one third of the heart's energy was supplied by carbohydrate oxidation. Cruickshank and his associates {4} suggested that "direct combustion" of fat, probably the blood fatty acids, met the rest of the heart's energy requirements. Thus, these early workers delineated carbohydrate and fatty acids as two of the most important myocardial fuels. From the biochemical point of view, glucose is of interest because factors controlling its uptake and utilization by glycolysis or glycogen synthesis have been extensively studied and an integrated scheme of the control of these processes has now been established (fig. 20-1). Therapeutically, glucose is of interest because of the possible use of glycolysis in maintaining anaerobic metabolism. Glucose is a component of the glucose-insulin-potassium solution now being evaluated for possible inclusion in one of the mass clinical trials of acute myocardial infarction.

Factors increasing glucose uptake

The rate of glucose uptake from the extracellular space into the heart cells is normally limited by the rate of transport of glucose across the cell membrane {5}, a process thought to involve a stereoscopic insulin-sensitive glucose transporter {6,7}.

Newsholme and Crabtree {8} have emphasized the crucial role of glucose transport as a "communication signal" in the metabolic control of glycolysis in muscle, because only glucose transport can "communicate" with both the glycolytic pathway and the circulating glucose concentration. Hence factors governing the transport of glucose are crucial in the regulation of glycolysis.

Three major factors that increase glucose uptake by the heart are insulin, hypoxia, and increased heart work (fig. 20-1). When insulin is added to the medium, it binds to

N. Sperelakis (ed.), Physiology and Pathophysiology of the Heart, Third Edition.
© *1995 Kluwer Academic Publishers. ISBN 0-7923-2612-1. All rights reserved.*

Table 20-1. Effect of nutritional state and exercise on fuel for oxidative metabolism of the human heart: Percentage of oxygen uptake accounted for, if various substrates are fully oxidized

Conditions	Glucose (OER percent)	Pyruvate (OER percent)	Lactate (OER percent)	Total CHO (OER percent)	FFA (OER percent)	TG (OER percent)	Ketones (OER percent)	Amino acids (OER percent)	RQ
Glucose and insulin	—	—	—	—	none	—	—	—	—
"Feeding"	—	—	—	92	5	—	—	—	Approaches 1.0
Postprandial, CHO meal[a]	68	4	28	100	—	—	—	—	0.94
Postprandial, lipid meal	10	—	10	20	30	50	—	—	—
Fasting, few hours[b]	31	2	28	61	34	—	5	0	—
Same during exercise	16	0	61	77	21	—	2	0	—
Same with recovery	21	2	36	59	36	—	3	0	—
Fasting overnight, resting	18	1	16	35	(67)[c]	—	5	6	—
	—	—	—	—	50[d]	—	—	—	—
	23	3	8	34	—	—	—	—	0.74
	—	—	—	30	58	—	—	—	—
	56	1	10	67	66	—	—	—	—
	15	1	13	29	70	—	9	—	—
	30	0	8	38	58	—	—	—	—
	22	1	8	31	53	14	—	—	—
	24	—	12	36	77	—	—	—	—
Mean values, fasting	27	1	11	38	62	14	7	—	0.74
Mean values, fasting corrected[e]	5	1	11	17	62	14	7	—	0.74
Mean values, fed (CHO)	68	4	28	96	5	—	—	—	0.94

[a] Subjects studied 2–3 h after a light low-fat breakfast.
[b] Subjects studied in the early afternoon after a light breakfast.
[c] Total fatty acid, includes triglyceride.
[d] Exact conditions not specified; overnight fast assumed.
[e] Corrected for actual oxidation rates of glucose.
OER = oxygen extraction ratio; CHO = carbohydrate; TG = triglyceride; RQ = respiratory quotient; — = absence of data.
Reproduced from Camici et al. {174}, with permission.

one or more insulin receptors {9} with acceleration of the activity of the glucose transporter. Acceleration of the rate of transsarcolemmal transport of glucose also occurs during the anoxic perfusion {4,10} or when the heart work is increased {11}; in either case, the rate of transport of glucose across the sarcolemma remains rate limiting {5}.

The mechanism of stimulation of the glucose transporter by hypoxia or increased heart work remains ill understood. Randle and Smith {10} proposed that the "entry of glucose ... is restrained ... by a process dependent on a supply of energy-rich phosphate." This mechanism must be different from the acceleration of glucose transport by insulin, which does not involve any changes in high-energy phosphate content and which relies on a complex intracellular signaling system {12}.

Factors decreasing glucose uptake

Conversely, glucose uptake is decreased by the diabetic state, by provision of fatty acids as alternate fuels, by decreased heart work, and by adequate myocardial oxygenation. The first two of these factors may act both by

direct inhibition of glucose transport and by inhibition of the glycolytic pathway, with a consequent increase in myocardial levels of glucose 6-phosphate and feedback inhibition of the enzyme hexokinase, which phosphorylates intracellular glucose. Hence free glucose accumulates in the cell to inhibit glucose transport.

GLYCOLYSIS

After uptake of glucose, its further metabolic pathway is that of glycolysis. By glycolysis is meant a pathway common to glucose and glycogen breakdown that converts glucose 6-phosphate to lactate in the absence of oxygen (*anaerobic glycolysis*). During normal oxidative metabolism, glycolysis yields pyruvate, which is then aerobically broken down in the citrate cycle of Krebs; conversion of glucose or glycogen to pyruvate in these circumstances may be termed *aerobic glycolysis*. Glycolysis produces ATP independently of oxygen. This process will happen whether the ultimate end point of glycolysis is the aerobic conversion of pyruvate to acetyl CoA with oxygen-

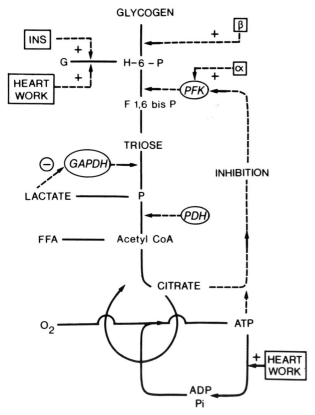

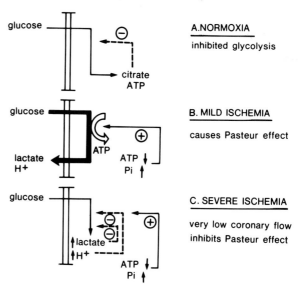

Fig. 20-2. **A:** In the normally oxygenated heart, tissue citrate and ATP are high and inhibit glycolysis. **B:** When coronary flow is mildly decreased (mild ischemia), the Pasteur effect results. **C:** In severe ischemia (severe deprivation of both oxygen and coronary flow), the accumulation of lactate and protons inhibits glycolysis despite any tendency to acceleration by a low cardiac content of ATP.

Fig. 20-1. Overall control of pathways of glycolysis, which is taken as the conversion of glucose 6-phosphate (G6P) to pyruvate (P): Ins = insulin; β = beta-adrenergic stimulation; α = alpha-adrenergic stimulation; PFK = phosphofructokinase; F 1,6bis P = fructose 1,6-diphosphate or fructose 1,6-bisphosphate; GAPDH = glyceraldehyde phosphate dehydrogenase. The basal inhibition of glycolysis at the level of phosphofructokinase is overcome by heart work (via changes in ATP/ADP and citrate) or by anoxia or mild ischemia (similar metabolic changes). During severe ischemia, when lactate accumulates in the tissue, glyceraldehyde 3-phosphate dehydrogenase is inhibited and the rate of glycolysis falls.

dependent production of ATP in the mitochondria or whether there is anaerobic glycolysis with production of only anaerobic ATP. During normal oxygenation, mitochondrial metabolism of pyruvate is the chief source of ATP from glycolysis, and the rather low rate of oxygen-independent production of ATP has not been shown to be critical. In contrast, in anaerobic circumstances, glycolysis is the sole source of ATP and therefore becomes a critical reaction. In response to anaerobiosis, glycolysis can be accelerated severalfold, a process often called the *Pasteur effect*.

"Pasteur effect"

Pasteur, working in France in 1876, discovered that unicellular microorganisms decreased their rate of "fermen-

tation" when exposed to oxygen gas. By "fermentation" he probably meant all the metabolic processes able to sustain life in the absence of oxygen {13}. Although these experiments are not directly applicable to the heart, they are often interpreted, perhaps incorrectly, to suggest that Pasteur established that glycolytic activity is increased during anaerobic conditions (fig. 20-2). The latter conclusion is now well established {3,10,14}.

Oxygen deprivation: Anaerobiosis, anoxia, hypoxia, or ischemia?

Each of the above conditions has been used to elucidate the effects of oxygen deprivation on glycolysis, but these terms are not all interchangeable. *Anoxia* is when an isolated heart is totally deprived of oxygen; the coronary flow then increases with an enhanced rate of washout of products of glycolysis, such as lactate and protons. As will be outlined, these products are potentially inhibitory to glycolysis, so that maintenance of coronary flow during anoxia ensures that there are peak rates of glycolysis and of production of anaerobic ATP {15}. Because it is difficult to ensure that the isolated heart is completely deprived of oxygen, the degree of oxygen deprivation may better be described as *hypoxia* (= too little oxygen) than as anoxia. None of these conditions, however, are directly relevant to the clinical situation in patients with coronary artery disease, where oxygen lack is almost always caused by an inadequate rate of delivery of blood to the myocardium, termed *ischemia*. The word *ischemia* is derived from two Greek words, *ischo* meaning "to hold back," and *haima* meaning "blood." Ischemia therefore means too little blood. The effects of ischemia are twofold: firstly, a reduced rate of delivery of oxygen, and secondly, a reduced rate of washout of metabolic products. Thus, in contrast to anoxia or hypoxia of the perfused heart, where coronary flow is maintained, in ischemia the coronary flow is reduced and the rate of glycolysis falls as products of glycolytic metabolism accumulate in the ischemic myocardium.

Anaerobiosis is a term that should strictly equate with anoxia (*an* = no; *aerobiosis* = presence of air, and therefore of oxygen). In practice, however, anaerobiosis is applied to any state of oxygen lack associated with the production of lactate by the myocardium, the process being termed *anaerobic glycolysis*.

PHOSPHOFRUCTOKINASE ACTIVITY

Much later the biochemical basis for these observations was laid by Randle et al. in Cambridge and Morgan's group in Nashville, Tennessee. They induced anoxia in isolated perfused hearts and established that the increased glycolytic flux was governed by a series of reactions, including acceleration of glucose transport into the cell and increased activity of the rate-limiting enzyme phosphofructokinase (which converts fructose 6-phosphate to fructose 1,6-bisphosphate). Fructose 6-phosphate is, in turn, derived by an equilibrium reaction from glucose 6-phosphate, the common meeting point of the pathways of glucose uptake and glycogen breakdown. In simplified form the equations from glucose uptake are

glucose + ATP → glucose 6-phosphate + ADP   (20-1)

glucose 6-phosphate ⇌ fructose 6-phosphate   (20-2)

fructose 6-phosphate + ATP →
$\qquad$ fructose 1,6-bisphosphate + ADP (20-3)

fructose 1,6-bisphosphate ⇌ glyceraldehyde
$\qquad$ 3-phosphate + dihydroxyacetone-P (20-4)

dihydroxyacetone-P ⇌ glyceraldehyde 3-phosphate (20-5)

The enzymes concerned are, respectively, hexokinase, hexosephosphate isomerase (= phosphoglucose isomerase), phosphofructokinase, aldolase, and triose phosphate isomerase. Only eqs. (20-1) and (20-3) are thought to have regulatory properties.

Evidence for control at the level of phosphofructokinase may be summarized as follows. First, the activity of the enzyme is low among the enzymes of glycolysis. Secondly, the mass action ratio of the reactants is far removed from the apparent equilibrium constant; hence, some factor is keeping the reactants from reaching equilibrium and that factor is probably the activity of the enzyme. Thirdly, flow through the enzyme can increase even when the tissue content of its substrate (fructose 6-phosphate) falls, as in anoxia. Fourthly, the enzyme has been isolated and has complex allosteric properties, including inhibition by ATP (and probably creatine phosphate), by citrate, and by a

low pH; on the other hand, there is relief of inhibition by products of ATP (such as adenosine diphosphate, inorganic phosphate, and adenosine monophosphate) or by a decreased citrate concentration or by alkalosis. Situations have been found where all these in vitro properties can be mimicked in the whole perfused heart, thus strongly supporting the controlling role of phosphofructokinase. An additional recently described, but not yet fully established, effector of the enzyme is fructose 2,6-bisphosphate {16}. Although a product of glycolysis, it is not an intermediate. It potently stimulates phosphofructokinase. It is produced from fructose 6-phosphate by an enzyme whose activity increases in response to some of the other effectors of PFK such as inorganic phosphate and AMP.

Glyceraldehyde 3-phosphate dehydrogenase

It has long been appreciated that control of glycolysis could pass from phosphofructokinase to other points down the line of glycolysis during extreme conditions, such as severe total ischemia {17} or an abrupt normoxic-anoxic transition {18}. Regulation of glycolysis at the site of

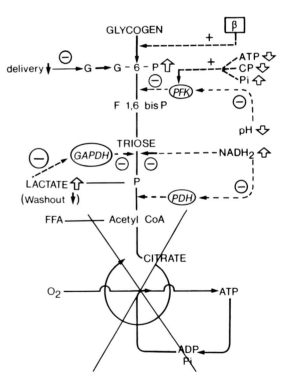

Fig. 20-3. Effect of severe ischemia in inhibiting glycolytic flux. Abbreviations as in fig. 20-1. Note inhibition of glycolysis by acidosis at level of phosphofructokinase and by NADH₂, and lactate accumulation at level of glyceraldehyde-3-phosphate dehydrogenase (GAPDH). In severe ischemia, the basic problem is lack of washout of inhibitory metabolites (protons, lactate). From Opie LH: The Heart: Physiology and Metabolism. Orlando, FL: Grune and Stratton, 1984, with permission.

the enzyme glyceraldehyde phosphate dehydrogenase (GAPDH) is probably the most important in explaining ischemic inhibition of glycolysis.

During severe total ischemia, glycolysis is inhibited rather than stimulated (fig. 20-3). In mild ischemia, the Pasteur effect accelerates glucose uptake and glycolytic flux through stimulation of glucose uptake and of phosphofructokinase; in severe ischemia, phosphofructokinase is inhibited by acidosis, while glyceraldehyde-3-phosphate dehydrogenase is inhibited by several products of glycolysis {19,20}. The molecular mechanisms involved are not known. The inhibitory powers of lactate are found on the crude enzyme preparation but not on the purified enzyme {20}. The inhibitory effect of lactate is independent of any pH effect, although protons also inhibit glyceraldehyde 3-phosphate dehydrogenase by a separate mechanism {21}. High concentrations of NADH (next section) strongly inhibit the enzyme {20}.

Anaerobic glycolysis will tend to slow down as tissue NADH and lactate rise to inhibit glyceraldehyde 3-phosphate dehydrogenase and as protons accumulate to inhibit phosphofructokinase. The tissue pH falls with increasing severity of ischemia {22}, one factor explaining greater glycolytic inhibition with increasing ischemia {23}. Such deceleration of glycolysis will slow down the rate of formation of protons, which are derived from ATP turnover (next section). Hence there appears to be a self-protective mechanism:

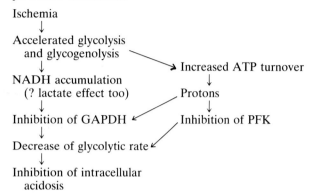

the enzyme glyceraldehyde phosphate dehydrogenase

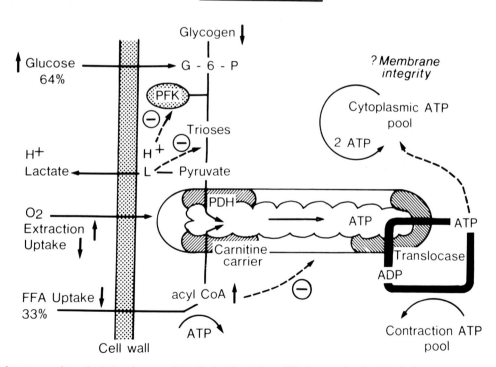

Cell wall

Fig. 20-4. Substrate supply to the ischemic zone of developing dog infarct 100 minutes after ligation {82}. Note the following changes. Although oxygen extraction is increased, there is decreased flow and net oxygen uptake is reduced. Free fatty acid extraction is reduced and, therefore, uptake is also reduced. Glucose extraction is increased but the uptake may be either unchanged or actually decreased because of the effect of reduced coronary flow. Although there is some output of lactate and protons, there is also intracellular accumulation with inhibition of phosphofructokinase (PFK) and of glyceraldehyde-3-phosphate dehydrogenase. An intracellular accumulation of acyl CoA may inhibit the translocase transporting ATP outwards from the mitochondria.

The complex interaction between carbohydrate and lipid metabolism in regional ischemia (developing myocardial infarction) is shown in fig. 20-4.

Proton production by anaerobic glycolysis

During anaerobic glycolysis, the reduced cofactor (NADH + H^+, which equals $NADH_2$) formed by the enzyme glyceraldehyde-3-phosphate dehydrogenase is reconverted to NAD during the formation of lactate. The overall reaction produces two molecules of ATP, independently of oxygen. Thus during anaerobic glycolysis protons are not formed. Why, then, is anaerobic glycolysis usually held to be proton producing and a potential source of intracellular acidosis?

Gevers {24} and Dennis et al. {25} have examined this question in detail. When all the charges are written into the individual glycolytic reactions, and allowance is made for the probable degree of interaction of ADP and ATP with Mg^{2+}, the following equations are derived:

$$\text{glucose} + 2\,MgADP^{1-} + 2\,Pi^{2-} \rightarrow$$
$$2\,\text{lactate}^{1-} + 2\,MgATP^{2-} \quad (20\text{-}6)$$

In anaerobic conditions, ATP will be broken down as fast as it is produced. Protons are produced by the breakdown of ATP:

$$2\,MgATP^{2-} \rightarrow 2\,MgADP^{1-} + 2\,Pi^{2-} + 2\,H^+ \quad (20\text{-}7)$$

These equations are only approximations and depend on a number of assumptions, including the concentration of free Mg^{2+} in the cytosol and the intracellular pH (the latter influencing the phosphate charge). Thus the turnover of glycolytically made ATP (and not the production of lactate) is the "source" of the protons produced during anaerobic glycolysis.

Glucose metabolism and glycolysis: Critical features

1. The rate of transport of glucose across the sarcolemma by the stereospecific glucose transporter is of major importance in controlling the rate of glucose uptake by the heart.
2. Glucose transport is accelerated by insulin, hypoxia, and increased heart work, which also increase the rate of flow through glycolysis by increasing the activity of the enzyme phosphofructokinase. Insulin increases glycolysis by stimulating the transporter, thereafter intracellular glucose is phosphorylated to glucose 6-phosphate and then converted to fructose 6-phosphate, which is the substrate for the enzyme phosphofructokinase. Anoxia and increased heart work both directly increase glucose transport. Anoxia also acts by breakdown of high-energy phosphate compounds that form products that relieve the inhibition that high levels of ATP exert on phosphofructokinase.
3. In aerobic conditions (normal oxygenation), the end point of glycolysis is pyruvate, which enters the citrate cycle of Krebs for further aerobic metabolism to form ATP.
4. In anaerobic conditions, the end point of glycolysis is

lactate; the rates of anaerobic glycolysis are not high enough to provide sufficient energy for the contracting heart but can provide for the needs of the potassium-arrested heart.
5. In ischemia, the coronary flow rate falls sufficiently to restrict both the supply of oxygen and the washout of metabolites.
6. In mild ischemia, the net effect of these processes is to stimulate glycolysis.
7. In severe ischemia, the products of glycolysis accumulate to inhibit glycolytic flux at the level of phosphofructokinase and glyceraldehyde-3-phosphate dehydrogenase. Hence, in severe ischemia, when glycolysis is most needed to produce anaerobic ATP, glycolysis is also least able to perform this vital function.

Thus far the input into glycolysis from the uptake of glucose from the circulation has been discussed. Another source of glycolysis is the breakdown of glycogen.

GLYCOGEN

Basic concepts

Glycogen is a polysaccharide (i.e., a combination of many molecules of glucose) that forms large storage granules in the cytoplasm of the heart. Although frequently thought of as a "storage" carbohydrate, the glycogen molecule is in a constant state of turnover as a result of variable rates of synthesis and degradation. In contrast to the very detailed understanding of the complex chemical signals controlling glycogen synthesis and breakdown, the physiologic function of cardiac glycogen remains poorly understood. Glycogen is not used as a reserve carbohydrate fuel for the heart during fasting, because the glycogen content of the heart rises during fasting and falls in the fed state. These changes in the glycogen content can be related to changes in blood free fatty acids. When blood free fatty acid concentrations are high, as during fasting, then glycolysis is inhibited with increased synthesis of cardiac glycogen {26} in response to an increased tissue content of glucose 6-phosphate. In the fed state, blood free fatty acid concentrations are low and so is cardiac glycogen, despite the high rates of glucose uptake and the activity of insulin that stimulates glycogen synthesis. The probable explanation is that in the fed state a high rate of glycogen turnover is accompanied by high rates of synthesis and breakdown of glycogen, especially the outer glycogen chains. The effects of insulin may explain at least some of these changes {27}.

Glycogen synthesis

The pathways of glycogen synthesis are separate from those of glycogen breakdown because there are two different enzyme systems (fig. 20-5). Glycogen synthesis starts with conversion of glucose 6-phosphate to glucose 1-phosphate. The critical step in glycogen synthesis is the transfer of glucose 1-phosphate to the end of a preexisting glycogen chain. The chief enzyme regulating this process is

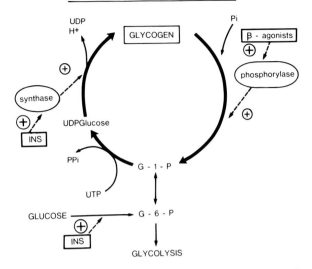

GLYCOGEN SYNTHESIS AND BREAKDOWN

Fig. 20-5. Control of glycogen metabolism. Note different pathways for synthesis, which is controlled by glycogen synthase (= synthetase), when compared with glucose breakdown, which is controlled by glycogen phosphorylase.

glycogen synthase (= glycogen synthetase = glycogen transferase), which exists in the more active *a* form and the less active *b* form. Glycogen synthesis requires the presence of high-energy phosphate — not as ATP, but as uridine triphosphate, derived from ATP. Hence glycogen synthesis cannot take place in a state of energy depletion.

The mode of action of insulin in stimulating glycogen synthesis is very complex {9} and not fully understood. Insulin increases the percentage of glycogen synthase in the more active *a* form, possibly by controlling the phosphatase enzyme that converts the interconversion of the two forms of the synthase. Thus glycogen synthesis is diminished as the activity of the synthase phosphatase falls {28}.

Besides the presence of insulin, the other major factor stimulating glycogen synthesis is a high cellular content of glucose 6-phosphate. Conditions increasing the cardiac contents of glucose 6-phosphate are (a) high circulating insulin and glucose, as after a meal; (b) inhibition of glycolysis, as when the heart is using fatty acids during fasting or in severe diabetes. In the latter two situations, the continued buildup of cardiac glycogen will eventually inhibit its own synthesis, which explains why a high level of glycogen is accompanied by a low rate of turnover. In contrast, during provision of glucose and insulin, glycolysis is accelerated and not inhibited, and the outer chains of glycogen that are formed are rapidly broken down, so that the overall level of glycogen does not rise despite the increased rate of synthesis.

Glycogen breakdown

The two major mechanisms for stimulating glycogen breakdown are mediated either by cyclic AMP or, in anoxia, by a fall in high-energy phosphate levels. Cyclic AMP promotes the cascade that eventually converts the inactive glycogen phosphorylase *b* to the highly active phosphorylase *a*. Thus

catecholamine stimulus → beta-adrenergic receptor → adenylate cyclase → cyclic AMP activation of protein kinase A → activation of phosphorylase *b* kinase → conversion of phosphorylase *b* to *a* → breakdown of glygogen.

Calmodulin, the intracellular calcium-binding receptor protein, is one of the subunits of phosphorylase *b* kinase; hence, calcium ions are required for the formation of phosphorylase *b*.

Another mechanism for promotion of glycogenolysis is by enhancing the activity of phosphorylase *b*, that is, without its conversion to the *a* form. This process, which occurs independently of adrenergic stimulation, is set in motion by the formation of adenosine monophosphate and inorganic phosphate from the breakdown of ATP {29}. Hence, in ischemia glycogenolysis is enhanced by both the cyclic AMP-dependent formation of phosphorylase *a* and the enhanced activity of phosphorylase *b* as ATP breakdown.

Function of cardiac glycogen

Cardiac glycogen is a potential source of glycolysis and hence of anaerobic ATP; yet the oxygen uptake of the heart is so avid that the cardiac glycogen content would have to be extremely high and glycogenolysis extremely rapid for glycogen to be the major fuel of the heart over a long period.

When there is a sudden severe spurt of work, very rapid glycogen breakdown within seconds may protect the heart from an acute lack of external fuel {30}. Many workers have thought that a measure of glycogen breakdown occurs with each cardiac cycle, but there is as yet no proof for this hypothesis. Glycogen may act as a storage "buffer" for carbon from glucose taken up from the circulation. In the fasted state in humans, the major part of the glucose uptake is not oxidized, but probably converted to glycogen with delayed oxidation {31}.

In total ischemia in the rat heart, glycogen breakdown may either help to preserve the myocardium {32} or to increase ischemic damage {33}. The major reason for these apparently conflicting results probably lies in the duration of total ischemia. After 30 minutes of total ischemia in the rat heart {33}, the tissue lactate values were about twice those found after 15 minutes {32}, so that more substantial inhibition of glycolysis could be expected when reperfusion follows more prolonged ischemia. It is, nevertheless, worth noting that glycogen depletion did not protect from 30 minutes of ischemia in the rabbit heart {34}. During postischemic recovery, enhanced glycogen resynthesis may account for the increased myocardial uptake of ^{18}F-fluorodeoxyglucose in patients {35}.

LACTATE

Competition of lactate with other substrates for myocardial oxygen uptake

The uptake of lactate can account for about 10% of the oxygen uptake of the heart of a resting, fasting person (table 20-1). When the blood lactate rises, as during vigorous exercise, lactate can account for about 60% of the myocardial oxygen uptake.

There is competition between lactate and free fatty acids for the myocardial oxygen uptake; either can be a major fuel, depending on the blood levels (table 20-1). The probable mechanism whereby lactate decreases free fatty acid metabolism is by inhibition of activation of thiokinase {36}; the probable mechanism whereby free fatty acids inhibit lactate metabolism is by inhibition of the enzyme complex pyruvate dehydrogenase {22,37}.

Pathways of lactate

The uptake of lactate by the heart depends on a stereo-specific transport mechanism. The sarcolemma is not entirely freely permeable to lactate, and a "permease" has been postulated {38}. The process appears to involve cotransport with protons. Once taken up, intracellular lactate is converted by lactate dehydrogenase to pyruvate, thereby joining the pyruvate derived from glycolysis.

Lactate dehydrogenase

The following reaction is freely reversible:

$$\text{lactate} + NAD^+ \rightleftharpoons \text{pyruvate} + NADH + H^+ \quad (20\text{-}8)$$

Thus, in conditions of adequate oxygenation and a high rate of lactate uptake, the equation proceeds toward pyruvate. In anaerobiosis, when NAD and H^+ accumulate and pyruvate cannot undergo dehydrogenation, the reaction proceeds toward lactate. The myocardial activity of lactate dehydrogenase is high enough to make it unlikely that it could be a rate-limiting enzyme. There are five LDH isoenzymes, named in order of rapidity of electrophoretic migration; each isoenzyme is a tetrameric unit composed of four subunits of the H or M type, where H is the form predominating in the heart and M in skeletal muscle. The major interest in the isoenzymes stems from their liberation into the bloodstream in patients with acute myocardial infarction.

Lactate discharge from the myocardium

When the heart is rendered ischemic, about 25% by mass must be ischemic before there is lactate discharge into the coronary sinus {11}. Such discharge is traditionally regarded as a good sign of myocardial anaerobic metabolism and hence of ischemia {39}. Decreased lactate extraction (without actual discharge) is not a reliable indicator of ischemia because lactate uptake can be inhibited by uptake of circulating free fatty acids {40}. An example of added knowledge gained by measurements of lactate discharge

across the heart, which requires coronary sinus catheterization, is in patients with thyrotoxicosis, in whom lactate-producing angina can occur even in the presence of normal coronary arteries {41}.

There are unusual circumstances in which lactate discharge occurs from the heart apparently in the absence of oxygen limitation: (a) the neonatal heart in situ; (b) experimental states in which the extracellular fluid contains little or no lactate, as in the isolated heart perfused with glucose as the only substrate; (c) sometimes in the transplanted heart; (d) intermittently in some apparently normal awake dogs with chronically implanted coronary sinus catheters; and (e) in some apparently normal patients (for references, see Opie {42}).

PYRUVATE

The circulating concentration of pyruvate is usually very low so that it only accounts for a small part of the myocardial oxygen uptake of the normal heart (table 20-1). The major pathways of pyruvate are either aerobic oxidation via pyruvate dehydrogenase and the citrate cycle, or anaerobic conversion to lactate. Anaerobic conversion to lactate helps to convert back to NAD^+, the NADH + H^+ accumulating during anaerobic glycolysis, and is therefore an essential part of the anaerobic pathway. Aerobic oxidation of pyruvate requires first the activity of pyruvate dehydrogenase.

Pyruvate dehydrogenase

Pyruvate dehydrogenase is a multienzyme compound with a very high molecular weight situated on the inner mitochondrial membrane. Pyruvate dehydrogenase can exist in either an active or inactive form. In the fed state only about 20% of the enzyme is in the active form, but increased provision of pyruvate from increased glycolytic flux can increase the activity up to 60–90% {43}. Increased heart work increases the percentage of the active form, acting at least in part through changes in the redox state of the mitochondria (fall of NAD^+ to NADH ratio {44–46}). Increased intramitochondrial calcium, as may occur with increased heart work, may also activate the enzyme {47} (for reservations, see Kobayashi and Neely {44}).

$$\text{pyruvate} + CoA + NAD^+ \overset{PDH}{\rightarrow}$$
$$\text{acetyl CoA} + CO_2 + NADH + H^+ \quad (20\text{-}9)$$

A specific kinase, pyruvate dehydrogenase kinase, phosphorylates and inactivates the enzyme. The kinase is activated by the end products, acetyl CoA and NADH, which, therefore, inactivate pyruvate dehydrogenase.

Furthermore, the active form of the enzyme is subject to end-product inhibition by acetyl CoA and NADH. Thus when NADH rises, as in anaerobiosis, then flux through pyruvate dehydrogenase is inhibited {44}. NADH also accumulates during the metabolism of fatty acids, a process that therefore inhibits pyruvate dehydrogenase {48}.

Transamination

In the anaerobic heart, there is formation of alanine from pyruvate by transamination. ATP is ultimately produced via GTP as succinate is formed. Of clinical significance is that infusion of glutamate improves the resistance of patients with effort angina to pacing {49}, presumably by production of GTP.

Transamination to replenish the citrate cycle

Another role of transamination may be as follows. If the citrate cycle suddenly speeds up due to a work jump, and glycolysis or lipolysis fails to deliver the required amount of acetyl CoA, the cardiac stores of amino acids can be used to form citrate-cycle intermediates by transamination. Such reactions, filling up the citrate cycle, are *anaplerotic reactions*. The potential effectiveness of this mechanism is seen by comparing the tissue value of aspartate (about $5\,\mu M$ fresh weight) with the mitochondrial oxaloacetate concentration, thought to be about $100\,pM/g$ in the working heart {45}. Thus only a very little aspartate is required to "top up" mitochondrial oxaloacetate. Asparate alone could not make a sustained contribution to the maintenance of sustained high rates of citrate cycle activity, which requires input from acetyl CoA from glycolysis or fatty acid metabolism.

COORDINATED CONTROL OF GLYCOLYSIS

The idea that there is a coordinated control of flow through glycolysis and through pyruvate dehydrogenase receives support from the many conjoint metabolic signals that act both on phosphofructokinase and on pyruvate dehydrogenase. Closest coordination of control of glycolysis is possible when the same closely related signals enhance the activities of these two major enzymes, as at the acute onset of increased heart work. Then glycolysis is accelerated by an increased glucose uptake with a greater supply of substrate for phosphofructokinase, and by transient changes in high-energy phosphate compounds only in some isolated heart models. Pyruvate dehydrogenase activity is accelerated by the decreased cellular NADH, by a fall in acetyl CoA, and possibly by an influx of Ca^{2+} into the mitochondria. Increased heart work directly stimulates transfer of glucose across the cell membrane, possibly acting by stretch receptors.

In the case of addition of insulin, glucose uptake is stimulated to increase formation of the substrates of phosphofructokinase and hence to increase flow through glycolysis. A third example of coordinated control is when the heart uses noncarbohydrate fuels such as fatty acids and ketone bodies; then phosphofructokinase is inhibited by a high level of citrate, while pyruvate dehydrogenase is both inhibited and inactivated, probably by the increased NADH and the rising level of acetyl CoA. Thus the whole flux through glycolysis is much decreased.

There is one important stimulus, anaerobiosis, which accelerates glycolysis but inhibits pyruvate entry into the citrate cycle. Anaerobiosis increases glucose transport into the cell and the activity of phosphofructokinase by changes in high-energy phosphates and by decreasing tissue citrate, whereas the accumulation of NADH inhibits active pyruvate dehydrogenase. The net result is acceleration of glycolysis with lactate output as its end result.

When anaerobiosis is part of severe ischemia, accumulated end products of glycolysis act to inhibit glycolytic flux.

FREE FATTY ACIDS

The importance of free fatty acids (FFA = nonesterified fatty acids = NEFA) as fuel for the human heart was originally stressed by the studies of Bing {50} and Bing et al. {51,52}, who found that carbohydrate only accounted for a minor part of the oxygen taken up by the heart, with the rest coming from fatty acid. Shipp et al. {26} found that free fatty acids inhibited the myocardial oxygenation of glucose. FFA inhibit the metabolism of glucose at several sites {43} and are the dominant fuel for the human heart, especially in the fasted state. The suppression of glycolysis by fatty acids must involve beta-oxidation, as shown by the improved glycolytic flux rate when crucial steps in fatty acid oxidation are inhibited {53}. Clinical interest in the metabolism of FFA has been stimulated by evidence that excess FFA can in certain circumstances be toxic to the heart and promote the severity of ischemia in some experiments.

Free fatty acid uptake by the heart: General factors

The general factors increasing the rate of uptake in the heart of FFA include (a) a high circulating concentration of FFA and (b) an increased circulating molar ratio of FFA to its carrier albumin.

That the rate of removal of products of FFA metabolism by oxidation can influence the uptake of FFA by the isolated rat heart is suggested because (a) there is a correlation between the rates of uptake and oxidation of FFA, (b) intracellular FFA and intermediates such as acyl CoA accumulate when fatty acid oxidation is blocked by the addition of acetoacetate {54} or by an alteration in the structure of the fatty acid chain, and (c) there is accumulation of intracellular FFA when the circulating concentration is high and the oxidative capacity of the system is blocked (for references, see Opie {55}).

FFA can also be released from the heart {36,56}. There is, however, no simple equilibrium between uptake and release because in vivo the type of FFA found in the intracellular and extracellular spaces is not the same {57}.

When the heart is perfused with equimolar mixtures of fatty acids, the molecular structure of fatty acid chain may regulate FFA uptake {58}. Differences between the various fatty acids may be explained by the varying affinity of the carrier albumin for the fatty acid and by the different intracellular rates of disposal.

Transport of FFA across the cell membrane

Contrary to the case of glucose, transport across the cell wall does not involve any hormonal-sensitive step, nor is it accelerated by anoxia {58}. The rate of transport of labeled FFA across the sarcolemmal membrane is rather similar to the rate across the capillary membrane and may simply be a physical process {36}.

Intracellular FFA and intracellular binding protein

The measured FFA values in the heart cell are very much lower than those in the circulation {59}, perhaps because there is a fatty acid binding protein (FABP) to which FFA binds with a high affinity. This 40-kDa protein is found both in endothelial cells and in the sarcolemma. The rate of interaction of FFA with the endothelial FABP may help regulate the uptake of FFA, which appears to occur by a nondiffusional process {58}. The sequence appears to be

albumin-bound FFA → free circulating FFA → interaction with FA binding protein of endothelial cells → binding with sarcolemmal FA binding protein → intracellular free FFA → some activated and metabolized; others remain bound.

Activation of intracellular FFA

Intracellular FFA can be activated by a reaction requiring ATP, reduced CoA, and Mg^{2+} (fig. 20-6). "Once the molecule has entered this reaction, it must proceed to be either esterified or oxidized" {36}. Using palmitate as an example,

$$\text{palmitate} + \text{CoA} + \text{ATP} \xrightarrow{Mg^{2+}}$$
$$\text{palmityl CoA} + \text{AMP} + \text{PPi} \quad (20\text{-}10)$$

Thus long-chain fatty acid is converted to long-chain acyl CoA. Pyrophosphate is enzymatically hydrolyzed to make the reaction irreversible:

$$\text{PPi} + H_2O \rightarrow 2\ \text{Pi} \quad (20\text{-}11)$$

The reaction rate is decreased by accumulation of acyl CoA and AMP, as in ischemia. During increased heart work, activation of citrate synthase {45} converts acetyl CoA to citrate and CoA. The increased CoA would help increase the rate of the fatty acid activation to help increase the uptake of FFAs required as fuel {60}.

Acyl CoA and carnitine

Acyl CoA has two possible fates: (a) transport into the mitochondria and (b) formation of triglyceride and other glycerides. The former mechanism depends on carnitine, which is a relatively simple compound of widespread distribution, with some properties resembling those of a vitamin. The structure is

$$(CH_3)_3N^+ \cdot CH_2 \cdot CH(OH) \cdot CH_2 \cdot COO^-.$$

How does carnitine act? Fritz {61} made the fundamental suggestion that the "presence of carnitine in muscle and other tissue may facilitate the transfer of long-chain fatty acids to the enzymatically active intramitochondrial sites for fatty acid oxidation." Carnitine reacts with acyl CoA:

$$\text{carnitine} + \text{acyl CoA} \xrightarrow{\text{CAT-I}} \text{acyl carnitine} + \text{CoA} \quad (20\text{-}12)$$

MALONYL CoA AND CAT-I

The cardiac form of CAT-I is very sensitive to inhibition by malonyl CoA, an intermediate in the pathway of elongation of exogenous fatty acids {62}. A speculative proposal is that during conditions of glucose loading of the heart, and when insulin is also present, formation of malonyl CoA from acetyl CoA is enhanced. This process occurs under the influence of the enzyme acetyl CoA carboxylase. Increased formation of malonyl CoA inhibits the activity of CAT-I {62}. Thus malonyl CoA may be a metabolic signal whereby promotion of carbohydrate metabolism could inhibit fatty acid metabolism in the heart.

CARNITINE ACYL TRANSFERASE-II

Fritz and Yue {63} made the further proposal that acyl carnitine "may function as a carrier to transport the acyl group from acyl CoA past mitochondrial barriers to the fatty acid oxidase system." They proposed that acyl CoA existed in two pools, one within the mitochondria and one in the cytoplasm. These pools were separated by the inner-mitochondrial membrane, and they proposed that acyl carnitine, but not acyl CoA, could cross that barrier. The intramitochondrial pool of acyl CoA is regulated by the reaction

$$\text{acyl carnitine} + \text{CoA} \xrightarrow{\text{CAT-II}}$$
$$\text{intramitochondrial acyl CoA} + \text{carnitine} \quad (20\text{-}13)$$

Specific antibodies have shown the existence of carnitine transferases localized, respectively, to the outer portion of the inner-mitochondrial membrane (carnitine acyl transferase-I or CAT-I) and to the inner portion of the membrane (carnitine acyl transferase-II or CAT-II). The carnitine formed intramitochondrially is transported outwards by carnitine-acyl-carnitine exchange mechanism {64–66}. The intramitochondrial acyl CoA enters the fatty acid oxidation spiral.

The above scheme explains how extramitochondrial FFA are transferred to acyl CoA within the mitochondria. The next step is beta-oxidation, with the ultimate production of acetyl CoA, which enters the citrate cycle. At this level, carnitine plays an additional, more subtle, and less immediately obvious role, because it can react with acetyl CoA to form acetyl carnitine.

The proposal is that transfer of acetyl carnitine across the inner mitochondrial membrane can help to couple rates of cytosolic fatty acid activation to mitochondrial oxidation rates {67}. Thus the end result of provision of excess fatty acids is that intramitochondrial acetyl CoA rises, acetyl carnitine is exported outwards, and cytosolic acetyl carnitine rises to form more cytosolic acetyl CoA with a fall in cytosolic CoA. Hence there is less CoA

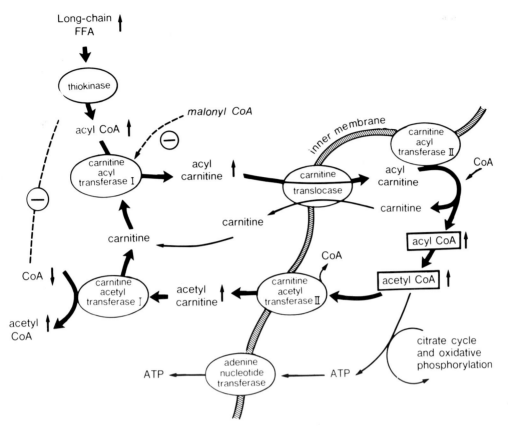

Fig. 20-6. Mechanism of feedback inhibition whereby excess circulating FFA (free fatty acid) increases acyl CoA and acetyl CoA levels in myocardial cells, with feedback inhibition to limit FFA activation. Scheme shows steps thought to be required to transport extramitochondrial acyl CoA to within the mitochondrion. The inner membrane represents the permeability barrier. The inner-mitochondrial enzymes are carnitine acyl transferase II, carnitine translocase (= carnitine acyl carnitine translocase), carnitine acetyl transferase II, and adenine nucleotide transferase. Such enzymes are required in transporting acyl carnitine inward and carnitine, acetyl carnitine, and ATP outward. The enzymes carnitine acyl transferase I and carnitine acetyl transferase I are held to be located on the outer part of the inner-mitochondrial membrane. The two carnitine acyl transferase may be in close physical opposition to the carnitine translocase. Note that the evidence for two carnitine acetyl transferases is disputed. The proposed reactions to an increased supply of blood free fatty acids are shown as an increase (↑) or decrease (↓) of intermediates. Modified from Opie {173} with permission of the *American Heart Journal.* For details, see Opie {173}.

available for fatty acid oxidation, which therefore falls (this sequence is shown in fig. 20-6). When mitochondrial oxidation increases, as during increased heart work, this series of reactions is thought to be reversed so that fatty acid activation is now enhanced.

Acyl CoA inhibition of adenine nucleotide translocase

Pande and Blanchaer {68} made the fundamental discovery that low concentrations of acyl CoA could instantly and reversibly inhibit heart mitochondria from using external ADP, which is required for oxidative phosphorylation to proceed. The inhibitory effect of acyl CoA resembled that of atractyloside, a known inhibitor of the adenine nucleotide translocase {69}, which acts by a "swing-door" mechanism to permit entry of ADP and exit of ATP from the nitochondria (ping-pong model).

Shug et al. {70} showed that myocardial ischemia, produced by coronary artery ligation in the dog, caused the twin changes of accumulation of long-chain acyl CoA and decreased activity of the adenine nucleotide translocase. Yet it is uncertain whether the inhibition of the translocase induced by acyl CoA has pathophysiologic significance {71,72}. A further question is whether the Klingenberg translocase model needs modification because some evidence suggests the formation of a carrier–nucleotide-ternary complex {73}.

Beta-oxidation

Beta-oxidation converts acyl CoA to acetyl CoA, passing through the fatty acid oxidation spiral, which removes two-carbon fragments as acetyl CoA from the carboxyl (—COOH) end of the chain. The enzymes of beta-

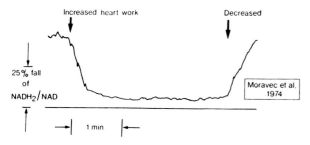

Fig. 20-7. Effect of increased heart work in isolated rat heart in increasing the fluorescence emission in the direction of NAD so that the ratio $NAD/NADH_2$ rises. The conditions selected are such that the fluorescence changes reflect chiefly the mitochondrial $NAD/NADH_2$ ratio. $NADH_2/NAD = (NAD^+)/(NADH)(H^+)$. Note that in the heart in situ these changes are controversial (see text) and some evidence suggests an increased rather than a decreased $NADH_2/NAD$ ratio. Modified from Moravec et al. {46} by permission of Academic Press.

oxidation are loosely organized into a multienzyme complex in which the intermediates never leave the complex, except for entering and departing, moving on to the next enzyme in the spiral {60}. The basic reactions are as follows:

1. Removal of two hydrogens from acyl CoA, with the conversion of FAD to $FADH_2$, to yield the alpha-beta-unsaturated acyl CoA.
2. Regaining of a hydroxyl group, derived from water, to give beta-hydroxyacyl CoA.
3. An important dehydrogenase reaction, converting NAD^+ to NADH and the hydroxyl group to a ketone group:

    beta-hydroxyacyl CoA + $NAD^+ \rightarrow$
    beta-ketoacyl CoA + NADH + H^+.

4. Finally, the beta-ketoacyl compound reacts with CoA to split off two carbons as acetyl CoA:

    beta-ketoacyl CoA + CoA $\rightarrow$
    acetyl CoA + (a shorter acyl CoA chain).

5. The shortened acyl CoA chain enters step 1 for a further turn of the spiral.

During *increased heart work* of the isolated rat heart, the mitochondria become more oxidized (fig. 20-7) {45,46} and intramitochondrial levels of $NADH_2$, and, presumably, of $FADH_2$ fall, and reactions 1 and 3 are accelerated; there is an increased turnover of the whole fatty acid oxidation spiral {74}.

Conversely, during *deprivation of oxygen*, intramitochondrial NADH rises {45} and probably so does $FADH_2$. The basic defect is probably impaired beta-oxidation due to decreased electron transport. Intermediates of fatty acid metabolism accumulate {75}. The rate of oxidation of beta-hydroxyacyl CoA (reaction 3 above) may be the rate-limiting step in fatty acid beta-oxidation by the oxygen-deficient heart.

FORMATION OF TRIGLYCERIDE AND GLYCERIDE

Triglyceride can be formed from acyl CoA and alpha-glycerophosphate, the latter derived from glycolysis by the process of *esterification*, as follows:
1. acyl CoA + alpha-glycerol-P $\rightarrow$ acyl glycerol-P + CoA
2. acyl glycerol-P + CoA $\rightarrow$
    diacylglycerol-P (phosphatidic acid) + CoA
3. diacylglycerol-P $\rightarrow$ diacylglycerol (diglyceride) + Pi
4. diglyceride + acyl CoA $\rightarrow$ triglyceride + CoA.

When the overall equation for triglyceride formation from FFA is written out, and allowance is made for the changes, we have {24}:

$$3 \text{ palmitate}^{1-} + 3 \text{ MgATP}^{2-} + 3 \text{ CoA}^{4-} \rightarrow$$
$$3 \text{ palmityl-CoA}^{4-} + 3 \text{ AMP}^{2-} + 6 \text{ Pi}^{2-} + 3\text{H}^+ +$$
$$3 \text{ Mg}^{2+} \quad (20\text{-}14)$$

$$\text{glycerol-3-phosphate}^{2-} + 3 \text{ palmityl-CoA}^{4-} \rightarrow$$
$$\text{triglyceride} + 3 \text{ CoA}^{4-} + \text{Pi}^{2-} \quad (20\text{-}15)$$

For every mole of triglyceride synthesized, there is the production of three protons, occurring at the stage of fatty acid activation. Continued triglyceride turnover in severe ischemia may, theoretically, be proton generating and be potentially harmful {24,25}.

Cardiac lipolysis

Lipolysis in the heart is under the influence of a hormonally sensitive lipase. When the heart is deprived of external fuels, there is lipolysis of endogenous triglycerides to provide energy {57}. Not all the triglyceride, however, is available for such energetic purposes because about one fifth remains even when the heart is exhausted by substrate depletion. For the normal heart in situ receiving an adequate supply of external substrate, endogenous lipid is not an energy source. There is indirect evidence for the existence of a "triglyceride-FFA cycle" {25,76}, the turnover of which is thought to be increased in ischemia {77}. There is an interesting paradox whereby in severe ischemia the turnover of this cycle is proton producing as expected, whereas in mild ischemia, when the AMP produced by the cycle may be resynthesized to ADP and thence to ATP by oxidative phosphorylation, the cycle may actually be proton consuming {25}. The proposed metabolic pathways can be summarized as

intracardiac FFA $\rightarrow$ intracardiac acyl CoA $\rightarrow$ acyl CoA combines with alpha glycerophosphate $\rightarrow$ glyceride, chiefly triglyceride, is formed $\rightarrow$ triglyceride breaks down under the stimulus of a catecholamine-sensitive lipase $\rightarrow$ intracardiac glycerol and FFA form $\rightarrow$ extracardiac glycerol and FFA form $\rightarrow$ intracardiac FFA recombines with intracardiac alpha glycerophosphate derived from glycolysis to remove triglyceride.

That lipolysis could give rise to FFA within the heart with the same effects of external FFA is suggested because stimulation of endogenous lipolysis by adrenaline increases the myocardial oxygen consumption in a way similar to the effects of exogenous FFA {78}. That the lipase system is sensitive to cholinergic stimulation is suggested because triglyceride accumulates after such stimulation {79}. Triglycerides are not normally a major energy source for the myocardium, except after a high-lipid meal (table 20-1), yet in the perfused heart triglyceride can provide about 10% of the energy requirement of the working rat heart {80}.

"FATTY ACID TOXICITY", CARNITINE, ACYL CARNITINE, AND LYSOPHOSPHOGLYCERIDES

Oliver and his colleagues {81} made the important observation that patients with acute myocardial infarction with complications were more likely to have high blood FFA levels than other patients and that mortality appeared to be related to the FFA level. In experimental developing myocardial infarction, there is still some continued uptake of FFA, albeit at a reduced rate {82}. The significance of this continued uptake of FFA lies in the possibility of accumulation of fatty acid intermediates "driving" the oxygen consumption of those mitochondria still receiving oxygen {83,84}, thereby aggravating ischemia.

Further evidence for "fatty acid toxicity" is provided by the development of arrhythmias {85}, depression of contractility and the aggravation of enzyme release {86}. In some preparations, excess external FFA can have toxic effects, even in the absence of oxygen deprivation {87}. Many of the observations have been made at highly unphysiological circulating FFA levels with extremely high

FFA-albumin molar ratios {76}. In other systems, "toxic" effects can be found with physiologic fatty acid levels. The earlier biochemical evidence on the effects of accumulation of acyl CoA (as already discussed) provided a reasonable basis for "fatty acid toxicity," although doubt has been cast on the significance of inhibition of the mitochondrial translocase by acyl CoA (see earlier), so that attention is turning to the possible role of acyl carnitine.

Acyl carnitine may be involved. In the normal heart, cytosolic concentration of this intermediate is very low. During ischemia the concentration increases much more than that of acyl CoA {88}. Furthermore, several drugs that inhibit the enzyme CAT-I (eq. 20-12) also lessen ischemic damage {53,88}. Long-chain acyl carnitine has potentially arrhythmogenic properties, including inhibition of the sodium current to cause inhomogeneity of the cardiac action potential {89}.

Whether *carnitine* itself may modify myocardial ischemic injury probably depends in part on whether or not circulating FFA are high, because L-carnitine is able to reduce FFA uptake by the mildly ischemic myocardium and to reduce levels of acyl CoA {90}. In addition, carnitine may inhibit fatty acid metabolism indirectly by promotion of glycolysis, acting indirectly in a way not fully understood {91}.

Lysophosphoglycerides are membrane-active fatty acids that are released from the phospholipids of the sarcolemma and other membranes during ischemia. The metabolic pathways and proposed regulatory signals in ischemia are shown in fig. 20-8. Accumulated lysophos-

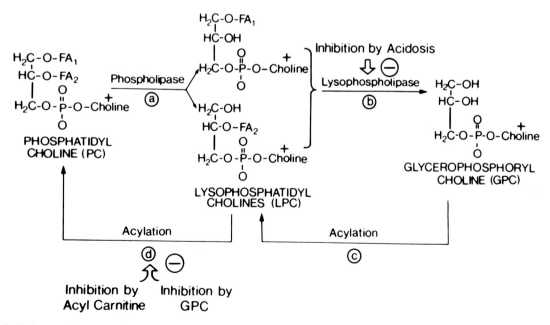

Fig. 20-8. Pathways of synthesis of major phospholipid compounds. In ischemia, lysophosphatidyl cholines may accumulate because of inhibition of lysophospholipase by acidosis (b on figure) and because pathway d is inhibited by accumulated acyl carnitine and glycerophosphoryl choline. Modified from Corr et al. {93} with permission.

phatidylcholine (LPC) has arrhythmogenic properties {92,93}. These proposals are controversial, although well argued {93}. If correct, there would be a vicious lipid circle in ischemia:

ischemia → membrane phospholipids →
lysophosphoglycerides → increasing membrane damage →
increasing ischemia

FREE FATTY ACID AND LIPID METABOLISM: CRITICAL FEATURES

Free fatty acids (FFA) are the major myocardial fuel of the normal heart, especially in the fasted state, and are able to inhibit the metabolism of glucose. FFA metabolism can, in turn, be inhibited by a high blood lactate, as occurs during exercise. That part of the FFA taken up that is not oxidized can form triglyceride and myocardial structural lipids, the latter by changes in the degree of saturation and chain length. Generally the heart does not synthesize lipid from glucose, nor from other nonlipid sources.

When excess FFA are provided to the myocardium, the rate of uptake exceeds the rate of disposal and intermediates of lipid metabolism, such as intracellular FFA, acyl CoA, and acyl carnitine accumulate. These changes also occur in the ischemic myocardium, despite the effect of ischemia itself in decreasing FFA uptake and in decreasing the oxidative contribution of FFA relative to that of glucose in the ischemic tissue. At least some of the lipid intermediates might be drived from endogenous lipolysis. The exact mechanism whereby these lipid intermediates exert their "toxic" effect still remains to be clarified. In the case of accumulated lysophophoglycerides (derived from membrane phospholipids), an arrhythmogenic potential has been found {92,94}. Derangements of fatty acid metabolism could, therefore, make a substantial contribution to myocardial ischemic injury (for review, see Katz and Messineo {95}).

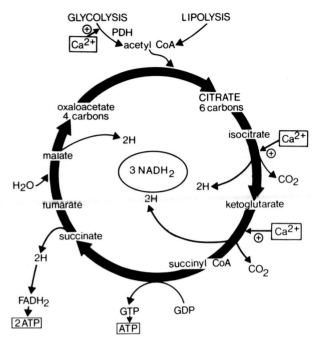

Fig. 20-9. The citrate cycle of Krebs. The following reactions are readily reversible: citrate → isocitrate; succinate → oxaloacetate via the intervening reactions. The most important potential sites of control are citrate synthase, isocitrate dehydrogenase, α-ketoglutarate dehydrogenase, and malate dehydrogenase (by regulating the supply of oxaloacetate). Of these, isocitric dehydrogenase and α-ketoglutarate dehydrogenase are calcium sensitive, as is pyruvate dehydrogenase (PDH). These dehydrogenases respond to a decreased mitochondrial $NADH_2$ during increased heart work by increased activity. From Opie LH: The Heart: Physiology and Metabolism. Orlando, FL: Grune and Stratton, 1984, with permission.

DISPOSAL OF NADH PRODUCED BY SUBSTRATE METABOLISM IN THE CITRATE CYCLE

Whatever the original substrate taken up from the coronary circulation, in each case there are pathways of substrate simplification to convert the original substrate ultimately to acetyl CoA, which can then enter the citrate cycle (fig. 20-9). In the process there are a variable number of dehydrogenations, which split off two H units from the substrate and reduce NAD^+ to $NADH + H^+$, i.e., NAD to $NADH_2$; further dehydrogenations in the citrate cycle produce more NADH. The reduction of FAD to $FADH_2$ also occurs, but is of much less quantitative importance. From $NADH_2$ ($NADH + H^+$), the reducing equivalents can pass through the mitochondrial membrane to form the proton gradient to help produce ATP and, then ultimately, to link with oxygen atoms to form water.

When $NADH + H^+$ is produced extramitochondrially, then there must be provision for such $NADH + H^+$ to be

transported into the mitochondria, or else accumulation of $NADH + H^+$ in the cytosol will inhibit the pathways of glycolysis (at the level of glyceraldehyde-3-phosphate dehydrogenase activity) and the uptake of lactate (which requires NAD^+ for conversion to pyruvate) so that only free fatty acids could act as fuel for the heart. Such cytosolic NADH is formed either by (a) glycolysis at the stage of glyceraldehyde-3-phosphate dehydrogenase or by (b) conversion of lactate taken up from the circulation to pyruvate before oxidation.

Malate-aspartate shuttle

During oxidative conditions, the chief mechanism for transfer of extramitochondrial NADH to intramitochondrial NADH is by the malate-aspartate shuttle (fig. 20-10). During anaerobic conditions, lactate cannot be taken up and conversion of cytosolic pyruvate to lactate disposes of glycolytically produced NADH. Malate and oxaloacetate occur both in cytosol and in the mitochondrial space,

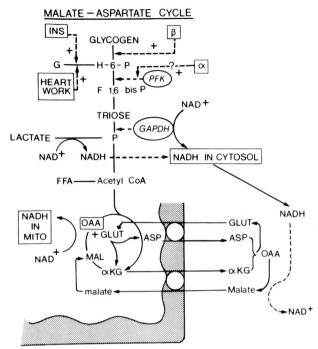

Fig. 20-10. The malate-aspartate cycle: OAA = oxaloacetate; Glut = glutamate; ASP = aspartate; MAL = malate; αKG = alpha-ketoglutarate. For other abbreviations see fig. 20-1 legend.

as does the enzyme malate dehydrogenase, which interconverts the two compounds

$$\text{oxaloacetate} + \text{NADH} + \text{H}^+ \rightleftharpoons \text{malate} + \text{NAD}^+ \quad (20\text{-}16)$$

During production of NADH + H$^+$ by glycolysis, oxaloacetate in the cytosol is converted to malate with the utilization of NADH + H$^+$ (the reformation of NAD$^+$ allows glycolysis to proceed). Malate then passes into the mitochondrial space as part of a complex transport system that "exports" alpha-ketoglutarate {96}. Once within the mitochondrial space, malate will reform oxaloacetate to enter the *citrate cycle*, NADH$_2$ (NADH + H$^+$) also reforms and is accessible to the electron transmitter chain, so that 3 ATP are formed for every 2 H entering:

$$\text{malate} + \text{NAD} \rightarrow \text{oxaloacetate} + \text{NADH} + \text{H}^+ \quad (20\text{-}17)$$

$$\text{NADH} + \text{H}^+ \rightarrow (\text{via proton pump}) \rightarrow 3\,\text{ATP} \quad (20\text{-}18)$$

The mitochondrial oxaloacetate formed from malate forms alpha-ketoglutarate and aspartate, via aspartate aminotransferase; the alpha-ketoglutarate leaves the mitochondrial space in exchange for malate, while the aspartate is transported to the extramitochondrial space {97} in exchange for uptake of glutamate. Once in the cytosol, aspartate reacts with alpha-ketoglutarate to reform oxaloacetate and glutamate. The oxaloacetate reenters [eq. (20-8) above] and the glutamate enters the mito-

chondrial space in exchange for aspartate; here too an antiport system is proposed.

Maximal possible rates of malate transport are about 40–45 nM/min/mg mitochondrial protein, or about 4 μM/min/g wet weight of heart {97,98}, only about double those required to cope with maximal rates of glucose oxidation of the "working" isolated rat heart in the presence of insulin {11,98,99}. Transient peak rates of glycolysis in isolated hearts during rapid increases of heart work may, therefore, exceed the peak capacity of the malate-aspartate system, and alternate means of disposal of cytosolic NADH are required. First, some glycolytic flux can form lactate, even in aerobic conditions during such very high rates of heart work; secondly, the alpha-glycerophosphate shuttle may play a role.

Glycerophosphate shuttle

The route of disposal of cytosolic NADH in many tissues is entry into mitochondria by way of the alpha-glycerophosphate (alpha-GP) shuttle:

$$\text{NADH} + \text{H}^+ + \text{DHAP} \rightarrow \text{NAD}^+ + \text{alpha-GP}, \quad (20\text{-}19)$$

where DHAP = dihydroxyacetone phosphate. The enzyme concerned is alpha-GP dehydrogenase. The alpha-GP enters the mitochondria to be oxidized by alpha-GP oxidase within the mitochondria. DHAP reforms, as does FADH$_2$; the former is transported outward and the latter enters the respiratory chain (fig. 20-10). It has been difficult to assess accurately the capacity of this system for transport of NADH$_2$ in the heart, and the malate-aspartate system may be more important. The chief reason for this conclusion is the relatively low rates of activities of the enzyme alpha-GP dehydrogenase {100}.

Unspanning of the citrate cycle

The activity of the citrate cycle in the rat heart can suddenly be accelerated by a surge of metabolic activity, as when glucose is replaced by acetate as the major fuel {101} when a substrate-free heart is perfused with glucose and insulin {102}. Using these instructive (but unphysiologic) situations, it appears that the citrate cycle can operate in two spans. The first span from the acetyl CoA to alpha-ketoglutarate is held to be regulated by citrate synthase, and the second span from alpha-ketoglutarate to oxaloacetate is regulated by alpha-ketoglutarate dehydrogenase. When acetyl CoA is suddenly formed by excess provision of glucose and insulin, the second part of the cycle is bypassed and the cycle is unspanned. Such unspanning may seem unlikely to occur during increased heart work, when the primary event driving the cycle is the removal of NADH$_2$ rather than the arrival of acetyl CoA. The computer calculations of Garfinkel {103}, however, show that alpha-ketoglutarate (and isocitrate dehydrogenase) increase in activity more than citrate synthase at the start of increased heart work, probably because the inhibition on alpha-ketoglutarate dehydrogenase is removed as NADH$_2$ falls abruptly. Hence unspanning of the cycle is possible at the start of increased heart work.

ENERGY PRODUCTION FROM VARIOUS SUBSTRATES

When *glucose* is the source of glycolysis, the whole glycolytic path uses 2 ATP and produces 4 ATP, i.e., the net production is 2 ATP. When *glycogen* is the source, ATP production is three per glucose molecule passing through glycolysis. An important point is that glycolytic ATP will be made whenever hexosephosphates are converted to pyruvate, even during oxidative metabolism when pyruvate enters the citrate cycle via acetyl CoA. The major source of energy from either glucose or glycogen lies in the citrate cycle, with ultimate conversion of pyruvate to CO_2 with the formation of intramitochondrial NADH.

Each molecule of *lactate* fully oxidized yields 18 molecules of ATP, of which three molecules result from the extramitochondrial production of NADH as lactate is converted to pyruvate; the 15 further ATP are the result of the further oxidation of pyruvate.

Although *pyruvate* is an insignificant external fuel in absolute terms, both glucose and lactate only produce the major part of their energy after conversion to pyruvate. Pyruvate dehydrogenation produces 1 molecule of NADH, which will give rise to 3 ATP molecules; the further 12 molecules are produced by one turn of the citrate cycle.

Fatty acid activation uses up 1 ATP per molecule. Taking the example of palmitate, seven turns of the fatty acid oxidation spiral will produce 7 $NADH_2$ = (NADH + H^+) and 7 $FADH_2$, all of these being intramitochondrial. The former will produce 21 ATP, the latter 14 ATP. Finally, 8 acetyl CoA will produce 96 ATP (12 ATP per acetyl CoA passing through the citrate cycle), with an overall energy yield of 130 ATP per palmitate molecule. (Previous calculations of 129 ATP per palmitate molecule are incorrect.)

Acetoacetate, when ultimately converted to 2 acetyl CoA, will have the usual yield of 24 ATP when ultimately oxidized. The simultaneous conversion of succinyl CoA to succinate when acetoacetyl CoA is formed, however, will deprive the heart of one substrate-level phosphorylation per 2 acetyl CoA units oxidized, with a net energy yield of 23 ATP per molecule of acetoacetate. When beta-hydroxybutyrate is being utilized, an additional $NADH_2$ (= NADH + H^+) will be formed during the initial dehydrogenation to acetoacetate, and a further 3 ATP will be formed, with a total energy yield of 26 ATP per molecule of beta-hydroxybutyrate. Such ketone bodies are only an important source of energy of myocardial energy when the circulating levels are very high, as in diabetic ketosis.

Phosphorylation-oxidation ratio

Each of the myocardial fuels yields a different amount of ATP per molecule. The highest yield of ATP per molecule is from a fatty acid such as palmitate. The fatty acid molecules contain little oxygen and therefore can yield more ATP per carbon atom. The disadvantage of fatty acids as fuel is that for each molecule of ATP produced, they need relatively more oxygen. Experimentally, a heart

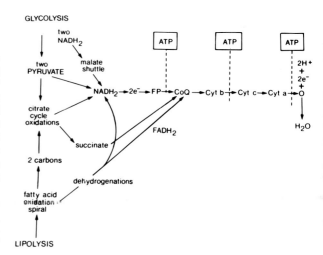

Fig. 20-11. Patterns of aerobic metabolism with intramitochondrial production of ATP.

using fatty acid alone would need about 17% more oxygen to produce the same amount of ATP than when using glucose.

The molecular explanation for the relatively poor ATP yield of fatty acids per oxygen taken up is that each turn of the fatty acid spiral yields equal amounts of $FADH_2$ and $NADH_2$. $FADH_2$ enters the respiratory chain "further along" than does $NADH_2$ and yields less ATP (fig. 20-11). Thus generation of $FADH_2$ accounts for part of the "oxygen-wasting" capacity of fatty acids; in addition, when fatty acids are presented in excess to the heart or when fatty acids cannot be fully oxidized as in ischemia, then fatty acids can waste even more oxygen through mechanisms that are still obscure {84}, but may include increased turnover of the intracellular FFA-triglyceride cycle {24,25}.

Glycolytic ATP

The amount of ATP generated by glycolysis in the normally oxygenated heart is negligible from the point of view of the normal energy requirements of the heart. In the ischemic myocardium, glycolysis from glucose is accelerated by the Pasteur effect in zones of moderate ischemia; even then the rate of production of anaerobic ATP is negligible when compared with the rate of ATP produced by the residual oxygen uptake {23}. Yet sustenance of glycolysis in ischemic hearts can (a) reduce the rate of enzyme release {104,105}, (b) help prevent reperfusion arrhythmias {104}, (c) maintain the action potential duration {106}, and (d) prevent ischemic contracture {107}. In the hypoxic heart, glycolytic inhibition increased the severity of ultrastructural damage {108}, in agreement with the previous findings. Entman et al. {109} have described a glycogenolytic-sarcoplasmic reticulum complex. They found that fragments of the sarcoplasmic reticulum possess their characteristic calcium-accumulating system in physical association with a series of glycogenolytic enzymes. Their proposal means that the arrival of Ca^{2+} would stimulate glycogenolysis and glycolysis, and hence, produce more glycolytic ATP. Our tentative proposal is that the rate of glycolysis limits the rate of Ca^{2+} uptake and hence the process of mechanical relaxation {110}.

Several of the above observations can be interpreted in terms of cytosolic compartmentation of ATP. It is, therefore, appropriate to examine some aspects of the metabolism of high-energy phosphate compounds in the myocardium.

ATP and phosphocreatine

The initial picture that emerged was that ATP was the immediate source of energy for contraction and other energy-consuming processes, with phosphocreatine as the reserve energy. A more recent proposal is that phosphocreatine has a transport role. As ATP is exported from the mitochondria, the proposal is that ATP is immediately converted to phosphocreatine by a mitochondrial creatine kinase (= creatine phosphokinase) isoenzyme {111}. Phosphocreatine may then be transported throughout the cytosol, presumably following a downhill gradient to a cytosolic site of utilization of energy where another creatine kinase isoenzyme liberates the high-energy phosphate required for energetic purposes:

$$PC + ADP \rightarrow ATP + creatine \qquad (20\text{-}20)$$

This transport role of phosphocreatine does not eliminate its alternate role as an energy reservoir, especially because the equilibrium constant of the above reaction favors the formation of ATP. During a sustained hypoxic stimulus, both ATP and phosphocreatine will fall; while ATP may fall before phosphocreatine, in the next phase phosphocreatine falls more, as it is the energy reservoir.

Breakdown products of phosphocreatine

Creatine may help stimulate the production of high-energy phosphate by the mitochondria {112}, probably by providing ADP by the action of the mitochondrial creatine kinase isoenzyme. Inorganic phosphate may stimulate glycolysis at the level of phosphofructokinase, because this regulatory enzyme is inhibited by phosphocreatine (as well as by ATP) and the inhibition is relieved by inorganic phosphate {113}. Inorganic phosphate may also play a complex role in regulation of Ca^{2+} transport into myocardial cells {114}.

HEART WORK AND HIGH-ENERGY PHOSPHATES

Confusion continues about the effects of mechanical heart work on high-energy phosphate compounds. An important proposal has been that the cytosolic phosphate potential, defined by the ratio of cytosolic (ATP)/(ADP)(Pi), drives respiration; 90% or more of ATP is found in the cytosol, whereas cytosolic ADP is very low {102}. Hence the ratio

ATP/ADP in the cytosol is 200–300 times greater than in the mitochondria. During acute heart work, it is expected that the cytosolic ATP is utilized and that cytosolic ADP rises to drive mitochondrial respiration according to classic concepts {102}. Phosphocreatine functions as a reserve energy at the acute onset of heart work {11,30}. As the oxygen uptake rises, phosphocreatine will tend to be restored so that at high workloads overall values of tissue high-energy phosphates are little changed despite a doubling of the cytosolic ratio of ATP/ADP.

The above concepts, based on theoretical calculations (see references in earlier editions of this book), are supported by direct measurements of mitochondrial and cytosolic adenine nucleotides in the isolated working guinea pig heart {115} using density gradient centrifugation of lyophilized myocardial homogenates.

Controversy and alternate interpretations

The concept that respiration during increased heart work is driven by ADP, Pi, and creatine has been challenged by Balaban {116}. While it is agreed that the role of phosphorylation potential and other energy changes may be valid in isolated mitochondria and in isolated perfused hearts, in vivo the cytosolic concentrations of ADP and Pi do not change significantly with increased work. Hence other regulatory processes must be at work, for example, increased stimulation of mitochondrial metabolism by calcium (fig. 20-9), or by the supply of oxygen {117}. Yet another possibility, recently considered, is that the rate of activity of the mitochondrial ATP synthase can respond to metabolic variations during increased heart work {118}.

NADH during increased heart work

Thus far it has been proposed that mitochondrial NADH falls during increased heart work {46}. This view is challenged by Balaban {116} and by Koretsky et al. {119}. The latter authors proposed that NADH rises rather than falls, and point out the number of problems in methodology involved in assessing the true change in mitochondrial NAD^+/NADH ratios. The topic is controversial. It can be seen how a primary change in the cytosolic ATP/ADP ratio could help drive citrate cycle activity, thereby increasing NAD^+ while NADH falls. Likewise, increased provision of oxygen will increase NAD^+ and decrease NADH. On the other hand, primary stimulation of the citrate cycle by, for example, increased cytosolic calcium, will increase NADH to drive respiration. It is possible that different mechanisms play a different role according to the model and the exact circumstances studied.

Beat-to-beat control?

Another explanation for failure to find changes in overall tissue values of high-energy phosphate compounds in some preparations is the possibility of beat-to-beat control. Morgan's group {120} found that there are small changes in the isolated rat heart, detectable by nuclear magnetic resonance techniques. Small overall changes can be trans-

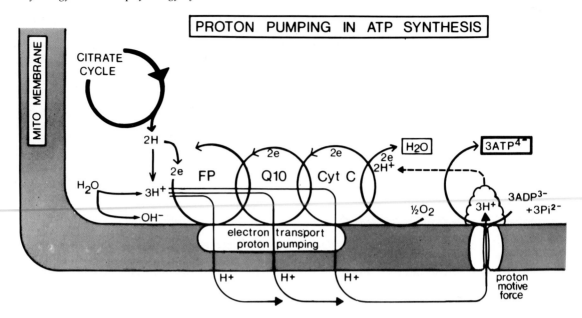

Fig. 20-12. Mitchell's chemiosmotic hypothesis, according to which the electron transfer components of the respiratory chain are arranged spatially and in sequence so that alternate electron and proton transfers occur. From Opie LH: *The Heart: Physiology and Metabolism.* Orlando, FL: Grune and Stratton, 1984, with permission.

lated into large changes in the cytosolic phosphate potential, as already discussed. Hence there may be cyclical variations in the mitochondrial oxygen uptake.

MITOCHONDIAL ENERGY PRODUCTION AND ELECTRON TRANSPORT*

Reducing equivalents, derived from $NADH_2$ ($NADH + H^+$), flow along the respiratory transport (or electron transmitter) chain as follows:

$$NADH + H^+ + \text{flavoprotein} \rightarrow$$
$$\text{reduced flavoprotein} + NAD^+ \quad (20\text{-}21)$$

$$\text{Reduced flavoprotein} + \text{coenzyme } Q \rightarrow$$
$$\text{reduced coenzyme } Q$$
$$(\text{ubiquinone, coenzyme } Q_{10} + \text{flavoprotein} \quad (20\text{-}22)$$

$$\text{Reduced coenzyme } Q + \text{cytochromes} \rightarrow$$
$$\text{reduced cytochromes} + \text{coenzyme } Q \quad (20\text{-}23)$$

$$\text{Reduced cytochromes} + \text{oxygen} \rightarrow$$
$$\text{cytochromes} + H_2O \quad (20\text{-}24)$$

Electrons are transferred through the cytochromes (b, c, and a), which are electron-transferring proteins containing iron porphyrin (heme) groups. The iron atoms undergo reversible changes in valency from the ferrous to the ferric form, and vice versa.

* This section was modified from pages 254 and 255 of Opie LH, The Heart: Physiology and Metabolism, New York: Raven Press, 1991, with permission.

The respiratory chain may be divided into three spans, each associated with the pumping of protons and with the production of ATP (fig. 20-12). Site I is the span between NADH and coenzyme Q, site 2 is the span between cytochrome *b* and cytochrome *c*, and site 3 is the span between cytochrome *c* and oxygen. Each of these sites yields one ATP via proton pumping. The mitochondrial oxidation of NADH produced by the citrate cycle, therefore, yields three molecules of ATP per atom of oxygen reduced (a phosphorylation/oxygen uptake ratio, or P/O ratio, of 3). Other reactions (e.g., pyruvate dehydrogenase) forming $NADH_2$ also will have a P/O ratio of 3, but reactions feeding into the chain at the level of coenzyme Q will have a P/O ratio of 2. The first step of the fatty acid oxidation spiral and also succinate dehydrogenase produce $FADH_2$, which reacts with coenzyme Q, and therefore has a P/O ratio of 2 and not 3.

Proton pumping

The actual mechanism for ATP manufacture is closely linked with the fate of protons rather than of electrons. Thus

$$\text{Hydrogen atom} = \text{proton} + \text{electron}$$
$$H = H^+ + e^- \quad (20\text{-}25)$$

There is thus an accompanying movement of protons together with electrons. It is simple to suppose that the 2 H^+ link up wih the two electrons and oxygen eventually to form water. According to Mitchell's theory of oxidative phosphorylation, protons are pumped outward across the inner mitochondrial membrane to yield a gradient of H^+ across the membrane {121}. This H^+ gradient is the driving force for phosphorylation of ADP because protons reenter the mitochondrial matrix through a complex of membrane proteins called *ATP synthetase*, which is a protein ionophore. Formation of ATP from ADP is driven by proton movements caused by the transmembrane proton gradient.

SUBSTRATE AND ENERGY METABOLISM IN ISCHEMIA

Is there a relation between overall level of ATP and ischemic injury?

When studying a variety of injuries to the cell, various other workers have concluded that the degree of fall of the total ATP to a "critical" level may help to indicate whether or not the cell could recover. Thus Kubler and Spieckermann {17} found that as myocardial ATP fell below $3.5\,\mu M/g$ wet weight in hearts arrested by ischemia at $15°C$, lactate production ceased because of lack of ATP for the conversion of fructose 6-phosphate to fructose 1,6-bisphosphate (phosphofructokinase reaction). The same ATP level also defined the limit of myocardial ischemia that could be associated with recovery of adequate cardiac function after rewarming the heart. Hearse {122} found a similar limit for recovery from whole-heart ischemia induced by aortic clamping. Gudbjarnason et al. {123}, however, found that in the noninfarcted zone after coronary ligation in the dog, ATP could drop as low as $1.5–2.0\,\mu M/g$ and the heart could contract and survive. Neely and Grotyohann {33} could also dissociate ATP levels from postischemic recovery. Loading the myocardium with deoxyglucose, which acts to trap ATP, can drop total ATP levels by about two thirds, while cardiac contractile activity is still about 75% of control values {124}. The pattern of recovery of the isolated rat hearts during postischemic reperfusion {33,125} shows that altered rates of ATP production are more important than absolute overall levels of ATP in determining postischemic recovery.

Glycolytic flux and reversibility of ischemic injury

During subtotal ischemia, maintenance of glycolysis prevents ischemic contracture {110}, possibly acting by maintenance of calcium homeostasis. The minimum rate of ATP production from glycolysis required to prevent ischemic contracture is about $5\,\mu M/min/g$ wet weight. This beneficial effect of glycolysis may seem to be inconsistent with the data of Neely and Grotyohann {33}, who showed that some products of glycolysis, such as protons and lactate, can promote the severity of ischemic damage. The results are not really in conflict. In our model, there was a maintained low rate of coronary flow (low-flow ischemia) and glycolysis was not totally inhibited. In the Neely model, there was a prolonged period of total global ischemia, during which products of glycolysis had to accumulate within the ischemic cells. Combining the observations of the two groups, we suggest that (a) cessation of glycolysis can be linked to irreversible ischemic damage {126} and (b) coronary flow must be sustained, albeit at a low level, to maintain glycolysis and to prevent the accumulation of adverse products of glycolysis. These arguments are more fully developed elsewhere {1}.

Proposed benefits of glycolysis and harm of lipolysis for ischemic myocardium

It now becomes reasonable to propose that inhibition of glycolysis and accumulation of products of lipolysis are harmful events for the ischemic myocardium, acting independently from the rate of fall of ATP. Inhibitors of glycolysis act, at least in part, through an increase of cytosolic calcium, whereas the products of lipolysis more directly interact with cellular membranes to enhance ischemic injury. In total or severe ischemia, glycolytic rates may not be high enough to prevent the accumulation of calcium, but continued accumulation of products of glycolysis, such as protons and lactate, can help promote ischemic damage.

ATP-SENSITIVE POTASSIUM CHANNEL

ATP-dependent potassium channel

The resting potential of the cardiac myocyte is basically dependent on a transmembrane gradient of potassium ions. The link between impaired cardiac energy metabolism and potassium release during ischemia can at least in part be explained by the existence of this potassium channel. An important problem is the discrepancy between the minute concentrations of ATP required in vitro to keep the channel closed and the relatively high overall tissue levels of ATP found at the time that the channel opens in vivo. That channel opening does occur at these relatively high ATP levels is shown by the effects of glibenclamide, a specific closer of the ATP-dependent potassium channel {127,128}.

The three major explanations for potassium channel opening at relatively high overall cellular levels of ATP are as follows. First, breakdown of even relatively small amounts of ATP can give rise to large changes in the breakdown products, such as ADP, adenosine, and magnesium. It may be that the levels of these breakdown products actually regulate the opening of this potassium channel {129,130}, or it could be that the ratio ATP/ADP is effective {131}. Another product of the glycolytic turnover of ATP is proton formation. When protons are washed out early in ischemia, then extracellular acidosis could enhance potassium channel activity {132}. Second, an important alternative hypothesis is that compartmentalization of ATP produced by glycolytic enzymes located in relation to the sarcolemma could help regulate the activity of this channel {131}. Third, it has now become evident that only a minute percentage of the potassium channels need to open to allow detectable potassium loss to occur {131}. Nevertheless, the discovery and elucidation of the pro-

ATP POOLS/COMPARTMENTS

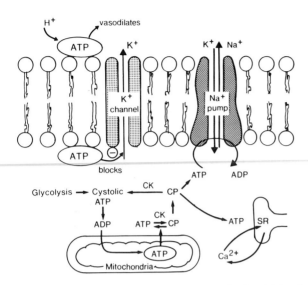

Fig. 20-13. The major ATP compartments are mitochondrial and cytosolic. Minor localized pools are associated with the potassium channel, the sodium pump, and the sarcoplasmic reticulum (SR). According to the concepts of Kuznetsov et al. {124}, the mitochondrial creatine kinase (CK) isoenzyme is situated between the inner and outer mitochondrial membranes to form creatine phosphate (CP) from creatine. The outer mitochondrial membrane is freely permeable to CP, which can then reform ATP from ADP generated by contraction. From Opie LH: *The Heart: Physiology and Metabolism*, 2nd ed. New York: Raven Press, 1991.

perties of this potassium channel support the general concept of cellular compartmentation of ATP (fig. 20-13).

REPERFUSION INJURY

Reperfusion injury may be defined as a group of events occurring as a consequence of reperfusion, which subtracts either transiently or permanently from the overall beneficial effect of reperfusion. Thus, reperfusion injury encompasses a spectrum of events, including reperfusion arrhythmias, reperfusion stunning, accelerated or new cell necrosis, and microvascular injury {133}. A similar grouping is described by Hearse {134}. Previously reperfusion injury was synonymous with and limited to increased cell necrosis as a result of reperfusion {135}.

Reperfusion stunning

Mechanical stunning is a temporary decrease of mechanical function in the reperfusion period, found in the absence of any cell necrosis {136}. Stunning is an alternate outcome to full recovery in short-lived ischemia {137–139}.

Stunning is currently being explained by two major hypotheses, namely, formation of free radicals and/or intracellular cytosolic calcium overload {133,140}. These two concepts are not mutually exclusive, because formation of free radicals leads to an increase of cytosolic calcium {140} and, conversely, increased cytosolic calcium leads to more formation of free radicals {141}. The concept of free radical-mediated damage as a cause of reperfusion injury was led by Hearse and his group in relation to arrhythmias {142} and by Bolli and his group {143} in relation to stunning.

Can reperfusion injury increase cell necrosis?

While it is true that early reperfusion limits the progress of severe ischemia to cell death, reperfusion can also accelerate cell death {135,144}. The problem is to know whether reperfusion merely accelerates myocardial cell necrosis, with the same number of cells eventually dying, or whether a greater total number of cells die. The former sequence is the "acceleration of the funeral events of cell death" {135}. Recently there has been new evidence favoring the proposal that reperfusion actually increases the total amount of cell necrosis, especially in zones of less severe ischemic injury {145}.

Reperfusion and free radicals

It was Guarnieri who in 1980 first reported that reoxygenation of the myocardium led to formation of free radicals {146}. Next the concept of oxygen toxicity was applied to the heart {147}. Formation of oxygen-derived free radicals during reperfusion explained at least in part the "oxygen paradox," whereby reoxygenation of the hypoxic heart had adverse effects {148}.

The sites of formation of free radicals may include mitochondria, neutrophils, and the blood-vessel endothelial walls. The harmful effects of free radicals are restrained by naturally occurring defense systems. One of the important defense systems involves glutathione peroxidase and the conversion of reduced glutathione (GSH) to the oxidized form (GSSG). Therefore, Ferrari and colleagues {149} used the ratio of GSH to GSSG in the blood leaving the heart during reperfusion after coronary bypass surgery to show that there had been oxidative stress.

Interaction of free radicals and calcium

Free radicals may not be the ultimate cause of manifestations of reperfusion damage such as arrhythmias {150} and stunning {151}. Furthermore, reperfusion injury as assessed by arrhythmias can be achieved by readmission of coronary flow without readmission of oxygen {152}. Rather, the radicals may initiate calcium-mediated damage {133,134,140}. For example, free radicals may act on the sarcoplasmic reticulum to liberate calcium {153}. Excess oscillations of cytosolic calcium may then be intimately involved with the generation of the abnormal currents thought to underlie postischemic ventricular arrhythmias and postischemic stunning {133}. Not only may free

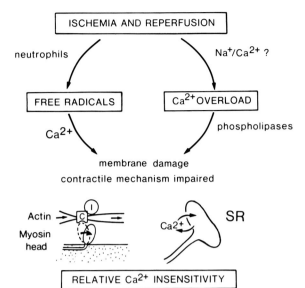

Fig. 20-14. Illustration of the two major mechanisms for reperfusion injury, formation of free radicals, and calcium overload. This scheme reconciles these apparently conflicting hypotheses, showing the proposed combined role of free radicals and calcium overload in causing membrane damage and relative calcium insensitivity of contractile mechanism (actin-myosin interaction on left and sarcoplasmic reticulum on right). From Opie {133}, with permission of the American Heart Association.

radicals lead to an increase of cytosolic calcium, but conversely an increased calcium can lead to increased formation of free radicals {141}, so that the noxious roles of these two agents, calcium and free radicals, may be interactive and additive (fig. 20-14) {151}.

Reperfusion and glycolysis

In isolated heart systems, glycolysis in the early reperfusion period is associated with improved recovery. The mechanism may involve better control of cytosolic calcium levels {154} or of internal free fatty acids {155}. Provision of nonglycolytic fuels leads to increased levels of calcium or of fatty acids.

Current status of reperfusion injury

Conflict still abounds about the exact mechanism of reperfusion injury {142,150,152}. Experimentally, the effects of several free radical scavengers on various manifestations of reperfusion injury, such as stunning and arrhythmias, are under study {134,142,156,157}. Free radical scavengers or calcium modulators have to be given at the onset of reperfusion or earlier {143,158}. An alternate approach might be to test the hypothesis that enhancement of endogenous myocardial antioxidant activity by vitamin E could be protective.

HIBERNATION: CHRONIC ISCHEMIA WITH BALANCED REDUCTION OF BLOOD FLOW AND CONTRACTILITY

Hibernation is yet another possible outcome of ischemia, not so well understood, whereby metabolism of the ischemic zone seems to be fixed in such a way that a certain level of relatively mild ischemia can be tolerated for days or months. An attractive explanation is that an increase of cytosolic calcium levels in the reperfusion period can lead to a variety of outcomes, including stunning, arrhythmias, hibernation, or cell necrosis. Which outcome is manifest may in part depend on the severity and duration of the ischemia.

Kloner et al. {159} and Ferrari and Visioli {160} have done an important service to cardiologists by pointing out that the end points of ischemia are no longer simply reversibility or irreversibility, but also stunning and hibernation. The latter is a phrase first used by Rahimtoola {161} to describe chronic left ventricular mechanical dysfunction relieved when the coronary blood flow is increased, whereas stunning is the temporary postischemic dysfunction precipitated by reperfusion. When there is a mild reduction in coronary flow, it is proposed that a proportionate reduction of the contractile activity maintains the oxygen supply/demand ratio {162,163}. It follows that the control of cytosolic calcium is maintained in this balanced state. The crucial question is how the decreased contractility in hibernation can be coupled to the fall in the oxygen supply. When the flow reduction becomes more severe, then hibernation changes to frank ischemia. The oxygen supply becomes insufficient for the demand, even of the ischemically arrested myocardium, and now there are definite tissue markers of metabolic impairment, such as decreased levels of ATP, creatine phosphate, a fall of tissue pH, and a rise in tissue lactate {163}.

Beside the balanced reduction of contractility and blood flow, another mechanism may contribute to the development of hibernation. During prolonged moderate ischemia in pig hearts, there is evidence for downregulation of the energy requirements of the ischemic tissue to below the rates of energy production {164}. Such an adaptive mechanism, currently unknown in its origin, suggests the possible existence of endogenous pathways for myocardial metabolic protection, speculatively involving *heat stress proteins* {165}.

PRECONDITIONING: SHORT-LIVED ISCHEMIA PROTECTS FROM SUBSEQUENT LONGER ISCHEMIA

Repetitive episodes of ischemia might be expected to produce cumulative metabolic damage. Not so, showed Swain et al. {166}; three separate 12-minute episodes of ischemia did not decrease ATP more than a single episode. Then Jennings' group {167} proposed and proved the hypothesis that repetitive episodes of ischemia were actually protective. They gave the name *preconditioning* to this phenomenon. Even one single episode of brief ischemia can precondition, so that stunning and preconditioning may coexist {168}. Experimentally, one major effect of preconditioning is a major reduction of infarct size {167}. In addition, preconditioning appears to extend to other aspects, such as protection against reperfusion arrhythmias or stunning {169}.

Mechanisms for preconditioning

One proposed explanation for preconditioning is that the stunned myocardium needs less ATP turnover for survival of its depressed contractile activity; however, stunning cannot be equated with preconditioning because in some models the duration of stunning may be prolonged beyond the time of occurrence of preconditioning {168}. A second explanation is that preconditioning requires glycolysis for its effects, so that inhibition of glycolysis by addition of pyruvate to the isolated heart can prevent preconditioning {170}.

Preconditioning may occur in patients undergoing percutaneous transluminal coronary angioplasty because transmyocardial release of lactate is less during the second than during the first balloon occlusion. The proposed clinical extrapolation of preconditioning is that repetitive episodes of ischemia might actually lessen the severity of subsequent cell necrosis, that is to say, diminish infarct size. A third possible explanation is that adenosine, by effects on the A_1-myocardial receptor, may be involved {171}. The adenosine proposal can be linked to a role for enhanced glycolysis because adenosine stimulates glycolytic flux via myocardial A_1 receptors {172}, consonant with the concept that glycolysis is required for preconditioning. The K^+-sensitive ATP channel might be more easily or more persistently opened to shorten the action potential duration, and thereby to lessen the inward flux of calcium {169}.

Thus several of the explanations for preconditioning involve modulation of high-energy phosphate metabolism, not through the absolute level of ATP but by its counter-regulatory breakdown product, adenosine {176}.

CONCLUDING COMMENTS

High rates of myocardial energy production are required to maintain the constant demand of the working heart for ATP, used largely for contractile purposes, but also for maintenance of ion gradients and other metabolic functions. A constant supply of oxygen to the myocardial cell is assured by the regulation of the coronary blood flow, which only fails when coronary arterial disease or spasm develops. The coronary flow also provides a more than adequate supply of external substrates: glucose, lactate, and free fatty acids. In the case of glucose, the complex uptake mechanism is sensitive to hormonal regulation chiefly by insulin and responds to the state of oxygenation of the myocardium. During hypoxia, tissue levels of ATP and phosphocreatine fall, while glucose uptake, glycogen breakdown, and anaerobic glycolysis are accelerated.

The pathways for fatty acid oxidation are complex. The transsarcolemmal uptake of FFA involves a fatty acid binding protein. Thereafter fatty acid activation is followed by formation of acyl carnitine, which is transported by a complex mechanism into the intramitochondrial space, where acyl CoA is reformed. The latter compound enters the fatty acid oxidation spiral to form acetyl CoA units while shedding 2H units to FAD and NAD, to form $FADH_2$ and $NADH_2$ (i.e., $NADH + H^+$). The acetyl CoA is oxidized via the citrate cycle of Krebs to yield more $NADH_2$. $NADH_2$ and $FADH_2$ are reoxidized by the electron transport chain to yield, respectively per molecule, three and two molecules of ATP. The overall energy yield of free fatty acid is 130 ATP per C16 molecule. This value seems substantially higher than that of glucose (three ATP per molecule anaerobically oxidized), but the advantage is bought at the cost of a lower P/O (phosphorylation-oxidation) ratio. Therefore, oxidation of free fatty acids is relatively oxygen wasting. With the very high circulating FFA values and high rates of uptake, additional ill-understood mechanisms for oxygen wastage come into play.

During myocardial ischemia, free fatty acid (FFA) uptake is decreased as the rate of mitochondrial oxidation falls. Probably an early step in this sequence is the accumulation of intramitochondrial $NADH_2$, which inhibits the oxidation of one of the intermediates of the fatty acid oxidation spiral (beta-hydroxyacyl CoA), thus explaining the accumulation of acyl CoA, acyl carnitine, and intracellular FFA in ischemia. Each of these metabolites has been postulated to have adverse effects in the setting of myocardial ischemia. A further potentially adverse change in lipid metabolism in ischemia is the formation of membrane-derived phospholipids, which may have arrhythmogenic potential.

During increased heart work, the mechanisms driving mitochondrial respiration are controversial. The proposal has been that an increased cytosolic phosphorylation potential or increase in creatine or other changes in high-energy phosphates drive mitochondrial respiration, so that the mitochondrial ratio $NADH_2/NAD$ falls (i.e., NAD^+ rises). That would be the converse of what happens in anoxia or ischemia. This increase in mitochondrial NAD/$NADH_2$ increases citrate cycle turnover, the activity of pyruvate dehydrogenase, the activity of the fatty acid oxidation spiral, and thereby, fatty acid activation. The acceleration of glycolysis produces increased cytosolic $NADH_2$, which requires the activity of the malate-aspartate cycle. Through additional regulatory mechanisms, the uptake of three primary substrates (glucose, lactate, FFA) can be accelerated. Which substrate becomes the major one for the working heart depends on the physiologic conditions.

According to a second and more recent proposal, there is no change in the levels of high-energy phosphate compounds nor in their breakdown products during increased heart work, at least in the heart in situ. Alternate mechanisms for stimulation of respiration include an increased cytosolic calcium with enhanced activity of mitochondrial dehydrogenases, an increase rather than a decrease in

NADH, an increase in the supply of oxygen, and increased activity of mitochondrial ATP synthase.

The currently favored view is that ATP is not only compartmentalized between the mitochondria and cytosol, with most in the cytosol, but that subcompartments of ATP in the cytosol exist as a result of cytosolic creatine kinase isoenzymes. According to this view, ATP produced in the mitochondria leaves by the ATP translocase and is then rapidly converted to phosphocreatine; the latter acts as a carrier of high-energy phosphates to the local cytosolic site where ATP is used. Thus ATP in the cytosol is replenished. Further evidence favoring the existence of cytosolic compartments of ATP is the apparent role of glycolysis in protecting from ischemic injury and ischemic contracture. Alternate points of view also merit attention. In ischemic injury, a relationship is claimed between the severity of loss of total tissue ATP and irreversibility; however, most data can be interpreted within the view favoring ATP subcompartmentation. The recent discovery of the ATP-sensitive potassium channel also supports the concept of cytosolic compartmentation of ATP.

New metabolic entities are reperfusion injury (including stunning), hibernation, and preconditioning.

Note added in proof:

Glucose transport in ischemia may be increased by translocation of the glucose transporter, GLUT 4, to myocyte membranes (Sun et al, *Circulation* 89:793–798, 1994.)

REFERENCES

1. Opie LH: Cardiac metabolism — emergence, decline, and resurgence. Part I. *Cardiovasc Res* 26:721–733, 1992.
2. Locke FS, Rosenheim O: Contributions to the physiology of the isolated heart. The consumption of dextrose by mammalian cardiac muscle. *J Physiol (Lond)* 36:205–220, 1907.
3. Evans CL: The effect of glucose on the gaseous metabolism of the isolated mammalian heart. *J Physiol (Lond)* 45:407–418, 1914.
4. Cruickshank EWH, Kosterlitz HW: The utilization of fat by the aglycaemic mammalian heart. *J Physiol (Lond)* 99:208–223, 1941.
5. Morgan HE, Neely JR, Brineaux JP, Park CR: Regulation of glucose transport. In: Chance B, Estabrook RW, Williamson JR (eds) *Control of Energy Metabolism*. New York: Academic Press, 1965, pp 347–355.
6. Park CR, Reinwein D, Henderson MJ, Cadenas E, Morgan HE: The action of insulin on the transport of glucose through the cell membrane. *Am J Med* 26:674–684, 1959.
7. Randle PJ, Morgan HE: Regulation of glucose uptake by muscle. *Vitam Horm* 20:199–243, 1962.
8. Newsholme EA, Crabtree B: Theoretical principles in the approaches to control of metabolic pathways and their application to glycolysis in muscle. *J Mol Cell Cardiol* 11:839–856, 1979.
9. Moller DE, Flier JS: Insulin resistance — mechanisms, syndromes, and implications. *N Engl J Med* 325:938–948, 1991.
10. Randle PJ, Smith GH: Regulation of glucose uptake by muscle. I. The effects of insulin, anaerobiosis and cell poisons on the uptake of glucose and release of potassium by isolated rat diaphragm. *Biochem J* 70:490–500, 1958.
11. Opie LH, Norris RM, Thomas M, Holland AJ, Owen P, van Noorden S: Failure of high concentrations of free fatty acids to provoke arrhythmias in experimental myocardial infarction. *Lancet* 1:818–822, 1971.
12. Bell GI, Kayano T, Buse JB, Burant CF, Takeda J, Lin D, et al.: Molecular biology of mammalian glucose transporters. *Diabetes Care* 13:198–208, 1990.
13. Burk D: A colloquial consideration of the Pasteur and neo-Pasteur effects. *Cold Spring Harb Symp Quant Biol* 7:420–459, 1939.
14. Neely JR, Morgan HE: Relationship between carbohydrate and lipid metabolism and the energy balance of heart muscle. *Ann Rev Physiol* 36:413–459, 1974.
15. Opie LH: Substrate utilization and glycolysis in the heart. *Cardiology* 56:2–21, 1971/72.
16. Lawson JWR, Uyeda K: Effects of insulin and work on fructose 2,6-bisphosphate content and phosphofructokinase activity in perfused rat hearts. *J Biol Chem* 262:3165–3173, 1987.
17. Kubler W, Spieckermann PG: Regulation of glycolysis in the ischemic and the anoxic myocardium. *J Mol Cell Cardiol* 1:351–377, 1970.
18. Williamson JR: Glycolytic control mechanisms. II. Kinetics of intermediate changes during aerobic-anoxic transition in perfused rat heart. *J Biol Chem* 241:5026–5036, 1966.
19. Neely JR, Whitmer JT, Rovetto MJ: Inhibition of glycolysis in hearts during ischemic perfusion. In: Harris P, Bing RJ, Fleckenstein A (eds) *Recent Advances in Studies on Cardiac Structure and Metabolism*, Vol 7. Biochemistry and Pharmacology of Myocardial Hypertrophy, Hypoxia and Infarction. Baltimore, MD: University Park Press, 1976, pp 243–248.
20. Mochizuki S, Neely JR: Control of glyceraldehyde-3-phosphate dehydrogenase in cardiac muscle. *J Mol Cell Cardiol* 11:221–236, 1979.
21. Rovetto MJ, Lamberton WF, Neely JR: Mechanism of glycolytic inhibition in ischemic rat hearts. *Circ Res* 37:742–751, 1975.
22. Apstein CS, Deckelbaum L, Mueller M, Hagopian L, Hood WB Jr: Graded global ischemia and reperfusion: Cardiac function and lactate metabolism. *Circulation* 55:864–872, 1977.
23. Opie LH: Effects of regional ischemia on metabolism of glucose and fatty acids. *Circ Res* 38(Suppl 1):52–74, 1975.
24. Gevers W: Generation of protons by metabolic processes in heart cells. *J Mol Cell Cardiol* 9:867–874, 1977.
25. Dennis SC, Gevers W, Opie LH: Protons in ischemia: Where do they come from, where do they go to? *J Mol Cell Cardiol* 23:1077–1086, 1991.
26. Shipp JC, Opie LH, Challoner D: Fatty acid and glucose metabolism in the perfused heart. *Nature* 189:1018–1019, 1961.
27. Bailey IA, Radda GK, Seymour AL, Williams SR: The effects of insulin on myocardial metabolism and acidosis in normoxia and ischaemia. *Biochim Biophys Acta* 720:17–27, 1982.
28. Miller TB: A dual role for insulin in the regulation of cardiac glycogen synthase. *J Biol Chem* 253:5389–5394, 1978.
29. Morgan HE, Parmeggiani A: Regulation of glycogenolysis in muscle. III. Control of muscle glycogen phosphorylase activity. *J Biol Chem* 239:2440–2445, 1964.
30. Achs MJ, Garfinkel D, Opie LH: Computer simulation of metabolism of glucose perfused rat heart in a work-jump. *Am J Physiol* 243:R389–R399, 1982.

31. Wisneski JA, Gertz EW, Neese RA, Gruenke LD, Morris DL, Craig JC: Metabolic fate of extracted glucose in normal human myocardium. *J Clin Invest* 76:1819–1827, 1985.

32. Schneider CA, Taegtmeyer H: Fasting in vivo delays myocardial cell damage after brief periods of ischemia in the isolated working rat heart. *Circ Res* 68:1045–1050, 1991.

33. Neely JR, Grotyohann LW: Role of glycolytic products in damage to ischemic myocardium. Dissociation of adenosine triphosphate levels and recovery of function of reperfused ischemic hearts. *Circ Res* 55:816–824, 1984.

34. Largerstrom CF, Walker WE, Taegtmeyer H: Failure of glycogen depletion to improve left ventricular function of the rabbit heart after hypothermic ischemic arrest. *Circ Res* 63:81–86, 1988.

35. Camici P, Araujo LI, Spinks T, Lammertsma AA, Kaski JC, Shea MJ, et al.: Increased uptake of ^{18}F-fluorodeoxyglucose in postischemic myocardium of patients with exercise-induced angina. *Circulation* 74:81–88, 1986.

36. Rose CP, Goresky CA: Constraints on the uptake of labeled palmitate by the heart: The barriers at the capillary and sarcolemmal surfaces and the control of intracellular sequestration. *Circ Res* 41:534–545, 1979.

37. Lassers BW, Kaijser L, Wahlqvist ML, Carlson LA: Relationship in man between plasma free fatty acids and myocardial metabolism of carbohydrate substrates. *Lancet* 2:448–450, 1971.

38. Dennis SC, Kohn MC, Anderson GJ, Garfinkel D: Kinetic analysis of monocarboxylate uptake into perfused rat hearts. *J Mol Cell Cardiol* 17:987–995, 1985.

39. Krasnow N, Neill WA, Messer JV: Myocardial lactate and pyruvate metabolism. *J Clin Invest* 41:2075–2085, 1962.

40. Gertz EW, Wisneski JA, Neese R, Houser A, Korte R, Bristow JD: Myocardial lactate extraction: Multi-determined metabolic function. *Circulation* 61:256–261, 1980.

41. Resnekov L, Falicov RE: Thyrotoxicosis and lactate-producing angina pectoris with normal coronary arteries. *Br Heart J* 39:1051–1057, 1977.

42. Opie LH: Lipid metabolism of the heart and arteries in relation to ischaemic heart disease. *Lancet* 1:192–195, 1973.

43. Randle PJ: Regulation of glycolysis and pyruvate oxidation in cardiac muscle. *Circ Res* 38(Suppl 1):8–12, 1976.

44. Kobayashi K, Neely JR: Mechanism of pyruvate dehydrogenase activation by increased heart work. *J Mol Cell Cardiol* 15:369–382, 1983.

45. Opie LH, Owen P: Assessment of mitochondrial free NAD$^+$/NADH ratios and oxaloacetate concentrations during increased mechanical work in isolated perfused rat heart during production or uptake of ketone bodies. *Biochem J* 148:403–415, 1975.

46. Moravec J, Corsin A, Owen P, Opie LH: Effect of increased aortic perfusion pressure on fluorescent emission of the isolated rat heart. *J Mol Cell Cardiol* 6:187–200, 1974.

47. Kohn MC, Achs MJ, Garfinkel D: Computer simulation of metabolism in pyruvate-perfused rat heart. III. Pyruvate dehydrogenase. *Am J Physiol* 237:R167–R173, 1979.

48. Bremer J: Pyruvate dehydrogenase, substrate specificity and product inhibition. *Eur J Biochem* 8:535–540, 1969.

49. Thomassen A, Nielsen TT, Bagger JP, Pedersen AK, Henningsen P: Anti-ischemic and metabolic effects of glutamate during pacing in patients with stable angina pectoris secondary to either coronary artery disease or Syndrome X. *Am J Cardiol* 68:291–295, 1991.

50. Bing RJ: Cardiac metabolism. *Physiol Rev* 45:171–213, 1965.

51. Bing RJ, Siegel A, Vitale A, Balboni F, Sparks E, Taeschler M, et al.: Metabolic studies on the human heart in vivo. I.

52. Bing RJ, Siegel A, Ungar I, Gilbert M: Metabolism of the human heart. II. Studies on fat, ketone and amino acid metabolism. *Am J Med* 16:504–515, 1954.

53. Lopaschuk GD, Spafford MA, Davies NJ, Wall SR: Glucose and palmitate oxidation in isolated working rat hearts reperfused after a period of transient global ischemia. *Circ Res* 66:546–553, 1990.

54. Menahan LA, Hron WT: Regulation of acetoacetyl-CoA in isolated perfused rat hearts. *Eur J Biochem* 119:295–299, 1981.

55. Opie LH: Metabolism of the heart. II. Metabolism of triglycerides. Substrates for oxidative metabolism. Mitochondrial metabolism. Synthetic reactions. Excitation coupling. *Am Heart J* 77:100–122, 1969.

56. Lassers BW, Kaijser L, Carlson LA: Myocardial lipid and carbohydrate metabolism in healthy, fasting men at rest: Studies during continuous infusion of ^{3}H-palmitate. *Eur J Clin Invest* 2:348–358, 1972.

57. Olson RE, Hoeschen RJ: Utilization of endogenous lipid by the isolated perfused rat heart. *Biochem J* 103:796, 1967.

58. Vyska K, Meyer W, Stremmel W, Notohamiprodjo G, Minami K, Machulla H-J, et al.: Fatty acid uptake in normal human myocardium. *Circ Res* 69:857–870, 1991.

59. Van der Vusse GJ, Roemen ThHM, Prinzen FW, Coumans WA, Reneman RS: Uptake and tissue content of fatty acids in dog myocardium under normoxic and ischemic conditions. *Circ Res* 50:538–546, 1982.

60. Hochachka DW, Neely JR, Driedzic WR: Integration of lipid utilization with Krebs cycle activity in muscle. *Fed Proc* 36:2009–2014, 1977.

61. Fritz IB: Action of carnitine on long-chain fatty acid oxidation by liver. *Am J Physiol* 197:297–304, 1959.

62. Awan MM, Saggerson ED: Malonyl-CoA metabolism in cardiac myocytes and its relevance to the control of fatty acid oxidation. *Biochem J* 1993, in press.

63. Fritz IB, Yue KTN: Long-chain carnitine acyltransferase and the role of acylcarnitine derivatives in the catalytic increase of fatty acid oxidation induced by carnitine. *J Lipid Res* 4:279–288, 1963.

64. Pande SV: A mitochondrial carnitine acylcarnitine translocase system. *Proc Natl Acad Sci USA* 72:883–887, 1975.

65. Ramsay RR, Tubbs PK: The mechanism of fatty acid uptake by heart mitochondria: An acylcarnitine-carnitine exchange. *FEBS Lett* 54:21–25, 1975.

66. Pande SV, Parvin R: Characterization of carnitine acylcarnitine translocase system of heart mitochondria. *J Biol Chem* 251:6683–6691, 1976.

67. Idell-Wenger JA, Grotyohann LW, Neely JR: Regulation of fatty-acid utilization in heart. Role of carnitine-acetyl-CoA transferase and carnitine-acetyl carnitine translocase system. *J Mol Cell Cardiol* 14:413–417, 1982.

68. Pande SV, Blanchaer MC: Reversible inhibition of mitochondrial adenosine disphosphate phosphorylation by long-chain acyl CoA esters. *J Biol Chem* 246:402–411, 1971.

69. Heldt HW, Jacobs H, Klingenberg M: Endogenous ADP of mitochondria, an early phosphate acceptor of oxidative phosphorylation as disclosed by kinetic studies with C^{14} labelled ADP and ATP and with atractyloside. *Biochem Biophys Res Commun* 18:174–178, 1965.

70. Shug AL, Shrago E, Bittar N, Folts JD, Kokes JR: Long-chain fatty acyl CoA inhibition of adenine nucleotide translocase in the ischemic myocardium. *Am J Physiol* 228:689–692, 1975.

71. Lochner A, Van Niekerk I, Kotze JCN. Mitochondrial acyl

CoA, adenine nucleotide translocase activity and oxidative phosphorylation in myocardial ischemia. *J Mol Cell Cardiol* 13:991–997, 1981.

72. La Noue KF, Watts JA, Koch CD: Adenine nucleotide transport during cardiac ischemia. *Am J Physiol* 241:H663–H677, 1981.

73. Barbour RL, Chan SHP: Characterization of the kinetics and mechanism of the mitochondrial ADP-ATP carrier. *J Biol Chem* 256:1940–1948, 1981.

74. Oram JF, Bennetch SL, Neely JR: Regulation of fatty acid utilization in isolated perfused rat hearts. *J Biol Chem* 248:5299–5309, 1973.

75. Moore KH, Radloff JF, Koen AE, Hull PE: Incomplete fatty acid oxidation by heart mitochondria: Beta-hydroxy fatty acid production. *J Mol Cell Cardiol* 14:451–459, 1982.

76. Opie LH: Metabolism of free fatty acids, glucose and catecholamines in acute myocardial infarction. Relation to myocardial ischemia and infarct size. *Am J Cardiol* 36:938–953, 1975.

77. Van Bilsen M, van der Vusse GJ, Willemsen PHM, Coumans WA, Roemen THM, Reneman RS: Lipid alterations in isolated, working rat hearts during ischemia and reperfusion: Its relation to myocardial damage. *Circ Res* 64:304–314, 1989.

78. Challoner DR, Steinberg D: Metabolic effect of epinephrine on the oxygen consumption of the perfused rat heart. *Nature* 205:602–663, 1965.

79. Glaviano VV, Goldberg JM, Pindok M, Wallick D, Aranis C: Cholinergic intervention on myocardial dynamics and metabolism in the non-working dog heart. *Circ Res* 41:508–514, 1977.

80. Saddik M, Lopaschuk D: Myocardial triglyceride turnover and contribution to energy substrate utilization in isolated working rat hearts. *J Biol Chem* 266:8162–8170, 1991.

81. Oliver MF, Kurien VA, Greenwood TW: Relation between serum free fatty acids and arrhythmias and death after acute myocardial infarction. *Lancet* 1:710–715, 1968.

82. Opie LH, Owen P, Riemersma RA: Relative rates of oxidation of glucose and free fatty acids by ischemic and non-ischemic myocardium after coronary artery ligation in the dog. *Eur J Clin Invest* 3:419–435, 1973.

83. Challoner DR, Steinberg D: Oxidative metabolism of myocardium as influenced by fatty acids and epinephrine. *Am J Physiol* 211:897–892, 1966.

84. Pearce FJ, Forster J, De Leeuw G, Williamson JR, Tutwiler GF: Inhibition of fatty acid oxidation in normal and hypoxic perfused rat hearts by 2-tetradecylglycidic acid. *J Mol Cell Cardiol* 11:893–915, 1979.

85. Kurien VA, Yates PA, Oliver MF: The role of free fatty acids in the production of ventricular arrhythmias after acute coronary artery occlusion. *Eur J Clin Invest* 1:225–241, 1971.

86. De Leiris J, Opie LH: Effect of substrates and of coronary artery ligation on mechanical performance and on release of lactate dehydrogenase and creatine phosphokinase in isolated working rat hearts. *Cardiovasc Res* 12:585–596, 1978.

87. Opie LH: Effect of fatty acids on contractility and rhythm of the heart. *Nature* 227:1055–1056, 1970.

88. Molaparast-Saless F, Liedtke AJ, Nellis SH: Effects of the fatty acid blocking agents, oxfenicine and 4-bromocrotonic acid, on performance in aerobic and ischemic myocardium. *J Mol Cell Cardiol* 19:509–520, 1987.

89. Sato T, Kiyosue T, Arita M: Inhibitory effects of palmitoylcarnitine and lysophosphatidylcholine on the sodium current of cardiac ventricular cells. *Pflügers Arch* 420:94–100, 1992.

90. Liedtke AJ, Nellis SH, Whitesell LF: Effects of carnitine

isomers on fatty acid metabolism in ischemic swine hearts. *Circ Res* 48:859–866, 1981.

91. Broderick TL, Quinney HA, Lopaschuk GD: Carnitine stimulation of glucose oxidation in the fatty acid perfused isolated working rat heart. *J Biol Chem* 267:3758–3763, 1992.

92. Sobel BE, Corr PB, Robison AK: Accumulation of lysophosphoglyceride with arrhythmogenic properties in ischemic myocardium. *J Clin Invest* 62:546–553, 1978.

93. Corr PB, Gross RW, Sobel BE: Arrhythmogenic amphiphilic lipids and the myocardial cell membrane. *J Mol Cell Cardiol* 14:619–626, 1982.

94. Man RYK, Choy PC: Lysophosphotidylcholine causes cardiac arrhythmia. *J Mol Cell Cardiol* 14:173–175, 1982.

95. Katz AM, Messineo FC: Lipid-membrane interactions and the pathogenesis of ischemic damage in the myocardium. *Circ Res* 48:1–16, 1981.

96. La Noue KF, Walajtys EI, Williamson JR: Regulation of glutamate metabolism and interactions with the citric acid cycle in rat heart mitochondria. *J Biol Chem* 248:7171–7183, 1973.

97. Digerness SB, Reddy WJ: The malate-aspartate shuttle in heart mitochondria. *J Mol Cell Cardiol* 8:779–785, 1976.

98. Puckett SW, Reddy WJ: A decrease in the malate-aspartate shuttle and glutamate translocase activity in heart mitochondria from alloxan-diabetic rats. *J Mol Cell Cardiol* 11:173–187, 1979.

99. Kobayashi K, Neely JR: Control of maximum rates of glycolysis in rat cardiac muscle. *Circ Res* 44:166–175, 1979.

100. McGinnis JF, De Vellis J: Glycerol-3-phosphate dehydrogenase isoenzymes in human tissues: Evidence for a heart specific form. *J Mol Cell Cardiol* 11:795–802, 1979.

101. Randle PJ, England PJ, Denton RM: Control of the tricarboxylic acid cycle and its interactions with glycolysis during acetate utilization in rat heart. *Biochem J* 117:677–695, 1970.

102. Williamson JR, Ford C, Illingworth J, Safer B: Coordination of citric acid cycle activity with electron transport flux. *Circ Res* 38(Suppl I):39–48, 1976.

103. Garfinkel D: Lactate permeation. In: Randle PJ (ed) Discussion of Regulation of Glycolysis and Pyruvate Oxidation in Cardiac Muscle. *Circ Res* 38(Suppl I):13–15, 1976.

104. Bricknell OL, Opie LH: Glycolytic ATP and its production during ischaemia in isolated Langendorff-perfused rat hearts. In: Kobayashi T, Sano T, Dhalla NS (eds) *Recent Advances in Studies of Cardiac Structure and Metabolism*, Vol 11. Heart Function and Metabolism. Baltimore, MD: University Park Press, 1978, pp 509–519.

105. Opie LH, Bricknell OL: Role of glycolytic flux in effect of glucose in decreasing fatty acid-induced release of lactate dehydrogenase from isolated coronary ligated rat heart. *Cardiovasc Res* 13:693–702, 1979.

106. Cowan JC, Vaughan Williams EM: The effects of palmitate on intracellular potentials recorded from Langendorff-perfused guinea-pig hearts in normoxia and hypoxia and during perfusion at reduced rate of flow. *J Mol Cell Cardiol* 9:327–342, 1977.

107. Bricknell OL, Daries PS, Opie LH: A relationship between adenosine triphosphate, glycolysis and ischaemic contracture in the isolated rat heart. *J Mol Cell Cardiol* 13:941–945, 1981.

108. Bing OHL, Fishbein MC: Mechanical and structural correlates of contracture induced by metabolic blockade in cardiac muscle from the rat. *Circ Res* 45:298–308, 1979.

109. Entman ML, Bornet EP, Van Winkle WB, Goldstein MA, Schwartz A. Association of glycogenolysis with cardiac

sarcoplasmic reticulum: II. Effect of glycogen depletion, deoxycholate solubilization and cardiac ischemia: Evidence for a phosphorylase kinase membrane complex. *J Mol Cell Cardiol* 9:515–528, 1977.

110. Owen P, Dennis S, Opie LH: Glucose flux rate regulates onset of ischemic contracture in globally underperfused rat hearts. *Circ Res* 66:344–354, 1990.

111. Saks VA, Kuznetsov AV, Kupriyanov VV, Miceli MV, Jacobus WE: Creatine kinase of rat heart mitochondria. *J Biol Chem* 260:7757–7764, 1985.

112. Seraydarian MW, Artaza L: Regulation of energy metabolism by creatine in cardiac and skeletal muscle cells in culture. *J Mol Cell Cardiol* 8:669–678, 1976.

113. Krzanowski J, Matchinsky FM: Regulation of phosphofructokinase by phosphocreatine and phosphorylated glycolytic intermediates. *Biochem Biophys Res Commun* 34:816–823, 1969.

114. Ponce-Hornos JE, Langer GA, Nudd LM: Inorganic phosphate: Its effects on Ca exchange and compartmentalization in cultured heart cells. *J Mol Cell Cardiol* 14:41–51, 1982.

115. Soboll S, Bunger R: Compartmentation of adenine nucleotides in the isolated working guinea-pig heart stimulated by adrenaline. *Hoppe Seylers Z Physiol* 362:125–132, 1981.

116. Balaban RS: Regulation of oxidative phosphorylation in the mammalian cell. *Am J Physiol* 258:C377–C389, 1990.

117. Clarke K, Willis RJ: Energy metabolism and contractile function in rat heart during graded, isovolumic perfusion using ^{31}P nuclear magnetic resonance spectroscopy. *J Mol Cell Cardiol* 19:1153–1160, 1987.

118. Das AM, Harris DA: Regulation of the mitochondrial ATP synthase in intact rat cardiomyocytes. *Biochem J* 266:355–361, 1990.

119. Koretsky AP, Katz LA, Balaban RS: The mechanism of respiratory control in the in vivo heart. *J Mol Cell Cardiol* 21(Suppl I):59–66, 1989.

120. Fossel ET, Morgan HE, Ingwall JS: Measurement of changes in high-energy phosphates in the cardiac cycle by using gated ^{31}P nuclear magnetic resonance. *Proc Natl Acad Sci USA* 77:3654–3658, 1980.

121. Mitchell P: *Chemiosmotic Coupling and Energy Transduction.* Bodmin, UK: Glynn Research, 1968.

122. Hearse DJ: Oxygen deprivation and early myocardial contractile failure: A reassessment of the possible role of adenosine triphosphate. *Am J Cardiol* 44:1115–1121, 1979.

123. Gudbjarnason S, Mathes P, Ravens KG: Functional compartmentation of ATP and creatine phosphate in heart muscle. *J Mol Cell Cardiol* 1:325–339, 1970.

124. Kupriyanov VV, Lakomkin VL, Kapelko VI, Steinschneider AY, Ruuge EK, Saks VA: Dissociation of adenosine triphosphate levels and contractile function in isovolumic hearts perfused with 2-deoxyglucose. *J Mol Cell Cardiol* 19:729–740, 1987.

125. Taegtmeyer H, Roberts AFC, Raine AEG: Energy metabolism in reperfused heart muscle: Metabolic correlates to return of function. *J Am Coll Cardiol* 6:864–870, 1985.

126. Opie LH: Hypothesis: Glycolytic rates control cell viability in ischemia. *J Appl Cardiol* 3:407–414, 1988.

127. Fosset M, De Weille JR, Green RD, Schmid-Antomarchi H, Lazdunski M: Antidiabetic sulfonylureas control action potential properties in heart cells via high affinity receptors that are linked to ATP-dependent K$^+$ channels. *J Biol Chem* 263:7933–7936, 1988.

128. Kantor PF, Coetzee WA, Carmeliet EE, Dennis SC, Opie LH: Reduction of ischemic K$^+$ loss and arrhythmias in rat hearts. Effect of glibenclamide, a sulfonylurea. *Circ Res* 66:478–485, 1990.

129. Lederer WJ, Nichols CG: Nucleotide modulation of the activity of rat heart ATP-sensitive K$^+$ channels in isolated membrane patches. *J Physiol* 419:193–211, 1989.

130. Kirsch GE, Codina J, Birnbaumer L, Brown AM: Coupling of ATP-sensitive K$^+$ channels to A$_1$ receptors by G-proteins in rat ventricular myocytes. *Am J Physiol* 259:H820–H826, 1990.

131. Weiss JN, Venkatesh N: Metabolic regulation of cardiac ATP-sensitive K$^+$ channels. *Cardiovasc Drugs Ther*, 1993, in press.

132. Coetzee WA: Effects of intra- and extracellular pH on current through ATP-sensitive potassium channels of isolated guinea-pig ventricular myocytes. *J Physiol* 446:543P, 1992.

133. Opie LH: Reperfusion injury and its pharmacological modification. *Circulation* 80:1049–1062, 1989.

134. Hearse DJ. Reperfusion-induced injury: A possible role for oxidant stress and its manipulation. *Cardiovasc Drugs Ther* 5:225–236, 1991.

135. Jennings RB, Reimer KA, Steenbergen C: Myocardial ischemia revisited. The osmolar load, membrane damage, and reperfusion. *J Mol Cell Cardiol* 18:769–780, 1986.

136. Bolli R: Mechanism of myocardial "stunning." *Circulation* 82:723–738, 1990.

137. Heyndrickx GR, Millard RW, McRitchie RJ, Maroko PR, Vatner SF: Regional myocardial functional and electrophysiological alterations after brief coronary artery occlusion in conscious dogs. *J Clin Invest* 56:978–985, 1975.

138. Heyndrickx GR, Baig H, Nellens P, Leusen I, Fishebein MC, Vatner SF: Depression of regional blood flow and wall thickening after brief coronary occlusions. *Am J Physiol* 234:H653–H659, 1978.

139. Braunwald E, Kloner RA: The stunned myocardium: Prolonged, postischemic ventricular dysfunction. *Circulation* 66:1146–1149, 1982.

140. Hearse DJ: Stunning: A radical re-view. *Cardiovasc Drugs Ther* 5:853–876, 1991.

141. Thompson-Gorman S, Maupoil V, Zweier J: The influence of extracellular calcium concentration on free radical generation in myocardial ischemia/reperfusion injury (abstr). *Circulation* 84(Suppl II):II254, 1991.

142. Bernier M, Hearse DJ, Manning AS: Reperfusion-induced arrhythmias and oxygen-derived free radicals. Studies with "anti-free radical" interventions and a free radical-generating system in the isolated perfused rat heart. *Circ Res* 58:331–340, 1986.

143. Bolli J, Jeroudi MO, Patel BS, Aruoma OI, Halliwell B, Lai EK, McCay PB: Marked reduction of free radical generation and contractile dysfunction by anti-oxidant therapy begun at the time of reperfusion: Evidence that myocardial "stunning" is a manifestation of reperfusion injury. *Circ Res* 65:607–622, 1989.

144. Jennings RB, Shen AC: Calcium in experimental myocardial ischemia. In: Bajusz E, Rona G (eds) *Myocardiology.* Baltimore, MD: University Park Press, 1972, pp 639–655.

145. Becker, Schaper J, Jeremy R, Schaper W: Severity of ischemia determines the occurrence of myocardial reperfusion injury (abstr). *Circulation* 84(Suppl II):II254, 1991.

146. Guarnieri C, Flamigni F, Caldarera CM: Role of oxygen in the cellular damage induced by re-oxygenation of hypoxic heart. *J Mol Cell Cardiol* 12:797–808, 1980.

147. Shattock MJ, Manning AS, Hearse DJ: Hydrogen peroxide effects on the isolated working rat heart. In: Caldarera CM, Harris P (eds) *Advances in Studies on Heart Metabolism.* Bologna, Italy: CLUEB, 1982, pp 468–474.

148. Hearse DJ, Humphrey SM, Bullock GR: The oxygen

paradox and the calcium paradox: Two facets of the same problem. *J Mol Cell Cardiol* 10:641–668, 1978.

149. Ferrari R, Alfieri O, Curello S, Ceconi C, Cargnoni A, Narzollo P, et al.: Occurrence of oxidative stress during reperfusion of the human heart. *Circulation* 81:201–211, 1990.

150. Coetzee WA, Owen P, Dennis SC, Saman S, Opie LH: Reperfusion damage: Free radicals mediate delayed membrane changes rather than early ventricular arrhythmias. *Cardiovasc Res* 24:156–164, 1990.

151. Opie LH: Postischemic stunning — the case for calcium as the ultimate culprit. *Cardiovasc Drugs Ther* 5:895–900, 1991.

152. Yamada M, Hearse DJ, Curtis MJ: Reperfusion and readmission of oxygen. Pathophysiological relevance of oxygen-derived free radicals to arrhythmogenesis. *Circ Res* 67:1211–1224, 1990.

153. Holmberg SRM, Cumming DVE, Kusama Y, Hearse DJ, Poole-Wilson PA, Shattock MJ, Williams AJ: Reactive oxygen species modify the structure and function of the cardiac sarcoplasmic reticulum calcium-release channel. *Cardioscience* 2:19–25, 1991.

154. Jeremy RW, Koretsune Y, Marban E, Becker LC: Relation between glycolysis and calcium homeostasis in postischemic myocardium. *Circ Res* 70:1180–1190, 1992.

155. de Groot MJM, Coumans WA, Willemsen PHM, van der Vusse GJ: Substrate-induced changes in the lipid content of ischemic and reperfused myocardium. Its relation to hemodynamic recovery. *Circ Res* 72:176–186, 1993.

156. Opie LH: Importance of glycolytically produced ATP for the integrity of the threatened myocardial cell. In: Piper HM (ed) *Pathophysiology of Severe Ischemic Myocardial Injury.* Dordrecht, The Netherlands: Kluwer Academic Publishers, 1989, pp 41–65.

157. Bolli R: Oxygen-derived free radicals and myocardial reperfusion injury: An overview. *Cardiovasc Drugs Ther* 5:249–268, 1991.

158. Du Toit J, Opie LH: Modulation of severity of reperfusion stunning in the isolated rat heart by agents altering calcium flux at onset of reperfusion. *Circ Res* 70:960–967, 1992.

159. Kloner RA, Przyklenk K, Rahimtoola SH, Braunwald E: Myocardial stunning and hibernation. Mechanisms and clinical implications. In: Braunwald E (ed) *Heart Disease Update.* Philadelphia: WB Saunders, 1990, pp 241–256.

160. Ferrari R, Visioli O: Stunning: Damaging or protective to the myocardium? *Cardiovasc Drugs Ther* 5:939–946, 1991.

161. Rahimtoola SH: The hibernating myocardium. *Am Heart J* 117:211–221, 1989.

162. Heusch G: The relationship between regional blood flow and contractile function in normal, ischemic, and reperfused myocardium. *Basic Res Cardiol* 86:197–218, 1991.

163. Keller AM, Cannon PJ: Effect of graded reductions of coronary pressure and flow on myocardial metabolism and performance: A model of "hibernating" myocardium. *J Am Coll Cardiol* 17:1661–1670, 1991.

164. Arai AE, Pantely GA, Anselone CG, Bristow J, Bristow JD: Active downregulation of myocardial energy requirements during prolonged moderate ischemia in swine. *Circ Res* 69:1458–1469, 1991.

165. Yellon DM, Latchman DS: Stress proteins and myocardial protection during ischaemia and reperfusion. In: Yellon DM, Jennings RB (eds) *Myocardial Protection. The Pathophysiology of Reperfusion and Reperfusion Injury.* New York: Raven Press, 1992, pp 185–195.

166. Swain JL, Sabina RL, Hines JJ, Greenfield JC, Holmes EW: Repetitive episodes of brief ischaemia (12 min) do not produce a cumulative depletion of high energy phosphate compounds. *Cardiovasc Res* 18:264–269, 1984.

167. Murry CE, Jennings RB, Reimer KA: Preconditioning with ischemia: A delay of lethal cell injury in ischemic myocardium. *Circulation* 74:1124–1136, 1986.

168. Jennings RB, Murry CE, Reimer KA: Preconditioning myocardium with ischemia. *Cardiovasc Drugs Ther* 5:933–938, 1991.

169. Reimer KA, Jennings RB: Preconditioning: Definitions, proposed mechanisms, and implications for myocardial protection in ischemia and reperfusion. In: Yellon DM, Jennings RB (eds) *Myocardial Protection. The Pathophysiology of Reperfusion and Reperfusion Injury.* New York: Raven Press, 1992, pp 165–183.

170. Omar BA, Hanson AK, Bose SK, McCord JM: Reperfusion with pyruvate eliminates ischemic preconditioning in the isolated rabbit heart: An apparent role for enhanced glycolysis. *Cor Art Dis* 2:799–804, 1991.

171. Thornton JD, Liu GS, Olsson RA, Downey JM: Intravenous pretreatment with A_1-selective adenosine analogues protects the heart against infarction. *Circulation* 85:659–665, 1992.

172. Wyatt DA, Edmunds MC, Rubio R, Berne RM, Lasley RD, Mentzer RM Jr: Adenosine stimulates glycolytic flux in isolated perfused rat hearts by A1-adenosine receptors. *Am J Physiol* 257:H1952–H1957, 1989.

173. Opie LH: Role of carnitine in fatty acid metabolism of normal and ischemic myocardium. *Am Heart J* 97:375–388, 1979.

174. Camici P, Ferrannini E, Opie LH: Myocardial metabolism in ischemic heart disease: Basic principles and application to imaging by positron emission tomography. *Prog Cardiovasc Dis* 32:217–238, 1989.

175. Kuznetsov AV, Khuchua ZA, Vassil'eva EV, et al.: Heart mitochondrial creatine kinase revisited: The outer mitochondrial membrane is not important for coupling of phosphocreatine production to oxidative phosphorylation. *Arch Biochem Biophys* 268:176–190, 1989.

176. Oliver MF, Opie LH: Effects of glucose and fatty acids on myocardial ischemia and arrhythmias. *Lancet* 343:155–158, 1994.

CHAPTER 21

Autonomic Neural Control of Cardiac Function

MATTHEW N. LEVY & PAUL J. MARTIN

INTRODUCTION

The heart is regulated by both divisions of the autonomic nervous system. The sympathetic division is facilitatory, whereas the parasympathetic division is inhibitory. The central nervous system controls the activity in each division, usually in a reciprocal fashion; that is, as sympathetic activity increases, parasympathetic activity diminishes, and vice versa. In certain regions of the heart, such as the nodal tissues, the parasympathetic effects tend to predominate over the sympathetic influences. However, in other regions, such as the ventricular myocardium, the effects of the sympathetic division usually dominate those of the parasympathetic division. The cardiac effects of each division are determined mainly by the relative abundance of nerve fibers and the density of ligand receptors associated with each division. When both divisions are active simultaneously, the sympathetic and vagal effects do not usually summate algebraically; instead, the summation is often highly nonlinear. Several detailed reviews of this subject have been published during the past decade {1–4}.

CARDIAC INNERVATION

Sympathetic innervation

Our knowledge of the cardiac innervation is based mainly upon studies in experimental animals, and substantial variations exist among mammals. The cell bodies of the preganglionic sympathetic fibers to the heart in most mammals are located in the intermediolateral columns of the upper eight thoracic and the lower two cervical segments of the spinal cord. These preganglionic fibers emerge through the white rami communicantes and enter the paravertebral chain of ganglia {5–7}. Most of the preganglionic cardiac sympathetic fibers ascend in the paravertebral chains and funnel through the stellate ganglia (fig. 21-1). The cardiac sympathetic fibers pass through the dorsal or ventral limbs of the ansa subclavia, and they converge at the caudal cervical ganglia.

The location of the synapses between the preganglionic and postganglionic cardiac sympathetic fibers varies among species. Synapses may be located in any of the upper thoracic ganglia, including the stellate, middle cervical, or superior cervical ganglia. In the cat, the synapses lie mainly in the stellate ganglia, whereas in the dog most of them lie in the caudal (or middle) cervical ganglia. Where most of these synapses are located in humans has not been established. In most mammals, however, the postganglionic fibers travel to the heart as a complicated plexus of mixed nerve trunks {5,7}, as shown in fig. 21-1.

Parasympathetic innervation

The preganglionic cardiac vagal neurons are located in the medulla oblongata, in either the nucleus ambiguus or the dorsal nucleus of the vagus, depending on the species {8,9}. After the preganglionic vagal fibers on each side exit from the skull, they travel down the neck in the carotid sheath. In some species, such as the dog, cervical vagal and sympathetic fibers form a common bundle, the vagosympathetic trunk. In other species, including humans, fibers from the two divisions lie in separate nerve trunks (fig. 21-1). In the thorax the efferent vagal fibers join the cardiac neural plexus, which is a complicated network of mixed nerve trunks. The individual nerves in the plexus contain preganglionic vagal and postganglionic sympathetic efferent fibers, and also many afferent nerve fibers from cardiopulmonary sensory receptors. The anatomical arrangement of the mixed nerves in the cardiac plexus differs considerably on the right and left sides {5,7}. Each nerve bundle in the plexus is distributed to a distinct cardiac region, but the various regions overlap substantially {10,11}.

The synapses between the preganglionic and postganglionic vagal neurons occur in intracardiac ganglia or in epicardial fat pads, usually close to the structures innervated by the postganglionic neurons {10–12}. The autonomic innervation of the atrioventricular (AV) and sinoatrial (SA) nodes appears to funnel through separate epicardial fat pads. Resection of a fat pad that lies at the junction of the inferior vena cava and the right atrium eliminated all vagal input to the AV node region in dogs, but it did not alter the vagal control of SA nodal function {13}. Electrical stimulation of a discrete fat pad can alter separately either SA or AV nodal function {14}. Administration of appropriate autonomic antagonists has shown that the

N. Sperelakis (ed.), Physiology and Pathophysiology of the Heart, Third Edition.

413

Right Side

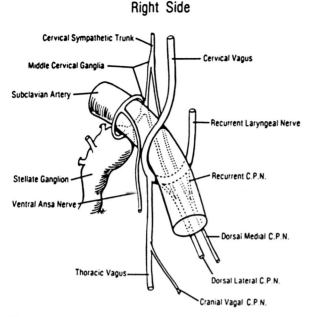

Fig. 21-1. The autonomic innervation (right side) of the heart in man. C.P.N. = cardiopulmonary nerves. From Janes et al. {7}, with permission.

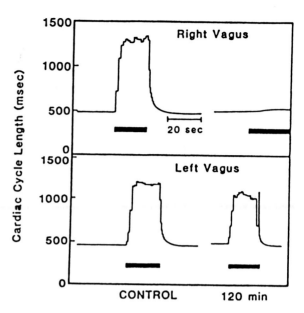

Fig. 21-2. Changes in cardiac cycle length evoked by stimulations (at the horizontal bars) of the right and left vagus nerves in an anesthetized dog. The responses on the left side of the figure were recorded under control conditions. The responses on the right side of the figure were recorded after 120 minutes of hemicholinium-3 infusion combined with intense right vagal stimulation. Adapted from Lang et al. {9}, with permission.

discrete distribution of neural fibers to the two nodal regions applies to the sympathetic as well as the parasympathetic divisions of the autonomic nervous system {15}.

Innervation of the sinoatrial node

The sympathetic fibers to the SA node approach the heart along the peripulmonary tissues, the pulmonary veins, and the superior vena cava {10,16}. The SA node receives many more sympathetic fibers from the right than from the left side of the body. The spatial distribution of sympathetic nerve fibers to the heart has been assessed by measuring the tissue concentrations of norepinephrine (NE). The NE concentration is two to four times higher in atrial and nodal tissues than in the ventricles {6}.

The two vagus nerves are usually considered to be distributed asymmetrically to the various cardiac structures. The right vagus nerve is thought to be consigned mainly to the SA node and the left vagus nerve mainly to the AV conduction system {6,10,16}. This asymmetry has been challenged, however. In certain experiments on anesthetized dogs, right vagal stimulation exerted a greater negative chronotrophic effect than did left vagal stimulation {17}. In other experiments {18}, however, the effects of right and left vagal stimulation on heart rate did not differ appreciably. Nevertheless, right vagal transection did increase heart rate more than did left-sided transection in these experiments {18}. These data suggest, therefore, that the right vagus nerve ordinarily restrains the SA node more than does the left vagus nerve.

Although the preganglionic fibers of the right and left vagus nerves control the activities of the SA and AV nodes, the extent of convergence of preganglionic fibers from the vagi on common postganglionic neurons is negligible {19}. In the experiment shown in fig. 21-2, for example, preganglionic stimulation of the right vagus nerve in an anesthetized dog increased the cardiac cycle length by 860 ms under control conditions, and preganglionic stimulation of the left vagus nerve increased cardiac cycle length by 720 ms. Thereafter, hemicholinium-3 was administered, and the right vagus nerve was stimulated intensely for 120 minutes in order to deplete the acetylcholine (ACh) from the preganglionic right vagal fibers and also from the postganglionic neurons innervated by those right vagal preganglionic neurons. Presumably, some of those postganglionic neurons were also innervated by preganglionic fibers from the left vagus nerve. Subsequent preganglionic stimulation of the right vagus nerve elicited only a negligible chronotropic response, which confirms that the depletion regimen was effective. However, this depletion regimen attenuated only slightly the response to preganglionic stimulation of the left vagus nerve (fig. 21-2). This finding indicates that very few of the postganglionic vagal neurons innervated by the left vagal preganglionic fibers are also innervated by preganglionic fibers of the right vagus nerve; the ACh would have been depleted in such bilaterally innervated postganglionic neurons.

ACh itself and some of the enzymes involved in its metabolism have been used to assess the density of distribution of the vagal fibers in the heart {1}. In the cat heart ACh is most concentrated in the SA node. The ACh concentration in the atria is about half that in the SA node, and the ACh concentration in the ventricles is only about one-third that in the atria. Acetylcholinesterase is also considerably more concentrated in the SA node than in the surrounding atrial tissue, and its concentration in the ventricular walls is considerably less than in the atria.

NEURAL CONTROL OF HEART RATE

Sympathetic control

The norepinephrine (NE) released from the sympathetic nerve endings increases the firing frequency of the automatic cells in the SA node. The sympathetic nerves from the right side of the body evoke greater increases in heart rate than do those from the left side {6,10}. The increases in heart rate are accomplished by augmenting the slope of slow diastolic depolarization in the automatic cells in the SA node {20,21}. The increased slope is achieved by the effect of the neurally released NE on several ionic currents. Catecholamines enhance the calcium current through L-type calcium channels and augment the so-called pacemaker current (i_f), which is mainly an inward Na^+ current {2,21,22}. Catecholamines may also diminish the rate of K^+ efflux from the automatic cell, and thereby accelerate the slow diastolic depolarization.

Sympathetic neural activity evokes a gradual cardiac acceleration (fig. 21-3B), rather than the abrupt change that characterizes the vagal response (fig. 21-3A). The latent period for the response to sympathetic stimulation is about 1 or 2 seconds, and the response does not reach a plateau until about 30–60 seconds after the beginning of neural stimulation {23–25}. One explanation for the long latency and the gradual rise to a plateau is that the process that transduces the signal from the β-adrenergic receptors involves a slow second messenger system, notably the adenylyl cyclase system {2,26,27}. This explanation is controversial, however, because recent evidence indicates that some of the β-adrenergic receptors are coupled to the ion channels directly via G proteins {28,29}. Such a coupling would be expected to hasten the cardiac response to sympathetic stimulation, and possibly allow beat-by-beat sympathetic regulation of the heart {28,29}.

However, the sluggish response to sympathetic stimulation might instead depend mainly on a relatively slow release of NE from the sympathetic nerve endings in the heart {25}. The amount of NE ordinarily released from the sympathetic nerve endings in the heart during one heart beat is probably too small to alter cardiac performance very much from one beat to the next. This slow rate of transmitter release may have evolved as a consequence of the very slow removal of the sympathetic neurotransmitter from the cardiac interstitium, as described below. If NE were released rapidly from the cardiac sympathetic nerves but removed too slowly from the cardiac intersti-

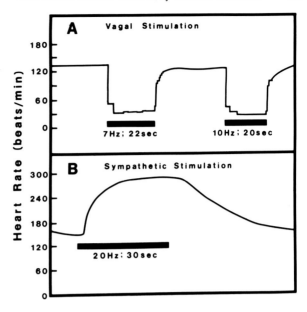

Fig. 21-3. The changes in heart rate (H.R.) evoked by stimulation (horizontal bars) of the vagal (A) and sympathetic (B) nerves in an anesthetized dog. Modified from Warner and Cox {23}, with permission.

tium, the concentration of NE in the cardiac tissues would often exceed noxious levels {25}.

After sympathetic activity ceases, the chronotropic response gradually decays back to the control level (fig. 21-3B). The principal mechanisms that remove the neuronally released NE in the heart are (a) the uptake of neurotransmitter by the sympathetic nerve endings and by the cardiac cells, and (b) diffusion of neurotransmitter away from the neuroeffector gap and into the coronary bloodstream {24,30–32}. When the neuronal reuptake mechanism is suppressed by drugs such as cocaine, the decay of the chronotropic response to sympathetic stimulation is markedly prolonged {33}. However, cocaine does not potentiate the chronotropic response to sympathetic neural stimulation, although it does potentiate the response to exogenous NE {34,35}.

Parasympathetic control

STEADY-STATE CONTROL

In contrast to the gradual development of the chronotropic response to sympathetic stimulation, the vagal response is much more rapid (fig. 21-3A). The latent period of the response to tonic vagal stimulation is about 150 ms, and the steady-state response is reached within one or two cardiac cycles (fig. 21-3A). The heart responds so quickly because many of the muscarinic receptors are coupled directly via G proteins to ACh-regulated K^+ channels in the automatic cell membranes; a slow second messenger system is not interposed {36–39}. The prompt response enables beat-by-beat regulation of heart rate {25}.

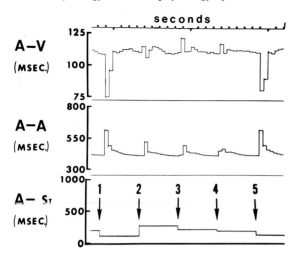

Fig. 21-4. Changes in atrioventricular conduction (A-V interval) and cardiac cycle length (A-A interval) elicited by five vagal stimuli (arrows) delivered at different phases of the cardiac cycle (as expressed by the A-St interval, which is the time from atrial depolarization to the vagal stimulus) in an anesthetized dog. Modified from Levy et al. {44}, with permission.

Furthermore, when vagal activity ceases, the response decays rapidly to the basal level {23,40}. The enzyme acetylcholinesterase is abundant in the nodal regions of the heart {1,6,41,42}, and therefore the ACh released into the cardiac tissues is quickly hydrolyzed.

BRIEF VAGAL STIMULI

The chronotropic effect of a brief vagal stimulus depends on its timing relative to the cardiac cycle {43–47}. In the experiment {44} shown in fig. 21-4, for example, a vagal stimulus (St) was applied at five different times (A-St intervals) after the beginning of atrial depolarization (A wave). The figure shows that the chronotropic responses (that is, the changes in A-A intervals) differ for each A-St interval, and that the response to each stimulus persists for several seconds. The changes in atrioventricular conduction time (A-V interval) also vary with the timing of the stimuli {45,47}; this will be discussed below.

The chronotropic responses to stimuli delivered at various times within the cardiac cycle can be combined to derive a so-called vagal response curve {43–47}. The curve is typically triphasic (fig. 21-5). A brief, pronounced slowing (ABC) is followed by a transient cardiac acceleration (CDE), which may be relative or absolute. This phase is then followed by a more prolonged, but slight, secondary deceleration (EFG).

Hyperpolarization of the automatic cells (fig. 21-6) is mainly responsible {46,47} for the primary phase of deceleration (ABC, fig. 21-5). The ACh released at the vagal endings very quickly activates the ACh-regulated K^+ channels, as stated above. This action augments the potassium conductance, and thereby hyperpolarizes the

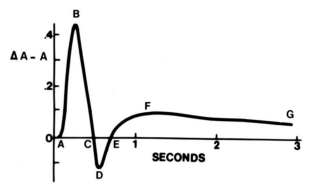

Fig. 21-5. Time course of the changes in cardiac cycle length (A-A interval) evoked by brief vagal stimuli in a dog. The curve was reconstructed from the responses to a number of identical vagal stimuli, but each stimulus was delivered at a different time in the cardiac cycle. Also, each stimulus was delivered after the response to the preceding stimulus had fully recovered. Modified from Iano et al. {45}, with permission.

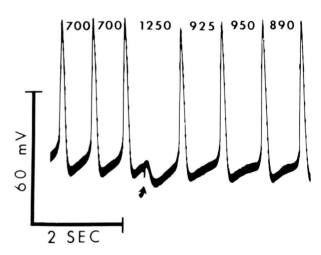

Fig. 21-6. The effects of a brief burst of vagal stimuli (at the arrow) on the transmembrane action potentials recorded from an automatic cell in the SA node of a cat. The numbers between the action potentials indicate the cardiac cycle lengths, in milliseconds. Modified from Jalife and Moe {46}, with permission of the American Heart Association, Inc.

automatic cells (just after the arrow in fig. 21-6). Activation of these K^+ channels requires a relatively high concentration of ACh {21,48}. However, the ACh is rapidly hydrolyzed because of the abundant acetylcholinesterase in the cardiac tissues. Therefore, the hyperpolarization disappears within one or two cardiac cycles (fig. 21-6).

The secondary phase of deceleration (EFG, fig. 21-5) is characterized by a diminished rate of diastolic depolarization (fig. 21-6, last two cardiac cycles); hyperpolarization is absent {46,47}. These small, secondary prolongations of cardiac cycle length are probably mediated by the action of ACh on the channels that conduct the so-called pacemaker current (I_f). These channels are affected by much lower ACh concentrations than are required to activate the ACh-regulated potassium channels {21,48}. Also, the cAMP second messenger system mediates the effect of ACh on the I_f channels {21,48}. Hence, the secondary deceleratory phase (EFG, fig. 21-5) is more gradual and sustained than is the first phase (ABC).

The two deceleratory phases of the vagal response are characteristically separated by a brief phase of relative or absolute acceleration (CDE, fig. 21-5). This phase, which is represented by the 925-ms cycle in fig. 21-6, is probably also mediated by the I_f channels. If the vagal stimulus is sufficiently strong and properly timed, the neurally released ACh might hyperpolarize the automatic cell membrane excessively near the beginning of slow diastolic depolarization. If the I_f current is activated strongly enough by the pronounced hyperpolarization, the slope of the pacemaker potential actually becomes sufficiently steep to abbreviate the cardiac cycle {46,49,50}.

REPETITIVE VAGAL BURSTS

The spontaneous neural activity in efferent cardiac vagal fibers tends to be clustered within a discrete phase of each cardiac cycle {51,52}, as illustrated in fig. 21-7. To mimic this pattern of neural activity, one supramaximal stimulus per cardiac cycle was delivered to the transected vagus nerves of anesthetized dogs {53}. The changes in cardiac cycle length (A-A interval) induced by the vagal stimuli depended on their timing within the cardiac cycle (fig. 21-8). When the vagal stimuli (St) were given 225 ms after the beginning of atrial depolarization (A wave), the cardiac cycle was prolonged maximally. However, when the stimuli were given somewhat later in the cardiac cycle (i.e., at A-St = 390), the increment in the A-A interval was substantially less. One reason that changes in the timing of the vagal stimuli can exert such pronounced effects on cycle length is that the neurally released ACh is hydrolyzed rapidly by the acetylcholinesterase in the cardiac tissues {6,41,42}. If this enzyme is inhibited by physostigmine, the phase dependency is much less pronounced {40}.

This phase dependency endows the vagus nerves with the ability to entrain the firing of the automatic cells in the SA node {53,54}. The schematic phase-response curve (graph of A-A intervals as a function of the stimulus timing) shown in fig. 21-9 illustrates how entrainment is achieved. Let stimuli (S) be delivered to the vagus nerves always at a constant frequency. Also, let the automatic cells fire temporarily at a rate that precisely equals the stimulation frequency. The A-S intervals will then remain constant from cycle to cycle; in fig. 21-9; therefore, A_1-S_1 = A_2-S_2 = A_3-S_3. Let such repetitive stimuli fall at time S_s (i.e., a time that yields a "stable" equilibrium). As shown below, S_s always lies on a region of the phase-response curve that has a positive slope.

Let the automatic cell misfire momentarily, such that the fourth A wave occurs slightly later than expected (at

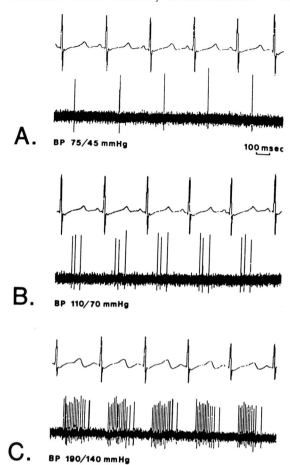

A.   BP 75/45 mmHg   100 msec

B.   BP 110/70 mmHg

C.   BP 190/140 mmHg

Fig. 21-7. Action potentials recorded from an efferent cardiac vagal fiber, along with the electrocardiogram, at three levels of arterial blood pressure (BP) in an anesthetized cat. The control blood pressure was 110/70 mmHg (**B**). The blood pressure was lowered by bleeding (**A**) and raised by injecting phenylephrine (**C**). Modified from Cerati and Schwartz {52}, with permission from the American Heart Association.

A_A rather than A_4 in fig. 21-9). The next stimulus (S_4) will then be delivered earlier in that cycle; i.e., the A_A-S_4 interval will be reduced. S_4 will then fall earlier than S_s on the phase-response curve, and hence the chronotropic response will be diminished. Therefore, the next cardiac cycle will not be as long as the preceding cycles; i.e., A_A-A_B < A_3-A_4. If the initial correction is only partial, then A_B will occur later than would the normally expected A wave (A_5). Hence, the A_B-S_5 interval would still be less than the control A-St intervals (e.g., A_1-S_1). Consequently, stimulation at interval A_B-S_5 would evoke a cycle length A_B-A_6 that is shorter than the control cycle length (e.g., A_1-A_2). This adjustment would continue until stable entrainment is resumed; i.e., until the A-A intervals equal the S-S intervals {53}.

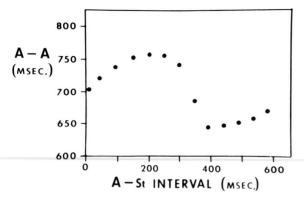

Fig. 21-8. The effects of vagal stimuli, delivered once each cardiac cycle, on the cardiac cycle length (A-A interval) in the dog. The stimuli (St) were delivered at various times (A-St intervals) after atrial depolarization (A wave). Modified from Levy et al. {53}, with permission of the American Heart Association.

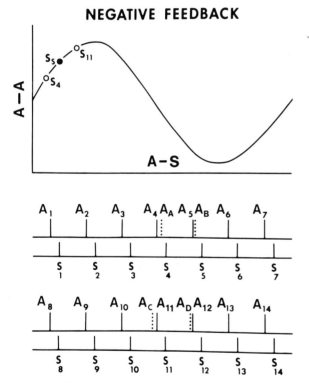

Fig. 21-9. Schematic phase-response curve and timing diagrams to illustrate the tendency for equally spaced vagal stimuli to entrain the firing of the cardiac pacemaker cells. The phase-response curve indicates how the chronotropic response (change in A-A interval) of the heart to vagal stimuli (S) varies with the time (A-S interval) that the stimulus is delivered after the beginning of atrial depolarization (A wave). S_S represents a stable equilibrium point; A_A and A_C represent momentary perturbations of the otherwise constant rhythm; A_B and A_D indicate the partial restoration of the regular rhythm. From Levy et al. {53}, with permission of the American Heart Association.

Because repetitive vagal stimuli exert such a strong synchronizing influence, the heart rate tends to equal the vagal stimulation frequency over a substantial frequency range. Within this range, a specific increase in vagal stimulation frequency will evoke an equal change in heart rate. This is a *paradoxical* response, considering that a greater frequency of stimulation of the *inhibitory* vagus nerves does not decrease the heart rate, but instead actually *increases* it.

As vagal activity increases, the number of action potentials in each burst of neural activity (fig. 21-7) recorded in efferent vagal fibers to the heart tends to rise {52}. As the number of action potentials per burst increases, the synchronizing tendency of the repetitive vagal activity is augmented {54}. In the experiment shown in fig. 21-10, the vagus nerves were stimulated with repetitive bursts of pulses, and the bursts were delivered at a gradually increasing frequency (bottom tracing). Overall, the increased stimulation frequency tended to prolong the cardiac cycle length (A-A interval). This conforms to the well-established tenet that the vagus nerves inhibit the SA nodal cells. However, the gradually increasing stimulation frequency certainly did not elicit a continuous, monotonic change in cycle length (fig. 21-10). Instead, the A-A interval tracing displayed several discontinuities, at each of which a small change in stimulation frequency was associated with a large change in cycle length. Between successive discontinuities (indicated by the arrows), the chronotropic response was paradoxical; i.e., the A-A interval diminished as the stimulation frequency increased.

The ratios of stimulus bursts to atrial depolarizations are denoted by the ratios (St:A) between the arrows. When the ratio was 1:1, a rise in the burst frequency from 0.76 to 1.33 bursts/s was associated with an increase in the heart rate (computed from the A-A intervals) from 0.76 to 1.33 beats/s (i.e., from 46 to 80 beats/min). The heart rate at each moment equaled the prevailing stimulation frequency. Entrainment also prevailed over other frequency ranges, but the St:A ratios were different (fig. 21-10).

In the S-A node, the cardiac impulse is probably not conducted effectively from one cluster of automatic cells to the next {55}. Furthermore, various subsidiary pacemaker sites exist in the right atrium. Such pacemaking centers, together with the SA node, constitute a multicentric pacemaker complex {56–58}. Therefore, communication among the clusters of SA node cells and among the various components of the multicentric complex may be hampered. The pronounced synchronizing tendency of repetitive vagal activity may help to coordinate the activity of such diverse centers of automaticity, and hence may stabilize the pacemaking function of the heart {59,60}.

SYMPATHETIC-PARASYMPATHETIC INTERACTIONS

Sympathetic and vagal nerve endings often lie close together in the cardiac tissues. This permits complex interactions to take place between the components of the two

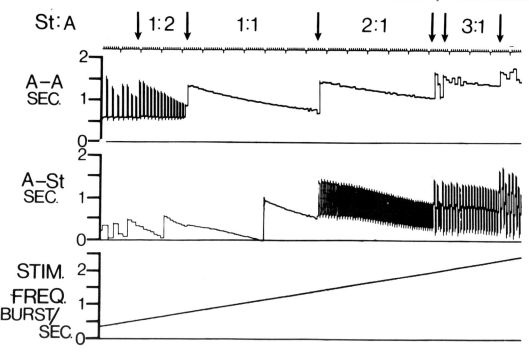

Fig. 21-10. Changes in cardiac cycle length (A-A interval) evoked by a progressive increase in the frequency of vagal stimulation in an anesthetized dog. The A-St interval denotes the time from the beginning of atrial depolarization (A wave) to the beginning of vagal stimulation (St). The ratios between the arrows indicate the ratio of vagal stimulus bursts to heart beats. Modified from Levy et al. {54}, with permission of the American Heart Association.

autonomic subdivisions {3,6,61}. One manifestation of the principal type of interaction, which has been called *accentuated antagonism*, is that augmented vagal activity may attenuate the ability of sympathetic activity to enhance cardiac function.

Sympathetic-vagal interactions prevail in many aspects of cardiac regulation, especially in the neural control of heart rate. A dramatic example {62} of accentuated antagonism in the control of heart rate is illustrated in fig. 21-11. In the absence of vagal stimulation (V = 0), an increase in the frequency of sympathetic stimulation to 4 Hz raised the heart rate by about 80 beats/min in an anesthetized dog. However, when the vagus nerves were being stimulated at a frequency of 8 Hz (V = 8), an increase in the sympathetic stimulation frequency to 4 Hz now barely altered the heart rate. Vagal stimulation at a frequency of 4 Hz (V = 4) had an intermediate influence on the response to sympathetic stimulation. Hence, the chronotropic response to sympathetic stimulation was progressively attenuated as the level of vagal activity was increased.

Accentuated antagonism is effected at prejunctional and postjunctional levels of the neuroeffector junction (fig. 21-12). Prejunctionally, the ACh released from vagal terminals inhibits the release of NE from the sympathetic nerve endings {63–65}, and NE and neuropeptide Y (NPY), both released from sympathetic nerve fibers, sup-

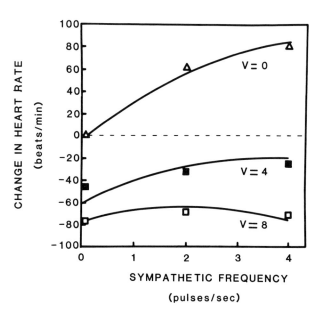

Fig. 21-11. The changes in heart rate evoked by cardiac sympathetic stimulation (from 0 to 4 Hz) at three different frequencies of vagal stimulation (V = 0, 4, and 8 Hz) in an anesthetized dog. Modified from Levy and Zieske {62}, with permission.

Cardiac Cell

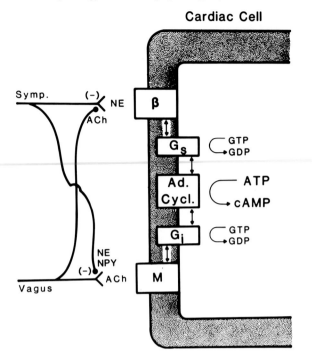

Fig. 21-12. Prejunctional and postjunctional mechanisms involved in cardiac sympathetic-parasympathetic interactions. ACh = acetylcholine; Ad. Cycl. = adenylyl cyclase; β = β-adrenergic receptor; cAMP = cyclic AMP; G_i and G_s = inhibitory and stimulatory G proteins; M = muscarinic receptors; NE = norepinephrine; NPY = neuropeptide Y. Modified from Levy {97}, with permission.

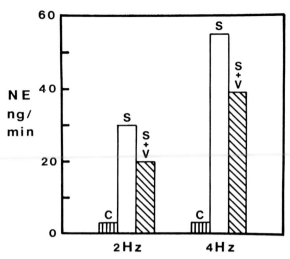

Fig. 21-13. The mean overflows of norepinephrine (NE) into the coronary sinus blood in a group of seven anesthetized dogs under control conditions (C), during supramaximal sympathetic stimulation (S) at 2 and 4 Hz, and during combined stimulation (S + V) of the sympathetic (2 and 4 Hz) and vagus (15 Hz) nerves. Modified from Levy and Blattberg {64}, with permission from the American Heart Association.

press the release of ACh from vagal nerve endings {66–69}. Postjunctionally, the adrenergic and cholinergic transmitters interact at the level of the effector cell itself {2,26,70}.

Prejunctional mechanisms

Various receptors that regulate neurotransmitter release are located on the postganglionic autonomic nerve endings in the heart {1,65,71}. Muscarinic receptors on postganglionic sympathetic endings (fig. 21-12) serve to inhibit the release of NE from those endings {1,65}, whereas alpha-adrenergic and NPY receptors on parasympathetic nerve endings act to inhibit the release of ACh {66,68,69}.

The NE overflow into the coronary sinus blood reflects the difference between the release of NE from the cardiac nerve endings and its uptake by the nerve endings and extraneuronal tissues {24,32,64,72}. If the uptake processes are not affected appreciably by the experimental procedures, the changes in NE overflow during an experiment reflect the changes in transmitter release. The NE overflow into the coronary sinus blood (fig. 21-13) of anesthetized dogs was measured under control conditions, during cardiac sympathetic stimulation alone, and during combined sympathetic and vagal stimulation {64}. During sympathetic stimulation (S) alone at frequencies of 2 and

4 Hz, the NE overflows were 30 and 55 ng/min, respectively. During combined sympathetic and vagal (S + V) stimulation, the NE overflows decreased by 33%. This inhibitory effect of vagal stimulation was abolished by atropine.

The second type of prejunctional autonomic interaction involves the inhibition of the release of ACh from vagal nerve endings by the NE and NPY released from neighboring sympathetic nerve endings (fig. 21-12). The inhibitory effects of NE on vagal neurotransmission are mediated by prejunctional α_1 receptors, and the inhibition wanes quickly after the sympathetic activity ceases {66}.

The NPY that is also released from the sympathetic nerve endings exerts a more sustained inhibition of ACh release from vagal terminals {68,69}. Potter {67} was the first to demonstrate the pronounced effect of this neuropeptide on vagal neurotransmission. She showed that a brief train of sympathetic stimulation at a frequency of 20 Hz (S20) could attenuate markedly the cardiac chronotropic responses to periodic vagal stimulations in anesthetized dogs (fig. 21-14, top tracing), and the attenuation could persist for about an hour. This inhibitory effect of sympathetic stimulation was mimicked by an intravenous injection of NPY (fig. 21-14, bottom tracing). Furthermore, neither neurally released nor exogenous NPY altered the chronotropic responses to muscarinic agonists. By exclusion, therefore, the most likely explanation is that NPY suppresses vagal neurotransmission by diminishing the release of ACh from the vagal nerve endings.

Warner and her coworkers {73–76} confirmed Potter's results, and also found that (a) the responses to neurally

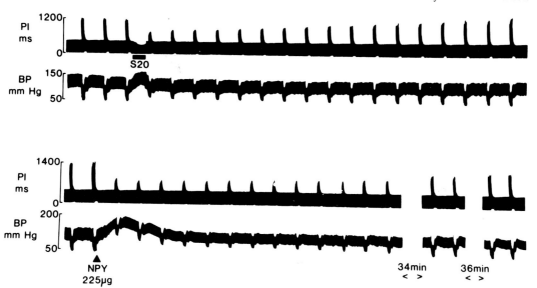

Fig. 21-14. The effects of sympathetic stimulation (**upper panel**) for 1 minute at a frequency of 20 Hz (S20) or of an injection of neuropeptide Y (NPY, **lower panel**) on the arterial blood pressure (BP) and on the chronotropic responses (changes in pulse intervals, PI) to repetitive 15-second trains of vagal stimulation, delivered once every 2 minutes. From Potter {67}, with permission.

released NPY can be detected even when sympathetic stimulation frequencies as low as 2 Hz are used, (b) the inhibitory effects on vagal neurotransmission depended on the frequency and duration of sympathetic stimulation, and (c) the overflow of NPY into the coronary sinus blood evoked by sympathetic stimulation varied directly with the sympathetic stimulation frequency and with the depression of vagal neurotransmission. These cardiovascular effects of NPY in dogs are mediated in cats by a different neuropeptide, namely, galanin {77,78}.

The sequence of sympathetic and vagal activation affects the nature of the autonomic interaction {79,80}. If the sympathetic nerves alone are stimulated, the responses to subsequent vagal stimuli will be suppressed for a long time (as shown in fig. 21-14), presumably because of the persistent action of the NPY released during the sympathetic stimulation. However, if the sympathetic and vagal stimulations are initiated simultaneously, then the vagal effects will predominate over the sympathetic effects. This confirms the experimental results shown above in fig. 21-11. Presumably, the ACh released from the vagal nerve endings quickly and effectively suppresses the release of NE and NPY from the sympathetic nerve endings. Conversely, the NE and NPY released from the sympathetic nerve endings do not act nearly as quickly or effectively to inhibit vagal neurotransmission. Therefore, when the two autonomic divisions are stimulated simultaneously and with approximately the same intensity, the rapidly acting ACh quickly suppresses the release of NE and NPY, and hence the vagal effects tend to preponderate. For the effects of sympathetic stimulation to preponderate over the effects of equally intense vagal stimulation, the sympa-

thetic activity must begin well in advance of the vagal activity.

Postjunctional mechanisms

Autonomic interactions are prominent not only when sympathetic and vagal nerves are stimulated, but also when adrenergic and cholinergic agonists are infused {61}. Hence, autonomic interactions must also take place at the level of the cardiac effector cell itself; that is, postjunctionally {2,26,70}.

The postjunctional interactions in the heart (fig. 21-12) are mediated principally by the adenylyl cyclase system {2,26,70,81,82}. Occupation of the beta-adrenergic receptors (β) by the adrenergic neurotransmitter (NE) stimulates the membrane-bound enzyme, adenylyl cyclase, which catalyzes the intracellular production of cyclic AMP (cAMP) from ATP. The coupling of the beta-adrenergic receptors to the adenylyl cyclase is mediated by a stimulatory protein, G_s. This coupling involves the hydrolysis of guanosine triphosphate (GTP) to guanosine diphosphate (GDP). The ACh released from vagal nerve endings antagonizes these adrenergic effects by occupying muscarinic receptors (M) on the effector cell surface (fig. 21-12). The muscarinic receptors inhibit adenylyl cyclase through an inhibitory protein, G_i, which also facilitates the hydrolysis of GTP to GDP. The principal postjunctional interaction thus operates through adenylyl cyclase. The facilitatory effects of sympathetic activity are mediated by raising the intracellular levels of cAMP. Concomitant vagal activity antagonizes this process by inhibiting adenylyl cyclase, and thereby attenuates the adrenergically induced rise in the cAMP concentration.

NEURAL CONTROL OF THE ATRIOVENTRICULAR JUNCTION

Steady-state control

The atrioventricular junction is sensitive to stimuli from both autonomic divisions. A recent comparison has indicated that automatic cells in the AV junction are actually more responsive than are those in the SA node to both sympathetic and vagal stimulations {83}. AV conduction velocities are also quite responsive to autonomic activity {6}, even though vagal activity affects AV automaticity differently than it affects AV conduction {84}.

Studies of the direct effect of vagal activity on AV conduction are best done with the heart paced at a constant cycle length, because a change in cardiac cycle length will, of itself, alter AV conduction time. An increase in cycle length can decrease the AV conduction time substantially, and a reduction in cycle length will have the opposite effect. Thus, in the unpaced heart vagal activity will increase the cardiac cycle length, and this will tend to decrease the AV conduction time. However, the direct vagal effect on the AV conducting fibers will tend to retard AV conduction. Because these direct and indirect influences are oppositely directed, their effects tend to cancel. Hence, during vagal stimulation the simultaneous changes in cycle length mask the direct neural effects on AV conduction. Thus, studies of the effects of vagal stimulation on AV conduction in the unpaced heart are liable to be misinterpreted.

The sympathetic control of AV conduction displays interactions that resemble those described above for vagal control. Thus, sympathetic activity tends to decrease cardiac cycle length, and this effect would tend to prolong AV conduction. However, if cycle length is held constant by artificial pacing, cardiac sympathetic stimulation decreases the AV conduction time. Thus, the direct effects of the adrenergic transmitter on the AV conduction fiber and the indirect effect of a concomitant reduction in cardiac cycle length exert opposite effects on AV conduction. The combined effects of the direct and indirect influences of sympathetic activity on AV nodal conduction can thus be complex {85,86}.

During a sustained vagal stimulation (fig. 21-15), the AV conduction response may display two phases {87,88}. The initial phase, when present, consists of a brief decline in the AV conduction time (fig. 21-15A). The secondary phase is more prolonged; during this phase, the AV conduction time may either increase, decrease, or remain constant. During the secondary phase, the chronotropic and atrial responses to the sustained vagal stimulation consistently decrease, or "fade" {88,89}. The mechanisms responsible for fade of the cardiac responses to vagal stimulation are complex; one important mechanism involves muscarinic receptor desensitization {90}. This mechanism is probably mainly responsible for the fade of

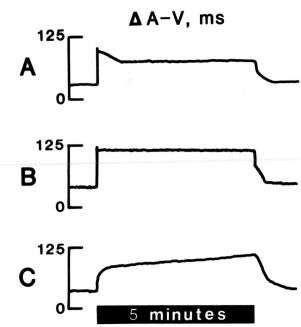

Fig. 21-15. The three types of long-term AV conduction responses to 5-minute vagal stimulations (horizontal bar). Tracings (unpublished) were recorded in experiments described in Martin {87}, with permission.

the chronotropic and inotropic responses to vagal stimulation, and for the fade of the dromotropic response as well when it is manifest. However, when the secondary phase consists of an increase in AV conduction, the mechanism may be an interaction between fade and the rate-responsive properties of the conduction fibers in the AV node {87}.

For both vagal and sympathetic activity, the interactions between the direct effects of the autonomic transmitters and the indirect effects of induced changes in cardiac cycle length on AV conduction are pronounced {85,87,91}. That is, when the separate direct and indirect effects are added, the alegebraic sums do not equal the magnitude of the physiological responses obtained when both influences operate simultaneously (as when the heart is not paced). The mechanisms responsible for these interactions are complex, but they probably involve vagally induced changes in atrial conduction patterns and in the functional properties of the AV node {91}.

Vagal activity is an important determinant of AV conduction, not only in experimental animals, but also in human subjects as well. The significant prolongation of AV conduction time observed in trained athletes is ascribable to their elevated vagal tone. When the heart was paced at a constant rate in human subjects, an increase in blood pressure reflexly prolonged the A-H interval (but not the H-V interval); a fall in blood pressure had the opposite effect {92}. These changes were blocked by atropine. Direct stimulation of the carotid sinus nerves in patients significantly prolonged the AV interval when the heart was paced {93}. This response appeared after a latency of about 1 second, reached a maximum in about 5 seconds, and then it declined gradually to attain a steady-state level after about 20 seconds. Again, the vagus nerves played a major role in this response, with only a minor contribution from the sympathetic system.

In experimental animals, supramaximal vagal stimulation prolonged the AV conduction time after a latency of less than 1 second, and it induced bradydysrhythmias with fixed or variable degrees of AV block {94}. The prolongation of AV conduction time was a monotonically increasing function of stimulus intensity. Complete AV block usually did not appear until the AV conduction time had been prolonged by more than 50%. The prolongation depended on the concomitant slowing of the sinus rate; that is, there was a strong interaction between the direct vagal inhibitory effect on the AV node and the indirect facilitatory effect on AV conduction of the concomitant decrease in heart rate. Furthermore, the vagal innervations of the SA node and AV junction are functionally and anatomically distinct {95}. Thus, the dynamic balance of vagal activity to both structures may change from moment to moment.

In conscious resting dogs, vagal control predominated in the regulation of AV conduction, but control by the sympathetic system was dominant during exercise {96}. The opposing effects of simultaneous activity in the two autonomic divisions on AV conduction were algebraically additive {62,86}. The change in conduction time in response to steady-state activity in one autonomic division was independent of the level of steady-state activity in the other, i.e., there was no significant vagal-sympathetic interaction with respect to AV conduction. This is in sharp contrast to the autonomic control of SA nodal function and of myocardial contractility, where such an interaction is pronounced {61,62,97}. However, AV conduction did display a significant vagal-sympathetic interaction when brief bursts of vagal activity were added to a steady level of sympathetic activity {98,99}.

When both autonomic divisions were blocked in human subjects and the heart rate was not controlled artificially, the AV conduction time did not change appreciably {100}. It appeared, therefore, that the effects of the two autonomic divisions were equally balanced in the control of AV conduction. However, the apparent balance may have been due in part to the concomitant changes in heart rate induced by the autonomic blockade, as discussed above.

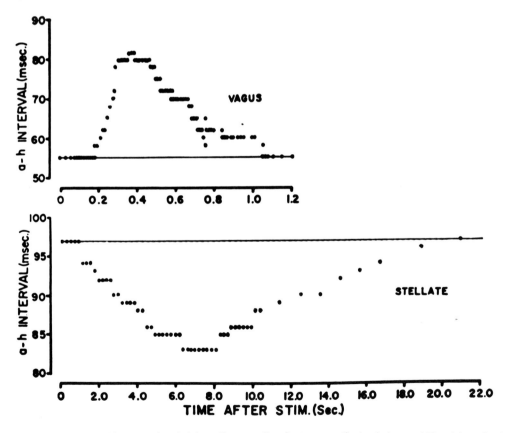

Fig. 21-16. The effects of left vagal (**top panel**) and right stellate ganglion (**bottom panel**) stimulation on AV nodal conduction (the a-h interval) in two representative experiments. Note the 10-fold difference in the scaling factor of the abscissae for the vagal and the stellate effects. From Spear and Moore {104}, with permission of the American Heart Association.

Dynamic control

Studies of the dynamic responses of AV conduction to autonomic stimulation have been focused mainly on the vagal effects. Cardiac electrophysiological responses to vagal stimuli are minimal in the neonate {101}, but muscarinic receptor responsiveness increases markedly with age {102}. Morphological and electrophysiological correlates of the AV nodal response to vagal stimuli indicate that both the density of nerve endings as well as the maximal depressant effect of acetylcholine are greatest in the midnodal (N cell) region of the AV node {103}.

A brief vagal stimulus burst given in one cardiac cycle can prolong the AV conduction time (a-h interval) on the very next cardiac cycle (fig. 21-16), and the effect quickly decays over the next several cycles {104}. The response to a single sympathetic stimulus burst has a longer latency, it takes several cycles to become fully manifest, and it requires many more cycles to decay (fig. 21-16). Thus dynamic responses to vagal stimulation may participate in arrhythmias on a beat-to-beat basis, whereas sympathetic responses are inherently too slow for such a role {25}.

When we studied the simultaneous responses of the SA and AV nodes to vagal stimulation, the AV nodal responses were very variable {44}. When identical stimulus bursts were given at different phases of the cardiac cycle, the AV responses varied in magnitude and direction (fig. 21-4). The change in AV conduction elicited by the vagal stimulus depended on the increase of the cardiac cycle length {44}. When the cycle length was held constant by pacing, vagal stimuli always prolonged the AV conduction time.

The phase of the cardiac cycle at which a vagal impulse arrives at the AV junction is also an important determinant of its efficacy {105}, just as it is for the vagal control of the SA node. This phase responsiveness is due mainly to the rapidity of the release, diffusion, and inactivation of ACh and to the speed with which the ACh-regulated K^+ channels in the cardiac cell membranes are able to transduce the vagal signals to the cardiac cells {25}. The corresponding features of sympathetic activity are much slower {25}. However, the phase-dependent characteristics of the dromotropic response seem to be unaffected by the spatial dispersion of ACh release from the vagal nerve endings {106}.

Additional factors that strongly influence AV conduction are the heart rate and level of sympathetic activity {91}. Figure 21-17 shows that the vagal effect becomes more pronounced as the cardiac cycle length (PP interval) is decreased. A decrease in heart rate exerts this effect probably because the relative refractory periods of the AV conduction system are longer than the associated action potential durations {107}. As the AV conduction time is prolonged (whether by vagal activity or otherwise), the action potentials and relative refractory periods of the critical conduction fibers in the AV node are prolonged because of electrotonic interactions {107}. This may lead to the following sequence of events when the heart beats at a constant rate: (a) a vagal stimulus given early in the cardiac cycle prolongs the AV conduction time and the

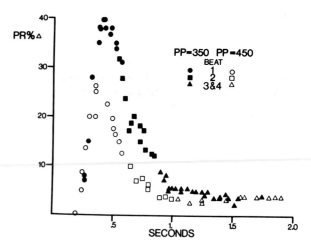

Fig. 21-17. Vagal effect curves recorded from an anesthetized dog at two different atrial pacing intervals. The abscissa indicates the elapsed time from a single vagal stimulus burst given at t = 0. The ordinates are the percent changes in AV conduction time over a sequence of consecutive cardiac cycles. The circles, squares, and triangles represent the changes that occurred in the first, second, and subsequent beats after the beat during which the stimulus was given. From Martin {105}, with permission.

AV nodal refractory period during the first beat after the stimulus, (b) the second atrial impulse after the vagal stimulus will arrive at the AV node when the conducting fibers are more refractory, and (c) this will evoke an additional increment in AV conduction time on the second beat, just as indicated in fig. 21-17. This mechanism may also be involved in the genesis of the AV nodal Wenckebach phenomenon {107}.

NEURAL CONTROL OF MYOCARDIAL EXCITABILITY

ACh significantly shortens the atrial action potential, and therefore vagal stimulation significantly reduces the atrial refractory period {108,109}. Sympathetic stimulation also shortens the effective refractory periods of the atria, and simultaneous activation of both autonomic divisions abridges the refractory period as the algebraic sum of the responses to the separate stimulations {109}.

The effects of acetylcholine and vagal stimulation on ventricular refractory periods are not so clear, however. In the dog {111} and in humans {112}, muscarinic blockade decreases the ventricular refractory periods. However, blockade of both autonomic divisions evokes negligible changes in refractory periods. Also, vagal stimulation in the dog significantly prolongs ventricular refractory periods, but not after sympathectomy {113}. These findings suggest that the ACh released from vagal nerve endings mainly acts indirectly, by antagonizing the sympathetic effects {111,113,114}. The vagi probably constitute the dominant efferent pathway for the reflex control of ventricular refractoriness in cats, and the vagal effect is prominent even when sympathetic activity is negligible {115}.

Such results {99,115} appear to contradict the view that ACh mainly acts indirectly, by antagonizing the sympathetic effects.

Studies in humans indicate that resting vagal tone significantly increases ventricular refractoriness, even in the absence of sympathetic influences {100}. Reflex vagal stimulation via neck suction or infusion of phenylephrine tended to confirm this contention {116}. These findings suggest that such vagally induced changes of refractoriness may exert a protective effect against the occurrence of sudden death in patients with ischemic heart disease {116}. Prolongation of AV junctional and ventricular refractory periods may also help terminate reentrant arrhythmias and suppress ventricular tachycardias {117}.

NEURAL CONTROL OF MYOCARDIAL CONTRACTILITY

Sympathetic effects

The sympathetic innervation of the atria is abundant but not uniform. Cardiac sympathetic stimulation produces profound effects on the heart. The increase in atrial con-

tractility evoked by sympathetic activity augments ventricular filling. The consequent rise in left ventricular end-diastolic pressure thus produces a greater increment in ventricular end-diastolic volume and in stroke volume. The adrenergic enhancement of atrial contractility also helps to maintain ventricular filling when heart rates are very high.

The sympathetic nervous system also richly innervates ventricular tissue. Cardiac sympathetic stimulation enhances ventricular contractility, and thereby increases left ventricular systolic pressure, the rate of change of ventricular pressure, the mean arterial pressure, and the arterial pulse pressure. Sympathetic stimulation also decreases the duration of ventricular systole. This helps to preserve ventricular filling time, despite the concomitant reduction of cardiac cycle length. Sympathetic stimulation also increases coronary blood flow, myocardial oxygen consumption, stroke volume, stroke work, and cardiac output. Furthermore, these effects are produced independently of changes in preload and afterload; i.e., they occur even when preload and afterload are held constant. However, excessive sympathetic activity for 10- to 30-minute periods actually depresses myocardial contractility in rabbit hearts {118}.

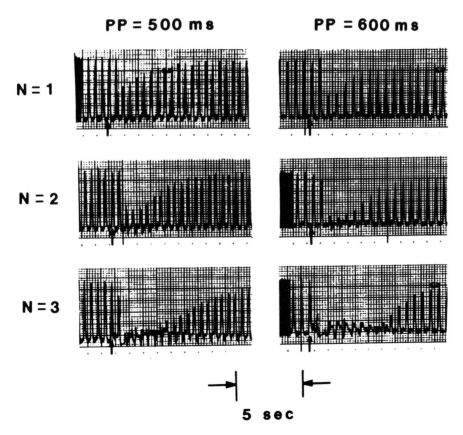

Fig. 21-18. The changes in pressure in an atrial balloon in response to one, two, or three stimuli (N) per vagal burst, given at the time marked by the arrows, at cycle lengths (PP) of 500 and 600 ms. From Martin {120}, with permission.

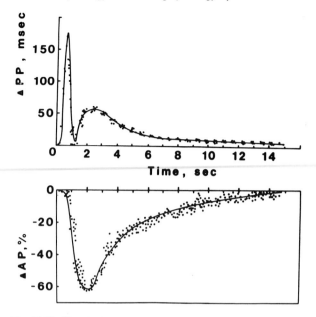

concentration than do the ventricles. Thus the diffusion distances for ACh are much shorter in the atria than in the ventricles, and the response to vagal stimulation is terminated more rapidly in the atria than in the ventricles.

In the early studies of the atrial responses to vagal activity in mammals, long trains of stimuli were used and steady-state responses were measured. More recently the transient inotropic responses of canine atria to single or brief vagal stimuli were studied {120}. Figure 21-18 shows the typical results of stimulating the vagi with a burst of one, two, or three pulses while the heart is paced at two different cycle lengths (PP intervals). Note that a single vagal stimulus pulse reduces atrial contraction (AP) by 62% when the cycle length is 600 ms. One burst of two or three pulses suppresses the atrial contractions entirely for 2–8 seconds. The depression of the inotropic response is less pronounced when the cycle length is diminished to 500 ms.

The inotropic responses may be quantified by means of vagal effect curves. Figure 21-19 shows the vagal effect curves for the simultaneous changes in cardiac cycle length (P-P interval) and atrial contractility (AP). The time course of the inotropic response is similar to that of the secondary peak of the chronotropic response. The similar time course suggests that the mechanisms responsible for these two responses may share a common component.

The response of the atrial myocardium to vagal stimulation also depends on the phase of the cardiac cycle at which the stimulus burst is given {121}, just as do the SA and AV nodes. A burst of vagal stimuli that occurs during one phase of the cardiac cycle may depress the next atrial contraction completely, whereas at a different phase of the cycle the same vagal stimulus may have little effect. Such effects of timing may influence the atrial contribution to ventricular filling.

The inotropic responses of the atria to vagal stimulation are greater when the heart rate is held constant than when it is allowed to vary {120}. This difference cannot

Fig. 21-19. Vagal effect curves for cardiac cycle length (PP) in an unpaced-heart preparation and for pressure (AP) in an atrial balloon in a paced-heart preparation. The data were obtained from a sequence of vagal stimulus bursts given at various P-St intervals in the same dog. From Martin {120}, with permission.

Vagal effects

Many decades ago, Wiggers {119} showed that the atria are very responsive to vagal influences, and his findings have been amply confirmed. The atria have a much richer parasympathetic innervation and a higher cholinesterase

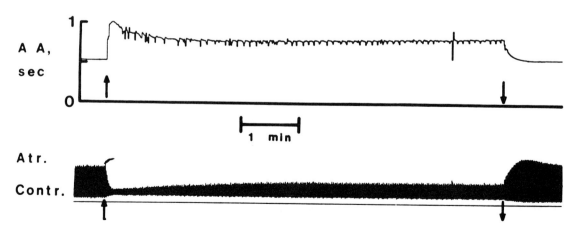

Fig. 21-20. Changes in cardiac cycle length (**top panel**) and atrial contractility (**bottom panel**) in response to a continuous train of vagal stimuli (between the arrows). Note that both the chronotropic and inotropic responses return back toward control from some initial maximal value, despite the continued vagal stimulation. From Martin et al. {89}, with permission.

be explained by changes of preload. The explanation may involve the dynamic frequency-force relationship, which probably differs from the traditional steady-state frequency-force relationship. In a recent study of the dynamic relation {121}, heart rate had a significant effect on the response to high vagal stimulation levels, but only a small effect at low levels.

In response to a sustained vagal stimulation (fig. 21-20), heart rate initially increases to some maximum value and contractile force initially declines to some minimum value {89}. Both responses then begin to fade back towards their control levels. The decline in heart rate back toward control reaches a steady state in about 15–20 seconds, whereas the recovery of contractile force back toward control requires 1–2 minutes. However, the AV conduction responses may or may not fade (fig. 21-15) during sustained vagal stimulation {87}. Thus different mechanisms may be responsible for the fade of the various cardiac responses. Although a progressive reduction in the neuronal release of ACh during the stimulus train cannot be excluded, the available evidence suggests that the muscarinic receptors desensitize {90}; that is, the receptors gradually lose their ability to bind the transmitter.

Until about two decades ago, it was commonly considered that the vagi had a negligible influence on ventricular function in mammals {6}. The neural control of myocardial contractility is difficult to study because contractility is influenced by so many variables in addition to the neural factors. In our laboratory three different experimental preparations were used to control certain critical experimental variables; namely, heart rate, preload, afterload, atrial transport function, and coronary perfusion pressure {122}. Trains of vagal stimuli caused reductions in ventricular contractility that varied inversely as the frequency of vagal stimulation. When the vagi were maximally stimulated, ventricular contractility was depressed by 15–25%.

The findings that vagal activity affects ventricular function have been confirmed in various other canine preparations and in other mammals, including humans. Vagal stimulation causes the ventricular function curves to be shifted to the right, it significantly reduces the maximum rate of rise of intraventricular pressure, and it diminishes ventricular contractile force {123}. In patients with heart failure, the severity of ventricular dysfunction was correlated with the level of parasympathetic neural activity {124}.

ACKNOWLEDGMENTS

This work was supported by U.S.P.H.S. grants HL 10951 and HL 22484.

REFERENCES

1. Löffelholz K, Pappano AJ: The parasympathetic neuroeffector junction of the heart. *Pharmacol Rev* 37:1–24, 1985.
2. Hartzell HC: Regulation of cardiac ion channels by catecholamines, acetylcholine and second messenger systems. *Prog Biophys Mol Biol* 52:165–247, 1988.
3. Levy MN: Sympathetic-parasympathetic interactions in the heart. In: Kulbertus HE, Franck G (eds) *Neurocardiology*. Mount Kisco, NY: Futura, 1988, pp 85–98.
4. Levy MN, Warner MR: Autonomic interactions in cardiac control: Role of neuropeptides. In: Zipes DP, Jalife J (eds) *Cardiac Electrophysiology: From Cell to Bedside*. Philadelphia: WB Saunders Co, 1990, pp 305–311.
5. Mizeres MJ: The origin and course of the cardioaccelerator fibers in the dog. *Anat Record* 132:261–279, 1958.
6. Levy MN, Martin PJ: Neural control of the heart. In: Berne RM, Sperelakis N (eds) *Handbook of Physiology, Section 2: Cardiovascular System; Vol. I.: Heart*. Bethesda, MD: American Physiological Society, 1979, pp 581–620.
7. Janes RD, Brandys JC, Hopkins DA, Johnstone DE, Murphy DA, Armour JA: Anatomy of human extrinsic cardiac nerves and ganglia. *Am J Cardiol* 57:299–309, 1986.
8. Spyer KM: Neural organisation and control of the baroreceptor reflex. *Rev Physiol Biochem Pharmacol* 88:23–124, 1981.
9. Machado BH, Brody MJ: Role of the nucleus ambiguus in the regulation of heart rate and arterial pressure. *Hypertension* 11:602–607, 1988.
10. Randall WC: Selective autonomic innervation of the heart. In: Randall WC (ed) *Nervous Control of Cardiovascular Function*. New York: Oxford University Press, 1984, pp 46–67.
11. Ardell JL, Randall WC: Selective vagal innervation of sinoatrial and atrioventricular nodes in canine heart. *Am J Physiol* 251:H764–H773, 1986.
12. Carlson MD, Geha AS, Hsu J, Martin PJ, Levy MN, Jacobs G, Waldo AL: Selective stimulation of parasympathetic nerve fibers to the human sinoatrial node. *Circulation* 85: 1311–1317, 1992.
13. Randall WC, Milosavljevic M, Wurster RD, Geis GS, Ardell JL: Selective vagal innervation of the heart. *Ann Clin Lab Sci* 16:198–208, 1986.
14. Furukawa Y, Wallick DW, Carlson MD, Martin PJ: Cardiac electrical responses to vagal stimulation of fibers to discrete cardiac regions. *Am J Physiol* 258:H1112–H1118, 1990.
15. Furukawa Y, Wallick DW, Martin PJ, Levy MN: Chronotropic and dromotropic responses to stimulation of intracardiac sympathetic nerves to sinoatrial or atrioventricular nodal region in anesthetized dogs. *Circ Res* 66:1391–1399, 1990.
16. Geis WP, Kaye MP, Randall WC: Major autonomic pathways to the atria and S-A and A-V nodes of the canine heart. *Am J Physiol* 224:202–208, 1973.
17. Parker P, Celler BG, Potter EK, et al.: Vagal stimulation and cardiac slowing. *J Auton Nerv Syst* 11:226–231, 1984.
18. Hamlin RL, Smith CR: Effects of vagal stimulation on S-A and A-V nodes. *Am J Physiol* 215:560–568, 1968.
19. Lang SA, Zieske H, Levy MN: Insignificant bilateral convergence of preganglionic vagal fibers on postganglionic neurons to the canine heart. *Circ Res* 67:556–563, 1990.
20. Noble D: *The Initiation of the Heartbeat*, 2nd ed. Oxford: Clarendon Press, 1979, p 109.
21. DiFrancesco D, Zaza A: The cardiac pacemaker current I_f. *J Cardiovasc Electrophysiol* 3:334–344, 1992.
22. Gadsby DC: Effects of β adrenergic catecholamines on membrane currents in cardiac cells. In: Rosen MR, Janse MJ, Wit AL (eds) *Cardiac Electrophysiology: A Textbook*. Mount Kisco, NY: Futura, 1990, pp 857–876.
23. Warner HR, Cox A: A mathematical model of heart rate control by sympathetic and vagus efferent information. *J Appl Physiol* 17:349–355, 1962.

24. Levy MN: The release and reuptake of noradrenaline during stimulation of the cardiac sympathetic nerves. In: Riemersma RA, Oliver MF (eds) *Catecholamines in the Nonischaemic and Ischaemic Myocardium.* Amsterdam: Elsevier Biomedical, 1982, pp 25–36.

25. Levy MN, Yang T, Wallick DW: Assessment of beat by beat control of heart rate by the autonomic nervous system: Molecular biology technics are necessary, but not sufficient. *J Cardiovasc Electrophysiol,* in press.

26. Watanabe AM, Lindemann JP, Fleming JW: Mechanisms of muscarinic modulation of protein phosphorylation in intact ventricles. *Fed Proc* 43:2618–2623, 1984.

27. Clapham D: Intracellular regulation of ion channels. In: Zipes DP, Jalife J (eds) *Cardiac Electrophysiology: From Cell to Bedside.* Philadelphia: WB Saunders, 1990, pp 85–93.

28. Yatani A, Brown AM: Rapid β-adrenergic modulation of cardiac calcium channel currents by a fast G protein pathway. *Science* 245:71–74, 1989.

29. Brown AM: Ion channels as G protein effectors. *News Physiol Sci* 6:158–161, 1991.

30. Cousineau D, Goresky CA, Bach GG, Rose CP: Effect of β-adrenergic blockade on in vivo norepinephrine release in canine heart. *Am J Physiol* 246:H283–H292, 1984.

31. Trendelenburg U: The metabolizing systems involved in the inactivation of catecholamines. *Naunyn-Schmiedebergs Arch Pharmacol* 332:201–207, 1986.

32. Esler M, Jennings G, Lambert G, Meredith I, Horne M, Eisenhofer G: Overflow of catecholamine neurotransmitters to the circulation: Source, fate, and functions. *Physiol Rev* 70:963–985, 1990.

33. Masuda Y, Levy MN: Heart rate as a determinant of the cardiac inotropic response to sympathetic nervous activity. *Can J Physiol Pharmacol* 61:1374–1381, 1983.

34. Matsuda Y, Masuda Y, Levy MN: The effects of cocaine and metanephrine on the cardiac responses to sympathetic nerve stimulation in dogs. *Circ Res* 45:180–187, 1979.

35. Inoue H, Zipes DP: Cocaine-induced supersensitivity and arrhythmogenesis. *J Am Coll Cardiol* 11:867–874, 1988.

36. Pfaffinger PJ, Martin JM, Hunter DD, et al.: GTP-binding proteins couple cardiac muscarinic receptors to a K channel. *Nature* 317:536–538, 1985.

37. Brown AM, Birnbaumer L: Direct G protein gating of ion channels. *Am J Physiol* 254:H401–H410, 1988.

38. Sorota S, Hoffman BF: Role of G proteins in the acetylcholine-induced potassium current of canine atrial cells. *Am J Physiol* 257:H1516–H1522, 1989.

39. Holmer SR, Homcy CJ: G proteins in the heart. *Circulation* 84:1891–1902, 1991.

40. Henning RJ, Masuda Y, Yang T, Levy MN: Rate of acetylcholine hydrolysis affects the phase dependency of cardiac responses to vagal stimulation. *Cardiovasc Res* 21:169–176, 1987.

41. Lindmar R, Löffelholz K, Weide W: Interstitial washout and hydrolysis of acetylcholine in the perfused heart. *Naunyn-Schmiedebergs Arch Pharmacol* 296:143–148, 1982.

42. Dexter F, Levy MN, Rudy Y: Mathematical model of the changes in heart rate elicited by vagal stimulation. *Circ Res* 65:1330–1339, 1989.

43. Brown GL, Eccles JC: The action of a single vagal volley on the rhythm of the heart beat. *J Physiol* 82:211–240, 1934.

44. Levy MN, Martin PJ, Iano T, Zieske H: Effects of single vagal stimuli on heart rate and atrioventricular conduction. *Am J Physiol* 218:1256–1262, 1970.

45. Iano TL, Levy MN, Lee MH: An acceleratory component of the parasympathetic control of heart rate. *Am J Physiol* 224:997–1005, 1973.

46. Jalife J, Moe GK: Phasic effects of vagal stimulation on pacemaker activity of the isolated sinus node of the young cat. *Circ Res* 45:595–607, 1979.

47. Spear JF, Kronhaus KD, Moore EN, Kline RP: The effect of brief vagal stimulation on the isolated rabbit sinus node. *Circ Res* 44:75–88, 1979.

48. DiFrancesco D, Ducouret P, Robinson RB: Muscarinic modulation of cardiac rate at low acetylcholine concentrations. *Science* 243:669–671, 1989.

49. Jalife J, Slenter VAJ, Salata JJ, Michaels DC: Dynamic vagal control of pacemaker activity in the mammalian sinoatrial node. *Circ Res* 52:642–656, 1983.

50. Yang T, Jacobstein MD, Levy MN: Sustained increases in heart rate induced by timed repetition of vagal stimulation in dogs. *Am J Physiol* 249:H703–H709, 1985.

51. Katona PG, Poitras JW, Barnett GO, Terry BS: Cardiac vagal efferent activity and heart period in the carotid sinus reflex. *Am J Physiol* 218:1030–1037, 1970.

52. Cerati D, Schwartz PJ: Single cardiac vagal fiber activity, acute myocardial ischemia, and risk for sudden death. *Circ Res* 69:1389–1401, 1991.

53. Levy MN, Martin PJ, Iano T, Zieske H: Paradoxical effect of vagus nerve stimulation on heart rate in dogs. *Circ Res* 25:303–314, 1969.

54. Levy MN, Iano T, Zieske H: Effects of repetitive bursts of vagal activity on heart rate. *Circ Res* 30:186–195, 1972.

55. Hariman RJ, Hoffman BF, Naylor RE: Electrical activity from the sinus node region in conscious dogs. *Circ Res* 47:775–791, 1980.

56. Boineau JR, Schuessler RB, Mooney CR, Wylds AC, Miller CB, Roger PE, Hudson RD, Borremans JM, Brockus CW: Multicentric origin of the atrial depolarization wave: The pacemaker complex. *Circulation* 58:1036–1048, 1978.

57. Randall WC, Rinkema LE, Jones SB, et al.: Functional characterization of atrial pacemaker activity. *Am J Physiol* 242:H98–H106, 1982.

58. Schuessler RB, Bromberg BI, Boineau JP: Effect of neurotransmitters on the activation sequence of the isolated atrium. *Am J Physiol* 258:H1632–H1641, 1990.

59. James TN: The sinus node as a servomechanism. *Circ Res* 32:307–313, 1973.

60. Yang T, Jacobstein MD, Levy MN: Synchronization of automatic cells in S-A node during vagal stimulation in dogs. *Am J Physiol* 246:H585–H591, 1984.

61. Levy MN: Sympathetic-parasympathetic interactions in the heart. *Circ Res* 29:437–445, 1971.

62. Levy MN, Zieske H: Autonomic control of cardiac pacemaker activity and atrioventricular transmission. *J Appl Physiol* 27:465–470, 1969.

63. Löffelholz K, Muscholl E: Inhibition by parasympathetic nerve stimulation of the release of the adrenergic transmitter. *Naunyn-Schmiedebergs Arch Pharmacol* 267:181–184, 1970.

64. Levy MN, Blattberg B: Effect of vagal stimulation on the overflow of norepinephrine into the coronary sinus during cardiac sympathetic nerve stimulation in the dog. *Circ Res* 38:81–85, 1976.

65. Muscholl E: Peripheral muscarinic control of norepinephrine release in the cardiovascular system. *Am J Physiol* 239:H713–H720, 1980.

66. Wetzel GT, Goldstein D, Brown JH: Acetylcholine release from rat atria can be regulated through an α_1-adrenergic receptor. *Circ Res* 56:763–766, 1985.

67. Potter EK: Prolonged non-adrenergic inhibition of cardiac vagal action following sympathetic stimulation: Neuromodulation by neuropeptide Y? *Neurosci Lett* 54:117–121, 1985.

68. Potter EK: Neuropeptide Y as an autonomic neurotransmitter. *Pharmacol Ther* 37:251–273, 1988.

69. Warner MR, Levy MN: Role of neuropeptide Y in neural control of the heart. *J Cardiovasc Electrophysiol* 1:80–91, 1990.

70. Stiles GL, Caron MG, Lefkowitz RJ: β-Adrenergic receptors: Biochemical mechanisms of physiological regulation. *Physiol Rev* 64:661–743, 1984.

71. Starke K, Göthert M, Kilbinger H: Modulation of neurotransmitter release by presynaptic autoreceptors. *Physiol Rev* 69:864–989, 1989.

72. Lavallée M, deChamplain J, Nadeau RA, Yamaguchi N: Muscarinic inhibition of endogenous myocardial catecholamine liberation in the dog. *Can J Physiol Pharmacol* 56:642–649, 1978.

73. Warner MR, Levy MN: Neuropeptide Y as a putative modulator of the vagal effects on heart rate. *Circ Res* 64:882–889, 1989.

74. Warner MR, Levy MN: Inhibition of cardiac vagal effects by neurally released and exogenous neuropeptide Y. *Circ Res* 65:1536–1546, 1989.

75. Warner MR, Levy MN: Sinus and atrioventricular nodal distribution of sympathetic fibers that contain neuropeptide Y. *Circ Res* 67:713–721, 1990.

76. Warner MR, Senanayake P, Ferrario CM, Levy MN: Sympathetic stimulation-evoked overflow of norepinephrine and neuropeptide Y from the heart. *Circ Res* 69:455–465, 1991.

77. Revington M, Potter EK, McCloskey DI: Prolonged inhibition of cardiac vagal action following sympathetic stimulation and galanin in anaesthetized cats. *J Physiol (Lond)* 431:495–503, 1990.

78. Ulman LG, Potter EK, McCloskey DI: Effects of sympathetic activity and galanin on cardiac vagal action in anaesthetized cats. *J Physiol (Lond)* 448:225–235, 1992.

79. Revington ML, McCloskey DI: Sympathetic-parasympathetic interactions at the heart, possibly involving neuropeptide Y, in anaesthetized dogs. *J Physiol (Lond)* 428:359–370, 1990.

80. Yang T, Levy MN: Sequence of excitation as a factor in sympathetic-parasympathetic interactions in the heart. *Circ Res* 71:898–905, 1992.

81. Evans DB: Modulation of cAMP: Mechanism for positive inotropic action. *J Cardiovasc Pharmacol* 8(Suppl 9):S22–S29, 1986.

82. Fleming JW, Strawbridge RA, Watanabe AM: Muscarinic receptor regulation of cardiac adenylate cyclase activity. *J Mol Cell Cardiol* 19:47–61, 1987.

83. Neely BH, Urthaler F: Quantitative effects of sympathetic and vagal nerve stimulations on sinus and AV junctional rhythms. *J Auton Nerv Syst* 37:109–120, 1992.

84. Mazgalev T, Miyagawa A, Dreifus LS, Michelson EL: Vagal control of the atrioventricular node — In vitro. II. Differential postganglionic vagal influence on anterograde atrioventricular nodal conduction and junctional pacemaker activity. In: Mazgalev T, Dreifus LS, Michelson EL (eds) *Electrophysiology of the Sinoatrial and Atrioventricular Nodes.* New York: Alan R. Liss, 1988, pp 155–167.

85. Loeb JM, deTarnowsky JM: Integration of heart rate and sympathetic neural effects on AV conduction. *Am J Physiol* 254:H651–H657, 1988.

86. Wallick DW, Martin PJ, Masuda Y, Levy MN: Effects of autonomic activity and changes in heart rate on atrioventricular conduction. *Am J Physiol* 243:H523–H527, 1982.

87. Martin P: Secondary AV conduction responses during tonic vagal stimulation. *Am J Physiol* 245:H584–H591, 1983.

88. Loeb JM, Dalton DP, Moran JM: Sensitivity differences of SA and AV node to vagal stimulation: Attenuation of vagal effects at SA node. *Am J Physiol* 241:H684–H690, 1981.

89. Martin P, Levy MN, Matsuda Y: Fade of cardiac responses during tonic vagal stimulation. *Am J Physiol* 243:H219–H225, 1982.

90. Jalife J, Hamilton AJ, Moe GK: Desensitization of the cholinergic receptor at the sinoatrial cell of the kitten. *Am J Physiol* 238:H439–H448, 1980.

91. Martin PJ: Paradoxical dynamic interaction of heart period and vagal activity on atrioventricular conduction in the dog. *Circ Res* 40:81–89, 1977.

92. Mancia G, Bonazzi O, Pozzoni L, Ferrari A, Gardumi M, Gregorini L, Perondi R: Baroreceptor control of atrioventricular conduction in man. *Circ Res* 44:752–758, 1979.

93. Borst C, Karemaker JM, Danning AJ: Prolongation of atrioventricular conduction time by electrical stimulation of the carotid sinus nerves in man. *Circulation* 65:432–434, 1982.

94. O'Toole MF, Ardell JL, Randall WC: Functional interdependence of discrete vagal projections to SA and AV nodes. *Am J Physiol* 251:H398–H404, 1986.

95. Thomas JX Jr, Randall WC: Autonomic influences on atrioventricular conduction in conscious dogs. *Am J Physiol* 244:H102–H108, 1983.

96. Hageman GR, Randall WC, Armour JA: Direct and reflex cardiac bradydysrhythmias from small vagal nerve stimulations. *Am Heart J* 89:338–348, 1975.

97. Levy MN: Sympathetic-parasympathetic interactions in the heart. In: Kulbertus HE, Franck G, (eds) *Neurocardiology.* Mt. Kisco, NY, Futura Publishing, 1988, pp 85–98.

98. Salata JJ, Gill RM, Gilmour RF Jr, Zipes DP: Effects of sympathetic tone on vagally induced phasic changes in heart rate and atrioventricular node conduction in the anesthetized dog. *Circ Res* 58:584–594, 1986.

99. Wallick DW, Stuesse SL, Masuda Y: Sympathetic and periodic vagal influences on antegrade and retrograde conduction through the canine atrioventricular node. *Circulation* 73:830–836, 1986.

100. Prystowsky EN, Jackman WM, Rinkenberger RL, Heger JJ, Zipes DP: Effect of autonomic blockade on ventricular refractoriness and atrioventricular nodal conduction in humans. *Circ Res* 49:511–518, 1981.

101. Yamasaki S, Stolfi A, Pickoff AS: Characterization of responses of neonatal sinus and AV nodes to critically timed, brief vagal stimuli. *Am J Physiol* 260:H459–H464, 1991.

102. Ferrari AU, Daffonchio A, Gerosa S, Mancia G: Alterations in cardiac parasympathetic function in aged rats. *Am J Physiol* 260:H647–H649, 1991.

103. Imaizumi S, Mazgalev T, Dreifus LS, Michelson EL, Miyagawa A, Bharati S, Lev M: Morphological and electrophysiological correlates of atrioventricular nodal response to increased vagal activity. *Circulation* 82:951–964, 1990.

104. Spear JF, Moore EN: Influence of brief vagal and stellate nerve stimulation on pacemaker activity and conduction within the atrioventricular conduction system of the dog. *Circ Res* 32:27–41, 1973.

105. Martin PJ: Dynamic vagal control of atrial-ventricular conduction: Theoretical and experimental studies. *Ann Biomed Eng* 3:275–295, 1975.

106. Yang T, Cheng J, Martin P, Levy MN: Effects of spatial dispersion of acetylcholine release on AV conduction responses to vagal stimulation in dogs. *Am J Physiol* 261:H392–H397, 1991.

107. Levy MN, Martin PJ, Zieske H, Adler D: Role of positive feedback in the atrioventricular nodal Wenckebach phenomenon. *Circ Res* 34:697–710, 1974.

108. Cagin NA, Kunstadt D, Wolfish P, Levitt B: The influence of heart rate on the refractory period of the atrium and A-V

conduction system. *Am Heart J* 85:358–366, 1973.

109. Zipes DP, Mihalick MJ, Robbins GT: Effects of selective vagal and stellate ganglion stimulation on atrial refractoriness. *Cardiovasc Res* 8:647–655, 1974.

110. Takei M, Furukawa Y, Narita M, Ren L-M, Karasawa Y, Murakami M, Chiba S: Synergistic nonuniform shortening of atrial refractory period induced by autonomic stimulation. *Am J Physiol* 261:H1988–H1993, 1991.

111. Schwartz PJ, Verrier RL, Lown B: Effect of stellectomy and vagotomy on ventricular refractoriness in dogs. *Circ Res* 40:536–540, 1977.

112. Vallin HO: Autonomous influence on sinus node and AV node function in the elderly without significant heart disease: Assessment with electrophysiological and autonomic tests. *Cardiovasc Res* 14:206–216, 1980.

113. Martins JB, Zipes DP: Effects of sympathetic and vagal nerves on recovery properties of the endocardium and epicardium of the canine left ventricle. *Circ Res* 46:100–110, 1980.

114. Kolman BS, Verrier RL, Lown B: Effect of vagus nerve stimulation upon excitability of the canine ventricle. Role of sympathetic-parasympathetic interactions. *Am J Cardiol* 37: 1041–1045, 1976.

115. Blair RW, Shimizu T, Bishop VS: The role of vagal afferents in the reflex control of the left ventricular refractory period in the cat. *Circ Res* 46:378–386, 1980.

116. Ellenbogen KA, Smith ML, Eckberg DL: Increased vagal cardiac nerve traffic prolongs ventricular refractoriness in patients undergoing electrophysiology testing. *Am J Cardiol* 65:1345–1350, 1990.

117. Waxman MB, Wald RW: Termination of ventricular tachycardia by an increase in cardiac vagal drive. *Circulation* 56:385–391, 1977.

118. Pilati CF, Clark RS, Gilloteaux J, Bosso FJ, Holcomb P, Maron MB: Excessive sympathetic nervous system activity decreases myocardial contractility. *Proc Soc Exp Biol Med* 193:225–231, 1990.

119. Wiggers CJ: The physiology of the mammalian auricle. II. The influence of the vagus nerves on the fractionate contraction of the right auricle. *Am J Physiol* 42:133–140, 1917.

120. Martin P: Atrial inotropic responses to brief vagal stimuli: Frequency-force interactions. *Am J Physiol* 239:H333–H341, 1980.

121. Martin PJ, Ishikawa S: Dynamic interaction between brief vagal stimulation and heart period on atrial contractility. *J Auton Nerv Syst* 17:249–262, 1986.

122. DeGeest H, Levy MN, Zieske H, Lipman RI: Depression of ventricular contractility by stimulation of the vagus nerves. *Circ Res* 17:222–235, 1965.

123. Randall WC, Wechsler JB, Pace JB, Szentivanyi M: Alterations in myocardial contractility during stimulation of the cardiac nerves. *Am J Physiol* 214:1205–1212, 1968.

124. Nolan J, Flapan AD, Capewell S, MacDonald TM, Neilson JMM, Ewing DJ: Decreased cardiac parasympathetic activity in chronic heart failure and its relation to left ventricular function. *Br Heart J* 67:482–485, 1992.

CHAPTER 22

Embryonic Development and Regulation of Cardiac Autonomic Responsiveness

JONAS B. GALPER, JOEY V. BARNETT, EDWARD J. KILBOURNE, & ALBERT P. GADBUT

INTRODUCTION

In this chapter we summarize recent insights gained into the embryonic development of autonomic responsiveness of the heart and mechanisms by which the balance between the sympathetic and parasympathetic responsiveness of the heart is regulated. Developmental studies will be presented not only for the insight they give into the ontogenesis of the cardiac autonomic response, but also for the understanding these data offer into the mechanism of interaction of autonomic receptors with guanine nucleotide binding proteins (G proteins) and effectors.

Vagal stimulation of the heart results in a decrease in the rate and force of contraction. These effects have been related to the ability of muscarinic stimulation to increase K^+ permeability of the heart cell membrane and to antagonize the elevation of cyclic AMP levels mediated by the sympathetic nervous system {1,2}. In addition, the response of the heart to muscarinic stimulation is also associated with a decrease in Ca^{2+} permeability {3}, increased levels of cyclic GMP {4}, and increased turnover of phosphatidyl inositol with production of diacylglycerol and inositol phosphates {5,6}.

Sympathetic stimulation of the heart results in an increase in the rate and force of contraction. These effects have been related to the ability of beta-adrenergic stimulation to increase cAMP levels and indirectly to activate Ca^{2+} channels {7,8}. In the embryonic heart, sympathetic and parasympathetic responses of the heart develop noncoordinately {9}. Thus, early in development embryonic chick hearts give a positive chronotropic response to norepinephrine but little negative chronotropic response to muscarinic stimulation.

Recent studies have demonstrated that transduction of muscarinic, beta-adrenergic and many other receptor-initiated signals across the cell membrane involves at least three components: binding of the hormone or neurotransmitter to a receptor, the coupling of the receptor-agonist complex to a G protein, and the GTP-dependent activation of an effector within the cell. Molecular biologic studies of muscarinic receptors and the G proteins that couple the receptor to a physiologic response in the cell demonstrate that muscarinic, beta-adrenergic, alpha-adrenergic, and other receptors and G proteins exist as multiple isoforms in the cell. Furthermore, the effector molecules to which these G proteins are coupled — the catalytic subunit of adenylate cyclase, phospholipase C, phospholipase D, and ion channels — also appear to exist as multiple isoforms. The specificity of interaction of receptor, G protein, and effector isoforms for a given tissue or a given physiologic response is not well understood. Furthermore, whether a given subtype of receptor, G protein, or effector is developmentally regulated and its expression is required for the appearance of specific second messenger pathways and physiologic responses is unclear.

In this chapter we will review classic studies of muscarinic and beta-adrenergic receptor function and mechanisms of parasympathetic and sympathetic modulation of cardiac function. We will also review more recent findings utilizing molecular biologic approaches to help understand the relationship between mechanisms of ontogenesis of autonomic responses and receptor effector coupling in the heart.

EFFECTS OF AUTONOMIC STIMULATION ON CARDIAC PHYSIOLOGY: HISTORICAL PERSPECTIVE

The parasympathetic system is characterized by a two-neuron chain. Bodies of primary preganglionic neurons are located in the central nervous system and send out axons to synapse with secondary postganglionic neurons, whose cell bodies are located in a peripheral autonomic ganglion. The postganglionic axons then pass into and innervate their target organs. The parasympathetic input to the vagus nerve originates in the dorsal motor and salivatory nuclei of the medulla oblongata. The dorsal motor nucleus is the principal source of preganglionic parasympathetic fibers destined to innervate the heart {10}. Fibers in the cardiac plexus synapse on ganglia that are located primarily in the atria, with a particularly high collection of ganglia in the region of the sinoatrial and atrioventricular nodes {10,11}. In the sympathetic nervous system the cell bodies that give rise to the sympathetic division lie in the thoracic and lumbar regions of the spinal cord in the small lateral horns. This intermedeal lateral

N. Sperelakis (ed.), Physiology and Pathophysiology of the Heart, Third Edition.

cell column receives input from the hypothalamus. These autonomic nuclei in the spinal cord send their axons to synapse on a second set of postganglionic cells that are found in collections of cell bodies in the paravertebral sympathetic trunk. It is fibers from these ganglia that enter the viscera, heart, and other smooth muscle organs.

In 1921, Otto Loewi described the release of a chemical substance from the vagus nerve, which he termed *vagusstoff* or *parasympathic* {12}. Vagusstoff was shown to be released by electrical stimulation of the vagus nerve and to slow the beat rate of the perfused heart. Feldberg and Krayer later determined that vagusstoff was acetylcholine {13}. The postsynaptic site on which acetylcholine exerted its effects was defined by Dale as the muscarinic receptor {14}. This receptor site was specifically stimulated by acetylcholine and selectively antagonized by the belladonna alkaloid atropine. Dale's description of the response of the heart to the mushroom alkaloid muscarine constitutes the classic definition of the muscarinic cholinergic receptor still in use today. However, drugs such as nicotine and dimethylphenylpiperazinium, which are selective nicotinic agonists, also suppressed sinoatrial pacemaker activity in isolated chick embryo hearts. Furthermore, acetylcholine was shown to be a neurotransmitter at both preganglionic and postganglionic parasympathetic fibers. This apparent discrepancy was resolved when it was determined that preganglionic cholinergic receptors are nicotinic, while postganglionic receptors in the heart are muscarinic {15}.

Langely and Lewandowsky {16,17} noted independently the similarity between the cardiostimulatory effects of injection of extracts of the adrenal gland and the stimulation of sympathetic nerves. Otto Loewi found that although in the winter the frog vagus preferentially released a cardioinhibitory substance, vagusstof; in the summer the frog vagus, a mixed nerve, liberated a cardioacceleration substance {12}. Cannon and Uvidil {18} demonstrated that stimulation of hepatic sympathetic nerves released an epinephrinelike substance that increased blood pressure and heart rate, which they called *sympathin*. However, as early as 1910, Barger and Dale {19} demonstrated that the injection of sympathomimetic amines more closely paralleled the effects of sympathetic neurostimulation than epinephrine. Although the possibility that demethylated epinephrine might be "sympathin" was recognized, evidence for its role as the sympathetic mediator was not obtained until von Euler identified it as the neurotransmitter of sympathetic nerves {20}. Catecholamines were also noted to mediate both excitatory and inhibitory effects on smooth muscle contraction. Ahlquist proposed the terms *alpha-* and *beta-adrenergic* receptors for sites on smooth muscle that gave excitatory and inhibitory responses, respectively {21}.

CLASSIC PHYSIOLOGIC RESPONSES OF THE HEART TO MUSCARINIC STIMULATION

Vagal stimulation of the heart or direct exposure of the heart to acetylcholine produces characteristic changes in both the sinus venosus and atrial muscle, which include hyperpolarization of the resting membrane potential and shortening of action potential duration. These changes are associated with increased K^+ permeability and decreased Ca^{2+} permeability.

Effects on K^+ permeability

Early studies by Hutter and Trautwein documented a hyperpolarization of the heart cell membrane in response to vagal stimulation and also accelerated repolarization of the action potential in atrial tissue and the sinoatrial node, resulting in decreased action potential duration {22}. These effects were found to be sensitive to extracellular K^+ concentration. Harris and Hutter documented that vagal stimulation of the heart or exposure to acetylcholine resulted in an increase in the rate of $^{42}K^+$ efflux from a sinus venosus preparation loaded with $^{42}K^+$ {23}. It is now widely accepted that the chronotropic response to muscarinic stimulation involves an increase in K^+ conductance of the heart cell membrane. This has been extensively quantified by Glitsch and Pott using voltage-clamp techniques {24}.

Effects of muscarinic stimulation on calcium currents

In electrically paced guinea pig atria, acetylcholine decreased contraction amplitude by 80%, concomitant with a 40% decrease in $^{45}Ca^{2+}$ uptake over 5 minutes {25}. These and other studies supported the conclusion that muscarinic stimulation decreased calcium flux in atrial preparations {26,27}. Modulation of cyclic GMP and cyclic AMP levels by muscarinic agonists appears to be the mechanism by which parasympathetic stimulation decreases Ca^{2+} uptake and contractile force. Increases in cyclic AMP levels have been shown to correlate with increases in slow inward current (I_{si}) and enhanced contractility. In addition, agents, including histamines and phosphodiesterase inhibitors, that increase intracellular cAMP levels independent of the effects of beta-adrenergic stimulation also increase I_{si} and contractility {7,8}. Hence cAMP, presumably acting through the stimulation of protein phosphorylation via cyclic AMP-activated protein kinase, is capable of increasing Ca^{2+} influx. It is now well established that the antagonistic effects of parasympathetic stimuli on the response to sympathetic stimulation are mediated, at least in part, by the ability of muscarinic agonists to lower intracellular cyclic AMP levels {28,29}.

DEVELOPMENT OF AUTONOMIC RESPONSIVENESS IN THE HEART

The ontogenesis of parasympathetic responsiveness of the heart has been most fully described in the chick embryo. Gestation of the chick embryo requires 21 days. In the chick embryo, vagal fibers appear in the region of the truncus arteriosus during the third day in ovo, reach the atria toward the end of the fourth day in ovo, and reach the interatrial septum on the fifth day in ovo {15,30}.

Innervation of the sinoatrial node and atrial wall has been demonstrated on days 6 and 7 in ovo, respectively. The atrial ventricular groove is reached by vagal fibers by the ninth day. Far less is known regarding the development of the parasympathetic innervation of the human heart. Nerve cells are known to be present at about 5 weeks of gestation, while ganglia appear to develop between the fifth and 12th weeks of gestation {31}.

In the chick heart, inhibitory transmission between postganglionic neurons and sinoatrial pacemaker cells appears on the 12th day in ovo {32}. Evidence indicates that muscarinic receptors are present in the embryonic chick heart for a substantial period prior to ingrowth of the vagus nerve {33–35}. However, exogenously added acetylcholine mediates only a very modest decrease in the beating rate of chick hearts 2–3 days in ovo. The sensitivity of beating to acetylcholine increases gradually between the 5th and 10th days in ovo, a time well after vagal innervation {33,36,37}. Although nerve cells derived from the sympathetic system first contact the embryonic chick heart on day 5 in ovo and catecholamines have been detected histochemically in the bulbus cordis at day 6 in ovo, catecholamine-containing nerve endings were not detected in the ventricle until day 16 in ovo. Pappano and Loffelholtz {32} and Pappano and Skowronek {38} were unable to demonstrate a positive chronotropic response to field stimulation or nicotine until day 21, just before hatching. However, prior to days 4 and 5 in ovo, beta-adrenergic stimulation by exogenous norepinephrine results in cardioacceleration {9}. Hence, autonomic responsiveness in the embryonic chick heart proceeds noncoordinately. Some of the molecular mechanisms that may be responsible for the noncoordinate development of the sympathetic and parasympathetic response of the heart are discussed below.

DEVELOPMENTAL CHANGES IN MUSCARINIC RESPONSIVENESS

The availability of ligands radiolabeled to high specific activity allowed the study of developmental changes in receptors and their coupling to physiologic responses in the heart. Several laboratories demonstrated that during embryonic development, chick hearts 2–4 days in ovo decreased beat rate by less than 10% in response to 1 mM carbamylcholine, while beat rates in embryos 5–6 days in ovo decreased by 90% at the same carbamylcholine concentration {32–34}. By days 7–12 in ovo beating was totally inhibited by 1 μM carbamycholine {33}. Although results from several laboratories are not fully in agreement, most investigators agree that muscarinic receptors are present prior to ingrowth of the vagus nerve, when these receptors are relatively insensitive to muscarinic agonists. For example, the number of muscarinic receptors per milligram of cell protein remained unchanged from days $2\frac{1}{2}$ to 12 in ovo, as measured by the binding of the labelled muscarinic antagonist (^{3}H)-quinuclidinylbenzilate (QNB) {33,39}. Although most investigators agree that muscarinic receptor number does increase prior to hatching

{39,40}, the negative chorotropic response to muscarinic stimulation has already reached a maximum before this increase in receptor number occurs. Thus, the development of sensitivity to muscarinic agonists following vagal innervation does not appear to be due to an alteration in receptor numbers, but rather to the changes in the coupling of these receptors to processes within the cell. The coupling of autonomic receptors to a physiologic response in the cell requires the interaction of the receptor with a G protein. This interaction of the receptor and G protein results in a shift of the receptor from a low- to high-affinity state.

Effects of GTP-binding proteins in determining the affinity state of muscarinic receptors: Evidence for a role of G proteins in the development of the parasympathetic response in the heart

Competition binding between carbamylcholine and [^{3}H]QNB to homogenates of embryonic chick heart cultures 10 days in ovo demonstrated at least two agonist binding sites: (a) High-affinity binding sites (R_H), constituting 26% of total sites with an IC_{50} for inhibition of [^{3}H]QNB binding of 3.9×10^{-7} M; (b) low-affinity sites (R_L) with an IC_{50} of 4.5×10^{-5} M for inhibition of [^{3}H]QNB binding {41}. Others have suggested that the receptor might exist in three affinity states, a super high-affinity, high-affinity and low-affinity state {42,43}.

Rosenberger and colleagues {44} found that guanine nucleotides and Na$^+$ decreased the affinity of the muscarinic receptor for agonist. In homogenates of cultures of embryonic chick heart cells, guanine nucleotides had no effect on the total number of receptors, but resulted in the conversion of the subset of 26% of high-affinity receptors to a low-affinity form {41}. Radiolabeled muscarinic agonist binding has also demonstrated the loss of high-affinity sites in response to guanine nucleotides. The muscarinic agonist [^{3}H] oxotremorine-M and the partial agonist [^{3}H]cis-dimethyldioxalane bind to cell homogenates and give high levels of specific binding to a high-affinity site (K_d, for [^{3}H]cis-methyldioxalane of a 1.6×10^{-9} M) and a low-affinity site (K_d, 4×10^{-7} M). Dissociation of labelled agonist is biphasic, with a rate constant of 0.09 ± 0.01 min and 1.9 ± 0.5 min for the high- and low-affinity states, respectively. Incubation with guanine nucleotides increased the fraction of [^{3}H]cis-methyldioxalane bound to the low-affinity form of the receptor with a half-maximal effect at 10^{-6} M Gpp(NH)p {45}. These findings are consistent with the view that muscarinic receptors exist in at least two forms, and that guanine nucleotides mediate the conversion of the high-affinity receptor to a low-affinity form {46,47}.

Ternary complex model for the interaction of muscarinic agonists, receptors, and guanine nucleotide binding proteins

The data cited above suggest the following model for the interaction of muscarinic agonist, high-affinity receptor, and G protein. This scheme parallels that presented by Delean et al. {48} for the beta-adrenergic receptor.

$$R_H G_i GDP + A \text{ (step 1)} \rightarrow AR_H G_i GDP + GTP \text{ (step 2)} \rightarrow$$
$$AR_H G_i GTP + GDP \text{ (step 3)} \rightarrow R_L + G_i GTP + A.$$

In this scheme R_H is a high-affinity form of the receptor, R_L is a low-affinity form of the receptor, G_i is an inhibitory G protein, and A is the agonist. According to this scheme, in the absence of agonist the high-affinity receptor-associated G protein complex is bound to GDP and hence is in the inactive form. Agonist binding results in release of GDP and binding of GTP. Whether $AR_H G_i GTP$ actually exists is unclear. The GTP-bound form of the G protein ($G_i GTP$) is the form that interacts with effectors. The conversion of R_H to R_L in the presence of GTP is associated with the release of the G protein (step 3). In support of this conclusion, Florio and Sternweiss {49} demonstrated that reconstitution of phospholipid vesicles containing muscarinic receptors in the low-affinity form with G_i resulted in the appearance of the high-affinity form of the receptor and the development of sensitivity of agonist binding to guanine nucleotides. Hence, regeneration of R_H from R_L is associated with the binding of a GDP-bound form of G protein ($G_i GDP$) to a low-affinity form of the receptor.

Changes in G protein α-subunits and affinity state of the muscarinic receptor during embryonic development of the chick heart

We have demonstrated that early in embryonic development ($3\frac{1}{2}$ days in ovo), at a time when muscarinic agonists are incapable of mediating a negative chronotropic response in embryonic chick atrial cells, guanine nucleotides have no effect on conversion of muscarinic receptors from the high-affinity to the low-affinity form {50}. Furthermore, growth of these cells in selected lots of serum resulted in an increase in the high-affinity form of the receptor and the development of the ability of guanine nucleotides to convert these receptors to a low-affinity form. These changes in coupling of G proteins to muscarinic receptors were associated with an increase in physiologic response of the cells to muscarinic stimulation as measured by the ability of carbamylcholine to augment K^+ permeability {50}. One interpretation of these data is that early in embryonic development, specific G proteins are either absent or markedly decreased in these cells.

Liang et al. demonstrated that during embryonic development of the chick heart between days $2\frac{1}{2}$ and 10 in ovo, the ability of carbamylcholine to inhibit isoproterenol-stimulated adenylate cyclase activity increased threefold from 7% to 20%, while the efficacy of carbamylcholine for inhibition of isoproterenol-stimulated adenylate cyclase activity increased 26-fold from an IC_{50} of $16 \pm 5\,\mu M$ to $0.4 \pm 0.1\,\mu M$ (n = 7). Over this same time course, levels of α_o and α_i, as measured by ADP ribosylation with pertussis toxin in the presence of ^{32}P-NAD (see below) and by immunoblotting, increased up to threefold {39}.

Furthermore, reconstitution of homogenates of hatched chick hearts in which both muscarinic receptors and adenylate cyclase had been inactivated with membranes from embryonic chick hearts $2\frac{1}{2}$ days in ovo enhanced the ability of muscarinic agonists to inhibit isoproterenol-stimulated adenylate cyclase activity {51}. The factor in the hatched chick homogenates responsible for reconstituting enhanced muscarinic inhibition of adenylate cyclase activity was inactivated by pretreatment of the hatched chick with pertussis toxin. This suggests that the factor that couples muscarinic receptors to inhibition of adenylate cyclase activity was a G protein. These data suggested that the embryonic development of a muscarinic response in the chick heart may require the appearance of increased levels of G proteins or expression of a new G protein isoform. Hence the multiplicity of isoforms of G proteins and receptors may play a role in the ontogenesis of the autonomic response in the heart. This would require the presence of a genetic program for the regulation of expression of specific isoforms at appropriate developmental stages. In the following sections, the various isoforms of muscarinic receptors and G proteins, and mechanisms for the regulation of their expression, will be discussed.

MULTIPLE SUBTYPES OF MUSCARINIC RECEPTORS

As mentioned previously, signal transduction requires the interaction of three components: the receptor, G protein, and effector. All of these exist in multiple isoforms. The physiologic function of each of these isoforms is not well understood, but existing data suggest that certain subtypes are specific for a given tissue or cell type, or appear to be specific for a given physiologic response. Furthermore certain subtypes of receptors, G proteins, or effectors might be expressed transiently during embryonic development in the heart. Data presented earlier suggested that changes in G protein receptor interaction might be critical for the development of autonomic responsiveness in the heart. A further explanation for the absence of a physiologic response to muscarinic agonists early in embryonic development is that muscarinic receptors exist in several isoforms and that development of the muscarinic response in the heart involves expression of isoforms not present at early embryonic ages. In recent years studies using both specific muscarinic ligands and molecular biological approaches have demonstrated the existence of at least five subtypes of muscarinic receptors.

Studies by Barlow et al. {52} in 1976 implied that different muscarinic receptors were present in atria and ilium. The antagonist, 4-DAMP (4-diphenyl-acetoxy-N-methyl-piperazine methiodide), demonstrated a 10-fold selectivity for binding to atrial muscarinic receptors compared to binding to the muscarinic receptors present in the ileum. Rattan and Goyal {53} demonstrated in 1978 that two subpopulations of muscarinic receptors are responsible for eliciting a rise, and subsequently a fall, in lower esophageal sphincter pressure in the opossum. These investigators determined that muscarinic receptors present on inhibitory neurons in the vagus nerve that innervates the sphincter muscle caused a fall in pressure by relaxing the sphincter muscle. This population of receptors was specifically activated by McN-A343 (4-hydroxy-2-butyl trimethylammonium chloride-m-chlorocarbinilate {53}), a compound now identified as a selective agonist for activating muscarinic receptors found in ganglia {54–56}. This subpopulation of muscarinic receptors that decreased lower esophageal pressure was termed M_1 *receptors* {59}. A different subpopulation of muscarinic receptors, which caused a rise in sphincter pressure and which were selectively activated by bethanacol and carbamylcholine, was located directly on the sphincter muscle itself and was termed M_2 *receptors* {57}. Data from other studies further supported the existence of multiple muscarinic receptor subtypes. For example, very low concentrations of pirenzepine, a muscarinic antagonist, were required to block gastric acid secretion compared to the doses required to block the effects of cholinergic agonists on smooth muscle and the heart {58–60}.

While these physiologic studies suggested multiple muscarinic receptor subtypes, the advent of radioligand binding made the examination of these receptor subtypes possible {61}. Comparison of the binding of two muscarinic antagonists, [^{3}H]-QNB and [^{3}H-pirenzipine], demonstrated that relatively few [^{3}H]QNB binding sites in rat heart, ileum, and cerebellum exhibited high-affinity binding for pirenzipine {60,62,63}. Luthin and Wolfe {64} demonstrated that these differences in the binding site densities for these two ligands, [^{3}H]-QNB and [^{3}H]-pirenzepine, were not due to differences in the rate of interconversion between two forms of the receptor ligand complex. Therefore, it appears that QNB and pirenzepine are recognizing functionally distinct stable receptor types, as opposed to transitory intermediates or conformational states of the same protein. Hence, studies with pirenzepine have confirmed the initial division of the muscarinic receptor into two subtypes.

The M_1 subtype muscarinic receptor has a high affinity for pirenzepine, K_d values of 5–20 nM, and is located primarily in cerebral cortex, hippocampus, striatum, and peripheral ganglia; whereas the M_2 subtypes have a low affinity for pirenzepine, with K_d values of 200–800 nM, and are located in peripheral tissues, such as smooth muscle and atria. Lambrecht et al. and others {65–68} developed novel cholinergic antagonists to further subclassify muscarinic receptors. In this scheme receptors are initially classified as M_1 or M_2 based on their affinity for pirenzepine. Within these groups the authors further subclassified the M_1 and M_2 receptors as $M_1\alpha$, $M_1\beta$, $M_2\alpha$, and $M_2\beta$, based on relative inhibition by pirenzepine and relative affinity for HHSID (hexahydrosiladifenidol) and methoctramine. Lambrecht further characterized the four forms of the receptor by site of localization. For example, $M_1\alpha$ is found in the hippocampus, $M_1\beta$ in ganglia and cortex, and $M_2\alpha$ in smooth muscle and exocrine glands. This classification closely parallels data from molecular biologic studies outlined below.

In several studies, attempts were made to link specific muscarinic receptor subtypes to specific biochemical responses. Gil and Wolfe {69} compared the ability of pirenzepine and atropine to inhibit muscarinic stimulation of IP_3 production or muscarinic inhibition of adenylate cyclase activity. They demonstrated a 15-fold difference in K_i for pirenzepine inhibition of muscarinic action on adenylate cyclase activity when compared to pirenzepine inhibition of phospholipase C activity. These results led Gil and Wolfe {69} to conclude that stimulation of phosphoinositide hydrolysis was mediated by an M_1 receptor that exhibits a low K_d value for pirenzepine, and inhibition of adenylate cyclase was mediated by an M_2 receptor that exhibits a higher K_d value for pirenzepine.

Molecular biological and biochemical approaches to receptors and receptor coupling: Identification and characterization of muscarinic receptor isoforms

Molecular biological approaches have confirmed the existence of multiple muscarinic receptor subtypes. Cloning of the muscarinic receptors involved initial purification of the receptor from porcine atrium {70}. The 80 K_d purified protein demonstrated a high affinity for the muscarinic antagonist QNB, with a binding capacity of 12.4 nM/mg of protein. Peralta et al. {71} determined the amino acid sequence of tryptic peptides derived from the receptor. Oligonucleotides corresponding to the deduced nucleotide sequence of these tryptic peptides were used to screen a cDNA library prepared from porcine atria. Analysis of the longest clone obtained demonstrated an open reading of 466 amino acids, giving a protein of molecular weight 51 K_d. The putative M_2 atrial receptor sequence gave a 30% amino acid identity with the beta-adrenergic receptor from the turkey erythrocyte. Hydropathicity analysis suggested that atrial muscarinic receptors had seven transmembrane-spanning domains of 27 amino acids, as suggested by the sequence homology with the beta-adrenergic receptor. Expression of this cDNA in Chinese hamster ovary cells (CHO) demonstrated high-affinity [^{3}H]QNB binding of 10 pmol/mg protein compared to less than 5 fmol/mg protein in nontransfected CHO cells. These transfected receptors bound QNB with high affinity and pirenzepine with a low affinity, consistent with the identity of the receptor as the M_2 type. The use of this cDNA probe to establish the structure of the atrial muscarinic receptor gene demonstrated that the coding region of this gene existed as a single exon.

Kubo et al. {72}, utilizing a partial amino acid sequence from an M_2 muscarinic receptor purified from bovine brain, cloned a muscarinic receptor with 38% homology overall with that cloned by Peralta et al. {72}. This clone had extensive local identities found in transmembrane domains (50–91%), as well as identities in small connecting loops (40–76%) with the porcine M_2. The porcine cerebral muscarinic receptor contained 460 amino acid residues, with a calculated molecular weight of 51,416. Hydropathicity studies also demonstrated the presence of seven hydrophobic segments. The gene coding for this cDNA was also demonstrated to be intronless, and ex-

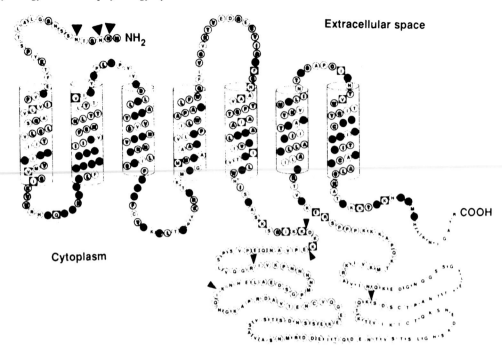

Fig. 22-1. Predicted transmembrane domain structure of the porcine M_2 myocardial muscarinic receptor. The seven membrane-spanning sequences and connecting loops are shown. Identities between the sequences of the M_2 porcine myocardial and M_1 cerebral muscarinic receptors are indicated by shaded circles. Identities between both muscarinic receptors and turkey or hamster beta-adrenergic receptors are indicated by a solid circle around each residue. Squares indicate identities between myocardial M_2 muscarinic receptor and avian or hamster beta-adrenergic receptors. Reprinted with permission from Peralta et al.: *Science* 236:600–605, 1987.

pression studies of the cDNA in *Xenopus* oocytes demonstrated the appearance of an inward current in response to acetylcholine that was abolished by 10 nM atropine. Extracts prepared from oocytes injected with the mRNA coding for this gene exhibited an [³H]QNB binding capacity ranging from 3.2 to 6.8 fmol/oocyte, whereas no measurable binding was observed with extracts derived from control oocytes. These binding sites demonstrated a high affinity for pirenzepine, as expected for an M_1 receptor. Hybridization analysis of poly A^+ RNA from different porcine tissues with this muscarinic acetylcholine receptor cDNA probe demonstrated high concentrations of the M_1 receptor mRNA in cerebral cortex, a somewhat decreased level in corpus striatum, and the complete absence of this mRNA in the medulla, pons, and atrium {72}.

Bonner et al. {73} screened a rat cerebral cortex cDNA library with a portion of cDNA taken from the beginning of the second transmembrane region of the porcine brain cDNA and obtained four different clones. The first clone was identical to the M_1 clone previously isolated by Kubo et al. {74} from the cerebral cortex; the second clone coded for a 586 amino acid protein with 98% identity to porcine M_2. The third clone isolated coded for a 589 amino acid protein, which differed from both the M_1 and M_2 clones, and was referred to by Bonner as M_3. The fourth

clone isolated coded for a protein containing 478 amino acids and was designated M_4.

Comparison of these sequences with those of the porcine receptor showed a high degree of conservation in the regions corresponding to postulated transmembrane regions with much less homology in the amino-terminal and carboxy-terminal regions. In addition, a large cytoplasmic loop between transmembrane regions 5 and 6, variable in size from 157 to 203 amino acids, showed little similarity among M_1 through M_4, except for a large fraction (17–20%) of basic residues. This loop is much smaller in the beta-adrenergic receptor and rhodopsin than it is in the muscarinic receptor. If one excludes this loop and the amino and carboxy-terminal ends from the comparison, the M_3 sequence has 79% identity with the M_1 sequence. The M_2 receptor sequence is 65% identical to M_3, but is more closely related to the porcine M_2 receptor, with 85% identity. The poor homology between the amino terminus and the large cytoplasmic loop of the M_2 receptor with the corresponding regions of the M_4 receptor indicates that the M_4 receptor is not the rat homologue of the porcine M_2 receptor. All four receptor genes appear to be intronless. More recently, a fifth muscarinic receptor has been cloned from human and rat, and expressed in mammalian cells {75}. The mammalian gene coded for a 532 amino acid protein with 89% sequence identity to the 531 amino acid rat protein and was most closely related to the M_3 receptor. Both the rat and human proteins are encoded by a single exon.

Recently three isoforms of the muscarinic receptor have been cloned from the chick. Tietje et al. {76,77} cloned both the M_4 and M_2 receptor from a chick genomic library. The M_4 clone coded for a protein with 490 amino acids and was 83% identical on the amino acid level with rat M_4 and 70% identical with porcine M_2 in regions not including the third cytoplasmic loop. The M_2 clone codes for a protein with 466 amino acids and was 92% identical on the amino acid level with porcine M_2 and 68% identical with rat M_4 in regions not including the third cytoplasmic loop. Expression of chick M_2 and M_4 in CHO and Y_1 cells demonstrated a high affinity for atropine and a low affinity for pirenzipine. We have recently cloned the chick M_3 receptor, which encodes a 640 amino acid protein with 83% identity with human M_3 and only 67% and 54% homology with chick M_2 and M_4, respectively. RNAse protection studies have demonstrated the presence of mRNA coding for all three of these receptors in the chick atrium {77a}.

Binding properties of cloned muscarinic receptor subtypes

All five muscarinic-cholinergic receptors were stably expressed in CHO-K_1 hamster ovary cells {73}. Studies with the selective antagonists pirenzepine, AFDX-116, methoctramine, and HHSID (hexahydrosiladifenidol) were used to differentiate receptor binding properties. Receptors could be divided into high-affinity pirenzepine-type receptors, low-affinity pirenzepine-type receptors, and receptors with intermediate affinity for pirenzepine of the type found in exocrine glands (glandular type). Expression of these genes in COS7 cells demonstrated that pirenzepine displaced ^{3}H-QNB binding with high affinity in cells transfected with M_1, and intermediate affinity to M_3 and M_4. The human M_2 transfectants had low affinity for pirenzepine, consistent with its M_2 classification {78}.

Specificity of coupling of a receptor subtype to different effector systems

In order to determine the specificity of coupling of a particular muscarinic receptor subtype to a given effector system, muscarinic receptors were expressed in CHO cells. The ability of the M_2 receptor from pig to mediate inhibition of adenylate cyclase activity and to stimulate phosphoinositide hydrolysis were compared {79}. Stimulation of phosphoinositide hydrolysis was significantly less efficient and more dependent on levels of receptors expressed in the transfected cells than the inhibition of adenylate cyclase activity.

Human embryonic kidney (HEK) cells were transfected with each of the four muscarinic receptor subtypes individually, and the effects of carbamylcholine on inhibition of adenylate cyclase activity and inositol phosphate production were compared {79}. It was determined that cells transfected with both HM_2 and HM_4 mediated a modest carbamylcholine stimulation of inositol phosphate production and an inhibition of forskolin-stimulated adenylate cyclase activity with an EC_{50} of 3×10^{-8} M. HM_1 and HM_3 cells actually stimulated cyclic AMP production in the presence of carbamylcholine, while producing a large stimulation of inositol phosphate production. These experiments suggested specificity of coupling of the M_2 and M_4 receptors to inhibition of adenylate cyclase and the M_1 and M_3 receptors to stimulation of phospholipase C activity. Expression of chick M_2 and M_4 in CHO and Y_1 cells demonstrated that both receptors coupled to inhibition of adenylate cyclase activity and stimulation of an inositol phosphate response {76,77}. The chick M_3 receptor in CHO cells was coupled to only a modest inhibition of adenylate cyclase activity and stimulation of a more robust inositol phosphate release {77a}. The finding of mRNAs coding for M_2, M_4, and M_3 forms of the muscarinic receptor in the embryonic chick atrium is unique since only the M_2 form has been demonstrated in atria of other species.

Data presented demonstrate that during embryonic development of the chick heart muscarinic responsiveness is converted from a robust inositol phosphate response with only minimal inhibition of adenylate cyclase activity at day 5 in ovo to a more modest stimulation of inositol phosphate production with a marked inhibition of adenylate cyclase activity at day 14 in ovo {39,80}. These data are consistent with the hypothesis that during embryonic development of the chick heart, a conversion from an M_1- or M_3-mediated response to an M_2-mediated response may be responsible for the changes in muscarinic coupling to second messenger production. The presence of mRNAs coding for all three of these muscarinic receptor isoforms in the embryonic chick atrium may be related to the mechanism by which muscarinic responsiveness develops in the embryonic chick heart.

MULTIPLICITY OF GTP-BINDING PROTEIN ISOFORMS: DO THEY PLAY A ROLE IN THE ONTOGENESIS OF THE PARASYMPATHETIC RESPONSE IN THE HEART?

The multiplicity of muscarinic receptors suggests that one mechanism for the developmental appearance of specific cholinergic functions in the heart could be related to changes in expression of muscarinic receptor subtypes. However, the finding of an even greater diversity of G-protein subunit subtypes suggests that regulation of expression of G-protein isoforms could also play a role in the development of the parasympathetic response. For this reason we will review the organization of the G-protein heterotrimers and the known subtypes of each subunit.

Characterization of G-protein α subunits

The physiology and biochemistry of G proteins has been extensively studied using bacterial toxins that catalyze the transfer of an ADP-ribose moiety from nicotinamide adenine dinucleotide (NAD) to the α subunit. A protein initially referred to as *islet activating protein* (IAP), isolated from cultures of *Bordetella pertussis*, was shown to potentiate the effects of various insulin secretagogues when incubated with pancreatic islet cells {81}. This effect was associated with an increase in cAMP levels. Hazeki and Ui demonstrated that levels of cAMP in isoproterenol-stimulated heart cells were significantly higher in cells preincubated with IAP {82}. Although muscarinic agonists markedly inhibited cAMP accumulation in isoproterenol-stimulated rat heart myocyte cultures, muscarinic agonists had no effect on isoproterenol-stimulated cAMP levels in cells pretreated with IAP. These data suggested that IAP interfered with the action of agonists that inhibited adenylate cyclase activity.

It is well established that both isoproterenol and GTP stimulate adenylate cyclase activity {83}. Katada and Ui {84} demonstrated that IAP (now referred to as *pertussis toxin*) enhanced the effect of GTP or GTP plus isoproterenol on cAMP production in membranes from cultured neural cells. Nicotinamide adenine dinucleotide (NAD) and ATP were required for this effect, and the reaction was shown to involve the transfer of an ADP ribose moiety from NAD to a C-terminal cysteine on a $41\text{-}K_d$ protein. Katada and Ui further demonstrated that pertussis toxin treatment converted the muscarinic receptor from a high-affinity to a low-affinity form by interfering with the interaction of the receptor and G protein. Hence not only is hormonal inhibition of adenylate cyclase activity prevented, but basal levels of adenylate cyclase activity are increased by release of adenylate cyclase from tonic inhibition by an inhibitory G protein.

Inhibitory G proteins have been termed *Gi* and have been shown to exist as heterotrimers composed of three subunits, designated α, β, and γ {85–88}. The α subunit has been shown to be a protein that varies in molecular weight from 39 to 41 kDa, binds GTP, catalyzes the hydrolysis of GTP to GDP, and is the substrate for pertussis toxin. The β subunit is a 35 kDa protein that is found in association with the 9 kDa γ subunit {89}.

A second toxin derived from *Vibrio cholera* has been shown to enhance the activity of adenylate cyclase by catalyzing the transfer of ADP-ribose from NAD to a cysteine at amino acid 200 in a 45 kDa GTP-binding protein designated α_s. The α_s subunit has been found to associate with a $\beta\gamma$ subunit identical to that associated with α_i and is responsible for coupling stimulatory receptors to adenylate cyclase {90}.

Families of GTP-binding proteins

Jones and Reed {91} cloned five G proteins from rat olfactory neuroepithelium. One clone encoded the α subunit of Gs, while the remaining clones encoded G proteins that were pertussis toxin substrates, $G_{\alpha o}$, a 39 kDa protein found in high levels in the brain, and three other proteins designated $G_{\alpha i\text{-}1}$, $G_{\alpha i\text{-}2}$, and $G\text{-}\alpha_{i\text{-}3}$. More recently, Strathmann et al. {92} cloned five new G proteins utilizing the polymerase chain reaction (PCR) with a template cDNA prepared from reverse-transcribed RNA from adult mouse brain and spermatids with oligonucle-

otide primers that were 95% identical to sequences in G_s, G_o, G_i, and transducin. These data suggested that the family of G proteins contained more than 15 members. Several of these family members — αq, lack the carboxy-terminal cysteine residue that is the site for pertussis-toxin-mediated ADP ribosylation. Hence they are GTP-binding proteins whose coupling to the receptor is insensitive to pertussis toxin. Although all of these α subunits are activated by binding GTP and are characterized by the hydrolysis of bound GTP to GDP via their intrinsic GTPase activity, different G-protein α subunits may have significantly different characteristic rates of GTP hydrolysis. αz has a very slow rate of GTPase activity and is found primarily in neurons. αq and $\alpha 11$ are 88% identical at the amino acid level, are widely distributed in the same cells, and differ primarily in the amino terminus. These differences in the amino terminus may be related to the specificity of these α subunits for $\beta\gamma$ interaction, since the amino terminus of α subunits is believed to be the site of interaction with $\beta\gamma$. Other members of the αq family include $\alpha 14$, found in stromal and epithelial cells, and $\alpha 15$ and $\alpha 16$, found in hematopoietic stem cells.

Other family members have been characterized as the products of alternate splicing of mRNAs coding for G-protein α subunits. Studies in Drosophila and in mammalian cells have demonstrated the presence of multiple isoforms of α_o, resulting from alternately spliced exons within the α_o gene {93–96}. Two forms of human α_o, α_{o1} and α_{o2}, were cloned from a human insulin-secreting tumor library {94}. α_{o1} is identical to bovine α_o on the amino acid level, while α_{o2} is identical up to and including animo acid 248, and differs thereafter in 26 of the remaining 106 amino acids of the carboxy terminus. In Drosophila two α_o proteins, which differ in the amino terminus, result from alternate splicing of the first exon within the α_o gene {95,96}. We {96a} have recently cloned a chick cDNA coding for an α subunit that is a chimera between α_o and α_{i3}, with the first 30 amino acids identical to rat α_o and the remaining amino acids identical to chick α_{i3}. RNA coding for this protein was demonstrated in brain, heart, lung, liver, and kidney by RNAse protection and PCR. In vitro translation of RNA transcribed from this cDNA resulted in the production of a GTP-binding protein of the appropriate molecular size.

β SUBUNITS

Four isoforms of the β subunit of the G protein have been described. β_1 is a 36 kDa protein, and β_2 a 35 kDa protein {97,98}. β_1, β_2, and β_3 {99} are ubiquitously expressed, while β_4 is abundant in brain and lung {100}. The β subunit is characterized by eight segments, each of which shares a repetitive 40 amino acid motif that is characterized by certain amino acids plus a tryptophan-aspartic acid pair.

γ SUBUNITS

The diversity of γ subunits may be even greater than that of β subunits. Molecular cloning studies have demonstrated at least five isoforms of the γ subunit {101,102}. Peptide sequences of purified proteins have suggested the presence of several other isoforms {102}. $γ_1$ is expressed only in photorecetors, $γ_2$ is expressed at various levels in all tissues, and $γ_3$ is expressed primarily in brain and testes {101}. The cDNA for $γ_4$ has been detected in bovine kidney and retina. The amino terminus of the proteins coded for by these cDNAs differ markedly, with a 43% identity between the first 15 amino acids of $γ_3$ and $γ_2$, and almost no identity between the first 15 amino acids of $γ_1$ and $γ_2$. The remaining portion of $γ_2$ and $γ_3$ were 82% identical. The amino-terminal portion of $γ_3$ had no homology with the first 15 amino acids of $γ_1$, and only a 36% identity to the remaining sequences of $γ_1$. Recently {104} a $γ_5$ with a 25% identity with $γ_1$ and 49% identity with $γ_2$ has been cloned from bovine and rat liver. All of the γ subunits have a carboxy terminus that ends in CAAX (where C is cysteine, A is an alanine, and X is any amino acid), except $γ_5$, which ends in CXXX {104,105}. Posttranslational modification results in geranylgeranylation or isoprenylation of the cysteine removal of the AAX, followed by carboxymethylation {105,106}.

If modification of the γ subunit by isoprenylation or geranylgeranylation is inhibited either by mutation of the C-terminus cystine or by inhibition of isoprenoid biosynthesis by mevinolin, an HMG CoA reductase inhibitor, the resulting γ subunits are still capable of forming a complex with β. However, the resulting βγ does not localize to the plasma membrane. Furthermore, β remains in the cytoplasm and the βγ complex is inactive {106,107}. This modification of γ most closely resembles the posttranslational modification of RAS {108}.

Role of diversity in isoforms of α, β, and γ subunits in determining the specificity of receptor-effector interaction

For some time it was assumed that the specificity of G-protein receptor-effector coupling resided in the localization and relative levels of expression of different G-protein α-subunits. The finding of multiple forms of β and γ subunits suggests that they also may play a role in determining the specificity of interaction. This view is reinforced by recent findings that βγ interacts directly with effectors such as adenylate cyclase, K^+ channels, and phospholipase C {109–111}.

RECEPTOR EFFECTOR COUPLING VIA G PROTEINS

Studies using reconstitution of purified receptors, G-protein subunits, and effectors, as well as antisense DNA to specific G-protein subunit subtypes, have begun to establish the specificity of receptor–G-protein–effector interaction. In the following sections data will be reviewed that demonstrate that specificity does exist between different isoforms of receptors, G-protein subunits, and effectors. Studies will be reviewed that support the hypothesis that innervation of the heart or exposure of the heart to growth factors may regulate autonomic responsiveness by altering the expression of different G-protein isoforms {112,113}.

Inhibition of adenylate cyclase activity

Although the identity of the specific G-protein isoform involved in the muscarinic inhibition of adenylate cyclase activity has not been unequivocally established, data have demonstrated that both the α subunit and βγ subunit play a role in the muscarinic inhibition of hormone-stimulated adenylate cyclase activity (fig. 22-2). Northrup et al. {90}

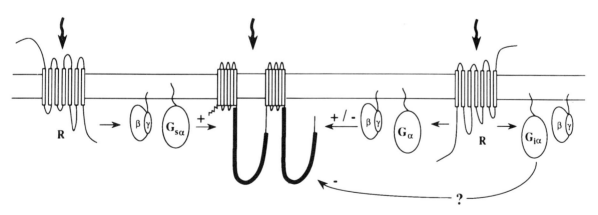

Fig. 22-2. Regulation of adenylyl cyclase activity by beta-adrenergic and muscarinic receptors. Beta-adrenergic receptor (R, left) stimulated activation of adenylyl cyclase (center) occurs through activation of G-protein $α_s$ subunits ($G_sα$). Muscarinic receptor (R, right) stimulated inhibition of adenylyl cyclase activity occurs through G-protein $α_i$ ($G_iα$) subunits. Different adenylyl cyclase subtypes are either stimulated (+), inhibited (−), or unaffected by released G-protein βγ dimers. Reprinted with permission from Tang WJ, Gilman AG: *Cell* 70:869–872, 1992.

demonstrated that the $\beta\gamma$ subunit is capable of inactivating GTP or fluoride-stimulated adenylate cyclase activity in the presence of α_s. These authors suggested that hormone receptor interaction resulted in release of $\beta\gamma$ from α_i, and that the association of free $\beta\gamma$ with α_s resulted in inhibition of the GTP or fluoride-dependent activation of adenylate cyclase {90}. Evidence has also been presented that suggests α_i alone is capable of exerting an inhibitory effect on adenylate cyclase activity {90}. Recently the catalytic subunit of adenylate cyclase has been purified and cloned, and the interaction of α_s, $\beta\gamma$, and α_i with the catalytic subunit of adenylate cyclase has been further studied.

Analysis of the cDNA encoding the catalytic subunit of adenylate cyclase demonstrates that this protein has a quasi-duplicated structure. There are two membrane-spanning domains, each with six putative transmembrane helices and two nucleotide-binding domains. Both halves of the molecule appear to be required for catalytic activity {109}. There are presumably at least five different subtypes of the catalytic subunit of adenylate cyclase. The subtypes differ in some cases in localization to a specific cell type and in the ability to interact with calmodulin and $\beta\gamma$. Thus the type I subunit is found in brain {109}, and the type II subtype {114} is found in brain, with low levels in lung. The type III {115} form is widely distributed in heart, liver, kidney, and lung. The type V form is found primarily in heart with lower levels in brain {116}. Only the type I and III forms are associated with calcium/calmodulin. The $\beta\gamma$ subunit of the G-protein heterotrimer has been shown to inhibit the activity of the type I isoform {117}, to stimulate the activity of the type II and type IV forms, and to have no effect on the type III form. Although no data are available on the specificity of $\beta\gamma$ isoforms for interaction with the various isoforms of the catalytic subunit, the developmental regulation of these isoforms could play a role in the ontogenesis of the control of adenylate cyclase activity. Furthermore, data suggest that in *Dictyostelium* the expression of different isoforms of the adenylate cyclase catalytic subunit may be developmentally regulated {118}.

Muscarinic-stimulated inositol phosphate production: Role of $\beta\gamma$ and specificity of α

The hydrolysis of membrane-bound phosphotidylinositol (4,5) P_2 has emerged as a major intracellular signaling pathway. Since the initial report of Hokin and Hokin in 1954 {119} describing the release of inositol phosphates from stimulated cells, phospholipase C activation resulting in inositol phosphate release has been demonstrated in many tissues and in response to stimulation by a large number of agonists {for a review, see 120}. The hydrolysis of phosphotidylinositol {4,5} P_2 yields both inositol (1,4,5) P_3, which releases Ca^{2+} from intracellular stores {121, 122}, and 1,2-diacylglycerol, which activates protein kinase C. Recently it has been suggested that phosphorylated metabolites of inositol (1,4,5) P_3 may be physiologically active. For example, inositol (1,3,4,5) P4 {123–125} may modulate calcium levels, and inositol P_5 and inositol P_6 may act as extracellular signals {126}. Muscarinic-

stimulated inositol phosphate production in the heart was demonstrated by Masters et al. {127} using chick ventricular cells 13-days in ovo cultured for 24 hours. The EC_{50} for carbamylcholine-stimulated inositol phosphate production in the ventricle was reported to be 20–30 µM which is in agreement with the value subsequently reported in chick atria. This study also demonstrated that inositol phosphate produced in response to muscarinic stimulation was insensitive to pertussis toxin. Jones et al. {128}, using chick ventricular cells 13 days in ovo cultured for 24 hours, also demonstrated that inositol phosphate production was stimulated by GTPγS in saponin-permeabilized chick ventricular cells. These data suggested that in ventricular cells a pertussis toxin insensitive G protein coupled the muscarinic receptor to phospholipase C activation.

Role of αq and $\beta\gamma$ in activation of phospholipase C activity. Purification of PLC from various tissues and molecular cloning have demonstrated the existence of at least eight isoforms of PLC divided into four classes: α, β, γ, and δ. The PLC-γ isoforms appear to be the target of the tyrosine kinases associated with growth factors. The PLCβ1 has been shown to be activated by GTP and has been copurified with the members of a subclass of G-protein α subunits, α_q and α_{11}, that lack the carboxy-terminal cysteine site for ADP ribosylation by pertussis toxin {129}. Specific antibodies to α_q and α_{11} have been shown to interfere with bradykinin, angiotensin, and histamine stimulation of PLC activity in various cell types {130}. The $\beta\gamma$ subunit plays a role in modulating activity of PLC β-1. GTP- or AlF_4-stimulated PLC activity was inhibited by $\beta\gamma$ {110}, while the stimulatory effect of the purinergic agonist 2-methylthioadenosine 5'-triphosphate on PLC was potentiated 50–100% in response to reconstitution with increasing amounts of $\beta\gamma$ subunits {131}.

Ontogenesis of muscarinic stimulated IP_3 production in the embryonic chick heart. Recent studies by Barnett et al. {132} have described the ontogenesis of muscarinic-stimulated inositol phosphate production in cultures of chick heart cells from both atria and ventricle. These studies demonstrated different mechanisms of coupling of muscarinic receptors to phospholipase C in atrium and ventricle. In agreement with the work of Masters et al. {127}, ventricular cells cultured from embryos 5, 7, 10, 12, and 14 days in ovo demonstrated a developmental decrease of 50% in the ability of muscarinic agonists to stimulate inositol phosphate production. Muscarinic stimulation of phospholipase C activity was insensitive to pertussis toxin at all ages studied {127}.

In atrial cells muscarinic-stimulated inositol phosphate production also decreased by 50% between days 5 and 14 in ovo. However, over this time course muscarinic-stimulated inositol phosphate production developed a partial sensitivity to pertussis toxin. Hence between days 5 and 14 in ovo pertussis toxin inhibition of muscarinic-stimulated inositol phosphate production increased from undetectable levels to 40% of total {132}.

In cultured chick heart cells from both atria and ventricle from hearts 5 days in ovo permeabilized with saponin, GTPγS stimulated pertussis-toxin-insensitive inositol phosphate production. In cultures of atria and ventricles 14 days in ovo permeabilized with saponin, pertussis toxin was able to inhibit a fraction of the response stimulated by GTPγS only in the atrium {78,132}. These data taken together suggest that in ventricle a pertussis-toxin-insensitive G protein couples the muscarinic receptor to phospholipase C activation. However, in atria phospholipase C activity is initially coupled to a pertussis-toxin-insensitive G protein, but during the course of development, coupling of phospholipase C to the muscarinic receptor occurs via two separate G proteins, one pertussis toxin sensitive and the other pertussis toxin insensitive. The time course of the development of pertussis-toxin-sensitive inositol phosphate production in chick atria parallels the time course of the developmental increase in the levels of pertussis toxin substrates α_o and α_i described previously {39}. This finding supports the hypothesis that developmental changes in responsiveness to muscarinic stimulation may be related to developmental increases in G proteins or the appearance of previously unexpressed isoforms of G-protein α subunits.

Inositol phosphate production in the mammalian heart is less well described. Poggioli et al. {133} demonstrated IP_3 production in intact rat heart in response to α_1-adrenergic, muscarinic cholinergic, and electrical stimulation. Schmitz et al. {134} have reported that both the α_1-adrenergic receptor mediated inotropic effect and α_1-adrenergic-stimulated IP_3 production are insensitive to pertussis toxin. In this study, IP_3 production was found to precede the inotropic effect of α_1-adrenergic receptor stimulation consistent with a role of IP_3 in mediating the inotropic effect of α_1-adrenergic stimulation of the heart. However, total inositol phosphate production in response to α_1-adrenergic stimulation in cultured rat cardiac myocytes has been reported by Steinberg et al. {135} to be partially sensitive to pertussis toxin.

Muscarinic stimulation of diacylglycerol formation

Recent studies {136} have suggested that although a fraction of diacylglycerol is produced via direct action of phospholipase C on phosphatidylinositol biophosphate to produce IP_3 and diacylglycerol, a large fraction of diacylglycerol is generated via the action of phospholipase D on phosphatidyl inositol. Phospholipase D has been shown to cleave the phosphodiester bond between the phosphate and polar head group of the phospholipid, releasing the polar moiety and phophatidic acid.

Muscarinic stimulation of chick atrial cells whose phospholipids have been labeled with [3H] arachidonic acid results in the initial appearance of phosphatidic acid, followed by an increase in diacylglycerol levels and a parallel decrease in phosphatidyl inositol, suggesting a role for phospholipase D in the hydrolysis of phosphatidyl inositol and the production of diacylglycerol. Furthermore, muscarinic stimulation of cultured chick heart cells labeled with [3H] choline resulted in increased release of both [3H] choline and [3H] phosphocholine in both cultured chick atrial and ventricular cells, consistent with phosphatidyl choline as a source of diacylglycerol in these cells.

Muscarinic stimulation of diacylglycerol production in cells labelled with [3H] arachidonic acid is partially sensitive to pertussis toxin in the atrium, but insensitive to pertussis toxin in the ventricle. Furthermore, the GTPγS-stimulated production of phosphatidic acid and diacylglycerol in the atrium were partially sensitive to pertussis toxin, consistent with the hypothesis that phospholipase D activity in the atrium is coupled to the muscarinic receptor via two separate G proteins.

Furthermore, in atrial cells labeled with [3H] myristate, which is incorporated primarily into phosphatidyl choline, muscarinic and GTPγS-stimulated diacylglycerol is fully sensitive to pertussis toxin inhibition. One likely interpretation of these data is that muscarinic stimulation of diacylglycerol formation from phosphatidyl choline and phosphatidyl inositol may be coupled to the receptor via different G proteins {136}.

Ontogenesis of diacylglycerol production in the embryonic chick heart.
Studies of the embryonic development of muscarinic stimulation of diacylglycerol in the chick heart demonstrate that although muscarinic stimulation of diacylglycerol production is present at the earliest ages studied (less than $3\frac{1}{2}$ days in ovo), development of this response is associated with changes in the mechanism of coupling of diacylglycerol production to the receptor and the appearance of new pathways for diacylglycerol (DG) production between days 5 and 14 in ovo. Thus in the ventricle muscarinic stimulation of both IP_3 and DG production decreased by 50% during development. In the atrium, however, muscarinic stimulation of IP_3 production decreased, while DG production remained constant throughout development. Since the action of PLC on phosphotidylinositol bisphosphate results in the formation of both DG and IP_3, a 50% decrease in IP_3 production during embryonic development of the atrium should result in a decrease in muscarinic-stimulated DG production in the atrium. However, the finding that muscarinic stimulation of DG production in the atrium was unchanged during cardiac development suggested that some other pathway might develop to compensate for the loss of DG due to decreased IP_3 production.

Stephan et al. {137} demonstrated that between days 5 and 14 in ovo muscarinic stimulation of phosphatidic acid production in the atrium increased threefold. Furthermore, in cells labeled with [3H] choline, muscarinic-stimulated release of [3H] choline and [3H] phosphocholine increased from undetectable levels above basal at day 5 in ovo to 35–40% above basal at day 14 in ovo. These data suggested that a pathway utilizing phosphatidyl choline as a source of DG developed in the atrium between day 5 and 14 in ovo.

Muscarinic stimulation of K^+ channel activity: Role of $\beta\gamma$ and α

We have previously outlined the classic studies of the effects of muscarinic stimulation on K^+ permeability and its relationship to changes in the chronotropic state of the heart. More recently, Martin et al. {138} demonstrated that pertussis toxin treatment of cultured embryonic chick heart cells interfered with muscarinic stimulation of $^{42}K^+$ uptake. Pfaffinger et al. {111} demonstrated that coupling of the muscarinic receptor in embryonic chick atrial cells to an inward rectifying potassium channel required intracellular GTP. Pretreatment of cells with pertussis toxin eliminated the acetylcholine-induced inward rectification {111}. Logothetis et al. {139} demonstrated that addition of the purified $\beta\gamma$ complex increased I_{k-Ach} in inside-out patches in which K^+ channels had been uncoupled from the muscarinic receptor by pertussis toxin catalyzed ADP ribosylation of endogenous α proteins. Neither a GTP-liganded α subunit nor a GTPγS-liganded α subunit were capable of activating this current. However, when the α subunits were added in excess over $\beta\gamma$, they inhibited activation of K^+ channels by $\beta\gamma$, presumably by binding the $\beta\gamma$ and rendering it unavailable for activation of the K^+ channel. Logothetis et al. {140} subsequently demonstrated that at a concentration of 200 pM, $\beta\gamma$ activated K^+ channels in patches from rat and chick atria 97% of the time. Activation was maximal at 10 nM. They further demonstrated that activated α subunits purified from human erythrocytes (α40-GTPγS) at concentrations of 10 pM or greater opened K^+ channels in 5 out of 27 chick atrial patches, and in 5 out of 11 rat atrial patches. Hence activation of the channel by both $\beta\gamma$ and α subunits appears to be possible. Recently a product of phospholipase A_2 activity has been implicated in the response of chick atrial patches to $\beta\gamma$ subunits via production of a lipoxygenase-derived second messenger {141,142}.

Yatani et al. {143} have demonstrated that activation of mammalian atrial muscarinic potassium channels by a human erythrocyte pertussis-toxin-sensitive G protein, G_k, which they have identified as α_{i3} {144}, is responsible for coupling muscarinic stimulation to activation of the acetylcholine-sensitive K^+ channel. Subsequent studies have demonstrated that α_{i1}, α_{i2}, and α_{i3} can all couple muscarinic receptors to K^+ channel activation {145} at picomolar concentrations of G_k, whereas nM concentrations of human red blood cell G_s were ineffective. In their hands, $\beta\gamma$ dimers at nanomolar concentrations had no effect on these K^+ currents. Recently the signaling pathway between atrial muscarinic receptors, G proteins, and K^+ channels has been shown to be interrupted by the presence of a low molecular weight G-protein ras-p21 and the GTPase activating proteins (GAPs). Although the mechanism is not well understood {146}, data suggest that ras p21-GAP does not interfere with the interaction of G_k with the K^+ channel, but interferes with coupling of the receptor to the G protein. Mutational studies of GAP suggest that this effect is dependent on the ability of GAP to interact with ras p21 and to bind phosphoproteins {147}.

Use of antisense DNA to establish the specificity of α, β, γ subunits in coupling specific receptors and effectors

One of the most effective ways to establish the function of a specific protein is to inhibit its expression and to observe the effect on receptor-effector coupling. Kleuss et al. {148} utilized antisense oligonucleotides injected into GH_3 cells to study the specificity of G-protein α, β, and γ subunits in coupling muscarinic and somatostatin receptors to the inhibition of voltage-dependent Ca^{2+} channels. Comparison of the effects of antisense cDNA to the alternate splice forms of α_o, α_{o1} and α_{o2}, demonstrated that only α_{o2} interfered with the somatostatin inhibition of the Ca^{2+} channel. The α_{o1} antisense cDNA interfered with the carbamylcholine inhibition of the Ca^{2+} channel {148}. A similar study comparing the effects of antisense to $\beta_{1,2,3}$ or β_4 on somatostatin and carbamylcholine inhibition of Ca^{2+} current demonstrated that anti-β_3 interfered with the carbamylcholine inhibition of the Ca^{2+} channel and anti-β_1 interfered with the somatostatin response. Antisense β_4 had no effect on either the somatostatin response or the carbamylcholine response, and β_3 antisense had no effect on the somatostatin response {149}.

In a more recent paper, comparison of the effects of antisense DNA to γ_1, γ_2, γ_3, or γ_4 injected into GH_3 cells demonstrated that anti-γ_3 interfered with the ability of somatostatin to inhibit voltage-sensitive calcium channels, while antisense-γ_4 interfered with the effects of carbamylcholine on this current {150}. These studies suggest that a high degree of specificity may occur in the coupling of receptors and G-protein α, β, and γ subunits to different effector systems. Thus the M_4 muscarinic receptor would appear to be coupled to L-type Ca^{2+} channels via an $\alpha_{o1}/\beta_3/\gamma_4$ heterotrimer, and the somatostatin receptor would appear to be coupled to the same effector via an $\alpha_{o2}/\beta_1/\gamma_3$ heterotrimer.

CONCLUSION: ROLE OF DEVELOPMENTAL REQULATION OF EXPRESSION OF RECEPTOR-G-PROTEIN-EFFECTOR ISOFORMS ON THE ONTOGENESIS OF AUTONOMIC RESPONSES IN THE HEART

If the degree of specificity for β, γ subunit isoforms suggested by these antisense studies can be demonstrated in other systems, one likely regulatory mechanism for the development of the autonomic response would be the activation, by growth factors or innervation of the heart (see below), of programmed gene expression, which determines the order of appearance for specific isoforms of receptors, G-protein subunits, and effectors.

Data presented previously demonstrated that in the developing chick heart, levels of α_o and α_i, measured either by Western blot analysis or ADP ribosylation with pertussis toxin, increased over time. This increase paralleled the developmental increase in muscarinic inhibition of adenylate cyclase activity, the development of a pertussis-toxin-sensitive muscarinic stimulation of IP_3 and DG production, and the development of a pertussis-toxin-sensitive negative chronotropic response to muscarinic stimulation. Thus the appearance of all of these pathways that involve coupling of muscarinic receptors to pertussis-toxin-sensitive G proteins could be related to changes in the expression of isoforms of receptors; $G_{\alpha i}$, G_β, or G_γ; or effectors expressed in the atrium.

Models for the study of cardiac autonomic development

Several studies have suggested that innervation of the heart may play a role in the induction of autonomic responsiveness. Steinberg et al. demonstrated that mixed cultures of neonatal rat ventricular cardiocytes with sympathetic ganglia resulted in the appearance of a negative inotropic response to α_2-adrenergic stimulation {112}. This group also suggested that this mixed culture mediated an increase in pertussis toxin substrate. However, because this was a mixed culture of sympathetic ganglion cells and cardiocytes, it was not possible to determine which cell type was responsible for the increase in G proteins {112}. Marvin et al. {151} demonstrated that coculture of both sympathetic and parasympathetic ganglia with rat heart cells resulted in an increase in the chronotropic and inotropic responses of these cells to sympathetic agonists. Recently a system for coculture of intact ciliary ganglia and heart cells in which ganglia could be removed following coculture was used to demonstrate that coculture induces a negative chronotropic response to muscarinic stimulation in heart cells $3\frac{1}{2}$ days in ovo. The development of this parasympathetic response was associated with a threefold increase in levels of α_o and α_i, as measured by ADP ribosylation with pertussis toxin {113}.

Media conditioned by growth of heart cells and ciliary ganglia was also capable of inducing a negative chronotropic response to muscarinic stimulation in heart cells $3\frac{1}{2}$ days in ovo and an increase in levels of α_o and α_i. These data demonstrate that a soluble factor released during coculture of heart cells and ciliary ganglia is capable of inducing muscarinic responsiveness in heart cells $3\frac{1}{2}$ days in ovo {113}. Recent studies using RNAse protection probes derived from clones of G-protein α subunits and muscarinic receptors have shown that following coculture of chick atrial cells $3\frac{1}{2}$ days in ovo with ciliary ganglia, levels of mRNAs encoding α_{i3} and the M_2 receptor increased in the postinnervated heart cells (Kilbourne and Galper, personal communication).

Further support for the concept that shifts in the expression of isoforms of receptors and G proteins might play a role in the development of the autonomic response in the heart has been obtained from studies of developmental changes in the muscarinic response of canine Perkinje fibers {152}. In young dogs, low-dose acetylcholine increased automaticity, while high-dose acetylcholine decreased automaticity. The decrease in automaticity was blocked by AFDX-116 an M_2 blocker, and the increase in automaticity was blocked by pirenzepine and M_1 blocker. In adult dogs only the AFDX-116-sensitive decrease in automaticity was seen, supporting the conclusion that only the M_2 response remained in the adult fibers. Hence developmental regulation of subtype expression of receptors, G proteins, or effectors might play a major role in the development of the cardiac autonomic response.

BETA-ADRENERGIC RECEPTORS

As discussed above, the two limbs of the autonomic nervous system develop noncoordinately. The ability of the heart to respond to catecholamines precedes the development of a negative chronotropic response to muscarinic agonists {9}. Furthermore, in the embryonic chick heart the positive chronotropic response to norepinephrine was demonstrated as early as $2\frac{1}{2}$–3 days in ovo {9}. Furthermore the K_D and B_{max} for isoproterenol stimulation of adenylate cyclase activity were unchanged between days $2\frac{1}{2}$ in ovo and 2 days posthatching {39}. However, several studies have suggested that components of the sympathetic response system do change during embryonic development. Thus in the embryonic chick heart beta-adrenergic receptor number, as demonstrated by the binding of [^{3}H] dihydroalprenalol (DHA) between days 4.5 and 7.5 in ovo, decreased from 6.36 pM/mg protein to 0.22 pM/mg protein by day 9 in ovo, and to 0.16 pM/mg protein by day 16 in ovo. Over the same time course, both isoproterenol and GppNHp stimulated adenylate cyclase activity and the K_D for [^{3}H] DHA binding remained constant {153}.

These data suggested that early in ontogeny of the chick heart, some beta-adrenergic receptors appear not to be coupled to adenylate cyclase, since their disappearance during development was not reflected in a decreased activation of the enzyme. The decrease in the number of DHA binding sites could be due to downregulation of beta-adrenergic receptors caused by increased availability of neurotransmitter at later stages of development. Data have been presented that suggest the content of norepinephrine in the chick heart increased markedly between the 7th and 10th day in ovo {155,156}, in parallel with decreased DHA binding {154}. Several studies, however, have suggested that the source of this early appearance of norepinephrine is extracellular {157, 158}.

Studies in rat hearts 5–28 days postpartum did not demonstrate a change in DHA binding {159}, while in mouse a fourfold increase in DHA binding was described between days 17 and 18 in utero until neonatal day 4 {160}. As described above, the interaction of receptor and G-protein α subunits is required to generate the high-affinity form of the receptor. Hence the relative distribution of receptors between high- and low-affinity states can be taken as a measure of receptor G-protein interaction. Competition binding studies between ^{125}I-pindolol and increasing concentrations of isoproterenol demonstrated high- and low-affinity states of the beta-adrenergic receptor (K_D 10^{-8} and 10^{-5} M, respectively) in homogenates of embryonic chick heart cells 10–12 days in ovo {154}, consistent with the presence of α_s in these cells. No study of developmental changes in the distribution of beta-adrenergic receptors between high- and low-affinity states have appeared.

Few studies of developmental changes in α_s have appeared. In a recent study {113} Barnett et al. demonstrated by Western blot analysis with specific antibody to α_s that at day $3\frac{1}{2}$ in ovo only a 52-kDa and 42-kDa band appeared, while at day 14 in ovo 42-kDa, 45-kDa and 52-

kDa bands could be demonstrated {161}. The significance of the developmental appearance of the 45-kDa band is unclear.

BETA-ADRENERGIC RECEPTOR SUBTYPES

In order to discuss the regulatory mechanisms of receptor and G-protein expression with respect to the development of cardiac autonomic response, it is first necessary to review the data on the cloning and characteristic properties of beta-adrenergic receptor subtypes. Three beta-adrenergic receptor subtypes, termed β_1, β_2, and β_3, have been characterized by pharmacology, tissue distribution, and primary structure. Lands et al. {162} characterized the rank order of potency of agonists as β_1: $(-)$ isoproterenol, $\gg$ epinephrine = norepinephrine; β_2 receptors: isoproterenol $\gg$ epinephrine $>$ norepinephrine. Thus epinephrine bears a much higher affinity for the β_2 receptor than does norepinephrine. Furthermore, norepinephrine appears to have a 10- to 100-fold greater affinity for the β_1 receptor than the β_3 receptor.

CLONING OF THE β_2-ADRENERGIC RECEPTOR

Affinity-purified hamster lung β_2-adrenergic receptor (AR) provided the starting material from which tryptic peptides were obtained and used to generate oligonucleotides for cloning the cDNA encoding the β_2AR {163}. They obtained an intronless gene with an open reading frame coding for a protein of 418 amino acids with a predicted molecular weight of 49 kDa containing the predicted seven hydrophobic segments corresponding to seven membrane-spanning domains.

The human β_2 receptor was cloned from a human epidermal cell line A431 genomic library using the hamster lung β_2AR cDNA as a probe. The genomic DNA contained an open reading frame coding for 413 amino acids {163}.

The cloning of the human β_1AR from a human placenta cDNA library was accomplished using a 5 hydroxytryptamine-1 A gene as a probe that gave a cDNA of 2.4 kb coding for a 477 amino acid protein with 54% identity to the human β_2AR. Expression of this cDNA in *Xenopus* oocytes resulted in a βAR with properties distinct from the β_2AR, with the rank order potency for activation of adenylate cyclase consistent with that for the β_1AR {165}. Northern blot analysis revealed a unique distribution for the β_1 and β_2 mRNAs in cell tissues studied. β_1-receptor mRNA was most highly expressed in the pineal gland and was present in lesser amounts in cerebral cortex, heart, lung, and adipose tissues. The β_2 receptor was found in the lung and prostate, with lower levels in the heart and cerebral cortex.

Based on the hypothesis that a unique form of the βAR might be associated with metabolic processes in the digestive tract and adipose tissues, Muzzin et al. {166} cloned a β_3-adrenergic receptor from a rat brown adipose tissue cDNA library. When expressed in CHO cells, this receptor displayed a low affinity for β-adrenergic antagonists and a high affinity for BRL 37344, an agonist that stimulated lipolysis in adipose tissue {166}. The rank order of potency for agonist-stimulated increases in cAMP levels was similar to that seen for agonist-stimulated lipolysis in brown adipocytes: BRL 32344 > zinterol (β_2-adrenergic agonist) > tazolol (β_1-adrenergic agonist) > $(-)$ isoproterenol $(-)$ epinephrine > norepinephrine. Emorine et al. {167} also cloned a β_3 receptor by screening a human cDNA library with a combination of the coding regions of the turkey β_1 and human β_2AR cDNAs. A 2.1-kb *Bam*HI-*Bgl*II fragment contained a region coding for a 402 amino acid polypeptide with a predicted molecular weight of 43 kDa. The sequence was 50% identical to human β_1AR and 49% identical to human β_2AR. Expression of β_3 in CHO cells demonstrated that most of the β_1 and β_2AR antagonists had no effect in blocking isoproterenol stimulation of cAMP. Pindolol and oxypindolol, antagonists of β_1 and β_2AR, behaved as agonists of cAMP production in CHO cells expressing β_3 receptors. The β_3 receptor was found to be expressed primarily in brown and white adipose tissues.

REGULATION OF BETA-ADRENERGIC RECEPTOR ACTIVITY

Exposure of cells to beta-adrenergic agonists causes rapid activation of the stimulatory G protein, G_s, activation of adenylate cyclase activity, and an increase in cyclic AMP levels. However, continuous exposure of cells to agonists results in a decrease in the enzymatic response within minutes.

Four major processes contribute to this functional desensitization:

1. Downregulation, a slow (minutes to hours) process, reflected in decreased binding of agonist due to internalization of receptors and subsequent loss of receptor binding sites.
2. Sequestration or translocation of β_2AR into a compartment where ligand binding is still detectable.
3. Generation of a state in which the receptor remains on the cell surface but is uncoupled from G_s. This appears to involve phosphorylation of the receptor, either via a cAMP-dependent protein kinase or a specific beta-adrenergic receptor kinase (βARK).
4. Finally, the level of beta-adrenergic receptors is regulated by factors that control rates of transcription and degradation of mRNAs coding for the receptor, as well as rates of translation of the message and posttranslational modifications.

Since all of these processes control the responsiveness of the heart to autonomic stimulation, and since the appearance of these mechanisms of receptor regulation could be developmentally regulated, the appearance of desensitization processes in the developing heart could play a role in the ontogenesis of the cardiac autonomic response.

Downregulation and sequestration of receptors

Both muscarinic and beta-adrenergic receptors, as well as many other receptors, are subject to sequestration and downregulation. Regulation of the muscarinic receptor will be discussed first.

A 3-hour exposure of cultured chick heart cells to carbamylcholine resulted in a 70% decrease in the number of muscarinic receptor sites, as judged by [³H]-QNB binding to heart cell homogenates {168}. The affinity of the remaining receptors for [³H]-QNB was unchanged, indicating that the reduced [³H]-QNB binding reflects a loss of binding sites.

The physiologic response to muscarinic stimulation of the heart requires the interaction of agonist with receptors on the cell surface. An assay for the binding of the muscarinic antagonist [³H] methyloscopolamine ([³H]MS) to intact cultured heart cells {41} was used to correlate cell-surface receptor number with physiologic responsiveness. Unlike QNB, [³H]MS is a highly charged muscarinic antagonist that does not enter the hydrophobic environment of the cell membrane and thus binds only to cell surface receptors. Binding of [³H]MS was saturable, of high affinity, and the relative potency of muscarinic ligands to compete with [³H]MS for binding to intact cells showed the order expected for binding to a muscarinic receptor.

In cells incubated with the muscarinic agonist carbamylcholine, a brief lag phase was followed by a 72% decrease in the number of [³H]MS binding sites over 6 hours with a half-time of 30 minutes {41}. Binding sites recovered over a 12-hour incubation period in the presence of fresh media, and recovery was inhibited by the protein synthesis inhibitor cycloheximide. A close correlation existed between the time course of the agonist-mediated decrease in binding of [³H]MS and the time course of the decrease in the ability of agonist to increase K^+ permeability and to decrease beating rate. All three of these parameters showed a 15-minute lag period followed by decreases that were maximal after 6 hours and were half-maximal at about 30 minutes {41,169}. This close relationship between the number of receptors on the surface of the intact cell and the physiologic responsiveness of the cell suggests that agonist modulation of receptor number constitutes a sensitive mechanism for the control of muscarinic responsiveness of the cultured heart cell.

In several well-studied systems, binding of a ligand to a receptor results in a process know as *receptor-mediated endocytosis* {83,168,170}. Agents, including colchicine and vinblastine, that inhibit microtubule function interfere with the process of endocytosis {171}. Intact cultured heart cells preexposed to muscarinic agonists in the presence of colchicine and vinblastine showed a marked decrease in the loss of receptors compared to cells exposed to agonist alone {168}. These findings are consistent with the hypothesis that agonist exposure causes a change in the configuration of the receptor in the cell membrane, or some other alteration in receptor state, which renders the receptor inaccessible to ligand binding and subject to endocytosis.

Although following prolonged agonist exposure, the receptor may not be capable of stimulating a physiologic response to agonist binding, it is possible that a hydrophobic radioligand might continue to bind specifically to such an altered form of the receptor. To test this hypothesis, studies compared the binding of [³H]MS and the more hydrophobic antagonist [³H]QNB to cells subjected to prior agonist exposure for various times {41}. The results of these experiments show that [³H]QNB continued to bind specifically to muscarinic receptors for 90 minutes after [³H]MS binding had essentially disappeared, long after the loss of a physiologic response. Analysis of these data suggested a sequential conversion of the receptor from a form (A) that gave a physiologic response to agonist and bound both [³H]QNB and [³H]MS to a form, B, that bound only [³H]QNB and did not give a physiologic response to agonist. B was converted to a form, C, presumably a degraded form of the receptor, that was unable to bind either [³H]MS or [³H]QNB. Thus B may constitute an intermediate state of the receptor formed during endocytosis that is more intimately associated with the cell membrane, but is inaccessibly to agonist and has not yet progressed to a degraded state.

Work by Harden et al. {172} demonstrated that following prolonged exposure to an agonist, muscarinic receptors in NG108 cells were translocated from the cell surface into a light vesicular fraction. Receptors from this fraction, although no longer present at the cell surface, continued to bind muscarinic antagonists.

Downregulation of beta-adrenergic receptors

Prolonged exposure of human 1321N1 astrocytoma cells to low concentrations of isoproterenol resulted in uncoupling of the receptor from adenylate cyclase, followed by the slow loss of measurable beta-adrenergic receptor binding sites {173}. Preincubation of turkey erythrocytes with low concentrations of isoproterenol resulted in conversion of the beta-adrenergic receptor from a form that bound [¹²⁵I] azido-benzyl carazolol (a beta-adrenergic antagonist, [¹²⁵I] PABC) to two peptides that migrate on SDS polyacrylamide gels with molecular weights of 38 and 50 kDa to a form that bound [¹²⁵I] PABC to two polypeptides of apparent molecular weight of 42 and 53 kDa {174}. Stadel et al. {175} demonstrated that following agonist exposure nearly 50–60% of sites assayed by binding of the beta-adrenergic agonist [¹²⁵I-] cyanopindolol were lost. Eighty-five percent of these receptors could be recovered in a light vesicle fraction obtained by centrifuging the cytosol at 158,000 ×g for 1 hour {176}. These vesicles contained little adenylate cyclase activity, and receptors in this fraction bound agonist with only low affinity. Furthermore, guanine nucleotides had no effect on agonist binding to these receptors, suggesting that the receptor was sequestered away from both the adenylate cyclase catalytic subunit and G protein. These receptors, when fused with *Xenopus* laevis erythrocytes, rendered adenylate cyclase activity in these cells sensitive to isoproterenol {176,177}. Hence it is likely that the receptors are uncoupled from adenylate cyclase due to physical separation rather than to some alteration of the receptor itself.

Phosphorylation of the receptor as a mechanism of desensitization

Use of a cell-free system has demonstrated that a 30-minute incubation of a turkey erythrocyte lysate with isoproterenol resulted in a 41% desensitization of catecholamine-stimulated adenylate cyclase activity and a 35% decrease in fluoride-stimulated adenylate cyclase activity. Addition of cAMP alone caused a 26% decrease in isoproterenol-stimulated adenylate cyclase activity and a 22% decrease in fluoride-stimulated activity {178}. In the presence of $[\gamma^{32}P]ATP$, desensitization by isoproterenol was found to be associated with phosphorylation of the receptor, as measured by incorporation of $[^{32}P]$, in a dose-dependent manner. The dose/response curve and time dependence paralleled that for the isoproterenol-mediated desensitization of adenylate cyclase. However, incubation with cAMP-activated cyclic AMP dependent protein kinase only partially mimicked the effect of isoproterenol on the phosphorylation of the receptor and desensitization of the adenylate cyclase response {179}. Furthermore, an inhibitor of cAMP-dependent protein kinase decreased the ability of isoproterenol to desensitize the cAMP response by only 50%. Hence some other mechanism must account for the remaining 50% of agonist-stimulated phosphorylation of the receptor and desensitization of the catecholamine-stimulated adenylate cyclase activity {180}.

Studies have demonstrated that desensitization of hormone receptor-coupled adenylate cyclase is divided into two categories. Homologous desensitization is characterized by the fact that only the response to the stimulatory hormone is attenuated. Heterologous desensitization is characterized by a decreased responsiveness to hormones other than the specific agonist, as well as decreased sensitivity of adenylate cyclase to activators such as guanine nucleotides and fluoride ion. Homologous desensitization has been associated with sequestration of the receptors and uncoupling of the receptor-adenylate cyclase interaction in the absence of cAMP generation, but is associated with phosphorylation of the receptor {181}. In contrast, heterologous desensitization is correlated with phosphorylation of the beta-adrenergic receptor, mediated in part by cAMP.

Using purified receptors reconstituted with G_s to study the effect of isoproterenol on phosphorylation of the receptor by protein kinase A revealed that isoproterenol caused an increase in the rate and extent of receptor phosphorylation and an increase in the rate of dephosphorylation of the receptor by phosphatase. Studies of the effect of phosphorylation on receptor function revealed that phosphorylation had no effect on agonist binding, but interfered with the ability of the receptor to interact with G_s and stimulate GTPase activity {182}.

The finding that homologous desensitization and beta-adrenergic receptor phosphorylation could be demonstrated in cAMP-dependent protein kinase deficient (kin⁻) S49 lymphoma cells suggested the presence of an agonist-dependent protein kinase. Such an enzyme was purified from the supernatant of kin⁻ mutant S49 lymphoma cells and was shown to induce a 5- to 10-fold increase in receptor phosphorylation in response to isoproterenol. The enzyme, which is serine specific, prefers the agonist-occupied form of the receptor {183}. The beta-adrenergic receptor kinase (β-ARK) phosphorylates multiple serine and threonine residues on the carboxy-terminal end of the receptor. Protein kinase A phosphorylates independent repeating sites with the sequence Arg-Arg-Ser-Ser on the carboxy-terminal intracytoplasmic tail of the receptor {184}. Low (nanomolar) concentrations of agonist induced phosphorylation at the protein kinase A sites, while higher (μM) doses induced phosphorylation at the β_2 ARK sites {185}. Phosphorylation of the site of cAMP-dependent phosphorylation interferes with receptor G-protein coupling.

Attempts to reproduce the inhibition of receptor function with purified protein components demonstrated that phosphorylation of the receptor with βARK resulted in a modest reduction of receptor function in comparison to a more crude homogenate. A similar modest reduction of function was seen with purified phosphorylated rhodopsin. Addition of a 48-kDa retinal protein, arrestin, potentiated the effects of β_2ARK-mediated phosphorylation of the β_2 receptor. However, high doses of arrestin were needed for this effect {186}. Subsequently a cDNA coding for a β-arrestin was cloned. Expression of this cDNA resulted in an activity that markedly potentiated the effects of phosphorylation of the beta-adrenergic receptor by β_2ARK on the receptor G-protein interaction. It has been subsequently shown that arrestin and β-arrestin display marked specificity for rhodopsin and the beta-adrenergic receptors, respectively. Furthermore, phosphorylation of the receptors by specific receptor kinases enhances the potency of β arrestin inhibition of β_2 receptor function 10-fold {187}.

The rate and extent of the agonist-dependent phosphorylation of beta-adrenergic receptors and rhodopsin by βARK are markedly enhanced by addition of G-protein βγ subunits. Data suggested that the βγ subunit interacts with the carboxy-terminal region of βARK with formation of a βγ-βARK complex. This results in the receptor-facilitated localization of the enzyme to the cell membrane {188}. Thus the cascade of events in the inactivation of the β_2-AR involves agonist binding, release of βγ from the G-protein heterotrimer, association of βγ with βARK, and its translocation to the cell membrane, phosphorylation of serine/threonine residues, followed by the binding of β-arrestin to the receptor, which prevents receptor G-protein coupling and interferes with beta-adrenergic stimulation of adenylate cyclase activity.

Agonist-induced phosphorylation of muscarinic receptors by specific kinases

Although data are far less complete, studies of the desensitization of muscarinic receptors also support the conclusion that agonist-stimulated phosphorylation by a βARK-like kinase plays a role in inactivation of the muscarinic receptor. Kwatra et al. {189,190} demonstrated that prior exposure of chick heart to muscarinic agonists resulted in the phosphorylation of serine and threonine residues in a 79-kDa protein, which was identified as a muscarinic receptor. They further suggested a parallel between this phosphorylation and the loss of the ability of the receptor to mediate a negative inotropic response to muscarinic agonists. These authors suggested that the phosphorylation of the cardiac muscarinic receptor required agonist occupancy and was related to muscarinic receptor desensitization. Muscarinic receptors were shown to be substrates for βARK. Haga and Haga {191} partially purified a protein kinase from cerebrum that phosphorylated atrial and cerebral muscarinic receptors in an agonist-dependent manner.

More recently $\beta\gamma$ subunits of G_s, G_o, and G_i were shown to increase the activity of this receptor kinase {191}, consistent with the findings with β_2ARK {188}.

Studies of human muscarinic M_1 and M_2 receptors expressed in SF9 insect cells demonstrated that only the M_2 receptor could undergo agonist-dependent phosphorylation by an endogenous insect kinase. Pertussis toxin, which inactivated the receptor-associated G proteins, had no effect on the phosphorylation and desensitization of the M_2 receptor by this insect kinase {192}.

Transcriptional control of autonomic receptor activity

The hypothesis that the ontogenesis of autonomic responsiveness in the heart is associated with a pattern of gene regulation that controls the expression of genes coding for the various isoforms of receptors, G-protein subunits, and effectors implies that a program exists in cardiac cells for the expression and organization of these components at the appropriate times during development. In this section we will briefly review data that demonstrate that the expression of receptors and G-protein subunits can be regulated by signals such as agonist binding, second messenger production thyroid hormones and glucocorticoids.

CONTROL OF mRNAS CODING FOR BETA-ADRENERGIC RECEPTORS BY cAMP

Cyclic AMP has been shown to enhance the expression of many genes. In most cases this increase is due to an increased rate of transcription, although effects on mRNA stability have also been reported. The enhancement of transcription by cAMP is mediated by a promoter element in the target gene, called a *cAMP response element* (CRE). Most CREs contain some variation of the motif TGACGTCA, which is the site for interaction with a cAMP response element binding protein (CREB). CREB binding to the CRE is markedly enhanced by cAMP-dependent phosphorylation. The 5′ upstream regulatory region of the β_2AR from hamster and human reveals the presence of putative CREs {193}. Using DDT$_1$-MF-2 cells, Collins et al. {193} demonstrated that a brief 30-minute exposure to epinephrine (100 nM) stimulated the rate of β_2AR gene transcription with a three- to fourfold increase in steady-state levels of mRNA. These effects were mimicked by cAMP analogues. The half-life of mRNA was unchanged over this period. Prolonged exposure to agonist, however, caused a 50% reduction of

β_2AR mRNA and β_2-adrenergic receptors. Transfection of the β_2AR promoter construct ligated to a chloramphenicol acetyl-transferase reporter (CAT) gene demonstrated a two- to fourfold induction of CAT activity by agents such as forskolin and phosphodiesterase inhibitors that increase cAMP levels {193}. Although the significance of the early cAMP-mediated rise in β_2 mRNA is unclear, these data demonstrate that second messengers like cAMP do play a role in regulating receptors that control their synthesis.

ROLE OF GLUCOCORTICOIDS IN REGULATION OF β_2-RECEPTOR mRNA

Hyperthyroidism and states that elevate glucocorticoids have been known to generate a hyperadrenergic state. Glucocorticoids have been shown to increase β_2-adrenergic receptor number twofold in DDT$_1$-MF-2 hamster smooth muscle cells. Steady-state levels of β_2-AR mRNA increased 2.4-fold within 1 hour and returned to control levels by 24 hours. The rate of gene transcription as measured by nuclear runoff assays increased 3.1-fold. Hadcock et al. {194} demonstrated that dexamethasone blunted the decrease in β_2AR mRNA due to prolonged agonist exposure. Nuclear runoff experiments demonstrated that dexamethasone had no effect on β_2AR mRNA stability but increased the rate of transcription fourfold. Conversely, in cells treated with isoproterenol, the transcription rate was unchanged, while the rate of β_2AR mRNA turnover increased from a half-life of 12 hours to a half-life of 5 hours in isoproterenol-treated cells {195,196}.

Differential regulation of mRNAs coding for different β-AR subtypes

Using β_1 and β_2AR ligands, Guest et al. {197} demonstrated that the relative levels of β_1 and β_2AR in differentiating 3T3-L$_1$ cells varied markedly during differentiation to adipocytes. While levels of β_1 and β_2AR were equal in the 3T3 fibroblast, following treatment with dexamethasone and isobutymethyl xanthine (IBMX, a phosphodiesterase inhibitor), total receptor level increased fourfold, while the ratio of β_1/β_2 decreased to 5/95. β_2AR mRNA increased threefold during development of the adipocyte phenotype, while β_1AR mRNA decreased 20-fold. Similarly, levels of expression of β_3AR mRNA could be increased 2.4-fold by surgical sympathectomy of interscapular brown adipose tissue, while β_1AR mRNA levels remained unchanged. Furthermore, increased sympathetic nerve stimulation increased β_3AR mRNA, while having no effect on β_1 mRNA {198}.

EFFECT OF AGONIST EXPOSURE ON LEVELS OF MRNA CODING FOR MUSCARINIC RECEPTORS

Habecker and Nathanson {199} demonstrated that prolonged agonist exposure resulted in a decrease in mRNAs coding for M_2 and M_4 muscarinic receptors in chick heart. They further suggested that protein kinase C and cAMP levels might play a role in the regulation of levels of M_2 mRNA {200}.

CROSSREGULATION OF AUTONOMIC
RECEPTORS AND G PROTEINS

A series of studies have suggested that autonomic receptors and their associated G proteins can be coordinately regulated and that stimulatory and inhibitory G proteins and receptors can be reciprocally regulated. It has been demonstrated that growth of chick atrial cells from hearts 14 days in ovo in medium supplemented by serum from which lipoproteins had been removed resulted in an increase in parasympathetic responsiveness {202} and a decrease in the positive inotropic response to beta-adrenergic stimulation {161}. These changes were associated with a twofold increase in levels of both muscarinic receptors and $G\alpha_o$ and $G\alpha_i$ {202}, a twofold decrease in beta-adrenergic receptor number, and a 67% decrease in $G\alpha_s$ {161}.

Parsons and Stiles demonstrated that chronic administration of adenosine agonists to rats resulted in a decrease in the level of adenosine receptors and α_i, and an increase in the levels of α_s {203}. Hence inhibition of adenylate cyclase was decreased and stimulation of adenylate cyclase was increased {202}.

Hadcock et al. {196} demonstrated that stimulation of S49 lymphoma cells with forskolin or isoproterenol enhanced somatostation inhibition of adenylate cyclase activity, increased levels of α_{i2} threefold, and decreased levels of α_s by 25%. Levels of mRNA coding for α_{i2} increased fourfold and mRNA coding for $G_{\alpha s}$ initially increased 25% but then decreased to 75% of control {203}. Thus components of the autonomic response system may be highly regulated. This is consistent with the existence of a program for the regulation of gene expression that could not only determine the balance between sympathetic and parasympathetic responsiveness in the heart following agonist exposure, but may regulate the relative appearance of specific receptor, G protein, and effector isoforms during ontogenesis of the parasympathetic response in the embryonic heart.

CLINICAL IMPLICATIONS OF ALTERATIONS IN MUSCARINIC RECEPTOR–G-PROTEIN EFFECTOR COUPLING, FACTORS THAT ALTER AUTONOMIC BALANCE

The balance between sympathetic and parasympathetic responsiveness in the heart plays an important role in establishing the inotropic and chronotropic state of the heart, and in the genesis of arrhythmias. Thus the association of certain pathologic states of the heart with changes in expression of genes coding for components of the autonomic response system could play an important role in the pathogenesis of cardiac disease.

Role of changes in guanine nucleotide binding proteins and receptors in congestive heart failure, and cardiomyopathy

Cardiomyopathic myocardium has been shown to respond abnormally to neurohumoral stimulation {204}. Colucci and others {205,206} have shown that the chronotropic response to graded isoproterenol infusion was depressed in patients with congestive heart failure. Studies in patients with idiopathic dilated cardiomyopathic hearts have demonstrated decreased numbers of surface beta-adrenergic receptors and a depressed adenylate cyclase response to isoproterenol and the nonhydrolyzable analogue of GTP, 5 guanylylimidodiphosphate (GppNHP) {207}.

However, in the same group of patients the response to forskolin, a direct activator of the catalytic subunit of adenylate cyclase, was preserved, suggesting a postreceptor modification of the adenylate cyclase receptor response.

These data are interpreted as suggesting an abnormal response of adenylate cyclase to guanine nucleotide stimulation in the cardiomyopathic human myocardium and further support the hypothesis that this decreased responsiveness may be due to an abnormality in one or more G proteins. Studies using cholera toxin in genetically cardiomyopathic Syrian hamsters have demonstrated a 50% decrease in Gs activity without a change in immunologically determined G-protein levels {208}. In tissues from idiopathic cardiomyopathic human hearts, pertussis toxin labeling has also demonstrated a 36% increase in levels of G_i associated with enhanced inhibition of adenylate cyclase activity by GppNHp {209}. These studies suggest that abnormalities in autonomic responsiveness in the failing heart are associated with abnormalities in receptor-effector coupling mediated by G proteins and altered G-protein and receptor levels.

Effect of cardiac denervation on autonomic responsiveness of the heart

Several groups have studied the effects of dernervation on the autonomic responsiveness of the heart. Using a model of total surgical cardiac denervation in dogs, Vatner et al. {210} have found that denervation leads to upregulation of beta-adrenergic receptor density, and hence isoproterenol-mediated adenylate cyclase activity, while there is downregulation of muscarinic receptor density. Osario et al. {211} have shown that sympathetic denervation of the heart leads to norepinephrine depletion and the development of adrenergic supersensitivity. Ono and Lindsey {212} have developed a rat model of heterotopic cardiac transplantation in the Lewis rat. Using the established method of Ono, Lurie et al. {213,214} have demonstrated that in membrane preparations from isographs of rabbit and rat cardiac transplanted myocardium, transplantation is associated with a twofold increase in beta-adrenergic receptor density and isoproterenol-stimulated adenylate cyclase activity for up to 4 weeks following transplantation.

Following orthotopic human cardiac transplantation, the physiologic responses to exercise and stress are impaired. Most striking of these changes is the delay in achieving peak heart rate and the maximum heart rate achieved in response to maximal exercise effort that is seen even years following transplantation {215}. In analyzing clinical responses to graded infusions of isoproterenol and exercise response and duration, these abnormalities appear to be due to the lack of sympathetic innervation {216}. Despite this finding in the denervated human transplanted myocardium, beta-adrenergic receptor density and the forskolin-stimulated adenylate cyclase response appears to be unchanged from normal human myocardium {217,204}. However, the response of adenylate cyclase to GppNHp was depressed in the transplanted myocardium. There is no evidence for beta-adrenergic receptor upregulation or supersensitivity in the denervated transplanted human myocardium. These findings suggest that the major abnormality responsible for decreased beta-adrenergic responsiveness may be related to alterations in levels of G proteins. Recently Loh et al. (submitted) demonstrated a decrease in the adenylate cyclase response of GppNHp and forskolin in transplanted human myocardium. This effect was associated with a decrease in levels of α_s and mRNAs coding for α_s.

Thus in several model systems in which changes in autonomic balance can be demonstrated, changes in the levels of receptors and G proteins may play a role.

SUMMARY

Muscarinic cholinergic stimulation of the heart has been associated with increasing potassium permeability and the development of a negative chronotropic response. Experiments have demonstrated the role of G proteins in coupling muscarinic receptors to potassium channels and to the enhancement of potassium permeability. During embryonic development of the chick heart, the absence of coupling of the muscarinic receptor to a G protein is associated with decreased ability of muscarinic agonist to both mediate a negative chronotropic response and inhibit adenylate cyclase activity. The development of muscarinic responsiveness in the embryonic chick heart is associated with the appearance of increased levels of G proteins, suggesting that developmental changes in the expression of G protein may be related to the appearance of parasympathetic responsiveness in the heart.

The association of the receptor and the G protein appears to be critical for the development of the high-affinity state of the muscarinic receptor and coupling the muscarinic receptor to physiologic responses. A ternary complex between muscarinic receptor, G proteins, and the agonist has been demonstrated. Treatment of cells with pertussis toxin results in uncoupling of the muscarinic receptor from inhibition of adenylate cyclase activity, enhancement of K^+ channel permeability, as well as activation of phosphatidyl inositol hydrolysis and diacylglycerol formation. A pertussis-toxin-insensitive G protein has also been shown to couple muscarinic receptors to phospholipase C activity.

A family of GTP binding proteins has been associated with the coupling of muscarinic receptors to various physiologic responses. The specificity of these G proteins for a given physiologic response has not been established. Furthermore, it has been determined that the β and γ subunits of G proteins also exist in multiple isoforms. The specificity of these isoforms for a given physiological response is not well established. Further data using anti-sense oligonucleotides have suggested that such specificity does exist. Recently studies have demonstrated that the relative levels of G protein subunits and receptors may be regulated at the level of both transcription and translation. Treatment of cells with agonist has been shown not only to regulate levels of receptors and their associated G proteins that inhibit adenylate cyclase activity, but also induce reciprocal increases in the receptors and their associated G proteins that stimulate adenylate cyclase activity. Furthermore, it has been shown that treatment of cells with glucocortoids and thyroid hormones also regulate relative levels of G proteins and their associated receptors.

The finding that these G proteins and isoforms of autonomic receptors may be regulated suggests that a program exists for the regulation of gene expression. These changes in expression may be due to stimuli such as innervation of the heart or the interaction with growth factors, and may play a role in the ontogenesis of the parasympathetic response in the embryonic heart and the pathogenesis of congestive heart failure. The elucidation of the molecular mechanisms that control levels of expression of components of the autonomic nervous system will aid in our understanding of cardiac development and in the treatment of myopathy.

REFERENCES

1. Levy MN: Sympathetic-parasympathetic interactions in the heart. *Circ Res* 29:437–445, 1971.
2. Hutter OF: In: Florey F (ed) *Nervous Inhibition*. Elmsford, NY: Pergamon Press, 1961, pp 114–123.
3. Ten Eick R, Nawrath H, McDonald TF, Trautwein W: On the mechanism of the negative inotropic effect of acetylcholine. *Pflügers Arch* 361:207–213, 1976.
4. George WJ, Polson JB, O'Toole AG, Goldberg ND: Elevation of guanosine $3'-5'$cyclic phosphate in rat heart after perfusion with acetyl-choline. *Proc Natl Acad Sci USA* 66:398–403, 1970.
5. Michell RH, Jafferji SS, Jones LM: In: Bazaan H, Brenner R, Giusto H (eds) *Advances in Experimental Medicine and Biology*. New York: Plenum Press 83:447–464, 1976.
6. Lindemann JP, Jones LR, Watanabe AM: Effect of muscarinic cholinergic agonist on beta receptor induced increases in membrane protein phosphorylation in intact ventricles. *Circ Res* 28:●●–●● 1980.
7. Watanabe AM, Besch Jr HR: Cyclic adenosine monophosphate modulation of slow calcium influx channels in guinea pig hearts. *Circ Res* 35:316–324, 1974.
8. Tsien RW: Cyclic AMP and contractile activity in the heart. In: Greengard P, Robison GA (eds) *Advances in Cyclic Nucleotide Research*. New York: Academic Press, 1977, pp 363–420.
9. Culver NG, Fishman DA: Pharmacological analysis of sympthetic function in the embryonic chick heart. *Am J Physiol* 232:R116–R123, 1977.
10. Carpenter MB: In: *Human Neuroanatomy*. Baltimore, MD: Williams and Wilkins, 1976.

11. Hirsch EF: The innervation of the vertebrate heart. Springfield, IL: Charles C. Thomas, 1970, pp 3–24.
12. Loewi O: Uber humorale Uebertragbarkeit der herznervenwirkung. *Pflügers Arch* 189:239–242, 1921.
13. Feldberg W, Krayer O: Das auftreten eines azetylcholin artigen stoffes in herzvenenblut von warmblutern bei biezung der nervi vagi. *Naunryn Scheidebergs Pharmackol* 172:170–193, 1933.
14. Dale HH: The action of certain esters and ethers of choline, and their relation to muscarine. *Pharmacol Exp Ter* 6:147–190, 1914.
15. Pappano AJ: Onset of chronotropic effects of nicotinic drugs and tyramine on the sino-atrial pacemaker in chick embryo heart: Relationship to the development of autonomic neuroeffector transmission. *J Pharmacol Exp Ther* 196:676–684, 1976.
16. Langley JN: Observations on the physiological action of extracts of the supra-renal bodies. *J Physiol (Lond)* 27:237–256, 1901.
17. Lewandowsky M: Ueber eine Wirkung des Nebennierenextractes auf des Auge. *Zentralbl Physiol* 12:599–600, 1989.
18. Cannon WB, Uvidil JE: Studies on the conditions of activity in endocrine glands VIII. Some effects on the denervated heart of stimulating the nerves of the liver. *Am J Physiol* 58:353–354, 1921.
19. Barger G, Dale HH: Chemical structure and sympathomimatic action of amines. *J Physiol (Lond)* 41:19–59, 1910.
20. von Euler US: Adrenaline and nonadrenaline distribution and action. *Pharmacol Rev* 6:15–22, 1954.
21. Alquist RP: A study of the adrenotropic receptors. *Am J Physiol* 1153:586–600, 1948.
22. Hutter DF, Trautwein W: Vagal and sympathetic effects on the pacemaker fibers in the sinus venosus of the heart. *J Gen Physiol* 89:715–733, 1956.
23. Harris EJ, Hutter OF: The action of acetylcholine on the movement of potassium ions in the sinus venosus of the heart. *J Physiol* 133:58–59, 1956.
24. Glitsch HG, Pott L: Effects of acetylcholine and parasympathetic nerve stimulation on membrane potential in quiescent guinea pig atria. *J Phyiol* 279:655–668, 1978.
25. Grossman A, Furchgott RF: The effects of various drugs on calcium exchange in the isolated guinea-pig left auricle. *J Pharmacol Exp Ther* 145:162–172, 1964.
26. Hoditz H, Lullmann H: Der enfluss von actylcholin auf den calcium satz ruhsender und Kontrahierender vonhofnuskulatur in vitro. *Experimentia* 20:279–280, 1964.
27. Prokopcznk A, Pytkowski B, Lawartowshi B: Effect of acetylcholine on calcium efflux from atrial myocardium. *Eur J Pharmacol* 70:1–6, 1961.
28. Jakobs KA: Inhibition of adenylate cyclase by hormones and neurotransmitters. *Mol Cell Endocrinol* 16:147–156, 1979.
29. Jakobs KA, Aktories K, Schultz G: GTP-dependent inhibition of cardiac adenylate cyclase by muscarinic cholinergic agonists. *Naunyn-Schmideborgs Arch Pharmacol* 310:113–119, 1979.
30. Abel W: Further observations on the development of the sympathetic nervous system in the chick. *J Anat Physiol* 47:35–72, 1912.
31. Gardner E, O'Rahilly R: The nerve supply and conducting system of the human heart at the end of the embryonic period proper. *J Anat* 121:571–187, 1976.
32. Pappano AJ, Loffelholz K: Ontogenesis of adrenergic and cholinergic neuroeffector transmission in chick embryo heart. *J Pharmacol Exp Ther* 191:468–478, 1974.
33. Galper JB, Klein W, Catterall WA: Muscarinic acetylcho-line receptors in developing chick heart. *J Biol Chem* 252:8692–8699, 1977.
34. Coraboeuf E, Le Douarin G, Obrecht-Coutris G: Release of acetylcholine by chick embryo heart before innervation. *J Physiol* 206:383–385, 1970.
35. Pappano AJ: Ontogenetic development of autonomic neuroeffector transmission and transmitter reactivity in embryonic and fetal hearts. *Pharmacol Rev* 29:3–33, 1977.
36. Pappano AJ, Skowronek CA: Reactivity of chick embryo hearts to cholinergic agonists during ontogenesis: Decline in desensitization at the onset of cholinergic transmission. *J Pharmacol Exp Ther* 191:109–118, 1974.
37. DuFour JJ, Pasternak JM: Effects chromotropex de l'acetylcholine sur le couer de l'embryon du poulet. *Helv Physiol Pharmacol Acta* 18:563–580, 1960.
38. Pappano AJ, Skowronek C: Nicotinic receptor development in autonomic neurons of the chick embryo heart. *Pharmacologist* 16:268–272, 1974.
39. Liang BT, Hellmick MR, Neer EJ, Galper JB: Development of muscarinic cholinergic inhibition of adenylate cyclase in embryonic chick heart. *J Biol Chem* 261:9011–9021, 1986.
40. Hosey MM, Fields JZ: Quantitative and qualitative differences in muscarinic cholinergic receptors in embryonic and newborn chick hearts. *J Biol Chem* 256:6395–6399, 1981.
41. Galper JB, Dziekan LC, O'Hara DS, Smith TW: The biphasic response of muscarinic cholinergic receptors in cultured heart cells to agonists. *J Biol Chem* 257:10344–10356, 1982.
42. Hosey MM, McMahon KK, Denckers AM, O'Callahan CM, Wong J, Green RD: Differences in the properties of muscarinic cholinergic receptors in the developing chick myocardium. *J Pharmacol Exp Ther* 232:795–801, 1985.
43. Sorota S, Adam LP, Pappano AJ: Comparison of muscarinic receptor properties in hatched chick heart atrium and ventricle. *J Pharmacol Exp Ther* 236:606–609, 1986.
44. Rosenberger LB, Yamamura H, Roeske WR: Cardiac muscarinic cholinergic receptor binding is regulated by Na^+ and guanine nucleotides. *J Biol Chem* 255:820–823, 1980.
45. Galper JB, Haigh LS, Hart AC, O'Hara DS, Livingston DJ: Muscarinic cholinergic receptors in the embryonic chick heart: Interaction of agonist, receptor, and guanine nucleotides studied by an improved assay for direct binding of the muscarinic agonist [^{3}H] cismethyldioxolane. *Mol Pharmacol* 32:320–240, 1987.
46. Ehlert FJ, Yamamura HI, Triggle D, Roeske WR: The influence of guanyl-5'-yl'imidodiphosphate and sodium chloride on the binding of the muscarinic agonist, [^{3}H] cismethyldioxalane. *Eur J Pharmacol* 61:317–318, 1980.
47. Birdsall NJM, Berrie CP, Burgeron ASU, Hulme EC: Modulation of binding properties of muscarinic receptors: Evidence for receptor effector coupling. In: Pepeu G, Kuhar MJ, Enna S (eds) *Receptors for Neurotransmitters and Peptide Hormones*. New York: Raven Press, 1980, pp 107–116.
48. DeLean A, Stadel JM, Lefkowitz RJ: A ternary complex model explains the agonist-specific binding properties of the adenylate cyclase-coupled β-adrenergic receptor. *J Biol Chem* 255:7108–7117, 1980.
49. Florio VA, Sternweiss PC: Reconstitution of resolved muscarinic cholinergic receptors with purified GTP-binding proteins. *J Biol Chem* 260:3477–3488, 1985.
50. Galper JB, Dziekan LC, Smith TW: The development of physiologic responsiveness to muscarinic agonists in chick embryo heart cell cultures: Role of high affinity receptors

and sensitivity to guanine nucleotides. *J Biol Chem* 259: 7382–7390, 1984.

51. Liang BT, Galper JB: Reconstitution of muscarinic cholinergic inhibition of adenylate cyclase activity in homogenates of embryonic chick hearts by membranes of adult chick hearts. *J Biol Chem* 262:2494–2501, 1987.

52. Barlow RB, Berry KJ, Glenton PAM, Nickolaou NM, Soh KS: A comparison of affinity constants for muscarinic-sensitive acetylcholine receptors in guinea pig atrial pacemaker cells at 29° and in ileum at 29° and 37°C. *Br J Pharm* 58:613–620, 1976.

53. Rattan S, Goyal RK: Evidence of 5-HT participation in vagal inhibitory pathway to opossum LES. *Am J Physiol* 234:E273–E276, 1978.

54. Roszkowski AP: Muscarinic receptor subtypes: An unusual type of sympathetic ganglionic stimulant. *J Pharmacol Exp Ther* 132:156–170, 1961.

55. Hammer R, Giachetti A: M_1 and M_2 biochemical and functional characterization. *Life Sci* 31:2991–2998, 1982.

56. Birdsall NJ, Burgen ASV, Holme EC, Stockton JM, Zigmond MH: The effect of McN-A343 on muscarinic receptors in the cerebral cortex and heart. *Br J Pharmacol* 78:257–259, 1983.

57. Goyal RK, Patton S: Neurohumoral, hormonal, and drug receptors from the lower esophageal sphincter. *Gastroenterology* 74:593–619, 1973.

58. Hammer R, Berrie CP, Birdsall NMJ, Burgen ASV, Hulme EC: Pirenzepine distinguishes between different subclasses of muscarinic receptors. *Nature* 283:90–92, 1980.

59. Strockbrugger RW, Jaup BH, Dotevall G: The effect of different doses of pirenzepine on gastric secretion stimulated by modified sham feeding in man. *Scand J Gastroenterol* 17(Suppl 72):111–116, 1982.

60. Strockbrugger RW, Jaup BP, Abrahamsson H, Dotevall G: Clinical pharmacology of muscarinic antagonists. *Trends Pharmacol Sci* 5(Suppl):74–77, 1984.

61. Patton WOM, Rang HP: The uptake of atropine and related drugs by intestinal smooth muscle of the quinea-pig in relation to acetylcholine receptors. *Proc R Soc Lond B* 163:1–44, 1965.

62. Watson M, Yamamura HI, Roeske WR: A unique regulatory profile and regional distribution of [^{3}H]-pirenzepine binding in the rat provide evidence for distinct M_1 and M_2 muscarinic receptor subtypes. *Life Sci* 32:3001–3010, 1983.

63. Luthin GR, Wolfe BB: Comparison of [^{3}H]-pirenzepine and [^{3}H]-quinuclidinylbenzilate binding to muscarinic cholinergic receptors in rat brain. *J Pharmacol Exp Ther* 228:648–655, 1984.

64. Luthin GR, Wolfe BB: [^{3}H]-pirenzepine and [^{3}H]-quinuclidinylbenzilate binding to rat brain muscarinic cholinergic receptors: Differences in measured receptor density not explained by differences in receptor isomerization. *J Mol Pharmacol* 26:164–169, 1984.

65. Lambrecht G, Linch H, Moser U, Mutschler E, Strecker M, Tacke R, Weiss J: In: Dahlbom R, Nilssan JLG (eds) *Proceedings of the VIIIth International Symposium on Medicinal Chemistry*, Vol 2. Stockholm: Swedish Pharmaceutical Press, 1985, pp 424–456.

66. Lambrecht G, Moser U, Muschler E, Wess J, Linch H, Strecker M, Tacke R: Hexahydro-sila difenidol: A selective antagonist of ileal muscarinic receptors; Naunyn Schmidebergs *Arch Pharmacol* 325(Suppl):1262, 1984.

67. Lambrecht G, Moser U, Wagner M, Wess J, Gonelin G, Rafeiner K, Strohmann C, Tacke R, Mutschler E: Pharmacological and electrophysiological evidence for muscarinic M_1 and M_2 receptor heterogeneity. In: *Third International Symposium on Subtypes of Muscarinic Receptors*. Sydney, Australia, 1987.

68. Lambrecht G, Mutschler E, Moser U, Riotte R, Wagner M, Wess J, Gmelin G, Tacke R, Zilch H: Heterogeneity in muscarinic receptors: Evidence from pharmacological and physiological studies with selective antagonists. In: Cohen S, Sokolovsky M (eds) *Muscarinic Cholinergic Mechanisms*. Tel Aviv: Freund Publishing House, 1987.

69. Gil DW, Wolfe BB: Pirenzepine distinguishes between muscarinic receptor-mediated phosphoinositide breakdown and inhibition of adenylate cyclase. *J Pharmacol Exp Ther* 232:608–616, 1985.

70. Peterson G, Herron G, Yamaki M, Fullerton D, Schimmerlik M: Purification of the muscarinic acetylcholine receptor from porcine atria. *Proc Natl Acad Sci USA* 81:4993–4998, 1984.

71. Peralta EG, Winslow JW, Peterson GL, Smith DH, Ashkenazi A, Ramachandran J, Schimerlik M, Capon DJ: Primary structure and biomechanical properties of an M_2 muscarinic receptor. *Science* 236:600–605, 1987.

72. Kubo T, Fukada K, Mikami A, Maeda A, Takahashi H, Mishina M, Haga T, Haga K, Ichiyama A, Kangawa K, Kojima M, Matsuo H, Hirose T, Numa S: Cloning, sequencing, and expression of complementary DNA encoding the muscarinic acetylcholine receptor. *Nature* 232:411–416, 1986.

73. Bonner TI, Buckley NJ, Young AC, Brann MR: Identification of a family of muscarinic acetylcholine receptor genes. *Science* 237:527–532, 1987.

74. Kubo I, Maeda A, Sugimoto K, Akiba I, Mikami A, Takahashi H, Haga T, Haga K, Ichiyama A, Kangawa K, Matsuo H, Hirose T, Numa S: Primary structure of porcine cardiac muscarinic acetylcholine receptor deduced from the cDNA sequence. *FEBS Lett* 209:367–377, 1986.

75. Bonner TI, Young AC, Brann MR, Buckley NJ: Cloning and expression of human and rat M_5 muscarinic acetylcholine receptor genes. *Neuron* 1:403–410, 1988.

76. Tietje KM, Goldman PS, Nathanson NM: Cloning and functional analysis of a gene encoding a novel muscarinic acetylcholine receptor expressed in chick heart and brain. *J Biol Chem* 265:2828–2834, 1990.

77. Tietje KM, Nathanson NM: Embryonic chick heart expresses multiple muscarinic acetylcholine receptor subtypes. *J Biol Chem* 266:17382–17387, 1991.

77a. Gadbut AP, Galper JB: A novel M_3 muscarinic Acetylcholine Receptor is Expressed in chick atrium and ventricle. *J Biol Chem*, in press.

78. Ashkenazi A, Winslow JW, Peralta EG, Peterson GL, Schimerlik MI, Capon DJ, Ramachandran J: An M_2 muscarinic receptor subtype coupled to both adenylyl cyclase and phosphoinositide turnover. *Science* 238:672–675, 1987.

79. Peralta EG, Ashkenzi A, Winslow JW, Ramachandran J, Capon DJ: Differential regulation of PI hydrolysis and adenylatecyclase by muscarinic receptor subtypes. *Nature* 334:434–437, 1988.

80. Barnett JV, Shamah SM, Griendling KK, Lasseugue B, Galper JB: Muscarinic cholinergic stimulation of inositol phosphate production in cultured embryonic chick atrial cells: Evidence for coupling via two independent G-proteins. Submitted.

81. Katada T, Ui M: Perfusion of the pancreas isolated from pertussis-sensitized rats: Potentiation of insulin secretory responses due to β-adrenergic stimulation. *Endocrinology* 101:1247–1252, 1977.

82. Hazeki O, Ui M: Modification by islet-activating protein of

receptor mediated regulation of cyclic AMP accumulation in isolated rat heart cells. *J Biol Chem* 256:28566–28572, 1981.

83. Lefkowitz R, Stadel J, Caron M: Adenylate cyclase-coupled beta-adrenergic receptors: Structure and mechanisms of activation and desensitization. *Annu Rev Biochem* 52: 159–186, 1983.

84. Katada T, Ui M: ADP-ribosylation of the specific membrane protein of C_6 cells by islet-activating protein associated with modification of adenylate cyclase activity. *J Biol Chem* 257:7210–7216, 1982.

85. Katada T, Bokoch GM, Northup J, Ui M, Gilman AG: The inhibitory guanine nucleotide-binding regulatory component of adenylate cyclase: Properties and function of the purified protein. *J Biol Chem* 259:3568–3577, 1984.

86. Katada T, Northup J, Bokoch GM, Ui M, Gilman AG: The inhibitory guanine nucleotide-binding regulatory component of adenylate cyclase: Subunit disassociation and guanine nucleotide-dependent hormonal inhibition. *J Biol Chem* 259:3578–3585, 1984.

87. Katada T, Bokoch GM, Smigel MD, Ui M, Gilman AG: The inhibitory guanine nucleotide-binding regulatory component of adenylate cyclase: Subunit disassociation and the inhibition of adenylate cyclase in S49 lymphoma cyc^- and wild type cell membranes. *J Biol Chem* 259:3586–3595, 1984.

88. Bokoch GM, Katada T, Northup JK, Ui M, Gilman AG: Purification and properties of the inhibitory guanine nucleotide-binding regulatory component of adenylate cyclase. *J Biol Chem* 259:3560–3567, 1984.

89. Hildebrandt JD, Codina J, Risenger R, Birnbaumer L: Identification of a gamma subunit associated with the adenylate cyclase regulatory proteins N_s and N_i. *J Biol Chem* 259:2039–2042, 1984.

90. Northup JK, Smigel MD, Sternweis PC, Gilman AG: The subunits of the stimulatory regulatory component of adenylate cyclase: Resolution of the activated 45,000 dalton (α) subunit. *J Biol Chem* 258:11369–11376, 1976.

91. Jones DT, Reed RR: Molecular cloning of five GTP-binding proteins cDNA from rat olfactory neuroepithelium. *J Biol Chem* 262:1424–1429, 1987.

92. Strathman M, Wilke JM, Simon MI: Diversity of the G-protein family: sequences from five additional α subunits in the mouse. *Proc Natl Acad Sci USA* 86:7407–7409, 1989.

93. Hsu WH, Rudolph U, Sanford J, Bertrand P, Olate J, Nelson C, Moss LG, Boyd AE III, Codina J, Birnbaumer L: Molecular cloning of a novel splice variant of the α subunit of the mammalian G_o protein. *J Biol Chem* 265:11220–11226, 1990.

94. Bertrand P, Sanford J, Rudolph U, Codina J, Birnaumer L: At least alternatively-spliced mRNAs encoding two α subunits of the G_o GTP-binding protein can be expressed in a single tissue. *J Biol Chem* 265:18576–18578, 1990.

95. M de Sousa S, Hoveland LL, Yarfitz S, Hurley JB: The Drosophila $G_o\alpha$-like protein gene produces multiple transcripts and is expressed in the nervous system and the ovaries. *J Biol Chem* 264:18544–18551, 1989.

96. Yoon J, Shortridge RD, Blooomquist BT, Schneuwly S, Perdew MH, Pak WL: Molecular characterization of Drosophila gene encoding G_{ao} subunit homolog. *J Biol Chem* 264:18536–18543, 1989.

96a. Kibourne EJ, Galper JB: Isolation and expression of a novel chick G-protein CDNNA coding for a $G\alpha_{i3}$ protein with a $G\alpha_0$ N-terminus. *Biochem J* 297:303–308, 1994.

97. Amatruda TT III, Narasimham G, Fong HKW, Northrup JK, Simon MI: The 35- and 36-kDa β subunits of GTP-binding regulatory proteins are products of separate genes. *J Biol Chem* 263:5008–5011, 1988.

98. Gao B, Gilman AG, Robishaw JD: A second form of the β subunit of signal-transducing G proteins. *Proc Natl Acad Sci USA* 84:6122–6125, 1987.

99. Levine MA, Smallwood PM, Moen PT, Helman LJ, Ahn TG: Molecular cloning of β3 subunit, a third form of the G protein β-subunit polypeptide. *Proc Natl Acad Sci USA* 87:2329–2333, 1990.

100. von Weizsacker E, Strathmann MP, Simon MI: Diversity among the beta subunits of heterotrimeric GTP-binding proteins: Characterization of a novel beta-subunit cDNA. *Biochem Biophys Res Commun* 183:350–356, 19●●.

101. Gautam N, Northrup J, Tamir H, Simon MI: G protein diversity is increased by associations with a variety of γ subunits. *Proc Natl Acad Sci USA* 87:7973–7977, 1990.

102. Tamir H, Fawzi AB, Tamin A, Evans T, Northup JK: G-protein βγ forms: Identity of β and diversity of γ subunits. *Biochemistry* 30:3929–3936, 1991.

103. Fisher KJ, Aronson NN Jr: Characterization of the cDNA and genomic sequence of a G protein γ subunit (γ_5). *Mol Cell Biol* 12:1585–1591, 1992.

104. Maltese WA, Robinshaw JD: Isoprotenylation of C-terminal cysteine in a G-protein γ subunit. *J Biol Chem* 265:18071–18074, 1990.

105. Mumby SM, Casey PJ, Gilman AG, Gutowski S, Sternweis PC: G-protein γ subunits contain a 20-carbon isoprenoid. *Proc Natl Acad Sci USA* 87:5873–5877, 1990.

106. Fukada Y, Tako T, Ohguro H, Yoshizawa T, Akmo T, Shimonishi Y: Farnesylated γ-subunit of photo receptor G-protein indispensible for GTP binding. *Nature* 346:11658, 1990.

107. Muntz KH, Sternweis PC, Gilman AG, Mumby SM: Influence of γ subunit prenylation on association of guanine nucleotide-binding regulatory proteins with membranes. *Mol Biol Cell* 3:49–61, 1992.

108. Casey PJ, Solski PA, Der CJ, Buss JE: p21ras is modified by a farnesyl isoprenoid. *Proc Natl Acad Sci USA* 86: 8323–8327, 1989.

109. Tang W-J, Gilman AG: Type-specific regulation of adenylyl cyclase by G protein βγ subunits. *Science* 254:1500–1503, 1991.

110. Waldo GL, Boyer JL, Morris AJ, Harden TK: Purification of an ALF-4 and G-protein βγ-subunit regulated phospholipase C-activating protein. *J Biol Chem* 266:14217–14225, 1991.

111. Pfaffinger PJ, Martin JM, Hunter DH, Nathanson NM, Hille B: GTP-binding proteins couple cardiac muscarinic receptors to a K channel. *Nature* 317:536–538, 1985.

112. Steinberg S, Drugge ED, Bilezkian JP, Robinson RB: Acquisition by innervated cardiac myocytes of a pertussis toxin-specific regulatory protein linked to the α_i-receptor. *Science* 230:186–188, 1985.

113. Barnett JV, Tanicchi M, Yang MB, Galper JB: Co-culture of embryonic chick heart cells and ciliary ganglia induces parasympathetic responsiveness in embryonic chick heart cells. *Biochem J* 292:395–399, 1993.

114. Bakalyar HA, Reed RR: Identification of a specialized adenylyl cyclase that may mediate odorant detection. *Science* 250:1403–1406, 1990.

115. Gao B, Gilman AG: Cloning and expression of a widely distributed (type IV) adenylyl cyclase. *Proc Natl Acad Sci USA* 88:10178–10182, 1991.

116. Ishikawa Y, Katsushika S, Chen L, Halnon NJ, Kawabe J-I, Homey CJ: Isolation and characterization of a novel cardiac adenylyl cyclase cDNA. *J Biol Chem* 287:13553–13557, 1992.

117. Tang WJ, Krupinski J, Gilman AG: Expression and charac-

terization of calmodulin-activated (type I) adenylyl cyclase. *J Biol Chem* 266:8595–8603, 1991.

118. Pitt GS, Milona N, Borleis J, Lin KC, Reed RR, Devreotes PN: Structurally distinct and stage-specific adenylyl cyclase genes play different roles in dictyostelium development. *Cell* 69:305–315, 1992.

119. Hokin MR, Hokin LE: Enzyme secretion and incorptatin of ³²P into phospholipids of pancreas slices. *J Biol Chem* 209:549–558, 1954.

120. Shears SB: Metabolism of the inositol phosphates produced upon receptor activation. *Biochem J* 260:313–329, 1989.

121. Berridge MJ: Metabolism of the inositol phosphates produced upon receptor activation. *Ann Rev Biochem* 56:159–193, 1987.

122. Downes CP, Michell RH: In: Cohen P, Houslay MD (eds) *Molecular Mechanisms of Transmembrane Signaling.* Amsterdam: Elsevier, 1985, pp 3–56.

123. Irvine RF, Moor RM: Micro-injection of inositol 1,3,4,5-tetrakisphosphate activates sea urchin eggs by a mechanism dependent on external Ca²⁺. *Biochem J* 240:917–920, 1986.

124. Morris AP, Gallacher DV, Irvine RF, Petersen OH: Synergism of inositol triphosphate and tetrakisphosphate in activating Ca⁺ dependent K⁺ channels. *Nature* 330:653–665, 1987.

125. Parker I, Miledi R: Injecting inositol 1,3,4,5-tetrakisphosphate into xenopus oocytes generates a chloride current dependent upon intracellular calcium. *Proc R Soc London Ser B* 232:59–70, 1987.

126. Vallejo M, Jackson T, Lightman S, Hanley MR: Occurrence and extracellular actions of inositol pentakis- and hexakisphosphate in mammalian brain. *Nature* 330:656–658, 1987.

127. Masters SB, Martin NW, Harden TK, Brown JH: Pertussis toxin does not inhibit muscarinic receptor-mediated phosphoinositide hydrolysis or calcium mobilization. *Biochem J* 227:933–937, 1985.

128. Jones LG, Goldstein D, Brown JH: Guanine nucleotide-dependent inositol trisphosphate for motion in chick heart cells. *Circ Res* 62:299–305, 1988.

129. Blank JL, Ross AH, Exton JH: Purification and characterization of two G-proteins that activate the β1 isozyme of phosphoinositide-specific phospholipase C. *J Biol Chem* 266:18206–18216, 1991.

130. Gutowski S, Smrcka A, Nowak L, Wu D, Simon M, Sternweis PC: Antibodies to the αq subfamily of guanine nucleotide-binding regulatory protein α subunits attenuate activation of phosphatidylinositol 4,5-bisphosphate hydrolysis by hormones. *J Biol Chem* 266:20519–20524, 1991.

131. Boyer JL, Waldo GL, Evans T, Northup JK, Downes CP, Harden TK: Modification of ALF-4- and receptor-stimulated phospholipase C activity by G-protein βγ subunits. *J Biol Chem* 264:13917–13922, 1989.

132. Barnett JV, Shamah SM, Griendling KK, Lasseugue B, Galper JB: The development of muscarinic-cholinergic stimulation of inositol phosphate production in cultured embryonic chick atrial cells: Evidence for a switch in G-protein coupling. *Biochem J* 271:443–448, 1990.

133. Poggioli J, Sulpice JC, Vassort G: Inositol phosphate production following β-adrenergic, muscarinic or electrical stimulation in isolated rat heart. *FEBS Lett* 206:292–298, 1986.

134. Schmitz W, Scholz H, Scholz J, Steinfath M, Lohse M, Purunen J, Schwabe U: *Eur J Pharm* 134:377–378, 1987.

135. Steinberg SF, Chow YK, Robinson RB, Bilezikian JB: A pertussis toxin substrate regulates alpha₁-adrenergic dependent phosphatidyl inositol hydrolysis in cultured rat myocytes. *Endocrinology* 120:1889–1895, 1987.

136. Stephan CC, Griendling KK, Galper JB: Muscarinic cholinergic stimulation of diacylglycerol production in cultured chick atrial cells: Evidence for a role of phospholipase D and coupling via two G-proteins. Submitted.

137. Stephan CC, Griendling KK, Getzen SG, Galper JB: Development of a pathway for muscarinic cholinergic stimulation of diacylglycerol production in cultured embryonic heart cells: Evidence for alternate pathways in atrium and ventricle and a role for phosphatichylcholine. Submitted.

138. Martin JM, Hunter DD, Nathanson NM: Islet activating protein inhibits physiological responsiveness evoked by cardiac muscarinic acetylcholine receptors; Role of guanosine triphosphate binding proteins in regulation of potassium permeability. *Biochemistry* 24:7521–7525, 1985.

139. Logothetis DE, Kurachi Y, Galper JB, Neer EJ, Clapham DE: The β subunits of GTP-binding proteins activate the muscarinic K⁺ channel in heart. *Nature* 325:321–326, 1987.

140. Logothetis DE, Kim D, Northup JK, Neer EJ, Clapham DE: Specificity of action of guanine nucleotide-binding regulatory protein subunits on the cardiac muscarinic K⁺ channel. *Proc Natl Acad Sci USA* 85:5814–5818, 1988.

141. Kim D, Lewis DL, Graziadei L, Neer EJ, Bar-Sagi D, Clapham DE: G-protein βα-subunits activate the cardiac muscarinic K⁺-channel via phospholipase A₂. *Nature* 337:557–560, 1989.

142. Kurachi Y, Ito H, Sugimoto T, Shimizu T, Miki I, Ui M: Arachidonic acid metabolites as intracellular modulators of the G-protein-gated cardiac K⁺ channel. *Nature* 337:555–557, 1989.

143. Yatani A, Codina J, Brown AM, Birnbaumer L: Direct activation of mammalian atrial muscarinic potassium channels by GTP regulatory protein Gₖ. *Science* 235:207–211, 1987.

144. Codina J, Olate J, Abramowitz J, Mattera R, Cook RG, Birnbaumer L: αᵢ₋₃ cDNA encodes the γ subunit of Gₖ, the stimulatory G-proteins of receptor-regulated K⁺ channels. *J Biol Chem* 263:6746–6750, 1988.

145. Yatani A, Mattera R, Codina J, Graf R, Okabe K, Padrell E, Iyengar R, Brown AM, Birnbaumer L: The G-protein-gated atrial K⁺ channel is stimulated by three distinct G-α subunits. *Nature* 336:680–682, 1988.

146. Yatani A, Okabe K, Polakis P, Halenbeck R, McCormick F, Brown AM: rasp21 and GAP inhibit coupling of muscarinic receptors to atrial K⁺ channels. *Cell* ●●:769–776, 1990.

147. Martin GA, Yatani A, Clark R, Conroy L, Polakis P, Brown AM, McCormick F: GAP domains responsible for Ras p21-dependent inhibition of muscarianic atrial K⁺ channel currents. *Science* 255:192–194, 1991.

148. Kleuss C, Hescheler J, Ewel C, Rosenthal W, Schultz G, Wittig B: Assignment of G-protein subtypes to specific receptors inducing inhibition of calcium currents. *Nature* 353:43–48, 1991.

149. Kleuss C, Scherubl H, Hescheler J, Schultz G, Wittig B: Different β-subunits determine G-protein interaction with transmembrane receptors. *Nature* 358:424–426, 1992.

150. Kleuss C, Scherubl H, Hescheler J, Schultz G, Wittig B: Selectivity in signal transduction determined by γ subunits of heterotrimeric G proteins. *Science* 259:832–834, 1993.

151. Marvin MJ, Atkins DL, Chittick UL, Land DD, Hemersmeryer K: In vitro adrenergic and cholinergic innervation of the developing rat myocyte. *Circ Res* 55:49–58, 1984.

152. Rosen MR, Steinberg SF, Danilo P Jr: Developmental changes in the muscarinic stimulation of canine Purkinje fibers. *J Pharmac Exp Ther* 254:356–361, 1990.

153. Alexander RW, Galper JB, Neer EJ, Smith TW: Non-coordinate development of β-adrenergic receptors and adenylate cyclase in chick heart. *Biochem J* 204:825–830, 1982.

154. Linden J, Patel A, Spanier AM, Weglicki WB: Rapid agonist-induced decrease of [^{125}I]-pindolol binding to β-adrenregic receptors. Relationship to desensitization of cyclic AMP accumulation in intact heart cells. *J Biol Chem* 259:15115–15122, 1984.

155. Stewart DE, Kirby ML, Aronstam RS: Regulation of β-adrenergic receptor density in the non-innervated and denervated embryonic chick heart. *J Mol Cell Cardiol* 18:469–475, 1986.

156. Ignarro LJ, Shideman FE: Appearance and concentrations of catecholamines and their biosynthesis in the embryonic and developing chick. *J Pharmacol Exp Ther* 159:38–48, 1968.

157. Higgins D, Pappano AJ: Development of transmitter secretory mechanisms by adrenergic neurons in the embryonic chick heart ventricle. *Dev Biol* 87:148–162, 1981.

158. Stewart DE, Kirby ML: Endogenous tyrosine hydroxylase activity in the developing chick heart: A possible source of extraneuronal catecholamines. *J Mol Cell Cardiol* 17:389–398, 1985.

159. Lincoln TM, Keeley SL: Effects of acetylcholine and nitroprusside on cGMP-dependent protein kinase in the perfused rat heart. *J Cyclic Nucleotide Res* 6:83–91, 19●●.

160. Roeske WR, Wildenthal K: Responsiveness to drugs and hormones in the murine model of cardiac ontongenesis. *Pharmacol Ther* 14:55–66, 1980.

161. Barnett JV, Haigh LS, Marsh JD, Galper JB: Effects of low density lipoproteins and mevinolin on sympathetic responsiveness in cultured chick atrial cells: Regulation of β-adrenergic receptors and α$_s$. *J Biol Chem* 264:10779–10786, 1989.

162. Lands HM, Arnold A, McAlff JP, Ludena FP, Brown IG: Differentiation of receptor systems activated by sympathomimetic amines. *Nature* 214:597–598, 1967.

163. Dixon RA, Kobilka BK, Strader DJ, Benovic JL, Dohlman HG, Frielle T, Bolanowski MA, Bennett CD, Rands E, Diehl RE, Mumford RA, Slater EE, Sigal IS, Caron MG, Lefkowitz RJ, Strader CD: Cloning of the gene and cDNA for mammalian β-adrenergic receptor and homology with rhodopsin. *Nature* 321:75–79, 1986.

164. Emorine LJ, Marullo S, Delavier-Klutchko C, Kaveri SV, Duriu-Trautmann O, Strosberg AD: Structure of the gene for human β$_2$-adrenergic receptor: Expression and promotor characterization. *Proc Natl Acad Sci USA* 84:6995–6999, 1987.

165. Frielle T, Collins S, Daniel KW, Caron MG, Lefkowitz RJ, Kobilka BK: Cloning of the cDNA for the human β$_1$-adrenergic receptor. *Proc Natl Acad Sci USA* 84:7920–7924, 1987.

166. Muzzin P, Revelli J-P, Kuhne F, Gocayne JD, McCombie WR, Venter JC, Giacobino J-P, Fraser CM: An adipose tissue-specific β-adrenergic receptor. *J Biol Chem* 266:24053–24058, 1991.

167. Emorine LJ, Marullo S, Briend-Sutren MM, Patey G, Tate K, Delavier-Klutchko C, Strosberg AD: Molecular characterization of the human β$_3$-adrenergic receptor. *Science* 245:1118–1121, 1989.

168. Galper JB, Smith TW: Agonist and guanine nucleotide modulation of muscarinic cholinergic receptors in cultured heart cells. *J Biol Chem* 255:9571–9579, 1980.

169. Galper JB, Dziekan LC, Miura DS, Smith TW: Agonist-induced changes in the modulation of K$^+$ permeability and

beating rate by muscarinic agonists in cultured heart cells. *J Gen Physiol* 80:231–256, 1982.

170. Goldstein JL, Anderson RGW, Brown MS: Coated pits, coated vesicles, and receptor-mediated endocytosis. *Nature* 279:679–685, 1979.

171. Wilson L, Bramburg JR, Mizel SB, Grisham LM, Creswell KM: Interaction of drugs with microtubule proteins. *Fed Proc* 33:158–166, 1974.

172. Harden KT, Petsh LA, Traynelis SF, Waldo GL: Agonist-induced alteration in the membrane form of the muscarinic cholinergic receptors. *J Biol Chem* 260:13060–13066, 1985.

173. Su Y-F, Harden TK, Perkins JP: Isoproterenol-induced desensitization of adenylate cyclase in human astrocytoma cells. *J Biol Chem* 254:38–41, 1979.

174. Stadel JM, Nambi P, Lavin TN, Heald SL, Caron MG, Lefkowitz RJ: Catecholamine-induced desensitization of turkey erythrocyte adenylate cyclase. *J Biol Chem* 257:9242–9245, 1982.

175. Stadel J, Strulovici B, Nambi P, Lavin TN, Briggs MM, Caron MG, Lefkowitz RJ: Desensitization of the β-adrenergic receptor of frog erythrocytes. *J Biol Chem* 258:3032–3038, 1983.

176. Strulovici B, Stadel JM, Lefkowitz RJ: Functional integrity of desensitized β-adrenergic receptors. *J Biol Chem* 258:6410–6414, 1983.

177. Toews ML, Waldo GL, Harden TK, Perkins JP: Relationship between an altered membrane form and a low affinity form of the β-adrenergic receptor occurring during catecholamine-induced desensitization. *J Biol Chem* 259:11844–11850, 1984.

178. Nambi P, Sibley DR, Stadel JM, Michel T, Peters JR, Lefkowitz RJ: Cell-free desensitization of catecholamine-sensitive adenylate cyclase. *J Biol Chem* 259:4629–4633, 1984.

179. Sibley DR, Peters JR, Mambi P, Caron MG, Lefkowitz RJ: Desensitization of turkey erythrocyte adenylate cyclase. *J Biol Chem* 259:9742–9749, 1984.

180. Nambi P, Peters JR, Sibley DR, Lefkowitz RJ: Desensitization of the turkey erythrocyte β-adrenergic receptor in a cell-free system. *J Biol Chem* 260:2165–2171, 1985.

181. Sibley DR, Strasser RH, Caron MG, Lefkowitz RJ: Homologous desensitization of adenylate cyclase is associated with phosphorylation of the β-adrenergic receptor. *J Biol Chem* 260:3883–3886, 1985.

182. Benovic JL, Pike LJ, Cerione RA, Staniszewski C, Yoshimasa T, Codina J, Caron MG, Lefkowitz RJ: Phosphorylation of the mammalian β-adrenergic receptor by cyclic AMP-dependent protein kinase. *J Biol Chem* 260:7094–7101, 1985.

183. Benovic JL, Strasser RH, Caron MG, Lefkowitz RJ: β-adrenergic receptor kinase: Identification of a novel protein kinase that phosphorylates the agonist occupied form of the receptor. *Proc Natl Acad Sci USA* 83:2797–2801, 1986.

184. Dohlman HG, Bouvier M, Benovic JL, Caron MG, Lefkowitz RJ: The multiple membrane spanning topography of the β$_2$-adrenergic receptor. *J Biol Chem* 262:14282–14288, 1987.

185. Hausdorff WP, Bouvier M, O'Dowd BF, Irons GP, Caron MG, Lefkowitz RJ: Phosphorylation sites on two domains of the β$_2$-adrenergic receptor are involved in distinct pathways of receptor desensitization. *J Biol Chem* 264:12657–12665, 1989.

186. Bouvier M, Collins S, O'Dowd BF, Campbell PT, de Blasi A, Kobilka BK, MacGregor C, Irons GP, Caron MG, Lefkowitz RJ: Two distinct pathways for cAMP-mediated

down-regulation of the β₂-adrenergic receptor. *J Biol Chem* 264:16786–16792, 1989.

187. Lohse MJ, Andexinger S, Pitcher J, Trukawinski S, Codina J, Faure JP, Caron MG, Lefkowitz RJ: Receptor-specific desensitization with purified proteins. *J Biol Chem* 267: 8558–8564, 1992.

188. Pitcher JA, Inglese J, Higgins JB, Arriza JL, Casey PJ, Kim C, Benovic JL, Kwatra MM, Caron MG, Lefkowitz RJ: Role of βγ subunits of G proteins in targeting the β-adrenergic receptor kinase to membrane-bound receptors. *Science* 257:1264–1267, 1992.

189. Kwatra, MM, Hosey MM: Phosphorylation of the cardiac muscarinic receptor in intact chick heart and its regulation by a muscarinic agonist. *J Biol Chem* 261:12429–12432, 1986.

190. Kwatra, MM, Leung E, Man AC, McMahon KK, Ptasienski J, Green RD, Hosey MM: Correlation of agonist-induced phosphorylation of chick heart muscarinic receptors with receptor desensitization. *J Biol Chem* 262:16314–16321, 1987.

191. Haga K, Haga T: Activation by G protein βγ subunits of agonist- or light-dependent phosphorylation of muscarinic acetylcholine receptors and rhodopsin. *J Biol Chem* 267: 2222–2227, 1992.

192. Richardson RM, Hosey MM: Agonist-induced phosphorylation and desensitization of human m2 muscarinic cholinergic receptors in Sf9 insect cells. *J Biol Chem* 267: 22249–22255, 1992.

193. Collins S, Bouvier M, Bolanowski MA, Caron MG, Lefkowitz RJ: cAMP stimulates transcription of the β-2-adrenergic receptor gene in response to short-term agonist exposure. *Proc Natl Acad Sci USA* 86:4853–4857, 1989.

194. Hadcock JR, Malbon CC: Regulation of β-adrenergic receptors by "permissive" hormones: Glucocorticoids increase steady-state levels of receptor mRNA. *Proc Natl Acad Sci USA* 85:8415–8419, 1988.

195. Collins S, Caron MG, Lefkowitz RJ: β-2-adrenergic receptors in hamster smooth muscle cells are transcriptionally regulated by glucocorticoids. *J Biol Chem* 263:9067–9070, 1988.

196. Hadcock JR, Wang H-Y, Malbon CC: Agonist-induced destabilization of β-adrenergic receptor mRNA. *J Biol Chem* 264:19928–19933, 1989.

197. Guest SJ, Hadcock JR, Watkins DC, Malbon CC: β₁- and β₂-adrenergic receptor expression in differentiating 3T3-L1 cells. *J Biol Chem* 265:5370–5375, 1990.

198. Granneman JG, Lahners KN: Differential adrenergic regulation of β₁- and β₃-adrenoreceptor messenger ribonucleic acids in adipose tissues. *Endocrinology* 130:109–114, 1992.

199. Habecker BA, Nathanson NM: Regulation of muscarinic acetylcholine receptor mRNA expression by activation of homologous and heterologous receptors. *Proc Natl Acad Sci USA* 89:5035–5038, 1992.

200. Habecker BA, Wang H, Nathanson NM: Multiple second messenger pathways mediate agonist regulation of muscarinic receptor mRNA expression. *Biochemistry* 32:4986–4990, 1992.

201. Renaud JF, Scanu AM, Kazazogloa T, Lombart A, Romey G, Lazdunski M: Normal serum and lipoprotein deficient serum give different expressions of excitability, corresponding to different stages of differentiation in chick cardiac cells in culture. *Proc Natl Acad Sci USA* 29:7768–7772, 1982.

202. Haigh LS, Leatherman GF, O'Hara DS, Smith TW, Galper JB: Effects of low density lipoproteins and mevinolin on cholesterol content and muscarinic cholinergic responsiveness in cultured chick atrial cells: Regulation of levels of muscarinic receptors and guanine nucleotide regulatory proteins. *J Biol Chem* 263:15608–15618, 1988.

203. Parson WJ, Stiles GL: Heterologous desensitization of the inhibitory A₂ adenosine receptor-adenylate cyclase system in rat adipocytes: Regulation of both Nₛ and Nᵢ. *J Biol Chem* 262:841–847, 1987.

204. Colucci WS, Denniss RA, Leatherman GF, Quigg RJ, Ludmer PL, Marsh JD, Gauthier DF: Intracoronary infusion of dobutamine to patients with and without severe congestive heart failure. *J Clin Invest* 81:1103–1110, 1988.

205. Colucci WS, Ribiero JP, Rocco MB, Quigg RJ, Creager MA, Marsh JD, Gauthier DF, Hartley LH: Impaired chronotropic response to exercise in patients with congestive heart failure: Role of postsynaptic β-adrenergic desensitization. *Circulation* 80:314–323, 1989.

206. Erne P, Lipkin D, Maseri A: Impaired beta-adrenergic receptors and normal postreceptor responsiveness in congestive heart failure. *Am J Cardiol* 61:1132–1134, 1988.

207. Denniss RA, Marsh JD, Quigg RJ, Gordon JB, Colucci WS: β-adrenergic receptor number and adenylate cyclase function in denervated transplanted and cardiomyopathic human hearts. *Circulation* 79:1028–1054, 1989.

208. Kessler PD, Cates AE, Van Dop C, Feldman AM: Decreased bioactivity of the guanine nucleotide-binding protein that stimulates adenylate cyclase in hearts from cardiomyopathic Syrian hamsters. *J Clin Invest* 84:244–252, 1989.

209. Feldman AM, Cates AE, Veazey WB, Hershberger RE, Bristow MR, Baughman KL, Baumgartner WA, Van Dop C: Increase of the 40,000 mol. wt. pertussis toxin substrate (G-protein) in the failing human heart. *J Clin Invest* 82: 189–197, 1988.

210. Vatner DE, Lavalle M, Amano J, Finizola A, Homcy CJ, Vatner SF: Mechanisms of supersensitivity to sympathomimetic amines in the chronically denervated heart of the conscious dog. *Circ Res* 57:55–64, 1985.

211. Osorio, ML, Stevano JFE, Langer SZ: Heteroptic heart transplanted in the cat. An experimental model for the study of the development of sympathetic denervators and of allograft rejection. *Naunyn Schmiedebergs Arch Pharmacol* 283:389–407, 1974.

212. Ono K, Lindsey ES: Improved technique of heart transplantation in the rat. *J Thorac Cardiovasc Surg* 57:225–229, 1969.

213. Luri KG, Bristow MR, Reitz BA: Increased β-adrenergic receptor density in an experimental model of cardiac transplantation. *J Thorac Cardiovasc Surg* 86:195–201, 1983.

214. Savin WM, Haskell SC, Schroeder JS, Stinson EB: Cardiorespiratory responses of cardiac transplant patients to graded, symptom-limited exercise. *Circulation* 62:55–60, 1980.

215. Pope SE, Stinson EB, Daughters GT, Schroeder JS, Ingels NB, Alderman EL: Exercise response of the denervated heart in long-term cardiac transplant recipients. *Am J Cardiol* 96:213–218, 1980.

216. Quigg RJ, Rocco MB, Gauthier DF, Creager MA, Hartley LH, Colucci WS: Mechanisms of the attenuated peak heart rate to exercise after orthotopic cardiac transplantation. *J Am Coll Cardiol* 14:338–344, 1989.

217. Gilbert EM, Eiswirth CC, Mealey P, Herrick C, Bristow MR: β-adrenergic supersensitivity of the human heart is presynoptic in origin. *Circulation* 79:344–349, 1989.

CHAPTER 23

Alpha-Adrenergic Modulation of Cardiac Rhythm in the Developing Heart

MICHAEL R. ROSEN, RICHARD B. ROBINSON, IRA S. COHEN,
SUSAN F. STEINBERG, & JOHN P. BILEZIKIAN

INTRODUCTION

For many years the role of the autonomic nervous system
in the control of cardiac rhythm was thought to be rather
straightforward {1}. The parasympathetic nervous system
and its mediator, acetylcholine, were thought to exert
an inhibitory function (depressing automaticity and atrioventricular conduction), and the sympathetic nervous
system, and epinephrine and norepinephrine, were thought
to be excitatory, enhancing automaticity and speeding
atrioventricular conduction. In the context of cardiac
rhythm modulation per se, the important sympathetic
actions were thought to be beta-adrenergic; only a minor
role, if any, was consigned to the alpha-adrenergic system.
The major complicating factor in the picture was that
of accentuated antagonism, whereby the parasympathetic
limb of the autonomic nervous system was shown to
have enhanced effects in the presence of preexisting sympathetic tone {1,2}.

A number of observations have occurred to modify this
view of autonomic control. Among these have been the
recognition of additional humoral substances that may
be neurally released, such as adenosine, serotonin, and
peptides such as neuropeptide Y, that have demonstrable
and important effects on cardiac rhythm; the recognition
of elaborate second messenger signaling mechanisms that
link receptors to distinct functional responses such that
under certain circumstances the effect of a given receptor
to modulate rhythm may be excitatory, whereas under
other conditions the response to the same receptor may be
inhibitory; and the recognition of an increasingly complex
set of interactions among the limbs and neurohumors of
the autonomic nervous system.

In this chapter we concentrate on the alpha-adrenergic
component of the cardiac-autonomic interaction. Recent work has used the alpha-adrenergic system as a
model for understanding the extensive qualitative and
quantitative changes that occur in the control of cardiac rhythm as a result of cardiac sympathetic innervation. In this chapter we shall discuss the role of cardiac
and sympathetic neuronal growth and development in
the modulation of alpha-adrenergic control of cardiac
rhythm.

CELLULAR PATHWAYS MEDIATING AUTONOMIC RESPONSIVENESS

The list of hormones and neurotransmitters known to
regulate cellular events by utilizing guanine nucleotide
binding proteins (G proteins) now numbers over 100. The
new family of odorant receptors could swell that number
to over 1000. G proteins to which receptors are linked
critically regulate an array of signal transduction systems
that include activation or inhibition of adenylyl cyclase,
stimulation of phosphatidylinositol turnover, stimulation
of cyclic GMP phosphodiesterase, and regulation of a
number of ion channels: sodium, calcium, and potassium
{3}. The family of G proteins also grows daily; 20 different
G proteins have already been isolated and characterized
{4–7}. G proteins involved in signal transduction are all
heterotrimers with α, β, and γ subunits. The individuality
of a given G protein appears to reside primarily in the α
subunit, which has distinctive properties that set it apart
from its relatives. However, the α subunits do share
similar properties. The usual molecular weight range is
39–45 kDa. They share a site for GTP binding, a locus that
is a critical activating domain of the protein. The α subunit
also contains a common region of GTPase activity, which
is a critical deactivating domain of the protein {8,9}. Some
α units, such as those belonging to the G proteins G_s,
G_i, G_t, and G_o, are substrates for an ADP-ribosylation
reaction catalyzed either by cholera or pertussis toxin
{10}. In the case of G_s, ADP ribosylation leads to persistent activation; in the case of G_i, ADP ribosylation
leads to inactivation. The ADP-ribosylation reaction has
been a very useful tool for assessing the functional properties of G proteins in the context of the biochemical
effector systems that they mediate. The ADP-ribosylation
reaction has also helped to assign a role for a particular G
protein(s) in the developing α_1-adrenergic response of the
neonatal heart (see below). The other components of G
proteins are β (approximately 35–36 kDa) and γ (approximately 8–10 kDa) subunits. In contrast to α subunits, the
β and γ subunits of G proteins are not necessarily unique.
However, they are not all the same either {3}. So far, five
distinct β subunits and 10 or more γ subunits have been
isolated. It is not known to what extent a given β or γ

457

N. Sperelakis (ed.), Physiology and Pathophysiology of the Heart, Third Edition.

subunit or β-γ subunit combination is necessarily associated with an α subunit. In fact, some of the complexity of the subunit structure of G proteins could relate to the many different permutations and combinations that could arise by simply considering the number of α, β, and γ subunits. One could have over 1000 different combinations of G-protein heterotrimers just on the basis of the number of subunits discovered so far.

Alpha-adrenergic modulation of pacemaker function

EFFECTS OF ALPHA-ADRENERGIC STIMULATION ON
PACEMAKER FUNCTION

In adult canine Purkinje fibers superfused with epinephrine or phenylephrine, only about one third show a sigmoid relationship between concentration and automatic rate such that automaticity uniformly increases. The other two thirds show a profound decrease in automaticity at low agonist concentrations and an increase at high concentrations (fig. 23-1) {11,12}. The decrease in automaticity at low epinephrine or phenylephrine concentrations is inhibited by prazosin or phentolamine, but not yohimbine,

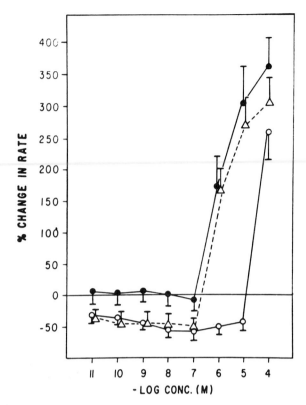

Fig. 23-2. Effects of phentolamine and of propranolol on the response to epinephrine of isolated human atrial tissues ($\bar{x} \pm$ SE). The vertical axis is percent change in automatic rate, with control set to 0; the horizontal axis is molar concentration of epinephrine. Control rates (beats/min) = epinephrine alone (Δ) 27 ± 7; epinephrine + phentolamine (●) 25 ± 6; epinephrine + propranolol (○) 27 ± 2. There is a negative chronotropic effect during exposure to low concentrations of epinephrine alone and a positive effect of high concentrations (Δ, n = 9). The negative chronotropic effect is abolished by phentolamine, $1 \times 10^{-7}\,M$ (●, n = 5) and is sustained through higher agonist concentrations by propranolol $2 \times 10^{-7}\,M$ (○, n = 7). This is consistent with the inhibition of automaticity being an alpha-adrenergic event. Modified after Mary-Rabine et al. {15}, with permission.

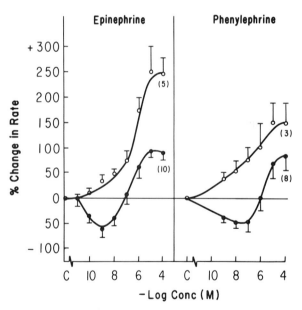

Fig. 23-1. The response of adult canine Purkinje fibers to epinephrine (**left panel**) and phenylephrine (**right panel**). The vertical axis is percent change in automatic rate with control arbitrarily set to 0. The actual control rate (all groups) was 12 ± 2 beats/min ($\bar{x} \pm$ SE). There were no significant differences among the subgroups. The horizontal axis is the drug concentration. The number of preparations incorporated in each curve is in parentheses. For both agonists the majority of preparations showed a biphasic curve (●), with automaticity decreasing at the low agonist concentrations and increasing at high concentrations. Fewer preparations showed a monophasic curve (○), with rate increasing at all concentrations. See text for discussion. Modified after Rosen et al. {11}, with permission.

and hence is α_1 adrenergic; the increase in automaticity at higher concentrations is blocked by propranolol, and hence is beta-adrenergic {11-14}. Studies of isolated human atrial tissue showed a result similar to those in ventricular specialized fibers; that is, automaticity is inhibited by low epinephrine concentrations, and the inhibition is blocked by phentolamine, but not propranolol (fig. 23-2) {15}. Posner et al. {12} studied transmembrane K^+ fluxes in ventricular specialized fibers and suggested the decrease in automaticity resulted from an epinephrine-induced increase in K^+ efflux that, in turn, was induced by activation of alpha-adrenergic receptors.

That the alpha-adrenergic inhibition of automaticity could occur in the heart in situ was shown in dogs in which complete heart block had been induced by injection of the

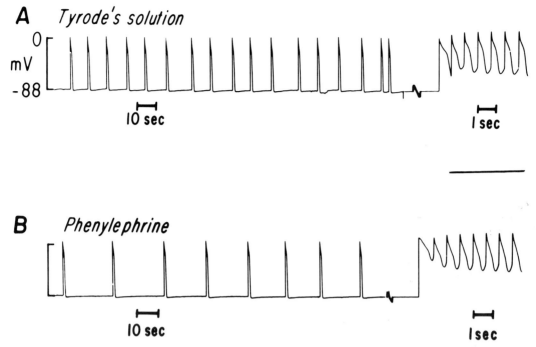

A *Tyrode's solution*

0
mV
-88

10 sec

1 sec

B *Phenylephrine*

10 sec

1 sec

Fig. 23-3. Effects of phenylephrine on Purkinje fiber automaticity at two levels of membrane potential. **Upper panel**: Control automaticity in a Purkinje fiber having a high maximum diastolic potential and following depolarization to a low membrane potential by intracellular current injection. **Lower panel**: The same protocol repeated in the presence of phenylephrine, 5×10^{-9} M. Note that at the high membrane potential automatic rate has slowed appreciably (the alpha-adrenergic effect). At the depolarized level of membrane potential, the slowing of automatic rate is not seen. Reprinted from Hewett and Rosen {17} by permission.

His bundle with formalin {16}. In these animals we determined the effects of infusion of epinephrine, in concentrations too low to alter arterial pressure, on both sinus and on idioventricular pacemaker rate. This was not decreased by epinephrine alone, but when animals were pretreated with the beta-blocker, propranolol, epinephrine infusion decreased ventricular (but not sinus) automaticity.

These observations suggested there might be a voltage-dependent aspect of the alpha-adrenergic effect; that is, since the sinus node has a significantly lower membrane potential and a different pacemaker mechanism than highly polarized fibers elsewhere in the atrium and in the Purkinje system, voltage dependence might provide a basis for the difference in the response seen. This possibility was tested further using adult rabbit sinus node and canine Purkinje fibers {17}.

No effect of alpha-adrenergic stimulation on the sinus node transmembrane potential was seen, nor was there a decrease in automaticity. Hence, in the isolated rabbit sinus node, as well as the canine sinus node, in situ alpha-adrenergic stimulation did not inhibit automaticity. Moreover, when canine Purkinje fibers were depolarized to approximately −60 mV with intracellular current injection, there was no longer any inhibition of automaticity, and in some instances automaticity increased (fig. 23-3). This same effect of alpha-adrenergic stimulation to increase

automaticity in depolarized preparations was demonstrated by Amerini et al. {18} in barium-depolarized fibers and by Han et al. in K^+-depolarized innervated ventricular myocytes {19}. These results confirmed that there is either a voltage-dependent component of alpha-adrenergic inhibition of automaticity or that alpha stimulation affects pacemaker currents occurring at high or low levels of membrane potential differently. The latter possibility has been borne out as follows: In experiments using voltage-clamped disaggregated Purkinje myocytes {20}, α_1-adrenergic agonist stimulated an outward current, providing an explanation for the decrease in automaticity. This effect was antagonized by prazosin and not propranolol, and did not occur following treatment with dihydroouabain. These results suggested α_1-adrenergic stimulation of the Na/K pump. Additional experiments using ion-sensitive microelectrodes have quantified a decrease in intracellular Na^+ activity induced by the actions of alpha agonists in canine Purkinje fibers {21}. This decrease occurs only in those fibers in which automaticity decreases, and is linearly proportional to the decrease. Moreover, prazosin, but not propranolol, blocks the effect of an alpha agonist on aNa_i. This body of evidence additionally favors the actions of alpha agonists to stimulate the Na/K pump.

In considering the effects of α_1 stimulation, one must take cognizance of the fact that at least two α_1-adrenergic receptor subtypes exist, which can be identified using the alkylating agent chloroethylclonidine (CEC) and the competitive antagonist WB 4101 {22}. The effect of an alpha agonist to decrease automaticity is blocked by CEC, but not WB 4101 {23}. Hence a subtype-selective action of α_1 agonist on the Na/K pump appears to explain the decrease in automaticity that is seen. What of the increase in automaticity occurring both at high and at low levels of membrane potential? Both types are blocked by WB 4101, which also inhibits alpha-receptor-dependent hydrolysis of phosphoinositides in heart muscle {23}. This had led to the hypothesis that the WB 4101-sensitive α_1-receptor pathway, perhaps through an IP_3 or DAG-dependent action to modulate $[Ca^{2+}]_i$, increases automaticity. Although available evidence suggests that $[Ca^{2+}]_i$ does *not* increase appreciably in the presence of an alpha agonist {24,25}, the observation that the effect of an alpha agonist to increase automaticity in fibers having high membrane potentials is blocked by ryanodine suggests that calcium-dependent processes may be contributory {26}. However, in depolarized fibers exposed to simulated "ischemic" solutions ($pO_2 < 25\,mmHg$; $pH = 6.8$; $[K^+]_o = 10\,mM$), alpha agonists induce an increase in automaticity that is blocked by WB 4101, and not CEC, but is unaffected by ryanodine {26}. Manipulations that increase (ACh) or decrease (Ba^{2+}) K^+ conductance, respectively, decrease or increase the alpha effect on automaticity in these depolarized fibers {27}. This has led to the thought that an action to decrease K conductance may be important to the α_1 effect on automaticity at low membrane potentials. This observation is supported by experiments in disaggregated Purkinje myocytes showing that α_1-adrenergic stimulation inhibits background g_K {20}, an action that would tend to enhance the pacemaker rate.

To summarize results to this point, there are at least two α_1-adrenergic linkages to automaticity. One, involving a receptor subtype blocked by CEC, stimulates the Na/K pump to decrease automaticity. A second, blocked by WB 4101, is linked via a ryanodine-sensitive mechanism to an increase in automaticity in normally polarized fibers and via a ryanodine-insensitive mechanism (perhaps related to a K conductance) to an increase in automaticity in depolarized or "ischemic" fibers.

DEVELOPMENTAL CHANGES IN ALPHA-ADRENERGIC EFFECTS ON AUTOMATICITY

As in adults, superfusion of neonatal canine Purkinje fibers with epinephrine induces two types of response: Automaticity either decreases or increases. However, the proportion of fibers showing the increase and decrease is consistently 1:1 (different from the proportion in adult fibers of 1:2 {11}). A comparison of the dose-response curves for epinephrine in neonatal and adult fibers is shown in fig. 23-4. Several factors are apparent here: First, the magnitude of the decrease in automaticity (left panel) is comparable in the neonates and adults; second, in that

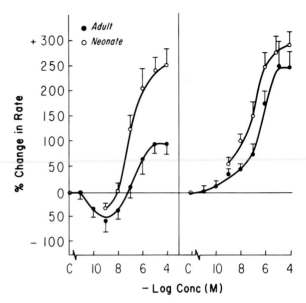

Fig. 23-4. Comparison of the effects of epinephrine on automaticity of adult and neonatal Purkinje fibers ($\bar{x} \pm SE$). Vertical and horizontal axes and curves for the adult fibers (●) are taken from fig. 23-1. Data for 19 neonatal fibers (○) are incorporated, 9 in the left panel and 10 in the right. Control rate for neonatal fibers = 10 ± 1 beats/min. Note that in the **left panel** (demonstrating alpha-adrenergic-induced inhibition of automaticity) the neonatal curve is upward and to the left of the adult; in the **right panel** (absence of alpha-adrenergic-induced inhibition) the curves are nearly superimposable. Modified from Rosen et al. {11}, with permission.

same group of fibers the increase in automaticity in the neonates at higher epinephrine concentrations is significantly greater than in the adults; third, in those fibers showing only an increase in automaticity (right panel), the neonatal and adult responses are comparable. Hence, it appeared that α_1-adrenergic stimulation was capable of inducing an increase in automaticity in the immature dog heart and that with development this response changed in the majority of the population to an inhibition of automaticity. Because of the immaturity of sympathetic nerve development in the neonate, studies were then performed to consider the relationship of sympathetic innervation to the alpha response.

The model used was the neonatal rat cardiac myocyte in tissue culture alone or in coculture with sympathetic ganglion cells. This model was viewed as appropriate because preliminary studies of adult and neonatal rat ventricles showed, respectively, an α_1-adrenergic-induced decrease and increase in automaticity {28}. That the myocyte cultures were nerve free and the cocultures were innervated was demonstrated in studies of ultrastructure — showing close nerve-muscle apposition in the latter — and in studies using tyramine, which induced the release of catecholamines in the latter but not the former {29}.

In pure muscle cultures, phenylephrine increased automaticity and this was blocked by prazosin {28}. In two thirds of the cocultures, phenylephrine decreased automaticity; in the other one third the rate increased. Both responses were blocked by prazosin. Neither propranolol, atropine, nor adenosine deaminase blocked the inhibition of automaticity, indicating the response was unrelated to an action at presynaptic α_1 receptors located on sympathetic, parasympathetic, or purinergic neurons. These results suggested that a factor released by sympathetic nerves during sustained innervation in some way modified the response to alpha stimulation, leading this to change qualitatively from excitation to inhibition of automaticity {28}.

To test whether the factor(s) released by nerve to muscle might be present in the bulk phase or, rather, was communicated to muscle directly or via the narrow space between nerve and muscle, experiments were done in which nerve-conditioned medium was used, rather than permitting direct contact between nerve and muscle cells {29}. Conditioned medium failed to reproduce the effect of innervation on alpha-adrenergic responsiveness. This suggested that either the factor(s) responsible for the maturation of the alpha response was released directly from nerve to muscle, or — if transferred via the bulk phase — the concentration was sufficiently high to modulate the alpha response only in the immediate vicinity of the nerve. That the factor was not norepinephrine was suggested by the absence of a correlation between the endogenous norepinephrine levels in cocultures plus the appearance of inhibition of automaticity {30}. We next tested whether neuropeptide Y (NPY), a peptide present in and released from cardiac sympathetic neurons {32,32}, could account for the action of innervation {33}. Sustained growth of cultures in the presence of 100 nM NPY resulted in expression of a negative chronotropic alpha-adrenergic response (fig. 23-5a), while acute exposure did not (fig. 23-5b). That this was the mechanism by which sympathetic innervation also altered alpha-adrenergic responsiveness was demonstrated in another series of experiments. In this case, innervated cultures were either acutely or chronically exposed to the NPY antagonist PYX-2 {34}. The chronically treated cultures failed to develop the inhibitory response to phenylephrine typical of the innervated preparation, but the acutely treated cells responded normally (fig. 23-5c). Thus the action of sympathetic neurons to alter alpha-adrenergic chronotropic responsiveness from excitatory to inhibitory appears to be mediated by neurally released NPY.

α_1 RECEPTOR AND GTP REGULATORY PROTEINS: RELATIONSHIP TO THE DEVELOPMENTAL CHANGE IN ALPHA-ADRENERGIC RESPONSIVENESS

The studies reviewed to this point indicate an association between the development of sympathetic innervation and the conversion of the response to alpha-adrenergic stimulation from excitation to inhibition of automaticity. Age-dependent differences in α_1-adrenergic receptor expression also have been considered in the sheep, rat, dog, and

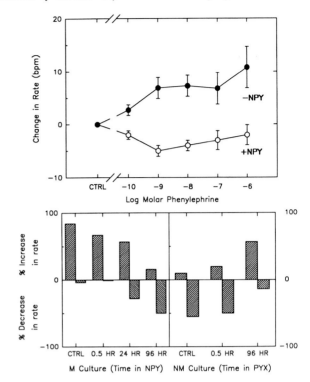

Fig. 23-5. Effect of NPY on the alpha-adrenergic chronotropic response in newborn rat ventricle cultures. **a:** Dose-response relation in muscle (M) cells grown in the presence (○) and absence (●) of NPY for 96 hours. Data are mean ± SEM; the curves differ significantly (p < 0.05). **b:** Percent of M cells exhibiting either an increase in rate (upward bars) or decrease in rate (downward bars) after exposure to NPY for the indicated periods of time. Those cells not responding with either a consistent increase or decrease in rate to successive doses of phenylephrine are excluded (and ranged from 11–35% of the cells studied). **c:** Percent of nerve-muscle (NM) cells exhibiting either an increase or decrease in rate after exposure to the putative NPY antagonist PYX-2 for the indicated periods of time. Modified after Sun et al. {33}, with permission.

mouse {35–37} heart. In each case, α_1-adrenergic receptor density decreases with development. Interestingly, the magnitude of the fall in α_1-adrenergic receptor density varies among species. For example, α_1-adrenergic density decreases about 50% and 10-fold with development in the rat and dog, respectively {23}. However, in these species studies using CEC to discriminate distinct α_1-adrenergic receptor subtypes indicate that the proportion of α_1-receptors identified by CEC is similar in the neonatal and adult heart, regardless of total α_1-adrenergic receptor density {23}.

Another factor that is of possible importance in the developmental modulation of alpha-adrenergic responsiveness is a G protein. In a number of models, we have associated a pertussis-toxin-sensitive G protein with the development of the mature (i.e., negative) chronotropic response to α_1-agonist stimulation {19}. In some models, such as the developing canine myocardium, prenatally and postnatally {14}, as well as in the rat myocyte-nerve coculture system {38}, there is a clear increase in this pertussis-toxin-sensitive G protein. Moreover, studies using NGF and NGF antibody in the intact rat support the notion that sympathetic innervation plays a key role in inducing an increase in the PT-sensitive G protein, which then functionally couples the α_1-adrenergic receptor to inhibition of automaticity {39}.

In other models, such as the neonatal and adult rat, the developmental maturation in α_1-adrenergic responsiveness is best appreciated as a change in the receptor-G protein linkage {40}. The experimental paradigm is as follows: G proteins regulate receptor affinity for agonists such that the receptor–G-protein complex binds agonists with higher affinity than the free form of the receptor. Binding of GTP to the G protein leads to a reduction in the affinity of the receptor for agonist, reflecting dissociation of the G protein from the receptor. The observation that agonist binding to the α_1-adrenergic receptor is best fit by a model describing a heterogenous population of high- and low-affinity receptors in the absence of GTP analogs, but a homogenous population of low-affinity sites in their presence in both adult and neonatal rat myocardial membranes {40}, is evidence that the α_1 receptor is linked to a G protein in both tissues. However, persistence of high-affinity binding, which can be modulated by GTP analogs in pertussis-toxin-treated neonatal, but not adult, myocardial membranes, supports the notion that the α_1-adrenergic receptor in the adult (but not the neonatal) heart is coupled to a pertussis-toxin-sensitive G protein. Finally, the functional importance of the α_1-receptor–pertussis-toxin-sensitive G-protein linkage is established by the observation that pertussis toxin reverts the mature negative chronotropic response to α_1-agonist stimulation to a positive chronotropic response in all experimental models tested to date {38,40,41}. Studies attempting to identify which of the candidate pertussis toxin substrates is linked to the α_1-adrenergic receptor and is responsible for the mature α_1-adrenergic response are ongoing.

Complementary observations have been made in intact Purkinje fiber bundles {41}. In adult Purkinje fibers not exposed to pertussis toxin, two thirds showed an alpha-adrenergic inhibition of automaticity, but in adult fibers exposed to toxin at a dose that completely ADP ribosylates and inactivates the endogenous G protein, there was a uniform increase in automaticity. At intermediate concentrations of toxin that only partially inactivate the endogenous G protein, the proportion of fibers showing a decrease in automaticity in response to alpha-adrenergic stimulation gradually shifted from two thirds to zero. In all instances where alpha-adrenergic stimulation increased automaticity, less G protein was detectable than in situations in which automaticity decreased. Both the increase in automaticity in the presence of pertussis toxin and that in the absence of toxin were blocked by prazosin.

These observations suggest that alpha-adrenergic stimulation is not only linked via a G protein to a mechanism that inhibits automaticity, but that when the G protein is functionally ablated (with pertussis toxin) an alpha effect persists, but this is now expressed as excitation of automaticity. Moreover, the prazosin-sensitive excitation of automaticity seen in a minority of adult fibers, in the absence of exposure to pertussis toxin {41}, may represent persistence of the condition characteristic of the newborn state into adulthood. Whether this represents incomplete development of sympathetic innervation remains to be tested. In any event, these observations suggest that the G protein is an integral control mechanism of the response to α_1-adrenergic stimulation through adult life.

The biochemical mechanisms linked to the α_1-adrenergic receptor through pertussis-toxin-sensitive and -insensitive G proteins has received considerable attention. There does not appear to be any linkage between the α_1-adrenergic receptor and either stimulation or inhibition of cAMP accumulation {38}. In contrast, α_1-receptors have an important effect to stimulate phosphoinositide hydrolysis. α_1-adrenergic receptor stimulation has been shown to lead to the generation of IP_3 {42} and diacylglycerol. Importantly, this pathway is guanine nucleotide sensitive, but is not attenuated in cells pretreated with pertussis toxin, indicating that the α_1-adrenergic receptor couples to phosphoinositide hydrolysis through a pertussis-toxin-insensitive G protein. Although α_1-agonist stimulation of phosphoinositide hydrolysis and excitation of automaticity both reflect the actions of a WB 4101-sensitive α_1-adrenergic receptor through a PT-insensitive pathway, the precise role of this biochemical response in the modulation of automaticity is not known.

On the other hand, the negative chronotropic response can be inhibited by CEC or pertussis toxin and may well be mediated by stimulation of the Na/K pump {20}. The evidence derives from studies of the ionic events underlying pacemaker function in disaggregated Purkinje myocytes. Here, the α_1-adrenergic enhancement of Na^+/K^+ pumping is prevented by pretreatment with pertussis toxin {20}. In addition, the α_1-adrenergic decrease in background g_K also was blocked by pertussis toxin. These observations suggest, then, that via a pertussis-toxin-sensitive G protein, pump current is stimulated and background g_K is suppressed. Hence, a link has been established that involves the G protein in ionic processes that have divergent effects on automaticity. Depending on which effect predominates and on the level of membrane potential, the result should be either a decrease, an increase, or no change in automaticity.

ALPHA-ADRENERGIC MODULATION OF REPOLARIZATION

That alpha agonists prolong repolarization has been known for over 20 years {43,44}. The voltage-time course of the repolarization change is such that in Purkinje fibers, which have a phase 1 notch, this may decrease somewhat in magnitude, but the major event appears to be a lengthening of the plateau and a delay in phase 3 repolarization.

Voltage-clamp studies of single myocytes have demonstrated a decrease in I_{to} {45–48} and/or a decrease in I_K {48–50} as the primary cause of the increase in repolarization. There is evidence from sufficient numbers of studies in a variety of species {45–48} that alpha agonists decrease I_{to}. What is less certain is the effect of a decrease in I_{to} on repolarization. It can be argued that by decreasing I_{to}, there would be longer maintenance of the plateau and persistence of Ca^{2+} entry. However, agents such as 4-aminopyridine, which block I_{to}, have the effect of elevating the plateau and accelerating repolarization, presumably via more rapid onset of I_K {51}. Hence, while the effect of alpha agonist to decrease I_{to} in atrial and ventricular tissues is not questioned, the relationship of this to action potential prolongation is open to question.

The effect of alpha agonist on the delayed rectifier has been studied in the guinea pig and rat {48–50}. In the former species, I_K is increased and the action potential is accelerated. In the latter species, I_K decreased and the action potential was prolonged. The effect of an alpha agonist on action potential repolarization has also been studied in canine Purkinje fiber {51}. Here, 4-aminopyridine was used to block the transient outward current, I_{to}. Nonetheless, alpha agonist still prolonged repolarization. In contrast, the I_K blocker, WY48986, completely attenuated the alpha-adrenergic prolongation of action potential duration. This observation is more consistent with an α_1-adrenergic decrease in I_K than any other single mechanism.

In some studies, alpha agonists increased inward Ca^{2+} current {52}. This has been attributed to an action on L-type Ca^{2+} channels via phosphorylation of channel protein. This effect is thought to be protein kinase C mediated. However, this action has varied extensively among preparations (whole tissue and single cells) and species {53}. It is neither as large an effect nor as consistent a finding as that with beta agonists. Furthermore, it is not consistently blocked by prazosin. Finally, studies using either aequorin or fura-2 as $[Ca^{2+}]_i$ indicators have shown either small or absent effects of alpha agonist on $[Ca^{2+}]_i$ {24,25}. Nonetheless, it appears that an effect of α_1-adrenergic receptor activation on cellular Ca metabolism still warrants consideration in evaluating the prolongation of repolarization that occurs.

Cellular electrophysiologic studies have suggested that the α_1-receptor subtype responsible for prolongation of repolarization is blocked by WB 4101 {54}. Moreover, the prolongation of repolarization occurs even in fibers from animals treated with pertussis toxin, according to a protocol that completely ADP ribosylates and inactivates endogenous G proteins {54}. In fact, following pertussis toxin treatment, the effect of alpha agonist to prolong repolarization increases in magnitude, suggesting that the alpha effect to stimulate the Na/K pump generates sufficient outward current to accelerate repolarization. This action, via a CEC-blocked receptor subtype and transduced by a pertussis-toxin-sensitive G protein, acts counter to the action of alpha agonist to prolong repolarization via the WB 4101-blocked receptor {54}.

Whether there are phosphorylation steps involved in the actions of alpha agonists on K conductance, and — indeed — what the intermediary steps beyond the level of the G protein are, has not yet been determined. It is clear that a pathway involving a WB 4101-blocked receptor and a pertussis-toxin-insensitive G protein *is* involved in alpha-adrenergic stimulation of phosphoinositide metabolism. However, it is unclear whether the latter event simply parallels or is causally involved in the alpha effect on repolarization.

INTACT ANIMAL STUDIES

When working with any isolated cell or tissue system, it is always useful to understand the extent to which one's findings are related to effects in the intact animal. Certainly, there is general agreement in the cellular electrophysiologic findings of an alpha effect to decrease Purkinje fiber automaticity and to decrease idioventricular pacemaker rate in the intact dog. Similarly, the absence of any α_1 action on isolated sinus node or on sinus node function in the intact heart provides useful negative data.

However, given the work in cell culture showing the relationship of sympathetic innervation to the functional acquisition of pertussis-toxin-sensitive G proteins that link the α_1 receptor to a decrease in automaticity, we felt it important to test the extent to which sympathetic innervation in the intact animal might alter α_1-adrenergic responsiveness {39}. Hence, neonatal rats were administered either nerve growth factor (NGF) or its antiserum (Ab) or placebo for the first 10 days of life. Electrocardiograms were recorded and the isolated hearts were then studied. The innervation pattern of the heart, tested via tyrosine hydroxylase staining, was such that the NGF-treated animals had many more sympathetic terminals than the placebo group. The Ab group had many nerve processes, but few terminals were seen. Moreover, measurement of tissue catecholamine levels demonstrated high norepinephrine and low dopamine levels in the NGF group and the reverse in the Ab group.

The level of pertussis-toxin-sensitive G protein paralleled the development of sympathetic innervation: It was highest in the NGF group, intermediate in the placebo group, and lowest in the Ab group. That the functional linkage of the G protein remained important in the intact animal was seen in the fact that 90% of the NGF-treated 10-day rats showed a decrease in automaticity (much like normal 3-week-old rats) and 70% of the Ab-treated rats showed increased automaticity (like 3- to 5-day rats). Hence, the implication of the cellular studies, linking the alpha receptor to the Na/K pump through a pertussis-toxin-sensitive G protein, was operative in the intact animal as well.

SUMMARY

There is a link between sympathetic innervation, a pertussis-toxin-sensitive G protein, and the response to α_1-adrenergic stimulation. The pertussis-toxin-sensitive protein links the α_1-receptor either directly or indirectly to the Na^+/K^+ pumping mechanism and to a background g_K, thereby providing an explanation for the modulation of automaticity in fibers that have mature innervation. The mechanisms responsible for the excitation of automaticity in the immature heart and in noninnervated myocytes remain to be identified.

ACKNOWLEDGMENTS

Certain of the studies referred to were supported by USPHS-NHLBI grant HL-28958.

REFERENCES

1. Pappano AJ: Ontogenetic development of autonomic neuro-effector transmission and transmitter reactivity in embryonic and fetal hearts. *Pharmacol Rev* 29:3–33, 1977.
2. Levy MN: Sympathetic-parasympathetic interactions in the heart. *Circ Res* 29:437–445, 1971.
3. Birnbaumer L: Transduction of receptor signal into modulation of effector activity by G proteins: The first 20 years or so. *FASEB J* 4:3068–3078, 1990.
4. Gilman AG: G Proteins: Transducers of receptor-generated signals. *Ann Rev Biochem* 56:615–647, 1987.
5. Bourne HR, Sanders DA, McCormick F: The GTPase superfamily: A conserved switch for diverse cell functions. *Nature* 348:125–132, 1990.
6. Simon MI, Strathmann P, Narasimhan G: Diversity of G proteins in signal transduction. *Science* 252:802–808, 1991.
7. Kaziro Y, Itoh H, Kozasa T, Nakafuku M, Satoh T: Structure and function of signal-transducing GTP-binding proteins. *Ann Rev Biochem* 60:349–400, 1991.
8. Johnson GL, Dhanasekaran: The G-protein family and their interaction with receptors. *Endocr Rev* 10:317–331, 1989.
9. Freissmuth M, Casey PJ, Gilman AG: G proteins control diverse pathways of transmembrane signaling. *FASEB J* 3:2125–2131, 1989.
10. Gilman AG: G proteins and regulation of adenylyl cyclase. *JAMA* 262:1819–1825, 1989.
11. Rosen MR, Hordof AJ, Ilvento J, Danilo P: Effects of adrenergic amines on electrophysiologic properties and automaticity of neonatal and adult canine cardiac Purkinje fibers. *Circ Res* 40:390–400, 1977.
12. Posner P, Farrar E, Lambert C: Inhibitory effects of catecholamines in canine cardiac Purkinje fibers. *Am J Physiol* 231:1415–1420, 1976.
13. Rosen MR, Weiss R, Danilo P Jr: Effect of alpha adrenergic agonists and blockers on Purkinje fiber transmembrane potentials and automaticity in the dog. *J Pharmacol Exp Ther* 231:566–571, 1984.
14. Rosen MR, Robinson RB: Neural influences on automaticity. In: Lown B, Malliani A, Prosdocimi M (eds) *Neural Mechanisms and Cardiovascular Disease*. Padova, Italy: Liviana Press, 1986, pp 335–358.
15. Mary-Rabine L, Hordof A, Bowman FO, Malm JR, Rosen MR: Alpha and beta-adrenergic effects on human atrial specialized conducting fibers. *Circulation* 57:84–90, 1978.
16. Hordof AJ, Rose E, Danilo P Jr, Rosen MR: Alpha and beta adrenergic effects of epinephrine on ventricular pacemakers in dogs. *Am J Physiol* 242:H677–H682, 1982.
17. Hewett K, Rosen MR: Developmental changes in the rabbit sinus node action potential and its response to adrenergic agonists. *J Pharmacol Exp Ther* 235:308–312, 1985.
18. Amerini S, Piazzesi G, Giotti A, Mugelli A: Alpha adreno-ceptor stimulation enhances automaticity in barium treated cardiac Purkinje fibers. *Arch Int Pharmacodyn Ther* 270:97–105, 1984.
19. Han H-M, Bilezikian JP, Robinson RB. Functional uncoupling of the inhibitory α_1-adrenergic response from a G protein in innervated cultured cardiac cells by K^+ depolarization. *J Mol Cell Cardiol* 22:49–56, 1990.
20. Shah A, Cohen IS, Rosen MR: Stimulation of cardiac alpha receptors increases Na/K pump current and decreases g_K via a pertussis toxin-sensitive pathway. *Biophys J* 54:219–225, 1988.
21. Zaza A, Kline R, Rosen M: Effects of alpha-adrenergic stimulation on intracellular sodium activity and automaticity in canine Purkinje fibers. *Circ Res* 66:416–426, 1990.
22. Minneman K: Alpha$_1$-adrenergic receptor subtypes, inositol phosphates, and sources of cell Ca^{2+}. *Pharmacol Rev* 40:87–119, 1988.
23. del Balzo U, Rosen MR, Malfatto G, Kaplan LM, Steinberg SF: Specific α_1-adrenergic receptor subtypes modulate catecholamine induced increases and decreases in ventricular automaticity. *Circ Res* 67:1535–1551, 1990.
24. Endoh M, Blinks JR: Actions of sympathomimetic amines on the Ca^{2+} transients and contractions of rabbit myocardium: Reciprocal changes in myofibrillar responsiveness to Ca^{2+} mediated through α- and β- adrenoceptors. *Circ Res* 62:247–265, 1988.
25. Terzic A, Puceat M, Clement O, Scamps F, Vassort G: Alpha$_1$-adrenergic effects on intracellular pH and calcium, and on responsiveness of myofilaments to calcium in single rat cardiac cell. *J Physiol* 447:275–292, 1992.
26. Anyukhovsky EP, Rybin VO, Nikashin AV, Budanova OP, Rosen MR: Positive chronotropic responses induced by α_1-adrenergic stimulation of normal and "ischemic" Purkinje fibers have different receptor-effector coupling mechanisms. *Circ Res* 71:526–534, 1992.
27. Anyukhovsky EP, Rybin VO, Nikashin AV, Budanova OP, Rosen MR: The α_1-adrenergic receptor-effector coupling pathway responsible for abnormal automaticity in "ischemic" canine Purkinje fibers. *Circulation* 84:II494, 1991.
28. Drugge E, Rosen MR, Robinson R: Neuronal regulation of the development of the alpha adrenergic chronotropic response in the rat heart. *Circ Res* 57:415–423, 1985.
29. Drugge ED, Robinson RB: Trophic influence of sympathetic neurons on the cardiac α adrenergic response requires close nerve-muscle association. *Dev Pharmacol Ther* 10:47–52, 1988.28.
30. Robinson RB: Models of cardiac development: Transplants, organ culture, cell dispersion and cell culture. In: Legato MJ (ed) *The Developing Heart*. Boston: Kluwer Academic, 1985, pp 69–94.13.
31. Furness JB, Costa M, Papka RE, Della NG, Murphy R: Neuropeptides contained in peripheral cardiovascular nerves. *Clin Exper Hypertens [A]* 6:1–2, 1984.
32. Rudehill A, Sollevi A, Franco-Cereceda A, Lundberg JM: Neuropeptide Y (NPY) and the pig heart: Release and coronary vasoconstrictor effects. *Peptides* 7:821–826, 1986.
33. Sun LS, Ursell PC, Robinson RB: Chronic exposure to neuropeptide Y determines cardiac α_1-adrenergic responsiveness. *Am J Physiol* 261:H969–H973, 1991.
34. Tatemoto K: Neuropeptide Y and its receptor antagonists: Use of an analog mixture-screening strategy. In: Allen JM, Koenig JI (eds) *Central and Peripheral Significance of Neuropeptide Y and its Related Peptides*. New York: New York Academy of Sciences, 1990, pp 1–6.
35. Cheny JB, Cornett LE, Goldfein A, Roberts JM: Decreased concentration of myocardial α adrenoceptors with increasing age in foetal lambs. *Br J Pharmacol* 70:515–517, 1980.

36. Noguchi A, Whitset JA, Dickman L: Ontogeny of myocardial α_1-adrenergic receptor in rat. *Dev Pharmacol* 3:179–188, 1981.
37. William RS, Dukes DF, Lefkowitz RJ: Subtype specificity of α-adrenergic receptors in rat heart. *J Cardiovasc Pharmacol* 3:522–531, 1981.
38. Steinberg SF, Drugge ED, Bilezikian JP, Robinson RB: Innervated cardiac myocytes acquire a pertussis toxin-specific regulatory protein functionally linked to the α_1-receptor. *Science* 230:186–188, 1985.
39. Malfatto G, Rosen TS, Steinberg SF, Ursell PC, Sun LS, Daniel S, Danilo P, Rosen MR: Sympathetic neural modulation of cardiac impulse initiation and repolarization in the newborn rat. *Circ Res* 66:427–437, 1990.
40. Han H-M, Robinson RB, Bilezikian JP, Steinberg SF: Developmental changes in guanine nucleotide regulatory proteins in the rat myocardial α_1-adrenergic receptor complex. *Circ Res* 65:1763–1773, 1989.
41. Rosen M, Steinberg S, Chow Y-K, Bilezikian J, Danilo P: The role of a pertussis toxin-sensitive protein in the modulation of canine Purkinje fiber automaticity. *Circ Res* 62:315–323, 1988.
42. Steinberg SF, Kaplan LM, Inouye T, Zhang JF, Robinson RB: Alpha$_1$-adrenergic stimulation of 1,4,5-inositol triphosphate formation in rat ventricular myocytes. *J Pharmacol Exp Ther* 250:1141–1148, 1990.
43. Giotti A, Ledda F, Mannaioni PF: Effects of noradrenaline and isoprenaline, in combination with α- and β-receptor blocking substances, on the action potential of cardiac Purkinje fibers. *J Physiol* 229:99–113, 1973.
44. Ledda F, Marchetti P, Manni A: Influence of phenylephrine on transmembrane potentials and effective refractory period of single Purkinje fibers of sheep heart. *Pharmacol Res Commun* 3:195–205, 1971.
45. Fedida DY, Shimoni Y, Giles WR: A novel effect of norepinephrine on cardiac cells is mediated by α_1-adrenoceptors. *Am J Physiol* 255:H1500–H1504, 1989.
46. Fedida D, Shimoni Y, Giles R: Alpha adrenergic modulation of the transient outward current in rabbit atrial myocyte. *J Physiol* 423:257–277, 1990.
47. Tohse N, Nakaya H, Mattori Y, Endou M, Kanno M: Inhibitory effect mediated by α_1-adrenoceptor on transient outward current in isolated ventricular cells. *Pflügers Arch* 415:575–581, 1990.
48. Apkon M, Nerbonne JM: Alpha$_1$-adrenergic agonists selectively suppress voltage-dependent K^+ currents in rat ventricular myocytes. *Proc Natl Acad Sci USA* 85:8756–8760, 1988.
49. Satoh H, Hashimoto K: Effects of α_1-adrenoceptor stimulation with methoxamine and phenylephrine on spontaneously beating rabbit sinoatrial node cells. *Naunyn-Schmeidebergs Arch Pharmacol* 337:415–422, 1988.
50. Ravens U, Wang XL, Wettauer E: Alpha adrenoceptor stimulation reduces outward currents in rat ventricular myocytes. *J Pharmacol Exp Ther* 250:364–370, 1989.
51. Lee JH, Rosen MR: Mechanism of α_1-adrenergic prolongation of canine Purkinje fiber action potentials (abstr). *Circulation* 1992, in press.
52. Bruckner R, Scholz M: Effects of α-adrenoceptor stimulation with phenylephrine in the presence of propranolol on force of contraction, slow inward current and cyclic AMP content in the bovine heart. *Br J Pharmacol* 82:223–232, 1984.
53. Endoh M: Myocardial α-adrenoceptors: Multiplicity of subcellular coupling processes. *Asia Pacific J Pharmacol* 6:171–188, 1991.
54. Lee JH, Steinberg SF, Rosen MR: A WB 4101-sensitive α_1-adrenergic receptor subtype modulates repolarization in canine Purkinje fibers. *J Pharmacol Exp Ther* 258:681–687, 1991.

CHAPTER 24

Mechanisms of Adrenergic and Cholinergic Regulation of Myocardial Contractility

JON P. LINDEMANN & AUGUST M. WATANABE

INTRODUCTION

The autonomic nervous system is the major system extrinsic to the heart that regulates myocardial contractility. This system can be subdivided on the basis of anatomy, functional effects, and neurotransmitters released from postganglionic nerves into two major divisions, sympathetic and parasympathetic nervous systems (fig. 24-1). In general, an increase in sympathetic nerve activity stimulates the heart (i.e., increases heart rate, conduction velocity through the specialized conducting tissues, and myocardial contractility), whereas augmentation of parasympathetic activity is inhibitory. The heart is innervated by sympathetic nerves and the vagus, which is the parasympathetic innervation. The neurotransmitter released from preganglionic nerves in both the sympathetic and parasympathetic nervous systems is acetylcholine. Norepinephrine is the neurotransmitter that is released from postganglionic sympathetic nerves that innervate the heart. The transmitter released from postanglionic parasympathetic (vagal) nerve endings is acetylcholine (fig. 24-1). Both norepinephrine and acetylcholine produce their effects locally in the immediate area into which they are released, that is, they function as neurotransmitters. Epinephrine is a catecholamine that is released from the adrenal medulla and travels via the circulation to the heart and thus functions as a hormone.

The sympathetic and parasympathetic nervous systems modify cardiac function by means of catecholamines and acetylcholine interacting with discrete proteins, referred to as receptors, located on the sarcolemma of cardiac cells (fig. 24-1). The receptors of the sympathetic nervous system have been broadly subdivided into alpha and beta, and both of these major types have been further subdivided into subclasses that have been designated α_1 and α_2, and β_1 and β_2. Norepinephrine stimulates alpha- and β_1-receptors; epinephrine stimulates alpha- and both subclasses of beta-receptors. Acetylcholine released from parasympathetic nerve endings interacts with muscarinic receptors.

In the intact animal or in conscious humans, the cardiac effects of activation of the autonomic nervous system are very complex and are dependent on multiple interrelating factors. Some of the most important of these factors are activation of reflexes, adrenergic-cholinergic interaction, and vascular effects. The nature and magnitude of interaction depend on how the autonomic nervous system is activated. For example, if the sympathetic nervous system is activated physiologically, such as by exercise, parasympathetic tone is likely to be reduced simultaneously, and activation of reflexes and adrenergic-cholinergic interaction may not be pronounced. On the other hand, if the sympathetic system is activated by administration of a drug, interaction of these modulatory factors becomes very important in determining the ultimate cardiovascular effect of the administered agent. If norepinephrine is infused into an intact animal or human being, it will activate β_1 receptors in the heart and also alpha-adrenergic receptors in the vasculature. The activation of alpha-adrenergic receptors will cause arteriolar vasoconstriction with resultant increases in peripheral vascular resistance and blood pressure. The norepinephrine-induced hypertension will cause activation of the baroreceptor reflex, with consequent increases in efferent vagal nerve activity. The resultant augmentation of acetylcholine stimulation of muscarinic receptors powerfully modulates the effects of the circulating norepinephrine, such that heart rate actually decreases rather than increases in response to β_1-receptor stimulation. Increases in myocardial contractility also are blunted. The vasoconstriction produced by alpha-adrenergic stimulation also modulates cardiac function because of the increased resistance to ventricular ejection (i.e., increased afterload). If the animal or subject is pretreated with atropine prior to the administration of norepinephrine, a pure sympathetic effect, free of cellular responses to activation of reflexes and adrenergic-cholinergic interaction, will be seen. In this situation, heart rate will increase and myocardial contractility will be augmented to a greater extent in response to the norepinephrine administration.

Thus, activation of reflexes, hemodynamic effects, and adrenergic-cholinergic interaction are very important factors in determining the cardiac response to autonomic stimulation. The sympathetic and parasympathetic nervous systems interact dynamically in a coordinated manner to regulate cardiac function. The highest level of interaction occurs in vasomotor regulatory centers in the brain, where afferent signals from the cardiovascular system are

N. Sperelakis (ed.), Physiology and Pathophysiology of the Heart, Third Edition.
© 1995 Kluwer Academic Publishers. ISBN 0-7923-2612-1. All rights reserved.

467

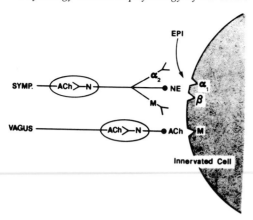

Fig. 24-1. Schematic representation of the relationship between sympathetic and vagal nerve terminals and the receptors with which their respective neurotransmitters interact. Acetylcholine (ACh) stimulates nicotinic (N) receptors in ganglia of both systems and muscarinic (M) receptors. Norepinephrine, released from sympathetic terminals and epinephrine (EPI), stimulate alpha₁ (α₁), alpha₂ (α₂), and beta (β) receptors. Symp = sympathetic.

received and processed, and efferent sympathetic and vagal nerve activities are regulated. In addition to this CNS level of integration, important interactions occur between the two systems at the level of the nerve terminals (fig. 24-1). Histological studies have shown that in some regions of the heart, terminals of sympathetic and vagal nerves are in apposition, one with the other. This physical relationship allows for interaction between the two systems at the nerve terminals. This interaction occurs both prejunctionally between nerves and postjunctionally at the level of membranes of innervated cells and within the cell. In the prejunctional level of interaction, acetylcholine released from parasympathetic nerve endings can stimulate muscarinic receptors on sympathetic terminals to inhibit release of norepinephrine (fig. 24-1) (for review, see Levy and Martin {1}). Thus vagal activity can modulate sympathetic effects by inhibiting norepinephrine release. In addition, stimulation of muscarinic receptors on the membranes of innervated cells can modulate the cellular response to norepinephrine that is released from sympathetic terminals and to circulating epinephrine.

This chapter discusses the cellular and subcellular mechanisms by which catecholamines and acetylocholine modify cardiac cell function and the cellular mechanisms of interaction between the sympathetic and parasympathetic nervous systems.

BETA-ADRENERGIC RECEPTORS

Evidence from both classical pharmacology experiments as well as radioligand studies suggests that there are both β₁- and β₂-adrenergic receptors in the heart (for reviews, see {2–4}). More recently, genes encoding for a third type of beta-adrenergic receptor have been described. This

receptor, termed the *β₃-adrenergic receptor*, does not appear to exist in human heart based on analysis of mRNA expression {5,6}. Moreover, the positive chronotropic effects of putative β₃-adrenergic selective agonists have been shown to be mediated by baroreflex mechanisms {7}.

There are important species differences in the relative amounts of the two beta-adrenergic receptor subtypes (β₁ and β₂) in ventricular myocardium. In most mammalian species, left ventricular beta-adrenergic receptors are predominantly (rabbit, cat, dog, human) or exclusively (rat, guinea pig) of the β₁ subtype {3}. By contrast, in the frog heart, nearly 80% of beta-adrenergic receptors are β₂ {9}. The ratio of β₁ to β₂ receptors also shows regional variation within the heart. Evidence from several pharmacologic studies using agonists with different selectivities for β₁ and β₂ receptors have shown that β₂-selective agonists produce a more prominent chronotropic than inotropic effect, whereas β₁-selective drugs produce equivalent inotropic and chronotropic effects {10}. These results were interpreted to indicate an increased proportion of β₂ receptors in the sinus node compared to the ventricular myocardium. More recently it was found that whereas β₂ receptors comprised only 25% of the total number of beta-adrenergic receptors in dog right atrium, they accounted fro 50% of the electrophysiologic (shortening of action potential duration) of catecholamines {11}. These results further support a role for β₂ receptors in mediating the electrophysiologic (and chronotropic?) effects of beta-adrenergic agonists in the atrium.

Beta-adrenergic receptors are located in the sarcolemma of myocardial cells. It became possible to prove this after the development of methods for preparing highly purified sarcolemma and internal membrane systems (including sarcoplasmic reticulum) from the heart {2,12,13}. By comparing the distribution of beta-adrenergic receptors with the distribution of marker enzymes known to be localized to sarcolemma, sarcoplasmic reticulum, and mitochondria, it was shown that beta receptors reside only on sarcolemma.

Studies with radiolabeled ligands have revealed differences in the molecular interactions of agonists and antagonists with beta-adrenergic receptors. The difference in the nature of agonist and antagonist binding is observed by analysis of the effects of guanine nucleotides on agonist competition curves. Addition of guanine nucleotides (GTP or Gpp[NH]p) to the assay medium decreases the affinity of beta-receptors for agonists without changing the affinity for agonists (fig. 24-2 and table 24-1) {2–4}. Partial agonists are affected in an intermediate manner proportional to their activity as agonists. This observation that was made originally in model systems subsequently has been extended to a variety of other tissues including heart (fig. 24-2 and table 24-1). In terms of their interaction with agonists, beta receptors can exist in two states {2–4}. Receptors in membranes depleted of guanine nucleotides exist in both high- and low-affinity states {2–4}. This coexistence of two affinity states of the receptor is manifested in radioligand binding studies as shallow agonist competition curves, nonlinear Scatchard plots, and slope factors less than unity (fig. 24-2 and table 24-1). The

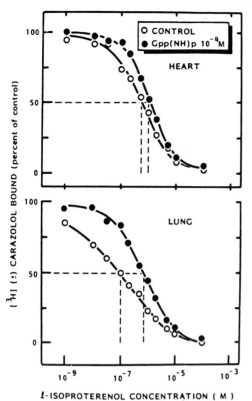

addition of exogenous guanine nucleotides to such preparations is thought to convert a majority (or all) of the receptors into a single low-affinity state, thus transforming the agonist competition curve to a form with a steeper slope and shifting the dissociation constants to higher values (lower affinity; fig. 24-2 and table 24-1) {2–4}. The data in fig. 24-2 are from cardiac membranes (panel A), which generally demonstrate only a small guanine-nucleotide-induced shift in slope and affinity, and lung (panel B). Although in heart the change in receptor affinity for agonists is small compared to that seen in some other systems, these changes are consistent and reproducible. Antagonist competition curves are always steep and uniphasic, regardless of the presence or obsence of guanine nucleotides, and these curves are not altered by the addition of guanine nucleotides (fig. 24-3 and table 24-1). The agonist-specific two-state receptor conformation appears to be an in vitro manifestation of receptor changes induced by agents with intrinsic activity, these changes resulting under appropriate conditions in activation of adenylate cyclase {3,4,8}. It is postulated that beta-receptor agonists can induce a high-affinity state of receptor, resulting in a receptor-agonist complex that then interacts with a third component, a coupling protein. This ternary complex of hormone, receptor, and coupling protein then interacts with regulatory guanine nucleotides, which leads to a return of the receptor to a low-affinity state and dissociation of the hormone-receptor complex, and at the same time activation of adenylate cyclase {3,4,8}. Antagonists (agents without intrinsic activity) cannot induce the high-affinity state and also do not activate adenylate cyclase. This concept is discussed in more detail in later sections of this chapter.

Beta-adrenergic receptors in the heart are not static but rather dynamic entities whose properties can change in response to physiologic stress, disease states, or administration of drugs {2–4}. The most readily detected and widely studied dynamic property of beta receptors is their density in plasma membranes. The number of beta receptors appears to vary according to the magnitude of their stimulation. As a broad generalization, the density of beta-receptors increases when stimulation is low (called *upregulation*) and decreases when stimulation is high (called *downregulation*) {2–4}. These changes in receptor

Fig. 24-2. Curves describing competition of l-isoproterenol with [^{3}H] (±) carazolol for binding to beta-adrenergic receptors in canine heart (upper panel) and lung (lower panel) membranes: ○—○, no added guanine nucleotide, ●—●, 10^{-4}M added Gpp(NH)p. Note that in both heart and lung membranes, addition of Gpp(NH)p shifts the isoproterenol competition curve to a steeper slope (slope factor shift from 0.73 to 0.86 in heart and 0.42 to 0.74 in lung) and lower affinity (K_d change from 0.17 to 0.29 μM in heart and 0.026 to 0.23 μM in lung). Because the curve in the absence of Gpp(NH)p was more shallow in lung than in heart, the guanine-nucleotide-induced shift is greater in the former than in the latter.

Table 24-1. Effect of guanine nucleotides on interaction of beta-adrenergic receptors with the antagonist propranolol and catecholamines

Drug	Slope factor		K_D	
	−Gpp(NH)p	+Gpp(NH)p	−Gpp(NH)p	+Gpp(NH)p
l-Propranolol	0.91	0.91	5.80	5.60
l-Isoproterenol	0.73	0.86	0.17	0.29
l-Epinephrine	0.81	0.90	3.30	4.70
l-Norepinephrine	0.76	0.82	2.20	3.20

Values are means from three to nine experiments. K_d for propranolol × 10^{-9}M and for catecholamines × 10^{-6}M.

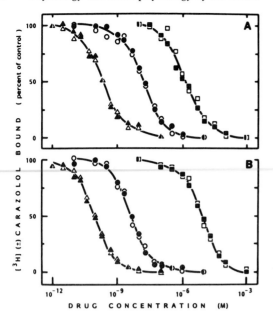

Fig. 24-3. Competition of beta-adrenergic antagonists with [³H](±)carazolol for binding to beta-adrenergic receptors present in membrane vesicles derived from canine ventricular myocardium (**A**) and canine lung (**B**); S(−)carazolol (△▲); (−)propranolol, (○●); (±)metoprolo (□■). Presence (filled symbols) or absence (unfilled symbols) of 0.1 μM Gpp(HN)p has no effect on the position or configuration of antagonist-radioligand competition curves. Reprinted with permission from Manalan et al. {193}.

density are one of what are probably multiple alterations that may occur in an organ that renders it either desensitized or supersensitized to catecholamine stimulation. Alterations in receptor density may occur with physiologic variations in sympathetic activity. For example, reductions in sympathetic nerve activity in humans by increasing sodium intake from 100 to 400 mEq daily resulted in a 50% increase in leukocyte beta-adrenergic receptors {14}. The functional significance of these changes in receptor density was suggested by the observation that the subject's sensitivity to the positive chronotropic effects of isoproterenol was also increased {14}. Reductions in the number of beta-adrenergic receptors in failing human myocardium obtained just prior to transplantation have also been reported {15}, a situation commonly associated with increased levels of circulating catecholamines {16}. More recent studies have shown that the reduction in beta-adrenergic receptor number in failing myocardium is due to a reduction in the number of β_1 receptors, with the number of β_2 receptors remaining unchanged {17}. Changes in receptor density may also occur in response to drugs {3}. Drugs that diminish beta-receptor stimulation by destroying sympathetic nerves and/or depleting catecholamine stores (e.g., 6-hydroxydopamine and guanethidine) cause upregulation. On the other hand, chronic pharmacologic stimulation of beta receptors causes a reduction in receptor density.

Beta-receptor density also changes with certain disease states. The most extensively studied such association is that seen with abnormal thyroid states. Patients with hyperthyroidism exhibit signs of a hyperactive sympathetic nervous system, whereas patients with hypothyroidism appear just the opposite. For example, hyperthyroid patients commonly have tachycardia, increased cardiac output, and tremulousness. Hypothyroid patients have bradycardia. Animal studies have shown that in hyperthyroidism the density of beta-adrenergic receptors is increased by 50–100%, whereas in hypothyroidism the density of beta-adrenergic receptors is reduced modestly {18,19}. The reduction in beta-adrenergic number in hypothyroidism produced by thyroidectomy is accompanied by a reduction in the expression of mRNA for both the β_1- and β_2-receptor subtypes, and is reversible by administration of thyroxin {20}. Clinical studies have shown that administration of triiodothyronine to normal subjects leads to an increase in density of beta-adrenergic receptors in leukocytes {21}. Thus, beta-receptor density in the heart is related to thyroid state, and changes in the receptors may explain, at least partially, the cardiovascular changes that accompany altered thyroid status.

Mechanisms underlying beta-adrenergic receptor desensitization have recently been elucidated (for review, see {22}). Homologous desensitization of beta receptors occurs in response to beta-adrenergic stimulation and results in decreased responsiveness of the tissue or cell type to beta-adrenergic agonists, but not other agonists linked to adenylate cyclase. Recent studies have shown that this form of desensitization is associated with phosphorylation of the beta-adrenergic agonist-receptor complex by a cAMP-independent protein kinase activity {23}. This phosphorylation results in the inability of the receptor to stimulate adenylate cyclase activity {23}. Subsequently, the phosphorylated receptor is "internalized" and is no longer accessible to agonists at the cell surface {22}. An actual loss of beta-adrenergic receptors (downregulation, in contrast to internalization of receptors described) may be mediated by intracellular modification of the internalized receptors, requiring protein synthesis of new receptors to regain responsiveness. Beta-adrenergic receptors may also be phosphorylated by other protein kinase activities, such as cAMP-dependent protein kinase and protein kinase C. Phosphorylation of beta-adrenergic receptors by cAMP-dependent protein kinase may play a role in heterologous desensitization, a condition in which responsiveness of adenylate cyclase to other stimulatory receptors is diminished {22}. Whether such mechanisms are operative in myocardium remains to be established.

Beta-adrenergic receptors belong to a class of membrane receptors linked to guanine nucleotide binding proteins (G proteins; for reviews, see {24,25}). It is now clear that the interaction of the beta-agonist-receptor complex with G proteins results in the modification of cellular function by two broad mechanisms: activation of adenylate cyclase or direct interaction of proteins with sarcolemmal ion channels. The mechanisms and consequences of the adenylate cyclase/cAMP pathway are discussed in detail in ensuing sections. Direct interactions between G proteins and sarcolemmal ion channels are discussed in other chapters of this book.

ADENYLATE CYCLASE

Hormone-regulated adenylate cyclase is comprised of at least three major units: receptors such as beta-adrenergic receptors, a catalytic unit that catalyzes the conversion of ATP to cyclic AMP (cAMP), and a guanine nucleotide binding protein (G protein), which couples the receptor to the catalytic unit. The details of the biochemistry and molecular biology of adenylate cyclase have been elucidated primarily in nonmammalian model systems (for general reviews of adenylate cyclase, see {4,8,27}). However, most of the properties of the enzyme described in these systems appear to hold true also for myocardial adenylate cyclase {28}. Adenylate cyclase is located in sarcolemma, as are beta receptors, and not in internal membranes such as sarcoplasmic reticulum {26}.

It is now clearly established that adenylate cyclase can be regulated in both a stimulatory and inhibitory manner, and that there are neurotransmitter and hormone receptors that can inhibit as well as those that can stimulate the enzyme {29–31}. α_2- and muscarinic receptors interact with the enzyme in a manner that leads to inhibition of activity {30,32}. A growing body of experimental evidence now suggests that the effects of stimulatory and inhibitory agonists on adenylate cyclase activity are mediated by the G proteins {4,8,27}.

Of the multiple G proteins described {33}, at least three major types of G proteins have been identified in myocardium {34}. G_s mediates the effects of stimulatory receptors, whereas G_i mediates the effects of inhibitory receptors. G_o (for other or unknown function) may be involved in mediating receptor modulation of inositol-containing phospholipid hydrolysis (see below). All four types are heterotrimers, comprised of alpha (α), beta (β), and gamma (γ) subunits. Differences between the three types reside in the α subunit. $G_s\alpha$ (α_s) has a molecular weight of 45 kDa, whereas $G_i\alpha$ (α_i) has a molecular weight of 41 kDa and $G_o\alpha$ has a molecular weight of 35 kDa. The β (35 kDa) and γ (8–10 kDa) subunits appear to be tightly coupled as a $\beta\gamma$ subunit. The α subunits also differ with respect to their ability of be ADP ribosylated by bacterial toxins (for review, see {35}). α_s is ADP ribosylated at a specific arginine residue in the presence of cholera toxin, whereas α_i and α_o are ADP ribosylated at asparagine residues by islet-activating protein, one of the pertussis toxins. ADP ribosylation of the α subunits results in a change in the affinity of the α subunits for $\beta\gamma$. The functional consequences of these changes in affinity are discussed below.

Reconstitution experiments utilizing purified stimulatory receptors, G proteins, and the catalyst of adenylate cyclase have yielded considerable insight into the molecular mechanisms of hormonal regulation of the catalytic activity of adenylate cyclase (fig. 24-4; for review, see {25}). The beta-agonist-receptor complex (β-R_β) binds to α_s and is associated with displacement of GDP by GTP from the guanine nucleotide binding site. The binding of GTP to α_s promotes the dissociation of α_s from $\beta\gamma$ (or activation of the G_s holoprotein). This activation results in the stimulation of the catalytic activity of adenylate cyclase. The nucleotide binding site possesses GTPase activity, which in the presence of the agonist-receptor-complex results in the hydrolysis of the bound GTP to GDP and a reduction of the stimulatory effect of α_s (or G_s) on the catalyst. α_s-GDP has a higher affinity for $\beta\gamma$, resulting in the reassociation of the heterotrimer. In a similar manner, binding of an appropriate agonist on inhibitory receptors (e.g., muscarinic) results in the dissociation of α_i from $\beta\gamma$. The

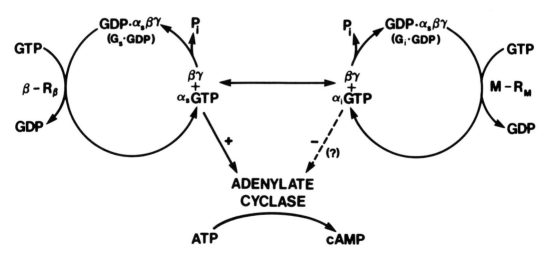

Fig. 24-4. Schematic representation of hypothetical mechanism by which G proteins mediate hormonal regulation of adenylate cyclase activity.

βγ complex appears to mediate inhibition of adenylate cyclase activity, presumably by association with α_s to form the inactive heterotrimer {36}. Whether direct interaction of α_i with adenylate cyclase occurs under physiologic conditions is unknown.

As mentioned previously, the α subunits of both G_s and G_i may be covalently modified by ADP ribosylation in the presence of specific bacterial toxins {35}. ADP ribosylation of α_s by cholera toxin results in inhibition of the GTPase activity and a reduction in the affinity of α_s for βγ. Thus, GTP remains bound to α_s, resulting in persistent activation of adenylate cyclase activity. By contrast, pertussis toxin-catalyzed ADP-ribosylation of α_i results in an increased affinity of α_i for βγ, promoting reassociation of α_i with βγ. The physiologic consequence of the effect of ADP ribosylation of G_i is abolition of the effects of inhibitory receptor stimulation on adenylate cyclase activity mediated by G_i.

As in most systems studied, guanine nucleotides are necessary for regulation of adenylate cyclase activity in the heart {37}. In cardiac membranes, guanine nucleotides themselves can stimulate enzyme activity (fig. 24-5). In addition, guanine nucleotides are required for hormonal regulation of enzyme activity. Catecholamines do not stimulate the enzyme unless guanine nucleotides (either

GTP or nonhydrolyzable analogues) are present (fig. 24-5) {27}. In like manner, GTP must be present for expression of muscarinic inhibition of cardiac adenylate cyclase activity {37}. Unlike beta-receptor stimulation of activity, which can occur in the presence of GTP or nonhydrolyzable analogues of GTP, muscarinic inhibition of the enzyme occurs only when GTP is the guanine nucleotide present (fig. 24-5) {27}. If nonhydrolyzable analogues are used, muscarinic inhibition of the enzyme does not occur (fig. 24-5) {27}. The selective effect of inhibitory stimuli (such as muscarinic agonists) on GTP-stimulated activity presumably arises from the fact that binding of nonhydrolyzable analogues of GTP result in a persistent reduction of the affinity of α_s for βγ and thereby sustained activation of adenylate cyclase.

Thus cardiac muscle sarcolemma contains both stimulatory (beta-adrenergic) and inhibitory (muscarinic) receptors, which interact with G proteins. When stimulatory or inhibitory receptors are activated by their respective agonists, the activity of the catalytic unit is either increased or reduced, this change in enzyme activity being mediated by the appropriate G protein (G_s or G_i). Intracellular cAMP levels then either increase or decrease.

Intracellular cAMP levels are controlled by the activity of two enzymes: adenylate cyclase and phosphodiesterase

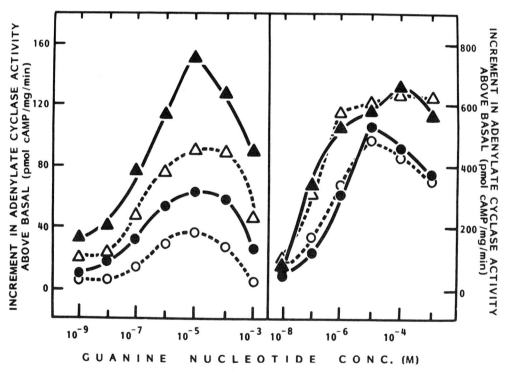

Fig. 24-5. Guanine nucleotide stimulation of adenylate cyclase activity in canine cardiac membrane vesicles. The guanine nucleotide added was GTP in the **left panel** and Gpp(NH)p in the **right panel**. Circles are values with guanine nucleotides alone and triangles with guanine nucleotides plus 10^{-7} M isoproterenol. Unfilled symbols designate the presence of 10^{-5} M methacholine in addition to guanine nucleotide alone or with isoproterenol. Note that methacholine significantly inhibits GTP or GTP plus isoproterenol activation of adenylate cyclase (left panel), but does not affect adenylate cyclase activity when the guanine nucleotide added is Gpp(NH)p (right panel).

(fig. 24-4). The latter enzyme converts cAMP into 5'-AMP, acting to restore cellular levels of the cyclic nucleotide to prestimulation values. There is as yet no direct evidence that activation of autonomic receptors alters the activity of phosphodiesterase in myocardium, but inhibition of this enzyme is a well-known important mechanism of action of certain drugs, most notably methylxanthines. Some of the new nonglycoside, non-catecholamine-positive inotropic agents, such as amrinone, may produce part of their contractile effects by inhibiting phosphodiesterase, thereby increasing tissue levels of cAMP.

PROTEIN PHOSPHORYLATION

cAMP-dependent protein kinase

When cAMP is increased within myocardial cells by the increased catalytic activity of adenylate cyclase, it then produces its effects on cellular function by interacting with another protein called cAMP-dependent protein kinase (for a review see {38}). This enzyme exists in sarcolemma as well as in soluble form in the cytosol. cAMP-dependent protein kinase is an enzyme that is composed of two units, which are referred to as the *regulatory* and *catalytic subunits*. When cAMP-dependent protein kinase exists as a holoenzyme, it is not catalytically active. The regulatory subunit is a receptor for cAMP, so that when cAMP is increased within the cell, it binds to the regulatory subunit, and this interaction then causes the regulatory and catalytic subunits to dissociate. When the catalytic subunit is released from the regulatory subunit, it becomes catalytically active and catalyzes the transfer of the terminal phosphate of ATP to various proteins within the myocardial cell. This phosphorylation results in a conformational change, which alters the properties of the protein in such a manner that its interaction with ions (i.e., Ca^{2+}) or other proteins is altered, and thus the functional properties of the heart are modified.

Evidence has been accumulated to show that cAMP-dependent protein kinase is compartmented within the myocardial cells: One portion of the total cellular protein kinase is associated with the particulate fractions (membranes) and the other with the cytosol {39}. Subsequent studies have shown that the membrane-bound cAMP-dependent protein kinase is located in the sarcolemma {12}. Since adenylate cyclase and beta-adrenergic receptors are located in the sarcolemma, it follows that in response to beta-adrenergic stimulation the sarcolemmal kinase might be activated prior to the cytosolic protein kinase activity. In both isolated perfused hearts {40} and isolated adult myocytes {41}, it has been shown that beta-adrenergic stimulation results in an increase in cAMP and a decrease in cAMP-dependent protein kinase in the particulate fraction. The decrease in particulate kinase activity was interpreted to indicate dissociation of the regulatory and catalytic subunits of cAMP-dependent protein kinase and diffusion of the catalytic subunits into the cytosol. By contrast, PGE_1, while increasing cytosolic

cAMP levels and the activity of soluble cAMP-dependent protein kinase activity, did not alter levels of either of these parameters in the particulate fraction, nor did the prostaglandin result in activation of glycogen phosphorylase or a positive inotropic effect {40,41}. These results suggest, therefore, that activation of sarcolemmal cAMP-dependent protein kinase is essential for mediating the cAMP-dependent cellular effects of beta-adrenergic stimulation.

The specific functional responses are determined by the proteins phosphorylated and their intracellular location. Various cytosolic and intrinsic membrane proteins in cardiac muscle have been shown in vitro to be substrates of cAMP-dependent protein kinase. Two broad classes of myocardial proteins are thought to play potential roles in the regulation of myocardial contractility. The first group is the contractile regulatory proteins, including the inhibitory subunit of troponin (TnI) and protein C. The second class includes membrane proteins located in the sarcolemma and sarcoplasmic reticulum, which are postulated to regulate transmembrane Ca influxes. In the ensuing sections, evidence for reversible phosphorylation of these proteins playing a role in the physiologic regulation of myocardial contractility will be considered.

Contractile proteins

Troponin-I (TnI) is a component of troponin, one of the regulatory proteins of the myofibrillar contractile protein complex. It has been shown that TnI can be phosphorylated by cAMP-dependent protein kinase in vitro or in intact myocardial preparations exposed to beta-adrenergic agonists {42}. The onset and development of increased contractile state correlated with phosphorylation of TnI, but the reversal of these processes could be dissociated {43}. Upon removal of catecholamines, TnI remained phosphorylated while contractile force returned to control values. Other agents (ouabain, increased Ca^{2+}, X537A) or maneuvers (reduced Na^+ in perfusion medium, Treppe) that produced positive inotropic effects but did not elevate cAMP levels did not cause phosphorylation of TnI {43}. Stimulation of TnI phosphorylation in intact myocardium is mediated by the particulate cAMP-dependent protein kinase activity {44}.

The functional significance of TnI phosphorylation has been suggested by in vitro studies. These studies have shown that cAMP-dependent phosphorylation of TnI results in reduced Ca^{2+} sensitivity of actomyosin ATPase activity {45}. This reduction is mediated by an increase in the rate of Ca^{2+} dissociation from the Ca^{2+} specific binding site of troponin-C in reconstituted whole cardiac troponin {45}. Computer modeling of the effect of TnI phosphorylation on the time course of Ca^{2+} binding to cardiac troponin indicated that this change was sufficient to account for the relaxant, but not the positive intropic effects of beta-adrenergic stimulation. It appears, therefore, that phosphorylation of TnI may be involved in the relaxant, but not the inotropic effects of beta-adrenergic stimulation. Since there are additional potential mechanisms for the relaxant effects of beta-adrenergic agonists in the myocardium (see below), the extent to which TnI phosphorylation is involved in this effect remains unknown.

C-protein is a 155–165 kDa protein associated with the thick filament of striated muscle. Although its function is not clearly defined, studies in intact tissue systems have shown that it is phosphorylated in response to beta-adrenergic stimulation of mammalian {46} and amphibian myocardium {47}. In both instances, phosphorylation of C protein was correlated with the positive inotropic effects of catecholamines. More recently, it has been shown that the time course of phosphorylation of C protein in amphibian myocardium is more closely paralleled by alterations in myocardial relaxation rather than the inotropic effects of beta-adrenergic stimulation {48}. In vitro studies have shown that this protein is a substrate of cAMP-dependent protein kinase, as well as a Ca^{2+}/calmodulin-dependent protein kinase activity, which copurifies with C protein in this preparation {49}. Further, phosphorylation of C protein by cAMP-dependent protein kinase attenuates the stimulation of actin-activated myosin ATPase activity by C protein {49}. This observation has led to the speculation that C-protein phosphorylation might affect relaxation by altering the interaction between actin and myosin {49}, presumably resulting in a decrease in the V_{max} of myosin ATPase activity. However, it recently has been shown that beta-adrenergic agonists result in stimulation of actin-activated ATPase activity in intact myocardial preparations {50}. Thus, what role phosphorylation of C protein plays in mediating the contractile effects of beta-adrenergic stimulation in intact myocardium remains to be established.

Sarcoplasmic reticulum proteins

In vitro studies on the role of phosphorylation in regulating sarcoplasmic reticulum function revealed that a major substrate for cAMP-dependent protein kinase was a 22 kDa protein, which appeared to be intrinsic to the sarcoplasmic reticulum membranes {51,52}. It was shown that addition of cAMP to sarcoplasmic reticulum membranes, with or without exogenous cAMP-dependent protein kinase, resulted in phosphorylation of this 22 kDa protein and, associated with this, increased Ca^{2+}-ATPase activity {50,51}. This protein, termed *phospholamban*, has been demonstrated to regulate the Ca^{2+} transport activity of sarcoplasmic reticulum {52}.

Phospholamban is a homopentameric protein, composed of five identical monomers, each containing specific phosphorylation sites for cAMP-dependent and Ca/calmodulin-dependent protein kinase activities {53–55}. Additional evidence has been obtained to support a role for cAMP-dependent phosphorylation of phospholamban in regulating sarcoplasmic reticulum Ca transport. Slow skeletal muscle, as does cardiac muscle, demonstrates increased rates of relaxation in response to beta-adrenergic stimulation, whereas fast skeletal muscle does not. Pretreatment of sarcoplasmic reticulum from slow, but not fast, skeletal muscle with cAMP-dependent protein kinase results in phosphorylation of phospholamban and stimulation of Ca transport {51}. These results suggest that phospholamban phosphorylation and stimulation of Ca

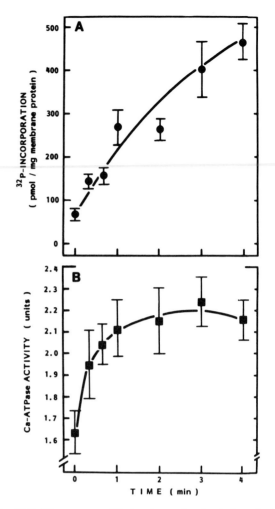

Fig. 24-6. Time course of beta-adrenergic stimulation of phospholamban phosphorylation (**A**) and Ca^{2+}-ATPase activity (**B**) in guinea pig ventricles. Hearts were perfused with buffer containing 1.1–1.8 mCi $^{32}P_i$ for 30 minutes. Isoproterenol was then administered by continuous infusion and hearts were frozen at the times indicated. Membrane vesicles were prepared and divided into aliquots for SDS-polyacrylamide gel electrophoresis or assay of Ca^{2+}-ATPase activity. After autoradiography, ^{32}P-incorporation into phospholamban was quantified by counting the radioactivity in the bands from the dried gel and dividing by the specific radioactivity of $[\gamma^{32}P]$ ATP determined for each heart. Values are mean ± SEM for 3–15 hearts. Reprinted with permission from Lindemann et al. {60}.

transport may mediate the relaxant effects of beta-adrenergic stimulation in slow skeletal muscle. The most direct evidence for a role of phospholamban phosphorylation in the regulation of sarcoplasmic reticulum Ca transport in mammalian myocardium is the observation that monoclonal antibodies to phospholamban inhibit cAMP-dependent stimulation of Ca transport in vitro {56}. More recent studies have shown that purified phospholamban forms Ca^{2+} channels in planar lipid bilayers {57}.

Several laboratories have demonstrated that phospholamban can be phosphorylated in intact hearts {58–60}. This phosphorylation occurs rapidly (within 20 seconds of onset of catecholamine infusion) and occurs with low concentrations of drug, as low as 3 nM isoproterenol (fig. 24-6A) {60}. Ca^{2+}-ATPase activity of the same sarcoplasmic reticulum vesicles in which phospholamban is phosphorylated (i.e., sarcoplasmic reticulum isolated from intact ventricles) is increased in a time and concentration dependence that parallels the time and concentration dependence of phospholamban phosphorylation (fig. 24-6B) {60}. Phospholamban phosphorylation and Ca^{2+}-ATPase activity closely parallel the onset and development of changes in relaxation parameters (i.e., reduction in $t_{1/2}$ of relaxation), leading to the hypothesis that phospholamban phosphorylation mediated the relaxant effects of beta-adrenergic stimulation {60}. These studies have been confirmed and extended in experiments with isolated myocytes in which beta-adrenergic stimulation was shown to enhance the rate of decay of Ca^{2+} transients {61}. This effect of beta-adrenergic stimulation was markedly attenuated by intracellular dialysis with antibodies raised to a peptide corresponding to the sequence of the cytoplasmic domain of phospholamban. (Studies with purified sarcoplasmic reticulum reveal that these antibodies maximally stimulate the rate of Ca^{2+} uptake). Loading the cells with antibodies alone markedly enhanced the rate of decline in the Ca^{2+} transients. Moreover, antibody loading also attenuated the increase in the peak Ca^{2+} transient while having no effect on I_{Ca} enhanced by beta-adrenergic stimulation. In that the peak Ca^{2+} transient was maximally stimulated in cells dialyzed with antibody, the failure of beta-adrenergic agonists to increase the Ca^{2+} transient further suggests that the peak Ca^{2+} transient is due in large part to release of Ca from sarcoplasmic reticulum {61}. These findings provide strong evidence that the positive inotropic effects of beta-adrenergic stimulation may be mediated by enhanced sarcoplasmic reticulum Ca^{2+} transport as a result of phosphorylation of phospholamban.

In isolated membrane vesicles, phospholamban is phosphorylated by a Ca^{2+}/calmodulin-dependent protein kinase activity, in addition to cAMP-dependent protein kinase {62–64}. Beta-adrenergic stimulation of phosphorylation of phospholamban in intact myocardium occurs at both cAMP- and Ca^{2+}/calmodulin dependent sites {65,72}. Interestingly, phosphorylation of these adjacent amino acid residues (serine 16 and threonine 17 for cAMP- and Ca^{2+}-calmodulin dependent kinases, respectively) appears to occur sequentially. The cAMP-dependent site is always phosphorylated prior to the Ca^{2+}/calmodulin-dependent site, suggesting that cAMP-dependent phosphorylation is essential for phosphorylation of the Ca^{2+}/calmodulin-dependent site {65}.

Sarcolemmal proteins

Beta-adrenergic stimulation may modulate a number of sarcolemmal ion currents, including Ca^{2+} {66,67}, K^+ {68}, Na^+ {69,70}, and Cl^- {71} currents. Additional experimental evidence has shown that beta-adrenergic modulation of ion currents are mediated by both direct and indirect mechanisms. These mechanisms include a direct interaction between G_s ($G_{s\alpha}$) and sarcolemmal ion channels, and indirect modification of ion channels by cAMP-dependent protein phosphorylation. Direct regulation is discussed elsewhere in this volume.

Functional studies strongly suggest that one of the subcellular mechanisms by which catecholamines modify cardiac function is by causing phosphorylation of Ca^{2+} channels (I_{Ca}) {72}. The role of cAMP-dependent mechanisms in mediating beta-adrenergic stimulation of I_{Ca} was first examined by studying so-called slow responses induced by various inotropic agents {73}. Intact cardiac tissue can be rendered inexcitably by inactivation of fast Na^+ channels, for example, by depolarization, administration of high concentrations of tetrodotoxin, or administration of buffer containing zero Na^+. Restoration of excitability in these tissues is mediated by increases in I_{Ca} and occurred in response to agents that increase cAMP levels {73}. This restoration can be blocked by Ca^{2+} antagonists, which do not alter catecholamine-induced elevation of cAMP levels. cAMP levels in these same hearts were increased by agents that induced slow responses (catecholamines, histamine, phosphodiesterase inhibitors, dibutyryl cAMP) {73}. Presumably agents that elevate cAMP levels increase I_{Ca} by causing phosphorylation of a protein component of sarcolemmal Ca^{2+} channels {74}. Voltage-clamp studies have also suggested that catecholamines produce part of their effects by causing phosphorylation of I_{Ca} channels. Direct administration of cAMP or analogues to cardiac fibers caused increases in I_{Ca} measured by voltage-clamp techniques {75}. Similar effects are observed in response to intracellular injection of the nonhydrolyzable analog of GTP, Gpp(NH)p, and cholera toxin (which activates adenylate cyclase) {76}.

The most direct evidence for cAMP-dependent protein phosphorylation in mediating beta-adrenergic effects on sarcolemmal Ca^{2+} channels in mammalian ventricular myocardium has come from analysis of Ca^{2+} channels in single cells {75}. Using this approach it was shown that in mammalian {77,78} and frog {79} ventricular myocytes that the intracellular injection of the catalytic subunit of cAMP-dependent protein kinase increased I_{Ca}. Subsequent studies have shown that the effects of intracellular addition of the catalytic subunit of cAMP-dependent protein kinase were not additive with those of extracellular isoproterenol or intracellular cAMP application, suggesting that all of these maneuvers acted by the same mechanism {80}. Additional studies have shown that the effects of isoproterenol can be inhibited by intracellular dialysis with the protein kinase inhibitor or the regulatory subunit of cAMP-dependent protein kinase {81}, or with a phosphoprotein phosphatase {82}. Substantial evidence exists, therefore, to suggest that sarcolemmal Ca^{2+} channels are another subcellular site that is modified by catecholamines to effect functional changes, and that this modification involves protein phosphorylation {74,75}.

In vitro studies using purified sarcolemmal preparations have revealed a number of sarcolemmal substrates for cAMP-dependent protein kinase (for review, see {83}). However, which of these multiple substrates mediates the effects of beta-adrenergic stimulation on I_{Ca} remains unknown. The most predominant sarcolemmal substrate of cAMP-dependent protein kinase is a 15-kDa protein {13,83}. However, cardiac sarcolemmal dihydropyridine receptors (putative sarcolemmal Ca^{2+} channels) purified by affinity chromatography do not contain a 15-kDa peptide {84}. Moreover, the molar stoichiometry of cAMP-dependent phosphorylation of the 15-kDa protein exceeds that of dihydropyridine receptors by at least an order of magnitude, further suggesting that the 15-kDa protein is not a component of sarcolemmal Ca^{2+} channels {83}. In all of the aforementioned physiological studies, the effects of beta-adrenergic stimulation or cAMP-dependent protein kinase were considered to suggest direct phosphorylation of sarcolemmal Ca^{2+} channels. These studies do not, however, exclude the possibility that these effects are not mediated by phosphorylation of a protein that is not a component of the Ca^{2+} channel and that modifies the Ca^{2+} channel by protein-protein interaction.

Studies conducted to determine sarcolemmal substrates of cAMP-dependent protein kinase in intact myocardial preparations have been reported {83}. Phosphorylation of either 27-kDa or 24-kDa proteins in perfused rat hearts have been correlated temporally with the positive inotropic effect of isoproterenol {85,86}. However, studies using membrane vesicles highly enriched in sarcolemma have shown that these substrates are intrinsic to the sarcoplasmic reticulum {83}. Additional studies have shown that beta-adrenergic stimulation of guinea pig ventricles results in the phosphorylation of a 15-kDa protein that is distinct from phospholamban and is localized to the cytoplasmic surface of the sarcolemma {87}. Phosphorylation of this protein was closely correlated with the inotropic effect of isoproterenol, whereas phosphorylation of phospholamban was delayed and correlated more closely with the relaxant effects of isoproterenol (fig. 24-7). Subsequent studies have shown that phosphorylation of this protein by either alpha- or beta-adrenergic agonists was associated with restoration of contractions in a 25-mM K^+-depolarized slow response model in perfused rat hearts ({88}, see below).

The 15-kDa protein has been cloned and sequenced {89}. The protein, named *phospholemman*, has a highly charged cytoplasmic domain, which contains phosphorylation sites for both cAMP-dependent protein kinase and protein kinase C. Incorporation of phospholemman mRNA into *Xenopus* oocytes results in the expression of Cl^--selective current, with differs from other reported cardiac Cl^- currents and is not sensitive to Ca^{2+} {90}. Although phospholemman appears to be an ion channel rather than a modulatory protein, the mechanism by which phosphorylation of phospholemman alters sarcolemmal ion currents in heart remains to be established.

Phosphorylation of all of the foregoing proteins discussed is reversed by the action of phosphoprotein phosphatases, which remove the phosphate and thereby return the protein to its basal state. Thus far there is no direct evidence that neurotransmitters or hormones can regulate

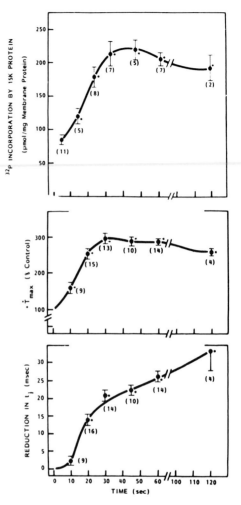

Fig. 24-7. Time course of the effects of 100 nM isoproterenol on phosphorylation of the 15-kDa sarcolemmal protein and contractile parameters in isolated perfused guinea pig ventricles. ^{32}P-perfused ventricles were exposed to isoproterenol for the indicated times, freeze clamped, and sarcolemmal vesicles were prepared two identically treated hearts. ^{32}P-incorporation into the 15-kDa protein was assessed in sarcolemmal vesicles as described for phospholamban in fig. 24-6. **Top**, ^{32}P incorporation into the 15-kDa protein; **middle**, maximal rate of developed tension ($+T_{max}$); **bottom**, reduction in time from peak tension to half-relaxation ($t_{1/2}$). Reprinted with permission from Presti et al. {87}.

phosphoprotein phosphatase activities and thereby influence protein phosphorylation in myocardium. However, such a mechanism of action is an attractive hypothesis for certain antiadrenergic agents, such as muscarinic agonists. This will be discussed in detail in later sections.

To summarize this section, it seems likely that agents that increase cellular cAMP levels, such as catecholamines, alter myocardial cell function by causng phosphorylation of proteins. Several proteins that have been shown in intact hearts to be phosphorylated in response to catecholamine treatment have been considered. There are gaps or deficiencies in the evidence for a functional role of this phosphorylation for each of the proteins considered. There is substantial in vitro evidence indicating probable roles for cAMP-dependent phosphorylation of TnI and phospholamban in mediating the relaxant effects of beta-adrenergic stimulation. Both are phosphorylated in intact myocardium in response to beta-adrenergic stimulation. In each case, however, reversal of phosphorylation appears to lag behind reversal of the relaxant effects of catecholamines. Finally, although substantial physiologic evidence suggests that sarcolemmal Ca^{2+} channels could be a substrate for cAMP-dependent protein kinase, which of the multiple sarcolemmal substrates of cAMP-dependent protein kinase mediates increases in I_{Ca} is not known. Thus much remains to be studied to establish the functional role of phosphorylation of these proteins in mediating the positive inotropic effects of catecholamines.

MECHANISMS OF ALPHA-ADRENERGIC EFFECTS

Although the existence and physiologic role of alpha-adrenergic receptors in the myocardium have been controversial for some time, it is now evident that alpha-adrenergic stimulation can result in functionally significant effects in myocardium (for reviews, see {91,92}). Functional studies have shown that alpha agonists can increase myocardial contractility in certain species, such as rat and rabbit. However, the magnitude of the contractile responses to alpha-receptor stimulation is small in comparison to those produced by beta-adrenergic stimulation. Further, the mechanical changes induced by alpha agonists are not associated with the relaxant effects of beta-receptor agonists, suggesting that different biochemical mechanisms mediate the contractile effects of these two types of adrenergic receptors.

The positive inotropic effects elicited by alpha-adrenergic stimulation are associated with increases in transarcolemmal Ca^{2+} influx as assessed by Ca^{2+}-dependent action potentials {93} and slow inward current (I_{si}, {94}). Although increases in I_{si} are usually attributed to elevations in I_{Ca}, alpha-adrenergic stimulation of I_{Ca} has never been documented in isolated myocytes using patch-clamp or whole-cell recording techniques {95}. Nevertheless, inotropic effects of alpha-adrenergic stimulation can be influenced by interventions that alter Ca^{2+} influx via sarcolemmal Ca^{2+} channels. Specifically, organic Ca^{2+} channel blockers antagonize the positive inotropic effects of alpha-adrenergic stimulation without altering agonist binding {96}. This suggests that alpha-adrenergic stimulation may enhance voltage-dependent Ca^{2+} influx by mechanisms other than a direct effect on Ca^{2+} channels. In fact, alpha-adrenergic stimulation inhibits I_{to} (the transient outward current that is involved in phase I of the cardiac action potential) and thereby prolongs action potential duration (APD) and increases the intracellular Ca^{2+} transient (see below). Indeed, there is a close correlation between alpha-adrenergic mediated prolongation of APD and increases in contractile force {97}.

Alpha-adrenergic stimulation has also been shown to affect a number of K^+ currents. More specifically, alpha-adrenergic stimulation decreases transient outward K^+ current (I_{to}) {98,99,132}, reduces delayed rectifier K^+ current (I_K) {99}, decreases inward rectifier current (I_{K1}) {100}, shifts holding current to more negative values {100}, and stimulates $Na^+,-K^+$ pump current {100,101}. These effects have not, however, been observed by all investigators, possibly because of differences in species {97} or tissues used {102}.

Alpha-adrenergic receptors

The presence of alpha-adrenergic receptors in the myocardium has now been demonstrated in multiple laboratories by radioligand binding techniques {103}. These studies reveal that the receptors are predominantly of the α_1 subtype {104,105}. However, recent studies in other tissues have distinguished several subtypes of α_1-adrenergic receptors (termed α_{1a}, α_{1b}, α_{1c}, and α_{1d}; for review see Minneman {106}, and the distribution of these subtypes in myocardium has not been well established. In fact, current knowledge is based primarily on experiments performed when it was assumed that there are only two α_1-receptor subtypes in the heart. Binding studies conducted in homogenates of rat ventricular myocardium with the antagonist [^3H]WB4101 revealed two populations of α_1-adrenergic receptors: 16% displaying high affinity (then termed the α_{1a} subtype) and 84% displaying low affinity (termed the α_{1b} subtype) {104,106}. In contrast, studies examining 10 µM chloroethylclonidine (CEC; then believed to be an irreversible antagonist of only α_{1b} receptors) inhibition of ^{125}IBE 2254 binding led investigators to propose that 8–27% of the α_1-adrenergic receptors are α_{1b} {106}. This disparity regarding α_{1a}- and α_{1b}-adrenergic receptor binding densities may have resulted from differences in radioligands, antagonist concentrations, assay conditions, or the membrane preparations utilized. Northern blot analysis of myocardium revealed higher levels of mRNA for the α_{1b} subtype than for the α_{1a} subtype {107}. Furthermore, a recent report by Lefkowitz and coworkers (*Clin Res* 41:188A, 1993) indicated that mRNA levels for the α_{1c}-adrenergic receptor are predominant in human heart, with minor levels of mRNA encoding the α_{1b} subtype. Thus it would appear that the heart may possess three or more α_1-receptor subtypes. The affinity of agonist binding to all previously identified α_1-adrenergic receptor subtypes was reduced by guanine nucleotides, suggesting that these receptors are linked to G proteins {104}. However, it has been hypothesized that the different α_1-adrenergic receptor subtypes are not linked to the same intracellular effector mechanisms {106}.

As is the case with beta-adrenergic receptors, the number of alpha-adrenergic receptors may also vary in disease states. In a rat model of chronic congestive heart failure, it has been shown that the number of alpha-adrenergic receptors (as well as beta-adrenergic receptors) is increased {108}. This model of CHF resulted in a reduction of myocardial catecholamine levels. More recent studies have shown that the reduced myocardial responsiveness to alpha-adrenergic stimulation in aging is associated with a decrease in α_1-receptor density and mRNA expression {109}.

Effector mechanisms

In contrast to the well-established role of cAMP in mediating the effects of beta-adrenergic stimulation, the mechanisms underlying alpha-adrenergic effects are poorly defined {91,92}. It is generally accepted that physiologic effects of alpha-adrenergic stimulation are not mediated by cAMP {91}. Moreover, alpha-adrenergic stimulation has been shown to decrease cAMP under basal conditions {110} and to antagonize the increases in cAMP elicited by beta-adrenergic stimulation or other hormones that activate adenylate cyclase activity {110–112}. There are two potential mechanisms by which alpha-adrenergic stimulation can attenuate cAMP levels: (a) inhibition of adenylate cyclase activity, or (b) activation of phosphodiesterase activity. Reported guanine nucleotide effects on agonist binding to alpha-adrenergic receptors raises the possibility that these receptors are coupled to adenylate cyclase by G_i. Indeed, studies have indicated that the predominant physiological effects of alpha-adrenergic stimulation on spontaneous depolarization are attenuated or abolished by pretreatment with pertussis toxin {113, 114}. However, studies in cardiac myocytes showed that alpha-agonist-induced effects on the cAMP accmulation elicited by beta-adrenergic stimulation are not altered by pertussis toxin pretreatment, whereas the inhibitory effects of muscarinic stimulation are abolished {115}. Furthermore, these investigators found that alpha-adrenergic agonists enhance the degradation of cAMP following beta-adrenergic stimulation, and that this effect is abolished by phosphodiesterase inhibitors. This suggests that alpha-adrenergic stimulation modulates cAMP levels by activation of a cAMP phosphodiesterase {115}.

As alluded to in the previous section, guanine nucleotide regulation of alpha-adrenergic receptor binding suggests that these actions may be mediated by G proteins. The negative chronotropic effects of alpha-adrenergic stimulation in canine Purkinje fibers {113} and neonatal rat ventricular myocytes {114} are associated with the presence of a 41-kDa pertussis toxin substrate. Pretreatment with pertussis toxin (or the absence of the substrate in neonatal myocardium) results in a positive chronotropic response to alpha-receptor stimulation. This bears a remarkable similarity to the effect of pertussis toxin pretreatment on the response to muscarinic cholinergic stimulation {116}, where toxin treatment changes the cholinergic response from hyperpolarization to depolarization and the negative inotropic effect to a positive inotropic effect. In contrast, other actions elicited by alpha-adrenergic stimulation, such as activation of phosphoinositide hydrolysis, are not altered by pertussis toxin {117} (see below). The occurrence of both pertussis-toxin-sensitive and -insensitive effects suggests that multiple G proteins may be involved in mediating these effects and that different G proteins may be linked to specific alpha-adrenergic receptor subtypes {106}.

Evidence from a number of cell types suggests that alpha-adrenergic effects are mediated by hydrolysis of inositol-containing phospholipids (for reviews see {106, 118}). In this proposed scheme, agonist-receptor binding stimulates the phosphodiesteric hydrolysis of phosphatidylinositol 4,5-bisphosphate, resulting in the formation of 1,2-diacylglycerol (DAG) and inositol 1,4,5-trisphosphate (InsP₃). Both compounds have been shown to function as intracellular second messengers. DAG stimulates the activity of protein kinase C, with the resultant phosphorylation of a number of cellular proteins {73}, while InsP₃ results in the mobilization of intracellular Ca^{2+} {118,119}.

A number of studies indicate that alpha-adrenergic stimulation results in increases in inositol phosphate production in the heart (for reviews see {106,120}). More recent studies suggest that the rapid formation of the 1,4,5-isomer of InsP₃ is associated with the rapid transient positive inotropic effect of alpha-adrenergic stimulation in rat papillary muscle {121}. This transient effect is not altered by nifedipine, suggesting that InsP₃ may mobilize Ca^{2+} from intracellular stores {121}. Studies in permeabilized {122} cardiac cells have shown that InsP₃ can release Ca^{2+} from the sarcoplasmic reticulum; however, these InsP₃-induced increases in Ca_i are relatively small, and it is not known if they are sufficient to mediate the functional effects of alpha-adrenergic stimulation.

Studies examining the relationship between phosphoinositide hydrolysis and the inotropic effects of alpha-adrenergic stimulation have produced variable results. Endoh and coworkers found no association between steady-state α_1-adrenergic stimulation of contractile force and the generation of inositol phosphates in rabbit papillary muscle {97}. However, the same laboratory subsequently reported that CEC pretreatment of the same preparation inhibited both the phosphoinositide hydrolysis and the positive inotropic effect, suggesting that both actions were mediated by a CEC-sensitive receptor {123}. Alpha-adrenergic stimulation of inositol phosphate production is generally insensitive to pretreatment with pertussis toxin {106} and, in contrast to results described above with CEC in rabbit papillary muscle {123}, has been suggested to be mediated by α_{1a} receptors in many other tissues. There are no published reports on the effects of pertussis toxin on the positive inotropic effects of alpha-adrenergic stimulation.

Myocardial effects of alpha-adrenergic stimulation may also be mediated by phosphorylation of sarcolemmal proteins by protein kinase C. Alpha-adrenergic stimulation is associated with translocation of protein kinase C activity from the cytosol to the particulate fraction {124}, a response generally associated with activation of protein kinase C-dependent processes {119}. In vitro studies have revealed the presence of an endogenous protein kinase C activity in highly purified canine cardiac sarcolemmal vesicles {125}. The only sarcolemmal protein phosphorylated by protein kinase C in this preparation is a 15-kDa protein {125}, which appears to be identical to the 15-kDa protein phosphorylated by cAMP-dependent protein kinase {13}. This same protein is phosphorylated in response to alpha-adrenergic stimulation of isolated perfused rat ventricles and is temporally associated with the de-

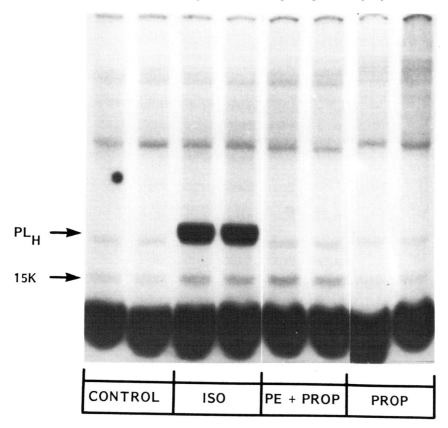

Fig. 24-8. Autoradiogram depicting beta- and alpha-adrenergic stimulation of in situ phosphorylation of membrane proteins. Isolated rat ventricles were perfused with $^{32}P_i$ for 30 minutes and then with nonradioactive buffer containing 25 mM K^+ for an additional 5 minutes. The hearts were then exposed an additional 5 minutes to buffer containing water alone (CONTROL, 1st and 2nd lanes), 0.1 μM isoproterenol (ISO, 3rd and 4th lanes), 10 μM phenylephrine + 3 μM propranolol (PE + PROP, 5th and 6th lanes), or 3 μM propranolol alone (PROP, 7th and 8th lanes). The hearts were then freeze-clamped and membrane vesicles were partially enriched in sarcolemma prepared from individual hearts. Membrane vesicles were then subjected to SDS-polyacrylamide gel electrophoresis and autoradiography. PL_H indicates the high M_r form of phospholamban; 15K denotes the 15-kDa sarcolemmal protein. Whereas β-adrenergic stimulation resulted in phosphorylation of both phospholamban and the 15-kDa protein, alpha-adrenergic stimulation resulted in phosphorylation of only the 15-kDa protein. Reprinted with permission from Lindemann {88}.

velopment of contractile slow responses {88}. These results have been confirmed and extended in isolated rabbit heart {126}, where alpha-adrenergic stimulation also resulted in translocation of protein kinase C and phosphorylation of a 28-kDa cytosolic protein. Since the 15-kDa protein is the only sarcolemmal protein phosphorylated in response to both alpha- and beta-adrenergic stimulation, it is tempting to speculate that phosphorylation of this protein mediates the contractile slow responses produced by both stimuli {88} (fig. 24-8).

Phorbol esters or synthetic diacylglycerols are frequently used to directly activate protein kinase C {119,127}. These compounds result in translocation of protein kinase C to the membrane and stimulation of phosphotransferase activity. Administration of these compounds to isolated myocardial tissues uniformly elicits negative, not positive, inotropic effects {126,128}. In isolated myocytes, phorbol esters decreased twitch amplitude and diminished the Ca_i

transient {128}. In additional studies, the same investigators found that Ca^{2+} loading of the cells (produced by increasing Ca_o) reversed the effects of alpha-adrenergic stimulation on both twitch amplitude and the Ca_i transient. This effect was mimicked by phorbol esters and inhibited by staurosporine, a protein kinase C antagonist {129}. These results suggest that the negative inotropic effect of alpha-adrenergic stimulation is mediated by protein kinase C {129}.

Detailed studies of the electrophysiologic effects of protein kinase C have only recently been reported, and the results have been variable. In isolated adult guinea pig ventricular cells, phorbol esters elicited a temperature-dependent increase in I_K while having no effect on I_{Ca} {130} or I_{K1} {131}. In adult rat myocytes, phorbol esters suppressed I_{to} {98}, mimicking the effects of alpha-adrenergic agonists {132,99}. By contrast, in *neonatal* rat ventricular cell preparations, phorbol esters were shown to increase I_{Ca} {133} and the activity of single Ca^{2+} channels {134}. It is interesting to note that this increase in I_{Ca} was observed only in neonatal preparations, since these cells have very low levels of pertussis toxin substrate and do not display muscarinic or angiotensin II receptor-mediated attenuation of isoproterenol-induced stimulation of cAMP accumulation. After 11 days in culture, these agonists potently inhibit cAMP accumulation in a pertussis-toxin-sensitive manner {135}. These results suggest that the failure to demonstrate phorbol ester-induced increases in I_{Ca} is possibly related to the presence of a pertussis-toxin-sensitive G-protein that links muscarinic and angiotensin II receptors to inhibition of cAMP accumulation. Whether this change in G-protein expression is a manifestation of other alterations in the protein composition of the sarcolemma that modify the ability of protein kinase C to alter I_{Ca} is unknown.

MECHANISMS OF CHOLINERGIC EFFECTS ON THE HEART

The importance of the parasympathetic nervous system in regulation of myocardial function is well established (for reviews see {1,136}). However, important differences exist in the functional responsiveness of the myocardium sympathetic and parasympathetic stimulation. One of the respects in which parasympathetic regulation of cardiac function differs from sympathetic regulation is that there is much more marked variability in response of different cardiac tissue to parasympathetic than to sympathetic stimulation {1}. All tissues of the heart respond similarly qualitatively and quantitatively to beta-adrenergic-receptor stimulation. By contrast, ventricular tissue is much less responsive to muscarinic agonists than is atrial tissue {1}. Choline esters potently decrease automaticity of spontaneously excitable atrial tissue and exert powerful negative inotropic effects on atrial muscle. By contrast, muscarinic agonists produce minimal negative inotropic and electrophysiologic effects on isolated ventricular tissues (in the absence of sympathetic stimulation). Muscarinic agonists may exert direct electrophysiologic effects on Purkinje fibers of some species. In both supraventricular and ventricular structures, muscarinic agonists antagonize the effects of beta-agonists. Because of the relatively minimal effects of muscarinic agonists alone in ventricular tissues, the muscarinic antiadrenergic effect is pronounced compared to the effect seen with muscarinic agonists alone. This magnification of muscarinic effect during simultaneous sympathetic stimulation, which can be observed in isolated cardiac tissues as well as in intact animals with normal sympathetic and vagal innervation, has been termed *accentuated antagonism* {137}. These differences in responsiveness of supraventricular and ventricular structures to muscarinic stimulation suggest (a) that multiple subcellular mechanisms mediate the cardiac effects of muscarinic stimulation, and (b) that only some of these subcellular mechanisms are shared by atrial and ventricular tissues. The various myocardial cell components that mediate muscarinic effects on the heart will be discussed in the following sections.

MUSCARINIC CHOLINERGIC RECEPTORS

Like adrenergic receptors, muscarinic receptors have also come to be studied directly with radioligand binding assays (for a general review of radioligand binding assays of muscarinic receptors, see {138,139}). These assays have demonstrated that muscarinic receptors exist in both atria and ventricules, and that the density of receptors is at least as great or greater than that in atria. Thus the differences in atrial and ventricular responses to muscarinic agonists cannot be explained by muscarinic-receptor distribution. Further, myocardial muscarinic receptors appear to be of the M_2 type {140}, with the exception of chick heart, which appears to be M_1 {141}. Binding studies indicate that muscarinic receptors are membrane associated and probably predominantly or exclusively located in the plasma membrane {13,142}. Muscarinic binding sites in purified sarcolemma and sarcoplasmic reticulum from dog hearts copurified with the sarcolemmal marker Na,K-ATPase and away from the sarcoplasmic reticulum marker Ca^{2+}-ATPase {13,142}. Muscarinic binding activity also copurified with beta-adrenergic binding sites. Therefore, both beta-adrenergic and muscarinic receptors are localized to the sarcolemma in myocardium. Such a location would be optimal for accessibility of neurotransmitters to the receptors and for intracellular interaction between the two branches of the autonomic nervous system at the level of the receptors and their effectors (fig. 24-1).

Similar to beta-adrenergic receptors, muscarinic receptors are also regulated by a variety of influences {138, 139}. Binding assays have revealed that the interaction of agonists with muscarinic receptors is much more complex than that of antagonists, similar to the situation with beta-adrenergic receptors. Muscarinic receptors exist in multiple states in terms of their interaction with agonists {138,139}. The same binding sites (i.e., muscarinic receptors) that interact with antagonists in a uniform manner interact with agonists heterogeneously. This is recognized by analysis of the curves relating the occupancy of muscarinic receptors to the concentration of muscarinic agonists added to the receptors. The binding curves relating antagonist occupation of receptors to antagonists concentration are of the form predicted by the law of mass action by the interaction of a ligand with a uniform set of binding sites (fig. 24-9). In contrast, the pattern of agonist binding curves deviates substantially from this simple mass-action relationship (fig. 24-9). These agonist curves are shallower than antagonist binding curves and have slope factors substantially less than 1.0. the most plausible explanation for this is that muscarinic receptors exist in multiple conformations in terms of their interaction with agonists {138,139}. Three different classes of muscarinic binding sites, each with different affinities for agonists, have been described in rat brain membranes {138}. At least two binding sites (high and low affinity) for agonists have been described in several other organs, including heart

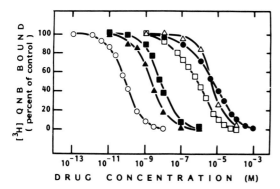

Fig. 24-9. Competition curves for [³H]QNB binding to muscarinic receptors in membrane vesicles derived from canine ventricular myocardium. Data from separate experiments performed in purified membrane preparations are presented, with binding expressed as a percent of control binding in the absence of competing drug. For all curves, [³H]QNB concentration was approximately 80 pM. Note that oxotremorine (□) and methacholine (●) slopes are shallow compared to the antagonist slopes. Drugs are QNB (○), dexetimide (▲), atropine (■), oxotremorine (□), methacholine (●), and levitimide (△). Reprinted with permission from Mirro et al. {194}.

{138,139}. These different affinity binding sites are non-interconvertible in the binding assay, and therefore the slopes describing occupancy as a function of agonist concentration represent the sum of the interaction of ligand with multiple binding sites.

Muscarinic receptors, like beta-adrenergic receptors, are regulated by guanine nucleotides {77}. Analysis of agonist competition with antagonist radioligands for binding to muscarinic receptors in cardiac membrane preparations from which endogeneous guanine nucleotides have been removed yields the shallow binding curves described above (fig. 24-9). If exogenous guanine nucleotides are added, however, the curves shift to a steeper form, a pattern compatible with the interaction of ligand with a single, homogenous class of binding sites {139}. At the same time the affinity of the receptor for agonists is reduced substantially. These data have been interpreted as showing a guanine-nucleotide-induced conversion of receptors in a high-affinity state for agonists into a low-affinity state {139}, analogous to the situation with guanine nucleotide regulation of beta-adrenergic receptors. Thus, with added guanine nucleotide binding curves are steeper (representing a single class of binding sites) and shifted to the right because most or all of the receptors are in a low-affinity state. The interaction of guanine nucleotides, presumably via G proteins, with muscarinic receptors might be a mechanism for coupling of the receptor to intracellular effectors, analogous to the situation for beta-adrenergic receptors (fig. 24-4). In recent studies, muscarinic receptors purified from brain have been reconstituted with G_o or G_i in phospholipid vesicles {143–145}.

Analogous to the situation with beta-adrenergic receptors, the density of muscarinic receptors varies depending

on the ambient concentration of muscarinic agonists. For example, cultured chick embryo heart cells exposed to carbamylcholine for various durations had a diminished negative chronotropic response to muscarinic agonists associated with a substantial reduction in receptor density {146}. Detailed analysis revealed a biphasic pattern to this agonist-induced receptor alteration, a rapid phase (occurring over 1 minute) associated with a reduced affinity of receptors for agonists, followed by a slower phase (occurring over several hours), reflecting a true reduction in measurable receptor binding {146}. By contrast, in a perfused rat heart system, low doses (4 µM) of carbachol reduced the affinity of atrial receptors with a much longer time course, while the number of receptors decreased only in the ventricles {147}. The agonist-induced reduction in cardiac muscarinic-receptor density has also been demonstrated in in-vivo studies. Carbachol was administered to chicks in ovo. The negative chronotropic response to carbachol of hearts removed from these chicks compared to that of hearts from control chicks, and the density of muscarinic receptors in homogenates of these hearts was reduced markedly {148}. More recent studies have shown that chronic administration of carbachol in vitro, conditions that result in the slow reduction in receptor number, also result in the stimulation of ³²P-incorporation into muscarinic receptors {149}.

Like beta-adrenergic receptors, the density of cardiac muscarinic receptors can vary depending on thyroid status. Thyroidectomy increased the density, whereas treatment with triiodothyronine resulted in a modest decrease in density of muscarinic receptors {150}. These effects of thyroid state on muscarinic receptors are exactly the opposite of the effects on beta-adrenergic receptors. Hyperthyroidism increases the density, whereas hypothyroidism decreases the density, of beta-adrenergic receptors in cardiac tissues {23,26}. Thus the tachycardia of hyperthyroid animals and the bradycardia of hypothyroid animals may reflect a reciprocal alteration in the density of receptors of both limbs of the autonomic nervous system.

INTRACELLULAR EFFECTORS COUPLED TO MUSCARINIC CHOLINERGIC RECEPTORS

Compared to the relatively detailed knowledge regarding the subcellular mechanisms by which beta agonists modify cardiac function, the intracellular mechanisms for producing muscarinic effects are sketchy. However, significant advances toward our understanding have occurred over the past several years. Several potential mechanisms will be discussed in this section.

Cation channels

The electrophysiologic and inotropic effects of muscarinic activation of mammalian atria appear to be mediated predominantly by alterations in the outward K^+ current (I_k) and the inward Ca^{2+} current (I_{Ca}) {136,151,152}. In atrial tissues, increases in I_k result in earlier repolarization of the membrane, shortening of the action potential duration, and decreases in contractility. The reduction in contractility is thought to be due to a secondary diminution in I_{Ca} {151}. Because action potential duration is shortened by increased outward currents, the plateau phase of the action potential during the time at which I_{Ca} occurs is abbreviated {151}. By contrast, cholinergic effects in ventricular myocardium appear to be limited to inhibition of I_{Ca}. For example, in chick atria muscarinic inhibition of I_{Ca} (assessed as slow action potentials) is associated with hyperpolarization and a reduction in resting membrane potential, effects not noted in ventricles {153}. Whether increases in I_k can account entirely for the negative inotropic effects of muscarinic activation or whether additional mechanisms (to be discussed in later parts of this section) are operative in atrial tissues remains to be established.

In mammalian atria, the effects of muscarinic activation on cation channels appears to depend on the concentration of muscarinic agonist used. With low concentrations of acetylcholine (sufficient to reduce twitch tension by 30–40%), the previously described effects of muscarinic activation on K^+ currents occurred {151}. At this concentration of acetylcholine, the changes in I_{si} were secondary or "indirect," i.e., these changes resulted from the shortening in plateau duration. With higher concentrations of acetylcholine (sufficient to reduce twitch tension by 70–90%), a direct effect on I_{si} also was observed with voltage-clamp studies {151}. Thus, with high concentrations of muscarinic agonists, I_k increased and I_{si} also decreased. These dual actions on ion flux would be expected to produce strong negative inotropic effects. As in the case of K^+ channels, the nature of the coupling between muscarinic receptors and I_{si} channels remains unknown.

Tissue differences also exist in muscarinic effects on I_{si}. In mammalian atria, high concentrations of acetylcholine directly reduced I_{si} {151}. However, in mammalian ventricular tissues, activation of muscarinic receptors, even with high concentrations of acetylcholine, did not appear to produce a direct effect on I_{si}.

Recent studies published in the last several years have provided substantial evidence for a role of G proteins in the coupling of muscarinic-receptor stimulation with alterations in I_k. The first evidence for the role of G proteins came from studies using pertussis toxin. In these studies pretreatment of atrial tissues with pertussis toxin resulted in inhibition of I_k, assessed either as radiolabeled K^+ efflux {154} or I_k {155–157}. Using excised patch-clamp techniques, it has been shown that G_i isolated from erythrocytes, when activated with GTPγS (G_i-GTPγS), can directly activate muscarinic K^+ channels in isolated guinea pig atrial myocytes {158}. Simultaneously, it has been reported that the purified βγ subunits of G protein alone could activate muscarinic K^+ channels in cultured embryonic chick atrial cells {159}. In contrast to {158}, the activated α subunits of several G proteins did not activate K^+ channels {159}. In both instances, however, the activation occurred in the absence of ATP or free GTP, suggesting that intracellular second messengers or protein phosphorylation could not mediate these effects. These studies provide strong evidence for direct activation of myocardial K^+ channels by activated G proteins (or subunits thereof). Additional studies will need to be done to resolve these somewhat disparate results, although it is

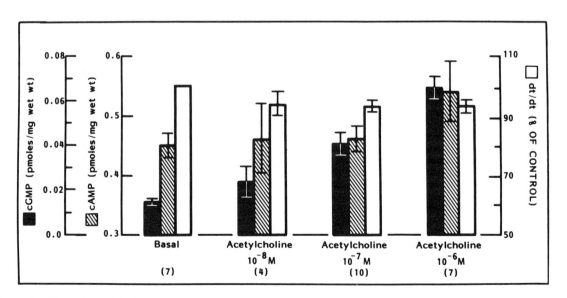

Fig. 24-10. Effect of acetylcholine on cGMP and cAMP levels in guinea pig ventricles. Acetylcholine was perfused for 2 minutes prior to freezing hearts. Note the concentration-dependent increase in cyclic GMP levels, without a change in cyclic AMP levels except at 10^{-6} M acetylcholine. At this highest concentration of acetylcholine, catecholamines may have been released to account for the small elevation in cAMP level. Note also the lack of any significant negative inotropic effect of acetylcholine. Reprinted with permission from Watanabe and Besch {166}.

possible that the differences arise from utilization of different tissues.

Thus, one well-established effect of muscarinic activation is alterations in the properties of ion channels located in the sarcolemma of myocardial cells.

Cyclic GMP

It was first shown in cardiac tissues that cyclic-GMP (cGMP) levels could be elevated by activation of muscarinic cholinergic receptors. This original observation of muscarinic-induced increases in cGMP levels in cardiac tissues was confirmed and extended by multiple subsequent studies done in hearts from a variety of different species (fig. 24-10; for review, see Goldberg and Haddox {160}). Thus, there is no question that, under appropriate conditions, activation of muscarinic receptors can result in increases in tissue cGMP levels (fig. 24-10), but whether this muscarinic-induced elevation in cGMP levels has any physiologic role remains an issue of controversy {160,161}. Moreover, the biochemical mechanisms by which changes in tissue cGMP might alter cardiac function are largely unknown {161}.

The original studies that attempted to demonstrate a physiologic role for cGMP correlated a physiologic response (e.g., contractile state) with tissue cGMP levels. In these studies, acetylcholine was given to cardiac preparations in various concentrations for different durations, the mechanical or physiologic responses of the hearts were observed, and cGMP levels were determined in the same tissues. Although there appeared to be a fairly good correlation between tissue cGMP levels and the measured physiologic response, these studies could be criticized as being inconclusive because a sufficiently detailed concentration-response analysis was not performed {161}.

Analogues of cGMP have been shown to mimic certain of the electrophysiologic effects of acetylcholine. Dibutyryl cGMP (Bt$_2$cGMP) slowed the spontaneous beating rate of isolated cultured rat heart cells, whereas Bt$_2$cGMP increased the spontaneous beating rate {162}. cGMP injected directly into sinoatrial nodal cells by iontophoresis decreased the slope of spontaneous diastolic depolarization {163}. Acetylcholine administered by this same route was without effect, presumably because the choline ester must interact with muscarinic receptors on the outside of the sarcolemma to produce its effects {163}. Like acetylcholine, 8-bromo-cGMP (8-Br-cGMP) inhibited atrial slow-response action potentials {164}, an indirect assessment of I$_{si}$. Associated with this inhibition of the slow-response action potential was a negative inotropic effect. 8-bromo-cGMP also mimicked the effects of acetylcholine on action potential configuration and contractile state in rat atria {165}. In this same study, 8-Br-cGMP decreased Ca^{2+} uptake by beating atrial preparations, but had no effect on K$^+$ content. It was concluded that cGMP might mediate the effects of muscarinic activation on I$_{si}$, but not on K$^+$ channels {165}.

Analogues of cGMP have also been used to assess the possible role of cGMP in the antiadrenergic effects of acetylcholine. Bt$_2$cGMP mimicked the effect of acetylcho-

line and antagonized the positive inotropic effects of catecholamines in isolated cardiac tissues {166}. These results have been confirmed by other laboratories. Like acetylcholine, Bt$_2$cGMP also attenuated the positive inotropic effects of isoproterenol in hearts from hyperthyroid rats {167}. cGMP analogues also mimic acetylcholine in antagonizing certain of the electrophysiologic effects of catecholamines or cAMP. Isoproterenol antagonized the inhibition by 8-Br-cGMP of slow responses in guinea pig atria {164}. This can be thought of as the reciprocal of cGMP antagonism of isoproterenol-induced augmentation of slow responses. cGMP analogues also mimicked the cholinergic antagonism of the cardiac metabolic effects of catecholamines {167}. Hearts from hyperthyroid rats were hyperresponsive to the metabolic effects of beta agonists compared to those from euthyroid animals {167}. Acetylcholine antagonized isoproterenol-induced activation of phosphorylase in such hearts. Bt$_2$cGMP mimicked these effects of acetylcholine without lowering cAMP levels. Thus it has been shown that analogues of cGMP can mimic the effects of acetylcholine in antagonizing the electrophysiologic, inotropic, and metabolic actions of beta agonists.

Another approach to test the cGMP hypothesis has been to elevate cGMP with drugs that do not interact with muscarinic receptors. Because of its potency in elevating tissue cGMP levels, Na nitroprusside has been widely used for such studies. It has been shown that Na nitroprusside did not mimic the inotropic, electrophysiologic, metabolic, or antiadrenergic effects of acetylcholine, even though it markedly increased cGMP levels (for a review, see {161}). However, because Na nitroprusside elevates cGMP levels in heart without producing physiologic effects, it does not necessarily follow that cGMP has no role in mediating the effects of acetylcholine. Immunohistochemical evidence in noncardiac {168} and cardiac {169} tissues has shown that cGMP can be compartmentalized within the cell and that muscarinic agonists and Na nitroprusside affect the concentrations of this nucleotide in different compartments. The observation that acetylcholine, but not Na nitroprusside, activates cGMP-dependent protein kinase in rat hearts provides further evidence for different compartments or pools of cGMP, each of which can be selectively regulated and has different intracellular effectors (see below). Analogous evidence has been provided for compartmentation of cAMP and differential regulation of cAMP levels in different pools in myocardial cells.

If cGMP is involved in mediating some of the effects of muscarinic-receptor stimulation in the heart, the biochemical mechanism by which this occurs remains unknown. One hypothesis is that, analogous to the cAMP-dependent protein kinase system, cGMP interacts with a specific protein kinase, which in turn phosphorylated certain substrates to alter protein function. A cGMP-dependent protein kinase has been identified in various tissues, including heart {170}. It has been shown that administration of acetylcholine to intact rat heart results in increases in cGMP-dependent protein kinase activity ratios associated with elevations in cGMP levels {170}. Both of these biochemical responses were associated with a negative inotropic effect in the same hearts. Na nitroprusside also increased cGMP levels, in fact, to much greater levels than that caused by acetylcholine. However, Na nitroprusside did not increase cGMP-dependent protein kinase activity ratios, nor did it change the force of contraction {170}. These results suggest several conclusions: (a) They suggest a possible mechanism by which cGMP, the levels of which are altered in response to muscarinic stimulation, might modify protein function and the physiologic properties of the heart; (b) they support the notion that cGMP and its intracellular effectors might be compartmentalized; and (c) they demonstrate the hazards of using agents other than muscarinic agonists to elevate cGMP levels and then drawing conclusions about the role of cGMP if these agents do not mimic the choline esters.

There is a body of evidence that has been interpreted to show that cGMP does not have any role in cardiac regulation {161}. The most convincing evidence against a role for cGMP in mediating certain physiologic effects are the observations that over a range of concentrations of muscarinic agonist, certain physiologic effects can be induced without changing tissue cGMP levels. Acetylcholine decreased automaticity and shortened action potential duration of guinea pig atria, and these changes appeared to occur without any relationship to tissue cGMP levels {171}. Muscarinic agonists antagonized the positive inotropic effects of agents that elevate cAMP levels (catecholamines, phosphodiesterase inhibitors, cholera toxin) without elevating cGMP levels {172}. These results could be interpreted as eliminating a role for cGMP in the electrophysiologic or antiadrenergic effects of muscarinic agonists. However, the following considerations should be kept in mind: (a) The aforementioned criticisms are based on studies conducted in atrial tissues where the predominant effects likely are mediated by changes in I_k, effects that are probably mediated directly by G proteins; (b) muscarinic receptors might be linked to multiple responses, of which only one or a few which are regulated by cGMP; each of these must be examined carefully before ruling out in a blanket fashion any physiologic role for cGMP; (c) cGMP might be compartmentalized, and small undetectable (by available assays) changes in levels might have occurred in experiments that appeared to show no change in the levels of the nucleotide.

Thus substantial evidence exists both in support of and against the concept that cGMP plays a role in mediating certain cardiac effects of muscarinic-receptor stimulation. It is clear that this is an unresolved issue. Further experiments must be done to establish or completely eliminate a role for this cyclic nucleotide in cardiac regulation.

cGMP levels are regulated by two enzymes: guanylate cyclase and cGMP phosphodiesterase {160}. Guanylate cyclase occurs as both a membrane and a soluble enzyme in cardiac tissues. The membrane-bound form of the enzyme is located in the sarcolemma, the same location of muscarinic receptors {173}. The two forms of the enzyme in cardiac muscle are differentially regulated: nonionic detergents stimulate the particulate enzyme without modifying the activity of the soluble enzyme, whereas Na nitroprusside stimulates only the soluble enzyme {173}.

These results showing both particulate and soluble forms of the enzyme provide further support for the notion of different intracellular pools of cGMP that can be modified selectively by certain agents. Acetylcholine presumably increases cGMP levels by stimulating guanylate cyclase. As noted, both muscarinic receptors and particulate guanylate cyclase are located in sarcolemma. Except for rare reports, however, investigators have failed to show any effect of muscarinic agonists on guanylate cyclase activity in broken cell preparations {150}. In intact tissues, Ca^{2+} is required for muscarinic-induced elevations in cGMP levels. The divalent cation ionophore A23187 increased cGMP levels in guinea pig ventricles, presumably by elevating Ca^{2+} in certain critical areas of the myocardial cell {174}. Ca^{2+} has been shown to stimulate particulate guanylate cyclase activity {175}. Based on these types of results, it has been suggested that Ca^{2+} might in some way function as an intermediary between the muscarinic receptor and guanylate cyclase. However, this conclusion remains to be established. Other studies have shown Ca^{2+} inhibition of guanylate cyclase {160}. In cardiac muscle, although Ca^{2+} is required for muscarinic-induced increases in cGMP levels, the physiologic response to muscarinic stimulation is either no change or a decrease in contractile state {166}. These mechanical effects suggest that muscarinic agonists do not produce a generalized increase in intracellular Ca^{2+} concentration. If activation of muscarinic receptors leads to mobilization of Ca^{2+}, this must occur in discrete intracellular pools (presumably in the region of guanylate cyclase) because contractile proteins and other intracellular enzymes (e.g., phosphorylase kinase) do not appear to be affected.

Phosphoinositide hydrolysis

A number of studies have appeared that show the administration of muscarinic agonists to intact myocardial preparations results in stimulation of phosphoinositide hydrolysis (for reviews see {120,166}). Early studies revealed that muscarinic stimulation increased labeling of PtdIns and phosphatidic acid in myocardial preparations incubated with $^{32}P_i$ or $[^3H]$-inositol {176,177}. Subsequent studies have revealed that cholinergic stimulation results in hydrolysis of phosphoinositides as measured by accumulation of inositol phosphates {178}. Studies of agonist sensitivities in chick heart have revealed that oxotremorine, while acting as a full agonist with respect to inhibition of adenylate cyclase activity and negative chronotropic response, produces only submaximal stimulation of inositol phosphate formation {179}. Thus the functional significance of phosphoinositide hydrolysis in mediating the effects of muscarinic stimulation remain to be established. Further, a mechanism by which phosphoinositide hydrolysis might mediate these effects is unknown. One potential role might be in the stimulation of guanylate cyclase activity through release of arachidonic acid {160,166}.

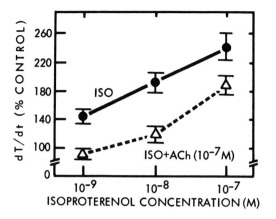

Fig. 24-11. Effect of acetylcholine (ACh) on the positive inotropic effect of isoproterenol (ISO) in isolated perfused guinea pig ventricles. Measurements were taken after hearts had reached a stable level of contractions after 2 minutes of continuous drug infusion. Note that the inotropic response to isoproterenol was markedly attenuated by acetylcholine. Values are mean ± SEM for 7–15 hearts. Reprinted with permission from Watanabe and Besch {166}.

Cellular (postjunctional) mechanisms of muscarinic modulation of adrenergic effects on the heart

In cardiac preparations from various mammalian species, it has been shown that choline esters antagonize the positive inotropic effects of beta-receptor agonists {166,180} (fig. 24-11). In most of these studies with isolated tissues, the negative inotropic effects of muscarinic agonists given alone were prominent and easily observed in the atria {180}, but were small or absent in the ventricles {166}. Muscarinic antagonism of the positive inotropic effects of catecholamines was seen in both atria and ventricles. Thus, it appears that in atrial tissues muscarinic agonists produce negative inotropic effects both by a direct action (presumably mediated by stimulation of I_k) and by antagonizing the effects of beta-receptor agonists. By contrast, in ventricles the predominant muscarinic effect appears to be inhibition of the inotropic effects of beta-agonists.

In isolated cardiac preparations, muscarinic agonists also antagonize the electrophysiologic effects of catecholamines. Choline esters attenuated the positive chronotropic effects of catecholamines on isolated atrial preparations, presumably by antagonizing the catecholamine-induced increase in spontaneous phase 4 depolarization. Muscarinic agonists antagonize the electrophysiologic effects of cate-

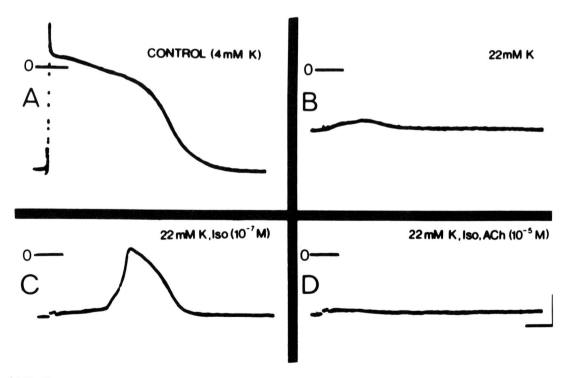

Fig. 24-12. The effects of acetylcholine on an isoproterenol-dependent slow response. **A:** Control Purkinje fiber action potential in 4 mM potassium. **B:** Generalized depolarization and loss of excitability produced by superfusion of Tyrode solution containing 22 mM potassium. **C:** Restoration of excitability by the addition of 10^{-7} M isoproterenol. **D:** The addition of acetylcholine (10^{-5} M) abolishes the "slow response" generated by the addition of isoproterenol. Zero potential indicated in each panel. Calibrations: horizontal bar = 50 ms; vertical bar = 25 mV. Reprinted with permission from Bailey et al. {181}.

cholamines on isolated Purkinje fibers or ventricular muscle. Acetylcholine inhibited isoproterenol-induced shortening of action potential duration in normally polarized paced cardiac Purkinje fibers. Acetylcholine also abolished isoproterenol-dependent slow responses in cardiac Purkinje fibers or guinea pig papillary muscles (fig. 24-12) {181,182}. More recent studies have shown that acetylcholine can markedly attenuate beta-adrenergic-induced increases in I_{Ca} in isolated ventricular myocytes {183,184}.

Thus, in isolated cardiac preparations there is abundant evidence for intracellular interaction of beta-adrenergic and muscarinic receptors. In isolated ventricular tissues, it appears that modulation of sympathetic effects is a major mechanism by which the parasympathetic nervous system exerts its effect. Choline esters alone produced little or no change in the inotropic, electrophysiologic, or metabolic properties of isolated ventricular tissues. Only when these physiologic or metabolic responses were stimulated by beta-adrenergic agonists did muscarinic cholinergic effects become readily apparent. In this situation, muscarinic agonists potently antagonized the beta-adrenergic alteration of these properties. The mechanisms for the intracellular interaction between the components of the sympathetic and parasympathetic systems are discussed in the next section.

MUSCARINIC INHIBITION OF ADENYLATE CYCLASE

A number of investigators using different types of cardiac preparations from various species have shown that muscarinic agonists can attenuate beta-agonist-induced increases in steady-state tissue cAMP levels {167,180,185}. When physiolgoic or metabolic responses were measured, the muscarinic attenuation of cAMP generation paralleled the inhibition of the myocardial response to catecholamines. Muscarinic agonists inhibited beta-adrenergic-induced increases in cAMP levels and concomitantly attenuated the positive inotropic effects {37,167,180}. Muscarinic agonists also antagonized beta-adrenergic-induced activation of phosphorylase while inhibiting cAMP generation {185}. These results are consistent with the conclusion that the muscarinic inhibition of cAMP generation is physiologically and metabolically important in cardiac cells, and that attenuation of cAMP generation might be a contributing mechanism for the antiadrenergic effects of muscarinic agonists.

A major mechanism for muscarinic attenuation of beta-adrenergic-induced cAMP generation involves inhibition of adenylate cyclase activity. It was first shown two decades ago, prior to any detailed knowledge regarding regulation of adenylate cyclase, that muscarinic agonists inhibited adenylate cyclase activity in crude preparations of dog myocardium {186}. Carbachol added to these preparations inhibited both basal and epinephrine-stimulated adenylate cyclase activity {186}. These results were confirmed in similar experiments that used a crude myocardial preparation from rabbit hearts {187}. As mentioned previously, adenylate cyclase activity in purified membranes from myocardial cells is not stimulated by hormones unless exogenous guanine nucleotides are added (fig. 24-5). Addition of exogenous guanine nucleotides stimulated the enzyme directly, as well as facilitating hormone stimulation of the enzyme {37} (fig. 24-5). Thus, guanine nucleotides can activate cardiac adenylate cyclase directly and are required for hormone activation of the emzyme. In purified membrane preparations, muscarinic agonists had no effect on basal adenylate cyclase activity, i.e., activation in the absence of added guanine nucleotides {37}. If GTP was added to the enzyme preparation, muscarinic agonists inhibited adenylate cyclase activity (fig. 24-5, left panel). This was true whether GTP was added alone or together with a catecholamine (fig. 24-5, left panel). In the earlier studies cited {186,187}, because the membrane preparations were crude, it is likely that endogenous GTP was present. Thus, in these earlier studies it is likely that muscarinic effects on adenylate cyclase activity were also dependent on GTP. This dependency of the muscarinic inhibitory activity on GTP was specific for this guanine nucleotide. Cardiac adenylate cyclase activity was also increased by the nonhydrolyzable guanine nucleotide Gpp(NH)p (fig. 24-5, right panel). However, muscarinic agonists had no effect on enzyme activity in the presence of this nucleotide {37} (fig. 24-5, right panel). Similarly, muscarinic agonists did not modify NaF stimulation of adenylate cyclase activity {37}. The effects of muscarinic agonists were blocked by atropine {37}. It was concluded that the interaction of both muscarinic and beta-adrenergic receptors with adenylate cyclase was regulated by the naturally occurring guanine nucleotide GTP. These studies have been confirmed subsequently.

Based on these findings and the data that show guanine nucleotide regulation of muscarinic-receptor affinity for agonists {138,139}, it is reasonable to hypothesize that a G protein is involved in "coupling" inhibitory muscarinic receptors to adenylate cyclase (fig. 24-4). Current evidence now indicates that muscarinic receptors are coupled to adenylate cyclase by G_i (fig. 24-4, see above). The fact that this inhibition does not occur when the nonhydrolyzable analog Gpp (NH) p is the guanine nucleotide present is due to the high affinity of $G_s\alpha$ for the nonhydrolyzable GTP analog. The physiologic relevance of this mechanism has recently been demonstrated in guinea pig ventricular myocytes, where acetylcholine failed to attenuate increases in I_{Ca} produced by intracellular dialysis with Gpp (NH) p {183}. Thus, a major mechanism by which muscarinic agonists can diminish tissue cAMP levels is by inhibiting catecholamine stimulation of adenylate cyclase.

In addition to inhibition of adenylate cyclase activity, there is at least one additional potential mechanism for muscarinic diminution of tissue cAMP levels, namely, stimulation of cAMP phosphodiesterase activity. However, results of studies examining this possibility in intact cellular preparations have been conflicting. It has recently been shown, for example, that intracellular injection of cGMP in frog ventricle can inhibit increases in I_{Ca} produced either by extracellular application of isoproterenol or by intracellular injection of cAMP {188}. By contrast,

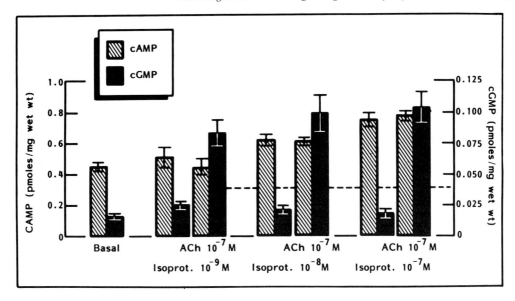

Fig. 24-13. Cyclic nucleotide levels in hearts receiving isoproterenol (Isoprot.) alone or in combination with acetylcholine (ACh) for 2 minutes of continuous infusion. Values are mean ± SEM for 7–16 hearts. The horizontal broken line is the mean value of cGMP found in hearts receiving 10^{-7} M acetylcholine alone for 2 minutes. Reprinted with permission from Watanabe and Besch {166}.

different results were obtained in guinea pig ventricular myocytes {183}. In these latter studies, neither extracellular acetylcholine nor intracellular cGMP had any effect on increases in I_{Ca} produced by intracellular injection of cAMP {183}. Whether these disparate findings were due to species or methodologic differences is not known.

MUSCARINIC MODULATION OF cAMP EFFECTS INDEPENDENT OF CHANGES IN cAMP LEVELS

The muscarinic attenuation of catecholamine-induced cAMP generation cannot account entirely for the muscarinic antagonism of the cardiac effects of beta agonists. Under certain condition, muscarinic agonists can potently inhibit the physiologic and metabolic effects of catecholamines without changing cAMP levels. Acetylcholine markedly antagonized the positive inotropic effects of isoproterenol in isolated perfused guinea pig ventricles {166} (fig. 24-11). cGMP levels in the acetylcholine-treated hearts were markedly elevated (fig. 24-13). However, cAMP levels in hearts receiving both acetylcholine and isoproterenol were not significantly different from those in hearts receiving isoproterenol alone {166} (fig. 24-13). These results have been confirmed subsequently by several other investigators. It has been shown either that muscarinic agonists attenuated a physiologic or metabolic response to catecholamine out of proportion to the magnitude of reduction in cAMP or that the inhibition of physiologic response occurred without any change in cAMP levels. Additional evidence for muscarinic antagonism of

catecholamine effects by mechanisms not involving cAMP reduction comes from studies in which cAMP levels are increased independently of stimulation of beta receptors. It was observed many years ago that acetylcholine blocked the positive inotropic effects of both epinephrine and theophylline in isolated turtle hearts {188}. Although cAMP levels were not measured, it is reasonable to conclude that the positive inotropic effects of both epinephrine and theophylline were mediated at least in part by cAMP {188}.

Subsequently, several investigators have utilized phosphodiesterase inhibitors to produce positive inotropic effects and elevate cAMP levels in cardiac preparations and then to examine the effects of muscarinic agonists on these parameters. Methylisobutylxanthine (MIX) elevated cAMP levels and augmented Ca^{2+}-dependent action potentials and contraction in chick ventricles {189}. Acetylcholine (1 μM) abolished the MIX-induced increase in tension without reducing tissue cAMP levels {189}. In isolated rat left atria, methacholine antagonized the positive inotropic effects of MIX without changing cAMP levels {180}. Myocardial cAMP levels also can be increased by treating the intact tissue with cholera toxin {172}. Cholera toxin, by ADP ribosylation of $G_s\alpha$, results in an increased affinity of $G_s\alpha$ for GTP and a decreased affinity for βγ. Cholera toxin elevated cAMP levels {172} and increased contractions of intact cardiac preparations. Muscarinic agonists inhibited the positive inotropic effect of cholera toxin without reducing cAMP levels {172}. These results thus provide additional evidence that muscarinic agonists can antagonize the effects of cAMP with the myocardial cell.

There are several potential sites beyond cAMP where muscarinic agonists could act to interfere with the intracellular effects of the nucleotide. One of these is cAMP activation of cAMP-dependent protein kinase. This has been examined in only a limited manner. However, the studies that have attempted to examine the relationship between cAMP levels and activation of cAMP-dependent protein kinase have failed to reveal any effect of acetylcholine on this relationship {190}. That is, for a given level of cAMP, cAMP-dependent protein kinase was proportionately activated in the presence or absence of muscarinic agonists. Muscarinic agonists thus do not appear to interfere with cAMP activation of protein kinase.

Another potential site where muscarinic agonists might interfere with the intracellular effects of cAMP is at the level of phosphorylation of proteins that are thought to mediate the effects of hormones or drugs that elevate cAMP concentrations. Because TnI and phospholamban have been shown to be phosphorylated in intact muscle in response to catecholamines, both proteins are good candidates for examining the effects of muscarinic agonists on protein phosphorylation. It has been shown in limited studies that acetylcholine reverses epinephrine-induced phosphorylation of TnI {43}. Acetylcholine also potently attenuated isoproterenol-induced increases in ^{32}P-incorporation into phospholamban while antagonizing the positive inotropic effects of catecholamines {191} (fig. 24-14). Thus muscarinic agonists can potently antagonize catecholamine-induced phosphorylation of myocardial cell proteins, which may be involved in mediating the positive inotropic effects of catecholamines. It is not yet known whether this attenuation of protein phosphorylation can be accounted for entirely by muscarinic attenuation in cAMP levels and thus in kinase activity. In view of the earlier studies mentioned, this seems unlikely. Rather, it seems more likely that cAMP may have been reduced somewhat and that this accounts partially for the reduced phosphorylation, but that some additional mechanism was also operative to produce the ultimate observed inhibition of ^{32}P-incorporation. One reasonable hypothesis is that

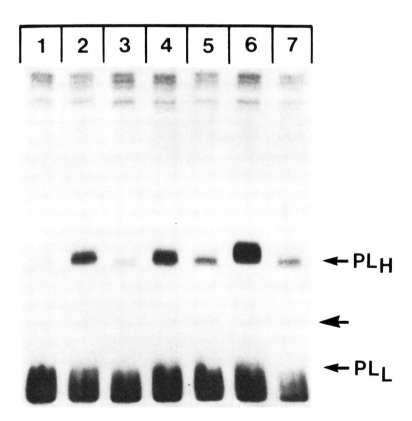

Fig. 24-14. Autoradiogram depicting muscarinic inhibition of beta-adrenergic stimulation of phospholamban phosphorylation in situ. Isolated guinea pig ventricles were perfused with buffer containing ^{32}P$_i$ and then with nonradioactive buffer containing 10 nM isoproterenol alone (lanes 2, 4, and 6) or in combination with 100 nM acetylcholine (lanes 3, 5, and 7). The hearts were freeze-clamped after 20 seconds (lanes 2 and 3), 40 seconds (lanes 4 and 5), or 60 seconds (lanes 6 and 7) of drug exposure and processed as described for fig. 24-6. The heart in lane 1 received no agonists (control). PL$_H$ and PL$_L$ refer to the high and low M$_r$ forms of phospholamban, respectively. PL$_L$ was not clearly resolved from the labeled phospholipids in this autoradiogram. Acetylcholine markedly antagonized stimulation of phospholamban phosphorylation by isoproterenol. Reproduced from Lindemann and Watanabe with permission {191}.

muscarinic agonists somehow activate a protein phosphatase. There are, however, not yet any data available that address this question specifically.

Thus, muscarinic agonists appear to act at more than one level in modulating the cascade of reactions mediating the intracellular effects of beta-receptor stimulation. They can inhibit adenylate cyclase activity by somehow reducing the efficacy of GTP. In addition, they appear to be able to interfere with the intracellular effects of cAMP. The mechanism for this latter effect is yet unknown.

SUMMARY

Catecholamines modify cardiac function by interacting with beta- and alpha-adrenergic receptors on myocyte cell surfaces. The intracellular effects of beta-adrenergic-receptor stimulation are mediated, at least partially, by the cAMP, cAMP-dependent protein kinase system. This ultimately involves cAMP-dependent-protein-kinase-dependent phosphorylation of proteins in myocardial cells to alter protein function and thereby change Ca^{2+} flux and binding to cellular components critical in regulating myocardial contractility. Several protein substrates of cAMP-dependent protein kinase, which are involved in Ca^{2+} regulation of the myofibrillar contractile protein complex or in membrane control of Ca^{2+} movements, have been identified and shown to be phosphorylated in intact hearts treated with catecholamines. Although it seems likely that phosphorylation of one or more of these proteins is involved in mediating the cellular effects of cAMP, additional studies are needed to establish this and to elucidate the detailed mechanisms for these effects. Additional proteins, not yet identified, may also be involved in mediating these effects. It is possible that stimulation of beta-adrenergic receptors leads directly to altered cellular Ca^{2+} handling independent of changes in the cAMP, cAMP-dependent protein kinase system. However, no convincing evidence regarding such a mechanism is available.

Alpha-adrenergic agonists increase myocardial contractility in some species by activating myocardial alpha-adrenergic receptors. The intracellular mechanisms by which alpha agonists modify myocardial cell function are not known. Altered Ca^{2+} handling by myocytes must be involved, but how this occurs is unknown. It is known that the cAMP, cAMP-dependent protein kinase does not mediate alpha-adrenergic effects on the heart.

The cellular mechanisms by which muscarinic agonists modify myocardial cell function are also less well elucidated than those for beta-adrenergic effects. Muscarinic activation in atria leads to increased K^+ flux. However, what "couples" muscarinic receptors to K^+ channels is unknown. cGMP levels can be elevated by muscarinic agonists, but the role of this nucleotide in modifying myocardial cell function remains questionable. One definite mechanism by which muscarinic agonists modify cardiac function is by modulating the cellular effects of beta agonists. This occurs by muscarinic inhibition of beta-adrenergic stimulation of adenylate cyclase and muscarinic attenuation of phosphorylation of proteins. The detailed mechanisms of both of these muscarinic effects remain to be elucidated.

Thus, while there is substantial information about the cellular and subcellular mechanisms by which autonomic transmitters modify myocardial cell function, much remains to be established and to be elucidated in more detail. Future investigation in these areas should be fruitful and rewarding.

ACKNOWLEDGMENTS

The authors' work cited in this chapter was supported by the Herman C. Krannert Fund; by grants HL06308, HL07182, and HL29208 from the National Heart Lung and Blood Institute, National Institutes of Health, Bethesda, Maryland; the Veterans Administration; and the American Heart Association, Indiana Affiliate.

REFERENCES

1. Levy MN, Martin PJ: Neural control of the heart. In: Handbook of Physiology — The Cardiovascular System. I. Berne RM and Sperelakis N, (eds). Bethesda, MD: American Physiological Society, 1979, pp 581–620.
2. Watanabe AM, Jones LR, Manalan AS, Besch HR Jr: Cardiac autonomic receptors: Recent concepts from radio-labelled ligand studies. *Circ Res* 50:161–174, 1982.
3. Stiles GL, Caron MG, Lefkowitz RJ: β-adrenergic receptors: Biochemical mechanisms of physiologic regulation. *Physiol Rev* 64:661–743, 1984.
4. Levitski A: β-adrenergic receptors and their mode of coupling to adenylyl cyclase. *Physiol Rev* 66:819–854, 1986.
5. Emorine LJ, Marullo S, Briend-Sutren M-M, Patey G, Tate K, Delavier-Klutchko C, Strosberg AD: Molecular characterization of the human β3-adrenergic receptor. *Science* 245:1118–1121, 1989.
6. Krief S, Lönnqvist F, Raimbault S, Baude B, Van Spronsen A, Arner P, Strosberg AD, Ricquier D, Emorine LJ: Tissue distribution of β3-adrenergic receptor mRNA in man. *J Clin Invest* 91:344–349, 1993.
7. Tavernier G, Galitzky J, Bousquet-Melou A, Montastruc JL, Berlan M: The positive chronotropic effect induced by BRL 37344 and CGP 12177, two beta-3 adrenergic agonists, does not involve cardiac beta adrenoceptors but baroreflex mechanisms. *J Pharmacol Exp Ther* 263:1083–1090, 1992.
8. Birnbaumer L, Codina J, Mattera R, Cerione RA, Hildebrandt JD, Sunyer T, Rojas F, Caron MG, Lefkowitz RJ, Iyengar R: Regulation of hormone receptors and adenylyl cyclases by guanine nucleotide binding N proteins. *Rec Prog Hormone Res* 41:41–99, 1985.
9. Hancock AA, De Lean AL, Lefkowitz RJ: Quantitative resolution of β-adrenergic receptor subtypes by selective ligand binding: Application of a computerized model fitting technique. *Mol Pharmacol* 16:1–9, 1980.
10. Carlsson E, Dahlof C, Hedberg A, Tangstrand B: Differentiation of cardiac chronotropic and inotropic of β-adrenoceptor agonists. *Naunyn-Schmiedebergs Arch Pharmacol* 300:101–105, 1977.
11. Liang BT, Frame LH, Molinoff PB: β2-adrenergic receptors contribute to catecholamine-stimulated shortening of action potential duration in dog atrial muscle. *Proc Natl Acad Sci USA* 82:4521–4525, 1985.

12. Jones LR, Maddock SW, Besch HR Jr: Unmasking effect of alamethicin on the (Na⁺,K⁺)-ATPase, β-adrenergic receptor-coupled adenylyl cyclase, and cAMP-dependent protein kinase activities of cardiac sarcolemmal vesicles. *J Biol Chem* 255:9971–9980, 1980.

13. Manalan AS, Jones LR: Characterization of the intrinsic cAMP-dependent protein kinase activity and endogenous substrates in highly purified cardiac sarcolemmal vesicles. *J Biol Chem* 257:10052–10062, 1982.

14. Fraser J, Nadeau J, Robertson D, Wood AJJ: Regulation of human leukocyte beta receptors by endogenous catecholamines: Relationship of leukocyte beta receptor density to the cardiac sensitivity to isoproterenol. *J Clin Invest* 67:1777–1784, 1981.

15. Bristow MR, Ginsburg R, Minobe W, Cunbicciotti RS, Sageman WS, Lurie K, Billingham ME, Harrison DC, Stinson EG: Decreased catecholamine sensitivity and β-adrenergic receptor density in failing human hearts. *N Engl J Med* 307:205–211, 1982.

16. Thomas JA, Marks BH: Plasma norepinephrine in congestive heart failure. *Am J Cardiol* 41:233–43, 1978.

17. Steinfath M, Danielsen W, Von der Leyen H, Mende U, Meyer W, Neumann J, Nose M, Reich T, Schmitz, Scholz H, Starbatty J, Stein B, Döring V, Kalmar P, Haverich A: Reduced α₁- and β-adrenoceptor-mediated positive inotropic effects in human end-stange heart failure. *Br J Pharmacol* 105:463–469, 1992.

18. McMonnaughey MM, Jones LR, Watanabe AM, Besch HR Jr, Williams LT, Lefkowitz RJ: Thyroxine and propylthiouracil effects on α- and β-adrenergic receptor number, ATPase activities, and sialic acid content of rat cardiac membrane vesicles. *J Cardiovasc Pharmacol* 1:609–623, 1979.

19. Williams LT, Lefkowitz RJ, Watanabe AW, Hathaway DR, Besch HR Jr: Thyroid hormone regulation of β-adrenergic receptor number. *J Biol Chem* 252:2767–2769, 1977.

20. Lazar Wesley E, Hadcock JR, Malbon CC, Kunos G, Ishac EJ: Tissue-specific regulation of α₁ᵦ, β₁, and β₂-adrenergic receptor mRNAs by thyroid state in the rat. *Endocrinology* 129:1116–1118, 1991.

21. Ginsberg AM, Clutter WE, Shah SD, Cryer PE: Triiodothyronine-induced thyrotoxicosis increases mononuclear leukocyte β-adrenergic receptor density in man. *J Clin Invest* 67:1785–1791, 1981.

22. Sibley DR, Lefkowitz RJ: Molecular mechanisms of receptor desensitization using the β-adrenergic receptor-coupled adenylyl cyclase system as a model. *Nature* 317:124–129, 1985.

23. Strasser RH, Sibley DR, Lefkowitz RJ: A novel catecholamine-activated adenosine cyclic 3′,5′-phosphate independent pathway for β-adrenergic receptor phosphorylation in wild-type and mutant S₄₉ lymphoma cells: Mechanism of homologous desensitization of adenylyl cyclase. *Biochemistry* 25:1371–1377, 1986.

24. Holmer SR, Homcy CJ: G proteins in the heart: A redundant and diverse transmembrane signaling network. *Circulation* 84:1891–1902, 1991.

25. Fleming JW, Wisler PL, Watanabe AM: Signal transduction by G proteins in cardiac tissues. *Circulation* 85:420–433, 1992.

26. Besch HR Jr, Jones LR, Fleming JW, Watanabe AM: Parallel unmasking of latent Na⁺,K⁺-ATPase and adenylyl cyclase activities in cardiac sarcolemmal vesicles: A new use of the channel-forming ionophore alamethicin. *J Biol Chem* 252:7905–7908, 1977.

27. Gilman AG: G proteins and regulation of adenylyl cyclase. *JAMA* 262:1819–1825, 1989.

28. Drummond GI: Resolution and properties of the catalytic subunit of cardiac adenylyl cyclase. *J Mol Cell Cardiol* 17:183–194, 1985.

29. Seamon KB, Daly JW: Guanosine 5′-(β,γ-imido) triphosphate inhibition of forskolin-activated adenylyl cyclase is mediated by the putative inhibitory guanine nucleotide regulatory protein. *J Biol Chem* 257:11591–11596, 1982.

30. Smith SK, Limbird LL: Evidence that human platelet α-adrenergic receptors coupled to inhibition of adenylyl cyclase are not associated with the subunit of adenylyl cyclase ADP-ribosylated by cholera toxin. *J Biol Chem* 257:10471–10478, 1982.

31. Hildebrandt JD, Hanoune J, Birhaumer L: Guanine nucleotide inhibition of cyc⁻ S49 mouse lymphoma cell membrane adenylyl cyclase. *J Biol Chem* 257:14723–14725, 1982.

32. Watanabe AM, McConnaughey MM, Strawbridge RA, Fleming JW, Jones LR, Besch HR Jr: Muscarinic cholinergic receptor modulation of β-adrenergic receptor affinity for catecholamines. *J Biol Chem* 253:4833–4836, 1978.

33. Birnbaumer L: G proteins in signal transduction. *Annu Rev Pharmacol Toxicol* 30:675–705, 1990.

34. Robishaw J, Foster KA: Role of G proteins in the regulation of the cardiovascular system. *Annu Rev Physiol* 51:229–244, 1989.

35. Ueda K, Hayaishi O: ADP-ribosylation. *Ann Rev Biochem* 54:73–100, 1985.

36. Cerione RA, Staniszewski C, Gierschick P, Codina J, Somers RL, Birnbaumer L, Spiegel AM, Caron MG, Lefkowitz RJ: Mechanism of guanine nucleotide regulatory protein-mediated inhibition of adenylyl cyclase. *J Biol Chem* 261:9514–9520, 1986.

37. Fleming JW, Strawbridge RA, Watanabe AM: Muscarinic receptor regulation of cardiac adenylyl cyclase activity. *J Mol Cell Cardiol* 19:47–61, 1987.

38. Krebs EG, Beavo JA: Phosphorylation-dephosphorylation of enzymes. *Ann Rev Biochem* 48:923–959, 1979.

39. Corbin JD, Sudgen PH, Lincoln TM, Keely SL: Compartmentalization of adenosine 3′:5′-monophosphate and adenosine 3′:5′-monophosphate-dependent protein kinase in heart tissue. *J Biol Chem* 252:3854–3861, 1977.

40. Hayes JS, Brunton LL, Mayer SE: Selective activation of particulate cAMP-dependent protein kinase by isoproterenol and prostaglandin E₁. *J Biol Chem* 255:5113–5119, 1980.

41. Buxton ILO, Brunton LL: Compartments of cyclic AMP and protein kinase in mammalian cardiomyocytes. *J Biol Chem* 258:10233–10239, 1983.

42. Stull JT, Mayer SE: Biochemical mechanisms of adrenergic and cholinergic regulation of myocardial contractility. In: Handbook of Physiology: The Cardiovascular System. Berne RM and Sperelakis N, (eds). Bethesda, MD: American Physiological Society, 1979, pp 741–774.

43. England PJ: Studies on the phosphorylation of the inhibitory subunit of troponin during modification of contraction in perfused rat heart. *Biochem J* 160:295–304, 1976.

44. Brunton LL, Hayes JS, Mayer SE: Hormonally specific phosphorylation of cardiac troponin I and activation of glycogen phosphorylase. *Nature* 280:78–80, 1979.

45. Robertson SP, Johnson JD, Holroyde MJ, Kranias EG, Potter JD, Solaro RJ: The effect of troponin I phosphorylation in the Ca²⁺-binding properties of the Ca²⁺-regulatory site of bovine cardiac troponin. *J Biol Chem* 257:260–263, 1980.

46. Jeacocke SA, England PJ: Phosphorylation of a myofibrillar protein of Mᵣ 150,000 in perfused rat heart, and the tentative identification of this as C-protein. *FEBS Lett* 122:129–132, 1980.

47. Hartzel, HC, Titus L: Effects of cholinergic and adrenergic

agonists on phosphorylation of a 165,000-Dalton myofibrillar protein in intact cardiac muscles. *J Biol Chem* 257: 2111–2120, 1982.

48. Hartzell HC: Phosphorylation of C-protein in intact amphibian cardiac muscle: Correlation between ^{32}P incorporation and twitch relaxation. *J Gen Physiol* 83:563–588, 1984.

49. Hartzell HC, Glass DB: Phosphorylation of purified cardiac muscle C-protein by purified cAMP-dependent protein kinase and endogenous Ca^{2+}-calmodulin-dependent protein kinases. *J Biol Chem* 259:15587–15596, 1984.

50. Winegrad S, Weisberg A, Lin LE, McClellan G: Adrenergic regulation of myosin adenosine triphosphatase activity. *Circ Res* 58:83–95, 1986.

51. Kirchberger MA, Tada M: Effects of adenosine 3′:5′-monophosphate-dependent protein kinase on sarcoplasmic reticulum isolated from cardiac and slow and fast contracting skeletal muscles. *J Biol Chem* 251:725–729, 1976.

52. Tada M, Katz AM: Phosphorylation of the sarcoplasmic reticulum and sarcolemma. *Annu Rev Physiol* 44:401–423, 1982.

53. Jones LR, Simmerman HKB, Wilson WW, Gurd FRN, Wegener AD: Purification and characterization of phospholamban from canine cardiac sarcoplasmic reticulum. *J Biol Chem* 260:7721–7730, 1985.

54. Simmerman HKB, Collins JH, Theibert JL, Wegener AD, Jones LR: Sequence analysis of phospholamban: Identification of phosphorylation sites and two major structural domains. *J Biol Chem* 261:13333–13341, 1986.

55. Fujii J, Ueno A, Katsuhiko K, Tanaka S, Kadoma M, Tada M: Complete complementary DNA-derived amino acid sequence of canine cardiac phospholamban. *J Clin Invest* 79:301–304, 1987.

56. Suzuki T, Wang JH: Stimulation of bovine sarcoplasmic reticulum Ca^{2+} pump and blocking of phospholamban phosphorylation and dephosphorylation by a phospholamban monoclonal antibody. *J Biol Chem* 261:7018–7023, 1986.

57. Kovacs RJ, Nelson MT, Simmerman HKB, Jones LR: Phospholamban forms Ca^{2+}-selective channels in lipid bilayers. *J Biol Chem* 263:18364–18368, 1988.

58. Le Peuch CJ, Guilleaux JC, De Maille JC: Phospholamban phosphorylation in the perfused rat heart is not solely dependent in beta adrenergic stimulation. *FEBS Lett* 114: 165–168, 1980.

59. Kranias EG, Solaro RJ: Phosphorylation of troponin I and phospholamban during catecholamine stimulation of rabbit heart. *Nature* 298:182–184, 1982.

60. Lindemann JP, Jones LR, Hathaway DR, Henry BG, Watanabe AM: β-adrenergic stimulation of phospholamban phosphorylation and Ca^{2+}-ATPase activity in guinea pig ventricles. *J Biol Chem* 258:464–471, 1984.

61. Sham JSK, Jones LR, Morad M: Phospholamban mediates the β-adrenergic-enhanced Ca^{2+} uptake in mammalian ventricular myocytes. *Am J Physiol* 261: H1344–H1349, 1991.

62. Tada M, Inui M, Yamada M, Kadoma M, Kuzuya T, Abe H, Kakiuchi S: Effects of phospholamban phosphorylation catalyzed by adenosine 3′, 5′-monophosphate- and calmodulin-dependent protein kinases on calcium transport ATPase of cardiac sarcoplasmic reticulum. *J Mol Cell Cardiol* 15:335–346, 1982.

63. Kirchberger MA, Antonetz T: Calmodulin-mediated regulation of calcium transport and (Ca^{2+} + Mg^{2+})-activated ATPase activity in isolated cardiac sarcoplasmic reticulum. *J Biol Chem* 257:5685–5691, 1982.

64. Lindemann JP, Watanabe AM: Phosphorylation of phospholamban in intact myocardium: Role of Ca^{2+}-calmodulin-dependent mechanisms. *J Biol Chem* 260:4516–4525, 1985.

65. Wegener AD, Simmerman HKB, Lindemann JP, Jones LR: Phospholamban phosphorylation in intact ventricles. Phosphorylation of serine 16 and threonine 17 in response to β-adrenergic stimulation. *J Biol Chem* 264:11468–11474, 1989.

66. Trautwein W, Hescheler J: Regulation of cardiac L-type calcium current by phosphorylation and G proteins. *Annu Rev Physiol* 52:257–274, 1990.

67. Brown AM, Birnbaumer L: Ionic channels and their regulation by G protein subunits. *Annu Rev Physiol* 52:197–213, 1990.

68. Szabo G, Otero AS: G protein mediated regulation of K$^+$ channels in heart. *Annu Rev Physiol* 52:293–305, 1990.

69. Schubert B, VanDongen AMJ, Kirsch GE, Brown AM: Inhibition of cardiac Na$^+$ currents by isoproterenol. *Am J Physiol (Heart Circ Physiol)* 258:H977–H981, 1990.

70. Matsuda JJ, Lee H, Shibata EF: Enhancement of rabbit cardiac sodium channels by β-adrenergic stimulation. *Circ Res* 70:199–207, 1992.

71. Harvey RD, Clark CD, Hume JR: Chloride current in mammalian cardiac myocytes. Novel mechanism for autonomic regulation of action potential duration and resting membrane potential. *J Gen Physiol* 95:1077–1102, 1990.

72. Mirro MJ, Bailey JC, Watanabe AM: Role of cyclic AMP in regulation of the slow inward current. In: *Role of the Slow Inward Current in Cardiac Electrophysiology*. The Hague: Matinus Nijhoff, 1980, pp 111–126.

73. Watanabe AM, Besch HR Jr: Cyclic adenosine monophosphate modulation of slow calcium influx channels in guinea pig hearts. *Circ Res* 35:316–324, 1974.

74. Sperelakis N: Phosphorylation hypothesis of the myocardial slow channels and control of Ca^{2+} influx. In: *Cardiac Electrophysiology and Arrhythmias*. New York: Grune and Stratton, 1985, pp 123–135.

75. Reuter H: Calcium channel modulation by neurotransmitters, enzymes and drugs. *Nature* 301:569–574, 1983.

76. Li T, Sperelakis N: Stimulation of slow action potentials in guinea pig papillary muscle cells by intracellular injection of cAMP, Gpp(NH)p, and cholera toxin. *Circ Res* 52:111–117, 1983.

77. Osterreider W, Brum G, Hescheler J, Trautwein W, Hofmann F, Flockerzi V: Injection of subunits of cyclic AMP-dependent protein kinase into cardiac myocytes modulates Ca^{2+} current. *Nature* 298:576–578, 1982.

78. Brum G, Flockerzi V, Hofmann F, Osterrieder W, Trautwein W: Injection of catalytic subunit of cAMP-dependent protein kinase into isolated cardiac myocytes. *Pflügers Arch* 398: 147–154, 1983.

79. Bean BP, Nowycky MC, Tsien RW: β-adrenergic modulation of calcium channels in frog ventricular heart cells. *Nature* 307:371–375, 1984.

80. Kameyama M, Hofmann F, Trautwein W: On the mechanism of β-adrenergic regulation of the Ca channel in the guinea-pig heart. *Pflügers Arch* 405:285–293, 1985.

81. Kameyama M, Hescheler J, Hofmann F, Trautwein W: Modulation of Ca current during the phosphorylation cycle in the guinea pig heart. *Pflügers Arch* 407:123–128, 1986.

82. Kameyama M, Hescheler J, Mieskes G, Trautwien W: The protein-specific phosphatase antagonizes the β-adrenergic increase of the cardiac Ca current. *Pflügers Arch* 407: 461–463, 1986.

83. Jones LR, Presti CF, Lindemann JP: Protein phosphorylation and the cardiac sarcolemma. In: *Protein Phosphorylation in Heart Muscle*. Solaro RJ (ed) Boca Raton, FL: CRC Press, 1986, pp 85–103.

84. Campbell KP, Lipshutz GM, Denney GH: Direct photo-affinity labeling of the high affinity nitrendipine-binding

site in subcellular membrane fractions isolated from canine myocardium. *J Biol Chem* 259:5384–5387, 1984.

85. Walsh DA, Clippinger MS, Sivaramakrishnan S, McCullough TE: Cyclic adenosine monophosphate depednent and independent phosphorylation of sarcolemmal proteins in perfused rat heart. *Biochemistry* 18:871–877, 1979.

86. Huggins JP, England PJ: Sarcolemmal phospholamban is phosphorylated in isolated rat hearts perfused with isoprenaline. *FEBS Lett* 163:297–302, 1983.

87. Presti CF, Jones LR, Lindemann JP: Isoproterenol-induced phosphorylation of a 15-kilodalton sarcolemmal protein in intact myocardium. *J Biol Chem* 260:3860–3867, 1985.

88. Lindemann JP: α-adrenergic stimulation of sarcolemmal protein phosphorylation and slow responses in intact myocardium. *J Biol Chem* 261:4860–4867, 1986.

89. Palmer CJ, Scott BT, Jones LR: Purification and complete sequence determination of the major plasma membrane substrate for cAMP-dependent protein kinase and protein kinase C in myocardium. *J Biol Chem* 266:11126–11130, 1991.

90. Moorman JR, Palmer CJ, John JE,III, Durieux ME, Jones LR: Phospholemman expression induces a hyperpolarization-activated chloride current in Xenopus oocytes. *J Biol Chem* 267:14551–14554, 1992.

91. Scholz H: Effects of β- and α-adrenoreceptor activators and adrenergic transmitter releasing agents on the mechanical activity of the heart. In: *Handbook of Experimental Pharmacology*, Vol 54/1. Berlin: Springer-Verlag, 1980, pp 651–733.

92. Benfey BG: Function of myocardial α-adrenoceptors. *Life Sci* 46:743–757, 1990.

93. Miura Y, Inui J: Multiple effects of α-adrenoceptor stimulation on the action potential of the rabbit atrium. *Naunyn-Schmiedebergs Arch Pharmacol* 325:47–53, 1984.

94. Bruckner R, Scholz H: Effects of α-adrenoreceptor stimulation with phenylephrine in the presence of propranolol on force of contraction, slow inward current and cyclic AMP content in the bovine heart. *Br J Pharmacol* 82:223–232, 1984.

95. Hescheler J, Trautwein W: Modulation of calcium currents of ventricular cells. In: Piper HM, Isenberg G (eds) *Isolated Adult Cardiomyocytes*, Vol 2: *Electrophysiology and Contractile Function*. Boca Raton, FL: CRC Press, 1989, pp 129–154.

96. Kushida H, Hiramoto T, Endoh M: The preferential inhibition of α₁- over β-adrenoceptor-mediated positive inotropic effect by organic calcium antagonists in the rabbit papillary muscle. *Naunyn-Schmiedebergs Arch Pharmacol* 341:206–214, 1990.

97. Endoh M, Hiramoto T, Ishihata A, Takanashi M, Inui J: Myocardial α₁-adrenoceptors mediate positive inotropic effect and changes in phosphatidylinositol metabolism. Species differences in receptor distribution and the intracellular coupling process in mammalian ventricular myocardium. *Circ Res* 68:1179–1190, 1991.

98. Apkon M, Nerbonne JM: α₁-adrenergic agonists selectively suppress voltage-dependent K^+ currents in rat ventricular myocytes. *Proc Natl Acad Sci USA* 85:8756–8760, 1988.

99. Ravens U, Wang XL, Wettwer E: Alpha-adrenoceptor stimulation reduces outward currents in rat ventricular myocytes. *J Pharmacol Exp Ther* 250:364–370, 1989.

100. Shah A, Cohen IS, Rosen MR: Stimulation of cardiac alpha receptors increases Na/K pump current and decreases gK via a pertussis toxin-sensitive pathway. *Biophys J* 54:219–225, 1988.

101. Zaza A, Kline RP, Rosen MR: Effects of α-adrenergic stimulation on intracellular sodium activity and automaticity in canine Purkinje fibers. *Circ Res* 66:416–426, 1990.

102. Ertl R, Jahnel U, Nawrath H, Carmeliet E, Vereecke J: Differential electrophysiologic and intropic effects of phenylephrine in atrial and venticular heart muscle preparations from rats. *Naunyn-Schmiedebergs Arch Pharmacol* 344:574–581, 1991.

103. Bode DC, Brunton LL: Adrenergic, cholinergic, and other hormone receptors on cardiac myocytes. In: Piper HM, Isenberg G (eds) *Isolated Adult Cardiomyocytes*, Vol I: *Structure and Metabolism*. Boca Raton, FL: CRC Press, 1989, pp 164–202.

104. Colucci WS, Gimbrone MA Jr, Alexander RW: Regulation of myocardial and vascular α-adrenergic receptor affinity: Effects of guanine nucleotides, cations, estrogen, and catecholamine depletion. *Circ Res* 55:78–88, 1984.

105. Karliner JS, Barnes P, Hamilton CA, Dollery CT: Alpha₁-adrenergic receptors in guinea pig myocardium: Identification by binding of a new radioligand, (^{3}H)-prazosin. *Biochem Biophys Res Commun* 90:142–149, 1979.

106. Minneman KP: α₁-adrenergic receptor subtypes, inositol phosphates, and sources of cell Ca^{2+}. *Pharmacol Rev* 40:87–119, 1988.

107. Lomasney JW, Cotecchia S, Lefkowitz RJ, Caron MG: Molecular biology of α-adrenergic receptors: Implications for receptor classification and for structure-function relationships. *Biochim Biophys Acta Mol Cell Res* 1095:127–139, 1991.

107a. Price DT, Schwinn DA, Caron MG, Lefkowitz RJ: Tissue specific expression of α₁-adrenergic receptor subtype mRNAs: Therapeutic implications for targeted receptor blockade (abstract). *Clin Res* 41:188A, 1993.

108. Karliner JS, Barnes P, Brown M, Dollery C: Chronic heart failure in the guinea pig increases cardiac α₁- and β-adrenoceptors. *Eur J Pharmacol* 67:115–118, 1980.

109. Kimball KA, Cornett LE, Seifen E, Kennedy RH: Aging: Changes in cardiac α₁-adrenoceptor responsiveness and expression. *Eur J Pharmacol* 208:231–238, 1991.

110. Watanabe AM, Hathaway DR, Besch HR Jr, Farmer BB, Harris RA: α-adrenergic reduction of cyclic adenosine monophosphate concentrations in rat myocardium. *Circ Res* 40:596–602, 1974.

111. Buxton ILO, Brunton LL: α-adrenergic receptors on rat ventricular myocytes: Characteristics and linkage to cAMP metabolism. *Am J Physiol* 251:H307–H313, 1986.

112. Keely SL, Corbin JD, Lincoln T: Alpha-adrenergic involvement in heart metabolism: Effects on adenosine cyclic 3′,5′-monophosphate, adenosine cyclic 3′,5′-monophosphate-dependent protein kinase, guanosine cyclic 3′,5′-monophosphate, and glucose transport. *Mol Pharmacol* 13:965–975, 1977.

113. Rosen MR, Steinberg SF, Chow YK, Bilezikian JP, Danilo P Jr: Role of a pertussis toxin-sensitive protein in the modulation of canine Purkinje fiber automaticity. *Circ Res* 62:315–323, 1988.

114. Steinberg SF, Druggee ED, Bilezikian JP, Robinson RB: Acquisition by innervated cardiac myocytes of a pertussis toxin-specific regulatory protein linked to the α₁-receptor. *Science* 230:186–188, 1985.

115. Buxton ILO, Brunton LL: Action of the cardiac α₁-adrenergic receptor: Activation of cyclic AMP degradation. *J Biol Chem* 260:6733–6737, 1985.

116. Tajima T, Tsuji Y, Brown JH, Pappano AJ: Pertussis toxin-insensitive phosphoinositide hydrolysis, membrane depolarization, and positive inotropic effect of carbachol in chick atria. *Circ Res* 61:436–445, 1987.

117. Del Balzo U, Rosen MR, Malfatto G, Kaplan LM, Steinberg

SF: Specific α-adrenergic receptor subtypes modulate catecholamine-induced increases and decreases in ventricular automaticity. *Circ Res* 67:1535–1551, 1990.

118. Berridge MJ: Inositol trisphosphate and diacylglycerol: Two interacting second messengers. *Ann Rev Biochem* 56: 159–193, 1988.

119. Nishizuka Y: The role of protein kinase C in cell surface signal transduction and tumour promotion. *Nature* 308: 693–698, 1984.

120. Brown JH, Jones LG: Phosphoinositide metabolism in the heart. In: Receptor Biochemistry and methodology. Venter JC, Harrison LC (eds) New York, Alan R. Liss, 1986, pp 245–270.

121. Otani H, Das DK: α₁-adrenoceptor-mediated phosphoinositide breakdown and inotropic response in rat left ventricular papillary muscles. *Circ Res* 62:8–17, 1988.

122. Nosek TM, Williams MF, Zeigler ST, Godt RE: Inositol trisphosphate enhances calcium release in skinned cardiac and skeletal muscle. *Am J Physiol* 250:C807–C811, 1986.

123. Takanashi M, Norota I, Endoh M: Potent inhibitory action of chlorethylclonidine on the positive inotropic effect and phosphoinositide hydrolysis mediated via myocardial alpha₁-adrenoceptors in the rabbit ventricular myocardium. *Naunyn-Schmiedebergs Arch Pharmacol* 343:669–673, 1991.

124. Henrich CJ, Simpson PC: Differential acute and chronic response of protein kinase C in cultured neonatal rat heart myocytes to α₁-adrenergic and phorbol ester stimulation. *J Mol Cell Cardiol* 20:1081–1085, 1988.

125. Presti CF, Scott BT, Jones LR: Identification of an endogenous protein kinase C activity and its intrinsic 15-kilodalton substrate in purified canine cardiac sarcolemmal vesicles. *J Biol Chem* 260:13879–13889, 1985.

126. Talosi L, Kranias EG: Effect of α-adrenergic stimulation on activation of protein kinase C and phosphorylation of proteins in intact rabbit hearts. *Circ Res* 70:670–678, 1992.

127. Shearman MS, Sekiguchi K, Nishizuka Y: Modulation of ion channel activity: A key function of the protein kinase C enzyme family. *Pharmacol Rev* 41:211–237, 1989.

128. Capogrossi MC, Kaku T, Filburn CR, Pelto DJ, Hansford RG, Spurgeon HA, Lakatta EG: Phorbol ester and dioctanoylglycerol stimulate membrane association of protein kinase C and have a negative inotropic effect mediated by changes in cytosolic Ca^{2+} in adult rat cardiac myocytes. *Circ Res* 66:1143–1155, 1990.

129. Capogrossi MC, Kachadorian WA, Gambassi G, Spurgeon HA, Lakatta EG: Ca^{2+} dependence of α-adrenergic effects on the contractile properties and Ca^{2+} homeostasis of cardiac myocytes. *Circ Res* 69:540–550, 1991.

130. Walsh KB, Kass RS: Regulation of a heart potassium channel by protein kinase A and C. *Science* 242:67–69, 1988.

131. Tohse N, Nakaya H, Hattori Y, Endou M, Kanno M: Inhibitory effect mediated by α₁-adrenoceptors on transient outward current in isolated rat ventricular cells. *Pflügers Arch* 415:575–581, 1990.

132. Fedida D, Shimoni Y, Giles WR: A novel effect of norepinephrine on cardiac cells is mediated by α₁-adrenoceptors. *Am J Physiol* 256:H1500–H1504, 1989.

133. Dösemeci A, Dhallan RS, Cohen NM, Lederer WJ, Rogers TB: Phorbol ester increases calcium current and stimulates the effects of angiotensin II on cultured neonatal rat heart myocytes. *Circ Res* 62:347–357, 1988.

134. Lacerda AE, Rampe D, Brown AM: Effects of protein kinase C activators on cardiac Ca^{2+} channels. *Nature* 335: 249–251, 1988.

135. Allen IS, Gaa ST, Rogers TB: Changes in expression of a functional Gi protein in cultured rat heart cells. *Am J Physiol* 24:C51–C59, 1988.

136. Loffelholz K, Pappano AJ: The parasympathetic neuroeffector junction of the heart. *Pharmacol Rev* 37:1–24, 1985.

137. Levy MN: Sympathetic-parasympathetic interactions in the heart. *Circ Res* 29:437–445, 1971.

138. Birdsall NJM, Hulme EC: Biochemical studies on muscarinic acetylcholine receptors. *J Neurochem* 27:7–16, 1976.

139. Ehlert FJ, Roeske WR, Yamamura HT: The nature of muscarinic receptor binding. In: Iversen LL, Iversen SD, Snyder SH (eds) *Handbook of Psychopharmacology*. New York: Plenum Press, 1983, pp 241–283.

140. Mattera R, Pitts BJR, Entman ML, Birnbaumer L: Guanine nucleotide regulation of a mammalian myocardial muscarinic receptor system. *J Biol Chem* 260:7410–7421, 1985.

141. Brown JH, Goldstein D, Masters SB: The putative M₁ muscarinic receptor does not regulate phosphoinositide hydrolysis. *Mol Pharmacol* 27:525–531, 1985.

142. Manalan AS, Werth DK, Jones LR, Watanabe AM: Enrichment, solubilization, and partial characterization of digitoninsolubilized muscarinic receptors derived from canine ventricular myocardium. *Circ Res* 52:664–676, 1983.

143. Florio VA, Sternweiss PC: Reconstitution of resolved muscarinic cholinergic receptors with purified GTP-binding proteins. *J Biol Chem* 260:3477–3483, 1985.

144. Kurose H, Katada T, Haga T, Haga K, Ichiyama A, Ui M: Functional interaction of purified muscarinic receptors with purified inhibitory guanine nucleotide regulatory proteins reconstituted in phospholipid vesicles. *J Biol Chem* 261: 6423–6428, 1986.

145. Haga K, Haga T, Ichiyama A, Katada T, Kurose H, Ui M: Functional reconstitution of purified muscarinic receptors and inhibitory guanine nucleotide regulatory protein. *Nature* 316:731–733, 1985.

146. Galper JB, Smith TW: Properties of muscarinic acetylcholine receptors in heart cell cultures. *Proc Natl Acad Sci USA* 75:5831–5835, 1978.

147. Roskoski R Jr, Reinhardt RR, Enseleit W, Johnson WD, Cook PD: Cardiac cholinergic muscarinic receptors: Changes in multiple affinity forms with down regulation. *J Pharmacol Exp Ther* 232:754–759, 1985.

148. Halvorsen SW, Nathanson NM: In vivo regulation of muscarinic acetylcholine receptor number and function in embryonic chick heart. *J Biol Chem* 256:7941–7948, 1981.

149. Kwatra MM, Hosey MM: Phosphorylation of the cardiac muscarinic receptor in intact chick heart and its regulation by a muscarinic agonist. *J Biol Chem* 261:12429–12432, 1986.

150. Sharma VK, Banerjee SP: Muscarinic cholinergic receptors in rat heart: Effect of thyroidectomy. *J Biol Chem* 252: 7444–7446, 1977.

151. Ten Eick R, Nawrath H, McDonald TF, Trautwein W: On the negative inotropic effect of acetylcholine. *Pflügers Arch* 361:207–213, 1976.

152. Trautwein W: Generation and conduction of impulses in the heart as affected by drugs. *Pharmacol Rev* 15:277–332, 1963.

153. Inoue D, Hachisu M, Pappano AJ: Acetylcholine increases resting membrane potassium conductance in atrial but not ventricular muscle during muscarinic inhibition of Ca^{2+}-dependent action potentials in chick heart. *Circ Res* 53:158–167, 1983.

154. Martin JM, Hunter DD, Nathanson NM: Islet activating protein inhibits physiological responses evoked by cardiac muscarinic acetylcholine receptors. Role of guanosine triphosphate binding proteins in regulation of potassium permeability. *Biochemistry* 24:7521–7525, 1985.

155. Breitwieser G, Szabo G: Uncoupling of cardiac muscarinic and β-adrenergic receptors from ion channels by a guanine nucleotide analogue. *Nature* 317:538–540, 1985.

156. Pfaffinger PJ, Martin JM, Hunter DD, Nathanson NM, Hille B: GTP-binding proteins couple cardiac muscarinic receptors to a K channel. *Nature* 317:536–538, 1985.

157. Kurachi Y, Nakajima T, Sugimoto T: Acetylcholine activation of K^+ channels in cell-free membrane of atrial cells. *Am J Physiol* 251:H681–H684, 1986.

158. Yatani A, Codina J, Brown AM, Birnbaumer L: Direct activation of mamalian atrial muscarinic potassium channels by GTP regulatory protein G_k. *Science* 235:207–211, 1987.

159. Logothetis DE, Kurachi Y, Galper J, Neer EJ, Clapham DE: The βγ subunits of GTP-binding proteins activate the muscarinic K^+ channel in heart. *Nature* 325:321–326, 1987.

160. Goldberg ND, Haddox MK: Cyclic GMP metabolism and involvement in biological regulation. *Annu Rev Biochem* 46:823–896, 1977.

161. Linden J, Brooker G: The questionable role of cyclic guanosine 3′:5′-monophosphate in heart. *Biochem Pharmacol* 28:3351–3360, 1979.

162. Krause EG, Halle W, Wollenberger A: Effect of direct dibutyryl cyclic GMP on cultured beating rat heart cells. *Adv Cyclic Nucleotide Res* 1:301–305, 1972.

163. Tuganowski W, Kopec P, Kopyta M, Wezowska J: Iontophoretic application of autonomic mediators and cyclic nucleotides in sinus node cells. *Naunyn-Schmiedebergs Arch Pharmacol* 299:65–67, 1977.

164. Kohlhardt M, Haap K: 8-bromo-guanosine-3′,5′-monophosphate mimics the effect of acetylcholine on slow response action potential and contractile force in mammalian atrial myocardium. *J Mol Cell Cardiol* 10:573–586, 1978.

165. Nawrath H: Does cyclic GMP mediate the negative inotropic effect of acetylcholine in the heart? *Nature* 267:72–74, 1977.

166. Watanabe AM, Besch HR Jr: Interaction between cyclic adenosine monophosphate and cyclic guanosine monophosphate in guinea pig ventricular myocardium. *Circ Res* 37:309–317, 1975.

167. Watanabe AM, Hathaway DR, Besch HR Jr: Mechanism of cholinergic antagonism of the effects of isoproterenol on hearts from hyperthyroid rats. In: Kobayashi T, Sano T, Dhalla N (eds) *Recent Advances in Studies on Cardiac Structure and Metabolism*, Vol 11. Baltimore, MD: University Park Press, 1978, pp 423–429.

168. Ong SH, Steiner AL: Localization of cyclic GMP and cyclic AMP in cardiac and skeletal muscle: Immunocytochemical demonstration. *Science* 195:183–185, 1977.

169. Mirro MJ, Harper JF, Steiner AL: Compartmentation of cGMP in sinus node: Subcellular localization by immunocytochemistry. *Circulation* 62:III239, 1980.

170. Lincoln TM, Keely SL: Regulation of the cardiac cyclic GMP-dependent protein kinase. *Biochem Biophys Acta* 676:230–244, 1981.

171. Mirro MJ, Bailey JC, Watanabe AM: Dissociation between the electrophysiological properties and total tissue cyclic GMP content of guinea pig atria. *Circ Res* 45:225–233, 1979.

172. Pappano AJ, Hartigen PM, Coutu MD: Acetylcholine inhibits the positive inotropic effects of cholera toxin in ventricular muscle. *Am J Physiol* 243:H434–H441, 1982.

173. Revtyak G, Jones LR, Watanabe AM, Besch HR Jr: Canine myocardial guanylate cyclase: Differential activation of sarcolemmal and cytoplasmic forms. *Pharmacologist* 20:147, 1978.

174. Lindemann JP, Besch HR Jr, Watanabe AM: Indirect and direct effects of the divalent cation inophore A23187 on guinea pig and rat ventricular myocardium. *Circ Res* 44:472–482, 1979.

175. Wallach F, Pastan I: Stimulation of membranous guanylate cyclase by concentrations of calcium that are in the physio-logical range. *Biochem Biophys Res Commun* 72:859–865, 1976.

176. Quist E: Evidence for a carbachol stimulated phosphatidylinositol effect in heart. *Biochem Pharmacol* 31:3130–3133, 1982.

177. Brown SL, Brown JH: Muscarinic stimulation of phosphatidylinositol metabolism in atria. *Mol Pharmacol* 24:351–356, 1983.

178. Brown JH, Buxton IL, Brunton LL: α₁-adrenergic and muscarinic cholinergic stimulation of phosphoinositide hydrolysis in adult rat cardiomyocytes. *Circ Res* 57:532–537, 1985.

179. Brown JH, Brown SL: Agonists differentiate muscarinic receptors that inhibit cyclic AMP formation from those that stimulate phosphoinositide metabolism. *J Biol Chem* 259:3777–3781, 1984.

180. Brown BS, Polson JB, Krzanowski JJ, Wiggins JR: Influence of isoproterenol and methylisobutylxanthine on the contractile and cyclic nucleotide effects of methacholine in isolated rat atria. *J Pharmacol Exp Ther* 212:325–332, 1980.

181. Bailey JC, Watanabe AM, Besch HR Jr, Lathrop DR: Acetylcholine antagonism of the electrophysiological effects of isoproterenol on canine cardiac Purkinje fibers. *Circ Res* 44:378–383, 1979.

182. Inui J, Imamura H: Effects of acetylcholine on calcium-dependent electrical and mechanical response in the guinea-pig papillary muscle partially depolarized by potassium. *Naunyn-Schmiedebergs Arch Pharmacol* 299:1–7, 1977.

183. Hescheler, J, Kameyama M, Trautwein W: On the mechanism of muscarinic inhibition of the cardiac Ca current. *Pflügers Arch* 407:182–189, 1986.

184. Hartzell HC, Fischmeister R: Opposite effects of cyclic GMP and cyclic AMP on Ca^{2+} current in single heart cells. *Nature* 323:273–275, 1986.

185. Gardner RM, Allen DO: The relationship between cyclic nucleotide levels and glycogen phosphorylase in isolated rat hearts perfused with epinephrine and acetylcholine. *J Pharmacol Exp Ther* 202:346–353, 1977.

186. Murad F, Chi YM, Rall TW, Sutherland EW: Adenyl cyclase. *J Biol Chem* 237:1233–1238, 1962.

187. La Raia PJ, Sonnenblick EH: Autonomic control of cardiac cAMP. *Circ Res* 28:377–384, 1971.

188. Meester WD, Hardman HF: Blockade of the positive inotropic actions of epinephrine and theophylline by acetylcholine. *J Pharmacol Exp Ther* 158:241–247, 1967.

189. Biegon RL, Epstein PM, Pappano AJ: Muscarinic antagonism of the effects of a phosphodiesterase inhibitor (methylisobutylxanthine) in embryonic chick ventricle. *J Pharmacol Exp Ther* 215:348–356, 1980.

190. Keely SL Jr, Lincoln TM, Corbin JD: Interaction of acetylcholine and epinephrine on heart cyclic AMP-dependent protein kinase. *Am J Physiol* 234:H432–H438, 1978.

191. Lindemann JP, Watanabe AM: Muscarinic cholinergic inhibition of β-adrenergic stimulation of phospholamban phosphorylation and Ca^{2+}-transport in guinea pig ventricules. *J Biol Chem* 260:13122–13129, 1985.

192. Iwasa Y, Hosey MM: Cholinergic antagonism of β-adrenergic stimulation of cardiac membrane protein phosphorylation in situ. *J Biol Chem* 258:4571–4575, 1983.

193. Manalan AS, Besch HR Jr, Watanabe AM: Characterization of [³H] (±) carazolol binding to β-adrenergic receptors: Application to study of β-adrenergic receptor subtypes in canine ventricular myocardium and lung. *Circ Res* 49:326–336, 1981.

194. Mirro MJ, Manalan AS, Bailey JC, Watanabe AM: Anticholinegic effects of disopyramide and quinidine on guinea pig myocardium: Mediation by direct muscarinic receptor blockade. *Circ Res* 47:855–865, 1980.

CHAPTER 25

Pharmacology of Cardiac Glycosides

TAI AKERA & THEODORE M. BRODY

INTRODUCTION

The term *cardiac glycosides* is commonly used to represent a wide variety of steroid derivatives that have the property of increasing the force of cardiac contraction and eliciting characteristic electrophysiological effects. These substances are contained in many plant and animal sources. The medicinal actions of the squill, or sea onion, were recognized as early as 1500 B.C. The glycosides most frequently used today are derived from the leaves of the foxglove, *Digitalis purpurea* and *D. lanata*. The classic study on the actions of digitalis was published in 1785 by William Withering, who described his experience with digitalis in *An Account of the Foxglove, and Some of Its Medicinal Uses: With Practical Remarks on Dropsy, and other Diseases* {1}. Withering recognized the efficacy of digitalis in reducing edema and its notorious tendency to produce arrhythmias. A second comprehensive monograph was published 14 years later by John Ferrier, who suggested that the beneficial effects of digitalis might stem from an action on the heart. Traube in 1850 recognized the effect of digitalis in promoting the efficiency of cardiac muscle and further suggested that the bradycardia observed was the result of vagal stimulation. The usefulness of digitalis preparations in atrial fibrillation was first established in the early 20th century. Following the purification of the digitalis glycosides, they became the mainstay of therapy for congestive heart failure.

Cattell and Gold demonstrated that cardiac glycosides increase the force of contraction in nonfailing as well as failing heart muscle preparations isolated from the cat {2}. They further raised the question of whether the positive inotropic (therapeutic) and toxic (arrhythmogenic) actions of the glycosides could be separated by modification of their chemical structures {3}. On the basis of the few compounds available at the time, they concluded that these actions of the glycosides were inseparable. This conclusion still holds true today after the synthesis and testing of a large number of compounds. The current theory is that both the inotropic and toxic effects of the glycosides are caused by an interaction of the drug with the same receptor, sarcolemmal Na,K-ATPase. This hypothesis provides the theoretical basis that therapeutic and toxic actions of glycosides cannot be completely separated by the modification of the chemical structure.

Because of its narrow margin of safety and because a given plasma glycoside concentration produces therapeutic effects in many patients and intoxication in others, toxic manifestations during clinical use of the glycosides are a common, serious, and potentially fatal complication. In recent years, efforts have been directed to (a) synthesizing newer and safer positive inotropic drugs and (b) developing alternative treatments of congestive heart failure using a combination of diuretics and vasodilators. Attempts to synthesize newer and safer positive inotropic drugs have met with only limited success.

It is important to understand how the glycosides produce their therapeutic and toxic effects. First, the glycosides enhance efficiency of the excitation-contraction coupling mechanism in cardiac muscle. Therefore, an understanding of the mechanism of action of the cardiac glycoside leads us to a better knowledge of cardiac muscle physiology that may be modulated by a new drug. Furthermore, digitalis toxicity results from Ca^{2+} overload of cardiac muscle. Therefore, understanding the mechanisms responsible for the expression of digitalis toxicity is essential to our understanding of the relationship between cardiotoxicity and Ca^{2+} overload. Myocardial Ca^{2+} overload also results from overdose of newer positive inotropic drugs or catecholamines, ischemia, and reperfusion, and toxicity caused by many other therapeutic agents including doxorubicin. Doxorubicin is a potent anticancer drug whose clinical usefulness is limited by cardiac toxicity. Finally, the cardiac glycosides are still widely used for the treatment of congestive heart failure and supraventricular arrhythmias.

CHEMISTRY

The chemistry of cardiotonic steroids and their structure-activity relationships have been studied extensively over the past 60 years. In 1960s, structural characteristics required for cardiotonic activity were considered to be well established {4}; however, more recent data suggest that earlier hypotheses no longer hold. A review by Thomas et al. {5} encompasses both the classic structure-activity relationship studies and some of the newer findings. In this

N. Sperelakis (ed.), Physiology and Pathophysiology of the Heart, Third Edition.

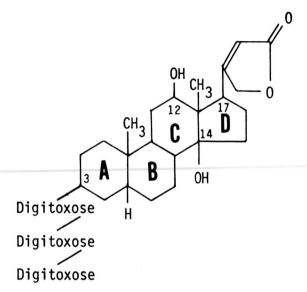

Fig. 25-1. Chemical structure of the cardiac glycoside, digoxin. The aglycone, digoxigenin, lacks the sugars (all three digitoxoses) in the 3-position. Digitoxin differs from digoxin by the absence of a hydroxyl group at the C-12 position. Ouabain, which has a rhamnose as a sugar and 5 hydroxyl groups on the steroid nucleus, is relatively water soluble and is frequently used for in vitro studies.

study, a model for the interaction of the inotropic drugs with the putative digitalis receptor is described. The model is consistent with the concept that the effects of these agents to increase force of contraction are closely related to their inhibitory effect on Na,K-ATPase.

The cardiac glycoside consists of an aglycone, or genin, and one or more sugar molecules. For example, digoxin, the glycoside most frequently used in the United States, possesses aglycone, digoxigenin, and three molecules of digitoxose attached at position 3 (see fig. 25-1). The aglycones are steroids containing an unsaturated lactone ring and are generally shorter acting and less potent as cardiotonic agents, but have the same therapeutic and toxic characteristics as the glycosides.

Classic structure-activity relationship studies of the digitalis-like compounds indicate that inotropic activity resides only in those derivatives with 14-hydroxysteroids substituted with a 17-unsaturated lactone ring and additionally possessing the stereochemical features of the digitalis steroids, specifically, a cis/trans/cis configuration at the ring junctions {4}. Corticosteroids, which have the trans fusion between the C and D rings, were considered to be devoid of digitalis-like activities. Subsequently, however, it was found that there are A-B trans compounds that are more potent than digoxin (e.g., asclepin). Neither the hydroxyl group at C-14 nor the double bond in the lactone ring and cis-fusion at the C-D junction are absolute requirements (e.g., prednisolone-3,20-bisguanyl-hydrazone and chlormadinone acetate). Substitution of a C-14 hydroxyl group by hydrogen, or saturation or

modification of the lactone ring, results in a considerable loss of potency, but not efficacy, for the inotropic effect {6}. The C-14 hydroxyl group appears to be important only for positioning the lactone ring at an optimal angle with the steroid nucleus. The receptor apparently has binding sites complementary to the unsaturated lactone ring at C-17 and the first sugar attached at the C-3 position. Alterations of these sites generally reduce the affinity of the molecule for its receptor site. These changes do not alter the efficacy of these compounds in eliciting a positive inotropic effect. The lack of strict structural requirements is not surprising because such diverse chemical structures as prednisolone-3,20-bisguanylhydrazone and cassaine share common pharmacological properties with the cardiac glycosides.

Among the various glycosides and aglycones, there is a difference in the number and position of hydroxyl groups. Apparently hydroxyl groups are important for determining lipid solubility, protein binding, biotransformation, and therefore the duration of action of a particular compound. Contrary to a common misunderstanding, digitoxose molecules attached to digoxigenin or digitoxigenin neither increase water solubility nor decrease lipid solubility {7}. Digitalis-like compounds containing a five-membered unsaturated lactone ring at C-17 are called *cardenolides*. The more common ones are digoxin, digitoxin, and ouabain.

PHARMACOKINETICS

Clinically, the most widely used preparations are digoxin and digitoxin. Their pharmacokinetics in humans have been extensively studied. In normal patients, the absorption of digoxin following oral administration varies from 45% to 85%, depending on the preparation used. Absorption of digoxin is more favorable from hydroalcoholic solutions, and variable and generally low with tablets. Differences in bioavailability among digoxin tablets pose problems. Although digoxin tablets must now meet a tablet dissolution test, physicians using a specific brand should probably maintain the patient on that preparation. Following oral administration, a peak level of digoxin is achieved at 45–60 minutes. Concentrations of digoxin in plasma then fall in a slowly declining phase 5–6 hours after drug administration. This latter phase represents a half-life ($t_{1/2}$) of approximately 35 hours, which results from metabolism and excretion of the drug.

Absorption of digitoxin, which is more lipid soluble than digoxin, is almost complete after oral administration. The biological half-life of digitoxin is about 5–6 days in humans. Avid tissue binding and the ensuing large apparent volume of distribution for digitoxin contribute to its long biological half-life.

The cardiac glycosides are widely distributed throughout tissue and fluid compartments of the body. Plasma proteins are a significant site for glycoside binding; about 25% of digoxin and 90% of digitoxin in plasma are bound to proteins. Both glycosides are distributed to all body tissues, with highest concentrations found in kidney, skeletal muscle, heart, liver, and adrenal. Most tissues have concentrations up to 100 times greater than that of the free drug concentration found in plasma at equilibrium, indicating avid binding of the glycosides to tissue protein. The importance of skeletal muscle has been emphasized as a distribution volume for digitalis glycosides in guinea pigs and human subjects.

Digoxin is removed from the body primarily by renal excretion. The fraction of unchanged digoxin excreted in urine varies from 40% to 90%, with the remainder probably consisting of polar, conjugated metabolites. The most important determinant of the fate of digoxin is renal function; clearance of this glycoside is directly proportional to creatinine clearance. A small amount of digoxin is secreted by the kidney, with some reabsorbed from the tubular lumen. Variable amounts of digoxin (5–50%) are metabolized in humans during chronic digoxin treatment.

Digitoxin is believed to be largely metabolized by liver, and renal function does not significantly alter the half-life of this glycoside. Up to 50–80% of that excreted in urine may be in the form of unchanged digitoxin. However, nearly 60% of a given dose of digitoxin is unaccounted for as unchanged digitoxin or its metabolites in urine and feces. Moreover, large individual variations exist in the ability of normal volunteers and patients to metabolize digitoxin. Cleavage of the sugar residues of digitoxin in liver is not by simple hydrolysis but involves the mixed-function oxidase system. Conjugation reactions with glucuronic or sulfuric acid may also occur following cleavage. Enzymatic 12β-hydroxylation of digitoxin to digoxin occurs in animals, but is a minor pathway in humans. Apparently, intestinal flora can play a significant role in the overall metabolism of digitoxin.

Cardiac glycosides are distributed relatively slowly throughout the body and have a large apparent volume of distribution. Their onset of action is slow, even in isolated heart muscle preparations exposed to a fixed concentration of glycoside. This slow onset of action results from slow binding of the drug to its pharmacological receptor. The rate of glycoside binding is dependent on the concentration of K^+ in the extracellular environment and also the intracellular Na^+ concentration {8,9}. Effects of these ions are similar to those on glycoside binding to Na,K-ATPase observed in vitro. For example, the rate of binding of digitalis to its receptor is enhanced, as is its rate of onset and degrees of pharmacological action in a hypokalemic animal, or in a patient with a low plasma K^+ concentration. Hyperkalemia retards the onset of the digitalis effect {10}. Na^+ influx across the cardiac cell membrane promotes binding of the cardiac glycoside to its receptor. Therefore, the extracellular Na^+ concentration, the presence of the Na^+ ionophore, such as monensin, or the number of contractions or depolarizations per unit time (which all tend to increase Na^+ influx) will influence the rate of onset of glycoside action {9}. In contrast, a reduction in rate of Na^+ influx does not delay the onset of glycoside action to a significant degree {11, also see below}.

The difference in sensitivity of the heart to the positive inotropic action of the cardiac glycosides is remarkable among various animal species and is unique among ino-tropic drugs. Part of these species-dependent differences in glycoside sensitivity result from differences in the rate of metabolism and elimination of the glycoside. The primary cause of these differences, however, is inherent in heart muscle. This is indicated by the observation that glycoside sensitivity is remarkably different in isolated heart muscle preparations obtained from various species. The isolated myocardium from human, dog, cat, cow, or sheep is highly sensitive to the inotropic and toxic actions of the glycoside, whereas that from guinea pig or rabbit is approximately an order of magnitude less sensitive. Glycoside concentrations needed to produce a marked positive inotropic effect in rat heart are two orders of magnitude higher than those required for guinea-pig or rabbit hearts, although a small positive inotropic effect may be observed with low concentrations of the glycoside (so-called low-dose inotropic effect) in rat ventricular muscle. These differences in glycoside sensitivity are apparently caused by variations in affinity of the receptor for glycoside {12}. A similar magnitude of inotropic effect can be obtained in each species when the myocardium is exposed to appropriate concentrations of the glycoside, i.e., dose-response curves are parallel (fig. 25-2).

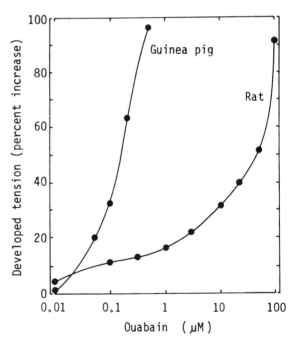

Fig. 25-2. Differences in response of rat and guinea pig heart to the positive inotropic effect of ouabain. Isolated ventricular muscle strips were incubated in Krebs–Henseleit bicarbonate buffer solution (pH 7.4) at 30°C and stimulated at 1.5 Hz. Each point represents the mean of five experiments. Rat heart is generally regarded to be "digitalis insensitive"; however, the difference is in the glycoside concentration required to produce the effect and not the magnitude of response. Rat heart has a small fraction of Na,K-ATPase that has high affinity for the glycoside. Corresponding to this, a small positive inotropic effect can be observed at low concentrations (0.1–1 µM) of ouabain.

Doses (expressed as mg/kg of body weight) of cardiac glycoside needed to produce an inotropic effect in neonates and young children are considerably larger than those in adults. This does not result from differences in metabolic disposition or excretion. Therefore, in younger individuals or animals, higher serum concentrations of drug are observed with no evidence of toxicity. Reasons for this tolerance to digitalis by younger patients are unclear; however, in ferret heart in which two isoenzymes of Na,K-ATPase are found, the high-affinity $\alpha(+)$ form is lacking in neonatal hearts, corresponding to a lack in the low-dose positive inotropic effect. As the ferret matures, the $\alpha(+)$ form of Na,K-ATPase appears and the low-dose effect of the glycoside becomes apparent.

PHARMACODYNAMICS

Digitalis has two useful clinical effects. These are (a) to increase the force of myocardial contraction in patients with congestive heart failure and (b) to slow the beating of the ventricle in atrial fibrillation or flutter. It was thought for many years that the beneficial effects of digitalis in congestive heart failure might result from slowing of the ventricular rate and a resulting increase in filling volume. It is now firmly established, however, that the primary beneficial effect results from the positive inotropic action caused by a direct action of digitalis on the heart. Its effect on the electrophysiological activity of the heart, including slowing of the ventricular rate, is either direct or indirect. The latter involves the autonomic nervous system. The cardiac glycosides have significant effects on sympathetic and parasympathetic function in both therapeutic and toxic concentrations. Changes in sympathetic and parasympathetic influence on the heart may be caused by alterations in baroreceptor sensitivity, direct actions of the drug on brain, or a modification of transmission at neuro-effector junctions. Thus, the overall pharmacodynamics of this class of compounds is complex, influenced by indirect as well as by direct effects on the target tissue.

Positive inotropic effects

The cardiac glycosides increase the force of contraction of both atrial and ventricular heart muscle. This is in contrast to some of the newer experimental positive inotropic drugs, which may be less efficacious in either atrial or ventricular muscle. The *positive inotropic effect* of the cardiac glycosides can be consistently observed in various isolated cardiac muscle preparations obtained from a variety of animals, including humans. The glycoside increases contractility in normal as well as the failing heart; however, the positive inotropic effect is not generally seen in normal patients or unanesthetized animals because of counterbalancing hemodynamic adjustments.

In isolated heart muscle preparations, cardiac glycosides increase peak developed tension without altering the time to peak tension or the rate of relaxation (fig. 25-3). With higher concentrations and after prolonged exposure, either a negative inotropic effect associated with an in-

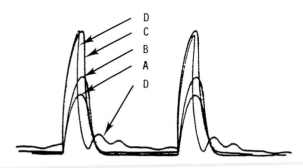

Fig. 25-3. Twitch-tension curves showing the positive inotropic and toxic effects of ouabain. An isolated papillary muscle preparation obtained from guinea pig heart was incubated in Krebs–Henseleit bicarbonate buffer solution (pH 7.4) at 30°C and stimulated at 0.6 Hz in the presence of 5 µM propranolol and 2 µM phentolamine. **A:** At the end of 60-minute equilibration (control). **B:** Four minutes after the addition of 3 µM ouabain. Developed tension increased without changes in time to peak tension. **C:** Eleven minutes after ouabain addition. Time to peak tension is slightly decreased. At 40 minutes, ouabain concentration was increased to 8 µM (= toxic concentration). **D:** Ten minutes after the increase in ouabain concentration. Resting tension was elevated and oscillatory aftercontractions developed. The tracings are provided by Dr. Yuk-Chow Ng, Department of Pharmacology and Toxicology, Michigan State University.

crease in resting tension (contracture) or oscillatory aftercontractions may be observed (fig. 25-3). The duration of twitch contraction may be shortened at this stage, probably resulting from enhanced catecholamine release from sympathetic nerve terminals.

During congestive heart failure, a number of pathophysiological events occur that are ultimately modified by digitalis treatment. The basic defect is the inability of the heart to adequately perfuse the tissues with blood. While the initial insult resulting in depression of myocardial contractility may vary, the pathological sequelae are similar. When the force of contraction of heart muscle becomes inadequate, several mechanisms are triggered in an attempt to compensate for the deficit. There is an increase in end-diastolic volume, resulting in the heart operating at a new point on the Frank–Starling ventricular function curve (fig. 25-4). This is followed by an increase in sympathetic nerve activity and, finally, a significant increase in ventricular size. Sympathetic activity is increased, responding to reduced cardiac output and blood pressure, stimulating the baroreceptor reflex. The result is a compensatory rise in heart rate, peripheral resistance, and blood pressure. This increase in sympathetic activity forces the heart to work harder to eject adequate blood to perfuse the tissues at the expense of decreased cardiac efficiency. Intravascular volume, and therefore preload, may also be increased by activation of the renin-angiotensin-aldosterone axis and the release of vasopressin.

An increase in sympathetic activity decreases energetic efficiency of the failing heart by the following mechanisms: (a) A shortening of the twitch contraction time of individual myocytes decreases the tension-time integral for

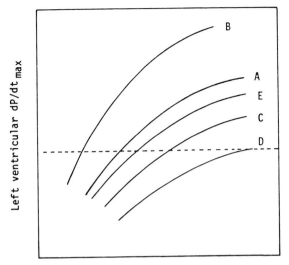

Fig. 25-4. Ventricular function curves. The first derivative of increase in ventricular pressure ($+dP/dt_{max}$) is an index of ventricular contractility. **A:** Normal. **B:** Normal heart in the presence of digitalis. Ventricular end-diastolic volume decreases until developed tension matches that needed for normal function. **C:** Compensated, hypertrophied heart. Ventricular end-diastolic volume increases until developed tension matches that needed for normal function. **D:** Failing heart. **E:** Failing heart during digitalis treatment. The broken line represents the level of ventricular contractility required for normal activity.

the amount of ATP hydrolyzed by the actin-myosin system. (b) An increase in total peripheral vascular resistance increases the work of heart muscle to achieve a given tissue perfusion. (c) An increase in heart rate reduces the efficiency of pumping resulting from decreased stroke volume. (d) In addition, an increase in ventricular diameter observed in failing heart further decreases energetic efficiency because a greater wall tension is required to develop the necessary intraventricular pressure as described by the law of LaPlace.

In compensated heart failure, an increased preload is necessary to maintain cardiac output at the expense of a reduced ventricular ejection fraction. Myocardial oxygen consumption is increased and vascular and pulmonary congestion may result from increased preload. An increase in pulmonary capillary wedge pressure indicating the pulmonary congestion is a reliable measure of congestive heart failure, together with a reduced ventricular ejection fraction. Ventricular hypertrophy is also a consequence of a decrease in myocardial contractility. The rise in ventricular pressure and ensuing stretching of the sarcolemma, or an increase in plasma angiotensin II concentrations, is postulated to promote an increase in the number of myofibrils in each ventricular muscle cell, thereby increasing heart muscle mass. These mechanisms act in concert in an attempt to maintain cardiac output at the expense of a reduced energetic efficiency of heart muscle. When underlying pathological changes progress further, however, uncompensated heart failure develops.

Intervention with digitalis is still a very effective treatment in the patient with compensated or uncompensated congestive heart failure when that patient is refractory to other therapeutic modalities. With cardiac glycosides, the heart now operates on a new ventricular function curve, indicative of a higher level of cardiac contractility (fig. 25-4). Thus at any ventricular filling pressure, greater force is generated. An enhanced shortening of muscle reduces the duration of systole, estimated from systolic time intervals.

The systolic time interval is that time between initiation of contraction (closing of the mitral valve) to opening of the aortic valve. It is a noninvasive method of estimating force of contraction in intact whole heart in vivo. This value correlates well with the maximal $+dP/dt$ (the first derivative of increase in intraventricular pressure during systole), observed only with the use of an intraventricular catheter. An increase in force of contraction by the cardiac glycoside decreases the time needed to develop an intraventricular pressure equal to aortic pressure (= systolic time intervals).

The effect of the glycosides to increase the force of contraction reverses the above-described changes, including increased sympathetic activity. Because the kidney is now more effectively perfused, more salt and water are excreted and edema is reduced. Peripheral vasoconstriction is diminished, plasma volume is lowered, cardiac preload is decreased, and the heart returns toward its normal size {13}. These changes are associated with a decrease in pulmonary wedge pressure and an increase in ventricular ejection fraction. In isolated papillary muscle preparations, oxygen consumption is increased by the cardiac glycosides, associated with their positive inotropic effect. In the failing heart in vivo, however, cardiac glycosides decrease net oxygen consumption because of improvement in hemodynamic efficiency. This improvement is not due to an action of the glycoside to improve energetic efficiency of heart muscle; instead, energetic efficiency is improved, resulting from a reversal of events that occur in the failing heart, as described above.

Similar beneficial effects may be obtained by a combination of diuretics and vasodilators. An angiotensin converting enzyme inhibitor is the drug of choice for a vasodilator because it does not depress the force of cardiac contraction. More recently, flosequinan has been claimed to be useful because of its well-balanced vasodilator activities. This *alternative therapy* of congestive heart failure is usually used in conjunction with digitalis therapy. The alternative therapy with diuretics and vasodilator alone, however, would appear as effective as the glycoside alone. This would indicate that chronic heart failure is a *relative* insufficiency of the force of myocardial contraction, and hence can be treated by either increasing force of contraction or decreasing demand. It is now well established that treatment of patients with chronic heart failure with diuretics and vasodilators improves the quality of life and prolongs life expectancy. These effects of digitalis therapy are less obvious.

Associated with cardiac hypertrophy, remodeling of

heart muscle occurs. This is characterized by shifts in isoforms of functional proteins, including myosin, creatine kinase, and Na,K-ATPase. Whether an adequate maintenance of patients on cardiac glycoside prevents remodeling is presently unknown.

Electrophysiological effects

The digitalis glycosides have both beneficial and toxic electrophysiological effects on the heart. In addition to increasing the force of cardiac contraction, glycosides are used therapeutically to correct rhythm disturbances of supraventricular origin. In high concentrations, however, the glycosides cause life-threatening rhythm and conduction disturbances that limit their therapeutic usefulness. Therefore, an understanding of the basic electrophysiology of the glycosides is important. Most of the pertinent experimental studies have been performed either in vitro on isolated preparations or in situ on species other than humans. Fortunately, there is a good correspondence between observations in experimental animals and in humans. Electrophysiological effects of the glycosides on specialized conducting tissues of the heart are somewhat different from those on atrial muscle or ventricular muscle proper.

DIRECT EFFECTS

The most extensively studied cardiac tissue from the viewpoint of the direct electrophysiological actions of digitalis is mammalian Purkinje fibers {14}. This tissue is especially relevant for electrophysiological studies because the arrhythmogenic action of the glycoside generally results from its direct action on cardiac Purkinje fibers, or its direct or indirect actions on the atrioventricular node. Among these, the action on Purkinje fiber is important because it may trigger life-threatening ventricular tachycardia.

Cardiac glycosides in high concentrations promote spontaneous firing of Purkinje fibers, which may disrupt normal rhythm of the heart. Although toxic concentrations of the glycosides cause a slight depolarization of resting membrane potential, more important are the development of oscillatory afterpotentials, also referred to as *transient depolarizations* or *delayed afterdepolarizations* (fig. 25-5). Glycoside-induced transient depolarizations can be observed more easily in Purkinje fibers when the frequency of electrical stimulation is high and when electrical stimulation is terminated for a brief period following a rapid train of stimuli. The transient depolarization reaching threshold potential induces repetitive volleys. These transient depolarizations have also been reported in atrial or ventricular muscle preparations using larger concentrations of cardiac glycosides and aglycones. In the whole heart in situ, however, they seem to originate from Purkinje fibers and propagate through the ventricle. Purkinje fibers have the highest sensitivity to the glycoside to produce this aberrant depolarization.

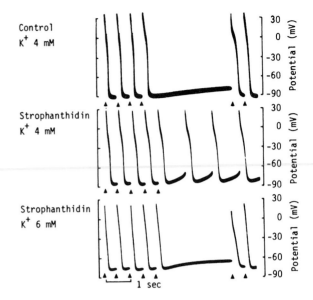

Fig. 25-5. Oscillatory afterpotentials caused by strophanthidin and their reversal by K$^+$. Feline Purkinje fibers were incubated in a modified Krebs–Henseleit bicarbonate buffer solution (pH 7.4) containing 4 mM K$^+$ at 30°C and stimulated at 2 Hz (electrical stimulation is shown by triangles). **Top panel:** Control tracing. **Middle panel:** Fifteen minutes after the addition of 0.6 μM strophanthidin. When electrical stimulation was stopped, afterpotentials reached the threshold potential and spontaneous activity continued. **Bottom panel:** Three minutes after raising K$^+$ concentration to 6 mM. Afterpotentials were suppressed and failed to reach the threshold potential.

INDIRECT EFFECTS

Both experimental and clinical studies have shown that efferent vagal activity is increased by glycosides and that the glycoside-induced slowing of heart rate can be largely blocked by atropine. Several sites have been implicated in slowing of the heart rate. The slowing is dependent on an intact autonomic nervous system. Both increases in parasympathetic nerve activity and inhibition of sympathetic nerve activity are involved.

At high doses of digitalis, sympathetic nerve activity may be enhanced instead of inhibited. Whether sympathetic stimulation originates within the central nervous system resulting from a central action of the glycoside or from peripheral sites (e.g., enhanced baroreceptor sensitivity coupled with hypotensive effects of toxic doses of glycoside) is still uncertain. The importance of sympathetic stimulation in the genesis of arrhythmias seen with larger doses of digitalis is also unknown. The role of the autonomic nervous system in the actions of digitalis has been reviewed by Gillis and Quest {15}.

EFFECTS ON VARIOUS CARDIAC TISSUES

Atrial tissue is very sensitive to the indirect actions of cardiac glycosides because of its well-known responsiveness to acetylcholine. Acetylcholine markedly decreases the effective refractory period (ERP), automaticity, and action potential duration (APD) associated with hyperpolarization. Although the direct effect of the glycosides tends to *depolarize* the resting membrane potential, the indirect vagal effects may predominate, causing hyperpolarization of atrial muscle. Therapeutic concentrations of digitalis may decrease ERP and APD in atrial muscle in situ with intact vagal innervation.

The atrioventricular (AV) nodal tissues are easily influenced by acetylcholine so that digitalis has a significant effect on this tissue. Both rate of rise and amplitude of action potentials in AV nodal tissue are decreased, resulting in depression of conduction through the AV node and a prolongation of ERP for AV nodal tissue (note: ERP of the ventricular muscle may be shortened). A 10–20% increase in PR interval can be seen on the ECG with therapeutic doses of glycoside. Toxic doses of glycosides can lead to AV block. The effects of glycosides on the AV node are important in the treatment of atrial fibrillation and atrial flutter.

Purkinje fibers and ventricular muscle are much less sensitive to acetylcholine and therefore are less influenced by the vagal effects of digitalis. As a result of the direct and indirect electrophysiological actions of the cardiotonic glycosides, the following changes may be observed on the ECG of patients treated with therapeutic doses of digitalis: Heart rate is decreased due to the depressed sinoatrial nodal automaticity. PR interval, the propagation through the AV node, is lengthened as a result of decreased AV nodal conduction velocity. QT interval, an estimate of the ERP of ventricular muscle, is shortened. ST segment and T wave may be depressed or inverted.

TREATMENT OF ARRHYTHMIAS

Cardiac glycosides are effective in the control of heart rate (frequency of ventricular contractions) in patients with atrial fibrillation, atrial flutter, or supraventricular paroxysmal tachycardia. In the treatment of atrial flutter, the aim is to reduce ventricular rate. This is brought about by the direct and indirect actions of digitalis on the AV node. Indirect actions result when the glycoside elevates blood pressure or the sensitivity of baroreceptors. This increases vagal activity and reduces sympathetic activity. The direct effect on the AV node is to prolong ERP of this tissue so that fewer impulses pass through the AV node to the ventricles. The increased vagal activity shortens the atrial ERP to further increase atrial rate. As a result, the AV node is bombarded at a greater frequency by impulses, but most are extinguished because the node is depressed and the ERP prolonged. Supraventricular paroxysmal tachycardias are generally relieved by maneuvers that enhance vagal activity; thus the use of digitalis is indicated. It is important to note, however, that digitalis overdose causes various types of arrhythmias, including supraventricular paroxysmal tachycardia with AV block. More common types of arrhythmias caused by digitalis overdose are partial or complete AV block and ventricular tachycardia.

DIGITALIS INTOXICATION

All glycosides produce similar toxic effects. In addition to cardiac rhythm disturbances, other untoward effects are frequently observed. These include gastrointestinal disturbances; anorexia, nausea, and vomiting; diarrhea; and abdominal pain. Gastrointestinal side effects (particularly nausea and vomiting) are apparently caused by stimulation of the chemoreceptor trigger zone in the area postrema of the medulla. Headache, malaise, and drowsiness are prominent central nervous side effects that occur early in digitalis intoxication. Visual disturbances are seen in patients intoxicated with digitalis, with blurring and color vision disturbances occurring most commonly.

The primary event that occurs most frequently in patients with digitalis overdose is arrhythmia. These include rhythm abnormalities of both atrial and ventricular origins, and disturbances of AV conduction. Diagnosis is complicated because underlying diseases may often cause arrhythmias. The diagnosis of digitalis-induced arrhythmias rests on patient history and an estimation of the concentration of digitalis glycoside in plasma. Because therapeutic and toxic ranges of the glycosides in plasma overlap, clinical evaluation is important.

Treatment

The digitalis-induced arrhythmias, once diagnosis is made, may be treated with antiarrhythmic drugs. Lidocaine, procainamide, or propranolol are frequently used and effective. Phenytoin is also useful to treat atrial arrhythmias; however, several instances of sudden death with this agent have been reported. Quinidine should not be used in patients with digoxin-induced arrhythmias because quinidine elevates plasma digoxin concentrations (see below). Procainamide or beta-adrenergic blockers can enhance digitalis-induced AV block.

Potassium administration is one of the most effective means of treating digitalis-induced arrhythmias when the plasma K^+ concentration is either low or normal. If the plasma K^+ concentration is high, however, a further increase in K^+ will enhance AV block and may induce cardiac arrest. The mechanism by which K^+ reverses digitalis-induced arrhythmias is not fully understood. The following explanations have been proposed: Potassium is known to reduce the glycoside binding to sarcolemmal Na,K-ATPase (fig. 25-6). [Inhibition of oscillatory afterpotentials (fig. 25-5) and ensuing reversal of arrhythmias, however, are too rapid for the shift in glycoside binding to occur]. Extracellular K^+ may stimulate the sodium pump and decrease intracellular Na^+, thereby reducing intracellular Ca^{2+} overload (see below). Alternatively, the effect of K^+ in altering membrane conductance may play an important role.

Drug interactions

Quinidine has long been contraindicated for the treatment of digitalis-induced arrhythmias. Subsequently, admini-

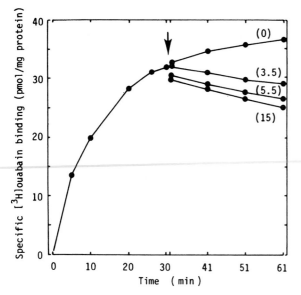

Fig. 25-6. The effect of K⁺ on [³H]ouabain binding. Partially purified Na,K-ATPase preparations obtained from dog heart were incubated at 37°C in the presence of 10 nM [³H]ouabain, 100 mM NaCl, 5 mM MgCl₂, 5 mM Tris-ATP, and 50 mM Tris-HCl buffer (pH 7.5). KCl was added at the time indicated by the arrow. Numbers in parentheses indicate the final KCl concentration in millimolar. KCl reduces both the association and dissociation rate constants; however, the association rate constant decreases more than dissociation rate constant, thereby the level of glycoside binding decreases. Significant changes in the glycoside binding, however, take more than several minutes.

stration of quinidine to patients receiving digoxin was found to increase digoxin concentration in plasma. The pharmacokinetic interaction is mutual: Quinidine increases plasma digoxin concentrations and digoxin increases plasma quinidine concentrations, apparently through competitive displacement at mutual binding sites. This binding site is distinct from the receptor site for the cardiac glycosides for their positive inotropic or toxic effects, and apparently is separate from the bulk of tissue binding sites for digitoxin. For this reason, and because digitoxin has a large apparent volume of distribution, pharmacokinetic interactions between quinidine and digitoxin are less obvious. Administration of quinidine to patients receiving digoxin may elevate plasma digoxin concentration to a dangerously high level, precipitating toxic manifestations {16}. Because mutual binding sites are separate from receptor sites, digoxin sensitivity of heart muscle is unchanged by quinidine.

When patients are treated with a combination of digoxin and quinidine, it is necessary to reduce the dose of digoxin such that the plasma digoxin concentration is within the normal range. Under these conditions (chronic treatment with a combination of quinidine and digoxin, instead of quinidine administration to patients who have been receiving digoxin alone), the pharmacokinetic interaction cannot

be explained from competition for mutual binding sites. This is because the plasma digoxin concentration during chronic treatment is determined by the rate of drug intake and the net clearance of digoxin. Theoretically, a decrease in apparent volume of distribution does not influence the clearance of digoxin. Under these conditions, an elevation of plasma digoxin concentration must result from the additional effect of quinidine to reduce clearance of the cardiac glycoside.

Plasma digitoxin concentrations are less affected by quinidine administration, whereas those for ouabain are apparently not influenced. More recently, pharmacokinetic interactions between digoxin and many drugs have been reported. These include amiodarone, nifedipine, and verapamil.

Clinically important drug interactions involving the cardiac glycosides occur with drugs that cause hypokalemia. This is important because it is a common practice to use a combination of digitalis and diuretics to treat patients with congestive heart failure and associated edema. Conversely, hyperkalemia will retard the glycoside binding to its receptor, and slow the onset and reduce the magnitude of the therapeutic action. Agents (e.g., monensin, veratridine, etc.) and conditions (e.g., increased heart rate) that increase the rate of Na⁺ influx reduce the tolerance of the heart to the toxic actions of the glycoside. Calcium ion potentiates the toxicity of the cardiac glycosides. All of these are pharmacodynamic interactions involving digoxin, digitoxin, and ouabain, and reduce the tolerance of the heart to the toxic actions of the glycoside by lowering the fractional occupancy of Na,K-ATPase required to precipitate arrhythmias. The beta-adrenergic agonists and cholinergic muscarinic agonists may promote or precipitate digitalis-induced arrhythmias. Other drugs that must be used judiciously with the cardiac glycosides are the beta-adrenergic antagonists and the Ca²⁺ channel blockers. These drugs may compromise the increased force of myocardial contraction induced by the glycoside and augment the glycoside-induced depression of the AV conduction.

MECHANISMS OF THERAPEUTIC ACTION

Although the cardiac glycosides have a proven efficacy of increasing the force of myocardial contraction, especially in the failing heart, their clinical use is compromised by their narrow margin of safety. Concentrations of digoxin in plasma observed in patients who are adequately treated with glycosides are generally in the range of 1–2 ng/ml. These concentrations are approximately one half of those observed in patients showing signs of digoxin toxicity, representing an extremely narrow margin of safety for this group of drugs. Clinical studies have indicated that the therapeutic and toxic concentrations of digoxin or digitoxin in plasma overlap {17}.

This narrow margin of safety of the cardiac glycosides has resulted in a high incidence of glycoside toxicity among patients on digitalis therapy. Because of this problem, it is necessary to understand the mechanism responsible for both therapeutic and toxic actions of the cardiac glycosides. The strategy to develop safer compounds and also the rational treatment of patients are largely dependent on whether the receptors for the two actions of the glycoside are the same or different.

Na,K-ATPase and the sodium pump

Among the numerous biochemical systems examined during the past 50 years, the sodium pump of the cardiac plasma membrane or sarcolemma, or its enzymatic representation, Na,K-ATPase, has been shown to be most sensitive to the cardiac glycosides. Various cardiac glycosides and their derivatives bind to Na,K-ATPase in a specific manner, and inhibit this enzyme activity {8,9}. The significant binding and ensuing substantial enzyme inhibition observed in vitro occur in a range of glycoside concentrations that produce positive inotropic effects in isolated heart preparations or in intact animals. Moreover, when heart muscle is exposed to a therapeutic concentration of a cardiac glycoside, and Na,K-ATPase or sodium pump activity is assayed under conditions in which release of the glycoside bound to the enzyme is negligible, a 20–40% inhibition of the enzyme or sodium pump activity can generally be observed. Finally, the cardiotonic steroids have been shown to increase intracellular Na^+ activity associated with an increase in developed tension. These findings suggest that the binding of cardiac glycosides to sarcolemmal Na,K-ATPase and the resulting sodium pump inhibition are involved in the mechanism of the positive inotropic action of these compounds.

Characteristics of the positive inotropic effect

The positive inotropic effect of the cardiac glycoside has many salient features. For example, the rate of onset of the inotropic effect is slow. This slow onset is apparently not due to a slow absorption or distribution of the glycoside. The slow onset of action can be observed even when the glycoside is injected intravenously, or in isolated heart muscle preparations that are exposed to a fixed concentration of glycoside. The rate of onset of the inotropic action can be accelerated by conditions that increase the rate of Na^+ influx into myocardial cells. These conditions include twin-pulse stimulation, or the presence of a Na^+ ionophore, monensin. When isolated heart muscle preparations are exposed to the glycoside at a relatively low temperature (e.g., 30°C), the rate of onset of the positive inotropic effect is strictly beat dependent. This phenomenon can also be explained from the fact that the rate of Na^+ influx is roughly proportional to the frequency of stimulation under these conditions. The rate of onset is delayed by elevating the extracellular K^+ concentration {9}.

The loss of positive inotropic effect of the cardiac glycosides in the intact animal is generally determined by the loss of the compound from the body, and therefore is dependent on the rate of metabolism and elimination. In isolated heart studies in which the glycoside concentration of extracellular fluid can be rapidly reduced to zero, the loss of the inotropic effect is dependent on the rate of release of the glycoside from the inotropic receptor. Under these conditions, the rate of loss of the positive inotropic effect is dependent on the chemical structure of compounds and the animal species. A slight change in the chemical structure of the active cardiac glycosides, e.g., saturation of the lactone ring, substitution of a hydroxyl group at the C-14 position with hydrogen, or removal of the sugar moiety from the glycosides, markedly reduces potency of the compound {4–6}. Generally, the greater the potency of compound or the sensitivity of the myocardium, the slower the washout of the inotropic effect {9}. This slow rate is further delayed by elevating the extracellular K^+ concentration.

These unique characteristics of the positive inotropic effect of the cardiac glycoside should be consistent with any proposed mechanism of inotropic action of the glycosides.

Binding of cardiac glycosides to Na,K-ATPase

Na,K-ATPase is a membrane-bound enzyme that is responsible for the coupled, active transport of Na^+ and K^+ across the cell membrane {8}. Apparently, the enzyme system spans the entire thickness of the cell membrane, binds Na^+ at its inner surface, and transports and releases Na^+ at the external surface. The enzyme system then binds K^+ at the external surface and releases it at the inner surface. Each cycle of the above reaction is accompanied by a cycle of phosphorylation and dephosphorylation of, and conformational changes in, the enzyme protein. The enzyme is phosphorylated from ATP, which is hydrolyzed to ADP and inorganic phosphate during the reaction cycle. The free energy released from ATP is used for active cation transport.

Cardiac glycosides bind to Na,K-ATPase at a site accessible from extracellular side {9}. The binding normally occurs when the enzyme has just completed the transport of Na^+, i.e., when the enzyme is in a Na^+-induced conformation. If K^+ induces a further conformational change in enzyme protein, the binding sites become less accessible to the glycoside. This means that the binding of the glycoside to Na,K-ATPase is promoted by conditions that either increase the intracellular Na^+ available to the sodium pump or reduce the extracellular K^+. Therefore, a higher heart rate, twin-pulse electrical stimulation, the presence of a Na^+ ionophore, or hypokalemia enhance the glycoside binding to Na,K-ATPase. Because glycoside binding occurs preferentially to the Na^+-induced form of the enzyme, and the enzyme spends only a short time in this form during each cycle of conformational change, the binding of cardiac glycosides to Na,K-ATPase is relatively slow. The slow binding results in a slow onset of glycoside action, even when the drug is given intravenously.

In contrast to an increase in Na^+ influx that promotes glycoside binding to Na,K-ATPase, a decrease in the rate of Na^+ influx does not appear to reduce the glycoside binding {11}. This results from the fact that the Na^+ activation curve for Na,K-ATPase activity or [^3H]ouabain binding is relatively flat between 4 and 10 mM Na^+. Decreases in intracellular Na^+ activity from the normal range of 7–8 mM to a lower value, therefore, do not affect the rate of glycoside binding to Na,K-ATPase.

Structure-activity relationship studies with various glycoside derivatives have shown that the ability of a compound to bind to and inhibit isolated Na,K-ATPase or the sodium pump is well related to its ability to produce positive inotropic effects in isolated heart muscle preparations {5}. Corresponding to the species-dependent differences in glycoside sensitivity, Na,K-ATPase preparations obtained from heart muscle of highly sensitive species have a high affinity for the glycoside, and those from relatively low-sensitivity species have a low affinity. Low affinity for a given combination of isolated Na,K-ATPase and the glycoside derivative is primarily the result of a large dissociation rate constant. Regardless of whether the source of the enzyme or chemical structure of the compound is responsible for the low affinity, the compounds are released rapidly from the binding sites on the enzyme {12}. Again, good correlation is observed between the rate of release of the compounds from isolated Na,K-ATPase and the rate of loss of the inotropic effect observed in isolated heart muscle preparations {18}.

Finally, when Na,K-ATPase is isolated from cardiac muscle exposed to a positive inotropic concentration of glycoside, one can generally observe that the enzyme is inhibited by 20–40% {9}. These results indicate that substantial glycoside binding to Na,K-ATPase must occur in heart muscle at a time when the inotropic effect of the glycoside is apparent.

Because of these impressive relationships between the binding of cardiac glycosides to Na,K-ATPase and their inotropic effects {9}, and because it is now well established that therapeutic concentrations of the glycoside cause a slight elevation in intracellular Na^+ concentrations {19}, it is now generally believed that Na,K-ATPase is the receptor molecule for the pharmacological action of the glycosides.

Events that connect Na,K-ATPase inhibition to inotropic effects

The binding of cardiac glycosides to Na,K-ATPase seems to be essential for their positive inotropic effect. There are, however, differences in opinion regarding the mechanisms by which glycoside binding leads to an increase in the force of myocardial contraction, or whether inhibition of Na,K-ATPase is the sole mechanism for the positive inotropic effect of the glycoside. In cardiac muscle, membrane excitation is characterized by a rapid Na^+ influx, causing membrane depolarization, followed by a delayed K^+ efflux, which causes membrane repolarization. Unlike the action potential in nerve cells, the time interval between membrane depolarization and repolarization in cardiac muscle (the plateau phase) is as long as 200–500 ms. During this time, Ca^{2+} channels open and Ca^{2+} ions enter the cell. These Ca^{2+} ions, combined with those released from intracellular sites, cause a transient increase in the intracellular free Ca^{2+} concentration (Ca^{2+} transient)

shortly following each membrane excitation. The increase in Ca^{2+} concentration activates troponin C, resulting in muscle contraction. Cardiac glycosides have been shown to enhance calcium transients, thereby increasing the force of contraction {20} (fig. 25-7). It may be concluded, therefore, that in some manner the glycosides increase the efficiency of events that connect membrane excitation to calcium transients.

There is no consensus as to precisely how the glycoside modifies the normal process of the coupling mechanism to increase the efficiency of coupling. One obvious consequence of the glycoside binding to Na,K-ATPase is an inhibition of sodium pump activity. Studies with Na^+-sensitive microelectrodes have shown that the positive inotropic effect of strophanthidin, a rapidly acting cardiotonic steroid, is associated with an increase in intracellular Na^+ ion activity {19}. These investigators claimed that developed tension is linearly related to intracellular Na^+ activity raised by the power of 6, and therefore a slight increase in intracellular Na^+ can account for a marked increase in developed tension observed with therapeutic concentrations of the cardiotonic steroid {21}. Results of Na^+-sensitive microelectrode studies, however, do not explain how an elevation of intracellular Na^+ observed during the diastolic phase of the cardiac function augments the calcium transient triggered by the subsequent membrane excitation.

Several investigators have proposed that sodium pump inhibition causes an elevation of the intracellular Na^+ concentration, which in turn elevates intracellular Ca^{2+} concentration by either stimulating a Ca^{2+}-influx/Na^+-efflux exchange reaction or inhibiting a Na^+-influx/Ca^{2+}-efflux exchange reaction {22}. These exchange reactions work bidirectionally {23}. During the systolic phase, Ca^{2+} influx is coupled with Na^+ efflux, presumably due to the relatively high Na^+ concentration at the inner surface of the cell membrane and reduced transmembrane potential. Because 3 Na^+ are exchanged with 1 Ca^{2+}, the Na^+/Ca^{2+} exchange is not electroneutral, and the loss of transmembrane potential favors Na^+ efflux coupled with Ca^{2+} influx. During the diastolic phase, Na^+ influx is coupled with Ca^{2+} efflux. Therefore, it is likely that sodium pump inhibition, with its augmented increase in Na^+ concentration at the inner surface of the cell membrane during the systolic phase, enhances Ca^{2+} influx. Alternatively, an increase in intracellular Na^+ concentration during the diastolic phase and ensuing reduction in transmembrane Na^+ gradient may reduce Ca^{2+} efflux.

Substantial inhibition of the sodium pump does not cause a matching increase in the intracellular Na^+ concentration. This must indicate that the remaining sodium pump units, now turning over faster in response to a slightly elevated intracellular Na^+ concentration, are adequate to pump out Na^+ entering the cell during a cycle of myocardial function (fig. 25-8). It would appear that the sodium pump has a reserve capacity. The presence of such a reserve capacity is also apparent from studies when the rate of Na^+ influx is increased by increasing the heart rate or by agents that increase Na^+ influx. Under these conditions the intracellular Na^+ concentration rises only

Control   Ouabain 0.5 μM

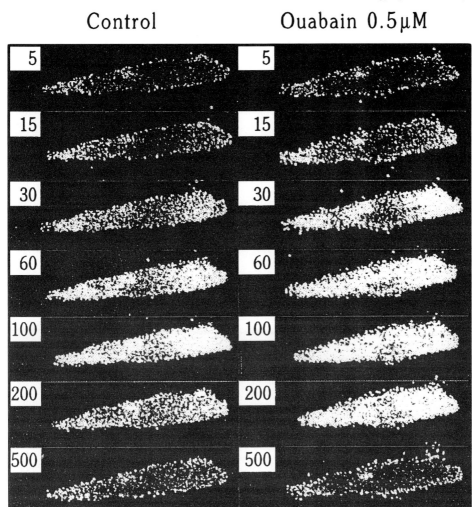

$$\longmapsto 50\,\mu m$$

Fig. 25-7. The effect of ouabain on intracellular Ca^{2+} transient. Myocyte isolated from guinea pig heart was loaded with fura-2. The cell was incubated at 30°C and electrically stimulated at 1 Hz. Images represent the 500-nm fluorescence intensity ratio recorded at 340- and 380-nm activation. Numbers indicate elapsed time in milliseconds after electrical stimulation. Ouabain augments transient increase in Ca^{2+} concentration without changing the pattern or time course of the Ca^{2+} transient. (For technical details, see Akera T, Temma K, Kondo H, Hagane K: Digital imaging system for recording rapid changes in intracellular Ca^{2+} concentrations triggered by electrical stimulation of cardiac myocytes. *Keio J Med* 39:168–172, 1990.)

minimally, indicating that the sodium pump is now turning over faster, resulting from the slight elevation of intracellular Na^+ concentration, and is adequate to handle the enhanced Na^+ influx. Therefore, one has to question whether the partial inhibition of a system that has a significant reserve capacity can have any physiological importance.

Two hypotheses have been advanced to explain why a partial inhibition of a system that has a significant reserve capacity would produce significant physiological effects. One hypothesis is that dynamic changes in the intracellular

Na^+ concentration are such that one cannot experimentally determine, with the currently available methods, the true changes in intracellular Na^+ concentration caused by a moderate sodium pump inhibition. During the early phase of membrane excitation, the rate of Na^+ influx suddenly increases. Such an increase may effectively elevate the Na^+ concentration at the inner surface of the cell membrane, thereby stimulating the sodium pump and also the Ca^{2+}-influx/Na^+-efflux exchange reaction {9}. During this period, individual sodium pump units may be turning over faster in response to an elevated intracellular

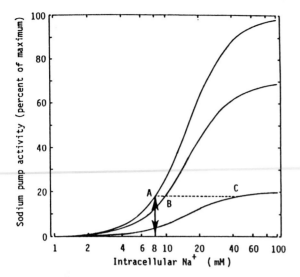

Fig. 25-8. Sodium pump activity and intracellular Na⁺ concentrations. **A:** Normal. Sodium pump activity is equivalent to the rate of Na⁺ influx (size of the vertical arrow below A). Intracellular Na⁺ concentration is approximately 8 mM, which is significantly lower than the K value of 16 mM for Na,K-ATPase activation. **B:** Moderate inhibition of the sodium pump by therapeutic concentrations of the glycoside. Intracellular Na⁺ concentration slightly increases until the activity of the remaining pump matches the rate of Na⁺ influx. **C:** Marked inhibition of the sodium pump by toxic concentrations of the glycoside. A marked increase in intracellular Na⁺ is required to activate the remaining sodium pump units so that pump activity matches the rate of Na⁺ influx. Due to the marked elevation of intracellular Na⁺, the rate of Na⁺ influx may decrease slightly.

Na⁺, and may be operating at close to their maximum capacity to extrude Na⁺. Therefore, an inhibition of the sodium pump by the glycoside may cause a significant difference in intracellular Na⁺ during this time period. More Na⁺ may be extruded by the Na⁺/Ca²⁺ exchange mechanism, resulting in an enhanced Ca²⁺ influx, and augmentation of Ca²⁺ transients. During the later phase of myocardial function, the rate of Na⁺ influx declines, providing an opportunity for the inhibited sodium pump to "catch up" before the next membrane excitation.

This explanation is consistent with most observations, such as the finding (a) that only a slight increase in intracellular Na⁺ is observed during the diastolic phase in cardiac muscle exposed to inotropic concentrations of the glycoside, (b) that Na⁺ accumulation occurs more easily when the glycoside-treated heart is stimulated at a higher frequency, (c) that agents or conditions that enhance transmembrane Na⁺ influx can increase the force of myocardial contraction, and (d) that the augmentation of the Ca²⁺ transient by the cardiac glycosides has a relatively minor effect on the diastolic Ca²⁺ concentration in the cytoplasm. In this regard, it should be noted that an enhancement of Na⁺ influx, which would produce a similar net result as would sodium pump inhibition, also

produces inotropic effects and toxicity remarkably similar to those caused by the cardiac glycosides.

Alternatively, a slight increase in intracellular Na⁺ concentration observed during the diastolic phase of the cardiac cycle described above may play an important role in the positive inotropic effect of the cardiac glycosides. During the diastolic phase, the Na⁺/Ca²⁺ exchange mechanism is most likely to be mediating Ca²⁺ efflux coupled with Na⁺ influx. A slight elevation of intracellular Na⁺, and a decrease in transmembrane Na⁺ gradient, would decrease Ca²⁺ efflux by this mechanism, causing more Ca²⁺ to be taken up by the sarcoplasmic reticulum. A decrease in Na⁺ concentration in the medium causes a marked increase in developed tension in isolated heart muscle preparations. This finding would indicate that changes in the transmembrane Na⁺ gradient affect Ca²⁺ movements. A moderate increase in Ca²⁺ loading of the sarcoplasmic reticulum may increase the amount of Ca²⁺ released from this organelle triggered by membrane excitation, and thereby could augment intracellular Ca²⁺ transients.

The faster turnover of the sodium pump, or utilization of the pump reserve capacity, is caused by a slight elevation of intracellular Na⁺ in cardiac muscle exposed to an inotropic concentration of glycoside. Studies with Na⁺-sensitive microelectrodes show that intracellular Na⁺ is elevated 1 or 2 mM by positive inotropic concentrations of the cardiotonic steroids {19,21} or by a sudden increase in stimulation frequency {24} associated with an increase in force of twitch contraction. This 1–2 mM increase in intracellular Na⁺ may be sufficient to cause a significant relative increase in intracellular Ca²⁺ concentration. The cytoplasmic free Ca²⁺ concentration is less than 0.001 mM. Therefore, even when a small fraction of elevated Na⁺ is exchanged with Ca²⁺ at a ratio of 3 Na⁺ to 1 Ca²⁺, it should have a great influence on the intracellular Ca²⁺ concentration.

The above two possible mechanisms are not mutually exclusive. Because the cardiac glycoside enhances developed tension observed under relatively high-frequency stimulation and also augments potentiated postrest contraction in atrial muscle preparations isolated from guinea-pig heart {25}, both mechanisms may be operating. This is because developed tension observed in this species under high-frequency stimulation is primarily determined by transmembrane Ca²⁺ influx, whereas potentiated postrest contraction is dependent on the amount of Ca²⁺ stored in the sarcoplasmic reticulum.

Additional hypotheses have been advanced attempting to explain the enhancement of myocardial contraction resulting from the glycoside binding to Na,K-ATPase in the apparent presence of the sodium pump reserve capacity. For example, the glycoside binding to Na,K-ATPase might alter properties of membrane lipids associated with the enzyme. The capacity and affinity of the Ca²⁺ binding sites within the cell membrane may be altered, favoring binding and release of Ca²⁺ associated with membrane excitation {26,27}. Such glycoside-enhanced Ca²⁺ binding sites may be either inside or outside the membrane lipid bilayer. In addition, several investigators claim that there are intracellular sites of action for the cardiac glycosides.

Cardiac glycosides are capable of producing positive inotropic effects by their direct action on the heart, probably by binding to sarcolemmal Na,K-ATPase and inhibiting sodium pump activity. There is, however, no a priori reason to believe that this is the only mechanism by which the glycosides modify the force of myocardial contraction. Some of the alternative mechanisms described above may play a secondary role. Moreover, various cardiac glycosides alter the configuration of the action potential of cardiac muscle cells. The effect is both concentration and time dependent. In low concentrations and at an early time, the glycosides prolong the action potential duration, and at higher concentrations and after prolonged exposure, they shorten the action potential duration. These changes cannot be the primary mechanism for the positive inotropic action of the glycoside. The inotropic effect can be observed at the time when the action potential is shortened, as well as when it is prolonged. Nevertheless, these changes undoubtedly modify the force of contraction, which is anticipated to be enhanced when the action potential duration is prolonged. It is possible that the positive inotropic effect of the cardiac glycosides is mediated by two or more parallel pathways.

Recording of the intracellular Ca^{2+} transient using Ca^{2+} indicators such as aequorin, indo-1, or fura-2 revealed that enhancement of the Ca^{2+} transient is indeed responsible for glycoside-induced increase in twitch contraction {20,28} (fig. 25-7). Other positive inotropic drugs, such as catecholamines, including xamoterol and denopamine, augment the Ca^{2+} transient. Newer positive inotropic drugs, such as amrinone, milrinone, enoximone, and vesnarinone, act primarily by inhibiting type III phosphodiesterase or K^+ channels, and thereby increasing the Ca^{2+} transient. In this regard, the usefulness of most positive inotropic drugs, including digitalis glycosides, may be limited because the Ca^{2+} transient in advanced failing human heart muscle shows the features of Ca^{2+} overload {29}. Pimobendan also enhances the Ca^{2+} transient. In addition, this drug has been claimed to increase Ca^{2+} sensitivity of troponin C. Whether the latter action of pimobendan makes this drug more useful compared to digitalis glycosides is presently unknown. Because inhibition of relaxation is a serious problem of failing heart, careful studies are needed to ascertain the usefulness of drugs that increase Ca^{2+} sensitivity of contractile proteins.

MECHANISM OF TOXICITY

Electrophysiological toxicity

Some of the toxic signs of cardiac glycosides, such as nausea, vomiting, fatigue, and yellow vision, are apparently caused by their actions on the central nervous system. The most important toxicity, cardiac arrhythmias, however, involves a direct action of the glycoside on the heart and indirect actions, i.e., those on the nervous system. Because the arrhythmogenic actions of the glycoside can be demonstrated with isolated heart preparations, glycosides are apparently capable of producing arrhythmias by their direct action on heart. Such a direct arrhythmogenic action of the glycoside is generally considered to result from inhibition of the sodium pump exceeding its reserve capacity {9}. In animal experiments with anesthetized dogs, cardiotoxicity of the glycoside is associated with a 60–80% inhibition of the sodium pump. At this level of sodium pump inhibition, the remaining sodium pump units are insufficient to extrude Na^+ entering the cell associated with membrane excitation (fig. 25-8). This would result in inability of myocardial cells to maintain a low intracellular Na^+ concentration. Myocardial cells accumulate Na^+ and lose K^+.

Cellular accumulation of Na^+ and loss of K^+ then cause partial depolarization. The transmembrane potentials become less negative, approaching the threshold potential for activation of Na^+ channels. The concept that the reduced difference between the resting membrane potential and the threshold potential is the primary cause of increased excitability, causing myocardial cells to fire more easily without being driven by the normal pacemaker cells and thereby causing arrhythmias, is not supported. An elevation of the extracellular K^+ concentration causes a further depolarization, yet reverses the glycoside-induced arrhythmias (fig. 25-5).

Electrophysiological studies indicate that ventricular tachycardia caused by toxic doses of cardiac glycoside originates, at least initially, from Purkinje fibers {30}. When these fibers are exposed to toxic concentrations of the glycoside, oscillatory afterpotentials can be observed immediately following repolarization (fig. 25-5). The oscillatory afterpotentials are apparently caused by fluctuations in membrane permeability to various cations during the short period that follows membrane repolarization. This increase in membrane permeability results in Na^+, and perhaps Ca^{2+}, flowing through the sarcolemma into the cell, generating transient inward currents. The inward currents make the membrane potential less negative. Subthreshold oscillatory afterpotentials do not propagate; however, when the size of the afterpotential becomes large enough to reach threshold potential, spontaneous firing occurs. This will originate in Purkinje fibers and propagate into ventricular muscle proper, causing arrhythmic contractions of the heart. In glycoside-poisoned Purkinje fibers, such firing may become repetitive, resulting in ventricular tachycardia.

The transient increase in membrane permeability seems to result from Ca^{2+} overload at the inner surface of the cell membrane. Toxic doses of the cardiac glycosides inhibit the sodium pump beyond its reserve capacity and cause intracellular Na^+ accumulation. This is followed by a Ca^{2+} overload through reduced Ca^{2+} extrusion, resulting from an inhibition of the coupled Na^+-influx/Ca^{2+}-efflux exchange. Ca^{2+} overload is speculated to cause oscillatory movements of Ca^{2+} between the sarcoplasmic reticulum and sarcoplasm with associated phasic changes in membrane conductance.

These phasic changes in membrane conductance and ensuing ventricular arrhythmias caused by oscillatory afterpotentials (triggered activity) should be distinguished from enhanced pacemaker (automatic) activity. Unlike pacemaker activity, triggered activity is difficult to overdrive. This is because triggered activity is enhanced by increasing the frequency of stimulation, whereas automatic activity is subject to postpacing depression. An elevation of the extracellular Ca^{2+} concentration tends to depress automatic activity by reducing the slope of phase-4 depolarization, whereas it enhances the glycoside-induced oscillatory afterpotentials.

Cardiac glycosides may cause many different types of arrhythmias. Among them, ventricular tachycardia is perhaps most important, as it poses the greatest danger to patients. Clinically, however, other types of arrhythmias are more frequently observed, with the use of digitalis glycosides resulting from suppression of atrioventricular (AV) conduction. A slight increase in PR intervals, i.e., first-degree AV block, can be seen in most patients treated with "therapeutic" doses of digitalis. As the dose of the cardiac glycoside is increased, more advanced AV block can be observed. Stimulation of the parasympathetic nerve, presumably due to action of the glycoside on the central nervous system and baroreceptors, is considered as the primary cause of the AV conduction block. The action of the glycosides on the AV node is easily reversed by atropine or vagotomy in experimental animals. There are, however, extravagal components that cannot be blocked by atropine.

The blockade of the sympathetic nervous system by various means also increases the dose of the cardiac glycoside needed to cause arrhythmias. It is uncertain, however, whether the glycoside-induced increase in sympathetic nerve activity plays an important role in the arrhythmogenic action of the glycoside, or if the basal activity of the sympathetic nervous system is required to maintain the susceptibility of the heart to glycoside-induced toxicity. The latter view is favored by the observation that sympathetic discharge is not always increased in experimental animals exposed to toxic concentrations of glycoside. As the baroreceptor is sensitized by the glycoside, sympathetic discharge becomes more phasic; a burst occurs during the diastolic phase, and the sympathetic discharge almost ceases during the systolic phase {31}. Overall activity, however, may be somewhat decreased until the glycoside-induced arrhythmias cause a significant decrease in the mean arterial blood pressure.

Of particular interest is the hypothesis that the glycoside causes a nonuniform discharge within the cardiac sympathetic nerve. The nonuniform discharge may cause nonuniform electrophysiological properties of cardiac muscle cells and might predispose the heart to arrhythmias {32}. If this were to occur, then sympathetic nerve activity contributes to the glycoside-induced arrhythmias, regardless of whether overall activity is decreased or increased. It should also be pointed out that whereas sympathectomy in experimental animals elevates the tolerance of animals to digitalis-induced arrhythmias, it decreases the dose of glycoside needed to cause cardiac arrest.

Thus, the arrhythmogenic action of the cardiac glycoside may involve a direct action of the glycoside on the myocardium and indirect actions on the nervous system. The latter action of the glycoside may result from alterations in sensitivity of the baroreceptor, central actions of the glycoside, or an effect on nerve terminals. It is not surprising that the glycosides affect various systems, because Na,K-ATPase is ubiquitous and is likely to play important roles in various tissues. It is easy to understand these actions of the cardiac glycoside as stemming from sodium pump inhibition, because they can be explained from either reduced transmembrane potentials or by modulation of the coupled Na^+/Ca^{2+} exchange.

Mechanical toxicity

Ventricular tachyarrhythmias are the most prominent toxic effect of the cardiac glycosides. In isolated heart muscle preparations, however, other types of toxicity, such as (a) an increase in diastolic tension, (b) a decrease in developed tension, and (c) oscillatory aftercontractions may be observed in addition to (d) oscillatory afterpotentials and tachyarrhythmias. Among these, the first three (mechanical toxicity), if they occur, could cause severe problems in patients with chronic heart failure because inadequate relaxation of the myocardium is one problem associated with this condition. A popular hypothesis is that a toxic concentration of the cardiac glycoside increases diastolic Ca^{2+} concentration in the cytoplasm, causes Ca^{2+} overload of the sarcoplasmic reticulum, and causes an uncontrolled and oscillatory release of Ca^{2+} from this intracellular storage site. Once this chain of events occurs, then a general increase in cytoplasmic Ca^{2+} elevates diastolic tension. Moreover, the sarcoplasmic reticulum may not be fully loaded with Ca^{2+} at the time of membrane depolarization if uncontrolled spontaneous and partial release of Ca^{2+} occurs. This would reduce developed tension, which is triggered by full membrane depolarization. It follows then that all four types of digitalis toxicity described above are caused by Ca^{2+} overload of the sarcoplasmic reticulum.

Although many investigators presently support the above view, whether all types of digitalis toxicity result from Ca^{2+} overload of the sarcoplasmic reticulum, and whether there is an intimate relationship between oscillatory afterpotentials and oscillatory aftercontractions are somewhat questionable. This is because the order of appearance and intensities of the four types of digitalis toxicity are not always uniform. Under conditions in which contracture is observed first, a decrease in developed tension follows; however, a severe contracture appears to inhibit the development of arrhythmias. Moreover, ryanodine, which impairs utilization of Ca^{2+} stored in the sarcoplasmic reticulum, effectively reverses oscillatory aftercontractions but has a relatively weak effect on arrhythmias. Nifedipine, which inhibits Ca^{2+} influx through slow channels, effectively reverses arrhythmias but fails to affect oscillatory aftercontractions. Finally, a train of rapid stimulations, which reduces Ca^{2+} loading of the sarcoplasmic reticulum, enhances oscillatory afterpotentials but reduces oscillatory aftercontractions. These results indicate that the relationship among the various manifestations of digitalis toxicity may not be as close as that suggested by the current hypothesis.

SUMMARY

Despite the fact that the digitalis glycosides have been clinically used for many decades, they have a notorious tendency to produce toxicity. While numerous efforts have been made to improve existing compounds or to develop newer and safer positive inotropic drugs, digoxin and digitoxin are still extensively used. These drugs produce their therapeutic (positive inotropic) effects by causing a 20–40% inhibition of sarcolemmal Na,K-ATPase. Na,K-ATPase inhibition and ensuing sodium pump inhibition augment the intracellular Ca^{2+} transient by elevating the intracellular Na^+ concentration and modulating the Na^+/Ca^{2+} exchange reaction. It is currently believed that increased Ca^{2+} loading of the sarcoplasmic reticulum is the mechanism responsible for the positive inotropic effect of digitalis glycosides. Greater inhibition of the sodium pump, exceeding its reserve capacity, causes toxic manifestations that are expressed as transient inward currents, oscillatory afterpotentials, and ultimately arrhythmias. Toxicity may also be expressed as an increase in diastolic tension, a decrease in developed tension, and oscillatory aftercontractions. The precise mechanisms by which excessive sodium pump inhibition elicits the several toxic manifestations are presently unknown.

REFERENCES

1. Withering W: An Account of the Foxglove, and Some of its Medicinal Uses: With Practical Remarks on Dropsy, and Other Diseases. London: GGJ and J Robinson, 1785.
2. Cattell M, Gold H: The influence of digitalis glycosides on the force of contraction of mammalian cardiac muscle. *J Pharmacol Exp Ther* 62:116–125, 1938.
3. Cattell M, Gold H: Studies on purified digitalis glucosides. III. The relationship between therapeutic and toxic potency. *J Pharmacol Exp Ther* 71:114–125, 1941.
4. Tamm C: The stereochemistry of the glycosides in relation to biological activity. In: Wilbrandt W, Lindgren P (eds) *Proceedings of the First International Pharmacological Meeting.* Vol 3: *Newer Aspects of Cardiac Glycosides*, Oxford: Pergamon, 1963, pp 11–26.
5. Thomas R, Brown L, Gelbart A: The digitalis receptor: Inferences from structure activity relationships. *Circ Res* 46(Suppl 1):167–172, 1980.
6. Guntert TW, Linde HHA: Chemistry and structure-activity relationships of cardioactive steroids. In: Greeff K (ed) *Handbook of Pharmacology*, Vol. 56, Part 1: *Cardiac Glycosides*. Berlin: Springer-Verlag, 1981, pp 13–24.
7. Akera T, Ng YC, Shieh IS, Bero E, Brody TM, Braselton WE: Effects of K^+ on the interaction between cardiac glycosides and Na,K-ATPase. *Eur J Pharmacol* 111:147–157, 1985.
8. Schwartz A, Lindenmayer GE, Allen JC: The sodium-potassium adenosine triphosphatase: Pharmacological, physiological and biochemical aspects. *Pharmacol Rev* 27:3–134, 1975.
9. Akera T: Effects of cardiac glycosides on Na,K-ATPase. In: Greeff K (ed) *Handbook of Experimental Pharmacology,*

Vol. 56, Part 1: *Cardiac Glycosides*. Berlin: Springer-Verlag, 1981, pp 288–336.
10. Goldman RH, Coltart DJ, Schweizer E, Snidow G, Harrison DC: Dose response in vivo to digoxin in normo- and hyperkalaemia-associated biochemical changes. *Cardiovasc Res* 9:515–523, 1975.
11. Berlin JR, Akera T, Brody TM: Lack of pharmacodynamic interactions between quinidine and digoxin in isolated atrial muscle of guinea pig heart. *J Pharmacol Exp Ther* 238:632–641, 1986.
12. Tobin T, Brody TM: The rate of dissociation of enzyme-ouabain complexes and $K_{0.5}$ values in $(Na^+ + K^+)$ adenosine-triphosphatase from different species. *Biochem Pharmacol* 21:1553-1560, 1972.
13. Mason DT: Regulation of cardiac performance in clinical heart disease: Interactions between contractile state mechanical abnormalities and ventricular compensatory mechanisms. *Am J Cardiol* 32:437–448, 1973.
14. Tsien RW, Weingart R, Kass RS: Digitalis: Inotropic and arrhythmogenic effects on membrane currents in cardiac Purkinje fibers. In: Morad M (ed) *Biophysical Aspects of Cardiac Muscle*. New York: Academic Press, 1978, pp. 345–368.
15. Gillis RA, Quest JA: The role of the nervous system in the cardiovascular effects of digitalis. *Pharmacol Rev* 31:19–97, 1979.
16. Doering W: Quinidine-digoxin interaction: Pharmacokinetics, underlying mechanism and clinical implications. *N Engl J Med* 301:400–404, 1979.
17. Beller GA, Smith TW, Abelmann WH, Haber E, Hood WB: Digitalis intoxication: A prospective clinical study with serum level correlations. *N Engl J Med* 284:989–997, 1971.
18. Akera T, Baskin SI, Tobin T, Brody TM: Ouabain: Temporal relationship between the inotropic effect and the in vitro binding to, and dissociation from, $(Na^+ + K^+)$-activated ATPase. *Naunyn Schmiedebergs Arch Pharmacol* 277:151–162, 1973.
19. Lee CO, Dagostino M: Effect of strophanthidin on intracellular Na ion activity and twitch tension of constantly driven canine cardiac Purkinje fibers. *Biophys J* 40:185–198, 1982.
20. Allen DG, Blinks JR: Calcium transients in aequorin-injected frog cardiac muscle. *Nature* 273:509–513, 1978.
21. IM WB, Lee CO: Quantitative relation of twitch and tonic tensions to intracellular Na^+ activity in cardiac Purkinje fibers. *Am J Physiol* 247:C478–C487, 1984.
22. Langer GA: The intrinsic control of myocardial contraction — ionic factors. *N Engl J Med* 285:1065–1071, 1971.
23. Mullins LJ: The generation of electric currents in cardiac fibers by Na/Ca exchange. *Am J Physiol* 236:C103–C110, 1979.
24. Cohen CJ, Fozzard HA, Sheu SS: Increase in intracellular sodium ion activity during stimulation in mammalian cardiac muscle. *Circ Res* 50:651–662, 1982.
25. Temma K, Akera T: Effects of inotropic agents on isolated guinea-pig heart under conditions which modify calcium pools involved in contractile activation. *Can J Physiol Pharmacol* 64:947–954, 1986.
26. Gervais A, Lane LK, Anner BM, Lindenmayer GE, Schwartz A: A possible molecular mechanism of the action of digitalis: Ouabain action on calcium binding to sites associated with a purified sodium-potassium-activated adenosine triphosphatase. *Circ Res* 40:3–14, 1977.
27. Lüllmann H, Peters T: Action of cardiac glycosides on the excitation-contraction coupling in heart muscle. *Prog Pharmacol* 2:1–57, 1977.
28. Morgan JP: The effects of digitalis on intracellular calcium

transients in mammalian working myocardium as detected with aequorin. *J Mol Cell Cardiol* 17:1065–1075, 1985.

29. Gwathmey JK, Copelas L, MacKinnon R, Shoen FJ, Feldman MD, Grossman W, Morgan JP: Abnormal intracellular calcium handling in myocardium with patients with end-stage heart failure. *Circ Res* 61:70–76, 1987.

30. Ferrier GR, Saunders JH, Mendez C: A cellular mechanism for the generation of ventricular arrhythmias by acetylstro-phanthidin. *Circ Res* 32:600–609, 1973.

31. Weaver LC, Akera T, Brody TM: Digoxin toxicity: Primary sites of drug action on the sympathetic nervous system. *J Pharmacol Exp Ther* 197:1–9, 1976.

32. Lathers CM, Kelliher GJ, Roberts J, Beasley AB: Nonuniform cardiac sympathetic nerve discharge: Mechanism for coronary occlusion and digitalis-induced arrhythmias. *Circulation* 57:1058–1065, 1978.

CHAPTER 26

Calcium Channels and the Mechanism of Action
of Calcium Antagonists

HELMUT A. TRITTHART

INTRODUCTION AND HISTORY

The term *calcium antagonism* was coined by A. Fleckenstein in the late sixties to describe the mode of action of a new group of compounds that apparently mimicked the effect of Ca^{2+} withdrawal on excitation and contraction of cardiac and smooth muscle fibers [1,2]. The initial, key observation was that verapamil blocked contraction of the myocardium and the high-energy phosphate utilization related to contraction but produced little change in the action potential [1,3,4]. This specific inhibition of cardiac contraction confirmed the early discovery by Mines in 1913 [5] that, although perfusion with Ca^{2+}-free solution stopped the contraction, the surface electrical activity of the heart was still present.

However, a great variety of compounds were known to exert a negative inotropic effect, resembling that of calcium withdrawal, e.g., beta-adrenoceptor blocking agents, membrane stabilizing and antiarrhythmic compounds, barbituric acid derivatives, etc. Hence, Fleckenstein's interpretation of these findings and the hypothesis of a new and selective calcium antagonistic mode of action for this new group of compounds was initially not widely accepted in pharmacology and physiology. It should be noted, however, that regenerative membrane depolarizations recorded from crustacean muscle in zero sodium solutions had, by 1953, led to the suggestion that voltage-gated calcium conductances exist [6].

That a variety of other chemical structures, at least at higher concentrations, also possess calcium blocking properties [for review see 7] was recognized early, and Fleckenstein's first classification of calcium antagonists was aimed at clearly distinguishing between nonspecific calcium antagonism and calcium antagonism by compounds having outstanding specificity (group A) or satisfactory specificity (group B) [8,9]. As shown in fig. 26-1, calcium antagonists of group A (verapamil, gallopamile, nifedipine, and diltiazem) are capable of inhibiting calcium-dependent excitation-contraction coupling in the mammalian ventricular myocardium by 90% or more before the fast Na^+ influx, which occurs during the rising phase of the action potential, is also affected, i.e., before $\dot{V}_{max}$ is diminished. Group B antagonists (prenylamine, fendiline, terodiline, perhexiline, and caroverine) are somewhat less

specific, and it was found that potent Na^+-antagonistic effects (decrease in $\dot{V}_{max}$) occurred at concentrations that reduced Ca^{2+}-dependent isometric tension development in papillary muscles by about 50–70% [8,9].

It was not known at the time of this first classification that a decrease in $\dot{V}_{max}$ is not a reliable measure of Na^+-current inhibition [10], that Na^+-current inhibition is usually not only dose but also strongly rate dependent [11,12], and that calmodulin inhibition, which was found to be an additional property of some calcium blockers such as fendiline flunarizine and bepridile [13,14], exerts a marked smooth muscle relaxing and Na^+-antagonistic effect [15,16].

Although these criteria for the classification of calcium antagonists were unrelated to their chemical constitution or to their binding efficacy, and did not include smooth muscle effects, the clinically, now widely established, agents diltiazem, nifedipine, and verapamil and closely related compounds all proved to belong to group A of Fleckenstein's first classification. Even more convincing was the pharmacological line of evidence for a highly specific mode of action of Ca antagonists and for the lack of beta-adrenoceptor blocking activities. Initially, these new compounds were considered to be beta-adrenoceptor blockers [17], but Fleckenstein [18] and others [19,20] presented evidence that calcium antagonists lack beta-adrenoceptor blocking effects. In fact, the relaxation and inhibition of excitation of the smooth muscle fibers of the myometrium by calcium antagonists [21] was the exact opposite effect of that of beta-adrenoceptor blockers (cf. fig. 26-2). It was found later that calcium antagonists relax more or less all smooth muscle fibers and also inhibit excitation. The most prominent effects were fortunately found to occur in the coronary system and in the peripheral vascular bed (see fig. 26-2).

At this early stage of defining a new Ca^{2+}-antagonistic principle (1972/73), the following data had already been documented by Fleckenstein's laboratory:

1. Inhibition of excitation and of excitation-contraction coupling of uterine and vascular smooth muscle [2,21–25]
2. Inhibition of [$^{45}Ca^{2+}$] uptake into the myocardium and of Ca^{2+} influx measured by sucrose gap voltage clamp [26–29]

511

N. Sperelakis (ed.), Physiology and Pathophysiology of the Heart, Third Edition.

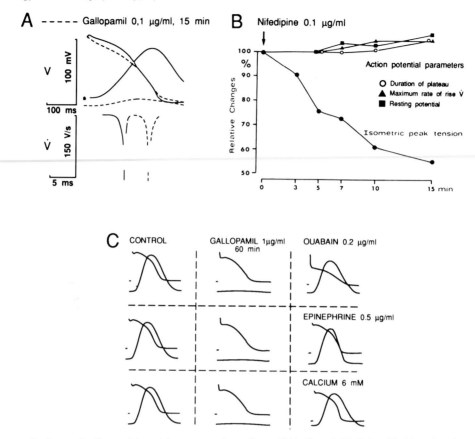

Fig. 26-1. The negative inotropic effects of the calcium antagonists gallopamil (**A,C**) and nifedipine (**B**). Note that the maximum rate of rise of the action potentials ($\dot{V}$ in lower half of A and ▲ in B) is not reduced by the calcium antagonists. A and B are experiments with guinea pig papillary muscles (35°C, rate of stimulation 2/s). In C the inhibition of tension development, due to antagonism of calcium, by gallopamil in cat ventricular myocardium is antagonized by the addition of either cardiac glycosides, by stimulation of beta-adrenoceptors with epinephrine, or by an increase in extracellular calcium concentration. Data from Fleckenstein et al. {1,30}; see Fleckenstein {8} for review.

3. Inhibition of contraction of ventricular myocardium and antagonism of this effect by Ca^{2+} ions, beta-adrenoceptor stimulation, or cardiac glycosides {1,4,8,18,27,30}
4. Inhibition of Ca^{2+}-dependent action potentials in partially depolarized ventricular myocardium by inhibitors of transmembrane Ca^{2+} inflow and antagonism of this effect by promotors of Ca^{2+} inflow {31–33}
5. Inhibition of cardiac pacemaker activity, of atrioventricular conduction velocity and prolongation of refractoriness {9,34}

Parallel with these studies, clinical testing of Ca^{2+}-antagonistic compounds started as early as 1963 in Europe and Japan and, up to 1972 covered the following topics: angina pectoris {35–52}, supraventricular tachyarrhythmias {53–61}, and hypertension {55,63–65}. There was one report on tocolytic effects {66} and one on asystole {67}. These early studies on the cardiovascular and smooth muscle effects of Ca^{2+} antagonists were well in line with Fleckenstein's hypothesis of specific inhibition of the permeation of Ca^{2+} ions through sarcolemnal calcium channels.

The notion of calcium-selective ion channels being receptor sites for the action of calcium antagonists became more and more accepted with further characterization of channel subtypes by a new technique called *patch clamp* that permitted the measurement of ionic currents through single membrane channels {68,69}. The term *calcium antagonists* could be extended to calcium entry or calcium channel blockers, to slow channel blockers, or more specifically, to L-type calcium channel blockers. It should be noted, however, that it is not irreversible block but rather reversible inhibition of calcium channel activities that is found in the presence of Ca^{2+} antagonists.

In addition, advances in the understanding of the genetic regulation of ion channels {70,71}, their amino acid sequences, and their probable configurations strongly promoted the concept of Ca^{2+} ion channels as likely key receptor sites for the modulation of cardiovascular functions {72}. The application of voltage and patch-clamp

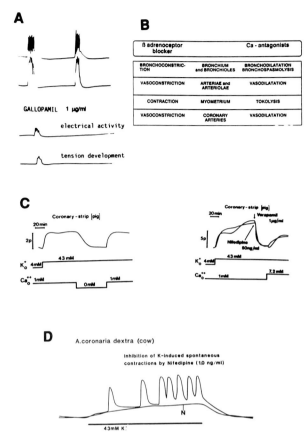

are ubiquitous features of other excitable cells. They have an important function not only in vertebrate smooth and cardiac muscle but also in embryonic skeletal muscle, neuron somata, synaptic terminals, sensory receptors, and a wide range of cells that secrete hormones, neuromodulators, or neurotransmitters. Calcium channels have also been shown to exist in a number of nonexcitable cells, such as glial cells {73}, myeloma cells {74}, osteoblasts {75}, and fibroblasts {76}, those of the latter being modulated by growth factors and oncogenes.

Calcium channels are not as highly conserved as, for instance, sodium channels, but vary rather widely between different tissues in properties such as their conductance; voltage dependence; inactivation mechanism; inhibition by ions, blockers, or toxins; and modulation by receptors, G proteins, or second messengers. Analogous to conventional pharmacological characterizations, the key criterion for the classification of voltage-dependent calcium channels (L, N, T types — see Chapter 9) is their pharmacological specificity and, where available, information concerning separate genetic control. T-channel expression can be inhibited by transforming genes without simultaneous modification of L-channel expression {76}. This chapter will focus on L- and, in part, on T-type channels only; for a review of calcium channels in a variety of cell membranes see other works {77–82}. A major monograph {9} and other reviews have shed light on the historical aspects of the discovery of drugs acting on calcium channels {7,83,84}.

CALCIUM ION CHANNELS

Julius Bernstein correctly hypothesized in 1902 that excitable cells maintain an intracellular potential as a result of their membranes being selectively permeable to potassium ions. Selective permeability exists because of aqueous pores, called *channels*, formed by protein macromolecules that span the membrane and through which ions can permeate the hydrophobic lipid membrane. The property of K^+ selectivity is related to the presence of just two amino acid residues in the ion channel protein {85}.

Selectivity is a distinct property of ion channels for which they are usually named, i.e., a calcium channel selects for Ca^{2+} ions and this preferred ion passes through the channel at least a hundred times more easily than rejected ions. Channels accomplish ion selectivity by either steric means (a narrow opening excluding larger ions) or by the binding strength of the selected ion to sites within the channel. Calcium channels do not simply repel other ions, such as Na^+, since large currents of Na^+ or of other alkaline ions flow through calcium channels in the absence of Ca^{2+} ions {86; for review see 87}, but these currents are blocked by micromolar amounts of Ca^{2+} ions.

Calcium channels are both very selective and highly permeable. During channel opening, fluxes of several thousand Ca^{2+} ions per millisecond have been observed {88–91}. The calcium channel is somewhat unique in its selectivity when compared to other ionic channels, e.g., in Na^+ channels K^+ permeability is 0.1 and Ca^{2+} is 0.05 of

Fig. 26-2. Calcium antagonists inhibit spontaneous transmembrane electrical activity (measured by sucrose gap technique) and tension development in rat myometrial strips (**A**, see Tritthart et al. {21}). Excitation and excitation-contraction coupling is inhibited by calcium antagonists throughout smooth muscle fibers, whereas beta-adrenoceptor blockers predominantly promote contractions (**B**). In **C** the relaxation of potassium-depolarized coronary strips is shown for Ca^{2+} withdrawal (left) or for calcium antagonist addition (right). In the presence of calcium antagonists, an increase in extracellular Ca^{2+} partially restores contractile tension. In freshly dissected coronary arteries, rhythmic spontaneous contractions of large amplitude are common or can be initiated or supported by a variety of factors (e.g., potassium, see D). Calcium antagonists are very effective on these spontaneous or induced vasospastic activities (**D**). Trace N was recorded 13 minutes after the addition of nifedipine. Potassium-induced contractile activities under control conditions and after the addition of nifedipine are superimposed.

techniques to isolated cardiac or smooth muscle cells, the use of fluorescent calcium-sensitive dyes, and, last but not least, the utilization of calcium channel blockers became very useful tools in studying the role of calcium ions in the normal cardiovascular system, including pathophysiological changes.

Dedication: In memoriam Albrecht Fleckenstein, who died in 1992.

However, it soon became evident that calcium channels

the Na$^+$ permeability {1}, whereas Na$^+$ permeability of Ca^{2+} channels is usually 0.001. Models that account for the ionic selectivity of calcium channels incorporate specific multiple binding properties of the channel for Ca^{2+} {92} and Ca^{2+}-induced transformation from strongly to weakly binding states {93}. These ion-channel interactions and conformational changes, which lead to a "fluctuating barrier" {94}, can model the permeability features of the calcium channel, but the physical picture of the reactions of a single-file, double-binding site model of the Ca^{2+} channel has yet to be developed.

Ca^{2+} is rather exceptional among permeant ions in that Ca^{2+} ions themselves serve crucial functions within the cell and inside the membrane, in addition to merely carrying electrical charge. Calcium ions are ubiquitous intracellular second messengers in an intracellular environment of very low calcium activity {95}, and the need for high selectivity and powerful transmembrane signaling via high Ca^{2+}-permeability pathways is obvious. Intracellular Ca^{2+} modulates other ion channels, such as Ca^{2+}-activated potassium, chloride, or nonselective channels, leading to complex electrical behaviors (see Chapter 5). Elevated Ca^{2+} levels in cardiac or smooth muscle cells play a role in various pathophysiological processes (see Chapters 31, 32). In addition, Ca^{2+}-dependent enzymes, such as protein kinase C or Ca^{2+}-calmodulin kinases, are most probably influenced by calcium channel openings, and, via modulation of other channels and receptors, these enzymes then contribute to the complexity of electrical and nonelectrical activities following modulation of calcium channel activity.

The macromolecules spanning the lipid membrane and forming the Ca^{2+} channel may conceptually be considered as enzymes that reduce the energy of transmembrane ion diffusion and, thus, enhance the rate of diffusion by a factor of 10^{20} to 10^{30}. In fact, like enzymes, channels display substrate specifity in the form of ionic selectivity. Furthermore, competitive inhibition by substrate analogues that are divalent ions or blockers for Ca^{2+} channels has been seen (see below). Like enzymes, calcium channels have the capability of undergoing rapid conformational changes, i.e., changes between open and conducting, or closed and nonconducting, states of the channel.

The conductivity of the single Ca channel has a constant value in the open state under constant experimental conditions. Hence, (a) the likelihood of the stochastic channel opening reactions, (b) the duration of channel opening, and (c) the density of active channels are the key factors governing the calcium current strength of individual cells. Very little is known about upregulation and downregulation of calcium channels in humans and, as a result, about normal homeostasis of calcium channel density {96}, or channel function during cardiac failure, hypertrophy, hypertension {97,98}, cardiomyopathy {99}, etc. After prolonged treatment with calcium channel blockers, only a few rebound effects following cessation of therapy have so far been reported {100}. This probably indicates that channel density is little affected during diseases or by therapy and is not the key site of action of Ca^{2+} antagonists. Hence, all agents or factors that modify activation or function of voltage-dependent calcium channels alter, predominantly, the probability of the open time of activated channels and, as a result, change the peak calcium current measurable under given experimental conditions (fig. 26-4). Prolonged treatment may, nevertheless, alter intracellular Ca^{2+} homeostasis and thus cause a variety of indirect effects and cellular adjustments.

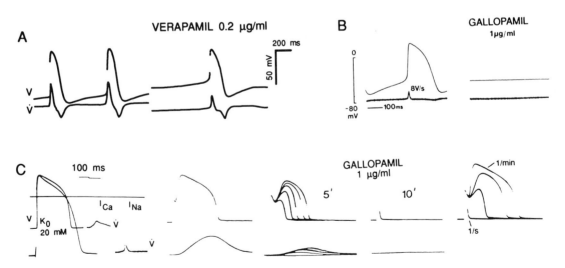

Fig. 26-3. The inhibitory effects of verapamil on the isolated AV-node of the rabbit {34}. Beat frequency decreases due to elevation of threshold potentials and retardation of slow diastolic depolarizations. In addition, the rate of rise ($\dot{V}$) and overshoot of AV action potentials are reduced by calcium antagonists (A). The electrical activity of embryonic chick heart cells resembles that of SA- and AV-nodal cells in adult hearts (see Chapter 37), and calcium antagonists completely inhibit the spontaneous discharge in these cells (B). Slow action potentials (see Chapter 13), recorded in 20 mM K^+_o, of guinea pig papillary muscles are blocked by calcium antagonists (C). This complete inhibition of slow and Ca^{2+}-dependent action potentials by gallopamil (C) is overcome by periods of rest of sufficient duration (right, change of stimulation rate from 1/s to 1/min).

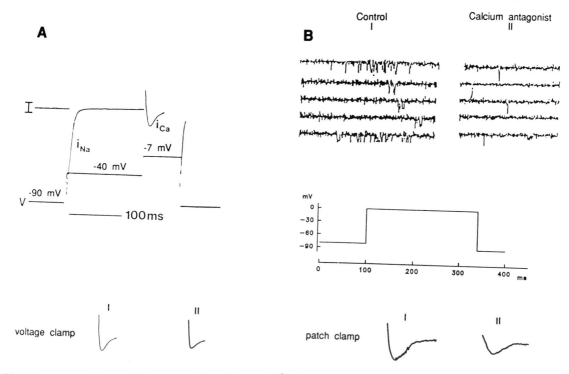

Fig. 26-4. The transmembrane calcium current through L-type Ca^{2+} channels. **A:** Whole-cell voltage clamp. The initial depolarization to -40 mV elicites a fast Na^+ current with rapid inactivation. The ensuing depolarization activates the calcium inward current. This whole-cell calcium current is the result of accumulated single-channel openings, as indicated in **B**, and can be resolved by patch-clamp experiments (B). Following depolarization, the probability of calcium channel opening, as well as the open duration in individual channels, is reduced by calcium antagonists. Thus, the depolarization-induced transmembrane Ca^{2+} current is diminished by Ca^{2+} antagonists.

VOLTAGE AND ION EFFECTS ON CALCIUM CHANNELS

The single-channel calcium current has been shown to flicker between on and off states with a time course that is considerably faster than that of activation of the macroscopic current {90,101}. These rapid transitions between open and closed states, although a somewhat stochastic equilibrium prevails, allows the investigator to lump them together into one state, the active state, which can be modulated by a comparatively slowly developing process that leads the channel to a temporarily inactive and non-conductive form different from the closed state of the activated channel. The complex kinetics of calcium channel activation can be modeled by assuming that activation starts from two inactivated states. Figure 26-5 shows that all transitions leading to the inactive state I_{Ca} are Ca^{2+} and voltage dependent, whereas other transitions are simply voltage dependent. This model {102, see also 80} also accounts for the voltage and Ca^{2+} dependency of the recovery from inactivation, for the biphasic inactivation time course, and for the Ca^{2+} dependency of the inactivation rate {103}. Voltage-dependent activation and inactivation of calcium channels implies that, at the molecular

level, charged groups ("gates") move in response to alteration of the transmembrane electrical field. Although gating currents could, so far, not be resolved at the single-channel level, it is likely that they contain components for activation and inactivation as well as for opening and closing of individual channels.

Voltage-sensitive calcium channels may either require a large amount of membrane depolarization to become activated (L, N, P, class) or are activated with minor amounts of depolarization (low threshold). These latter channels are called T (for transient) channels. Transient T-type calcium channels inactivate rapidly, whereas long-lasting L-type channels exhibit a slow, time-dependent inactivation. However, due to the Ca^{2+} dependency of inactivation (see below) L channels may inactivate quite rapidly under physiological conditions, i.e., when Ca^{2+} ions are present, instead of the more permeable Ba^{2+} ions used experimentally as charge carrier (half-times of 20–100 ms).

Inactivation of T channels develops monoexponentially, is complete and appears to be strictly voltage dependent, and is thus independent of the type of charge-carrying ion or the amount of Ca^{2+} entry into the cell. Maximal slope conductances in cell-attached patches were found to be 6.8 and 3.4 pS (100 mM Ca^{2+}_o) with T channels being equally permeable to Ca^{2+} and Ba^{2+} {104–106}. In contrast, the high-voltage activated L-type calcium channels carry Ba^{2+} nearly twice as effectively as they do Ca^{2+} ions {104} and have a much higher conductance: 22–28 pS, in 110 mM Ba^{2+}, in cardiac fibers; 20–25 pS, in 110 mM Ba^{2+}, in smooth muscle fibers {107,108}.

T channels are somewhat dominant in embryonic cells {109} and since pacemaker discharge activities are characteristic for embryonic heart cells (see Chapter 37), it is not so surprising that T channels are predominantly found in those atrial and ventricular cells that exhibit an automatic discharge capability, such as pacemaker cells {110}. T channels are also found in smooth muscle cells {108,111–113}. T channels, at resting membrane potentials, are probably inactivated, but they may be activated following hyperpolarization and, thus, may modulate the discharge rate of pacemaker cells, and excitability, as well as oscillatory and bursting activities in smooth muscle. However, there is no doubt that excitation-contraction coupling in cardiac and in smooth muscle in governed by L-type channel activity, as are suprathreshold slow inward currents in pacemaker or other cardiac cells and in smooth muscle cells.

Calcium channels greatly prefer Ca^{2+}, Ba^{2+}, and Sr^{2+} over all other alkaline ions for which a permeant ratio as low as 0.001 or less has been calculated. The different types of calcium channels share a similar permeability for alkaline earth ions, with the exception of the Mg^{2+} ion being nearly impermeant. The T channel is equally permeable to Ca^{2+} and Ba^{2+}, with a small preference for Sr^{2+} {114}, whereas the L-type calcium channel has a clear preference for Ba^{2+} ions {104}. This first category of inorganic cations carries current through the calcium channel. Competitive inhibitors of calcium currents are La^{3+}, Co^{2+}, Ni^{2+}, and Cd^{2+}. T channels are potently blocked by Ni^{2+} and are less potently blocked by Cd^{2+}. Cadmium is a much more potent blocker of the L-type channel {115–117}. Mn^{2+}, Zn^{2+}, and Mg^{2+} also act as competitive inhibitors of calcium currents but can carry current in some cells. The blockade of calcium currents by Mg^{2+} was discovered early {118} and could be attributed to reduced mean open times {115}, most probably due to the entry of Mg^{2+} ions. When Ca^{2+} ions are lacking, Mg^{2+} ions can occupy the channel for some time, preventing the passage of the permeant ions and, thus, resembling in part the blocking action of Ca^{2+} ions, which opposes the passage of Na^+ or Li^+ ions through calcium channels. Increase in the concentration of intracellular Mg^{2+} to the millimolar range inhibits L-type calcium channels {118, 119}. A phosphorylation-independent, direct activation of calcium channels by Mg^{2+} nucleotide complexes has recently been reported {120}. Addition of adenosine triphosphate (ATP) to the intracellular solution reduces the rate of irreversible rundown of calcium current in dialyzed cells {121} and increases calcium current when endogenous ATP production is inhibited {122}.

In guinea pig ventricular myocytes, alkaline pH enhanced L-type calcium current and acidic pH reduced it to about 60–70% of that at pH 7.5 {123}. These findings are consistent with the titration of negatively charged groups in the inner or outer membrane surface, which control not only gating, but also ion permeation of the channel. Lowering pH inside the cell caused both activation and inactivation curves to be shifted toward less negative potentials as well as a decrease in channel opening probability {124}.

CHANNEL INHIBITORS

The compounds and agents that affect the activity of voltage-dependent calcium channels can conveniently be grouped into three categories: (A) inorganic ions, (B) channel inhibitors and openers, and (C) naturally occurring regulators. The main focus of this chapter will be on groups A and B of calcium channel modulators. Group C will be discussed in other chapters of this book.

Corpora non agunt nisi fixata, i.e., compounds act only when bound to some structure (Paul Ehrlich, 1912). This receptor concept raises many questions with regard to the location and type of binding sites for Ca^{2+} antagonists, access to these sites, structure-activity relations, binding and allosteric modulation of channel function and of affinity to binding sites, etc. The first question is whether calcium channels act as true receptors, or only have some features that resemble those of receptors. The chemical heterogeneities of the most widely used Ca^{2+} antagonists — nifedipine, verapamil, and diltiazem — are very obvious, and a common receptor for their inhibitory action appeared highly unlikely. Consequently, Fleckenstein's intention to introduce the new pharmacological principle of Ca^{2+} antagonism was seriously hampered by the fact that it was necessary to have a group of different receptor sites that were all responsible for the same mode of action. In addition, indirect evidence attributed a calcium-blocking property to a very large number of other structures {for review see 7}, and this contributed to the confusion. That a multiplicity of binding sites are found on the L channel is today not so surprising, since the α_1-subunit of the calcium channel, the site of binding of Ca^{2+} antagonists, has a sequence highly homologous with that of the sodium channel, which exhibits at least five distinct binding sites {125}. Nevertheless, it is surprising that evidence for the existence of endogenous ligands for calcium channels is still missing. There are only few reports of calcium channel modulation by endogenous peptides {7,126,127}, but no specific inhibition of Ca^{2+}-antagonist binding has been reported for any of the known neurotransmitters or peptide hormones.

There are only few compounds, all of them not very specific {81}, that will block T channels. These include octanol {128}, amiloride {129}, and diphenylhydantoin {130}. Among Ca^{2+} antagonists, flunarizine and nicardipine were reported to inhibit T channels in vascular smooth muscle {131}, as do felodipine and cinnarizine in atria {132,133}. In a similar fashion as in sodium channels, T-channels are inhibited by almost all compounds that inhibit L-type channels, provided that the concentration is high enough. There are no specific toxins {but see 134} or calcium antagonists available that block T channels only

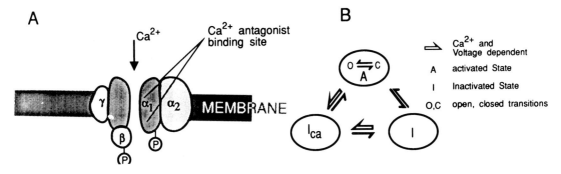

Fig. 26-5. Schematic model of the L-type Ca^{2+} channel. The part forming the transmembrane pore and water conduit is the α_1 subunit, which is also the site of binding of calcium antagonists. Models of kinetic channels transitions usually include open, closed, activated, and inactivated states in order to describe channel functions. The extremely fast transition between open and closed states of activated channels allows the separation of these fast transitions from the slow processes of Ca^{2+}-channel activation and inactivation, both being voltage and/or Ca^{2+} dependent (see text).

with sufficient selectivity to study T-channel function. Hence, no extensive pharmacology for T channels has yet been developed, and the contribution of T channels to normal and disturbed cardiovascular functions is not at all well defined. We therefore focus in this chapter on Ca^{2+} antagonists that bind to and have the capability to modulate L-type calcium channels.

L-TYPE CALCIUM CHANNELS: STRUCTURE, LIGANDS, BINDING, FUNCTION

Calcium channel ligands are compounds that act by binding directly to voltage-sensitive calcium channels and not to some nearby or distant receptor. This binding will decrease (or increase) the movement of Ca^{2+} ions through the channel without alteration of the intrinsic permeability in the open state, but modulation of the open-state probability and duration. The overall calcium current through channels in a cell (I) is simply the product of active channel number (n), the probability of a channel being in the open state (P), and the unitary current through a single calcium channel (i), i.e.,

$$I = n \cdot P \cdot i.$$

These unitary currents (i) are probably events that are mediated by the α_1-subunit of the channel molecule, since calcium currents can be reconstituted by the dihydropyridine receptor α_1 subunit alone {71,72,134}. Reconstitution experiments showed that the purified dihydropyridine binding site is the functional calcium transmembrane pore {135,136}. The linings of the conduction pores are probably formed by localized stretches of only 20–25 amino acid residues repeated in each subunit. Point mutations can lead to alterations of ion selectivity, conductance, and affinity for blocking agents. Hence, binding sites for Ca^{2+} antagonists are most likely to be located in close proximity to the channel outer and inner mouth, and to the calcium binding sites within the core of the channel. The number

of discrete binding sites for Ca^{2+} antagonists are, most likely, not only linked allosterically, one to another, but also to the structures of the channel governing permeation and gating.

Figure 26-5 shows the main components of the L-type calcium channel. The α_1 subunit contains the channel-forming structures {72,137} as well as various binding sites of Ca^{2+}-antagonistic compounds. The cytoplasmic site of the α_1 subunit is a good substrate for protein kinase A phosphorylation {138} and the beta subunit may also be a site of cAMP-dependent phosphorylation {139} (see other chapters of this book for second-messenger and G-protein mediated alterations of channel function). Four tightly coupled subunits — α_1, α_2, β, and γ — form the channel complex (fig. 26-5); the primary structure of each subunit has been determined; and α_1, α_2, and β cDNAs have been used to characterize transcripts expressed in various tissues {140}.

The calcium channel likely has at least seven separate binding sites for Ca^{2+} antagonists of structurally distinct chemical classes {141}, including the sites for 1,4-dihydropyridines, phenylalkylamines, and benzothiazepines, as well as for the classical compounds nifedipine, verapamil, and diltiazem. Depending on the position of the binding site, different avenues of access may be used by ligands: (a) directly from the extracellular aqueous environment, (b) using the waterconduit of the open channel, (c) by lateral diffusion after partitioning into the membrane bilayer, and (d) after crossing the cell membrane from the intracellular aqueous environment. Most calcium antagonists are some 100 times more concentrated in the cell membrane than in the aqueous environment and are usually more potent when added to the external side of the cell membrane.

Divalent cations have very marked effects on binding of calcium channel ligands {142,143}. Electrophysiological and binding studies indicate that the affinity increases with membrane depolarization {144–146}, indicating preferential binding to the inactivated states of the channel.

The "modulated receptor" hypothesis (see Chapter 31) was the first to depict the binding of a channel inhibitor to a receptor in a transmembrane channel as being modulated by the state of the channel. Diltiazem as well as verapamil and other members of the phenylalkylamine group exert a strongly rate-dependent inhibition of calcium currents (see Chapter 13, this book) {147–152}. In contrast to the uncharged 1,4-dihydropyridines at normal pH, these compounds are charged and their access to the binding site is not predominantly via the lipophilic membrane pathway but rather through the open channels. These observations of dependency on the rate of excitation may be attributed either to preferential binding to the open state or to easier access, through open channels, to preferential binding sites in the inactivated state.

Calcium antagonists bound to their receptor site in the channel-forming α_1 subunit do not alter the amplitude of the unitary channel current but allosterically affect the activation of channels and, hence, decrease the probability of channel opening. Positive and negative allosteric interactions between different binding sites, as well as between binding sites and the calcium pore, have also been found, e.g., diltiazem and ($-$) devapamil inhibit or increase 1,4-dihydropyridine binding depending on the temperature {153}. The S-enantiomer of 5-nitro-1,4-dihydropyridine acts as a channel activator, increasing opening probability and open state duration {154}, but can also act as a channel inhibitor depending on the membrane potential {155,156}. The transformation of the mode of action of this calcium channel activating compound into an inhibitory action was recently also observed during allosteric interactions from another binding site, i.e., by fendiline binding {157}.

THERAPEUTIC ASPECTS OF CALCIUM CHANNEL LIGANDS

As described in detail in other chapters of this book, the most important therapeutic sites of action of calcium antagonists are the L-type channels in both vascular smooth muscle and cardiac cells. Effects on other calcium channels as well as on other receptors and channels, at dosages employed in the clinic, rarely reach borderline clinical significance. This statement applies only to the first generation of calcium antagonists; the actions of second-generation compounds reach beyond the cardiovascular system, e.g., nimodipine is used in the treatment of neurological deficits during subarachnoid hemorrhage {158}, and future drug developments are aimed at channel, tissue, and/or disease selectivity. Among the borderline effects of classical Ca^{2+} antagonists is nifedipine inhibition of aldosterone secretion {159}. Also, a mild but significant reduction of platelet aggregation and prolongation of bleeding time, which is likely due to inhibition of the transmembrane Ca^{2+} inflow in thrombocytes, has been reported {160}. Beneficial effects of calcium channel blockers in arterial thrombosis, deep vein thrombosis, pulmonary emboli, vasculities, thrombotic thrombo-

cytopenic purpurea, and thrombocythemia have been reported {161}.

Experiments on smooth muscle cells without intact membranes, so-called skinned fibers, indicated that some calcium antagonists have intracellular sites of action {15}. Fendiline, bepridile; and flunarizine are potent inhibitors of calmodulin {13,14} and, thus, of smooth muscle contraction, regardless of the source of calcium activating the contraction {15}. To what extent calmodulin antagonism of some calcium channel blockers contributes to the therapeutically important, smooth muscle relaxation needs to be evaluated. This intracellular site of action of Ca^{2+} channel blockers is, in every pharmacokinetic and pharmacodynamic aspect, different from the membrane site of action.

In cancer therapy calcium antagonists have beneficial effects when used in combination with certain anticancer compounds. This action is probably related to inhibition of the multidrug resistance phenotype {162,163}. A similar mechanism may be responsible for the verapamil-induced reversal of chloroquine resistance in malaria {164}. The features of the classical Ca^{2+} antagonists relevant to the acute and chronic treatment of cardiovascular diseases, as well as their clinical efficacy, have been reviewed extensively {7,9,165–168}, and here only selected aspects related to physiology and pathophysiology will be briefly summarized.

The inhibitory effects of Ca^{2+} antagonists on excitation and excitation-contraction coupling in vascular smooth muscle fibers engendered the successful and widespread use of Ca^{2+} antagonists against hypertension, in hypertensive crisis, in angina, and in Prinzmetal angina against coronary vasospasm. Nifedipine has a high affinity for Ca^{2+} channels at low membrane potential and, probably, for the inactivated state of the channel. Smooth muscle cells have a lower membrane potential than heart muscle cells and nifedipine, due to the low membrane potential, and to the composition of the smooth muscle membrane being more favorable for partitioning, is about twice as effective in the vascular bed as in the heart. Verapamil and diltiazem are about equieffective. In vascular smooth muscle cells, all Ca^{2+} antagonists exhibit the highest efficacy against vasospastic activities (fig. 26-6), are effective against depolarization-induced contractions, and are least effective against receptor-operated channel activities and the resultant transmitter-induced vasoconstrictions. Accordingly, in the coronary system Ca^{2+} antagonists are very effective against vasospastic activities, they dilate large extramurally coronary vessels but do not alter peripheral coronary resistance or even cause coronary steal effects {169,170}. More than 90% of patients with angina pectoris have parts of the large extramural vessels narrowed to less than half the normal diameter {171}, and hence, vasodilatation in these areas of increased resistance will be effective in increasing blood supply, and the concomitant reduction in myocardial oxygen demand will effectively reduce myocardial ischemia.

The cardiac effects of Ca^{2+} antagonists administered into coronary blood vessels differ thoroughly from those following systemic administration. When administered

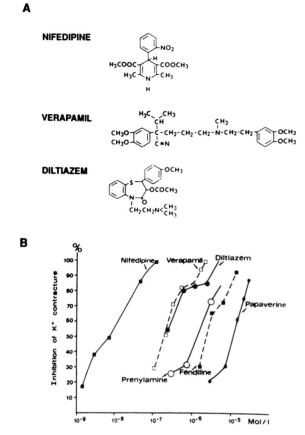

A

NIFEDIPINE

VERAPAMIL

DILTIAZEM

B

Ca2+ antagonists applied	in vitro or intracoronary	in vivo
sinus rate	decrease: N, V, D	at rest N: +, V, D: -/+ during exercise N:-/+, V,D:-
sinus node recovery time	prolongation: N, V, D: ++	N, V, D: -/+ sik sinus node syndrome: N, V, D: +++
Atrio-ventricular conduction time (AH duration)	VD: strongly rate dependent prolongation of AH duration, Wenckebach type blocks N: no rate dependency of prolongation of AH duration almost no blocks	VD: prolongation of AH duration Wenckebach type blocks N: no or minor AH prolongation noblocks
effective refractory period of AV conduction	VD: ++ prolongation N: minor or no prolong- ation	VD: prolongation Wenckebach type blocks N: no prolongation, no blocks
Nifedipine N,	Verapamil V,	Diltiazem D

Fig. 26-7. The generation and conduction of the cardiac impulse is influenced by calcium antagonists. Only in in-vitro experiments or following intracoronary administration do these direct inhibitory effects of calcium antagonists become evident. Baroreceptor reflex control of cardiac activities is stimulated by the vascular effects of calcium antagonists and significantly modifies these direct, inhibitory effects.

Fig. 26-6. **A:** Chemical structures of compounds in the classical first generation of calcium antagonists (not shown is gallopamil, a methoxy derivative of verapamil). **B:** Calcium antagonists suppress the potassium-induced contractions of pig coronary strips. The tension induced by 43 mM KCl within 40 minutes is taken as 100%, and the dose-dependent decrease of tension is shown for different calcium antagonists and for papaverine (average values from 15 individual experiments for each concentration) {9}.

systemically Ca^{2+} antagonists lower vascular resistance and blood pressure {9,165–167,172} and interfere with autoregulative vasoconstrictions and, thus, alter the circulatory reflex control of the heart. Diltiazem and verapamil have been reported to reduce baroreceptor reflex sensitivity {173}. Stimulation of beta-adrenoceptors in the myocardium physiologically opposes the inhibitory effects of Ca^{2+} antagonists. Agents that stimulate adenylate cyclase in cardiac cells, or cAMP and its analogs, all stimulate cardiac L current by increasing the probability and duration of channel opening {174, for review see 168}, whereas inhibitors of adenylate cyclase or muscarinic agonists decrease calcium current {175}. The direct cardiac effects of Ca^{2+} antagonists on impulse generation (heart rate) and conduction (SA- and AV-nodal conduction) are therefore significantly modified in vivo by the vegetative nervous system (see fig 26-7) and the negative inotropic

cardiodepressant effects are self-limiting. Whenever a decrease in myocardial contractility leads to a disproportionate fall in blood pressure, the reflex release of sympathetic transmitters will counteract the drug's effect and make the drug safe to use in vivo. The reduction of contractility to the minimum level necessary for normal pump function in combination with a reduced heart rate during workload, reduced afterload and preload, and improved oxygen supply makes the pumping activity of the heart more economical and reduces the risk of angina. In this way, together with their potent vasodilator properties, Ca^{2+} antagonists improve cardiac function, even in patients with failing left ventricles {175}. Even more surprising, patients with stable angina receiving oral beta-adrenoceptor blockers showed an increased cardiac output with nifedipine but no change in cardiac output after verapamil {177}.

The direct effects of all Ca^{2+} antagonists when given by the intracoronary route are a decrease in heart rate and a slowing of sinoatrial conduction. Among heart cells, the sinus-node cells have the lowest membrane potential and, accordingly, the most prominent inhibitory effect of nifedipine is in the sinus node. Less marked effects are seen in the AV node. In healthy people, nifedipine leaves heart rate unchanged, or even, by baroreceptor reflexes, slightly increased, indicating a complete compensation, or even an overcompensation, of the direct and inhibitory effects of nifedipine on the sinus node. This reflex increase in heart rate is not advantageous in patients with angina pectoris. In the sick sinus-node syndrome, compensation by beta-adrenoceptor stimulation is no longer effective and, accordingly, all Ca^{2+} antagonists may lead to life-threatening bradycardia or asystole, and are therefore strictly counterindicated.

The inhibitory effects of nifedipine are not dependent on the rate of activity or on channel opening as are those of verapamil and diltiazem. Thus, the effects of nifedipine may be completely compensated by cAMP-mediated activation of calcium channels, whereas the rate-dependent part of the overall inhibitory action of verapamil or diltiazem is unlikely to be compensated for by baroreceptor reflex responses. The direct and antiarrhythmic effects of the Ca^{2+} antagonists, verapamil and diltiazem, prolong the intranodal conduction time (AH duration) and lengthen the antegrade and retrograde effective and functional refractory periods in a strongly dose- and rate-dependent manner, finally causing Wenckenbach-type block of conduction {34,178}. As a rational basis for the clinical use of Ca^{2+} antagonists in the management of supraventricular arrhythmias, Singh et al. {20,180} have proposed that among their fourth class of antiarrhythmic action, there exists a type-1 group of drugs, which includes verapamil and diltiazem, that prolongs AV-nodal conduction and refractoriness, and is comprised of moderate vasodilators; in addition, a type-2 group, which includes nifedipine, with almost no direct electrophysiological effects in the heart, causes potent peripheral vasodilation. Clinicians need to be aware of the complex nature of action of Ca^{2+} antagonists, which is, in fact, more a mosaic of effects in vivo than just a simple L-type channel blockade. Also, in physiology and pathophysiology, the systemic effects following cellular and molecular modification of Ca^{2+} channels warrant deeper understanding.

SUMMARY AND CONCLUSIONS

Transsarcolemnic Ca^{2+}-ion movements play a key role in excitation-contraction coupling in heart and in smooth muscle fibers. They participate in the transmembrane currents initiating action potentials or during action potentials, and give rise to transmembrane signals that start a variety of nonelectrical cell activities. The pioneering work of Fleckenstein was the first indication that modulation of transsarcolemmic Ca^{2+} currents is possible in a very selective way. The introduction of calcium antagonistic compounds strongly improved the understanding of the Ca^{2+} dependency of many physiological functions of the heart, as well as of some cardiovascular diseases. Hence, many clinical studies were initiated and their results confirmed the new pharmacological principle of calcium antagonism. These new compounds were also very helpful tools in the study of transmembrane Ca^{2+} currents throughout biology and medicine. In this chapter the history of the discovery of calcium antagonists is briefly outlined.

The verification of Ca^{2+}-selective membrane channels as receptor sites for calcium antagonists and new methods to study single-channel opening heralded a new molecular dimension of the physiology and pharmacology of Ca^{2+} channels, that comprises the analysis of structure, function, ligand binding, and channel modulation by receptors or second messengers. The distinct features of L-type and T-type channels, both of which are present in the cardiovascular system, such as conductivity, activation, and inactivation processes, are described. The two channels differ significantly in their ion preference, inhibition by divalent ions or blockers, and voltage dependence. The lack of highly specific blockers of T channels has strongly inhibited the analysis of T-channel dependent functions in heart and smooth muscle.

The present concepts of structure and function of L-type channels, their ionic selectivity, and their modulation by other ions, including Mg^{2+}, and by pH, give an interesting view on the likely sites and the mode of action of calcium antagonists. Ligand binding is necessarily dependent on the pathway of access to the binding site and on affinity to the binding site, which may be different depending on the state of the channel. There are a number of distinct sites for the different chemical classes of calcium antagonists on the α_1 subunit, and modulation of channel activity likely takes place by allosteric interactions with the key structures of channel function (activation, gating). In this way the molecular mode of action of calcium antagonists can be analyzed very precisely, and the decrease in the total transmembrane current of a cell can be attributed to a reduction in the probability and duration of the open state of Ca^{2+} channels without any simultaneous changes of the unitary current amplitude in the individual open channel.

All direct effects of calcium antagonists on cardiac cells are significantly modified by baroreceptor reflex activities in the heart due to concurrent effects on the blood pressure and the peripheral vascular bed that follow systematic administration of these compounds. Beta-adrenoceptor stimulation is the physiological opponent of calcium antagonistic effects, and because of this, the pumping function, even of failing hearts, is not endangered by the direct negative inotropic effects of calcium antagonists. In a similar fashion, the direct and bradycardic effect of calcium antagonists is not detectable in vivo (exception: sick sinus-node syndrome). Calcium antagonists have proven to be most effective against vasospastic activities and against depolarization-induced contractions of smooth muscle, and least effective against transmitter-induced smooth muscle contractions. Nifedipine is about twice as effective as verapamil and diltiazem.

There are some interesting effects of calcium antagonists that are not related to effects on L-type channels (e.g., in cancer treatment). However, the future trend of the steadily increasing spectrum of clinical applications for the next generation of calcium antagonists will be focused on the refined selectivities of such compounds with respect to channel types and subtypes, tissue-specific expression of channels, and specific changes during cardiovascular diseases.

REFERENCES

1. Fleckenstein A, Tritthart H, Fleckenstein B, Herbst A, Grün G: A new group of competitive Ca antagonists (Iproveratril, D600, Prenylamine) with highly potent inhi-

bitory effects on excitation-contraction coupling in mammalian myocardium. *Pflügers Arch* 307:25, 1969.

2. Grün G, Fleckenstein A, Tritthart H: Excitation-contraction uncoupling on the rats uterus by some "musculotropic" smooth muscle relaxants. *Pflügers Arch* 264:239, 1969.

3. Fleckenstein A: Die Bedeutung der energiereichen Phosphate für Kontraktilität und Tonus des Myokards. *Verh Dtsch Ges Inn Med* 70:81–89, 1964.

4. Fleckenstein A, Döring HJ, Kammereier H, Grün G: Influence of prenylamine on the utilization of high energy phosphates in cardiac muscle. *Biochim Applic* 14(Suppl 1):323–344, 1968.

5. Mines GR: On functional analysis by the action of electolytes. *J Physiol (Lond)* 46:188–235, 1913.

6. Fatt P, Katz B: The electrical properties of crustacean muscle fibers. *J Physiol* 120:171–204, 1953.

7. Janis RA, Silver P, Triggle DJ: Drug action and cellular calcium regulation. *Adv Drug Res* 16:309–591, 1987.

8. Fleckenstein A: Specific inhibitors and promotors of calcium action in the excitation-contraction coupling of heart muscle and their role in the prevention of production of myocardial lesions. In: Harris P, Opie LH (eds) *Calcium and the Heart*. New York: Academic Press, 1971, pp 135–188.

9. Fleckenstein A: *Calcium Antagonism in Heart and Smooth Muscle*. Experimental Facts and Therapeutic Prospects. New York: John Wiley, 1983.

10. Hondeghem LM: Validity of $\dot{V}_{max}$ as a measure of the sodium current in cardiac and nervous tissues. *Biophys J* 23:147–152, 1978.

11. Chen CM, Gettes LS, Katzung BG: Effects of lidocaine and quinidine on steady state characteristics and recovery kinetics $(dV/dt)_{max}$ in guinea pig ventricular myocardium. *Circ Res* 37:20–29, 1975.

12. Hondeghem LM, Katzung BG: Time and voltage dependent interaction of antiarrhythmic drugs with cardiac sodium channels. *Biochim Biophys Acta* 472:373–398, 1977.

13. Bayer R, Mannhold R: Fendiline: A review of its basic pharmacological and clinical properties. *Pharmacotherapy* 5:103–136, 1987.

14. Lugner C, Follenius A, Gerard D, Stoclet JC: Bepridil and flunarizine as calmodulin inhibitors. *Eur J Pharmacol* 98:157–161, 1984.

15. Metzger H, Stern HO, Pfitzer GU, Ruegg JC: Calcium antagonists affect calmodulin-dependent contractility of a skinned smooth muscle. *Arnzeim Forsch/Drug Res* 32:1425–1427, 1982.

16. Ichikawa M, Urayama M, Matsumoto G: Anticalmodulin drugs block the sodium gating current of squid axons. *J Membr Biol* 120:211–222, 1991.

17. Haas H, Busch E: Vergleichende Untersuchungen der Wirkungen von α-Isopropyl-α-(N-methyl-N-homoveratryl)-γ-aminopropyl-3,4-dimethoxyphenyl-acetonitril, seiner Derivate sowie einiger anderer Coronardilatatoren und β-Receptor-affiner Substanzen. *Arzneim Forsch/Drug Res* 17:257–271, 1967.

18. Fleckenstein A, Kammermeier H, Döring HJ, Freund HJ: Zum Wirkungsmechanismus neuartiger Koronardilatatoren mit gleichzeitig Sauerstoff-einsparenden Myokardeffekten, Prenylamin und Iproveratril. *Z Kreislaufforsch* 56:716–744, 839–853, 1967.

19. Nayler WG, McInnes I, Swann JB, Prive JM, Garson V, Race D, Lowe TE: Some effects of iproveratril (Isoptin) on the cardiovascular system. *J Pharmacol Exp Ther* 161:247–261, 1968.

20. Sing BN, Vaughan Williams EM: A fourth class of antiarrhythmic action. Effects of verapamil on ouabain toxicity on

atrial and ventricular intracellular potentials and other features of cardiac function. *Cardiovasc Res* 6:109–119, 1972.

21. Tritthart H, Grün G, Byon YK, Fleckenstein A: Influence of Ca-antagonistic inhibitors of excitation-contraction coupling in isolated uterine muscle, studies with the sucrose gap method. *Pflügers Arch* 319:117, 1970.

22. Fleckenstein A, Grün G: Reversible blockade of excitation-contraction coupling in rat uterine smooth muscle by means of organic calcium antagonists (iproveratril, D600, prenylamine). *Pflügers Arch* 307:26, 1969.

23. Fleckenstein A, Grün G, Tritthart H, Byon YK: Uterus-Relaxation durch hochaktive Ca-antagonistische Hemmstoffe der elektromechanischen Koppelung wie Isoptin (Verapamil, Iproveratril), Substanz D600 und Segontin (Prenylamin). *Klin Wschr* 49:32–41, 1971.

24. Grün G, Fleckenstein A, Byon YK: Hemmung der Motilität isolierter Uterus-Streifen aus gravidem und nicht-gravidem menschlichem Myometrium durch Ca^{2+}-Antagonisten und Sympathomimetica. *Arzneim Forsch/Drug Res* 21:1585–1590, 1971.

25. Grün G, Fleckenstein A, Byon YK: Blockierung der Ca^{2+}-Effekte auf Tonus und Autoregulation der glatten Gefäßmuskulatur durch Ca^{2+}-Antagonisten (Verapamil, D600, Prenylamin, Bay a 1040 u.a.). In: Betz E (ed) *Vascular Smooth Muscle. Procceedings of the 25th International Congress of International and Physiological Sciences*. Berlin: Springer Verlag, 1972, pp 69–70.

26. Janke J, Fleckenstein A, Jaedike W: Hemmung der Isoproterenol-induzierten Ca^{2+}-45 Netto-Aufnahme in das Ventrikelmyokard durch Ca^{2+}-antagonistische Hemmstoffe der elektromechanischen Koppelung (Isoptin-Verapamil, Iproveratril und Substanz D600). *Pflügers Arch* 316:10, 1970.

27. Fleckenstein A: Specific inhibitors and promoters of calcium action in the excitation contraction coupling of heart muscle and their role in the production or prevention of myocardial lesions. In: Harris P, Opie L (eds) *Calcium and the Heart*. London: Academic Press, 1971, pp 135–188.

28. Tritthart HA, Kaufmann R, Volkmer HP: The influences of Ca^{2+}-antagonistic compounds on the electrical and mechanical activities of the mammalian myocardium measured in voltage clamp experiments. *Naunyn-Schmiedebergs Arch Pharmacol* 274:117, 1972.

29. Kohlhardt M, Bauer B, Krause H, Fleckenstein A: Differentiation of the transmembrane Na- and Ca-channel in mammalian cardiac fibres by the use of specific inhibitors. *Pflügers Arch* 335:309–322, 1972.

30. Fleckenstein A, Tritthart H, Döring HJ, Byon YK: BAY a 1040 — ein hochaktiver Ca^{2+}-antagonistischer Inhibitor der elektromechanischen Kopplungsprozesse im Warmblüter-Myokard. *Arzneim Forsch/Drug Res* 22:22–33, 1972.

31. Volkmann R, Weiss R, Tritthart HA, Fleckenstein A: Susceptibility of Ca-carried action potentials in partially depolarized cardiac fibers to changes in external Ca or to inhibitors and promotors of transmembrane Ca-movements. *Pflügers Arch* 339:6, 1973.

32. Volkmann R, Tritthart HA, Fleckenstein A: The inhibition of Ca-dependent action potentials in mammalian myocardium by Ca-antagonistic compounds (Verapamil, D600). *Naunyn-Schmiedebergs Arch Pharmacol* 277:85, 1973.

33. Tritthart HA, Volkmann R, Weiss R, Fleckenstein A: Calcium mediated action potentials in mammalian myocardium: Alteration of membrane response as induced by changes of Ca or by promoters and inhibitors of transmembrane Ca-inflow. *Naunyn-Schmiedebergs Arch Pharmacol* 280:239–252, 1973.

34. Tritthart HA, Fleckenstein B, Fleckenstein A: Some fundamental actions of antiarrhythmic drugs on excitability and contractility of single myocardial fibers. *Naunyn-Schmiedebergs Arch Pharmacol* 169:2–4, 212–219, 1971.

35. Tshirdewahn B, Klepzig H: Klinische Untersuchungen über die Wirkung von Isoptin und IsoptinS bei Patienten mit Koronarinsuffizienz. *Dtsch Med Wochenschr* 88:1702–1707, 1963.

36. Straessle B, Burckhardt D: Isoptin (D-365), klinische Untersuchungen zur Behandlung coronarer Herzkrankheit. *Schweiz Med Wochenschr* 95:667–672, 1965.

37. Wette K, Heimsoth V, Jansen FK: Einfluß von Iproveratril auf EKG-Veränderungen bei Hochdruckpatienten mit Angina pectoris. *Münch Med Wochenschr* 108:1238–1242, 1966.

38. Neumann M, Luisada AA: Double blind evaluation of orally administered iproveratril in patients with angina pectoris. *Am J Med Sci* 251:552–556, 1966.

39. Sandler G, Clayton GA, Thornicroft SG: Clinical evaluation of verapamil in angina pectoris. *Br Med J* 1968:224–227, 1968.

40. Hofmann H: Klinische Untersuchungen zur Wirkung von Iproveratril bei Koronarinsuffizienz und zur sympathikolytischen Beeinflussung der Myokardfunktion. *Z Inn Med* 23:357–364, 1968.

41. Kaltenbach M, Zimmermann D: Zur Wirkung von Iproveratril auf die Angina pectoris und die adrenergischen β-Rezeptoren des Menschen. *Dtsch Med Wochenschr* 93:25–28, 1968.

42. Kaltenbach M: Medikamentöse Therapie der Angina pectoris. Prüfung verschiedener Medikamente mit Hilfe von Arbeitsversuchen. *Arnzeim Forsch/Drug Res* 20:1304–1310, 1970.

43. Cardoe N: A 2-year study of the efficacy and tolerability of prenylamine in the treatment of angina pectoris. *Postgrad Med J* 46:708–711, 1970.

44. Cardoe N: The treatment of angina pectoris over a two-year period. A double blind study of prenylamine (Synadrin, Segontin) in outpatients. *Clin Trials J* 8(1):18–23, 1971.

45. Winsor T, Bleifer K, Cole S, Goldman IR, Karpman H, Kaye H, Oblath R, Stone SH: Prenylamine (Synadrin) in angina pectoris. A double-blind, double crossover trial. *Clin Trials J* 8(1):24–34, 1971.

46. Sepaha GC, Jain SR, Jain P: The treatment of angina pectoris. A double blind study of prenylamine (Synadrin, Segontin). *Clin Trials J* 8:43–46, 1971.

47. Rudolph W, Kriener J, Meister W: Die Wirkung von Verapamil auf Coronardurchblutung, Sauerstoffutilistation und Kohlendioxydproduktion des menschlichen Herzens. *Klin Wochenschr* 49:982–988, 1971.

48. Rowe GG, Stenlund RR, Thomsen JH, Corliss RJ, Sialer S: The systemic and coronary hemodynamic effects of iproveratril. *Arch Int Pharmacodyn Ther* 193:381–390, 1971.

49. Raff WK, Kosche F, Lochner W: Untersuchungen mit Nifedipine, einer coronargefäßerweiternden Substanz mit schneller sublingualer Wirkung. *Arzneim Forsch/Drug Res* 22:33–39, 1972.

50. Loos A, Kaltenbach M: Die Wirkung von Nifedipine (BAY a 1040) auf das Belastungs-Elektrokardiogramm von Angina-pectoris Kranken. *Arzneim Forsch/Drug Res* 22:358–362, 1972.

51. Hayase S, Hirakawa S, Hosokawa S, Mori N, Kanyama S, Iwasa M: Hemodynamic and therapeutic effects of BAY a 1040 on the patients with ischemic heart disease. *Arzneim Forsch/drug Res* 22:370–373, 1972.

52. Kobayashi T, Ito Y, Tawara I: Clinical experience with a new coronary active substance (BAY a 1040). *Arzneim Forsch/Drug Res* 22:380–389, 1972.

53. Bender F: Isoptin zur Behandlung der tachykarden Form des Vorhofflatterns. *Med Klin* 62:634–636, 1967.

54. Haas H, Busch E: Antiarrhythmische Wirkungen von Verapamil und seinen Derivaten im Vergleich zu Propranolol, Pronethanol, Chinidin, Procainamid und Ajmalin. *Arzneim Forsch/Drug Res* 18:401–407, 1968.

55. Bender F: Die Behandlung der tachykarden Arrhythmien und der arteriellen Hypertonie mit Verapamil. *Arzneim Forsch/Drug Res* 20:1310–1316, 1970.

56. Brichard G, Zimmermann P: Verapamil in cardiac dysrhythmias during anaesthesia. *Br J Anaesth* 42:1005–1011, 1970.

57. Hanna C, Schmid JR: Antiarrhythmic actions of coronary vasodilator agents papaverine, dioxyline and verapamil. *Arch Int Pharmacol* 185:228–233, 1970.

58. Neuss H, Schlepper M: Der Einfluß von Verapamil auf die atrio-ventrikuläre Überleitung. Lokalisation des Wirkortes mit His-Bündel Elektrogrammen. *Verh Dtsch Ges Kreisl Forsch* 37:433–438, 1971.

59. Schamroth L: Immediate effects of intravenous verapamil on atrial fibrillation. *Cardiovasc Res* 5:419–424, 1971.

60. Schamroth L, Krikler DM, Garett S: Immediate effects of intravenous verapamil in cardiac arrhythmias. *Br Med J* 1972:660–662, 1972.

61. Sacks H, Kennelly BM: Verapamil in cardiac arrhythmias. *Br Med J* 2:716, 1972.

62. Boothby CB, Garrard CS, Pickering D: Verapamil in cardiac arrhythmias. *Br Med J* 2:348–349, 1972.

63. Roskamm H, Froehlich GJ, Reindell H: Die Wirkung verschiedener Koronardilatoren auf den Sauerstoffverbrauch, die Herzfrequenz und den Blutdruck bei standardisierter Belastung auf dem Ergometer. *Arzneim Forsch/Drug Res* 16:835–841, 1966.

64. Brittinger WD, Schwarzbeck A, Wittenmeier KW, Twittenhoff WD, Stegaru B, Huber W, Ewald RW, v Henning GE, Fabricius M, Strauch M: Klinisch-experimentelle Untersuchungen über die blutdrucksenkende Wirkung von Verapamil. *Dtsch Med Wochenschr* 95:1871–1877, 1970.

65. Vaughan-Neil EF, Snell NJC, Bevan G: Hypotension after verapamil. *Br Med J* 2:529, 1972.

66. Weidinger H, Wiest W: Die Behandlung der vorzeitigen Wehentätigkeit mit einem neuen Tokolytikum und Isoptin. *Z Fortschr Medizin* 89:1380–1381, 1971.

67. Krikler D, Spurell RA: Asystole after verapamil. *Br Med J* 2:405, 1972.

68. Hamill OP, Marty A, Neher E, Sakmann B, Sigworth FJ: Improved patch-clamp techniques for high-resolution current recording from cells and cell-free membrane patches. *Pflügers Arch* 391:85–100, 1981.

69. Sakmann B, Neher E: *Single Channel Recording.* New York: Plenum Press, 1983.

70. Salkoff LB, Tanouye MA: Genetics of ion channels. *Physiol Rev* 66:301–329, 1986.

71. Tanabe T, Beam KG, Powell JA, Numa S: Restoration of excitation-contraction coupling and slow calcium current in dysgenic muscle by dihydropyridine receptor complementory DNA. *Nature* 336:134–139, 1988.

72. Mikami AK, Imoto T, Tanabe T, Niidome Y, Mori H, Takeshima S, Narumiya S, Numa S: Primary structure and functional expression of the cardiac dihydropyridine-sensitive calcium channel. *Nature* 340:230–233, 1989.

73. Barres BM, Chan LLY, Corey DP: Ion channel expression by white matter glia I. Type 2 astrocytes and oligodendro-

cytes. *Glia* 1:10–30, 1988.

74. Fukushima Y, Hagiwara S: Voltage gated Ca^{2+}-channels in mouse myeloma cells. *Proc Natl Acad Sci USA* 80:2240–2243, 1983.
75. Chesnoy-Marchai D, Fritsch J: Voltage gated sodium and calcium currents in rat osteoblasts. *J Physiol* 398:291–311, 1988.
76. Chen C, Corbley MJ, Roberts TM, Hess P: Voltage-sensitive calcium channels in normal and transformed 3T3 fibroblasts. *Science* 239:1024–1026, 1988.
77. Tsien RW: Calcium channels in excitable cell membranes. *Ann Rev Physiol* 45:341–358, 1983.
78. Tsien RW: Calcium currents in heart cells and neurons. In: Kaczmarek LK, Levitan IB (eds) *Neuromodulation.* New York: Oxford University Press, 1987, pp 206–242.
79. Kostyuk PG: Diversity of calcium ion channels in cellular membranes. *Neuroscience* 28:253–261, 1989.
80. Bean BP: Classes of calcium channels in vertebrate cells. *Ann Rev Physiol* 51:367–384, 1989.
81. Hess P: Calcium channels in vertebrate cells. *Ann Rev Neurosci* 13:337–356, 1990.
82. Fox AP, Hirning LD, Mogul DJ, Artalejo CR, Penington NJ, Scroggs RS, Miller RJ: Modulation of calcium channels by neurotransmitters, hormones and second messengers. In: Hurwitz L, Partridge LD, Leach JK (eds) *Calcium Channels: Their Properties, Functions, Regulation, and Clinical Relevance.* Boca Raton, FL: CRC Press, 1991, pp 251–263.
83. Godfraind T, Miller R, Wibo M: Calcium antagonism and calcium entry blockade. *Pharmacol Rev* 38:321–416, 1986.
84. Triggle DJ, Lang DA, Janis RA: Ca^{2+}-channel ligands: Structure-function relationship of the 1,4-dihydropyridines. *Med Res Rev* 9:123–180, 1989.
85. Heginbotham L, Abramson T, MacKinnon R: A functional connection between the pores of distantly related ion channels as revealed by mutant K^+-channels. *Science* 258:1152–1155, 1992.
86. Kostyuk PG, Krishtal OA: Effects of calcium and calcium chelating agents on the inward and outward current in the membrane of mollusc neurones. *J Physiol* 270:569–580, 1977.
87. Tsien RW, Hess P, McCleskey EW, Rosenberg RL: Calcium channels: Mechanism of selectivity, permeation and block. *Ann Rev Biophys Chem* 16:265–290, 1987.
88. Lux HD, Nagy K: Single channel Ca^{2+} currents in "Helix pomatia" neurons. *Pflügers Arch* 391:252–254, 1981.
89. Isenberg G, Klöckner U: Calcium currents of isolated bovine ventricular myocytes are fast and of large amplitude. *Pflügers Arch* 395:30–41, 1982.
90. Reuter H, Stevens CF, Tsien RW, Yellen G: Properties of single calcium channels in cardiac cell culture. *Nature* 297:501–504, 1982.
91. Matsuda H, Noma A: Isolation of calcium current and its sensitivity to monovalent cations in dialysed ventricular cells of guinea pig. *J Physiol* 357:553–573, 1984.
92. Hess P, Tsien RW: Mechanism of ion permeation through calcium channels. *Nature* 309:453–456, 1984.
93. Lux HD, Carbone E, Zucker H: Na^+ currents through low voltage activated Ca^{2+} channels of chick sensory neurones; block by external Ca^{2+} and Mg^+. *J Physiol* 430:159–188, 1990.
94. Läuger P: Conformational transitions of ionic channels. In: Sakmann B, Neher E (eds) *Single Channel Recording.* New York: Plenum Press, 1983, pp 177–189.
95. Carafoli E: Intracellular calcium homeostasis. *Ann Rev Biochem* 56:395–433, 1987.
96. Gengo P, Skattebol A, Moran JF, Gallant S, Hawthorn M,

Triggle DJ: Regulation by chronic drug administration of neuronal and cardiac calcium channel, beta-adrenoceptor and muscarinic receptor levels. *Biochem Pharmacol* 37:627–633, 1988.
97. Chatelain P, Demol D, Roba J: Comparison of H^3-nitrendipine binding to heart membranes of normotensive and spontaneously hypertensive rats. *J Cardiovasc Pharmacol* 6:220–223, 1984.
98. Garthoff B, Bellemann P: Effects of salt loading and nitrendipine on dihydropyridine receptors in hypertensive rats. *J Cardiovasc Pharmacol* 10(Suppl 10):36–39, 1987.
99. Finkel MS, Patterson RE, Roberts WC, Smith TD, Keiser HR: Calcium channel binding characteristics in the human heart. *Am J Cardiol* 62:1281–1284, 1988.
100. Tiggle DJ, Janis RA: Calcium channel ligands. *Ann Rev Pharmacol Toxicol* 27:347–369, 1987.
101. Lux HD, Brown AM: Activation of single neuronal calcium channels. In: *Proceedings of the 16th FEBS Congress,* 1985, p 407.
102. Carbone E, Swandulla D: Neuronal calcium channels: Kinetics blockade and modulation. *Prog Biophys Mol Biol* 54:31–58, 1989.
103. Campbell DL, Giles WR, Hume JR, Shibata EF: Inactivation of calcium current in bullfrog atrial myocytes. *J Physiol* 403:287–315, 1988.
104. Bean BP: Two kinds of calcium channels in canine atrial cells. Differences in kinetics, selectivity and pharmacology. *J Gen Physiol* 86:1–30, 1985.
105. Fedulov SA, Kostyuk PG, Veselovsky NS: Two types of calcium channels in the somatic membrane of newborn rat dorsal root ganglion neurons. *J Physiol* 359:431–446, 1985.
106. Nilius B, Hess P, Lansmann JB, Tsien RW: A novel type of cardiac calcium channel in ventricular cells. *Nature* 316:443–446, 1985.
107. Benham CD, Tsien RW: Noradrenaline modulation of calcium channels in single smooth muscle cells from rabbit ear artery. *J Physiol* 404:767–784, 1988.
108. Yatani A, Seidel CL, Allen J, Brown AM: Whole cell and single-channel calcium currents of isolated smooth muscle cells from saphenous vein. *Circ Res* 60:523–533, 1987.
109. McCobb DP, Best PM, Beam KG: Development alters the expression of calcium currents in chick limb motoneurons. *Neuron* 2:1633–1643, 1989.
110. Tseng GN, Boyden PA: Multiple types of Ca^{2+}-currents in single canine Purkinje cell. *Circ Res* 65:1735–1750, 1989.
111. Bean BP, Sturek M, Puga A, Hermsmeyer K: Calcium channels in muscle cells isolated from rat mesenteric arteries. Modulation by dihydropyridine drugs. *Circ Res* 59:229–235, 1986.
112. Friedmann E, Suarez-Kurtz G, Kaczorowski GJ, Katz GM, Reuben JP: Two calcium currents in a smooth muscle cell line. *Am J Physiol* 250:H699–H703, 1986.
113. Aaronson PI, Benham CD, Bolton TB, Hess P, Lang RJ, Tsien RW: Two types of single-channel and whole-cell calcium or barium currents in single smooth muscle cells of rabbit ear artery and the effects of noradrenaline. *J Physiol* 377:36, 1986.
114. Carbone E, Lux HD: Kinetics and selectivity of a low-voltage activated calcium current in chick and rat sensory neurons. *J Physiol* 386:547–570, 1987.
115. Lansman JB, Hess P, Tsien RW: Blockage of current through single calcium channels by cadmium, magnesium and calcium. *J Gen Physiol* 88:321–347, 1986.
116. Jmari K, Mironneau C, Mironneau J: Selectivity of calcium channels in rat uterine smooth muscle. Interaction between

sodium, calcium and barium ions. *J Physiol* 384:247–261, 1987.

117. Hagiwara S, Irisawa H, Kameyama M: Contribution to two types of calcium channels to the pacemaker potentials of rabbit sino atrial node cells. *J Physiol* 395:233–253, 1988.

118. Hartzell HC, White RE: Effects of magnesium on inactivation of the voltage gated calcium current in cardiac myocytes. *J Gen Physiol* 94:745–767, 1989.

119. Agus ZS, Kelepouris E, Dukes I, Morad M: Cytosolic magnesium modulates Calcium channel activity in mammalian ventricular cells. *Am J Physiol* 256:C452–C455, 1989.

120. O'Rourke B, Backx PH, Marban E: Phosphorylation-independent modulation of L-type calcium channels by magnesium-nucleotide complexes. *Science* 257:245–248, 1992.

121. Belles B, Malécot CO, Hescheler J, Trautwein W: "Run down" of the Ca current during long whole-cell recordings in guinea pig heart cells, role of phosphorylation. *Pflüger Arch* 411:353–360, 1988.

122. Taniguchi J, Noma A, Irisawa H: Modification of the cardiac action potential by intracellular injection of adenosine triphosphate and related substanzes in guinea pig single ventricular cells. *Circ Res* 53:131–139, 1983.

123. Prod'hom B, Pietrobon D, Hess P: Direct measurement of proton transfer rates to a group controlling dihydropyridine sensitive Ca-channel. *Nature* 329:243–246, 1987.

124. Kaibara M, Kameyama M: Inhibition of the calcium channel by intracellular protons in single ventricular myocytes of the guinea pig. *J Physiol* 403:621–640, 1988.

125. Strichartz G, Rando T, Wang GR: An integrated view of the molecular toxicology of sodium channel gating in excitable cells. *Ann Rev Neurosci* 10:237–267, 1987.

126. Callewaert G, Hanbauer I, Morad M: Modulation of calcium channnels in cardiac and neuronal cells by an endogenous peptide. *Science* 243:663–666, 1989.

127. Hallström S, Koidl B, Müller U, Werdan K, Schlag G: A cardiodepressant factor isolated from blood blocks Ca^{2+} current in cardiomyocytes. *Am J Physiol* 260:H869–H876, 1991.

128. Llinas R, Yarom Y: Specific blockage of the low threshold calcium channel by high molecular weight alcohols. *Soc Neurosci Abs* 12:49.3, p. 174, 1986.

129. Tang CM, Presser F, Morad M: Amiloride selectively blocks the low theshold (T) calcium channel. *Science* 240:213–215, 1988.

130. Twombly DA, Yoshii M, Narahashi T: Mechanism of calcium channel block by phenytoin. *J Pharmacol Exp Ther* 246:189–195, 1988.

131. Kuga T, Sadoshima J, Tomoike H, Kanaide N, Nakamura M: Action of Ca^{2+} antagonists on two types of Ca^{2+} channels in rat aorta smooth muscle cells in primary culture. *Circ Res* 67:469–480, 1990.

132. Van Skiver DM, Spires S, Cohen CJ: Block of T-type Ca channels in guinea pig atrial cells by cinnarizine. *Biophys J* 53:233, 1988.

133. Van Skiver DM, Spires S, Cohen CJ: High affinity and tissue specific block of T-type Ca-channels by felodipine. *Biophys J* 55:593, 1985.

134. Furukawa I, Ito H, Nitta J, Tsujino M, Adachi S, Hiroe M, Maramo F, Sawanobori T, Hiraoka M: Endothelin 1 enhances calcium entry through T-type calcium channels in cultured neonatal rat ventricular myocytes. *Circ Res* 71:1242–1253, 1992.

135. Perez-Reyes E, Kim SH, Lacerda AE, Horne W, Wei X, Rampe D, Campbell KP, Brown AM, Birnbaumer L: Induction of calcium currents by the expression of the alpha$_1$-subunit of the dihydropyridine receptor from skeletal muscle. *Nature* 340:233–236, 1989.

136. Talvenheimo JA, Worley JF, Nelson MT: Heterogeneity of calcium channels from a purified dihydropyridine receptor preparation. *Biophys J* 52:891–899, 1987.

137. Hymel L, Striessnig J, Glossmann H, Schindler H: Purified skeletal muscle 1–4 dihydropyridine receptor forms phosphorylation-dependent oligomeric calcium channels in planar bilayers. *Proc Natl Acad Sci USA* 85:4290–4294, 1988.

138. Mori Y, Friedrich T, Kim MS, Mikami A, Nakai J, Ruth P, Bosse E, Hofmann F, Flockerzi V, Furuichi T, Mikoshiba K, Imoto K, Tanabe T, Numa S: Primary structure and functional expression from complementary DNA of a brain calcium channel. *Nature* 350:398–402, 1991.

139. Catterall WA: Structure and function of voltage sensitive ion channels. *Science* 242:50–61, 1988.

140. Nastainczky W, Röhrkasten W, Sieber M, Rudolph C, Schächtele C, Marme D, Hofmann F: Phosphorylation of the purified receptor for calcium channel blockers by cAMP kinase and protein kinase C. *Eur J Biochem* 169:137–142, 1987.

141. Miller RJ: Voltage sensitive Ca^{2+} channels. *J Biol Chem* 267:1403–1406, 1992.

142. King VF, Garcia ML, Shevell JL, Slaughter RS, Kaczorowski GJ: Substituted diphenylbutylpiperidines bind to a unique high affinity site on the L-type calcium channel. *J Biol Chem* 264:5633–5641, 1989.

143. Glossmann H, Striessnig J: Calcium channels. *Vitam Horm* 49:155–328, 1988.

144. Hosey MM, Lazdunski M: Calcium channels: Molecular pharmacology, structure and regulation. *J Membr Biol* 104:81–105, 1988.

145. Schilling WP, Drewe JA: Voltage-sensitive nitrendipine binding in isolated cardiac sarcolemma preparation. *J Biol Chem* 261:2750–2758, 1986.

146. Kokubun S, Prod'hom B, Becker C, Prozig H, Reuter H: Studies on Ca^{2+} channels in intact cardiac cells: Voltage-dependent effects and cooperative interactions of dihydropyridine enantiomers. *Mol Pharmacol* 30:571–584, 1986.

147. Wei XY, Ruledge A, Triggle DJ: Voltage dependent binding of 1,4-dihydropyridine Ca^{2+} channel antagonists and activators in cultured neonatal rat ventricular myocytes. *Mol Pharmacol* 35:541–552, 1989.

148. Tritthart HA, Volkmann R, Weiss R, Fleckenstein A: Calcium mediated action potentials in mammalian myocardium: Alteration of membrane responses as induced by changes of Ca^{2+} or by promotors and inhibitors of the transmembrane Ca^{2+}-inflow. *Naunyn-Schmiedebergs Arch Pharmacol* 280:239–252, 1973.

149. Tritthart HA: Frequency dependence of verapamil-induced inhibition of the Ca^{2+}-inflow during excitation of papillary muscles. *Can Physiol* 6:62, 1975.

150. Nawrath H, Teneick RE, McDonald TF, Trautwein W: On the mechanism underlying the action of D600 and slow inward current and tension in mammalian myocardium. *Circ Res* 40:408–414, 1977.

151. Ehara T, Kaufmann R: The voltage- and time-dependent effects of verapamil on the slow inward current in isolated rat ventricular myocardium. *J Pharmacol Exp Ther* 207:49–55, 1978.

152. Bayer R, Ehara T: Comparative studies on calcium antagonists. *Prog Pharmacol* 2:31–37, 1978.

153. Kanaya S, Katzung BG: Rate- and voltage-dependent block of slow responses and calcium current by diltiazem. *Circulation* 64(4,II):IV274, 1981.

154. Reynolds IJ, Snowhan AM, Snyder SH: (−)-[⁻³H]Demethyl-oxyverapamil labels multiple calcium channel modulator receptors in brain and skeletal muscle membranes: Differentiation by temperature and dihydropyridines. *J Pharmacol Exp Ther* 237:731–738, 1986.

155. Bechem M, Hebisch S, Schramm M: Ca²⁺-agonists: New, sensitive probes for Ca²⁺-channels. *Topics Pharm Sci* 9:257–261, 1988.

156. Wei XY, Luchowski EM, Rutledge A, Su CM, Triggle DJ: Pharmacologic and radioligand binding analysis of the actions 1,4-dihydropyridine activator-antagonist pairs in smooth muscle. *J Pharmacol Exp Ther* 239:144–153, 1986.

157. Kass RS: Voltage-dependent modulation of cardiac calcium channel current by optical isomers of Bay K8644. Implications for channel gating. *Circ Res* 61:11–15, 1987.

158. Schreibmayer W, Tripathi O, Tritthart HA: Kinetic modulation of guinea-pig cardiac L-type calcium channels by fendiline and reversal of the effects of Bay K8644. *Br J Pharmacol* 106:151–156, 1992.

159. Pickard JD, Murray GD, Illingworth R, Shaw MDM, Teasdale GM, Foy PM, Humphrey PRD, Lang DA, Nelson R, Richards P, Sinar J, Bailey S, Skene A: Effect of oral nimodipine on cerebral infarction and outcome after subarachnoid haemorrhage: British aneurysm nimodipine trial. *Br Med J* 298:636–642, 1989.

160. Hiramatsu K, Yamagishi F, Kubota T, Yamada T: Acute effects of the calcium antagonist, nifedipine, on blood pressure, pulse rate and the renin-angiotensin-aldosterone system in patients with essential hyertension. *Am Heart J* 104:1346–1350, 1982.

161. Dale J, Landmark K, Myhre E: The effects of nifedipine, a calcium antagonist, on platelet function. *Am Heart J* 105:103–105, 1983.

162. Ahn YS, Jy W, Harringstone WJ, Shanbaky N, Fernandez LF, Haynes DH: Increased platelet calcium in thrombosis and related disorders and its correction by nifedipine. *Thromb Res* 45:135–143, 1987.

163. Baeyens JM: Interactions between calcium channel blockers and noncardiovascular drugs: Interaction with anticancer drugs. *Pharmacol Tox* 63:1–7, 1988.

164. Naito M, Tsuruo T: Competitive inhibition by verapamil of ATP-dependent high affinity vincristine binding to the plasma membrane of multidrug-resistant K562 cells without calcium ion involvement. *Cancer Res* 49:1452–1455, 1989.

165. Martin SK, Oduola AM, Milhous WK: Reversal of chloroquine resistance in *Plasmodium falciparum* by verapamil. *Science* 235:899–901, 1987.

166. Sperelakis N, Caulfield JB: *Calcium Antagonists*. Boston: Martinus Nijhoff, 1985.

167. Opie LH: Calcium channel antagonists, part II. Use and comparative properties of the three prototypical calcium antagonists in ischemic heart disease, including recommendations based on an analysis of 41 trials. *Cardiovas Drugs Ther* 1:461–491, 1988.

168. Nayler WG: *Calcium Antagonists*. New York: Academic Press, 1988.

169. Triggle DJ: Calcium antagonists. In: Antonaccio M (ed) *Cardiovascular Pharmacology*. New York: Raven Press, 1990, pp 107–160.

170. Braunwald E: Coronary artery spasm as a cause of myocardial ischemia. *J Lab Clin Med* 97:299–312, 1981.

171. Kimura E, Kishida H: Treatment of variant angina with drugs. A survey of 11 cardiology institutes in Japan. *Circulation* 63:844–848, 1981.

172. Lenegre J, Himbert J: Critical study of the relationship between angina pectoris and coronary arteriosclerosis. *Am Heart J* 58:539–551, 1959.

173. Bolli P, Erne P, Hulthen UL, Ritz R, Kiowski W, Ji BH, Buhler FR: Parallel reduction of calcium influx dependent vasoconstriction and platelet-free calcium concentration with calcium entry and β-adrenoceptor blockade. *J Cardiovasc Pharmacol* 6:996–1001, 1984.

174. Millard RW, Gabel M, Fowler NO, Schwartz A: Baroreceptor reflex sensitivity reduced by diltiazem and verapamil. *Fed Proc* 41:57959, 1982.

175. Trautwein W, Pelzer D: Kinetics and beta-andrenergic modulation of cardiac Ca²⁺-channels. In: Morad M, Nayler W, Kazda W, Schramm S (eds) *The Calcium Channel: Structure, Function and Implications*. New York: Springer Verlag, 1988, pp 39–53.

176. Reuter H: Calcium channel modulation of neurotransmitters, enzymes and drugs. *Nature* 301:569–574, 1983.

177. Ferlinz J: Effects of verapamil on normal and abnormal ventricular functions in patients with ischemic heart disease. In: Zanchetti A, Krickler M (eds) *Calcium Antagonism in Cardiovascular Therapy*. Amsterdam: Excerpta Medica, 1981, pp 92–105.

178. Winniford M, Markham R, Firth B, Nicod P, Hillis D: Hemodynamic and electrophysiologic effects of verapamil and nifedipine in patients on propranolol. *Am J Cardiol* 50:704–710, 1982.

179. Wit AL, Cranefield PF: Effects of verapamil on sino-atrial and atrio-ventricular nodes of the rabbit and the mechanism by which it terminates AV nodal reentrant tachycardia. *Circ Res* 35:413–425, 1974.

180. Sing BN, Baky S, Koonlawee N: Second-generation calcium antagonists: Search for greater selectivity and versatility. *Am J Cardiol* 55:214B–221B, 1985.

CHAPTER 27

Lipid-Derived Amphiphiles and their Contribution to Arrhythmogenesis During Ischemia

PETER B. CORR, JANE McHOWAT, GAN-XIN YAN, & KATHRYN A. YAMADA*

INTRODUCTION

Sudden cardiac death claims over 300,000 deaths per year in the United States alone, most often due to malignant ventricular arrhythmias, which lead to the development of ventricular fibrillation {1–5}. Results at autopsy demonstrate a high incidence of coronary artery disease and intracoronary thrombi, with little evidence of a recent highly defined myocardial infarct in most patients {6,7}. These findings suggest that the likely event leading to malignant ventricular arrhythmias and sudden cardiac death in humans is transient myocardial ischemia secondary to intracoronary arterial thrombi.

Myocardial ischemia in vivo leads to dramatic electrophysiologic alterations within minutes of cessation of coronary flow {8}. These rapid and heterogeneous electrophysiologic alterations are seen very early after the onset of ischemia and are totally reversible if reperfusion occurs within the first 7–10 minutes, with no evidence of any cellular damage, with the exception of significant depletion of glycogen. These findings suggest that some subtle, biochemical alterations within or near the sarcolemma occur in response to brief ischemia and account for the rapidity and reversibility of the electrophysiologic derangements. Previous studies have shown that venous blood obtained from the ischemic region in vivo can elicit electrophyisologic derangements in normoxic tissue in vitro suggesting, albeit indirectly, that the ischemic cells or vasculature or both may release factors that dramatically alter the electrical activity of the myocardium {9}. Although factors including reduced pO_2 (hypoxia), acidosis, and elevated extracellular K^+ certainly contribute to the electrophysiologic alterations during ischemia, their presence, even in combination, does not completely replicate some of the unique electrophysiologic alterations induced by venous blood obtained from ischemic regions {9}. Therefore, it is likely that other factors contribute as well.

Our laboratory and others have been investigating the electrophysiologic effects of two amphipathic metabolites,

long-chain acylcarnitine and lysophosphatidylcholine (LPC), both of which have been shown to increase rapidly in ischemic tissue in vivo and to elicit electrophysiologic derangements in vitro and in vivo {for previous review see 10}. The results of the CAST trial demonstrate that class IC agents, which depress the sarcolemmal ion channel function nonspecifically, are not effective in reducing mortality in patients with coronary artery disease and may actually increase the incidence of lethal arrhythmias {11}. The ultimate goal is the development of effective therapeutic approaches to decrease the incidence of sudden cardiac death in patients with ischemic heart disease. However, approaches designed to develop effective therapeutic agents will require an understanding of both the biochemical as well as the electrophysiologic alterations that contribute to arrhythmogenesis in the ischemic heart. This brief review will examine both the electrophysiologic and biochemical alterations that occur during early ischemia, their interrelationship, and possible therapeutic approaches to modify the arrhythmias responsible for sudden cardiac death in patients with ischemic heart disease.

ELECTROPHYSIOLOGIC ALTERATIONS DURING EARLY MYOCARDIAL ISCHEMIA

Transmembrane action potentials recorded from the epicardial surface of the ischemic heart exhibit within 1–2 minutes a marked decrease in resting membrane potential and a decrease in upstroke velocity of phase 0 depolarization with a reduction in both action potential amplitude as well as duration {8,12}. Studies performed in the isolated perfused ventricle preparation exposed to brief intervals of ischemia have revealed that similar alterations occur in the subendocardium {13}.

The most striking event during early myocardial ischemia is the marked degree of heterogeneity of the electrophysiologic alterations even within closely adjacent regions. In addition, there is spatial and temporal dissociation in the development of conduction delay within the ischemic zone and marked differences in the alterations in the refractory periods between the endocardium and epicardium of the ischemic zone {14}. Conduction velocity through the endocardium appears to remain near normal

* This article has been updated from a recently published review (McHowat et al., J Cardiovasc Electrophys 4:288–310, 1993) with any duplication through permission of Futura Publishing Company.

527

N. Sperelakis (ed.), *Physiology and Pathophysiology of the Heart, Third Edition.*

at a time when epicardial conduction velocity slows and the wavefront of propagation becomes fractionated {15–18}. This marked difference between endocardium and epicardium occurs despite a similar degree of ischemia. Although differences between the endocardium and epicardium contribute importantly to the underlying heterogeneity and, therefore arrhythmogenesis, the most dramatic differences occur at the border zone between ischemic and nonischemic tissue {19,20}.

Several of the electrophysiologic alterations that occur during myocardial ischemia are consistent with the development of reentry as the mechanism underlying arrhythmias during early ischemia. Using detailed three-dimensional mapping from 232 simultaneous intramural sites throughout the left ventricle, right ventricle, and septum of the feline heart in vivo, we have shown that premature ventricular contractions and the initial beats of ventricular tachycardia occur by intramural reentry in 76% of cases {21}. In all but one case, initiation occurred in the subendocardium, adjacent to the site of delayed subendocardial and midmyocardial activation of the preceding sinus beat. The marked conduction delay of the preceding sinus beat in the subendocardium and midmyocardium, distal to the unidirectional block, could lead to reactivation of adjacent subendocardial tissue proximal to the block, a region in which cells had recovered their excitability. In the remaining 24% of cases, initiation of the first beat of ventricular tachycardia arose in either the subendocardium or subepicardium by a nonreentrant or focal mechanism. This was defined as initiation of a ventricular ectopic beat distant from the site of the preceding (sinus) beat with no intervening electrical activity {21}. A complex interaction between reentrant and nonreentrant mechanisms existed such that ventricular tachycardia could be spontaneously initiated by one mechanism and maintained or terminated by the other {21}. In addition, both mechanisms could occur during initiation of the same beat and during the same tachycardia {21}. Thus it is likely that therapeutic strategies to inhibit or prevent these malignant arrhythmias will require interruption of both mechanisms.

AMPHIPATHIC METABOLITES AND MEMBRANE DYSFUNCTION DURING ISCHEMIA

The sarcolemma contains transmembrane ion channels and pumps that determine the electrophysiologic function of cardiac cells. The sarcolemma is comprised predominantly of phospholipids, cholesterol, and proteins. Phospholipids are amphipathic in nature and are composed of a charged polar headgroup region and a nonpolar long-chain aliphatic hydrocarbon region. To provide maximal thermodynamic stability in aqueous solutions, the individual phospholipids spontaneously form a bilayer where the polar headgroup regions interface with either the aqueous cytosol or extracellular space, and the hydrophobic hydrocarbon fatty acids are directed inwards to form the nonpolar interior of the membrane, "the lipid bilayer" (see fig. 27-1 for a diagramatic representation of the phospholipid species present in the sarcolemma).

Sarcolemma Structure and Phospholipid Composition

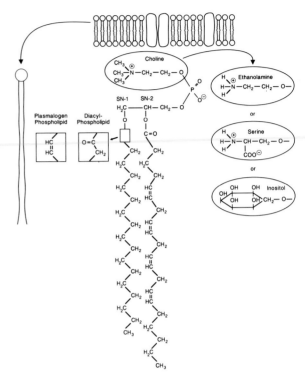

Fig. 27-1. Diagrammatic representation of the structure of the sarcolemma. The packing of membrane phospholipids to form the lipid bilayer together with two integral membrane proteins are shown in the top portion of the figure, with the individual structure of the phospholipids shown below. The structures to the right indicate the different polar headgroups, and the structural variations for the covalent attachment of the sn-1 fatty acid to the phospholipid polar headgroup, are shown on the left. Reproduced with permission from Creer et al. {10}.

Integral membrane proteins within the sarcolemma determine the metabolic characteristics and the active and passive transport functions of the myocytes. These proteins include ion channels, transport proteins, receptors, proteins involved in signal transduction, structural proteins, surface antigens, and a variety of enzymes. Modulation of the activity of these proteins may arise through interaction of amphiphilic metabolites with adjacent membrane phospholipids or via direct interactions with the membrane protein per se. Alterations in the composition of membrane phospholipids and corresponding changes in the bulk biophysical properties of the membrane could affect the activity of receptors and other membrane proteins involved in signal transduction due to changes in the "fluidity" of the phospholipid bilayer. Likewise, insertion of charged amphiphiles into the sarcolemma could directly influence ion channel function through a surface charge effect due to the polar head group or directly within the ion channel protein subunits to alter channel conductance.

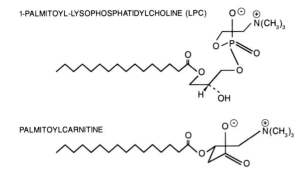

1-PALMITOYL-LYSOPHOSPHATIDYLCHOLINE (LPC)

PALMITOYLCARNITINE

Fig. 27-2. A comparison of the structures of long-chain acylcarnitine and lysophosphatidylcholine. Reproduced with permission from Pogwizd and Corr {206}.

During ischemia, due to their amphipathic nature (fig. 27-2), both long-chain acylcarnitines and lysophosphatidylcholine (LPC), a catabolic product of the major membrane phospholipid, phosphatidylcholine, incorporate into the phospholipid bilayer of the sarcolemma. The effects of these amphiphiles on membrane phospholipid dynamics, as well as the conformation of the phospholipids, appear to contribute to altering the function of transmembrane ion channels, as well as modification of ligand-receptor coupling and the activity of several membrane-bound enzymes. For example, modest changes in amphiphile content within the sarcolemma have effects on the physical characteristics of the sarcolemma. Electron spin resonance studies using isolated canine myocardial sarcolemma have demonstrated that as little as 1.5 mole% of either LPC or long-chain acylcarnitine incorporation into the membrane

resulted in significant changes in the molecular dynamics of the sarcolemmal membrane with a marked increase in membrane fluidity {22}. Using quantitative electron microscopic autoradiography to localize ^{3}H-LPC in isolated ventricular muscle in vitro, we have demonstrated that incorporation of 1–2 mole% LPC into the sarcolemmal membrane results in reversible electrophysiologic derangements similar to those seen in ischemic tissue in vivo {23,24}. It is also very likely that both long-chain acylcarnitines and LPC can directly alter ion channel function, either due to direct interaction with channel protein subunits or secondary to alteration in membrane surface charge {25}, both of which could markedly influence ion channel conductance. Under normoxic conditions, the concentrations of both of these amphiphilic metabolites within the myocyte are tightly controlled. However, during ischemia the mechanisms for maintaining low levels of both metabolites are disrupted, leading to an abrupt increase in both long-chain acylcarnitine and LPC (see below).

METABOLISM OF PHOSPHOLIPIDS AND MECHANISMS CONTRIBUTING TO THE INCREASE IN LYSOPHOSPHATIDYLCHOLINE DURING ISCHEMIA

The principal pathways responsible for the synthesis of LPC in myocardial tissue are shown in fig. 27-3. Lysophosphatidylcholine (LPC) is generated by the hydrolytic cleavage of one of the covalently bound aliphatic hydrocarbon groups of phosphatidylcholine (PC). Removal of the fatty acid at the sn-1 position is catalyzed by either phospholipase A$_1$ {26} or plasmalogenase, which cleaves the ester or the vinyl ether linkage of diacyl or plasmalogen PC to produce 2-monoacyl LPC (fig. 27-3). Hydrolysis of the sn-2 fatty acid to produce 1-monoacyl-LPC and free fatty acid is catalyzed by at least three distinct classes of phospholipase A$_2$ (PLA$_2$) in the heart. One PLA$_2$ is maximally active at acidic pH, is of lysosomal origin, acts on diacyl-PC as the substrate, and exhibits a positive Ca^{2+} dependence {27}. Another PLA$_2$ is maximally active at neutral pH, is Ca^{2+} dependent, and has been partially purified and characterized in rabbit myocardium and cardiac myocytes obtained from chick embryos {26}. Finally, a plasmalogen-selective PLA$_2$ has been identified in canine myocardium {28}. In contrast to PLA$_2$ which uses diacyl-PC as a substrate, the activity of this plasmalogen-selective PLA$_2$ is not influenced by Ca^{2+} {28}. The plasmalogen-selective PLA$_2$ is active at neutral pH and is present in the cytosol of the cardiac cell. The majority of LPC in myocardial tissue is derived by hydrolysis of the sn-2 fatty acid of diacyl-PC catalyzed by PLA$_2$. However, plasmalogens are the predominant species in the sarcolemma, and it is possible that relatively large increases in the concentration of lysoplasmalogens within the sarcolemma per se could occur during ischemia and result in significant electrophysiologic alterations, without a large change in the total cellular content, since the total sarcolemma comprises only 5–8% of total cellular phospholipid.

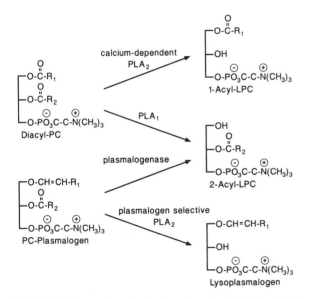

Fig. 27-3. Pathways of synthesis of lysophosphatidylcholine (LPC) and lysoplasmalogen from phosphatidylcholine (PC) and PC plasmalogen, respectively. R$_1$ and R$_2$ are long-chain aliphatic hydrocarbon groups at the sn-1 and sn-2 positions, respectively.

Several studies have reported that the activity of PLA$_2$ is increased during ischemia, resulting in an increase in LPC. Recent evidence suggests that the activity of a membrane-associated, Ca^{2+}-independent, plasmalogen-selective PLA$_2$ is increased dramatically after short intervals of ischemia in the isolated, perfused rabbit heart {29,30}. This activation of the plasmalogen-selective PLA$_2$ was rapidly reversible during reperfusion following short intervals of ischemia {29}. Since the PLA$_2$ that is activated during ischemia is highly selective for the plasmalogen substrate, and since the capacity of myocardium for the metabolism of lysophosphatidylcholine vastly exceeds that for lysoplasmenylcholine {31}, these results suggest that activation of this plasmalogen-selective PLA$_2$ may directly enhance the production of lysoplasmalogens within the sarcolemma and thereby contribute to the electrophysiologic derangements observed during ischemia (see below). However, it is not known whether LPC derived from choline plasmalogens has the same or similar electrophysiologic effects compared to LPC derived from diacyl-PC. In contrast, a recent study by Schwertz and Halverson {32} using globally ischemic rat hearts indicated a 15% reduction in PLA$_2$ activity during early ischemia and suggested that this reduction could serve a protective role by attenuating LPC accumulation during an ischemic event. However, in this latter study {32} the authors used phosphatidylethanolamine as the substrate to measure PLA$_2$ and therefore did not estimate plasmalogen-selective PLA$_2$ activity in the ischemic myocardium nor LPC derived from diacyl PC. Since Ford and colleagues {29} have demonstrated a 10-fold increase in the plasmalogen-selective PLA$_2$, this could easily override any reduction in other species of PLA$_2$ in the ischemic myocardium.

During short intervals of ischemia, we have reported that LPC increases in venular and lymphatic effluents from ischemic tissue {33,34}. Most importantly, recent results from Sedlis and colleagues have shown a marked increase in LPC in the coronary sinus effluent of patients with pacing-induced ischemia with no change in LPC in normal control patients without evidence of ischemic heart disease {35}. Although this could be a reflection of increased efflux of LPC from ischemic myocytes per se to the vascular space, these increases are observed early after the onset of ischemia before there is evidence of irreversible cell damage and significant disruption of the sarcolemma. The appearance of LPC extracellularly in both blood and lymph would suggest a vascular site of origin, possibly endothelial or smooth muscle cells. Since myocardial ischemia in humans usually occurs secondary to the formation of a coronary thrombus, it is possible that a factor, such as thrombin, released from or near the thrombus may act upon a component of the vasculature and lead to an increase in the extracellular production of LPC. Although isolated platelets have been shown to produce LPC in response to thrombin stimulation {36}, the production is relatively low and it is doubtful that the relatively small number of platelets present in the coronary circulation could contribute substantially to increased extracellular accumulation of LPC during ischemia. However, the interaction of thrombin with vascular cells may be an important mechanism whereby LPC accumulates extracellularly.

We have demonstrated recently that following stimulation by thrombin, cultured canine aortic endothelial cells increase LPC production, resulting in release of LPC into the surrounding media {37,38}. The response is completely blocked by inhibitors that block thrombin's proteolytic activity, including PPACK and DAPA, and is also induced by a thrombin-like 14 amino acid peptide, which directly stimulates the thrombin receptor. This effect appears to be mediated through the activation of protein kinase C. These results suggest that thrombin-specific stimulation of endothelial cells could contribute to the increase in LPC observed extracellularly in ischemic myocardium. Whether this contribution by endothelial cells is sufficient to account for the twofold increase in LPC in venous and lymphatic effluents from ischemic myocardium remains to be elucidated. These findings would also suggest that the presence of an intracoronary thrombus, with its attendant release of thrombin or generalized activation of the coagulation system during ischemia, may be potentially arrhythmogenic in part through the extracellular production and accumulation of LPC. More recently, we have demonstrated that thrombin can directly increase the accumulation of LPC in isolated adult canine ventricular myocytes, an effect that was significantly enhanced in the presence of acidosis and hypoxia {39}. The effect of thrombin appears to be mediated directly through the thrombin receptor, based on a similar response with the thrombin-like 14 amino acid peptide. Therefore, if the thrombin receptor on cardiac myocytes is activated during early ischemia, this could elicit a rapid increase in LPC, which would likely contribute to the associated electrophysiologic derangements and resulting malignant arrhythmias. This influence of thrombin and potentially other coagulation factors being activated during ischemia may necessitate evaluation of arrhythmias during ischemia in experimental preparations in which blood cell elements are present.

In summary, the increase in LPC in both ischemic myocardium and effluents from ischemic regions may arise via multiple mechanisms that stimulate LPC production, and the relative importance of each mechanism in the intact organ has yet to be determined.

MECHANISMS RESPONSIBLE FOR THE ACCUMULATION OF LONG-CHAIN ACYLCARNITINE DURING EARLY ISCHEMIA

Oxidation of fatty acids accounts for 60–80% of the energy requirements of the myocardium {40}. Metabolism of fatty acids begins with the uptake of free fatty acids by the cardiac myocyte, followed by binding to an intracellular fatty acid binding protein and transport to the mitochondria {10,41–43}.

At the outer mitochondrial membrane, fatty acids are thioesterified with free CoA to produce acyl CoA (fig. 27-4) {44}. Since the inner mitochondrial membrane is impermeable to acyl CoA, it is transesterified to free carnitine to form long-chain acylcarnitine and free CoA by the action of the enzyme, carnitine acyl transferase-I (CAT-I)

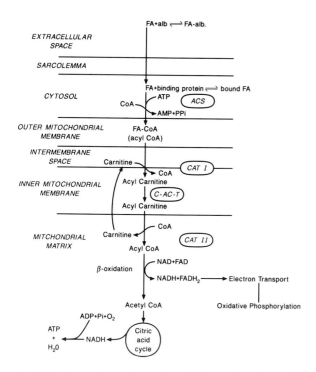

EXTRACELLULAR SPACE

SARCOLEMMA

CYTOSOL

OUTER MITOCHONDRIAL MEMBRANE

INTERMEMBRANE SPACE

INNER MITOCHONDRIAL MEMBRANE

MITCHONDRIAL MATRIX

Fig. 27-4. Metabolite pathway for oxidation of free fatty acids (FA) in cardiac myocytes. alb = albumin; CoA = "free" (non-esterified) coenzyme A; FA-CoA = fatty acyl-CoA; ACS = acyl-CoA synthetase; CAT I = carnitine acyltransferase I; CAT II = carnitine acyltransferase II; C-AC-T = carnitine-acylcarnitine translocase.

{45,46}. After crossing the inner mitochondrial membrane in exchange for free carnitine via carnitine-acylcarnitine translocase {47,48}, long-chain acylcarnitine is transesterified back to free CoA to form acyl CoA in a reversible reaction catalyzed by another distinct enzyme, carnitine acyltransferase II (CAT-II). The acyl CoA, now within the matrix of the mitochondria, undergoes β-oxidation to form acetyl CoA and the reduced forms of nicotinamide and flavin adenine dinucleotides (NADH and $FADH_2$). NADH and $FADH_2$ are closely coupled to electron transport and oxidative phosphorylation to maintain high rates of fatty acid oxidation in the mitochondria. Cytochrome oxidase, the terminal enzyme of electron transport, has an absolute requirement for oxygen. During ischemia, the abrupt interruption of coronary flow rapidly lowers the pO_2 in the involved tissue to near 0 mmHg. Electron transport is inhibited and results in an increase in NADH and $FADH_2$, which in turn leads to an inhibition of flux through the β-oxidation pathway by a negative feedback mechanism. A marked increase in both acyl CoA and long-chain acylcarnitine occurs {40,49–52}. Long-chain acylcarnitines can readily diffuse back across the mitochondrial membrane to gain access to most myocytic subcellular membrane compartments, including the sarcolemma, via the

cytosol {51}. Acyl CoA remains predominantly in the mitochondrial matrix during the reversible phase of ischemia because of its inability to traverse the inner mitochondrial membrane {51}.

There are two additional mechanisms that also contribute to the increase in the cytosolic level of long-chain acylcarnitine. First, as acyl CoA accumulates in the mitochondrial matrix, the free carnitine concentration in the matrix is reduced by reversal of the CAT-II reaction. This reduction in free carnitine at the matrix leads to a decrease in the rate of translocation of long-chain acylcarnitine from the cytosol to the matrix by carnitine-acylcarnitine translocase. Second, the activity of the translocase enzyme is decreased under ischemic conditions as a result of modification of protein sulfhydryl groups {53}. Inhibition of carnitine-acylcarnitine translocase and depletion of matrix free carnitine are the critical events responsible for the increase in long-chain acylcarnitine in the cytosol of the ischemic myocyte.

The magnitude of the increase in long-chain acylcarnitine during ischemia is limited by several mechanisms. First, the increase in long-chain acylcarnitine inhibits CAT-I, which catalyzes the formation of long-chain acylcarnitine at the outer portion of the inner mitochondrial membrane {54}. Second, the uptake of free fatty acids decreases rapidly following a reduction in coronary flow {40}. Third, acylcarnitine hydrolase, an enzyme that catalyzes the hydrolysis of long-chain acylcarnitine to form free fatty acid and carnitine, is present in myocardial tissue {55}. Despite these three mechanisms to limit the increase in long-chain acylcarnitines during ischemia, we have demonstrated that this amphiphile increases 3.5-fold within the first 2 minutes of ischemia in vivo {56}.

We and others have demonstrated that long-chain acylcarnitine levels increase in both ischemic tissue in vivo {49,51,52,56,57} and hypoxic myocytes in vitro {58–61}. For example, regional ischemia in the cat in vivo led to a 3.5-fold increase in long-chain acylcarnitine levels within 2 minutes in the ischemic compared to the corresponding nonischemic region of the left ventricle {56}. This marked increase in long-chain acylcarnitine is rapid enough to contribute, at least in part, to the electrophysiologic derangements seen early after the onset of ischemia. We have also shown that long-chain acylcarnitine increases ninefold within 10 minutes of hypoxia in isolated adult canine myocytes, which can be reversed by reoxygenation or blocked by pretreatment with the carnitine acyltransferase-I blocker, sodium 2-[5-(4-chlorophenyl)-pentyl]-oxirane-2-carboxylate (POCA) {59,61}. Most importantly, in isolated adult canine myocytes, electron microscopic autoradiography of cells prelabeled with ^{3}H-carnitine demonstrates that hypoxia of only 10 minutes duration elicits a 100-fold increase in long-chain acylcarnitine content within the sarcolemma, achieving a value of 1 mole% of membrane phospholipid, a concentration sufficient to elicit electrophysiologic derangements {61}. These findings are analogous to those shown previously from our laboratory in neonatal rat ventricular myocytes exposed to hypoxia {58}.

The marked increase in long-chain acylcarnitines in

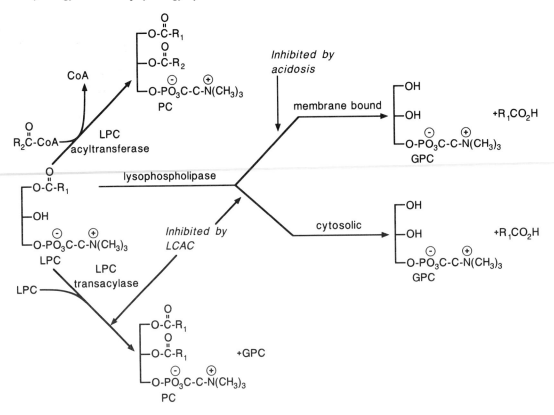

Fig. 27-5. Pathways of catabolism of lysophatidylcholine (LPC) to either phosphatidylcholine (PC) or glycerophosphorylcholine (GPC) in heart tissue.

ischemic myocardium may also contribute to the increase or retention of LPC in subcellular compartments through several mechanisms. LPC is usually present in small concentrations within cardiac cells because of the relatively high activity of several catabolic enzymes (fig. 27-5). Catabolism of LPC occurs through at least three different pathways, mediated by four separate enzymes. Lysophospholipase catalyzes the hydrolysis of LPC to glycerophosphoryl choline (GPC) and fatty acid (fig. 27-5). There are at least two distinct lysophospholipases, one found in the cytosol and one membrane bound, which is highly pH dependent {62–64}. Coenzyme A-LPC acyltransferase catalyzes the reacylation of LPC with acyl CoA to form diacyl-PC. Lysophospholipase-transacylase catalyzes a disproportionation reaction between two molecules of LPC to form diacyl-PC and GPC. The reactions catalyzed by lysophospholipase and lysophospholipase-transacylase have been shown to account for 70% of the total capacity for catabolism of LPC in homogenates of rabbit myocardium {65,66}. Under normoxic conditions, the capacity for catabolism of LPC is more than 100-fold greater than the capacity for production of LPC through activation of PLA$_2$. Thus, the accumulation of LPC is precluded. However, under ischemic conditions, the membrane bound lysophospholipase is almost completely inhibited by a

decrease in pH, and cytosolic lysophospholipase and lysophospholipase transacylase are both inhibited by long-chain acylcarnitine at concentrations that are readily achieved in ischemic tissue {65,66}. Thus, irrespective of whether LPC is produced within the myocyte membrane or at an extramyocytic source and delivered into myocyte sarcolemma, the simultaneous accumulation of long-chain acylcarnitine can have a profound effect on the accumulation of LPC within the sarcolemma and other subcellular compartments. These mechanisms may also explain the enhanced accumulation of LPC in isolated adult ventricular myocytes exposed to thrombin when acidosis and hypoxia are present simultaneously {39}.

In the in situ cat heart, we have demonstrated a twofold increase in LPC, a threefold increase in long-chain acylcarnitine, and a 64% incidence of ventricular tachycardia or fibrillation following 5 minutes of ischemia {57}. Pretreatment with POCA to inhibit carnitine acyltransferase I completely prevented the increase in both long-chain acylcarnitine and LPC, as well as the incidence of malignant arrhythmias, including ventricular tachycardia and fibrillation {57}. Thus inhibition of carnitine acyltransferase-I effectively reduced the increase in both amphiphiles, together with the incidence of lethal arrhythmias during the first 5 minutes of ischemia in vivo.

CONTRIBUTION OF LONG-CHAIN ACYLCARNITINE AND LYSOPHOSPHATIDYLCHOLINE TO ARRHYTHMOGENESIS DURING ISCHEMIA

Lysophosphatidylcholine and palmitoyl carnitine induce concentration-dependent and reversible reductions in maximum diastolic potential, total amplitude, and $\dot{V}_{max}$ of phase 0 depolarization of the transmembrane action potential, as well as a reduction in repolarization time in normoxic tissue at concentrations similar to those observed in ischemic myocardium {67–70}. The electrophysiologic effects of both LPC and palmitoyl carnitine are enhanced two- to threefold in the presence of extracellular acidosis (pH = 6.8), analogous to that which occurs in ischemic tissue in vivo {67}. The effects of both amphiphiles are not due to catabolites of LPC and long-chain acylcarnitine, since these failed to elicit significant electrophysiologic derangements at similar or even higher concentrations {67}. LPC and long-chain acylcarnitine in combination induced electrophysiologic derangements similar to those induced by comparable concentrations of either amphiphile alone, indicating an additive but not synergistic effect {67}. This, together with the fact that the effects of LPC and long-chain acylcarnitine on membrane molecular dynamics, as determined by electron spin resonance {22}, are additive, would suggest that the pathophysiologic effects of the accumulation of these amphiphiles are mediated, at least in part, by alterations in the biophysical properties of the sarcolemmal membrane, including an increase in membrane fluidity. However, the additive electrophysiologic effects of both amphiphiles could also be mediated through direct interactions with ion channel protein subunits or through an additive effect on membrane surface charge completely independent of membrane fluidity.

In studies performed several years ago in our laboratory, isolated neonatal rat myocytes exposed to hypoxia developed significant electrophysiologic derangements, the severity dependent on the magnitude of long-chain acylcarnitine accumulation in these myocytes {58}. With marked elevations of endogenous long-chain acylcarnitine (3.5 mole% of sarcolemmal membrane phospholipid), the cells became unresponsive to electrical field stimulation. Most importantly, exposure of these hypoxic cells to POCA prior to induction of hypoxia prevented the increase in long-chain acylcarnitine and markedly attenuated, but did not completely prevent, the associated electrophysiologic alterations. These findings add further support to the hypothesis that endogenous accumulation of long-chain acylcarnitines in the sarcolemma is an important contributor to the associated electrophysiologic alterations during ischemia.

Since hypoxia in isolated adult myocytes does not result in a measurable increase in LPC, it is likely that other factors may be involved in the increase in LPC observed during ischemia, including the extramyocytic sources discussed above. In isolated superfused neonatal rat myocytes, the depressant effects of LPC on contractility were found to be potentiated by acidosis and the presence of superoxide radicals {71}, both of which are prominent in ischemic tissue in vivo. Man and colleagues {72} have demonstrated that incubation of myocytes with LPC results in preferential incorporation into the outer leaflet of the sarcolemma. In concert, these results suggest that the electrophysiologic derangements induced by an increase in LPC during ischemia occur via its sarcolemmal accumulation but may in large part be from an extracellular rather than an intracellular source.

Although hypoxia does in fact simulate one major component of ischemia in vivo, additional factors are absent in this type of system. To evaluate the direct arrhythmogenic properties of an amphiphile such as LPC requires not only assessing its presence in the tissue, its subcellular site of accumulation, and its effects on membrane properties, but cause-effect relationships require inhibition of its accumulation with corresponding effects on modifying arrhythmogenesis. For example, in isolated rat hearts perfused with low concentrations of LPC (5 μM), a direct relation between the tissue content of LPC and the severity of arrhythmias has been observed {73}. No consistent alteration in total phospholipid, phosphatidylcholine, or cholesterol content was observed, suggesting that the arrhythmogenic effects of the LPC were not mediated through major alterations in lipid components of the heart {73}. Interestingly, the isolated rat heart appears to be more susceptible to the arrhythmogenic effects of LPC compared to the rabbit and guinea pig heart {74}. Perfusion with radiolabeled LPC indicated that the severity of arrhythmias was directly related to incorporation of LPC into the microsomal membrane fraction, which includes not only the sarcolemma but intracellular membranes as well {74}. However, an evaluation of the extent of *sarcolemmal* incorporation of LPC in the ischemic heart and its direct relation to the associated electrophysiologic alterations and resulting arrhythmias has not yet been achieved. This is due to technical limitations because conventional cellular fractionation to isolate the sarcolemmal fraction of ischemic or normal cardiac tissue results in both translocation to other subcellular compartments and catabolism of the LPC.

In summary, both LPC and long-chain acylcarnitine increase during short periods of ischemia and are capable of contributing to arrhythmogenesis. Studies in vitro demonstrate that both amphiphiles cause dramatic and reversible alterations in electrophysiologic indices. The similarity of the electrophysiologic derangements induced by these amphiphiles suggests that the effects are mediated, at least in part, by the amphipathic properties common to both moieties.

EFFECTS OF LPC AND LONG-CHAIN ACYLCARNITINES ON INDIVIDUAL IONIC CURRENTS IN CARDIAC CELLS

Our knowledge of the precise mechanisms whereby either of these amphiphiles alters specific ionic currents in cardiac cells is still incomplete. The voltage-sensitive rapid Na$^+$ inward current (I_{Na}) is decreased by both amphiphiles, not only as a result of a direct decrease in the peak magnitude of the current, but also secondary to a reduction in the resting membrane potential. Arnsdorf and Sawicki demonstrated that LPC decreased the conductance of I_{Na}, resulting in biphasic effects on excitability, with an initial increase followed by a decrease in excitability, and often development of complete inexcitability {75}.

Interestingly, this type of biphasic response on excitability occurs in ischemic myocardium in vivo {76}. In a recent study by Burnashev and colleagues {77}, LPC actually induced prolonged open times of Na^+ channels, and a subsequent study by Undrovinas and colleagues {78} demonstrated that this influence of LPC is secondary to clustering of Na^+ channels within the membrane with a marked delay in inactivation of Na^+ channels. This influence of LPC during ischemia could contribute to the marked slowing in conduction and conduction block, reduction in resting membrane potential due to potential increase in intracellular Na^+ (even at membrane potentials negative to $-90\,mV$), and development of both early and delayed afterdepolarizations, as discussed in detail below. We have recently demonstrated that palmitoyl carnitine also activated Na^+ channels, resulting in prolonged open times with a marked delay in inactivation {79}, potentially leading to an increase in intracellular Na^+. Sato and colleagues {80} have recently demonstrated that both palmitoyl carnitine and LPC had inhibitory effects on the rapid Na^+ inward current (I_{Na}) in isolated ventricular myocytes. Both amphiphiles retarded the time course of activation and inactivation of I_{Na}, suggesting that palmitoyl carnitine and LPC decrease the maximum Na^+ conductance and alter the surface negative charge of the membrane due to incorporation of the amphiphile into the phospholipid bilayer. Palmitoyl carnitine appears to have an additional effect of direct and reversible incorporation within the integral membrane proteins comprising the Na^+ channel and may thereby lead to activation of a slowly inactivating Na^+ current ($I_{Na(s)}$), as discussed above.

The influence of either LPC or palmitoyl carnitine on K^+ currents has not been completely delineated. However, Clarkson and Ten Eick {81} demonstrated that the reduction in membrane potential in response to LPC was secondary to a decreased K^+ conductance at negative membrane potentials. This was also shown by Kiyosue and Arita {82}, who reported that LPC decreased conductance through inward rectifier K^+ channels (I_{K1}) and thereby decreased the resting membrane potential of isolated guinea pig ventricular myocytes. It is likely that the reduction in resting membrane potential may be mediated not only by a decrease in I_{K1}, but also potentially due to an increase in $[Na^+]_i$ secondary to sustained activation of $I_{Na(s)}$. However, definitive data are not yet available.

The voltage-dependent Ca^{2+} current ($I_{Ca(L)}$) in cardiac cells not only contributes to the action potential duration {83}, and thereby influences the refractory period in ventricular muscle cells, but Ca^{2+} ions entering the myocyte through these channels are essential for excitation-contraction coupling, since they initiate normal cardiac contraction by triggering Ca^{2+} release from the sarcoplasmic reticulum {84–86}. The direct influence of long-chain acylcarnitine and LPC on $I_{Ca(L)}$ has only recently been evaluated. Previous studies have suggested that long-chain acylcarnitines may activate or enhance $I_{Ca(L)}$, not only in cardiac tissue {87} but in smooth muscle cells as well {88,89}. This conclusion was supported by indirect findings wherein palmitoyl carnitine increased action potential duration, amplitude, and maximal rate of rise of the action potential in isolated avian ventricular myocytes that were depolarized with elevated extracellular K^+ and were therefore dependent exclusively on $I_{Ca(L)}$ for inward current {87}. Likewise, in isolated guinea pig myocytes, Meszaros and Pappano {69} demonstrated that palmitoyl carnitine could induce delayed afterdepolarizations, suggesting indirectly that palmitoyl carnitine increased intracellular Ca^{2+}, thereby activating the transient inward current (I_{ti}).

However, we have recently used whole-cell voltage-clamp procedures in isolated guinea pig myocytes to assess the direct effects of palmitoyl carnitine on $I_{Ca(L)}$ {90}. Both extracellular and intracellular delivery of palmitoyl carnitine inhibited rather than stimulated $I_{Ca(L)}$ by approximately 50% (fig. 27-6). Despite the marked decrease in $I_{Ca(L)}$, palmitoyl carnitine induced both early and delayed afterdepolarizations with triggered activity, which likely contributes to the arrhythmogenic effect of long-chain acylcarnitines during ischemia (fig. 27-7). Although the direct effects of LPC on $I_{Ca(L)}$ are not known, LPC has been shown to decrease the magnitude of action potentials dependent solely on $I_{Ca(L)}$ for membrane depolarization, suggesting indirectly that $I_{Ca(L)}$ is decreased {81}. Despite the fact that LPC likely decreases $I_{Ca(L)}$, there is a simultaneous positive ionotropic effect {81,91}, which is likely a result of an increase in intracellular Ca^{2+}, although the precise mechanisms are unknown. We have shown that LPC induces delayed afterdepolarizations and triggered rhythms in isolated tissue {92}, an effect that is coupled to an increase in intracellular Ca^{2+}. Delayed afterdepolarizations induced by LPC persisted even in the presence of acidosis and increased extracellular K^+ {92}, analogous to those changes seen in ischemic tissue in vivo. Therefore, a critical question is, how do these amphiphiles increase $[Ca^{2+}]_i$?

ACCUMULATION OF AMPHIPHILES AND ALTERATIONS IN $[Ca^{2+}]_i$

Primary abnormalities in the regulation of intracellular Ca^{2+} in ischemic myocardium may contribute significantly to arrhythmogenesis, including the development of ventricular fibrillation. Several studies have demonstrated that ischemia results in a rapid increase in cytosolic Ca^{2+} {93–96}, although others have suggested that the increase is delayed for approximately 10 minutes {97–99}. It is possible that either long-chain acylcarnitine or LPC could mediate a primary role in the increase in $[Ca^{2+}]_i$ in response to early ischemia. These amphiphiles may produce membrane-perturbing effects, which could lead to nonspecific leakage of Ca^{2+} into myocytes. Alternatively, the amphiphiles may influence specific cellular Ca^{2+} transport

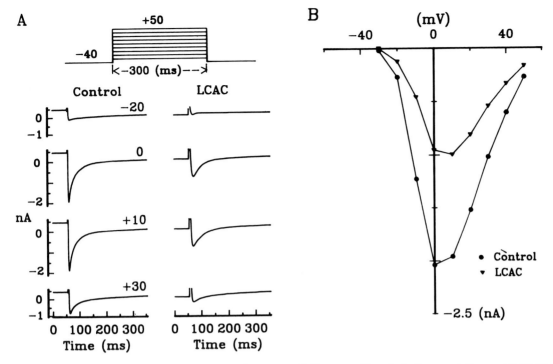

Fig. 27-6. Influence of long-chain acylcarnitine (LCAC) on L-type Ca^{2+} current ($I_{Ca(L)}$). **A:** Representative current traces are shown under control conditions and in the presence of LCAC ($5\,\mu M$) for 10 minutes. The cell was clamped from -30 to $+50\,mV$ at 10-mV steps from a holding potential of $-40\,mV$. Numbers on traces at left indicate selected membrane voltage-clamp potentials. Note that holding currents in the presence of LCAC were shifted inward due to a decrease in the resting membrane potential to less negative potentials. **B:** Current-voltage (I-V) relationship under control conditions and in the presence of LCAC ($5\,\mu M$) for 10 minutes. Data for I-V curves were obtained from the same cell as in A. Reproduced Wu and Corr {90} with permission from the American Physiological Society.

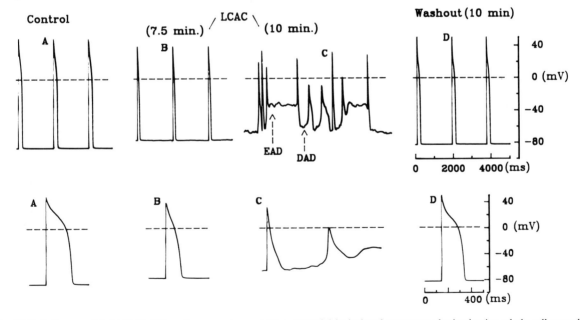

Fig. 27-7. Influence of LCAC ($5\,\mu M$) on transmembrane action potential in isolated myocytes obtained using whole-cell recording procedure with Axoclamp-2A in bridge mode. Alterations in membrane potential by LCAC are shown under control conditions (**A**), during exposure to LCAC for 7.5 minutes (**B**) and 10 minutes (**C**), and after washout (**D**). The cell was stimulated constantly at $1850\,ms$. In the bottom portion of each panel, selected action potentials are shown at faster sweep speeds. EAD and DAD represent early and delayed afterdepolarizations, respectively. Voltage and time scales in A, B, and C are the same as shown in D. Reproduced from Wu and Corr {90}, with permission from the American Physiological Society.

processes directly, as discussed below. Amphiphiles delivered at high concentrations, however, will likely exert nonspecific, irreversible effects, in addition to any reversible effects they may have on specific membrane transport mechanisms. Furthermore, amphiphile-induced increases in intracellular Ca^{2+} may activate phospholipases, which would augment LPC production and thereby the electrophysiologic effects of LPC. Additionally, catecholamine stimulation, particularly during hypoxia or ischemia, can increase intracellular Ca^{2+} via beta-adrenergic receptor activation, which may in turn activate PLA_2 {100,101}.

There is considerable indirect evidence to support the hypothesis that long-chain acylcarnitine and LPC produce an increase in intracellular Ca^{2+} in cardiac myocytes based primarily on the effects of these agents to enhance contractility and induce early and delayed afterdepolarizations {69,87,92}. The precise mechanisms responsible for the increase in intracellular Ca^{2+} have not yet been elucidated. Liu and colleagues {102} have demonstrated that LPC ($20\,\mu M$) markedly enhances cell shortening, produces spontaneous contractile activity, and increases intracellular Ca^{2+}, leading to contracture in isolated guinea pig ventricular myocytes. Woodley and colleagues {103} recorded increases in intracellular Ca^{2+}, also measured directly, in embryonic chick myocytes exposed to $10-100\,\mu M$ LPC. Unfortunately, the effects reported in both studies were not reversible. Thus, one cannot determine whether Ca^{2+} overload induced by LPC might also be responsible for the reversible electrophysiologic derangements observed during early ischemia or during pathophysiological levels ($1-2$ mole% of total membrane phospholipids) attained after exogenous delivery of LPC.

One possible mechanism responsible for the increase in $[Ca^{2+}]_i$ in response to LPC or long-chain acylcarnitines may be secondary to the activation of the slow inactivating Na^+ current ($I_{Na(s)}$) discussed above. We have recently obtained preliminary data demonstrating reversible increases in intracellular Ca^{2+} in response to $10\,\mu M$ palmitoyl carnitine in indo-1 free acid-loaded adult ventricular myocytes {104}, a response similar to that elicited with LPC {105}. The activation of $I_{Na(s)}$ by either LPC {78} or palmitoylcarnitine {79} may result in an increase in $[Na^+]_i$, thereby activating the Na^+/Ca^{2+} exchanger, leading to an increase in $[Ca^{2+}]_i$. This concept is supported by recent data {106} indicating that exposure of isolated myocytes to severe hypoxia leads to an increase in $[Na^+]_i$, a response that is blocked by pretreatment with R56,865, an agent that appears to attenuate $I_{Na(s)}$. Interestingly, R56,865 also significantly attenuated the increase in $[Ca^{2+}]_i$ induced by LPC in isolated cardiac myocytes {105}. Despite these findings, additional data will be required to absolutely confirm this sequence of events.

Data obtained by several groups of investigators indicate that long-chain acylcarnitine and LPC exert nonspecific detergent effects within the sarcolemma and other subcellular membranes if the concentration within the membrane is sufficient. This conclusion has been based largely on experimental protocols using high concentrations of either amphiphile, the effects of which are not comparable to the specific cellular derangements induced

by lower concentrations of the amphiphile. The reversibility of the response to these amphiphiles is a critical event that is unfortunately not always demonstrated in studies pertaining to these amphiphiles {102,103}. Similarly, palmitoyl carnitine ($5-25\,\mu M$) has been shown to inhibit sarcolemmal Ca^{2+} permeability in vitro {107}. Subsequently, these investigators concluded that there was no correlation between ischemia-induced accumulation of long-chain acylcarnitine and Ca^{2+} transport alterations in the sarcolemma or sarcoplasmic reticulum {108}. Isolation of subcellular membrane fractions using the procedures outlined in these studies would very likely lead to both translocation of the amphiphile as well as intrapreparative catabolism or synthesis of the amphiphile, as discussed above. Only studies in intact cell systems in which simultaneous direct measurements of intracellular Ca^{2+} in addition to other cellular transport mechanisms under conditions of known, reversible amphiphile incorporation will yield meaningful data on whether accumulation of amphiphiles plays a critical role in altering intracellular Ca^{2+} during early ischemia.

Several potential mechanisms for increasing intracellular Ca^{2+} during ischemia, including inhibition of sarcolemmal Na,K-ATPase and sarcoplasmic reticulum Ca-ATPase, may be evoked by accumulation of either of these amphiphiles. The Na,K-ATPase pump normally removes Na^+ ions from cells and returns K^+ ions in a $3:2$ ($Na^+:K^+$) exchange utilizing the hydrolysis of ATP and eliciting a net outward current {for review see 109}. The amount of long-term, restorative electrochemical work performed by the cardiac Na,K-ATPase pump is considerable. The Na,K-ATPase pump maintains the intracellular Na^+ ion concentration at a low level to maintain a large, inwardly directed electrochemical potential gradient for Na^+ that not only sustains electrical excitability, but also supplies the energy for several cotransport and countertransport systems. Among these is the Na^+/Ca^{2+} exchanger, which helps maintain the cytoplasmic Ca^{2+} ion concentration at a low level during diastole ($75-150\,nM$) {110-112}.

Whether intracellular Na^+ increases during early ischemia remains a subject of controversy. The apparent discrepancy between studies appears to arise from the species studied rather than the techniques used. Kléber {113} measured intracellular Na^+ activity from subepicardial layers of blood-perfused and ischemic guinea pig hearts and found no significant increase of intracellular Na^+ in the first 15 minutes of ischemia. A subsequent study in isolated superfused guinea pig papillary muscles demonstrated that combined severe hypoxia, substrate withdrawal, and acidosis did significantly increase intracellular Na^+ activity after $9-10$ minutes, an effect that was abolished by the increase in extracellular K^+ {114}. Several other studies in hypoxic, but not ischemic, myocardium have shown that the increase of intracellular Na^+ did not exceed $3\,mM$ in the first 10 minutes of hypoxia {115-117}. In contrast, determinations of intracellular Na^+ in ischemic rat hearts {118} showed an increase in intracellular Na^+, starting almost immediately after the arrest of perfusion and reaching 240% after 12 minutes.

This result supports a previous study by Fiolet and colleagues {119} demonstrating a threefold increase in intracellular sodium after 10–15 minutes of hypoxia in the rat heart and agrees with recent data in isolated myocytes exposed to severe hypoxia {106}.

It is known that *prolonged* ischemia causes a considerable decrease in sarcolemmal Na,K-ATPase activity {120,121} and that this decrease is further exacerbated during reperfusion {122}. However, during *early* ischemia Na,K-ATPase activity does not appear to be decreased significantly, and it is only after periods of greater than 15 minutes of ischemia that an inhibition is observed {123,124}. There is considerable evidence that both palmitoyl carnitine and LPC inhibit Na,K-ATPase (see below), but further studies examining this enzyme's activity following brief intervals of ischemia will be necessary to determine the role of accumulation of these amphiphiles on Na,K-ATPase in vivo.

Palmitoyl carnitine has been shown to inhibit Na,K-ATPase activity and to reduce the binding of [^{3}H]-ouabain to cardiac membranes {125}. These effects occurred within the concentration range of long-chain acylcarnitine that accumulates during acute ischemia. Na,K-ATPase is a transmembrane protein that is dependent upon structurally associated phospholipids of the sarcolemma for its activity and for binding of digitalis. Perturbation of the phospholipid bilayer by incorporation of long-chain acylcarnitine into the sarcolemma could thereby result in inhibition of enzyme activity as well as the binding of digitalis to Na,K-ATPase {126}. These studies support data reported by Wood and colleagues in bovine heart {127} and data obtained subsequently by Abe and colleagues in canine heart {128}, all demonstrating inhibition of Na,K-ATPase by palmitoyl carnitine. In one conflicting report, however, Owens and colleagues analyzed the susceptibility of Na,K-ATPase in highly enriched cardiac sarcolemma to perturbation by LPC, palmitoyl CoA, and palmitoyl carnitine {129}. Palmitoyl carnitine at a ratio of up to 10 μmol/mg of sarcolemmal protein did not produce significant inhibition of Na,K-ATPase, even after preincubation at 37°C {129}.

It is interesting to note that the sarcolemma used in the latter study was prepared from isolated canine ventricular myocytes. It is possible that enzymatic digestion required for myocyte isolation altered Na,K-ATPase responsiveness to palmitoyl carnitine in this later study. In contrast, LPC produced a 40% inhibition of Na,K-ATPase at a concentration of 0.6 μmol/mg protein {129}, a finding in agreement with other investigators at other even lower concentrations of LPC (10–30 μM) {130}. At much higher concentrations of LPC (above 2 mM), stimulation of Na,K-ATPase was observed, very likely due to the nonspecific detergent effects of the amphiphile {128}. Thus there is good evidence in isolated membranes that both LPC and palmitoyl carnitine can inhibit Na,K-ATPase at low concentrations. However, future studies will be required to examine the effects of these amphiphiles on Na,K-ATPase in intact cells and to assess the extent of membrane incorporation and the reversibility of the response.

If Na,K-ATPase is actually inhibited by either or both amphiphiles, there would be a net increase in intracellular Na$^+$, which could contribute to membrane depolarization, accumulation of extracellular K$^+$, and increase in intracellular Ca^{2+} via enhanced Na$^+$/Ca^{2+} exchange. Although Bersohn and coworkers reported that very high concentrations of LPC (0.3 μmol LPC/mg protein) resulted in a 50% inhibition of Na$^+$/Ca^{2+} exchange in normal canine sarcolemmal vesicles {131}, the amount of LPC incorporated into the sarcolemma in these experiments would be very high compared to the range found in ischemic tissue. Palmitoyl carnitine (30 μM) has also been reported to inhibit the initial rate of Na$^+$/Ca^{2+} exchange in sarcolemmal vesicles {132}. Although the concentration of LPC required to inhibit Na,K-ATPase is lower than that which will modulate other membrane-bound enzymes, the concentration of palmitoyl carnitine required to inhibit Na,K-ATPase is higher than that needed to alter Ca^{2+} and Na$^+$ permeability. As stated previously, whether inhibition of Na,K-ATPase is a critical event in the electrophysiologic alterations during ischemia will require additional study in carefully defined intact cell systems.

Inhibition of Ca-ATPase activity in the sarcoplasmic reticulum (SR) by amphiphiles may also contribute to an increase in intracellular Ca^{2+}. This may be a particularly important mechanism, since inhibition of SR Ca-ATPase may lead to a delay in reuptake of cytosolic Ca^{2+}, leading to activation of I$_{ti}$ and thereby triggered rhythms. Calcium-dependent ATPase from the SR pumps Ca^{2+} against a concentration gradient at the expense of hydrolysis of ATP. Palmitoyl carnitine has been shown to produce a concentration-dependent, biphasic effect on SR Ca-ATPase activity with an increase in activity at low concentrations of palmitoyl carnitine and inhibition of Ca-ATPase activity at higher concentrations {126}. In contrast, Pitts and coworkers reported that palmitoyl carnitine only inhibited Ca^{2+} binding and Ca-ATPase activity in sarcoplasmic reticulum, regardless of concentration {133}. Similarly, LPC (50 μM) has been shown to inhibit Ca^{2+} transport in SR and to uncouple Ca^{2+} transport and ATP hydrolytic activities, possibly via interaction of LPC with the Ca^{2+} pump itself or with its membrane environment {134}. Therefore, it is possible that modulation of Ca-ATPase in the SR by either or both amphiphiles may be important in arrhythmogenesis, but assessment in intact cell systems will be required.

Cytosolic protein kinase C (PKC) binds free Ca^{2+}, causing it to translocate to the cell membrane, where it interacts with phospholipids and binds diacylglycerol with high affinity. Because the enzyme can be active in the absence of diacylglycerol if it is fully integrated into the membrane, simply raising intracellular Ca^{2+} levels can be sufficient to activate the enzyme. The effects of PKC on cardiac L-type Ca^{2+} channels have not yet been completely resolved. For example, phorbol esters, which produce direct, persistent activation of PKC, have been shown to stimulate I$_{Ca(L)}$ in neonatal rat myocytes {135} and canine Purkinje cells and ventricular muscle cells {136}. LPC has been shown to stimulate PKC at low concentrations (<20 μM) and to inhibit PKC at higher concentrations (>30 μM) {137}. However, since I$_{Ca(L)}$ appears to be inhibited by both long-chain acylcarnitines and LPC, as discussed above, it is unlikely that modulation of the activity of PKC by either amphiphile is critical for the increase in intracellular Ca^{2+} in the intact ventricular muscle cell.

Another amphiphile, the plasmalogen metabolite 1-0-alkyl-1'-enyl-2-acyl-sn-glycerol (AAG), has been shown recently to be a potent activator of protein kinase C and to accumulate in ischemic myocardium {138,139}. Accumulation of AAG in ischemic myocardium in conjunction with increases in intracellular free Ca^{2+} may synergistically activate protein kinase C and thereby modulate phosphorylation of other membrane channel proteins that are critical to the electrophysiologic alterations and resulting arrhythmias in the ischemic heart. However, this sequence of events has not yet been addressed experimentally.

Finally, LPC and analogs of LPC have been shown to induce Ca^{2+} efflux from mitochondria isolated from liver {140,141}. Although this effect has not been tested in mitochondria isolated from heart, it may be yet another means by which LPC may contribute to arrhythmogenesis secondary to an increase in $[Ca^{2+}]_i$.

Therefore, both long-chain acylcarnitines and LPC are capable of increasing intracellular Ca^{2+} by at least three potential mechanisms: (a) delay in inactivation of a Na^+ channel, leading to an increase in intracellular Na^+ and enhanced Na^+, Ca^{2+} exchange; (b) inhibition of Na, K-ATPase, leading to an increase in $[Na^+]_i$ and thereby activating Na^+/Ca^{2+} exchange; and (c) inhibition of Ca-ATPase activity in the sarcoplasmic reticulum, leading to a reduction in net Ca^{2+} uptake and resulting in an increase in the intracellular concentration of Ca^{2+}.

ACCUMULATION OF EXTRACELLULAR K^+ DURING EARLY MYOCARDIAL ISCHEMIA

A small fraction of total intracellular K^+ is lost during early ischemia {142,143}. This K^+ loss begins within seconds after the onset of ischemia, and extracellular K^+ gradually increases from about 4 mM to 10–15 mM during the first 4–6 minutes of ischemia {144–150}. An increase in extracellular K^+ would be expected to decrease the resting membrane potential, shift the threshold potential to more positive potentials, reduce the maximum rate of rise of the action potential upstroke ($\dot{V}_{max}$), lower the action potential amplitude and plateau potential, shorten the plateau duration, accelerate the slope of rapid repolarization, suppress the oscillatory afterpotentials induced by an increase in intracellular Ca^{2+}, and decrease the rate of spontaneous diastolic depolarization in Purkinje fibers {151–153}. In brief, an increase in extracellular K^+ can potentially elicit many of the electrophysiologic alterations associated with early myocardial ischemia.

Studies of unidirectional K^+ flux indicate that the early K^+ depletion and extracellular accumulation is due to an increased rate of efflux of K^+ out of the cell. The mechanisms responsible for the enhanced K^+ efflux during early ischemia are not completely understood. It is feasible that factors such as LPC or long-chain acylcarnitines could

lead to membrane depolarization secondary to an increase in intracellular Na^+, as discussed above, and that K^+ efflux occurs secondarily as a result of a new, more positive membrane potential, and hence new equilibrium potential for K^+.

Extracellular K^+ accumulation may be a result of release of K^+ from the cell to maintain charge neutrality during ischemia when weak acids accumulating intracellularly are released from the ischemic cell {149,154}. Activation of the ATP-dependent K^+ channel may also contribute to K^+ loss from the myocyte {155}. This channel is activated by a fall in ATP. However, the total intracellular level of ATP does not fall rapidly during early ischemia to a level sufficient to activate this channel, at a time when extracellular K^+ increases markedly {156,157}. It is possible that activation of as little as 1% of the ATP-dependent channels, as may occur with modest falls in ATP, could be sufficient to account for the increase in extracellular K^+ and thereby elicit the electrophysiologic effects indicated above {158}. In addition, subcellular sites near the membrane ATP-dependent K^+ channel may sense a different pool of ATP than the rest of the cytoplasm, and this may be sufficient to activate this channel and thereby increase extracellular K^+ {159–163}. Sulfonylureas, including glibenclamide and tolbutamide, have been shown to block the ATP-dependent K^+ channel, reduce ischemia- or hypoxia-induced extracellular K^+ accumulation, and prevent the shortening in action potential duration {164–166}. However, the actions of these agents are diverse and include inhibition of carnitine acyltransferase {167}, decrease in coronary flow and stimulation of lactate production during normoxia {168}, and inhibition of the increase in lactate production during hypoxia {169}. Thus an alternative action of the sulfonylureas, other than inhibition of ATP-regulated K^+ channels, may be responsible for reducing intracellular K^+ loss and extracellular K^+ accumulation. Although LPC or long-chain acylcarnitines could potentially activate the ATP-sensitive K^+ channel during ischemia, initial evidence would suggest that LPC actually suppresses rather than activates this channel {170}.

ACCUMULATION OF AMPHIPATHIC METABOLITES AND THEIR INFLUENCE ON CELL-TO-CELL COUPLING

Individual cells communicate with each other via specialized membrane structures, the gap junctions. Chemical and electrical coupling by means of gap junctions is essential in a number of biological processes, including development {171}, growth {172}, secretion {173,174}, and impulse propagation {175–177}. Gap junctions form low-resistance pathways between adjacent myocytes, which permit the rapid and uniform flow of current from cell to cell, and thereby uniform and rapid conduction of the wavefront of electrical propagation {178–180}. A reduction in gap junctional conductance could contribute to slow conduction and ultimately conduction block, particularly in the presence of altered active membrane properties (i.e., decreased I_{Na}).

Studies using isolated cardiac preparations have shown that the transfer properties of gap junctions are modulated by cytosolic cations such as H^+, Ca^{2+}, and Mg^{2+} {181–183}. Besides this ionic control, intercellular current flow is also influenced by organic substances. Lipophilic substances such as general anesthetics {184–186}, alkanols (heptanol, octanol) {181,184,187,188}, or fatty acids (doxyl stearic acids, arachidonic acid, oleic acid) {189–191}, decrease the conductance through gap junctions. Interestingly, a recent report by Ovadia and Burt {192} utilizing adult myocytes suggests that the effect of free fatty acids on junctional conductance is much less marked and requires much higher concentrations to produce a similar uncoupling response compared to that in neonatal myocytes. Although cations and lipophilic agents decrease junctional conductance, cyclic adenosine monophosphate increases junctional conductance {193,194}. Conceivably, junctional conductance may be modified directly by acting on channel proteins or indirectly via interference with membrane phospholipids. We have recently demonstrated that palmitoyl carnitine (5 µM) induced a rapid and progressive decrease in gap junctional conductance in adult canine myocyte pairs {195}. The effect was reversible after washout of the amphiphile {195}. In addition, electron microscopic autoradiographic studies in isolated canine myocytes demonstrated a sevenfold preferential incorporation of endogenous long-chain acylcarnitines into the junctional as opposed to nonjunctional regions of the sarcolemma during 10 minutes of hypoxia, resulting in a concentration of 4 mole % of the total phospholipid content in the junctional regions {195}. These results suggest that during early ischemia, selective accumulation of long-chain acylcarnitines in junctional regions of the sarcolemma could contribute to a reduction in cellular coupling between adjacent myocytes (see below).

Previous studies have demonstrated that internal longitudinal resistance and intracellular resistivity (r_i) increase markedly in ischemic or hypoxic myocardium {196–201}. The specific cause of this increase in r_i is generally considered to be due to cellular uncoupling at gap junctions {193,202}. We have shown irreversible cellular uncoupling occurs after 30 minutes of hypoxia in canine myocardium, likely due to a decrease in the number of open gap junctional channels {201}. In the isolated blood perfused rabbit papillary muscle, Kléber and coworkers have shown rapid cellular uncoupling after 15–20 minutes of in vitro ischemia {150,198}. Coincident with cellular uncoupling was the development of ischemic contracture and a secondary rise in extracellular K^+ {150}. We have recently shown in this same blood-perfused papillary muscle exposed to ischemia that inhibition of the accumulation of long-chain acylcarnitines markedly delayed both cellular uncoupling (i.e., increase in r_t) and ischemic contracture {203}.

It is conceivable that slow conduction observed in vivo during ischemia is often caused by a high degree of cellular uncoupling {204}. Quan and Rudy {205} have demonstrated the importance of cellular uncoupling in the genesis of unidirectional block and reentry. The likelihood of induction of unidirectional block was proportional to the degree of cellular uncoupling. In addition, myocardium with increased cellular uncoupling was found to be vulnerable to unidirectional block and reentry induced by ectopic foci {206}. Thus, since the basis for the genesis of reentry in the initiation of ventricular tachycardia is the slow conduction and block present even during normal sinus rhythm early after the onset of ischemia {21}, it is likely that accumulation of an amphiphile such as long-chain acylcarnitine during ischemia that actually decreases junctional conductance will contribute importantly to the genesis of malignant arrhythmias dependent on reentry. This is particularly likely when active membrane properties are also altered in a direction that would depress conduction velocity (i.e., decreased I_{Na}). In addition, the fact that these amphiphiles appear to increase $[Ca^{2+}]_i$ likely contributes to the activation of I_{ti} and the appearance of both early and delayed afterdepolarizations, leading to triggered arrhythmias. This may explain the appearance of nonreentrant contributions to arrhythmogenesis during ischemia {21}, particularly in border regions where $[K^+]_o$ is near normal.

CONCLUSIONS

In conclusion, the above findings indicate that both long-chain acylcarnitine and LPC can contribute to membrane dysfunction early after ischemia and thereby to development of both reentrant and nonreentrant arrhythmias through a wide variety of mechanisms. Additional investigations will be required to ascertain the precise role of these amphiphiles in arrhythmogenesis and the dominant cellular and subcellular mechanisms whereby these moieties influence the electrophysiologic behavior of the heart. Since the observation that inhibition of carnitine acyltransferase-I (CAT-I) results in both inhibition of the accumulation of these amphipathic metabolites and a significant antiarrhythmic effect {57}, it would be expected that development of a specific CAT-I inhibitor would be of considerable therapeutic benefit for the prevention of sudden cardiac death in patients with ischemic heart disease. In addition, development of PLA_2 inhibitors is another potential therapeutic target, although this approach would only block the increase in LPC and would likely not affect the increase in long-chain acylcarnitines.

Although this review has focused on two amphipathic metabolites, it is clear that many other factors contribute to the development of arrhythmogenesis during ischemia. The critical challenge is to understand how all of these factors integrate in the ischemic heart and lead to the marked electrophysiologic derangements and lethal arrhythmias underlying sudden cardiac death in humans.

ACKNOWLEDGMENTS

Research from the authors' laboratory was supported by National Institutes of Health grants HL-17646, SCOR in Ischemic Heart Disease, grant HL-28995, and the American Heart Association, Missouri Affiliate.

REFERENCES

1. Bayés de Luna A, Coumel P, Leclercq JF: Ambulatory sudden cardiac death: Mechanisms of production of fatal arrhythmia on the basis of data from 157 cases. *Am Heart J* 117:151–159, 1989.
2. Cobb LA, Werner JA, Trobaugh GB: Sudden cardiac death. 1. A decade's experience with out-of-hospital resuscitation. *Med Concepts Cardiovasc Dis* 49:31–36, 1980.
3. Nikolic G, Bishop RL, Singh JB: Sudden death during Holter monitoring. *Circulation* 66:218–225, 1982.
4. Panidis IP, Morganroth J: Sudden death in hospitalized patients: Cardiac rhythm disturbances detected by ambulatory electrocardiographic monitoring. *J Am Coll Cardiol* 2:798–805, 1983.
5. Wang FS, Lien WP, Fond TE, Lin JL, Cherng JJ, Chen JH, Chen JJ: Terminal cardiac electrical activity in adults who die without apparent cardiac disease. *Am J Cardiol* 58:491–495, 1986.
6. Lie JT, Titus JL: Pathology of the myocardium and the conduction system in sudden coronary death. *Circulation* 52(Suppl III):41–52, 1975.
7. Davies MJ, Thomas A: Thrombosis and acute coronary artery lesions in sudden cardiac ischemic death. *N Engl J Med* 310:1137–1141, 1984.
8. Downar E, Janse MJ, Durrer D: The effect of acute coronary artery occlusion on subepicardial transmembrane potentials in the intact porcine heart. *Circulation* 56:217–224, 1977.
9. Downar E, Janse MJ, Durrer D: The effect of "ischemic" blood on transmembrane potentials of normal porcine ventricular myocardium. *Circulation* 55:455–462, 1977.
10. Creer MH, Dobmeyer DJ, Corr PB: Amphipathic lipid metabolites and arrhythmias during myocardial ischemia. In: Zipes DP, Jalife J (eds) *Cardiac Electrophysiology: From Cell to Bedside*. Philadelphia: WB Saunders, 1990, 417–433.
11. The Cardiac Arrhythmia Suppression Trial (CAST) Investigators: Preliminary report: Effect of encainide and flecainide on mortality in a randomized trial of arrhythmia suppression after myocardial infarction. *N Engl J Med* 321:406–412, 1989.
12. Kléber AG, Janse MJ, van Capelle FJL, Durrer D: Mechanism and time course of S-T and T-Q segment changes during acute regional myocardial ischemia in the pig heart determined by extracellular and intracellular recordings. *Circ Res* 42:603–613, 1978.
13. Kimura S, Bassett AL, Saoudi NC, Cameron JS, Kozlovskis PL, Myerburg RJ: Cellular electrophysiologic changes and "arrhythmias" during experimental ischemia and reperfusion in isolated cat ventricular myocardium. *J Am Coll Cardiol* 7:833–842, 1986.
14. Kimura S, Bassett AL, Kohya T, Kozlovskis PL, Myerburg RJ: Simultaneous recording of action potentials from endocardium and epicardium during ischemia in the isolated cat ventricle: Relation of temporal electrophysiologic heterogeneities to arrhythmias. *Circulation* 74:401–409, 1986.
15. Boineau JP, Cox JL: Slow ventricular activation in acute myocardial infarction: A source of reentrant premature ventricular contraction. *Circulation* 48:702–713, 1973.
16. Ruffy R, Lovelace DE, Mueller TM, Knoebel SB, Zipes DP: Relationship between changes in left ventricular bipolar electrograms and regional myocardial blood flow during acute coronary occlusion in the dog. *Circ Res* 45:744–770, 1979.
17. Scherlag BJ, El-Sherif N, Hope RR, Lazzara R: Characterization and localization of ventricular arrhythmias resulting from myocardial ischemia and infarction. *Circ Res* 35:372–383, 1974.
18. Williams DO, Scherlag BJ, Hope RR, El-Sherif N, Lazzara R: The pathophysiology of malignant ventricular arrhythmias during acute myocardial ischemia. *Circulation* 50:1163–1172, 1974.
19. Hearse DJ, Yellon DM: The "border zone" in evolving myocardial infarction: Controversy or confusion. *Am J Cardiol* 47:1321–1334, 1981.
20. Janse MJ, Cinca J, Morena H, Fiolet JWT, Kléber AG, de Vries GP, Becker AE, Durrer D: The "border zone" in myocardial ischemia: An electrophysiological, metabolic, and histochemical correlation in the pig heart. *Circ Res* 44:576–588, 1979.
21. Pogwizd SM, Corr PB: Reentrant and nonreentrant mechanisms contribute to arrhythmogenesis during early myocardial ischemia: Results using three-dimensional mapping. *Circ Res* 61:352–371, 1987.
22. Fink KL, Gross RW: Modulation of canine myocardial sarcolemmal membrane fluidity by amphiphilic compounds. *Circ Res* 55:585–594, 1984.
23. Gross RW, Corr PB, Lee BE, Saffitz JE, Crafford WA Jr, Sobel BE: Incorporation of radiolabeled lysophosphatidylcholine into canine Purkinje fibers and ventricular muscle: Electrophysiological, biochemical and autoradiographic correlation. *Circ Res* 51:27–36, 1982.
24. Saffitz JE, Corr PB, Lee BI, Gross RW, Williamson EK, Sobel BE: Pathophysiological concentrations of lysophosphoglycerides quantified by electron microscopic autoradiography. *Lab Invest* 50:278–286, 1984.
25. Mészàros J, Villanova L, Pappano A: Calcium ions and l-palmitoylcarnitine induce erythrocyte electrophoretic mobility: Test of a surface charge hypothesis. *J Mol Cell Cardiol* 20:481–492, 1988.
26. Franson RC, Waite M, Weglicki W: Phospholipase A activity of lysosomes of rat myocardial tissue. *Biochemistry* 11:472–476, 1972.
27. Franson RC, Weir DL, Thakkar J: Solubilization and characterization of a neutral-active, calcium-dependent, phospholipase A_2 from rabbit heart and isolated chick embryo myocytes. *J Mol Cell Cardiol* 15:189–196, 1983.
28. Wolf RA, Gross RW: Identification of neutral active phospholipase C which hydrolyzes choline glycerophospholipids and plasmalogen selective phospholipase A_2 in canine myocardium. *J Biol Chem* 260:7295–7303, 1985.
29. Ford DA, Hazen SL, Saffitz JE, Gross RW: The rapid and reversible activation of a calcium-dependent plasmalogen-selective phospholipase A_2 during myocardial ischemia. *J Clin Invest* 88:331–335, 1991.
30. Hazen SL, Ford DA, Gross RW: Activation of a membrane-associated phospholipase A_2 during rabbit myocardial ischemia which is highly selective for plasmalogen substrate. *J Biol Chem* 266:5629–5633, 1991.
31. Gross RW: Myocardial phospholipases A_2 and their membrane substrates. *Trends Cardiovasc Med* 2:115–121, 1992.
32. Schwertz DW, Halverson J: Changes in phosphoinositide-specific phospholipase C and phospholipase A_2 activity in ischemic and reperfused rat heart. *Basic Res Cardiol* 87:113–127, 1992.
33. Snyder DW, Crafford WA Jr, Glashow JL, Rankin D, Sobel BE, Corr PB: Lysophosphoglycerides in ischemic myocardium effluents and potentiation of their arrhythmogenic effects. *Am J Physiol* 243:H700–H707, 1981.
34. Akita H, Creer MH, Yamada KA, Sobel BE, Corr PB: Electrophysiologic effects of intracellular lysophosphoglycerides and their accumulation in cardiac lymph with myo-

cardial ischemia in dogs. *J Clin Invest* 78:271–280, 1986.

35. Sedlis SP, Sequeira JM, Altszuler HM: Coronary sinus lysophosphatidylcholine accumulation during rapid atrial pacing. *Am J Cardiol* 66:695–698, 1990.

36. Broekman MJ, Ward JW, Marcus AJ: Phospholipid metabolism in stimulated human platelets. Changes in phosphatidylinositol, phosphatidic acid, and lysophospholipids. *J Clin Invest* 66:275–283, 1980.

37. McHowat J, Corr PB: Thrombin-induced release of lysophosphatidylcholine from endothelial cells. *J Biol Chem* 268:15605–15610, 1993.

38. McHowat J, Corr PB: Mechanisms underlying the thrombin induced increase in lysophosphatidylcholine in endothelial cells (abstr). *Circulation* 86(Suppl I):740, 1992.

39. McHowat J, Corr PB: Thrombin induced increases in lysophosphatidylcholine in adult ventricular myocytes (abstr). *Circulation* 86(Suppl I):821, 1992.

40. Whitmer JT, Idell-Wenger JA, Rovetto MJ, Neely JR: Control of fatty acid metabolism in ischemic and hypoxic hearts. *J Biol Chem* 253:4305–4309, 1978.

41. Corr PB, Saffitz JE, Sobel BE: What is the contribution of altered lipid metabolism to arrhythmogenesis in the ischemic heart? In: Hearse D, Manning A, Janse M (eds) *Life-Threatening Arrhythmias During Ischemia and Infarction*. New York: Raven Press, 1987, pp 91–114.

42. van der Vusse GJ, Roemen Th HM, Prizen FW, Couman WA, Reneman RS: Uptake and tissue content of fatty acids in dog myocardium under normoxic and ischemic conditions. *Circ Res* 50:538–546, 1982.

43. van der Vusse GJ, Glatz JFC, Stam HCG, Reneman RS: Fatty acid homeostasis in the normoxic and ischemic heart. *Physiol Rev* 72:881–940, 1992.

44. Oram JF, Wenger JI, Neely JR: Regulation of long chain fatty acid activation in heart muscle. *J Biol Chem* 250:73–78, 1975.

45. Haddock BA, Yates DW, Garland PB: The localization of some coenzyme A-dependent enzymes in rat liver mitochondria. *Biochem J* 119:565–573, 1970.

46. Brosnan JT, Fritz IB: The permeability of mitochondria to carnitine and acetylcarnitine. *Biochem J* 125:94P–95P, 1971.

47. Pande SV: A mitochondrial carnitine acylcarnitine translocase system: Carnitine acylcarnitine transport/exchange diffusion/acyl(+)carnitine inhibition/fatty acyl transport. *Proc Natl Acad Sci USA* 72:883–887, 1975.

48. Ramsey RR, Tubbs PK: The mechanism of fatty acid uptake by heart mitochondria: An acylcarnitine-carnitine exchange. *FEBS Lett* 54:21–25, 1975.

49. Shug AL, Thomsen JH, Folts JD, Bittar N, Klein MI, Koke JR, Huth PJ: Changes in tissue levels of carnitine and other metabolites during myocardial ischemia and anoxia. *Arch Biochem Biophys* 187:25–33, 1978.

50. Hochachka PW, Neely JR, Driedzic WR: Integration of lipid utilization with Krebs cycle activity in muscle. *Fed Proc* 36:2009–2014, 1977.

51. Idell-Wenger JA, Grotyohann LW, Neely JR: Coenzyme A and carnitine distribution in normal and ischemic hearts. *J Biol Chem* 253:4310–4318, 1978.

52. Liedtke AJ, Nellis S, Neely JR: Effects of excess free fatty acids on mechanical and metabolic function in normal and ischemic myocardium in swine. *Circ Res* 43:652–661, 1978.

53. Pauly DF, Yoon SB, McMillin JB: Carnitine-acylcarnitine translocase in ischemia: Evidence for sulfhydryl modification. *Am J Physiol* 253:H1557–H1565, 1987.

54. Kopec B, Fritz IB: Properties of a purified carnitine palmitoyltransferase, and evidence for the existence of other carnitine acyltransferases. *Can J Biochem* 49:941–948, 1971.

55. Moore KH, Bonema JE, Solomon FJ: Long-chain acyl-CoA and acylcarnitine hydrolase activities in normal and ischemic rabbit heart. *J Mol Cell Cardiol* 16:905–913, 1984.

56. DeTorre SD, Creer MH, Pogwizd SM, Corr PB: Amphipathic lipid metabolites and their relation to arrhythmogenesis in the ischemic heart. *J Mol Cell Cardiol* 23(Suppl I):11–22, 1991.

57. Corr PB, Creer MH, Yamada KA, Saffitz JE, Sobel BE: Prophylaxis of early ventricular fibrillation by inhibition of acylcarnitine accumulation. *J Clin Invest* 83:927–936, 1989.

58. Knabb MT, Saffitz JE, Corr PB, Sobel BE: The dependence of electrophysiological derangements on accumulation of endogenous long-chain acylcarnitine in hypoxic neonatal rat myocytes. *Circ Res* 58:230–240, 1986.

59. Heathers GP, Yamada KA, Kanter EM, Corr PB: Long-chain acylcarnitines mediate the hypoxia-induced increase in α_1-adrenergic receptors on adult canine myocytes. *Circ Res* 61:735–746, 1987.

60. Priori SG, Yamada KA, Corr PB: Influence of hypoxia on adrenergic modulation of triggered activity in isolated adult canine myocytes. *Circulation* 83:248–259, 1991.

61. McHowat J, Yamada KA, Saffitz JE, Corr PB: Subcellular distribution of endogenous long chain acylcarnitines during hypoxia in adult canine myocytes. *Cardiovasc Res* 27:1237–1243, 1993.

62. Gross RW, Sobel BE: Lysophosphatidylcholine metabolism in the rabbit heart. Characterization of metabolic pathways and partial purification of myocardial lysophospholipase-transacylase. *J Biol Chem* 257:6702–6708, 1982.

63. Gross RW, Ahumada GG, Sobel BE: Cytosolic lysophospholipase in cardiac myocytes and its inhibition by L-palmitoyl carnitine. *Am J Physiol* 246:C266–C270, 1984.

64. Gross RW: Purification of rabbit myocardial cytosolic acyl CoA hydrolase, identity with lysophospholipase, and modulation of enzymic activity by endogenous cardiac amphiphiles. *Biochemistry* 22:5641–5646, 1983.

65. Gross RW, Sobel BE: Rabbit myocardial cytosolic lysophospholipase: Purification, characterization, and competitive inhibition by L-palmitoyl carnitine. *J Biol Chem* 258:5221–5226, 1983.

66. Gross RW, Drisdel RC, Sobel BE: Rabbit myocardial lysophospholipase-transacylase: Purification, characterization and inhibition by endogenous cardiac amphiphiles. *J Biol Chem* 258:15165–15172, 1983.

67. Corr PB, Snyder DW, Cain ME, Crafford WA Jr, Gross RW, Sobel BE: Electrophysiological effects of amphiphiles on canine Purkinje fibers. Implications for dysrhythmia secondary to ischemia. *Circ Res* 49:354–363, 1981.

68. Corr PB, Cain ME, Witkowski FX, Price DA, Sobel BE: Potential arrhythmogenic electrophysiological derangements in canine Purkinje fibers induced by lysophosphoglycerides. *Circ Res* 44:822–832, 1979.

69. Mészàros J, Pappano AJ: Electrophysiological effects of L-palmitoylcarnitine in single ventricular myocytes. *Am J Physiol* 258:H931–H938, 1990.

70. Aomine M, Arita M, Shimada T: Effects of L-propionylcarnitine on electrical and mechanical alterations induced by amphiphilic lipids in isolated guinea pig ventricular muscle. *Heart Vessels* 4:197–206, 1988.

71. Sedlis SP, Sequeira JM, Altszuler HM: Potentiation of the depressant effects of lysophosphatidylcholine on contractile properties of cultured cardiac myocytes by acidosis and superoxide radical. *J Lab Clin Med* 115:203–216, 1990.

72. Man RYK, Kinnaird AAA, Bihler L, Choy PC: The association of lysophosphatidylcholine with isolated cardiac myocytes. *Lipids* 25:450–454, 1990.

73. Man RYK: Lysophosphatidylcholine-induced arrhythmias and its accumulation in the rat perfused heart. *Br J Pharmacol* 93:412–416, 1988.

74. Giffin M, Arthur G, Choy PC, Man RYK: Lysophosphatidyl choline metabolism and cardiac arrhythmias. *Can J Physiol* 66:185–189, 1988.

75. Arnsdorf MF, Sawicki GJ: The effects of lysophosphatidylcholine, a toxic metabolite of ischemia, on the components of cardiac excitability in sheep Purkinje fibers. *Circ Res* 49:16–30, 1981.

76. Elharrar V, Foster PR, Jirak TL, Gaum WE, Zipes DP: Alterations in canine myocardial excitability during ischemia. *Circ Res* 40:98–105, 1977.

77. Burnashev NA, Undrovinas AI, Fleidervish IA, Makielski JC, Rosenshtraukh LV: Modulation of cardiac sodium channel gating by lysophosphatidylcholine. *J Mol Cell Cardiol* 23(Suppl I):23–30, 1991.

78. Undrovinas AI, Fleidervish IA, Makielski JC: Inward sodium current at resting potentials in single cardiac myocytes induced by the ischemic metabolite lysophosphatidylcholine. *Circ Res* 71:1231–1241, 1992.

79. Wu J, Corr PB: Two distinct inward currents underlie the development of oscillatory membrane potentials by long-chain acylcarnitines in adult ventricular myocytes (abstr). *Circulation* 86(Suppl I):565, 1992.

80. Sato T, Kiyosue T, Arita M: Inhibitory effects of palmitoylcarnitine and lysophosphatidylcholine on the sodium current of cardiac ventricular cells. *Pflügers Arch* 420:94–100, 1992.

81. Clarkson CW, Ten Eick RE: On the mechanism of lysoposphatidylcholine-induced depolarization of cat ventricular myocardium. *Circ Res* 52:543–556, 1983.

82. Kiyosue T, Arita M: Effects of lysophosphatidylcholine on resting potassium conductance of isolated guinea pig ventricular cells. *Pflügers Arch* 406:296–302, 1986.

83. Dörr T, Denger R, Dörr A, Trautwein W: Ionic currents contributing to the action potential in single ventricular myocytes of the guinea pig studied with action potential clamp. *Pflügers Arch* 416:230–237, 1990.

84. Fabiato A: Rapid ionic modificaton during the aequorin-detected calcium transient in a skinned canine cardiac Purkinje cell. *J Gen Physiol* 85:189–246, 1985.

85. Fabiato A: Time and calcium dependence of activation and inactivation of calcium-induced release of calcium from the sarcoplasmic reticulum of a skinned canine cardiac Purkinje cell. *J Gen Physiol* 85:247–290, 1985.

86. Fabiato A: Stimulated calcium current can both cause calcium loading in and trigger calcium release from the sarcoplasmic reticulum of a skinned canine Purkinje cell. *J Gen Physiol* 85:291–320, 1985.

87. Inoue D, Pappano AJ: L-palmitylcarnine and calcium ions act similarly on excitatory ionic currents in avian ventricular muscle. *Circ Res* 52:625–634, 1983.

88. Spedding M, Mir AK: Direct activation of Ca^{2+} channels by palmitoyl carnitine, a putative endogenous ligand. *Br J Pharmacol* 92:457–468, 1987.

89. Spedding M: Activators and inactivators of Ca^{2+} channels: New perspectives. *J Pharmacol* 16:319–343, 1985.

90. Wu J, Corr PB: Influence of long chain acylcarnitines on the voltage-dependent calcium current in adult ventricular myocytes. *Am J Physiol* 263 *(Heart Circ Physiol 32)*: H410–H417, 1992.

91. Hajdu S, Weiss H, Titus E: The isolation of a cardiac active principle from mammalian tissue. *J Pharmacol Exp Ther* 120:99–113, 1957.

92. Pogwizd SM, Onufer JR, Kramer JB, Sobel BE, Corr PB: Induction of delayed afterdepolarizations and triggered activity in canine Purkinje fibers by lysophosphoglycerides. *Circ Res* 59:416–426, 1986.

93. Lee HC, Smith N, Mohabir R, Clusin WT: Cytosolic calcium transients from the beating mammalian heart. *Proc Natl Acad Sci USA* 84:7793–7797, 1987.

94. Lee HC, Mohabir R, Smith N, Franz MR, Clusin WT: Effect of ischemia on calcium-dependent fluorescence transients in rabbit hearts containing Indo-1. Correlation with monophasic action potentials and contraction. *Circulation* 78:1047–1059, 1988.

95. Allen DG, Lee JA, Smith GL: The consequences of simulated ischaemia on intracellular Ca^{2+} and tension in isolated ferret ventricular muscle. *J Physiol* 410:297–323, 1989.

96. Lee JA, Allen DG: Changes in intracellular free calcium concentration during long exposures to simulated ischemia in isolated mammalian ventricular muscle. *Circ Res* 71:58–69, 1992.

97. Marban E, Kitakaze M, Koretsune Y, Yue D, Chacko VP, Pike MM: Quantification of $[Ca^{2+}]_i$ in perfused hearts: Critical evaluation of 5F-BAPTA and nuclear magnetic resonance method as applied to the study of ischemia and reperfusion. *Circ Res* 66:1255–1267, 1990.

98. Marban E, Kitakaze M, Kusuoka H, Porterfield JK, Yue DT, Chacko VP: Intracellular free calcium concentration measured with ^{19}F NMR spectroscopy in intact ferret hearts. *Proc Natl Acad Sci USA* 84:6005–6009, 1987.

99. Steenbergen C, Murphy E, Levy L, London RE: Elevation in cytosolic free calcium concentration early in myocardial ischemia in perfused rat heart. *Circ Res* 60:700–707, 1987.

100. Kawaguchi H, Shoki M, Iizuka K, Sano H, Sakata Y, Yasuda H: Phospholipid metabolism and prostacyclin synthesis in hypoxic myocytes. *Biochim Biophys Acta* 1094:161–167, 1991.

101. Yamada KA, Corr PB: Effects of β-adrenergic receptor activation on intracellular calcium and membrane potential in adult cardiac myocytes. *J Cardiovasc Electrophsyiol* 3:209–224, 1992.

102. Liu E, Goldhaber JI, Weiss JN: Effects of lysophosphatidylcholine on electrophysiological properties and excitation-contraction coupling in isolated guinea pig ventricular myocytes. *J Clin Invest* 88:1819–1832, 1991.

103. Woodley SL, Ikenouchi H, Barry WH: Lysophosphatidylcholine increases cytosolic calcium in ventricular myocytes by direct action on the sarcolemma. *J Mol Cell Cardiol* 23:671–680, 1991.

104. Fischbach PS, Corr PB, Yamada KA: Long-chain acylcarnitine increases intracellular Ca^{2+} and induces afterdepolarizations in adult ventricular myocytes. *Circulation* 86(Suppl I):748, 1992.

105. Ver Donck L, Verellen G, Geerts H, Borgers M: Lysophosphatidylcholine-induced Ca^{2+}-overload in isolated cardiomyocytes and effect of cytoprotective drugs. *J Mol Cell Cardiol* 24:977–988, 1992.

106. Haigney MCP, Miyata H, Lakatta EG, Stern MD, Silverman HS: Dependence of hypoxic cellular calcium loading on Na^+-Ca^{2+} exchange. *Circ Res* 71:547–557, 1992.

107. Lamers JMJ, Stinis HT, Montfoort AD, Hülsmann WC: The effect of lipid intermediates on Ca^{2+} and Na^+ permeability and $(Na^+ + K^+)$-ATPase of cardiac sarcolemma. *Biochim Biophys Acta* 774:127–137, 1984.

108. Lamers JMJ, de Jonge-Stinis JT, Verdouw PD, Hülsmann WC: On the possible role of long chain fatty acylcarnitine accumulation in producing functional and calcium permeability changes in membranes during myocardial ischaemia. *Cardiovasc Res* 21:313–322, 1987.

109. Gadsby DC: The Na/K pump of cardiac myocytes. In: Zipes DP, Jalife J (eds) *Cardiac Electrophysiology: From Cell to Bedside*. Philadelphia: WB Saunders, 1990, pp 35–51.

110. Mullins LJ: *Ion Transport in Heart*. New York: Raven Press, 1981.

111. Reuter H: Na-Ca countertransport in cardiac muscle. In: Martonosi AN (ed) *Membranes and Transport*, Vol 1. New York: Plenum Press, 1982.

112. Reeves JP: The sarcolemmal sodium-calcium exchange system. In: Shamoo A (ed) *Regulation of Calcium Transport Across Muscle Membranes*. New York: Academic Press, 1985.

113. Kléber AG: Resting membrane potential, extracellular potassium activity and intracellular sodium activity during acute global ischemia in the isolated guinea pig heart. *Circ Res* 52:442–450, 1983.

114. Wilde AAM, Kléber AG: The combined effects of hypoxia, high K$^+$, and acidosis on the intracellular sodium activity and resting potential in guinea pig papillary muscle. *Circ Res* 58:249–256, 1986.

115. Ellis D, Noireaud J: Intracellular pH in sheep Purkinje fibers and ferret papillary muscles during hypoxia and recovery. *J Physiol (Lond)* 383:125–141, 1987.

116. Guarnieri T: Intracellular sodium-calcium dissociation in early contractile failure in hypoxic ferret papillary muscles. *J Physiol (Lond)* 388:449–465, 1987.

117. Nakaya H, Kimura S, Kanno M: Extracellular potassium activity and intracellular sodium activity under hypoxia, acidosis, and no glucose in dog hearts. *Am J Physiol* 249:H1078–H1085, 1985.

118. Balschi JA, Frazer JC, Fetters JK, Clarke K, Springer CS, Smith TW, Ingwall JS: Shift reagent and Na-23 nuclear magnetic resonance discriminates between extra and intracellular sodium pools in ischemic heart. *Circulation* 72(Suppl 3):355, 1985.

119. Fiolet JWT, Baartscheer A, Schumacher CA, Coronel R, Ter Welle HF: The change of the free energy of ATP hydrolysis during global ischemia and anoxia in the rat heart. Its possible role in the regulation of the transsarcolemmal sodium and potassium gradients. *J Mol Cell Cardiol* 16:1023–1036, 1984.

120. Bersohn MM, Philipson KD, Fukushima JY: Sodium-calcium exchange and sarcolemmal enzymes in ischemic rabbit hearts. *Am J Physiol* 242:C288–C295, 1982.

121. Daly MJ, Elz JS, Nayler WG: Sarcolemmal enzymes and Na$^+$-Ca^{2+} exchange in hypoxic, ischemic, and reperfused rat hearts. *Am J Physiol* 247:H237–H243, 1984.

122. Dhalla NS, Panagia V, Singal PK, Makino N, Dixon IM, Eyolfson DA: Alterations in heart membrane calcium transport during the development of ischemia-reperfusion injury. *J Mol Cell Cardiol* 20:3–13, 1988.

123. Vrbjar N, Slezak J, Ziegelhoffer A, Tribulova N: Features of the (Na,K)-ATPase of cardiac sarcolemma with particular reference to myocardial ischaemia. *Eur Heart J* 12(Suppl F):149–152, 1991.

124. Winston DC, Spinale FG, Crawford FA, Schulte BA: Immunocytochemical and enzyme histochemical localization of Na$^+$,K$^+$-ATPase in normal and ischemic porcine myocardium. *J Mol Cell Cardiol* 22:1071–1082, 1990.

125. Adams RJ, Pitts BJR, Wood JM, Gende DA, Wallick ET, Schwartz A: Effect of palmitoyl carnitine on ouabain binding to Na,K-ATPase. *J Mol Cell Cardiol* 11:941–959, 1979.

126. Adams RJ, Cohen DW, Gupte S, Johnson JD, Wallick ET, Wang T, Schwartz A: In vitro effects of palmitylcarnitine on cardiac plasma membrane Na,K-ATPase, and sarcoplasmic

127. reticulum Ca^{2+}-ATPase and Ca^{2+} transport. *J Biol Chem* 254:12404–12410, 1979.

127. Wood JM, Bush B, Pitts BJR, Schwartz A: Inhibition of bovine heart Na$^+$,K$^+$-ATPase by palmitylcarnitine and palmityl-CoA. *Biochem Biophys Res Comm* 74:677–684, 1977.

128. Abe M, Yamazaki N, Suzuki Y, Kobayashi A, Ohta H: Effect of palmitoyl carnitine on Na$^+$,K$^+$-ATPase and adenylate cyclase activity of canine myocardial sarcolemma. *J Mol Cell Cardiol* 16:239–245, 1984.

129. Owens K, Kennett FF, Weglicki WB: Effects of fatty acid intermediates on Na$^+$-K$^+$-ATPase activity of cardiac sarcolemma. *Am J Physiol* 242:H456–H461, 1982.

130. Karli JN, Karikas GA, Hatzipavlov PK, Levis GM, Moulopoulos SN: The inhibition of Na$^+$ and K$^+$ stimulated ATPase activity of rabbit and dog heart sarcolemma by lysophosphatidylcholine. *Life Sci* 24:1869–1876, 1979.

131. Bersohn MM, Philipson KD, Weiss RS: Lysophosphatidylcholine and sodium-calcium exchange in cardiac sarcolemma: Comparison with ischemia. *Am J Physiol* 260:C433–C438, 1991.

132. Philipson KD, Nishimoto AY: Stimulation of Na$^+$-Ca^{2+} exchange in cardiac sarcolemmal vesicles by proteinase pretreatment. *Am J Physiol* 243:C191–C195, 1982.

133. Pitts BJ, Tate CA, Van Winkle WB, Wood JM, Entman ML: Palmitylcarnitine inhibition of the calcium pump in cardiac sarcoplasmic reticulum: A possible role in myocardial ischemia. *Life Sci* 23:391–401, 1978.

134. Ambudkar IS, Abdallah E-S, Shamoo AE: Lysophospholipid-mediated alterations in the calcium transport systems of skeletal and cardiac muscle sarcoplasmic reticulum. *Mol Cell Biochem* 79:81–89, 1988.

135. Dosemeci A, Dhallan RS, Cohen NM, Lederer WJ, Rogers TB: Phorbol ester increases calcium current and stimulates the effects of angiotensin II on cultured neonatal rat heart myocytes. *Circ Res* 62:347–357, 1988.

136. Tseng GN, Boyden PA: Different effects of intracellular calcium and protein kinase C on the cardiac T and L Ca currents. *Am J Physiol* 261:H364–H379, 1991.

137. Oishi K, Raynor RL, Charp PA, Kuo JF: Regulation of protein kinase C by lysophospholipids. *J Biol Chem* 263:6865–6871, 1988.

138. Ford DA, Gross RW: Activation of myocardial protein kinase C by plasmalogenic diglycerides. *Am J Physiol* 258:C30–C36, 1990.

139. Ford DA, Miyake R, Glaser PE, Gross RW: Activation of protein kinase C by naturally occurring ether-linked diglycerides. *J Biol Chem* 264:13818–13824, 1989.

140. Lenzen S, Görlich J-K, Rustenbeck I: Regulation of transmembrane ion transport by reaction products of phospholipase A$_2$. I. Effects of lysophospholipids on mitochondrial Ca^{2+} transport. *Biochim Biophys Acta* 982:140–146, 1989.

141. Rustenbeck I, Eibl H, Lenzen S: Structural requirements of lysophospholipid-regulated mitochondrial Ca^{2+} transport. *Biochim Biophys Acta* 1069:99–109, 1991.

142. Case RB: Ion alterations during myocardial ischemia. *Cardiology* 56:245–262, 1971.

143. Harris AS: Potassium and experimental coronary occlusion. *Am Heart J* 71:797–802, 1966.

144. Hill JL, Gettes LS: Effect of acute coronary occlusion on local myocardial extracellular K$^+$ activity in swine. *Circulation* 61:768–778, 1980.

145. Weiss J, Shine KI: Extracellular K$^+$ accumulation during myocardial ischemia in isolated rabbit heart. *Am J Physiol* 242:H619–H628, 1982.

146. Kléber AG: Resting membrane potential, extracellular

potassium activity, and intracellular sodium activity during acute global ischemia in isolated perfused guinea pig hearts. *Circ Res* 52:442–450, 1983.

147. Kléber AG: Extracellular potassium accumulation in acute myocardial ischemia. *J Mol Cell Cardiol* 16:389–394, 1984

148. Wiegand V, Güggi M, Meesmann W, Kessler M, Greitschuss F: Extracellular potassium activity changes in the canine myocardium after acute coronary occlusion and the influence of beta-blockade. *Cardiovasc Res* 13:297–302, 1979.

149. Kléber AG, Riegger CB, Janse MJ: Extracellular K⁺ and H⁺ shifts in early ischemia: Mechanisms and relation to changes in impulse propagation. *J Mol Cell Cardiol* 19(Suppl V):35–44, 1987.

150. Cascio WE, Yan G-X, Kléber AG: Passive electrical properties, mechanical activity, and extracellular potassium in arterially perfused and ischemic rabbit ventricular muscle. Effects of calcium entry blockade or hypocalcemia. *Circ Res* 66:1461–1473, 1990.

151. Gettes LS, Surawicz B, Shiue JD: Effect of high K⁺, low K⁺ and quinidine on QRS duration and ventricular action potential. *Am J Physiol* 203:1135–1140, 1963.

152. Weidmann S: The effect of the cardiac membrane potential on the rapid availability of the sodium-carrying system. *J Physiol* 27:213–224, 1955.

153. Weidmann S: Shortening of the action potential due to brief injections of KCl following the onset of activity. *J Physiol* 132:156–163, 1956.

154. Skinner RB Jr, Kunze DL: Changes in extracellullar potassium activity in response to decreased pH in rabbit atrial muscle. *Circ Res* 39:678–683, 1976.

155. Noma A: ATP-regulated K⁺ channels in cardiac muscle. *Nature* 305:147–148, 1983.

156. Elliott AC, Smith GL, Allen DG: Simultaneous measurements of action potential duration and intracellular ATP in isolated ferret hearts exposed to cyanide. *Circ Res* 64:583–591, 1989.

157. Yan G-X, Yamada KA, Kléber AG, McHowat J, Corr PB: Dissociation between cellular K⁺ loss, reduction in repolarization time, and tissue ATP levels during myocardial hypoxia and ischemia. *Circ Res* 72:560–570, 1993.

158. Nichols CG, Ripoll C, Lederer WJ: ATP-sensitive potassium channel modulation of the guinea pig ventricular action potential and contraction. *Circ Res* 68:280–287, 1991.

159. Baumgarten CM, Cohen CJ, McDonald TF: Heterogeneity of intracellular potassium activity and membrane potential in hypoxic guinea pig ventricle. *Circ Res* 49:1181–1189, 1981.

160. Mercer RW, Dunham PB: Membrane-bound ATP fuels the Na/K pump. *J Gen Physiol* 78:547–568, 1981.

161. Paul RJ: Functional compartment of oxidative and glycolytic metabolism in vascular smooth muscle. *Am J Physiol* 244:C399–C409, 1983.

162. Jones DP: Intracellular diffusion gradients of O₂ and ATP. *Am J Physiol* 250:C663–C675, 1986.

163. Weiss JN, Lamp ST: Cardiac ATP-sensitive K⁺ channels. *J Gen Physiol* 94:911–937, 1989.

164. Kantor PF, Coetzee WA, Carmeliet EE, Dennis SC, Opie HL: Reduction of ischemic K⁺ loss and arrhythmias in rat hearts: Effect of glibenclamide, a sulfonylurea. *Circ Res* 66:478–485, 1990.

165. Gasser RNA, Vaughan-Jones RD: Mechanisms of potassium efflux and action potential shortening during ischemia in isolated mammalian cardiac muscle. *J Physiol* 431:713–741, 1990.

166. Deutsch N, Klitzner TS, Lamp ST, Weiss JN: Activation of

167. Cook GA: The hypoglycemic sulfonylureas glyburide and tolbutamide inhibit fatty acid oxidation by inhibiting carnitine palmitoyltransferase. *J Biol Chem* 262:4968–4972, 1987.

168. Wilde AAM, Escande D, Schumacher CA, Thuringer D, Mestre M, Fiolet JWT, Janse MJ: Potassium accumulation in the globally ischemic mammalian heart: A role for the ATP-sensitive potassium channel, *Circ Res* 67:835–843, 1990.

169. Venkatesh N, Lamp ST, Weiss JN: Sulfonylureas, ATP-sensitive K⁺ channels, and cellular K⁺ loss during hypoxia, ischemia, and metabolic inhibition in mammalian ventricle. *Circ Res* 69:623–637, 1991.

170. Kim D, Duff RA: Regulation of K⁺ channels in cardiac myocytes by free fatty acids. *Circ Res* 67:1040–1046, 1990.

171. Guthrie SC: Intercellular communication in embryos. In: De Mello WC (ed) *Cell-to-Cell Communication*. New York: Plenum Press, 1987, pp 223–244.

172. Sheridan JD: Cell communication and growth. In: De Mello WC (ed) *Cell-to-Cell Communication*. New York: Plenum Press, 1987, pp 187–222.

173. Peterson OH: Importance of electrical cell-to-cell communication in secretory epithelia. In: Bennett MVL, Spray DC (eds) *Gap Junctions*. Cold Spring Harbor, NY: Cold Spring Harbor Laboratory, 1985, pp 315–324.

174. Meda P, Bruzzone R, Chanson M, Bosco D, Orci L: Gap junctional coupling modulates secretion of exocrine pancreas. *Proc Natl Acad Sci USA* 84:4901–4904, 1987.

175. Fozzard HA: Conduction of the action potential. In: *Handbook of Physiology 1*, Section 2, *Cardiovascular System*. Bethesda. MD: American Physiological Society, 1979, pp 335–356.

176. Daniel EE: Gap junctions in smooth muscle. In: De Mello WC (ed) *Cell-to-Cell Communication*. New York: Plenum Press, 1987, pp 149–185.

177. Jaslove SW, Brink PR: Electrotonic coupling in the nervous system. In: De Mello WC (ed) *Cell-to-Cell Communication*. New York: Plenum Press, 1987, pp 103–147.

178. Weidmann S: The diffusion of radiopotassium across intercalated disks of mammalian cardiac muscle. *J Physiol* 187:323–342, 1966.

179. Weidmann S: Electrical constants of trabecular muscle from mammalian heart. *J Physiol* 210:1041–1054, 1970.

180. Cranefield PF: *The Conduction of the Cardiac Impulse.* Mount Kisco, NY: Futura, 1975.

181. White RL, Spray DC, Campos de Carvalho AC, Wittenberg BA, Bennett MVL: Some electrical and pharmacological properties of gap junctions between adult ventricular myocytes. *Am J Physiol* 249:C447–C455, 1985.

182. Maurer P, Weingart R: Cell pairs isolated from adult guinea pig and rat hearts: Effects of [Ca²⁺]ᵢ on nexal membrane resistance. *Pflügers Arch* 409:394–402, 1987.

183. Noma A, Tsuboi N: Dependence of junctional conductance on proton, calcium and magnesium ions in paired cardiac cells of guinea pig. *J Physiol (Lond)* 382:193–211, 1987.

184. Niggli E, Rüdisüli A, Maurer P, Weingart R: Effects of general anesthetics on current flow across membranes in guinea pig myocytes. *Am J Physiol* 256:C273–C281, 1989.

185. Burt JM, Spray DC: Volatile anesthetics block intercellular communication between neonatal rat myocardial cells. *Circ Res* 65:829–837, 1989.

186. Terrar DA, Victory JGG: Influence of halothane on electrical coupling in cell pairs isolated from guinea-pig ven-

tricle. *Br J Pharmacol* 94:509–514, 1988.

187. Jalife J, Sicouri S, Delmar M, Michaels DC: Electrical uncoupling and impulse propagation in isolated sheep Purkinje fibers. *Am J Physiol* 257:H179–H189, 1989.

188. Rüdisüli A, Weingart R: Electrical properties of gap junction channels in guinea-pig ventricular cell pairs revealed by exposure to heptanol. *Pflügers Arch* 415:12–21, 1989.

189. Burt JM, Spray DC: Arachidonic acid uncouples cardiac myocytes. *Biophys J* 55:217a, 1989.

190. Burt JM, Massey KD, Minnich BN: Uncoupling of cardiac cells by fatty acids: Structure-activity relationships. *Am J Physiol* 260:C439–C448, 1991.

191. Fluri GS, Rüdisüli A, Willi M, Rohr S, Weingart R: Effects of arachidonic acid on the gap junctions of neonatal rat heart cells. *Pflügers Arch* 417:149–156, 1990.

192. Ovadia M, Burt JM: Developmental modulation of susceptibility to arrhythmogenesis in myocardial ischemia: Reduced sensitivity of adult vs. neonatal heart cells to uncoupling by lipophilic substances (abstr). *Circulation* 84(Suppl II):II324, 1991.

193. DeMello WC: Intercellular communication in cardiac muscle: Physiological and pathological implications. In: Zipes DP (ed) *Cardiac Electrophysiology and Arrhythmias.* New York: Grune & Stratton, 1985.

194. Burt JM, Spray DC: Inotropic agents modulate gap junctional conductance between cardiac myocytes. *Am J Physiol* 254:H1206–H1210, 1988.

195. Wu J, McHowat J, Saffitz JE, Yamada KA, Corr PB: Inhibition of gap junctional conductance by long-chain acylcarnitines and their preferential accumulation in junctional sarcolemma during hypoxia. *Circ Res* 72:879–889, 1993.

196. Hiramatsu Y, Buchanan JW, Krisley SB, Gettes LS: Rate-dependent effects of hypoxia on internal longitudinal resistance in guinea pig papillary muscles. *Circ Res* 63:923–929, 1988.

197. Ikeda K, Hiraoka M: Effects of hypoxia on passive electrical properties of canine ventricular muscle. *Pflügers Arch* 393:45–50, 1982.

198. Riegger CB, Alperovich G, Kléber AG: Effect of oxygen withdrawal on active and passive electrical properties of arterially perfused rabbit ventricular muscle. *Circ Res* 64:532–541, 1989.

199. Streit J: Effects of hypoxia and glycolytic inhibition on electrical properties of sheep cardiac Purkinje fibers. *J Mol Cell Cardiol* 19:875–885, 1987.

200. Wojtczak J: Contractures and increase in internal longitudinal resistance of cow ventricular muscle induced by hypoxia. *Circ Res* 44:88–95, 1979.

201. Hoyt RH, Cohen ML, Corr PB, Saffitz JE: Alterations of intercellular junctions induced by hypoxia in canine myocardium. *Am J Physiol* 258:H1439–H1448, 1990.

202. Reber WR, Weingart R: Ungulate cardiac Purkinje fibers: The influence of intracellular pH on the electrical cell-to-cell coupling. *J Physiol* 328:87–104, 1982.

203. Yamada KA, McHowat J, Yan G-X, Donahue K, Peirick J, Kléber AG, Corr PB: Cellular uncoupling induced by accumulation of long-chain acylcarnitine during ischemia. *Circ Res* 74:83–95, 1994.

204. Dillon S, Allessi M, Ursell P, Wit A: Influences of anisotropic tissue structure on reentrant circuits in the epicardial border zone of subacute canine infarcts. *Circ Res* 63:182–206, 1988.

205. Quan W, Rudy Y: Unidirectional block and reentry of cardiac excitation: A model study. *Circ Res* 66:367–382, 1990.

206. Pogwizd SM, Corr PB: Electrophysiologic and biochemical mechanisms underlying malignant ventricular arrhythmias during early myocardial ischemia. In: Heusch G (ed) *Pathophysiology and Rational Pharmacotherapy of Myocardial Ischemia.* Darmstadt: Steinkopff Verlag, 1990, pp 137–173.

CHAPTER 28

Cellular Electrophysiology and Ischemia

EUGENE PATTERSON, BENJAMIN J. SCHERLAG, & RALPH LAZZARA

INTRODUCTION

The study of the cellular electrophysiologic effects of ischemia has been frustrated by the difficulty of evaluating the properties of individual myocytes in the beating heart. Intracellular recordings are exceedingly difficult both to obtain and maintain in actively contracting tissues. Studies of individual cells within the intact heart are further complicated by the low-resistance, intercellular connections of the multicellular matrix and the inhomogeneity of injury observed with myocardial ischemia. The difficulties imposed by in vivo cellular electrophysiologic studies have been successfully endured or conquered by few investigators, compelling other investigators to use less direct approaches to the study of cellular electrophysiology and myocardial ischemia.

A common experimental approach has been to "simulate ischemia" in superfused myocardial tissue preparations in vitro using hypoxia or "ischemic" superfusion solutions designed to mimic the extracellular milieu of acute ischemia. Although lactic acidosis, respiratory acidosis, hypoxia, and hyperkalemia reproduce some of the metabolic abnormalities associated with acute ischemia, the entire spectrum of changes produced by acute ischemia can not be accurately simulated in nonperfused tissue preparations. The approach also suffers from defects in our present knowledge concerning relevant changes in the extracellular milieu occurring at various times during the ischemic process.

Another experimental approach has been to produce myocardial ischemia or infarction in vivo and to study the superfused isolated tissue or enzymatically dispersed myocytes in vitro. Conclusions based upon observations and interventions performed under these circumstances require the assumption that the electrophysiologic changes caused by ischemic injury in vivo persist during prolonged periods of superfusion in vitro, even though the superfusate contains adequate oxygen and substrates. An inherent presumption of the method is that the electrophysiologic alterations in the isolated tissue are lasting and stable, and independent of any continuing myocardial ischemia.

The ensuing discussion will concentrate on four different models of myocardial ischemic injury studied using intracellular recordings: (a) simulated ischemia or hypoxia, (b) acute global or regional ischemia in blood-perfused or buffer-perfused mammalian hearts, (c) isolated mammalian tissues studied in vitro following extended periods of coronary artery ligation in vivo, and (d) enzymatically dispersed myocytes obtained from the endocardial or epicardial border zones of mammalian hearts previously subjected to coronary artery ligation.

RESTING POTENTIAL

Acute myocardial ischemia

A reduction in the resting potential of myocardial cells is observed within 1–2 minutes following coronary artery occlusion {1,2}. The extent (but not the rate) of depolarization observed in ischemic myocardium during the early minutes of ischemia is consistent with the loss of membrane potential observed following either hypoxia {3,4} or a disruption of oxidative metabolism {5}. Membrane potential is reduced in concert with the transsarcolemmal movement of potassium ions from the intracellular to the extracellular compartment {6–8}. The rise in extracellular potassium ion concentrations can be quantified using extracellular potassium ion-specific electrodes inserted at varying depths into the left ventricular free wall {9–16}. The rise in extracellular potassium is greatest and most rapid in subendocardium and is least in epicardium. Extracellular concentrations of potassium in midmyocardium attain 8–10 mM within 5–10 minutes following coronary artery occlusion {11–16}, with the resting membrane potential following 10 minutes of ischemia corresponding closely to the potential predicted by the transmural potassium gradient {13,14}. Because intracellular space is three times greater than extracellular space and intracellular potassium concentrations greatly exceed extracellular potassium ion concentrations, a large change in extracellular potassium ion concentrations and a physiologically important reduction in the resting potential can be observed despite only minor decreases in intracellular potassium ion concentrations. Intracellular sodium ion accumulation is small {13} or not observed {14} during the early stages of myocardial ischemia {13}, suggesting

N. Sperelakis (ed.), Physiology and Pathophysiology of the Heart, Third Edition.

547

that a dramatic reduction of Na,K-ATPase activity is not an important contributor to early potassium efflux.

The mechanisms responsible for the transsarcolemmal movement of potassium in the early stages of acute myocardial ischemia are not well described. Potassium ion efflux occurs in association with both phosphate and lactate efflux {14,17}. The anion loss is smaller than the total potassium ion loss and suggests a possible contribution of a variety of potassium ion channels to the aggregate potassium efflux.

1. In the isolated, perfused guinea pig heart, the potassium potential, E_k, is more negative than the resting membrane potential, V_m, in the normal state, but equalizes following a 10-minute period of myocardial ischemia. The finding suggests that relative potassium ion permeability increases during acute ischemia, with depolarization accompanying the rise in K_o^+ {13}.

2. Hypoxia produces an increase in K^+ conductance, which can be prevented by the maintenance of intracellular ATP {19}. An increase in the inwardly rectifying potassium current, I_{K1}, may also be important during the earliest minutes of myocardial ischemia, before the depletion of intracellular ATP is sufficient to prevent the activation of the ATP-dependent potassium channels {20,21}. One potential mechanism for an increase in I_{K1} is acidosis. Extracellular pH in the guinea pig myocardium decreases by approximately -0.8 units following 15 minutes of global ischemia {22}. When extracellular pH is reduced, I_{K1} (the inward rectified potassium current) is reduced in both superfused feline myocardium {23} and in isolated myocytes from guinea pig hearts {24}.

3. Potassium ion efflux is only partially suppressed by glibenclamide in ischemic rat hearts without any reduction of lactate efflux {19}. Although glibenclamide and other sulfonylurea drugs inhibit the opening of ATP-dependent potassium channels in individual cardiac myocytes {25}, and prevent the increased potassium ion permeability and loss of membrane potential accompanying ATP depletion {25,26}, the efficacy of the sulfonylureas may, however, be limited by an intracellular accumulation of ADP and ADP-induced opening of the ATP-dependent potassium channels {26}.

4. Verapamil and diltiazem, inhibitors of calcium entry through L-type calcium channels, partially reverse transsarcolemmal potassium efflux {10,27} and antagonize the loss of membrane potential {28,29} in the early minutes of myocardial ischemia. Potassium loss {30} and depolarization {29} during acute myocardial ischemia are also decreased with the reduction in extracellular calcium ion concentrations. Conversely, Bayer K8644 increases L-type calcium current and potentiates the loss of membrane potential accompanying acute myocardial ischemia in the rabbit {28}. It is intriguing to speculate that part of the transsarcolemmal potassium movement accompanying acute myocardial ischemia occurs through activation of calcium-sensitive potassium channels {31,32} activated by the increased intracellular calcium concentrations observed during myocardial ischemia {33,34}.

Although the activation of various potassium ion channels during ischemia often has been implicated in the net loss of intracellular potassium during ischemia, it is not immediately obvious that the opening of potassium ion channels should lead to potassium efflux in the absence of anion loss or the activation of other cation channels leading to increased Na_i^+ or Ca_i^{2+}. In the absence of anion loss or background inward currents, one might expect a more negative membrane potential with increased potassium ion permeability.

Transsarcolemmal potassium ion movement may not be the only basis for the loss in membrane potential observed with acute myocardial ischemia. During the first minutes of myocardial ischemia, rapid heart rates produce a greater decrease in the transmembrane potential than slow heart rates, despite the absence of differential K_o^+ accumulation {35,36} (fig. 28-1). A depolarizing (inward) current has been hypothesized to be present during the initial minutes of acute ischemia {35}, corresponding to a depolarizing current recorded in cultured myocytes exposed to metabolic inhibitors {36,37}. The current is unrelated to potassium efflux {37} and fails to reverse when the cells are clamped to potentials negative to E_k {36}. The depolarizing current is observed immediately following the administration of metabolic inhibitors and can be prevented by the removal of either sodium or calcium ions from the extracellular milieu {36}. One possible carrier of the depolarizing current is a calcium-activated nonselective cation channel described in myocytes from the guinea pig {37}. The current carried by this channel is smaller than the depolarizing current carried through the ATP-dependent channel, but may predominate during early ischemia if activated prior to ATP depletion and $I_{K(ATP)}$ activation.

Chronic ischemic injury

If coronary artery occlusion is maintained in excess of 30 minutes, even with a restoration of blood flow to the ischemic myocardium, myocardial necrosis (infarction) will be present on the subendocardial surface. Prolonged alterations in the electrical properties of surviving myocardial cells can be observed in isolated, superfused myocardial tissues more than 30 days following coronary artery ligation {39–43}, and are maintained in enzymatically dispersed myocytes during short-term culture (1–3 days) {44–46}. At both 1 and 4 days postinfarction, there is a good correlation between the electrophysiologic properties of surviving epicardial border zone cells studied as intact, superfused tissue preparations and as enzymatically dispersed epicardial myocytes {46}. This is observed despite the conspicuous possibilities for (a) the biased selection of an inappropriate subpopulation of injured cells through enzymatic dispersion/cell isolation and (b) cellular impairment with the enzymatic dispersion/isolation procedure.

Despite the presence of a normal extracellular milieu in vitro, cells in both ischemically injured Purkinje {39–41} and ventricular epicardial {42,46} tissue preparations demonstrate a reversible loss of membrane potential. The reversal of a loss of membrane potential can be observed

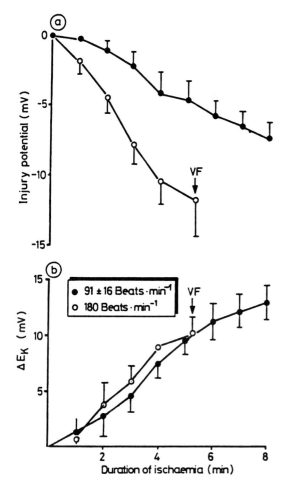

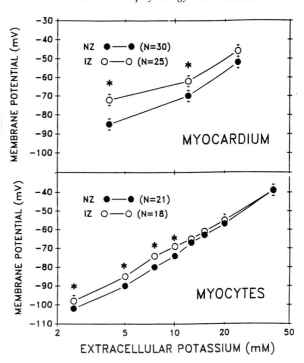

Fig. 28-2. The relationship between extracellular potassium ion concentrations and membrane potential in cells of normal and ischemically injured epicardial tissue and in enzymatically dispersed myocytes from normal epicardium and the epicardial border zone, 4 days after myocardial infarction. The differential in membrane potential between normal and injured cells, intact within tissue and isolated by enzymatic dispersion, is shown. The loss of membrane potential is most prominent at low concentrations of potassium and high levels of membrane potential (*$p <$ 0.05).

Fig. 28-1. Rate-dependent depolarization of ischemic myocardium independent of potassium efflux. Injury potentials (proportional to the loss of membrane potential) and extracellular potassium concentrations were determined before and during coronary artery occlusion in the isolated dog heart. Rapid atrial pacing increased the loss of membrane potential without increasing the rate of potassium efflux from ischemic tissue. From Blake et al. {35}, with permission from the authors and the British Medical Association.

in ventricular epicardium over a recovery period of 14–30 days in vivo {42} with a partial recovery of membrane potential of cells from 1-day-old infarcts observed over a period of several hours in superfused endocardial tissue preparations {39–41,47}. The recovery can occur in the presence of hypoxia and in the absence of oxidative/glycolytic substrates, and has suggested that washout of a depressant substrate or product of myocardial ischemia formed in vivo may provide for the prolonged recovery period observed in vitro {48}. A significant loss of membrane potential remains when enzymatically dispersed Purkinje fibers {44} or myocytes {47} bordering myocardial infarction are removed 1–4 days following coronary artery occlusion and maintained in culture medium. A

comparison of membrane potentials over a wide range of extracellular potassium concentrations can be observed for normal and ischemically injured myocardium/isolated myocytes in fig. 28-2. Although the reduction in the resting membrane potential present 24 hours following coronary artery occlusion is somewhat larger for normal and ischemically injured epicardial tissues vs. isolated myocytes, the reduced resting potential is preserved for myocytes maintained in short-term cell culture.

The basis for the prolonged loss of membrane potential unrelated to increased K_o^+ is unknown. At 24 hours following canine myocardial infarction, intracellular potassium activity is reduced and intracellular sodium ion activity is only slightly increased (ion-specific microelectrode determinations). The potassium reversal potential is reduced {47}. With prolonged superfusion, over a period of hours, the values partially recover but still remain significantly different from control values. Similar changes in intracellular potassium and sodium activity were measured in border-zone endocardial cells (but not cells underlying myocardial infarction) as late as 2–6 months following myocardial infarction in the cat {49}. As observed at 24 hours, prolonged superfusion with normal Tyrode's solution produced an increased resting potential, increased intracellular potassium ion activity, and decreased intracellular sodium accumulation {49}. Although the increased ratio of sodium ion to potassium ion permeability with ischemic injury could result from an increased sodium permeability, the observed increase in input resistance {44,45} and the altered steady-state current voltage relationship {44,45} is more consistent with a loss of sarcolemmal potassium ion permeability. In addition, reduced sodium-potassium ATPase activity cannot be directly implicated as a basis for membrane depolarization in ischemically injured subendocardial Purkinje fibers {50}. It is conceivable that a small background inward current may contribute to the decreased resting potential in canine tissues, as recently suggested for injured myocardial tissues obtained from diseased human ventricles {51}.

The resting potentials of cells from diseased human ventricular tissue are depolarized (approximately -80 to -50 mV) {52–54} and are relatively insensitive to changes in K_o^+ over the range of $2-10$ mM {52}. This finding suggested to the investigators that a dramatic decrease in potassium conductance was present and the cell failed to function as a potassium-specific electrode. Later studies have suggested that potassium permeability remains intact, with little difference between normal and ischemically injured cells at potassium concentrations above 20 mM. Instead, a Mn^{2+}-sensitive inward current may be present, depolarizing the cell {51}. The magnitude of the differences observed in diseased human ventricle and lesser findings described in the ischemically injured canine heart {46} (fig. 28-2) are dramatic and suggest fundamental differences in the underlying electrophysiology of ischemic injury or in the overall disease processes in humans and experimental animal models. Ischemic heart disease in humans is a long-term process, progressing relentlessly over a period of two or more decades. Myocardial infarction most commonly occurs in the presence of continuing coronary artery disease and relative myocardial ischemia. The disease process accumulates from repeated and continuing bouts of myocardial ischemia, with compensatory alterations of myocardial metabolism and ultrastructure. Repair may proceed slowly, interpolated between repeated bouts of reversible and irreversible injury. Our present experimental models of myocardial ischemia/infarction are performed in healthy animals, in the absence of coronary artery disease and with the rapid development of collateral circulation to the infarct border zone. The normal dog, cat, pig, or rabbit may poorly simulate the severity and incessant nature of the pathologic process in humans, and may underestimate the degree and/or the extent of protracted electrophysiologic injury present in the diseased human heart.

ACTION POTENTIAL UPSTROKE: EXCITATORY CURRENT

Acute myocardial ischemia

A pronounced depression of excitatory current (V_{max}) is observed early following coronary artery ligation {2,28, 55,56}. This observation should not be surprising in light of the potassium efflux and reduced membrane potentials observed with acute myocardial ischemia. Depolarization produces both a reduction in V_{max} by increasing the steady-state inactivation of V_{max}/I_{Na} {44–46,57} as well as modestly prolonging the time-dependent recovery of V_{max}/I_{Na} from inactivation {45,46,57}. The depression of V_{max} and conduction velocity is, however, greater than could be predicted simply from the observed change in resting potential and suggests that mechanisms additional to transsarcolemmal potassium movement and membrane depolarization are responsible for the reduction in excitatory current. At least three other factors (hypoxia, substrate depletion, and acidosis) are known to act in concert with increased extracellular potassium to alter V_{max} {14,58–60}.

As a single intervention in superfused tissue preparations, hypoxia produces rather mild effects upon both the resting potential and V_{max} of Purkinje and ventricular muscle tissue. In nonworking tissue and myocyte preparations, a prolonged hypoxia (greater than 30 minutes) or anoxia is needed to produce significant changes in resting potential and V_{max} {58,60,62,63}. The electrophysiologic effects of hypoxia are more prominent in the absence of glucose and can be partially reversed with an increase in extracellular glucose concentrations {62,63}. Acidosis also profoundly diminishes both the resting potential and V_{max} when superimposed upon increased K_o^+ {58,60,64}, but fails to further alter the mild electrophysiologic alterations observed with hypoxia {60}.

In the squid axon {65} and the frog node of Ranvier {66}, increased K_o^+ enhances voltage-dependent inactivation of i_{Na} and produces slow inactivation of sodium channels in the frog node of Ranvier {66}. Both processes may have profound effects upon excitatory current I_{Na} in acutely ischemic myocardium. Neither a shift in the voltage-dependent inactivation curve nor a prolonged recovery of V_{max} from inactivation is present in normal guinea pig myocardium with increases in K_o^+ {67}. Extracellular acidosis (pH 6.5), however, decreases V_{max} and shifts the membrane responsiveness curve in the depolarizing direction {68} without altering the recovery of V_{max} from inactivation {69}. Beta-adrenergic receptor agonists and other agents that increase cAMP shift the steady-state inactivation curve of I_{Na} to more negative potentials in mammalian cardiac cells {70}, similar to the shift in activation of I_{Na} produced by phosphorylation of the alpha subunit of the sodium channel in rat brain {71}.

Hypoxia produces both contracture and an increase in intercellular resistance in bovine Purkinje fibers. The increase occurs in conjunction with myocardial contracture and a presumed increase in intracellular calcium ion concentrations {62}. The loss of effective cellular coupling occurs only after $15-30$ minutes of acute myocardial ischemia {72}. An early increase ($0-15$ minutes) in extracellular resistance, R_o, coincides with a loss of perfusion pressure, while a later increase in internal resistance, R_i, produces effective uncoupling of the myocardium. Although the basis for the delayed rise in R_i is unknown, an increase in internal proton or calcium ion concentrations, both of which rise with acute ischemia {22,33}, could be responsible for the delayed uncoupling of individual myocardial cells.

Excitability changes may also play an important role in altering myocardial conduction velocity with acute ischemia and in altering cardiac impulse formation {73}. Following coronary artery occulusion, there is an initial increase in myocardial excitability, accompanying a small loss in membrane potential, bringing the membrane potential closer to the threshold potential {73}. The initial changes in excitability with myocardial ischemia correspond with changes observed with altered K_o^+ {74}. An initial decrease in the excitability threshold is followed by a prolonged decrease in excitability. The prolonged decrease in excitability observed in the central zone following the intial 3–5 minutes of coronary artery occlusion may contribute to slow conduction and prolonged refractoriness {16,73}. In the border zone, however, only small increases in K_o^+ may be observed and a decreased excitability may be prolonged and may facilitate impulse formation in the border zone {16}.

Chronic ischemic injury

During the first 2 weeks following myocardial infarction, there is a significant reduction in V_{max} present in surviving tissues of the epicardial {42,43} and endocardial border zones {39–41,75}. The reduction of V_{max} is maintained during prolonged periods of superfusion with oxygenated Tyrode's solution containing physiologic concentrations of electrolytes. Both the resting potential and V_{max} recover slowly during the subacute phase of myocardial infarction. Resting potential and V_{max} in the epicardial {42,75} border zones do not differ from normal tissues when studied in vitro, after 2 weeks of recovery in vivo, following myocardial infarction. The investigators did not examine the consequences of increased heart rates upon the electrophysiologic properties of epicardial cells and limited their reported observations to a paced rate of 1 Hz. Purkinje tissue from the subendocardial border zone demonstrate more prolonged electrophysiologic alterations than epicardial tissues with a 4 mV loss of membrane potential and a 150-V/s (30% decrease) in V_{max} observed as late as 7 weeks following coronary artery ligation in the dog {41}. Similar results may be observed as late as 6 months following coronary artery ligation in the feline heart {43}.

Little information is available examining the relationship between excitatory current and membrane potential in injured myocardial tissues following coronary artery occlusion, as voltage control of individual myocardial cells during excitation is exceedingly difficult. Whole-cell sodium current cannot be accurately determined at physiologic temperature, even in individual cardiac myocytes. Our current knowledge is based upon microelectrode measurements of V_{max} performed in enzymatically dispersed myocardial cells from the endocardial {44} or epicardial {45,46} border zones following myocardial infarction or upon membrane potential changes produced by alterations in K_o^+ {46}. Fortunately, there is good agreement between the alterations observed following ischemic injury in superfused epicardium in vitro and enzymatically dispersed myocytes from the epicardial border zone studied following short-term culture {46}.

Individual cells from superfused epicardium overlying

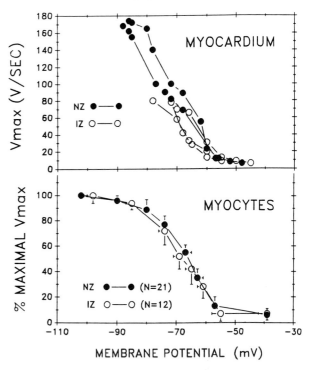

Fig. 28-3. The relationship between V_{max} and membrane potential, 1 day following myocardial infarction. In the **upper panel**, the relationship between V_{max} and membrane potential is shown for two normal epicardial cells and three ischemically injured epicardial cells, 1 day following anterior myocardial infarction in the dog. Reduced membrane potentials were produced by the addition of 24 mM potassium chloride to the superfusion solution. There is no clear distinction between the two groups in the relationship between V_{max} and membrane potential. The lack of distinction between groups is also present in enzymatically dispersed myocytes isolated from normal and ischemically injured epicardium (**lower panel**). The fractional inactivation of V_{max} with depolarization is not different for normal and injured myocardium.

myocardial infarction {42,46} and enzymatically dispersed myocytes from the epicardial border zone {46} are modestly depolarized both 24 hours and at 4–5 days following myocardial infarction (fig. 28-2). V_{max} is also moderately depressed at both intervals following myocardial infarction (figs. 28-3 and 28-4). Despite the similar changes in membrane potential and V_{max} observed at 1 and 4–5 days postinfarction in superfused subepicardial tissues and enzymatically dispersed myocytes, the electrophysiologic mechanisms responsible for the reduced membrane responsiveness may differ at the two time periods following canine myocardial infarction. At 24-hour postinfarction, V_{max} is smaller for ischemically injured versus normal myocytes at each K_o^+ concentration. The recovery of V_{max} from inactivation is also reduced (fig. 28-5). When the relationship is corrected for observed differences in resting potentials, however, the differences between normal and ischemically injured tissues are decreased and the differences between normal and ischemically injured cells can

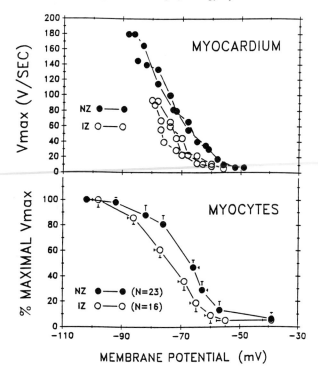

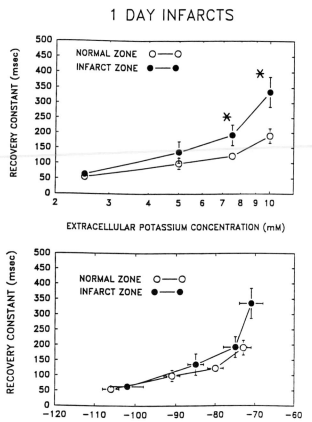

1 DAY INFARCTS

Fig. 28-4. The relationship between V_{max} and membrane potential, 4 days following myocardial ischemia. In the **upper panel**, the relationship between V_{max} and membrane potential is shown for two normal epicardial cells and three ischemically injured epicardial cells, 4 days following anterior myocardial infarction in the dog. There is a small (8 ± 2 mV; $p < 0.05$) shift in inactivation to more negative membrane potentials in the relationship between V_{max} and membrane potential with ischemic injury. The distinction between groups is also present in enzymatically dispersed myocytes isolated from normal vs. ischemically injured epicardium (**lower panel**). The fractional inactivation of V_{max} is shifted to more negative membrane potentials in injured epicardium, 4 days following myocardial infarction.

Fig. 28-5. The relationship between extracellular potassium ion concentration/membrane voltage and the first-order recovery constant for V_{max} from inactivation for myocytes isolated from normal and ischemically injured epicardium, 1 day following myocardial infarction in the dog. In the **upper panel**, at 7.5 and 10 mM, the recovery constant is significantly prolonged ($p < 0.05$) in epicardial myocytes from ischemically injured versus normal myocardium. When the differences in membrane potential at each extracellular potassium ion concentration are assessed (**lower panel**), there is no difference in the relationship between membrane voltage and first-order recovery constants from inactivation for the two treatment groups (*$p < 0.05$).

be largely explained by the reduced resting potentials observed in the ischemically injured group (figs. 28-3 and 28-5) {46}. Depolarization was the predominant, but not the only, cause for the depressed V_{max} observed in both epicardial tissue and isolated myocytes studied 24 hours following coronary artery ligation.

A second injury pattern was observed in a minority of ischemically injured cells/myocytes studied 24 hours post-infarction, and was observed in almost all of the injured cells/myocytes studied at 4 days. At 4 days, there was a (-8 ± 2 mV) shift in the steady-state inactivation curve for V_{max} with an increase in the Boltzmann constant (3.4 ± 0.5 vs. 2.9 ± 0.3; $p < 0.05$) compared to normal subepicardium. Both mild depolarization as well as increased inactivation provide for a decrease in the V_{max} observed at 4 days {46} and 5 days {45} following canine myocardial infarction. The similarities in the results were observed despite differences in the mechanisms used to produce a

change in membrane potential (current injection {45}; altered K_o^+ {46}).

Investigators have demonstrated a prolongation in the recovery of V_{max} from inactivation in enzymatically dispersed myocytes from the epicardial border zone both at both 4 days {46} (fig. 28-6) and 5 days {45} following myocardial infarction in the dog. The recovery of V_{max} from inactivation is prolonged more at depolarized membrane potentials {46} or with less negative repriming voltages {45} in both normal and ischemically injured myocytes. There is, however, a much greater prolongation of the recovery constant for V_{max} at reduced membrane potentials {45,46}. The mechanism for the prolongation of

FOUR DAY INFARCT

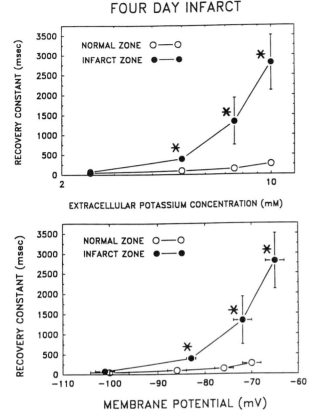

Fig. 28-6. The relationship between extracellular potassium ion concentration/membrane potential and the first-order recovery constant for V_{max} from inactivation for myocytes isolated from normal and ischemically injured epicardium, 4 days following myocardial infarction in the dog. In the **upper panel**, at 5.0, 7.5, and 10 mM, the recovery constant is significantly prolonged (*$p < 0.05$) in epicardial myocytes from ischemically injured versus normal myocardium. Unlike the recovery costant on day 1 post-infarction, when the differences in membrane potential at each extracellular potassium ion concentration are assessed (**lower panel**), a difference between the two groups in the relationship between membrane voltage and first-order recovery constants from inactivation is maintained for the two treatment groups.

recovery with ischemic injury as well as the basis for the enhanced prolongation with depolarization in the ischemically injured hearts is unknown. Both a shift in the inactivation curve as well as a prolongation of recovery of V_{max} from inactivation would be consistent with the altered conduction/refractoriness observed in ischemically injured tissues. The latter property may be essential for the observation of postrepolarization refractoriness.

The reduced membrane potentials and V_{max} observed with ischemic injury have suggested the possible involvement of slow-channel (L-type calcium channel) current as an excitatory current. The lack of any substantial contribution of L-type calcium current as an excitatory current

has been suggested by the efficacy of the selective sodium channel antagonist, tetrodotoxin, but not the L-type calcium channel antagonists, verapamil or gallopamil (methoxyverapamil), to depress excitatory current in ischemically injured epicardium overlying anterior myocardial infarction in dogs {76}. An example can be observed in fig. 28-7. Direct determinations of L-type calcium current have been performed at 5 days following canine myocardial infarction and have been determined to be significantly reduced in ischemically injured epicardial myocytes {77}. Endocardial cells with markedly depressed excitatory current from human ventricular aneurysms have demonstrated selective sensitivity to the sodium channel antagonist, tetrodotoxin, as well as selective sensitivity to calcium channel blockers {53,76}. The mere presence of slow-channel-dependent action potentials in ischemically injured tissues does not, however, imply an important role for such potentials in producing ventricular arrhythmia. The low safety factor and the high likelihood for conduction block/inexcitability would preclude any critical role of slow potentials in mediating reentrant ventricular arrhythmia.

Heterogeneity of resting potential, action potential amplitude, and V_{max} are hallmarks of cells in the epicardial border zone. An illustration of this phenomenon is shown in figs. 28-7 and 28-8. Figure 28-8 displays action potentials generated from a single ischemically injured subepicardial cell. Such a phenomenon might derive from heterogeneity of fast channels on a microscale — groups of channels in the vicinity of the microelectrode with different fundamental kinetics and voltage dependence. Differences between action potentials in panels A and B in fig. 28-8 were produced by alteration of stimulus intensity (less in panel B). It is likely that the stimulus current affected the wavefront rather than the cell itself, since the cell was activated 15–20 ms after the stimulus. The greater stimulus intensity (fig. 28-8A) was followed by an irregular upstroke, but the lesser intensity stimulus resulted in a long-step potential preceding a more regular upstroke. It has been shown that the sequence of activation in ischemically injured tissues may be irregular, especially at rapid rates when regions of refractoriness are encountered {77–79}.

Fractionated electrograms are common in subepicardium overlying myocardial infarction {80}, even as late as 3 months following coronary artery ligation. These observations have been made at a time when the resting potential, action potential amplitude, and V_{max} of subepicardial cells have returned to control values {42}. The asynchrony of activation was attributed to partial uncoupling of individual cells by interspersed fibrosis {39,80}, with a possible additional contribution of increased electrical resistance at gap junctions. Other investigators have noted irregularities of depressed upstrokes and irregularities of repolarization, in keeping with electrotonic interaction of the cells with neighboring cells {75}. Measurement of electrotonic voltage spread in ischemically injured subepicardium {81} demonstrates a reduced space constant, indicative of reduced electrical communication between individual cells. Input resistance, membrane resistance, and axial resistance are decreased with a significant decrease in membrane

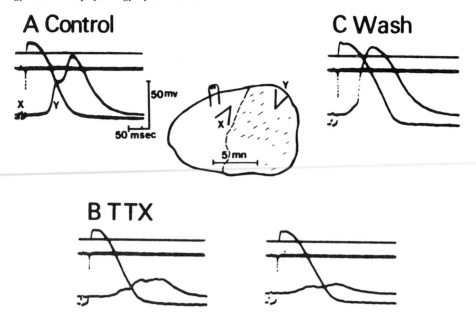

Fig. 28-7. The influence of tetrodotoxin (TTX) on the severely depressed upstroke of an ischemic myocardial cell (Y) from an epicardial preparation isolated 3 days after coronary occlusion in the dog. Action potentials recorded from a cell bordering the ischemic zone (X) are also shown along with the upstroke velocity (middle trace) of the border cells. TTX added to the superfusate greatly depressed the response of the cell in the ischemic zone, while depressing modestly (approximately 25%) V_{max} of the cell in the normal zone. A = control recording, B = TTX administration, C = After TTX washout.

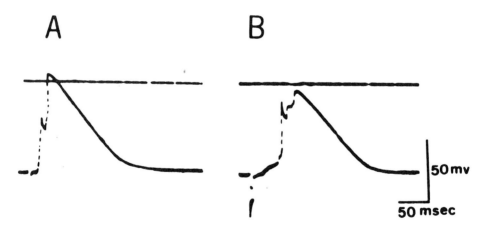

Fig. 28-8. Irregular upstroke of a myocardial cell in the ischemic zone of an epicardial preparation isolated 2 days after coronary artery occlusion in the dog. Stimulus intensity in panel **A** was higher than that in panel **B**, as shown by the differing amplitudes of the stimulus artifact. There was greater irregularity of the upstroke at the lower stimulus intensity (panel B).

capacitance {82}. The data are consistent with electrical uncoupling of ischemically injured cells at gap junctions, with additional changes in membrane resisitivity and capacitance, possibly from changes in membrane phospholipid content {82}.

REPOLARIZATION AND REFRACTORINESS

Acute ischemia

Acute ischemia shortens the plateau phase of the action potential and decreases action potential duration {1,2, 28,55}. Hypoxia produces a similar acceleration of repolarization as observed with ischemia, except the shortening of action potential develops more slowly {4,23,26,60}. An inhibition of oxidative metabolism with cyanide also shortens action potential duration {20,26}. The shortening of action potential duration can be attributed to the following alterations in membrane currents:

1. There is an increased potassium efflux and an increase in a time-independent outward potassium current associated with hypoxia {21,23,26}, ischemia {26}, and an inhibition of oxidative metabolism {19,20,26}. The efflux may be accompanied by both an increase in I_{K1} {21,23} and in $I_{K(ATP)}$ {19,20,26}. An increase in both currents can be observed simultaneously, suggesting that the two currents are not mediated by the same potassium ion channels, but are distinct and separate entities {83}. The increase in I_{K1} may be associated with an increase in a_{ca}^i {31,32} $I_{K(ATP)}$ is believed to be activated by a reduction in intracellular ATP below 1 mM {19,20,26} or a fall in intracellular ATP below 4 mM if internal ADP concentrations exceed 1 mM {26,84}. The interplay of the two potassium currents may vary during different times following the initiation of myocardial ischemia, being dependent upon changes in intracellular ATP, ADP, and calcium ion concentrations.

2. Hypoxia reduces a delayed outward current (I_K) in cat ventricular muscle subjected to hypoxia {23}. The current is too small during early repolarization to provide for a significant reduction in action potential amplitude. Any intracellular accumulation of Na^+ or Ca^{2+} following the onset of myocardial ischemia could reduce action potential duration by increasing I_K. A 20-mM increase of a_{ca}^i will increase I_K in myocytes from normal rabbit Purkinje fibers {85} over a wide range of potentials. Intracellular calcium ion concentration of 10^{-6} M shift the activation curve for I_K and increase the magnitude of I_K {32,85}. Intracellular concentrations of both cations are known to increase with acute myocardial infarction, although the mild increases of both cations seen with myocardial ischemia, as well as the small effect of I_K early in the action potential, suggest only an unimportant effect of I_K upon potassium efflux during acute myocardial ischemia, with little effect of I_K current on action potential duration.

3. Calcium ion currents (both T type and L type) may be

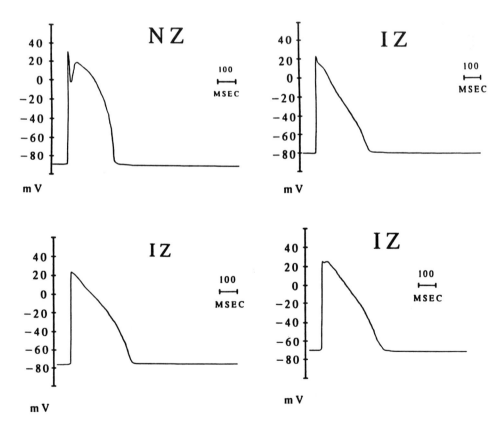

Fig. 28-9. Intracellular recordings from enzymatically dispersed myocytes of normal and ischemically injured epicardium, 4 days following myocardial infarction in the dog (paced rate = 1 Hz). In the upper left-hand panel, the typical "spike-and-dome" pattern of normal (NZ) canine epicardium is observed. The remaining three intracellular potentials were recorded from isolated myocytes from the ischemically injured epicardial border zone (IZ). There is a loss of the "spike-and-dome" pattern. Action potential duration (50%) is shortened, and there is a resultant "triangularization" of the action potential.

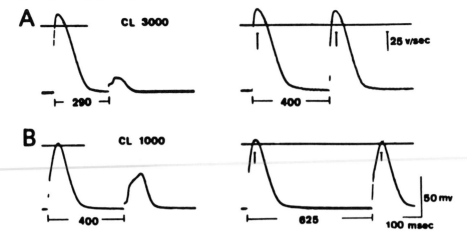

Fig. 28-10. Anomalous refractory properties of ischemically injured epicardial cells. On the left are shown the earliest responses of an injured cell at a cycle length (CL) of 3000 ms (**A**) and 1000 ms (**B**). The absolute refractory period extends well into diastole and is longer at the shorter basic cycle length. Also shown are later responses that are nearly equivalent to the driven responses at the respective cycle lengths, marking the approximate end of the relative refractory periods. The upstroke velocities of the refractory periods are long in comparison with the relative refractory period associated with the terminal portion of repolarization in normal cells, and the durations of the relative refractory periods are longer at the shorter cycle length. The intracellular recordings were made from a cell in the ischemic zone of an epicardial preparation isolated 3 days after coronary occlusion in the dog.

EPICARDIUM

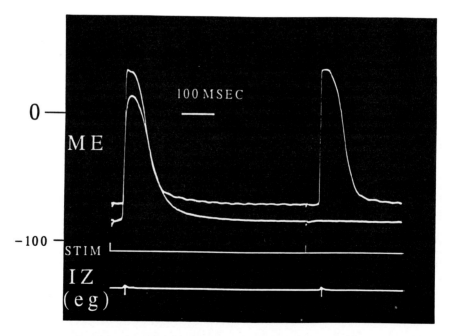

Fig. 28-11. Intracellular recordings (ME) for two epicardial cells from ischemically injured epicardial tissue. The preparation is paced at a basic cycle length of 1000 ms. A bipolar electrogram has been recorded from ischemically injured tissue. When a premature stimulus (two times diastolic threshold) is introduced at an interval of 600 ms, only one of the two cells is responsive to the late-diastolic interval stimulus. Iz = ischemically injured epicardial border zone.

reduced with acute myocardial ischemia. Hypoxia has been reported both to reduce {86,87} and to not alter $I_{Ca(L)}$ {23}. Three physiologic alterations known to occur with myocardial ischemia are also known to alter L-type calcium current. A reduction in intracellular ATP from 5 to 2 mM can decrease calcium current {19}. The amplitude and kinetics of L-type calcium current can be altered by acidosis, with internal protons inhibiting L-type calcium current more effectively than extracellular protons {88}. The rise in intracellular calcium ion concentrations may depress L-type calcium currents. A persistent increase in intracellular calcium reduces L-type calcium current {89}.

4. Although there are substantial differences in action potential morphology (and in both I_{k1} and I_k currents) between subepicardial myocytes and subendocardial myocytes in the feline heart {90}, there is little difference in the response to simulated ischemia (hypoxia, acidosis, hyperkalemia, and glucose deprivation) between the two groups of cells. The response to lysophosphatidylcholine is also not quantitatively or qualitatively different in the two myocardial tissues {91}.

Although there are a number of currents that may contribute to a shortening of action potential duration with acute myocardial ischemia, a practical definition of refractoriness in acutely ischemic tissue bears little relationship to action potential duration. Effective refractory periods determined using strength-interval curves are shortened in accordance with the shortening of action potential duration only when suprathreshold currents are applied {92,93}. The shortening of refractoriness is, however, dependent upon a dramatic decrease in myocardial excitability {73,92,93}. Myocardial tissue may be inexcitable or demonstrate prolonged refractoriness when stimulus strength is restricted to twice diastolic threshold for the tissue before coronary artery occlusion. Two to one, 3:1, and Wenckebach-like patterns of conduction block of normally conducted beats are commonly observed in conjunction with the development of acute arrhythmia soon after coronary artery occlusion {94,95}. It must be stressed that refractoriness is a composite property of myocardial tissue, dependent upon the size and duration of the current source, the resistance and capacitance of myocardial tissue, and the threshold potential, in addition to action potential duration {96}. When the current source (V_{max}) is reduced {1–3,28,55,56,60}, myocardial excitability is decreased {73,74}, and the recovery of excitable current from inactivation is delayed {57,67}, despite the return of membrane potential with accelerated repolarization, the cell may be capable of responding only to unrealistically large current sources. This is probably the basis for the observation of postrepolarization refractoriness with normally conducted sinus beats during acute ischemia {94,95}.

Chronic ischemic injury

Chronic ischemic injury and myocardial infarction have a variable and heterogeneous effect upon repolarization in surviving subepicardial {42,45,46,73} and subendocardial {39–41,43,47} cardiac tissues. The response may depend

upon (a) the location (subepicardial vs. subendocardial), (b) the proximity to the center of the infarct zone, and (c) the time interval following myocardial infarction. In canine {41} and feline {43} subendocardial tissue in the central infarct region, there is an initial prolongation (approximately 100 msec) of action potential duration (100% of repolarization) at 4 days following myocardial infarction with a significant (75 ms) shortening of action potential duration (100%) at later time intervals. Early changes are associated with lipid deposition, and recovery is associated with a lessening of ultramicroscopic changes and lipid deposition. Subendocardial cells at the lateral border of

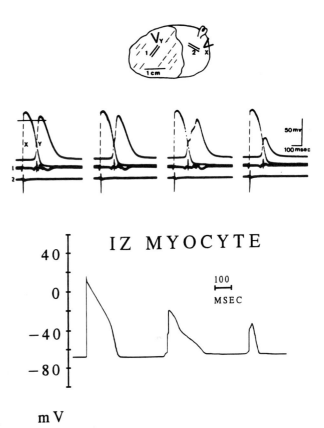

Fig. 28-12. Progressive beat-by-beat depression of the upstroke of the action potential with ischemic injury. The progressive beat-by-beat depression of the action potential of an injured epicardial cell (Y) following myocardial infarction in the dog is shown in the upper panel. Also shown are action potentials recorded from a cell in the normal zone (X) and electrograms recorded from the injured zone (1) and normal zone (2) in the vicinity of the respective action potential recordings. An enzymatically dispersed myocyte from ischemically injured ventricular epicardium overlying anterior myocardial infarction in the dog is shown 4 days following coronary artery occlusion (**lower panel**). The paced cycle length is 450 ms at 1.3x diastolic threshold using 2-ms duration stimulus. With the second and third beats, there is decremental generation of action potential amplitude and excitatory current (V_{max}). The excitation pattern was stable over a period of 30 seconds, with a repeating 3:1 pattern.

surviving endocardium demonstrate only a prolongation of repolarization (100%) lasting up to 6 months following coronary artery occlusion in the cat {43}. Ischemic injury, however, produces only a shortening of early repolarization (50% of repolarization), both early and late, in both the center and lateral border zone, in both the dog {41} and the cat {43}. This leads to a "triangularization" of the action potential (fig. 28-9).

Surviving cells within the epicardial border zone overlying myocardial infarction fail to demonstrate a profound change in action potential duration at 100% of repolarization, although the early phase of repolarization (30–50% of repolarization) is accelerated. The acceleration is maintained for at least 2 weeks following myocardial infarction {42,46,61}. The changes in action potential duration and shape are maintained in short-term cell culture following enzymatic dispersion, and allow the measurement of individual currents contributing to repolarization of the action potential.

Action potentials recorded from ischemically injured subendocardial myocytes overlying infarction lack the prominent notch (phase 1) characteristic of subendocardial ventricular cells {45,46}. Transient outward current in conspicuously absent in most subepicardial cells isolated 5 days following coronary artery occlusion. Even when the current in present, I_{to} is dramatically reduced in density without major changes in its kinetics {45}. There is also a reduction in $L_{Ca(L)}$ in the same group of cells {97}. Information is not available for other currents providing for repolarization in ischemically injured subepicardial cells.

Refractoriness in ischemically injured myocardium sur-viving myocardial infarction corresponds poorly with action potential duration in the tissue, with refractoriness outlasting repolarization {25,46,61}. The period of in-excitability in diastolic can be due both to alterations in absolute refractory period as well as relative refractory period, with conduction dependent upon a greater requirement for excitatory current. Because the recovery of excitatory current from inactivation rather than the recovery of membrane potential determines refractoriness, refractoriness increases rather than decreases with an increase in heart rate. This feature of postrepolarization refractoriness can be observed in ischemically injured tissue in figs. 10 and 11, and in a single myocyte isolated from ischemically injured myocardium, 4 days following myocardial infarction (fig. 28-12).

The anomalous refractoriness of ischemically injured cells, like the refractoriness of normal cells, has a rate dependence with a temporal evolution. An adjustment to a new rate is incomplete within a single cycle. The time required for a new equilibrium and the magnitude of change over time may be greater with anomalous refractoriness than normal refractoriness. Moreover, there is a cycle-length dependence of the response that is superimposed on the refractory properties of a single cycle and that manifests also a temporal evolution to a new equilibrium state. In fig. 28-10, at a cycle length of 3000 ms, the refractory period of the injured cell approximated 400 ms. When the basic cycle length is reduced to 1000 ms, the refractory period of the single cycle prolonged to approximately 650 ms, and the basic response, although outside the refractory period, was further depressed. The time

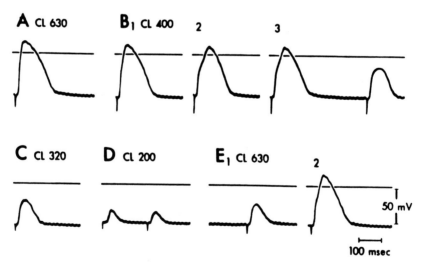

Fig. 28-13. Rate-dependent and time-dependent (fatigue) depression of response in ischemically injured myocardium from the epicardial border zone following myocardial infarction in the dog. Action potentials at various driven cycle lengths (CL) are shown in panels **A–D** with return to the original driving cycle in **E**. Panel B1 shows the response to an immediate change from a cycle length of 630 ms to a cycle length of 400 ms, whereas panel B2 was recorded 20 seconds later and panel B3 was recorded 40 seconds later. In panel B3 there were alternating responses of greater and lesser magnitude. Immediately upon a return to a cycle length of 630 ms in panel E1, the response improved only slightly, but 15 seconds later (panel E2) there was considerable improvement. The changes in responses occurred in the absence of appreciable changes in resting membrane potential. The recordings were made from a cell in the ischemically injured zone of an epicardial preparation isolated 5 days after coronary occlusion in the dog.

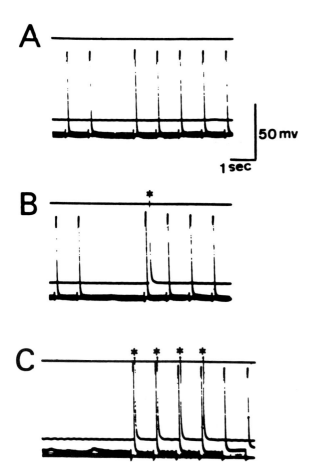

50 mv

1 sec

Fig. 28-14. Restoration of excitation of a cell in the ischemic zone by the introduction of a pause. Action potentials were recorded from two cells of ischemically injured epicardium excised 4 days following myocardial infarction in the dog. Driving the preparation at a cycle length of 1 second resulted in quiescence of one cell after a 10–15 second drive period. The introduction of a 2-second pause (panel **A**) was not followed by a response in the quiescent cell, but the introduction of a 3-second pause (panel **B**) was followed by a single response indicated by the asterisk. The introduction of an 8-second pause (panel **C**) resulted in four consecutive responses, followed by quiescence.

dependence and cycle-length dependence of the response are illustrated in figs. 28-13 and 28-14. When a more rapid rate is abruptly imposed, there is deterioration over time in the response, sometimes culminating in quiescence. The introduction of a long cycle produces a deterioration over time in the response, sometimes culminating in quiescence. The introduction of a long cycle produces a response to the subsequent stimulus. This behavior has been termed *fatigue* {48}. This temporal evolution often is not dependent on changes in resting potential, but sometimes higher heart rates may be accompanied by progressive depolarization. This type of response is shown in fig. 28-14. During short-term changes in rate, the loss of resting membrane

potential is not seen as often as simple depression of response. Apparently there is accumulation of depressant factors with time, these factors acting on the excitatory current. The greatly prolonged recovery times of excitatory current following an excitation apparently reflect delay in the recovery from inactivation of the depressed fast channel.

The combination of heterogeneous repolarization and variable postrepolarization recovery times of the excitatory current conspire to greatly disperse the refractory periods in injured myocardium. Moreover, a special feature of postrepolarization refractoriness is anomalously long refractory periods, periods during which even more depressed responses are generated with greater disarray of the activation sequence. The likelihood of reentry in this environment is greatly enhanced. Detailed mapping of the sequences of activation at the formation of reentrant excitation have documented the crucial role of abnormal refractory properties in producing the disordered activation sequence that culminates in reentry.

AUTOMATIC AND TRIGGERED FIRING

Diastolic depolarization in ischemically injured Purkinje fibers is more rapid, and the rate spontaneous depolarization is increased {39–41,43}. This disorder does not occur in the early phases of myocardial infarction, but is prominent after 6–12 hours and subsides over several days. During prolonged superfusion of ischemically injured endocardium over several hours, even with solutions low in oxygen and glucose, the rate of diastolic depolarization diminishes towards normal {39}. The enhanced rate is sensitive to (but not dependent upon) beta-adrenergic receptor stimulation {39,98}. Diastolic depolarization is less affected by lidocaine {99,100} than diastolic depolarization of normal Purkinje fibers and is more affected by moricizine {100}. Accumulated byproducts of phospholipid metabolism, such as lysophosphoglycerides, enhance the rate of diastolic depolarization of normal Purkinje fibers {101}.

Both enhanced diastolic depolarization {39–41,47, 98,102} and triggered afterpotentials {103,104} have been universally observed in Purkinje tissues subjacent to myocardial infarction during the initial 48–72 hours following coronary artery ligation. Diastolic depolarization and triggered afterpotentials have also been observed in surviving epicardial tissues at 24 hours following coronary artery ligation {105}. The slower rates of abnormal rhythm formation present in superfused subendocardial tissue preparations (60–120 beats/min) versus the more rapid rates observed (150–200 beats/min) in vivo have confused the interpretations of studies performed in vitro, with both mechanisms touted as the primary arrhythmia mechanism at 24 and 48 hours {39–41,100,102–104}. Most evidence, however, favors automaticity as the predominant mechanisms for the accelerated ventricular rhythm observed 24 and 48 hours following myocardial infarction.

1. Triggering of afterdepolarizations in superfused endocardial tissue preparations underlying myocardial in-

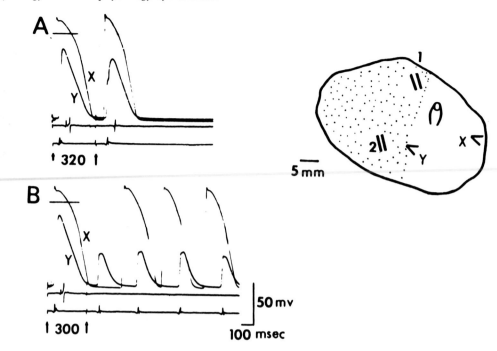

Fig. 28-15. Induction of repetitive firing (tachyarrhythmia) in an epicardial preparation containing normal and injured (stippled) regions isolated 4 days after coronary occlusion in the dog. Action potentials are recorded from a cells by the border (Y) and in the normal zone (X). Electrograms are also recorded from the normal (1) and injured zones (2). With a premature beat at a coupling interval of 320 ms (panel **A**), all sites responded to the premature stimulus in a manner similar to the driven responses. At a coupling interval of 300 ms (panel **B**), site 1 failed to respond and site Y responded with a diminutive action potential. Site X responded late with a full action potential, followed by repetitive responses at site 2, X, and Y (diminutive response at site Y). The tachycardia was accompanied by continuous block of propagation into site 1.

farction is commonly observed only when lowering the temperature of the tissue bath 3°C below normal body temperature in the dog {100,102–104}. The same intervention also lowers the rate of spontaneous impulse formation {100,103} from ischemically injured subendocardial tissues.

2. The anticancer antibiotic doxorubicin inhibits the formation of delayed afterdepolarization and triggering in vitro, while failing to inhibit abnormal automaticity in vitro or to slow the accelerated ventricular rhythm present 24 hours following myocardial infarction in the intact dog {100}.

3. Single premature ventricular beats and rapid pacing produce a resetting of spontaneous ventricular rhythms present 24 hours following myocardial infarction and in abnormal automaticity present in ischemically injured subendocardial tissue preparations. Triggered rhythms in vitro do not demonstrate this response, but can be initiated, terminated, or accelerated, responses not uniformly observed in vivo {100}.

4. The calcium entry blocker verapamil {102} or diltiazem {103} suppresses afterdepolarization formation and triggered rhythms in vitro, with only a mild reduction in the rate of spontaneous ventricular arrhythmia at 24 hours {106}.

The response to beta-agonists and beta-adrenergic blockade provides little information, as both triggered firing and abnormal automaticity may be enhanced by beta-agonists, with little suppression by beta-adrenergic receptor antagonists.

REENTRY

Reentry is a frequent basis for arrhythmia initiated in ischemically injured subendocardium and subepicardium. It is not the purpose of the present chapter to review reentry as an arrhythmia mechanism. The scope of the subject is too large. The cellular bases capable of facilitating localized reentry, slow conduction, and prolonged refractoriness have been discussed, and it is important to document the ability to sustain reentry in the tissues selected for the study of cellular properties. An example of reentry in a small epicardial tissue preparation overlying myocardial tissue can be observed in fig. 28-15. The premature stimulation impinges on regions with different refractory periods, demonstrating block (quiescence) in one region and a greatly diminished response in the other. Because this reentry circuit was not mapped, it cannot be stated that the quiescent region provided any essential component of the reentry circuit. Nonetheless, it is clear that in quiescent regions, block can be created from the abnormal refractoriness of ischemically injured tissue and is associated with the formation of reentrant rhythms.

REFERENCES

1. Kardesh M, Hogancamp CE, Bing RJ: Effect of complete ischemia on the intracellular electrical activity of the whole mammalian heart. *Circ Res* 6:715–725, 1958.
2. Samson WE, Scher AM: Mechanism of S-T segment alteration during acute myocardial injury. *Circ Res* 8:780–787, 1960.
3. Trautwein W, Gottstein U, Dudel J: Der aktionsstrom der myokardfaser un sauerstoffmangel, *Pflügers Arch* 260:40–60, 1954.
4. Coraboeuf E, Gargouil YM, Laplaud J, Desplaces A: Action de l'anoxie sur les potentiels electriques des cellules cardiaque de mammiferes actives et enertes (tissu ventriculaire isole de cobaye). *C R Acad Sci (D) (Paris)* 246:3100–3103, 1976.
5. Webb JL, Hollander PB: Metabolic aspects of the relationship between the contractility and membrane potentials of the right atrium. *Circ Res* 4:618–626, 1956.
6. Moore DJ: Potassium changes in the functioning heart under conditions of ischemia and congestion. *Am J Physiol* 123:443–447, 1938.
7. Harris AS, Bisteni A, Russel RA, Brigham JC, Firestone JE: Excitatory factors in ventricular tachycardia resulting from myocardial ischemia: Potassium a major excitant. *Science* 119:200, 1954.
8. Jennings RB, Crout JR, Smetters GW: Studies on distribution and localization of potassium in early myocardial ischemic injury. *Arch Pathol* 63:586, 1957.
9. Watanabe I, Johnson TA, Graebner CA, Engle CL, Noneman JW, Gettes LS: Effects of graded coronary flow reduction on ionic, electrical, and mechanical consequences of ischemia in the pig. *Circulation* 76:1127–1134, 1987.
10. Watanabe I, Johnson TA, Engle CL, Graebner C, Jenkins MG, Gettes LS: Effects of verapamil and propranolol on changes in extracellular K$^+$, pH, and local activation during graded coronary flow in the pig. *Circulation* 79:939–947, 1989.
11. Weigand M, Guggi W, Meesman W, Kessler M, Greitschus F: Extracellular potassium activity changes in the canine myocardium after acute coronary occlusion and the influence of beta-blockade. *Cardiovasc Res* 13:297–302, 1979.
12. Hill JL, Gettes LS: Effect of acute coronary artery occlusion on local myocardial extracellular K$^+$ activity in swine. *Circulation* 61:768–778, 1980.
13. Kleber AG: Resting membrane potential, extracellular potassium activity, and intracellular sodium activity during acute global ischemia in isolated perfused guinea pig hearts. *Circ Res* 52:442–450, 1983.
14. Wilde AAM, Kleber AG: The combined effects of hypoxia, high K$^+$, and acidosis on the intracellular sodium activity and resting potential in guinea pig papillary muscle. *Circ Res* 58:249–256, 1986.
15. Mori H, Sakuri K, Miyazaki T, Ogawa S, Nakamura Y: Local myocardial electrogram and potassium concentrations in superficial and deep intramyocardium and their relations with early ischaemic ventricular arrhythmias. *Cardiovasc Res* 21:447–454, 1987.
16. Coronel R, Fiolet JW, Wilms-Schopman FJG, Schaapherder

17. Coronel R, Wilms-Schopman FJG, Opthof T, van Capelle FJL, Janse MJ: Injury current and gradients of diastolic stimulation threshold, TQ potential, and extracellular potassium concentration during acute regional ischemia in the isolated perfused pig heart. *Circ Res* 68:1241–1249, 1991.
18. Mathur PP, Case RB: Phosphate loss during reversible myocardial ischemia. *J Mol Cell Cardiol* 5:375–393, 1973.
19. Noma A, Shibasaki T: Membrane current through adenosine-triphosphate-regulated potassium channels in ginea pig ventricular cells. *J Physiol* 366:365–385, 1985.
20. Elliot AC, Smith GL, Allen DG: Simultaneous measurements of action potential duration and intracellular ATP in isolated ferret hearts exposed to cyanide. *Circ Res* 64:583–591, 1989.
21. Ruiz-Petrich E, de Lorenzi F, Chartier D: Role of the inward rectifier I_{k1} in the myocardial response to hypoxia. *Cardiovasc Res* 25:17–26, 1991.
22. Kleber AG, Rieger CB, Janse MJ: Extracellular K$^+$ and H$^+$ shifts in early ischemia: Mechanisms and relation to changes in impulse propagation. *J Mol Cell Cardiol* 19(Suppl):34–44, 1987.
23. Vluegels A, Vereecke J, Carmeliet E: Ionic currents during hypoxia in voltage-clamped cat ventricular muscle. *Circ Res* 47:501–508, 1980.
24. Sato R, Noma A, Kurachi Y, Irisawa H: Effects of intracellular acidification on membrane currents in ventricular cells of the guinea pig. *Circ Res* 57:553–561, 1985.
25. Kantor PF, Coetzee WA, Carmeliet EE, Dennis SC, Opie LH: Reduction of ischemic K$^+$ loss and arrhythmias in rat hearts: Effect of glibenclamide, a sulfonylurea. *Circ Res* 66:478–485, 1990.
26. Venkatesh N, Lamp ST, Weiss JN: Sulfonylureas, ATP-sensitive K$^+$ channels, and cellular K$^+$ loss during hypoxia, ischemia, and metabolic inhibition in mammalian ventricle. *Circ Res* 69:623–637, 1991.
27. Fleet WF, Johnson TA, Graebner CA, Engle CL, Gettes LS: Effects of verapamil on ischemia-induced changes in extracellular K$^+$, pH, and local activation in the pig. *Circulation* 73:837–846, 1986.
28. Kabell G: Modulation of conduction showing in ischemic rabbit myocardium by calcium channel activation and blockade. *Circulation* 77:1385–1394, 1988.
29. Clusin WT, Buchbinder M, Ellis AK, Kernoff RS, Giacomini JC, Harrison DC: Reduction of ischemic depolarization by the calcium channel blocker diltiazem: Correlation with improvement of ventricular conduction and early arrhythmias in the dog. *Circ Res* 54:10–20, 1984.
30. Weiss J, Shine KI: Extracellular K$^+$ accumulation during myocardial ischemia in the isolated rabbit heart. *Am J Physiol* 242:H619–H628, 1982.
31. Mazzanti M, DiFrancesco D: Intracellular Ca modulates K-inward rectification in cardiac myocytes. *Pflügers Arch* 413:322–324, 1986.
32. Tohse N, Kameyama M, Irisawa H: Intracellular Ca^{2+} and protein kinase C modulate K$^+$ current in guinea pig heart cells. *Am J Physiol* 253:H1321–H1324, 1987.
33. Steenbergen C, Murphy E, Levy L, London RE: Elevation in cytosolic free calcium concentration early in myocardial ischemia in perfused rat heart. *Circ Res* 60:700–707, 1987.
34. Lee HC, Hohabir R, Smith N, Franz MR, Clusin WT: Effects of ischemia on calcium-dependent fluorescence transients in rabbit hearts containing indo 1: Correlation with

AFM, Johnson TA, Gettes LS, Janse MJ: Distribution of extracellular potassium and its relation to electrophysiologic changes during acute myocardial ischemia in the isolated perfused porcine heart. *Circulation* 77:1125–1138, 1988.

monophasic action potentials and contraction. *Circulation* 78:1047–1059, 1988.

35. Blake K, Smith NA, Clusin WT: Rate dependence of ischaemic myocardial depolarization: Evidence for a novel membrane current. *Cardiovasc Res* 20:557–562, 1986.

36. Clusin WT: Mechanism by which metabolic inhibitors depolarize cultured cardiac cells. *Proc Natl Acad Sci USA* 80: 3865–3868, 1983.

37. Hasin Y, Barry WH: Myocardial metabolic inhibition and membrane potential, contraction, and potassium uptake. *Am J Physiol* 247:H322–329, 1984.

38. Ehara T, Noma A, Ono K: Calcium activated non-selective cation channel in ventricular cells isolated from guinea pig hearts. *J Physiol* 403:117–133, 1986.

39. Lazzara R, El-Sherif N, Scherlag BJ: Electrophysiological properties of canine Purkinje cells in one-day-old myocardial infarction. *Circ Res* 33:722–734, 1973.

40. Lazzara R, El-Sherif N, Scherlag BJ: Early and late effects of coronary artery occlusion on canine Purkinje fibers. *Circ Res* 25:391–399, 1974.

41. Friedman PL, Fenoglio JJ Jr, Wit AL: Time course for reversal of electrophysiological and ultrastructural abnormalities in subendocardial Purkinje fibers surviving extensive myocardial infraction in dogs. *Cir Res* 36:127–144, 1975.

42. Ursell PC, Gardner PI, Albala A, Fenoglio JJ Jr, Wit AL: Structural and electrophysiological changes in the epicardial border zone of canine myocardial infarcts during infarct healing. *Circ Res* 56:436–451, 1985.

43. Myerburg RJ, Gelband H, Nilsson, Sung RJ, Thurer RJ, Morales AR, Bassett AL: Long-term electrophysiological abnormalities resulting from experimental myocardial infarction in cats. *Circ Res* 41:73–84, 1977.

44. Boyden PA, Albala A, Dresdner KP Jr: Electrophysiology and ultrastructure of canine subendocardial Purkinje cells isolated from control and 24-hour infarcted hearts. *Circ Res* 65:955–970, 1989.

45. Lue WM, Boyden PA: Abnormal electrical properties of myocytes from chronically infarcted canine heart: Alterations in Vmax and transient outward current. *Circulation* 85:1175–1188, 1992.

46. Patterson E, Scherlag BJ, Lazzara R: Rapid inward current in ventricular epicardium and epicardial myocytes following myocardial infarction. *J Cardiovasc Electrophysiol* 4:9–22, 1993.

47. Dresdner HP, Kline RP, Wit AL: Intracellular K$^+$ activity, intracellular Na$^+$ activity and maximal diastolic potential of canine subendocardial Purkinje cells from one-day-old infarcts. *Circ Res* 60:122–132, 1987.

48. Lazzara R, El-Sherif N, Scherlag BJ: Disorders of cellular electrophysiology produced by ischemia of the canine Hisbundle. *Circ Res* 36:444–453, 1975.

49. Kimura S, Bassett AL, Gaide MS, Kozlovskis PL, Myerburg RJ: Regional changes in intracellular potassium and sodium activity after healing of experimental myocardial infarction in cats. *Circ Res* 58:202–208, 1986.

50. Boyden PA, Dredsner K: Electrogenic Na-K pump in Purkinje myocytes from control, non-infarcted, and infarcted hearts. *Am J Physiol* 250:H766–H772, 1990.

51. McCullough JC, Chua WT, Rasmussen HH, Ten Eick RE, Singer DH: Two stable levels of diastolic potential at physiological K$^+$ concentrations in human ventricular myocardial cells. *Circ Res* 66:191–201, 1990.

52. Spear JF, Horowitz LN, Hodess AB, MacVaugh H, Moore EN: Cellular electrophysiology of human myocardial infarction: I. Abnormalities of cellular activation. *Circulation* 59:247–256, 1979.

53. Ten Eick RE, Baumgarten CM, Singer DH: Ventricular dysrhythmia: Membrane basis of currents, channels, gates, and cables. *Prog Cardiovasc Dis* 25:157–188, 1981.

54. Gilmour RF, Heger JJ, Prystowsky EN, Zipes DP: Cellular electrophysiologic abnormalities of diseased human ventricular myocardium. *Am J Cardiol* 51:137–144, 1983.

55. Downar E, Janse MJ, Durrer D: The effect of acute coronary artery occlusion on subepicardial transmembrane potentials in the intact porcine heart. *Circulation* 56:217–224, 1977.

56. Czarnecka M, Lewartowski B, Prokopcyk A: Intracellular recordings from the in situ working heart in physiological conditions and during acute ischemia and fibrillation. *Acta Physiol Pol* 24:331–337, 1973.

57. Gettes LS, Reuter H: Slow recovery from inactivation of inward currents in mammalian myocardial fibres. *J Physiol* 240:703–724, 1974.

58. Kodama I, Wilde AAM, Janse MJ, Durrer D, Yamada K: Combined effects of hypoxia, hyperkalemia and acidosis on membrane action potential and excitability of guinea-pig ventricular muscle. *J Mol Cell Cardiol* 16:247–259, 1984.

59. Wilde AAM, Kleber AG: The combined effects of hypoxia, high K$^+$, and acidosis on the intracellular sodium activity and resting potential in guinea pig papillary muscle. *Circ Res* 58:249–256, 1986.

60. Morena H, Janse MJ, Fiolet JWT, Krieder WJG, Crijns H, Durrer D: Comparison of the effects of regional ischemia, hypoxia, hyperkalemia, and acidosis on intracellular and extracellular potentials and metabolism in the isolated porcine heart. *Circ Res* 46:634–646, 1980.

61. Lazzara R, Hope RR, El-Sherif N, Scherlag BJ: Effects of lidocaine on hypoxic and ischemic cardiac cells. *Am J Cardiol* 41:872–879, 1978.

62. Wojtczak J: Contractures and increase in internal longitudinal resistance of cow ventricular muscle induced by hypoxia. *Circ Res* 44:88–95, 1979.

63. McDonald TF, MacLeod DP: Metabolism and the electrical activity of anoxic ventricular muscle. *J Physiol (Lond)* 229:559–582, 1973.

64. Kagiyama Y, Hill JL, Gettes LS: Interaction of acidosis and increased extracellular potassium on action potential characteristics and conduction in guinea pig ventricular muscle. *Circ Res* 51:614–623, 1982.

65. Adelman WJ, Palti Y: The influence of external potassium on the inactivation of sodium currents in the giant axon of the squid, *Loglio pealei*. *J Gen Physiol* 53:685–703, 1969.

66. Peganov EM, Khodorov BI, Shishkova LD: Slow sodium inactivation in the Ranvier node membrane: Role of external potassium. *Bull Exp Biol Med* 76:1014–1017, 1973.

67. Clarkson CW, Matsubara T, Hondeghem LM: Slow inactivation of Vmax in guinea pig myocardium. *Am J Physiol* 247:H645–H654, 1984.

68. Van Bogaert PP, Carmeliet E: Sodium inactivation and pH in cardiac Purkinje fibers. *Arch Int Physiol Biochem* 80: 833–835, 1988.

69. Grant AO, Strauss LJ, Strauss HC: The influence of pH on the electrophysiologic effects of lidocaine in guinea pig ventricular myocardium. *Circ Res* 47:542–550, 1980.

70. Ono K, Kiyosue T, Arita M: Isoproterenol, DBcAMP, and forskalin inhibit cardiac sodium current. *Am J Physiol* 256:C1131–C1137, 1989.

71. Coombs J, Scheuer T, Rossie S, Catterall W: Evidence that cAMP dependent phosphorylation promotes inactivation in embryonic rat brain cells in primary culture. *Biophys J* 53:542, 1989.

72. Kleber AG, Riegger CB, Janse MJ: Electrical uncoupling and increase of extracellular resistance after induction of ischemia in isolated, arterially perfused rabbit papillary

muscle. *Circ Res* 61:271–279, 1987.

73. Elharrar V, Foster PR, Jirak TL, Gaum WE, Zipes DP: Alterations in myocardial excitability during ischemia. *Circ Res* 40:98–105, 1977.

74. Dominguez G, Fozzard HA: Influence of extracellular K$^+$ concentrations on cable properties and excitability of sheep cardiac Purkinje fibers. *Circ Res* 26:656–574, 1970.

75. Spear JF, Michelson EL, Moore EN: Cellular electrophysiologic characteristics of chronically infarcted myocardium in dogs susceptible to sustained ventricular tachyarrhythmias. *J Am Coll Cardiol* 4:1099–1110, 1983.

76. Lazzara R, Scherlag BJ: The role of the slow current in the generation of arrhythmias in ischemic myocardium. In: Zipes DP, Bailey JC, Elharrar V (eds) *The Slow Inward Current and Cardiac Arrhythmias*. The Hague: Martinius Nijhoff, 1980, pp 399–416.

77. Richards DA, Blake GJ, Spear JF, Moore EN: Electrophysiologic substrate for ventricular tachycardia: Correlation of properties in vitro and in vivo. *Circulation* 69:369–381, 1984.

78. El-Sherif N, Smith RA, Evans K: Canine ventricular arrhythmias in the late myocardial infraction period. 8. Epicardial mapping of reentrant circuits. *Circ Res* 49:255–265, 1981.

79. Wit AL, Alessie MA, Bonke FIM, Lamemrs W, Smeets J, Fenoglio JJ Jr: Electrophysiologic mapping to determine the mechanism of experimental ventricular tachycardia initiated by premature impulses. Experimental approach and initial results demonstrating reentrant excitation. *Am J Cardiol* 49:166–185, 1982.

80. Gardner PI, Ursell PC, Fenoglio JJ Jr, Wit AL: Electrophysiologic and anatomic basis for fractionated electrograms recorded from healed myocardial infarcts. *Circulation* 72:596–611, 1985.

81. Spear JF, Michelson EL, Moore EN: Reduced space constant in slowly conducting regions of chronically infarcted canine myocardium. *Circ Res* 53:176–185, 1983.

82. Argentieri TM, Frame LH, Colatsky TJ: Electrical properties of canine subendocardial Purkinje fibers surviving in 1-day-old experimental myocardial infarction. *Circ Res* 66:123–134, 1990.

83. Belles B, Hescheler J, Trube G: Changes of membrane currents in cardiac cells induced by long whole cell recordings and tolbutamide. *Pflügers Arch* 409:582–588. 1987.

84. Dunne MJ, West-Jordan JA, Abraham RJ, Edwards RHT, Petersen OH: The gating of nucleoside-sensitive K$^+$ channels in insulin secreting cells can be modulated by changes in both the ration of ATP^{4-}/ADP^{3-} and by non-hydrolyzable derivatives of both ATP and ADP. *J Memb Biol* 104:165–177, 1988.

85. Scamps F, Carmeliet E: Delayed K current and external K in single Purkinje cells. *Am J Physiol* 275:C1086–C1092, 1989.

86. Ruiz-Ceretti E, Ragault P, LeBlanc N, Ponce Zumino AZ: Effects of hypoxia and altered K$_o$ on the membrane potential of rabbit ventricle. *J Mol Cell Cardiol* 15:845–854, 1983.

87. Payet MD, Schanne OF, Ruiz-Ceretti E, Demes JM: Slow inward current and outward currents of rat ventricular fibers under anoxia. *J Physiol (Paris)* 74:31–55, 1978.

88. Irisawa H, Sato R: Intra- and extracellular actions of proton on the calcium current of isolated guinea pig ventricular cells. *Circ Res* 59:348–355, 1986.

89. Kokubun S, Irisawa H: Effects of various intracellular Ca ion concentrations on the calcium current of guinea pig single ventricular cells. *Jpn J Physiol* 34:599–611, 1984.

90. Furukawa T, Kimura S, Furukawa N, Bassett AL, Myerburg RJ: Potassium rectifier currents differ in myocytes of endocardial and epicardial origin. *Circ Res* 70:91–103, 1992.

91. Kimura S, Bassett AL, Furukawa T, Cuevas J, Myerburg RJ: Electrophysiological properties and responses to simulated ischemia in cat ventricular myocytes of endocardial and epicardial origin. *Circ Res* 66:469–477, 1990.

92. Brooks CM, Gilbert JL, Greenspan ME, Lange G, Mazzalla HM: Excitability and electrical response of ischemic heart muscle. *Am J Physiol* 198:1143–1147, 1960.

93. Tsuchida T: Experimental studies of the excitability of ventricular muscle in infarcted region. *Jpn Heart J* 6:152–164, 1965.

94. Williams DO, Scherlag BJ, Hope RR, El-Sherif N, Lazzara R: The pathophysiology of malignant ventricular arrhythmias during acute myocardial ischemia. *Circulation* 50:1163–1172, 1974.

95. El-Sherif N, Scherlag BJ, Lazzara R: Electrode catheter recordings during malignant ventricular arrhythmias following experimental acute myocardial ischemia. *Circulation* 51:1003–1014, 1975.

96. Arnsdorf M: A matrical perspective of cardiac excitability, cable properties, and inpulse propagation. In: Sperelakis N (ed) *Physiology and Pathophysiology of the Heart*. Boston: Kluwer Academic Publishers, 1989.

97. Aggarwal R, Boyden PA: Calcium currents in canine myocytes from the epicardial border zone of the infarcted heart. *Circulation* 84:II549A, 1991.

98. Cameron JS, Han J: Effects of epinephrine on automaticity and the incidence of arrhythmias in Purkinje fibers surviving myocardial infarction. *J Pharmacol Exp Ther* 223:573–579, 1982.

99. Allen JD, Brennan JF, Wit AL: Actions of lidocaine on transmembrane potentials of subendocardial Purkinje fibers surviving in infarcted canine hearts. *Circ Res* 43:470–478, 1978.

100. Le Marec H, Dangman KH, Danilo P Jr, Rosen MR: An evaluation of automaticity and triggered activity in the canine heart one to four days after myocardial infarction. *Circulation* 71:1224–1236, 1985.

101. Arnsdorf MF, Sawicki GJ: The effects of lysophosphatidylcholine, a toxic metabolite of ischemia, on the components of cardiac excitability in sheep Purkinje fibers. *Circ Res* 49:16–30, 1981.

102. Le Marec H, Spinelli W, Rosen MR: The effects of doxorubicin on ventricular tachycardia. *Circulation* 74:881–886, 1986.

103. El-Sherif N, Gough WB, Zeiler RH, Mehra R: Triggered ventricular rhythms in 1-day-old myocardial infarction in the dog. *Circ Res* 52:566–579, 1983.

104. Gough WB, Zeiler RH, El-Sherif N: Effects of diltiazem on triggered activity in canine one day old infarction. *Cardiovasc Res* 18:339–343, 1984.

105. Dangman KH, Dresdner KP, Zaim S: Automatic and triggered initiation in canine subepicardial ventricular muscle cells from border zones of 24-hour transmural infarcts. *Circulation* 78:1020–1030, 1988.

106. Hashimoto K, Satoh H, Shibuya T, Imai S: Canine effective plasma concentrations of antiarrhythmic drugs on the two-stage coronary ligation arrhythmia. *J Pharmacol Exp Ther* 223:801–810, 1982.

CHAPTER 29

Basic Principles of Pharmacokinetics: Antiarrhythmic Drugs

DONALD C. HARRISON & MICHAEL B. BOTTORFF

INTRODUCTION

The leading cause of death and disability in patients with heart disease continues to be cardiac arrhythmias. In spite of the development of new antiarrhythmic drugs and new technologies for terminating arrhythmias, sudden cardiac death, which is generally due to ventricular arrhythmias or asystole, remains the leading cause of death in the United States and in many western countries. Because of the failure of existing antiarrhythmic drugs to prevent sudden death, as demonstrated in the Cardiac Arrhythmia Suppression Trail (CAST) {1–4}, there is a continued need for the development of new arrhythmic drugs. Other modes of therapy for arrhythmias have also been developed because of a better understanding of the cardiac conduction system and the electrophysiology of arrhythmias during the past decade. These new approaches include catheter ablation techniques with radiofrequency energy for arrhythmias in which electrophysiologic studies demonstrate abnormal pathways of conduction or abnormal function in the AV node {5,6}. In addition, the surgical implantation of devices that terminate ventricular tachycardia and fibrillation when they occur, known as Automatic Implantable Cardioverter Devices (AICD), have been shown to prevent sudden death in patients with drug-resistant arrhythmias {7,8}. In this review we will not focus on these new technologies for the prevention and treatment of arrhythmias, but on the scientific basis for the treatment and prevention of arrhythmias with drugs.

Much of the scientific investigation on sudden death in the past two decades has been directed to determining whether or not premature ventricular depolarizations were responsible for initiating ventricular fibrillations and sudden death, and whether or not this could be used as a marker to determine patients needing therapy. The CAST trial suggests that this concept is no longer viable and that other mechanisms for preventing sudden death must be developed {1–4}. On the other hand, electrophysiologic studies have suggested that arrhythmias that predispose sudden cardiac death may have a different mechanism and pathophysiology from those producing frequent premature ventricular beats {9,10}. This has led to the studies on agents that effect the duration of the cellular action potential and His-Purkinje and ventricular muscle tissue and

cellular refractoriness by blocking potassium channels. These agents have been suggested to alter the likelihood of sudden cardiac death. Recent basic pharmacologic investigations have produced a number of new agents that block potassium channels that are now under clinical study {11–13}.

At this time all clinical evidence available suggests that new antiarrhythmic compounds with improved or different mechanisms of electrophysiologic action to combat the frequency of symptomatic cardiac arrhythmias, and the mortality that results from the arrhythmias, need to be developed. In addition, pharmacologically sound principles on which antiarrhythmic drugs can be administered to patients need further elucidation as the pharmacologic basis for treatment is developed. Thus the purpose of this chapter is to provide the pharmacologic basis for drug therapy of cardiac arrhythmias and scientific rationale, which can be converted into clinical concepts for the correct use of antiarrhythmic drug therapy. The following chapter by Hondeghem and Katzung (Chapter 30) on the biophysics of cardiac activation and conduction, basic cellular electrophysiology, and the electrophysiologic actions of several therapeutic agents serves as companion reading for this chapter.

The three specific purposes for this chapter are
1. To outline a rational classification proposal for antiarrhythmic drugs and its scientific basis
2. To present basic pharmacokinetic principles for using antiarrhythmic drugs in clinical practice
3. To present the most relevant pharmacokinetic concepts for each important antiarrhythmic agent or class now available in the United States

BASIS FOR CLASSIFICATION OF ANTIARRHYTHMIC DRUGS

A number of classifications of antiarrhythmic drugs have been proposed based on the chemical structure of the compounds used for suppression of arrhythmia, the intracellular physiologic properties of the drug, and the electrophysiologic properties of agents in the intact heart {14–16}. More recently, an initiative entitled "The Sicilian Gambit" succinctly described the scientific advances in our

N. Sperelakis (ed.), Physiology and Pathophysiology of the Heart, Third Edition.

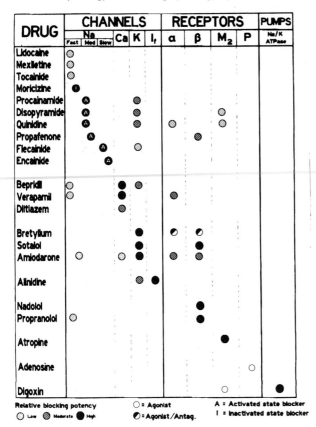

DRUG	CHANNELS						RECEPTORS				PUMPS
	Na Fast|Med|Slow			Ca	K	I_f	α	β	M_2	P	Na/K ATPase
Lidocaine	◎										
Mexiletine	◎										
Tocainide	◎										
Moricizine	●										
Procainamide		Ⓐ			◎						
Disopyramide		Ⓐ			◎				○		
Quinidine		Ⓐ			◎		○		○		
Propafenone		Ⓐ						◎			
Flecainide			Ⓐ		◎						
Encainide			Ⓐ								
Bepridil	◎			●	◎						
Verapamil	◎			●				◎			
Diltiazem				◎							
Bretylium					●		◑	◑			
Sotalol					●			●			
Amiodarone	○			○	●		◎	◎			
Alinidine					◎	●					
Nadolol								●			
Propranolol	○							●			
Atropine									●		
Adenosine										○	
Digoxin										○	●

Relative blocking potency   ○ = Agonist   A = Activated state blocker
○ Low ◎ Moderate ● High   ◑ = Agonist/Antag.   I = Inactivated state blocker

Fig. 29-1. Sicilian Gambit proposed classification of antiarrhythmic drugs by their action on membrane channels, receptors, and ion pumps in the heart. The order of drugs (rows) correlates with the columns for actions so that the chart forms a diagonal. Drugs with multiple actions depart strikingly from this (e.g., amiodarone). The actions of drugs on sodium, calcium, and potassium (I_k), and I_f channels are indicated. Sodium channel blockade is subdivided into three groups: fast (<300 ms), medium (med) (200–1500 ms), and slow (>1500 ms) time constants for recovery from block. The rate constant for onset of block might be more relevant. Blockade in the inactive (I) or activated (A) state is indicated. Information on the state of dependency of the block caused by moricizine, propafenone, encainide, and flecainide is limited. Drug interaction with receptors (α, β, muscarinic subtype 2 (M_2), and A_1 purinergic (P) and drug effect on Na,K-ATPase are indicated. Filled circles indicate antagonist or inhibitory action; unfilled circles indicate direct or indirect acting agonists or stimulators. The darkness of the symbol increases with the intensity of the action.

understanding of antiarrhythmic drugs, their molecular and cellular targets in the heart, their effects on the conduction systems within the heart, the interaction of electrophysiology and the nervous system, and the observed actions of specific drugs in clinical cardiology {17}. This new classification, as presented in fig. 29-1, is an extremely valuable contribution for basic pharmacologists but, as suggested earlier, is not practical for clinical application {18}.

Each classification proposal has its proponents and opponents among investigators and clinicians. The most widely used classification scheme as proposed by Vaughn-Williams in 1970 has provided a basis for discussion and planning for investigators studying new antiarrhythmic drugs {14}. This classification was based on intracellular electrophysiologic studies of isolated cardiac tissue exposed to drugs that had antiarrhythmic action. Drugs that act on the fast sodium channels were placed in Class I. The prototypical drug with Class I action is quinidine. Class II drugs are those that block beta-adrenergic receptors, although at the time the proposal was made the biochemical definition of a beta-receptor had not been determined. Propranolol was the prototype for this class of drugs. Drugs that selectively prolong the duration of the intracellular action potential, the refractoriness of atrial ventricular muscle, and the His-Purkinje system were placed in Class III. Amiodarone was the classic example proposed by Vaughn-Williams at the time. Class IV agents were calcium channel blocking drugs, of which verapamil was the only available candidate in 1970.

In 1979 at an international conference on arrhythmias at Stanford University, a proposal for three subdivisions of Class I compounds was made based on clinical observations, microelectrode studies in cardiac and specialized conducting tissues, and clinical electrophysiologic studies {15,19,20}. Scientific evidence for this proposal was incomplete initially and the proposal was considered empiric, since it depended on differences among the effects of the three subclasses of drugs, at commonly observed clinical concentration in specialized conduction tissue of the heart, and the effects of these drugs on ventricular refractoriness and repolarization. This modification of the original classification is presented in table 29-1 and has been widely accepted during the past decade. In addition, basic science evidence to support the concept has been developed {21,22}. Since all Class I agents block fast sodium channels in cardiac cell membranes, it was postulated that the difference between the three subclasses is in the concentration necessary for the attachment to the sodium channel

Table 29-1. Harrison modification of Class I antiarrhythmic agents

Class	Actions	Agents
Ia	Slows dV/dt of phase O Moderate prolongation of repolarization Prolongs PR, QRS, and QT intervals	Quinidine Procainamide Disopyramide Cibenzoline
Ib	Limited effect on dV/dt of phase O Shortens repolarization Shortens QT in clinical doses Elevates fibrillation thresholds	Lidocaine Tocainide Mexiletine
Ic	Markedly slows dV/dt Little effect on repolarization Markedly prolongs PR and QRS on electrocardiogram	Encainide Diprafenone Flecainide Propafenone Ajmeline

From Harrison {20}, with permission.

receptor and the rate of release from these same sodium channel receptors. This would imply there is not a fundamental difference in the cellular action of the agent, but the difference is based on binding characteristics to ion channels. Electrophysiologic studies recently published lend support to the subclassification to the Class I agents {21,22}.

In order to understand these principles, it is necessary to know that sodium channels and His-Purkinje cells exist in at least three physiologic states. They are closed when they are near the resting potential of the cell, but are available to be opened by stimulation or depolarization. Once channels are open, they let sodium ions pass selectively across the membrane. When they close, they are no longer available to be opened and are thus classified as inactive {22,23}. More recently, investigators have suggested that antiarrhythmic drugs attached to the sodium channel in its inactive state {22,23}, thus interfering with the recovery of the properties of the membrane after repolarization. Further studies have demonstrated that the maximal rate of depolarization (MRD) is altered by drugs on stimulation at increasingly frequent intervals after depolarization {23}. An approximate measure of the number of channels that have recovered can be estimated using this concept. The effects of a drug on the electrical threshold of activity can be developed by estimating the percentage of channels permanently eliminated and the percentage of channels with no drug attached. This concept is that antiarrhythmic drug actions are frequency dependent and their effect on reducing the MRD and conduction velocity may be a function of the frequency of the trains of stimuli used in the isolated cell experiments {23}. When steady-state MRD depression is achieved, recovery is exponential and can be determined by the administration of a single stimulus given after depolarization. Thus it is possible to differentiate Class I antiarrhythmic drugs and to demonstrate that Class Ib drugs, such as lidocaine, have rapid disassociation from sodium channels, with rapid recovery of the MRD. Class Ic drugs, such as flecanide and encainide, have very long recovery times and slow disassociation. The Harrison-classified Ia drugs show intermediate recovery times {15,16}.

Onset study kinetics for drugs in these three subclasses provides a similar grouping possibility. Lidocaine, mexiletine, and tocainide (Class Ib) had time constants for attachment to the channels of less than 0.5 second, and steady-state depression of the MRD was achieved within a few beats after starting a train of stimuli in isolated cell preparations. In contrast, Class Ic drugs, such as flecinide and encainide, showed a delayed onset of depression of MRD for more than 20 stimuli delivered in a train to isolated cells. It is possible to classify antiarrhythmic drugs into Class I subdivisions based on their onset and offset kinetics determined by electrophysiologic study in vitro. However, it has been shown that the fundamental action of all Class I agents is similar, involving attachment to sodium channels in their inactivated state, but that quantitative differences in the attachment and detachment from the sodium channels accounts for the different electrophysiologic profiles.

More recently, in an attempt to be more comprehensive in providing a rational scientific basis for classification of antiarrhythmic drugs, a group of electrophysiologists have proposed the Sicilian Gambit. Much of the data needed to fill in the charts provided in the Sicilian Gambit are not available scientifically at this time (fig. 29-1). As cellular electrophysiology and basic receptor kinetics are better understood, it should be possible to fill in the gaps in the data needed to make the Sicilian Gambit more successful. The hypothetical explanations suggested above provide for some of the differences in the clinical, electrophysiologic, and electrocardiographic observations in patients with these drugs. The classification schemes provide a reference for communication among basic scientists and clinicians considering new, pharmacologic agents. This common basis for discussion among colleagues aids in the design of rational, new agents for therapy. They also suggest that further modifications of classification schemes will be necessary. With the rapid development of agents that block potassium channels and the multiplicity of potassium channels that have been shown to exist, it seems likely that a subclassification of potassium channel blocking agents will be forthcoming. Since there are at least three major potassium channels in cardiac tissue that have been identified to date, the onset and offset of binding to these channels, and the effect of one channel versus another, may provide a rational basis for subclassification of potassium channel blocking drugs in the future.

Several agents have been shown to have more than one mechanism of action, and confusion in the classification of compounds of this type has occurred. Amiodarone, for example, has not only Class III action, but has Class I sodium channel blocking actions. Another example is sotalol, which is a Class II beta-adrenergic blocking drug but has recently been shown to have Class III potassium channel blocking actions, by which it prolongs the duration of the action potential and the refractoriness of cardiac tissue. Generally, a drug has been classified according to their predominant action when one or more action was identified as its mechanism.

PHARMACOKINETIC PRINCIPLES FOR ANTIARRHYTHMIC DRUGS

Pharmacokinetics are defined as the study of the time course of processes involved in the absorption, distribution, metabolism, and elimination of drugs from the body. Clinical pharmacokinetics are usually defined as the application of these basic processes for treating diseases with drugs. The terms and abbreviations used are outlined in table 29-2. Studies of pharmacokinetics provide better understanding of drug uptake, transport, binding, and metabolism, and frequently lead to development of models for explaining drug distribution and accumulation. These models have been independently important in developing new information about antiarrhythmic drugs. Our purpose is to provide basic pharmacokinetic principles that may be useful in understanding the action of these drugs. A

Table 29-2. Definitions of pharmacokinetic terms

AUC_o	Area under the concentration time curve, from zero to infinite time
A_b	Amount of drug in the body
C	Drug concentration
$\bar{C}$	Average drug concentration during a dosing interval
C^{ss}	Drug concentration at steady state
CL_H	Hepatic clearance
CL_{int}	Intrinsic clearance
CL_T	Total body clearance
E	Extraction ratio
F	Systemic availability
f_B	Fraction of drug unbound in blood
Q	Hepatic blood flow
R	Rate of drug administration
$\bar{R}$	Average rate of drug administration
t_0, t_1, etc.	Time zero, time one, etc.
$t_{1/2} (\alpha\beta)$	Half-life (α phase, β phase)
τ	Dosing interval
V_d	Volume of distribution
V_c	Volume of distribution of the central compartment
V_β	Volume of distribution at pseudoequilibrium
V_d^{ss}	Volume of distribution at steady state

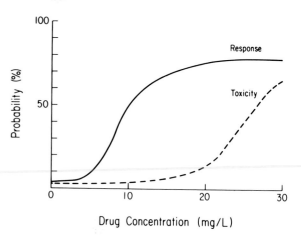

Fig. 29-2. Graph of a theoretical drug showing the probability of a therapeutic response and toxicity with a given serum drug concentration. Reproduced with permission from Applied Pharmacokinetics: Principles of Therapeutic Drug Monitoring {32}.

number of reviews of this subject have been published {24–31}.

Therapeutic range and dosing of drugs

The therapeutic and toxic actions of antiarrhythmic drugs depend on drug concentration at the sites of action, usually related to the binding of a specific drug to a receptor site in a specific cell in the heart. At present, the receptor site binding is not known for most antiarrhythmic drugs. Furthermore, it is assumed that at steady state, the concentration of the drug in plasma is in equilibrium with its concentration at the active receptor site. Drug concentrations in body fluids such as plasma or whole blood do frequently correlate with pharmacologic response. This relationship may be either linear or nonlinear, but it is the concept that forms the basis for measuring plasma concentration of drugs as a practical measure. Therefore, it is possible to define therapeutic plasma concentrations for antiarrhythmic drugs that produce designated, electrophysiologic effects and pharmacologic action in many arrhythmias. Concentrations within an accepted plasma range correlate with drug effect, and when concentrations rise above a certain level, toxicity occurs with increasing frequency. Furthermore, when the plasma concentrations falls below a therapeutic range, little clinical effect may be noted. Thus, it is relatively important to determine the range of plasma concentration for an antiarrhythmic drug when initial studies are conducted because the therapeutic range cannot be used as the only indication for administering an appropriate dose in an individual patient. It does, however, permit establishing a therapeutic level that should be effective in a large percentage of patients. Thus using pharmacokinetic principles enables the physician to estimate a higher probability of pharmacologic effect,

while at the same time avoiding toxicity from many antiarrhythmic drugs (fig. 29-2) {32}.

To determine dosing, pharmacokinetic principles can be used in three specific steps — first, to determine an initial loading dose; second, to determine a maintenance dose to provide a steady-state desired plasma concentration; and third, to adjust the dose in patients with alterations in hepatic, renal, and other organ function in order to produce the desired response while avoiding long-term toxicity. In many patients drugs show little intersubject variability in their disposition, and thus standard initial loading and maintenance doses will usually be appropriate. In other cases with disease of the cardiovascular system, this is not possible because of alterations in distribution and clearance resulting from the disease.

Plasma concentration

Generally there is no exact way to determine the total amount of an antiarrhythmic drug in the body (Ab). On the other hand, the concentration of the drug in blood or plasma can be determined by numerous new analytical technologies. The volume into which the drug is distributed (V_d) is a proportionality constant that relates plasma concentration (C_p) to the amount of drug in the body at a specific time:

$$Ab = V_d C_p. \tag{29-1}$$

V_d is a proportionality constant that does not have specific physiological significance as an actual space or volume. Once V_d is known and the desired therapeutic plasma concentration is identified, the initial amount of the drug that is required to achieve the C_p can be estimated using eq. (29-1) if the body is assumed to be a single compartment, and if all parts of the compartment are assumed to be in rapid equilibrium. Such an approach can be used to determine the initial dose for an antiarrhythmic

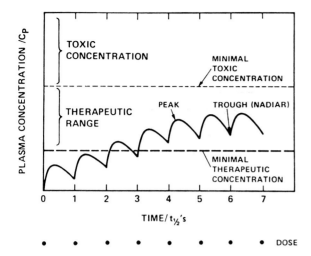

Fig. 29-3. Graph of plasma half-lives ($t_{1/2}$) versus plasma concentration for oral administration of antiarrhythmic drug with administration at half-life intervals. Steady state is achieved after five half-lives, and peak and trough levels occur in each dosing interval.

drug, but other factors are necessary to estimate a maintenance dose. The clearance (Cl), or volume of plasma from which the drug is irreversibly removed per unit of time, either by metabolism or excretion, is one such parameter. Clearance can be used to calculate the rate at which antiarrhythmic drugs must be given to maintain the desired C_p. For this reason, clearance becomes the single most useful information obtained for a particular drug with a particular disease process. After the drug is administered several times at constant intervals, the rate at which the drug enters and leaves the body is constant and the C_p fluctuates between a constant maximum (peak level) and the constant minimum (trough level) (fig. 29-3). Maintaining a C_p between the peak and trough levels is generally referred to as *steady state* and occurs at approximately four to five half-lives after multiple administration for most drugs. This permits the following relationship to be established:

Drug input = drug elimination

$$ \text{or} \qquad (29\text{-}2) $$

Drug dose rate = $C_p \cdot Cl.$

Once clearance is known, the maintenance dose necessary to keep a steady-state plasma at C_p can be calculated. Since most drugs are eliminated by renal excretion and/or hepatic metabolism, the upper limits of Cl relate to the blood flow to these organs. This is referred to as the total body clearance and approximates 1.5 l/min for hepatic blood flow, and 1.2 l/min for renal blood flow. When both processes are involved, the total body clearance is their sum, and in this model clearance is independent of distribution and does not require assumption of a single- or multiple-compartment model. In general, clearance provides information necessary for adjusting dose in many patients, since for antiarrhythmic drugs there is direct

proportionality between dosage size and steady-state C_p. If Cl is constant, doubling the dose will double C_p after steady state is again achieved or after a time interval of five half-lives for the drug.

On the other hand, clearance frequently changes with different clinical situations in advanced cardiovascular disease. Thus it becomes necessary to monitor C_p frequently with many antiarrhythmic drugs. The concepts, however, require intelligent use of the measurement of C_ps. First, the patient must be at or near steady state for correct interpretation. Second, if only limited C_p measurement can be made, it is preferable to obtain them at the end of a dosing interval, where artifacts due to absorption are likely to be avoided. The use of these two guides enables individual differences in drug disposition due to cardiovascular, hepatic, or renal disease, and genetic differences in degradation of the agent to be considered appropriately.

Pharmacokinetic models

Mathematical models of pharmacokinetics provide a conceptual framework for understanding drug disposition. For this presentation, only one and two compartment models are considered.

ONE-COMPARTMENT MODEL

This model assumes the body to be homogeneous with respect to drug concentration; that is, drug distribution is instantaneous or at least extremely rapid when compared with drug elimination. Using a one-compartment model, fig. 29-4 shows the time course of drug concentration in the plasma or blood after an intravenous bolus. If the dose is such that the initial concentration at time zero (T_0) is 100

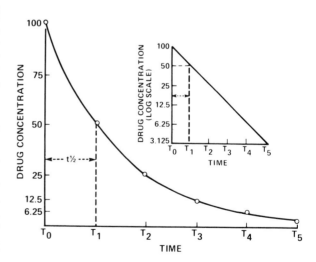

Fig. 29-4. Drug concentrations at various times following a bolus dose, when the body has the characteristics of a one-compartment model. The inset shows the same information with concentration plotted on a logarithmic scale. Used with the permission of Harrison et al. {24}.

concentration units, then at time 1 (T_1) the concentration has fallen to half this value, and at the end of each succeeding equal time interval (T_1, T_2, etc.), the concentration has fallen to half the concentration present at the start of each interval. Such a process, in which an equal fraction of the drug remaining in the body is eliminated per unit of time, is called a *first-order process*. The particular time interval defined above, in which the concentration falls to half its initial value, is called the *half-life*. In contrast to the constant fraction of the drug remaining in the body that is removed per unit of time, increasingly smaller fractions of the initial concentration or the dose are removed (fig. 29-4), and in theory, an infinite time would be required to remove all of the drug from the body. It is useful to remember that approximately 90% of the dose is removed in three half-lives, or approximately 97% in five half-lives. The first-order, or exponential decay of drug concentration, can be linearized by plotting the logarithm of the concentration versus time, or plotting the data on semilogarithmic graph paper (fig. 29-4, inset). The half-life of a drug in the body is important in determining an appropriate dosage regimen for a patient and is one of the factors that contributes to the duration of drug action.

Since the concept of volume of distribution assumes uniform distribution, a fictitious volume many times that of the body is required to account for the small concentrations observed in the plasma. The volume of distribution can be estimated after an intravenous bolus into a one-compartment model, using eq. (29-1), by extrapolating drug concentration data to time zero. Immediately after the dose is given, distribution, which is assumed to be instantaneous, is complete and no elimination has yet taken place; thus the amount of drug in the body is known. Such extrapolations are most easily performed from the semilog plots rather than from plots of concentration versus time.

TWO-COMPARTMENT MODEL

One-compartment models consider the body to be a homogenous unit into which a drug is distributed instantaneously. Generally, few cardioactive drugs can be studied and understood with this model. For most drugs, a two-compartment model is more appropriate for understanding cardiovascular drugs and considers drug distributions such that time is required before all parts of the body are in pseudoequilibrium. Pseudoequilibrium means that parallel changes, rather than identical drug concentrations, occur in all parts of the body. Figure 29-5 illustrates a two-compartment model, and the volume of the central compartment relates the amount of drug in the body to the concentration in the rapidly equilibrating compartments.

From a physiologic point of view, the rate at which a particular organ takes up drug depends on the rate of perfusion of the organ and the drug affinity of the organ tissue. Thus, there may be a large number of distribution processes taking place in various parts of the body. When viewed from the perspective of changes in the plasma concentration, these multiple processes tend to be averaged

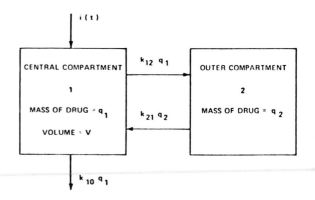

Fig. 29-5. Two-compartment model of drug disposition: i (t) is dose per time, q is mass of drug, and k is transfer constant.

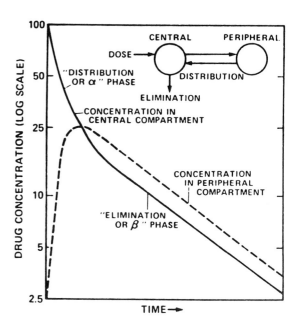

Fig. 29-6. A model in which the body is represented as consisting of two compartments, one that equilibrates rapidly (central compartment), and the other slowly (peripheral compartment) with drug plasma. The drug concentrations in each compartment following an intravenous bolus are also shown {24}.

into fast and slow processes. For many drugs, most of the distributive processes are faster than drug elimination, and thus, the nonexact terms of *distributive* or α phase or half-life, and *elimination* or β phase or half-life have been widely adopted (fig. 29-5). Although this approach inadequately describes the physiologic events taking place, it greatly enhances the use of compartmental models for describing and predicting blood concentrations.

Figure 29-6 is the conceptual representation of a two-compartment model, in which drug elimination is assumed to take place from the central compartment only, together with the drug concentrations in the central and peripheral compartments at various times following an intravenous bolus. Initially, all the drug is in the central compartment, with which it rapidly equilibrates. This compartment consists of the plasma and those rapidly perfused tissues, such as the liver and kidney, central nervous system, and myocardium. Distribution takes place from the rapidly equilibrating, or central, compartment into a more slowly equilibrating, or peripheral, compartment at a rate that is a function of the concentration (strictly the amount) of drug in the compartment. As drug concentration in the central compartment falls because of elimination, there is a transfer of drug from the peripheral compartment back to the central compartment. The reversible transfer of drugs between compartments is the sum of two first-order processes. In the postdistributive or β phase, the rate of drug loss from the central and peripheral compartments is the same, and a pseudoequilibrium is established in which the concentrations in the two compartments decline in parallel (fig. 29-6). Prior to distributional pseudoequilibrium, the relationship between the drug concentration in the plasma and in the slowly equilibrating compartment is constantly changing; whereas after pseudoequilibrium is established, there is a constant relationship between the plasma concentration and the concentration in other parts of the body. For a drug whose site of action is located in the peripheral compartment, plasma concentrations obtained shortly after the administration of a dose may correlate poorly with a pharmacologic response.

Because drug distribution is time dependent, a number of terms describing volume of distribution have come into use with the multicompartmental models. These relate the amount of drug in the body or a given compartment to blood or plasma concentrations at various times. Immediately after an intravenous bolus, all of the drug is in the central compartment, and no elimination or distribution from this compartment has taken place. In a manner analogous to a one-compartment model, the volume of the central compartment (V_c) can be defined as dose divided by the concentration at zero time. The volume of the central compartment is important in defining maximum concentrations immediately following a dose. On the other hand, when dealing with long-term infusions or multiple oral doses, one needs to know the volume through which the drug is ultimately distributed, or the volume of distribution at steady state (V_d^{ss}). A third term (V_β) is obtained by extrapolating the terminal log linear portion of a log plasma concentration time plot to time zero and dividing the intercept into the dose. This volume term is used to describe the volume through which the durg is distributed after the establishment of pseudoequilibrium.

The half-life of the slowest step, $t_{1/2\beta}$, governs the rate at which the drug leaves the body and also the rate at which a steady state is approached during continuous drug administration. $t_{1/2}\beta$ is a composite term resulting from the various processes of distribution and elimination that take place during distributional pseudoequilibrium and should not be confused with the half-life for elimination from the central compartment. As with the single-compartment model discussed previously, clearance can be estimated

by dividing a dose by the total area under the drug concentration-time curve.

PLASMA HALF-LIFE

By understanding compartmental analysis, the plasma half-life of a drug can be defined. The time interval in which the C_p of a drug falls to half its initial value is defined as its half-life ($t_{1/2}$). Thus for each interval, an increasingly smaller fraction of the initial C_p is removed, and theoretically an infinite time would be required to remove all drugs from the body (fig. 29-4). Practically, for most drugs it should be remembered that approximately 90% of a dose is removed in three $t_{1/2}$s, and 97% in five $t_{1/2}$s. This exponential decay of C_p can be linearized by plotting the logarithm of C_p versus time or using semilog graph paper (fig. 29-4). The $t_{1/2}$ of a drug in multiple-compartmental drug distribution is the result of several phases (fig. 29-6). The initial rapid phase $t_{1/2}$ represents the distribution of the drug when given in a single injection. The alpha, or flow distributional phase (fig. 29-6), and the elimination $t_{1/2}$ of the drug are related to its degradation and removal (Cl). Simple procedures for calculating initial and maintenance doses for a drug are presented in eqs. (29-1) and (29-2) and are based on the V_d or V_d^{ss} and plasma Cl. In physiologic terms, the plasma Cl of a drug and the volume through which it is distributed determines its $t_{1/2}$, that is,

$$t_{1/2} = V_d \, (144/Cl). \qquad (29\text{-}3)$$

Thus, if the V_d were reduced and the Cl remained constant, the $t_{1/2}$ would decrease. It is possible for both Cl and V_d to decrease simultaneously, as with lidocaine in severe congestive heart failure, with the result of only a small change in the elimination $t_{1/2}$. Clinically, knowing the $t_{1/2}$ for specific antiarrhythmic drugs is the most important fact that a clinician can use in practical drug dosing terms. First, it permits estimation of the time required to produce steady-state conditions during mutiple dosing (that is, four or five $t_{1/2}$s); and second, to determine the dosing interval necessary to achieve peak and trough C_p within the therapeutic range.

As pointed out above in the two-compartment system, which represents the majority of cardioactive drugs, distribution processes are faster than elimination phase processes, and the inexact term *distributive* or *alpha* or *fast* half-life, and the *elimination* or *beta* (*terminal* or *slow* half-life) are widely used.

SYSTEMIC AVAILABILITY

When considering the oral administration of a drug, knowing its systemic availability (F) is necessary for compartmental modeling and for understanding the specific use of the drug in clinical situations. When a drug is administered orally, a number of factors may prevent the entire dose from reaching the systemic circulation, through which most drugs must pass to reach their sites of action. The drug may not be released from its dose form, it may not be soluble in the gastrointestinal fluids, it may be chemically or enzymatically degraded in the gastrointestinal tract or in mucosal cells, or there may be insufficient time for all of the drug to be absorbed before it is excreted in the stools. Drugs absorbed from the gastrointestinal tract must pass through the liver in order to reach the systemic circulation. Drugs with high nonrenal or hepatic clearances will have a significant fraction of the total dose removed during the first passage through the liver. This "first-pass" effect is a major reason why lidocaine cannot be used orally and is also an important factor to be considered in the oral administration of propranolol. Systemic availability (sometimes called *bioavailability*) of a drug is usually estimated by comparing the area under the plasma or blood concentration time curve (AUC) for an oral dose with that obtained after an intravenous dose (where systemic availability is by definition 1.0):

$$F = \frac{AUC_0^\infty(oral)}{AUC_0^\infty(i.v.)} \cdot \frac{dose\ (i.v.)}{dose\ (oral)}. \qquad (29\text{-}4)$$

DRUG DOSING

Intravenous infusions

Most patients receive a drug over a period of time, either as multiple doses or by continuous administration by intravenous infusion. Figure 29-7 illustrates the time course of plasma concentrations during and after two constant infusions, one given at twice the rate of the other. The drug concentrations gradually increase to a plateau level at a rate that is determined by the half-life for the drug. During one half-life, both infusions reach 50%, and in approximately three half-lives reach 90% of their respective plateau values. It will be observed that the rate of drug

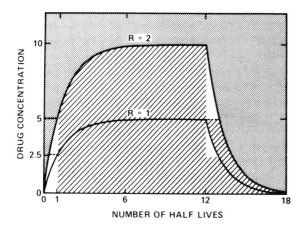

Fig. 29-7. Drug concentrations during and subsequent to constant drug infusions given at rate R and 2R. The time required to reach plateau concentrations is determined by the half-life for the drug and is independent of infusion rate. The magnitude of the plateau concentration is proportional to the infusion rate {24}.

administration does not influence the rate at which the final plateau concentration is reached, but it does determine its value. At the plateau, a steady-state situation occurs, where the rate of drug administration (R) is equal to the rate of drug elimination, and there is no net change in drug concentration. Drug concentration at steady state (C^{ss}) is determined by the following relationship:

$$\text{Infusion rate (R)} = C^{ss} \cdot CL_T$$
$$= \text{rate of elimination.} \qquad (29\text{-}5)$$

When the infusion is stopped, the concentration declines in a manner analogous to that after the intravenous bolus (fig. 29-4).

Multiple oral doses

Drugs are more commonly administered by multiple oral doses at regular intervals than by intravenous infusion. Such a dosage regimen can be considered, from a pharmacokinetic point of view, to be equivalent to an intermittent infusion. Because of the intermittent nature of drug administration, plasma concentrations fluctuate between a maximum and a minimum value during a dosage interval, as shown in fig. 29-3. The magnitude of these between-dose fluctuations increases as the absorption rate of the drug increases and the half-life decreases. In many situations, it is convenient to consider the average drug concentration ($\bar{C}$) during a dosage interval (τ). In a similar fashion, drug administration can be calculated as an average rate ($\bar{R}$). For example, 300 mg every 6 hours would be equivalent to an average rate of 50 mg/hr. Allowing for systemic availability, one may write, as for eq. (29-5):

$$\text{Dose rate } \bar{R} = \text{elimination rate}$$

$$\frac{F\ dose}{\tau} = C \cdot CL_T$$

or

$$\bar{C} = \frac{F\ dose}{CL_T \cdot \tau}. \qquad (29\text{-}5)$$

When a plateau is reached, one may use eq. (29-5) to calculate total body clearance (more strictly, $F \cdot CL_T$) for a particular patient, on the basis of the mean plasma concentration during a dosing interval. As can be seen in figs. 29-6 and 29-7, the time course of drug concentration and the factors governing them are essentially similar for a constant intravenous infusion and intermittent oral administration at fixed intervals. The time required to approach the mean plateau concentration is determined by the half-life of the drug, and the magnitude of the average plateau concentration is determined by the average dosing rate.

The fluctuations in plasma concentrations during a dosing interval and time required to reach plateau levels have clinically important implications. For drugs with long half-lives, or in situations where it is necessary to rapidly reach a therapeutic concentration, administration of the drug at a given constant rate may be unsatisfactory, be-

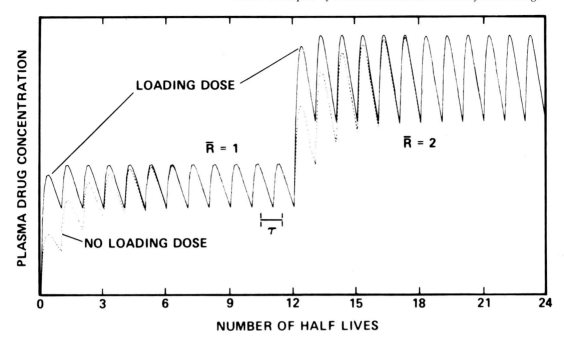

Fig. 29-8. Plasma drug concentrations during a multiple oral dosage regimen in which drug is administered with dosage interval (γ) equal to the half-life at an average rate of $\bar{R}$ and $2\bar{R}$. The solid line shows the effect of an initial loading dose, equal to twice the usual dose, on the time required to reach plateau concentrations {24}.

cause three to five half-lives are required to reach plateau concentrations. In such cases, one must give a large initial or loading dose, which rapidly produces the desired plasma concentration previously decided upon (fig. 29-7). The magnitude of the dose can be calculated using eq. (29-1). This concentration can then be maintained by administering the drug at such a rate that it replaces the drug lost from the body. By definition, half of the drug in the body will be eliminated during one half-life. Thus, if one gives half the initial dose every half-life, plasma concentration will fluctuate between the initial concentration and a minimum, half this value. This technique is illustrated in fig. 29-8, which also shows the same dosage regimen with, and in the absence of, the loading dose. It will be noted that when doubling the dose, an additional loading dose must be given if one desires to arrive rapidly at the new plateau. This is a convenient strategy for drugs with half-lives in the range of 4–24 hours. Drugs with half-lives shorter than 4 hours are impractical to administer with such a regimen because of inconvenience to the patient. This is also true of drugs to be administered less frequently than once a day. Antiarrhythmic drugs generally have low therapeutic-to-toxic ratios (therapeutic indices), and it is often undesirable to allow drug concentrations to fluctuate through more than a two- to threefold range during a dosing interval. For these reasons, drugs with narrow therapeutic indices and short half-lives are usually given by intravenous infusions (e.g., lidocaine).

Thus the choice of a particular dosage interval depends on the half-life of the drug, its therapeutic index, and

considerations of patient convenience. Figure 29-8 shows drug concentrations resulting from a dosage regimen in which half the loading dose is given every half-life, together with the concentrations resulting from the same dose rate but with a dosing interval of two half-lives. The larger dosing interval results in periods when the probability of toxicity is high shortly after the dose is given, and a period towards the end of the dosing interval when antiarrhythmic control may be poor. On the other hand, an initial loading dose and dosing every half-life rapidly attains and maintains effective antiarrhythmic concentrations at all times. Consistent with eq. (29-5), the average concentrations resulting from these two regimens are the same (fig. 29-8).

It is a common impression that some drugs accumulate in the body during multiple oral dosing, whereas others do not. It should be apparent from the foregoing discussion that the accumulation of a drug in such situations is a function of both its half-life and the dosing interval. Thus any drug will accumulate when given at a rate that exceeds its rate of removal from the body. The degree to which a drug accumulates is given by the relationship:

$$\frac{\bar{C} \text{ plateau}}{C(\text{first dose})} = \frac{1.44\ t_{1/2}}{\tau}. \qquad (29\text{-}6)$$

NONLINEAR PHARMACOKINETICS

One of the consequences of first-order kinetics (removal of a constant fraction of the amount of drug in the body per

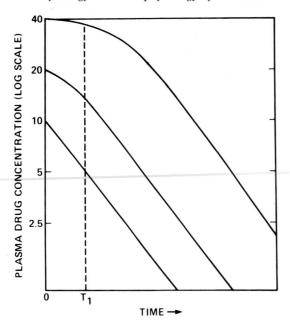

Fig. 29-9. Plasma drug concentrations at various times during three separate doses of D, 2D, and 4D of a drug showing nonlinear pharmacokinetics. The concentrations are nonsuperimposable when normalized for dose, and there is more than a proportional increase in the area under the concentration time curve. The half-life changes with concentration, with approximately 50% of D, 30% of 2D, and 20% of 4D being eliminated in the period O-T {24}.

unit time) is that drug concentrations are proportional to the amount of drug administered, as shown, for example, in figs. 29-4 and 29-6. Thus if drug concentrations are normalized by dividing by dose, they are superimposable. When concentrations can be superimposed in this way, the system is said to follow *linear kinetics*. Conversely, when this is not so, the system is said to be *nonlinear*.

The various processes of drug elimination, such as hepatic metabolism and (in some cases) renal excretion, are carried out by enzymes, and as such, obey Michaelis–Menten kinetics. In the cases discussed so far, the concentrations of drug are well below the maximum capacities of these systems, and under these conditions first-order kinetics are approximated. If drug concentrations become sufficiently high or the capacity of the enzyme system is sufficiently low, then the enzyme system may become saturated and a constant amount of drug is removed in a given time. This type of behavior is called *zero-order kinetics*. More commonly, a situation intermediate between first- and zero-order kinetics is observed, where there is less drug removed than would be expected from a first-order process, but the system is not completely saturated. Figure 29-9 illustrates plasma concentrations of a drug, showing nonlinear kinetics for various times after three separate single doses of magnitude; D, 2D, and 4D.

At the highest dose, one can see that there is a greater than proportional increase in the area (log scale) under the concentration-time curve. Furthermore, the half-life increases as the actual value of the concentration increases. Thus, at T_1, half of the smallest dose, but only approximately 30% of the medium dose and 20% of the highest dose, have been eliminated. Half-life has no precise meaning when applied to such data and should be reserved for first-order processes. The consequences of administering a second equal dose at T_1 are obviously quite different in each case. These phenomena have two important clinical consequences when such drugs are given in multiple doses. First, an increase in dose may produce a more than proportional increase in plasma concentration. Second, because the proportion of the dose that is eliminated in a given time decreases with dose, the half-life is increased and the time required to reach a plateau becomes progressively longer as the dose increases. In a true zero-order situation, as a constant amount rather than a constant fraction of the dose is removed in a given time, if the dosing rate exceeds the rate of removal, the concentrations will increase indefinitely. Two commonly used antiarrhythmic drugs, phenytoin and disopyramide, display nonlinear characteristics at normally prescribed doses.

INFLUENCE OF DISEASE ON DRUG DISPOSITION

The dosage regimens of antiarrhythmic drugs are well established and are usually based on a combination of clinical experience and general pharmacokinetic principles. For the majority of patients who, apart from their cardiac arrhythmia, are otherwise healthy, the general guideline will usually suffice. Patients with altered drug disposition as a result of disease may pose a problem for the physician. These patients form the group to which clinical pharmacokinetics can most fruitfully be applied {24–30}.

Although there are no useful correlates, such as those that exist between creatine clearance and the ability of the kidney to eliminate drugs, which would enable the individualization of drug dosage in patients with hepatic and cardiovascular dysfunction, some general trends have been demonstrated that may help to identify patients in whom dosage may need to be adjusted. Since the degree to which drug disposition is altered as a result of hepatic or cardiovascular dysfunction cannot be quantitated in a given individual, one must identify groups of patients in whom changes may be expected and indicate the anticipated direction of the change. This approach must be used exclusively for antiarrhythmic drugs, since generally used antiarrhythmic drugs, with the exception of procainamide, are not eliminated primarily by renal mechanisms. Even in the case of procainamide, a quantitative treatment is difficult because of the formation of an active metabolite. The strategy for the administration of antiarrhythmic drugs to such patients should involve the use of general guidelines in estimating initial dosage, followed by careful clinical observation, and in some cases, blood level monitoring.

Renal disease {24–30}

The effect of renal dysfunction on drug disposition has been the subject of several recent articles and reviews. The potential for alteration in drug disposition in renal disease increases with the fraction of the dose that is normally eliminated unchanged in the urine. It is possible, by using common indices of renal function, to establish guidelines for adjusting the dosage regimens of patients who have renal dysfunction and receive drugs eliminated predominantly by renal mechanisms. A number of antiarrhythmic drugs that are not significantly dependent on renal elimination undergo changes in disposition when given to patients with renal dysfunction.

Cardiac failure

On the basis of the discussion previously presented, it could be anticipated that those drugs with high hepatic (blood-flow-sensitive) clearances, such as lidocaine and propranolol, would show the greatest changes in disposition as a result of cardiac failure. Other effects of cardiac failure, such as visceral congestion and altered regional blood flows, may produce changes in the intrinsic clearance of drugs and in their volumes of distribution. The effects of cardiac failure on drug disposition have been reviewed by Benowitz and Meister {26}.

Hepatic dysfunction

The effects of hepatic disease on drug disposition and their likely therapeutic implications have been the subject of a number of recent reviews that attempt to evaluate existing data on the subject in terms of the physiologic model of drug disposition previously outlined {24}. Rowland and others {27} used this model to formulate guidelines for drug administration, resulting from a consideration of the likely outcome of changes in drug disposition due to hepatic disease in commonly encountered clinical situations. Based on an extensive review of the literature, these authors concluded that after single oral or intravenous doses, it is unlikely that doses would need to be altered because of hepatic disease. For an intravenous infusion reaching steady state, the unbound concentration (and hence the intensity of effect) of highly cleared drugs will be elevated when either hepatic blood flow is depressed or binding is diminished. For poorly cleared drugs, the unbound steady-state concentration is only sensitive to changes in drug-metabolizing activity, and although altered binding will alter blood concentration, the unbound steady-state drug concentration should remain the same.

Steady-state blood concentration for all drugs used for chronic oral dosing, whether highly or poorly cleared, depends on intrinsic clearance and should be independent of blood flow. More importantly, for all drugs given orally, the unbound concentration at steady state should depend solely on the drug metabolism activity of the liver (CL_{int}) and should be independent of both hepatic blood flow and binding. The above analysis was based on the assumption that the liver was the sole organ of elimination, and it was concluded that where nonhepatic mechanisms of elimination occurred, changes in drug disposition would be less pronounced. It was concluded that none of the available liver function tests provided a sufficiently reliable index to enable the adjustment of dosage. However, in chronic liver disease, serum albumin might serve as a crude index of drug metabolism activity. The situation with acute viral hepatitis is even less clearly defined, the clearance of some drugs being depressed and remaining unchanged in others. At this time, there does not appear to be even a rough guide available to indicate how to appropriately adjust dosage regimens during acute viral hepatitis.

Protein binding

The free concentration of drug unbound to plasma proteins is considered to be the concentration that most closely reflects the concentration at the receptor site and the pharmacologic response. For most drugs (for example, phenytoin) in patients without renal or hepatic dysfunction, the free concentration is a constant fraction of the total concentration (the concentration measured by usual analytical methods), with little intersubject variability. Small changes in the percent bound can make large differences in the free-drug concentrations of highly (>90%) bound drugs, such as phenytoin. For example, a decrease in the percent bound from 95% to 90% will increase the free fraction by twofold.

Age

Finally, although patient age can influence the disposition of some drugs, such as phenytoin, little is known about the effect of age on the kinetics of disposition of the antiarrhythmic drugs.

The fnal purpose of this chapter is to present the most relevant pharmacokinetic concepts for each of the important antiarrhythmic agents currently available in the United States. The relevant pharmacokinetic data will also be presented for a select few of the investigational agents likely to be marketed soon. It should be noted that, although the pharmacokinetic profile is well defined for most of the available antiarrhythmic drugs, there are very few studies that adequately describe the relationship between drug concentration in serum (the most readily accessible site for measuring drug) and the most appropriate end point for drug therapy, i.e., prevention of sudden cardiac death and/or alleviation of arrhythmia-related symptoms. Several clinical trials that attempted to relate plasma concentration to efficacy have shown higher levels in the nonresponders than in responders. This should not be interpreted to mean there is no relationship between drug plasma concentration and effect, but reflects that some patients' arrhythmias are refractory to the specific drug being studied, and larger doses have been administered trying to reach a therapeutic effect (threshold). These patients may well respond to a different drug or may have totally drug refractory arrhythmias. On the other hand, some patients can be identified as drug responders, and a target therapeutic plasma concentration can be identified to have a desired antiarrhythmia effect {33,34}. If this method of monitoring serum drug concentrations for antiarrhythmic drugs continues to prove useful in the future, then a complete understanding of the important pharmacokinetic principles for the available antiarrhythmic agents will assist the clinician in more rapidly achieving effective therapeutic drug concentrations and will aid the clinician in predicting alterations in drug concentrations as a response to drug-drug interactions or changing disease states.

CLASS I ANTIARRHYTHMIC DRUGS

Class Ia agents

QUINIDINE

Quinidine is the oldest antiarrhythmic agent still in use and remains one of the most commonly prescribed antiarrhythmic drugs. Approximately 80% of a quinidine dose is absorbed following oral administration. Peak serum concentrations occur in 90 minutes for regular-release forms of quinidine, with delayed peak serum concentrations occurring from 3 to 4 hours for the sustained-release forms of the drug. Quinidine plasma half-life ranges from 5 to 8 hours. The therapeutic range in plasma is approximately 1.5–5 μg/ml.

Quinidine is approximately 80–90% bound to serum proteins, primarily alpha-1-acid glycoprotein (AAG). The amount of free (unbound) quinidine in plasma decreases with increasing amounts of AAG and has been shown to rise in response to acute stress such as myocardial infarction {35}. This is not of clinical importance.

Quinidine is extensively metabolized in the liver to several known cardioactive metabolites. The most studied is 3-hydroxyquinidine. Although plasma concentrations of 3-hydroxyquinidine are usually far less than those of the parent compound, recent evidence suggests that unbound 3-hydroxyquinidine concentrations meet or exceed unbound quinidine concentrations and therefore may substantially contribute to the overall effects seen with quinidine therapy {36}.

Quinidine is rapidly distributed to many extravascular sites with a distribution half-life of approximately 7 minutes. The pharmacokinetics are described by a two-compartment open model with a volume of distribution of approximately 3 l/kg. Quinidine total body clearance averages 4.5 ml/min/kg; however, there is wide intersubject variability.

Although the presence of congestive heart failure does not increase serum half-life, binding to AAG is reduced, resulting in an increased volume of distribution and reduced clearance. Liver disease, primarily cirrhosis, can result in quinidine accumulation in plasma, requiring dosage reductions, and cautious monitoring for adverse effects. Patients with chronic ischemic heart disease and survivors of prehospital cardiac arrest have been shown to have reduced unbound concentrations of quinidine in serum due to higher AAG concentrations and higher protein binding {37}.

Quinidine has the narrow therapeutic range of 1.5–5 μg/ml in serum. Most of the data concerning quinidine serum concentration-effect relationships were obtained in the early 1970s, when "effects" were defined as changes in surface electrocardiogram intervals (QT, QRS) or reductions in PVC frequency, effects now known to not necessarily be related to prevention of sudden cardiac death. In addition, early assays for quinidine in serum were nonspecific, resulting in a somewhat higher therapeutic range than used today. Nevertheless, these early studies did define a clinically useful range of serum concentrations that reduced the likelihood of quinidine toxicity and did provide reasonable predictions of desired therapeutic effects.

Drugs inducing hepatic metabolism, such as phenobarbital, rifampin, and phenytoin, may enhance quinidine total body clearance and reduce the desired therapeutic effect. Conversely, enzyme inhibition with cimetidine or amiodarone may result in quinidine accumulation of 50–75% over baseline and an increased incidence of toxicity.

The major limitation to quinidine therapy is a relatively high incidence of adverse effects. The most common adverse effects of quinidine therapy are gastrointestinal, with diarrhea occurring in up to 30% of patients. Allergic responses may be manifest as rash, fever, hemolytic anemia, or thrombocytopenia. The most severe adverse effect of quinidine therapy is its ability to induce "quinidine syncope," a proarrhythmic response characterized by a polymorphic ventricular tachycardia (torsade de pointes). The generation of this proarrhythmic event is thought to be due to early afterdepolarizations and is commonly preceded by QT prolongation. Quinidine syncope is seen in approximately 0.5–2% of patients early in the course of therapy, may be associated with concomitant digitalis therapy, and its occurrence appears unrelated to quinidine plasma concentrations {38}.

PROCAINAMIDE

Procainamide has been used an antiarrhythmic since the 1950s and continues to be a useful agent for ventricular and supraventricular arrhythmias. Procainamide is metabolized through N-acetylation to an active metabolite, N-acetylprocainamide (NAPA), which has Class III electrophysiologic effects that differ from those of the parent compound. This may result in variable electrophysiologic effects in a given patient due to differences in hepatic N-acetyl-transferase activity and serum procainamide/NAPA ratios.

Procainamide is well absorbed after oral administration. Regular-release capsules produce peak serum concentrations in 1–2 hours; however, procainamide is more commonly administered in a sustained-release form due to a short (3–4 hour) elimination half-life. The sustained-release forms of procainamide provide peak serum concentrations in 3–4 hours. Approximately 50–70% of procainamide is excreted unchanged in urine, with the remainder being N-acetylated in the liver to NAPA. This form of hepatic metabolism is under genetic control, with approximately 45% of white and black populations and 10–20% of Oriental populations having "slow acetylator" status {39}. Over 90% of NAPA is then excreted unchanged in urine.

Procainamide pharmacokinetics follow a two-compartment open model with an initial distribution half-life of about 5 minutes and an elimination half-life of approximately 3–4 hours. The volume of distribution at steady state averages 2 l/kg. Procainamide and NAPA are bound less than 20% to serum proteins. Systemic clearance averages 8–9 ml/min/kg.

There is a linear relationship between decline in creatinine clearance and a reduction in both procainamide and NAPA total body clearance. Procainamide half-life averages 3–4 hours in patients with normal renal function and increases to 13–15 hours in anephric patients {40}. For NAPA, renal clearance is a higher proportion of total body clearance, and therefore NAPA serum concentrations will accumulate disproportionately to procainamide as renal function declines. This can result in alterations of the procainamide/NAPA ratio in serum and possibly lead to dosage reductions, resulting in loss of antiarrhythmic efficacy {41}.

As with quinidine, much of what is known about procainamide serum concentration-effect relationships was generated in the early 1970s, which resulted in a proposed therapeutic range of 4–10 µg/ml. Myerburg et al. have shown that, on average, higher serum concentrations of procainamide are necessary for 85% PVC suppression compared to those needed to prevent ventricular tachycardia in the same patients {42}. In addition, lower procainamide serum concentrations were required for 85% PVC suppression in patients with myocardial infarction than in patients with either chronic ischemic heart disease or recurrent ventricular tachycardia. These same investigators have also shown that maintenance of procainamide serum concentrations in the therapeutic range is associated with a lower recurrence of sudden cardiac death, compared to patients with variable and unstable serum concentrations, thus providing supporting evidence for the use of "therapeutic" serum concentrations in the absence of other surrogate end points to prevent the recurrence of sudden cardiac death {34}.

In addition to glomerular filtration, procainamide and NAPA are secreted across renal tubules by an active transport system for weak bases. This process has several known competitive inhibitors, including trimethoprim, ranitidine, and cimetidine. Concomitant therapy with these agents results in a reduction in procainamide renal clearance and increases of approximately 20–50% in serum concentrations {43}. Effects on NAPA renal secretion are less consistent.

The major limitations to procainamide therapy are its proarrhythmic effects and the induction of the lupus syndrome. Drug-induced lupus following procainamide therapy occurs in approximately 20% of patients and is characterized by fever, arthralgias, and myalgias. Although at least 80% of patients receiving procainamide for more than 1 year will convert to a positive serum anti-nuclear antibody (ANA) test, conversion does not require interruption of procainamide therapy unless the patient experiences SLE symptoms. A positive ANA and the lupus syndrome develop more slowly in rapid acetylators (7 months) compared to slow acetylators (3 months), implying that procainamide and not NAPA alters autoimmune function {44}. In fact, NAPA therapy alone only rarely induces a positive ANA and is not associated with development of the lupus syndrome. On the other hand, it is a rather poor antiarrhythmic drug. Therefore, the relative ratio of procainamide to NAPA in serum is an indicator of an individual patient's acetylator status and may be used to predict the likelihood of early versus late drug-induced lupus.

DISOPYRAMIDE

Disopyramide was synthesized in the 1954 in a search to find a safer antiarrhythmic than quinidine and procainamide. The drug has been in use in France since 1969 and in the United States since 1977; however, an association with significant myocardial depression has limited its clinical use. Disopyramide has one chiral center, and therefore is administered as a racemic mixture of equal amounts of $R(-)$ and $S(+)$ disopyramide. These enantiomers exhibit substantial differences in protein binding, renal clearance, and therapeutic/toxic effects.

Disopyramide is well absorbed following oral administration and has a systemic bioavailability averaging 85%, with a range of 50–90%. Disopyramide is extensively bound to serum proteins, primarily AAG, with unbound fractions in serum that range from 20% to 90%. This wide variability in unbound serum concentrations is a result of saturable, nonlinear protein binding that decreases as total serum disopyramide concentrations increase. This nonlinearity makes interpretation of serum levels for effectiveness or toxicity difficult. Approximately 50% of disopyramide can be recovered in urine unchanged, while the other half is N-dealkylated in the liver. Elimination half-life averages about 6 hours, necessitating every 6-hour dosing with regular release formulations. A sustained-release product may be administered every 8–12 hours.

Disopyramide pharmacokinetics are usually described by a two-compartment or three-compartment open model. At steady state, the volume of distribution for unbound disopyramide is approximately 1 l/kg. Total body clearance for unbound drug averages about 3 ml/min/kg. The unbound renal clearance for $S(+)$ disopyramide is approximately twice that of the $R(-)$ enantiomer, suggesting the involvement of stereoselective tubular secretion {45}.

There is little evidence that the presence of liver disease requires alterations in disopyramide dosage. Total (bound plus unbound) serum concentrations of disopyramide do not significantly change in patients with renal dysfunction; however, there is an increase in the ratio of unbound to total disopyramide serum concentrations at creatinine clearances less than 30–40 ml/min, necessitating a dosage reduction of 25–50%.

Unfortunately, only a few studies have evaluated disopyramide serum concentration-effect relationships using unbound disopyramide concentrations. This is necessary due to the substantial variability in protein binding at a given total disopyramide serum concentration. The reported therapeutic range for total disopyramide is 2–5 µg/ml. Several investigators have established a better concentration-effect relationship when using unbound disopyramide concentrations and changes in electrocardiographic intervals; however, no studies to date have evaluated the relationship between unbound disopyramide concentrations and antiarrhythmic efficacy.

Although not well studied in a classic concentration-effect fashion, the enantiomers of disopyramide differ in their pharmacologic effects. The anticholinergic effects seen with disopyramide therapy are more closely associated with the metabolite and R(−) disopyramide {46}. QTc prolongation is due exclusively to the presence of the S(+) isomer. However, the isomers appear to have similar potency for inhibition of sodium ion channels, indicating that binding to sodium channels is not stereoselective. S(+) disopyramide is predominantly associated with the negative inotropic effects of the drug. Hepatic enzyme induction due to rifampin or phenytoin can reduce total disopyramide serum concentrations and produce loss of the antiarrhythmic effect.

PIRMENOL

Pirmenol is a newer antiarrhythmic currently being evaluated in the United States. Its electrophysiologic effects are similar to that of other Class Ia antiarrhythmic in that conduction and refractoriness are prolonged. Unlike other agents in this class, however, pirmenol's effectiveness is independent of extracellular potassium concentrations.

Pirmenol is rapidly absorbed and produces peak serum concentrations in 1–1.5 hours; however, this may be erratic and produce second and third peaks in some patients {47}. Bioavailability averages 83–87%. The volume of distribution averages 2 l/kg, indicating extensive distribution to extravascular tissues. Pirmenol is approximately 85% bound in serum and shows AAG-dependent protein binding. Approximately 30% of a dose is excreted unchanged in the urine, with the remainder being hepatically metabolized to two biologically active metabolites. The half-life in serum averages 7–9 hours, but may range from 4 to 17 hours.

Following intravenous administration, pirmenol pharmacokinetics are described by a two-compartment open model. The distribution half-life was approximately 10 minutes, with a volume of distribution of 1–2 l/kg. Total body clearance averages 2–3 ml/min/kg, with renal clearance averaging 0.7–0.9 ml/mim/kg.

Little data are available on serum concentration-effect relationships with pirmenol. Based on arrhythmia recurrence following drug withdrawal, the minimally effective serum concentration has been suggested as 1.0 µg/ml {47}. Data from PES studies indicate somewhat higher "therapeutic" concentrations of 2.6–3.7 µg/ml {48,49}. These data together suggest a tenuous therapeutic range of 1–4 µg/ml.

Rifampin has been show to induce the hepatic metabolism of pirmenol, resulting in reduced serum concentrations. Although not yet reported, hepatic enzyme inhibitors (cimetidine, amiodarone) should be cautiously added to pirmenol therapy with careful monitoring for adverse effects due to the potential for reduced hepatic clearance.

Class Ib agents

LIDOCAINE

Lidocaine was first used in 1948 as a local anesthetic and was utilized as an antiarrhythmic in the 1950s. It is now the most widely used intravenous antiarrhythmic drug, although its use is primarily limited to ventricular arrhythmias.

Although well absorbed upon oral administration, lidocaine is extensively metabolized upon first pass through the liver, producing a low systemic bioavailability of about 35%. The metabolites formed upon first pass, which include MEGX and GX, have additive CNS toxicity to lidocaine itself, making oral administration unacceptable. Blood concentrations of lidocaine fall rapidly following intravenous administration, which may result in loss of initially achieved arrhythmia control. For this reason, several investigators have proposed lidocaine intravenous loading regimens designed to prevent this "subtherapeutic" dip in lidocaine serum concentrations. These loading regimens vary from single repeat IV bolus doses in 10–15 minutes to more complex, computer-designed, logarithmically declining infusions {50}.

Lidocaine is approximately 70% bound to serum proteins, primarily AAG and, to a lesser extent, albumin. Lidocaine is extensively metabolized in the liver to several metabolites, two of which have some antiarrhythmic activity (MEGX and GX). MEGX has been shown to have 80–90% of the activity of lidocaine in animal models of arrhythmia, with mean MEGX/lidocaine concentrations in serum of patients being 30% {51}. Thus, MEGX may contribute to the pharmacologic activity of lidocaine, but generally is not considered clinically important, and blood levels of lidocaine are used extensively by clinicians. Only 2% of an administered intravenous dose of lidocaine is excreted unchanged in the urine.

Lidocaine pharmacokinetics follow a two-compartment open model. The volume of distribution is approximately 2–2.5 l/kg. Total body clearance is heavily dependent on liver blood flow and averages 9–12 ml/mim/kg in patients with myocardial infarction. Serum elimination half-life is reported to average about 90 minutes in normal volunteers, but is closer to 4 hours in patients with relatively uncomplicated myocardial infarction {52}.

Lidocaine clearance has been shown to gradually decline as the duration of the infusion increases, such that prolonged infusions require monitoring of serum concentrations and dosage reductions if necessary.

Congestive heart failure and the resulting loss in hepatic

perfusion reduces lidocaine clearance by approximately 50% below clearance values for patients with uncomplicated myocardial infarction {53}. On the other hand, acute increases in AAG concentrations reduce unbound lidocaine concentrations in serum and may reduce efficacy. Chronic liver disease also results in a 40–50% reduction in lidocaine clearance, through impairment of liver blood flow and/or a reduction in hepatic metabolizing enzyme activity {54}.

Lidocaine serum concentrations of 2–2.5 μg/ml are needed to achieve 75% suppression of PVC frequency, while prophylaxis studies show that lidocaine serum concentrations of greater than 2 μg/ml are needed for the prevention of ventricular fibrillation post myocardial infarction {55,56}. More recent data show that objective signs of lidocaine toxicity (tinnitus, visual disturbances) occur at concentrations beginning at 6–8 μg/ml, suggesting a therapeutic range of 2–6 μg/ml to provide efficacy with minimal toxicity {57}.

Propranolol is reported to reduce lidocaine clearance by 40–50% {58}. Cimetidine and amiodarone also reduce lidocaine clearance. Enzyme inducers, such as rifampin and phenobarbital, have been reported to increase lidocaine clearance and result in reductions in serum concentrations.

TOCAINIDE

The synthesis of tocainide was the result of modifications to the basic lidocaine structure, which resulted in enhanced oral bioavailability and prolonged elimination half-life. Tocainide is well absorbed orally and essentially exhibits 100% bioavailability. Peak serum concentrations are achieved in 0.5–2 hours. Oral administration with food reduces peak serum concentrations by 40%; however, total absorption remains complete {59,60}. This suggests that tocainide should be administered with food to prevent dose-related side effects attributed to excessive peak concentrations. Tocainide is approximately 50% bound to serum proteins, and therefore protein binding interactions are of no clinical consequence. Elimination half-life in serum is approximately 13 hours in healthy volunteers, and tocainide may be administered two or three times a day to patients. Approximately 30–45% of an administered dose is excreted unchanged in the urine. The remainder is hepatically metabolized through glucuronidation to inactive metabolites, which are then eliminated renally. Urinary alkalinization reduces renal clearance by as much as 75% {58}.

Following intravenous administration, tocainide pharmacokinetics are well described by a two-compartment open model. Total body clearance ranges from 154 to 184 ml/min. In patients with renal disease, tocainide clearance is reduced to 35–94 ml/min and is associated with a prolonged elimination half-life of 22 hours {61}. As a result, tocainide doses can be reduced and given at longer dosing intervals. Interestingly, standard hemodialysis removes as much as 25% of tocainide in the body, which requires patients to receive a supplemental tocainide dose.

There are no data to support the need for dosage reduction in patients with hepatic dysfunction.

Arrhythmia suppression is associated with serum concentrations of approximately 3–9 μg/ml. In one study, Emax modeling was used to describe the relationship between PVC suppression and serum tocainide concentrations following tocainide withdrawal in patients with frequent PVCs. PVC suppression was negligible at concentrations below 4 μg/ml, while no further PVC suppression was seen at concentrations above 10 μg/ml {62}.

The relative balance between renal and nonrenal routes of elimination makes tocainide elimination relatively insensitive to drug-induced changes in hepatic metabolizing activity. Combination therapy with tocainide and a Class Ia antiarrhythmic may provide for synergistic antiarrhythmic effects with lower doses, thus lowering the incidence of intolerable toxicity. In one study by Barbey et al., the combination of tocainide and quinidine allowed for lower doses of both agents, reducing the occurrence of minor toxicities and increasing the numbers of patients responsive to antiarrhythmic therapy {63}.

MEXILETINE

Mexiletine was originally investigated as an anticonvulsant agent and was noted to possess significant antiarrhythmic properties. The minor difference in structure from lidocaine provides mexiletine with better oral absorption and a longer elimination half-life in serum.

Mexiletine is well absorbed orally and has a systemic bioavailability of 80–90%. Food delays the rate of absorption, but does not reduce the extent of absorption; thus, administration with food is recommended to reduce transient adverse effects associated with excessive peak concentrations. Peak serum concentrations occur between 2 and 4 hours, with an elimination half-life between 9 and 12 hours. Mexiletine is approximately 70% bound to serum proteins. The drug is widely distributed throughout skin, muscle, and fat tissues, with a large volume of distribution of 5.5–9.5 l/kg. Mexiletine undergoes extensive hepatic metabolism, with less than 25% of a dose excreted unchanged in the urine. The major metabolites of mexiletine — parahydroxymexiletine, hydroxymethylmexiletine, and their alcohols — are not cardioactive.

Mexiletine pharmacokinetics have been described using a three-compartment model. The first two exponents represent rapid and slow distribution to body tissues, with the terminal exponent representing elimination from the body. Total body clearance is approximately 7 ml/min/kg and is largely dependent on hepatic metabolic enzyme activity. The volume of distribution is extensive, with only 1% of total body stores of mexiletine present in serum.

Mexiletine absorption has been reported to be delayed in patients with acute myocardial infarction, although the extent of absorption is essentially unaltered. The mechanism of delayed absorption appears to be reduced gastric emptying caused by either transient reductions in gastrointestinal blood flow or coadministration of narcotic analgesics {64}.

Mexiletine clearance is significantly reduced in patients

with congestive heart failure. Patients with cirrhosis are reported to have markedly higher elimination half-lives that can exceed 28 hours, with clearance reduced from 8.3 to 2.3 ml/kg, compared to normal controls {65}.

Renal insufficiency has no apparent affect on mexiletine clearance. However, changes in urinary pH can have marked effects on mexiletine renal clearance. In one study, a urine pH of 8.0 increased steady-state serum mexiletine concentrations by 39% compared to a urinary pH of 5.0 {66}.

The therapeutic range for mexiletine is 0.5–2.0 μg/ml. Serum concentrations below 0.5 μg/ml are rarely effective and concentrations above 2.0 μg/ml are associated with an unacceptably high incidence of gastrointestinal and CNS side effects. However, there is considerable overlap in serum concentrations that produce efficacy and intolerable side effects.

Mexiletine absorption following oral administration is delayed during coadministration with cimetidine, antacids, and atropine. Conversely, metoclopramide enhances gastirc emptying and promotes mexiletine oral absorption. Hepatic enzyme inducers (rifampin, phenobarbital, phenytoin) are reported to increase mexiletine clearance, while enzyme inhibitors (cimetidine, amiodarone) can reduce mexiletine clearance.

One study has reported an additional 35% of patients will respond to combination therapy with mexiletine and a type Ia antiarrhythmic in patients not responding to mexiletine therapy alone {67}.

Class Ic agents

When originally developed, the Class Ic agents were recognized as some of the most potent antiarrhythmic drugs for suppressing supraventricular and ventricular arrhythmias. During development, these agents were compared to more standard therapies, usually quinidine, and were more effective at therapeutic doses for achieving both PVC suppression and prevention of episodes of nonsustained ventricular tachycardia.

FLECAINIDE

Flecainide is well absorbed orally (>95% bioavailability) and produces peak serum concentrations in 2–4 hours. Flecainide is only 30–40% bound to plasma proteins, primarily AAG. Approximately 25% of a dose is excreted unchanged in the urine. The remaining flecainide is extensively metabolized in the liver to inactive metabolites and their sulfate or glucuronide conjugates, which have substantially less antiarrhythmic activity and are unlikely to contribute to overall flecainide response. Serum elimination half-life averages 14 hours in normal volunteers, but increases to 20 hours during chronic oral dosing in patients.

Flecainide pharmacokinetics follow a two-compartment open model, with a rapid distribution phase and a slower elimination phase following intravenous administration. The volume of distribution is large, averaging 9 l/kg, and indicates extensive extravascular distribution. In some studies, total body clearance averages 355 ml/min, with a renal clearance of 170 ml/min (47% of total body clearance). Others have shown renal clearance to be a smaller component of total body clearance (23%).

Flecainide serum concentrations may accumulate to potentially toxic levels in patients with significant hepatic dysfunction. In patients with hepatic cirrhosis, flecainide half-life was significantly prolonged to 49 hours, compared to 9.5 hours in controls {68}. Plasma AUC values were approximately fourfold higher in patients with cirrhosis and volumes of distribution were 32% lower.

In patients with renal dysfunction, flecainide renal clearance was strongly correlated with creatinine clearance {69}. Elimination half-life averaged 38 hours, with a slight reduction in renal clearance to 300 ml/min. These data suggest than careful monitoring of flecainide therapy is warranted in patients with creatinine clearances below 20 ml/min. Flecainide serum concentrations were not significantly altered by hemodialysis.

The presence of congestive heart failure appears to have little effect on flecainide pharmacokinetics. Although renal clearance was slightly reduced, its contribution to overall body clearance was not significant enough to warrant alterations in flecainide dose.

Recently, flecainide hepatic metabolism has demonstrated genetic polymorphism, such that 5–10% of the Caucasian population have a genetic alteration in the hepatic P-450 isozyme (CYP2D6) responsible for flecainide metabolism, resulting in reduced or "poor metabolism" (PM) {70}. Thus flecainide metabolism cosegregates with that of debrisoquine, sparteine, and other known substrates for the CYP2D6 isozyme. In PM subjects, flecainide nonrenal clearance is reduced from 726 ml/min in EMs to 292 ml/min, a 2.5-fold reduction. The observed proarrhythmic effects of flecainide are, in part, due to elevated serum concentrations, and therefore PMs of flecainide may be particularly prone to adverse arrhythmogenic effects of the drug.

The therapeutic range for flecainide is 0.2–1.0 μg/ml. Greater than 95% suppression of PVCs can be achieved with serum concentrations in this range. The risk for serious proarrhythmia and significant reductions in left ventricular performance are greatly increased at serum concentrations above 1.0 μg/ml.

ENCAINIDE

The pharmacokinetics of encainide are complex and are dependent on a genetically determined ability to metabolize the parent compound. In a fashion similar to that observed with flecainide, approximately 90–95% of Caucasian populations extensively metabolize encainide (EMs), which results in significant first-pass removal of the drug and a bioavailability of about 30%. These patients have relatively low encainide concentrations in serum and severalfold higher concentrations of the active metabolites O-desmethyl encainide (ODE) and 3-methoxy-ODE (MODE). These metabolites are cardioactive and possess more potent, and electrophysiologically different, antiarrhythmic activity {71}. In EMs, the elimination half-life for encainide is between 1 and 3 hours. ODE elimination half-life ranges from 5 to 37 hours; MODE concentrations tend to plateau and make determinations of elimination half-life difficult. ODE, MODE, and their conjugates are then excreted renally, with only 5% recovered as intact encainide.

In PMs, oral bioavailability is over 80%. Encainide is the prevalent compound found is serum, with an elimination half-life of 11–22 hours. ODE, but not MODE, is detectable in serum. Almost 40% of a dose is recovered as unchanged encainide {72}. In spite of genetic variations in metabolism of encainide, the dosing schedule for both groups of patients is quite similar because of the active metabolites.

Intravenous encainide administration produces serum concentrations that may be fit by a two-compartment open model. Systemic clearance is 113 l/hr in EMs and 11 l/hr in PMs {72}. Steady-state volume of distribution is 270 l, with approximately 70–75% of encainide bound to serum proteins.

In patients with hepatic cirrhosis, encainide concentrations accumulate three-fold; however, ODE and MODE concentrations are unaltered and no change in electrocardiographic intervals were noted {73}. Thus no dose adjustments are recommended in these patients. In patients with renal failure, ODE and MODE serum concentrations were increased by 80% and 167%, respectively {74}, which would necessitate lower doses to prevent ODE and MODE toxicity.

Due to the presence of several cardioactive metabolites, serum concentration-effect relationships for encainide and metabolites are difficult to determine. Therefore, no "therapeutic range" is currently recommended. Nevertheless, in EMs receiving encainide therapy, it has been established that withdrawing encainide therapy results in arrhythmia return within 16 hours, long after encainide concentrations are undetectable in serum {75}. This supports a more important antiarrhythmic role for ODE and MODE, whose serum concentrations averaged 58 ng/ml and 152 ng/ml, respectively. Others have shown that PVC suppression and prolongation of electrocardiographic intervals (QRS, QT) correlates more strongly with ODE concentrations {76}.

Use of cimetidine has been reported to increase the serum AUC of encainide (31%), ODE (43%), and MODE (36%) {77}. The clinical significance of this is unknown.

Kazierad et al. have shown that diltiazem increases serum encainide concentrations; however, there were no significant alterations in ODE and MODE concentrations, nor were any significant changes noted in surface electrocardiographic intervals {78}.

Recently quinidine, in doses as small as 50 mg four times a day, has been shown to selectively inhibit the hepatic isozyme responsible for encainide metabolism in EMs, resulting in a "chemical" conversion of EMs to PMs {78}. Thus, quinidine-treated EMs thus have pharmacokinetic and pharmacologic profiles similar to those seen in genetically determined PMs.

PROPAFENONE

Propafenone differs from other Class Ic agents in that it also possesses some Class II and Class IV actions. Propafenone is structurally similar to propranolol and other beta-blockers, and has approximately 1/40th the beta-blocking potency of propranolol. The beta-blockade potential of propafenone may be of clinical significance in patients with extreme elevations in propafenone serum concentrations.

Propafenone is slowly absorbed after oral administration and produces peak serum concentrations in 2–4 hours. Propafenone undergoes substantial presystemic metabolism in most patients, with a low systemic bioavailability of approximately 12%. Propafenone metabolism is known to cosegregate with that of encainide {80}. As such, substantial differences exist in pharmacokinetic parameters between EMs and PMs of the substrate. EMs have a shorter propafenone half-life (5.5 vs. 17 hours) and a higher oral clearance (1115 vs. 264 ml/min). Plasma protein binding exceeds 95%. Less than 1% of the dose is excreted unchanged in the urine. Propafenone is extensively metabolized in the liver. Although the complete metabolic fate is not known, the primary metabolite, 5-hydroxypropafenone, has antiarrhythmic and beta-blocking properties, although the beta-blocking properties appear less potent than that of the parent compound {81}. In EMs, 5-hydroxypropafenone may contribute to the antiarrhythmic actions; however, the metabolite is undetectable in PMs. Beta-blockade is more likely to be evident in PMs due to higher serum propafenone concentrations {82}.

Propafenone is extensively bound to serum proteins and is widely distributed throughout the body. The ratio of 5-hydroxypropafenone/propafenone concentration approaches unity in myocardial tissue, suggesting an important role for the metabolite in pharmacologic response {83}.

There are little data concerning the effects of disease states on propafenone pharmacokinetics, although one trial has shown reduced systemic clearance and increased bioavailability in patients with hepatic dysfunction {84}.

There appears to be a wide discrepancy between effective and toxic serum propafenone concentrations. Arrhythmia suppression has occurred at trough propafenone concentrations ranging from 64 to 3271 ng/ml {85,86}. Suppression of complex ventricular ectopy (pairs, ventricular tachycardia) is achieved at lower serum concentrations than those needed to suppress simple PVCs {87}. Central nervous system toxicity is more commonly seen in PM subjects (67% vs. 14% in EMs), suggesting dependence on elevated propafenone concentrations {80}.

In EMs, propafenone AUC in serum increases by 147% when coadministered with food {88}. The effects of low-dose quinidine on propafenone metabolism have produced similar results to those seen with encainide. Funck-Brentano et al. administered quinidine and propafenone to 5 EMs, which resulted in a reduction of propafenone oral clearance of 58% and a twofold increase in steady-state propafenone serum concentrations {89}. 5-Hydroxypropafenone concentrations were reduced from 242 to 125 ng/ml.

Miscellaneous class I agents

CIBENZOLINE

Cibenzoline is a new compound with a chemical structure unrelated to other antiarrhythmic agents. Cibenzoline is well absorbed following oral administration, with a bioavailability of approximately 85%. More than one half of the drug is eliminated by glomerular filtration and tubular secretion. Elimination half-life ranges from 5 to 22 hours and is directly related to renal function and age {90}. Cibenzoline is partially metabolized in the liver to an inactive metabolite.

Following intravenous administration, cibenzoline serum concentrations conform to a two-compartment open model. The distribution phase is rapid and complete within 30 minutes {91}. Approximately 60% of cibenzoline is bound to serum proteins. The elimination half-life varies more than fourfold and is directly related to creatinine clearances.

Little is known about the effects of disease states on cibenzoline pharmacokinetics. Because elimination of cibenzoline from the body is primarily dependent on renal function, dosage reductions are necessary in patients with reduced creatinine clearance.

Following intravenous administration, cibenzoline produces dose-related increases in HV, QRS, QT, and AH intervals {92}. Prolongation of QRS best correlates with serum cibenzoline concentrations. In patients with frequent ventricular ectopy, the cibenzoline serum concentration associated with a 90% reduction in PVC frequency ranged from 215 to 405 ng/ml {93}. During electrophysiologic testing, cibenzoline serum concentrations of 1.3–3.19 μg/ml were observed following cibenzoline infusion {91}. Termination of the rhythm disorder was seen in 9 of 12 patients at these serum concentrations; however, these higher concentrations probably were obtained during the distribution phase. Tentatively, a therapeutic range of 200–400 ng/ml has been proposed.

MORICIZINE

Moricizine is a phenothiazine derivative originally developed in the Soviet Union. In electrophysiologic evaluations, moricizine has been demonstrated to possess Class Ia, Ib, and Ic activity. Moricizine is well absorbed orally, yet extensive first-pass metabolism results in a systemic bioavailability of approximately 30–40%. Peak serum concentrations are observed in about 1.5 hours. Moricizine undergoes extensive and complex hepatic metabolism, with only 1% of a dose excreted in the urine or feces. Over 40 metabolites have been isolated in animal studies, with approximately 14 of these metabolites identified. In animal models, the metabolite moricizine sulfoxide has been shown to possess pharmacologic activity similar to that of the parent compound; however,

it is not known whether any of the metabolites contribute to the pharmacologic response seen in humans {94}.

Moricizine serum concentration-time curves conform to a two-compartment model. Distribution is rapid, and moricizine readily penetrates most tissues, including the blood-brain barrier. Moricizine is approximately 92–95% bound to serum proteins, primarily albumin, AAG, and beta-lipoprotein. Moricizine's volume of distribution is 8–11 l/kg and total body clearance averages 38 ml/min/kg. Elimination half-life ranges from 2 to 4 hours, although single-dose studies may indicate a much higher elimination half-life {94}. This is consistent with auto-induction of hepatic metabolizing enzymes during chronic dosing, a concept now confirmed by at least one investigator {95}.

Little has been published on the effects of disease states on moricizine pharmacokinetics. One report indicated that no alteration in moricizine pharmacokinetics is seen in patients with congestive heart failure {96}.

Most studies have failed to show any significant correlation between moricizine serum concentration and effect. Some investigators have noted a delay of up to 24 hours in the onset of moricizine antiarrhythmic activity, suggesting delayed penetration to active sites or contribution of metabolites to the overall pharmacologic response {94,97}. At least in the short-term evaluation period, this delay in onset of activity makes difficult the determination of concentration-effect relationships.

Cimetidine has been shown to reduce moricizine clearance by approximately 50%, although no changes were noted in surface electrocardiographic intervals {98}.

CLASS II ANTIARRHYTHMIC DRUGS

In addition to their established efficacy in the treatment of hypertension, angina, and selected noncardiac disorders such as migraine headaches, the beta-blockers have proven antiarrhythmic effects, mediated through reductions in the electrophysiologic effects produced by excessive adrenergic stimulation {99}. These effects are manifest as (a) a reduction in catecholamine-induced increases in automaticity and (b) a "quinidine-like" effect to stabilize the membranes of cardiac cells, thereby reducing the rate of rise of the action potential. Sotalol is unique in that it possesses additional Class III antiarrhythmic properties (see below).

The pharmacokinetics of beta-blockers are varied and are dependent on the lipophilic properties of the agent. All beta-blockers share the ability to inhibit exercise or stress-related increases in heart rate, and thus clinically the pulse (and to some extent, blood pressure) is used to guide dosing. In addition, there is a discrepency between the biologic half-life of elimination and the pharmacodynamic half-life of elimination, in part due to the affinity of beta-blocking drugs for beta-receptors. Therefore, individual pharmacokinetic parameters will not be discussed and the major pharmacokinetic parameters of the available beta-blocking drugs are presented in table 29-3 {100}.

Table 29.3. Pharmacokinetic paramaters of beta blockers {99}

Drug	Bioavailability (%)	Protein binding (%)	Total clearance (l/hr/kg)	V_d (l/kg)	$t_{1/2}$ (hr)	Major route of elimination[a]	Drug accumulation in renal disease
Acebutolol	35–40	15	0.29	1.2	11	HM/RE (40% unchanged)	Yes (Diacetolol)
Atenolol	50–60	<5	0.16	1.2	6.9	RE	Yes
Betaxolol	80–90	55	0.28	8.7	14	HM	No
Esmolol	N/A	55	17	3.4	0.15	Esterases in RBCs	No
Labetalol	30–40	50	1.3	5.6	4	HM	No
Metoprolol	40–50	12	0.97	4.2	2.8–7.6	HM	No
Nadolol	30–50	20	0.1	2.0	20	RE	Yes
Penbutolol	95	90–95	0.34	0.6	18–27	HM	No
Pindolol	87	40–60	0.46	2.0	2–4	HM/RE (40% unchanged)	No
Propranolol	30–40	90	0.9	3.3	3–6	HM	No
Timolol	75	10	0.46	2.0–2.5	4	HM	No

[a] RE = renal excretion; HM = hepatic metabolism; RBCs = red blood cells.

CLASS III ANTIARRHYTHMIC DRUGS

Amiodarone

This agent was initially developed as an antianginal agent when pharmacologists were attempting to develop iodinated benzofuran derivatives that add activity to block the metabolic action of thyroxine. When the drug was shown to increase the duration of the action potential in the 1960s, it was studied as an antiarrhythmic drug and has been shown to be effective in treating a wide spectrum of cardiac arrhythmias. The drug's primary action is on potassium channels, but it has also been shown to have effects on sodium channels and calcium channels, and to have antiadrenergic activity. Thus amiodarone has properties of all four classes of drugs in the Vaughn-Williams classification. For the most part, however, it is classified as a Class III antiarrhythmic agent.

The oral bioavailability of amiodarone is low, ranging from 22% to 50%, with wide intersubject variation {100}. The limit in its systemic bioavailability is due to incomplete absorption across the gastrointestinal mucosa. Once administered, oral absorption continues for up to 15 hours, with maximum absorption occurring between 5 and 6 hours, and peak plasma concentration measurements occurring between 3 and 7 hours {101}.

More than six major metabolites of amiodarone have been identified in plasma and tissues of patients during long-term oral treatment. The concentration of these metabolites is low, and it is not known whether the metabolites contribute significantly to the parent drug's antiarrhythmic effects {102}.

Using ^{131}I-labelled drug, it has been shown that amiodarone accumulates extensively in skin, subcutaneous fat, and muscle. The metabolites distribute in the same general pathway as the parent compound. The largest concentrations of amiodarone are found in the liver, but high concentrations are found in the myocardium and skeletal muscle {100}. It has been tempting to relate the extensive tissue accumulation of this compound to some of its adverse effects on the eye and lung. The accumulated compound and its metabolites have been shown to produce changes in lysozymes and to have constituents of the cell membrane. These changes may contribute to the side effects and long-lasting accumulation of the compound in body tissues {103}.

Renal excretion of both amiodarone and its metabolites is small. It has been speculated that degradation of the compound by the liver is its most important metabolic pathway. An entrohepatic recirculation apparently occurs, since after a single intravenous dose secondary peaks in plasma concentration time curves are noted {104}.

Numerous studies on the disposition kinetics of amiodarone have been reported {105,106}. Considerable confusion about compartmental analysis has been reported because of the wide intrasubject variability. Siddoway et al. have proposed a three-compartment model in which amiodarone in the central compartment rises to reach steady-state concentrations within one day, with the accumulation of drug in the peripheral compartment being much slower and requiring several days or weeks to reach steady-state concentration {105}.

Amiodarone has a very large apparent volume of distribution and a comparatively low total body clearance. The elimination half-life of amiodarone is similar in normal subjects and cardiac patients, and has been described as being greater than 50 hours. Considerable discrepancy in the elimination half-life has been reported following a single dose, ranging from 3 hours to 25 days. When this is compared with measurements made following discontinuation of long-term oral therapy, elimination half-lifes of 13–55 days have been reported. Perhaps the best report from Holt et al. describes a 25-day half-life in normal subjects receiving a single 400-mg intravenous bolus of amiodarone {100}. Much of the confusion relating to amiodarone results from widely variable technology used to measure the compound and its metabolite.

A variety of mechanisms for administering amiodarone

to achieve early therapeutic plasma concentrations have been described. Using available pharmacokinetic data, a delay of up to 28 days between institution of therapy and antiarrhythmic effects might be expected. Initial loading with large doses of amiodarone at the beginning of therapy has been suggested to shorten the lag time to effective plasma concentrations to 10 days. No advantage of intravenous therapy over high-dose oral therapy has been demonstrated. The relationship between pharmacodynamic effects and plasma concentration has been shown to be 2–3 weeks in most studies, with a reduction in heart rate and a lengthening of the QTC interval on the electrocardiogram occurring at that time {107}. It is at this time that the drug has been thought to be effective in supressing atrial and ventricular arrhythmias. Studies have evaluated the relationship between amiodarone's steady-state plasma concentration and its therapeutic effects. The demonstrated level of effectiveness appears to be from 0.5 to 3.0 µg/ml. In another study by Haffajee, mean plasma amiodarone concentrations did not differ significantly between responders and nonresponders. However, they did note that arrhythmias recurred in nine responders when their concentrations fell below 1.0 µg/ml, suggesting this was the lower limit for activity {108}.

On the other hand, the adverse effects of amiodarone seem more common when plasma concentrations exceed 2.5 µg/ml, but adverse reactions can occur over a wide range of plasma concentrations.

Sotalol

Numerous physiologic studies and biochemical receptor binding experiments have demonstrated sotalol to be a specific beta-adrenergic blocking drug that is noncardioselective and lacks local anesthetic properties and intrinsic sympathomimetic action. Sotalol exists as a racemic mixture, and when resolved the d-isomer has minor beta-blocking properties, but still maintains unique Class III electrophysiologic properties, thus establishing that they are independent of its beta-blocking actions. It has recently been recommended by the Cardiorenal Advisory Committee of the FDA for use as an antiarrhythmic agent of the Class III type.

Studies have demonstrated that sotalol conforms pharmacokinetically to an open linear two-compartment model {109}. The absolute bioavailability of sotalol administered orally is 100%. The absorption is not altered by antacids, but may be reduced by the ingestion of food, particularly that containing high concentrations of calcium ions {110}.

The absorption of sotalol is generally slower than other beta-blocking drugs, reaching peak plasma concentrations after oral administration in 2–3 hours. No active metabolites of the drug have been identified {111}. Urinary excretion by glomerular filtration accounts for 75% of the drug administered, with recovery in the urine within 72 hours.

After oral dosing, the apparent volume of distribution for sotalol is greater than total body weight. Protein binding of the drug is small. Sotalol is one of the most hydrophilic

drugs in the beta-adrenergic blocking drug series. Its entry into the central nervous system is low, being only 10% of the concentration in plasma after a single oral dose. This compares favorably with atenolol {112}. The elimination half-life of sotalol has been shown to be approximately 15.5 hours {113}.

In comparison of pharmacokinetics of sotalol in young versus elderly patients with hypertension, it has been shown that the half-life of the drug is prolonged in elderly patients, and the renal clearance of the drug is reduced. There were increased serum concentrations of the drug in elderly patients {114}. On the other hand, in pregnancy, where sotalol is used in the treatment of hypertension, the elimination half-life and bioavailability of sotalol are not altered. The drug does cross the human placenta and is found in fetal blood. During pregnancy there is a more rapid clearance of sotalol due to an increased glomerular filtration rate {115}.

Sotalol is not metabolized by the liver, and its plasma concentration is not affected by hepatic dysfunction. On the other hand, sotalol is excreted by the kidney through glomerular filtration. Reduced creatinine clearance, in an almost linear way, reduces the clearance of sotalol, raises its plasma concentration, and prolongs its disposition half-life. Dose adjustment, based upon clinical response to the drug, is necessary in patients with diminished renal function {116,117}.

As with other beta-blocking drugs, there is only a rough correlation of plasma concentration-effect relationships. Pharmacodynamic studies, however, have shown that with increasing dose there is a further reduction in heart rate increase due to graded exercise. In general, the measurement of plasma concentration is not necessary, except in patients with moderate levels of renal impairment {118}.

REFERENCES

1. Cardiac Arrhythmia Suppression Trial (CAST) Investigators: Preliminary report: Effect of encainide and flecainide on mortality in a randomized trial of arrhythmia suppression after myocardial infarction. *N Engl J Med* 321:406–412, 1989.
2. Podrid PJ, Marcus FI: Lessons to be learned from the Cardiac Arrhythmia Suppression Trial. *Am J Cardiol* 64:1189–1191, 1989.
3. Woosley RL: CAST: Implications for drug development. *Clin Pharmacol Ther* 47:558–556, 1990.
4. Task Force of the Working Group on Arrhythmias of the European Society of Cardiology: CAST and beyond: Implications for the cardiac arrhythmia suppression trial. *Circulation* 81:1123–1127, 1990.
5. Newman D, Evans GT, Scheinman MM: Catheter ablation of cardiac arrhythmias. *Curr Probl Cardiol* 14:117–164, 1989.
6. Langberg JJ, Chin MC, Rosenqvist M, Cockrell J, Dullet N, Van Hare G, Griffin JC, Scheinman MM: Catheter ablation of the antrioventricular junction with radiofrequency energy. *Circulation* 80:1527–1535, 1989.
7. Winkle RA: The implantable defibrillator: Progression from first-to third-generation devices. In: Zipes DP, Jalife J (eds) *Cardiac Electrophysiology.* Philadelphia: WB Saunders, 1990, pp 963–969.
8. Mirowski M, Reid PR, Winkel RA: Mortality in patients with

implanted automatic defibrillators. *Ann Intern Med* 98:585–588, 1983.

9. Hondeghem LM, Snyders DJ: Class III antiarrhythmic agents have a lot of potential but a long way to go. *Circulation* 81:686–690, 1990.

10. Hoffman BF, Rosen MR: Cellular mechanisms for cardiac arrhythmias. *Circ Res* 49:1–15, 1981.

11. Cobbe SM: Modification of class III antiarrhythmic activity in abnormal myocardium. *Cardiovasc Res* 22:847–854, 1988.

12. Lynch JJ, Heaney LA, Wallace AA, Gehret JR, Selnick HG, Stein RB: Supression of lethal ischemic ventricular arrhythmias by the class III agent E4031 in a canine model of previous myocardial infarction. *J Cardiovasc Pharmacol* 15:764–775, 1990.

13. Nezasa Y, Kodama I, Toyama J: Effects of OPC-88177, a new antiarrhythmic agent, on the electrophysiological properties of rabbit isolated hearts. *Br J Pharmacol* 98:186–191, 1989.

14. Vaughan Williams EM: Classification of antiarrhythmic drugs. In: Sandoe E, Flensted-Jensen E, Oleson K (eds) *Cardiac Arrhythmias*. Sodertalje, Sweden: Ad Astra, 1970, pp 449–473.

15. Harrison DC, Winkle RA, Sami M, Mason JW: Encainide: A new and potent antiarrhythmic agent. In: Harison DC (ed) *Cardiac Arrhythmias: A Decade of Progress*. Boston: GK Hall, 1981, pp 315–330.

16. Harrison DC: Antiarrhythmic drug classification: New science and practical applications. *Am J Cardiol* 56:185–187, 1985.

17. Task Force of the Working Group on Arrhythmias of the European Society of Cardiology: The Sicilian gambit, a new approach to the classification of antiarrhythmic drugs based on their actions on arrhythmogenic mechanisms. *Circulation* 84:1831–1851, 1991.

18. Harrison DC: The Sicilian gambit: Reasons for maintaining the present antiarrhythmic drug classification. *Cardiovasc Res* 26:566–567, 1992.

19. Harrison DC: Introduction. Symposium on perspectives on the treatment of ventricular arrhythmias. *Am J Cardiol* 52:1C–2C, 1983.

20. Harrison DC: Antiarrhythmic drugs, current classification as a guide to rational clinical use. *New Ethicals* ●●:21–25, 1986.

21. Campbell TJ: Kinetics on onset of rate-dependent effects of class I antiarrhythmic drugs are important in determining their effects on refractoriness in guinea-pig ventricle, and provide a theoretical basis for their subclassification. *Cardiovasc Res* 17:344–352, 1983.

22. Campbell TJ: Kinetics on onset of rate-dependent depression of maximum rate of depolarization (V_{max}) in guinea-pig ventricular action potential by mexiletine, disopyramide and encainide. *J Cardiovasc Pharmacol* 5:291–296, 1983.

23. Hondeghem LM: Antiarrhythmic agents: Modulated receptor applications. *Circulation* 75:514–520, 1987.

24. Harrison DC, Meffin PJ, Winkle RA: Clinical pharmacokinetics of antiarrhythmic drugs. *Prog Cardiovasc Dis* 20:217–242, 1977.

25. Fabre J, Ballant L: Renal failure, drug pharmacokinetics and drug action. *Clin Pharmacokinet* 1:99–120, 1976.

26. Benowitz NL, Meister W: Pharmacokinetics in patients with cardiac failure. *Clin Pharmacokinet* 1:389–405, 1976.

27. Rowland M, Blaschke TF, Meffin PJ, et al.: Pharmacokinetics in disease states modifying hepatic and metabolic function. In: Benet LZ (ed) *The Effect of Disease States on Drug Pharmacokinetics*. Washington, DC: American Pharmaceutical Association Academy of Pharmaceutical Sciences, 1976, chap. 4.

28. Triggs EJ, Nation RL: Pharmacokinetics in the aged: A review. *J Pharmacokinet Biopharm* 3:387–418, 1976.

29. Wright JT Jr: Practical pharmacokinetics of ventricular antiarrhythmic therapy. *Am Heart J* 123:1148–1152, 1992.

30. Michelson EL, Dreifus LS: Newer antiarrhythmic drugs. *Med Clin North Am* 72:275–319, 1988.

31. Harrison DC, Bottorff MB: Advances in antiarrhythmic drug therapy. *Adva Pharmacolo* 23:179–225, 1992.

32. Evans WE: General principles of applied pharmacokinetics. In: Evans WE, Schentag JJ, Jusko WJ (eds) *Applied Pharmacokinetics: Principles of Therapeutic Drug Monitoring*, 3rd ed. Vancouver, WA: Applied Therapeutics, 1992, pp 1–3.

33. McCollam PL, Bauman JL, Beckman KJ, Hariman RJ: A simple method of monitoring antiarrhythmic drugs during short- and long-term therapy. *Am J Cardiol* 63:1273–1275, 1989.

34. Myerburg RJ, Conde C, Sheps DS: Antiarrhythmic drug therapy in survivors of pre-hospital cardiac arrest: Comparison of effects on chronic ventricular arrhythmias and recurrent cardiac arrest. *Circulation* 59:855–865, 1979.

35. Barchowsky A, Shand DG, Stargel WW: On the role of alacid glycoprotein in lignocaine accumulation following myocardial infarction. *Br J Clin Pharmacol* 13:411, 1982.

36. Wooding-Scott RA, Slaughter RL: Total and unbound concentrations of quinidine and 3-hydroxyquinidine at steady state. *Am Heart J* 113:302–206, 1987.

37. Kessler KM, Lisker B, Conde C, Silver J, Ho-Tung P, Hamburg C, Myerburg RJ: Abnormal quinidine binding in survivors of prehospital cardiac arrest. *Am Heart J* 107:665–669, 1984.

38. Roden DM, Woosley RL, Primm RK: Incidence and clinical features of the quinidine-associated long QT syndrome: Implications for patient care. *Am Heart J* 111:1088–1093, 1986.

39. Ellard GA: Variations between individuals and populations in the acetylation of isoniazid and its significance for the treatment of pulmonary tuberculosis. *Clin Pharmacol Ther* 19:610, 1976.

40. Gibson TP, Lowenthen DT, Nelson HA: Elimination of procainamide in end-stage renal failure. *Clin Pharmacol Ther* 17:321, 1975.

41. Bottorff MB, Kuo CS, Batenhorst RL: High dose procainamide in chronic renal failure. *Drug Intell Clin Pharm* 17:279–81, 1983.

42. Myerburg RJ, Kessler JM, Kiem I: Relationship between plasma levels of procainamide, suppression of premature ventricular complexes and prevention of recurrent ventricular tachycardia. *Circulation* 64:280–290, 1981.

43. Christain CD Jr, Meredith CG, Speeg KV: Cimetidine inhibits renal procainamide clearance. *Clin Pharmacol Ther* 36:221–227, 1984.

44. Woosley RL, Drayer DE, Reidenberg MM: Effect of acetylator phenotype on the rate at which procainamide induces antinuclear antibodies and the lupus syndrome. *N Engl J Med* 298:1157, 1978.

45. Lima JJ, Boudoulas H, Shields BJ: Stereoselective pharmacokinetics of disopyramide enantiomers in man. *Drug Metab Disp* 13:572–577, 1985.

46. Lima JJ, Boudoulas H: Stereoselective effects of disopyramide enantiomers in humans. *J Cardiovasc Pharmacol* 9:594–600, 1987.

47. Garg DC, Jaddad NS, Singh S, Ng KF, Weidler DJ: Efficacy and pharmacokinetics of oral pirmenol, a new antiarrhythmic drug. *J Clin Pharmacol* 28:812–817, 1988.

48. Easley AR, Mann DE, Reiter JJ: Electrophysiologic evaluation of pirmenol for sustained ventricular tachycardia secondary to coronary artery disease. *Am J Cardiol* 58:86–89, 1986.

49. Estes NAM, Gold R, Cameron J: Electrocardiographic and

electrophysiologic effects of pirmenol in ventricular tachycardia. *Am J Cardiol* 59:20H–26H, 1987.

50. Riddell JG, McAllister CB, Wilkinson GR: Constant plasma drug concentrations — a new technique with application to lidocaine. *Ann Intern Med* 100:25, 1984.

51. Burney RG, DiFazio CA, Peach MJ: Antiarrhythmic effects of lidocaine metabolites. *Am Heart J* 88:765–769, 1974.

52. Prescott LF, Adjepon-Yamoah KK, Talbot RG: Impaired lidocaine metabolism in patients with myocardial infarction. *Br Med J* 1:939–941, 1976.

53. Thomson PD, Melmon KL, Richardson JA: Lidocaine pharmacokinetics in advanced heart failure, liver disease and renal disease in humans. *Ann Intern Med* 78:499–508, 1973.

54. Zito RA, Reid PA: Lidocaine pharmacokinetics predicted by indocyanine green clearance. *N Engl J Med* 298:1160–1163, 1978.

55. Lie KI, Wellens HJ, van Capelle FJ: Lidocaine in the prevention of primary ventricular fibrillation. *N Engl J Med* 291:1324–1326, 1974.

56. Sheridan DJ, Crawford J, Rawlins MD: Antiarrhythmic action of lidocaine in early myocardial infarction. *Lancet* 1:824–825, 1977.

57. Pieper JA, Rodman JH: Lidocaine. In: Evans WE, Schentag JJ, Jusko WJ (eds) *Appied Pharmacokinetics*, 2nd ed, Spokane, WA: Applied Therapeutics, 1986, pp 639–681.

58. Conrad KA, Byers JM, Finley PR: Lidocaine elimination: Effects of metoprolol and of propranolol. *Clin Pharmacol Ther* 33:133–138, 1983.

59. Lalka D, Meyer MB, Duce BR, Elvin AT: Kinetics of the oral antiarrhythmic lignocaine congener, tocainide. *Clin Pharmacol Ther* 19:757, 1976.

60. Graffner C, Conradson T, Horvendahl S, Ryden L: Tocainide kinetics after intravenous and oral administration in health subjects and in patients with acute myocardial infarction. *Clin Pharmacol Ther* 27:64, 1980.

61. Wiegers U, Hanrath P, Kuck KH: Pharmacokinetics of tocainide in patients with renal dysfunction and during haemodialysis. *Eur J Clin Pharmacol* 24:503–507, 1983.

62. Meffin PJ, Winkle RA, Blaschke TF, Fitzgerald J, Harrison DC: Response optimization of drug dosage: Antiarrhythmic studies with tocainide. *Clin Pharmacol Ther* 22:42–57, 1977.

63. Barbey JT, Thompson KA, Echt DS, Woosley RL, Roden DM: Combination of low dose quinidine and tocainide in the treatment of ventricular arrhythmias in man (abstr). *J Am Coll Cardiol* 7:108, 1986.

64. Prescott LF, Pottage A, Clements JA: Absorption, distribution and elimination of mexiletine. *Postgrad Med J* 53(Suppl 1):50, 1977.

65. Pentikainen PJ, Hietakorpi S, Halinen MO, Lampinen LM: Cirrhosis of the liver markedly impairs the elimination of mexiletine. *Eur J Clin Pharmacol* 30:83–88, 1986.

66. Mitchell BC, Clements JA, Pottage A, Prescott LF: Mexiletine disposition: Individual variation in response to urine acidification and alkalinisation. *Br J Clin Pharmacol* 16:281–284, 1983.

67. Greenspan AM, Speilman SR, Webb CR, Sokoloff NM, Horowitz LN: Efficacy of combination therapy with mexiletine and a type 1A agent for inducible ventricular tachyarrhythmias secondary to coronary artery disease. *Am J Cardiol* 56:277, 1985.

68. McQuinn RL, Pentikainen PJ, Chang SF, Conard GJ: Pharmacokinetics of flecainide in patients with cirrhosis of the liver. *Clin Pharmacol Ther* 44:566–572, 1988.

69. Forland SC, Cutler RE, McQuinn RL, Kvam DC, Miller AM, Conard GJ, Parish S: Flecainide pharmacokinetics after multiple dosing in patients with impaired renal function. *J Clin Pharmacol* 28:727–735, 1988.

70. Gross AS, Mikus G, Fischer C, Hertrampf R, Gundert-Remy U, Eichelbaum M: Stereoselective disposition of flecainide in relation to sparteine/debrisoquine metabolism phenotype. *Br J Clin Pharmacol* 28:555–556, 1988.

71. Gomoll AW, Byrne JE, Mayol RF: Comparative antiarrhythmic actions of encainide and its major metabolites. *Arch Int Pharmacodyn* 281:277–297, 1986.

72. Wang T, Roden DM, Wolfenden HT, Woosley RL, Wood AJJ: Influence of genetic polymorphism on the metabolism and disposition of encainide in man. *J Pharmacol Exp Ther* 228:605, 1984.

73. Bergstrand RH, Wang T, Roden DM, Avant GR, Sutton WW, Siddoway LA, Wolfenden H, Woosley RL, Wilkinson GR, Wood AJJ: Encainide disposition in patients with chronic cirrhosis. *Clin Pharmacol Ther* 40:148–154, 1986.

74. Bergstrand RH, Wang T, Roden DM, Stone WJ, Wolfenden HT, Woosley RL, Wilkinson GR, Wood AJJ: Encainide disposition in patients with renal failure. *Clin Pharmacol Ther* 40:64–70, 1986.

75. Winkle RA, Peters F, Kates RE, Harrison DC: Possible contribution of encainide metabolites to the long-term antiarrhythmic efficacy of encainide. *Am J Cardiol* 51:1182–1186, 1983.

76. Carey EL Jr, Duff HJ, Roden DM, Primm RK, Wilkinson GR, Want T, Oates JA, Woosley RL: Encainide and its metabolites: Comparative effects in man on ventricular arrhythmia and electrocardiographic intervals. *J Clin Invest* 73:539–547, 1984.

77. Quart BD, Gallo DG, Sami MH, Wood AJJ: Drug interaction studies and encainide use in renal and hepatic impairment. *Am J Cardiol* 58:104C, 1986.

78. Kazierad DJ, Lalonde RL, Hoon TJ, Mirvis DM, Bottorff MB: The effect of diltiazem on the disposition of encainide and its active metabolites. *Clin Pharmacol Ther* 46:668–673, 1989.

79. Funck-Brentano C, Turgeon J, Woosley RL, Roden DM: Effect of low dose quinidine on encainide pharmacokinetics and pharmacodynamics. Influence of genetic polymorphism. *J Pharmacol Exp Ther* 249:134–142, 1989.

80. Siddoway LA, Thompson KA, McAllister CB, Want T, Wilkinson GR, Roden DM, Woosley RL: Polymorphism of propafenone metabolism and disposition in man: Clinical and pharmacokinetic consequences. *Circulation* 75:785–791, 1987.

81. von Philipsborn G, Hofmann GJ: Pharmacological studies on propafenone and its main metabolite 5-hydroxypropafenone. *Arzneimittelforschng* 34:1489–1497, 1984.

82. Lee JT, Kroemer HK, Silberstein DJ, Funck-Brentano C, Lineberry MD, Wood AJJ, Roden DM, Woosley RL: The role of genetically determined polymorphic drug metabolism in the beta-blockade produced by propafenone. *N Engl J Med* 322:1764–1768, 1990.

83. Latini R, Marchi S, Riva E, Cavalli A, Cazzaniga MG, Maggioni AP, Volpi A: Distribution of propafenone and its active metabolite, 5-hydroxypropafenone, in human tissues. *Am Heart J* 113:843–844, 1987.

84. Lee JT, Yee Y, Dorian P, Kates RE: Influence of hepatic dysfunction on the pharmacokinetics of propafenone. *J Clin Pharmacol* 27:384–389, 1987.

85. Connolly S, Kates R, Lebsack C, Harrison D, Winkle R: Clinical pharmacology of propafenone. *Circulation* 68:589–596, 1983.

86. Salerno DM, Granrud G, Sharkey P, Asinger R, Hodges M: A controlled trial of propafenone for treatment of frequent and repetitive ventricular premature complexes. *Am J Cardiol* 53:77–83, 1984.

87. Zoble RG, Kirsten EB, Brewington J, Propafenone Research

Group: Pharmacokinetic and pharmacodynamic evaluation of propafenone in patients with ventricular arrhythmia. *Clin Pharmacol Ther* 45:535–541, 1989.

88. Axelson JE, Chan GLY, Kirsten EB, Mason WD, Lanman RC, Kerr CR: Food increases the bioavailability of propafenone. *J Clin Pharmac* 23:735–741, 1987.

89. Funck-Brentano C, Kroemer HK, Pavlou H, Woosley RL, Roden DM: Genetically-determined interaction between propafenone and low dose quinidine: Role of active metabolites in modulating net drug effect. *Br J Clin Pharmac* 27:435–444, 1989.

90. Brazzell RH, Colburn WA, Aogaichi K, Szuna AJ, Somberg JC, Carliner N, Heger J, Morganroth J, Winkle RA, Block P: Pharmacokinetics of oral cibenzoline in arrhythmia patients. *Clin Pharmacokinet* 10:178–186, 1985.

91. Waleffe A, Dufour A, Aymard MF, Kulbertus H: Electrophysiologic effects, antiarrhythmic activity and pharmacokinetics of cibenzoline studied with programmed stimulation of the heart in patients with supraventricular reentrant tachycardias. *Eur Heart J* 6:253–260, 1985.

92. Touboul P, Atallah G, Kirkorian G, de Zuloaga C, Dufour A, Aymard MF, Lavaud P, Moleur P: Electrophysiologic effects of cibenzoline in humans related to dose and plasma concentration. *Am Heart J* 112:333, 1986.

93. Brazzell RK, Aogaichi K, Heger JJ, Somberg JC, Carliner NH, Morganroth J: Cibenzoline plasma concentration and antiarrhythmic effect. *Clin Pharmacol Ther* 35:307–316, 1984.

94. Woosley RL, Morganroth J, Fogoros RN, McMahon FG, Humphries JO, Mason DT, Williams RL: Pharmacokinetics of moricizine HCl. *Am J Cardiol* 60:35F–39F, 1987.

95. Pieniaszek HJ, Benedek IH, Davidson AF: Enzyme induction by moricizine: Time course and extent in health volunteers (abstr). *J Clin Pharmacol* 29:842, 1989.

96. Podrid PJ, Beau SL: Antiarrhythmic drug therapy of congestive health failure with focus on moricizine. *Am J Cardiol* 65:56D–64D, 1990.

97. Morganroth J: Dose-effect of moricizine on suppression of ventricular arrhythmias. *Am J Cardiol* 65: 26D–31D, 1990.

98. Biollaz J, Shaheen O, Wood AJJ: Cimetidine inhibition of ethmozine metabolism. *Clin Pharmacol Ther* 37:665–668, 1985.

99. Kazierad DJ, Schlanz DJ, Bottorff MB: Beta blockers. In: Evans WE, Schentag JJ, Jusko WJ (eds) *Applied Pharmacokinetics Principles of Therapeutic Drug Monitoring*, 3rd ed. Vancouver, WA: Applied Therapeutics, 1992.

100. Holt DW, Tucker GT, Jackson PR, Storey GCA: Amiodarone pharmacokinetics. *Am Heart J* 106:840–846, 1983.

101. Gillis AM, Kates RE: Clinical pharmacokinetics of the newer antiarrhythmic agents. *Clin Pharmacokin* 9:475–403, 1984.

102. Latini R, Connolly SJ, Kates RE: Myocardial disposition of amiodarone in the dog. *J Pharmacol Exp Ther* 224:603–608, 1983.

103. Lullmann H, Plosch H, Ziegler A: Ca replacement by cationic amphiphilic drugs from lipid monolayers. *Biochem Pharmacol* 29:2969–2974, 1980.

104. Andreasen F, Agerback H, Bjerregaard P, Gotzsche H: Pharmacokinetics of amiodarone after intravenous and oral administration. *Eur J Clin Pharmacol* 19:293–299, 1981.

105. Siddoway LA, McAllister CB, Wilkinson GR, Roden DM, Woosley RL: Amiodarone dosing: A proposal based on its pharmacokinetics. *Am Heart J* 106:951–956, 1983.

106. Heger JJ, Prystowsky EN, Zipes DP: Relationships between amiodarone dosage, drug concentrations, and adverse side effects. *Am Heart J* 106:931–935, 1983.

107. Nademanee K, Kannan R, Wagner R, Intarachot V, Hendrickson J, Singh B: Role of amiodarone desethylamiodarone and reserve T_3 serum levels in monitoring antiarrhythmic efficacy and toxicity: Superiority of rT_3 and desethylamiodarone levels. *Circulation* 68(Suppl III):278, 1983.

108. Haffajee CI, Love JC, Canada AT, Lesko LJ, Asdourian GK, Alpert JS: Clinical pharmacokinetics and efficacy of amiodarone for refractory tachyarrhythmias. *Circulation* 67: 1347–1355, 1983.

109. Ritschel WA: Compilation of pharmacokinetic parameters of beta-adrenergic blocking agents. *Drug Intell Clin Pharm* 14:746–756, 1980.

110. Kahela P, Anttila M, Sundquist H: Antacids and sotalol absorption. *Acta Pharmacol Toxicol* 49:181–183, 1981.

111. Schnelle K, Klein G, Schinz A: Studies on the pharmacokinetics and pharmacodynamics of the beta-adrenergic blocking agent sotalol in normal man. *J Clin Pharmac* 19: 516–522, 1979.

112. Taylor PJ, Cruickshank JM: Distribution coefficients of atenolol and sotalol. *J Pharm Pharmacol* 36:118–119, 1984.

113. McDevitt DG, Shanks RG: Evaluation of once daily sotalol administration in man. *Br J Clin Pharmacol* 4:153–156, 1977.

114. Ishizaki T, Hirayama H, Tawara K, Nakaya H, Sato M: Pharmacokinetics and pharmacodynamics in young normal and elderly hypertensive subjects: A study using sotalol as a model drug. *J Pharmacol Exp Ther* 212:173–181, 1980.

115. O'Hare MF, Leahey W, Murnaghan GA, McDevitt DG: Pharmacokinetics of sotalol during pregnancy. *Eur J Clin Pharmacol* 24:521–524, 1983.

116. Meier J: Pharmacokinetic comparison of pindolol with other beta-adrenoceptor-blocking agents. *Am Heart J* 104: 364–373, 1982.

117. Berglund G, Descamps R, Thomis JA: Pharmacokinetics of sotalol after chronic administration to patients with renal insufficiency. *Eur J Clin Pharmacol* 18:321–326, 1980.

118. Singh BN, Deedwania P, Koonlawee N, Ward A, Sorkin EM: Sotalol: A review of its pharmacodynamic and pharmacokinetic properties, and therapeutic use. *Drugs* 34: 311–349, 1987.

CHAPTER 30

Mechanism of Action of Antiarrhythmic Drugs

LUC M. HONDEGHEM & BERTRAM G. KATZUNG

INTRODUCTION

In this chapter we describe the modulated receptor theory for the action of certain antiarrhythmic drugs. We briefly review the work that led to this theory, present a detailed description of the mechanism, and apply it to a group of antiarrhythmic agents and the arrhythmias in which they are used.

A large number of drugs, e.g., antimalarials, local anesthetics, antiadrenergics, anticholinergics, antihistaminics, and antiepileptics, have antiarrhythmic effects. The search for a mechanism of action for such a diverse group of chemicals has led to several hypotheses. These hypotheses have had utility primarily as methods of classifying the drugs; few, if any, have come to grips with the basic question: How do useful antiarrhythmic drugs suppress abnormal electrical activity without similarly suppressing normal electrogenesis?

The application of electrophysiologic methods for studying the membrane actions of drugs has made it possible to identify some of the properties that appear to be associated with suppression of abnormal electrical activity.

The first property to be clearly defined as an important correlate of antiarrhythmic action was local anesthesia {1}. This action, associated with block of sodium channels, is now recognized as the major action of the most commonly used antiarrhythmic agents, e.g., quinidine, lidocaine, and their congeners. In nerve, impulse propagation is blocked in healthy as well as injured fibers at the relatively high concentrations of local anesthetics used for infiltration anesthesia. In the heart, abnormal conduction (e.g., from heart beats that conduct too slowly or occur too frequently) is suppressed but normal conduction is relatively less impaired, unless toxic doses are given. In other words, these drugs, at the concentrations used for the treatment of arrhythmias, selectively suppress abnormal conduction in the heart. This selectivity is probably most important in abolishing reentry arrhythmias {2}.

Two other effects of antiarrhythmic drugs can be at least partially ascribed to block of sodium channels. Block of sodium channels is important in the increase in refractoriness that is produced by some of these drugs. Block of sodium channels also plays a role in the suppression of abnormal pacemaker activity occurring at more negative diastolic potentials {3}.

The calcium-channel blocking agents were developed as vasodilators, but some members of this group also have antiarrhythmic effects. These drugs relax normal vascular smooth muscle and cause moderate or little depression of the normal heart. Some of them, however, very markedly depress abnormal activity in myocardium, e.g., slow responses in ischemic and depolarized tissues {4}. There is some evidence indicating that the response of vascular smooth muscle to the calcium-channel blockers is also modulated by the membrane potential. Thus, some members of this class of drugs also seem to induce a selective block of the channels with which they interact.

The action of antiarrhythmic agents that act by lengthening the action potential duration is also frequency dependent. Unfortunately, most agents have more of an effect upon the normal beat than upon a tachycardia beat (reverse use dependence {5}). Agents that prolong action potential duration in a use-dependent fashion might make antiarrhythmic agents with great selectivity (see below).

Recently it has been shown that the action of a blocker of i_f (a pacemaker current) is also frequency dependent {6}.

Selective depression of membranes at one frequency but less at another thus appears to be an effect common to at least four important subgroups of antiarrhythmic drugs. The mechanism for such selective depression is, at the present time, best explained by the modulated receptor theory {7,8}. This theory postulates that the binding of a blocking drug to the receptor of a transmembrane channel is modulated by the state of the channel, which in turn is governed by the voltage-time profile across the cell membrane.

BACKGROUND

The modulated receptor hypothesis explains the selective action of antiarrhythmic drugs on the basis of the differences between membrane electrogenesis in normal and abnormal tissue. Such differences may include disparities in resting potential, in action potential shape and duration, and in recovery time between successive action potentials.

N. Sperelakis (ed.), Physiology and Pathophysiology of the Heart, Third Edition.

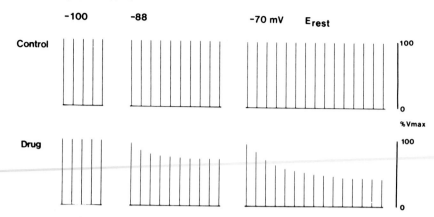

Fig. 30-1. Voltage dependence of $\dot{V}_{max}$ reduction by procainamide (180 μM). After a 20-second rest period, guinea pig papillary muscles were stimulated at 3.3 Hz. The resting membrane potential was altered by current injection. Note that the reduction of $\dot{V}_{max}$ is accentuated by depolarization (−70 mV) and that hyperpolarization (−100 mV) attenuates are procainamide effect. (Unpublished data, Dr. Ehring.)

Earlier work supporting these ideas is conveniently considered from the standpoint of the major variables involved: voltage and time.

Antiarrhythmic drug action is voltage dependent

In 1955 Weidman {1} showed that in sheep Purkinje fibers cocaine reduced $\dot{V}_{max}$ of the action potential without significantly changing the resting potential. ($\dot{V}_{max}$, or maximum upstroke velocity of the cardiac action potential, is commonly used as an indicator of the inward sodium current.) In addition, he made the important observation that hyperpolarization, even in the continued presence of the drug, restored $\dot{V}_{max}$. He interpreted these observations as indicating that cocaine inactivates the system responsible for carrying sodium through the membrane. Jensen and Katzung {9} showed that therapeutic concentrations of phenytoin, which had little or no effect upon $\dot{V}_{max}$ in low-potassium solution, markedly reduced $\dot{V}_{max}$ when the membrane was depolarized by elevating the concentration of extracellular potassium. The same effect was observed for lidocaine {20} (also see fig. 30-1). Hondeghem et al. {2} and Hope et al. {11} proposed that a major mechanism of action of some antiarrhythmic drugs is to selectively block sodium channels that are depolarized by hypoxia or ischemia. This proposal has since been confirmed in several laboratories {12–16}.

Antiarrhythmic drug action is time dependent

Johnson and McKinnon {17} and Heistracher {18} showed that repetitive activation enhances sodium-channel block by quinidine (also see fig. 30-2). From studies of local anesthetic action in nerves, Strichartz {19} and Courtney {20} proposed that each time the channels were used (activated and inactivated) a fraction of them became blocked. In studies of quinidine and lidocaine, Chen et al. {21} showed that during the interval between action potentials, sodium channels recover from block. In addi-

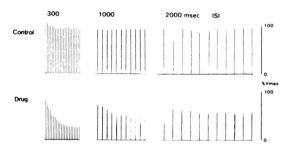

Fig. 30-2. Time dependence of $\dot{V}_{max}$ reduction by aprindine (14 μM). After a 20-second rest period, guinea pig papillary muscles were stimulated at 3.3, 1.0, or 0.5 Hz. Note that the depression of $\dot{V}_{max}$ is more marked at faster stimulus rates (less time at negative potentials; and more activations and more time at depolarized potentials). (Unpublished data, Dr. Moyer.)

tion, they demonstrated that the rate of recovery is strongly voltage dependent: Recovery is faster in well-polarized tissue than in partially depolarized tissue.

Antiarrhythmic drug action is state dependent

Hille {7} and Hondeghem and Katzung {8} proposed that the voltage- and time-dependent block of sodium channels caused by local anesthetic and antiarrhythmic drugs could be accounted for by a model based on the three channel states (fig. 30-3A) described by Hodgkin and Huxley {22}. At negative potentials the rested state is preferred; upon depolarization the channels rapidly pass through the activated state into the inactivated state, where they remain until the membrane is repolarized.

Data collected with protocols that measure the kinetics of block development as well as steady-state block suggest that most useful antiarrhythmic drugs have a different set of association and dissociation rate constants for each of the three states (resting, activated, and inactivated), i.e.,

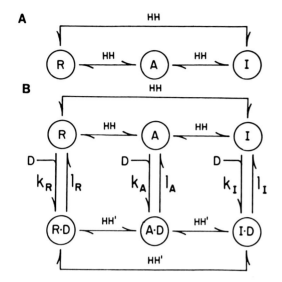

A

HH

B

HH

Fig. 30-3. Schematic representation of the modulated receptor. **A:** Drug-free. Sodium channels can exist in three states: rested (R; predominant at negative membrane potentials), activated (A; upon depolarization the channels open transiently), and inactivated (I; predominant at more positive potentials). The transitions between the three states have been described by Hodgkin and Huxley (HH) {31}. **B:** In the presence of drug. Drug molecules (D) can associate (down arrow) or dissociate (up arrow) with the channels in all three states. Drug-associated channels (R·D, A·D, and I·D) behave as if they are at a less negative transmembrane potential, i.e., their Hodgkin–Huxley parameters are shifted to more positive potentials (HH'). Drug-associated channels are also blocked, i.e., they do not conduct ionic current.

the drug interacts with a receptor that is modulated by the state of the channel (fig. 30-3B) {23,24}. Channels that have drug bound to their receptors behave as if the relationship between voltage and inactivation is shifted toward more negative potentials; in addition, they may not conduct ionic current. The reasons for these assumptions are as follows.

Interaction of drug with the channel in the activated state is required to account for the fact that for many drugs the block becomes more marked as the frequency of channel opening is increased {19}. Since development of some block and recovery can occur at rest {20,21,24}, the channels need not be open for some interactions to occur. However, since the rested state receptor frequently has a much lower affinity for the drug than the receptor in the inactivated state {8}, it is necessary that these states have different rate constants. The voltage shift of the inactivation relation is suggested because blocked channels behave as if they are at a potential less negative than the measured membrane potential {1,20,25,26}.

In 1977 quantitative aspects of the modulated receptor hypothesis were formulated in a set of differential equations that describe the interactions of drugs with channels as a function of time and membrane voltage {8}. By the early eighties, several laboratories had tested the model

and used it successfully to explain the effects of many antiarrhythmic drugs under various experimental conditions {23,27–57}.

In our laboratory we utilize a laboratory computer to solve the set of equations. The method provides an estimate of the proportion of channels in each of the Hodgkin–Huxley states — resting, activated, and inactivated — and the fraction of channels in each state that is complexed with drug. The total number of channels available is normalized to 1.0. All of the estimates provided below are normalized in this way.

Mechanisms of state-dependent drug-receptor interactions

The modulated receptor model can provide a dynamic "moving picture" of the changes in state of membrane channels, changes brought about by the physiologic effect of time and membrane voltage, as well as the pharmacologic binding of drug molecules to channel receptors. To diagram these changes in static illustrations, we have combined the basic Hodgkin–Huxley drug interaction diagram of fig. 30-3B with a semi-quantitative plot of the major fractions of the total pool of channels against time in figs. 30-4 to 30-8. Each graph shows the results computed for one or more action potentials elicited after a rest of 20 seconds, plotted with the total number of channels normalized to 1.0 (ordinate), and the fraction of channels residing in each state designated by shades. Throughout this series of figures rested channels are the lightest shade, activated channels are striped and inactivated channels are darker shades. The lightly shaded areas represent drug-free channels and the darker shades represent blocked channels.

Figure 30-4 illustrates the behavior of the model in the absence of drugs: Hodgkin–Huxley kinetics apply. When the cell membrane is maintained at a normal resting potential (e.g., −85 mV), all channels are in the rested state (R in fig. 30-4). Upon depolarization the channels become activated but the activated state is so brief (less than 2 ms) that it cannot be resolved in fig. 30-4A. This is indicated in the first subpicture above the graph by a heavy arrow from R (rested) via A (activated) to I (inactivated). Only when the time scale is greatly expanded can the transient activated state be visualized (O in fig. 30-4B). Although the activated state is very brief, it is the time during which current flows. This current is proportional to the magnitude of the activated state; drugs that have a high affinity for the activated state can cause development of substantial block during this time. Activated channels quickly become inactivated (I in fig. 30-4A and B) for the duration of the plateau. Upon repolarization, the channels recover rather promptly (I → R transition in fig. 30-4A).

Consequences of state-dependent affinity

To illustrate the significance of varying affinities for the three channel states, we first consider a set of three hypothetical drugs, each with a high affinity (small dissociation constant, $K_d = 10^{-6}$ M) for one channel state, and low affinity (large $K_d = 10^{-3}$ M) for the other two

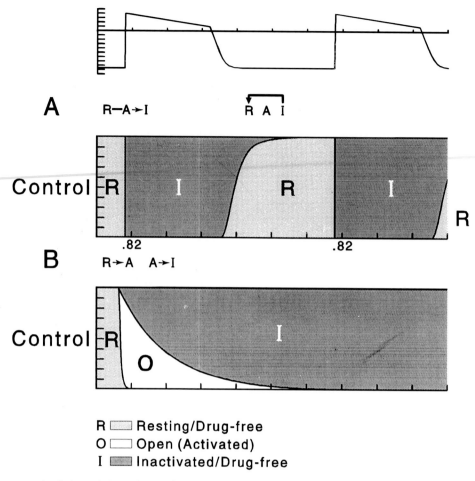

R ☐ Resting/Drug-free
O ☐ Open (Activated)
I ▨ Inactivated/Drug-free

Fig. 30-4. Computer simulations of channel states in the absence of drugs. The trace at the top shows two action potentials, at a frequency of 3.3 Hz, elicited after a 20-second rest period. The horizontal axis represents 500 ms. The distribution and shifts of channels from one state to another during these action potentials is shown in the panel below (**A**). The pool diagram at the top of A (R — A → I) shows the rapid shift of channels from the rested, through the activated, to the inactivated state at the time of the first upstroke. The thickness of the arrow connecting R to I indicates the relative rate of conversion from one state to the other. The somewhat slower recovery of channels is indicated during repolarization of the first action potential (I → R).

The graph diagrams these conversions quantitatively. In this figure and figures 30-5 to 30-8, R represents channels in the rested, drug-free state and I represents channels in the inactivated, drug-free state. The sum of all the channel states is unity. As indicated in A, during the 500-ms duration of the sequence, the conversion of channels from the rested state to the inactivated state is so rapid that the activated state can be detected only by greatly expanding the time scale. In **B**, the horizontal axis represents 2.4 ms during the upstroke of the first action potential of A. O represents the fraction of channels in the open or activated state. The maximum normalized sodium conductance achieved during the upstroke of each of the two action potentials is 0.82, indicated below the upstroke in panel A. This value is less than unity, even in the absence of blocking drug, because a few channels inactivated before the rest of the channels open.

states (table 30-1). The rate constants k and l were chosen to provide the K_d required for each state and a time constant in the range found for real drugs. To obtain a realistic degree of channel block, binding of the drugs is assumed to shift the inactivation curve 25 mV in the hyperpolarizing direction. This means that channels in which drug is bound to the receptor behave as though the membrane potential is 25 mV less negative than the measured potential. The effect of the voltage shift is discussed below.

EFFECTS OF A HYPOTHETICAL DRUG WITH HIGHEST AFFINITY FOR CHANNEL RECEPTORS IN THE ACTIVATED STATE

As shown in fig. 30-5A, a long rest period permits accumulation of nearly all the channels in the unblocked rested state (R area), since neither the receptors in inactivated channels nor those in the rested channels have sufficient affinity for the drug. At the time of the action potential upstroke (channel activation), affinity increases 1000-fold

Table 30-1. Kinetic parameters for the hypothetical drugs discussed in the text and displayed in figs. 30-4 through 30-8. Rate constants were selected to provide high (1 uM) or low (1 mM) affinities and realistic time constants for each drug. Time constants are calculated as: $1/(k \cdot dose + 1)$; dissociation constants (K_d) are calculated from $K_d = 1/k \cdot dose$ (8)

State	Rate Constants				Time constant (ms) For drug concentrations 10^{-5} M
	High Affinity $(K_d = 10^{-6} M)$		Low Affinity $(K_d = 10^{-3} M)$		
	k assoc. $(ms^{-1}M^{-1})$	1 dissoc. (ms^{-1})	k assoc. $(ms^{-1}M^{-1})$	1 dissoc. (ms^{-1})	
Rested	10^4	10^{-2}	10^2	10^{-1}	~10
Activated	1.5×10^5	0.15	1.5×10^3	1.5	~0.6
Inactivated	4×10^2	4×10^{-4}	4	4×10^{-3}	~230

Example: A hypothetical drug with highest affinity for the activated channel would be simulated using the high-affinity rate constants for the activated state (1.5×10^5 and 0.15) and the low-affinity constants for the rested and inactivated states (10^2, 10^{-1}; 4, 4×10^{-3}, respectively).

and about 30% of the channel receptors bind drug. This shift from A to A·D (indicated in the first subpicture above fig. 30-5A) is not seen in the graph because it occurs too quickly, but the result — an abrupt increase in blocked-inactivated channels (I·D) — follows immediately. The predicted sodium channel availability for the first action potential (0.77) is slightly less than control (0.82, fig. 30-4) because a few channels enter the I·D pool during rest, and because some channels block during the first part of the upstroke of the action potential.

During the ensuing plateau phase, channels equilibrate between the I and I·D pools (second subpicture above fig. 30-5A); since drug affinity for the inactivated channel is low, there is a slow exponential decrement of the I·D pool in favor of the I pool. At the end of the first plateau there is a rapid shift of drug-free inactivated channels (I pool) to the rested state (R pool) as the membrane potential returns to the resting level. However, the blocked channels (I·D pool) do not recover much and only slowly (time constant of I → I·D transition is about 230 ms) since the voltage shift associated with binding of drug makes them behave as though they were 25 mV more positive, i.e., −60 mV rather than −85 mV (thus the faster R → R·D → R transition, having a time constant of only 10 ms, is not available). At the time of the second action potential, 30% of the remaining unblocked channels become trapped in the I·D state. In a train of action potentials, this process would be repeated with each action potential, until a steady-state level of block was reached, (in this case 30%).

EFFECTS OF HYPOTHETICAL DRUG WITH HIGHEST AFFINITY FOR THE CHANNEL RECEPTOR IN THE INACTIVATED STATE

As shown by the pool diagrams in the upper part of fig. 30-5B, and by the slow increase in the I·D pool in the graph, most of the binding of this drug to receptor occurs during the plateau of the action potential, not during the upstroke. Repolarization at the end of the plateau reverses this process: The inactivated unblocked channels (I) are

rapidly shifted to the rested state (R). However, the inactivated blocked channels (I·D) "see" a membrane potential of only −60 mV (because of the voltage shift), and therefore most of the channels do not reactivate to the R·D state. Instead, they unblock slowly with the time-constant characteristic of I → I·D kinetics (time constant of about 230 ms). As a result, the sodium channel availability of the second action potential (0.49) is markedly reduced compared to the first action potential (0.76). The computed steady-state availability for a long train of action potentials under these conditions is 0.33. Note that recovery from block by this drug occurs only during the diastolic interval. Therefore, the steady-state block caused by a drug with high affinity for the inactivated state will be dependent on the ratio of the action potential duration to the diastolic interval. In contrast, block caused by the drug with a high affinity only when the channel is activated (fig. 30-5A) decreases during both plateau and diastole; thus net steady-state block will be influenced by rate, but not by action potential duration.

EFFECTS OF A DRUG WITH HIGHEST AFFINITY FOR THE CHANNEL RECEPTOR IN THE RESTED STATE

As indicated in fig. 30-5C, a drug with these characteristics would cause a large fraction of the channels to bind drug in the rested state (R·D). Because of the voltage shift, however, many of these move to the inactivated blocked (I·D) state — thus the preponderance of R·D and I·D in the graph. Consequently, sodium channel availability of the first action potential is maximally reduced after a long rest period. In the example shown, $\dot{V}_{max}$ of the second action potential is unchanged. It is theoretically possible to reduce the degree of block by very rapid stimulation (to minimize the diastolic interval) with this type of drug. Thus a drug with a high affinity for channels in the rested state would be a cardiac poison, depressing normal, rested cells, rather than selectively depressing abnormal cells. Such drugs will be considered no further in this chapter.

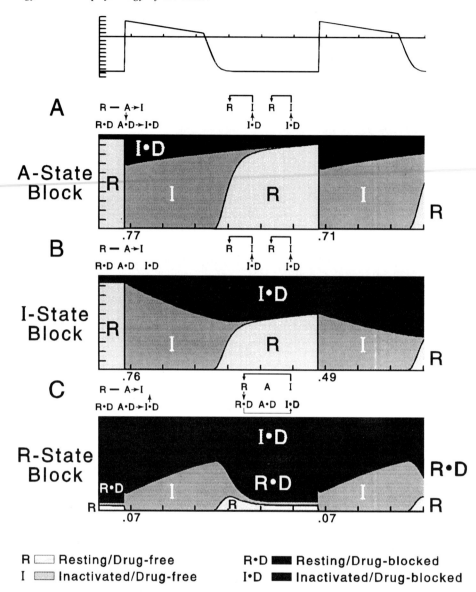

Fig. 30-5. Channel states in the presence of an activated-state blocker (**A**), inactivated-state blocker (**B**), or rested-state blocker (**C**). Simulated action potentials (top trace) and drug-free channels (light colors) are as defined in fig. 30-4. R-D: Rested drug-associated channels; I-D: inactivated blocked channels. Activated blocked channels (A · D) are not resolved in the time resolution of the figure. Kinetic parameters for these hypothetical drugs were taken from table 30-1 (see text). In **A**, block develops exclusively during activation, i.e., at the time of the upstroke of the action potential (A → A · D). Throughout the plateau and diastolic phase the channels unblock (I · D → I). Depending upon the unblocking rate and the time that elapses before the next action potentials, some block may persist to attentuate the $\dot{V}_{max}$ of the next upstroke. In **B**, no block is associated with activation; instead it develops throughout the plateau of the action potential. Unblocking occurs only during diastole. The combination of more block development and less recovery time in B results in a substantial reduction of $\dot{V}_{max}$ from 0.76 to 0.49. In **C**, most of the rested channels are blocked, i.e., very few are available to become activated; hence the very low $\dot{V}_{max}$ (0.07). Channels only unblock during the plateau, i.e., when they are inactivated. Thus, the channels are either blocker or inactivated, and can never conduct the sodium current.

Voltage dependence of channel block

The comparisons below are made using the inactivated-channel blocking drug introduced in fig. 30-5B. However, similar comparisons could be made for the activated-channel blocking drug.

SIGNIFICANCE OF DRUG-INDUCED SHIFT OF INACTIVATION

The hypothetical drugs described thus far (fig. 30-5) incorporate a voltage-shift effect. The importance of this shift can be appreciated by comparing fig. 30-6A with fig. 30-5B.

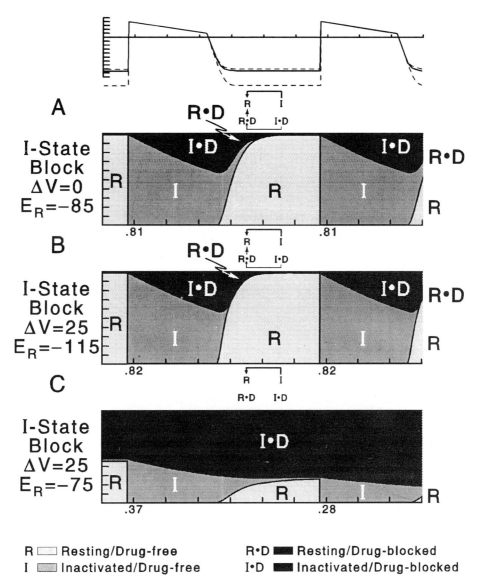

R ☐ Resting/Drug-free   R·D ■ Resting/Drug-blocked
I ▨ Inactivated/Drug-free   I·D ■ Inactivated/Drug-blocked

Fig. 30-6. Effects of the omission of a voltage shift (**A**), hyperpolarization (**B**), and depolarization (**C**) upon the channel states. Except for the indicated changes in voltage parameters, the conditions are identical to those in fig. 30-5B. In **A**, lack of voltage shift provides for recovery from the I·D block during repolarization through two routes: the slow I·D → I transition and the faster I·D → R·D transition. Since the latter is so much faster, most of the I·D channels quickly unblock to R via R·D, and the I·D to I path becomes relatively unimportant. In **B**, the same result is obtained in the presence of a voltage shift, by hyperpolarization of the cell membrane to −115 mV resting potential. In **C**, the cell membrane is slightly depolarized. Depolarization accentuates the effectiveness of the voltage shift, i.e., further closes the fast I·D → R·D route; and also promotes the I state, which in turn leads to block (cf., fig. 30-5B). Comparison of B and C clearly illustrates how an antiarrhythmic drug can *selectively* block depolarized tissue.

The hypothetical drug modeled in fig. 30-6A is identical to that of fig. 30-5B, except that it lacks a voltage shift. As a result, channels bind drug while they are inactivated and accumulate in the $I \cdot D$ pool as before. However, in contrast to the drug of fig. 30-5B, the channels in fig. 30-6A can level the $I \cdot D$ pool during diastole by two routes: the relatively fast Hodgkin–Huxley recovery from inactivation $(I \cdot D \rightarrow R \cdot D)$ as well as the slower unbinding of drug $(I \cdot D \rightarrow I)$. Since $R \cdot D \rightarrow R$ also occurs relatively fast, recovery from block is completed rather quickly. Therefore, in the absence of a voltage shift, even a short diastolic interval is sufficient to allow all the channels to unblock and no accumulation of block occurs; the sodium channel availability for the second action potential is identical to that of the first.

SIGNIFICANCE OF RESTING MEMBRANE POTENTIAL

It can be easily shown that even for a drug that induces a significant inactivation voltage shift, e.g., the 25 mV shift of fig. 30-5B, sufficient hyperpolarization, say from -85 to -115 mV (fig. 30-6B), will overcome the 25 mV voltage shift, causing the $I \cdot D$ channels to recover $(I \cdot D \rightarrow R \cdot D)$ and then quickly unblock $(R \cdot D \rightarrow R)$ or $(R \cdot D \rightarrow A \cdot D \rightarrow A \rightarrow R)$ {25,26}. Conversely, a moderately depressed resting potential, e.g., -75 mV, markedly potentiates cumulative block by causing more trapping in the $I \cdot D$ state. This effect is shown in fig 30-6C for the same hypothetical inactivated-channel blocking drug of fig. 30-5B. Note that the sodium channel availability for the first action potential is much more inhibited in the depolarized preparation and that repetitive activation leads to even more block. The predicted steady-state availability of sodium channels for the depolarized cell of fig. 30-6C is 0.13 compared to 0.33 for the cell of fig. 30-5B.

Time-dependent aspects of modulated receptor block

It has already been shown in fig. 30-5A and B that the increment of block with successive action potentials is limited by the degree of recovery that occurs between periods of maximum drug-receptor affinity. Therefore, steady-state block at slow heart rates (other factors being constant) will be less than that achieved at fast heart rates. Figure 30-7 shows the first two action potentials of a train at 1 Hz using the same hypothetical inactivated-state

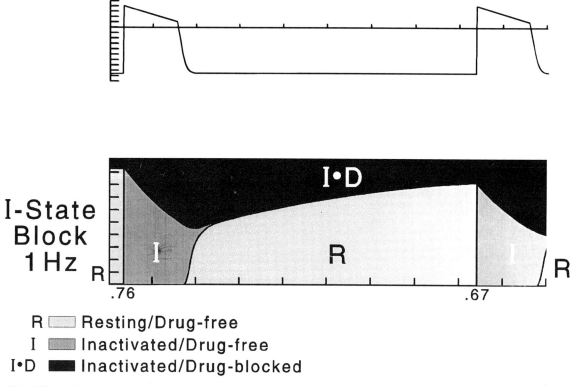

Fig. 30-7. Effect of inactivated-state blocker at 1 Hz. All parameters in this figure are identical to those of fig. 30-5B, except that heart rate was slowed from 3.3 Hz to 1 Hz and the horizontal axis represents 1.25 seconds. Thus, during the plateau of the first action potential the same amount of block develops as in fig. 30-5B. Upon repolarization, unblocking occurs at exactly the same rate, but because of the slower heart rate, unblocking occurs for a longer time the hence recovery from block is more complete. As a result the upstroke of the second action potential is 0.67 as compared to 0.49 in fig. 30-5B.

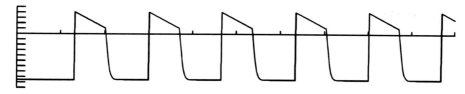

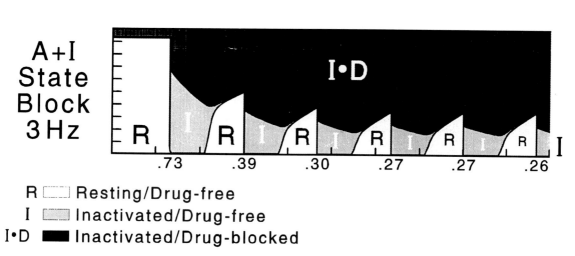

R ⬜ **Resting/Drug-free**
I ▥ **Inactivated/Drug-free**
I•D ⬛ **Inactivated/Drug-blocked**

Fig. 30-8. Cumulative block with a drug of high affinity for both the activated and inactivated states. The top trace shows a train of action potentials at 3.3 Hz (horizontal axis = 1.8 seconds). Note that block develops with each activation as well as during each inactivated (plateau) period. Sicne only the rested-state channel has a low affinity for the drug, recovery only proceeds when the membrane potential is negative, i.e., approaching or at the resting potential.

blocking drug displayed in fig. 30-5B at 3.3 Hz. The steady-state availability of sodium channels predicted at 1 Hz is 0.66 compared to the 0.33 predicted for 3.3 Hz. The same analysis applied to the effects of drugs on early extrasystoles shows that such depolarizations manifest greater depression of sodium current than for that of the preceding regular action potential for both activated-state and inactivated-state blocking drugs. The earlier the extrasystole, the less time for recovery and thus the more the inward current is reduced.

With continuous stimulation at a constant rate, sodium channel availability declines until it approaches a steady-state value slowly or rapidly, depending on the time constants of its interactions. This point has been discussed in some detail in a previous publication {23}. As shown in fig. 30-8, a hypothetical drug with high affinity for the channel receptor in both the activated and inactivated states, and with the time constants indicated in table 30-1, will approach steady state within 5–8 cycles.

Effects of action potential configuration on modulated receptor block

Some antiarrhythmic drugs depress the sodium current in atrial as well as Purkinje fibers and ventricular cells (e.g.,

quinidine), while others have much less effect on atrial cells (e.g., lidocaine) {58}. The modulated receptor theory provides a mechanistic explanation for these observations based on the relatively short action potential plateau exhibited by atrial cells as compared to Purkinje and ventricular fibers.

Referring to fig. 30-5A, it is apparent that a 50% change in action potential duration would have only a moderate effect on the depression of the sodium current of the second action potential of the train shown (as long as the rate is not changed), since recovery from block occurs at about the same rate during the plateau as during the diastolic interval. Therefore, a drug with high affinity only for the activated state will have the same effect regardless of action potential duration, i.e., the same effect on atrial as on Purkinje or ventricular cells. In contrast, a drug with high affinity for the inactivated channel (fig. 30-5B) would have much greater effect on a cell with a long plateau than on one with a short plateau since block continues to develop during the plateau period and diminishes only during diastole.

The predicted steady-state block caused by the two hypothetical agents (activated- and inactivated-channel blockers) as a function of action potential duration is given in table 30-2. Note that for the range of durations given,

Table 30-2. Relation of action potential duration to depression of steady-state $\dot{V}_{max}$ caused by pure activated channel and inactivated channel blocking drugs

Drug[a]	$\dot{V}_{max}$ for Action Potential Duration of					
	20	50	100	150	200	300 ms[b]
Activated-channel blocker	0.71	0.71	0.70	0.70	0.69	0.58
Inactivated-channel blocker	0.64	0.56	0.45	0.35	0.26	0.08

[a] Kinetic parameters taken from table 24-1. Action potential frequency 3.3 Hz. Drug-free normalized $\dot{V}_{max}$ for all action potential durations was 0.82.
[b] Action potential duration measured at 100% repolarization.

the decrement in $\dot{V}_{max}$ produced by the activated-channel blocking drug (from 0.71 to 0.58) is much less than the decrement produced by the blocker of inactivated channels (from 0.64 to 0.08). Since the plateau of atrial action potentials is typically 50 ms or less, while that of Purkinje fibers is 200 ms or more, it is apparent that a drug with high affinity only for inactivated channels would have a much greater effect in Purkinje tissue.

ACTIONS OF REAL ANTIARRHYTHMIC DRUGS

To be clinically useful, an inward-channel blocking drug must have significant affinity for the activated or for the inactivated channel (or for both), and preferentially have a lower affinity for rested channels. A meaningful classification of channel-blocking antiarrhythmic drugs should therefore be based on some measure of their affinities, e.g., dissociation constants, for each of the three channel states. To obtain such data requires experimental techniques that permit independent control of duration and membrane potential during each state. Obviously, the voltage-clamp technique is best for achieving such control. Because of the difficulty of voltage clamping cardiac tissue, only limited data for a few drugs are available: quinidine {23,50,51,56}, lidocaine {23,24,50,51,57,59}, procainamide {50,59}, amiodarone {60}, aprindine {60}, and some others {61}. Similarly, the data for the calcium-channel blockers is limited but most complete for verapamil and its analogue D600 {32,62,63}, diltiazem {63,64}, and nifedipine {65,66}. With the advent of single-cell voltage clamping, numerous more accurate studies have become available, but most of these are executed in reduced sodium current or at reduced temperature. Both these latter are known to significantly modify drug action.

Modulated receptor mechanism of action of sodium-channel blocking drugs

Of the sodium-channel blocking antiarrhythmic drugs that we have studied, amiodarone appears to have the purest affinity for the inactivated state. This is shown by the

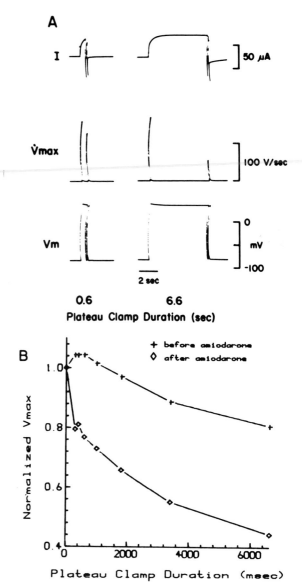

Fig. 30-9. Time-dependent inactivated-channel block by amiodarone (8.8×10^{-5} M) is illustrated. **A**, recorded during superfusion with amiodarone, shows current (upper trace), $\dot{V}_{max}$ (middle trace), and intracellular potential (lower trace) during a 600-ms (left) and a 6600-ms (right) conditioning plateau clamp to +28 mV, followed by a test stimulus. The $\dot{V}_{max}$ of the rest stimulus was mildly depressed after the short conditioning clamp and severely depressed by the long clamp. A plot of $\dot{V}_{max}$ in this experiment, normalized to the control value, against duration of the plateau clamp before and after amiodarone administration is shown in **B**. Reproduced with permission from Mason et al.: Pflügers Arch 396:80, 1983.

following results: Application of a fast pulse train of brief voltage clamps to the plateau level results in little or no block (fig. 30-9A). In contrast, a single long-plateau clamp pulse causes block to develop in an exponential fashion (fig. 30-9B). Application of clamps to different plateau voltages from −20 to +40 mV indicates no voltage dependence in this range for the development of block by amiodarone {60}. Of course, in sufficiently high concentrations, other states of the channel would ultimately also become blocked.

Similar studies have been carried out for lidocaine and a number of its analogues {59}. Bean et al. {24} studied lidocaine, utilizing the full voltage-clamp technique in rabbit Purkinje fibers. Both of these studies have obtained convincing evidence for predominantly inactivated-state block by lidocaine. However, lidocaine also blocks activated sodium channels {67}. Aprindine and a series of its analogues also show a marked affinity for the inactivated state {68}. However, like lidocaine, aprindine appears to have a higher affinity for the activated-channel receptor than does amiodarone. Quinidine also appears to have some affinity for the inactivated state, but not enough to account for all the block that develops during a pulse train {23,56}. It is tempting to speculate that the "extra" block that develops with each action potential represents block of the activated state. Thus most of the currently used clinical agents have mixed effects on activated and inactivated channels {61}. Figure 30-8 shows the effect of a drug with high affinity for both the activated and inactivated states.

Modulated receptor mechanism of action of organic calcium-channel blocking drugs

Ehara and Kaufmann {62} showed that verapamil has a strongly use-dependent blocking effect on the slow inward (calcium) current and that recovery from block is potential dependent. McDonald et al. {32} showed that D600 has a similar pattern of use-dependent onset of slow-channel block and voltage-dependent recovery from block. Results from this laboratory show that diltiazem also produces a use-dependent block (fig. 30-10); furthermore, the affinity for inactivated channels is much higher than for open (activated) channels {63}.

Nifedipine, a very potent calcium-channel blocking

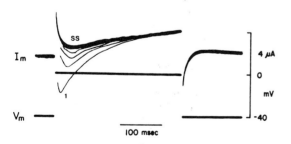

Fig. 30-10. Effect of diltiazem, 4.4 µM on slow inward current (Im) in voltage-clamped ferret papillary muscle. The drug had been present for 30 minutes. The numeral 1 indicates the first pulse of a train of clamps at 2 Hz after a rest period of several minutes; SS denotes the twentieth clamp. Traces for the first 20 clamp pulses are superimposed. Note that the current rapidly diminished toward a steady-state level with successive pulses.

drug with little antiarrhythmic usefulness {69}, appears to produce much less use-dependent block {66}, suggesting that the time constant of recovery from block must be short compared to the normal diastolic interval. These observations are further supported by comparison of the negative inotropic effects of verapamil and nifedipine. Verapamil has a markedly use-dependent negative inotropic action, manifested by reversal of the usual positive force-frequency relationship {70}. Furthermore, this effect is voltage dependent {71}. In contrast, nifedipine has negative inotropic effects at supratherapeutic doses that are relatively independent of stimulus frequency {72}. Unfortunately, little voltage-clamp information is available regarding the kinetics of nifedipine action on the slow inward current.

Modulated receptor mechanism of action for agents that lengthen action potential duration

Lengthening action potential duration can be achieved either by reducing an outward current or by augmenting an inward current. In order for such an agent to have more effect upon a tachycardia than upon a normal sinus beat, it must bind during each depolarization and dissociate during diastole. Binding during the plateau would, however, result in a positive feedback: the longer the plateau, the more binding, the longer the plateau, etc. This could quickly lead to repolarization disturbances, excessively long action potential durations, or perhaps non-repolarization. Therefore, it is mandatory that use-dependent agents bind only during the upstroke of the action potential and not during the plateau. Dissociation may occur during diastole and/or the plateau.

Unfortunately, most clinical agents that act by lengthening action potential duration lengthen the action potential primarily at slow heart rates (class III_b, b from bradycardia), but at fast heart rates they yield little prolongation. This may result from binding during diastole and unbinding during the plateau. Such reverse use dependence {5} is far from ideal. To the contrary, when lengthening becomes excessive after a long diastolic interval, it may lead to repolarization disturbances, early after depolarizations or even torsades de pointes.

It is remarkable that the drug that is generally considered to be the most effective antiarrhythmic agent, amiodarone, lengthens action potential duration to the same extent at fast and slow heart rates {73}. The fact that it is virtually devoid of torsades de pointes may be related in part to the fact that it does not cause excessive lengthening of the action potential following long diastolic intervals.

Optimal selectivity would, however, be achieved by drugs that lengthen action potential duration primarily during tachycardia and leave the normal sinus beat undisturbed. Such agents have been referred to as Class III_a, because they lengthen the action potential primarily upon acceleration of the heart {74}.

CLINICAL CORRELATIONS

While it is not yet possible to predict exactly which drugs will be the most effective in a given patient's cardiac arrhythmia, it is now possible to predict whether new drugs will be useful in atrial arrhythmias and to explain why some established agents are more useful for certain types of arrhythmias than for others.

Atrial tachycardia

The action potential of ordinary atrial muscle cells is characterized by a short plateau, which shortens even more in tachycardia. Therefore, inactivated-channel blockers will cause relatively less sodium-channel block in atrial tissue. If the inactivated-channel blocker also has relatively fast recovery kinetics during diastole (e.g., lidocaine and phenytoin) the drug will have a low efficacy against atrial tachycardia. If, on the other hand, diastolic recovery is slowed by depolarization (e.g., digitalis toxicity), the blocked inactivated channels will accumulate and the drug may be expected to be more effective. This provides an explanation for the clinical observation that lidocaine is not very effective for atrial arrhythmias except those caused by digitalis toxicity {58}. It is important to note that amiodarone, which appears to act almost exclusively upon inactivated channels, is nevertheless more effective than lidocaine in atrial arrhythmias {75}. There are several possible explanations for this. Amiodarone has a slower diastolic recovery from block. Moreover, amiodarone lengthens the action potential duration, thus potentiating its inactivated-state block. Finally, amiodarone has additional effects, including calcium-entry block and anti-adrenergic activity.

Quinidine is more effective as the number of action potentials per unit time is increased {23}, while action potential duration is of relatively less importance in determining the fraction of channels blocked. Quinidine has a relatively slow time constant of recovery from block during diastole so block accumulates, especially at fast rates; hence the drug's effectiveness against atrial tachycardias.

AV nodal arrhythmias

Numerous conditions exist in which slow conduction through the atrioventricular (AV) node contributes to reentry arrhythmias. Since the major inward current in the AV node is a calcium current {76}, it is not surprising that calcium-entry blockers can be quite effective against these arrhythmias. Like most of the sodium-channel blockers, these drugs have a high affinity for depolarized (i.e., inactivated) channels. Recovery from block proceeds slowly in depolarized cells and faster in cells with more negative resting potentials {32}. Therefore, in reciprocating rhythms involving an accessory pathway, these drugs will usually block the calcium-dependent pathway, especially if it is depolarized. Thus the node is more likely to be blocked than the accessory bundle.

Ventricular arrhythmias

Ventricular and Purkinje fibers have long action potentials, hence inactivation block is much more important in these cells than in atrial tissue. Another important feature of healthy ventricular and nonpacemaker Purkinje cells is their fairly negative diastolic potential (−85 to −90 mV). Thus, although lidocaine blocks a large fraction of the sodium channels during each plateau phase, the fast diastolic recovery (at −90 mV) ensures that most channels are unblocked by the time of the next normal action potential. There are, however, two exceptions: (a) V_{max} of early extrasystoles occurring before the drug-receptor complexes have dissociated are strongly suppressed, and (b) in tissues depolarized by disease, diastolic recovery from block proceeds much more slowly or not at all (compare figs. 30-5B and 30-6C). Hence in depolarized tissue, and especially for early extrasystoles, channels will be significantly blocked by a concentration of lidocaine that has no remarkable effect on conduction of the normal sinus impulse through healthy tissue.

Drugs that act on channels only when they are in the activated state are not assisted by the long plateau duration of Purkinje and ventricular cells. Only when a tachycardia develops will they succeed in blocking a substantial fraction of the sodium channels. It is then not surprising that lidocaine-like drugs appear more effective than quinidine {77} in suppressing premature depolarizations, while quinidine may be more effective in suppressing regular ventricular tachycardias {78}.

Drugs like flecainide and encainide are potent suppressors of PVCs. Perhaps because of their slow kinetics, they can reduce the inward pacemaker current throughout diastole, and hence effectively reduce automaticity. However, because of these slow kinetics the concentration that depresses a tachycardia must also interfere with the normal sinus beat, i.e., is proarrhythmic. Another possibility is that the concentration that does not interfere with the normal sinus beat will also not effectively suppress a tachycardia. Based upon these kind of computations, one of us {79} computed that these agents would be ineffective against tachycardias and that their proarrhythmic properties could render them unsafe. A few years later, encainide and flecainide had to be dropped from the CAST trial because they were found to be ineffective and to more than double mortality {80}.

Other clinical applications

As indicated in an earlier publication {23}, the combination of two antiarrhythmic drugs with different kinetic parameters may be considerably more effective than either drug alone, independent of dosage. In clinical tests {81,82} this prediction has been confirmed: Patients who were resistant to both disopyramide alone and mexiletine alone were successfully managed with a combination of these two dissimilar drugs; and combination of quinidine and mexilitine yielded greater therapeutic efficacy with fewer toxic side effects.

Another predictable drug interaction results from the

state-dependent model. If drug A lengthens the action potential duration and if drug B is an inactivated-state blocker, then at any given rate A will lengthen the effective time for inactivated-state block to develop and shorten the time for recovery from it. For example, amiodarone lengthens the action potential duration and terefore will enhance its own effect (see above), as well as that of any other inactivated-state blocker, e.g., lidocaine. Conversely, drugs that shorten action potential duration (e.g., acetylcholine in the atria) would be expected to reduce the effect of an inactivated-state blocker. Similarly, if a drug were found that safely and reliably reduced Purkinje or ventricular action potential duration, then such a drug might be useful in reversing conduction block induced by an overdose of an inactivated-state blocker.

At this stage in the development of the modulated receptor hypothesis, more extensive application to clinical drug selection would be premature. More information is needed on the cellular physiology of the cardiac tissue responsible for the abnormal rhythm. Especially valuable would be information on the resting potential in vivo. Unfortunately, this variable is more difficult to measure in patients.

CONCLUSIONS

We have discussed the modulated receptor hypothesis of sodium, calcium, and potassium channel block (and activators of inward currents) and applied it to various types of drugs used in the treatment of arrhythmias. The model provides a mechanism by which useful antiarrhythmic drugs can selectively suppress abnormal electrical activity. A better understanding of the voltage- and time-dependent actions of antiarrhythmic drugs will allow a more rational selection of a drug for a particular arrhythmia, as well as the development of new drugs with optimized voltage-time characteristics.

ACKNOWLEDGMENTS

The authors wish to thank Drs. Clarkson, Malecot, and Moyer for their critical suggestions. We are grateful to Dr. Moyer for his programming contributions, and Mr. Cotner and Mr. Cowan for their assistance with the graphic illustrations.

REFERENCES

1. Weidmann S: Effects of calcium ions and local anaesthetics on electrical properties of Purkinje fibres. *J Physiol (Lond)* 129:568–582, 1955.
2. Hondeghem L, Grant AO, Jensen RA: Antiarrhythmic drug action: Selective depression of hypoxic cardiac cells. *Am Heart J* 87:602–605, 1974.
3. Grant AO, Katzung BG: The effects of quinidine and verapamil on electrically induced automaticity in the ventricular myocardium of guinea pig. *J Pharmacol Exp Ther* 196:407–419, 1976.
4. Fleckenstein A: Specific inhibitors and promotors of calcium action in the excitation-contraction coupling of heart muscle and their role in the prevention of production of myocardial lesions. In: Harris P, Opie LH (eds) *Calcium and the Heart.* New York: Academic Press, 1971, pp 135–188.
5. Hondeghem LM, Snyders DJ: Class III antiarrhythmic agents have a lot of potential, but a long way to go: Reduced effectiveness and dangers of reverse use-dependence. *Circulation* 81:686–690, 1990.
6. van Bogaert PP, Goethals M, Simoens C: Use- and frequency-dependent blockade by UL-FS 49 of i_f pacemaker current in sheep cardiac Purkinje fibres. *Eur J Pharmacol* 187:241–256, 1990.
7. Hille B: Local anesthetics: Hydrophilic and hydrophobic pathways for the drug-receptor reaction. *J Gen Physiol* 69:497–515, 1977.
8. Hondeghem LM, Katzung BG: Time- and voltage-dependent interaction of antiarrhythmic drugs with cardiac sodium channels. *Biochim Biophys Acta* 472:373–398, 1977.
9. Jensen RA, Katzung BG: Electrophysiological action of diphenylhydantoin on rabbit atria: Dependence on stimulation frequency, potassium, and sodium. *Circ Res* 26:17–27, 1970.
10. Singh BN, Vaughan Williams EM: Effect of altering potassium concentration on the action of lidocaine and diphenylhydantoin on rabbit atrial and ventricular muscle. *Circ Res* 29:286–295, 1971.
11. Hope RR, Williams DO, El-Sherif N, Lazzara R, Scherlag BJ: The efficacy of antiarrhythmic agents during acute myocardial ischemia and the role of heart rate. *Circulation* 50:507–514, 1974.
12. Kupersmith J, Antman EM, Hoffman BF: In vivo electrophysiologic effects of lidocaine in canine acute myocardial infarction. *Circ Res* 36:84–91, 1975.
13. Michelson EL, Spear JF, Moore EN: Effects of procainamide on strength-interval relations in normal and chronically infarcted canine myocardium. *Am J Cardiol* 47:1223–1232, 1981.
14. Lamanna V, Antzelevitch C, Moe GK: Effects of lidocaine on conduction through depolarized canine false tendons and on a model of reflected reentry. *J Pharmacol Exp Ther* 221:353–361, 1982.
15. Wong SS, Myerburg RJ, Ezrin AM, Gelband H, Bassett AL: Electrophysiologic effects of encainide on acutely ischemic rabbit myocardial cells. *Eur J Pharmacol* 80:323–329, 1982.
16. Okumura K, Horio Y, Tokuomi H: Effects of lidocaine on conduction in normal and acutely ischemic ventricular myocardium of dogs. *Arch Int Pharmacodyn* 256:269–282, 1982.
17. Johnson EA, McKinnon MG: Differential effect of quinidine and pyridamine on the myocardial action potential at various rates of stimulation. *J Pharmacol Exp Ther* 120:460–465, 1957.
18. Heistracher P: Mechanism of action of antifibrillatory drugs. *Naunyn-Schmiedebergs Arch Pharmacol* 269:199–212, 1971.
19. Strichartz G: The inhibition of sodium currents in myelinated nerve by quaternary derivatives of lidocaine. *J Gen Physiol (Lond)* 62:37–57, 1973.
20. Courtney KR: Mechanism of frequency-dependent inhibition of sodium currents in frog myelinated nerve by the lidocaine derivative GEA 968. *J Pharmacol Exp Ther* 195:225–236, 1975.
21. Chen C-M, Gettes LS, Katzung BG: Effect of lidocaine and quinidine on steady-state characteristics and recovery kinetics of $(dV/dt)_{max}$ in guinea pig ventricular myocardium. *Circ Res* 37:20–29, 1975.
22. Hodgkin AL, Huxley AF: The dual effect of membrane potential on sodium conductance in the giant axon of Loligo. *J Physiol (Lond)* 116:497–506, 1952.

23. Hondeghem LM, Katzung BG: Effect of quinidine and lidocaine on myocardial conduction. *Circulation* 61:1217–1224, 1980.

24. Bean BP, Cohen CJ, Tsien RW: Lidocaine block of cardiac sodium channels. *J Gen Physiol* 81:613–642, 1983.

25. Snyders DJ, Hondeghem LM: Effects of quinidine on the sodium current of guinea pig myocytes: Evidence for a drug-associated rested state with altered kinetics. *Circ Res* 66:565–579, 1990.

26. Anno T, Hondeghem LM: Interactions of flecainide with guinea pig cardiac sodium channels: Importance of activation unblocking to the voltage dependence of recovery. *Circ Res* 66:789–803, 1990.

27. Sada H: Effect of phentolamine, alprenolol, and prenylamine on maximum rate of rise of action potential in guinea-pig papillary muscles. *Naunyn-Schmiedebergs Arch Pharmacol* 304:191–201, 1978.

28. Sada H, Kojima M, Ban T: Effect of procainamide on transmembrane action potentials in guinea-pig papillary muscles as affected by external potassium concentration. *Naunyn-Schmiedebergs Arch Pharmacol* 309:179–190, 1979.

29. Courtney KR: Interval-dependent effects of small antiarrhythmic drugs on excitability of guinea pig myocardium. *J Mol Cell Cardiol* 12:1273–1286, 1980.

30. Courtney KR: Antiarrhythmic drug design: Frequency-dependent block in myocardium. In: Fink RB (ed) *Molecular Mechanisms of Anesthesia. Progress in Anesthesiology*, Vol 2. New York: Raven Press, 1980, pp 111–118.

31. Kohlhardt M, Seifert C: Inhibition of $\dot{V}_{max}$ of the action potential by propafenone and its voltage-, time-, and pH-dependence in mammalian ventricular myocardium. *Naunyn-Schmiedebergs Arch Pharmacol* 315:55–62, 1980.

32. McDonald T, Pelzer D, Trautwein W: On the mechanisms of slow calcium channel block in heart. *Pflügers Arch* 385:175–179, 1980.

33. Oshita S, Sada H, Kojima M, Ban T: Effects of tocainide and lidocaine on the transmembrane action potentials as related to external potassium concentrations in guinea-pig papillary muscles. Naunyn-Schmiedebergs Arch Pharmacol 314:67–82, 1980.

34. Sada H, Ban T: Effects of acebutolol and other structurally related beta adrenergic blockers on transmembrane action potential in guinea-pig papillary muscles. *J Pharmacol Exp Ther* 215:507–514, 1980.

35. Arlock P: Actions of lofepramine, a new tricyclic antidepressant, and despiramine on electrophysiological and mechanical parameters of guinea pig atrial and papillary muscles. *Acta Pharmacol Toxicol* 49:248–258, 1981.

36. Catterall WA: Inhibition of voltage-sensitive sodium channels in neuroblastoma cells by antiarrhythmic drugs. *Mol Pharmacol* 20:356–362, 1981.

37. Cardinal R, Janse MJ, Van Eeden I, Werner G, Naumann d'Alnoncourt C, Durrer D: The effects of lidocaine on intracellular and extracellular potentials, activation and ventricular arrhythmias during acute regional ischemia in the isolated procine heart. *Circ Res* 49:792–806, 1981.

38. Carson DL, Dresel PE: Effects of lidocaine on conduction of extrasystoles in the normal canine heart. *J Cardiol Pharmacol* 3:924–935, 1981.

39. Cordova MA, Bagwell EE, Lindenmayer GE: Studies on the interaction of propranolol and tetrodotoxin on dV/dt_{max} of canine Purkinje fiber action potentials. *J Pharmacol Exp Ther* 219:187–191, 1981.

40. Courtney KR: Comparative actions of mexiletine on sodium channels in nerve, skeletal and cardiac muscle. *Eur J Pharmacol* 74:9–18, 1981.

41. Courtney KR: Significance of bicarbonate for antiarrhythmic drug action. *J Mol Cell Cardiol* 13:1031–1034, 1981.

42. Gilmour RF, Ruffy R, Lovelace DE, Mueller TM, Zipes DP: Effect of ethanol on electrogram changes and regional myocardial blood flow during acute myocardial ischemia. *Cardiovasc Res* 15:47–58, 1981.

43. Gilmour RF, Chikharev VN, Jurevichus JA, Zacharow S, Zipes DP: Effect of aprindine on transmembrane currents and contractile force in frog atria. *J Pharmacol Exp Ther* 217:390–396, 1981.

44. Kolhardt M, Haap K: The blockade of V_{max} of the atrioventricular action potential produced by the slow channel inhibitors verapamil and nifedipine. *Naunyn-Schmiedebergs Arch Pharmacol* 316:178–185, 1981.

45. Nattel S, Elharrar V, Zipes DP, Bailey JC: pH-dependent electrophysiological effects of quinidine and lidocaine on canine cardiac Purkinje fibers. *Circ Res* 48:55–61, 1981.

46. Rudiger HJ, Homburger H, Antoni H: Effects of a new antiarrhythmic compound {2-benzol-1-(2′ diisopropyl-aminoethoxy-imino)-cycloheptome hydrogen fumarate} on the electrophysiological properties of mammalian cardiac cells. *Naunyn-Schmiedebergs Arch Pharmacol* 317:238, 1981.

47. Sada H, Ban T: Time-independent effects on cardiac action potential upstroke velocity (resting block) and lipid solubility of beta adrenergic blockers. *Experientia* 37:171–172, 1981.

48. Sada N, Ban T: Effects of various structurally related beta-adrenocepter blocking agents on maximum upstroke velocity of action potential in guinea-pig papillary muscles. *Naunyn-Schmiedebergs Arch Pharmacol* 317:245–251, 1981.

49. Campbell TJ, Vaughan Williams EM: Electrophysiological and other effects on rabbit hearts of CCI22277, a new steroidal antiarrhythmic drug. *Br J Pharmacol* 76:337–345, 1982.

50. Carmelier E, Saikawa T: Shortening of the action potential and reduction of pacemaker activity by lidocaine, quinidine, and procainamide in sheep cardiac Purkinje fibers: An effect on Na or K current? *Circ Res* 50:257–272, 1982.

51. Colatsky TJ: Mechanisms of action of lidocaine and quinidine on action potential duration in rabbit cardiac Purkinje fibers. *Circ Res* 50:17–27, 1982.

52. Connors BW, Prince DA: Effects of local anesthetic OX314 on the membrane properties of hppocampal pyramidal neurons. *J Pharmacol Exp Ther* 220:476–481, 1982.

53. Grant AO, Trantham JL, Brown KK, Strauss HC: pH-dependent effects of quinidine on the kinetics of dV/dt_{max} in guinea pig ventricular myocardium. *Circ Res* 50:210–217, 1982.

54. Kojima M, Ban T, Sada H: Effects of disopyramide on the maximum rate of rise of the potential ($\dot{V}_{max}$) in guinea-pig papillary muscles. *Jpn J Pharmacol* 32:91–102, 1982.

55. Hohnloser S, Weirich J, Antoni H: Effects of mexiletine on steady-state characteristics and recovery kinetics of $\dot{V}_{max}$ and conduction velocity in guinea pig myocardium. *J Cardiovasc Pharmacol* 4:232–239, 1982.

56. Weld FM, Coromilas J, Rothman JN, Bigger JT Jr: Mechanisms of quinidine-induced depression of maximum upstroke velocity in ovine cardiac Pukinje fibers. *Circ Res* 50:369–376, 1982.

57. Payet MD: Effect of lidocaine on fast and slow inactivation of sodium current in rat ventricular cells. *J Pharmacol Exp Ther* 223:235–240, 1982.

58. Rosen MR, Hoffman BF, Wit AL: Electrophysiology and pharmacology of cardiac arrhythmias. V. Cardiac antiarrhythmic effects of lidocaine. *Am Heart J* 89:526–536, 1975.

59. Ehring GR, Moyer JW, Hondeghem LM: Implications from electrophysiological differences resulting from small structural changes in antiarrhythmic durgs. *Proc West Pharmacol Soc* 25:65–67, 1982.

60. Mason JW, Hondeghem LM, Katzung BG: Amiodarone blocks inactivated cardiac sodium channels. *Pflügers Arch* 396:79–81, 1983.

61. Kodama I, Toyama J, Takanaka C, Yamada K: Block of activated and inactivated sodium channels by class I antiarrhythmic drugs studied by using the maximum upstroke velocity ($\dot{V}_{max}$) of action potential in guinea-pig cardiac muscles. *J Mol Cell Cardiol* 19:367–377, 1987.

62. Ehara T, Kaufmann R: The voltage- and time-dependent effects of (−)-verapamil on the slow inward current in isolated cat ventricular myocardium. *J Pharmacol Exp Ther* 207:49–55, 1978.

63. Kanaya S, Arlock P, Katzung BG, Hondeghem LM: Diltiazem and verapamil preferentially block inactivated calcium channels. *J Mol Cell Cardiol* 15:145–148, 1983.

64. Morad M, Tung L, Greenspan AM: Effect of diltiazem on calcium transport and development of tension in heart muscle. *Am J Cardiol* 49:595–601, 1982.

65. Kolhardt M, Fleckenstein A: Inhibition of the slow inward current by nifedipine in mammalian ventricular myocardium. *Naunyn-Schmiedebergs Arch Pharmacol* 298:267–272, 1977.

66. Bayer R, Ehara T: Comparative studies with calcium antagonists. In: Van Zwieten PA, Schonbaum E (eds) *The Action of Drugs on Calcium Metabolism.* Stuttgart: Fischer Verlag, 1978, pp 31–37.

67. Matsubara T, Clarkson C, Hondeghem L: Lidocaine blocks open and inactivated cardiac sodium channels. *Naunyn-Schmiedebergs Arch Pharmacol* 336:224–231, 1987.

68. Moyer J, Hondeghem LM: Characterization of activation and inactivation block in a series of aprindine derivatives using voltage clamp technique. *Fed Proc* 42:634, 1983.

69. Kawai C, Konishi T, Matsuyama E, Okazaki H: Comparative effects of three calcium antagonists, dilitiazem, verapamil, an nifedipine, on the sinoatrial and atrioventricular nodes: Experimental and clinical studies. *Circulation* 63:1035–1042, 1981.

70. Bayer R, Hennekes R, Kaufmann R, Mannhold R: Inotropic and electrophysiological actions of verapamil and D-600 in mammalian myocardium. I. Patterns of inotropic effects of racemic compounds. *Naunyn-Schmiedebergs Arch Pharmacol* 290:49–68, 1975.

71. Linden J, Brooker G: The influence of resting membrane potential on the effect of verapamil on atria. *J Mol Cell Cardiol* 12:325–331, 1980.

72. Bayer R, Rodenkirchen R, Kaufmann R, Tec JH, Hennekes R: The effect of nifedipine on contraction and monophasic action potential of isolated cat myocardium. *Naunyn-Schmiedebergs Arch Pharmacol* 301:29–37, 1977.

73. Anderson KP, Walker R, Dustman T, Lux RL, Ershler PR, Kates RE, Urie PM: Rate-related electrophysiologic effects of long-term administration of amiodarone on canine ventricular myocardium in vivo. *Circulation* 79:948–958, 1989.

74. Hondeghem LM: Ideal antiarrhythmic agents: Chemical defibrillators. *J Cardiovasc Electrophysiol* 2:169–177, 1991.

75. Rowland E, Krikler DM: Electrophysiological assessment of amiodarone in treatment of resistant supraventricular arrhythmias. *Br Heart J* 44:82–90, 1980.

76. Kokubun S, Nishimura M, Noma A, Irasawa H: Membrane currents in the rabbit atrioventricular node cell. *Pflügers Arch* 393:15–22, 1982.

77. Sami M, Harrison DC, Kraemer H, Houston N, Shimasaki C, De Busk RF: Antiarrhythmic efficacy of encainide and quinidine: Validation of a model of drug assessment. *Am J Cardiol* 48:147–156, 1981.

78. Mason JW, Winkle RA: Electrode-catheter arrhythmia induction in the selection and assessment of antiarrhythmic drug therapy for recurrent ventricular tachycardia. *Circulation* 58:971–985, 1978.

79. Hondeghem LM, Snyders DJ: Class III antiarrhythmic agents have a lot of potential, but a long way to go: Reduced effectiveness and dangers of reverse use-dependence. *Circulation* 81:686–690, 1990.

80. CAST Investigators: Preliminary report: Effect of encainide and flecainide on mortality in a randomized trial of arrhythmia suppression after myocardial infarction. *N Engl J Med* 321:406–412, 1990.

81. Breithardt G, Seipel L, Abendroth RR: Comparison of antiarrhythmic efficacy of disopyramide and mexiletine against stimulus-induced ventricular tachycardia. *J Cardiovasc Pharmacol* 3:1026–1037, 1981.

82. Duff JH, Roden D, Primm RK, Oates JA, Woosley RL: Mexiletine in the treatment of resistant ventricular arrhythmias: Enhancement of efficacy and reduction of dose-related side effects by combination with quinidine. *Circulation* 67:1124–1128, 1983.

CHAPTER 31

Role of Calcium in Cardiac Cell Damage and Dysfunction

NARANJAN S. DHALLA, VIJAYAN ELIMBAN, HEINZ RUPP,
NOBUAKIRA TAKEDA, & MAKOTO NAGANO

INTRODUCTION

It is now well established that Ca^{2+} is essential for the excitation-contraction coupling process, regulation of metabolism, and maintenance of cellular integrity of cardiomyocytes. Under normal conditions the extracellular concentration of ionized Ca^{2+} is about 1.25 mM, whereas the intracellular (cytoplasmic) concentration of ionized Ca^{2+} varies in the range of $0.1-10 \mu M$, and thus cardiomyocytes can be seen to maintain a large Ca^{2+} concentration gradient across their cell membrane. This task is primarily achieved by the presence of different Ca^{2+}-influx and Ca^{2+}-efflux mechanisms as well as regulatory systems in the sarcolemmal membrane. Furthermore, the low level of Ca^{2+} in the cytoplasm is maintained by the presence of Ca^{2+}-pump mechanisms in the sarcoplasmic reticulum under physiological conditions. On the other hand, mitochondria are involved in accumulating a large amount of Ca^{2+}, mainly under situations where the cell is faced with high concentrations of Ca^{2+} and thus prevent the cell from the toxic effects of the elevated levels of cytoplasmic Ca^{2+} (intracellular Ca^{2+} overload). In this article we have attempted to describe briefly the functions of various membrane structures that participate in lowering and raising the intracellular concentration of free Ca^{2+} in the myocardium. Possible mechanisms that are considered to induce membrane defects for the occurrence of intracellular Ca^{2+} overload and subsequent heart dysfunction will be identified. Since Ca^{2+} in low concentrations is required for cardiac function, whereas high concentrations of intracellular Ca^{2+} are known to result in cardiotoxicity, it is planned to discuss the paradoxical effects of this cation in some detail. It is also our objective to describe the involvement of intracellular Ca^{2+} overload in the pathogenesis of cardiac cell damage and dysfunction in situations such as catecholamine-induced cardiomyopathy, genetically linked cardiomyopathy, and ischemia-reperfusion injury.

Ca^{2+}-translocating systems in cardiocytes

Sarcolemma has not only been shown to play an important role as a source of activator Ca^{2+} during the process of excitation-contraction coupling in the heart but is also considered to be intimately involved in lowering the cytoplasmic level of Ca^{2+} for the occurrence of relaxation {1–5}. Electrophysiological, biochemical, and pharmacological studies have revealed that the magnitude of sarcolemmal Ca^{2+} stores and opening of Ca^{2+} channels determine the amount of Ca^{2+} that enters the cell upon excitation of the myocardium, whereas Ca^{2+} efflux is carried out by the Na^{2+}-Ca^{2+} exchange and Ca^{2+}-pump mechanisms in the sarcolemmal membrane. ATP-independent Ca^{2+} binding (passive Ca^{2+} binding) with isolated sarcolemmal preparations has been suggested to represent the sarcolemmal superficial Ca^{2+} stores and has been shown to be due to the presence of sialic acid residues, proteins, and phospholipids in the membrane {6,7}. Although a lipoprotein component with a high Ca^{2+} binding capacity has been isolated from the heart plasma membrane {8} information with respect to its relation with sarcolemmal Ca^{2+} stores and Ca^{2+} channels is lacking, and thus no conclusion can be made for its functional role. Sarcolemmal preparations have been demonstrated to exhibit ATP-dependent Ca^{2+} uptake, Ca^{2+}-stimulated ATPase, and Na^+-Ca^{2+} exchange activities {1–5}. The heart sarcolemmal Ca^{2+}-stimulated ATPase, which may serve as a Ca^{2+} pump at the cell membrane, has been partially purified with a major band of 140 kDa {9}. The Ca^{2+}-stimulated ATPase has been shown to utilize MgATP as substrate and is activated by micromolar concentrations of Ca^{2+} with an apparent Ka of $0.2 \mu M$. The Na^+-Ca^{2+} antiporter, which is believed to carry out Na^+-Ca^{2+} exchange, has also been isolated in a partially purified form from the heart cell membrane {10}. Thus it can be appreciated that several Ca^{2+}-related activities have now been demonstrated in sarcolemmal preparations obtained by different methods, and various investigators have attempted to isolate different components for the Ca^{2+} influx and Ca^{2+} efflux mechanisms for establishing their exact function and significance in different phases of the cardiac contraction and relaxation cycle.

In addition to Ca^{2+}-stimulated ATPase, heart sarcolemmal preparations have also been shown to contain Na,K-ATPase and Ca^{2+}/Mg^{2+} ecto-ATPase activities {1–4}. While Na,K-ATPase has been demonstrated to serve as a pump for Na^+ and K^+ across the cell membrane, the function of Ca^{2+}/Mg^{2+} ecto-ATPase is far from clear. It should be pointed out that Ca^{2+}/Mg^{2+} ecto-ATPase

N. Sperelakis (ed.), Physiology and Pathophysiology of the Heart, Third Edition.
© *1995 Kluwer Academic Publishers. ISBN 0-7923-2612-1. All rights reserved.*

being referred to here is distinctly different from the Ca^{2+}-stimulated ATPase of heart sarcolemma or sarcoplasmic reticulum because it utilizes CaATP or MgATP as a substrate and requires millimolar concentrations of Ca^{2+} or Mg^{2+} for activation. Various divalent cations, such as Ni^{2+}, Co^{2+}, and Mn^{2+} which are known to block calcium currents, were found to decrease the sarcolemmal Ca^{2+} ecto-ATPase activity [11]. Furthermore, cyclic AMP-protein kinase dependent phosphorylation, which is considered to mediate the increase in Ca^{2+} influx due to hormone action, has been shown to increase the sarcolemmal Ca^{2+} ecto-ATPase activity [12]. The sarcolemmal Ca^{2+} ecto-ATPase activity was found to be altered in diseased hearts in which contractile force development was impaired [13–19]. Several cardiodepressants, such as a plasma factor, quinidine, lidocaine, procainamide, propranolol, pentobarbital, volatile anesthetic agents, and La^{3+}, have been reported to decrease the sarcolemmal Ca^{2+} ecto-ATPase activity [21–25]. These results clearly indicate that Ca^{2+}/Mg^{2+} ecto-ATPase in sarcolemma is a viable site for drug actions and is altered due to pathophysiological manipulations, and thus support the view that this enzyme system may be involved in the regulation of heart function.

According to a current concept of excitation-contraction coupling, depolarization of the cardiac muscle increases the permeability of the cell membrane and permits the entry of Ca^{2+} along the concentration gradient [1–5]. Electrophysiological evidence indicates the opening of Ca^{2+} channels in a voltage- and time-dependent manner when membrane permeability is increased upon depolarization, but it is not clear how exactly these Ca^{2+} channels open by an electrical stimulus and how these channels close upon the disappearance of the electrical impulse. Since opening of Ca^{2+} channels can be conceived to involve the physical movements of proteins, we have suggested that this process is a highly regulated event in which Ca^{2+}/Mg^{2+} ecto-ATPase may be involved for opening Ca^{2+} gates in the sarcolemmal membrane [1–3]. It is pointed out that opening of the slow channels through which the inward Ca^{2+} current during the action potential plateau traverses the heart sarcolemma has been shown to require metabolic energy in the form of ATP [26]. If this is the case, then an ATPase system similar to the sarcolemmal Ca^{2+}/Mg^{2+} ecto-ATPase can be seen to be involved in opening the Ca^{2+} channels in myocardium. It is noteworthy that several energy-yielding agents, including ATP, have been shown to produce an increase in contractile force of the cardiac muscle [27,28]. Thus it appears that Ca^{2+}/Mg^{2+} ecto-ATPase may represent a biochemical correlate of the electrophysiologically defined Ca^{2+} channels in heart sarcolemma, and it may be intimately involved in opening these gates by phosphorylating these proteins in the cell membrane. Schoffeniels has suggested a similar model for sodium channels in nerve membranes in which a cycle of phosphorylation and dephosphorylation is considered to be responsible for opening and closing these gates [29]. It is emphasized that the involvement of the sarcolemmal Ca^{2+}/Mg^{2+} ecto-ATPase in opening Ca^{2+} channels and subsequent Ca^{2+} entry

into the myocardium upon depolarization or hormonal activation should not be viewed as a phenomenon analogous to active Ca^{2+} transport. On the contrary, the movement of Ca^{2+} from the extracellular fluid into the cell is a passive process in the conventional sense, but it is the opening of Ca^{2+} channels that requires energy through participation of the sarcolemmal Ca^{2+}/Mg^{2+} ecto-ATPase system. In fact, nanomolar concentrations of ATP have been shown to activate Ca^{2+} channels in snail neurons [30]. It is pointed out that Ca^{2+}/Mg^{2+} ecto-ATPase has been demonstrated to be present in the heart sarcolemmal membrane by cytochemical techniques [31], and its activation by Ca^{2+} has been shown to exhibit a linear relationship with contractile force development in the myocardium [3,32].

By employing the heart sarcolemmal preparations containing the plasma membrane, basement membrane, and cell surface material, we were able to solubilize an ATPase by trypsin treatment [33]; this enzyme (Ca^{2+}-dependent ecto-ATPase) was purified as having Mr = 67,000 (two subunits of 55,000 and 12,000) and was found to be sensitive to Na^+ [34]. This enzyme was shown to be of contractile protein in nature, as it was found to exhibit some of the properties similar to that of myosin and has been proposed to serve as a Na^+-sensitive Ca^{2+}-entry mechanism in the cell membrane [35]. The Ca^{2+}/Mg^{2+} ecto-ATPase activity remaining in the sarcolemmal membrane after treatment with trypsin was characterized, solubilized, and purified [36–38]. The sarcolemmal Ca^{2+}/Mg^{2+} ecto-ATPase has Mr = 250,000 and is considered to serve as a gating mechanism for the voltage entry of Ca^{2+} into the myocardium. The Ca^{2+}/Mg^{2+} ecto-ATPase has been shown to differ from Ca^{2+}-dependent ecto-ATPase and Ca^{2+}-stimulated ATPase (Ca^{2+} pump) in the sarcolemmal membrane and was found to be regulated by ATP and lectinlike substances in the cell surface material [39,40]. Phospholipids were found to be required for the Ca^{2+}/Mg^{2+} ecto-ATPase activity [41], and phospholipid N-methylation was shown to depress the enzyme activities [42].

Our studies have shown that sulfhydryl groups are essential for the Ca^{2+}/Mg^{2+} ecto-ATPase activities, but these are embedded in the membrane bilayer [43]. We have observed that gramacidin S, an antibiotic agent, exerted a potent inhibitory action on the sarcolemmal Ca^{2+}-Mg^{2+} ecto-ATPase and produced a marked cardiodepressant effect [44]. Furthermore, electrical stimulation of the sarcolemmal membranes was found to activate Ca^{2+}/Mg^{2+} ecto-ATPase, an effect that was blocked by Ca^{2+} antagonists [45,46]. It should be pointed out that heart plasma membranes prepared by the sucrose density gradient were found to exhibit 10–15 times more active Ca^{2+}/Mg^{2+} ecto-ATPase than the sarcolemmal preparations obtained by the hypotonic shock-LiBr treatment method. We have now been able to solubilize the Ca^{2+}/Mg^{2+} ecto-ATPase from the heart plasma membranes without prior treatment with trypsin and have been successful in purifying this enzyme (specific activity 4000 µmol Pi/mg protein/hr) [47,48]. It is possible that there is a family of Ca^{2+}-related ATPases in the cell membrane and that these may have some specific roles in cellular function. It should also be noted that two types of Ca^{2+} channels have now been identified electrophysiologically on the basis of their activation threshold, inactivation kinetics, and response to different interventions in myocardium {49}, and it is likely that Ca^{2+}-dependent ecto-ATPase and Ca^{2+}/Mg^{2+} ecto-ATPase may serve as gating mechanisms for these channels. It is pointed out that the Ca^{2+}/Mg^{2+} ecto-ATPase complex in different cell types, including myocardium, has not only been implicated as a gating mechanism for the entry of divalent cations but has also been suggested to be involved in the regulation of extracellular ATP {50,51}.

Recent research has indicated that Ca^{2+} entry into the cardiac cell not only occurs through Ca^{2+} channels in sarcolemma, but Na^+-Ca^{2+} exchange may also participate in this process {52,53}. It is also known that Ca^{2+} influx through the sarcolemmal membrane is modulated by the sympathetic nervous system via the release of nor-epinephrine and by adrenergic receptors {1,54,55}. The activation of beta-receptors leads to the formation of cyclic AMP through G proteins and adenylyl cyclase, and this then results in cyclic AMP-dependent protein kinase mediated phosphorylation of Ca^{2+} channels and increased Ca^{2+} entry into the cell {1}. On the other hand, alpha-adrenergic receptors have been shown to stimulate phosphatidylinositol turnover in the sarcolemmal membrane due to the activation of phospholipase C, and the resultant activation of protein kinase C mediated phosphorylation of the sarcolemmal membrane may be associated with an increase in Ca^{2+} entry {56,57}. Although calmodulin-mediated phosphorylation has also been demonstrated to enhance Ca^{2+} movements across the sarcolemmal membrane {3}, the exact site of its action is less clear. The entry of Ca^{2+} in myocardium has also been shown to be increased by ATP, and this is associated with increased contractile force development {58,59}. It needs to be pointed out that ATP is released as a cotransmitter with norepinephrine {60}. The positive inotropic effect of ATP has been reported to be independent of the cyclic AMP-dependent mechanisms and is associated with increased inositol-lipid metabolism {61,62}. Furthermore, pharmacological studies {63} and biochemical experiments involving radioligand binding {64} have provided evidence concerning the presence of ATP receptors in the heart sarcolemmal membrane. Accordingly, it is proposed that ATP receptors in the sarcolemmal membrane may also modulate Ca^{2+} entry into the myocardium.

In addition to the sarcolemma, other membrane systems, such as the sarcoplasmic reticulum and mitochondria, are known to regulate the intracellular concentration of Ca^{2+} {1–3,65,66}. It is now well established that the sarcoplasmic reticular network contains Ca^{2+} sequestration, storage, and release systems, and is intimately involved in the delivery of Ca^{2+} to the contractile apparatus upon excitation of the cell. Ca^{2+} release from the sarcoplasmic reticulum is carried out by the activation of Ca^{2+}-release channels (450 kDa protein), which are affected by ryanodine and thus are called *ryanodine receptors* {67–70}. Although the exact mechanisms for the release of Ca^{2+} from the cardiac sarcoplasmic reticulum are not fully defined, the existing evidence support the view of Ca^{2+}-induced Ca^{2+} release for the occurrence of cardiac contraction {71–73}. On the other hand, the cytoplasmic level of ionized Ca^{2+} is lowered by the activation of Ca^{2+}-stimulated ATPase in the sarcoplasmic reticulum. This energy-dependent Ca^{2+} uptake in the sarcoplasmic reticulum is primarily responsible for the relaxation of the myocardium. The Ca^{2+}-pump ATPase is a 100 kDa protein and has been shown to represent 50–90% of the total protein content of the sarcoplasmic reticulum {74}. This high-affinity Ca^{2+}-stimulated ATPase (Ka of about 0.5 μM) requires MgATP as a substrate. It has now been shown that cyclic-AMP-dependent as well as calmodulin-dependent protein kinases phosphorylate phospholamban, a sarcoplasmic reticular-bound protein {75}, and thus increase the Ca^{2+}-stimulated ATPase activity. A different mode of regulation of the sarcoplasmic reticular Ca^{2+}-stimulated ATPase involving protein kinase C-mediated phosphorylation has also been demonstrated {76}.

Ca^{2+} accumulated across the sarcoplasmic reticular membrane is then bound to calsequestrin, a high-capacity and moderate-affinity Ca^{2+}-binding protein {77,78}, and is stored in the lumen of this tubular network. In contrast to sarcoplasmic reticulum, the mitochondria are known to possess a low-affinity (Ka of about 10 μM Ca^{2+}) Ca^{2+}-uptake system {65}. However, it is noteworthy that these organelles have the capacity to accumulate a large quantity of Ca^{2+} and thus can be seen to serve as a cytoplasmic Ca^{2+} buffer system. Mitochondrial Ca^{2+} uptake in normal myocardium is considered to be balanced by electroneutral exchange for H^+ so that a slow dynamic equilibrium of Ca^{2+} is achieved {79}. On the other hand, extramitochondrial Na^+ has been shown to play a role in the release of Ca^{2+} from the mitochondrial stores {80}. Evidence for the existence of both H^+-Ca^{2+} exchange and Na^+-Ca^{2+} exchange in the mitochondrial membrane have been put forward by several investigators {65}; however, their significance in terms of the regulation of cytoplasmic Ca^{2+} under normal conditions is not clear at present. Various subcellular structures concerned with the regulation of intracellular Ca^{2+} in the myocardial cell, including those present in sarcolemma, sarcoplasmic reticulum, and mitochondria, as well as their putative functions, are given in table 31-1.

MEMBRANE DEFECTS AND THE OCCURRENCE OF INTRACELLULAR Ca^{2+} OVERLOAD

Earlier work from different laboratories has identified a wide variety of sarcolemmal defects, including changes in Na,K-ATPase, adenylyl cyclase, phospholipid N-methylation, beta-adrenergic receptors, alpha-adrenergic receptors, and G-protein associated processes in different models of cardiomyopathies, ischemic heart disease, and heart failure {2,3,81–95}. Recent work by some investigators {81,96–112} has demonstrated marked changes in sarcolemmal Ca^{2+}-pump and Na^+-Ca^{2+} exchange activities in ischemic myocardium, catecholamine-induced

Table 31-1. Different membrane structures and their putative functions with respect to Ca^{2+} handling in cardiocytes

Membrane sites	Putative function
A. *Sarcolemmal mechanisms*	
1. Superficial Ca^{2+} stores	Availability of Ca^{2+} for Ca^{2+} influx
2. Voltage-sensitive Ca^{2+} channels	Ca^{2+} influx
3. Na^+-Ca^{2+} exchanger	Ca^{2+} influx and Ca^{2+} efflux
4. Ca^{2+}-pump ATPase	Ca^{2+} efflux
5. Ca^{2+}/Mg^{2+} ecto-ATPase	Gating system for Ca^{2+} influx
6. ATP receptors	Ca^{2+} influx
7. Na,K-ATPase	Regulation of Ca^{2+} influx
8. Alpha-adrenergic receptors	Regulation of Ca^{2+} influx
9. Beta-adrenergic receptors	Regulation of Ca^{2+} influx
B. *Intracellular mechanisms*	
1. Sarcoplasmic reticulum	
a. Ca^{2+} channels	Ca^{2+} release in the cytoplasm
b. Ca^{2+}-pump ATPase	Ca^{2+} uptake in the cytoplasm
c. Calsequestrin	Ca^{2+} storage in the lumen
2. Mitochondria	
a. Low-affinity Ca^{2+}-uptake system	Removal of Ca^{2+} from the cytoplasm
b. Na^+-Ca^{2+} exchanger	Release of Ca^{2+} in the cytoplasm

cardiomyopathy, diabetic cardiomyopathy, aging myocardium, and Ca^{2+} paradox. Since the sarcolemmal Ca^{2+} pump and Na^+-Ca^{2+} exchange activities are believed to determine the Ca^{2+}-efflux activity of the myocardial cell under normal conditions {1–4}, it is becoming evident that these abnormalities participate in the genesis of intracellular Ca^{2+} overload and subsequent cell damage associated with ischemic and cardiomyopathic hearts.

In view of the suspected role of the sarcolemmal Na^+-Ca^{2+} exchange system in the entry of Ca^{2+} into the cardiac cell under certain conditions associated with elevated levels of cytoplasmic Na^+ {50}, the participation of Na^+-Ca^{2+} exchange in altering the influx of Ca^{2+} in diseased hearts cannot be ruled out at present. Depression in the number of sarcolemmal Ca^{2+} channels has also been reported to occur during congestive heart failure in cardiomyopathic hamsters as well as due to myocardial infarction in rats {113,114}. Most of the literature on sarcolemmal defects in heart disease has been reviewed earlier {2,3,66,115}. However, virtually nothing is known about the pathophysiology of sarcolemmal defects leading to abnormal Ca^{2+} handling by the myocardium in different types of diseased hearts. Nonetheless, marked changes in membrane permeability to Ca^{2+} would remove the barrier between the extracellular and intracellular compartments of the cardiocytes and the cell can be seen to be flooded with Ca^{2+}.

The intracellular overload of Ca^{2+} can also occur when the Ca^{2+}-handling abilities of both the sarcoplasmic reticulum and mitochondria are impaired. In such situations, the total Ca^{2+} content may not change but the cytoplasmic concentration of free Ca^{2+} is markedly elevated. Several studies have demonstrated varying degrees of abnormalities in the sarcoplasmic reticular Ca^{2+}-uptake activities in failing hearts {116–120}. Although depressed Ca^{2+} uptake in the sarcoplasmic reticulum is usually associated with a depression in Ca^{2+}-stimulated ATPase activity, decrease in Ca^{2+} uptake without any changes in the Ca^{2+}-stimulated ATPase activity was also observed in certain types of failing hearts {121,122}. Nonetheless, several studies have reported a defect at the level of gene transcription, as mRNA levels for Ca^{2+}-stimulated ATPase were depressed in the failing hearts {123–125}. Defective Ca^{2+}-pump activity of the sarcoplasmic reticulum has been shown to result in intracellular Ca^{2+} overload in different types of failing hearts {126–128}. Likewise, depressed Ca^{2+} uptake by mitochondria in different types of failing hearts, particularly at late stages, has been reported by various investigators {2,3}. Increase in mitochondrial Ca^{2+} release due to elevated levels of intracellular Na^+ as a consequence of the inhibition of sarcolemmal Na,K-ATPase can also be seen to cause intracellular Ca^{2+} overload. It is likely that excessive Ca^{2+} release may occur through the sarcoplasmic reticular Ca^{2+} channels, and this may contribute towards the occurrence of intracellular Ca^{2+} overload in myocardium, but no such abnormality has yet been documented.

From the foregoing discussion it is evident that defects in different membrane systems may cause intracellular Ca^{2+} overload in the cardiocyte, and this may lead to functional abnormalities. However, the pathogenesis of membrane defects needs to be clearly defined in different types of heart diseases. Since the basement membrane is considered to serve as a protective coat for the sarcolemmal membrane, any changes in the basement membrane can be seen to increase the permeability of the cell to Ca^{2+}, and this will favor the occurrence of Ca^{2+} overload. Likewise, alterations in the cholesterol/phospholipid level, which is known to determine membrane fluidity, would result in the occurrence of intracellular Ca^{2+} overload. In fact the oxidation of membrane cholesterol has been shown to be associated with dramatic alterations in

Ca^{2+}-influx and Ca^{2+}-efflux mechanisms {129}. Incorporation of excessive amounts of free fatty acids or accumulation of long-chain acyl derivative and lysophospholipids in the cell would also result in the occurrence of intracellular Ca^{2+} overload {130–133}. An increase in Ca^{2+} influx has also been demonstrated upon deleting ATP stores of the myocardial cells {134}, and this may represent another mechanism for the occurrence of intracellular Ca^{2+} overload.

Reports from various laboratories have indicated that oxygen free radicals are intimately involved in the genesis of myocardial cell damage and subsequent contractile dysfunction under a wide variety of pathological situations {135–140}. Some investigators have demonstrated the generation of oxygen free radicals, by employing electron paramagnetic resonance spectroscopy, upon reperfusion of the ischemic hearts {141–143}, whereas others have shown beneficial effects of some scavengers of the oxygen free radicals on reperfusion injury {144,145}. Since intracellular Ca^{2+} overload is considered to play a crucial role in ischemia-reperfusion injury {2,3,146,147}, it is possible that different mechanisms, which are involved in the regulation of Ca^{2+} movements in the myocardial cell, are altered by oxygen free radicals. In this regard, it is pointed out that Ca^{2+}-channel density has been reported to decrease in ischemic heart disease {148,149} as well as upon treatment of the sarcolemmal membranes with oxygen free radicals {150}. Likewise, the activities of both Na^+-Ca^{2+} exchange and Ca^{2+} pump were depressed following hypoxia/ischemia reperfusion {96,99,100,110,151} as well as exposure of heart membranes to oxygen free radicals {152–155}. Oxygen free radicals have also been shown to affect other sarcolemmal activities such as Na,K-ATPase {155–157}, which is known to affect Ca^{2+} movements in the cell indirectly, and Ca^{2+},Mg^{2+} ecto-ATPase and the superficial store of Ca^{2+} {158}. Thus it appears that increased formation of oxygen free radicals in ischemic hearts upon reperfusion may induce sarcolemmal defects with respect to mechanisms related to Ca^{2+} movements, and this may result in the development of intracellular Ca^{2+} overload, myocardial cell injury, and functional abnormalities. It should be pointed out that oxygen free radical generating systems have been shown to result in heart dysfunction and myocardial cell damage {159–163}. Furthermore, oxygen free radicals have been reported to alter the activities of the sarcoplasmic reticulum {164, 165}. It is thus apparent that oxygen free radicals may be intimately involved in inducing membrane defects and subsequent intracellular Ca^{2+} overload in cardiomyocytes.

INTRACELLULAR Ca^{2+} OVERLOAD AND THE GENESIS OF CELLULAR DYSFUNCTION

It is now clear that low concentrations of Ca^{2+} are required for normal functioning of the heart and the involvement of various systems that regulate the movements of Ca^{2+} in cardiocytes is known in sufficient detail {1–5,65,167–169}. On the other hand, high concentrations of Ca^{2+} in the cell have been shown to exert toxic effects, such as derange-

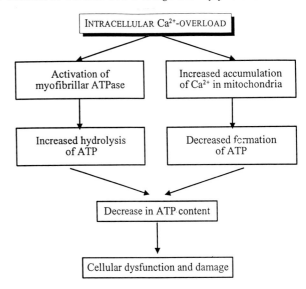

Fig. 31-1. Role of ATP depletion in inducing cardiac cell dysfunction and damage due to the occurrence of intracellular Ca^{2+} overload.

ment of metabolism, electrophysiological abnormalities, disruption of membrane integrity, leakage of intracellular enzymes, ultrastructural changes, cellular damage, and heart dysfunction {170–172}. It is generally believed that intracellular Ca^{2+} overload causes overstimulation of energy utilization processes, such as activation of myofibrillar ATPase, and this then leads to decreased ATP content. Elevated level of cytoplasmic concentration of Ca^{2+} can be seen to cause overloading of mitochondria, and this may result in depression of energy production and decreased ATP content. The cardiocytes with ATP insufficiency are then unable to maintain their structure and function. These events are described schematically in fig. 31-1. Excessive ATP hydrolysis and depressed ATP production are commonly seen to be associated with the occurrence of intracellular Ca^{2+} overload, which is usually reflected as increased tissue Ca^{2+} content. However, it needs to be recognized that the intracellular Ca^{2+} overload may not necessarily be associated with increased tissue Ca^{2+} content, and sufficient Ca^{2+} overloading of mitochondria may not occur for inducing depressed energy production. It should also be pointed out that maximal stimulation of myofibrillar Ca^{2+}-stimulated ATPase is seen at about $10\,\mu M$ Ca^{2+}, and a further increase in the concentration of Ca^{2+} is found to depress the enzyme activity. Thus it is difficult to explain the mechanism of cell damage due to intracellular Ca^{2+} overload on the basis of increased ATP hydrolysis and depressed ATP production. When the cytoplasmic concentration of Ca^{2+} is increased without any changes in the tissue Ca^{2+} content, the activation of phospholipase and proteases by high levels of cytoplasmic Ca^{2+} would result in membrane defects and disruption of proteins, respectively {3}. These changes then can cause contractile dysfunction and myocardial cell damage (fig.

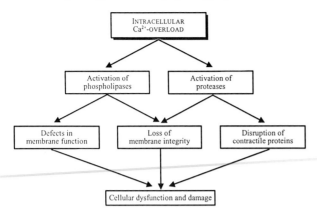

Fig. 31-2. Cellular dysfunction and damage as a consequence of subcellular defects due to intracellular Ca^{2+} overload in myocardium.

31-2). It is again emphasized that intracellular Ca^{2+} overload without any change in the tissue Ca^{2+} content can occur due to some specific defect in Ca^{2+}-handling properties of sarcoplasmic reticulum and/or mitochondria. On the other hand, intracellular Ca^{2+} overload associated with increased tissue Ca^{2+} content usually occurs upon changes in the sarcolemmal membrane with respect to excessive Ca^{2+} entry or insufficient Ca^{2+} removal from the cytoplasm.

OCCURRENCE OF INTRACELLULAR Ca^{2+} OVERLOAD IN Ca^{2+}-PARADOX PHENOMENON

When heart is perfused with Ca^{2+}-free medium, it loses its ability to generate contractile force within seconds. Reperfusion of the heart with medium containing Ca^{2+}, after a brief perfusion with Ca^{2+}-free medium, results in an irreversible loss of active tension generation, contracture, and severe ultrastructural damage {173–175}. This Ca^{2+}-paradox phenomenon has been postulated to be the result of an excessive accumulation of Ca^{2+} in the cell during reperfusion of the Ca^{2+}-depleted heart with Ca^{2+}-containing medium. Various mechanisms have been proposed for the development of an abnormal intracellular Ca^{2+} level due to the Ca^{2+} paradox {176,177}. Although sarcoplasmic reticular and mitochondrial defects with respect to Ca^{2+} accumulation have been reported {178}, these seem to be the effect rather than the cause of Ca^{2+} paradox. On the other hand, changes in sarcolemmal Na^+-Ca^{2+} exchange and Ca^{2+}-pump activities seem to contribute to the occurrence of intracellular Ca^{2+} overload in this condition {112,179,180}.

The participation of the Na^+-Ca^{2+} exchange system in the development of Ca^{2+}-paradoxic change is supported by the fact that an increase in the intracellular concentration of Na^+ is evident upon perfusing the hearts with Ca^{2+}-free medium, which then leads to the development of intracellular Ca^{2+} overload {181,182}. Furthermore,

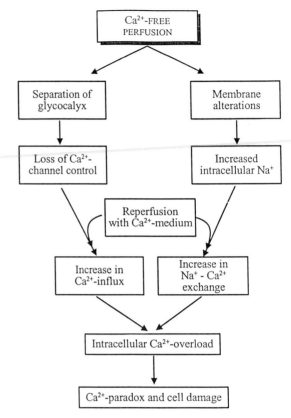

Fig. 31-3. Proposed mechanisms for the occurrence of intracellular Ca^{2+} overload in Ca^{2+} paradox.

lowering the concentration of Na^+ in the Ca^{2+}-free medium was found to prevent the occurrence of the Ca^{2+} paradox {112,174,176}. Changes in the permeability of the sarcolemmal membrane due to the separation of basement membrane as well as entry through voltage-sensitive Ca^{2+} channels have been suggested as routes for the uncontrolled entry of Ca^{2+} during the development of the Ca^{2+} paradox {183–186}. A scheme depicting a chain of events upon perfusing the hearts with Ca^{2+}-free medium, leading to the development of intracellular Ca^{2+} overload and cell damage upon reperfusion with Ca^{2+}-containing medium, is given in fig. 31-3. However, it is emphasized that the mechanisms described here for the occurrence of intracellular Ca^{2+} overload may not represent the complete picture, as other pathways such as those associated with phosphoinositide/phospholipase C activation have been recently implicated in the induction of the Ca^{2+} paradox {187}.

INTRACELLULAR Ca^{2+} OVERLOAD AND CATECHOLAMINE-INDUCED CARDIOMYOPATHY

Low concentrations of circulating catecholamines exert a positive inotropic action on the myocardium and thus are considered beneficial in regulating heart function. On the other hand, high concentrations of these hormones over a prolonged period produce deleterious effects on the cardiovascular system and are known to induce cardiomyopathy {188}. Since catecholamines in high doses have been demonstrated to produce hemodynamic changes, coronary insufficiency, increased myocardial oxygen demand, alterations in lipid and carbohydrate metabolism, and accumulation of free fatty acids and lipid intermediates, it is difficult to determine whether catecholamines do in fact exert a direct toxic influence on the myocardium or whether myocardial cell damage is in some way secondary to other actions of catecholamines {189–194}. In view of the fact that catecholamines by acting on beta-adrenergic receptors have been shown to increase the entry of Ca^{2+} through cyclic AMP-dependent mechanisms, it was proposed that myocardial cell damage due to high levels of circulating catecholamines is mediated through the occurrence of intracellular Ca^{2+} overload {195,196}. This concept was supported by the fact that tissue Ca^{2+} content was increased by high doses of catecholamines. Furthermore, different pharmacological, hormonal, and metabolic interventions, which reduce the occurrence of intracellular Ca^{2+} overload, were found to promote the catecholamine induced cell damage. In contrast to these findings, Bloom and Davis {197} observed that myocardial Ca^{2+} content increased in a manner well correlated to isoproterenol doses in the range from 0.1 to 10 µg/kg but did not further increase with higher doses of catecholamine required to produce myocardial cell damage. Thus it appears that some other derangement, possibly a defect in the regulation of intracellular Ca^{2+} metabolism, is required before the occurrence of cardiac necrosis as a consequence of intracellular Ca^{2+} overload. Indeed, marked alterations in the Ca^{2+}-handling ability of the sarcoplasmic reticulum and sarcolemmal membrane have been observed due to high doses of catecholamines {198,199}. The data in table 31-2 indicate impairment of the sarcolemmal ATP-dependent Ca^{2+} uptake and Na^+-dependent Ca^{2+} uptake as well as sarcoplasmic reticulum ATP-dependent Ca^{2+}

uptake activities. Such derangements can be seen to further contribute to the occurrence of intracellular Ca^{2+} overload.

Since beta-adrenergic receptors in the heart are downregulated upon injecting high doses of catecholamines {200}, it is difficult to reconcile the sole participation of beta-adrenergic mechanisms in the genesis of intracellular Ca^{2+} overload in catecholamine-induced cardiomyopathy. Furthermore, perfusing the hearts with high concentrations of catecholamines did not result in contractile failure or myocardial cell damage as long as the oxidation of catecholamines was prevented, whereas oxidized catecholamines, including adrenochrome, were found to cause cardiotoxic effects {201,202}. Adrenochrome was also shown to produce marked constriction of the coronary arteries as well as arrhythmias {203–205}. In addition to impairing the Ca^{2+}-transport activities of the sarcoplasmic reticulum and mitochondria {206,207}, adrenochrome was reported to depress sarcolemmal Na,K-ATPase activity {208}. The data given in table 31-3 indicate that perfusion of the heart with adrenochrome was found to decrease sarcolemmal ATP-dependent Ca^{2+} uptake and Na^+-dependent Ca^{2+} uptake, as well as sarcoplasmic reticular ATP-dependent Ca^{2+} uptake activities. These results show that adrenochrome is capable of inducing membrane defects with respect to Ca^{2+} handling and thus can be seen to be involved in the genesis of catecholamine-induced cardiomyopathy.

Although marked elevation in the levels of aminochrome (measured as aminoleutin) has been reported upon injecting high doses of catecholamines {209}, it should be noted that oxidation of catecholamines is associated with the generation of free radicals, which are known to be highly toxic. In fact, the involvement of free radicals in the development of catecholamine-induced cardiomyopathy has been proposed on the basis of observations that catecholamine-induced myocardial cell damage was prevented by pretreatment of animals with an antioxidant such as vitamin E {210}. Pretreatment of animals with vitamin E was also found to prevent the catecholamine-induced membrane defects with respect to Ca^{2+}-transport (table

Table 31-2. Effect of vitamin E on the isoproterenol-induced changes in rat heart Ca^{2+}-transport systems

	Control	Isoproterenol	Vitamin E + Isoproterenol
Sarcolemmal ATP-dependent Ca^{2+} uptake (nmol Ca^{2+}/mg/5 min)	25.3 ± 1.4	$14.8 \pm 1.2^*$	23.2 ± 1.7
Sarcolemmal Na^+-dependent Ca^{2+} uptake (nmol Ca^{2+}/mg/5 min)	40.7 ± 2.6	$25.9 \pm 2.3^*$	35.8 ± 2.8
Sarcoplasmic reticular Ca^{2+} uptake (nmol Ca^{2+}/mg/5 min)	203 ± 6.8	$151 \pm 5.7^*$	188 ± 6.5

Each value is the mean ± SE of four experiments. The animals were treated with or without vitamin E (25 mg/kg; i.p., daily) for 3 days before injecting 80 mg/kg (i.p.) isoproterenol. Control animals received saline injection. Animals were sacrificed 24 hours following saline or isoproterenol injection, and ventricular tissue was removed. Both sarcolemmal and sarcoplasmic reticular vesicles were isolated and their calcium transport activities were determined as described before {198,199}.
* Significantly different from the respective control value (p < 0.05).

Table 31-3. Alterations in Ca^{2+}-transport activities in isolated rat hearts upon perfusion with adrenochrome

	Control	Adrenochrome
Sarcolemmal ATP-dependent Ca^{2+} uptake (nmol Ca^{2+}/mg/5 min)	23.6 ± 1.2	$15.2 \pm 1.3^*$
Sarcolemmal Na^+-dependent Ca^{2+} uptake (nmol Ca^{2+}/mg/5 min)	37.8 ± 2.8	$24.7 \pm 2.2^*$
Sarcoplasmic reticular Ca^{2+} uptake (nmol Ca^{2+}/mg/5 min)	195 ± 5.6	$138 \pm 4.7^*$

Each value is the mean ± SE of six experiments. Hearts were perfused with or without 100 μg/ml adrenochrome for 30 minutes, and the ventricular tissue was processed for the isolation of sarcolemmal and sarcoplasmic reticular vesicles {198,199}. The Ca^{2+} transport activities were determined according to procedures indicated in table 31-2.
* Significantly different from the respective control value (p < 0.05).

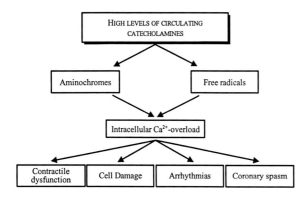

Fig. 31-4. Proposed mechanisms for the occurrence of intracellular Ca^{2+} overload in catecholamine-induced cardiomyopathy.

31-2). In this regard, it is noteworthy that the oxygen free radical generating system has also been reported to depress the sarcolemmal Ca^{2+} pump and Na^+-Ca^{2+} exchange as well as sarcoplasmic reticular Ca^{2+}-pump activities {152,154,164}. Thus it appears that formation of both free radicals and aminochromes during the oxidation of catecholamines may be intimately involved in inducing membrane defects, intracellular Ca^{2+} overload, and subsequent cardiomyopathy. A scheme depicting the events leading to the development of cardiotoxic effects of high levels of circulating catecholamines is shown in fig. 31-4.

INTRACELLULAR Ca^{2+} OVERLOAD AND GENETICALLY LINKED HAMSTER CARDIOMYOPATHY

Various strains of Syrian hamsters have been reported to exhibit cardiomyopathy {211–215}. Myocardial necrosis in these cardiomyopathic hamsters begins to appear at 30–40 days and reaches a maximum at 60–75 days of age. This necrotizing phase is followed by cardiac hypertrophy at 90–120 days of age, and thereafter varying degrees of congestive heart failure are seen in these cardiomyopathic hamsters. On the basis of clinical signs and general characteristics of cardiomyopathic hamsters, these animals at the age of 120–160 days, 160–200 days, and 200–280 days are considered to be at early, moderate, and severe stages of heart failure, respectively. Dramatic alterations with respect to heart function, structure, and metabolism in the cardiomyopathic hamsters are considered to be the consequence of increased sympathetic activity {216,217}, microangiopathy {218,219}, and the occurrence of intracellular Ca^{2+} overload {220,221}. The contention that the occurrence of intracellular Ca^{2+} overload may be of crucial importance in the genesis of cardiomyopathy in these hamsters was substantiated by the observations that verapamil, a Ca^{2+} antagonist, was found to prevent cardiac necrosis, microangiopathy, and metabolic changes {219,222,223}. Determination of myocardial cation con-

Table 31-4. Myocardial Ca^{2+} and Mg^{2+} content in cardiomyopathic hamsters (UM-X7.1) at different stages of congestive heart failure

	Ca^{2+} content (μmol/g wet wt)		Mg^{2+} content (μmol/g wet wt)	
	Control	Failing	Control	Failing
Prefailure	1.8 ± 0.21	$21.2 \pm 1.74^*$	10.5 ± 0.03	11.2 ± 0.65
Early failure	1.7 ± 0.32	$26.5 \pm 2.13^*$	9.6 ± 0.78	10.9 ± 0.86
Moderate failure	1.8 ± 0.27	$29.6 \pm 2.24^*$	9.8 ± 0.74	10.1 ± 0.77
Severe failure	1.9 ± 0.18	$27.8 \pm 1.96^*$	9.5 ± 0.81	9.8 ± 0.69

Each value is the mean ± SE of six experiments. The cardiomyopathic animals at prefailure, early failure, moderate failure, and severe failure stages were 90–120, 120–160, 160–200, and 200–280 days of age, respectively. Healthy hamsters of comparable age were used as controls in each group. Ca^{2+} and Mg^{2+} contents were determined according to the method described elsewhere {176}.
* Significantly different from the respective control value (p < 0.05).

tents by atomic absorption spectrophotometry {176} revealed a dramatic increase in tissue Ca^{2+} without any significant change in Mg^{2+} level in cardiomyopathic hearts (table 31-4).

In order to understand the mechanisms of intracellular Ca^{2+} overload in cardiomyopathy, several investigators have employed different strains of cardiomyopathic hamsters at various stages of disease. In view of the elevated levels of circulating catecholamines in these hamsters {216,217}, increased activity of the sympathetic nervous system results in excessive entry of Ca^{2+} through a wide variety of mechanisms, including those described earlier in this chapter. Enhanced alpha-adrenergic receptor mechanisms in cardiomyopathic heart will also promote the development of intracellular Ca^{2+} overload {224–226}. Furthermore, membrane defects seen in the cardiomyopathic hearts {81,84,97,107,111} can be viewed to

contribute towards the occurrence of intracellular Ca^{2+} overload. Impaired ability of the sarcoplasmic reticulum and mitochondria to accumulate Ca^{2+} {121} would also favor the occurrence of elevated levels of cytoplasmic Ca^{2+}. Marked depression in Ca^{2+} accumulation by sarcoplasmic reticular vesicles from the UM-X7.1 strain of cardiomyopathic hamster hearts, in the absence or presence of oxalate, a permanent anion, was observed (table 31-5). Although an increase in the density of Ca^{2+} channels has been reported by some investigators {113}, others have failed to observe such a change in cardiomyopathic hamsters {227}. The results described in table 31-6 reveal biphasic changes in the Ca^{2+}-channel density without any change in the Ca^{2+}-channel affinity at different stages of cardiomyopathy. The increased density of Ca^{2+} channels would be associated with an excessive entry of Ca^{2+} at early stages of cardiomyopathy, whereas decreased density can be seen to reflect reduced entry of Ca^{2+} at late stages and may contribute to the genesis of contractile failure in this type of heart disease.

The sarcolemmal Na, K-ATPase activity in the UM-X7.1 strain of cardiomyopathic hamster hearts was depressed in comparison to the age-matched control preparations (table 31-7). Such a change in the Na,K-ATPase activity in the cardiomyopathic preparations is not due to differences in the sidedness of the sarcolemmal vesicles, since no difference in the sensitivities of the enzyme to oubain in control and experimental preparations was seen (table 31-7). Furthermore, the sarcolemmal preparations from control and experimental animals showed an equal degree of purification with respect to heart homogenates. The depressed sarcolemmal Na,K-ATPase activity has been observed in these cardiomyopathic hearts at about 25–30 days of age, whereas necrotic lesions were seen at 30–40 days of age in hamsters {81}. Since depressed Na,K-ATPase activity would increase the level of intracellular Na^+ and produce a subsequent increase in Ca^{2+} influx through the Na^+-Ca^{2+} exchange system, it is possible that such a change in the sarcolemmal membrane could account for the occurrence of myocardial necrosis in these

Table 31-5. Sarcoplasmic reticular Ca^{2+}-uptake activities in cardiomyopathic hamsters (UM-X7.1) at different stages of congestive heart failure

| | ATP-dependent Ca^{2+} uptake (nmol Ca^{2+}/mg/5 min) | | | |
| | Absence of oxalate | | Presence of 5 mM oxalate | |
	Control	Failing	Control	Failing
Prefailure	48 ± 4.4	$33 \pm 3.2^*$	439 ± 24	426 ± 18
Early failure	53 ± 3.6	$30 \pm 3.1^*$	460 ± 23	$365 \pm 16^*$
Moderate failure	51 ± 3.9	$24 \pm 2.5^*$	475 ± 31	$301 \pm 25^*$
Severe failure	45 ± 1.9	$21 \pm 1.9^*$	486 ± 21	$268 \pm 17^*$

Each value is the mean $\pm$ SE of six experiments. The ages of cardiomyopathic hamsters at different stages of failure were the same as described in table 31-4. Sarcoplasmic reticular vesicles were isolated and the Ca^{2+}-uptake activity was determined as described before {198}.
* Significantly different from the respective control value (p < 0.05).

Table 31-6. Sarcolemmal Ca^{2+}-channels in cardiomyopathic hamsters (UM-X7.1) at different stages of congestive heart failure

| | ^{3}H-nitrendipine binding | | | |
| | K_d (nM) | | B_{max} (fM/mg) | |
	Control	Failing	Control	Failing
Prefailure	0.52 ± 0.04	0.44 ± 0.03	142 ± 7.8	$204 \pm 11.2^*$
Early failure	0.45 ± 0.04	0.49 ± 0.05	138 ± 9.4	$181 \pm 6.7^*$
Moderate failure	0.51 ± 0.03	0.46 ± 0.04	145 ± 6.8	$123 \pm 4.5^*$
Severe failure	0.48 ± 0.05	0.48 ± 0.04	150 ± 9.9	$107 \pm 8.8^*$

Each value is the mean $\pm$ SE of four experiments. The ages of cardiomyopathic hamsters at different stages of failure were the same as described in table 31-4. The purified sarcolemmal preparation was isolated according to the method described earlier {112} and the Ca^{2+}-channel activities were determined as before {150}.
* Significantly different from the respective control value (p < 0.05).

Table 31-7. Sarcolemmal Na^+-K^+-ATPase activity in cardiomyopathic hamsters (UM-X7.1) at different stages of congestive heart failure

	Na^+-K^+ ATPase (umol/mg/hr)		Ouabain sensitivity (%)	
	Control	Failing	Control	Failing
Prefailure	17.5 ± 1.0	$13.2 \pm 0.7^*$	14 ± 1.7	17 ± 1.9
Early failure	18.0 ± 1.6	$10.4 \pm 1.8^*$	16 ± 2.0	18 ± 2.0
Moderate failure	19.4 ± 0.8	$9.6 \pm 0.5^*$	15 ± 1.4	15 ± 1.6
Severe failure	19.8 ± 0.5	$9.5 \pm 0.4^*$	16 ± 1.8	15 ± 1.3

Each value is the mean $\pm$ SE of three to four experiments. The ages of cardiomyopathic hamsters at different stages of failure were the same as described in table 31-4. Light sarcolemmal preparations were employed. The purity factor, calculated as the ratio of Na,K-ATPase activity in sarcolemma and heart homogenate, varied between 11 and 12 in both control and failing preparations. The methods for the isolation of sarcolemma and determination of Na,K-ATPase activity were the same as described before {110}. The concentration of ouabain used was 1 mM.
* Significantly different from the respective control value (p < 0.05).

animals. Although the exact reason for the low specific activity of the sarcolemmal Na,K-ATPase in cardiomyopathic hearts is not clear, a genetic defect in this regard seems most likely. It should be noted that sarcolemmal Na^+-dependent Ca^{2+} uptake was not depressed until the animals showed clinical signs of congestive heart failure (table 31-8). Similar results were seen with respect to depression in sarcolemmal ATP-dependent Ca^{2+}-ATPase and Ca^{2+}-stimulated ATPase activities in cardiomyopathic hamster hearts (fig. 31-5). These data on sarcolemmal Na^+-Ca^{2+} exchange and Ca^{2+}-pump activities confirm those available in the literature {81,97,107}. Although depression in sarcolemmal Na^+-Ca^{2+} exchange and Ca^{2+}-pump activity will favor the occurrence of intracellular Ca^{2+} overload in failing hearts, these alterations do not appear to contribute to the pathogenesis of cardiomyopathy in these hamsters at early stages. A chain of events leading to the development of intracellular Ca^{2+} overload and myocardial cell damage at early stages of hamster cardiomyopathy is described in fig. 31-6.

INTRACELLULAR Ca^{2+} OVERLOAD AND ISCHEMIA-REPERFUSION INJURY

Since the observation of Shen and Jennings {228} regarding the association of gain in tissue Ca^{2+} with postischemic reperfusion injury to the myocardium, various investigators have confirmed this phenomenon by using different types of preparations {170,229–233}. The role of Ca^{2+} overload in the pathophysiology of contractile dysfunction and myocardial cell damage due to ischemic-reperfusion injury is further evident from the fact that different Ca^{2+}-channel entry blocking agents, such as verapamil and dilitazem, have been shown to exert beneficial effects in this condition {234–240}. Although the exact mechanisms responsible for intracellular Ca^{2+} overload due to ischemia-reperfusion injury are not fully understood, several suggestions have been made by different investigators. In view of the lack of oxygen in the ischemic myocardium, acidification of the cytoplasm and accumulation of free fatty acids and lipid metabolites can be seen to occur. The cytoplasmic acidification will stimulate Na^+-H^+ exchange, which may in turn increase the Na^+-Ca^{2+} exchange process and thus may lead to the development of intracellular Ca^{2+} overload. On the other hand, incorporation of lipids into heart membranes will increase their permeability and result in the occurrence of intracellular Ca^{2+} overload. These events are depicted in fig. 31-7.

Myocardial ischemia is also known to decrease energy production and deplete ATP stores. The insufficiency of available ATP may depress the functions of different cation pumps, such as sarcolemmal Na,K-ATPase and Ca^{2+}-pump ATPase, as well as sarcoplasmic reticular Ca^{2+}-pump ATPase. All these changes may then produce intracellular Ca^{2+} overload in the ischemic myocardium

Table 31-8. Sarcolemmal Na^+-Ca^{2+} exchange activity in cardiomyopathic hamsters (UM-X7.1) at different stages of congestive heart failure

	Nonspecific Ca^{2+} binding (nmol Ca^{2+}/mg/min)		Na^+-dependent Ca^{2+} uptake (nmol Ca^{2+}/mg/min)	
	Control	Failing	Control	Failing
Prefailure	2.5 ± 0.32	3.0 ± 0.41	38.4 ± 2.1	35.9 ± 1.7
Early failure	2.3 ± 0.24	2.7 ± 0.31	37.8 ± 2.5	$24.2 \pm 1.4^*$
Moderate failure	2.5 ± 0.40	2.9 ± 0.27	40.1 ± 1.5	$19.6 \pm 1.3^*$
Severe failure	2.6 ± 0.28	2.7 ± 0.22	38.8 ± 1.9	$13.9 \pm 0.8^*$

Each value is the mean $\pm$ SE of three to four experiments. The ages of cardiomyopathic hamsters at different stages of failure were the same as described in table 31-4. The methods for the isolation of sarcolemmal preparations and determination of nonspecific and specific Na^+-depdendent Ca^{2+}-uptake activities were the same as described earlier {110}. The concentration of Ca^{2+} was $40\,\mu M$.
* Significantly different from the respective control value (p < 0.05).

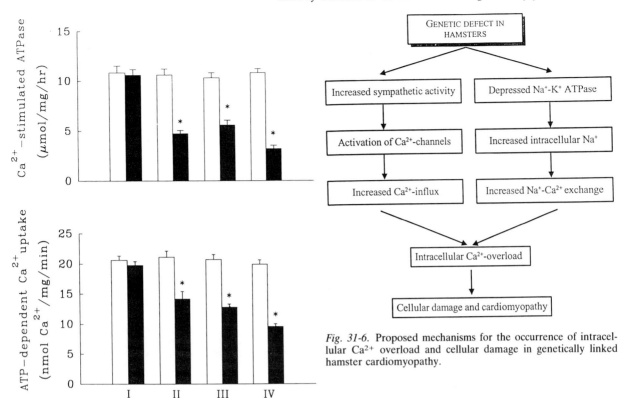

Fig. 31-5. Sarcolemmal Ca^{2+}-stimulated ATPase and ATP-dependent Ca^{2+} uptake in UM-X7.1 strain of cardiomyopathic hamsters at prefailure (I), early failure (II), moderate failure (III), and severe failure (IV) stages. The methods for the isolation of sarcolemma and determination of Ca^{2+}-pump activities were the same as described earlier. Each value is the mean ± SE of four experiments. The concentration of Ca^{2+} was 10 μM. *$p < 0.05$.

Fig. 31-6. Proposed mechanisms for the occurrence of intracellular Ca^{2+} overload and cellular damage in genetically linked hamster cardiomyopathy.

(fig. 31-8). On the other hand, as indicated earlier in this chapter, reperfusion of the ischemic myocardium will release norepinephrine from the nerve ending as well as increase the generation of free radicals. These alterations will result in the occurrence of intracellular Ca^{2+} overload (fig. 31-9). Although there is considerable evidence that a large uptake of extracellular Ca^{2+} in the reperfused heart is mediated by the participation of both alpha- and beta-adrenergic receptor mechanisms {241–243}, the role of intracellular organelles in raising the cytoplasmic level of Ca^{2+} cannot be overlooked {242}. Furthermore, the direct participation of defects in different membranous systems, such as the sarcolemma and sarcoplasmic reticulum, in raising the intracellular concentration of ionized Ca^{2+} due to ischemia-reperfusion injury of the myocardium seems likely. In this regard it is pointed out that depressed Ca^{2+}-uptake activities of the sarcoplasmic reticulum as well as Na^+-Ca^{2+} exchange and Ca^{2+}-pump activities of the sarcolemmal vesicles have been observed (as indicated previously) in different experimental models of ischemia-

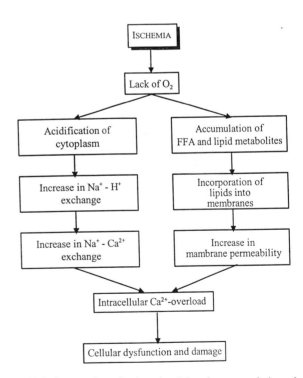

Fig. 31-7. Proposed mechanisms involving the accumulation of H^+, FFA, and lipid metabolites in the ischemic myocardium for the occurrence of intracellular Ca^{2+} overload and cell damage.

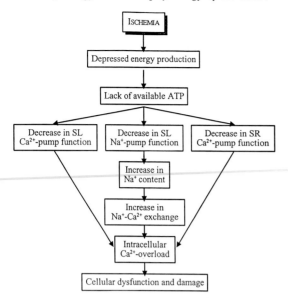

Fig. 31-8. Proposed mechanisms involving depressed function of different cation pumps for the occurrence of intracellular Ca^{2+} overload in the ischemic myocardium.

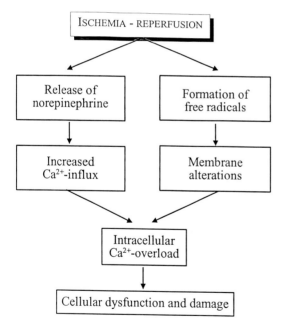

Fig. 31-9. Proposed mechanisms of intracellular Ca^{2+} overload and subsequent cell damage due to ischemia-reperfusion injury in the myocardium.

reperfusion injury. Thus it is essential to improve the Ca^{2+}-handling capabilities of different membrane systems if we have to prevent the occurrence of intracellular Ca^{2+}-overload and subsequent cell damage due to ischemia-reperfusion injury.

CONCLUDING REMARKS

It is now well established that Ca^{2+} flows into the cardiocyte down a sharp electrochemical gradient from an extracellular Ca^{2+} concentration of about 1.25 mM to an intracellular Ca^{2+} concentration in the range of 0.1–10 μM. The rise of intracellular Ca^{2+} in response to excitation is transient in nature and is terminated by closure of the sarcolemmal Ca^{2+} channels as well as sequestration of Ca^{2+} by the sarcoplasmic reticulum and removal of Ca^{2+} from the cytoplasm by Ca^{2+}-efflux mechanisms in the sarcolemmal membrane. Excessive entry of Ca^{2+} due to inappropriate functioning of Ca^{2+} channels, overdrive of adrenergic influences, inhibition of Na,K-ATPase with subsequent stimulation of the Na$^+$-Ca^{2+} exchange system, and/or inability of Ca^{2+}-efflux mechanisms lead to the development of intracellular Ca^{2+} overload as well as increased tissue Ca^{2+} content. Malfunction of the sarcoplasmic reticular Ca^{2+} pump and/or Ca^{2+}-release systems also results in the occurrence of intracellular Ca^{2+} overload, but in this case the tissue Ca^{2+} content may not change. A defect in the mitochondrial membrane or an increased level of cytoplasmic Na$^+$ and subsequent release of Ca^{2+} from mitochondria may also induce intracellular Ca^{2+}, but again this may not be associated with increased tissue Ca^{2+} content. Thus it is emphasized that the term *intracellular Ca^{2+} overload* should refer to the situation in which different membrane systems are unable to maintain the homeostasis of intracellular Ca^{2+} within the physiological range (0.1–0.2 μM) and the resting level of free Ca^{2+} in the cytoplasm remains high for a prolonged period. Previously intracellular Ca^{2+} overload was considered to cause overstimulation of energy utilization systems and to result in ATP depletion and subsequent cardiac dysfunction. However, on the basis of recent information, it appears that intracellular Ca^{2+} overload activates phospholipases and proteases, and these may then result in membrane defects with respect to Ca^{2+} handling and heart dysfunction.

Under a wide variety of pathological situations, mitochondria, by virtue of their ability to accumulate a large quantity of Ca^{2+}, serve as a buffer system for preventing the occurrence of intracellular Ca^{2+} overload; however, by doing so these organelles end up impairing their main function of generating ATP. This then sets up a chain of events that leads to the disruption of various organelles in the cell and results in irreversible injury and cellular death. In view of the role of the sarcoplasmic reticular system to raise and lower the concentration of Ca^{2+} in the cytoplasm for the occurrence of cardiac contraction and relaxation, respectively, any abnormality in this organelle can be seen to result in impaired heart function and arrhythmias as a consequence of the occurrence of intracellular Ca^{2+} overload. Although our efforts have been directed toward understanding the occurrence of intracellular Ca^{2+} overload in terms of increased Ca^{2+} influx at the sarcolemmal membrane, in the past it should be pointed out that impairment of mechanisms involved in the removal of Ca^{2+} from the cytoplasm has also been shown to cause intracellular Ca^{2+} overload. Therefore it is a real challenge not only to improve the site-specific blockade of Ca^{2+} entry but also to find ways and means to promote Ca^{2+} efflux from the myocardial cell faced with intracellular Ca^{2+} overload. Likewise, appropriate Ca^{2+} antagonists have to be discovered that may specifically affect the intracellular sites if we have to improve heart function under pathological conditions associated with the occurrence of intracellular Ca^{2+} overload in the cardiocytes.

Perfusion of heart in the absence of Ca^{2+} and subsequent occurrence of the Ca^{2+} paradox upon reperfusion are fine examples of the role of Ca^{2+} in both heart function and dysfunction. It is now well known that different cardiomyopathies, such as those associated with high levels of circulating catecholamines or in some genetic strains of hamsters, develop as a result of intracellular Ca^{2+} overload. Likewise, the reperfusion injury in ischemic myocardium occurs as a consequence of intracellular Ca^{2+} overload. Catecholamine-induced cardiomyopathy seems to be due to oxidation stress, in which the formation of toxic substances, such as aminochrome and free radicals, plays an important role in the pathogenesis of intracellular Ca^{2+} overload and cardiac dysfunction. Hamster cardiomyopathy seems to be a sequence of membrane defects that is superimposed upon the toxic effects of high levels of circulating catecholamines. Ischemia-reperfusion injury, on the other hand, appears to result from the accumulation of different metabolites as well as the formation of oxygen free radicals and subsequent membrane defects. While the pathophysiology of cardiac dysfunction in cardiomyopathies as well as ischemia-reperfusion injury appears to be different, it is becoming clear that intracellular Ca^{2+} overload in these situations plays a determinant role. Therefore the control of intracellular Ca^{2+} overload by pharmacologic interventions affecting the sarcolemmal sites for Ca^{2+} influx and Ca^{2+} efflux, as well as the intracellular sites in the sarcoplasmic reticulum and mitochondria, is critical for improving the therapy of different types of heart disease.

ACKNOWLEDGMENTS

The research reported in this article was supported by a grant from the Medical Research Council of Canada under MRC Group in Experimental Cardiology.

REFERENCES

1. Dhalla NS, Ziegelhoffer A, Harrow JAC: Regulatory role of membrane systems in heart function. *Can J Physiol Pharmacol* 55:1211–1234, 1977.
2. Dhalla NS, Das PK, Sharma GP: Subcellular basis of cardiac contractile failure. *J Mol Cell Cardiol* 10:363–385, 1978.
3. Dhalla NS, Pierce GN, Panagia V, Singal PK, Beamish RE: Calcium movements in relation to heart function. *Basic Res Cardiol* 77:117–139, 1982.
4. Sulakhe PV, St. Louis PJ: Passive and active calcium fluxes across plasma membranes. *Prog Biophys Mol Biol* 35:135–195, 1980.
5. Langer GA: Calcium at the sarcolemma. *J Mol Cell Cardiol* 16:147–153, 1984.
6. Takeo S, Daly MG, Anand-Srivastava MB, Dhalla NS: Influence of neuraminidase on rat heart sarcolemma. *J Mol Cell Cardiol* 12:211–217, 1980.
7. Matsukubo MP, Singal PK, Dhalla NS: Negatively charged sites and calcium binding in the isolated rat heart sarcolemma. *Basic Res Cardiol* 76:16–28, 1981.
8. Feldman DA, Weinhold PA: Calcium binding to rat heart plasma membranes: Isolation and purification of a lipoprotein component with a high calcium binding capacity. *Biochemistry* 16:3470–3475, 1977.
9. Caroni P, Carafoli E: The Ca^{2+}-pumping ATPase of heart sarcolemma. Characterization, calmodulin dependence and partial purification. *J Biol Chem* 256:3263–3270, 1981.
10. Soldati L, Longoni S, Carafoli E: Solubilization and reconstitution of the Na^+/Ca^{2+} exchanger of cardiac sarcolemma. Properties of the reconstituted system and tentative identification of the protein(s) responsible for the exchange activity. *J Biol Chem* 260:13321–13327, 1985.
11. Harrow JAC, Das PK, Dhalla NS: Influence of some divalent cations on heart sarcolemmal bound enzymes and calcium binding. *Biochem Pharmacol* 27:2605–2609, 1978.
12. Ziegelhoffer A, Anand-Srivastava MB, Khandelwal RL, Dhalla NS: Activation of heart sarcolemmal Ca^{2+}/Mg^{2+} ATPase by cyclic AMP-dependent protein kinase. *Biochem Biophys Res Commun* 84:1073–1081, 1979.
13. Singh JN, Dhalla NS, McNamara DB, Bajusz E, Jasmin G: Membrane alteration in failing hearts of cardiomyopathic hamsters. In: Fleckenstein A, Rona G (eds) *Recent Advances in Studies on Cardiac Structure and Metabolism*, Vol 6. Baltimore, MD: University Park Press, 1975, pp 259–268.
14. Dhalla NS, Jasmin JN, Bajusz E, Jasmin E: Comparison of heart sarcolemmal enzyme activities in normal and cardiomyopathic (UMX7.1) hamsters. *Clin Sci Mol Med* 51:233–242, 1976.
15. Tomlinson CW, Lee SL, Dhalla NS: Abnormalities in heart membranes and myofibrils during bacterial infective cardiomyopathy in the rabbit. *Circ Res* 39:82–92, 1976.
16. Dhalla NS, Ziegelhoffer A, Singal PK, Panagia V, Dhillon KS: Subcellular changes during cardiac hypertrophy and heart failure due to bacterial endocarditis. *Basic Res Cardiol* 75:81–91, 1980.
17. Moffat MP, Dhalla NS: Heart sarcolemmal ATPase and calcium binding activities in rats fed a high cholesterol diet. *Can J Cardiol* 1:194–200, 1985.
18. Dhalla NS, Smith CI, Pierce GN, Elimban V, Makino N, Khatter JC: Heart sarcolemmal cation pumps and binding sites. In: Rupp H (ed) *Regulation of Heart Function*. New York: Thieme, 1986, pp 121–136.
19. Heyliger CE, Dhalla NS: Sarcolemmal Ca^{2+} binding and Ca^{2+}-ATPase activities in hypertrophied heart. *J Appl Cardiol* 1:447–467, 1986.
20. Utsunomiya T, Krausz MM, Dunham B, Shepro D, Hechtman HB: Depression of myocardial ATPase activity by plasma obtained during positive end-expiratory pressure. *Surgery* 91:322–328, 1982.
21. Dhalla NS, Harrow JAC, Anand MB: Actions of some antiarrhythmic agents on heart sarcolemma. *Biochem Pharmacol* 27:1281–1283, 1978.
22. Dhalla NS, Lee SL, Anand MB, Chauhan MS: Effects

of acebutolol, practolol and propranolol on the rat heart sarcolemma. *Biochem Pharmacol* 26:2055–2060, 1977.

23. Khatter JC, Hoeschen RJ, Dhalla NS: Effects of sodium pentobarbital on rat heart sarcolemma. *Res Commun Chem Pathol Pharmacol* 24:57–66, 1979.

24. Lee SL, Alto LE, Dhalla NS: Effects of some volatile anesthetic agents on rat heart sarcolemma. *Life Sci* 24:1441–1446, 1979.

25. Takeo S, Duke P, Taam GML, Singal PK, Dhalla NS: Effects of lanthanum on heart sarcolemmal ATPase and calcium binding activities. *Can J Physiol Pharmacol* 57:496–503, 1979.

26. Sperelakis N, Schneider JA: A metabolic control mechanism for calcium ion influx that may protect the ventricular myocardial cell. *Am J Cardiol* 37:1079–1085, 1976.

27. Antoni H, Engstfeld G, Fleckenstein A: Inotropic effect of ATP and adrenalin on hypodynamic frog myocardium after electro-mechanical decoupling by calcium ion withdrawal. *Pflügers Arch* 272:91–106, 1960.

28. Saks VA, Rosenschtraukh LV, Smirnov VN, Chazov EI: Role of creatine phosphokinase in cellular function and metabolism. *Can J Physiol Pharmacol* 56:691–706, 1978.

29. Schoffeniels E. In: Lahbou B (ed) *Epithelial Transport in Lower Vertebrates.* Cambridge, UK: Cambridge University Press, 1980, pp 125–160.

30. Yatani A, Tsada Y, Akaike N, Brown AM: Nanomolar concentrations of extracellular ATP activate membrane Ca channels in snail neurones. *Nature* 296:169–171, 1982.

31. Malouf NN, Meissner GJ: Cytochemical localization of a "basic" ATPase to canine myocardial surface membrane. *Histochem Cytochem* 28:1286–1294, 1980.

32. Vornanen M: Activation of contractility and sarcolemmal Ca^{2+}-ATPase by Ca^{2+} during postnatal development of the rat heart. *Comp Biochem Physiol* 78A:691–695, 1984.

33. Dhalla NS, Anand-Srivastava MB, Tuana BS, Khandelwal RL: Solubilization of a calcium dependent adenosine triphosphatase from rat heart sarcolemma. *J Mol Cell Cardiol* 13:413–423, 1981.

34. Tuana BS, Dhalla NS: Purification and characterization of a Ca^{2+}-dependent ATPase from rat heart sarcolemma. *J Biol Chem* 257:14440–14445, 1982.

35. Elimban V, Zhao D, Dhalla NS: A comparative study of the rat heart sarcolemmal Ca^{2+}-dependent ATPase and myosin ATPase. *Mol Cell Biochem* 77:143–152, 1987.

36. Anand-Srivastava MB, Dhalla NS: Characteristics of Ca^{2+}/Mg^{2+} ATPase in heart sarcolemma treated with trypsin. In: Dhalla NS, Pierce GN, Beamish RE (eds) *Heart Function and Metabolism.* Boston: Martinus Nijhoff, 1987, pp 191–203.

37. Tuana BS, Dhalla NS: Solubilization of a divalent cation dependent ATPase from dog heart sarcolemma. *Mol Cell Biochem* 77:79–87, 1987.

38. Tuana BS, Dhalla NS: Purification and characterization of a Ca^{2+}/Mg^{2+} ecto-ATPase from rat heart sarcolemma. *Mol Cell Biochem* 81:75–88, 1988.

39. Zhao D, Dhalla NS: Characterization of rat heart plasma membrane Ca^{2+}/Mg^{2+} ATPase. *Arch Biochem Biophys* 263:281–292, 1988.

40. Zhao D, Makino N, Dhalla NS: Specific stimulation of heart sarcolemmal Ca^{2+}/Mg^{2+} ATPase by concanavalin A. *Arch Biochem Biophys* 268:40–48, 1989.

41. Anand-Srivastava MB, Dhalla NS: Alterations in Ca^{2+}/Mg^{2+} ATPase activity upon treatment of heart sarcolemma with phospholipases. *Mol Cell Biochem* 77:89–96, 1987.

42. Panagia V, Elimban V, Ganguly PK, Dhalla NS: Decreased Ca^{2+}-binding and Ca^{2+}-ATPase activities in heart sarcolemma upon phospholipid methylation. *Mol Cell Biochem* 78:65–71, 1987.

43. Elimban V, Zhao D, Dhalla NS: Effect of sulfhydryl group modification on Ca^{2+}-dependent ATPase activity of heart sarcolemma. *J Mol Cell Cardiol* 19(Suppl IV):S.38, 1987.

44. Zhao D, Dhalla NS: Influence of gramicidin S on cardiac membrane Ca^{2+}/Mg^{2+} ATPase activities and contractile force development. *Can J Physiol Pharmacol* 67:546–552, 1989.

45. Dhalla NS, Ziegelhoffer A, Makino N: Biochemical mechanisms of calcium fluxes across sarcolemma upon excitation of myocardium. In: Stone HL, Weglicki WB (eds) *Pathobiology of Cardiovascular Injury.* Boston: Martinus Nijhoff, 1985, pp 222–231.

46. Ziegelhoffer A, Dhalla NS: Activation of Ca^{2+}/Mg^{2+} ATPase in heart sarcolemma upon electrical stimulation. *Mol Cell Biochem* 77:135–141, 1987.

47. Zhao D, Dhalla NS: Purification and composition of Ca^{2+}/Mg^{2+} ATPase from rat heart plasma membrane. *Mol Cell Biochem* 107:135–149, 1991.

48. Zhao D, Elimban V, Dhalla NS: Characterization of the purified rat heart plasma membrane Ca^{2+}/Mg^{2+} ATPase. *Mol Cell Biochem* 107:151–160, 1991.

49. Mitra R, Morad M: Two types of calcium channels in guinea pig ventricular myocytes. *Proc Natl Acad Sci USA* 83:5340–5344, 1986.

50. Dhalla NS, Zhao D: Cell membrane Ca^{2+}/Mg^{2+} ATPase. *Prog Biophys Mol Biol* 52:1–37, 1988.

51. Dhalla NS, Zhao D: Possible role of sarcolemmal Ca^{2+}/Mg^{2+} in heart function. *Magnesium Res* 2:161–172, 1989.

52. Sheu SS, Sharma VK, Uglasity A: $Na^{+}-Ca^{2+}$ exchange contributes to increase of cytocolic Ca^{2+} concentration during depolarization in heart muscle. *Am J Physiol* 250:C651–C656, 1986.

53. Leblanc N, Hume JR: Sodium current-induced release of calcium from cardiac sarcoplasmic reticulum. *Science* 248:372–376, 1990.

54. Reuter H: Calcium movements through cardiac cell membranes. *Med Res Rev* 5:427–440, 1985.

55. Tsien RW: Calcium channels in excitable cell membranes. *Ann Rev Physiol* 45:341–358, 1983.

56. Lindemann JP: Alpha-adrenergic stimulation of sarcolemmal protein phosphorylation and slow responses in intact myocardium. *J Biol Chem* 261:4860–4867, 1986.

57. Berridge MJ: Inositol triphosphate and diacylglycerol: Two interacting second messengers. *Ann Rev Biochem* 56:159–193, 1987.

58. DeYoung MB, Scarpa A: Extracellular ATP induces Ca^{2+} transients in cardiac myocytes which are potentiated by norepinephrine. *FEBS Lett* 223:53–58, 1987.

59. Danziger RS, Raffaeli S, Moreno-Sanchez R, Sakai M, Capagrossi MC, Spurgeon HA, Hanford RG, Lakata EG: Extracellular ATP has a potent effect to enhance cytosolic calcium and contractility in single ventricular myocytes. *Cell Calcium* 9:193–199, 1988.

60. Burnstock G: Purinergic nerves. *Pharmacol Rev* 24:509–581, 1972.

61. Scamps F, Legssyer A, Mayoux E, Vassort G: The mechanism of positive inotropy induced by adenosine triphosphate in rat heart. *Circ Res* 67:1007–1016, 1990.

62. Legssyer A, Poggioli J, Renard D, Vassort G: ATP and other adenine compounds increase mechanical activity and inositol triphosphate production in rat heart. *J. Physiol* 401:185–199, 1988.

63. Williams M: Purine receptors in mammalian tissues: Pharmacology and functional significance. *Ann Rev Pharmacol Toxicol* 27:315–345, 1987.

64. Zhao D, Dhalla NS: [^{35}S]ATPγS binding sites in purified heart sarcolemma membrane. *Am J Physiol* 258:C185–C188, 1990.

65. Carafoli E: Intracellular calcium homeostasis. *Ann Rev Biochem* 56:395–433, 1987.
66. Dhalla NS, Dixon IMC, Beamish RE: Biochemical basis of heart function and contractile failure. *J Appl Cardiol* 6:7–30, 1991.
67. Sutko JL, Thompson LJ, Kort AA, Lakatta EG: Comparison of effects of ryanodine and caffeine on rat ventricular myocardium. *Am J Physiol* 250:H786–H795, 1986.
68. Beuckelmann DJ, Wier WG: Mechanism of release of calcium from sarcoplasmic reticulum of guinea-pig cardiac cells. *J Physiol* 405:233–255, 1988.
69. Hansford RG, Lakatta EG: Ryanodine releases calcium from sarcoplasmic reticulum in calcium-tolerant rat cardiac myocytes. *J Physiol* 390:453–467, 1987.
70. Imagawa T, Smith JS, Coronado R, Campbell KP: Purified ryanodine receptor from skeletal muscle sarcoplasmic reticulum is the Ca^{2+}-permeable pore of the calcium release channel. *J Biol Chem* 262:16636–16643, 1987.
71. Fabiato A: Time and calcium dependence of activation and inactivation of calcium-induced release of calcium from the sarcoplasmic reticulum of a skinned cardiac Purkinje cell. *J Gen Physiol* 85:247–289, 1985.
72. Valdeolmillos M, O'Neill SC, Smith GL, Eisner DA: Calcium-induced calcium release activates contraction in intact cardiac cells. *Pflügers Arch* 413:676–698, 1989.
73. Nabauer M, Morad M: Ca^{2+}-induced Ca^{2+}-release as examined by photolysis of caged Ca^{2+} in single ventricular myocytes. *Am J Physiol* 258:C189–C193, 1990.
74. Inesi G: Mechanisms of calcium transport. *Ann Rev Physiol* 47:573–601, 1985.
75. Inui M, Chamberlain BK, Saito A, Fleischer S: The nature of the modulation of Ca^{2+} transport as studied by reconstitution of cardiac sarcoplasmic reticulum. *J Biol Chem* 261:1794–1800, 1986.
76. Movesian MA, Nishikawa M, Adelstein RS: Phosphorylation of phospholamban by calcium-activated, phospholipid-dependent protein kinase. *J Biol Chem* 259:8029–8032, 1984.
77. Jorgensen AD, Shen AVY, Campbell KP: Ultrastructural localization of calsequestrin in adult rat atrial and ventricular muscle cells. *J Cell Biol* 101:257–268, 1985.
78. Jorgensen AD, Broderick R, Somlyo AP, Somlyo AV: Two structurally distinct calcium storage sites in rat cardiac sarcoplasmic reticulum. An electron microprobe analysis study. *Circ Res* 63:1060–1069, 1988.
79. Vercosi A, Reynaforje B, Lehninger AL: Stoichiometry of H^+ ejection and Ca^{2+} uptake coupled to electron transport in rat heart mitochondria. *J Biol Chem* 253:6379–6385, 1978.
80. Carafoli E, Tiozzo R, Luigi G, Crovetti F, Kratzing C: The release of calcium from heart mitochondria by sodium. *J Mol Cell Cardiol* 6:361–371, 1974.
81. Panagia V, Singh JN, Anand-Srivastava MB, Pierce GN, Jasmin G, Dhalla NS: Sarcolemmal alterations during the development of genetically determined cardiomyopathy. *Cardiovasc Res* 18:567–572, 1984.
82. Ganguly PK, Rice KM, Panagia V, Dhalla NS: Sarcolemmal phosphatidylethanolamine N-methylation in diabetic cardiomyopathy. *Circ Res* 55:504–512, 1984.
83. Daly MJ, Dhalla NS: Alterations in the cardiac adenylate cyclase activity in hypothyroid rat. *Can J Cardiol* 1:288–293, 1985.
84. Okumura K, Panagia V, Jasmin G, Dhalla NS: Sarcolemmal phospholipid N-methylation in genetically determined hamster cardiomyopathy. *Biochem Biophys Res Commun* 143:31–37, 1987.
85. Daly MJ, Dhalla NS: Sarcolemmal Na^+-K^+ ATPase activity in hypothyroid rat heart. *J Appl Cardiol* 2:105–119, 1987.
86. Panagia V, Okumura K, Shah KR, Dhalla NS: Modification of sarcolemmal phosphatidylethanolamine N-methylation during heart hypertrophy. *Am J Physiol* 253:H8–H15, 1987.
87. Okumura K, Panagia V, Beamish RE, Dhalla NS: Biphasic changes in the sarcolemmal phosphatidylethanolamine N-methylation activity in catecholamine-induced cardiomyopathy. *J Mol Cell Cardiol* 19:357–366, 1987.
88. Lefkowitz RJ, Caron MG, Stiles GL: Mechanisms of membrane-receptor regulation. Biochemical, physiological and clinical insights derived from the studies of the adrenergic receptors. *N Engl J Med* 310:1570–1579, 1984.
89. Denniss AR, Colucci WS, Allen PD, Marsh JD: Distribution and function of human ventricular beta adrenergic receptors in congestive heart failure. *J Mol Cell Cardiol* 21:651–660, 1989.
90. Gilson N, Houda NE, Covsin A, Crozatier B: Left ventricular function and beta-adrenoreceptors in rabbit failing heart. *Am J Physiol* 258:H634–H641, 1990.
91. Horn EM, Bilezikian JP: Mechanisms of abnormal transmembrane signalling of the beta-adrenergic receptor in congestive heart failure. *Circulation* 82(Suppl I):26–34, 1990.
92. Bristow MR, Hershberger RE, et al.: Beta-adrenergic pathways in non-failing and failing human ventricular myocardium. *Circulation* 82(Suppl I):12–25, 1990.
93. Newmann J, Schnitz W, Scholz H, Meyerinck L, Dosing V, Kalmar P: Increase in myocardial G_i-proteins in heart failure. *Lancet* II:936–937, 1988.
94. Vago T, Bevliacqua M, Norbiato G, Baldi G, Chebat E, Bertora P, Baroldi G, Accinni R: Identification of alpha 1-adrenergic receptors on sarcolemma from normal subjects and patients with idiopathic dilated cardiomyopathy: Characteristics and linkage to GTP-binding protein. *Circ Res* 64:474–481, 1989.
95. Leier CV, Brinkley PF, Cody RJ: Alpha-adrenergic component of the sympathetic nervous system in congestive heart failure. *Circulation* 82(Suppl I):68–76, 1990.
96. Chemnitius JM, Sasaki Y, Burger W, Bing RJ: The effect of ischemic and reperfusion on sarcolemmal function in perfused canine hearts. *J Mol Cell Cardiol* 17:1139–1140, 1985.
97. Kuo TH, Tsang W, Wiener J: Defective Ca^{2+}-pumping ATPase of heart sarcolemma from cardiomyopathic hamster. *Biochim Biophys Acta* 900:10–16, 1987.
98. Mallov S: Effect of cardiotoxic concentrations of catecholamines on Na^+-Ca^{2+} exchange in cardiac sarcolemmal vesicles. *Exp Mol Pathol* 40:206–213, 1984.
99. Bersohn MM, Philipson KD, Fukushima JY: Sodium-calcium exchange and sarcolemmal enzymes in ischemic rabbit hearts. *Am J Physiol* 242:C288–C295, 1982.
100. Daly M, Elz JS, Nayler WG: Sarcolemmal enzymes and Na^+-Ca^{2+} exchange in hypoxic, ischemic and reperfused rat hearts. *Am J Physiol* 247:H237–H243, 1984.
101. Heyliger CE, Prakash A, McNeill JH: Alterations in cardiac sarcolemmal Ca^{2+} pump activity during diabetes mellitus. *Am J Physiol* 252:H540–H544, 1987.
102. Narayanan N: Differential alterations in ATP-supported calcium transport activities of sarcoplasmic reticulum and sarcolemma of aging myocardium. *Biochim Biophys Acta* 678:442–459, 1981.
103. Narayanan N: Comparison of ATP-dependent calcium transport and calcium activated ATPase activities of cardiac sarcoplasmic reticulum and sarcolemma from rats of various ages. *Mech Aging Dev* 38:127–143, 1987.
104. Dhalla NS, Dzurba A, Pierce GN, Tregaskis MG, Panagia V, Beamish RE: Membrane changes in myocardium during catecholamine-induced pathological hypertrophy. *Persp Cardiovasc Res* 7:527–534, 1983.
105. Makino N, Dhruvarajan R, Elimban V, Beamish RE, Dhalla

NS: Alterations of sarcolemmal Na⁺-Ca²⁺ exchange in catecholamine-induced cardiomyopathy. *Can J Cardiol* 1: 225–232, 1985.

106. Heyliger CE, Takeo S, Dhalla NS: Alterations in sarcolemmal Na⁺-Ca²⁺ exchange and ATP-dependent Ca²⁺-binding in hypertrophied heart. *Can J Cardiol* 1:328–339, 1985.

107. Makino N, Jasmin G, Beamish RE, Dhalla NS: Sarcolemmal Na⁺-Ca²⁺ exchange during the development of genetically determined cardiomyopathy. *Biochem Biophys Res Commun* 133:491–497, 1985.

108. Daly MJ, Dzurba A, Tuana BS, Dhalla NS: Sarcolemmal Ca²⁺-binding and enzyme activities in myocardium from hypothyroid rat. *Can J Cardiol* 2:356–361, 1986.

109. Makino N, Dhalla KS, Elimban V, Dhalla NS: Sarcolemmal Ca²⁺ transport in streptozotocin-induced diabetic cardiomyopathy in rats. *Am J Physiol* 253:E202–E207, 1987.

110. Dixon IMC, Eyolfson DA, Dhalla NS: Sarcolemmal Na⁺-Ca²⁺ exchange activity in hearts subjected to hypoxia reoxygenation. *Am J Physiol* 253:H1026–H1034, 1987.

111. Dhalla NS, Panagia V, Makino N, Beamish RE: Sarcolemmal Na⁺-Ca²⁺-pump activities in cardiomyopathies due to intracellular Ca²⁺-overload. *Mol Cell Biochem* 82: 75–79, 1988.

112. Makino N, Panagia V, Gupta MP, Dhalla NS: Defects in sarcolemmal Ca²⁺ transport in hearts due to induction of calcium paradox. *Circ Res* 63:313–321, 1988.

113. Wagner, JA, Weisman HF, Snowman AM, Reynold IJ, Weisfeldt ML, Snyder SH: Alterations in calcium antagonist receptors and sodium-calcium exchange in cardiomyopathic hamster tissue. *Circ Res* 65:205–214, 1989.

114. Dixon IMC, Lee SL, Dhalla NS: Nitrendipine binding in congestive heart failure due to myocardial infarction. *Circ Res* 66:782–788, 1990.

115. Carafoli E, Bing RJ: Myocardial failure. *J Appl Cardiol* 3:3–18, 1988.

116. Gertz EW, Hess ML, Lain RF, Briggs FN: Activity of vesicular calcium pump in the spontaneously failing heart-lung preparation. *Circ Res* 20:477–484, 1967.

117. Harigaya S, Schwartz A: Rate of calcium binding and uptake in normal animal and failing human cardiac muscle. *Circ Res* 25:781–794, 1971.

118. Sordahl LA, Wood WG, Schwartz A: Production of cardiac hypertrophy and failure in rabbits with ameroid clips. *J Mol Cell Cardiol* 1:341–354, 1970.

119. Ito Y, Suko J, Chidsey CA: Intracellular calcium binding and myocardial contractility. V. Calcium uptake of sarcoplasmic reticulum fractions in hypertrophied and failing hearts. *J Mol Cell Cardiol* 6:237–247, 1974.

120. McCollum WB, Crow C, Harigaya S, Bajusz E, Schwartz A: Calcium binding by cardiac relaxing system isolated from myopathic Syrian hamsters. *J Mol Cell Cardiol* 1:447–457, 1970.

121. Sulakhe PV, Dhalla NS: Excitation-contraction coupling in heart. VIII. Calcium accumulation in subcellular particles in congestive heart failure. *J Clin Invest* 50:1019–1027, 1971.

122. Tomlinson CW, Lee SL, Dhalla NS: Abnormalities in heart membrane and myofibrils during bacterial infective cardiomyopathy in the rabbit. *Circ Res* 39:82–92, 1976.

123. Komuro I, Kurabayashi M, Shibazaki Y, Takaku F, Yazaki Y: Molecular cloning and characterization of a Ca²⁺ or Mg²⁺-dependent adenosine triphosphatase from rat cardiac sarcoplasmic reticulum. *J Clin Invest* 83:1102–1108, 1989.

124. Nagai R, Zarain-Herzberg A, Brandl CJ, Fujii J, Tada M, MacLennan DH, Alpert N, Periasamy M: Regulation of myocardial Ca²⁺-ATPase and phospholamban mRNA expression in response to pressure overload and thyroid hormone. *Proc Natl Acad Sci USA* 86:2966–2970, 1989.

125. Mercadier JJ, Lompre AM, Duc P, Boheler KR, Fraysse JB, Wisnewsky C, Allen PK, Komajda M, Schwartz K: Altered sarcoplasmic reticulum Ca²⁺-ATPase gene expression in the human ventricle during end-stage heart failure. *J Clin Invest* 85:305–309, 1990.

126. Gwathmey JK, Morgan JP: Altered calcium handling in experimental pressure-overload hypertrophy in the ferret. *Circ Res* 57:836–843, 1985.

127. Gwathmey JK, Copelas L, MacKinnon R, Schoen FJ, Feldman MD, Grossman W, Morgan JP: Abnormal intracellular calcium handling in myocardium from patients with end-stage heart failure. *Circ Res* 61:70–76, 1987.

128. Gwathmey JK, Slawsky MT, Hajjon RJ, Briggs GM, Morgan JP: Role of intracellular calcium handling in force-interval relationships of human ventricular myocardium. *J Clin Invest* 85:1599–1613, 1990.

129. Kutryk MJB, Maddaford TG, Ramjiawan B, Pierce GN: Oxidation of membrane cholesterol alters active and passive transsarcolemmal calcium movements. *Circ Res* 68:18–26, 1991.

130. Philipson KD, Ward R: Effects of fatty acids on Na⁺-Ca²⁺ exchange and Ca²⁺ permeability of cardiac sarcolemmal vesicles. *J Biol Chem* 260:9666–9671, 1985.

131. Wu J, Corr PB: Influence of long chain acylcarnitines on voltage-dependent calcium current in adult ventricular myocytes. *Am J Physiol* 253:H410–H417, 1992.

132. Donck LV, Verellen G, Geerts H, Bogers M: Lysophosphatidylcholine-induced Ca²⁺ overload in isolated cardiomyocytes and effect of cytoprotective drugs. *J Mol Cell Cardiol* 24:977–988, 1992.

133. Dhalla NS, Elimban V, Rupp H: Paradoxical role of lipid metabolism in heart function and dysfunction. *Mol Cell Biochem* 116:3–9, 1992.

134. Clague JR, Post JA, Langer GA: Cationic amphiphiles prevent calcium leak induced by ATP depletion in myocardial cells. *Circ Res* 72:214–218, 1993.

135. Freeman BA, Crapo JD: Biology of disease: Free radicals and tissue injury. *Lab Invest* 47:412–426, 1982.

136. Dhalla NS, Pierce GN, Innes IR, Beamish RE: Pathogenesis of cardiac dysfunction in diabetes mellitus. *Can J Cardiol* 1:263–281, 1985.

137. Singal PK (ed): *Oxygen Radicals in the Pathophysiology of Heart Disease*. Boston: Kluwer Academic Publishers, 1988.

138. Godin DV, Wahaieb SA, Garnett ME, Gounmeniouk AD: Antioxidant enzyme alterations in experimental and clinical diabetes. *Mol Cell Biochem* 84:223–231, 1988.

139. Opie LH: Reperfusion injury and its pharmacologic modification. *Circulation* 80:1049–1062, 1989.

140. Hammond B, Hess ML: The oxygen free radical system: Potential mediator of myocardial injury. *J Am Coll Cardiol* 6:215–220, 1985.

141. Flaherty JT, Weisfeldt ML: Reperfusion injury. *Free Radic Biol Med* 5:409–419, 1988.

142. Arroyo CM, Kramer JH, Dickens BF, Weglicki WG: Identification of free radicals in myocardial ischemia/reperfusion by spin trapping with nitrone DMPO. *FEBS Lett* 221: 101–104, 1987.

143. Zweier JL, Flaherty JT, Weisfeldt ML: Direct measurement of free radical generation following reperfusion of ischemic myocardium. *Proc Natl Acad Sci USA* 84:1404–1407, 1987.

144. Jolly SR, Krane WJ, Bailie MB, Abrams GD, Lucchesi BR: Canine myocardial reperfusion injury. Its reduction by the combined administration of superoxide dismutase and catalase. *Circ Res* 54:277–285, 1984.

145. Ambrosio G, Becker LC, Hutchins GM, Weisman HF, Weisfeldt ML: Reduction in experimental infarct size by recombinant human superoxide dismutase: Insights into the

pathophysiology of reperfusion injury. *Circulation* 74: 1424–1433, 1986.

146. Murphy JG, Smith TW, Marsh JD: Mechanism of reoxygenation-induced calcium overload in cultured chick embryo hearts. *Am J Physiol* 254:H1133–H1141, 1988.

147. Nayler WG, Panagiotopoulos S, Elz JS, Daly MJ: Calcium-mediated damage during post-ischemic reperfusion. *J Mol Cell Cardiol* 20(Suppl II):41–54, 1988.

148. Matucci R, Bennardini F, Sciammarella ML, Baccaro C, Stendardi I, Franconi F, Giotti A: [^{3}H]-nitrendipine binding in membranes obtained from hypoxic and reoxygenated heart. *Biochem Pharmacol* 36:1059–1062, 1987.

149. Nayler WG, Dillon JS, Elz JS, McKelvie M: An effect of ischemia on myocardial dihydropyridine binding sites. *Eur J Pharmacol* 115:81–89, 1985.

150. Kaneko M, Lee SL, Wolf CM, Dhalla NS, Reduction of calcium channel antagonist binding sites by oxygen free radicals in rat heart. *J Mol Cell Cardiol* 21:935–943, 1989.

151. Meno H, Jarmakani JM, Philipson KD: Effect of ischemia on sarcolemmal Na^+-Ca^{2+} exchange in neonatal hearts. *Am J Physiol* 256:H1615–H1620, 1989.

152. Kaneko M, Beamish RE, Dhalla NS: Depression of heart sarcolemmal Ca^{2+}-pump activity by oxygen free radicals. *Am J Physiol* 256:H368–H374, 1989.

153. Kaneko M, Elimban V, Dhalla NS: Mechanisms for depression of heart sarcolemmal Ca^{2+} pump by oxygen free radicals. *Am J Physiol* 257:H804–H811, 1989.

154. Hata T, Kaneko M, Beamish RE, Dhalla NS: Influence of oxygen free radicals on heart sarcolemmal Na^+-Ca^{2+} exchange. *Cor Art Dis* 2:397–407, 1991.

155. Xie Z, Wang Y, Askari A, Huang WH, Klaunig JE: Studies on the specificity of the effects of oxygen metabolites on cardiac sodium pump. *J Mol Cell Cardiol* 22:911–920, 1990.

156. Kramer JH, Mak IT, Weglicki WB: Differential sensitivity of canine cardiac sarcolemmal and microsomal enzymes to inhibition by free radical-induced lipid peroxidation. *Circ Res* 55:120–124, 1984.

157. Kim MS, Akera T: O_2 free radicals: Cause of ischemia-reperfusion injury to cardiac Na^+-K^+ ATPase. *Am J Physiol* 252:H252–H257, 1987.

158. Kaneko M, Singal PK, Dhalla NS: Alterations in heart sarcolemmal Ca^{2+}-ATPase and Ca^{2+}-binding activities due to oxygen free radicals. *Basic Res Cardiol* 85:45–54, 1990.

159. Basu DK, Karmazyn M: Injury to rat hearts produced by an exogenous free radical generating system. Study into the role of arachidonic acid and eicosanoids. *J Pharmacol Exp Ther* 242:673–685, 1987.

160. Burton KP, McCord JM, Ghai G: Myocardial alterations due to free radical generation. *Am J Physiol* 246: H776–H783, 1984.

161. Gupta M, Singal PK: Time course of structure, function and metabolic changes due to an exogenous source of oxygen metabolites in rat heart. *Can J Physiol Pharmacol* 67: 1549–1559, 1989.

162. Kaminishi K, Yanagishita T, Kako KJ: Oxidant injury to isolated heart cells. *Can J Cardiol* 5:168–174, 1989.

163. Eley DW, Korecky B, Fliss H: Dithiothreitol restores contractile function to oxidant-injured cardiac muscle. *Am J Physiol* 257:H1321–H1325, 1989.

164. Rowe GT, Manson NH, Caplan M, Hess ML: Hydrogen peroxide and hydroxyl radical mediation of activated leukocyte depression of cardiac sarcoplasmic reticulum. Participation of the cyclooxygenase pathway. *Circ Res* 53:584–591, 1983.

165. Losser KE, Kukreja RC, Kazziha SY, Jesse RL, Hess ML: Oxidative damage to the myocardium: A fundamental mechanism of myocardial injury. *Cardioscience* 2:199–216, 1991.

166. Kukreja RC, Hess ML: The oxygen free radical system. From equations through membrane-protein interactions to cardiovascular injury and protection. *Cardiovasc Res* 26: 641–655, 1992.

167. Balke CW, Gold MR: Calcium channels in the heart: An overview. *Heart Dis Stroke* 1:398–403, 1992.

168. Langer GA: Calcium and the heart: Exchange at the tissue, cell and organelle levels. *FASEB J* 6:893–902, 1992.

169. Carafoli E: The Ca^{2+}-pump of the plasma membrane. *J Biol Chem* 267:2115–2118, 1992.

170. Nayler WG, Daly MJ: Calcium and the injured cardiac myocytes. In: Sperelakis N (ed) *Physiology and Pathophysiology of the Heart*, 2nd ed. Boston: Kluwer Academic Publishers, 1989, pp 527–540.

171. Billman GE, McIlroy B, Johnson JD: Elevated myocardial calcium and its role in sudden cardiac death. *FASEB J* 5:2386–2592, 1991.

172. Bjua LM, Fattor RA, Miller JC, Chien KR, Willerson JT: Effects of calcium loading and impaired energy production on metabolic and ultrastructural features of cell injury in cultured neonatal rat cardiac myocytes. *Lab Invest* 63: 320–331, 1990.

173. Zimmerman ANE, Hulsmann WG: Paradoxical influence of calcium ions on the permeability of cell membranes of the isolated rat heart. *Nature* 211:646–647, 1966.

174. Yates JC, Dhalla NS: Structural and functional changes associated with failure and recovery of hearts after perfusion with Ca^{2+}-free medium. *J Mol Cell Cardiol* 7:91–103, 1975.

175. Ruigrok TJC, Bergerdijk FJA, Zimmerman ANE: The calcium paradox: A reaffirmation. *Eur J Cardiol* 3:59–63, 1972.

176. Alto LE, Dhalla NS: Myocardial cation content during induction of the calcium paradox. *Am J Physiol* 237: H713–H719, 1979.

177. Nayler WG, Perry SE, Elz JS, Daly MJ: Calcium, sodium and the calcium paradox. *Circ Res* 55:227–237, 1984.

178. Alto LE, Dhalla NS: Role of changes in microsomal calcium uptake in the effects of reperfusion of Ca^{2+}-deprived hearts. *Circ Res* 48:17–24, 1981.

179. Dhalla NS, Alto LE, Singal PK: Role of Na^+-Ca^{2+} exchange in the development of cardiac abnormalities due to calcium paradox. *Eur Heart J* 4(Suppl II):51–56, 1983.

180. Goshima K, Wakabayashi S, Masuda A: Ionic mechanisms of morphological changes of cultured myocardial cells on successive incubation with media without and with Ca^{2+}. *J Mol Cell Cardiol* 12:1135–1157, 1980.

181. Ruano-Arroyo G, Gerstenblith G, Lakatta EG: Calcium paradox in the heart is modulated by cell sodium during the calcium-free period. *J Mol Cell Cardiol* 16:783–793, 1984.

182. Turnstall J, Busselen P, Rodrigo GC, Chapman RA: Pathways for the movements of ions during Ca^{2+}-free perfusion and the induction of Ca^{2+}-paradox. *J Mol Cell Cardiol* 18:241–254, 1986.

183. Dhalla NS, Tomlinson CW, Singh JN, Lee SL, McNamara DB, Harrow JAC, Yates JC: In: Roy PE, Dhalla NS (eds) *The Sarcolemma*. Baltimore, MD: University Park Press, 1976, pp 377–394.

184. Post JA, Nievelstein PEEM, Leunissen-Bijvelt J, Verkleij AJ, Ruigrok TJC: Sarcolemmal disruption during the calcium paradox. *J Mol Cell Cardiol* 17:265–273, 1985.

185. Hearse DJ, Baker JE, Humphrey SM: Verapamil and the calcium paradox. *J Mol Cell Cardiol* 12:733–740, 1980.

186. Dhalla NS, Singal PK, Takeo S, McNamara DB: Mechanism of the beneficial effects of some Ca^{2+} antagonists on the

Ca^{2+} paradox in myocardium. In: Sperelakis N, Caulfield J (eds) *Calcium Antagonists and Heart Disease*. Boston: Martinus Nijhoff Publishing, 1984, pp 219–227.

187. Persaud S, Vrbanova A, Meij JTA, Panagia V, Dhalla NS: Possible role of phospholipase C in the induction of Ca^{2+}-paradox in the rat heart. *Mol Cell Biochem* 121:181–190, 1993.

188. Dhalla NS, Yates JC, Naimark B, Dhalla KS, Beamish RE, Ostadal B: Cardiotoxicity of catecholamines and related agents. In: Acosta D Jr (ed) *Cardiovascular Toxicology*, 2nd ed. New York: Raven Press, 1992, pp 239–282.

189. Rona G, Chappel CI, Balazs T, Gaudry R: An infarct like myocardial lesion and other toxic manifestations produced by isoproterenol in the rat. *Arch Pathol* 67:443–455, 1959.

190. Rona G, Boutet M, Huttner I, Peter H: Studies on infarct-like myocardial necrosis produced by isoproterenol: A review. *Rev Can Biol* 22:241–255, 1963.

191. Handforth CP: Isoproterenol-induced myocardial infarction in animals. *Arch Pathol* 73:161–165, 1962.

192. Sobel B, Jequier E, Sjoersdma A, Lovenberg W: Effect of catecholamines and adrenergic blocking agents on oxidative phosphorylation in rat heart mitochondria. *Circ Res* 19:1050–1061, 1966.

193. Rona G: Catecholamine cardiotoxicity. *J Mol Cell Cardiol* 17:291–306, 1985.

194. Ostadal B, Beamish RE, Barwinsky J, Dhalla NS: Ontogenetic development of cardiac sensitivity to catecholamines. *J Appl Cardiol* 4:467–486, 1989.

195. Fleckenstein A: Specific inhibitors and promoters of calcium action in the excitation-contraction coupling of heart muscle and their role in the prevention and production of myocardial lesions. In: Harris P, Opie LH (eds) *Calcium and the Heart*. London: Academic Press, 1971, pp 135–188.

196. Fleckenstein A, Janke J, Doering HJ: Myocardial fiber necrosis due to intracellular Ca^{2+} overload. A new principle in cardiac pathophysiology. In: Dhalla NS (ed) *Recent Advances in Studies on Cardiac Structure and Metabolism*, Vol 4. Baltimore, MD: University Park Press, 1974, pp 563–580.

197. Bloom S, Davis D: Isoproterenol myocytolysis and myocardial calcium. In: Dhalla NS (ed) *Recent Advances in Studies on Cardiac Structure and Metabolism*, Vol 4. Baltimore, MD: University Park Press, 1974, pp 581–590.

198. Panagia V, Pierce GN, Dhalla KS, Ganguly PK, Beamish RE, Dhalla NS: Adaptive changes in subcellular calcium transport during catecholamine-induced cardiomyopathy. *J Mol Cell Cardiol* 17:411–420, 1985.

199. Dhalla NS, Ganguly PK, Panagia V, Beamish RE: Catecholamine-induced cardiomyopathy: Alterations in Ca^{2+} transport systems. In: Kawai C, Abelman WH (eds) *Pathogenesis of Myocarditis and Cardiomyopathy*. Tokyo: University of Tokyo Press, 1987, pp 135–147.

200. Corder D, Heyliger CE, Beamish RE, Dhalla NS: Defect in the adrenergic receptor-adenylate cyclase system during development of catecholamine-induced cardiomyopathy. *Am Heart J* 107:537–542, 1984.

201. Yates JC, Dhalla NS: Induction of necrosis and failure in the isolated perfused rat heart with oxidized isoproterenol. *J Mol Cell Cardiol* 7:807–816, 1975.

202. Yates JC, Beamish RE, Dhalla NS: Ventricular dysfunction and necrosis produced by adrenochrome metabolite of epinephrine: Relation to pathogenesis of catecholamine cardiomyopathy. *Am Heart J* 102:210–221, 1981.

203. Karmazyn M, Beamish RE, Fliegel L, Dhalla NS: Adrenochrome-induced coronary artery constriction in the rat heart. *J Pharmacol Exp Ther* 219:225–230, 1981.

204. Singal PK, Dhillon KS, Beamish RE, Dhalla NS: Myo-

cardial cell damage and cardiovascular changes due to I.V. infusion of adrenochrome in rats. *Br J Exp Pathol* 63:167–176, 1982.

205. Beamish RE, Dhillon KS, Singal PK, Dhalla NS: Protective effect of sulfinpyrazone against catecholamine metabolite adrenochrome-induced arrhythmias. *Am Heart J* 102:149–152, 1981.

206. Takeo S, Taam GML, Beamish RE, Dhalla NS: Effects of adrenochrome on calcium accumulating and adenosine triphosphatase activities of the rat microsomes. *J Pharmacol Exp Ther* 214:688–693, 1980.

207. Takeo S, Taam GML, Beamish RE, Dhalla NS: Effect of adrenochrome on calcium accumulation by heart mitochondria. *Biochem Pharmacol* 30:157–163, 1981.

208. Takeo S, Fliegel L, Beamish RE, Dhalla NS: Effects of adrenochrome on rat heart sarcolemmal ATPase activities. *Biochem Pharmacol* 29:559–564, 1980.

209. Dhalla KS, Ganguly PK, Rupp H, Beamish RE, Dhalla NS: Measurement of adrenolutin as an oxidation product of catecholamines in plasma. *Mol Cell Biochem* 87:85–92, 1989.

210. Singal PK, Kapur N, Dhillon KS, Beamish RE, Dhalla NS: Role of free radicals in catecholamine-induced cardiomyopathy. *Can J Physiol Pharmacol* 60:1390–1397, 1982.

211. Bajusz E, Baker J, Nixon CW, Hamburger F: Spontaneous hereditary myocardial degeneration and congestive heart failure in a strain of Syrian hamsters. *Ann NY Acad Sci* 156:105–129, 1969.

212. Gertz EW: Cardiomyopathic Syrian hamster: A possible model of human disease. *Prog Exp Tumor Res* 16:242–260, 1972.

213. Paterson RA, Layberry RA, Nadkarni BB: Cardiac failure in the hamster. A biochemical and electron microscopic study. *Lab Invest* 26:755–766, 1972.

214. Colgan JA, Lazarus ML, Sachs HG: Post-natal development of the normal and cardiomyopathic Syrian hamster heart. A quantitative electron microscopic study. *J Mol Cell Cardiol* 10:43–54, 1978.

215. Jasmin G, Proschak L: Hereditary polymyopathy and cardiomyopathy in Syrian hamster: I. Progression of heart and skeletal muscle lesions in the UM-X7.1 line. *Muscle Nerve* 5:20–25, 1982.

216. Sole MJ, Lo CM, Laird CW, Sonnenblick EH, Wurtman RJ: Norepinephrine turnover in the heart and spleen of the cardiomyopathic Syrian hamster. *Circ Res* 41:855–862, 1975.

217. Sole MJ, Kamble AB, Hussain MN: A possible change in the rate-limiting step for cardiac norepinephrine synthesis in the cardiomyopathic Syrian hamster. *Circ Res* 41:814–817, 1977.

218. Factor S, Sonnenblick EH: Microvascular spasm as a cause of cardiomyopathies. *Cardiovasc Rev Rep* 4:1177–1182, 1983.

219. Factor SM, Minase T, Cho S, Dominita R, Sonnenblick EH: Microvascular spasm in cardiomyopathic Syrian hamsters: A preventable cause of focal myocardial necrosis. *Circulation* 66:342–345, 1982.

220. Lossnitzer K, Bajusz E: Water and electrolyte alterations during the life course of the BIO 14.6 Syrian Golden hamsters. A disease model of hereditary cardiomyopathy. *J Mol Cell Cardiol* 6:163–177, 1974.

221. Jasmin G, Proschek L: Calcium and myocardial cell injury. An appraisal in the cardiomyopathic hamster. *Can J Physiol Pharmacol* 62:891–898, 1984.

222. Jasmin G, Solymoss B: Prevention of hereditary cardiomyopathy in the hamster by verapamil and other agents. *Proc Soc Exp Biol Med* 149:193–198, 1975.

223. Wikman-Coffelt J, Sievers R, Parmley WW, Jasmin G: Verapamil preserves adenine nucleotide pool in cardiomyopathic Syrian hamsters. *Am J Physiol* 250:H22–H28, 1986.

224. Sen L, Liang BT, Colucci WS, Smith TW: Ehanced α_1-adrenergic responsiveness in cardiomyopathic hamster cardiac myocytes. Relation to the expression of pertussis toxin-sensitive G proteins and α_1-adrenergic receptors. *Circ Res* 67:1182–1192, 1990.

225. Kagiya T, Hori M, Iwakura K, Iwai K, Watanabe Y, Uchida S, Yoshida H, Kitabatake A, Inoue M, Kamada T: Role of increased α_1-adrenergic activity in cardiomyopathic Syrian hamsters. *Am J Physiol* 260:H80–H88, 1991.

226. Kawaguchi H, Shoki M, Sano H, Kuda T, Sawa H, Okamoto H, Sakata Y, Yasuda H: Phospholipid metabolism in cardiomyopathic hasmter heart cells. *Circ Res* 69:1015–1021, 1991.

227. Bazan E, Sole MJ, Schwartz A, Johnson CL: Dihydropyridine receptor binding sites in the cardiomyopathic hamster heart are unchanged from control. *J Mol Cell Cardiol* 23:111–117, 1991.

228. Shen AC, Jennings RB: Myocardial calcium and magnesium in acute ischemic injury. *Am J Pathol* 67:417–440, 1972.

229. Nayler WG: The role of calcium in the ischemic myocardium. *Am J Pathol* 102:126–134, 1981.

230. Peng CF, Kane JJ, Murphy ML, Straub KD: Abnormal mitochondrial oxidative phosphorylation of ischemic myocardium reversed by Ca^{2+}-chelating agents. *J Mol Cell Cardiol* 9:897–908, 1977.

231. Shen AC, Jennings RB: Kinetics of calcium accumulation in acute myocardial ischemic injury. *Am J Pathol* 67:441–452, 1972.

232. Shine KI, Douglas AM, Ricchiuti NV: Calcium, strontium and barium movements during ischemia-reperfusion in rabbit ventricle. Implications for myocardial preservation. *Circ Res* 43:712–720, 1978.

233. Chien KR, Engler R: Calcium and ischemic myocardial injury. In: Langer GA (ed) *Calcium and the Heart.* New York: Raven Press, 1990, pp 333–354.

234. Bush LR, Li VP, Schlafer M, Jolly SR, Lucchesi BR: Protective effects of diltiazem during myocardial ischemia in isolated cat hearts. *J Pharmacol Exp Therap* 218:653–661, 1981.

235. Nayler WG, Ferrari R, Williams A: Protective effect of pretreatment with verapamil, nifedipine and propranolol on mitochondrial function in the ischemic and reperfused myocardium. *Am J Cardiol* 46:242–248, 1980.

236. Bersohn MM, Shine KI: Verapamil protection of ischemic isolated rabbit heart: Dependence on pretreatment. *J Mol Cell Cardiol* 15:659–671, 1983.

237. Watts JA, Maiorano LJ, Mairoramo PC: Comparison of the protective effects of verapamil, diltiazem, nifedipine and buffer containing low Ca^{2+} upon global myocardial ischemic injury. *J Mol Cell Cardiol* 18:255–263, 1986.

238. Ichihara K, Ichihara M, Abiko Y: Effect of verapamil and nifedipine on ischemic myocardial metabolism in dogs. *Drug Res* 29:1539–1544, 1979.

239. Lange R, Ingwall J, Hale SL, Akler KJ, Braunwald E, Kloner RA: Preservation of high energy phosphates by verapamil in reperfused myocardium. *Circulation* 70:734–741, 1984.

240. Reimer KA, Lowe JE, Jennings RB: Effect of the calcium antagonist verapamil on necrosis following temporary coronary artery occlusion in dogs. *Circulation* 55:581–587, 1977.

241. Sharma AD, Saffitz JE, Lee BI, Sobel BE, Corr PB: Alpha adrenergic-mediated accumulation of calcium in reperfused myocardium. *J Clin Invest* 72:802–818, 1983.

242. Mukherjee A, Wong TM, Buja LM, Lefkowitz RL: Beta-adrenergic and muscarinic cholinergic receptors in canine myocardium. Effects of ischemia. *J Clin Invest* 64:1423–1428, 1979.

243. Corr PB, Shayman JA, Kramer JB, Kipnis RJ: Increased alpha-adrenergic receptors in ischemic cat myocardium. A potential mediator of electrophysiological derangements. *J Clin Invest* 67:1232–1236, 1981.

244. Lee JA, Allen DG: Mechanisms of acute ischemic contractile failure of the heart. Role of intracellular calcium. *J Clin Invest* 88:361–367, 1991.

CHAPTER 32

Cell Coupling and Healing-Over in Cardiac Muscle

WALMOR C. DE MELLO

INTRODUCTION

As in many other tissues the internal milieu of cardiac fibers is separated from the extracellular fluid by an insulating surface layer characterized by a high electrical resistance.

When the surface cell membrane is injured an electrical potential difference appears between damaged and non-damaged cells (*injury potential*). In 1877. Engelmann demonstrated that when the cardiac muscle is injured the injury potential soon vanishes (fig. 32-1). An explanation for this interesting phenomenon (healing-over) is that the cells located near damage are depolarized and consequently the flow of injury current is interrupted. This is not the case, however, because the injury potential can be reestablished by damaging the cells located near the previous lesion {1}.

In many types of cells the injury of the surface cell membrane is immediately followed by an extrusion of protoplasm through the damaged area. This healing process, which avoids the loss of intracellular material, is based on the formation of a new membrane at the injured area and has been described in protozoa, marine eggs, and skeletal muscle {2}.

If a skeletal muscle fiber is immersed in a Ca-free Ringer solution and ulteriorly lesioned film formation does not occur and disintegration inevitably follows, the formation of a new membrane at the site of damage is dependent on Ca {2}. The establishment of this membrane has been ascribed to a chemical reaction (surface precipitation reaction) involving a substance, *ovothrombin*, formed from some precursor in the cell in the presence of Ca^{2+} {2}.

Is myocardial healing-over due to the establishment of a new membrane at the site of damage? To answer this question we must enquire if the *surface precipitation reaction* provides a good electrical sealing. It is known that healing-over as described in cardiac muscle does not exist in skeletal muscle where the injury currenrs spread along the muscle fiber, rendering it wholly depolarized {3}. In isolated sarrorius muscle fibers, small lesions produced by punching the cell membrane with a microelectrode depolarize the fiber irreversibly (fig. 32-2) {4}.

Thus, under normal conditions the establishment of a

plug at the area of cell damage is not enough to provide an electrical sealing. Of some interest in this context is that in skeletal muscle fibers immersed in isotonic Ca solution, the depolarization of the muscle fibers elicited by small lesions is completely reversed in a few seconds {4}. Some observations suggest that membrane lipids are involved in this process. Thus, calcium is known to induce coalescence of phospholipid films {5} and phospholipase C impairs the sealing process in high-Ca solution {4}.

As the formation of a new membrane at the damage area does not represent an effective ionic barrier under normal conditions, it seems reasonable to conclude that the healing-over of cardiac muscle is not explained by a surface precipitation reaction. The other plausible alternative is that a high-resistance barrier is established between damaged and nondamaged cells.

In frog ventricular muscle the depolarization caused by lesion is quickly reversed regardless of the size of the preparation. This finding led Rothschuh {3} to postulate the hypothesis that cardiac muscle is composed of small functional units — *mikroelementen* — separated by polarized ionic barriers.

Ulterior studies by Weildmann {6} demonstrated that in cardiac Purkinje fibers the core resistivity is quite low ($105\,\Omega\,cm$) and the space constant high ($1.9\,mm$) compared with the length of a single cell (about $125\,\mu m$). This certainly rules out the possibility that cardiac cells are separated by preestablished ionic barriers.

Evidence is, indeed, available that cardiac cells are electrically coupled {6–9}. When one half of a bundle of ventricular fibers is exposed to radioactive K and the other half is continuously washed with non-radioactive Tyrode, a steady state with respect to tissue ^{42}K is reached in about 6 hours {10}. At the end of this time an appreciable amount of ^{42}K is found in the half of the bundle not exposed to radioactive potassium. The exponential decay of radioactivity along the muscle has a length constant of $1.55\,mm$, which clearly indicates that the longitudinal movement of ^{42}K is not hindered by the intercellular junctions {10}. The quantitative analysis of these results led to the conclusion that the permeability of the intercellular junctions is about 5000 times greater than that of the nonjunctional membrane.

The intercellular channels are also permeable to dif-

N. Sperelakis (ed.), Physiology and Pathophysiology of the Heart, Third Edition.

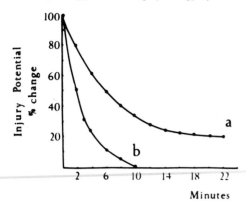

Fig. 32-1. Healing-over of toad ventricular muscle immersed in normal Ringer solution (**b**). Curve (**a**) shows the influence of Ca-free solution on the healing-over process. From De Mello et al. {18}, with permission.

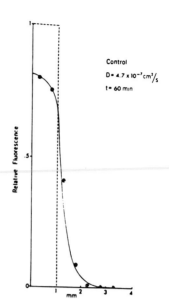

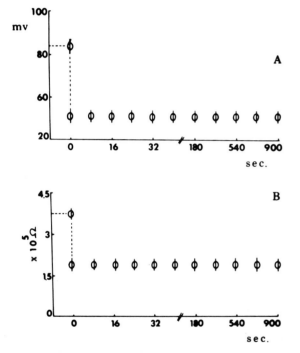

Fig. 32-2. Lack of sealing in frog skeletal muscle fibers immersed in normal Ringer solution. Irreversible drop of resting potential (*A*) and input resistance (**B**) produced by puncture of the cell membrane with a micropipette (about 4 μm in diameter). Each curve is the average from 25 fibers. Vertical dotted line indicates moment of lesion. Vertical line at each point indicates SE of the mean. From De Mello {4}, with permission.

ferent molecules. Cell-to-cell diffusion of Procion Yellow (Mw 697) {11}, tetraethyl-ammonium (Mw 130) {12}, ^{14}cAMP (Mw 328) {13}, and fluorescein (Mw 330) {14,15} has been reported in cardiac tissues.

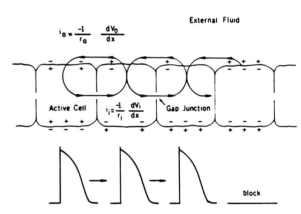

Fig. 32-3. **Top:** Longitudinal distribution of Lucifer Yellow along travecula dissected from right atrium of dog's heart. D = diffusion coefficient; t = diffusion period. From De Mello and van Loon {42}, with permission. **Bottom:** Diagram illustrating the flow of local circuit current in a cardiac fiber and the role of gap junctions in the spread of propagated activity. From De Mello {45}, with permission.

Recently, a new compound, Lucifer Yellow (Mw 473) was introduced by Stewart {16} as a fluorescent probe and proved extremely valuable in studies of cell-to-cell communication. Lucifer Yellow is *sui generis* — it does not diffuse through the nonjunctional membrane, but crosses the gap junctions in several tissues {16,17}. Studies carried out in our laboratory showed that the dye diffuses longitudinally along dog trabeculae after its introduction into the cell with cut-end method {11}. As is shown in fig. 32-3, the dye can be detected by spectrofluorometric methods 4 mm away from the rubber partition $1\frac{1}{2}$ hours after its introduction into the cell.

The question of whether the longitudinal movement of

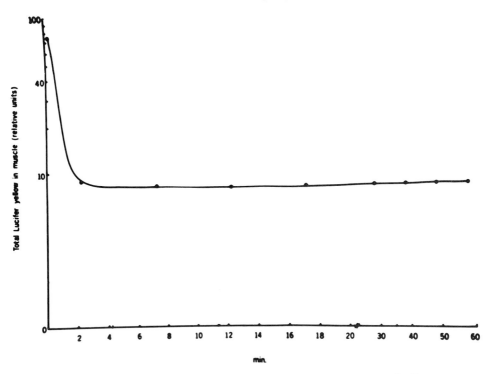

Fig. 32-4. Loss of Lucifer Yellow from a dog trabecula. The washout curve shows a first rapid component t$\frac{1}{2}$, 1^{48} min) and an extremely slow second component (t$\frac{1}{2}$, 2 × 10^3 mim). Temperature, 37°C. From De Mello and Castillo, unpublished.

the dye is due to intracellular diffusion can be answered by performing washout studies. Figure 32-4 shows that the washout curve for Lucifer Yellow consists of a first rapid component $\left(\dfrac{48}{t_{1/2} = 1 - \text{min}} \right)$, which represents the loss of Lucifer Yellow from the extracellular space and a second slow component that correlates to the outward movement of the dye through the surface cell membrane. The second component has an extremely long half life ($t_{1/2}$ = 2 × 10^3 min), supporting the view that the permeability of the surface cell membrane to Lucifer Yellow CH is, indeed, negligible. The meaning of these results is that the dye diffuses longitudinally along cardiac fibers through the intercellular channels.

Since cardiac cells are connected through low-resistance channels it might be reasonable to think that following damage the junctional conductance can be markedly reduced suppressing the flow of injury currents from damaged to nondamaged cells {18}. On the other hand, it is known that Ca ions are essential for the healing-over porcess {18–20}. These findings led to the hypothesis that the junctional conductance in heart might be modulated by variations in free {Ca^{2+}}$_i$ {20}. In order to check this idea, I injected Ca iontophoretically inside a cardiac cell and searched for possible changes in cell-to-cell coupling. The results show that the electrical coupling of the heart cells is gradually reduced and cell decoupling is finally achieved in about 600 seconds {9,20} (fig. 32-5). Concur-

rently with fall in intercellular communication the input resistance (V$_o$/I$_o$) of the injected cell increases appreciably (fig. 32-5). Both effects of Ca are completely reversible. Rose and Loewenstein {21}, using aequorine, demonstrated that the injection of Ca ions into salivary gland cells of *Chironomus* produces a quick decline of the electrical coupling when the light emission is seen to spread all the way to the intercellular junctions.

These findings are indicative that healing-over can be ascribed to a marked increase in electrical resistance of the intercellular junctions located between normal and damaged cells and due to a rise in free Ca.

The mechanism by which Ca ions change the junctional conductance is not known. Two hypotheses seem worth consideration: (a) Ca ions bind to negative polar groups of gap junction phospholipids and abolish the permeability of the hydrophilic channels. Phospholipids and proteins are normal constituents of gap junctions {22}. (b) Ca activates enzyme reactions that lead to closure of the intercellular channels through a conformational change in gap junction proteins. As the intracellular injection of La^{3+} causes a quick suppression of cell-to-cell coupling {23}, it seems reasonable to think that the binding of the cation to negative sites at the gap junctions might, indeed, alter the channel permeability.

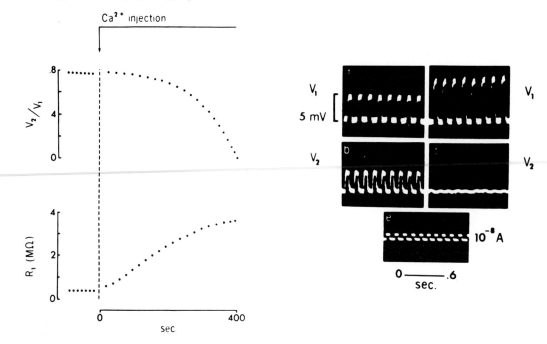

Fig. 32-5. Effect of intracellular Ca injection on the electrical coupling of cardiac Purkinje cells. **Left:** Typical effect of Ca injection on coupling coefficient (V_2/V_1) and input resistance (R_1) (average from six experiments). **Right:** (a) and (b) show V_1 and V_2 controls; (c) and (d) recorded after 410 seconds of Ca injection showing cell decoupling. From De Mello, unpublished.

INFLUENCE OF NA-CA EXCHANGE ON CELL-TO-CELL COUPLING

In cardiac muscle, like in nerve fibers, the extrusion of Ca ions is dependent upon the energy provided by the Na concentration gradient across the nonjunctional membrane {24,25}. The Na-K pump produces a sodium electrochemical gradient across the nonjunctional membrane that is used to energize the Ca extrusion from the cell. The Na-Ca exchange can be reversed if the intracellular Na concentration is increased with consequent increase in Ca influx {26}.

As a rise in $\{Na^+\}_i$ reverses the Na-Ca exchange the obvious question is, can the injection of Na ions into the cell impair the cell-to-cell coupling? The answer is yes. When Na is injected iontophoretically into a cardiac cell, the intracellular longitudinal resistance is increased and cell decoupling is produced {27,28} (fig. 32-6). The suppression of the electrical coupling elicited by high $\{Na^+\}_i$ is dependent on the extracellular Ca concentration. So when $\{Ca^{2+}\}_o$ is low, the effect of Na injection on cell-to-cell communication is negligible {28}, supporting the view that the abolishment of the electrical coupling is accomplished by the activation of the Na-Ca exchange and ulterior rise in free $\{Ca^{2+}\}_i$.

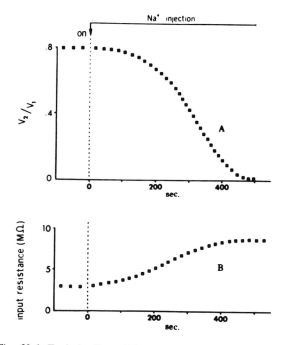

Fig. 32-6. Typical effect of intracellular Na injection on the electrical coupling (V_2/V_1) (**A**) and input resistance (**B**) of a canine Purkinje fiber. Modified from De Mello {28}, with permission.

COST OF CELL-TO-CELL COMMUNICATION

Since the enhancement of $\{Na^+\}_i$ impairs or even abolishes the electrical coupling of cardiac cells, it seems logical that the inhibition of the Na-K pump can also change intercellular communication. Indeed, when cardiac fibers are exposed to certain concentrations of ouabain, the intracellular longitudinal resistance increases appreciably and finally cell decoupling is produced {28,29}. The effect of the glycoside on cell-to-cell coupling is greatly due to the increase in free $\{Ca^{2+}\}_i$. So, in fibers exposed to ouabain, the time required for cell decoupling was dependent upon the extracellular Ca concentration {29}.

In cardiac Purkinje cells partially depolarized by recent dissection, the activation of the Na-K pump with norepinephrine increases the resting potential and the electrical coupling of the heart cells {30}.

The conclusion drawn from these observations is that the Na extrusion exerts a remarkable influence on the transference of electrical and chemical signals between cells. The changes in junctional permeability brought about by alterations of $\{Na^+\}_i$ are due to the rise or fall in free $\{Ca^{2+}\}_i$, which are related to the rate of Na-Ca exchange.

Rapidity of sodium transport across the nonjunctional membrane is also essential for the maintenance of conduction velocity.

It is known that the conduction velocity (θ) is proportional to: $\theta \propto 1/\sqrt{a r_i}$, where a is the fiber diameter and r_i the intracellular longitudinal resistance. Contrary to previous ideas, the intracellular longitudinal resistance is now considered a variable parameter that depends, among other things, on the free $\{Ca^{2+}\}_i$ {9,31}. Therefore, an increase in r_i reduces the conduction velocity in cardiac fibers.

The maintenance of a high junctional permeability, however, is not free. The cell must spend energy on the extrusion of Na ions and in keeping the free $\{Ca^{2+}\}_i$ low. ATP is supplied from metabolism solely by oxidative phosphorylation in mitochondria and by glycolisis. Metabolic inhibition decreases the rates of active ion transport by reducing the rate of ATP production. 2–4 dinitrophenol, for instance, an uncoupler of oxidative phosphorylation, increases the intracellular longitudinal resistance in cardiac fibers and abolishes the electrical coupling and the cell-to-cell diffusion of fluorescein {15}. These effects of dinitrophenol are related to the elevation of free $\{Ca^{2+}\}_i$ {15}. Indeed, when EDTA is injected into the heart cells exposed to dinitrophenol, the electrical coupling is partly recovered. Although the evidence available from these studies is that the modulation of junctional permeability is a smooth process, it is not clear whether the number of active channels varies with the changes in free $\{Ca^{2+}\}_i$ or whether all the channels are simultaneously involved.

IS THE JUNCTIONAL PERMEABILITY INFLUENCED BY INTRACELLULAR PH?

In 1977, Turin and Warner {32} demonstrated that the exposure of embryonic cells of *Xenopus* to 100% CO_2 not only reduces the pH_i but also depolarizes the cells and abolishes the cell-to-cell coupling.

More recently it has been shown that the intracellular injection of H^+ ions into cardiac cells increases the intracellular longitudinal resistance and causes cell decoupling {33,34}. In sheep Purkinje fibers exposed to 100% CO_2, a similar increase in r_i has been reported {35}.

The question remains as to whether the effect of low pH_i on the electrical coupling is due to a rise in free $\{Ca^{2+}\}_i$. In *Chironomus* salivary gland cells {36} or in barnacle muscle {37}, the changes in pH_i caused by high P_{CO_2} are seen concurrently with an increase in free $\{Ca^{2+}\}_i$. The exposure of sheep Purkinje fibers to high P_{CO_2} reduces pH_i but the free $\{Ca^{2+}\}_i$ also falls {38}. Myocardial healing-over, a phenomenon related to a drastic increase in junctional resistance {20}, can be accomplished in the absence of Ca if the pH_o is reduced to 5 {39}.

The evidence reviewed above suggests that H ions have a direct effect on junctional resistance in cardiac fibers. In embryonic cells of Fundulus, acidification of the cytosol causes cell decoupling — an effect due to a direct interaction of protons with gap-junction molecules {40}.

As the buffer capacity of heart cells is quite high {41}, it is not clear whether pH_i plays a role in the control of junctional resistance under physiologic conditions. During myocardial ischemia, however, when the pH_i and pH_o are reduced, it is easy to visualize that H ions contribute to the healing-over process, avoiding the spread of injury currents and the flow of metabolites between injured and normal cells {31}.

CYCLIC AMP AND JUNCTIONAL PERMEABILITY: THE PHOSPHORYLATION HYPOTHESIS

Evidence is available that cAMP increases junctional permeability {42} and conductance in isolated heart cell pairs {43}. Using the cut-end method, heart fibers were loaded with Lucifer Yellow CH, and its longitudinal diffusion along the fibers was followed under control conditions and after administration of isoproterenol (10^{-5} M). The results indicated that the diffusion coefficient (D) was increased from $4.7 \times 10^{-7} cm^2/s$ in controls to $2.4 \times 10^{-6} cm^2/s$. Similar results were obtained with dibutyryl cAMP (5×10^{-4} M) {42}. The nexus permeability (P-nexus) was estimated to be $3 \times 10^{-4} cm/s$ in the controls and $9.1 \times 10^{-4} cm/s$ in muscles treated with dibutyryl-cAMP {42}.

More recently, cell pairs isolated from the ventricle of adult rats have been used to measure the influence of isoproterenol on junctional conductance {43}. Gigaohm sealing was obtained in both cells, the cell membrane was broken, and a whole-cell voltage clamp was achieved for each cell. By holding the membrane potential of both cells at -40 mV followed by applying a clamp pulse large enough to depolarize one of the cells to 0 mV, but maintaining the membrane potential of the other cell constant, the junctional current can be measured. Knowing the transjunctional voltage (V1) and the junctional current (I2), the junctional conductance can be determined (fig. 32-7). As shown in fig. 32-8, the administration of a

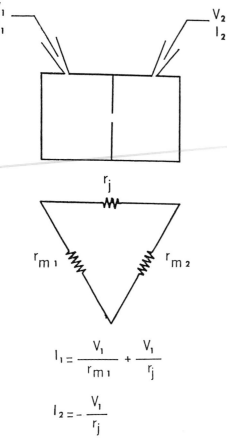

$$I_1 = \dfrac{V_1}{r_{m_1}} + \dfrac{V_1}{r_j}$$

$$I_2 = -\dfrac{V_1}{r_j}$$

Fig. 32-7. **Top:** Diagram of the experimental arrangement showing each cell of the pair connected to a voltage-clamp circuit through a pipette. The whole-cell clamp made it possible to apply to voltage steps (V_1 and V_2) to each cell and record the current (I_1, I_2). **Center and bottom:** The equivalent electrical circuit used for data analysis is shown. rm_1 and rm_2 are the nonjunctional membrane resistances of cells 1 and 2, and rj represents the junctional membrane resistance. From De Mello {44}, with permission.

phosphodiesterase inhibitor (methylxanthine) (10^{-6} M) increased gj within 20 seconds {44}.

The mechanism by which cAMP increases junctional conductance has been investigated in isolated heart cell pairs, and the hypothesis has been proposed that cAMP activates a cAMP-dependent protein kinase, with consequent phosphorylation of gap junction proteins, and hence an increase in gj {43–45}. To test this hypothesis the cAMP-dependent protein kinase inhibitor (PKI) was dialyzed in both cells of a pair, and its influence on the effect of methylxanthine on gj was tested. Figure 32-8 shows that the action of methylxanthine on gj was totally suppressed by PKI. It is interesting to note that PKI alone reduced gj by 18%, indicating that the basal levels of cAMP inside the cells contribute to the modulation of junctional conductance (phosphorylation tonus) {44}. The

conclusion of these studies is that cAMP is a fast modulator of gj in heart muscle and activation of a cAMP-dependent protein kinase is an essential step in the effect of cAMP on gj.

The effect of protein kinase C on gj seems to be different from cAMP-dependent protein kinase because inhibitors of PKC, such as staurosporine, increase gj {46}.

Recently it was found that the renin-angiotensin system plays an important role in control of cell communication in the heart. Indeed, angiotensin II reduces and enalapril — an angiotensin converting enzyme inhibitor — increases gj in isolated heart cell pairs {47} (fig. 32-9). The effect of angiotensin II on gj is dependent on protein kinase C activation, and the peptide reduces gj through activation of specific receptors {47}.

These findings suggest that the antiarrhythmic effect of enalapril, as well its effect in congestive heart failure, are related to the increase in electrical synchronization. Indeed, the heart contractions depend not only on activation of contractile proteins, but also on synchronized depolarization of thousands of heart cells. Cell decoupling elicited by hypoxia, ischemia, or other pathological processes might contribute to heart failure.

PHYSIOLOGIC AND PATHOLOGIC IMPLICATIONS OF CELL-TO-CELL COMMUNICATION

The organization of cardiac muscle is based on isolated functional units connected through low-resistance intercellular channels. This morphologic arrangement enables the electrical impulse to travel without delay throughout the cardiac fibers, allowing the heart cells to beat synchronously. Contrary to skeletal muscle in which the intracellular longitudinal resistance is provided by the myoplasm only, in heart the junctional resistance represents an important regulatory factor of the spread of the electrical impulse. When the junctional conductance is increased, as for example when the concentration of cyclic AMP is enhanced, the spread of electrical activity is greatly augmented. On the other hand, when the free $\{Ca^{2+}\}_i$ is elevated or the intracellular pH is reduced, the conductance of the intercellular channels declines, impairing the impulse conduction. Consequently, slow conduction is produced, which facilitates the generation of cardiac arrhythmias. The finding that the junctional resistance is highly dependent on metabolic energy, which is necessary to pump Na out of the cell and maintain a low free $\{Ca^{2+}\}_i$, indicates that parameters such as conduction velocity are also dependent upon cell metabolism and ATP synthesis. Changes in cardiac rhythm elicited by digitalis toxicity or myocardial ischemia are in part due to the rise in free $\{Ca^{2+}\}_i$ or the fall in pH_i. In both situations the electrical coupling is greatly impaired or abolished, in part due to membrane depolarization, but also because the intracellular resistance is markedly enhanced {3}.

In the atrioventricular node the size and number of gap junctions is smaller than in the atrium or ventricle {48,49} and the intracellular longitudinal resistance is normally

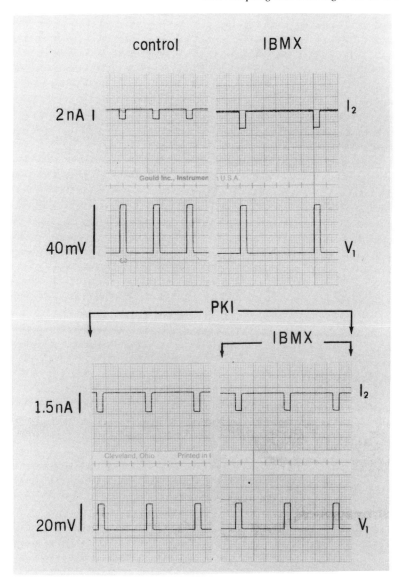

Fig. 32-8. **Top:** Increase in gj caused by isobutylmethylxanthine (IBMX; 10^{-6} M) in a single cell pair immersed in normal Krebs solution. The holding potential in both cells was -40 mV. Cell 1 was pulsed to 0 mV, and the membrane potential of cell 2 was kept unchanged. **Bottom:** Suppression of the effect of IBMX (10^{-6} M) on gj caused by previous intracellular dialysis of protein kinase inhibitor (20 μg/ml) for 2 minutes **(left)**. IBMX was added to the bath **(right)**. I_2 = junctional current; V_1 = transjunctional voltage; pulse duration 100 ms for all experiments. From De Mello {44}, with permission.

high {50}. This explains, in part, the delay of impulse conduction typical of this cardiac area. Here, more than in atrial or ventricular muscle, the impulse conduction is extremely vulnerable to further enhancement of intracellular resistance. The so-called fatigue phenomenon of the atrioventricular node is known to be frequency dependent. A reasonable explanation for this phenomenon is the increase in intracellular resistance produced by stimulation at high rate and probably related to the increment in free $\{Ca^{2+}\}_i$. As the number of hydrophilic channels connecting the node cells is small and the generation of action

potentials is dependent upon a slow current carried by Ca and Na {51}, it is expected that in the atrioventricular node the impulse propagation is highly dependent on frequency of stimulation.

Evidence has been provided, indeed, that in myocardial fibers the intracellular longitudinal resistance is increased by stimulation at high rate {52}.

Thanks to the compartmentalized structure of cardiac muscle "death of a cell does not necessarily mean the death of adjacent cells." The lesion of the surface cell membrane enhances the free $\{Ca^{2+}\}_i$, markedly suppres-

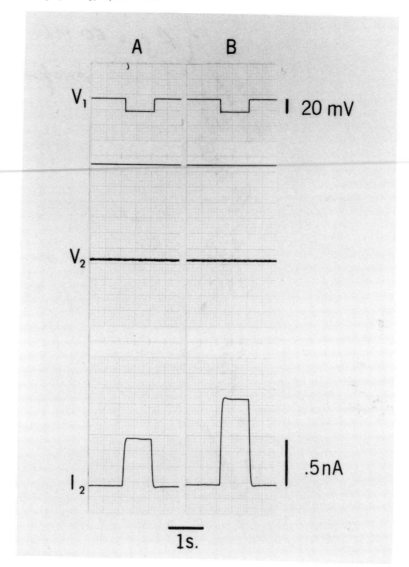

Fig. 32-9. Effect of enalapril (1 µg/ml) on junctional conductance of a single cell pair. **A:** Control; **B:** Increase in junctional conductance elicited by enalapril and recorded 4 minutes after its addition to the bath. V_1 = transjunctional voltage; I_2 = junctional current. Pulse duration is 1 second. From De Mello and Altieri {47}, with permission.

sing cell communication and the flow of injury current that would depolarize large masses of normal cardiac cells. The healing-over process represents, indeed, an important mechanism of preservation of heart function during injury.

UNCOUPLING LEADS TO DECREASED. STRENGTH OF HEARTBEAT

The strength of heart contraction is dependent not only on activation of contractile proteins, but also on electrical synchronization, which enables large populations of cells to contract simultaneously. Electrical uncoupling produced by anoxia, ischemia, or even by drugs can lead to lack of mechanical synchronization and a decline in the strength of muscle contraction.

The possibility that cardiac failure can be produced by impairment of electrical synchronization has not been emphasized in clinical cardiology and is a subject for further investigation.

REFERENCES

1. Engelmann TW: Vergleichende untersuchungen zur lehre von der muskel- und nervenelektricität. *Pflügers Arch* 15:116–148, 1877.
2. Heilbrunn LV: Dynamics of living protoplasm. Heilbrunn LV (ed) New York: Academic Press, 1956.
3. Rothschuh KE: Ueber den funktionellen aufbau des herzens aus elektrophysiologischen elementen und ueber den mechanisms der erregungsleitung in herzen. *Pflügers Arch* 253:238–251, 1951.
4. De Mello WC: Membrane sealing in frog skeletal muscle fibres. *Proc Natl Acad Sci USA* 70:982–984, 1973.
5. Blioch ZL, Glagoleva JM, Lieberman EA, Nenashev VA: A study of the mechanism of quantal transmitter release at a chemical synapse. *J Physiol (Lond)* 199:11–35, 1968.
6. Weidmann S: The electrical constants of Purkinje fibres. *J Physiol (Lond)* 118:348–360, 1952.
7. Woodbury JW, Crill WE: On the problem of impulse conduction in the atrium. In: Florey E (ed) *Nervous Inhibition.* Oxford: Pergamon, 1961, pp 124–125.
8. Barr L, Dewey MM, Berger W: Propagation of action potentials and the nexus in cardiac muscle. *J Gen Physiol* 48:797–823, 1965.
9. De Mello WC: Effect of intracellular injection of calcium and strontium on cell communication in heart. *J Physiol* 250:231–245, 1975.
10. Weidmann S: The diffusion of radiopotassium across intercalated discs of mammalian cardiac muscle. *J Physiol (Lond)* 187:323–342, 1966.
11. Imanaga I: Cell-to-cell diffusion of Procion Yellow in sheep and calf Purkinje fibres. *J Membr Biol* 16:381–388, 1974.
12. Weingart R: The permeability to tetraethylammonium ions of the surface membrane and the intercalated disks of the sheep and calf myocardium. *J Physiol (Lond)* 240:741–762, 1974.
13. Tsien R, Weingart R: Inotropic effect of cyclic AMP in calf ventricular muscle studied by a cut end method. *J Physiol* 260:117–141, 1976.
14. Pollack GH: Intercellular coupling in the atrioventricular node and other tissues of the heart. *J Physiol* 255:275–298, 1976.
15. De Mello WC: Effect of 2–4 dinitrophenol on intercellular communication in mammalian cardiac fibres. *Pflügers Arch* 380:267–276, 1979.
16. Stewart WC: Functional connections between cells as revealed by dye-coupling with a high fluorescent naphthalimide tracer. *Cell* 14:741–759, 1978.
17. Bennett MVL, Spira ME, Spray DC: Permeability of gap junctions between embryonic cells of *Fundulus*: A reevaluation. *Dev Biol* 65:114–125, 1978.
18. De Mello WC, Motta G, Chapeau M: A study on the healing-over of myocardial cells of toads. *Circ Res* 24:475–487, 1969.
19. Délèze J: Calcium ions and the healing-over of heart fibres. In: Taccardi B, Marchetti G (eds) *Electrophysiology of the heart.* London: Pergamon, 1965, pp 147–148.
20. De Mello WC: The healing-over process in cardiac and other muscle fibers. In: De Mello WC (ed) *Electrical Phenomena in the Heart.* New York: Academic Press, 1972, pp 323–351.
21. Rose B, Loewenstein WR: Calcium ion distribution in cytoplasm visualized by aequorin: Diffusion in cytosol restricted by energized sequestering. *Science* 190:1204–1206, 1975.
22. Griepp EB, Revel JP: Gap junctions in development. In: De Mello WC (ed) *Intercellular Communication.* New York: Plenum Press, 1977, pp 1–32.
23. De Mello WC: Effect of intracellular injection of La^{3+} and Mn^{2+} on electrical coupling of heart cells. *Cell Biol Int Rep* 3:113–119, 1979.
24. Reuter H, Seitz N: The dependence of calcium efflux from cardiac muscle on temperature and external ion composition. *J Physiol* 195:451–470, 1968.
25. Baker PF, Blaustein MP, Hodgkin AL, Steinhardt RA: The influence of calcium on sodium efflux in squid axons. *J Physiol* 200:431–458, 1969.
26. Blaustein MP, Hodgkin AL: The effect of cyanide on the efflux of calcium from squid axons. *J Physiol* 200:497–527, 1969.
27. De Mello WC: Electrical uncoupling in heart fibres produced by intracellular injection of Na or Ca. *Fed Proc* 17:3, 1974.
28. De Mello WC: Influence of the sodium pump on intracellular communication in heart fibres: Effect of intracellular injection of sodium ion on electrical coupling. *J Physiol* 263:171–197, 1976.
29. Weingart R: The action of ouabain on intercellular coupling and conduction velocity in mamalian ventricular muscle. *J Physiol* 264:341–365, 1977.
30. De Mello WC: Factors involved on the control of junctional conductance in heart. *Proc Int Union Physiol Sci* 12:319, 1977.
31. De Mello WC: Intercellular communication in cardiac muscle. *Cir Res* 50:2–35, 1982.
32. Turin L, Warner AE: Carbon dioxide reversibly abolishes ionic communication between cells of early amphybian embryon. *Nature (Lond)* 270:56–57, 1977.
33. De Mello WC: On the decoupling action of ouabain in cardiac fibers. *Fed Proc* 22:4, 1979.
34. De Mello WC: Influence of intracellular injection of H$^+$ on the electrical coupling in cardiac Purkinje fibres. *Cell Biol Int Rep* 4:51–57, 1980.
35. Weingart R, Reber W: Influence of internal pH on r_i of Purkinje fibres from mammalian heart. *Experientia* 35:929, 1979.
36. Rose B, Rick R: Intracellular pH, intracellular free Ca, and junctional cell-cell coupling. *J Membr Biol* 44:377–415, 1978.
37. Lea TJ, Ashley CC: Increase in free Ca^{2+} in muscle after exposure to CO$_2$. *Nature (Lond)* 275:236–238, 1978.
38. Hess P, Weingart W: Intracellular free calcium modified by pH$_i$ in sheep Purkinje fibres. *J Physiol* 307:60, 1980.
39. De Mello WC: The influence of pH on the healing-over of mammalian cardiac muscle. *J Physiol* 339:299–307, 1983.
40. Spray DC, Harris AL, Bennett MVL: Gap junctional conductance is a simple and sensitive function of intracellular pH. *Science* 211:712–715, 1981.
41. Ellis D, Thomas RC: Direct measurements of the intracellular pH of mammalian cardiac muscle. *J Physiol* 262:755–771, 1976.
42. De Mello WC, van Loon P: Further studies on the influence of cyclic nucleotides on junctional permeability in heart. *J Mol Cell Cardiol* 19:763–771, 1989.
43. De Mello WC: Increase in junctional conductance caused by isoproterenol in heart cell pairs is suppressed by cAMP-dependent protein kinase inhibitor cAMP-dependent protein kinase inhibitor. *Biochem Biophys Res Commun* 154:509–514, 1988.
44. De Mello WC: Effect of isoproterenol and 3-isobutyl-1-methylxanthine on junctional conductance in heart cell pairs. *Biochim Biophys Acta* 1012:291–298, 1989.
45. De Mello WC: The role of cAMP and Ca on the modulation of junctional conductance: An intergrated hypothesis. *Cell Biol Int Rep* 7:1033–1040, 1983.
46. De Mello WC: Effect of vasopressin and protein kinase C inhibitors on junctional conductance in isolated heart cell

pairs. *Cell Biol Int Rep* 15:467–477, 1991.

47. De Mello WC, Altieri P: The role of the renin-angiotensin system in the control of cell communication in the heart; effects of angiotensin II and enalapril. *J Cardiovasc Pharmacol* 20:643–651, 1992.

48. James TN, Scherf L: Ultrastructure of the atrioventricular node. *Circulation* 37:1049–1070, 1968.

49. Masson-Pevet M: The fine structure of cardiac pace-maker cells in the sinus node and in tissue culture. Thesis.

Amsterdam: Rodopi.

50. De Mello WC: Passive electrical properties of the atrioventricular node. *Pflügers Arch* 371:135–139, 1977.

51. Mendez C, Moe GK: Atrioventricular transmission. In: De Mello WC (ed) *Electrical Phenomena in the Heart*. New York: Academic Press, 1972, pp 263–291.

52. Bredikis J, Bukauskas F, Veteikis R: Decreased intercellular coupling after prolonged rapid stimulation in rabbit atrial muscle. *Circ Res* 49:815–820, 1981.

CHAPTER 33

Interactions of Natural Toxins with Ion Channels in Heart

KENNETH M. BLUMENTHAL

INTRODUCTION

Naturally occurring toxins have for many years been essential ingredients in the arsenal of pharmacologists, physiologists, and biochemists interested in identifying the macromolecules involved in transmembrane ion fluxes and in characterizing their mechanisms of action at the molecular level. These toxins have proven to be especially valuable reagents because of a remarkable degree of specificity for their molecular targets. The purpose of this chapter is to briefly describe certain of these toxins, their target molecules, and their physiologic effects. I shall attempt to focus on similarities and differences in the chemical nature of these toxins and also to describe in detail our present knowledge of their binding site interactions. As most of the toxins to be discussed have as their site of action the voltage-sensitive sodium channel, a description of structure-function relationships in this macromolecular complex will also be provided in order to place the information into its proper context; the structural similarities between this channel and those for Ca^{2+} and K^+ should be borne in mind during this discussion.

With respect to the toxins themselves, their chemical diversity is astonishing, including alkaloids of diverse structures, guanidinium heterocycles, and a wide array of homologous and nonhomologous polypeptides isolated from both marine invertebrates and terrestrial arthropods. As we shall see, these toxins are targeted at a variety of channel functions, including blockade of transmembrane ion fluxes, alterations in the membrane potential dependence of channel activation and inactivation, and reduction in its ionic selectivity. Clearly, the information available from the use of such agents extends well beyond their obvious utility as probes for channel purification.

MOLECULAR CHARACTERIZATION OF VOLTAGE-DEPENDENT SODIUM CHANNELS

The sodium channel is responsible for the depolarization phase of the cardiac action potential. Although the neuronal and cardiac channels differ in a number of functionally significant properties, certain unifying themes are readily evident. Because our knowledge of structure-

function relationships in the neuronal sodium channel is more highly developed than for the cardiac version, the former will be discussed first, and then contrasted with information presently available on the cardiac channel.

The initial purification and characterization of mammalian voltage-sensitive sodium channels from rat brain was described by Catterall and coworkers in a series of papers culminating in 1984 {1–3}. With the availability of the purified channel, the essentiality for both ion fluxes and toxin binding of a 260,000 molecular weight subunit (designated α) was demonstrated. As we shall see, these α subunits from nerve, heart, and skeletal muscle have homologous amino acid sequences and all are well described by the same model for transmembrane organization of the protein (fig. 33-1).

The rat brain sodium channel, isolated as a macromolecular complex of molecular weight approximately 330 kDa, contains three subunits, designated α (260 kDa), β_1 (35 kDa), and β_2 (33 kDa), in 1:1:1 stoichiometry. Based on toxin binding, photoaffinity labeling, reconstitution of functional properties from purified components {4,5}, and expression of its microinjected mRNA in *Xenopus* oocytes {6}, the α subunit alone is capable of recapitulating most of the properties of the intact complex. Nonetheless, because the inactivation kinetics of channels containing only the α subunit are abnormal {6}, and because this abnormality can be overcome by coexpression of low molecular weight brain mRNAs in the same oocytes {7}, a role for at least one of the β subunits in neuronal channel function is indicated. Very recently, cDNA clones for the β_1 subunit have been sequenced and coexpressed with α in oocytes {8}. These studies indicate that β_1 is important in defining the magnitude of the peak sodium current, in addition to its ability to accelerate channel inactivation and to hyperpolarize its potential dependence. It should be noted, however, that these studies involve the neuronal channel, and that in non-neuronal tissues, such as rat skeletal muscle and chick cardiac sarcolemma, the existence of β subunits is less well established than in brain {9,10}.

The α subunit of the voltage-sensitive sodium channel from *E. electricus* was initially cloned and sequenced by Noda and coworkers {11}, using oligonucleotide probes designed by reverse translation of the amino acid sequences of peptides isolated from the purified channel. Later,

N. Sperelakis (ed.), Physiology and Pathophysiology of the Heart, Third Edition.

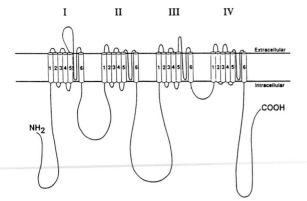

Fig. 33-1. Proposed structure of the voltage-sensitive sodium channel. The channel consists of four homologous domains (I–IV), each consisting of six transmembrane segments (S1–S6). Cytoplasmic loop III–IV has been implicated in both activation and inactivation of the channel, while residues lying between S5 and S6 are involved in both ionic selectivity and binding of specific channel blockers such as TTX. From McClatchey et al. {19}, with permission.

Table 33-1. Toxins acting on the Na^+ channel

Toxin class	Representative	Effect
Guanidinium heterocycles	Tetrodotoxin	Channel blocker
Alkaloid toxins	Batrachotoxin	Persistent activation
α-Scorpion toxins; anemone toxins	*Leiurus* toxin; *Anthopleura* toxin	Delay inactivation
β-Scorpion toxins	*Centruroides* toxin	Alter potential dependence of activation
Pyrethroids	RU 15525	Prolong action potential
Goniopora toxin	GPT	Delay inactivation
Brevetoxins		Shift potential dependence of activation to more hyperpolarized values
Ciguatoxin		Persistent activation

cDNAs encoding three isoforms of the rat brain channel were isolated, using the homologous eel clones as probes, and sequenced. The deduced amino acid sequence of the voltage-dependent sodium channel is organized into four homologous repeat domains, presumably derived via gene duplication and fusion. Application of various predictive algorithms {12,13} to this sequence has been interpreted in the context of a model containing six transmembrane α helices per domain, one of which (S4) is likely to be involved in voltage sensing, based on its content and distribution of cationic side chains. The sequences of voltage-sensitive potassium and calcium channels are also well fit by this model, the major features of which have thus far withstood the test of time. The most significant refinement incorporated into the model is the inclusion of two nonhelical, partially transmembrane sequences, designated SS1 and SS2, postulated to lie between the putative S5 and S6 helices {14}. Analyses of this region by site-directed mutagenesis of both sodium and potassium channels strongly suggests that this region provides the inner lining of the pore itself and is intimately involved in binding of a variety of toxins. A model depicting the transmembrane organization of the sodium channel is shown in fig. 33-1.

Structure-function relationships in the sodium channel have been probed by both site-directed mutagenesis and site-specific antibodies. That voltage-sensitive sodium and potassium channels are structurally homologous has been of great value in these studies, allowing results obtained in one system to be extrapolated to the other. Such studies have established the involvement of residues within the cytoplasmic linker joining domains III and IV in channel inactivation {15–17}, and of transmembrane helix S4 {15–17} in activation {17,18}. It is interesting that the genetic disease Paramyotonia congenita, which appears

to involve gating aberrancies, also maps to the domain III–IV linker {19}. Very recent data arising from analysis of the homologous *shaker* potassium channels suggest that the four domains of the sodium channel interact via their N-terminal sequences {20}. In a subsequent section, I shall discuss the use of mutagenesis to identify specific elements of the toxin binding sites.

In an elegant series of experiments carried out mainly in Catterall's laboratory {21–23}, the presence of a minimum of four independent classes of toxin binding sites on the rat brain sodium channel was first established. These sites include those for alkaloid activators of the channel, exemplified by batrachotoxin and veratridine; guanidinium inhibitors, such as tetrodotoxin (TTX) and saxitoxin (STX); polypeptide toxins (α toxins) from scorpion and sea anemone venoms, which delay channel inactivation; and a distinct set of scorpion β toxins, which alter the voltage dependence of channel activation. More recently, Angelides and coworkers, using fluorescently labeled derivatives of these toxins, have demonstrated that these sites, while independent, appear to be conformationally coupled to one another (24). The known classes of sodium channel-specific toxins are summarized in table 1; each of these sites will be discussed in turn below.

GUANIDINIUM HETEROCYCLES: TETRODOTOXIN AND SAXITOXIN

Tetrodotoxin (TTX) is perhaps the best known of this group of toxins. The presence of a paralytic toxin in pufferfish, newts, and other organisms has been well known since prior to 1950, and the structure of this compound (fig. 33-2) was independently described by four groups in 1964 (cited in Mosher {25}). At about the same time, Narahashi and coworkers showed the high toxicity of TTX was due to its ability to block the transient increase in sodium conductance associated with the rising phase of the

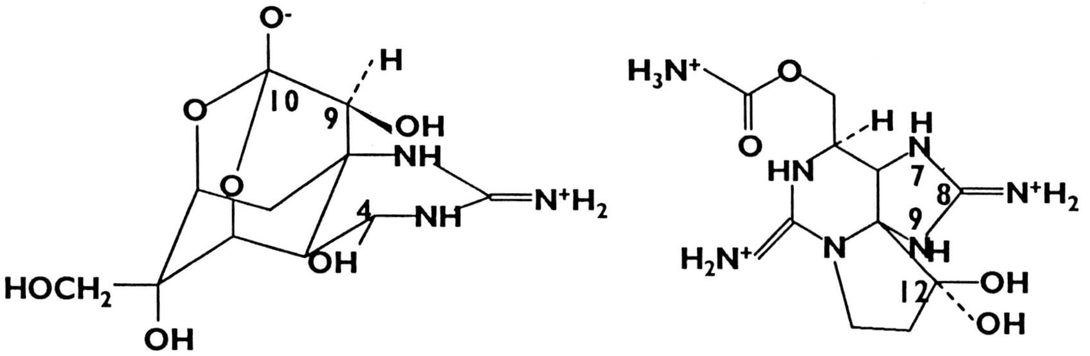

Fig. 33-2. The structures of tetrodotoxin (**left**) and saxitoxin (**right**). For TTX the guanidinium group and the C4, 9, and 10 hydroxyls are important for activity, while in saxitoxin the C12 hydroxyl and the 7,8,9 guanidinium group are essential.

action potential in frog muscle {26}. In parallel with these studies, Schantz and collaborators succeeded in purifying a related compound, saxitoxin, from dinoflagellates {27} and establishing its structure {28} (fig. 33-2), while Kao and Nishiyama demonstrated that saxitoxin (STX) and TTX had essentially the same mechanism of action {29}. Because both these toxins bind to neuronal channels reversibly and with high affinity (1–5 nM), and because this property is essentially unaltered upon detergent solubilization of the channel, the purification and characterization of these toxins were essential for the subsequent biochemical purification of the channel protein. It is safe to say that without the availability of TTX and STX, the explosive growth in our knowledge of sodium channels that has occurred over the past 10 years would have been impossible.

TTX and STX are heterocyclic guanidinium compounds that interact with a site accessible from the external face of neuronal and muscle sodium channels, and the K_ds measured biochemically with the tritiated toxins are in excellent agreement with estimates of affinity obtained by titration of functional effects. This correlation between binding and blockade of the sodium current was originally thought to involve interaction of both STX and TTX with the ionized form of a channel carboxylate associated with the selectivity filter of the channel {30}. Although more recent analyses have corroborated the importance of channel carboxylates in TTX binding, the idea that these groups were also involved in ionic selectivity was abandoned when it was shown that chemical modification of the carboxylate(s) important for TTX binding with trimethyloxonium salts or via carbodiimide-mediated nucleophilic attack was without effect on selectivity {31,32}. Classical structure-activity studies of TTX and STX have established that the guanidinium group of TTX, and the corresponding 7,8,9 guanidinium of STX, are essential for activity, while the C4, C9, and C10 hydroxyl groups of TTX and the C12 hydroxyl of STX are also required {33}. Current models for the action of these toxins propose that the guanidinium groups interact with channel carboxylates (but see below), while the hydroxyl functions form hydrogen bonds with as yet unidentified channel acceptor

sites. Consistent with this model, conversion of Glu-387 of the rat brain channel (Glu-376 in heart numbering) to Gln by site-directed mutagenesis increases the K_d for both TTX and STX by at least 1000-fold {34}, suggesting that Glu-387 is one of the sites with which the guanidinium toxins interact; Glu-387 is located within the SS1-SS2 region described above.

A cDNA encoding the α subunit of the "tetrodotoxin-insensitive" sodium channel of human heart has also been cloned and sequenced, providing the deduced amino acid sequence of the channel protein {35}. It should be noted that *TTX insensitivity* is a relative term: Sodium fluxes in cardiac cells remain TTX sensitive, albeit with a much higher TTX concentration dependence. In its overall features, this sequence is very similar to isoforms characterized in brain and skeletal muscle; indeed, the nucleotide sequence of the muscle channel was used to design probes for isolation of the cardiac clone. The cDNA encodes a protein containing 2016 amino acid residues (calculated molecular weight = 227,159), and predictive algorithms indicate that the essential features of the model discussed above are retained in the cardiac channel. Interestingly, sequence conservation is highest within the repeat domains and in the interdomain region (III–IV) previously identified as being somehow involved in channel inactivation. Microinjection of in vitro transcribed mRNA from this clone into *Xenopus* oocytes results in expression of voltage-dependent channels with a slope conductance of 22 pS that are blocked by TTX with an IC$_{50}$ of 6 μM; as noted below, these channels are therefore referred to as being TTX insensitive. The gating kinetics of these channels are similar to those measured in mammalian heart by patch clamp.

Cardiac sodium channels are much less sensitive to TTX and STX than their neuronal and skeletal muscle counterparts. Electrophysiologic analysis of the rate of rise of the action potential indicates that concentrations of TTX in excess of 1 μM are required for inhibition {36}. Although a number of other studies have reported the existence in cardiac homogenates of TTX/STX sites displaying affinities in the nanomolar range {37}, convincing evidence exists that these higher affinity sites are associated with autonomic nerve endings present in the extracts rather than with the endogenous cardiac channel {38}. Direct analysis of TTX binding to cultured rat heart cells is consistent with a dissociation constant in the micromolar range {39}; however, the magnitude of this K_d is highly temperature dependent.

As mentioned previously, the advent of site-directed mutagenesis has greatly facilitated analysis of the molecular nature of the TTX binding site. In addition to identifying Glu-387 of the type II rat brain channel as being important for TTX binding, this technique has also been used to probe for the structural difference underlying the relative insensitivity of the cardiac channel to TTX blockade. Although comparison of the sequences of the cardiac and neuronal channels reveals a large number of differences, most investigators have focused on substitutions within the SS1–SS2 region of domain I, which is now well accepted to be intimately involved in channel function. Numa's group had originally proposed that the replacement of Arginine-377 of the cardiac channel by asparagine (R377N) in the neuronal form was responsible for the increased sensitivity to TTX displayed by the latter; this would of course imply that charge-charge repulsion between channel and ligand guanidinium groups was at the heart of the effect. However, characterization of STX and TTX binding to a mutated cardiac channel containing the R377N replacement shows increases of two- to eightfold in K_d, respectively {40}. Because the wild-type cardiac and neuronal channels differ by approximately 1000-fold in their sensitivities to these agents, it is considered unlikely that R377 is a major factor in determining TTX sensitivity. Attention has therefore been shifted to neighboring residues that differ between the two channels, leading to the surprising discovery that replacement of Cysteine-374 of the cardiac channel by tyrosine (C374Y), found in the neuronal version, increases the affinity for STX and TTX by 14- and 700-fold, respectively {40}. Analysis of other properties of the wild-type and mutated channels is fully consistent with the conclusion that position 374 is a major determinant of TTX/STX sensitivity. It has been suggested that tyrosine at this position facilitates binding of the guanidinium toxins because of the ability of its pi-electron cloud to interact with the fixed positive charge on the ligand. Analogous models have been put forward to account for binding of acetylcholine to its receptor {41}, and of tetraethylammonium ion to potassium channels, lending additional credence to this suggestion {42}.

While the importance of positions 374 and 376 to TTX binding thus seem to be well established, it seems intuitively likely that binding of these and other ligands to the channel most probably involves combinatorial effects. While the sites identified above lie in the SS1 region, mutagenesis of anionic sites in SS2 has implicated these regions in interaction with TTX as well {43}. Neutralizing replacements of Aspartate-384 and Glutamate-387 (to

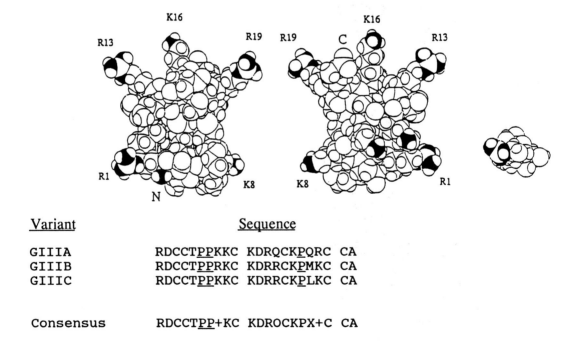

Variant	Sequence
GIIIA	RDCCTP̲P̲KKC KDRQCKP̲QRC CA
GIIIB	RDCCTP̲P̲RKC KDRRCKP̲MKC CA
GIIIC	RDCCTP̲P̲KKC KDRRCKP̲LKC CA
Consensus	RDCCTP̲P̲+KC KDROCKPX+C CA

Fig. 33-3. μ-Conotoxin structures. **Top:** A space-filling model of the three-dimensional structure of μ-GIIIA, as deduced from two-dimensional nuclear magnetic resonance data. Black spheres indicate side-chain nitrogens of Arg, Lys, and the N-terminal group. **A** and **B** depict different faces of the molecule, while the structure of tetrodotoxin is shown in scale in **C** for comparison. From Lancelin et al. {47}, with permission. **Bottom:** Amino acid sequences of three μ-conotoxin variants are shown in the single-letter code, with P designating hydroxyproline. Disulfide bonds link Cys3-Cys15, Cys4-Cys20, and Cys10-Cys21. In the consensus sequence, + = cationic residue; X = ambiguous character.

asparagine and glutamine, respectively) of the rat brain channel result in thousandfold decreases in affinity for both TTX and STX; independent studies have implicated D384 as being an important determinant of single channel conductance {44}. In the cardiac channel, neither site is occupied by an ionizable residue. Coupled with the results discussed above, these data implicate multiple channel carboxylate functions in TTX binding, and also demonstrate the criticality of non-ionic interactions. Finally, the four homologous domain model of sodium channel structure must also be borne in mind. In this context, photolabeling of the electroplax channel with a diazirine derivative of TTX has shown that the SS1–SS2 region from domains III and IV may also be involved in binding of the natural ligand {45}.

A structurally unrelated toxin designated as μ-conotoxin or geographutoxin, functions as a high-affinity sodium channel blocker in muscle, but not nerve, and its binding is competitive with TTX/STX {reviewed in 46}. Isolated from piscivorus snails, μ-conotoxin is a 22-residue polypeptide that contains hydroxyproline and is tightly cross-linked by three disulfide bonds. Its structure (fig. 33-3), recently solved by two-dimensional nuclear magnetic resonance {47}, contains a series of tight turns within the N-terminal region, and a short stretch of right-handed α helix; the core of the peptide encompasses what the authors refer to as a disulfide cage. An apparently important feature of this structure lies in the orientation of the six cationic side chains, all of which project into solution. Of these, Arg-13 has been shown to be essential for activity: even the very conservative replacement by lysine reduces μ-conotoxin activity by an order of magnitude {48}. TTX-resistant sodium channels are likewise resistant to the action of μ-conotoxin.

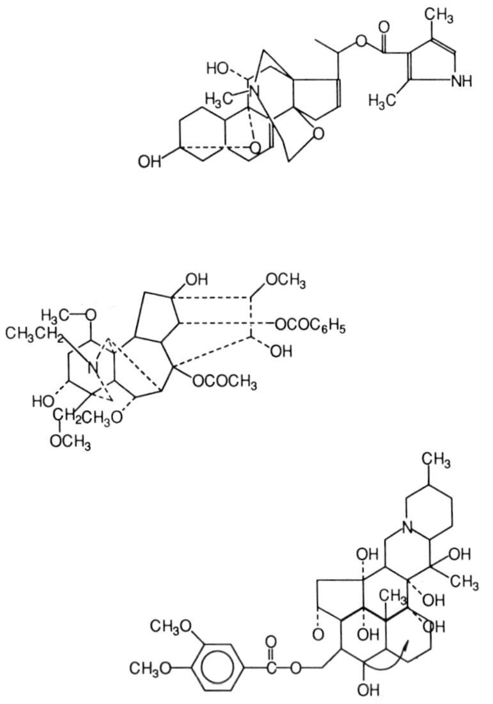

LIPID-SOLUBLE ALKALOIDS: BATRACHOTOXIN AND VERATRIDINE

The structures of well-characterized alkaloids known to have profound effects on the gating and selectivity properties of the sodium channel are shown in fig. 33-4. Because of their highly apolar character, these alkaloids are generally lipid soluble and have the ability to pass freely through biological membranes. They thus have the potential to interact with receptor sites on the channel that are on either side of, or buried within, the membrane bilayer; clearly, this distinguishes them from both TTX and STX. The alkaloids discussed below are in general toxic to excitable cells {reviewed in 49}; the two used most commonly are batrachotoxin, derived from skin secretions of the frog *Phyllobates aurataenia*, and veratridine, obtained from plants of the genera Lilaceae and Ericaceae. Despite their different biological origins and concentration-effect relationships (the IC_{50} values for batrachotoxin and veratridine differ by roughly two orders of magnitude, with the former being in the submicromolar range), both molecules display very similar effects on channel function, causing persistent activation, which leads ultimately to membrane depolarization {reviewed in 50}. Batrachotoxin

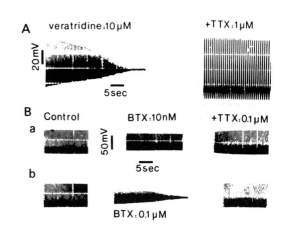

Fig. 33-4. Structures of some major alkaloid agonists of the voltage-sensitive sodium channel. **Top**, batrachotoxin; **center**, aconitine; **bottom**, veratridine.

Fig. 33-5. The effects of alkaloids on cultured 3-day aggregates. In panel **A**, electrical activity is blocked within 2 minutes by 10 μM veratridine, and subsequently restored in the presence of 1 μM TTX. In panel **B**, activity is likewise blocked by batrachotoxin at 0.1 μM (lower middle) and restored by the same concentration of TTX.

is among the most toxic substances known to humans, and its lethal effects are most likely due to its ability to induce cardiac arryhthmias {51}.

The effects of veratridine and batrachotoxin on embryonic chicken cardiac cells are depicted in fig. 33-5.

Depolarization of the membranes of excitable cells by batrachotoxin or veratridine is attributable to the ability of both compounds to activate sodium channels at the resting potential and to maintain these channels in the activated conformation {52,53}, and is sensitive to TTX blockade {54}. The alkaloids have been shown to share a common binding site by functional assays {21}, and direct measurements of batrachotoxin binding to rat brain synaptosomes have been reported, with binding site densities that correlate well with those for TTX and STX {55}. In order to account for the physiologic effects of these toxins described above, this site must be coupled to structural features of the channel important for both its activation and inactivation. Additional evidence supporting this conclusion exists in the literature. For example, Angelides and coworkers, using resonance energy transfer between fluorescently labeled derivatives of batrachotoxin and tetrodotoxin, have measured the distance between the respective binding sites and also have shown that this distance is altered by binding of other channel ligands that affect gating {56}. Moreover, alkaloid-treated channels are known to display a less stringent ionic selectivity than do their naive counterparts, treatment with veratridine resulting in relative permeability increases for guanidinium, potassium, and rubidium by factors of 2.7-, 4.5-, and 10-fold, respectively {57}. Catterall has proposed that the alkaloids act by binding preferentially to the channel in its open conformation, thus shifting a preexisting equilibrium between active and inactive states. In this formulation, toxin action would obey the allosteric model of Monod, in which the binding energy for a given alkaloid is expressed as a shift in the voltage dependence of activation {50}.

In a variety of cardiac preparations, low concentrations of either veratridine or batrachotoxin prolong the repolarization phase of the action potential in a TTX-sensitive fashion {reviewed in 58}, while higher concentrations of either agent result in abolition of the membrane potential. As alluded to above, batrachotoxin is significantly more active than veratridine in this assay. Analogous results have been obtained from measurements of TTX-sensitive sodium fluxes in cultured chick embryonic cardiac cells {59}. In a pharmacologic sense, batrachotoxin would thus be classified as a full, and veratridine a partial, agonist for the channel.

The ability of the alkaloids discussed above, as well as others, to cause persistent activation of the cardiac sodium channel is related to their dose-dependent production of a reversible, TTX-sensitive positive inotropic effect {58}. In this respect, each alkaloid displays its own unique specific activity, but in all cases the maximum attainable increase in force of contraction is essentially the same. Because the cardiac action potential is calcium, rather than sodium, dependent, it is essential to understand whether this positive inotropic effect is a direct or an indirect one. Available evidence indicates strongly that the latter mechanism is correct. Apparently, the persistent activation of the sodium channel caused by the alkaloids in turn leads to activation of a Na^+-Ca^{2+} exchanger, as demonstrated both electrophysiologically and biochemically {59,60}. It should be intuitively obvious that the indirect nature of

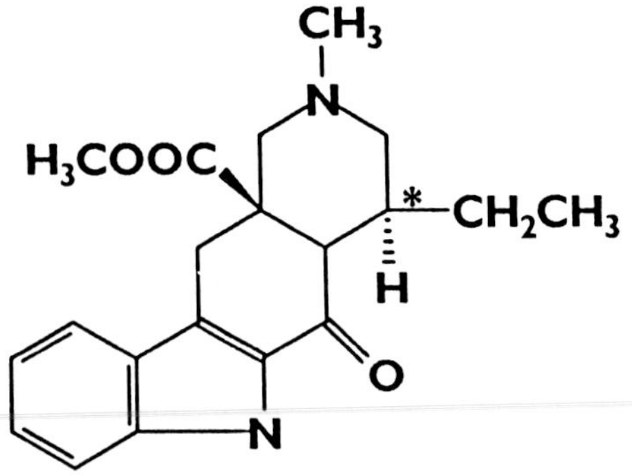

Fig. 33-6. The structure of ervatamine is depicted. In epiervatamine, the stereochemistry of the hydrogen and the ethyl group at the carbon, indicated by the asterisk, is inverted.

this effect allows the signal to be amplified, and analysis of the respective ion fluxes in tissue culture systems indicates that the extent of this amplification is approximately fivefold {59}. It should be noted that evidence has been presented that veratridine and batrachotoxin block slow calcium channels in neuroblastoma cells {61}, although whether they also display this effect in cardiac cells is not known at present.

Ervatamine, another plant alkaloid, and its derivative epiervatamine block neuroblastoma voltage-dependent sodium channels at micromolar (or slightly lower) concentrations {62}. Analysis by both voltage-clamp and ion flux methods indicates that these toxins act as competitive inhibitors of batrachotoxin action {63}. The authors interpret this as competition for the batrachotoxin binding site, but direct evidence for such competition is lacking. What is clear from the binding analyses is that ervatamine and its relatives are unable to compete at the classical TTX site. The effects of ervatamine on heart channels are qualitatively similar, but their sensitivity to ervatamine is at least an order of magnitude less than in nerve. The structures of ervatamines are shown in fig. 33-6.

POLYPEPTIDE TOXINS

The ability of scorpion venom to alter sodium conductance in nerve was first noted over 25 years ago {64,65}. In the intervening years, toxins active on sodium channels have been purified and sequenced from the venoms of *Androctonus*, *Leiurus*, *Centruroides*, and *Tityus* spp., and their interactions with target channels have been measured. Although all these toxins have certain structural features in common, including size, isoelectric point, and a common disulfide core, there is a good deal of diversity at the level of amino acid sequence. Moreover, two functionally distinct classes of scorpion toxins, designated α- and β-toxins, exist {66}. α-Toxins, typically derived from *Androctonus* and *Leiurus* venoms, delay or abolish channel inactivation, thus prolonging repolarization by binding to the channel in a membrane-potential dependent fashion {67}. In con-

Representative α-Toxins:

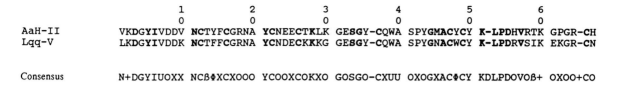

	10	20	30	40	50	60
AaH-II	VKDGYIVDDV	NCTYFCGRNA	YCNEECTKLK	GESGY-CQWA	SPYGMACYCY	K-LPDHVRTK	GPGR-CH
Lqq-V	LKDGYIVDDK	NCTFFCGRNA	YCNDECKKKG	GESGY-CQWA	SPYGNACWCY	K-LPDRVSIK	EKGR-CN
Consensus	N+DGYIUOXX	NCBΦXCXOOO	YCOOXCOKXO	GOSGO-CXUU	OXOGXACΦCY	KDLPDOVOβ+	OXOO+CO

Representative ß-Toxins:

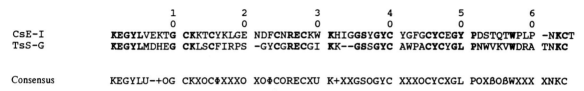

	10	20	30	40	50	60
CsE-I	KEGYLVEKTG	CKKTCYKLGE	NDFCNRECKW	KHIGGSYGYC	YGFGCYCEGY	PDSTQTWPLP	-NKCT
TsS-G	KEGYLMDHEG	CKLSCFIRPS	-GYCGRECGI	KK--GSSGYC	AWPACYCYGL	PNWVKVWDRA	TNKC
Consensus	KEGYLU-+OG	CKXOCΦXXXO	XOΦCORECXU	K+XXGSOGYC	XXXOCYCXGL	POXβOβWXXX	XNKC

Fig. 33-7. Primary structures of representative α- and β-scorpion toxins. Sequences are shown in the single-letter code, and disulfide bonds link half-cystines 12 and 63, 16 and 36, 22 and 46, and 26 and 48 in both groups. Numbering is based on the sequence of AaH-II. Residues shown in boldface are invariant within the α or β subgroup. In the consensus sequence, the coding is as follows: +, cationic residue; O, polar residue; X, character undefined; U, nonpolar residue; Φ, aromatic residue; β, branched side chain. AaH, *Androctonus australis* Hector; Lqq, *Leiurus quinquestriatus quinquestriatus*; CsE, *Centruroides sculpturatus* Ewing; TsS, *Tityus serrulatus*.

trast, the β-toxins, generally obtained from *Centruroides* and *Tityus* venoms, shift the voltage dependence of activation to more negative potentials upon binding to a different receptor subsite on the same polypeptide; binding of β-toxins is independent of membrane potential {66}. Most of the α-toxins exhibit K_ds in the nanomolar range, while the affinity of the β-toxins is usually somewhat weaker.

The primary structures of the most thoroughly studied of the α- and β-toxins are shown in fig. 33-7; these are only representatives of the more than two dozen scorpion toxins of known sequence. Shared features amongst all long scorpion toxins include their molecular weight, the positions of the disulfides, limited sequence homology, and a good deal of similarity in backbone structure at the three-dimensional level {68,69}. It is at least possible, and perhaps likely, that the sequence homology observed in the scorpion toxins exists chiefly to impose folding constraints, rather than serving to identify residues directly responsible for interaction with receptor. However, this statement remains conjecture due to our lack of extensive knowledge of the atomic details of the binding site. Within the scorpion toxin family, only Lys-56 of *Androctonus* toxin has been clearly identified as being essential for toxicity {70}. While it is true that additional sites have been implicated in activity by treatment of one or more other scorpion toxins with group-specific reagents, overall patterns have not yet emerged. It is anticipated that this situation will be remedied with the relatively recent addition of site-directed mutagenesis to the armamentarium of scientists interested in understanding the structure and function of these polypeptides. Because the actions of β-toxins on cardiac channels have not been well charac-

terized, this group will not be discussed further, although it should be noted that at least one such toxin is known to bind to this channel with very high affinity {10}.

The three-dimensional structures of at least four scorpion toxins are now known, including representatives of both classes. As shown in fig. 33-8 for *Centruroides* toxin, these proteins have in common a dense core of secondary structure containing three strands of antiparallel β-pleated sheet (residues 1–4, 37–41, and 46–50) and two disulfide bonds. A short strand of α-helix (residues 23–32) is linked to this core by a third disulfide. Structural differences between the α- and β-toxins are largely restricted to several loops that protrude from the core. In addition to the aforementioned features, a relatively nonpolar surface region containing many conserved aromatic residues is present. Because chemical modification of sites external to this surface is generally without significant effect on toxin function, and because Lys-56, discussed above, lies within it, Fontecilla-Camps and coworkers have argued that this region is essential for receptor binding. Interestingly, this surface is fairly well conserved in both the α- and β-toxins.

A structurally distinct group of polypeptide toxins shares the scorpion α-toxin binding site: Representative of these proteins are a diverse family of sea anemone toxins derived from *Anemonia*, *Anthopleura*, *Stichodactyla*, and *Radianthus* spp. As will be discussed in a subsequent section, under certain conditions these polypeptides can function as cardiac stimulants. While basic and disulfide rich, the anemone toxins differ from scorpion toxins in being smaller (46–50 residues vs. 60–65) and having three, rather than four, disulfide bonds. Comparisons of

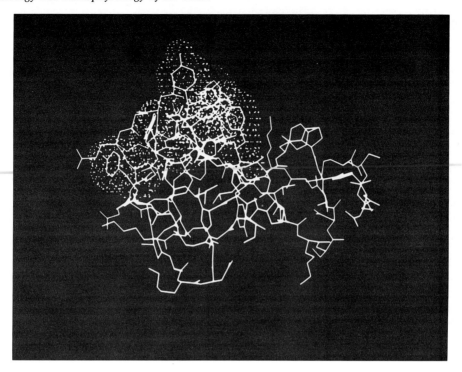

Fig. 33-8. Three-dimensional structure of *Centruroides* toxin variant 3. Structural coordinates were obtained from the Brookhaven Protein Database, with permission. Although variant 3 is a β-toxin, the overall folding patterns of the α- and β-toxins are highly similar {69}. The hydrophobic surface proposed to be important in toxin-receptor interactions is shown as a dotted surface.

Representative Anemone Toxin Sequences

```
               1           2           3           4
               0           0           0           0
AsI       GAPCKCKSDG  PNTRGNSMSG  TIWV--FGCP  SGWNNCEGRA  --HGYCCKQ
AsII      GVPCLCDSDG  PSVRGNTLSG  IIWL--AGCP  SGWHNCKKHG  PTIGWCCKQ
AsV       GVPCLCDSDG  PSVRGNTLSG  ILWL--AGCP  SGWHNCKKHK  PTIGWCCK
ApA       GVSCLCDSDG  PSVRGNTLSG  TLWLYPSGCP  SGWHNCKAHG  PTIGWCCKQ
ApB       GVPCLCDSDG  PRPRGNTLSG  ILWFYPSGCP  SGWHNCKAHG  PNIGWCCKK
ShI       -AACKCDDEG  PDIRTAPLTG  TVDL--GSCN  AGWEKCASYY  TIIADCCRKKK
RpII      -ASCKCDDDG  PDVRSATGTG  TVDF--WNCN  EGWEKCTAVY  TPVASCCRKK


Consensus XUXCXCOODG  POXROOOUOG  βUXUXXXOCX  OGWOOCOOXX  XXXOXCC+O
```

Fig. 33-9. Primary structures of representative sea anemone toxins. Sequences are shown in the single-letter code, with the numbering based on the sequence of Anthopleurin A. Disulfide bonds link Cys4-Cys46, Cys6-Cys36, and Cys29-Cys47. Residues shown underlined are invariant. In the consensus sequence, the coding is +, cationic residue; O, polar residue; X, character undefined; U, nonpolar residue; Φ, aromatic residue; β, branched side chain. As, *Anemonia sulcata*; Ap, *Anthopleura xanthogrammica*; Sh, *Stichodactyla helianthus*; Rp, *Radianthus paumotensis*.

anemone (fig. 33-9) and scorpion toxin sequences reveal no homology.

The solution structures of four distinct anemone toxins have been reported within the past few years, all being determined by multidimensional NMR {71}. While these structures display obvious differences in positioning of side chains, their backbone structures are remarkably similar (fig. 33-10). A key feature of all is the presence of four strands of a twisted, antiparallel β-pleated sheet (residues 2–4, 18–23, 31–34, and 42–47 in the Anthopleurin A numbering), which is unrelated to any structural motifs seen in the scorpion toxins. Nonetheless, as it is known

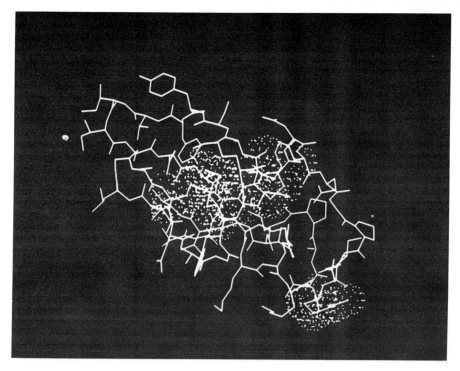

Fig. 33-10. Three-dimensional structure of *Stichodactyla helianthus* toxin I, a representative anemone toxin. Structural coordinates {71} were obtained from the Brookhaven Protein Database, with permission. The overall folding patterns for anemone toxins of known structure are similar. The positions of the disulfide bonds are indicated by the dotted surfaces. A dotted surface also identifies the invariant arginine residue, which is essential for activity (lower right portion of the structure).

that anemone toxins compete with scorpion α-toxins for binding {72}, one might anticipate the existence of limited structural similarities that remain to be elucidated. In this context, demonstration by NMR of a small hydrophobic patch on the surface of homologous anemone toxins (this patch includes Trp 45 and Ile-43 in Anthopleurin A) may be significant. Chemical modification of an *Anemonia* toxin has demonstrated the essentiality of Arg-14 for biological activity {73}. This residue, located in a highly flexible region of the polypeptide chain {74}, is conserved in all anemone toxins sequenced to date. Recent success in bacterial expression of wild-type and mutant forms of anemone toxins {75} affords hope of greatly expanding our knowledge of the structure and function of these polypeptides.

Both anemone and scorpion α-toxins function by dramatically slowing sodium channel inactivation, and photoaffinity labeling of channel preparations with a derivative of *Leiurus* toxin has demonstrated binding of this toxin to channel sequences lying between the S5 and S6 helices (i.e., the SS1–SS2 domain described above {76}). Because binding of anemone and scorpion toxins is competitive, it is assumed that the anemone toxins interact with this same region of the channel. Both classes of toxins bind to a site accessible from the extracellular face and in 1:1:1 stoichiometry with the sites discussed previously.

A number of different scorpion and anemone toxins

have been tested for effects on cardiac channels, both as tissue preparations and in cell culture. Invariably, these experiments result in a significant prolongation of the cardiac action potential, which is inhibited by TTX {77–80}. The ensuing positive inotropic effect is produced at very low toxin concentrations, in the low nanomolar range for the most active *Anemonia* and *Anthopleura* toxins {81,82}. With the notable exception of the *Radianthus* toxins, which in general display rather poor specific activities, the anemone toxins are roughly 10-fold more active than the scorpion toxins, both in their measured effects on alkaloid-stimulated, TTX-sensitive sodium fluxes and in their generation of inotropic effects.

Data on cardiac concentration-effect relationships for a variety of polypeptide toxins are presented in table 33-2, while the effects of selected toxins on sodium fluxes and contractility are depicted in fig. 33-11; it should be re-emphasized that toxin-dependent uptake of calcium, which drives the action potential in these cells, is two to five times greater than that of sodium {79}. The most active anemone toxin in either assay has been named AX_{II} and ApB by different groups; it has an ED_{50} for sodium uptake of 2 nM in cultured cardiac cells and displays a maximum inotropic effect at 0.3 nM. It is important to note that the maximum inotropic effects are consistently obtained at toxin concentrations below the ED_{50} for ion flux and also below the concentration at which arrhythmias are

Table 33-2. Functional properties of polypeptide toxins

Genus	Toxin	Na$^+$ uptake, $K_{0.5}$	Inotropic effect, maximum	Arrhythmia onset
Anemonia	II	15	1–3	10–30
	V	1.5	3	4–6
Anthopleura	I (A)	3	1	2–3
	II (B)	2	0.3	10
Radianthus	III	4000	300	3000
Androctonus	II	30	3	10
Leiurus	V	200	n.d.	n.d.
Tityus	γ	200	10–30	100–300

Effects of toxins on ion fluxes were measured in cultured rat cardiac cells in the presence of 0.2 mM veratridine as coeffector. Inotropic effects and arrhythmias were measured in rat atria. All values are expressed in nanomolar concentrations. n.d. = not done.

observed {83}. Because ApB is the most active of the polypeptide toxins characterized to date, and also because it displays the smallest ratio of concentration required for maximum inotropic effect to concentration at the onset of

arrhythmia, the potential utility of this polypeptide, and related ones, as cardiotonic agents is under active investigation.

The salient features of the foregoing discussion are that (a) these toxins induce long action potentials and increases in both amplitude and duration of cardiac contractions; (b) cellular uptake of both sodium and calcium is enhanced in toxin-treated cells, and both uptakes are sensitive to TTX; (c) toxin-induced contractions are insensitive to verapamil or D-600, which are well-characterized blockers of the slow calcium channel in cardiac tissues. More recently, however, evidence has been presented that *Anemonia* toxin II also diminishes the ability of cardiac myocytes to reactivate following an action potential {84}. The authors suggest that this may be due to indirect toxin-induced increases in inwardly rectifying potassium currents.

Most current models for sodium channel function postulate the existence of open, closed, and inactivated conformations, with openings directly from the latter state not being permitted {85}. Recent data suggest that *Anemonia* toxin II reduces the transition from the open to the inactivated state without altering the rates of other conformational transitions in the channel {86}.

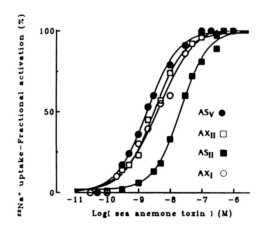

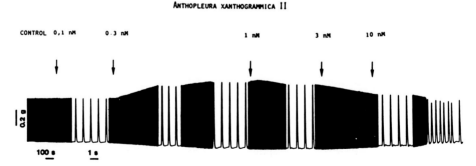

Fig. 33-11. The action of sea anemone toxins on the rat cardiac sodium channel. The upper panel depicts the effects of toxins II (■) and V (●) of *Anemonia sulcata*, and I (Ax$_I$ ○) and II (AX$_{II}$ □) of *Anthopleura xanthogrammica* on sodium uptake stimulated by 200 μM veratridine. The effect of Ap-B on contractile response of rat left atria is shown in the lower panel.

OTHER SODIUM CHANNEL TOXINS

A potpourri of other organic molecules, mostly lipid soluble, have been shown to affect functions of the voltage-sensitive sodium channels. These include the pyrethroid insecticides, toxins derived from corals (*Goniopora* spp.), and toxins from dinoflagellates (ciguatoxin, maitotoxin, and brevetoxin). While many of these agents have not as yet been completely characterized, it is important that the reader be aware of their existence and current hypotheses as to their mechanism of action.

Pyrethroids comprise a group of synthetic chrysanthemic acid derivatives that are widely used as insecticides. These compounds have been examined mostly in nerve and in cell lines of neuronal origin. In neuroblastoma cells, pyrethroids interact synergistically with veratridine to stimulate TTX-sensitive sodium uptake {87}. In a functional sense, this effect mimics those of the scorpion and anemone toxins discussed above. The pyrethroids also display synergism with scorpion and anemone toxins, in this case mimicking the effect of alkaloids like veratridine. In the absence of any coeffector, pyrethroids do not have measurable effects on sodium fluxes. Although direct measurements of pyrethroid binding have not been reported, the functional results cited above suggest the presence on sodium channels of distinct receptor sites for alkaloids, polypeptides, and pyrethroids, with the likelihood that these sites are conformationally linked.

Goniopora toxins comprise a group of proteinaceous substances isolated from corals. While structural characterization of these toxins remains incomplete at present, it seems likely from estimations of their molecular weight (values of 10,000–19,000 have been reported for different preparations) that multiple toxins exist and that these toxins are distinct from the other known polypeptide effectors of sodium channels. In addition, the lack of complete structural characterization renders it difficult to draw unambiguous conclusions as to the molecular targets of *Goniopora* toxin(s), since it is not clear in all cases that the same protein is being analyzed. Such problems notwithstanding, at least some of the *Goniopora* toxins (described as having molecular weights in the 10-kDa range) are related to anemone and scorpion toxins in a functional sense, interacting synergistically with veratridine to enhance the persistent activation of neuronal channels {88}. Although *Goniopora* toxin competes with *Leiurus* toxin in direct binding studies, much higher concentrations of the coral toxin are required for competition than for production of physiologic effects, leading to the conclusion that *Goniopora* toxin interacts at a unique binding site. In rabbit myocardium, *Goniopora* toxin produces a positive inotropic effect, which is inhibited by TTX and attenuated by verapamil {89}. Finally, characterization of a 19-kDa *Goniopora* toxin that stimulates nitrendipine-sensitive uptake of calcium into cultured cardiac cells has been reported {90}. Binding of this toxin to rabbit T-tubules is competed by the calcium channel antagonist (+)-PN 200-110, suggesting its molecular target to be the slow calcium channel.

Ciguatoxin (CTX) is an 1100 molecular weight dinoflagellate-derived substance whose structure has been described in general terms as being an oxygenated polyether {91}. In neuroblastoma cells, this compound produces TTX-sensitive membrane depolarization {92} and interacts synergistically with alkaloids, pyrethroids, or anemone and scorpion toxins. Its effects on skeletal muscle, while less completely characterized, appear to be similar.

Brevetoxins comprise yet another family of lipid-soluble dinoflagellate toxins that interact with sodium channels; eight distinct brevetoxins have been isolated to date {93}. These toxins depolarize nerve and muscle preparations by shifting the voltage dependence of sodium channel activation to more negative potentials {94}. Brevetoxin-activated channels also display very slow opening kinetics and do not show rapid inactivation. Brevetoxins bind reversibly and with high affinity to sodium channels at a site distinct from those for the toxins described previously in this chapter, although evidence has been presented for cooperative interactions between the brevetoxin and alkaloid binding sites {95,96}. Recent studies indicate similar effects of brevetoxins on the cardiac sodium channel and, in addition, indicate that these compounds induce a variety of different open states of the channel {97}.

TOXINS SPECIFIC FOR THE CALCIUM CHANNEL

Calcium channels are more complex than sodium channels, having a total of five subunits, ranging in size from 30 to about 170 kDa {103}. Despite this, at least one of the calcium channel polypeptides, designated α_1, is strikingly similar to the α subunit of the sodium channel, the two being 29% identical in amino acid sequence and fitting equally well the model already described for transmembrane organization. As is true for the sodium channel, this α_1 subunit by itself is capable of facilitating transmembrane ion fluxes and functioning as the receptor for a variety of agonists and antagonists of the channel.

Voltage-sensitive calcium channels, which are responsible for the plateau phase of cardiac action potentials, have been extensively studied in the past, primarily by application of dihydropyridines and antiarrhythmics. Because these agents would not be classified as toxins, their actions will not be discussed further here. However, a number of other toxic compounds do have the calcium channel as their site of action, and these will be discussed in the next section.

Maitotoxin, a water-soluble, nonproteinaceous agent isolated from dinoflagellates, is among the most toxic substances known. Maitotoxin was initially shown to activate verapamil-sensitive calcium channels in the rat pheochromocytoma line PC12 {98}. This activation is not dependent on external sodium and occurs at maitotoxin concentrations of 0.1–1 μg/ml. Maitotoxin also induces calcium-dependent contraction of skeletal muscle {99} and at very low concentrations (of the order of ng/ml) induces a positive inotropic effect in cardiac muscle that is calcium dependent {100,101}. Paradoxically, the maitotoxin-induced calcium current seems not to flow through calcium channels, but rather appears to create a channel pore that is a pharmacologic mimic of these entities. Either maitotoxin itself creates a transmembrane pore through which calcium can pass and that is inhibited by calcium channel antagonists, or it functions by converting an endogenous membrane protein into a calcium-selective pore. The first possibility is readily testable, and because maitotoxin fails to increase calcium uptake by liposomes {98}, this model has fallen into disfavor. The alternative mechanism is clearly more difficult to test experimentally, although analogies drawn with palytoxin are intriguing. It has been hypothesized that palytoxin, a depolarizing agent, which also seems not to function via either existing ion channels or as an ionophore, acts by converting the Na,K-ATPase into a potassium permeability pathway {102}; this would be analogous to the second model for maitotoxin action discussed above.

A new family of peptide toxins that has received a great deal of attention is the conotoxins, isolated from piscivorus snails. Conotoxins {reviewed in 46} directed at the acetylcholine receptor, muscle sodium channels,

vasopressin, and NMDA receptors, and voltage-sensitive calcium channels have been described. While the ω-conotoxins described to date are all specific for neuronal channels {46}, the complexities of the *Conus* venoms suggests that a host of additional biologically interesting compounds remain to be characterized. Conotoxins specific for calcium channels are designated *omega-conotoxins* (hereafter abbreviated as CgTX).

To date, seven CgTX variants have been described in the literature. All contain three disulfide bonds and a large number of hydroxylated amino acid residues, including hydroxyproline; all are highly cationic in nature; and all have amidated C-terminal residues. Sequences of CgTXs are shown in fig. 33-12A. Although two basic classes of CgTXs exist, and homology between these groups amounts to about 40%, it appears that conservation of the positions of the disulfide bonds is the major constraint placed on the sequences of these peptides. CgTXs were first identified based on their ability to prevent transmitter release at presynaptic terminals {104}, and the mechanism of the conotoxin designated GVIA was subsequently examined in greater detail. Analysis of its action on voltage-

Sequences of ω-Conotoxins:

```
                 1          2
                 0          0
GVIA    CKSPGSSCSP TSYNCCR-SC NPYTKRCY
GVIB    CKSPGSSCSP TSYNCCR-SC NPYTKRCYG
GVIIA   CKSPGTPCSR GMRDCCT-SC LLYSNKCRRY
GVIIB   CKSPGTPCSR GMRDCCT-SC LSYSNKCRRY
MVIIA   CKGKGAKCSR LMYDCCTGSC R--SGKC
MVIIB   CKGKGASCHR TSYDCCTGSC N--RGKC
```

Sequences of Spider Toxins:

```
                1          2          3
                0          0          0
μAga-I     ECVPENGHC RDWYDE-CCE GFYCSCRQPP KCICRNNN
μAga-II    ECATKNKRC ADWAGPWCCD GLYCSCRSYP GCMCRPSS
μAga-III   ADCVGDGQRC ADWAGPYCCS GYYCSCRSMP YCRCRSDS
μAga-IV    ACVGENQQC ADWAGPHCCD GYYCTCRYFP KCICRNNN
μAga-V     ACVGENKQC ADWAGPHCCD GYYCTCRYFP KCICRNNN
μAga-VI    DCVGESQQC ADWAGPHCCD GYYCTCRYFP KCICVNNN
CuTX-I     SCVGEYGRC RSAYED-CCD GYYCNCSQPP YCLCRNNN
CuTX-II    ADCVGDGQRC ADWAGPYCCS GYYCSCRSMP YCRCRSDS
CuTX-III   ADCVGDGQKC ADWFGPYCCS GYYCSCRSMP YCRCRSDS
```

```
            1          2          3          4          5          6          7
            0          0          0          0          0          0          0
ωAga-IA   AKALPPGSVC DGNESDCKCY GKWHKCRCPW KWHFTGEGP- CTCEKGMKHT CITKLHCPNK AEQGLNW
ωAga-IB   ERGLPEGAEC DGNESDCKCA GAWIKCRCPP MWHING
ωAga-IIA  -GCIEIGGDC DGYQEKSYCQ CCRNNGFCS
ωAga-IIIA -SCIDIGGDC DGEKD--DCQ CCRRNGYCSC YSLFGYLKSG CKCVVGTSAE FQGICRRKAR QCYNSDPDKC ESHNKPKRR
```

```
            1          2          3          4
            0          0          0          0
ωAga-IVA  KKKCIAKDYG RCKWGGFPCC RGRGCICSIM CECKPRLIME GLGLA
```

Fig. 33-12. **a:** Primary structures of omega-conotoxin variants. The sequences are shown in the single-letter code, with invariant residues shown in boldface. Disulfide bonds link Cys1-Cys16, Cys15-Cys27, and Cys8-Cys20. **b:** Primary structures of representative spider toxins specific for Ca channels. Residues shown in boldface are invariant within a group. Where complete sequences have not been determined (omega agatoxins IB, IIA, and IVA), N-terminal sequences are shown. Disulfide pairings are not known. Aga, agatoxins; CuTX, curtatoxins.

clamped chick dorsal root ganglion preparations has shown that ω CgTX irreversibly blocks about 95% of the calcium current {105}, with the remaining 5% being ascribed to T-channels. A binding constant was estimated as being at most 1 nM. Based on analyses of the biochemistry, pharmacology, and physiology of ω CgTX binding, non-calcium channel sites of action have been excluded {cited in 46}.

More recently, emphasis has been placed on identifying the channel subtype with which the ω-conotoxins interact. T, N, and L subtypes of calcium channels have been defined in neuronal tissue and, of these, the T type is most clearly unaffected by conotoxins. Data on the remaining subtypes are not definitive, but do show a profound inhibition of N-type channels in virtually all preparations tested, while effects on L channels display variability from one tissue source to another {106,107}.

Another group of polypeptides that has recently been shown to act presynaptically to prevent transmitter release is the agatoxins, isolated from funnel-web spider venom. Agatoxins exist in two general groupings {108–110}. Long, or ω-agatoxins, are similar in both size and charge to the scorpion toxins (65–75 residues), but contain six, rather than four, disulfides. The short, or μ-agatoxins, contain 36–38 amino acid residues and have four disulfide bonds; in addition, they are somewhat less cationic in nature than the omega toxins. Sequences of agatoxins are shown in fig. 33-12b, emphasizing their unrelatedness to the CgTX family at the level of primary structure.

Unfractionated funnel web spider venom blocks a dihydropyridine and CgTX-insensitive calcium current {111}, which can also be measured in *Xenopus* oocytes upon expression of microinjected rat brain mRNA {112}. More recent experiments have focused on characterizing purified components of this venom. Evidence has been presented that the ω-agatoxins have the ability to discriminate amongst calcium channel subtypes. For example, ω-Aga-IIA and IIIA are able to block entry of calcium into depolarized chick synaptosomes with mean effective doses in the nanomolar range, while ω-Aga-IA is ineffective in this assay up to 1 μM. Moreover, binding competition studies have demonstrated that ω-Aga-IIA is able to inhibit CgTX binding to synaptosomes, while ω-Aga-IA and -IB are not {113}. A newly discovered agatoxin, ω-Aga-IVA, has recently been found to target a dihydropyridine and CgTX-resistant calcium channel in synaptosomes; this channel is of the P type {114,115}. Thus, although development of agatoxins as pharmacologically useful reagents is still at a relatively early stage, and most have thus far only been characterized in neuronal tissues, the biochemical and physiological diversity of the venom offers great promise that it will soon become another source of valuable probes.

POTASSIUM CHANNELS

The existence of a variety of potassium channels in excitable tissues has been demonstrated over the years, and a brief discussion of these is warranted, even though these channels have not been analyzed in cardiac preparations. These may be distinguished from one another by their ability to be activated by voltage or calcium ions, and by their unit conductance (BK vs. SK channels). A large number of voltage-activated potassium channels, all related to the *shaker* locus originally identified as a behavioral mutant in *Drosophila*, have been cloned and their properties studies in oocyte preparations. Although they lack the four-domain structure described earlier, the *shaker* channels are structurally homologous to voltage-gated sodium and calcium channels, and the six-helix model seems to be an excellent predictor of their properties as well. Convincing evidence has been presented that the functional unit for these channels is a noncovalent tetramer. As of this date, only one calcium-activated potassium channel has been cloned; in *Drosophila* this protein is encoded by the *slowpoke* locus. While its transmembrane organization is likely to be closely related to the channels already described, the degree of homology between *shaker* and *slowpoke* channels is too low for them to be detectable by crosshybridization.

During the past 5 years it has become apparent that scorpion venom contains small peptides that block potassium channels, and two excellent reviews on this subject have appeared recently {116,117}. These toxins, which display no sequence homology with scorpion toxins directed at the sodium channel, include charybdotoxin, iberiotoxin, and scyllatoxin. Miller and his coworkers {118,119}, using analysis of the blocking kinetics of mutated forms of charybdotoxin, have begun to develop a picture of the binding surface of the toxin, with the intention of using this information to infer a structure for the complementary surface of the channel itself. This work offers the exciting prospect of beginning to understand what the outer vestibule of the channel looks like to an approaching ion.

Analysis of the three-dimensional structure of charybdotoxin {120} has nonetheless revealed a significant degree of similarity between the backbone structure of this polypeptide and previously analyzed scorpion toxins. This rather unexpected observation becomes even more surprising when one considers that the potassium channel toxins are blocking agents, rather than modulators of channel gating. Other polypeptides that function as potassium channel blockers include the dendrotoxins, derived from mamba venom, and apamin, obtained from honeybees. Neither of these toxins is structurally related to each other, or to the scorpion toxins discussed above.

SUMMARY AND CONCLUSIONS

Based on the material presented in the preceding sections, it is clear that toxins acting on cardiac ion channels can be subdivided into two groups based on their molecular target: those specific for sodium and calcium channels. The former family can be subdivided into a minimum of six groups, based primarily upon the functional consequences of their interaction with the channel. These include the guanidinium channel blockers TTX and STX;

the alkaloid activators, typified by batrachotoxin; the scorpion α- and sea anemone toxins, which enhance activation by the alkaloids; scorpion β-toxins, which shift the voltage dependence of channel activation; the brevetoxins, whose effects mimic to some extent those of scorpion β-toxins; ciguatoxin, which functions analogously to the alkaloid activators to cause persistent channel activation; and the pyrethroids and *Goniopora* toxins, which delay inactivation and thus prolong the action potential. It should be emphasized that despite the functional similarities outlined above, there is absolutely no evidence in the literature for binding competition between toxins of different families. Clearly, the channel comprises a complex and fascinating molecular structure, well worth the expenditure of scientific ingenuity and resources that it has absorbed in the past.

Calcium channels, which until recently have been targetted only by synthetic drugs, are now also known to be the target of natural toxins. Since analysis of the components of *Conus* and *Agelenopsis* venoms is presently at a rather early state, one cannot state with confidence that, for example, toxins from these sources will aid in uncovering new channel subtypes or in furthering our understanding of how already known channels function. What can be said with assurance is that history strongly indicates that such will ultimately prove to be the case.

The toxins that have been discussed, and those that remain to be discovered, have over the years been of the utmost importance in our ability to both purify and analyze the structure and function of voltage-sensitive ion channels. It is to be anticipated that the fact that the world is indeed a poisonous place will continue to be both the good news and the bad news for scientists intrigued by the problem of how ion channels function in excitable membranes.

REFERENCES

1. Catterall WA, Morrow CS, Hartshorne RP: Neurotoxin binding to receptor sites associated with voltage-sensitive sodium channels in intact, lysed and detergent-solubilized brain membranes. *J Biol Chem* 254:11379–11387, 1979.
2. Hartshorne RP, Catterall WA: Purification of the saxitoxin receptor of the sodium channel from rat brain. *Proc Natl Acad Sci USA* 78:4620–4624, 1981.
3. Hartshorne RP, Catterall WA: The sodium channel from rat brain: Purification and subunit composition. *J Biol Chem* 259:1667–1675, 1984.
4. Hartshorne RP, et al.: Functional reconstitution of the purified brain sodium channel in planar lipid bilayers. *Proc Natl Acad Sci USA* 82:240–244, 1985.
5. Tamkun MM, Talvenheimo JA, Catterall WA: The sodium channel from rat brain: Reconstitution of neurotoxin-activated ion flux and scorpion toxin binding from purified components. *J Biol Chem* 259:1676–1688, 1984.
6. Goldin AL, et al.: Messenger RNA coding for only the α subunit of the rat brain Na⁺ channel is sufficient for expression of functional channels in *Xenopus* oocytes. *Proc Natl Acad Sci USA* 83:7503–7507, 1986.
7. Krafte DS, et al.: Evidence for the involvement of more than one mRNA species in controlling the inactivation process of rat and rabbit brain Na⁺ channels expressed in *Xenopus* oocytes. *J Neurosci* 8:2859–2868, 1988.
8. Isom LL, et al.: Primary structure and functional expression of the β₁ subunit of the rat brain sodium channel. *Science* 256:839–842, 1992.
9. Casadei JM, et al.: Monoclonal antibodies against the voltage-sensitive Na⁺ channel from mammalian skeletal muscle. *Proc Natl Acad Sci USA* 81:6227–6231, 1984.
10. Lombet A, Lazdunski M: Characterization, solubilization, affinity labeling and purification of the cardiac Na⁺ channel using *Tityus* toxin. *Eur J Biochem* 141:651–660, 1984.
11. Noda M, et al.: Primary structure of *Electrophorus electricus* sodium channel deduced from cDNA sequence. *Nature* 312:121–127, 1984.
12. Chou PY, Fasman GD: Empirical predictions of protein conformation. *Ann Rev Biochem* 47:251–276, 1978.
13. Kyte J, Doolittle RF: A simple method for displaying the hydropathic character of a protein. *J Mol Biol* 157:105–132, 1982.
14. Durell SR, Guy HR: Atomic scale structure and functional models of voltage-gated potassium channels. *Biophys J* 62:238–250, 1992.
15. Vassilev PM, Scheuer T, Catterall WA: Identification of an intracellular peptide segment involved in sodium channel inactivation. *Science* 241:1658–1661, 1988.
16. Moorman JR, et al.: Changes in sodium channel gating produced by point mutations in a cytoplasmic linker. *Science* 250:688–691, 1990.
17. Stuhmer W, et al.: Structural parts involved in activation and inactivation of the sodium channel. *Nature* 339:597–603, 1989.
18. Auld VJ, et al.: A neutral amino acid change in segment IIS4 dramatically alters the gating properties of the voltage-dependent sodium channel. *Proc Natl Acad Sci USA* 87:323–327, 1990.
19. McClatchey AI, et al.: Temperature-sensitive mutations in the III–IV cytoplasmic loop region of the skeletal muscle sodium channel gene in paramyotonia congenita. *Cell* 68:769–774, 1992.
20. Li M, Jan YN, Jan LY: Specification of subunit assembly by the hydrophilic amino-terminal domain of the shaker potassium channel. *Science* 257:1225–1230, 1992.
21. Catterall WA: Cooperative activation of action potential Na ionophore by neurotoxins. *Proc Natl Acad Sci USA* 72:1782–1786, 1975.
22. Catterall WA, Beress L: Sea anemone toxin and scorpion toxin share a common receptor site associated with the action potential sodium ionophore. *J Biol Chem* 253:7393–7396, 1978.
23. Jover E, Couraud F, Rochat H: Two types of scorpion neurotoxins characterized by their binding to two separate receptor sites on rat brain synaptosomes. *Biochem Biophys Res Commun* 95:1607–1614, 1980.
24. Angelides KJ, Nutter TJ: Mapping the molecular structure of the voltage-dependent sodium channel. *J Biol Chem* 258:11958–11967, 1983.
25. Mosher HS: The chemistry of tetrodotoxin. In: Kao CY, Levinson SR (eds) *Ann NY Acad Sci* 479:32–43, 1986.
26. Narahashi T, Moore JW, Scott WR: Tetrodotoxin blockage of sodium conductance increase in lobster giant axons. *J Gen Physiol* 47:965–974, 1984.
27. Schantz EJ, et al.: Paralytic shellfish poison. VI. A procedure for the isolation and purification of the poison from toxic clam and mussel tissues. *J Am Chem Soc* 79:5230, 1957.
28. Schantz EJ, et al.: The structure of saxitoxin. *J Am Chem Soc* 97:1238, 1975.

29. Kao CY, Nishiyama N: Actions of saxitoxin on peripheral neuromuscular systems. *J Physiol* 180:50, 1965.

30. Hille B: The receptor for tetrodotoxin and saxitoxin, a structural hypothesis. *Biophys J* 15:615–619, 1975.

31. Baker PF, Rubinson KA: Chemical modification of crab nerves can make them insensitive to the local anaesthetics tetrodotoxin and saxitoxin. *Nature* 257:412–414, 1975.

32. Shrager P, Profera C: Inhibition of the receptor for tetrodotoxin in nerve membranes by reagents modifying carboxyl groups. *Biochim Biophys Acta* 318:141–146, 1973.

33. Kao CY: Structure-activity relations of tetrodotoxin, saxitoxin, and analogs. *Ann NY Acad Sci* 479:52–67, 1986.

34. Noda M, et al.: A single point mutation confers tetrodotoxin and saxitoxin insensitivity on the sodium channel II. *FEBS Lett* 259:213–216, 1989.

35. Gellens ME, et al.: Primary structure and functional expression of the human cardiac tetrodotoxin-insensitive voltage-dependent sodium channel. *Proc Natl Acad Sci USA* 89:554–558, 1992.

36. Cohen CJ, et al.: Tetrodotoxin block of sodium channels in rabbit Purkinje fibers. *J Gen Physiol* 78:383–411, 1981.

37. Tanaka JC, Doyle DD, Barr L: Sodium channels in vertebrate hearts. Three types of saxitoxin binding sites in heart. *Biochim Biophys Acta* 775:203–214, 1984.

38. Catterall WA, Coppersmith J: High-affinity saxitoxin receptor sites in vertebrate heart. Evidence for sites associated with autonomic nerve endings. *Mol Pharmacol* 20:526–532, 1981.

39. Catterall WA, Coppersmith J: Pharmacological properties of sodium channels in cultured rat heart cells. *Mol Pharmacol* 20:533–542, 1981.

40. Satin J, et al.: A mutant of TTX-resistant cardiac sodium channels with TTX-sensitive properties. *Science* 256:1202–1205, 1992.

41. Dougherty DA, Stauffer DA: Acetylcholine binding by a synthetic receptor: Implications for biological recognition. *Science* 250:1558–1560, 1990.

42. Kavanaugh MP, et al.: Interaction between tetraethylammonium and amino acid residues in the pore of cloned voltage-dependent potassium channels. *J Biol Chem* 266:7583–7587, 1991.

43. Terlau H, et al.: Mapping the site of block by tetrodotoxin and saxitoxin of sodium channel II. *FEBS Lett* 293:93–96, 1991.

44. Heinemann SH, et al.: Calcium channel characteristics conferred on the sodium channel by single mutations. *Nature* 356:441–443, 1992.

45. Nakayama H, et al.: Photolabeled sites with a tetrodotoxin derivative in the domain III and IV of the electroplax sodium channel. *Biochem Biophys Res Commun* 184:900–907, 1992.

46. Gray WR, Olivera BM: Peptide toxins from venomous *Conus* snails. *Ann Rev Biochem* 57:665–700, 1988.

47. Lancelin J-M, et al.: Tertiary structure of conotoxin GIIIA in aqueous solution. *Biochemistry* 30:6908–6916, 1990.

48. Soto K, et al.: Active site of μ-conotoxin GIIIA, a peptide blocker of muscle sodium channels. *J Biol Chem* 266:16989–16991, 1991.

49. Lazdunski M, Renaud J-F: The action of cardiotoxins on cardiac plasma membranes. *Ann Rev Physiol* 44:463–473, 1982.

50. Catterall WA: Neurotoxins that act on voltage-sensitive sodium channels in excitable membranes. *Ann Rev Pharmacol Toxicol* 20:15–43, 1980.

51. Albuquerque EX, Daly JW: Batrachotoxin: A selective probe for channels modulating sodium conductances in electrogenic membranes. In: Chapman and Hall (eds) *The Specificity and Action of Animal, Bacterial and Plant Toxins*, 1976.

52. Khodorov B, Revenko SV: Further analysis of the mechanisms of action of batrachotoxin on the membrane of myelinated nerve. *Neuroscience* 4:1315–1330, 1979.

53. Ulbricht W: The effect of veratridine on excitable membranes of nerve and muscle. *Erg Physiol* 61:18–71, 1969.

54. Narahashi T: Chemicals as tools in the study of excitable membranes. *Physiol Rev* 54:813–889, 1974.

55. Catterall WA, et al.: Binding of batrachotoxinin A 20-α-benzoate to a receptor site associated with sodium channels in synaptic nerve ending particles. *J Biol Chem* 256:8922–8927, 1981.

56. Angelides K, Terakawa S, Brown GB: Spatial relations of the neurotoxin binding sites on the sodium channel. *Ann NY Acad Sci* 479:221–237, 1986.

57. Frelin C, Vigne P, Lazdunski M: The specificity of the sodium channel for monovalent cations. *Eur J Biochem* 119:437–442, 1981.

58. Honerjager P: Cardioactive substances that prolong the open state of sodium channel. *Rev Physiol Biochem Pharmacol* 92:1–74, 1981.

59. Fosset M, et al.: Analysis of molecular aspects of Na^+ and Ca^{2+} uptakes by embryonic cardiac cells in culture. *J Biol Chem* 252:6112–6117, 1977.

60. Horackova M, Vassort G: Ionic mechanism of inotropic effect of veratridine on frog heart. *Pflügers Arch* 341:281–284, 1973.

61. Romey G, Lazdunski M: Lipid-soluble toxins thought to be specific for Na^+ channels block Ca^{2+} channels in neuronal cells. *Nature* 297:79–80, 1982.

62. Knox JR, Slobbe J: Three novel alkaloids from *Ervatamina orientalis*. *Tetrahedron Lett A* 26:2149–2151, 1971.

63. Frelin C, et al.: The interaction of ervatamine and epiervatamine with the action potential Na^+ ionophore. *Mol Pharm* 20:107–112, 1981.

64. Adam KR, et al.: Effect of scorpion venom on single myelinated nerve fibers of the frog. *Br J Pharmacol* 26:666–677, 1966.

65. Koppenhofer E, Schmidt H: Die wirkung von skorpiongift auf die ionenstrome des ranvierschen schnurrings I. Die permeabilitaten P_{Na} und P_K. *Pflügers Arch* 303:133–149, 1968.

66. Jover E, Couraud F, Rochat H: Two types of scorpion neurotoxins characterized by their binding to two separate receptor sites on rat brain synaptosomes. *Biochem Biophys Res Commun* 95:1607–1614, 1980.

67. Catterall WA: Membrane potential-dependent binding of scorpion toxin to the action potential Na^+ ionophore. *J Biol Chem* 252:8660–8667, 1977.

68. Fontecilla-Camps JC, et al.: Three-dimensional structure of a protein from scorpion venom: A new structural class of neurotoxins. *Proc Natl Acad Sci USA* 77:6496–6500, 1980.

69. Fontecilla-Camps JC, Habersetzer-Rochat C, Rochat H: Orthorhombic crystals and three-dimensional structure of the potent toxin II from the scorpion *Androctonus australis* Hector. *Proc Natl Acad Sci USA* 85:7443–7447, 1988.

70. Sampieri F, Habersetzer-Rochat C: Structure-function relationships in scorpion neurotoxins. *Biochim Biophys Acta* 535:100–109, 1978.

71. Fogh RH, Kem WR, Norton RS: Solution structure of neurotoxin I from the sea anemone *Stichodactyla helianthus*. *J Biol Chem* 265:13016–13028, 1990.

72. Catterall WA, Beress L: Sea anemone toxin and scorpion toxin share a common receptor site associated with the

action potential sodium ionophore. *J Biol Chem* 253: 7393–7396, 1978.

73. Barhanin M, et al.: Structure-function relationships of sea anemone toxin II from *Anemonia sulcata*. *J Biol Chem* 256:5764–5769, 1981.

74. Gould AR, Mabbutt BC, Norton RS: Structure-function relationships in the polypeptide cardiac stimulant anthopleurin A. *Eur J Biochem* 189:145–153, 1990.

75. Gallagher MJ, Blumenthal KM: Cloning and expression of wild-type and mutant forms of the cardiotonic polypeptide anthopleurin B. *J Biol Chem* 267:13958–13963, 1992.

76. Vassilev PM, Scheuer T, Catterall WA: Identification of an intracellular peptide fragment involved in sodium channel inactivation. *Science* 241:1658, 1988.

77. Coraboeuf E, Deroubaix E, Tazieff-Depierre P: Effect of toxin II isolated from scorpion venom on action potential and contraction of mammalian heart. *J Mol Cell Cardiol* 7:643–653, 1975.

78. Ravens U: Electromechanical studies of an *Anemonia sulcata* toxin in mammalian cardiac muscle. *Naunyn-Schmiedebergs Arch Pharmacol* 296:73–78, 1976.

79. Romey G, et al.: Pharmacological properties of the interaction of sea anemone polypeptide toxins with cardiac cells in culture. *J Pharm Exp Ther* 213:607–615, 1980.

80. Shibata S, et al.: Further studies of the positive inotropic effect of the polypeptide anthopleurin A from a sea anemone. *J Pharmacol Exp Ther* 205:685–692, 1978.

81. Alsen C, et al.: The action of a toxin from the sea anemone *Anemonia sulcata* upon mammalian heart muscles. *Naunyn-Schmiedebergs Arch Pharmacol* 295:55–62, 1976.

82. Shibata S, et al.: A polypeptide (ApA) from sea anemone (*Anthopleura xanthogrammica*) with potent positive inotropic action. *J Pharmacol Exp Ther* 199:298–309, 1976.

83. Couraud F, et al.: The interaction of polypeptide neurotoxins with tetrodotoxin-resistant Na$^+$ channels in mammalian cardiac cells. *Eur J Pharmacol* 120:161–170, 1986.

84. Isenberg G, Ravens U: The effects of the *Anemonia sulcata* toxin (ATX II) on membrane currents of isolated mammalian myocytes. *J Physiol* 357:127–149, 1984.

85. Schreibmayer W, Kazerani H, Tritthart HA: A mechanistic interpretation of the action of toxin II from *Anemonia sulcata* on the cardiac sodium channel. *Biochim Biophys Acta* 901:273–282, 1987.

86. El-Sharif N, Fozzard HA, Hanck DA: Dose-dependent modulation of the cardiac sodium channel by sea anemone toxin ATX II. *Circ Res* 70:285–301, 1992.

87. Jacques Y, et al.: Interaction of pyrethroids with the Na$^+$ channel in mammalian neuronal cells in culture. *Biochim Biophys Acta* 600:882–897, 1980.

88. Gonoi T, et al.: Mechanism of action of a polypeptide neurotoxin from the coral *Goniopora* on sodium channels in mouse neuroblastoma cells. *Mol Pharmacol* 29:347–354, 1986.

89. Fujiwara M, et al.: Effects of *Goniopora* toxin, a polypeptide isolated from coral, on electromechanical properties of rabbit myocardium. *J Pharmacol Exp Ther* 210:153–157, 1979.

90. Qar J, et al.: A polypeptide toxin from the coral *Goniopora*. Purification and action on calcium channels. *FEBS Lett* 202:331–335, 1986.

91. Murakami Y, Oshima Y, Yasumoto T: Identification of okadaic acid as a toxic component of a marine dinoflagellate *Prorocentrum lima*. *Bull Jpn Soc Sci Fish* 48:69–72, 1982.

92. Bidard JN, et al.: Ciguatoxin is a novel type of sodium channel toxin. *J Biol Chem* 259:8353–8357, 1984.

93. Poli MA, Mende TJ, Baden DG: Brevetoxins, unique activators of voltage-sensitive sodium channels, bind to specific sites in rat brain synaptosomes. *Mol Pharmacol* 30:129–135, 1986.

94. Huang JMC, Wu CH: Mechanism of the toxic action of T17 brevetoxin on nerve membranes. In: Anderson DM, et al. (eds) *Toxic Dinoflagellates*. New York: Elsevier, 1985, pp 351–356.

95. Catterall WA, Risk M: Toxin T4$_6$ from *Ptychodiscus brevis* enhances activation of voltage-sensitive sodium channels by veratridine. *Mol Pharmacol* 19:345–348, 1981.

96. Catterall WA, Gainer M: Interaction of brevetoxin A with a new receptor site on the sodium channel. *Toxicon* 23: 497–504, 1985.

97. Schreibmayer M, Jeglitsch G: The sodium channel activator brevetoxin-3 uncovers a multiplicity of different open states of the cardiac sodium channel. *Biochim Biophys Acta* 1104: 233–242, 1992.

98. Takahashi M, et al.: Calcium channel activating function of maitotoxin, the most potent marine toxin known, in clonal rat pheochromocytoma cells. *J Biol Chem* 258:10944–10949, 1983.

99. Ohizumi Y, Yasumoto T: Contractile response of the rabbit aorta to maitotoxin. *J Physiol* 337:711–721, 1983.

100. Kobayashi M, Ohizumi Y, Yasumoto T: The mechanism of action of maitotoxin in relation to calcium movements in guinea-pig and rat cardiac muscles. *Br J Pharmacol* 86: 385–391, 1985.

101. Kobayashi M, et al.: Cardiotoxic effects of maitotoxin, a principal toxin of seafood poisoning, on guinea pig and rat cardiac muscle. *J Pharmacol Exp Ther* 238:1077–1083, 1986.

102. Chatwal GS, Hessler HJ, Habermann E: The action of palytoxin on erythrocytes and resealed ghosts. Formation of small, nonselective pores linked with Na$^+$,K$^+$-ATPase. *Naunyn-Schmiedebergs Arch Pharmacol* 323:261–268, 1983.

103. Catterall WA: Structure and function of voltage-sensitive ion channels. *Science* 242:50–61, 1988.

104. Kerr LM, Yoshikami D: A venom peptide with a novel presynaptic blocking mechanism. *Nature* 308:282–284, 1984.

105. Feldman DM, Olivera BM, Yoshikami D: Omega *Conus geographus* toxin: A peptide that blocks calcium channels. *FEBS Lett* 214:295–300, 1987.

106. McCleskey EW, et al.: Omega-conotoxin: Direct and persistent blockade of specific types of calcium channels in neurons but not muscle. *Proc Natl Acad Sci USA* 84: 4327–4331, 1987.

107. Leonard JP, et al.: Calcium channels induced in xenopus oocytes by rat brain mRNA. *J Neurosci* 7:875–881, 1987.

108. Llinas R, et al.: Blocking and isolation of a calcium channel from neurons in mammals and cephalopods utilizing a toxin fraction (FTX) from funnel-web spider poison. *Proc Natl Acad Sci USA* 86:1689–1693, 1989.

109. Skinner WS, et al.: Purification and characterization of two classes of neurotoxins from the funnel web spider, *Agelenopsis aperta*. *J Biol Chem* 265:2150–2155, 1990.

110. Adams ME, et al.: Omega-agatoxins: Novel calcium channel antagonists of two subtypes from funnel web spider venom. *J Biol Chem* 265:861–867, 1990.

111. Bowers CW, et al.: Identification and purification of an irreversible presynaptic neurotoxin from the venom of the spider *Hololena curta*. *Proc Natl Acad Sci USA* 84: 3506–3510, 1987.

112. Lin J-W, Rudy B, Llinas R: Funnel-web spider venom and a toxin fraction block calcium current expressed from rat brain

mRNA in *Xenopus* oocytes. *Proc Natl Acad Sci USA* 87: 4538–4542, 1990.

113. Venema VJ, et al.: Antagonism of synaptosomal calcium channels by subtypes of omega-agatoxins. *J Biol Chem* 267:2610–2615, 1992.

114. Mintz IM, et al.: P-type calcium channels blocked by the spider toxin, omega-aga-IVA. *Nature* 355:827–829, 1992.

115. Lundy PM, Hong A, Frew R: Inhibition of a dihydropyridine, omega-conotoxin insensitive Ca^{2-} channel in rat synaptosomes by venom of the spider *Hololena curta*. *Eur J Pharmacol* 225:51–56, 1992.

116. Moczydlowski E, Lucchesi K, Ravindran A: The emerging pharmacology of peptide toxins targeted against potassium channels. *J Membr Biol* 105:95–111, 1988.

117. Garcia ML, et al.: Use of toxins to study potassium channels. *J Bioenerg Biomemb* 23:615–646, 1991.

118. Park C-S, Miller C: Mapping function to structure in a channel-blocking peptide: Electrostatic mutants of charybdotoxin. *Biochemistry* 31:7749–7755, 1992.

119. Park C-S, Miller C: Interaction of charybdotoxin with permeant ions inside the pore of a K^+ channel. *Neuron* 9:307–313, 1992.

120. Bontems F, et al.: Analysis of side-chain organization on a refined model of charybdotoxin: Structural and functional implications. *Biochemistry* 31:7756–7764, 1992.

CHAPTER 34

Cellular Electrical Activity of the Myocardium: Possible Electrophysiological Basis for Myocardial Contractility Changes

STEVEN R. HOUSER, ROBERT E. TENEICK, & ARTHUR L. BASSETT

INTRODUCTION

The myocardial cell hypertrophies in response to a sustained increase in workload, including pressure overload due to valvular stenosis or systemic hypertension; volume overload because of an AV fistula, other defects in the heart pump, or hypervolemia; and sustained increase in heart rate. It can also be subsequent to regional damage brought about by acute or chronic ischemia and infarction, by nutritional and hormonal disturbances, and by dynamic {1} and isometric exercise {2}. There are numerous changes concomitant, and perhaps associated, with myocardial hypertrophy, including recently described electrophysiological alterations. Hypertrophy may be compensatory, allowing the heart to normalize the increased workload per unit of myocardium. If hypertrophy is insufficient, pump failure ensues {3,4}. This review is limited to an examination of changes occurring in a common well-studied form of hypertrophy, that provoked by pressure overload. We describe and emphasize the electrophysiologic and ionic changes associated with this form of hypertrophy that might be involved in the altered contractile properties of the heart. We also consider pertinent mechanical, structural, and biochemical findings. We refer to other models and to naturally occurring disease-induced hypertrophy when relevant.

STRUCTURAL CHANGES IN HYPERTROPHY

Ultrastructural and structural changes occurring in dilated and hypertrophic heart may provide a partial explanation for altered contractile properties. Changes in sarcomere length and sarcomere banding patterns, including slippage of fibrils and enlargement of the cross-sectional area of muscle cells, occur in hypertrophy {15}, but substantial changes are usually only found in the failing heart. This enlargement reflects changes in subcellular structures and compartments involved in excitation and excitation-contraction coupling, including sarcolemma and T tubules, interstitial "extracellular space," sarcoplasmic reticulum, and mitochondria {6}. Increase in sarcoplasmic volume is associated with an extensive vesiculation of the sarcolemmal membranes {5}, described as *cardiac villi* or arcade-

like diverticulae. Multiple pinocytotic vesicles in close approximation to either surface of sarcolemmal membranes may reflect a need of hypertrophied cells to increase membrane surface area. Mitochondria tend to congregate near the sarcolemma, suggesting that during hypertrophy they provide energy to ion transport processes occurring at or near surface membranes {7}.

Hypertrophy-induced changes that are expected to alter cell-to-cell impulse conduction occur in the low-resistance pathways of the intercalated discs. In response to prolonged exercise, there are focal increases in the width of the gap junctions of intercalated discs, and vesicles exhibiting a moderately dense matrix appear in the gap region. The vesiculation serves to increase both the volume and surface area of the gap region involved in the intercellular transfer of ions and cell-to-cell communication {5}. Whether these focal increases in gap junctional width actually affect either impulse conduction or contraction is unclear. Gap junctions in intercalated discs of human hearts with mitral stenosis, congenital heart disease, myocardial fibrosis {8}, and idiopathic cardiomyopathy can separate {9}, but whether this structural change correlates with electrophysiologic disturbances in such hearts remains to be determined {10}.

Hypertrophy is characterized by an increase in the number of mitochondria, but there is controversy concerning the ratio of myofibrils to mitochondria. It has been suggested that hypertrophy evokes an increase in the relative amount of contractile material to be supplied with energy by mitochondria such that an imbalance of energy relationships can develop {11}. However, other studies fail to show a change in the ratio of these two structures {5}. Mitochondrial degeneration is evident in end-stage hypertrophy and idiopathic cardiomyopathy {9}. While there are indications that mitochondria and mitochondrial function and internal ultrastructure are altered in hypertrophy, the relation of changes in energy "status" to electrical and contractile changes is still unclear at present.

Dilatation of the transverse-tubule (T-tubule) system and the appearance of a fine granular material within the T tubules has been noted in hypertrophied, anoxic, hypoxic, and ischemic hearts {5}. During hypertrophy the T system expands markedly, dilating {12} as well as enlarging longitudinally. In clinical cases of idiopathic cardiac hyper-

653

trophy with or without muscular aortic stenosis, T tubules are particularly enlarged and expanded longitudinally {9,12}. Although the T system has an important role in the transmission of the surface action potential and the associated membrane current into the depths of the sarcomere, it is not clear if and to what extent changes in T-system morphology contribute to contractility changes associated with hypertrophy.

Because the significance of changes in ultrastructural morphology with respect to functional changes in hypertrophy remains to be elucidated, several animal models of cardiac hypertrophy have received attention. The rat heart has been used for numerous studies of mechanical, and more recently, electrical alterations associated with hypertrophy (see below). Concomitant changes in cellular anatomy and ultrastructure are of particular interest. A detailed examination of pressure-overload-induced changes in ultrastructure of rat ventricular cells using quantitative morphometry was accomplished by Page and McCallister {11}. Chronic partial constriction of the ascending aorta produced left ventricular systolic hypertension and progressively increased myocardial cell size. Ten or more days after aortic constriction, the fraction of cell volume occupied by myofibrils was uniformly increased, while the fraction of cell volume composed of mitochondria decreased. The volume and cross-sectional diameter and area of hypertrophied rat ventricular cells increase {11}. Yet hypertrophied cells have a smaller than normal surface area to volume ratio. The ratio change may affect the ability of hypertrophic cells to maintain homeostasis because of increased demand on the plasma membrane to perform vital functions, including uptake of metabolic nutrients from the blood and interstitial spaces, outward transport of waste products and metabolic intermediates into the interstitial space and blood, and finally, movements of ions associated with electrical excitation. However, Page and McCallister suggest that pressure-overloaded hypertrophied rat ventricular cells compensate for the decrease in surface-to-volume ratio by increasing the area of plasma membrane lining the T system. As cells expand in diameter, additional T-system membrane is generated so that the ratio of sarcolemmal membrane enclosing both the external and internal cell volumes remains constant, the cells becoming honeycombed with T-system channels that presumably contain extracellular fluid {11}.

Wendt-Gallitelli and Jacob {13} evaluated morphologic changes in heart tissue of Goldblatt rats during the compensatory stage of gradually provoked pressure-induced cardiac hypertrophy. Marked increases in myocardial cell size occurred within the first 4 weeks after renal artery coarctation; particularly evident was an enlargement of the T-tubule system. Their observation that the transverse tubular system and the sarcoplasmic reticulum increased in parallel with the enlarging cell volume and myofibrillar mass agrees with Page and McCallister {11}. Using aortic constriction, Goldstein et al. {14} also described ultrastructural changes in the left ventricle after gradual aortic constriction in the rabbit. Distortions of intercalated discs and widening of the Z bands were noted.

The significance of these morphologic changes with respect to altered cellular electrical activity noted by Aronson {15} in the Goldblatt rat model is considered below.

The nature of the stimulus provoking enlargement of the T-tubular space is unclear. Acute exercise, anoxic cardiac arrest, and ischemia produce T-tubule enlargement {16}. Transmitter-induced efflux of Cl$^-$ produces T-tubule dilation in crayfish skeletal muscle, and it is known that intracellular Cl$^-$ activity (a_i^{Cl}) decreases significantly in skeletal muscle during exhaustive work (see Tomanek and Banister {16} for a review). A number of papers (e.g., Horwood and Beznak {17}) document myocardial fluid and electrolyte shifts after imposition of aortic coarctation, but whether efflux of cellular Cl$^-$ is altered in the chronically pressure-overloaded ventricle is not known.

Anversa et al. {18} and Weiner et al. {19} have evaluated hypertrophic changes induced by experimental renal hypertension by examining morphometrically endocardial and epicardial myocytes in rat left ventricle. In normal ventricle, endocardial regions contain 30% more myocytes, but less interstitial space and capillary volume than epicardium, while capillary length per unit of tissue volume is similar. The cytoplasmic composition and surface areas of normal endocardial and epicardial myocytes are nearly identical. After 1–4 weeks of hypertension, endocardial myocytes enlarged 26% and epicardial myocytes enlarged 37%, while the number of myocytes and total length of capillaries remained constant in both areas. In the epicardial region, interstitial volume increased proportionately, whereas in the endocardium there was a disproportionate 55% increase in interstitial components. Hypertrophy of epicardial myocytes was accompanied by a reduced mitochondria to myofibril ratio and proportionately large increases (2–3×) in smooth endoplasmic reticulum and T-system volume and surface area. Regional differences also developed in rats with banded aortas {20}, the morphometric characteristics of myocytes from hypertensive rats are significantly different from normal, and significant differences occur between the inner and outer layers of the myocardium. These changes may have functional significance. Gulch {21} believes cell location (endocardial vs. epicardial) during pressure overload to be a factor in determining the degree of action potential changes associated with hypertrophy.

Marino et al. have described the effects of right ventricular hypertrophy on the cellular anatomy of a cat preparation extensively used for mechanical and electrophysiological studies {22}. Two weeks after partial chronic pulmonary artery occlusion, significant increases in myocyte cross-sectional area and diameter occurred with a concurrent increase in the volume density of interstitial tissue; there were no alterations in the volume density of organelles in hypertrophied myocytes. The authors suggest that a substantial increase in the proportion of connective tissue and a decrease in the surface area to volume ratio may represent early structural changes that directly relate to the abnormal contractile function found in this hypertrophy model {22}.

In summary, it appears from detailed ultrastructural studies that both sarcolemmal surface area and the surface area and volume of the T-tubule system increase in response to hypertrophy. Thus, total membrane area, including the area contiguous with the cell surface and that in abutment with the sarcoplasmic reticulum, increases. Enlargement of the T-tubule system in hypertrophic cells may reflect, in part, an adaptation intended to maintain normal excitation-contraction coupling as the cell enlarges. It is via these invaginations that penetrate the cell interior that the action potential "reaches" efficiently into the enlarged cell; also the lumenal membrane of the T-tubule canals may serve as a carrier system for cations, especially Ca^{2+}.

STIMULUS TO HYPERTROPHY

There are probably several signals linking physiologic stress to biochemical responses during hypertrophy {4,23–27}. Recently, this has been an area of active research and will not be reviewed extensively here. It has been suggested that hypertrophy may be provoked by norepinephrine via activation of protein kinase C {27} or pressure per se, perhaps by fiber stretch {26}. The stimulus may act directly on the myocardial nucleus or may act indirectly by a sequence of events such as the following: Increased Ca^{2+} from the sarcoplasmic reticulum would enhance the activation of PKC and protein phosphorylation, and, in turn, protein synthesis. In addition, nuclear cyclic AMP, which controls the synthesis of certain proteins in a variety of tissues, may be an important regulator in hypertrophy {28}. These hypotheses are currently being actively investigated.

Meerson {3} has described three states or stages of hypertrophy in the mammalian ventricle after chronic partial aortic or pulmonary artery occlusion. Stage 1 is a period of developing hypertrophy, often with contractile dysfunction. Stage 2 is stable hypertrophy with "normal" or even enhanced contractility. During stage 3, the hypertrophied heart demonstrates gradual contractile impairment and eventual "failure." Hatt et al. {29} have reviewed the structural characteristics of hypertrophy in terms of Meerson's scheme and have found that degenerative changes are more frequent when the load is more severe {30}. Factors related to the development of physiologic (stage 2) versus pathologic hypertrophy (stage 3) have been reviewed by Wikman-Coffelt et al. {4}. Major determinants include the degree and duration of ventricular wall stress, the nature of the inciting stimulus, the specific ventricle affected, as well as the species, age, and health of the animal. Most inducers of hypertrophy appear to act via a common mechanical-biochemical coupling mechanism. Work overload causes increased wall tension and pressure on myocardial cells, and stretches the muscle fibers. Mediated or modulated by norepinephrine release, the stretch and associated increased fiber strain augment RNA transcription and protein synthesis. Then, depending on the severity of the workload, secondary factors, such as increased tissue pCO_2 or low O_2, determine whether the heart can adjust to an elevation in workload by developing the characteristics of either physiologic or pathologic hypertrophy, i.e., does the force developed during contraction remain the same or even increase, or does a major deficit in ventricular function and contractility ensue? The role of cytokines, released from nonmyocytes during hypertrophy, on myocardial contractility has not yet been evaluated.

A number of studies indicate that hypertrophy in the well-characterized pressure overloaded cat right ventricle is a "local response" to an increased load. In an extensive series of experiments on cat heart, Cooper et al. {31} have surgically "unloaded" right ventricular papillary muscle after a period of chronically overloading the right ventricle; in other experiments, epicardial denervation and then pressure overloading was employed to assess the role of local neurogenic catecholamines in the genesis of hypertrophy. Their data suggest that catecholamines are not the major stimulus to hypertrophy under these conditions. The role of circulating catecholamines in these experiments is less clear. Cardiac hypertrophy appears to occur only in those cells in which stress and/or strain are increased. However, the molecular biology of the processes underlying myocardial hypertrophy remains to be clarified. Interestingly, a recent study by Sadoshima et al. {26} shows that myocyte stretch can activate PKC and produce hypertrophy. This finding suggests that both myocyte stretch and alpha-adrenergic stimulation {27} may produce hypertrophy by activation of PKC.

ELECTROMECHANICAL CHANGES IN HYPERTROPHY

The temporal stages of contractile function following pressure overload (ventricular systolic hypertension) have been studied using isolated ventricular muscles and single isolated myocytes from mammals and appear to vary both with the degree and duration of pressure overload, and the species used. An important advance toward understanding the pathophysiology of hypertrophic heart was development of chronic pressure-overload-induced cardiac hypertrophy failure in a cat model {32}. Active force and the force-velocity relation were markedly decreased in right ventricular muscles isolated from cats with overt chronic right heart failure (Meerson, stage 3, depressed contractility). The contractility of the intact cat right ventricle also was depressed {32,33}. Depression of active force has been confirmed by others {34,35}. Several groups have established that chronic pressure overload of the right ventricle in cat without cardiac failure (via sudden imposition of partial pulmonary artery occlusion) results in depression of the force-velocity relationship in isolated right ventricular muscles studied in vitro {32,33}. Active force and the maximum rate of development of force also are reduced {36}, and significant differences in the force-interval relation, as demonstrated by changes in the responses to altered rhythms, including postextrasystolic potentiation, are seen {37,38}. There has been some concern that the contractile changes noted in this animal model are related to the acute onset of the pressure overload, possibly because of transient ischemia {38}.

However, Cooper et al. {39} have produced right ventricular hypertrophy in cat by a nonacute progressive overload and have documented depressed velocity of shortening and active force, while time to peak force is prolonged. Recently, Bailey and Houser have found similar mechanical derangements in left ventricular myocytes induced by slow progressive pressure overload {38}. It seems reasonable to suggest that passive stiffness increases in hypertrophied right ventricular papillary muscles from cats with pulmonary artery constriction {40,41}, but this may depend on the mode of constriction {42}.

Most of the early electrophysiologic studies of pressure-overload induced hypertrophy used the cat model of right ventricular hypertrophy (pulmonary artery coarctation). Although Kaufman et al. {34} reported no differences in the electrophysiologic properties of normal vs. hypertrophied papillary muscles despite decreased velocity of shortening, a later study by the same group revealed prolonged action potentials, decreased resting potential, and reduced upstroke velocity after 3 weeks of exposure to pressure overload {43}. Right ventricular muscles studied 3 days after partial pulmonary artery occlusion and without congestive heart failure exhibited action potentials, with a rather depressed voltage during the plateau phase associated with decreased active force and rate of force development and increased time to peak force {44,45}. Ten Eick et al. {46,47} and Nuss and Houser {48} reported that in specimens of right ventricle, hypertrophied by PA banding 5–7 months prior to study, plateau voltage was depressed and action potential duration was significantly prolonged. Thus, action potential changes may persist for at least several months following initiation of pressure overload. Recent studies of isolated myocytes support these data {38,48}.

Possible reasons for the somewhat conflicting results of previous studies include different degrees of hypertrophy and slightly different experimental protocols. Bassett and Gelband {44} examined the action potentials at a single stimulus rate of 30/min in moderate hypertrophy, while Ten Eick et al. {46} used several stimulus rates ranging from 12 to 240 beats/min in more severe hypertrophy. Ten Eick and Bassett {47,49}, therefore, examined the possibilities that the magnitude of the changes in the action potential were determined by either the severity of the hypertrophy or by the stimulus rate. In general, the more hypertrophied the right ventricle, the greater was the depression of the plateau voltage and the more prolonged was the action potential duration. At a stimulus rate of 30/min in mildly hypertrophied muscle, however, the action potentials were indistinguishable from normal, except for a very slight decrease in the repolarization rate during phase 3. This finding confirmed the earlier data {44}. Interestingly, even in mildly hypertrophic preparations, when stimulated at rates of 60 beats/min or greater, it was possible to detect some prolongation of the duration associated with a slowing of the repolarization rate during phase 3. In moderately and severely hypertrophic muscles, at all stimulus rates, plateau voltage was depressed, repolarization rate during phase 3 was slowed, and duration was increased, particularly during the latter portion of

phase 3. The plateau depression was about 5–8 mV, ranging from 4 mV to as much as 15 mV. The implications of such a change in plateau voltage with regard to depression of cardiac contractility will be discussed later. These results have led Ten Eick and Bassett {47} to suggest that (a) the changes in the action potentials of cat heart subjected to pressure overload do not normalize with time, instead they persist; (b) the changes become more intensified as the severity of the hypertrophy becomes more severe; and (c) the extent of the changes is more evident at heart rates of 60/min or more than at slower rates.

Regional variation in the transient depression of the plateau voltage in cat right ventricular pressure overloaded for 3 days also has been documented {49,50} and may correlate with the area of greatest mechanical stress evoked by the ventricular pressure overload. Cameron et al. {51} monitored the regional variation in plateau voltage following partial pulmonary artery occlusion. The degree of hypertrophy, as indicated by the right ventricular free wall weight to body weight ratio, appears to be a factor determining the number of cells with an abnormal plateau voltage in the pressure-overloaded ventricle. Regional alterations in this study were most apparent on the right ventricular free wall near the tricuspid valve, an area perhaps the most stressed or dilated by sudden outflow tract occlusion. Regional variations in the action potential changes also are found in cat right ventricle after pressure overload for 5–7 months {48}. Regional variation is not restricted to this model. Aronson {52} has indicated that action potentials recorded from endocardial and epicardial sites in the Goldblatt rat model of hypertrophy also have a much wider variation in action potential configuration than in normal rat heart. These results are again consistent with the notion that action potential changes are related to the severity of the hypertrophy and/or the inciting stress.

Right ventricular hypertrophy induced by partial pulmonary artery occlusion in the rabbit {53–55} is associated with decreased velocity of shortening; decreased rate of force development, but without change in active force; and an increase in the time to peak force. In an electrophysiologic study of long-term (>5 months) pressure overload induced by pulmonary artery of aortic constriction, also in rabbits, Konishi {56} reported no change in ventricular resting potential, and action potential duration and amplitude. However, inspection of those data reveals a depression in action potential plateau voltage similar to that noted by Ten Eick et al. {46–48}. Using a rabbit volume-overload model of ventricular hypertrophy produced by experimentally induced hyperthyroidism, Sharp {57} has recently reported depression of the plateau voltage and slowing of repolarization during phase 3. These studies suggest action potential alteration is common to many species with hypertrophy.

Recently, Cameron et al. {58} have characterized cellular morphologic and electrical abnormalities occurring in cats with partial supracoronary aortic occlusion. The durations of randomly sampled action potentials recorded from left ventricular myocardium outside of patchy fibrotic areas were prolonged. This latter finding in nonfibrotic tissues is similar to that obtained from the hypertrophic right ventricle of cat {47}.

Capasso et al. {59} report resting left ventricular muscle compliance in rat is unaltered by renovascular hypertension-induced hypertrophy. Others have reported decreased cardiac distensibility 24 weeks after renal occlusion in the same model {60,61}, which may be related to an increase in the collagen content of the heart {62}. However, the renal hypertensive rat model of gradually induced myocardial hypertrophy does not appear to develop a phase of severe cellular damage and loss of myocardial contractility. Thus, the phase 1 stage of hypertrophy (depressed contractility with a suddenly imposed overload) described by Meerson {3} may not be applicable to all models. Studies of the mechanical properties of rat left ventricle during hypertrophy induced by aortic constriction report a decrease {37} or no change {63–66} in developed force, an increase {59,64} or no change {37,67} in time to peak force, an increase in time to peak shortening {65}, and a decrease in the velocity of shortening {37,63,64}. Gradual pulmonary artery constriction in young rats also produced significant hypertrophy with no impairment of force-generation or shortening velocity {67}. Unfortunately, these studies include no electrical data.

Electrophysiologic changes brought about by pressure overload of the rat left ventricle have been studied by Aronson {15} and Gulch {21,69,70}; and Capasso et al. {59} have summarized the electrophysiological and contractile alterations in hypertrophied rat ventricle. When left ventricle hypertrophy was gradually induced by renal hypertension, developed tension increased {59,60,68,71} or was not affected {59,67}, time to peak tension increased {21,59,63,64,71}, maximum velocity of shortening decreased {60,63,71}, and action potential duration {15, 21,69} invariably increased without significant changes in resting potential, action potential amplitude, overshoot, or maximum rate of rise of the upstroke. Moreover, Gulch et al. {69,70} observed a prolongation of action potential duration, which became more marked as the degree of hypertrophy became more severe. Thus, changes in cellular electrical activity associated with hypertrophy in rat heart are qualitatively quite similar to those observed in hypertrophic cat right ventricle {46–49}. Similar results were also seen in ventricular muscle from spontaneously hypertensive rats {73–75}.

Lengthening of action potential duration in rat and cat is not restricted only to hypertrophy induced by pressure overload. Tibbits et al. {72} noted that left ventricular papillary muscles from female rats run on a treadmill had altered electrical and mechanical properties when studied in tissue bath. Muscles from the trained rats generated greater peak isometric twitch tension per unit cross-sectional area than the control group. At the same time, while the action potentials were unchanged with respect to resting potential, action potential amplitude or overshoot, and APD_{90}, there was a significant prolongation of the action potential measured as time to repolarize to $-50\,mV$.

Aronson {52} has examined, using the renal hypertensive rat model, oscillations in membrane potential (which

have been termed *afterdepolarizations*) thought to be involved in arrhythmiagenesis {76,77}. Afterpotentials could be selectively induced in hypertrophied rat myocardium. Thus afterpotentials and associated triggered activity in pressure-overloaded myocardium may be factors underlying arrhythmia in these hearts.

Keung and Aronson {78} showed that the ventricular hypertrophy induced by renal hypertension in rats that is associated with a generalized lengthening of the action potential duration also causes a reproducible decrease in T-wave amplitude. The change in T-wave configuration of the ECG may result from a difference in the duration of endocardial and epicardial action potentials because there is good correlation between the cellular epicardial to endocardial repolarization gradient (as measured by action potential duration in isolated muscle preparations) and the change in T-wave morphology associated with cardiac hypertrophy {79}.

Action potentials recorded from ventricular tissue taken from the heart of a 42-year-old female with hypertrophic cardiomyopathy have been reported to have longer durations than action potentials recorded from "normal" papillary muscles taken from patients undergoing mitral valve replacement {82}. While this finding has been confirmed by Singer and Ten Eick and their coworkers, it is evident that changes in cellular electrical activity in hypertrophic diseased human heart are much more extensive and intensive {83,84} than those described in animal models of human disease. As in exercised rats {72}, the right atrial monophasic action potential obtained during cardiac catheterization increases in amplitude and duration after physical training in healthy human volunteers {85}. Although not reported even though chest x-rays were taken, it may be that exercise and training led to hypertrophy of the right atrium.

MEMBRANE BASIS OF ACTION POTENTIAL PROLONGATION

An almost universal finding in ventricular cells exposed to chronic pressure overload is increased action potential duration. The ionic basis for this was the subject of several studies using multicellular preparations. Aronson {15} has evaluated the responses of hypertrophied rat myocardium (Goldblatt procedure) to changes in extracellular fluid composition and during exposure to ionic channel blockers. They found that in pressure-overloaded and sham-operated control ventricles, the action potential changes brought about by various testing treatments differed quantitatively. Exposure to high Ca^{2+}-containing or low-Na^+ Tyrode's solution produced greater decreases in action potential duration in hypertrophic myocardium than in normal myocardium. Exposure to D-600, an inhibitor of Ca current, also produced a greater shortening, but its effect in pressure-overloaded muscles was limited to APD_{50}. In contrast, exposure to either Sr^{2+} or TEA instead of Ca^2 in Tyrode's produced an increase in APD_{50} and ADP_{75}, with the effect being similar in both "pressure-overloaded" and "sham-operated" myocardial action potentials. Exposure to Ca^{2+}-free Tyrode's solution had little effect on the action potential duration of either group. None of the treatments had significantly different effects on resting membrane potential or action potential amplitude in either group. One explanation for these results is that the prolongation of action potential duration in hypertrophied rat myocardium was due to slowing of the inactivation of a Ca^{2+}-inactivated inward current {15}. This notion has not been supported by recently obtained voltage-clamp data to be discussed below.

Gulch and coworkers also have manipulated the extracellular environment in hypertrophied (Goldblatt procedure) rat myocardium {69}. After depression of the fast Na^+ inward current by either tetrodotoxin, depolarization produced by augmentation of extracellular K^+ concentration, or by reduction of the extracellular Na^+ concentration, action potentials prolonged by hypertrophy remain prolonged. They concluded that Na current did not contribute importantly to the prolongation of APD. This idea has yet to be tested in detail in single hypertrophy myocytes. Gulch also manipulated the extracellular Ca^{2+} concentration after inhibiting fast Na^+ channel conductance and suggested that in the hypertrophied cells slow inward current was primarily carried by Ca^{2+} ions. From this report {70}, it appears that prolongation of APD could result from either an augmentation of either phasic or steady-state net Ca current or a decrease in either a time-dependent or time-independent net outward repolarizing current.

Ten Eick et al. {48}, using the single sucrose gap technique, examined voltage-clamping membrane current recorded from fine papillary muscles that had been isolated from the right ventricles of cats both with normal hearts and with hearts subjected to right ventricular pressure overload for 5–7 months. Their analysis suggests that, while the overall time course of the membrane current was qualitatively unchanged by hypertrophy, several parameters quantifying the total current and its component parts were altered. Slow inward current amplitude appeared to be reduced at all levels of membrane potential, but neither its voltage dependence nor time course of decay (inactivation rate) were affected. The notion that ventricular hypertrophy can reduce the Ca-dependent slow inward current {48} has received indirect support. Hemwall and Houser {99} have found that the amplitude and duration of slow-response, catecholamine-facilitated, calcium-dependent action potentials were smaller and had shorter durations in hypertrophic cat right ventricular myocardium than in normals. Although this finding can be interpreted as suggesting that hypertrophy can affect Ca current, it also can be explained by findings that cardiac beta-receptor number appears to decrease during hypertrophy {100–102}. Some of these findings have been verified in studies using single cells to be discussed later.

The time course for the development of time-dependent outward-rectifying potassium current was prolonged and its amplitude was reduced at all voltages; its voltage dependence was also shifted positively by about 10 mV {48}. However, the shift in the current-voltage relation does not account for the entire reduction in this component of membrane current. The shape of the current-voltage curve for the instantaneous background current was strikingly altered, having developed a region of negative slope between about −30 and 0 mV {48,49}. It should be mentioned that while inward rectification is seen in the instantaneous background current of normal cat papillary muscle, a negative slope region has never been reported {103}.

In order to extrapolate from the effects of hypertrophy on any of the components of the membrane current to effects on the membrane conductances for each of the currents, one assumes that the transmembrane concentration gradient for the involved ion species is unaltered by either the experimental intervention or the voltage-clamping pulse {104}. The latter is certainly not true in these studies using multicellular preparations, and there are compelling reasons to believe that hypertrophy and failure also affect the ionic concentration gradients {105}. Fluid and electrolyte shifts occur in pressure-overloaded dog and rat ventricle {106,107}. Martin et al. {105} studied electrogenic Na^+ pumping in failing cat papillary muscle. They noted that papillary muscles from the failing hearts had slightly lower resting potentials than those from normal animals and, when the muscles were cooled, resting potentials in both groups depolarized to low levels. However, after 2 hours of hypothermia, upon rewarming to 37°C in 10 mM K^+, the muscles from normal cat hearts abruptly hyperpolarized to −82 mV, a voltage about 14 mV negative to E_K, and then slowly leveled off at −66 mV. Muscles from animals in heart failure also hyperpolarized during rewarming, but to a lesser extent; steady-state potential also leveled off at −66 mV. They suggested that the electrogenic Na^+ pump is depressed in hearts from cats with pulmonary-artery-constriction-induced heart failure. These data can also support other hypotheses. For instance, simple Na-proton exchange could have been depressed (causing a more prolonged but smaller peak Na load), or electrogenic Na-Ca exchange could have been enhanced, offsetting a "normal" Na-pump-induced hyperpolarization.

MEANING AND BASIS FOR THE ELECTROMECHANICAL CHANGES

Several generalizations about hypertrophy emerge from the currently available data. Both the wave shape of the action potential and the contraction are altered in hypertrophy. Most studies on isolated cardiac muscle mechanics in rats and rabbits with cardiac hypertrophy produced by ventricular pressure overload report normal or increased developed tension, decreased velocity of shortening, and increased time to both peak tension and maximal shortening; in the rat model of left ventricular hypertrophy induced by renal hypertension or spontaneous hypertension, action potential duration is prolonged. In cats with right ventricular hypertrophy, developed tension is reduced, velocity of shortening and maximal rate of tension development are decreased, and these mechanical changes are generally associated with depression of plateau voltage, reduced rate of repolarization, and prolonged action potential duration.

The idea that there is a direct causal relationship between the prolongation of the action potential duration and slowing and prolongation of the isometric contraction has recently been evaluated {Nuss and Houser, in review}. There are several studies that demonstrate that the characteristics of the normal isometric contraction can be influenced by the voltage-time course of the membrane depolarization {86–89}. The nature of the relationship between contraction and membrane depolarization is complex and varies with species and experimental conditions, but it is not unreasonable to speculate that despite decreased shortening velocity and rate of tension development, normal levels of developed tension apparently can be maintained in rats and rabbits with left ventricular hypertrophy, at least partly because the duration of contraction is increased, possibly mediated by the prolongation of the plateau phase of the action potential {15,69}. Aronson {15} has shown for rat ventricular muscle that correlation between contraction and duration of depolarization was best for APD_{50} when muscles exhibited relatively short action potentials (sham and pressure-overload relieved muscles), yet the correlation virtually disappeared in hypertrophied muscles that had very long action potentials. Since maximum force development in rat ventricular muscle is affected very little by depolarizations lasting more than 100 ms {90}, it may be that once the action potential has reached a certain duration, active force is no longer influenced by this parameter {15}.

Alternatively, the long-duration action potentials noted in hypertrophied ventricle may be either secondary to or caused by altered contraction. Mechanical deformation can affect cardiac cellular electrical activity in frog heart {91}. Kaufmann et al. {34} have proposed that the duration of the myocardial action potential is influenced by the mode of contraction; isotonic shortening of cat papillary muscle prolongs action potential duration, while isometric force development tends to shorten it. Although extrapolation of these findings in isolated muscle to in situ behavior of muscle fibers in the hypertrophying heart is uncertain, especially in view of pressure-overload-induced or dilatation-induced changes in the connective tissue of the cardiac skeleton {92}, they clearly have implications for physiologic function. The length of various fiber bundles may vary within the walls of a particular chamber, not only during phasic ventricular contraction but also during pressure overload {93; reviewed by Wikman-Coffelt et al. 4}. Wall stress and therefore location of fibers also apparently determine the degree of their hypertrophy {18,19} and, in turn, the degree of prolongation of the action potential duration.

Gulch has noted that left ventricular action potentials in normal rat are prolonged in comparison to the right ventricle. This phenomenon is not specific for the rat, since in cat and guinea pig heart action potentials elicited by papillary muscles from the left ventricle are also prolonged compared to those of the right ventricle. Gulch {70} suggests that the differences between left and right ventricular action potentials are attributed to the differing mechanical loading to which the corresponding myocardial cells are subjected in situ, the left ventricle cells being more loaded. If this is the case, one must likewise propose that differences in the durations of action potentials of subendocardial cells will be prolonged relative to subepicardial cells because of the higher wall stress to which cells in wall layers located in the endocardial region are subjected. Indeed, Gulch {70} noted that action potentials in subendocardium are prolonged compared to subepicardial cells. It is also possible that in vivo loading induces AP changes that do not permanently alter membrane properties. This idea is supported by a study showing no differences in AP wave shape between normal right and left ventricular feline myocytes {94}. Thus, degree of pressure overload, and indirectly the cell location, particularly with respect to the ventricular chamber in which it is located, may be highly significant factors defining the duration of the action potential.

A third possibility is that while both the action potential and contraction change during hypertrophy, there is no direct causal relationship between these alterations. This idea is supported by recent studies in one of our laboratories (Houser, unpublished observations) that showed contractile properties of hypertrophied myocytes were different from normal, even when voltage was controlled with voltage-clamp techniques. These findings suggest that changes in other cell properties, such as regulation of cell Ca^{2+} by the sarcoplasmic reticulum {95,96}, are altered in hypertrophy and produced abnormal contractions.

Changes in collagen synthesis and content accompany ventricular pressure overload in dog {97} and rat {98}. One might speculate about whether they can alter cellular electrical coupling and inhibit propagation of the repolarization wave. Keung and Aronson {78} attempted to assess whether an alteration in cellular electrical coupling contributes to the electrophysiologic changes associated with hypertrophy. They analyzed the steady-state electrotonic voltage profile produced by intracellularly applied constant-current pulses, and found the effective input resistance was unaffected by hypertrophy in rat ventricular cells. They also demonstrated that the action potential prolongation accompanying hypertrophy was not uniform throughout the heart. While the entire time course of repolarization was prolonged in endocardial and papillary muscle fibers, only the latter half of repolarization was prolonged in epicardial fibers. They concluded that altered electrotonic coupling between cells was not an important factor contributing to the prolonged action potential durations seen in hypertrophied myocardium. Therefore, logically one should expect change in membrane ionic channel function to underlie any change in the action potential configuration. As stated above, alterations associated with hypertrophy may affect the intracellular concentration of Ca^{2+} and thus may modulate calcium-dependent membrane properties and ionic gradients or both, and even dissociate the action potential time course from contractile performance.

Martin et al. {105} also studied drive-related changes in extracellular K^+ activity (a_o^K) in muscles from hypertrophied hearts. Ion-selective microelectrodes and morphometric techniques were used. Upon the imposition of a higher driving rate, the a_o^K in the extracellular space reached a maximum and then returned toward a lower steady-state level. This pattern of extracellular K^+ accumulation took significantly longer to unfold in failing muscles than in normal muscles, and the steady-state concentration of K accumulated in the interstitial spaces of failing tissue was significantly higher. However, maximum a_i^K obtained in failing muscles was found to be slightly lower than that in normal muscles. These changes are consistent with previously reported differences in the patterns of drive-related changes in resting potentials measured in normal and failing muscles, and were explained by a decrease in the volume of the interstitial space of hypertrophic heart and an increase in the ionic load on a depressed Na^+-K^+ exchange pump. All of the studies reviewed above are difficult to interpret because of the complex nature of intact cardiac muscle, which makes it difficult to adequately control extracellular ion concentrations and membrane potential (in voltage-clamp studies). These problems have been overcome in studies employing single isolated myocytes.

ELECTROPHYSIOLOGY OF SINGLE HYPERTROPHY MYOCYTES

Until recently the ionic basis for the action potential changes in hypertrophy were not well understood because intact cardiac muscle is not well suited for voltage-clamp studies. With the advent of single isolated myocyte {108} and patch-clamp {109} technologies, these studies could be undertaken. A number of laboratories have examined the status of L-type {110} Ca^{2+} current (I_{ca}) in hypertrophy myocytes. In general these studies have shown no change in I_{ca} density in compensated hypertrophy {111,112}. Kleiman and Houser {111} found that I_{ca} density was unchanged in hypertrophied (without failure) feline RV myocytes, but the rate of I_{ca} inactivation was slowed. Similar results were observed in hypertrophied rat myocytes induced by either pressure overload {112} or growth hormone {113}. These results show that changes in action potential wave shape or contractility in myocytes from hearts with *compensated* hypertrophy probably do not involve alterations in the sarcolemmal density of Ca^{2+} channels. One of these studies {112} showed that while I_{ca} density was unchanged in hypertrophy myocytes, the ability of beta-adrenergic stimulation to increase I_{ca} was reduced. Since sympathetic nerve terminals in the hypertrophied heart have reduced amounts of norepinephrine, I_{ca} may be less than normal in hypertrophied myocardium during times of increased hemodynamic demand that require activation of sympathetic nerves. It should be noted that a single study by Keung {114} has shown that Ca current density is markedly increased in hypertrophy myocytes from animals with renovascular hypertension. The reason for this increase is not clear at present.

The idea that changes in K^+ currents are involved in action potential prolongation in hypertrophy also has recently been studied. Kleiman and Houser {115} showed

that delayed rectifier K currents were reduced in RV hypertrophy myocytes. It is unclear, at present, what the molecular basis for these changes involve. Another K current that is under investigation in our laboratories is the transient outward current (i_{To}) {116}. Ten Eick et al. have found that the fraction of RV cells that express I_{To} is increased and that the average magnitude of I_{To} is also increased in hypertrophy. These changes were associated with reduction in AP plateau height and AP prolongation. These studies suggest, therefore, that alterations in the number and properties of I_{To} channels may be involved in the AP wave shape changes of hypertrophied myocardium {116}.

Recently one of our laboratories has begun studies of single LV myocytes from animals with hypertrophy with or without congestive failure, which is induced by slow progressive pressure overload {38}. One study {48} using severely hypertrophied myocytes showed that I_{ca} density was significantly reduced while the voltage dependence of contraction (discussed below) was not changed. The fact that I_{ca} density is unchanged in hearts with compensatory hypertrophy and is decreased in myocytes from severely hypertrophied hearts with signs of decompensation suggests that a reduced Ca current may be involved in the transition from compensated hypertrophy to congestive failure. This idea deserves further study.

REGRESSION OF HYPERTROPHY

Hypertrophy-induced changes regress rapidly when excessive pressure or volume load on the heart are relieved by decreasing systemic hypertension or operative correction of aortic regurgitation or ventricular septal defect. Whether regression will be complete seems to depend on the degree and duration of hypertrophy, whether heart failure has occurred, as well as the age and health of the animal. Although ventricular hypertrophy regresses after correction of experimental or clinical hemodynamic overload, contractility usually remains depressed. Failure of contractility to return to normal may be related to the fact that connective tissue changes apparently do not regress as readily as do changes in myocardial mass, suggesting that the half-life for myofibrillar material is shorter than that for interstitial collagenous material. Investigations using the cat model have delineated the temporal aspects of regression in right ventricular hypertrophy after release of chronic pulmonary artery occlusion {117,118}. Coulson et al. noted that relief of pressure overload allows reversal of the depression of velocity of shortening and ability to develop force, although catecholamine depletion is still present. A study of intermittent pressure overloading on the development of right ventricular hypertrophy in the cat demonstrates that the regression of hypertrophy is a slower process than its progression {119}.

Little data exist on reversibility of the electrophysiologic changes. This question bears on the hypothesis that electrophysiologic changes partially underlie the contractility changes. Capasso et al. {59,120} have evaluated the electrical and mechanical changes brought about by reversal of pressure overload induced by renal hypertension in rats. Removal of the stimulus for hypertension consists of surgical excision of the left kidney of rats that previously had undergone clipping of the left renal artery. Capasso et al. {120} simultaneously recorded mechanical and electrical activity in sham and hypertrophied papillary muscles. Mechanical and electrical abnormalities described in their earlier studies were reversed in muscles from rats made normotensive for 10 weeks subsequent to 10 weeks of hypertension. The story, however, is far from clear. In one study on a rat model, anomalous contractile properties were reported to persist even after regression of hypertrophy induced by banding the aorta for 5–15 days {64}; in addition, various biochemical abnormalities also are not completely reversed {121}. In contrast, in a cat model of right ventricular pressure overload causing failure and doubling of right ventricular mass, the contractile changes after unloading could be dissociated from hypertrophy; following return of right ventricular pressure to "normal," muscle contractile function returned to normal yet hypertrophy persisted {122}. Pharmacologically induced regression of cardiac hypertrophy in animal models has been reviewed {123}.

AN ELECTROPHYSIOLOGIC BASIS FOR DECREASED CONTRACTILITY

Hypertrophy of the myocardium is associated with and appears to set into motion events at the molecular level that can culminate in depression of contractility and altered sarcolemmal electrophysiologic function. The alterations in electrophysiologic function manifest changes in the membrane action potential and transmembrane current. Voltage-clamp studies of the excitation-contraction process in normal sheep {88,124,125}, beef {89}, and cat {126} hearts indicate that at least one change in the action potential and one in the membrane current of hypertrophic heart could predictably reduce the force of contraction. Force of contraction is strongly influenced both by plateau voltage and by the strength of the Ca current. The relationships between contractile force and these two parameters are intimately intertwined. Membrane potential during the plateau of the action potential also influences the magnitude of the Ca current, and plateau voltage is influenced by the size of the Ca current; both are required to initiate excitation contraction coupling and both influence the force of the twitch.

The relationship between membrane potential and the force of contraction during the myocardial twitch is an S-shaped function that has a threshold near $-40\,\text{mV}$ and reaches a maximum at approximately $+10$ to $+20\,\text{mV}$ when defined with 250- to 800-ms long voltage-clamp pulses {97,126}. Inspection of the voltage-tension relationship reveals that any significant loss of membrane potential during the action potential plateau would exert a negative inotropic effect on twitch force. If the average level of potential during the plateau is reduced from $0\,\text{mV}$ to about $-10\,\text{mV}$, which we have indicated is not atypical for severely hypertrophic myocardium, the force of con-

traction would be expected to be reduced by about 15% from normal just by virtue of this reduction in plateau height and the function defining the relationship between peak twitch force and membrane potential. The reduction of twitch force by 15%, however, is predicted, assuming that hypertrophy does not affect the voltage-tension relationship. This assumption may or may not be valid. Ten Eick et al. {48}, using a sucrose gap voltage-clamp method, have defined the voltage-tension relationships of papillary muscles from both normal and hypertrophic right ventricles of cat. In the voltage range of the plateau, the position of the voltage-tension curve for hypertrophic heart was found to be about $10\,\text{mV}$ positive to that of the curve for normal heart. The voltage threshold for tension development was not much changed by hypertrophy, but the maximal tension in hypertrophic myocardium occurred when membrane potential was about $+30\,\text{mV}$. This shift of $10\,\text{mV}$ in the voltage-tension relationship, if real, means that even if the plateau voltage were unchanged by hypertrophy, twitch force would be reduced by about 15%. Add the 15% reduction in twitch force due to the shift in the voltage-tension relationship to the 15% reduction due to the putative loss of plateau voltage, and the loss of twitch force due to hypertrophy-induced electrophysiologic changes can account for a sizable, functionally significant decrease in myocardial contractility. However, a recent study using single cells from normal and hypertrophied feline left ventricles failed to confirm the above-stated finding {48}. This study showed that the voltage-contraction relationship was unchanged in hypertrophy myocytes. In addition there was no significant change in the plateau height. Importantly, these myocytes had the usual contractile alterations of hypertrophied myocardium, but they were unrelated to an altered voltage dependence of contraction. Other factors, discussed below, appear to be responsible for the reduced contractions of these hypertrophy myocytes. It is unclear at present why these different results have been obtained. However, the possibility of artifacts associated with tissue complexities should not be ignored in older sucrose gap voltage-clamp experiments.

It may be useful to consider that the prolongation of the action potential duration in hypertrophic myocardium is a compensation that helps prolong the contractile duration and thereby ensures adequate ejection in the face of increased afterload. Because of the apparent hypertrophy-related reduction in Ca current {48,111}, it is fortunate that the late (delayed rectifying) repolarizing outward current is also reduced, because if it were not the plateau in hypertrophied myocardium would be rather abbreviated and even greater loss of twitch force would occur.

We speculate that initially, as myocytes hypertrophy, I_{ca} density is maintained and contractile slowing and prolongation occurs by changes in other processes, possibly alterations in cellular Ca^{2+} homeostasis involving the sarcoplasmic reticulum {38,95,96}. As hypertrophy becomes more severe, however, there appears to be a reduction in density of the Ca current. This could be the result of (a) a reduction in the number of conducting Ca channels per cell or per unit area of sarcolemmal membrane (i.e., the same number of channels has to serve a larger membrane area in hypertrophied cells), or (b) hypertrophic-induced change in the probability that Ca channels will conduct under a particular set of conditions, or both. Reduction in density of the Ca current would be expected to cause the amount of activator Ca^{2+} released from the sarcoplasmic reticulum (SR) to be less than normal (if release is graded and not regenerative). In addition, the extent of SR Ca^{2+} loading should be less. Both of these should reduce the systolic level of activator Ca^{2+}. This result has been observed recently in single hypertrophied feline myocytes {38}.

A number of recent studies have shown that Ca homeostasis is altered in hypertrophy. These studies were recently reviewed by Morgan {127}. In general these studies have shown that the Ca^{2+} transient is prolonged in hypertrophy {38,128,129}. In addition, some studies have shown that peak systolic Ca^{2+} is reduced {38}. These changes in activator Ca^{2+} can explain the altered mechanical state of the hypertrophied heart. In particular, such changes can explain the reduced rate and magnitude of force generation (or shortening) and the general prolongation of contraction. The cellular basis for these changes probably involves changes in Ca^{2+} influx (via Ca^{2+} channels {48,111}), SR Ca^{2+} uptake and subsequent release {95,96}, and sarcolemmal Na/Ca exchange {130}. Studies currently underway in a number of laboratories should help resolve the cellular basis of AP and contractile changes in hypertrophy. It will then be necessary to define the molecular basis of these changes.

Extrapolation to intact in situ heart

We and others {38,48,127} have speculated that alterations in Ca^{2+} homeostasis occur in hypertrophy, but what might this mean to cardiac function? Do these changes affect the operation of the heart in situ with an intact sympathetic innervation? It is well known that contractility of the normal heart can be modulated by the level of sympathetic nervous activity playing on the myocardium. It is also well known that Ca current and SR function can be enhanced by norepinephrine and other beta-receptor agonists. Therefore one might wonder whether it matters if hypertrophy alters Ca current and SR function when they can be greatly enhanced by catecholamines in the intact in situ heart. The answer is not clear and may be paradoxical. It is well known that during Meerson's stage 3 of hypertrophy, the in situ myocardium can be moderately to severely depleted of its intrinsic catecholamines. In addition, hypertrophic myocardium has been found to have, relative to normal heart, a reduced number of beta-receptors capable of binding catecholamines {100–102, 131}. This situation is quite different from that found in hearts depleted of catecholamines by chronic sympathectomy. Denervated hearts have an increased number of beta-receptors and are supersensitive to the effects of catecholamines on both electrical and mechanical activity. Hypertrophied cat heart, on the other hand, appears to be subsensitive to catecholamines, as judged by their effects on the twitch and Ca-dependent, slow upstroke action potentials {99}.

Subsensitivity probably reflects a decrease in the number of beta receptors, since receptor ligand binding affinity is either unchanged {101} or increased {102}. However, recent studies {131} suggest that changes in cardiac beta-receptor number and characteristics during the progression of hypertrophy depend on species, the model of pressure overload, and the duration and magnitude of the workload increase. It may be that the effectiveness of the extrinsic neurally mediated compensatory mechanisms to modulate cardiac function is blunted in hypertrophic heart. In any case, because the effects of catecholamines on Ca current seem intimately related to their effects on cellular level of cyclic AMP, this question will not be resolved until more complete information is available on the effect of hypertrophy on the coupling mechanisms between beta-receptor activation and cyclic-AMP generation and metabolism, between cyclic-AMP level and Ca current enhancement, and between Ca current and the release of activator calcium. A recent study by Scamps et al. {112} has addressed these issues to some extent. These authors showed beta-adrenergic enhancement of I_{ca} is reduced in hypertrophy myocytes. These results further support the notion that altered Ca^{2+} homeostasis is centrally involved in the contractile derangements of the hypertrophied hearts.

HYPERTROPHY, ISCHEMIA, AND SUDDEN CARDIAC DEATH

As noted elsewhere in this chapter, a number of clinical conditions may cause or be associated with hypertrophy. The presence of hypertrophied myocardium has been identified as an independent risk factor in sudden cardiac death. It may be that ventricular hypertrophy underlies a tendency to develop potentially lethal arrhythmias {132}. Prior myocardial infarction also may be a risk factor for sudden cardiac death. There are studies indicating that mechanical activity may be altered in infarcted hearts, demonstrating regional hypertrophy {133}. Kozlovskis et al. {134} have shown that areas surrounding healed myocardial infarction in the cat heart are hypertrophied but have diminished norepinephrine concentration. In similarly prepared cats, Gaidee et al. {135} demonstrated enhanced shortening of the ventricular refractory period in fibers proximal to a healed infarction during stellate stimulation. The possibility of enhanced interaction between the autonomic nervous system and factors in locally hypertrophied areas to facilitate production of arrhythmias needs further evaluation. Hypertrophied myocardium or a healed infarct in a chronically pressure-overloaded heart may provide a "substrate" for electrophysiologic alterations that occur during acute ischemia and infarction. Failing hearts may be particularly susceptible; isolated ventricle from cat with right heart failure exhibited decreased resting potential, overshoot, and upstroke velocity (and presumably impaired conduction {47}). Consistent with this notion, Anversa et al. {136} recently reviewed the structural changes in the myocardium during ventricular hypertrophy induced by pressure overload and concluded that hypertrophied myocardium can exhibit structural abnormalities that are expected to increase its vulnerability to ischemia.

As noted above, cat myocardium exposed to long-term left ventricular pressure overload {48,111} shows long-lasting cellular electrophysiological abnormalities. It has also been demonstrated that acute infarction in the presence of long-term pressure overload (with fibrosis) is more "arrhythmogenic" than acute infarction in otherwise normal heart {138}. The mechanisms of these ischemic electrophysiologic disturbances probably involve both transitory ischemia and/or reperfusion phenomena interacting with long-duration action potentials and afterpotentials induced by pressure overload. Another study {139} using Langendorff-perfused hypertrophied rat hearts gives further evidence that pressure-overloaded myocardium is at increased risk to heart rhythm and other electrophysiological disturbances during acute ischemia. Rat hearts made severely hypertrophic by aortic constriction for 6–8 weeks and then studied during Langendorff perfusion show more severe acute ischemia-induced rhythm disturbances and greater tendency towards ventricular fibrillation compared to hearts with mild hypertrophy or normal or sham-operated hearts. Other studies indicate that the ventricular fibrillation threshold is less than normal in hypertrophied hearts, irrespective of whether hypertrophy is induced by aortic constriction-induced ventricular pressure overload {140} or by sustained elevated blood pressure in spontaneously hypertensive rats {141}. Thus interactions between the electrophysiologic abnormalities of the hypertrophied myocardium and its concomitant hemodynamic abnormalities appear to have important implications, but this is still unresolved.

CONCLUSIONS

It is now clear that the electrophysiological and contractile properties change in hypertrophied myocardium and that these changes are proportional to the inciting hemodynamic stress. The cellular basis for these alterations have in part been determined. They include maintenance of I_{ca} density in mild hypertrophy, with a subsequent reduction with severe hypertrophy and heart failure. Changes in K^+ currents also occur and together produce action potentials with somewhat reduced plateau phases and prolonged durations. Changes in the function of the sarcoplasmic reticulum and sarcolemmal Ca^{2+} channels appear to cause a reduction in peak systolic Ca^{2+} and a prolongation of the Ca^{2+} transient. These changes in the Ca^{2+} transient can explain the reduced contractile force and prolongation of contraction, which are characteristic of hypertrophied myocardium.

REFERENCES

1. Sheuer J, Tipton CM: Cardiovascular adaptation to physical training. *Annu Rev Physiol* 39:221–251, 1977.
2. Muntz KH, Gonyea WJ, Mitchell JH: Cardiac hypertrophy in response to an isometric training program in the cat. *Circ Res* 49:1092–1101, 1981.
3. Meerson FZ: The myocardium in hyperfunction, hypertrophy and heart failure. *Circ Res* 25(Suppl 2):1–163, 1969.
4. Wikman-Coffelt J, Parmely WW, Mason DJ: The cardiac hypertrophy process: Analyses of factors determining pathological vs. physiological development. *Circ Res* 45:697–707, 1979.
5. Leyton RA, Sonnenblick EH: Ultrastructure of the failing heart. *Am J Med Sci* 258:304–327, 1969.
6. Bishop SP, Cole CR: Ultrastructural changes in the canine myocardium with right ventricular hypertrophy and congestive heart failure. *Lab Invest* 20:219–229, 1969.
7. Lin HL, Katele KV, Grimm AF: Functional morphology of the pressure- and the volume-hypertrophied rat heart. *Circ Res* 41:830–836, 1977.
8. Kawamura K, Konishi T: Symposium on function and structure of cardiac muscle. 1. Ultrastructure of the cell junction of heart muscle with special reference to its functional significance in excitation, conduction and to the concept of "disease of intercalated disc." *Jpn Circ J* 31:1533–1543, 1967.
9. Sekiguchi M: Electron microscopical observation of the myocardium in patients with idiopathic cardiomyopathy using endomyocardial biopsy. *J Mol Cell Cardiol* 6:111–122, 1974.
10. Kawamuar K, Konishi T: Symposium of function and structure of cardiac muscle. 1. Ultrastructure of the cell junction of heart muscle with special reference to its functional significance in excitation, conduction and to the concept of "disease of intercalated disc." *Jpn Circ J* 31:1533–1543, 1967.
11. Page E, McCallister LP: Quantitative electron microscopic description of heart muscle cells. *Am J Cardiol* 31:172–181, 1973.
12. Meersen H: Ultrastructure of the myocardium: Its significance in myocardial disease. *Am J Cardiol* 22:319–327, 1968.
13. Wendt-Gallitelli MF, Jacob R: Time course of electron microscopic alterations in the hypertrophied myocardium of Goldblatt rats. *Basic Res Cardiol* 73:209–213, 1977.
14. Goldstein MA, Sordahl LA, Schwartz A: Ultrastructural analysis of left ventricular hypertrophy in rabbits. *J Mol Cell Cardiol* 6:265–273, 1974.
15. Aronson RS: Characteristics of action potentials of hypertrophied myocardium from rats with renal hypertension. *Circ Res* 47:443–454, 1980.
16. Tomanek RJ, Banister EW: Myocardial ultrastructure after acute exercise stress with special reference to transverse tubules and intercalated discs. *Cardiovasc Res* 6:671–679, 1972.
17. Horwood DM, Beznak M: Fluid and electrolyte shifts relating cardiac hypertrophy with normal growth. *Can J Physiol Pharmacol* 49:951–958, 1971.
18. Anversa P, Loud AV, Giacomelli F, Wiener J: Absolute morphometric study of myocardial hypertrophy in experimental tension. II. Ultrastructure of myocytes and interstitium. *Lab Invest* 38:597–609, 1978.
19. Weiner J, Giacomelli F, Loud AV, Anversa P: Morphometry of cardiac hypertrophy induced by experimental renal hypertension. *Am J Cardiol* 44:919–929, 1979.
20. Kuribayshi T, Furokuwa K, Katsume H, Ijichi H, Ibata Y: Regional differences of myocardial hypertrophy and three-dimensional deformation of the heart. *Am J Physiol* 250: H378–H388, 1986.
21. Gulch RW: The effect of chronic loading on the action potential of mammalian myocardium. *J Mol Cell Cardiol* 12:415–420, 1980.
22. Marino TA, Houser SR, Cooper G IV: Early morphological

alterations of pressure-overloaded cat right ventricular myocardium. *Anat Res* 207:417–426, 1983.

23. Cohn JN, Nath KA: What is the stimulus to myocardial hypertrophy? In: Tarazi RC, Dunbar JB (eds) *Perspectives in Cardiovascular Research*, Vol 8. New York: Raven Press, 1983, pp 21–26.

24. Rabinowitz M: Protein synthesis and turnover in normal and hypertrophied heart. *Am J Cardiol* 31:202–210, 1973.

25. Schreiber SS, Rotheschild MA, Oratz M: Investigation into the causes of increased protein synthesis in acute hemodynamic overload. In: Rona G, Ito Y (eds) *Recent Advances in Studies on Cardiac Structure and Metabolism*, Vol 12. Baltimore, MD: University Park Press, 1978, pp 49–60.

26. Sadoshima J, Takahaski T, John L, Isumo S: Roles of mechano-sensitive ion channels, cytoskeleton and contractile activity in stretch-induced intermediate-early gene expression and hypertrophy of cardiac myocytes. *Proc Natl Acad Sci USA* 89:9905–9909, 1992.

27. Simpson PC, Kariya K, Karns LR, Long CS, Farliner JS: Adrenergic hormones and control of cardiac myocyte growth. *Mol Cell Biochem* 104:35–43, 1991.

28. Yabe Y, Abe H: Change in DNA synthesis in significantly hypertrophied human cardiac muscle. In: Tajddin M, Das PK, Tarig M, Dhalla MS (eds) *Advances in Myocardiology*, Vol 1. Baltimore, MD: University Park Press, 1980, pp 553–564.

29. Hatt PY, Berjal G, Moraver J, Swynghedauw B: Heart failure: An electron microscopic study of the left ventricle papillary muscle in aortic insufficiency in the rabbit. *J Mol Cell Cardiol* 1:235–247, 1970.

30. Hatt PY: Cellular changes and damage in mechanically overloaded hearts. In: Fleckenstein A, Rona G (eds) *Recent Advances in Studies on Cardiac Structure and Metabolism*, Vol 6. Baltimore MD: University Park Press, 1975, pp 325–334.

31. Cooper G IV, Kent RL, Uboh CE, Thompson EW, Marino TA: Hemodynamic versus adrenergic control of cat right ventricular hypertrophy. *J Clin Invest* 75:1403–1414, 1986.

32. Spann JF, Buccino RA, Sonnenblick EH, Braunwald E: Contractile state of cardiac muscle obtained from cats with experimentally produced ventricular hypertrophy and heart failure. *Circ Res* 21:341–354, 1962.

33. Spann JF, Covell JW, Eckberg DL, Sonnenblick EH, Ross J, Braunwald E: Contractile performance of the hypertrophied and chronically failing cat ventricle. *Am J Physiol* 233:1150–1157, 1972.

34. Kaufman FR, Homburger H, Wirth H: Disordar in excitation-contraction coupling of cardiac muscle from cats with experimentally produced right ventricular hypertrophy. *Circ Res* 28:346–357, 1971.

35. Gelband H, Bassett AL: Depressed transmembrane potentials during experimentally induced ventricular failure in cats. *Circ Res* 32:625–634, 1973.

36. Cooper G IV, Satavan M Jr, Harrison CE, Coleman HN III: Mechanisms for the abnormal energetics of the pressure induced hypertrophy of the cat myocardium. *Circ Res* 33:213–223, 1973.

37. Meerson FZ, Kapelko VI: The contractile function of the myocardium in two types of cardiac adaptation to a chronic load. *Cardiology* 57:183–199, 1972.

38. Bailey BA, Houser SR: Calcium transients in feline left ventricular myocytes with hypertrophy induced by slow progressive pressure overload. *J Mol Cell Cardiol* 24:365–373, 1992.

39. Cooper G IV, Tomanek RJ, Ehrhardt JC, Marcus ML:

Chronic progressive pressure overload of the cat right ventricle. *Circ Res* 48:488–497, 1981.

40. Natarajan G, Bove AA, Coulson RL, Carey RA, Spann JF: Increased passive stiffness of short term pressure overload hypertrophied myocardium in cat. *Am J Physiol* 337:H676–H680, 1979.

41. Williams JF Jr, Porter RD: Passive stiffness of pressure induced hypertrophied cat myocardium. *Circ Res* 49:211–215, 1981.

42. Williams JF Jr, Mathew B, Hern DL, Potter RD, Deiss WP Jr: Myocardial hydroxyproline and mechanical response to prolonged pressure loading followed by unloading in the cat. *J Clin Invest* 72:1910–1917, 1983.

43. Tritthart H, Laudcke H, Bayer R, Sterle H, Kauffman R: Right ventricular hypertrophy in the cat: An electrophysiological anatomical study. *J Mol Cell Cardiol* 7:163–174, 1975.

44. Bassett AL, Gelband H: Chronic partial occlusion of the pulmonary artery in cats: Change in ventricular action potential configuration during early hypertrophy. *Circ Res* 32:15–26, 1973.

45. Bassett AL, Gelband H: Electrical and mechanical properties of cardiac muscle during chronic right ventricular pressure overload. In: Dhalla NS (ed) *Myocardial Biology. Recent Advances in Studies on Cardiac Structure and Metabolism*, Vol 4. Baltimore, MD: University Park Press, 1973, pp 3–20.

46. Ten Eick RE, Gelband H, Kahn J, Bassett AL: Changes in outward currents of papillary muscles of cats with right ventricular hypertrophy. *Circulation* 56:III46, 1977.

47. Ten Eick RE, Bassett AL, Robertson LL: Possible electrophysiological basis for decreased contractility associated with myocardial hypertrophy in cat: A voltage clamp approach. In: Alpert N (ed) *Perspectives in Cardiovascular Research*, Vol 7: *Myocardial Hypertrophy and Failure*. New York: Raven Press, 1983, pp 245–259.

48. Nuss HB, Houser SR: Voltage dependence of contraction and calcium current in severely hypertrophied feline ventricular myocytes. *J Mol Cell Cardiol* 23:717–726, 1992.

49. Ten Eick RE, Gelband H, Good M, Bassett AL: Increased inward rectifying potassium current in cat ventricular subjected to chronic pressure overload. *Circulation* 56:II77, 1978.

50. Bassett AL, Gelband H, Nilsson K, Myerburg RJ: Localized transmembrane action potential abnormalities in right ventricles subjected to pressure overload. *Circulation* 47:II47, 1977.

51. Cameron JS, Gaide MS, Epstein K, Gelband H, Myerburg RJ, Bassett AL: Regional distribution of action potential abnormalities induced by subacute right ventricular pressure overload. *J Mol Cell Cardiol* 16:321–330, 1984.

52. Aronson RS: Afterpotentials and triggered activity in hypertrophied myocardium from rats with renal hypertension. *Circ Res* 48:720–727, 1981.

53. Alpert NR, Hamrell BB, Halpern W: Mechanical or biochemical correlates of cardiac hypertrophy. *Circ Res* 34/35:71–82, 1974.

54. Hamrell BB, Alpert NR: The mechanical characteristics of hypertrophied rabbit cardiac muscle in the absence of congestive heart failure: The contractile and series elastic elements. *Circ Res* 40:20–25, 1977.

55. Alpert NR, Mulieri LA: Increased myothermal economy of isometric force generation in compensated cardiac hypertrophy induced by pulmonary artery constriction in the rabbit: A characterization of heat liberation in normal and

hypertrophied right ventricular papillary muscles. *Circ Res* 50:491–500, 1982.

56. Konishi T: Electrophysiological study on the hypertrophied cardiac muscle experimentally produced in the rabbit. *Jpn Circ J* 29:491–503, 1965.

57. Sharp NA: Alterations in ventricular action potentials in pressure overload and thyrotoxic hypertrophy. In: Alpert N (ed) *Perspectives in Cardiovascular Research, Vol 7: Myocardial Hypertrophy and Failure.* New York: Raven Press, 1983, pp 245–259.

58. Cameron JS, Myerburg RJ, Wong SS, Gaide MS, Epstein K, Alvarez TR, Gelband H, Guse PA, Bassett AL: Electrophysiologic consequences of chronic experimentally-induced left ventricular pressure overload. *Am J Cardiol* 2:481–487, 1983.

59. Capsso JM, Strobeck JE, Sonnenblick EH: Myocardial mechanical alterations during gradual onset long term hypertension in rats. *Am J Physiol* 10:H435–H441, 1981.

60. Wendt-Gallitelli MF, Ebrecht G, Jacob R: Morphological alterations and their functional interpretation in the hypertrophied myocardium of Goldblatt hypertensive rats. *J Mol Cell Cardiol* 11:275–287, 1979.

61. Jacob R, Brenner B, Ebrecht G, Holubarsch C, Medugorac I: Elastic contractile properties of the myocardium in experimental cardiac hypertrophy of the rat: Methodological and pathophysiological considerations. *Basic Res Cardiol* 75:253–261, 1980.

62. Holubarsch CH: Contractive type and fibrosis type of decreased myocardial distensibility: Different changes in elasticity of myocardium in hypertension and hypertrophy. *Basic Res Cardiol* 75:244–252, 1980.

63. Bing OHL, Matsushita S, Fanburg BL, Levine HJ: Mechanical properties of rat cardiac muscle during experimental hypertrophy. *Circ Res* 28:234–245, 1971.

64. Jouannot P, Hatt PY: Rat myocardial mechanics during pressure induced hypertrophy development and reversal. *Am J Physiol* 299:355–364, 1975.

65. Bing OHL, Fanburg BL, Brooks WW, Matsushita S: The effect of the lathyrogen β-aminoproprionitrile (BAPN) on the mechanical properties of experimentally hypertrophied rat cardiac muscle. *Circ Res* 43:632–637, 1978.

66. Heller LJ: Augmented aftercontractions in papillary muscles from rats with cardiac hypertrophy. *Am J Physiol* 237:H649–H654, 1979.

67. Julian FJ, Morgan DL, Moss RL, Gonzalez M, Dwivedi P: Myocyte growth without physiological impairment in gradually induced rat cardiac hypertrophy. *Circ Res* 49:1300–1310, 1981.

68. Jacob R, Ebrecht G, Kammereit A, Medugorac L, Wendt-Gallitelli MF: Myocardial function in different models of cardiac hypertrophy: An attempt at correlating mechanical, biochemical and morphological parameters. *Basic Res Cardiol* 72:160–167, 1977.

69. Gulch RW, Baumann R, Jacob R: Analysis of myocardial action potential in left ventricular hypertrophy of the Goldblatt rats. *Basic Res Cardiol* 74:69–82, 1979.

70. Gulch RW: Alterations in excitation of mammalian myocardium as a function of chronic loading and their implications in the mechanical events. *Basic Res Cardiol* 75:73–80, 1980.

71. Kammereit A, Jacob R: Alterations in rat myocardial mechanics under Goldblatt hypertension and experimental aortic stenosis. *Basic Res Cardiol* 74:389–405, 1979.

72. Tibbits GF, Barnard RJ, Baldwin DM, Cugalj N, Roberts NK: Influence of exercise on excitation contraction coupling in rat myocardium. *Am J Physiol* 240:H472–H480, 1981.

73. Hayashi H, Shibata S: Electrical properties of cardiac cell membrane of spontaneously hypertensive rat. *Eur J Pharmacol* 27:355–359, 1974.

74. Heller LJ: Cardiac muscle mechanics from doca- and aging spontaneously hypertensive rats. *Am J Physiol* 235:H82–H86, 1978.

75. Heller LJ, Stauffer EK: Altered electrical and contractile properties of hypertrophied cardiac muscles. *Fed Proc* 38:975, 1979.

76. Ferrier GR, Moe GK: Effect of calcium on acetylstrophanthidin-induced transient depolarizations in canine Purkinje tissue. *Circ Res* 33:508–515, 1973.

77. Ferrier GR, Saunders JH, Mendez C: A cellular mechanism for the generation of ventricular arrhythmias by acetylstrophanthidin. *Circ Res* 32:600–609, 1973.

78. Keung ECH, Aronson RS: Non-uniform electrophysiological properties and electrotonic interaction in hypertrophied rat myocardium. *Circ Res* 49:150–158, 1981.

79. Keung ECH, Aronson RS: Transmembrane action potentials and the electrocardiogram in rats with renal hypertension. *Cardiovasc Res* 15:611–614, 1981.

80. Langer GA, Brady AJ, Tan ST, Serena SD: Correlation of the glycoside response, the force staircase, and the action potential configuration in the neonatal rat heart. *Circ Res* 36:744–752, 1975.

81. Charlemagne D, Maixent J-M, Preteseille M, LeLievre LG: Ouabain binding sites and (Na^+,K^+)-ATPase activity in rat cardiac hypertrophy. *J Biol Chem* 261:185–189, 1986.

82. Coltart DJ, Meldrum SJ: Hypertrophic cardiomyopathy an electrophysiological study. *Br Med J* 4:217–218, 1970.

83. Singer DH, Baumgarten CM, Ten Eick RE: Cellular electrophysiology of ventricular and other dysrhythmias: Studies on diseased and ischemic hearts. *Prog Cardiovasc Dis* 24:97–156, 1981.

84. Ten Eick RE, Baumgarten CM, Singer DH: Ventricular dysrhythmias: Membrane basis of currents, channels, gates and cables. *Prog Cardiovasc Dis* 24:157–188, 1981.

85. Brorson L, Conradson TB, Olsson B, Varnaukas E: Right atrial monophasic action potential and effective refractory periods in relation to physical training and maximum heart rate. *Cardiovasc Res* 10:160–168, 1976.

86. Kavaler F: Membrane depolarization as a cause of tension development in mammalian ventricular muscle. *Am J Physiol* 196:968–970, 1959.

87. Morad M, Trautwein W: The effect of the duration of the action potential on contraction in the mammalian heart muscle. *Pflügers Arch* 299:66–82, 1968.

88. Wood EH, Heppner RL, Weidmann S: Inotropic effects of electrical currents. I. Positive and negative constant electrical currents or current pulses applied during cardiac action potentials. II. Hypotheses: Calcium movements, excitation contraction coupling and inotropic effects. *Circ Res* 24:409–445, 1969.

89. Beeler GW Jr, Reuter H: Relation between membrane potential, membrane current and activation of contraction in ventricular myocardial fibers. *J Physiol* 207:211–229, 1970.

90. Leoty C: Membrane currents and activation of contraction in rat ventricular fibers. *J Physiol* 239:237–249, 1974.

91. Lab MJ: Mechanically dependent changes in action potentials recorded from the intact frog ventricle. *Circ Res* 42:519–528, 1978.

92. Spotnitz HM, Sonnenblick EH: Structural conditions in the hypertrophied and failing heart. *Am J Cardiol* 32:398–406, 1973.

93. Morady F, Laks MM, Parmely WW: Comparison of sarco mere lengths from normal and hypertrophied inner and middle canine right ventricle. *Am J Physiol* 225:127–1259, 1973.

94. Kleiman RB, Houser SR: Electrophysiologic and mechanical properties of single feline ventricular myocytes. *J Mol Cell Cardiol* 20:973–982, 1988.

95. Schwartz K, Carrier L, Lompre AM, Mercadier JJ, Boheler KR: Contractile protein and sarcoplasmic reticulum calcium ATPase gene expression in the hypertrophied and failing heart. *Bas Res Cardiol* 87(Suppl 1):285–290, 1992.

96. Schwartz K, Boheler KR, de la Bastie D, Lompre AM, Mercadier JJ: Switches in cardiac muscle gene expression as a result of pressure and volume overload. *Am J Physiol* 262:R364–R369, 1992.

97. Bonnin CM, Sparrow MP, Taylor RR: Collagen synthesis and content in right ventricular hypertrophy in the dog. *Am J Physiol* 241:H708–H713, 1981.

98. Medugorac I: Characteristics of the hypertrophied left ventricular myocardium in Goldblatt rats. *Basic Res Cardiol* 72:262–267, 1977.

99. Hemwall EL, Houser SR: Alterations of slow response action potentials in right ventricular hypertrophy. *Circulation* 66:II77, 1982.

100. Limas C, Limas CJ: Reduced number of β-adrenergic receptors in the myocardium of spontaneously hypertensive rats. *Biochem Biophys Res Commun* 83:710–714, 1978.

101. Woodcock EA, Funder JW, Johnston CI: Decreased cardiac beta-receptors in deoxycorticosterone-salt and renal hypertensive rats. *Circ Res* 45:560–565, 1979.

102. Cervoni P, Herzlinger H, Lai FM, Tanikella T: A comparison of cardiac reactivity and β-adrenoceptor number and affinity between aorta-coarcted hypertensive and normotensive rats. *Br J Pharmacol* 74:517–523, 1981.

103. McDonald TF, Trautwein W: Membrane currents in cat myocardium: Separation of inward and outward components. *J Physiol* 274:193–216, 1978.

104. DiFrancesco D, Noble D: A model of cardiac electrical activity incorporating ionic pumps and concentration changes. *Phil Trans R Soc Lond B* 307:353–398, 1985.

105. Martin FG, Freeman AR, Marino JA, Houser SR: Potassium measurements in the extracellular spaces of normal and failing cat myocardium. *Cardiovasc Res* 17:642–648, 1983.

106. Moulder PV, Eichelberger L, Daily PO: Segmental water and electrolyte distribution in canine hearts with right ventricular hypertrophy. *Fed Proc* 26:382, 1967.

107. Nachev P: The effect of aortic coarctation on the concentration of water and electrolytes in cardiac muscle. *Proc Soc Exp Biol Med* 147:137–139, 1974.

108. Silver LH, Hemwall EL, Marino TA, Houser SR: Isolation and morphology of calcium tolerant feline ventricular myocytes. *Am J Physiol* 245 (*Heart Circ Physiol* 14): H891–H896, 1983.

109. Sakman B, Trube G: Conductance properties of single inwardly rectifying potassium channels in ventricular cells from guinea-pig heart. *J Physiol (Lond)* 347:641–657, 1984.

110. Nilius B, Hess P, Lansman JB, Tsien RW: A novel type of cardiac calcium channel in ventricular cells. *Nature (Lond)* 316:443–446, 1985.

111. Kleiman RB, Houser SR: Calcium currents in normal and hypertrophied isolated feline ventricular myocytes. *Am J Physiol* 255 (*Heart Circ Physiol* 24):H1434–H1442, 1988.

112. Scamps F, Mayoux E, Charlemagne D, Vassort G: Calcium current in single-cells isolated from normal and hypertrophied rat heart. Effects of beta-adrenergic stimulation. *Circ Res* 67:199–208, 1990.

113. Xu X, Best PM: Decreased transient outward K^+ current in ventricular myocytes from acromegalic rats. *Am J Physiol* 260:H935–H942, 1991.

114. Keung EC: Calcium current is increased in isolated adult myocytes from hypertrophied rat myocardium. *Circ Res* 64:753–763, 1989.

115. Kleiman RB, Houser SR: Outward currents in normal and hypertrophied feline ventricular myocytes. *Am J Physiol* H1450–H1461, 1989.

116. Ten Eick RE, Whalley DW, Rasmussen H: Connections: Heart disease, cellular electrophysiology and ion channels. *FASEB J* 6:2568–2580, 1992.

117. Cooper G IV, Marino TA: Complete reversibility of cat ventricular chronic progressive pressure overload. *Circ Res* 54:323–331, 1984.

118. Cooper G IV, Satava R, Harrison CE, Coleman HN III: Normal myocardial function and energetics after reversing pressure overload hypertrophy. *Am J Physiol* 226:1158–1165, 1974.

119. Coulson RL, Yazdanfar S, Rubio E, Bove AA, Lemole GM, Spann JF: Recuperative potential of cardiac muscle following relief of pressure overload hypertrophy and right ventricular failure on the cat. *Circ Res* 40:41–49, 1977.

120. Capasso JM, Strobeck JE, Malohotra A, Scheuer J, Sonnenblick EH: contractile behavior of rat myocardium after reversal of hypertensive hypertrophy. *Am J Physiol* 242:H882–H889, 1982.

121. Cutilletta AF, Dowell RT, Rudnik M, Arcilla RA, Zak R: Regression of myocardial hypertrophy. I. Experimental model, changes in heart weight, nucleic acids and collagens. *J Mol Cell Cardiol* 7:767–781, 1975.

122. Wisenbaugh T, Allen P, Cooper G IV, O'Connor WN, Mezaros L, Streter F, Bahinski A, Houser S, Spann JF: Hypertrophy without contractile dysfunction after reversal of pressure overload in the cat. *Am J Physiol* 247:H146–H154, 1984.

123. Sen S: Regression of cardiac hypertrophy. Experimental animal model. *Am J Med* 75(Sept Suppl):87–93, 1983.

124. Gibbons WR, Fozzard HA: Voltage dependence and time dependence of contraction in sheep cardiac Purkinje fibers. *Circ Res* 28:446–460, 1971.

125. Gibbons WR, Fozzard HA: Relationships between voltage and tension in sheep cardiac Purkinje fibers. *J Gen Physiol* 63:345–366, 1975.

126. Trautwein W, McDonald TF, Tripathi O: Calcium conductance and tension in mammalian ventricular muscle. *Pflügers Arch* 354:55–74, 1976.

127. Morgan JP: Abnormal intracellular modulation of calcium as a major cause of cardiac contractile dysfunction. *N Engl J Med* 325:625–632, 1991.

128. Bing OH, Brooks WW, Conrad CH, Sen S, Perreault CL, Morgan JP: Intracellular calcium transients in myocardium from spontaneously hypertensive rats during the transition to heart failure. *Circ Res* 68:1390–1400, 1991.

129. Gwathmey JK, Slawsky MT, Hajjar RJ, Briggs GM, Morgan JP: Role of intracellular calcium handling in force-interval relationships of human ventricular myocardium. *J Clin Invest* 85:1599–1613, 1990.

130. Nakanishi H, Hakino N, Hata T, Matsui H, Yano K, Yanaga T: Sarcolemmal Ca^{2+} transport activities in cardiac hypertrophy caused by pressure overload. *Am J Physiol* 257:H349–H356, 1989.

131. Vatner DE, Homcy CJ, Sit SP, Manders WT, Vatner SF: Effects of pressure overload, left ventricular hypertrophy on beta-adrenergic receptors, and responsiveness to catecholamines. *J Clin Invest* 73:1473–1482, 1984.

132. Anderson KP: Sudden death, hypertension and hypertrophy. *J Cardiovasc Pharmacol* 6:S498–S503, 1984.

133. Bing OHL, Brooks WW, Conrad CH, Weinstein KB, Spadaro J, Radvany S: Myocardial mechanics of infarcted and hypertrophied non-infarcted myocardium following coronary artery occlusion. In: Steinkopff D (ed) *Cardiac Adaptation to Hemodynamic Overload, Training and Stress.* New York: Springer-Verlag, 1983, pp 235–244.

134. Kozlovskis PL, Fieber LA, Bassett AL, Cameron JS, Kimura S, Myerburg RJ: Regional reduction in ventricular nore-pinephrine after healing of experimental myocardial infarction in cats. *J Mol Cell Cardiol* 18:413–422, 1986.

135. Gaide MS, Myerburg RJ, Kozlovskis PL, Bassett AL: Elevated sympathetic response of epicardium proximal to healed myocardial infarction. *Am J Physiol* 245:H646–H652, 1983.

136. Anversa P, Ricci R, Olivetti G: Quantitative structural analysis of the myocardium during physiologic growth and induced cardiac hypertrophy: A review. *J Am Coll Cardiol* 7:1140–1149, 1986.

137. Goldstein MA, Sordahl LA, Schwartz A: Ultrastructural analysis of left ventricular hypertrophy in rabbits. *J Mol Cell Cardiol* 6:265–273, 1974.

138. Cameron JS, Bassett AL, Gaide MS, Wong SS, Lodge NJ, Kozlovskis PL, Myerburg RJ: Cellular electrophysiological effects of coronary artery ligation in chronically pressure overloaded cats hearts. *Int J Cardiol*, in press.

139. Kohya T, Kimura S, Myerburg RJ, Bassett AL: Ventricular fibrillation during acute ischemia in hypertrophied rat hearts. *Circulation* 74:(II)344, 1986.

140. Kohya T, Kimura S, Myerburg RJ, Bassett AL: Spontaneous ventricular fibrillation and ventricular fibrillation threshold in normal and hypertrophied rat hearts. *Fed Proc* 45:779, 1986.

141. Versailles JT, Verscheure Y, Le Kim A, Pourrias B: Comparison between the ventricular fibrillation thresholds of spontaneously hypertensive and normotensive rats — Investigation of antidysrhythmic drugs. *J Cardiovasc Pharm* 4:430–435, 1982.

CHAPTER 35

Developmental Changes in Membrane Electrical Properties of the Heart

NICHOLAS SPERELAKIS & GEORGE E. HADDAD

INTRODUCTION

Important physiologic, electrophysiologic, pharmacologic, biochemical, and ultrastructural changes occur during the embryonic development of avian and mammalian hearts. For example, striking changes occur in the electrical properties of ventricular myocardial cells during embryonic development of chick heart. In many mammalian hearts, some of the changes extend into the early postnatal period. These changes affect and determine the functional behavior and properties of the heart at each stage of development and differentiation. Therefore, it is the purpose of this chapter to review and summarize many of these changes in properties. The attention of the reader will be called to a number of recent review articles that summarize these properties, as well as go into greater detail.

Studies of the electrophysiologic properties of embryonic heart cells are useful, not only to elucidate the changes during differentiation, but also to obtain clues for understanding the complex electrophysiology of adult hearts. Most of the data presented are for the chick and rat, although some data are presented for developing mammalian hearts. Some findings on organ-cultured hearts and cultured heart cells will be presented for comparison. Since the electrical properties may be affected by morphologic and biochemical properties, relevant changes in these properties are also discussed.

DEVELOPMENTAL CHANGES IN CARDIAC MORPHOLOGY

The early embryo (up to one somite) possesses cells that are destined to form the heart. These cells migrate through the early embryo and congregate bilaterally into the so-called precardiac areas (mesoderm) of the anterior half of the flattened 16- to 17-hour (head process) blastoderm {1}.

Explants of the blastodermal and precardiac areas, after several days in culture, develop spontaneous action potentials (APs) of about 50-mV amplitude {2}. In culture, a tubular heart develops within a vesicle and it beats spontaneously for several days, but further differentiation does not proceed in vitro. The precardiac area can be treated with trypsin to facilitate mechanical separation of the three germ layers, and culture of the precardiac mesoderm gives rise to a solid mass of cells that fire spontaneous APs and contract {3}. If the postnodal piece (posterior third of blastoderm) is dissected from the 19-hour chick blastoderm and placed into culture, it does not normally give rise to heart tissue. If, however, the postnodal piece is cultured in the presence of an RNA-enriched fraction obtained from adult chicken hearts, a typical spontaneously beating tubular heart forms within a vesicle, as in the case of the precardiac areas described above {4}. The beating cells in the induced hearts were shown to possess some myofilaments. In addition, the induced tubular hearts exhibit spontaneous APs {5}. Thus it appears that either RNA or some other material within the extract obtained from the adult heart can induce cells in the postnodal piece, normally not destined to form the heart, to take on many of the properties of cardiac myoblasts.

Subsequently, in development in situ, twin tubular primordia form bilaterally from the precardiac mesoderm, and they fuse to form a single tubular heart. This fusion begins from the head end and proceeds posteriorly by a zipperlike process, such that the first region fused (ventricle) begins contracting first; the atria are added posteriorly later. The tubular heart begins contracting spontaneously at 30–40 hours (9–19 somite state). Cutting the 2-day heart into bulbus, ventricle, and sinoatrium regions shows that each region has a characteristic automaticity, the sinoatrium region being the fastest.

The tubular heart begins to propel blood shortly after it starts to beat. The blood pressure is very low (1–2 mmHg) at this stage, and it increases progressively during embryonic development (approximately 30 mmHg by day 18) and during postembryonic life {6,7}. The velocity of propagation of the peristaltic contraction wave in 3-day hearts is approximately 1 cm/s {7}.

The heart rate of the chick embryo increases from about 50 beats/min at day 1.5 to the maximal value of about 220 beats/min by day 8; it has been suggested that the increase in beating rate may result from the concomitant rise in blood pressure {7}. The influence of temperature on heart rate decreases markedly during development {7}. The Q_{10} decreases from about 3.6 on day 3

N. Sperelakis (ed.), *Physiology and Pathophysiology of the Heart, Third Edition.*

Table 35-1. Summary of data obtained from E_m versus long $[K]_o$ curves and from input resistance (r_{in}) measurments for chick embryonic hearts (ventricular cells) at various stages of development

Embryonic age (days)	E_m (mV)	Slope (mV/decade)	Extrapolated $[K]_i$ (mM)	E_K (rnV)	P_{Na}/P_K ratio	r_{in} (MΩ)
2	−40	30	125	−100	0.21	13.0
3	−51	40	130	−101	0.17	8.5
4	−57	46	140	−103	0.08	6.5
5–6	−58	50	130	−101	0.08	5.5
7–9	−71	51	145	−104	0.07	5.5
11–13	−80	53	145	−104	0.07	4.7
14–20	−78	52	155	−106	0.05	4.5

The resting potential (E_m) values are given for a $[K]_o$ of 2.7 mM. The slope is the average at $[K]_o$ levels between 10 and 100 mM. $[K]_i$ was estimated from the extrapolation of fitted curves to zero potential. The P_{Na}/P_K ratios were calculated from the Goldman constant-field equation at every $[K]_o$ level for which E_m was measured, and an average value was calculated for each heart; some individual values for hearts in the 14- to 20-day age group were as low as 0.02. Data were taken from Sperelakis and Shigenobu {14}, and Sperelakis et al. {54}. Similar values for slope and $[K]_i$ were obtained by Pappano {22} for embryonic chick atrium at 4, 6, and 12 days; the 18-day values were −59 mV/decade and 125 mM $[K]_i$, respectively.

to about 2.0 on day 18 for the same temperature range {8}. Breaks in the Arrhenius plots (of spontaneous heart rate vs. temperature) also occur at different temperatures in young hearts compared to old hearts.

For the rat, the gestation period is 21–22 days {9}. The transition from the embryonic to fetal period occurs between the 13th and 15th day of gestation. The heart primordia first appear about the middle of the 9th day, and the gross shape of the heart is complete by the end of the 13th day. Septation of the atria and ventricles is accomplished by day 15. From this time onward, the heart grows in size, but no new structures are added.

RESTING MEMBRANE AND K$^+$ PERMEABILITY

Resting potentials

The resting potential (E_m), measured by intracellular microelectrodes, of the ventricular portion of chick and rat hearts increases during embryonic development {10–16}. In embryonic chick heart (table 35-1), the greatest changes occur between days 2 and 7, and thereafter the increase is smaller. For example, in a 2-day-old heart, the mean resting E_m is about −40 mV, and this increases to about −51 mV on day 3. The resting potential is close to −80 mV by day 12, nearly the final adult value. Furthermore, current clamp experiments with a low-resistance, patch electrode showed similar hyperpolarization of the resting potential during the first postnatal weeks of the developing freshly isolated {17} and cultured (see fig. 35-9A) {18} rat ventricular myocytes. As discussed below, the large increase in resting E_m during the first few days may be due mainly to an increase in K$^+$ permeability (P_K) and not in K$^+$ equilibrium potential (E_K; or in $[K]_i$). However, some investigators {2} have reported larger values of resting E_m

for young hearts, i.e., less of a change during development, and have attributed low recorded potentials in young hearts to current leakage around the electrode tip due to improper sealing of the microclectrode. (This effect would be most prominent in cells having a high input resistance.)

RESTING POTENTIAL VERSUS LOG $[K]_o$ CURVES

The relationship between resting E_m and external K$^+$ concentration ($[K]_o$) was determined for embryonic hearts of different ages {15,19}. Data for 3-day, 5-day, and 15-day-old embryonic chick hearts are shown in fig. 35-1. $[K]_i$ was estimated by extrapolation of the curves to zero potential, and the values varied between 125 mM (for 2-day hearts) and 155 mM (for 14- to 20-day hearts; table 35-1). Also plotted in fig. 35-1 are the theoretical curves (calculated from the Goldman constant-field equation given in the inset) for five different ratios of P_{Na}/P_K: 0.001, 0.01, 0.05, 0.1, and 0.2. As indicated in the figure, it was assumed that $[Na]_i$ was 30 mM and $[K]_i$ was 150 mM for these calculations. The data points for the 3-day hearts most closely fit the theoretical curve for a P_{Na}/P_K ratio of 0.2, those for the 5-day hearts fit the curve for a P_{Na}/P_K of 0.1, and those for the 15-day hearts most closely fit between the 0.05 and 0.01 curves. These data suggest that the P_{Na}/P_K ratio is very high in young hearts and that this accounts for the low measured resting E_m: that is, the low resting E_m is not due to a greatly lower $[K]_i$ and E_K. As shown in table 35-1, only a very small increase in the calculated E_K occurs during development: from about −100 mV on day 2 to −106 mV on days 14–20. Thus, in the young hearts the resting E_m is far from E_K due to the high P_{Na}/P_K ratio. In this respect, the myocardial cells in young embryonic hearts resemble sinoatrial (SA) nodal cells in adult hearts. In newborn rat ventricular myocytes,

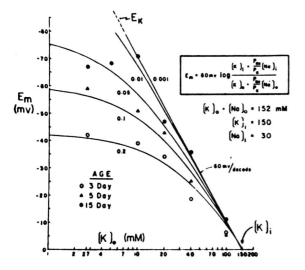

Fig. 35-1. Resting potential (E_m) plotted as a function of $[K]_o$ on a logarithmic scale for representative hearts of three different ages. $[K]_o$ was elevated by substitution of K^+ for equimolar amounts of Na^+. Continuous lines give theoretical calculations from the constant-field equation (inset) for P_{Na}/P_K ratios of 0.001, 0.01, 0.05, 0.1, and 0.2. Calculations were made assuming $[K]_i$ and $[Na]_i$ values shown. For a P_{Na}/P_K ratio of 0.001, the curve is linear over the entire range, with a slope of 60 mV/decade, i.e., it closely follows E_K. Symbols give representative data obtained from embryonic chick hearts at days 3 (○), 5 (△), and 19 (●). The data for the 3-day heart follow the curve for a P_{Na}/P_K ratio of 0.2, those for the 5-day heart follow the curve for 0.1, and those for 15-day heart fail between the curves for 0.01 and 0.05. The estimated intracellular K^+ activities ($[K]_i$) obtained by extrapolation to zero potential are nearly the same for all ages. Taken from Sperelakis and Shigenobu {14}, with permission.

$[K]_i$ did not change significantly, while P_{Na}/P_K decreased between day 1 and 7 after birth {20,21}.

In old embryonic chick or adult hearts, the E_m versus log $[K]_o$ curve is nearly linear above 10 mM K^+, with a slope approaching the theoretical 61 mV/decade (from the Nernst equation). If the slope were exactly 61 mV/decade, then E_m would be equal to E_K, and the membrane would be completely K^+ selective in high $[K]_o$. The data in fig. 35-1 and table 35-1 show that the slope for hearts 7–20 days old is 51–53 mV/decade, whereas the average slopes (curves continually bend) for 4-day, 3-day, and 2-day hearts are 46, 40, and 30 mV/decade, respectively. Similar values for $[K]_i$ and slope were found for embryonic chick atrial cells at various stages of development {22}. Similar results were found for 1- and 7-day-old rat ventricular myocytes with slopes of 44 and 47 mV/decade, respectively {20,21}. Since flattening of the resting potential versus log curve at lower $[K]_o$ levels is much more prominent for young hearts, i.e., they are depolarized less by a given increment in $[K]_o$ (see fig. 35-1), young hearts should be less affected by elevation of $[K]_o$. Young hearts are indeed less affected by elevation of $[K]_o$ than are older hearts {14,23}. This is true for both inhibition of automaticity of

the whole heart as well as for loss of excitability of the ventricle to electrical stimulation {14}.

MEMBRANE RESISTANCE

In order to ascertain whether the P_{Na}/P_K ratio is high in young embryonic chick hearts because of high Na^+ permeability or because of a low K^+ permeability, input resistance (r_{in}) was determined from steady-state voltage-current curves. The r_{in} of the ventricular cells is high (13 MΩ) in young 2-day-old hearts and rapidly declines over the next few days, reaching the final adult value of about 4.5 MΩ by day 14 (table 35-1). If the average cell size and the degree of electrical coupling between the cells remains unchanged during this period, the high r_{in} of the young hearts would suggest that membrane resistivity (R_m) is very high. The latter would be consistent with a low K^+ conductance and K^+ permeability in the young hearts. These results suggest that the P_{Na}/P_K ratio is high in young hearts because P_K is low, and not because P_{Na} is high.

Consistent with the interpretation that P_K is low in hearts is the finding that the chronaxie of young hearts (2-day-old) is about fourfold higher than that of 9- to 16-day-old hearts {10}. This indicates that the membrane time constant is about fourfold higher in young hearts and, if membrane capacitance remains constant, membrane resistivity must be fourfold higher.

Carmeliet et al. {24} have reported, on the basis of ^{42}K flux measurements, that P_K is about two- to threefold lower in 6- to 8-day hearts than in 18- to 20-day hearts, consistent with the conclusions from the electrical studies described above. (Although they reported that the calculated P_K for 3- to 5-day hearts was nearly as high as that for the 18- to 20-day hearts, which disagrees with the electrical measurements, they did not control for spontaneous beating and APs, and hence increased K^+ efflux, that occurs in the 3- to 5-day hearts; this might cause them to calculate an erroneously high P_K.) The values for the P_K coefficients were 13.2×10^{-8} cm/s for 7-day hearts and about 27.5×10^{-8} cm/s for 19-day hearts (at a $[K]_o$ of 2.5–5.0 mM). P_K was greatly reduced in 0 mM $[K]_o$. The P_{Na}/P_K ratios calculated from the constant-field equation were 0.018 for the 19-day hearts and 0.037 for the 7-day hearts. The P_{Na} coefficient, as calculated from the P_K and P_{Na}/P_K ratio, did not change during development (constant at about 0.50×10^{-8} cm/s).

LACK OF EFFECT OF ACETYLCHOLINE ON P_K

The young ventricular cells are not hyperpolarized by acetylcholine (ACh), even though a large hyperpolarization is theoretically possible because the resting E_m is much below E_K {14}. Therefore it is likely that ACh does not significantly increase P_K in ventricular cells. In ventricular muscle of old embryonic chick, ACh has little or no effect on shortening the AP also, whereas the atrial AP is markedly shortened. The artial cells of young hearts are slightly depolarized by ACh in normal medium and slightly hyperpolarized in Na^+-free medium, suggesting that ACh increases both Na^+ conductance and K^+ conductance in young hearts {22,25,26}. Pappano {22} interpreted the small hyperpolarization produced by ACh in Na^+-free solution to be consistent with a low P_K, namely, that few K^+ channels are available to be opened by ACh.

ION CONTENT

Sodium

Tissue electrolyte analyses in chick embryonic hearts (ventricles) show that the total tissue content of Na^+ in young hearts is very high and that it decreases gradually until about day 13, after which the level remains constant {11,27}. Sodium ion exchangeability is low in young hearts and rises gradually during development to about 70% near hatching. Thus, there may be a great amount of bound Na^+ in young hearts, including in the nucleus {28} and in the extracellular (subendocardial) mucopolysaccharide cardiac jelly (which serves a valvelike function) {29}. The data from electrophysiologic studies {11,14} indicated that the thermodynamically active free intracellular Na^+ concentration must not be extremely high because the Na^+-dependent APs already overshoot to $+11$ mV in day-2 hearts; the overshoot increases rapidly, reaching $+28$ mV by day 8; the latter value is the same as the adult value. McDonald and De Haan {15} reported that the Na^+ content of the chick heart did not change during development. Carmeliet et al. {24} measured $[Na]_i$ values of 16 mM and 15 mM for 7-day and 19-day embryonic chick hearts, respectively. Harsch and Green {30} reported that the $[Na]_i$ levels remained relatively constant (23–38 mM) between days 8 and 18. Thus there seems little doubt that the free $[Na]_i$ relatively low in young hearts.

Extracellular space: Chloride

There is a decrease in extracellular space during development of embryonic chick heart. The inulin space was reported to decrease from 39% at day 8 to 19% at day 18 {30}. The extracellular space determined by radioactive chromium EDTA decreased from 34% on days 6–8 to 27% on days 18–20 {24}.

The estimates of intracellular Cl^- for days 8–18 were 36–45 mM {30}. These values are too high to be consistent with the measured resting potentials (of -70 mV to -80 mV) if Cl^- were passively distributed. There is hardly any compelling evidence for a Cl^- pump in myocardial cells (see Sperelakis {31}).

Potassium

The K^+ content of chick hearts was reported to gradually increase during development, from about 68 mM/kg on days 2–3 to a plateau level of about 86 mM/kg on day 13 {27}. However, it was reported that the calculated $[K]_i$ levels may actually decrease during development: from 145 mM on day 8 to 91 mM on day 18 {30}. Similarly,

McDonald and De Haan {15} reported that $[K]_i$ changed from 167 mM on day 2 to 118 mM on days 14–18, and Carmeliet et al. {24} calculated $[K]_i$ values of 151 mM and 122 mM for chick hearts on days 6–8 and days 18–20, respectively. The electrophysiologic data from resting E_m versus log $[K]_O$ curves {14} indicate that $[K]_i$ is about 125 mM on day 2 and that it increases gradually to about 155 mM on days 14–20 (table 35-1). The calculated E_K increases from about -100 mV at day 2 to -106 mV at days 14–20 (table 35-1). Pappano {22} also reported high values of $[K]_i$ (145 mM) on day 4 for chick atrial cells. Similarly, Haddad et al. {20,21} calculated an $[K]_i$ of 148 mM and 141 mM in 1- and 7-day-old rat ventricular myocytes, respectively. Thus, $[K]_i$ is already high in young hearts, and so the cardiac cells must actively transport cations before day 1.

Na,K-ATPASE ACTIVITY

The specific activity of the Na,K-ATPase is low in young embryonic chick hearts and rises during development {32}. The average value on day 4 is about 35% of that on day 16 $(7.4 + 0.7 M P_i/hmg\ protein)$, that on day 6 is about 42%, that on day 9 is about 57%, and that on day 13 is about 77%. This enzyme activity is highest on day 20, about 144% of that on day 16. The adult level is about equal to that on embryonic day 16.

Thus while P_K is increasing during development, and hence the outward passive leak of K^+ and inward leak of Na^+ (due to the increased electrochemical driving force), the capability of the Na^+-K^+ pump is increasing correspondingly; that is, the increased cation pump capability tends to compensate for the increased demand on the pump due to increased cation leak. However, the pumping capacity of the very young hearts must be sufficient to maintain the relatively high $[K]_i$ and low $[Na]_i$ already present in the young cells.

When the ventricular myocardial cells from 16-day hearts are placed into monolayer cell culture, the specific activity of the Na,K-ATPase decreases by more than threefold {33}. The lower Na^+-K^+ pumping capability of the cultured cells is consistent with the lower K^+ permeability and somewhat lower $[K]_i$ generally observed in these cells {32}.

ELECTROGENIC PUMP POTENTIAL

The energy-dependent pump located in the cell membrane, which maintains the ionic gradients for Na^+ and K^+ ions across the cell membrane, becomes electrogenic when the ratio of Na^+ ions pumped out to K^+ ions pumped in is greater than 1; that is, the pump directly produces a potential (V_{ep}) that contributes to the measured resting potential, usually by between 2 and 15 mV, depending on the type of cell and the physiologic conditions (see reviews by Thomas {34} and Sperelakis {31}). An electrogenic Na^+ pump potential has been demonstrated in various tissues of the heart {35–40}.

Using flux studies, Lieberman et al. {41} found evidence for an electrogenic pump in cultured embryonic chick (11-day-old) myocardial cells. Pelleg et al. {42} observed an electrogenic pump potential of a few millivolts in cultured embryonic heart cell reaggregates derived from early (3-day-old) and late (16-day-old) stages of development that were subjected to overdrive stimulation. These studies indicate that electrogenic transport is present in early stages of ontogenesis and that this ability is retained in vitro. If $[Na]_i$ is somewhat higher in young hearts and if the pump coupling ratio (Na/K) is a function of $[Na]_i$, V_{ep} might be expected to be higher in young hearts, especially in view of the higher membrane resistance, but there is no evidence for this. This lack of a larger V_{ep} might be partly explained on the basis of a lower density of pump sites in the young hearts.

POSTDRIVE HYPERPOLARIZATION AND OVERDRIVE SUPPRESSION OF AUTOMATICITY

When automatic heart cells are driven at a faster rate than their intrinsic rate, upon termination of the drive there is a transient pause followed by a gradual recovery to the predrive firing rate {37,42}. This phenomenon of overdrive suppression of automaticity is caused by a small transient hyperpolarization of a few millivolts; this transient hyperpolarization is the cause of the suppression of the automaticity. Vassalle {37} presented evidence that the hyperpolarization was due to stimulation of an electrogenic Na^+ pump potential, presumably resulting from an increase in $[Na]_i$ and in $[K]_o$ during the drive. The high frequency of APs during the overdrive, with the accompanying increased Na^+ influx and K^+ efflux, initially overwhelm the Na-K pump capability, leading to elevation of $[Na]_i$ and $[K]_o$. This, in turn, stimulates the Na-K pump, and perhaps increases the Na/K coupling ratio of the pump, thus increasing V_{ep} and hyperpolarizing.

Overdrive suppression was observed in intact young 3-day-old hearts (prior to innervation of the heart) and was attributed to the release of an ACh-like substance from within the heart cells {43}. However, it was recently demonstrated by Pelleg et al. {42} that cultured heart cells (ventricular and atrial), isolated from both young and old embryonic chick hearts, which are automatic in vitro, exhibit the phenomena of postdrive hyperpolarization and overdrive suppression of automaticity that are blocked by ouabain but not by atropine. These findings support the view that stimulation of an electrogenic pump is the cause of this behavior. These results also indicate that young embryonic heart cells are capable of exhibiting electrogenic Na-K pumping.

AUTOMATICITY

Requirements for automaticity include (a) a low Cl^- conductance (g_{Cl}), as is generally true for myocardial cells, and (b) a low K^+ conductance (g_K). A low g_K enhances membrane inductance in series with one type of K^+

channel (the inward-rectifying anomalous rectification channel having a negative slope conductance region) and tends to cause oscillations in E_m. The low g_K also is responsible for the low resting potential (moves the resting E_m farther from E_K) and places E_m in the region that can support pacemaker oscillations.

Pronounced changes in automaticity of the ventricular cells also occur during development, as could be predicted from the changes in P_K. The incidence of hyperpolarizing afterpotentials and pacemaker potentials is very high {80–100} in young hearts, and this incidence decreases to 0% in the old embryonic hearts {14}. If a portion of the ventricle is cut and isolated to remove drive from the nodal cells, the incidence of pacemaker potentials is 100% for embryos up through day 10, whereas the incidence is 0% in embryos day 12 or older. These results indicate that the ventricular myocardial cells possess automaticity capability when they are young but that this capability diminishes as the cells age.

However, old ventricular cells again become automatic when they are trypsin dispersed and placed into monolyer cell culture. For example, ventricular myocardial cells dispersed from 16-day-old chick embryos and cultured as monolayers usually revert back toward the young embryonic state with respect to their electrical properties, including gain of automaticity {14}. When the cells are allowed to reaggregate into small spheres, however, they often retain their highly differentiated electrical properties, including lack of automaticity {44,45}. Some reaggregates exhibit automaticity, even though the APs are relatively fast rising and tetrodotoxin (TTX) sensitive. The gain in automaticity of cultured cells appears to reflect a decrease in P_K {46–48}. In some cases, isolated single ventricular cells in culture have such a low P_K that they are depolarized too far and do not normally exhibit automaticity or excitability {49}. However, if these cells are hyperpolarized by intracellular application of current pulses, spontaneous APs and contractions occur {49}.

It has been suggested that mechanical stretch of the wall of the tubular heart of the young chick embryo, by the gradual buildup of the blood volume and blood pressure, may play a role in the initiation of the heartbeat and in the gradual increase in the heart rate during development {50}. However, it is difficult to reconcile this view with other facts, such as (a) the demonstration that the precardiac tissue of the chick blastoderm can develop in vitro into spontaneously contracting heartlike tubes, vesicles, or cell clusters {2,4,5,51,52}, with no evidence of an intraluminal buildup of pressure and (b) the retention of automaticity of cultured, isolated single heart cells or monolayers.

ACTION POTENTIAL CHANGES

Rate of rise and overshoot

The action potentials (APs) of the cells of intact chick hearts undergo sequential changes during development in situ {14,53,54}, as shown in fig. 35-2. There is a progressive

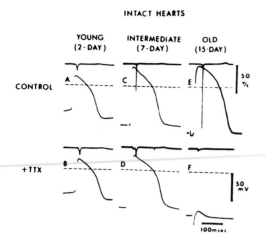

INTACT HEARTS

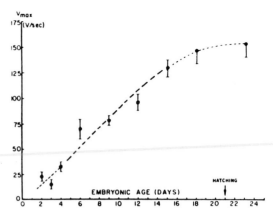

Fig. 35-2. Characteristics of the action potentials in intact embryonic chick hearts at different stages of development. **A,B:** Intracellular recordings from a 2-day-old heart before (A) and 20 minutes after (B) the addition of tetrodotoxin (TTX; 20 µg/ml). **C,D:** Recordings from a 7-day-old heart before (C) and 2 minutes after (D) the addition of TTX (2 µg/ml). Note the depression of the rate of rise in D. **E,F:** Records from a 15-day-old heart prior to (E) and 2 minutes after (F) the addition of TTX (1 µg/ml). The APs were abolished and excitability was not restored by strong field stimulation in F. Thus, the hearts became progressively more responsive to TTX during development, i.e., the effect of TTX increased with increasing embryonic age. The upper traces give dV/dt; this trace has been shifted relative to the V-t trace to prevent obscuring dV/dt. The horizontal broken line in each panel represents zero potential. dV/dt calibration (in E) and voltage and time calibrations (in F) pertain to all panels. Modified from Sperelakis and Shigenobu {14}, with permission.

Fig. 35-3. Evidence for two types of Na^+ channels. Data illustrating changes in the maximal rate of rise of the AP (dV/dt max) as a function of membrane potential (E_m) for representative hearts of three different embryonic ages (3, 5, and 13 days). The membrane potential was changed by applying rectangular polarizing current pulses of long duration (several seconds). The circles give the mean resting potential (polarizing pulses not applied). Note that complete inactivation for the 13-day heart occurs at about $-55\,mV$, whereas complete inactivation does not occur until about $-25\,mV$ for the 3-day and 5-day hearts. For the 3-day and 13-day hearts, there appears to be only one type channel: slow and fast, respectively. The data for the 5-day heart (transition period) suggest that there are two sets of channels, one set inactivating at about $-55\,mV$ and the other set at $-25\,mV$. Modified from Sperelakis and Shigenobu {14}, with permission.

increase in the maximal rate of rise (dV/dt max; fig. 35-2) and overshoot of the AP (fig. 35-2), as well as an increase in resting potential. The overshoot averaged $+11\,mV$ on day 2 and increased progressively over the next few days, reaching the maximal value of about $+28\,mV$ by day 8. The duration (at 50% repolarization) was hardly changed during development, the average value being 110 ms. The time course of the increase in dV/dt max was not parallel to the increase in resting E_m, the increase in resting E_m preceding the increase in dV/dt max by several days; that is, in young hearts it was not unusual to find a cell with a large resting potential but with a low dV/dt max.

Young embryonic (2–3 days in ovo) myocardial cells possess slowly rising (10–40 V/s). APs preceded by pacemaker potentials (fig. 35-2A). Hyperpolarization does not greatly increase the rate of rise (fig. 35-3), thus indicating that the low dV/dt max is not due to inactivation of fast Na^+ channels at the low resting potential, but rather to a low density of fast Na^+ channels. Excitability is not lost until the membrane is depolarized to less than $-20\,mV$ (fig. 35-3), thus indicating the preponderance of slow channels. The AP upstroke in young hearts is generated by Na^+ influx through (TTX-insensitive) slow Na^+ channels, as indicated by the dependence of the AP overshoot and

rate of rise (fig. 35-4) on the external Na^+ concentration. The reactivation kinetics for the inward currents contributing to the upstroke of the AP in 3-day-old hearts have been examined {55}.

Kinetically fast Na^+ channels are substantial in number by day 4. Circulation is established to the chorioallanoic membrane for gas exchange on day 5. On day 5, dV/dt max is about 50–70 V/s (table 35-2). During this intermediate stage of development (from about day 5–7), a large number of slow channels still coexist with the fast Na^+ channels in the membrane.

By day 8, depolarization to less than $-50\,mV$ abolishes excitability (fig. 35-3). This indicates that the AP-generating Na^+ channels now consist predominantly of fast Na^+ channels. The dependence of the inward current on $[Na]_o$ during the AP in old embryonic hearts is also shown in fig. 35-4. The density of fast Na^+ channels continues to increase until about day 18, when the adult maximal rate of rise of about 150 v/s is achieved (fig. 35-3). This conclusion has been strengthened by confirmatory observations reported by Iijima and Pappano {56} and Marcus and Fozzard {57}. A large fraction of the slow Na^+ channels appear to have been lost functionally, and insufficient numbers remain to support regenerative excitation. (However, the simultaneous increase in resting potential during development might render propagation more difficult for any given density of slow channels because of the greater critical depolarization required to reach

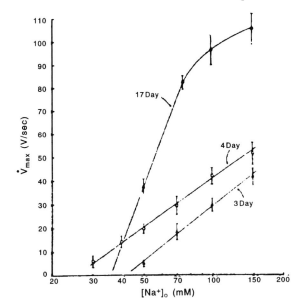

Fig. 35-4. Evidence that Na$^+$ is the predominant carrier of inward current in both young and old embryonic chick hearts. The effect of variation of [Na]$_o$ on maximum rate of rise of the action potential (dV/dt max) is shown. [Na]$_o$ was lowered by replacing the NaCl with equimolar amounts of choline-Cl. Plotted are the mean dV/dt max ($\pm$SE) values for 3-day, 4-day, and 17-day-old hearts. The curve for the old heart is linear at lower [Na]$_o$ levels and flattens at higher levels; for the young hearts, the curves are linear over the entire range. Modified from Sperelakis and Shigenobu {14}, with permission.

Table 35-2. Effect of tetrodotoxin (TTX) on the action-potential maximal rate of rise (dV/dt max) of chick embryonic hearts (ventricular muscle) as a function of development age

Embryonic age (days)	dV/dt max (V/s)		
	Control	+TTX	TTX sensitivity
2–3	15–35	10–30	Little or none
5–6	50–70	10–30	Partial
8–10	75–90	0	Complete
12–16	90–140	0	Complete
17–21	140–170	0	Complete

Data taken from Sperelakis and Shigenobu {14}, with permission.

threshold and because of the increased K$^+$ conductance.) Addition of some positive inotropic agents rapidly increases the number of slow Ca^{2+}-Na$^+$ channels available in the membrane and leads to the regaining of excitability in cells whose fast Na$^+$ channels have been voltage inactivated or blocked {58–60}.

Sensitivity to TTX and to calcium antagonistic drugs

Tetrodotoxin (TTX), a specific blocker of fast Na$^+$ channels, has no effect or only little effect on the AP rate of rise or overshoot of the young (2- to 3-day-old) hearts (fig. 35-2B; table 35-2). During the intermediate stage (days 5–7), TTX causes a reduction in dV/dt max to about 10–20 V/s, but the APs and accompanying contractions persist (figs. 35-2C and 35-2D; table 35-2). After day 8, the APs are completely abolished by TTX despite increased stimulation intensity (figs. 35-2E and 35-2F; table 35-2).

The Ca^{2+}-antagonist drugs, verapamil and D-600, block the APs of the young embryonic hearts {61,62}. This indicates that these agents block slow Na$^+$ channels as well as slow Ca^{2+} and slow Ca^{2+}-Na$^+$ channels, and so are not specific for blockade of Ca^{2+} current. In contrast, Mn^{2+} at 1 mM does not depress the APs of young hearts, although it does block the contractions, indicating a greater specificity for slow Ca^{2+} channels and not for the slow Na$^+$

channels {14}. The inward current during the AP is carried predominantly through TTX-insensitive slow Na$^+$ channels. The slow Na$^+$ channels are blocked by verapamil, D-600, and nifedipine, but not by 1 mM Mn^{2+}, diltiazem, bepridil, or mesudipine {63}.

In experiments on 3-day-old chick embryonic hearts, it was confirmed that verapamil and D-600 depress and block the AP {64}. Elevation of [Ca]$_o$ did not antagonize this blocking effect of the drugs, whereas elevation of [Na]$_o$ (starting from 50% of normal [Na]$_o$) did antagonize, consistent with the channel being a slow Na$^+$ rather than a slow Ca^{2+} channel. In addition, it was found that nifedipine also blocked, whereas diltiazem, bepridil, and mesudipin did not. The slow Na$^+$ channels found in 3-day-old hearts are stimulated by the Ca agonist drug, Bay-K-8644 {65}.

Galper and Catterall {66} reported that the early embryonic chick heart was insensitive to TTX (with no regard to contractions) but was sensitive to D-600. During subsequent development, the sensitivity to TTX increased and the sensitivity to D-600 decreased in a reciprocal manner. Kasuya et al. {67} also reported that the slowly rising APs of 3-day-old embryonic chick hearts involved cation channels that were pharmacologically different from those of old embryonic hearts. Nathan and De Haan {68} found that TTX-sensitive fast Na$^+$ conductance channels were absent or nonfunctional in cultured cell reaggregates derived from 3-day-old embryonic chick hearts. Ishima {69} reported that the contractions of 3- to 5-day-old embryonic chick hearts were not affected by TTX.

IONIC CHANNELS CHANGES

Fast sodium channels

Several laboratories reported from electrophysiologic experiments that there is a large increased in number of fast Na$^+$ channels during development. It was demonstrated by Renaud et al. {70} that the number of specific TTX-binding sites (using ^{3}H-ethylenediamine-TTX) is very low in 3-day-old embryonic chick hearts, and increases four- to fivefold during embryonic development (fig. 35-5). They also confirmed that the APs in the 2- to 3-day hearts were

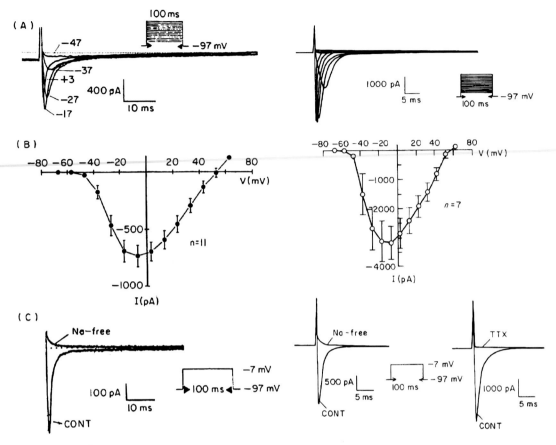

Fig. 35-5. Binding of [^{3}H]en-TTX to chicken embryonic heart cells. Evolution of the properties of TTX receptors during in ovo development of embryonic chicken heart ventricles. ●, maximum number of TTX binding sites; ○, K_d values. Modified from Renaud et al. {70}, with permission.

insensitive to TTX. Iijima and Pappano {56} and Marcus and Fozzard {57} reported that there are some fast Na$^+$ channels detectable on day 3 and that the sensitivity of the fast Na$^+$ channels to blockade by TTX does not change during development. Fujii et al. {73}, in voltage-clamp studies on isolated single ventricular cells from 2- to 7-day-old embryonic chick hearts, found that the fast Na$^+$ current density increased about eightfold (fig. 35-6) and the time constant of inactivation (τ_h) decreased from 2 to 1 ms. They concluded that the small, fast Na$^+$ current normally makes no contribution to the AP in the 2-day-old hearts because of their inactivation at the low resting potential or maximum diastolic potential at that stage of development. Other than the magnitude of the current, there was no difference in the activation kinetics, voltage dependence, or TTX sensitivity of the fast Na$^+$ current in 2-day versus 7-day hearts.

On the other hand, studying the developmental changes in the characteristics of the fast Na$^+$ current between 18-day-old fetal and 1-day-old neonatal rat ventricular myocytes, Conforti et al. {71} showed that (a) although the ion selectivity and sensitivity to TTX were identical at all de-

velopmental stages, the current density increased fivefold (196 pA/pF vs. 39.0 pA/pF) with development (fig. 35-7). In these experiments, the inward current was completely abolished by removing Na$^+$ from the external solution (replaced by choline) or in the presence of 50 μM TTX. The potentials for threshold and peak current in the fetal cells were comparable in the neonatal cells, but 10–20 mV more depolarized compared with those in adult cells {72}. These differences may arise from the difference in steady-state activation curve between the two age groups, whereas the h_∞ curve was not different at both developmental stages (fig. 35-8). (b) The recovery from complete inactivation of the Na$^+$ current in fetal cells was slower than in neonatal and adult cells {72}. This suggests that the fetal cells have a longer functional refractory period than the neonatal and adult cells. It may be related to the lower heart rate and longer APD$_{50}$ recorded at this fetal age compared to neonatal and adult rat hearts {74,75}. (c) Values of $V_{1/2}$ and k, for both steady-state activation and inactivation, were comparable to those reported for the fetal heart (table 35-3), giving a comparable overlap and window current. However, the fetal cells had a very slow

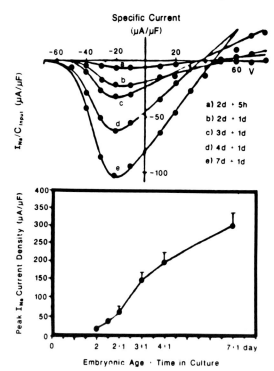

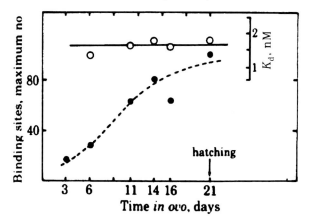

Fig. 35-7. Fast sodium current recorded from 18-day-old fetal (left) and 1-day-old (right) rat ventricular cardiomyocytes. Currents were recorded in Ca^{2+}/K^{+}-free external and internal solutions with 143 mM $[Na]_o$ and 20 mM $[Na]_i$. **A:** Na currents, uncorrected for capacitive or leakage currents, in response to several depolarizing steps. Only the first 70 ms of the 100-ms depolarizing pulse are shown. Holding potential was $-97\,mV$; test pulses, in 10-mV increments, were applied from $-67\,mV$ to 63 mV (**inset**) **B:** I-V relationship for the peak Na^{+} current. The curve represents the mean $\pm$ SE of 11 (left) or 7 (right) cells, and the measured reversal potential was (left) 51 $\pm$ 3 mV and (right) 53.3 $\pm$ 3 mV (calculated from individual I-V curves). **C:** Superimposed current traces showing fast Na^{+} current recorded during the control period (CONT) and after exposure to an external solution containing 0 mM $[Na]_o$ (Na^{+} completely replaced by choline) or 50 μM TTX. Only part of the 100-ms pulse is displayed. Dotted lines in A and C represent the zero current level. Modified from Conforti et al. {71}, with permission.

Fig. 35-6. Increase in density of fast Na^{+} channels during development of the heart. **Upper part:** I/V curves obtained from isolated single embryonic chick heart cells at different stages of embryonic development: (a) 2 days (+5 hours in culture), (b) 2 days (+1 day in culture), (c) 3 days (+1 day in culture), (d) 4 days (+1 day in culture), and (e) 7 days (+1 day in culture). Note the increase in intensity of the inward Na^{+} current with development. Current normalized for unit membrane capacitance, i.e., current density. **Lower part:** Plot of peak inward current density as a function of embryonic age. Note the very low current density on day 2 and the nearly linear increase up through day 8. Reproduced by permission from Fujii et al. {182}, with permission.

INWARD RECTIFIER POTASSIUM CHANNELS

The inwardly rectifying K^{+} current (I_{K1}) has been shown to play an important role in the electrogenesis of the atrial and ventricular action potential {80}. One function of I_{K1} is to maintain a stable resting potential, near E_K (the K^{+} equilibrium potential). Conversely, the virtual absence of I_{K1} in SA and AV nodal cells may contribute to the genesis of automaticity. During the first postnatal week, the action potential of the rat ventricular myocyte shortens markedly with concomitant regression of the plateau phase, increase in the rate of repolarization, and hyperpolarization of the resting potential (fig. 35-9; table 35-4). These changes may be related to developmental changes in the repolarizing current (mainly I_{K1}). Studying the developmental changes in I_{K1} between cultured 1-day- and 7-day-old rat ventricular myocytes, Haddad et al. {20} showed that with respect to the younger hearts: (a) I_{K1} was more sensitive to Ba^{2+} block; (b) I_{K1} channel density did not change; (c) E_{rev} of I_{K1} was more hyperpolarized, along with a lower P_{Na}/P_K; (d) the steady-state probability of opening of I_{K1} was higher in the 7-day- than in the 1-day-old cells (0.57 vs. 0.45, respectively, at $V_m = -130\,mV$); (e) the amplitude of the current density at $V_m < E_{rev}$ is significantly lower (fig. 35-9), relating this fact to the more negative E_{rev} of

decay process compared with the neonatal (table 35-3) and the adult cells {72}. This slow decay process accounts for the small, but significant, Na^{+} inward current ($I_{Na(si)}$), even at 100 ms, during the voltage-clamp pulse (fig. 35-7). This sustained current was observed over much wider potential ranges than expected from the window current (table 35-3). Similar kinetics of the fast Na^{+} current were observed in chick embryonic (3-day-old) heart cells, which was attributed to the burstlike mode of Na^{+} channel activity {76}. Although the burstlike mode was also reported in adult rat {77} and guinea pig {78,79}, the frequency of occurrence of this mode was lower than that in chick embryo. Therefore, very slow decay of the Na^{+} current may be a characteristic property of the fetal period. Thus the contribution of the Na^{+} current to the plateau phase is expected to be much smaller in adult compared to fetal ventricular cells.

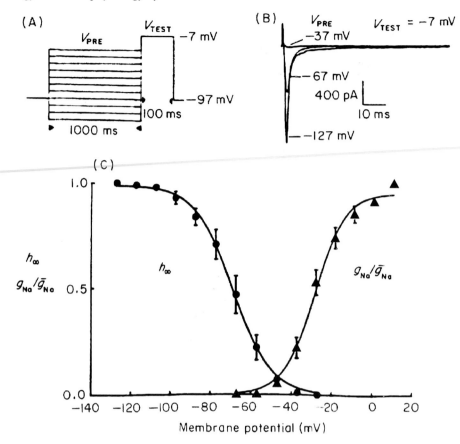

Fig. 35-8. Activation ($g_{Na}/\bar{g}_{Na}$) and steady-state inactivation (h_∞) curves for the fast Na^+ current recorded in fetal rat cardiomyocytes. Steady-state inactivation: The prepulse test program is shown in panel **A**. The prepulse potential (V_{PRE}) was changed from -127 to -27 mV in 10-mV increments, with the test voltage (V_{TEST}) at -7 mV. Representative currents are shown in panel **B**. The corresponding V_{PRE} values are indicated. Capacitive and leakage currents were subtracted. The test pulse current is expressed as a fraction of the maximum at -127 mV and plotted against the membrane potential in panel C for eight cells, giving the mean h_∞ curve (●). The points were best fitted to the Boltzmann equation: $max/[1 + exp([V_{PRE} - V_{1/2}]/k)]$. The slope factor (k) is 9.5 mV and the half-inactivation potential ($V_{1/2}$) is -69 mV. Activation is expressed as normalized Na^+ conductance (g_{Na}) calculated from the equation: $g_{Na} = I_{Na}/(V - V_{Na})$. I_{Na} was measured after subtraction of capacitive and leakage currents (in Na^+-free solution). The normalized g_{Na} ($= g_{Na}/\bar{g}_{Na}$) for eight cells is plotted against the membrane potential in panel C (●). The points are best fitted to the equation: $max/[1 + exp([V - V_{1/2}]/k)]$. The slope factor (k) is -8.4 mV and the half-activation potential ($V_{1/2}$) is -27 mV. h_∞ and $g_{Na}/\bar{g}_{Na}$ curves overlap between the potential range of -60 to -30 mV, giving a substantial window current. Taken from Conforti et al. {71}, with permission.

I_{K1} and stronger voltage-dependent steady-state inactivation of I_{K1} in the 7-day-old myocytes. This latter fact was supported with the findings of Kilborn and Fedida {18}, who used cultured cells as well. On the other hand, whole-cell recording in freshly isolated rat ventricular myocytes showed very small I_{K1} on fetal day 12 {81}. At this stage, a different type of I_{K1} channel that has a small conductance (11 pS) was observed. However, there was a marked increase in whole-cell I_{K1} between day 12 and neonatal day 5, concomitant with the appearance of a large-conductance (31 pS) channel (fig. 35-10); that is, in later stages of development, the small-conductance channel disappears, and there was an increase in the open probability of the large-conductance channel. The ratio

of (neonatal day 5)/(fetal day 18) for whole-cell current density and for single-channel open probability were well matched, namely, 2.5 in each case (table 35-5). Thus, the increase in whole-cell I_{K1} is likely due to the appearance and increase in open probability of the large-conductance channel. The small conductance may be an immature type of I_{K1} channel that disappears during development. A parallel conclusion was made by Wahler {17}, showing that the appearance of a large-conducting channel contributes to the developmental increase in I_{K1} of freshly dissociated neonatal and adult rat ventricular myocytes. In the same line, the magnitude of the macroscopic I_{K1} conductance was very small in the 3-day-old, but increased fivefold in the 17-day-old, embryonic chick ventricular

A

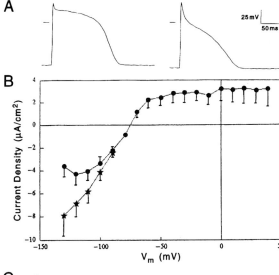

25mV |
‾‾‾‾‾
50ms

B

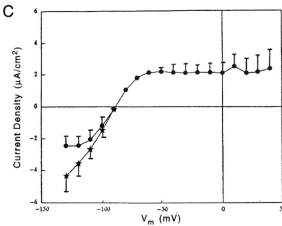

Table 35-3. Characteristics of fast sodium current recorded in 18-day-old fetal and 1-day-old neonatal rat ventricular cardiomyocytes

	18-day fetal rat	1-day neonatal[a]
I_d (pA/pF)	39 ± 7 (9)	196 ± 47
τ_{if} (ms)	1.3 ± 0.1	0.8 ± 0.1
τ_{is} (ms)	14 ± 2	5 ± 1
A_{if} (pA)	538 ± 10^5	3266 ± 440
A_{is} (pA)	110 ± 19	360 ± 95
A_{is}/A_{if}	0.24 ± 0.06	0.11 ± 0.03
τ_{rf} (ms)	10.5 ± 1.5 (5)	4.2 ± 1.2 (4)
τ_n (ms)	307 ± 44 (5)	74 ± 14 (4)

Mean $\pm$ SE (n).
[a] $p < 0.01$.
n is equal to 8 for fetal and 6 for neonatal myocytes unless otherwise indicated (parentheses).
All parameters were obtained at -7 mV.
Taken from Conforti et al. {71}, with permission.

C

Fig. 35-9. **A:** Stimulated action potentials of 1-day- (left) and 7-day (right) old rat ventricular cardiomyocytes, acquired during current-clamp experiments. Horizontal lines indicate the zero potential level. The stimulation frequency was 0.1 Hz with a 3-ms pulse, whose amplitude was set to 1.5 times the threshold. **B,C:** I-V relationship of the Ba^{2+}-sensitive steady-state (●) and initial peak (★) currents (I_{K1}) in 1-day- (B) and 7-day- (C) old rat ventricular cardiomyocytes. $[K]_o = 6$ mM and $[K]_i = 120$ mM. Corrections were made for the respective holding currents. Data points are means $\pm$ SE (n = 6 and 20 in B and C, respectively). Modified from Haddad {21}, with permission.

TRANSIENT OUTWARD CHANNELS

Kilborn and Fedida {18} reported that the transient outward current (I_{to}) in rat heart cells is mainly a time- and voltage-dependent current. They showed a progressively greater effect of 4-aminopyridine (blocker of I_{to}) on the action potential of the 5-day- and 10-day-old than the 1-day-old rat ventricular myocytes. They related that to the fourfold increase in the current density of I_{to}. Its steady-state inactivation kinetics did not change during development; however, its selectivity for K^+ increased, relating it to the more negative reversal potential in 10-day-old rats with respect to the 1-day-old animal. On the other hand, Conforti and Sperelakis {84} discovered and characterized an early fast component of I_{to} [$I_{to(f)}$] in ventricular cardiomyocytes freshly isolated from neonatal rats. I_{to} is blocked by 4-AP {85}, whereas $I_{to(f)}$ is insensitive to 4-AP but sensitive to 1 mM diphenyl-amine-2-carboxylate (Cl^- current blocker) and 50% inhibited by 10 μM TTX (Na^+ current blocker). Both currents were sensitive to K^+ removal; however, they were Ca^{2+} insensitive. $I_{to(f)}$ seems to be carried by Na^+, K^+, and Cl^-, contributing to the initial repolarization (phase 1) of the action potential. Its current density is 64 ± 7 pA/pF with a time to peak of 1.1 ± 0.1 ms, compared to 5 ms for the regular I_{to}.

CALCIUM CHANNELS

Using the patch-clamp method, two types of Ca^{2+} channels having different single-channel conductances have been found in myocardial cells {86–89}. The dihydropyridine (DHP)-sensitive L-type Ca^{2+} channel contributes to long-lasting current at large depolarizations (high threshold). The T-type Ca^{2+} channel produces a transient current activated at small depolarizations (low threshold) and is insensitive to DHPs. The L-type channels inactivate much more slowly that the T-type channels. L-type current is

myocytes {82}. This was related to an increase in the number of functional channels per unit membrane, an increase in the conductance per channel, and an increase in the probability of opening of single channel. In addition, Huynh et al. {83} showed that in rabbit ventricular myocytes, I_{K1} current density increases rapidly between day 21 and the perinatal period, and to a lesser extent after birth.

Table 35-4. Action potential characteristics of cardiomyocytes from 1-day- and 7-day-old rats

Age (days)	RP (mV)	APA (mV)	OS (mV)	APD (ms) 25	50	95
1	-73.1 ± 1.9	109.9 ± 4.7	38.2 ± 4.6	73.5 ± 20.0	118.2 ± 17.3	215.2 ± 12.4
7	-79.0 ± 1.1	113.8 ± 3.5	34.8 ± 3.4	32.6 ± 7.7	77.9 ± 9.5	165.8 ± 11.7

Mean $\pm$ SE.
n is equal to 9 for 1-day- and 14 for 7-day-old rat ventricular myocytes.
[a]$p < 0.05$; [b]$p < 0.01$, with respect to the younger heart cells.
Modified from Haddad {21}, with permission.

dominant in adult ventricular myocytes. In rat myocytes, the atrial T-current density increased by 70% from 3 to 14 postnatal weeks rat myocytes {90}. On the other hand, the gating of the cardiac L-type Ca^{2+} channel is characterized by brief openings that occur during rapid bursts (model 1) {91,92}. Recently, using guinea pig and frog heart cells, Hess et al. {92} showed a different form of gating behavior (mode 2), in addition to the conventional model 1. In mode 2, channel openings tend to be long lasting and channel closings tend to be brief. They also showed that the DHP Ca^{2+}-channel agonist, BAY K 8644, facilitated mode 2 behavior. In cultured embryonic chick (3-day-old) cardiomyocytes, Tohse and Sperelakis {93} demonstrated the occurrence of the long-lasting openings of the slow calcium channels in the absence of added Ca^{2+}-channel agonist, with a high frequency of observation (20.7%) of high-P_o sweeps ($P_o > 0.65$). This current was inhibited by 8Br-cGMp (fig. 35-11), which is a membrane-permeable derivative of cGMP known to block $I_{Ca,L}$ in cardiomyocytes (figs. 35-11 and 35-12). Recently, Tohse et al. {96} showed that the peak current density of $I_{Ca,L}$ was significantly higher in 3-day- than in 17-day-old embryonic cells, with no change in the window current during development (table 35-6). In single-channel recordings, the peak amplitude of the ensemble-averaged currents was 2.7-fold larger in 3-day cells than 17-day cells. This difference corresponds to the difference in the whole-cell current density and in the open probability (for all sweeps) with the naturally occurring mode 2 behavior disappearing during development (table 35-7).

A novel type of Ca^{2+} current was reported by Tohse et al. {97} in rat fetal cardiomyocytes, called the *fetal-type calcium current* [$I_{Ca(fe)}$]. This current was not blocked by DHPs, even at relatively high concentrations (fig. 35-13). Its activation threshold, potential for maximal amplitude, and inactivation time constants were similar to the L-type current. However, the steady-state inactivation curve for $I_{Ca(fe)}$ was shifted to more negative potentials with respect to the L current (fig. 35-14). They reported that the adult cells possess only the L-type Ca^{2+} current ($I_{Ca,L}$), and $I_{Ca(fe)}$ disappears during development and its channels may be replaced by newly synthesized DHP-sensitive channels.

In cultured single rat ventricular myocytes, Cohen and Lederer {98} compared the properties of $I_{Ca,L}$ at neonatal days 2–7 with those of the adult (6–8 weeks). They reported that the density of $I_{Ca,L}$ in neonatal cells was larger than that seen in the adult. They suggested that the larger transient and steady-state component of $I_{Ca,L}$ seen in the neonatal cells may reflect a greater Ca^{2+} channel density. The Ca^{2+} channel window current in adult cells was smaller than in neonatal cells, due to the steady-state inactivation curve (f_∞) shift in the hyperpolarizing direction by 15 mV (shift in V_h), whereas there was almost no shift in the steady-state activation curve (d_∞).

BIOCHEMICAL CHANGES

Cyclic nucleotides levels

Pronounced changes in cyclic AMP content occur during embryonic development of the chick heart {54,99,100}. The cyclic AMP level is highest in young hearts and it decreases during development. McLean et al. {99} found a cyclic AMP level of 116 pM/mg protein on day 4, and this decreased sharply by day 5 to about 41; there was a gradual further decline to 9.4 pM/mg protein, which is about the adult level, by day 16. Renaud et al. {100} found a cyclic AMP level of 33.6 pM/mg protein on day 4 and 11.7 on day 16.

In contrast to cyclic AMP levels, the cyclic GMP level was reported by Thakkar and Sperelakis {101} to be very low in young embryonic chick hearts and to increase during development (fig. 35-15). The cyclic GMP content was 45.5 ± 2.3 fM/mg protein in 3-day-old hearts and 338 ± 15.0 in 14- to 19-day hearts. Therefore there was a reciprocal relationship between the basal cyclic AMP and cyclic GMP levels. Nitroprusside (5×10^{-5} M) and hydrogen peroxide (0.1%), agents known to stimulate guanylate cyclase and elevate cyclic GMP, increased cyclic GMP level (in 3 minutes) in embryonic chick hearts 5 days old or older, but not in 3-day-old hearts. In young 3-day-old embryonic chick hearts, ACh (50 μM) and Ado (50 μM) increased cyclic GMP concentration only slightly, whereas these substances produced a large increase (e.g., about twofold) in cyclic GMP level in hearts 5 days old and older {101}. Therefore, it appears that the guanylate cyclase activity is very low in young 3-day-old hearts.

The relationship between changes in membrane pro-

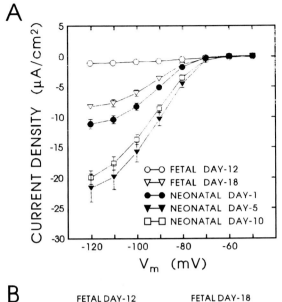

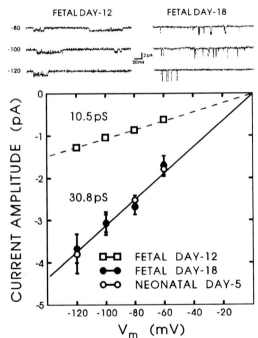

Table 35-5. Comparison of the whole-cell and single-channel data ($V_m = -80\,mV$)

	Whole-cell I_{K1} (pA/pF)	Single-channel P_o
Fetal day 18	1.4	2.8
Neonatal day 5	3.2	6.9
B/A ratio	2.5	2.5

Taken from Masuda and Sperelakis {81}, with permission.

Fig. 35-10. Developmental changes of I_{K1} in rat ventricular myocytes. **A:** Current/voltage relations at the different developmental stages (from fetal day 12 to neonatal day 10). Currents were elicited from a HP of $-40\,mV$. Data points are shown as mean ± SEM (n = 5–10). **B:** Current/voltage relations for single I_{K1} channels in different developmental stages. **Upper panel:** Single-channel current recording from typical fetal ventricular myocytes (days 12 and 18). **Lower panel:** Current/voltage relations for single I_{K1} channel in the three different developmental stages: fetal days 12 and 18, and neonatal day 5. Note the lower single-channel conductance at fetal day 12. Modified from Masuda and Sperelakis {81}, with permission.

perties and changes in cyclic AMP levels during development of heart remains to be clarified. In cultured skeletal muscle, however, the cyclic AMP level decreases sharply as the myoblasts fuse into myotubes, i.e., when the cells further differentiate {102}. In addition, the increase in cyclic AMP level is associated with an increase in the number of available slow channels. Therefore, it is tempting to speculate that the decrease in the number of available slow channels during development of chick heart, as described above, results from the concomitant drop in cyclic AMP level. This would allow positive inotropic agents that increase the cyclic AMP level to increase the number of available slow channels transiently back toward the density present in young embryonic hearts. In other words, the developmental change in steady-state level of cyclic AMP allows the fraction of slow channels that are available for activation to be modulated by inotropic agents.

It appears that the cyclic AMP level in cultured heart cells is either about the same (e.g., 16 pM/mg protein in cells derived from 16-day hearts) {99} or reduced (e.g, 4.5 pM/mg protein) {100}. A reduction in cyclic AMP was observed in cell cultures prepared from 4-day-old chick hearts. The cyclic AMP level of young (4-day) hearts placed into organ culture for 2 weeks declines (to 5.6 pM/mg protein), even though the cells do not further differentiate electrically or ultrastructurally {100}. A similar decline in cyclic AMP level (to 5–3 pM/mg protein) was observed in organ-cultured 16-day-old chick hearts. Isoproterenol was capable of markedly elevating the cyclic AMP level in all cases — young or old, cultured or noncultured – thus demonstrating the presence of functional beta-adrenergic receptors.

In rat heart, the cyclic AMP level was reported to increase during the period from just before birth to postnatal day 10 {103}. The changes in cyclic AMP in rat skeletal muscle were similar to those for the heart. Likewise, in embryonic chick skeletal muscle there was an increase in cyclic AMP level between days 7 and 15 {104,105}.

In mouse hearts, Haddox et al. {106} found that there was an increase in activity of the cyclic AMP-dependent protein kinase from prenatal day 16 to postnatal day 10, following which activity gradually declined to the adult level (fig. 35-16, squares). Chen et al. {107} found that the basal adenylate cyclase activity was very low at prenatal day 14 and progressively increased through postnatal day 45 (fig. 35-16, filled circles). The isoproterenol ($10^{-6}\,M$)-stimulated adenylate cyclase activity increased in parallel to the basal activity (fig. 35-16, unfilled circles). Au et al.

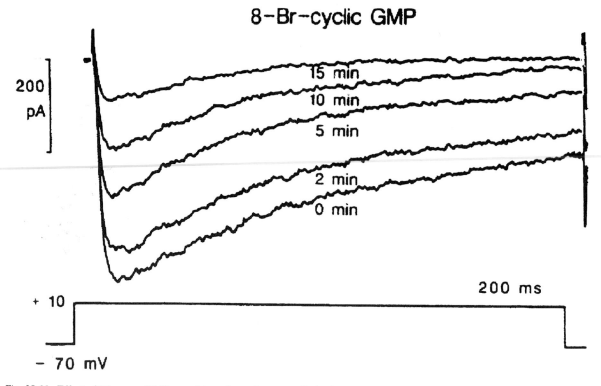

Fig. 35-11. Effect of 8-bromo-cGMP on calcium channel currents (I_{Ca}). Currents were elicited in cultured embryonic chick ventricular myocytes by depolarizing pulses from -70 to $+10\,mV$ in the control bath solution (0 minute), and following 2, 5, 10, and 15 minute superfusion with a solution containing $1\,mM$ 8-bromocyclic GMP. Modified from wahler et al. {94}, with permission.

Table 35-6. Summary of the developmental changes in characteristics of whole-cell L-type Ca^{2+} current in embryonic chick heart cells

	3-day cells	17-day cells	p
$I_{Ca(L)}$ density ($\mu A/cm^2$)	-8.1 ± 0.2	-5.1 ± 0.3	<0.01
τ_f (ms)	15.3 ± 0.3	6.7 ± 0.6	<0.01
τ_s (ms)	65.6 ± 1.5	33.2 ± 0.9	<0.01
V_h act (mV)	-12.4	-11.6	—
V_h intact (mV)	-25.7	-26.8	—

$I_{Ca(L)}$, L-type Ca^{2+} current at $10\,mV$; τ_f, fast time constant; τ_s, slow time constant. V_h, potential at which steady-state activation (act)- and inactivation (inact)-voltage relations are half maximum. Values are mean $\pm$ SEM. n = 5.
Taken from Tohse et al. {96}, with permission.

Table 35-7. Summary of the developmental changes in characteristics of the single Ca^{2+} (L-type) channels in embryonic chick heart cells

	3-day cells	17-day cells	p
Open probability (all sweeps)	0.15 ± 0.04 (14)	0.05 ± 0.01 (9)	<0.05
Mean open time (ms)	7.6 ± 1.5 (14)	4.5 ± 2.3 (8)	NS
Mode 2 (% of sweeps)	20.2	3.7	—
Mode 0 (% of sweeps)	33.8	46.3	—

Mode 2, open probability >0.25.
Mode 0, open probability of 0.
NS, not significant.
Numbers in parentheses given the number of cells.
Values are mean $\pm$ SEM for open probability and mean open time.
Taken from Tohse et al. {96}, with permission.

{108} found that the cAMP content (pM/mg tissue) of the hearts decreased from 0.82 ± 0.08 in 2-day-old rats to 0.51 ± 0.07 in 20-day-old rats. The younger heart was more sensitive to epinephrine than was the older heart. They indicated that there is a lack of functional linking between cAMP level and force in 2-day-old hearts, but an efficient link between them in 20-day-old hearts. Kithas et al. {109} showed that the V_{max} of the of phosphodiesterase-IV (inhibitor of cAMP) activity in the adult (6–8 months) was fivefold higher than in newborn (1–2 days) and threefold higher than that in the immature (14–16 days) rabbit ventricular myocytes {109}.

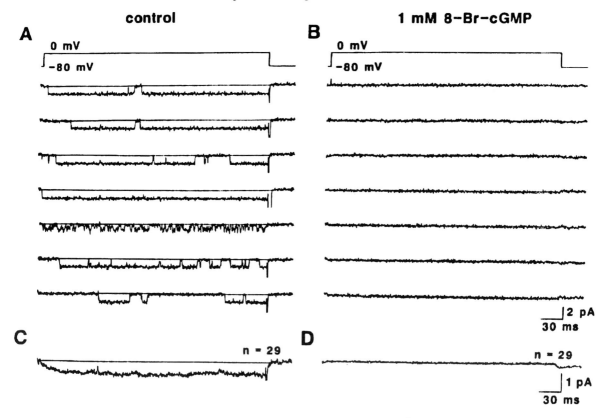

Fig. 35-12. Current recordings showing effect of 8-bromo-cGMP (8-Br-cGMP) on the Ca^{2+} slow channel activity in single myocardial cells isolated from 3-day-old embryonic chick hearts. Cell-attached patch configuration was used. Single-channel currents were evoked by depolarizing voltage pulses to 0 mV from a holding potential of -80 mV, at a repetition rate of 0.5 Hz and duration of 300 msec. **A,B:** Examples of original current recordings from the same patch before (A) and after (B) superfusion with 1.0 mM 8-bromo-cGMP. **C,D:** Ensemble averaged currents calculated from the original current recordings (n = 29). The current tracings were low-pass filtered at 1 kHz and corrected for leakage and capacitive currents. Current and time calibrations are given at the lower right. Taken from Tohse and Sperelakis {95}, with permission.

Protein kinase levels

According to the studies of Novak et al. {110} in rat hearts, the cAMP-protein kinase (PKA) activity was highest in fetal hearts and decreased rapidly by birth. At that time, its activity increased up to postnatal day 10 and remained relatively constant thereafter. In addition, they found that cAMP levels increased rapidly before birth and continued to increase to a maximum on postnatal day 10. Therefore, it appears that there is no close relationship between developmental changes in cAMP levels and PKA activity. Noguchi et al. {111} have reported a similar developmental pattern of PKA between 17 days gestation and 28 days postpartum.

Furthermore, Kuo {112} measured the levels of PKA and the cGMP-dependent protein kinase (PKG) at various stages of development in guinea pig hearts. The PKG activity was highest in the fetus and declined during development, whereas the PKA activity was lower initially and increased with age. Therefore, the ratio of PKG/PKA

levels decreased during development: 0.32 at 10 days before birth, 0.14 at 5 days postpartum, and 0.07 at 310 days. On the other hand, Noguchi et al. {111} found that the activity of the Ca^{2+}-activated phospholipid-dependent protein kinase (PKC) was generally higher in the neonatal period, but was not correlated with the α_1-adrenergic receptor and muscarinic receptor ontogeny in the rat hearts. In addition, they found no correlation between PKC and PKA.

Glucose uptake, amino acid uptake, and membrane fluidity

Changes in other membrane properties also occur during development. For example, glucose uptake is very high in young hearts and decreases during development. A carrier-mediated saturable glucose transport system appears on about day 7, and an enhancement of glucose uptake by insulin can be first demonstrated shortly thereafter {113}. Thus, insulin had no effect on glucose uptake of 5-day-old embryonic chick hearts but did affect 7-day-

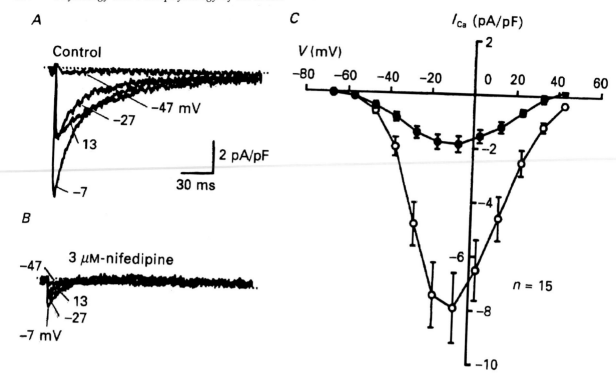

A

Control

−47 mV

−27

13

−7

2 pA/pF

30 ms

B

−47

3 μM-nifedipine

13

−27

−7 mV

C

I_{Ca} (pA/pF)

V (mV)

−80   −60   −40   −20   0   20   40   60

2

−2

−4

−6

−8

−10

$n = 15$

Fig. 35-13. Effects of 3 μM-nifedipine on the Ca^{2+} current in fetal rat cardiomyocytes. **A,B:** selected current tracings elicited by 300-ms depolarizing pulses to −47, −27, −7, and 13 mV from a holding potential of −87 mV; only the 150-ms segment is shown. Capacitive and leakage currents were subtracted by tracings in presence of Co^{2+} (2 mM). The current calibration is given as current density. In the presence of 3 μM-nifedipine, small inward currents remained at each potential. **C:** Current-voltage (current density) relationship of data from 15 cells. Data points are shown as means ± SEM. As shown nifedipine (3 μM) did not completely block the Ca^{2+} current (at all potentials; ○, control; ●, nifedipine). The nifedipine-resistant current had a threshold potential and a potential for maximal current similar to those of the control current. Taken from Tohse et al. {97}, with permission.

old hearts. Glucose uptake by hearts 5 days old and younger seems to be by simple diffusion across the membrane {114,115}. Ouabain stimulates glucose uptake in 10-day-old hearts but not in 5-day hearts {116}. As development proceeds, the heart myocytes also become progressively less permeable to sorbitol.

Amino acids are actively transported against concentration gradients in 5-day-old embryonic chick hearts, and insulin enhances the rate of amino acid transport {117}. The amino acid uptake decreases with development.

There are also changes in membrane fluidity (microviscosity) during development of chick hearts {115}. There is a trend toward increase in fluidity as development proceeds. The cholesterol-phospholipid ratio of the sarcolemma increases during development, concomitant with an increase in the number of unsaturated fatty acid residues. In general, the changes seem to be too complex to correlate with changes in the electrical properties, as, for example, with changes in K^+ permeability. The membrane fluidity of cultured chick skeletal myoblasts increases concomitant with fusion and myotube formation {118}.

Metabolic changes

Young (2- to 3-day-old) embryonic chick hearts have large pools of glycogen, and their metabolism is mainly by anaerobic glycolysis. The circulation to the chorioallantoic membrane under the eggshell for gas exchange is not established until day 5. Following this event, there is a shift toward aerobic metabolism, accompanied by changes in various enzymes. For example, there is an increase in pyruvate kinase activity {119,120}. Many of the biochemical changes that occur in hearts during development have been summarized in a review by Harary {121}.

Hearts of young chick embryos utilize the phosphogluconate pathway to a greater extent, relative to the tricarboxylic acid cycle pathway, than do hearts of older embryos or adults {122}. Proliferating cells in general are characterized by the high activity of pentose cycle enzymes {123}. Enzymes of the pentose shunt pathway, such as glucose-6-P dehydrogenase and 6-P-gluconic dehydrogenase, decrease from day 4 to day 20, whereas enzymes of the Krebs cycle, such as isocitric dehydrogense and α-

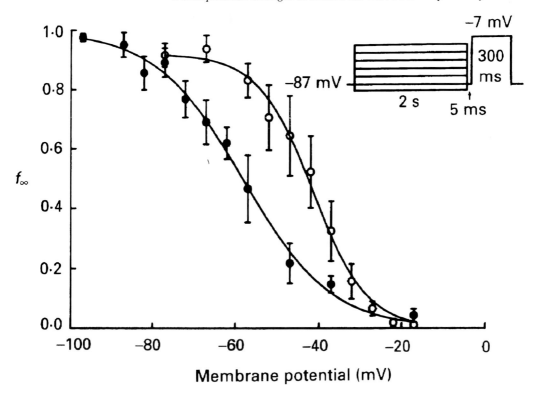

Fig. 35-14. Steady-state inactivation (f_∞) curves of the DHP-sensitive current ($\bigcirc$) and the DHP-resistant current ($\bullet$). Nifedipine (3 μM) was used for analysis. The inset shows the voltage protocol for measuring f_∞. Conditioning pulse duration was 2 seconds; test pulse duration was 300 ms. Test pulses were applied to −7 mV from various conditioning pulse levels. There was a 5-ms interval between the end of the conditioning pulse and the beginning of the test pulse in which the membrane potential was returned to the holding potential of −87 mV. Data are shown as mean ± SEM (n = 5–8). Both curves were fitted by the Boltzmann equation: $f_\infty = 1/[1 + (\exp[V - V_{0.5}]k)]$. The half-inactivation potential ($V_{0.5}$) was −42.0 and −58.4 mV for DHP-sensitive current and DHP-resistant current, respectively. The slope factors (k) were 6.8 (DHP sensitive) and 10^{-7} (DHP resistant). Note the 16-mV shift of the curve in the hyperpolarized direction compared with that for the DHP-sensitive current. Taken from Tohse et al. {97}, with permission.

ketoglutaric dehydrogense, increase during development {124}. In addition, hexokinase activity increases several-fold. The capacity to metabolize long-chain fatty acids appears late in development (after day 12) {125}.

In rat hearts, lactic dehydrogenase (LDH) shifts from the embryonic M-form isoenzyme (which catalyzes the reduction of pyruvate to lactate) to the adultlike H form (which facilitates pyruvate oxidation to CO_2 and H_2O) {126}. Similar changes were shown to occur in embryonic chick skeletal muscle {127}. When old embryonic chick myocardial cells are cultured in monolayers, they begin to synthesize the early embryonic M-LDH {128}. Isoenzyme transformation also occurs during rat heart development with respect to creatine phosphokinase {129}.

Consistent with the fact that young embryonic hearts have a low rate of aerobic metabolism, being mainly dependent on glycolysis, the young hearts are relatively resistant to metabolic interventions. For example, hypoxia does not block the slow APs of young embryonic chick hearts {130}. Similarly, ventricular cells of 7-day-old chick embryonic hearts are much less sensitive than those of 15-

day-old hearts to a variety of metabolic poisons {131}. In mammalian atrial muscle, which has a high glycogen content, the isoproterenol-induced slow APs are only slightly depressed by hypoxia {132}.

REGULATION OF Ca^{2+} MYOCARDIAL SLOW CHANNELS BY CYCLIC NUCLEOTIDE AND PHOSPHORYLATION

Action of positive inotropic agents

A number of positive inotropic agents exert an effect on the myocardial cell membrane to increase the number of available slow channels, and this action may at least partly explain their effect on increasing cardiac contractility. It is through the slow channels that Ca^{2+} influx occurs during the cardiac AP, and the amount of Ca^{2+} ion entering the myocardial cell controls the force of contraction. The Ca^{2+} entering also indirectly helps to elevate $[Ca]_i$ by bringing about the further release of Ca^{2+} from the intracellular

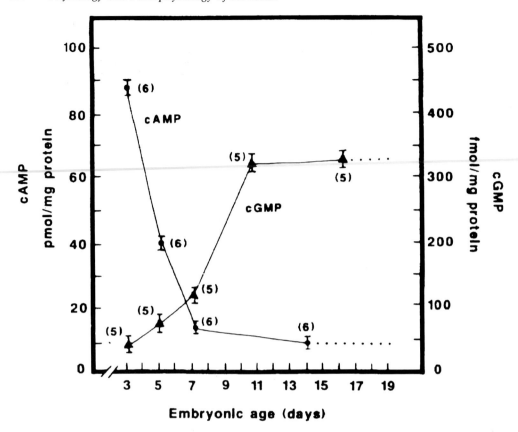

Fig. 35-15. Changes in the basal levels of cyclic AMP and cyclic GMP as a function of embryonic age. Hearts from chick embryos were removed, incubated in MEM, and cyclic nucleotide levels were determined as described in the methods: Cyclic AMP (O-O), cyclic GMP (Δ-Δ). The data point plotted at 10.5 days represents the average of cyclic GMP levels from days 9–12, and the data point plotted at 16.5 days represents the average from days 14–19. The average of cyclic AMP levels from days 9–19 is represented as a data point plotted at day 14. Reproduced from Thakkar and Sperelakis {101}, with permission.

stores in the SR {133}. Blockade of the slow channels, and hence Ca^{2+} influx, by Ca^{2+}-antagonistic agents, such as verapamil, D-600, nifedipine, Mn^{2+}, Co^{2+}, and La^{3+}, depresses or abolishes the contractions without greatly affecting the normal fast AP, i.e., contraction is uncoupled from excitation.

The positive inotropic agents that have been shown to affect the number of available slow channels include catecholamines (beta-adrenergic receptor agonists), histamine (H_2 receptor), methylxanthines, angiotensin II, and fluoride ion. The action of most of these agents is very rapid, the peak effect often occurring within 1–3 minutes.

Relationship to cyclic AMP

Histamine and beta-adrenergic agonists, subsequent to binding to their specific receptors, are known to lead to rapid stimulation of adenylate cyclase with resultant elevation of cyclic AMP levels {134,135}. The methylxanthines enter into the myocardial cells and inhibit phosphodiesterase, thus causing an elevation of cyclic

AMP {134}. These positive inotropic agents also rapidly induce the slow APs by making more slow channels available in the membrane. Hence, cyclic AMP is somehow involved in the functioning of the slow channels {59,134, 136–138}.

Consistent with this, cyclic AMP itself and its dibutyryl derivative also induce the slow APs, but only after a much longer lag period (peak effect in 15–30 minutes), as would be expected from slow penetration through the membrane {59,136}. Another test of the cyclic AMP hypothesis was done by using a GTP analog (5′-guanylimidodiphosphate [GPP (NH)P]), an agent known to directly activate adenylate cyclase in a variety of broken cell preparations. The addition of GPP(NH)P (10^{-5} to 10^{-3} M) induced the slow APs in cultured reaggregates of chick heart cells within 5–30 minutes {139}. These results support the hypothesis that the intracellular level of cyclic AMP controls the availability of the slow channels in the myocardial sarcolemma.

In another test of the cyclic AMP hypothesis, cyclic AMP was microinjected intracellularly into dog Purkinje

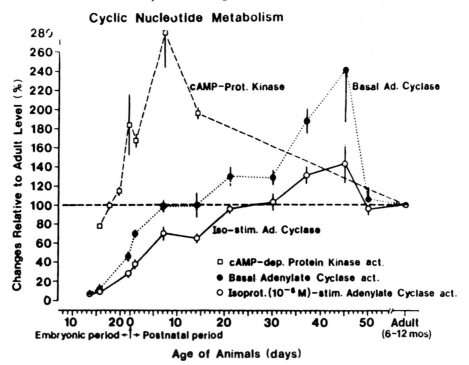

Fig. 35-16. Developmental changes in cyclic-AMP-dependent protein kinase and adenylate cyclase activity in mouse hearts. The ordinate shows percent changes (expressed as percent of adult level 6- to 12-months old) in total cyclic-AMP-dependent protein kinase activity (type I and type II [□]) and basal (●) and isoproterenol (10^{-6} M)-stimulated adenylate cyclase activities (○). Values for cyclic AMP-dependent protein kinase were recalculated from the values given in the papers by Haddox et al. {106}, and those for the basal and ISO-stimulated adenylate cyclase activity from Chen et al. {107}. The authors thank Dr. Michio Kojima for preparation of this figure by recalculation of data in the original articles.

fibers and guinea pig ventricular muscle {140}. It was found that cyclic AMP injections induced the slow APs in the injected cell for a transient period of 0.5–1 minutes; the amplitude and duration of the induced slow AP was a function of the amount of cyclic AMP injected. When a slow AP was induced by theophylline, cyclic AMP injections increased their rate of rise and amplitude also for a transient period. The responses were evident within 1–2 seconds after the injection was stopped, and the responses disappeared within about 30 seconds. These studies indicate that the average life span of the phosphorylated Ca^{2+} slow channels must be less than 30 seconds, and most likely is on the order of a few seconds at most. It is possible that the Ca^{2+} slow channels are phosphorylated and dephosphorylated during each cardiac cycle. Cyclic AMP injection into cultured heart cells by the phosphatidylcholine liposome method confirmed the results obtained by iontophoretic and pressure injections {141}.

Treatment with cholera toxin for 1–3 hours increased adenylate cyclase activity, cyclic AMP content, and contractility in embryonic chick ventricles {142}. Li and Sperelakis {143} showed that intracellular injection of GPP(NH)P and cholera toxin produced rapid and prolonged stimulation of the inward slow current. These

results support the hypothesis that the intracellular level of cyclic AMP controls the availability of the Ca^{2+} slow channels.

Metabolic dependence

The induced slow APs are blocked by hypoxia, ischemia, and metabolic poisons (including cyanide, dinitrophenol, and valinomycin), accompanied by a lowering of the cellular ATP level {60}. This suggests that interference with metabolism somehow leads to blockade of the slow channels. This effect is relatively rapid; for example, the blockade occurs within 5–15 minutes. In contrast, the fast APs are unaffected, thus indicating that the fast Na^+ channels are essentially unaffected. Thus there is a dependence of the functioning of the slow channels on metabolic energy. The contractions accompanying the fast APs are depressed or abolished, indicating that contraction is uncoupled from excitation, as expected if the slow channels were blocked.

In addition to the effect of metabolism on the slow channels, with prolonged metabolic intervention, e.g., 60–120 minutes of hypoxia, there is a gradual shortening of the duration of the normal fast AP, until a relatively brief spikelike component only remains, but which is still rapidly rising {60,131}. Thus, metabolic interference exerts a second, but much slower effect on the membrane, namely, to increase the kinetics of g_K turn-on, thereby shortening the AP. This effect could be mediated by a gradual rise in $[Ca]_i$, since a steady-state elevation in $[Ca]_i$ can cause an increase in g_K, by turning on the Ca^{2+}-activated g_K {144}.

The myocardial slow channels are selectively blocked by acidosis {145}. For example, the slow APs induced by isoproterenol (in 25 mM $[K]_o$) are depressed in rate of rise, amplitude, and duration as the pH of the perfusing solution is lowered below 7.0 {146}. Complete block occurs at about pH 6.1, and 50% inhibition occurs at about pH 6.6. The contractions are depressed in parallel with the slow APs. Acidosis has little or no effect on the fast APs, but the accompanying contractions become depressed and abolished as a function of the degree of acidosis {147}; that is, excitation-contraction uncoupling occurs, as expected from a selective blockade of the slow channels. Since the myocardium becomes acidotic during ischemia and hypoxia, it is likely that the effects of these metabolic interventions on the slow channels are partly mediated by the accompanying acidosis {147}.

PHOSPHORYLATION HYPOTHESIS

Because of the relationship between cyclic AMP and the number of available slow channels, and because of the dependence of the functioning of the slow channels on metabolic energy, it has been postulated that a membrane protein must be phosphorylated in order for the slow channel to become available for voltage activation {59, 60,137,143,148–151} (fig. 35-17). Elevation of cAMP by a positive inotropic agent activates a PKA, which phosphorylates a variety of proteins in the presence of ATP.

The protein that is phosphorylated might be a constituent of the slow channel itself. Phosphorylation could make the slow channel available for activation by causing a conformational change that allows the activation gate to be opened upon depolarization. The phosphorylated form of the slow channel would be the active (operational) form, and the dephosphorylated form would be the inactive (inoperative) form; that is, only the phosphorylated form would be available to become activated upon depolarization to threshold. The dephosphorylated channels would be electrically silent. Thus, agents that act to elevate the cyclic AMP level, either by stimulating the adenylate cyclase or by inhibiting the phosphodiesterase, would increase the fraction of the slow channels that are in the phosphorylated form and hence available for voltage activation.

Cyclic GMP was shown to have opposite effects of those of cyclic AMP in the heart. Bath application of 8-Br-cGMP produced a relatively slow inhibition of ongoing slow APs, and intracellular pressure injection of cyclic GMP produced a relatively rapid, transient depression of Ca^{2+}-dependent slow APs {152}. Similar results were obtained by liposome injection of cyclic GMP into cultured chick heart cells {153}. In addition, 8-Br-cGMP was

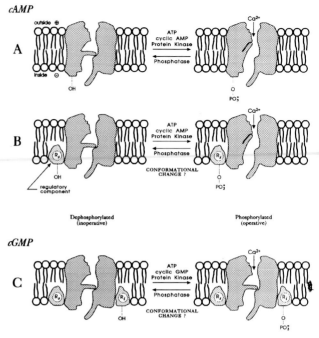

Fig. 35-17. Schematic model for a Ca^{2+} slow-channel myocardial cell membrane in two hypothetical forms: dephosphorylated (or electrically silent) form (left diagrams) and phosphorylated form (right diagrams). The two gates associated with the channel are an activation gate and an inactivation gate. The phosphorylation hypothesis states that a protein constituent of the slow channel itself (**A**) or a regulatory protein associated with the slow channel (**B**) must be phosphorylated in order for the channel to be in a state available for voltage activation. Phosphorylation of a serine or threonine residue occurs by a cAMP-dependent protein kinase (PK-A) in the presence of ATP. Phosphorylation may produce a conformational change that effectively allows the channel gates to operate. The slow channel (or an associated regulatory protein) may also be phosphorylated by a cGMP-PK (**C**), thus mediating the inhibitory effects of cGMP on the slow Ca^{2+} channel. Modified from Sperelakis and Schneider {137}, with permission.

shown to block the inward slow current in voltage-clamp experiments on single ventricular cells from old embryonic chick hearts (fig. 35-11).

In preliminary whole-cell voltage clamp experiments on single ventricular cardiomyocytes from 17-day embryonic chick, it was demonstrated that the stimulation of $I_{Ca,L}$ produced by 1 mM 8Br-cAMP added to the bath could be completely reversed by the addition of 1 mM 8Br-cGMP (figs. 35-18B and 35-18D) {Hadded et al., unpublished}. In addition, the basal $I_{Ca,L}$ (not previously stimulated by an agonist) was inhibited by 8Br-cGMP as well (figs. 35-18A and 35-18C). The I/V curves showed that cGMP did not alter the voltage for maximum current or the reversal potential of $I_{Ca,L}$. The concentration-response curves for 8Br-cGMP in the presence or absence of different concentrations of 8Br-cAMP were shifted showing antagonism between the two cyclic nucleotides (figs. 35-19). Similar

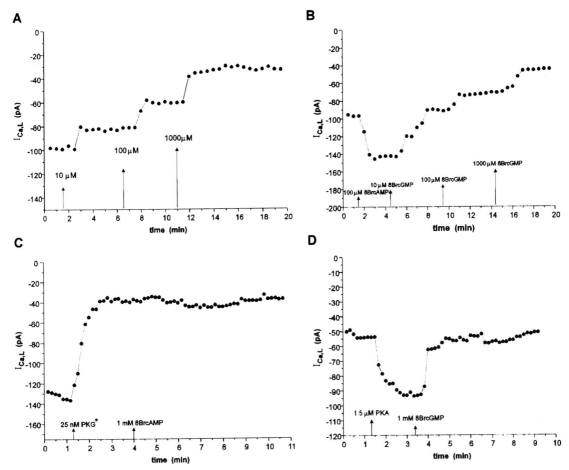

Fig. 35-18. Time courses for the modulation of the basal (**left panels**) and stimulated (**right panels**) $I_{Ca,L}$ by second messengers in the 18-day-old embryonic chick heart cells. $I_{Ca,L}$ was evoked by a test pulse of 200 ms from a holding potential of -45 mV to a test potential of $+10$ mV at a rate of 1/30 second in A–B and 1/10 second in C–D. **A:** Inhibition of the basal $I_{Ca,L}$ by 10, 100, and 1000 µM [8Br-cGMP] on the same cell. **B:** Stimulation of $I_{Ca,L}$ by 8Br-cAMP (100 µM) with subsequent inhibition of the stimulated $I_{Ca,L}$ with increasing [8Br-cGMP] on the same cell. **C:** Rapid inhibition of $I_{Ca,L}$ by intracellular perfusion with activated PKG (PKG*); 0.1 µM cGMP was added to the pipette solution for proper activation of PKG (0.1 µM cGMP in the pipette had no effect by itself on $I_{Ca,L}$). Subsequent addition of 8Br-cAMP (1 mM) was inefficient in reversing the effect of PKG*. **D:** Stimulation of $I_{Ca,L}$ by intracellular perfusion with the 1.5 µM PKA (the catalytic subunit), with the subsequent inhibition of the stimulated $I_{Ca,L}$ by 1 mM 8Br-cGMP. From Haddad et al. {unpublished}.

results were obtained on early neonatal (2-day) rat ventricular myocytes {Masuda et al., unpublished}. Therefore, it appears that the ratio of cAMP/cGMP determines the degree of stimulation of $I_{Ca,L}$, and that even the basal $I_{Ca,L}$ is inhibited by cGMP, at least in the case of the chick. Thus cGMP regulates the functioning of the myocardial Ca^{2+} slow channels in a manner that is antagonistic to that of cAMP. It is possible that the Ca^{2+} slow channel protein has a second site that can be phosphorylated by PKG and that, when phosphorylated, inhibits the slow channel. Another possibility is that there is a second type of regulatory protein that is inhibitory when phosphorylated.

In further preliminary studies in 17-day embryonic chick myocytes, the protein kinase was added to the patch pipette for diffusion into the cell during whole-cell voltage clamp. It was found that $I_{Ca,L}$ was promptly (<90 seconds) increased to $203.3 \pm 20.9\%$ by PKA, while the subsequent addition of 8Br-cGMP (1 mM) decreased it back to $129.9 \pm 24.9\%$ of the control value. On the other hand, the basal $I_{Ca,L}$ was inhibited markedly ($55.1 \pm 6.6\%$) and rapidly (<90 seconds) by PKG (25 nM); however, subsequent addition of 8Br-cAMP (1 mM; fig. 35-20) or isoproterenol (1 µM) failed to reverse the effect of PKG {Haddad et al., unpublished}. The control with no PKG demonstrated the lack of significant rundown within the 5–10 minutes tested. Thus these findings indicate that the effects of cAMP and cGMP on $I_{Ca,L}$ are mediated by activation of PKA and PKG, respectively. Nevertheless, it seems plausible that PKG phosphorylation of its respective site or regulatory protein hinders the phosphorylation of

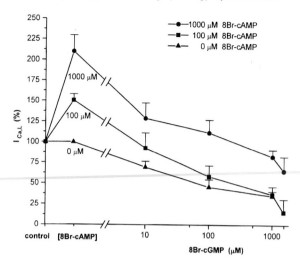

the Ca^{2+} slow channel PKA-related site or regulatory protein; however, the opposite is not true.

The developmental changes in the autonomic receptors of mouse hearts are summarized in fig. 35-22. Changes in the adrenergic receptors (beta-adrenergic and α_1-adrenergic) are given in panel A, and changes in the cholinergic muscarinic receptors are given in panel B. The details of the developmental changes in the autonomic receptors in chick and mouse hearts are summarized in Chapter 23.

It was suggested that the slow Na^+ channels may need to be phosphorylated like the slow Ca^{2+} channels. In addition, the pharmacology of these two types of slow channels, i.e., the slow Na^+ channel and the slow Ca^{2+} channel, appears to be similar. For example, the calcium antagonistic drugs have similar effects on both types {62,63}. In addition, the local anesthetics (lidocaine, procaine, procainamide, and quinidine) blocked the slow Na^+ channels of young embryonic chick hearts at concentrations similar to those for blockade of fast Na^+ channels in adult hearts {154}. It was shown that the local anesthetics also block the Ca^{2+} slow channels in concentrations similar for blockade of fast Na^+ channels {155,156}.

Fig. 35-19. The effects on $I_{Ca,L}$ amplitude of different concentrations of 8Br-cGMP in the absence or presence of different concentrations of 8Br-cAMP (100 or 1000 µM) on 18-day-old embryonic chick ventricular cardiomyocytes. Data points are mean ± SE (n = 5–9). Note the effect of 8Br-cGMP on the stimulated as well as on the basal $I_{Ca,L}$. From Haddad et al. {unpublished}.

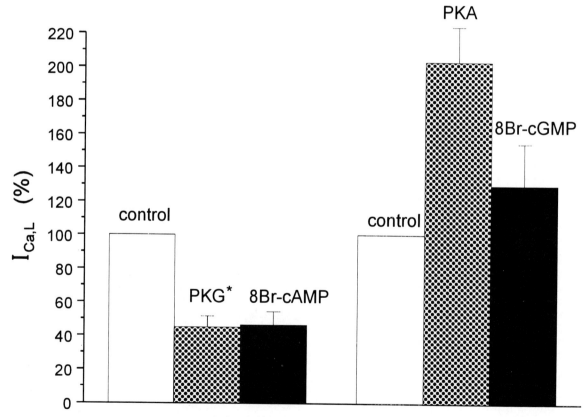

Fig. 35-20. Modulation of $I_{Ca,L}$ amplitude by PKG* or PKA, and the subsequent effect of 8Br-cAMP (1 mM) or 8Br0cGMP (1 mM), respectively, in 18-day-old embryonic chick ventricular myocytes. Note that 8Br-cAMP did not restore $I_{Ca,L}$ to the control level, while 8Br-cGMP reduced $I_{Ca,L}$ toward the control value. From Haddad et al. {unpublished}.

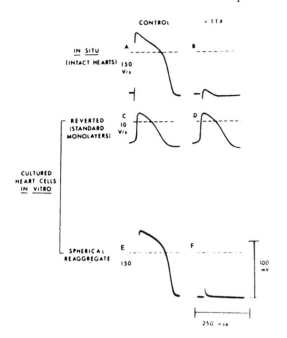

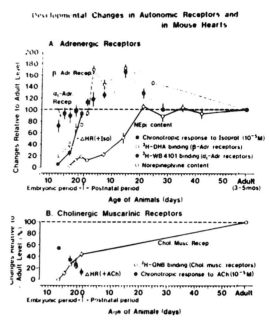

Fig. 35-21. Comparison of the electrophysiologic properties of the intact old (16-day) embryonic chick heart in situ (A and B) and those of trypsin-dispersed old ventricular myocardial cells in cultures prepared by three different methods (C–H). **A,B:** Intact heart; control AP (A) was rapidly rising (150 V/s), had a high stable resting potential (about −80 mV), and was completely abolished by tetrodotoxin (TTX; 0.1 g/ml) (B). **C,D:** Standard reverted monolayers; control AP was slowly rising (10 V/s) and was preceded by a pacemaker potential; the resting potential was low (about −50 mV; C), and TTX did not alter the AP (D). **E,F:** Highly differentiated cells in spherical reaggregate culture; control APs were rapidly rising (150 V/s), the resting potentials were high (−80 mV; E), and TTX abolished the APs (F). Taken from Sperelakis et al. {54} and Sperelakis and McLean {183,184}.

ULTRASTRUCTURAL CHANGES

Thin myofilaments are clearly present at 30 hours, and they begin to collect into groups at about 36 hours {157}. Thin filaments are found without thick filaments, but thick filaments usually occur in association with thin filaments. The myofibrils in the 2- to 3-day hearts are relatively sparse and in various stages of formation. The myofibrils are not aligned, and they run in all directions, including perpendicular to one another. Bundles of myofilaments attached to one Z line often radiate in several directions. The sarcomeres are usually incomplete early in their formation, and the myofibrils are short. H zones first become obvious at day 8, and M lines do not appear until about day 18. Free cyctoplasmic polyribosomes are abundant, and rough ER tubules lined with ribosomes are frequently in close association with the developing myofibrils. Large pools of glycogen are observed in the young (2- to 3-day-old) hearts.

With respect to the ultrastructure of rat cardiac cells, an

Fig. 35-22. Summary of developmental changes in autonomic receptors in mouse hearts relative to the adult level. **A:** Changes in cardiac adrenergic receptors, norepinephrine content, and chronotropic response to isoproterenol. Changes in number of α_1-adrenergic receptors (●), β-adrenergic receptors (○), norepinephrine content (○), and heart rate responses (as a percent of the control level) to isoproterenol (10^{-5} M; ■) are plotted. The abscissa gives developmental age in days prenatal (10–22 days) and postnatal (0–55 days and adult). α_1-adrenergic receptors were determined by ^{3}H-WP4101 (^{3}H-2-N [2,6-dimethoxyphenoxyethyl] amino ethyl-1,4 benzodioxane) binding, and the beta-adrenergic receptors by ^{3}H-DHA (^{3}H-dehydroalprenolol) binding. Values plotted are mean ± SE. (The SE was not shown when it was smaller than the size of a symbol.) There was no change in binding affinity for the antagonists, ^{3}H-WB4101 and ^{3}H-DHA, during this period (not shown). Values for α_1-adrenergic binding studies and norepinephrine content were recalculated from the data given in Yamada et al. {185}, and those for the beta-adrenergic binding studies and for the chronotropic response to ISO are from Chen et al. {186}. **B:** Changes in cholinergic muscarinic receptors and chronotropic response to acetylcholine (ACh). Changes in muscarinic receptor density (○) and heart rate response to ACh (10^{-5} M; ●), expressed as percent of the adult level and control level, respectively. The cholinergic muscarinic receptors were assayed by ^{3}H-QNB (^{3}H-quiniclidinyl benzilate) binding. Values plotted are mean ± SE. There was no change in binding affinity for the antagonist ^{3}H-QNB during development (not shown). The values were recalculated from the data given in Roeske and Yamamura {187}. The authors wish to thank Dr. Michio Kojima for preparation of this figure by recalculation of data in the original articles.

electron microscopic study of the heart from the 14th gestational day to the 31st postnatal day was done by Scheibler and Wolf {158}. Before birth, the round shaped myocyte has a primitive ultrastructure appearance, with a large nucleus occupying the bulk of the cell volume, scarce immature mitochondria with primitive small cristea, randomly scattered isolated myofilaments, and undeveloped transverse tubules that are not yet in smooth continuity with the sarcomere due to the absence of diads or triads. From the 20th gestational day onward into the postnatal period, alignment of the cells occurs. The longitudinal sarcoplasmic reticulum is formed during the first day of birth, whereas the transverse tubular system is formed between the 14th and 20th neonatal day. The amount of glycogen gradually decreases, until it finally reaches the normal adult level at about postnatal 13. The nucleus progressively regresses in size as the rate of protein synthesis declines with age {159}, the mitochondria are fully matured at about the 16th neonatal day, and their cellular distribution is completed by the 24th day. At this time, the differentiation, orientation, and density of the myofibrils are also complete. By the 31st neonatal day, the transverse-tubule system shows its typical structure and intercalated discs exhibit their characteristic interdigitation. At day 31, the ultrastructure is hardly distinguishable from that of the adult heart. Those ultrastructural changes result in an improved contractile ability in terms of pressure and tension development. Thus it seems that the myocyte changes towards maturity from a mainly protein-synthesizing to a force-developing machine.

ORGAN-CULTURED EMBRYONIC HEARTS

Cultivation of embryonic hearts in vitro aids in the analysis of the changes that occur during normal development in situ. When young (3-day-old) embryonic chick hearts, which have not yet become innervated by either cholinergic or adrenergic fibers, are placed into organ culture, they fail to gain TTX-sensitive fast Na^+ channels {160,161}. Instead, the APs continue to be generated by TTX-insensitive slow Na^+ channels, the rates of rise remain slow, and pacemaker potentials precede the APs. These APs resemble those recorded from 3-day-old hearts in situ. Similar findings were obtained when young hearts were grafted onto the chorioallantoic membrane of host chicks for blood perfusion {162}. Thus, organ-cultured young hearts do not differentiate further in vitro, but appear to be arrested in the young embryonic state.

When young hearts that have been arrested in the early developmental state are treated with RNA-enriched fractions obtained from adult chicken hearts, they gain fast Na^+ channels and become completely sensitive to TTX {163–165}; that is, young hearts in vitro can be induced to undergo further membrane differentiation.

However, slow Ca^{2+} channels were found to develop in young embryonic hearts during organ culture {166}. Three-day-old embryonic chick hearts having slowly rising spontaneous APs dependent on TTX-insensitive slow Na^+ channels were placed into organ culture for 5–11 days. AP duration was markedly increased, and a notch appeared in some hearts between the initial spike phase and the plateau phase. Spike amplitude was mainly dependent on $[Na]_o$, whereas the plateau amplitude was dependent on $[Ca]_o$. The spike phase and plateau phase of the slow APs are mainly dependent on currents through slow Na^+ channels

and through slow Ca^{2+} channels, respectively. Mn^{2+} (0.5 mM; a specific blocker of slow Ca^{2+} channels) and verapamil (5 μM; a blocker of both slow Na^+ channels and slow Ca^{2+} channels) depressed the plateau duration and overshoot. High concentrations (10–30 μM) of verapamil depressed the AP amplitude and dV/dt max, and abolished automaticity. These results indicate that slow Ca^{2+} channels appear de novo during organ culture of young embryonic hearts, while the slow Na^+ channels are retained. Thus when young embryonic hearts are placed into organ culture, they gain slow Ca^{2+} channels, but fail to gain a large number of fast Na^+ channels. These findings suggest that differentiation of slow Ca^{2+} channels and of fast Na^+ channels during embryonic development in situ is controlled by different mechanisms.

Organ-cultured intermediate (5- to 7-day-old) hearts have both fast and slow Na^+ channels, just as in situ {160–162}. The APs have moderate rates of rise (40–70 V/s), and TTX reduces the maximal rate of rise of the AP to about 10 V/s. Cultured 17-day hearts tend to retain their fast-rising APs and complete sensitivity to TTX, but survival is limited to a few days. Thus in organ culture the embryonic hearts tend to retain the state of differentiation achieved at the time of placement into culture.

CULTURED HEART CELLS

Various stages of cardiac electrical differentiation can be simulated in vitro using cell cultures, and their study may facilitate elucidation of the mechanisms operating during normal cardiogenesis. The electrophysiologic properties observed depend to a large extent on the age of the hearts from which the cells are isolated and on the method of cell culture.

OLD EMBRYONIC HEARTS

Monolayer cultures

When cells are dispersed from old embryonic hearts using trypsin, and standard monolayer cultures are prepared, the cells are found to possess slowly rising TTX-insensitive APs with pacemaker potentials (figs. 35-21C and 35-21D); that is, the APs are similar to those recorded in young (2- to 3-day-old) hearts, rather than in old hearts from which the cells were taken (figs. 35-21A and 35-21B). It thus appears that cell separation results in a rapid reversion toward the young embryonic state {3,61, 167–170}.

This reversion can be partially prevented (or reversed) by separating the cells in trypsinizing solutions containing elevated K^+ concentrations (12–60 mM; by isomolar substitutions of K^+ for Na^+) and 5 mM ATP {44}. The mechanism whereby elevated K^+ and ATP helps to minimize reversion of the cultured cell is not known, although $[K]_i$ is reduced in the reverted cells to about 90–100 mM, and this does not occur in highly differentiated cultured cells.

Jones et al. {171} reported that multilayer-cultured

ventricular cells can be made to exhibit highly differentiated morphology, as well as advanced electrical properties, if the fetal calf serum concentration is lowered from 10% to 0.1% after the first few days, presumably to remove growth-promoting factors, and the cells are subsequently allowed to age in vitro for several weeks.

Renaud et al. {172} recently demonstrated that monolayer hearts cells maintained in a lipoprotein-deficient serum differentiate electrically compared to cells cultured in normal media. The cells in lipoprotein-deficient media had greater resting potentials and faster rising APs that were greatly decreased by TTX, and muscarinic agonists now blocked automaticity. The authors found that the cholesterol content of the cell membranes was decreased in monolayer culture and that the lipoprotein-deficient medium returned it to normal levels. It was also reported that the TTX receptor and muscarinic receptor remained stable for over 25 hours after protein synthesis was blocked in the highly differentiated cells, whereas in the reverted cells these receptors were rapidly degraded (with half-times of 9–14 hours).

Spherical reaggregate cultures

Reaggregation is achieved either by gyrotation for 24–48 hours or by plating the cells on cellophane to which the cells adhere poorly. Action potentials recorded from cells in such reaggregates possess rapid rates of rise (up to 200 V/s) and are initiated from high stable resting potentials (about −80 mV), and TTX completely abolishes all excitability (figs. 35-21E and 35-21F). The intracellular records are indistinguishable from those made from the intact 16-day ventricle (figs. 35-21A and 35-21B). As in the case of the intact old embryonic hearts, positive inotropic agents induce slowly rising APs in the highly differentiated cultured cells following blockade of the fast Na^+ channels with TTX {44,173,174}. Acetylcholine was without noticeable effect on the APs of cultured ventricular cells, both reverted {175} and highly differentiated {44}.

YOUNG EMBRYONIC HEARTS

When young (2- to 3-day-old) embryonic hearts are trypsin dispersed and the cells are allowed to reaggregate in vitro, the cells retain electrical activity characteristic of the intact young heart; that is, the cells have low resting potentials, and they fire spontaneous slowly rising APs that are unaffected by TTX. As observed in the case of young organ-cultured intact hearts, however, the addition of RNA-enriched extracts from adult chicken hearts to the reaggregated young myocardial cells induces the appearance of rapidly rising (e.g., 100 V/s) APs, which fire from high stable resting potentials (−70 mV to −80 mV) and which are completely sensitive to TTX {162,163}. The mechanism of action of the active principle in the extract remains to be elucidated. Nathan and De Haan {68} reported that they can achieve further differentiation of young cells in reaggregate culture without the addition of special extracts.

MEANING OF VERATRIDINE DEPOLARIZATION

It was first shown by Sperelakis and Pappano {176} that veratridine depolarizes the reverted cultured (monolayer) heart cells and that TTX prevents this depolarization, even though TTX had no obvious effect on the APs. They interpreted these findings to suggest that veratridine opens up a resting-type (i.e., time-independent) Na^+ channel (i.e., resting is increased by veratridine) and that TTX blocks this action. (Since veratridine actually hyperpolarized the cells in the presence of TTX, they concluded that veratridine also increases the resting K^+ permeability, P_K.) Other investigators subsequently saw similar effects of veratridine and related toxins (such as batrachotoxin and grayanotoxin) on neurons and myocardial cells (see the review by Sperelakis {177}). Because veratridine depolarized and increased influx in monolayer culture heart cells that were reverted (i.e., exhibited slowly rising TTX-insensitive APs), it was suggested that there must be "silent" (i.e., inoperable) fast Na^+ channels present in the reverted cells that could be opened by veratridine {70,178}. However, this conclusion is based on the premise that veratridine can only act on fast Na^+ channels, which seems to be an assumption that is equivocal. In support of their conclusion, Renaud et al. {70} reported that there was some specific TTX binding in the young hearts (the number of such binding sites increased about sixfold during embryonic development), i.e., that there were some silent fast Na^+ channels in young hearts.

However, Pang and Sperelakis {179} showed that the veratridine-stimulated ^{45}Ca influx into the heart cells, which should reflect a parallel Na^+ influx because of the Ca-Na exchange system, was independent of embryonic age of the developing chick, i.e., the curve was flat. These investigators therefore concluded that veratridine must act on a second channel (in addition to the fast Na^+ channel) to increase Na^+ and Ca^{2+} influx and depolarize, since the number of TTX binding sites increases during embryonic development {70}, as does the rate of rise of the APs {8,14,167}, reflecting the number of fast Na^+ channels; that is, more and more fast Na^+ channels were available to be opened as a function of embryonic age, and yet the veratridine effect on Ca^{2+} influx was independent of embryonic age. The second channel opened by veratridine could be the resting P_{Na} channel and/or the voltage-dependent slow Na^+ channel.

Relevant to the evidence presented above that veratridine is not a specific opener of fast Na^+ channels in myocardial cells, Romey and Lazdunski {180} have now shown that veratridine, aconitine, batrachotoxin, and grayanotoxin are not specific for the fast Na^+ channels of neuroblastoma cells either, but also act to block the voltage-dependent slow Ca^{2+} channels, at the same or even lower concentrations.

SUMMARY AND CONCLUSIONS

Striking changes occur in the electrical properties of the myocardial cell membrane during embryonic development of the chick hearts. The young tubular hearts (2–3 days old) have a low resting potential of about $-40\,mV$ to $-50\,mV$, even though $[K]_i$ is nearly as high as the adult value. The low resting potential is caused by low K^+ permeability (P_K). The low P_K can also account for the high degree of automaticity observed in the ventricular cells of young embryonic hearts. P_K increases rapidly during development, attaining nearly the final adult value by day 12; the resting potential increases to about $-80\,mV$, and automaticity of the ventricular cells is suppressed. The young heart has a low Na,K-ATPase activity, and this enzyme activity increases during development along with P_K.

The young (2- to 3-day-old) hearts have action potentials (APs) with slow maximal rates of rise (dV/dt max) of $10-30\,V/s$. The slowly rising APs are not affected by tetrodotoxin (TTX), and hyperpolarization does not greatly increase the rate of rise. The APs are dependent mainly on $[Na]_o$. Thus it appears the fast Na^+ channels are absent or relatively few in number in young hearts, the inward current during the AP being carried predominantly through TTX-insensitive slow Na^+ channels. The slow Na^+ channels are blocked by verapamil, but not by $1\,mM$ Mn^{2+}. Mn^{2+} does block the contractions, presumably by blockade of the Ca^{2+} influx during the AP. This Ca^{2+} influx presumably occurs through some slow Ca^{2+} channels that are likely to be present. In many respects, the young tubular hearts resemble pulsating blood vessels, and their electrical properties are somewhat similar to those of vascular smooth muscle.

There is a progressive increase in dV/dt max of the AP during devlopment. By day 5, dV/dt max is about $50-80\,V/s$, and TTX now reduces dV/dt max to $10-30\,V/s$, i.e., to the value observed in 2- to 3-day-old hearts. Thus, the TTX-sensitive fast Na^+ channels progressively increase in number until they attain the final adult level by day 18. Between days 5 and 7, fast Na^+ channels and a high density of slow Na^+ channels coexist. After day 8, TTX completely abolishes excitability, suggesting that the number of functional slow channels has decreased sufficiently so as not to support regenerative excitation.

On the level of ionic channels, the TTX-sensitive fast Na^+ current density increased fivefold, with a significant faster decay and recovery from inactivation during development between the 18-day-old fetal and 1-day-old neonatal chick heart cells. Changes in the whole-cell current density of I_{K1} in rat ventricular cardiomyocytes during development may be due to the appearance and increase in the open probability of a large-conductance ($31\,pS$) and the disappearance of a small-conductance ($11\,pS$) channel. In addition, during the first 10 postnatal days of the rat, I_{to} increased fourfold with an increase in its K^+ selectivity. On the other hand, in the adult heart $I_{Ca,L}$ gating is characterized by burst openings (mode 1); while long openings (mode 2) are favored by the DHP-Ca^{2+} channel agonist. This mode 2 is the naturally occurring behavior in 3-day-old embryonic chick and is replaced by mode 1 with development; thus accounting, by and large, for the decrease in $I_{Ca,L}$. In the same line, the novel fetal type Ca^{2+} channel seems to disappear during development of the fetal rat ventricular cardiomyocytes.

The cyclic AMP level is very high in young hearts and decreases during development. The high cyclic AMP level in young hearts may keep most or all of the slow channels in a phosphorylated state, and hence available for voltage activation. Decrease in the cyclic AMP level during development allows control to be exercised over the number of available slow channels. The fact that isoproterenol can elevate the cyclic AMP level in even young (4-day-old) hearts (that already have high levels of cyclic AMP) indicates that functional beta-adrenergic receptors are present prior to innervation.

On the other hand, although cGMP content increases markedly during early embryonic stages of the chick heart cells, PKG activity was reported to decline with development in guinea pig hearts. If it is not for species difference, an increase in the phosphodiesterase activity would be a good candidate for explaining this discrepancy. Furthermore, PKC activity declines with development of the rat heart as well.

The slow channels in young hearts are predominantly of the slow Na^+ type, whereas those slow channels induced by some positive inotropic agents, e.g., isoproterenol, in older hearts are of the slow Ca-Na type.

Young embryonic rat hearts also have slowly rising TTX-insensitive APs. The major difference from the embryonic chick is that the slow channels that pass the inward current for the AP appear to be predominantly of the slow Ca^{2+} type rather than of the slow Na^+ type.

Young embryonic chick hearts (3 day old), removed prior to innervation and placed into organ culture for 2 weeks or grafted on the chorioallantoic membrane of a host chick for blood perfusion, do not gain fast Na^+ channels or otherwise differentiate. This suggests that something in the in situ condition, such as neurotrophic or other factors, is required for triggering further differentiation. If, however, these young organ-cultured hearts are exposed for several days to an RNA-enriched fraction obtained from adult chicken hearts, they do gain TTX-sensitive fast Na^+ channels. This induction is blocked by inhibitors of protein synthesis, such as cyclohexamide. Thus the synthesis of specific membrane proteins controls the appearance of fast Na^+ channels. Hence, cardiac myoblasts whose development, with respect to some membrane electrical properties, has been arrested in vitro can be induced to differentiate further. Trypsin-dispersed myocardial cells obtained from young embryonic chick hearts and placed in cell culture for several weeks also do not proceed with differentiation in vitro, unless exposed to the RNA extract from adult heart.

Monolayer cultures of heart cells prepared from old embryonic heart (ventricles) rapidly revert back to the young embryonic state; that is, they lose most or all of their fast Na^+ channels, gain slow and Na^+ channels, gain automaticity because of a low P_K; they also lose many of their myofibrils. If, however, the cells are allowed to reaggregate into small spheres and incubate for a period of 1–3 weeks, they often will regain highly differentiated electrical properties. These cells also retain their membrane receptors for catecholamines, histamine, and angiotensin. The cultured ventricular (and atrial) cells possess receptors for acetylcholine {181}. Thus, highly differentiated myocardial cells can be maintained in cell culture under appropriate conditions. Exposure of monolayer cultures possessing reverted electrical properties to media containing lipoprotein-deficient serum caused the cells to gain highly differentiated electrical characteristics concomitant with an increase in cholesterol content of the cell membrane.

Based on veratridine-induced depolarization of and stimulation of Na^+ and Ca^{2+} influx into monolayer cultured heart cells that possess reverted electrical properties, and TTX block of the veratridine effect, it has been postulated that there are some silent (nonfunctional) fast Na^+ channels in the reverted cells that can be opened by veratridine. Consistent with this view, there are some binding sites for a ^3H-TTX analog (for assessing specific binding sites, presumably on fast Na^+ channels) in the young (3-day-old) embryonic chick hearts. However, the number of ^3H-TTX binding sites increases about sixfold during embryonic development in ovo in parallel with the increase in dV/dt max of the AP, thus confirming by a different approach the fact that the number of fast Na^+ channels increases during development. The fact that the degree of veratridine stimulation of ^{45}Ca uptake is independent of embryonic age argues against the concept of silent fast Na^+ channels in the young hearts and for the likelihood that veratridine exerts effects on other types of channels, e.g., on slow channels or resting channels, as well as on fast Na^+ channels.

Positive inotropic agents, such as norepinephrine, histamine, and methylxanthine, rapidly induce slow Ca-Na channels in old embryonic myocardial cells. Following blockade of the fast Na^+ channels with TTX, these agents rapidly allow the production of slowly rising APs by increasing the number of slow channels available for voltage activation. Since norepinephrine, histamine, and methylxanthines rapidly elevate intracellular cyclic AMP levels, these results suggest that cyclic AMP controls the number of operational slow channels. Exogenous cyclic AMP produces the same effect but much more slowly, whereas intracellular injection of cyclic AMP increases the number of available slow channels within seconds.

The myocardial slow channels induced by the positive inotropic agents are very sensitive to blockade by metabolic poisons, hypoxia, and ischemia. In contrast, the fast Na^+ channels are essentially unaffected; however, the contractions accompanying the fast APs are depressed or abolished, i.e., contraction is uncoupled from excitation, as expected from the slow-channel blockade. Therefore, the slow channels are metabolically dependent, whereas the fast Na^+ channels are not. The slow channels are also selectively sensitive to blockade by acid pH.

Because of the dependence of the myocardial slow channels on cyclic AMP level and on metabolism, phosphorylation of a membrane protein constituent of the slow channel — by a cyclic AMP-dependent protein kinase and ATP — may be required to make it available for voltage activation. By virtue of these special properties of the slow channels, the Ca^{2+} influx of the myocardial cell can be controlled by extrinsic factors, such as by autonomic nerve stimulation or circulating hormones, or by intrinsic factors, such as intracellular pH or ATP level.

ACKNOWLEDGMENTS

The work of the authors summarized and reviewed in this chapter was supported by grants from the National Institutes of Health (HL-18711). The authors wish to acknowledge the collaborative efforts with his colleagues, particularly Drs. K. Shigenobu, M.J. McLean, J.-F. Renaud, and I. Josephson.

REFERENCES

1. Rosenquist G, De Haan RL: Migration of precardiac cells in the chick embryo: A radioautographic study. *Contrib Embryol Carnegie Inst Wash* 263:113–121, 1966.
2. LeDouarin G, Obrecht G, Coraboeuf E: Determinations regionales dans l'air cardiaque presomptive mises en evidence chez L'embryon de poulet par la methode microelectrophysiologique. *J Embryol Exp Morphol* 15:153–167, 1966.
3. Renaud D: Etude Electrophysiologique de la Differentiation Cardiaque chez L'embryon de Poulet. Thesis, University of Nantes, 1973.
4. Niu MC, Deshpande AK: The development of tubular heart in RNA-treated postnodal pieces of chick blastoderm. *J Embryol Exp Morphol* 29:485–501, 1973.
5. McLean MJ, Renaud JF, Sperelakis N: Cardiac-like action potentials recorded from spontaneously-contracting structures induced in post-nodal pieces of chick blastoderm exposed to an RNA-enriched fraction from adult heart. *Differentiation* 11:13–17, 1978.
6. Girard H: Arterial pressure in the chick embryo. *Am J Physiol* 224:454–460, 1974.
7. Romanoff A: In: *The Avian Embryo: Structure and Functional Development*. New York: Macmillan, 1960.
8. Sperelakis N: Changes in membrane electrical properties during development of the heart. In: Zipes DP, Bailey JC, Elharrar V (eds) *The Slow Inward Current and Cardiac Arrhythmias*. Boston: Martinus Nijhoff, 1980, pp 221–262.
9. Kojima M, Sperelakis N, Sada H: Ontogenesis of transmembrane signaling systems for control of cardiac Ca^{2+} channels. *J Dev Physiol* 14:181–219, 1990.
10. Shimizu Y, Tasaki K: Electrical excitability of developing cardiac muscle in chick embryos. *Tohoku J Exp Med* 88:49–56, 1966.
11. Yeh BK, Hoffman BF: The ionic basis of electrical activity in embryonic cardiac muscle. *J Gen Physiol* 52:666–681, 1967.
12. Couch JR, West TC, Hoff HE: Development of the action potential of the prenatal rat heart. *Circ Res* 24:19–31, 1969.
13. Boethius J, Knutsson E: Resting membrane potential in chick muscle cells during ontogeny. *J Exp Zool* 174:281–286, 1970.
14. Sperelakis N, Shigenobu K: Changes in membrane properties of chick embryonic hearts during development. *J Gen Physiol* 60:430–453, 1972.
15. McDonald TF, De Haan RL: Ion levels and membrane potential in chick heart tissue and cultured cells. *J Gen Physiol* 61:89–109, 1973.
16. Bernard C: Establishment of ionic permeabilities of the myocardial membrane during embryonic development of the rat. In: Lieberman M, Sano T (eds) *Developmental and*

Physiological Correlates of Cardiac Muscle. New York: Raven Press, 1976, pp 169–184.

17. Wahler GM: Developmental increase in the inwardly-ectifying potassium current of rat ventricular myocytes. *Am J Physiol* 262:C1266–C1272, 1992.

18. Kilborn M, Fedida D: A study of the developmental changes in outward currents of rat ventricular myocytes. *J Physiol* 430:37–60, 1990.

19. Sperelakis N: Pacemaker mechanisms in myocardial cells during development of embryonic chick hearts. In: Bouman LN, Jongsma JH (eds) *Developments in Cardiovascular Medicine*, Vol 17: *Cardiac Rate and Rhythm: Physiological, Morphological, and Developmental Aspects*. The Hague: Martinus Nijhoff, 1982, pp 129–165.

20. Haddad G, Ruiz-Petrich E, Schanne O: Background currents in ventricular myocytes of newborn and 7-day old rats. *FASEB J* (#4, part 1):A979 (abstr 246), 1992.

21. Haddad G: Metabolic Inhibition and the Background K^+ Current in 1-day and 7-day old Rat Ventricular Myocytes. Ph.D. thesis, University of Sherbrooke, 1992.

22. Pappano AJ: Sodium-dependent depolarization of non-innervated embryonic chick heart by acetylcholine. *J Pharmacol Exp Ther* 180:340–350, 1972.

23. De Haan RL: The potassium-sensitivity of isolated embryonic heart cells increases with development. *Dev Biol* 23:226–240, 1970.

24. Carmeliet EE, Horres CR, Lieberman M, Vereecke JS: Developmental aspects of potassium flux and permeability of the embryonic chick heart. *J Physiol (Lond)* 254:673–692, 1976.

25. Löffelholz K, Pappano AJ: Increased sensitivity of sinoatrial pacemaker to acetylcholine and to catecholamines at the onset of autonomic neuroeffector transmission in chick embryo heart. *J Pharm Exp Ther* 191:479–486, 1974.

26. Pappano AJ: Action potentials in chick atria: Ontogenic changes in the dependence of tetrodotoxin-resistant action potentials on calcium, strontium, and barium. *Circ Res* 39:99–105, 1976.

27. Klein RL: Ontogenesis of K and Na fluxes in embryonic chick heart. *Am J Physiol* 199:613–618, 1970.

28. Klein RL, Horton CR, Thureson-Klein A: Studies on nuclear amino acid transport and cation content in embryonic myocardium of the chick. *Am J Cardiol* 25:300–310, 1970.

29. Thureson-Klein A, Klein RL: Cation distribution and cardiac jelly in early embryonic hearts: A histochemical and electron microscopic study. *J Mol Cell Cardiol* 2:31–40, 1971.

30. Harsch M, Green JW: Electrolyte analyses of chick embryonic fluids and heart tissue. *J Cell Comp Physiol* 62:319–326, 1963.

31. Sperelakis N: Origin of the cardiac resting potential. In: Berne RM, Sperelakis N (eds) *Handbook of Physiology: The Cardiovascular System*, Vol 1: *The Heart*. Bethesda, MD: *American Physiological Society*, 1979, pp 187–267.

32. Sperelakis N: (Na^+-K^+)-ATPase activity of embryonic chick heart and skeletal muscles as function of age. *Biochim Biophys Acta* 266:230–237, 1972.

33. Sperelakis N, Lee EC: Characterization of (Na^+-K^+)-ATPase isolated from embryonic chick hearts and cultured chick heart cells. *Biochim Biophys Acta* 233:562–579, 1971.

34. Thomas RC: Electrogenic sodium pump in nerve and muscle cells. *Physiol Rev* 52:563–594, 1972.

35. Deleze J: Possible reasons for drop of resting potential of mammalian heart preparations during hypothermia. *Circ Res* 8:553–557, 1960.

36. Page E, Storm SR: Cat heart muscle in vitro. VIII. Active transport of sodium in papillary muscles. *J Gen Physiol* 48:957–972, 1965.

37. Vassalle M: Electrogenic suppression of automaticity in sheep and dog Purkinje fibers. *Circ Res* 27:361–377, 1970.

38. Glitsch HG: An effect of the electrogenic sodium pump on the membrane potential in beating guinea pig atria. *Pflügers Arch* 344:169–180, 1973.

39. Isenberg G, Trautwein W: The effect of dihydroouabain and lithium ions on the outward current in cardiac Purkinje fibers: Evidence for electrogenicity of active transport. *Pflügers Arch* 350:41–54, 1974.

40. Noma A, Irisawa H: Contribution of an electrogenic sodium pump to the membrane potential in rabbit sinoatrial node cells. *Pflügers Arch* 358:289–301, 1975.

41. Lieberman M, Horres CR, Aiton JF, Johnson EA: Active transport and electrogenicity of cardiac muscle in tissue culture. In: *27th Proceedings of the International Congress of Physiological Sciences*, Paris, Vol 13, 1977, p 446.

42. Pelleg A, Vogel S, Belardinelli L, Sperelakis N: Overdrive suppression of automaticity in cultured chick myocardial cells. *Am J Physiol* 238:H24–H30, 1980.

43. Coraboeuf E, Le Douarin G, Obrecht-Coutris G: Release of acetylcholine by chick embryo heart before innervation. *J Physiol (Lond)* 206:383–395, 1970.

44. McLean MJ, Sperelakis N: Retention of fully differentiated electrophysiological properties of chick embryonic heart cells in culture. *Dev Biol* 50:134–141, 1976.

45. Jongsma HJ, Masson-Pevet M, De Bruyne J: Synchronization of the beating frequency of cultured rat heart cells. In: Lieberman M, Sano T (eds) *Developmental and Physiological Correlates of Cardiac Muscle*. New York: Raven Press, 1976, pp 185–196.

46. Sperelakis N, Lehmkuhl D: Effect of current on transmembrane potentials in cultured chick heart cells. *J Gen Physiol* 47:895–927, 1964.

47. Sperelakis N, Lehmkuhl D: Ionic interconversion of pacemaker and non-pacemaker cultured chick heart cells. *J Gen Physiol* 49:867–895, 1966.

48. Sperelakis N: Electrophysiology of cultured chick heart cells. In: Sano T, Mizuhira V, Matsuda K (eds) *Electrophysiology and Ultrastructure of the Heart*. Tokyo: Bunkodo, 1967, pp 81–108.

49. Pappano AJ, Sperelakis N: Low K^+ conductance and low resting potentials of isolated single cultured heart cells. *Am J Physiol* 217:1076–1082, 1969.

50. Rajala GM, Pinter MJ, Kaplan S: Response of the quiescent heart tube to mechanical stretch in the intact chick embryo. *Dev Biol* 61:330–337, 1977.

51. Rosenquist GC: Localization and movement of cardiogenic cells in the chick embryo: Heart-forming portion of the primitive streak. *Dev Biol* 22:461–475, 1970.

52. Deshpande AK, Siddiqui MAQ: A reexamination of heart muscle differentiation in the postnodal piece of chick blastoderm mediated by exogenous RNA. *Dev Biol* 58:230–247, 1977.

53. Shigenobu K, Sperelakis N: Development of sensitivity to tetrodotoxin of chick embryonic hearts with age. *J Mol Cell Cardiol* 3:271–286, 1971.

54. Sperelakis N, Shigenobu K, McLean MJ: Membrane cation channels: Changes in developing hearts, in cell culture, and in organ culture. In: Lieberman M, Sano T (eds) *Developmental and Physiological Correlates of Cardiac Cells*. New York: Raven Press, 1976, pp 209–234.

55. Sada H, Sada S, Sperelakis N: Reactivation processes of three inward current systems involved in the rising phase of the action potentials in embryonic chick hearts. *Can J Physiol Pharmacol* 64:125–132, 1986.

56. Iijima T, Pappano AJ: Ontogenetic increase of the maximal rate of rise of the chick embryonic heart action potential:

Relationship to voltage, time and tetrodotoxin. *Circ Res* 44:358–367, 1979.

57. Marcus NS, Fozzard H: Tetrodotoxin sensitivity in the developing and adult chick heart. *J Mol Cell Cardiol* 13:335–340, 1981.

58. Pappano AJ: Calcium-dependent action potentials produced by catecholamines in guinea pig atrial muscle fibers depolarized by potassium. *Circ Res* 27:379–390, 1970.

59. Shigenobu K, Sperelakis N: Ca^{2+} current channels induced by catecholamines in chick embryonic hearts whose fast Na^+ channels are blocked by tetrodotoxin or elevated K^+. *Circ Res* 31:932–952, 1972.

60. Schneider JA, Sperelakis N: The demonstration of energy dependence of the isoproterenol-induced transcellular Ca^{2+} current in isolated perfused guinea pig hearts: An explanation for mechanical failure of ischemic myocardium. *J Surg Res* 16:389–403, 1974.

61. McLean MJ, Shigenobu K, Sperelakis N: Two pharmacological types of slow Na^+ channels as distinguished by verapamil blockade. *Eur J Pharmacol* 26:379–382, 1974.

62. Shigenobu K, Schneider JA, Sperelakis N: Blockade of slow Na^+ and Ca^{2+} currents in myocardial cells by verapamil. *J Pharmacol Exp Ther* 190:280–288, 1974.

63. Kojima M, Sperelakis N: Calcium antagonistic drugs differ in ability to block the slow Na^+ channels by young embryonic chick hearts. *Eur J Pharmacol* 94:9–18, 1983.

64. Kojima M, Sperelakis N: Calcium antagonistic drugs differ in ability to block the slow Na^+ channels of young embryonic chick hearts. *Eur J Pharmacol* 94:9–18, 1983.

65. Sada H, Sada S, Sperelakis N: Actions of the slow channel activator, Bay-K-8644, on the electrical activity of 3-day-old embryonic chick hearts. *Clin Exper Pharm Physiol* 12:521–525, 1985.

66. Galper JB, Catterall WA: Developmental changes in the sensitivity of embryonic heart cells to tetrodotoxin and D-600. *Dev Biol* 65:216–227, 1978.

67. Kasuya Y, Matsuki N, Shigenobu K: Changes in sensitivity to anoxia of the cardiac action potential plateau during chick embryonic development. *Dev Biol* 58:124–133, 1977.

68. Nathan RD, De Haan RL: In vitro differentiation of a fast Na^+ conductance in embryonic heart cell aggregates. *Proc Natl Acad Sci USA* 75:2776–2780, 1978.

69. Ishima Y: The effect of tetrodotoxin and sodium substitution on the action potential in the course of development of the embryonic chicken heart. *Proc Jpn Acad* 44:170–175, 1978.

70. Renaud JF, Romey G, Lombet A, Lazdunski M: Differentiation of the fast Na^+ channels in embryonic heart cells: Interaction of the channel with neurotoxin. *Proc Natl Acad Sci USA* 78:5248–5352, 1981.

71. Conforti L, Tohse N, Sperelakis N: Tetrodotoxin-sensitive sodium current in rat fetal ventricular muocytes — contribution to the plateau phase of action potential. *J Mol Cell Cardiol* 25:159–173, 1993.

72. Brown AM, Lee KS, Powell T: Voltage clamp and internal perfusion of single rat heart muscle cells. *J Physiol (Lond)* 318:455–477, 1981.

73. Fujii S, Ayer RJ Jr, Dehaan RL: Development of the fast sodium current in early embryonic chick heart cells. *J Membr Biol* 101:209–223, 1988.

74. Kojima M, Sada H, Sperelakis N: Developmental changes in β-adrenergic and cholinergic interactions on calcium-dependent slow action potentials in rat ventricular muscles. *Br J Pharmacol* 99:327–333, 1990.

75. Adolph EF: Ranges of heart rates and their regulation at various ages (rat). *Am J Physiol (Lond)* 212:595–602, 1967.

76. Josephson IR, Sperelakis N: Tetrodotoxin differentially blocks peak and steady-state sodium currents in early embryonic chick ventricular myocytes. *Pflügers Arch* 414:354–359, 1989.

77. Patlak JB, Oritiz M: Slow currents through single sodium channels of the adult rat heart. *J Gen Physiol* 86:89–104, 1985.

78. Kiyosue T, Arita M: Late sodium current and its contribution to action potential configuration in guinea-pig ventricular myocytes. *Circ Res* 64:389–397, 1989.

79. Nilius B: Modal gating behavior of cardiac sodium channels in cell-free membrane patches. *Biophys J* 53:857–862, 1988.

80. Noble DA: *The Initiation of the Heart Beat*. Oxford: Oxford Press, 1979, Chap. 9.

81. Masuda H, Sperelakis N: Inwardly-rectifying potassium current in rat fetal and neonatal ventricular cardiomyocytes. In press, 1993.

82. Josephson IR, Sperelakis N: Developmental increases in the inwardly-rectifying K^+ current of embryonic chick ventricular myocytes. *Biochim Biophys Acta* 1052:123–127, 1990.

83. Huynh TV, Chen F, Wetzel GT, Friedman WF, Klitzner TS: Development changes in membrane Ca^{2+} and K^+ currents in fetal, neonatal, and adult rabbit ventricular myocytes. *Circ Res* 70:503–515, 1992.

84. Conforti L, Sperelakis N: A novel fast component of transient outward current in rat ventricular carciomyocytes. In press, 1993.

85. Josephson IR, Sanchez-Chapula J, Brown AM: Early outward current in rat single ventricular cells. *Circ Res* 54:157–162, 1984.

86. Bean BP: Two kinds of calcium channels in canine atrial cells: Differences in kinetics, selectivity, and pharmacology. *J Gen Physiol* 86:1–30, 1985.

87. Mitra R, Morad M: Two types of calcium channels in guinea pig ventricular myocytes. *Proc Natl Acad Science USA* 83:5340–5344, 1986.

88. Hirano Y, Fozzard HA, January CT: Characteristics of L- and T-type Ca^{2+} currents in canine cardiac Purkinje cells. *Am J Physiol* 256:H1478–H1492, 1989.

89. Hess P: Cardiac calcium channels. In: Zipes DP, Jalife J (eds) *Cardiac Electrophysiology From Cell to Bedside*. Philadelphia: WB Saunders, 1990, pp 10–17.

90. Xu X, Best PM: Postnatal changes in T-type calcium current density in rat atrial myocytes. *J Physiol* 454:657–672, 1992.

91. Cavalie A, Ochi R, Pelzer D, Trautwein W: Elementary currents through Ca^{2+} channels in guinea-pig myocytes. *Pflügers Arch* 308:284–297, 1983.

92. Hess P, Lansman JB, Tsien RW: Different modes of Ca channel gating behavior favoured by dihydropyridine Ca agonists and antagonists. *Nature (Lond)* 311:538–544, 1984.

93. Tohse N, Sperelakis N: Long-lasting openings of single slow (L-type) Ca^{2+} channels in chick embryonic heart cells. *Am J Physiol* 259:H639–H642, 1990.

94. Wahler G, Rusch N, Sperelakis N: 8-Bromo-cyclic GMP inhibits the calcium channel current in embryonic chick ventricular myocytes. *Can J Physiol Pharmacol* 68:531–534, 1990.

95. Tohse N, Sperelakis N: cGMP inhibits the activity of single calcium channels in embryonic chick heart cells. *Circ Res* 69:325–331, 1991.

96. Tohse N, Meszaros J, Sperelakis N: Developmental changes in long-opening behavior of L-type Ca^{2+} channel in embryonic chick heart cells. *Circ Res* 71:376–384, 1992.

97. Tohse N, Masuda H, Sperelakis N: Novel isoform of Ca^{2+} channel in rat fetal cardiomyocytes. *J Physiol (Lond)* 451:295–306, 1992.

98. Cohen NM, Lederer WJ: Changes in the calcium current of rat heart ventricular myocytes during development. *J Physiol (Lond)* 406:115–146, 1988.

99. McLean MJ, Lapsley RA, Shigenobu K, Murad R, Sperelakis N: High cyclic AMP levels in young embryonic chick hearts. *Dev Biol* 42:196–201, 1975.

100. Renaud J-F, Sperelakis N, Le Douarin G: Increase of cyclic AMP levels induced by isoproterenol in cultured and non-cultured chick embryonic hearts. *J Mol Cell Cardiol* 10:281–286, 1978.

101. Thakkar JK, Sperelakis N: Changes in cyclic nucleotide levels during embryonic development of chick hearts. *J Dev Physiol* 9:497–505, 1987.

102. Reporter M: An ATP pool with rapid turnover, within the cell membrane. *Biochem Biophys Res Commun* 48:598–604, 1972.

103. Novak E, Drummond GI, Skala J, Hahn P: Development changes in cyclic AMP, protein kinase, phosphorylase kinase, phosphorylase in liver, heart and skeletal muscle of the rat. *Arch Biochem Biophys* 150:511–518, 1972.

104. Zalin RJ, Montague W: Changes in cyclic AMP, adrenylate cyclase and protein kinase levels during the development of embryonic chick skeletal muscle. *Exp Cell Res* 93:55–62, 1975.

105. Sperelakis N, Pappano AJ: Physiology and pharmacology of developing heart cells. In: Papp JG (ed) *International Encyclopedia of Pharmacology and Therapeutics*, Vol 22. Oxford: Pergamon Press, 1983, pp 1–39.

106. Haddox MK, Roeske WR, Russell DH: Independent expression of cardiac type I and II cyclic AMP-dependent protein kinase during murine embryogenesis and post-natal development. *Biochim Biophys Acta* 585:527–534, 1979.

107. Chen F-CM, Yamamura HI, Roeske WR: Adenlyate cyclase and beta adrenergic receptor development in the mouse heart. *J Pharmacol Exp Ther* 222:7–13, 1982.

108. Au TLS, Collins GA, Walker MJA: Rate, force and cyclic adenosine 3′,5′-monophosphate responses to (−)adrenaline in neonatal rat heart tissue. *Br J Pharmacol* 69:601–608, 1980.

109. Kithas PA, Artman M, Thompson WJ, Strada SJ: Subcellular distribution of high-affinity type IV cyclic AMP phosphodiesterase activities in rabbit ventricular myocardium: Relations to post-natal maturation. *J Mol Cell Cardiol* 21:507–517, 1989.

110. Novak E, Drummond GI, Skala J, Hahn P: Developmental changes in cyclic AMP, protein kinase, phosphorylase kinase, and phosphorylase in liver, heart, and skeletal muscle of the rat. *Arch Biochem Biophys* 150:511–518, 1972.

111. Noguchi A, deGuire J, Zanaboni P: Protein kinase C in the developing rat liver, heart and brain. *Dev Pharm Thera* 11:37–43, 1988.

112. Kuo JF: Changes in relative levels of guanosine-3′,5′-monophosphate-dependent protein kinases in lung, heart and brain of developing guinea-pig. *Proc Natl Acad Sci USA* 72:2256–2259, 1975.

113. Guidotti G, Kanemeishi D, Foa PP: Chick embryo heart as a tool for studying cell permeability and insulin action. *Am J Physiol* 201:863–868, 1961.

114. Guidotti G, Loreti L, Gaja G, Foa PP: Glucose uptake in the developing chick embryo heart. *Am J Physiol* 211:981–987, 1966.

115. Kutchai H, King SL, Martin M, Daves ED: Glucose uptake by chicken embryo hearts at various stages of development. *Dev Biol* 55:92–102, 1977.

116. Guidotti G, Foa PP: Development of an insulin-sensitive glucose transport system in chick embryo hearts. *Am J Physiol* 201:869–872, 1961.

117. Elsas LJ, Wheeler FB, Dannes DJ, De Haan RL: Amino acid transport by aggregates of cultured chicken hearts: Effect of insulin. *J Biol Chem* 250:9381–9390, 1975.

118. Herman BA, Fernandez BS: Developmental changes in membrane fluidity of cultured myogenic cells (abstr). *Physiologist* 19:223, 1976.

119. Harris W, Days R, Johnson C, Flinkelstein I, Stallworth J, Hubert C: Studies on avian heart pyruvate kinase during development. *Biochem Biophys Res Commun* 75:1117–1121, 1977.

120. Cardenas JM, Bandman E, Strohman RC: Hybrid isozymes of pyruvate kinase appear during avian cardiac development. *Biochem Biophys Res Commun* 80:593–599, 1978.

121. Harary I: Biochemistry of cardiac development: In vivo and in vitro studies. In: Berne RM, Sperelakis N (eds) *Handbook of Physiology: The Cardiovascular System*, Vol 1: *The Heart*. Bethesda, MD: American Physiological Society, 1979, pp 43–60.

122. Coffey R, Chendelin V, Newburgh R: Glucose utilization by chick embryo heart homogenates. *J Gen Physiol* 48:105–112, 1964.

123. Paul J: In: Wilmer ED (ed) *Cells and Tissue in Culture*, Vol 1. New York: Academic Press, 1965, pp 239–276.

124. Seltzer JL, McDougal DB: Enzyme levels in chick embryo heart and brain from 1–21 days of development. *Dev Biol* 42:95–105, 1975.

125. Warshaw JB: Cellular energy metabolism during fetal development. IV. Fatty acid activation, acyl transfer and fatty acid oxidation during development of the chick and rat. *Dev Biol* 28:537–544, 1972.

126. Fine IH, Kaplan NV, Kuftinec D: Developmental changes of mammalian lactic dehydrogenase. *Biochemistry* 4:116–124, 1963.

127. Cahn RD, Kaplan NO, Levine L, Zwilling E: Nature and development of lactic dehydrogenase. *Science* 136:962–969, 1962.

128. Cahn RD: Developmental changes in embryonic enzyme patterns: The effect of oxidative substrates on lactic dehydrogenase in beating chick embryonic heart cell cultures. *Dev Biol* 9:327–346, 1964.

129. Ziter FA: Creatine kinase in developing skeletal and cardiac muscle of the rat. *Exp Neurol* 43:539–546, 1974.

130. Sperelakis N, Lehmkuhl D: Effects of temperature and metabolic poisons on membrane potentials of cultured heart cells. *Am J Physiol* 213:719–724, 1967.

131. Vleugels A, Carmeljet E, Bosteds S, Zaman M: Differential effects of hypoxia with age on the chick embryonic hearts: Changes in membrane potential, intracellular K and Na, K efflux and glycogen. *Pflügers Arch* 365:159–166, 1976.

132. Thyrum PT: Reduced transmembrane calcium flow as a mechanism for the hypoxic depression of cardiac contractility. *J Int Res Commun* 1:1b, 1973.

133. Fabiato A, Fabiato F: Calcium and cardiac excitation-contraction coupling. *Am Rev Physiol* 41:473–484, 1979.

134. Watanabe AM, Besch HR Jr: Cyclic adenosine monophosphate modulation of slow calcium influx channels in guinea pig hearts. *Circ Res* 35:316–324, 1974.

135. Pappano AJ, Biegon RL: Mechanisms for muscarinic inhibition of calcium-dependent action potentials and contractions in developing ventricular muscle: The role of cyclic AMP. In: Hoffman BF, Lieberman M, Paes de Carvalho AP (eds) *Normal and Abnormal Conduction of the Heartbeat*. Mt Kisco, NY: Futura, 1983, pp 461–482.

136. Schneider JA, Sperelakis N: Slow Ca^{2+} and Na^+ current channels induced by isoproterenol and methylxanthines in

isolated perfused guinea pig hearts whose fast Na$^+$ channels are inactivated in elevated K$^+$. *J Mol Cell Cardiol* 7: 249–273, 1975.

137. Sperelakis N, Schneider JA: A metabolic control mechanism for calcium ion influx that may protect the ventricular myocardial cell. *Am J Cardiol* 37:1079–1085, 1976.

138. Reuter H: Localization of beta adrenergic receptors, and effects of noradrenaline and cyclic nucleotides on action potentials, ionic currents and tension in mammalian cardiac muscle. *J Physiol (Lond)* 242:429–451, 1974.

139. Josephson I, Sperelakis N: 5′-guanylimidodiphosphate stimulation of slow Ca^{2+} current in myocardial cells. *J Mol Cell Cardiol* 19:1157–1166, 1978.

140. Vogel S, Sperelakis N: Induction of slow action potentials by microiontophoresis of cyclic AMP into heart cells. *J Mol Cell Cardiol* 13:51–64, 1981.

141. Bkaily G, Sperelakis N: Injection of guanosine 5′-cyclic monophosphate into heart cells blocks calcium slow channels. *Am J Physiol* 248 (*Heart Circ Physiol* 17):H745–H749, 1985.

142. Pappano AJ, Hartigan PM, Coutu MD: Acetylcholine inhibits the positive inotropic effect of cholera toxin in ventricular muscle. *Am J Physiol* 243 (*Heart Circ Physiol* 12): H343–H441, 1982.

143. Li T, Sperelakis N: Stimulation of slow action potentials in guinea pig papillary muscle cells by intracellular injection of cyclic AMP, Gpp(NH)p, and cholera toxin. *Circ Res* 52:111–117, 1983.

144. Isenberg G: Is potassium conductance of cardiac Purkinje fibers controlled by [Ca^{2+}]$_i$? *Nature* 243:273–274, 1975.

145. Chesnais JM, Coraboeuf E, Sauviat MP, Vassas JM: Sensitivity to H, Li and Mn ions of the slow inward sodium current in frog atrial fibres. *J Mol Cell Cardiol* 7:627–642, 1975.

146. Vogel S, Sperelakis N: Blockade of myocardial slow inward current at low pH. *Am J Physiol* 233:C99–C103, 1977.

147. Belardinelli L, Vogel SM, Sperelakis N, Rubio R, Berne RM: Restoration of inward slow current in hypoxic heart muscle by alkaline pH. *J Mol Cell Cardiol* 11:877–892, 1979.

148. Sperelakis N: Regulatin of calcium slow channels in myocardial cells by cyclic nucleotides and phosphorylation. In: Solaro RJ (ed) *Protein Phosphorylation in Heart Muscle*. Boca Raton, FL: CRC Press, 1986, pp 55–83.

149. Tsien RW, Giles W, Greengard P: Cyclic AMP mediates the effects of adrenaline on cardiac Purkinje fibers. *Nature (New Biol)* 240:181–183, 1972.

150. Reuter H, Scholz H: The regulation of the calcium conductance of cardiac muscle by adrenaline. *J Physiol* 264: 49–62, 1977.

151. Sperelakis N, Belardinelli L, Vogel SM: Electrophysiological aspects during myocardial ischemia. In: *Proceedings of the 8th World Congress of Cardiology (Tokyo, 1978)*. Amsterdam: Excerpta Medica, 1979, pp 229–236.

152. Wahler GM, Sperelakis N: Intracellular injection of cyclic GMP depresses cardiac slow action potentials. *J Cyclic Nucleotide Protein Phosphoryl Res* 10:83–95, 1985.

153. Bkaily G, Sperelakis N: Injection of guanosine 5′-cyclic monophosphate into heart cells blocks calcium slow channels. *Am J Physiol* 248 (*Heart Circ Physiol* 17):H745–H749, 1985.

154. Riccioppo-Neto F, Sperelakis N: Effects of lidocaine, procaine, procainamide and quinidine on electrophysiologic properties of cultured embryonic chick hearts. *Br J Pharmacol* 86:817–826, 1986.

155. Coyle DE, Sperelakis N: Bupivacaine and lidocaine blockade of calcium mediated action potentials in guinea pig ventricular muscle. *J Pharmacol Exp Ther*, 1987, in press.

156. Josephson I, Sperelakis N: Local anesthetic blockade of Ca^{2+}-mediated action potentials in cardiac muscle. *Eur J Pharmacol* 40:201–208, 1976.

157. Hibbs RG: Electron microscopy of developing cardiac muscle in chick embryos. *Am J Anat* 99:17–52, 1956.

158. Schiebler TH, Wolff HH: Elektronenmikroskopische untersuchungen am herzmuskel der ratte wahrend der entwicklung. *Histochemie* 14:328–334, 1968.

159. Legato MJ: Ultrastructure characteristics of the rat ventricular cell grown in tissue culture, with special reference to sarcomerogenesis. *J Mol Cell Cardiol* 4:299–317, 1972.

160. Sperelakis N, Shigenobu K: Organ-cultured chick embryonic hearts of various ages. I: Electrophysiology. *J Mol Cell Cardiol* 16:449–471, 1974.

161. Shigenobu K, Sperelakis N: Failure of development of fast Na$^+$ channels during organ culture of young embryonic chick hearts. *Dev Biol* 39:326–330, 1976.

162. Renaud JF, Sperelakis N: Electrophysiological properties of chick embryonic heart grafted and organ cultured in vitro. *J Mol Cell Cardiol* 8:889–900, 1976.

163. McLean MJ, Renaud JF, Sperelakis N, Niu MC: mRNA induction of fast Na$^+$ channels in cultured cardiac myoblasts. *Science* 191:297–299, 1976.

164. Sperelakis N, McLean MJ, Renaud JF, Niu MC: Membrane differentiation of cardiac myoblasts induced in vitro by an RNA-enriched fraction from adult heart. In: Niu MC, Chuang HH (eds) *The Role of RNA in Development and Reproduction (Second International Symposium, Peking, China, 23–30 April, 1980)*. New York: Science Press; Beijing: Van Nostrant Reinhold, 1981, pp 730–771.

165. McLean MJ, Renaud JF, Niu MC, Sperelakis N: Membrane differentiation of cardiac myoblasts induced in vitro by an RNA-enriched fraction from adult heart. *Exp Cell Res* 110:1–14, 1977.

166. Kojima M, Sperelakis N: Development of slow Ca^{2+}-Na$^+$ channels during organ culture of young embryonic chick hearts. *J Dev Physiol* 7:355–363, 1985.

167. Sperelakis N: Electrical properties of embryonic heart cells. In: De Mello WC (ed) *Electrical Phenomena in the Heart*. New York: Academic Press, 1972, pp 1–61.

168. Sperelakis N, Lehmkuhl D: Effect of current on transmembrane potentials in cultured chick heart cells. *J Gen Physiol* 47:895–927, 1964.

169. Sperelakis N: Cultured heart reaggregate model for studying cardiac toxicology. Proceedings of the Conference on Cardiovascular Toxicology, Washington, DC. *Environ Health Perspect* 26:243–267, 1978.

170. Sperelakis N, Bkaily G: Cultured cell models for studying problems in cardiac toxicology. In: Atterwill CK, Steele CE (eds) *In Vitro Methods in Toxicology*. Cambridge, UK: Cambridge University Press, 1987, pp 77–113.

171. Jones JK, Paull K, Proskauer CC, Jones R, Lepeschkin E, Rush S: Ultrastructural changes produced in cultured myocardial cells by electric shock (abstr). *Fed Proc* 34:972, 1975.

172. Renaud JF, Scana AM Kazazoglou T, Lombet A, Romez G, Lazdunski M: Normal serum and lipoprotein-deficient serum give different expressions of excitability, corresponding to different stages of differentiation, in chick cardiac cells in culture. *Proc Natl Acad Sci USA* ●●:7768–7772, 1983.

173. Josephson I, Renaud JF, Vogel S, McLean M, Sperelakis N: Mechanisms of the histamine-induced positive inotropic action in cardiac muscle. *Eur J Pharmacol* 35:393–398, 1976.

174. Vogel S, Sperelakis N, Josephson I, Brooker G: Fluoride stimulation of slow Ca^{2+} current in cardiac muscle. *J Mol Cell Cardiol* 9:461–475, 1977.

175. Sperelakis N, Lehmkuhl D: Insensitivity of cultured chick heart cells to autonomic agents and tetrodotoxin. *Am J Physiol* 209:693–698, 1965.

176. Sperelakis N, Pappano AJ: Increase in P_{Na} and P_K of cultured heart cells produced by veratridine. *J Gen Physiol* 53:97–114, 1969.

177. Sperelakis N: Effects of cardiotoxic agents on the electrical properties of myocardial cells. In: Balazs I (ed) *Cardiac Toxicology*, Vol 1. Boca Raton, FL: CRC Press, pp 39–108, 1981.

178. Catterall WA: Activation of the action potential Na^+ ionophore of cultured neuroblastoma cells by veratridine and batrachotoxin. *J Biol Chem* 250:4053–4059, 1975.

179. Pang DC, Sperelakis N: Veratridine stimulation of calcium uptake by chick embryonic hearts cell in culture. *J Mol Cell Cardiol* 14:703–709, 1982.

180. Romey G, Lazdunski M: Lipid-soluble toxins thought to be specific for Na^+ channels block Ca^{2+} channels in neuronal cells. *Nature* 297:79–80, 1982.

181. Sperelakis N, Pappano A: Physiology and pharmacology of developing heart cells. In: Papp JG (ed) *International Encyclopedia of Pharmacology and Therapeutics*. Oxford: Pergamon Press; and in Pharm Thera 22:1–39, 1983.

182. Fujii S, Ayer RK Jr, De Haan RL: Differentiation of transmembrane ionic currents in the early embryonic chick heart. *Prog Dev Biol (Part A)*, 1986, pp 353–356.

183. Sperelakis N, McLean MJ: The electrical properties of embryonic chick cardiac cells. In: Longo LD, Reneau DD (eds) *Fetal and Newborn Cardiovascular Physiology*. Vol 1: Developmental Aspects. New York: Garland, 1978, pp 191–236.

184. Sperelakis N, McLean MJ: Electrical properties of cultured chick heart cells. In Dhalla NS, Sano T (eds) *Recent Advances in Studies on Cardiac Structure and Metabolism*, Vol 12. Baltimore, MD: University Park Press, 1978, pp 645–666.

185. Yamada S, Yamamura HI, Roeske WR: Ontogeny of α_1-adrenergic receptors in the mammalian myocardium. *Eur J Pharmacol* 68:217–221, 1980.

186. Chen F-CM, Yamamura HI, Roeske WR: Ontogeny of mammalian myocardial β-adrenergic receptors. *Eur J Pharmacol* 58:255–264, 1979.

187. Roeske WR, Yamamura HI: Maturation of mammalian myocardial muscarinic cholinergic receptors. *Life Sci* 23:127–132, 1978.

CHAPTER 36

Aging of the Adult Heart

EDWARD G. LAKATTA

INTRODUCTION

Both quantitative and qualitative assessments of normal cardiovascular function differ with age of the organism studied {1–4}. Thus functional studies of the normal heart at a single age are incomplete and represent only a point on a continuum. A full understanding of heart function in stressful or pathologic states must consider that age-related changes modify the substrate upon which the stress or disease process is superimposed and that the expression of a given pathologic state is not solely due to the disease per se but represents an age-disease interaction. Striking examples of this interaction can be observed in cardiac overload states {5} or in the effect of adaptation of the myocardium to chronic physical conditioning {6}.

The present chapter summarizes the results of studies that have investigated the effect of aging on some aspects of cardiac function discussed elsewhere in this volume. This approach appears optimal for integration of the aging variable into our current understanding of the function of the heart in normal and pathologic states. Primary emphasis is given to studies of cardiac function over the adult range, i.e., from adulthood to senescence; in addition, since the majority of these studies have been implemented in the rat aging model, this species is the main focus of discussion.

CARDIAC STRUCTURE

An increase in cardiac mass has been noted to occur with advancing age in many species, including humans {2,7}. In humans the gradual increase in aortic impedance and reflected pulse waves, due to progressive stiffening of the central arteries, and the resultant increase in systolic arterial pressure, are apparent causes of the modest cardiac hypertrophy that occurs with advancing age {3}. In some rodent strains, while hypertension is present in advanced age and may be causally related to cardiac hypertrophy, in other strains hypertrophy occurs even in the absence of an elevated blood pressure at rest {7,8}. In the Wistar strain, in which several aspects of cardiac biochemistry and physiology have been studied with respect to advanced age, the extent of left ventricular hypertrophy occuring

between adulthood (6 months) and senescence (24 months) is 20–30%, depending on whether heart mass is referenced to body size, i.e., tibial length, or to body weight (fig. 36-1A). Since body weight decreases during senescence, the 30% hypertrophy assessed by the left ventricular/body weight is probably an overestimate {9}. Absolute left ventricular weight increases 20%. There is no change in water content, and while hydroxyproline concentration nearly doubles {10}, the absolute amount can account for only a small part of the increase in mass. The average cell volume increases approximately 20% between adulthood and senescence (fig. 36-1B), and thus nearly all of the increase in heart mass is due to an increase in cell mass {9,11}. While cell length increases progressively throughout life (about 20% from 2 to 8 to 24 months) in the Wistar rat heart, the slack sarcomere length is not age related. Thus with increasing age, additional sarcomeres are added in series and in parallel {11}.

In hearts of males, Fischer 344 rats LV collagen increases from 5.5% of total protein at 1–4 months to approximately 12–16% at 22 and 26 months {12,13}; in the right ventricle (RV) collagen increases from 7% to 8% at 1 month to approximately 19.5–22% at 22–26 months {12,13}. Collagen accumulates in intrinsic collagenous structures, including perimysial weaves, coiled perimysial fibers, and struts, where the preexisting fibers are thickened and are more extensive. Regions of fibrosis also increase in size and volume in older animals, with predominant subendocardial localization {12,13}. In this rat strain an apparent (19%) reduction in the *number* of cardiac myocytes (muscle) has been estimated to occur in both ventricles between 4 and 12 months of age {12}. While at 20 months this reduction in cell number persists in the LV, it is reversed in the RV. Moreover, from 20 to 29 months, an apparent 59% increase in the *number* of cells has been inferred to occur in the RV with only a 3% estimated in the LV {12}. While this has been interpreted to indicate cardiac myocyte hyperplasia, i.e., an increase in the number of cardiac myocytes, more direct evidence of cell hyperplasia seems to be required to substantiate this provocative notion.

The density of subcellular organelles has not been precisely quantitated in senescence. Coronary atherosclerosis is not present in rats, and under light microscopy the age

N. Sperelakis (ed.), Physiology and Pathophysiology of the Heart, Third Edition.
© *1995 Kluwer Academic Publishers. ISBN 0-7923-2612-1. All rights reserved.*

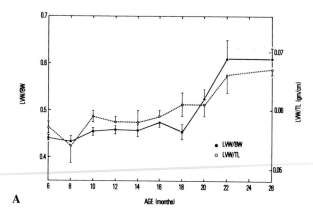

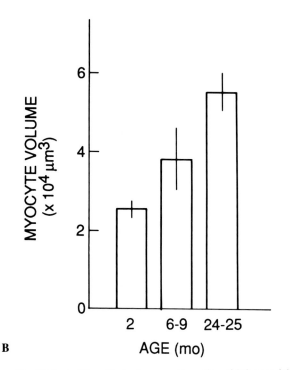

Fig. 36-1. **A:** The effect of age on the ratios of left ventricle to body weight (LVW/BW) and to tibial length (LVW/TL) in the Wistar rat. From Yin et al. {9}, with permission. **B:** Left ventricular cell volume (single cells, isolated via collagenase dissection of hearts), measured via the Coulter counter technique, increases with age. From Fraticelli et al. {11}, with permission.

of the hearts cannot be determined on the basis of coronary artery appearance {10}. Quantitative studies of capillary density and fiber densities have demonstrated a decrease in the former and a reduction in their ratio {14,15}. As in most other tissues, lipofuscin granules within the cell increase with advancing age {16}, but these have no apparent functional significance.

CARDIAC FUNCTION

Many functional aspects of the senescent heart resemble those in younger adult hearts that have hypertrophied in response to an experimentally increased work load {17,18}. These include changes in myocardial catecholamine content, action potential configuration, contraction duration, viscoelastic properties, the time course of the myoplasmic Ca^{2+} transient upon excitation, velocity of sarcoplasmic reticulum Ca^{2+} accumulation, myosin isozyme composition, myofibrillar and myosin ATPase activity, and protein synthesis {1,4}. Some of these changes have been linked to altered gene expression.

EXCITATION-CONTRACTION

Action potential

The effect of adult age on cardiac action-potential characteristics has been studied in rat atria and ventricles, guinea pig ventricles, canine Purkinje fibers, and individual ventricular myocytes. Resting membrane potential does not vary with age {19–27}. In unstretched rat atria {19,20}, a substantial increase in action-potential duration occurs during maturation from the neonatal period (2 months) to adulthood (6–12 months), with no further change through senescence (28 months). Similarly, in unloaded rat ventricular endocardium, no changes were observed in action-potential duration or the refractory period between adult and senescent heart {21}, and a similar effect of age on the duration of unstretched canine Purkinje fiber action potential has been observed {22}. The AP is prolonged in unloaded, single (and thus unstretched) LV myocytes isolated from senescent hearts compared to that in cells from younger hearts {25}.

The characteristics of the cardiac action potential are not fixed, but vary with many experimental factors. One such factor is the feedback interaction between excitation and contraction, i.e., mechanical factors of Ca^{2+} loading of the cell may modulate the action-potential duration {23}. To examine the relation between the action potential and contraction, the two must be studied simultaneously. In isolated guinea-pig right ventricular papillary muscles {24}, simultaneous measurements of the isometric twitch and transmembrane action potential made over a wide range of stimulation frequencies (30–400/min) indicate that both the plateau phase of the action potential and the contraction duration are prolonged in muscles from 3- to 4-month versus 26- to 40-month animals. With respect to the consideration of adult aging, it cannot be determined whether the age changes observed in this study occur over the adult to senescent period or, like the studies in unloaded rat cardiac tissues {19}, occur mainly over the maturational period in this species. In right ventricular papillary muscles contracting isometrically at the peak of their length-tension curve, prolongation of both action potential and contraction duration were observed in muscles from senescent (24 months) versus adult (6–8 month) rats {26,27}. Representative action potentials from senescent and adult muscle

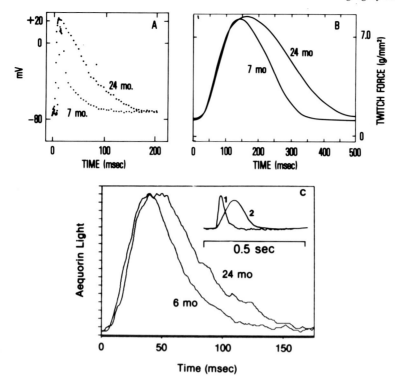

Fig. 36-2. **A:** Typical transmembrane action potentials measured in right ventricular papillary/muscles isolated from adult (7-month) and senescent (24-month) rat hearts. Muscles were stimilated to contract regularly at 24/min at 29°C in Krebs-Rigner solution containing 2.5 mM [Ca^{2+}]. The length of the muscles was that at which optimal force development in response to excitation occurred (L_{max}). **B:** Typical isometric contractions in right ventricular papillary muscles isolated from adult and senescent rat hearts and measured under conditions as in A. Redrawn from Wei et al. {27}, with permission. **C:** Aequorin luminescence in representative cardiac muscles from adult (6-month) and senescent (24-month) rats. Aequorin was injected into 30–100 cells of a right ventricular papillary muscle from a 6- and a 24-month Wistar rat. Muscles were bathed in 2 mM Ca^{2+}. The luminescence transient is the average of 100 consecutive steady-state contractions at 0.33 Hz at 30°C at L_{max}. Note that the light transient is prolonged in the 24-month muscle. The average time for aequorin luminescence to decay 50% in 11 young and 7 senescent muscles was 21.3 ± 1.5 and 32.9 ± 4.3 ms, respectively. Time to peak force in those same muscles in which light was measured was 88.8 ± 3.1 ms and 110.4 ± 6.8 ms, and the half-relaxation time was 54.9 ± 2.3 ms and 73.4 ± 4.4 ms in young and senescent muscles, respectively. From Orchard and Lakatta {32}, with permission.

are illustrated in fig. 36-2A, and typical isometric contractions are illustrated in fig. 36-2B. Greater overshoot and substantially greater area above 0 mV and repolarization times were observed in the senescent versus adult {27} muscles, and these differences persisted across a wide range of perfusate [Ca^{2+}].

Recent studies have begun to address the ionic basis of the AP prolongation with aging. The magnitude of the "inward going rectifier" K current does not change with age {28}. The peak L-type Ca^{2+} current in single ventricular myocytes (measured via the whole-cell patch clamp) normalized for cell capacitative area does not change with aging, suggesting that the density of this Ca^{2+} channel is not markedly altered in myocytes from older hearts {25}. However, a reduction in the inactivation rate of the Ca^{2+} current has been observed {25}. This, and an age-associated decrease in the magnitude of I_{To} (an outwardly directed K current), contribute to the prolonged

AP with aging {28}. The prolongation of the AP duration with aging may also relate to a prolonged cytosolic Ca^{2+} (Ca_i) transient (see below), as Ca^{2+} extrusion via the Na/Ca exchanger *during the AP* repolarization produces an inward current and prolongs AP duration of rat cells {29}.

ISOMETRIC CONTRACTION

Prolongation of the isometric twitch with advancing age (fig. 36-2B) has been observed in a variety of preparations from several species {21,30,31}. The precise relationship between the prolongation of the action potential and contraction duration in the senescent heart remains to be established. Plausible explanations include that with advancing age (a) prolonged depolarization retards the restitution of myoplasmic Ca^{2+} transient, (b) a prolonged Ca^{2+}

transient causes a delay in outwardly directed currents, or (c) prolongation of the electrical and mechanical parameters are unrelated and independently reflect prolonged restitution of preexcitation ionic gradients at the cell membrane and within the myoplasmic space. The transient increase in Ca_i concentration that results from excitation can be estimated by measuring the luminescence of a Ca^{2+}-sensitive protein, aequorin, which is pressure injected into multiple cells comprising the bulk muscle. Recent studies have indicated that while the amplitude of the Ca_i transient is not age related under some conditions, the decay of the Ca^{2+} transient back to the resting level is 50% prolonged in senescent versus younger adult rat cardiac muscle (fig 36-2C).

Increasing the stimulation rate or varying the stimulation pattern places a stress upon excitation-contraction mechanisms. In physiologic bathing $[Ca^{2+}]$ (Ca_o) in the absence of drugs, the amplitude of the twitch force and Ca_i transient in rat cardiac muscle decline as the stimulation frequency is increased, but the magnitude of this decline does not differ with age {32}. In contrast, in higher Ca_o muscles from younger adults are able to maintain the amplitude of twitch force and of Ca_i transient as the stimulation frequency increases, but senescent muscles cannot {32}. The postextrasystolic potentiation of contraction amplitude during continual paired stimulation at low rates is also preserved in senescent muscles bathed in low $[Ca_o]$ and stimulated at 24 pairs/min {33}. However, when the coupling interval of paired stimuli is decreased from 200 to 100 ms, senescent, but not adult, muscles fail to generate a twitch response to the second stimulus (fig

36-3). Additionally muscles from senescent rats show a greater likelihood to exhibit contractions of alternating amplitude at high frequencies of stimulation {34}. Thus, under the experimental stress of altered stimulation patterns during which the restitution time is decreased, the reduced kinetics of ionic channel restitution or of Ca^{2+} cycling in the senescent myocardium are associated with contractions of smaller amplitude.

SARCOPLASMIC RETICULUM

Although any mechanism that can alter the flux of Ca^{2+} into or out of the cytosol might affect the duration of the Ca_i transient, its decay is thought to largely depend upon the rate of Ca^{2+} removal by the SR Ca^{2+} pump {32}. The prolongation of the Ca_i transient in senescent muscle, as noted above, may be related, in part, to a diminished SR Ca^{2+} pumping rate. Early studies (fig. 36-4) have demonstrated that the rate of Ca^{2+} uptake into SR vesicles isolated from senescent Wistar rat hearts is less than that from vesicles from younger adult hearts {35}. The net Ca^{2+} uptake in studies of this sort depends upon the Ca^{2+} pumped into vesicles and any Ca^{2+} efflux that may occur during the experiment. The latter can result from a passive, nonspecific leak, or from an efflux via Ca^{2+} channels (ryanodine receptors) through which Ca^{2+} release is thought to occur following excitation. The passive leaking of Ca^{2+} from membrane vesicles derived from cardiac homogenate preparations has been found not to differ with age {36}. The rate of SR Ca^{2+} pumping into the SR

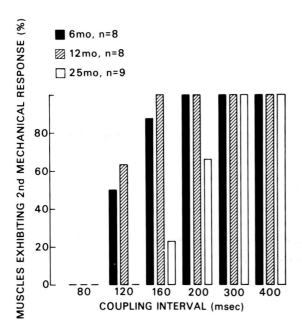

Fig. 36-3. The effect of adult age on the mechanical response to a reduction in the interval between successive stimuli. Redrawn from Lakatta et al. {21}, with permission.

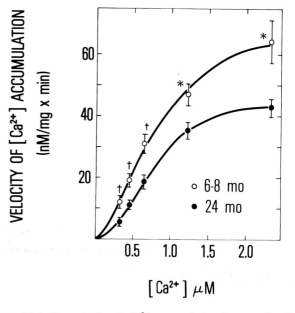

Fig. 36-4. The velocity of Ca^{2+} accumulation in sarcoplasmic reticulum isolated from 6- to 8-month (○) and 24- to 25-month (●) rat hearts. The curves are different at the $p < 0.001$ by analysis of variance. From Froehlich et al. {35}, with permission.

depends upon the cytosolic [Ca$_i$] concentration (or in isolated vesicles, on the [Ca^{2+}] of the medium bathing the vesicles; fig. 36-4). The reduction in the SR Ca^{2+} uptake rate with aging applies to the entire range of Ca$_i$ that occurs in cardiac cells from diastole to systole (fig. 36-4). More recent studies in SR isolated from other rat strains (Fischer 344 and Sprague Dawley) have produced very similar results {36–39} to those in the Wistar strain depicted in fig. 36-4. In the Fischer 344 strain, the diminished SR Ca^{2+} uptake rate persisted in the presence of calmodulin {40}. A decrease in constitutive levels of phosphorylation of phospholamban, an SR protein membrane that modulates the Ca^{2+} pump activity, has also been reported in native cardiac microsomes obtained from senescent rats {41}. As unphosphorylated phospholamban inhibits Ca^{2+} uptake by the Ca^{2+}-ATPase pump of the cardiac SR, it is possible that lower levels of phosphorylated phospholamban are a factor in the decreased rate of Ca^{2+} uptake by cardiac SR from older animals observed in the absence of cAMP-dependent stimulation in the above studies {35,36,39,42}. In one study in isolated membrane preparations from senescent Fischer 344 rats, although the Ca^{2+} uptake rate was found to be depressed, Ca^{2+}-induced stimulation of SR pump enzyme (i.e., the SR Ca^{2+}-ATPase) was not found to be reduced by aging {36}. Accordingly, it was suggested that there is an age difference in the efficiency of coupling between ATP splitting and Ca^{2+} pumping {36}. In contrast, another study in SR isolated from Fischer 344 rat hearts {43} did find about a 25% age-associated reduction in the maximum rate of SR Ca^{2+}-ATPase activity, accompanied by reductions of similar magnitude in the formation of acylphosphate formation and in Ca^{2+} uptake and SR vesicles from the senescent versus younger adult heart {43}. The reduction in the rate of Ca^{2+} pumped into the SR is likely due to a reduction in the total SR pump protein (Ca^{2+}-ATPase) activity {43}. The diminished Ca^{2+}-ATPase activity and rate at which the SR from senescent hearts pumps Ca^{2+} may be related to a reduction in mRNA coding for the SR Ca^{2+}-ATPase observed in some {44,45} but not all {46} studies, possibly reflecting a decrease in the relative density of SR pump sites with aging. This conclusion is further supported by the observations that gel electrophoresis shows a 40% reduction in the SR Ca^{2+}-ATPase *protein* without a concomitant reduction in calsequestrin, a Ca^{2+} binding protein within SR {43}. The mRNA levels of calsequestrin, likewise, do not decline with adult aging {44}.

A reduced rate of sarcoplasmic-reticulum Ca^{2+} sequestration could result in a prolonged Ca$_i$ transient (fig. 36-2C) and in delayed relaxation in a given contraction (fig. 36-2B), and may also affect a subsequent premature stimulus (fig. 36-3), since the extent of Ca^{2+} reloading within the sarcoplasmic reticulum might not be sufficient to respond to a trigger for its release {47}. Thus both prolonged contraction duration and delayed restitution of the excitation-contraction cycle in the senescent heart could be explained by age differences in the rate of sarcoplasmic Ca^{2+} transport or in requirements for its release.

Cardiac relaxation is also dependent upon the mechanical load borne by the myocardial fibers. The load-dependent aspects of relaxation of posterior papillary muscles from the left ventricle (LV) and right ventricle (RV) of Fischer and Sprague-Dawley rats have been studied at 4, 10, and 20 months of age {48}. In the Fischer 344 strain, the RV muscle was found completely load independent, whereas the LV muscle was fully load dependent at all physiological afterloads, Aging reduced the load independence of the RV and the load dependence of the LV in Fischer rats. In other words, the role of Ca^{2+} in modulating relaxation of LV relative to that of mechanical load increased with age. In contrast, no aging effect on the properties of afterloaded isotonic relaxation was observed in muscle from Sprague-Dawley rats {48}.

MYOFILAMENT PROPERTIES

While one major function of cardiac muscle is to stiffen to produce force, the other major, and ultimate function, is to shorten in order to eject blood. The speed of shortening, according to the crossbridge, sliding-filament theories of muscle contraction, is ultimately determined by the kinetics of crossbridge cycling. The velocity of shortening is inversely related to the load that the filaments bear. At very light loads (or zero load if this experiment were feasible), the maximum velocity of shortening will occur and will reflect the maximum crossbridge cycling rate. The maximum velocity of shortening also depends on the level of myofilament Ca^{2+} activation, which is not constant, but varies with time during the twitch. Studies of the effect of age on the velocity of shortening have documented a decline over the maturational period {31,49,50} and with advanced age {30–50}. It is important to note that the interpretation of these measurements of the effect of age on shortening velocity have not taken into consideration that the time course of Ca^{2+} activation is altered with age (fig. 36-2C). Thus differences in shortening velocity observed in muscles from different-aged rats following a release (i.e., permitted to shorten) at a given time following stimulation may, in part, be due to age-related differences in Ca^{2+} activation at that time rather than be indicative of specific age-related differences of intrinsic crossbridge kinetics.

In addition to the extent of Ca^{2+} binding to troponin C, the "ATPase activity" of myofilament proteins is a determinant of contraction characteristics. The *myofibrillar* ATPase activity, in preparations prepared using detergents, exhibits the identical Ca^{2+} dependence ($K_m = 0.6 \mu m$; Hill coefficient $\simeq 4.5$) as does force (see fig. 36-6A) {51}. Although the Ca^{2+} sensitivity of myofibrillar ATPase activity does not change with adult age, the maximum ATPase activity declines during maturation and then remains stable from 6 months of age through senescence {4,51}. The Ca^{2+}-activated ATPase activity in *actomyosin* preparations (i.e., actin plus myosin in the absence of troponin and tropomyosin) declines during maturation but also shows a further decline with age {52–54}.

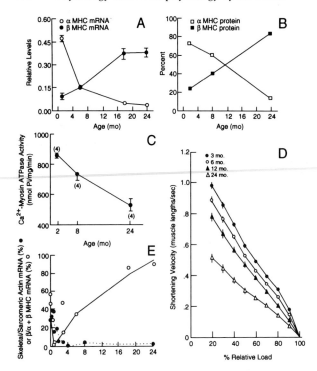

Fig. 36-5. **A:** Average values for α and β myosin heavy chain m rRNA/mRNA18S of individual hearts measured by dot blot analysis (n = 11, 6, 10, and 10 for ages 6 weeks and 6, 18, 24 months, respectively). From O'Neill et al. {59}, with permission. **B:** The α and β myosin heavy chain proteins (V_1 and V_3 isoforms) of hearts of the same rate strain. From Effron et al. {56}, with permission. **C:** Ca^{2+}-activated myosin ATPase activity of Wistar rat hearts decreases with age. From Effron et al. {56}, with permission. **D:** The velocity of shortening during lightly loaded isotonic contractions in isolated cardiac muscle from younger and older rats decreases with aging. From Capasso et al. {26}, with permission. **E:** Left ventricular actin isoforms (cardiac versus skeletal) do not change with aging in the Wistart rat. From Carrier et al. {63}, with permission.

The Ca^{2+}-*activated* ATPase activity of purified isolated *myosin* preparations (fig. 36-5C) in the rat declines progressively throughout the entire age range of 1–14 months {43,52,55,56}. This ATPase activity is modulated, in part, by the muscle MHC isoform composition {57}. The content of the αMHC isoform (often referred to as the V_1 isoform), which has a rapid ATPase activity, also decreases progressively with age (fig. 36-5B). The lower level of the αMHC protein in preparations isolated from senescent hearts {46,52,54,56,58} appears to be a major factor that underlies the decreased myosin ATPase activity. The mRNA coding for αMHC also declines with age in the myocardium of Wistar (fig. 36-5A) and Fischer 344 rats {46,58–60}, and the diminished expression of this gene with aging may account, in large part, for the reduction in the αMHC content with aging (fig. 36-5B). Conversely, with aging the mRNA coding for the βMHC isoform (sometime referred to as the V_3 isoform), which has a

lower ATPase activity than the αMHC, exhibits a several-fold increase {46,58,59,61} (fig. 36-5A) and is the apparent mechanism for an increase in the βMHC protein content with aging (fig. 36-5B). Thus the pattern of expression of MHC genes in the senescent heart resembles that which occurs around the time of birth {59}. In this regard a marked increase in mRNA coding for atrial natriuretic factor occurs in the LV with advancing adult age {62}. In contrast, the expression of genes coding for actin isoforms (i.e., cardiac and skeletal) does not shift with aging (fig. 36-5E) and thus does not resemble the fetal pattern {63}.

The switching of the MHC genes with advancing adult age may, in part, underlie the decline in the velocity of shortening in lightly loaded isotonic contractions (fig. 36.5D) with aging {49,52} and may also be related to the prolongation of time to peak tension in isometric contractions (fig. 36-2) and prolonged time to peak shortening in isotonic contractions in cardiac muscle from adult versus older animals {26, 52}. It is noteworthy that the βMHC or V_3 isoform is energy efficient in that a given level of tension develops in hearts with predominately the αMHC (V_1) isoform {64}.

Alterations of thyroid status can produce alterations in the variables depicted in figs. 36-2 to 36-5. In this regard the changes observed in the aging heart mimic, to some extent, those observed in the *hypo*thyroid state {57,58,65–69}. Whether a relative hypotyroid state accompanies aging is uncertain. An age-associated decline in plasma levels of thyroid hormones (T_3 or T_4) occurs in at least two rat strains {45,46,56,66,70}, but the magnitude of the decline is small. It has been reported that replacement of sufficient thyroxine to restore plasma levels in older rats to those levels occurring in younger rats can abolish the age-associated decline in myosin ATPase activity {66}. Administration of T_3 or T_4 to senescent rats also decreases the βMHC mRNA levels {58}. However, complete reversal of the MHC isoform profile did not occur with smaller doses of thyroxine {66}. Also, very high doses of thyroxine administered for a short period of time have been noted to increase the myosin αMHC (V_1 isoform) content of senescent hearts, but do not fully restore this level to that in the younger heart (fig. 36-6) {56}. Thus a failure of myocardial cells to response to thyroxine (e.g., due to deficits in nuclear thyroid receptors or changes of the binding properties of thyroid regulatory elements on the MHC and on other genes) may occur with aging and, in part, underlie the pattern of change depicted in figs. 36-2 to 36-5.

PASSIVE MYOCARDIAL STIFFNESS PROPERTIES

Data arising from studies in animal models are often cited as being indicative of a change in "passive" mechanical myocardial properties with advancing age. Passive mechanical properties of myocardial cells and tissue, i.e., those properties that are determined by the amount and composition of matrix (interstitial) proteins, e.g., collagen and cytoskeletal proteins, affect the contraction amplitude and relaxation of cardiac muscle and the filling properties of

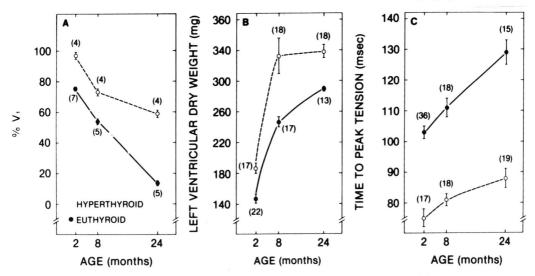

Fig. 36-6. **A:** The effect of age on the maximum rate of myofibrillar ATPase activity, time to peak twitch force (TPT), and maximum rate of twitch force development (dT/dt). Myofibrillar ATPase activity was measured in detergent-purified myofibrils at pCa of 5.8. Mechanical parameters were measured at L_{max} at $[Ca^{2+}]^o$. = 2.5 mM in right ventricular papillary muscles stimulated to contract regularly at 24/min at 29°C. Reprinted from Bhatnagar et al. {51}, with permission. **B:** The effect of age and thyroxine on the percent of V_1 myosin (left), left ventricular weight (center), and time to peak isometric twitch (right). From Effron et al. {56}, with permission.

the cardiac ventricle. An estimation of the elastic or viscoelastic modulus is a more meaningful method of assessing passive muscle properties than are measurements of the passive length-tension curve {71}. In isolated, unstimulated rat trabecular muscles, using small sinusoidal length perturbations across a range of muscle lengths, several studies have failed to demonstrate an age-associated alteration in the passive viscoelastic stiffness moduli {6,7,72}. In contrast, no generalization can be made from studies of the intact, isolated heart as the passive viscoelastic modulus was found to increase in the beagle dog {73}, to not change in the hamster {74}, and to decrease in the rat {75} with aging.

In addition to the variable results of different studies, more fundamental considerations underlie the ambiguity of the effect of age on passive myocardial properties, among which is the assumption of classic muscle mechanics that Ca^{2+} activation of myofilaments does not contribute to passive force, i.e., force measured in the absence of electrical stimulation. In the rat, in which most aging studies have been performed, the passive force in the isolated heart and cardiac muscle may indeed be influenced by asynchronous spontaneous Ca^{2+} oscillations that occur asynchronously among myocardial cells of unstimulated rat cardiac muscle (see below) when the Ca_o is in the range of 2.5 mM or less, i.e., over the range where most mechanical measurements have been made {76–78}. Furthermore, in isolated cardiac cells from rats, and from other species as well, a tonic, Ca^{2+}-dependent myofilament interaction is also present at rest and modulates the slack cell length {79}.

STEADY FORCE-CALCIUM RELATION

Under conditions in which the active properties of muscle might be measured, precise characterization of myofilament activation from force and stiffness measurements requires modeling of the geometric arrangement or linkage of myofilaments and passive viscoelastic structures. Measurement of force or stiffness over a range of Ca^{2+} activation rather than at a single level can circumvent this problem to a certain extent and may provide information regarding myofilament interaction. In muscle preparations chemically skinned with detergent, steady-state force production across the range of pCa that is likely to occur subsequent to excitation is not altered by age (fig. 36-7A). That the shape of the relative force-pCa curve is not age related fig. 36-7B) also suggests that sensitivity of troponin C to Ca^{2+} also may not be age related.

In muscles with intact membranes, because of the sarcolemmal barrier and sequestration of Ca^{2+} within the cell, force production in response to an excitation varies over a higher range of Ca_o than in skinned preparations. In intact adult rat cardiac muscle, force development varies over a relatively narrow range of Ca_o compared to most other species (fig. 36-8). This marked shift of the Ca_o developed force relationship in the rat to lower Ca_o cannot result from a difference in the force pCa^{2+} relationship, as in fig. 36-7, because this is fairly constant among species {47}. Rather it is most likely attributable to a species difference in cellular Ca^{2+} loading.

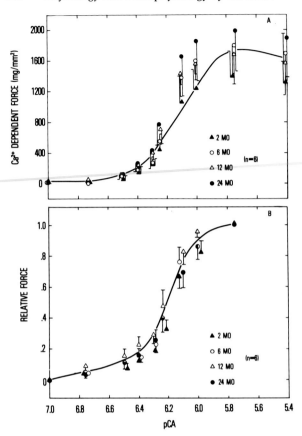

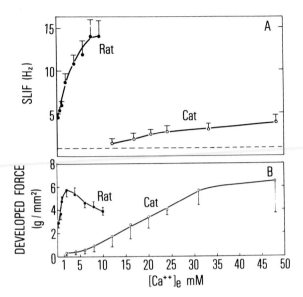

Fig. 36-8. The effect of Ca_o on **A**: *Scattered Light Intensity Fluctuations* (SLIF) caused by spontaneous diastolic cellular Ca^+ oscillations measured prior to an excitation. **B**: Force developed in response to that excitation in isolated rat (n = 3) and cat (n = 3) cardiac muscles. Stimulus frequency was 2/min and temperature was 29°C. It is important to note that the curves in the figure are not unique but vary with stimulation frequency, particularly in the cat. Also, the frequency of scattered light fluctuations is greater than the frequency of the underlying cellular Ca^{2+} oscillations because the amplitude of cellular motion caused by the Ca^{2+} oscillations is up to severalfold greater than the wavelength of the laser beam (0.5 nm) used to detect the microscopic motion {78}.

Fig. 36-7. **A:** The effect of age from the neonatal to senescent period on steady levels of force across a range of PCa. **B:** The data in each preparation have been normalized to their maximal level. From Bhatnagar et al. {51}, with permission.

SPONTANEOUS SR Ca^{2+} CYCLING

In mechanically skinned cell fragments of isolated cardiac cells, a small increase in Ca_i affects the release of Ca^{2+} from the sarcoplasmic reticulum {80,81}, referred to as Ca^{2+}-induced Ca^{2+} release. Once initiated, the cycle of Ca^{2+} release and reuptake can perpetuate itself without requiring additional Ca^{2+} input into the cell, or without a preceding sarcolemmal depolarization, i.e., under some Ca^{2+}-loading conditions *spontaneous* Ca^{2+}-induced-Ca^{2+} release can occur {80,81}. Since the frequency and amplitude of spontaneous SR generated Ca_i oscillations vary with the extent of cell Ca^{2+} loading, changes in the later can be monitored by changes in *Scattered Light Intensity Fluctuations* (SLIF), which result from microscopic tissue motion due to the Ca^{2+}-myofilament interactions produced from spontaneous Ca^{2+} oscillations. Rat cardiac muscle, in particular, demonstrates SLIF during the absence of or during the interbeat interval at low rates of stimulation {78,82,83} under experimental conditions

similar to those in figs. 36-2 and 36-3, i.e., those usually employed in studies of excitation-contraction mechanisms in cardiac muscle in vitro. An age difference in the extent to which this occurs {84} can pose problems with regard to studies of aging because the presence of spontaneous diastolic Ca^{2+} release can affect not only resting force but twitch force in the subsequent twitch as well {85–88}. Adjusting the stimulation frequency can, in many instances, suppresse the spontaneous release {82,88}.

As illustrated in fig. 36-8A, a marked shift in Ca^{2+} loading, as monitored by this technique, is observed in the rat and likely determines the shift in the twitch force-Ca_o relationship observed in this species (fig. 36-8B). It is also important to note that in isolated cardiac muscle, when Ca_o exceeds a maximum, force production falls (see rat in fig. 36-8B), and this is attributable, at least in part, to spontaneous diastolic Ca^{2+} release from the SR into the myoplasm {82,85,86}. This is spatiotemporally heterogeneous within and among cells comprising the muscle and can, as discussed above, be monitored as SLIF (fig. 36-8). Thus studies of the effect of Ca_o on cell Ca^{2+} loading should be performed over the optimal range of Ca_o i.e., less than 3 mM in the rat muscle stimulated at low frequencies at moderately low temperatures; increasing

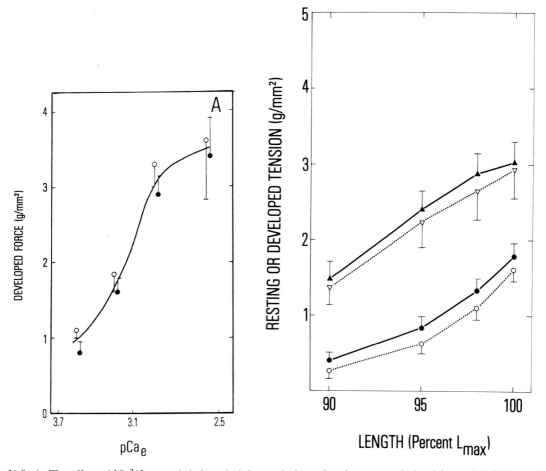

Fig. 36-9. **A:** The effect of $[Ca^{2+}]_o$ on twitch force in left ventricular trabeculae carneae isolated from adult (6–8 month; ●) and senescent (25 month; 0) Wistar rats. Muscles were stimulated to contract isometrically at 24/min at 29°C. From Lakatta and Yin {4}, with permission. **B:** The effect of resting muscle length on resting force (circles) and twitch force (triangles) in left ventricular trabeculae carneae from adult (closed symbols) and senescent (open symbols) rat hearts. Stimulation rate was 24/min and $[Ca^{2+}]_e$ was 2.5 mM. L_{max} is that length at which twitch force was optimal. Redrawn from Yin et al. {7}, with permission.

the stimulation frequency at low states of Ca^{2+} loading will suppress the spontaneous Ca^{2+} release {82,86,88}.

When Ca_o is kept low, the response in rat cardiac muscle to inotropic perturbations is qualitatively similar to that of other species {30,33,77}. Over the adult range, aging does not affect the Ca_o-developed force relationship over the optimal range of Ca_o (fig. 36-9A). In addition, at optimal Ca_o the effect of resting muscle length, which also modulates the extent of myofilament activation at a given Ca_o {89,90}, on developed force production is not altered by age (fig. 36-9B).

The cytosolic $[Na^+]$ regulates the cell Ca^{2+} load by affecting Ca^{2+} flux through the Na-Ca exchanger. It has been suggested that the Na-Ca exchanger is more active in ejecting Ca^{2+} from cells of older versus hearts during diastole {36,91}. Cytosolic $[Na^+]$ is primarily regulated by the Na-K pump. While Na-K ATPase activity has been

reported to decrease with aging, the cytosolic $[Na^+]$ measured via Na^+ selective microelectrodes does not appear to change with age, either at rest or during rapid stimulation {92}. In this regard, it is of interest to note than an age-associated decline in the contractile response to digitalis glycosides, which act via Na-K pump inhibition, occurs in the absence of an age difference in the relative extent of glycoside-induced Na,K-ATPase inhibition in both the rat and beagle dog models {33,93}.

The multiple changes in cardiac excitation, myofilament activation, and contraction mechanisms that occur with aging are interrelated. Many of these changes can be interpreted as adaptive in nature, as they also occur in the hypertrophied myocardium of younger animals that have adapted to experimentally induced chronic hypertension {17,36,94–98} (fig. 36-10).

Figure 36.11 summarizes the changes in specific gene

Chronic Alterations in Excitation-Contraction Coupling Mechanisms in Various Models

Functional Measure Measure	Experimental LV Pressure Loading (Rodent)	Normotensive Aging (Rodent)
Twitch Duration	↑	↑
Myosin Isozyme Composition	↓ V_1 ↑ V_3	↓ V_1 ↑ V_3
SR Ca^{2+} Pumping Rate	↓	↓
Ca Transient Duration	↑ (Ferret)	↑
Myofilament Ca^{2+} Sensitivity	↔	↔
Action Potential Repolarization Time	↑	↑
β-adrenergic Intropic Response	↓	↓
Cardiac Glycoside Response	↓	↓
Threshold for Ca^{2+} Overload	↓	↓

Fig. 36-10. Chronic alterations in excitation-contraction coupling mechanisms in various models. From Lakatta {3}, with permission.

Altered Myocardial Gene Expression in Advanced Age, Hypertension, Heart Failure or After Growth Factors*

	Rodent Aging	Rodent Hypertension	TGFβ	FGF acidic	FGF basic
SR Ca^{2+}-ATPase	↓	↓	↓	↓	↓
Calsequestrin	↔	↔			
Phospholamban		↑ (rabbit)			
α MHC	↓	↓	↓	↓	↓
β MHC	↑	↑	↑	↑	↑
β Tropomyosin	↓	↑ ***			
α Skeletal Actin	↓	↑ ***	↑	↓	↑
ANF	↑	↑	↑	↑	↑
Proenkephalin	↑				

*In neonatal cultured cardiocytes
**In atrial tissue
***Only transient changes occur *in situ* following cardiac pressure loading

Fig. 36-11. Altered myocardial gene expression in advanced age, hypertension, heart failure, or after growth factors. From Lakatta {3}, with permission.

expression that occur in the pressure-overloaded myocardium and aging. Note that a similar pattern occurs in both hypertensive young animals and with aging in normotensive animals, and in neonatal heart cells exposed to growth factors. It is tempting to speculate that, because a nearly identical *pattern* of change in cell mechanisms occurs both in experimental pressure overload and aging, and after growth factors in neonatal heart cells, this pattern may reflect a "logic" within the genome, i.e., that a common set of transcription factors regulates the expression of multiple genes, resulting in cellular adaptation. This particular constellation of apparent shifts in gene expression appears to be adaptive, in that it allows for an energy-efficient and prolonged contraction. In the hypertensive rodent heart, it can be inferred that these changes in gene expression permit functional adaptations in response to an increased vascular "afterload."

However, the stimulus for the age-associated changes is not presently known. Arterial stiffness dose not appear to increase with adult age in rats {4}. Unlike the hypertensive heart, the increased LV mass that occurs in the Wistar rat strain with aging is largely due to an increase in LV cavity size, i.e., the wall thickness appears to remain normal with aging {99}. However, as is the case in the young hypertensive rodent, cardiac myocytes become enlarged in the senescent heart, as noted above. It may be argued that mechanical or hormonal stimuli that initiate and maintain the cardiac hypertrophic response in the hypertensive heart are also present within the aging heart. It has been hypothesized that the apparent "dropout" of some myocardial cells with aging {12,100} leads to augmented stretch upon the remaining cells, this being the stimulus of cellular hypertrophy and of the accompanying changes in gene expression and biophysical mechanisms that lead to a prolonged contraction. On the other hand, prolonged contraction in older hearts persists when these hearts are transplanted, mechanically unloaded, and atrophied {101}. Also, the prolonged AP, Ca_i transient, and contraction occurs with aging in RV muscle {6,10} in which ventricular myocyte number may not be reduced in senescence {100}. Additionally, unlike the LV, the RV does not hypertrophy with age in the Wistar rat strain {9}.

EFFECTS OF CHRONIC EXERCISE ON MYOCARDIAL FUNCTION

Chronic exercise in senescent rats abolishes prolonged isometric contraction (fig. 36-12) in isolated LV trabeculae measured across a range of Ca_o and also reduces the active dynamic stiffness {6}. The type of chronic exercise (5-month duration, mild wheel exercise protocol) employed was insufficient to alter the body or heart weight in adult (6–9 months) and senescent (24–26 months) rats at sacrifice, and did not alter the twitch amplitude at any age. In the younger animals, this exercise protocol was ineffective in altering the duration of contraction (fig. 36-12) or dynamic stiffness measured during contraction in muscles. Since physical conditioning does not alter the collagen content in the heart {102,103}, reversal of prolonged contraction duration and altered active stiffness properties in the senescent heart {6} suggest that these properties of the senescent heart are not attributable to enhanced collagen content {11}. Additionally, that cardiac mass was not affected by this exercise protocol suggests that age-associated

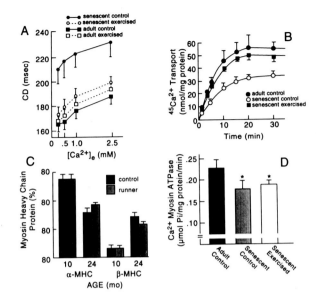

Fig. 36-12. Chronic exercise training decreases the isometric contraction duration in isolated right ventricular papillary muscles of senescent Wistar rats (**A**) and increases the velocity of Ca^{2+} accumulation in sarcoplasmic reticulum isolated from Fischer 344 rats (**B**). In contrast, chronic exercise neither alters age-associated decreases in the myosin heavy chain isoform content (**C**) nor age-associated changes in myosin ATPase activity (**D**). Panel A from Spurgeon et al. {6}; panels B and D from Tate et al. {39}; panel C from Farrar et al. {54}, with permission.

changes in dynamic stiffness or contraction duration cannot be directly attributed to an increase in cardiac mass with aging. This point is also clearly illustrated by the results of another study, which created the same extent of hypertrophy present in the senescent heart in middle-aged adult rats by banding the aorta {7}. Although muscles from the hypertrophied left ventricles of the banded animals exhibited a prolonged twitch and increased dynamic stiffness compared to controls, the magnitudes of these were not as great as those observed in the senescent heart. The reduction in both the active stiffness coefficient and duration of contraction would be consistent with an effect of exercise to reduce the duration of the Ca_i transient. Indeed, subsequent studies show that the duration of the Ca_i transient in senescent cardiac muscle is reduced following chronic exercise {104}. The AP prolongation in isolated muscle of senescent hearts is not reversed by exercise, however {104}. The reduced rate of SR Ca^{2+} sequestration (fig. 36-10) and SR Ca^{2+}-ATPase and mRNA levels in the senescent heart {39,43} can also be reversed by chronic physical conditioning. The progressive decline in myocardial Ca^{2+}-activated actomyosin ATPase activity, which begins during maturation (after 1 month in the rat) and progresses with advancing adult age, can be retarded by a chronic (3-month) period of exercise but the beneficial effects of exercise, however, are relatively small throughout 12–15 months {105}. Moreover,

in older animals that began exercise at 17–22 months, and were sacrificed at 20–25 months, a decline in actomyosin ATPase occurred {105}. The altered MHC isoform profile with aging (fig. 36-12) or myosin or myosin ATPase activities (fig. 36-12) in the senescent heart are not affected by chronic physical conditioning {39,54}.

β-ADRENERGIC STIMULATION

The convergence of several lines of evidence clearly indicates that advancing age in both healthy humans and animals is accompanied by a deterioration of the communication between the nervous system and the heart and vasculature {106}. Specifically, the efficacy of beta-adrenergic modulation of cardiovascular function decreases with aging. As circulatory catecholamine levels do not decline or are increased with aging, particularly during stress, the age-associated deficit in the effectiveness of beta-adrenergic control is largely postsynaptic in nature.

The precise role of beta-adrenergic modulation during dynamic exercise in the upright posture in humans has been ascertained by exercising individuals in the presence of beta-adrenergic blockade. When younger individuals exercise in the presence of propranolol, their heart rate increase to a lesser extent, but their end-diastolic volume (EDV) increases substantially, and a greater stroke volume is achieved than in the absence of beta blockade {107}. Additionally, the LV end-systolic volume (ESV) reduction that normally accompanies exercise is blunted. The hemodynamic profile during upright cycle exercise in healthy older men has been observed to differ from that in younger men in a way that resembles the profile observed during beta-adrenergic blockade. Specifically, during exercise in healthy, sedentary older individuals, the heart rate increase is blunted, the EDV and ESV and enhanced, and the LV ejection fraction is blunted relative to younger individuals {108,109}. Thus, the blunted cardiac responses in older men to an infusion of a beta-adrenergic agonist at rest {106} has "naturally occurring" counterparts during acute exercise stress. Moreover, when older and younger men exercise in the presence of beta-adrenergic blockade affected by propranolol, the age-associated decline in heart rate is markedly reduced (because of a greater drug-induced reduction in younger than in older men during beta blockade), and the age-associated ventricular dilatation is abolished because of greater ventricular dilatation in younger than in older men during beta blockade {110}. The age-associated decrease in the peak LV filling rate is also abolished during exercise in the presence of propranolol {111}. Additional studies have shown that the cardiac output differences between older and younger subjects during exercise also become attenuated in the presence of beta-adrenergic blockade {112}.

Studies in isolated tissue demonstrate a diminished postsynaptic component of the beta responsiveness with age {113–115}. In isolated LV muscle (fig. 36-13A) {116,117} and in individual rat ventricular cardiocytes (fig. 36-13B), a reduced contractile response to β-AR stimulation occurs with aging. This is due to a failure of the

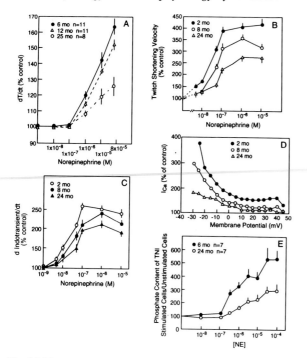

Fig. 36-13. **A:** The effect of norepinephrine on the maximum rate of isometric tension development in isolated trabeculae from hearts of varying age. From Lakatta et al. {113}, with permission. **B:** Velocity of cell shortening and (**C**) the maximum rate of increase of the indo-1 fluorescence transient, an index of sarcoplasmic reticulum Ca^{2+} release into the cytosol, during the electrically stimulated twitch in single cardiac myocytes isolated from the hearts of rats of varying ages and loaded with the fluorescent probe, indo-1. From Xiao et al. {116}, with permission. **D:** The effect of norepinephrine on increasing the L-type sarcolemmal channel current (I_{Ca}) measured via whole-cell patch-clamp technique in single cells isolated as in panels B and C. From Xiao et al. {116}, with permission. **E:** The effect of norepinephrine on increasing the phosphorylation of troponin I (TNI) in suspensions of heart cells isolated from hearts of rats of varying age as in the above panels. From Danziger et al. {117}, with permission. In panels B–E norepinephrine stimulated beta-receptors, as prazosin had no effect on the results.

intracellular Ca^{2+} transient to increase in cells of senescent hearts to the same extent to which it increases in cells from younger adult hearts {118} (fig. 36-13C). The blunted increase in the Ca^{2+} transient in cells from the aged heart is attributed to a decrease in the ability of β-AR stimulation to increase L-type sarcolemmal Ca^{2+} channel availability in cells from the senescent versus the younger adult hearts {118} (fig. 36-13D). As recent studies indicate the presence of functional $β_2$-adrenergic receptors within the myocardium, additional investigation of selective beta-receptor subtype responses in heart tissue or cells from adult and senescent animals, as in fig. 36-13, seems warranted.

The richly documented age-associated reduction in the postsynaptic response of the cardiovascular system to β-AR stimulation in human and animal tissues and cells

appears to be due to multiple changes in molecular and biochemical receptor-coupling and postreceptor mechanisms, rather than to a major modification of a single rate-limiting step, as might occur, for example, in a genetic defect. One change within the β-AR system is a decrease in the receptor affinity for agonists {119–126} without substantial changes in β-AR density being observed in most {114,120,121,127,128}, but not all {129}, studies. However, there is little information available regarding changes of β-AR subtype density, affinity, or functional regulation in aging. The postreceptor changes with aging include decreases in the activities of the G_s-protein adenylate-cyclase catalytic unit and a decrease in the cAMP-dependent PK activity (PKA) induced protein phosphorylation {67,120,121,123,130–134} (fig. 36-13E).

It has long been recognized that prolonged exposure of myocardial tissue to β-AR agonists modifies the β-AR responsiveness. A rapid heterologous desensitization of β-AR receptors occurs upon their phosphorylation by cAMP-dependent PK. In contrast, a rapid homologous pattern of the desensitization is mediated primarily by phosphorylation of the β-AR by a newly described cAMP-independent enzyme, β-adrenergic kinase (β-ARK) {135–138}. A comparison of such β-AR desensitization and the reduced efficacy of β-AR stimulation with aging suggests that the age-associated alterations may, at least in part, be caused by a desensitization of the β-AR adenylase cyclase system.

PARASYMPATHETIC STIMULATION

There is some evidence to indicate that parasympathetic control of cardiovascular function changes with age, but the evidence is conflicting. Some studies in rats suggest a more efficient cholinergic modulation with aging. The threshold of the negative chronotropic effects of vagus nerve stimulation and concentrations of acetylcholine required to cause changes in myocardial contractility are decreased with advancing age in rats {139–140}. Additionally, significantly greater increases in cyclic GMP in response to submaximal doses of acetylcholine have been observed in hearts of 24- to 26-month rats compared to 6- to 8-month rats. This difference persists in the presence of acetylcholinesterase blockade, suggesting that the mechanisms of the age-associated differences are at or distal to the receptor {141}. Other studies have observed an enhanced sensitivity to the direct chronotropic action of acetylcholine in right atria isolated from aged versus younger Fischer rats but have attributed to this an age-associated reduction in cholinesterase activity {142}. In contrast, other observations indicate an age-associated reduction in the response to parasympathetic agonists. In one such study a decrease in the heart rate reduction in old rats to both vagal nerve stimulation and to bolus injections of methacholine was observed {143}. More recent studies have indicated that the number of cholinergic receptors in the LV decreases with age in rats, as does the response to acetylcholine {129}. Finally, a marked *reduction* in acetylcholine content of atrial tissue from senescent rats has been demonstrated {144}. In humans, as noted above, a decrease in heart rate variability at rest or in response to a postural stress in older individual has been attributed, in part, to a reduction in parasympathetic tone with aging.

O₂ CONSUMPTION AND OXIDATIVE METABOLISM

Whereas the most instructive studies of excitation-contraction mechanisms with aging have been implemented in isolated cardiac muscle or cardiac cells, similar studies of energy metabolism have been conducted in intact hearts and isolated mitochondria. The maximum myocardial substrate oxidation rates in working heart preparation from Sprague–Dawley declines about 20% from adulthood to senescence {145}. However, the energy production rates are appropriate for the reduced work performed by the older hearts {for reviews see 4 and 146}. More recent studies in isolated, working hearts from Fischer 344 rats found cardiac work and efficiency to decline with age, particularly at high aortic pressures {147, 148}. This latter study, in which the workload on the heart was twofold greater than in prior studies {5}, clearly shows that the capacity for energy production in the heart of the Fischer 344 rat does not decline from adulthood to advanced old age {147}. This is indicated by the lack of an age-associated decline in maximum activities of rate-limiting enzymes in both the glycolytic pathway and Krebs cycle, or in the concentrations of cytochromes in the mitochondrial respiratory chain. In this study {147}, appropriate measurements that allowed for the calculation of the free energy of hydrolysis of ATP (ΔG_{ATP}) indicated that ΔG_{ATP} was not affected by aging under conditions where heart pumping performance had declined strongly. This suggests that the capacity of the aged heart (in isolation) to pump blood is not limited by bioenergetic factors {147}. An additional observation of this study was that, while chronic exercise conditioning did not affect the maximum aerobic energy production capacity, it did enhance other performance measurements of the isolated hearts of aged animals {147,148}. This dissociation of performance and energetics also indicates that non-energetic mechanisms (perhaps a primary decrease in coronary flow or a shift in MHC isoform types) determine performance of the senescent heart by chronic exercise training.

In contrast to the aforementioned studies in intact hearts, those in isolated mitochondria have observed that oxidation of certain substrates is diminished in senescent versus adult rat hearts {149–151}. ADP-stimulated (state 3) respiration of myocardial mitochondria was found to be diminished in Fischer 344 rats aged 20–24 months versus that in those 12–16 months when glutamate pyruvate, glutamate malate, and palmitylcarnitine were used as substrates. However, no age-associated differences were observed when succinate and ascorbate were employed as substrates {149}. In mitochondria isolated from hearts of Wistar rats, a 40% decline in palmitylcarnitine oxidation was also observed between 6 and 24 months of age {150};

further studies showed that the mitochondria from aged hearts retained less carnitine than did young ones and that this limited the rate of translocation, and thus the rate of oxidation of palmitate in the senescent mitochondria. In addition to these findings, it was observed that, as in the study of the intact working heart of the Fischer 344 rat {5}, tissue concentrations of both carnitine and acetylcarnitine are reduced in the senescent versus the adult myocardium {150}. However, why isolated mitochondria show declines in oxidation rates with aging, whereas isolated heart preparations do not, remains an enigma. An explanation sometimes offered to explain this enigma is that the maximum energy demand of isolated cardiac preparations is insufficient to stress the maximum energy production rates in situ. However, alternative interpretations are plausible.

PROTEIN METABOLISM

The effect of age on myocardial protein turnover has been studied in mouse and rat strains, in intact animals, isolated hearts, and cell-free systems. All studies in either species have demonstrated that a decrease in protein synthesis rate occurs from the maturational or growth phase to the adult period {152–157}. In hearts from 3-month versus 24-month animals, the older group had a diminution in myocardial RNA synthesis and a 359 reduction in protein synthesis {157}. The results suggested that with aging the number of ribosomes decreased, and since RNA degradation in the aged hearts was also decreased to 40% of that observed in the maturational animals, the rate of transcription is also reduced. Since exogenous transfer RNA was without effect at 3 months but increased the rate of protein synthesis in cell sap preparations from the senescent hearts by 40–50%, a slowing down at the translational step was also suggested. In toto, these studies clearly demonstrate that the rate of protein synthesis

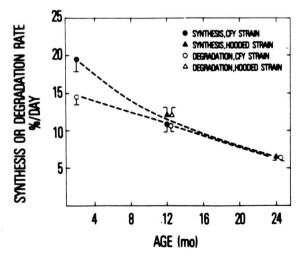

Fig. 36-14. The effect of age on in vivo protein synthesis in two strains of rats. Redrawn from Crie et al. {152}, with permission.

decreases after the growth phase and suggest that this is attributable to decreases in the rate of both transcription and translation. The question of whether protein synthesis or degradation is altered with adult aging in rats has been addressed more recently in a study that compared the rate of protein synthesis and degradation at three points across a broad age range {152}. Note that between 12 and 24 months an approximately 4590 decrease was observed in the rates of both protein synthesis and degradation (fig. 36-14). In the mouse model, a 25% decrease in the rate of protein synthesis was also observed between 7 and 26 months; thyroid injections enhanced the rate of synthesis in the older animals to levels near those in younger animals {151}. Thus, even after the growth phase ends, a further reduction in the rate of protein turnover occurs between adulthood and senescence in both mice and rats. The diminution in protein turnover rates suggests that the life span of cardiac proteins is increased in the senescent heart, but no effects of the rates of protein synthesis and degradation on contractile or metabolic function are currently known. It is noteworthy that in cardiac hypertrophy in younger animals caused by left ventricular pressure overload, the rate of protein synthesis and degradation were, as in the aging heart, also diminished, and this has led to the hypothesis that this form of hypertrophy represents accelerated aging {154–157}. However, additional studies are required to substantiate this hypothesis {4,17,18}.

REFERENCES

1. Gerstenblith G, Lakatta EG, Weisfeldt ML: Age changes in myocardial function and exercise response. *Prog Cardiovas Dis* 19:1–21, 1976.
2. Lakatta EG: Alterations in the cardiovascular system that occur in advanced age. *Fed Proc* 38:163–167, 1979.
3. Lakatta EG: Heart and Circulation. In: Schneider EL, Rowe J (eds) *Handbook of the Biology of Aging*, 3rd ed. New York: Academic Press, 1990, pp 181–216.
4. Lakatta EG, Yin FCP: Myocardial aging: Functional alterations and related cellular mechanisms. *Am J Physiol* 242: H927–941, 1982.
5. Walford GD, Spurgeon HA, Lakatta EG: Diminished cardiac hypertrophy and muscle performance in older compared with younger adult rats with chronic atrioventricular block. *Circ Res* 63:502–511, 1988.
6. Spurgeon HA, Steinbach MF, Lakatta EG: Chronic exercise prevents characteristic age-related changes in rat cardiac contraction. *Am J Physiol* (Heart Circ Physiol 13):H513–H518, 1983.
7. Yin FCCP, Spurgeon HA, Weisfeldt ML, Lakatta EG: Mechanical properties of myocardium from hypertrophied rat hearts; a comparison between hypertrophy induced by senescence and by aortic banding. *Circ Res* 46:292–300, 1980.
8. Rothbaum DA, Shaw DJ, Angell CS, Shock NW: Cardiac performance in the unanesthetized senescent male rat. *J Gerontol* 28:287–292, 1973.
9. Yin FCP, Spurgeon HA, Rakusan K, Weisfeldt ML, Lakatta EG: Use of tibial length to quantify cardiac hypertrophy: Application in the aging rat. *Am J Physiol* 243 (*Heart Circ Physiol* 12):H941–H947, 1982.
10. Weisfeldt ML, Loven EA, Shock NW: Resting and active mechanical properties of trabeculae carneae from aged male rats. *Am J Physiol* 220:1921–1972, 1971.
11. Fraticelli A, Josephson R, Danziger R, Lakatta E. Spurgeon HA: Morphological and contractile characteristics of rat cardiac myocytes from maturation to senescence. *Am J Physiol* 257:H259–H265, 1989.
12. Anversa P, Palackal T, Sonnenblick EH, Olivetti G, Meggs LG, Capasso JM: Myocyte cell loss and myocyte cellular hyperplasia in the hypertrophied aging rat heart. *Circ Res* 67:871–885, 1990.
13. Eghbali M, Eghbali M, Robinson TF, Seifter S, Blumenfeld OO: Collagen accumulation in heart ventricles as a function of growth and aging. *Cardiovasc Res* 23:723–729, 1989.
14. Rakusan K, Poupa O: Capillaries and muscle fibers in the heart of old rats. *Gerontologia* 9:107–112, 1964.
15. Tomanek RJ: Effects of age and exercise on the extent of the myocardial capillary bed. *Anat Rec* 167:55–62, 1970.
16. Travis DF, Travis A: Ultrastructural changes in the left ventricular rat myocardial cells with age. *J Ultrastruct Res* 39:124–148, 1972.
17. Lakatta EG: Do hypertension and aging similarly affect the myocardium? Circulation 75(Suppl I):169–177, 1987.
18. Lakatta EG: Cardiac muscle changes in senescence. *Ann Rev Physiol* 49:519–531, 1987.
19. Cavoto FV, Kelliher GJ, Robert J: Electrophysiological changes in the rat atrium with age. *Am J Physiol* 226:1293–1297, 1974.
20. Roberts J, Goldberg PB: Changes in cardiac membranes as a function of age with particular emphasis on reactivity to drugs. In: Cristofalo VJ, Roberts J, Adelman RC (eds) *Advances in Experimental Medicine and Biology*, Vol 61: *Explorations in Aging*. New York: Plenum Press, 1975, pp 119–148.
21. Lakatta EG, Gerstenblith G, Angell CS: Prolonged contraction duration in aged myocardium. *J Clin Invest* 55: 61–68, 1975.
22. Rosen MR, Reder RF, Hordof AJ, Davies M, Danilo P Jr: Age-related changes in Purkinje fiber action potentials of adult dogs. *Circ Res* 43:931–938, 1978.
23. Gulch RW: The effect of elevated chronic loading on the action potential of mammalian myocardium. *J Mol Cell Cardiol* 12:415–420, 1980.
24. Rumberger E, Timmermann J: Age changes of the force-frequency-relationship and the duration of action potential isolated papillary muscles of guinea pig. *Eur J Appl Physiol* 34:277–284, 1976.
25. Walker KR, Houser SR: Intracellular calcium buffers affect age-related calcium current decay (abstr). *Circulation* 82:III746, 1990.
26. Capasso JM, Malhotra A, Remily RM, Scheuer J, Sonnenblick EH: Effects of age on mechanical and electrical performance of rat myocardium. *Am J Physiol* 245 (*Heart Circ Physiol* 14):H72, 1983.
27. Wei JY, Spurgeon HA, Lakatta EG: Excitation-contraction in rat myocardium: Alteration with adult aging. *Am J Physiol* 246 (*Heart Circ Physiol*) 15:H784-H791, 1984.
28. Walker KE, Lakatta EG, Houser SR: Alterations in transient outward current prolong action potential duration in aged rat myocardium (abstr). *Biophys J* 59:558, 1991.
29. duBell WH, Boyett WH, Spurgeon HA, Talo A, Stern MD, Lakatta EG: The cytosolic calcium transient modulates the action potential of rat ventricular myocytes. *J Physiol* 436:347–369, 1991.

30. Lakatta EG: Excitation-contraction. In: Weisfeldt ML (ed) *Aging*, Vol 12: *The Aging Heart; its Function and Response to Stress*. New York: Raven Press, 1980, pp 77–100.

31. Urthaler F, Walker AA, James TN: The effect of aging on ventricular contractile performance. *Am Heart J* 96:481–485, 1978.

32. Orchard CH, Lakatta EG: Intracellular calcium transients and developed tensions in rat heart muscle. A mechanism for the negative interval-strength relationship. *J Gen Physiol* 86:637–651, 1985.

33. Gerstenblith G, Spurgeon HA, Froehlich JP, Weisfeldt ML, Lakatta EG: Diminished inotropic responsiveness to ouabain in aged rat myocardium. *Circ Res* 44:517–523, 1979.

34. Frolkis VV, Frolkis RA, Mkhitarian LS, Shevchuk VG, Fraifeld VE, Vakulenko LG, Syrovy I: Contractile function and Ca^{2+} transport system of myocardium in ageing. *Gerontology* 34:64–74, 1988.

35. Froehlich JP, Lakatta EG, Beard E, Spurgeon HA, Weisfeldt ML, Gerstenblith G: Studies of sarcoplasmic reticulum function and contraction duration in young adult and aged rat myocardium. *J Mol Cell Cardiol* 10:427–438, 1978.

36. Narayanan N: Differential alterations in ATP-supported calcium transport activities of sarcoplasmic reticulum and sarcolemma of aging myocardium. *Biochim Biophys Acta* 678:442–459, 1981.

37. Heyliger CE, Prakash AR, McNeill JH: Effect of calmodulin on sarcoplasmic reticular Ca^{2+}-transport in the aging heart. *Mol Cell Biochem* 85:75–79, 1989.

38. Kalish MI, Katz MS, Pineyro MA, Gregerman RI: Epinephrine- and glucagon-sensitive adenylate cyclases of rat liver during aging. Evidence for membrane instability associated with increased enzymatic activity. *Biochim Biophys Acta* 483:452–466, 1977.

39. Tate CA, Taffet GE, Hudson EK, Blaylock SL, McBride RP, Michael LH. Enhanced calcium uptake of cardiac sarcoplasmic reticulum in exercise-trained old rats. *Am J Physiol* 258:H431–H435, 1990.

40. Hallock P, Benson IC: Studies on the elastic properties of human isolated aorta. *J Clin Invest* 16:595–602, 1937.

41. Kirchberger MA, Zhen E, Kasinathan C, Kirchberger MA: Altered phospholamban phosphorylation in cardiac microsomes obtained from senescent rats (abstr). *Biophys J* 57:504, 1990.

42. Kadoma M, Sacktor B, Froehlich JP: Stimulation by cAMP and protein kinase of calcium transport in sarcoplasmic reticulum from senescent rat myocardium (abstr). *Fed Proc* 39:2040, 1980.

43. Taffet GE, Tate CA: The sarcoplasmic reticulum calcium ATPase from rat heart is decreased in senescence (abstr). *Gerontologist* 30:111A, 1990.

44. Lompre AM, Lambert F, Lakatta EG, Schwartz K: Expression of sarcoplasmic reticulum Ca^{2+}-ATPase and calsequestrin genes in rat heart during ontogenic development and aging. *Circ Res* 69:1380–1388, 1991.

45. Maciel LMZ, Polikar R, Rohrer D, Popovich BK, Dillmann WH: Age-induced decreases in the messenger RNA coding for the sarcoplasmic reticulum Ca^{2+}-ATPase of the rat heart. *Circ Res* 67:230–234, 1990.

46. Buttrick P, Malhotra A, Factor S, Greenen D, Leinwand L, Scheuer J: Effect of aging and hypertension on myosin biochemistry and gene expression in the rat heart. *Circ Res* 68:645–652, 1991.

47. Fabiato A: Calcium release in skinned cardiac cells: Variations with species, tissues, and development. *Fed Proc* 41:2238–2244, 1982.

48. Capasso JM, Puntillo E, Olivetti G, Anversa P: Differences in load dependence of relaxation between the left and right ventricular myocardium as a function of age in rats. *Circ Res* 65:1499–1507, 1989.

49. Alpert NR, Gale HH, Taylor N: The effect of age on contractile protein ATPase activity and the velocity of shortening. In: Tanz RD, Kavaler F, Robert J (eds) *Factors Influencing Myocardial Contractility*. New York: Academic Press, 1976, pp 27–133.

50. Heller LJ, Whitehorn WV: Age-associated alterations in myocardial contractile properties. *Am J Physiol* 222:1613–1619, 1972.

51. Bhatnagar GM, Walford GD, Beard ES, Humphreys S, Lakatta EG: ATPase activity and force production in myofibrils and twitch characteristics in intact muscle from neonatal, adult, and senescent rat myocardium. *J Mol Cell Cardiol* 16:203–218, 1984.

52. Capasso JM, Malhotra A, Scheuer J, Sonnenblick EH: Myocardial biochemical, contractile and electrical performance after imposition of hypertension in young and old rats. *Circ Res* 58:445–460, 1986.

53. Chesky JA, Rockstein M: Reduced myocardial actomyosin adenosine triphosphatase activity in the ageing male Fischer rat. *Cardiovasc Res* 11:242–246, 1977.

54. Farrar RP, Starnes JW, Cartee GD, Oh PY, Sweeney HL: Effects of exercise on cardiac myosin isozyme composition during the aging process. *J Appl Physiol* 64:880–993, 1988.

55. Bhatnagar GM, Effron MB, Ruano-Arroyo G, Spurgeon HA, Lakatta EG: Dissociation of myosin Ca^{2+}-ATPase activity from myosin isoenzymes and contractile function in rat myocardium (abstr). *Fed Proc* 44:826, 1985.

56. Effron MB, Bhatnagar GM, Spurgeon HA, Ruano-Arroyo G, Lakatta EG: Changes in myosin isoenzymes, ATPase activity, and contraction duration in rat cardiac muscle with aging can be modulated by thyroxine. *Circ Res* 60:238–245, 1987.

57. Hoh JFY, McGrath PA, Hale PT: Electrophoretic analysis of multiple forms of rat cardiac myosin: Effects of hypophysectomy and thyroxine replacement. *J Mol Cell Cardiol* 10:1053–1076, 1978.

58. Schuyler GT, Yarbrough LR: Comparison of myosin and creating kinase isoforms in left ventricles of young and senescent Fischer 344 rats after treatment with triiodothyronine. *Mech Ageing Dev* 56:39–48, 1990.

59. O'Neill L, Holbrook NJ, Fargnoli J, Lakatta EG: Progressive changes from young adult age to senescence in mRNA for rat cardiac myosin heavy chain genes. *Cardioscience* 2:1–5, 1991.

60. Florini JR, Ewton DZ: Skeletal muscle fiber types and myosin ATPase activity do not change with age or growth hormone administration. *J Gerontol Biol Sci* 44:B110–B117, 1989.

61. Amery A, Bossaert H, Verstraete M: Muscle blood flow in normal and hypertensive subjects. Influence of age, exercise, and body position. *Am Heart J* 78:211–216, 1969.

62. Boluyt MO, O'Neill L, Lakatta EG, Crow MT: Progressive elevation of atrial natriuretic factor mRNAs in rat heart with advancing age (abstr). *J Mol Cell Cardiol* 24(Suppl III):s.35, 1992.

63. Carrier L, Boheler KR, Chassagne C, de la Bastie D, Wisnewsky C, Lakatta EG, Schwartz K: Expression of the sarcomeric actin isogenes in the rat heart with development and senescence. *Circ Res* 70:999–1005, 1992.

64. Alpert NR, Mulieri LA: Increased myothermal economy of isometric force generation in compensated cardiac hyper-

trophy induced by pulmonary artery constriction in the rabbit. A characterization of heat liberation in normal and hypertrophied right ventricular papillary muscles. *Circ Res* 50:491–500, 1982.

65. Alpert NR, Blanchard EM, Mulieri LA: The quantity and rate of Ca^{2+} uptake in normal and hypertrophied hearts. In: Dhalla N, Singel P, Beamish RE (eds) *Pathophysiology of Heart Disease*. New York: Raven Press, 1983.

66. Carter WJ, Kelly WF, Faas FH, Lynch ME, Perry CA: Effect of graded doses of triiodothyronine on ventricular myosin ATPase activity and isomyosin profile in young and old rats. *Biochem J* 247:329–334, 1987.

67. Ericsson E, Lundholm L: Adrenergic β-receptor activity and cyclic AMP metabolism in vascular smooth muscle; variations with age. *Mech Ageing Dev* 4:1–6, 1975.

68. Hoh JFY, McGrath PA, Hale PT: Electrophoretic analysis of multiple forms of rat cardiac myosin: Effects of hypophysectomy and thyroxine replacement. *J Mol Cell Cardiol* 10:1053–1076, 1978.

69. Izumo S, Nadal-Ginard B, Mahdavi V: All members of the MHC multigene family response to thyroid hormone in a highly tissue-specific manner. *Science* 231:597–600, 1986.

70. Bramwell JC, Hill AV: The velocity of the pulse wave in man. *Proc R Soc (Series B)* 93:298–306, 1922.

71. Mirsky I, Laks MM: Time course of changes in the mechanical properties of the canine right and left ventricles during hypertrophy caused by pressure overload. *Circ Res* 46:530–542, 1980.

72. Spurgeon HA, Thorne PR, Yin FCP, Shock NW, Weisfeldt MF: Increased dynamic stiffness of trabeculae carneae from senescent rats. *Am J Physiol* 232:H373–H380, 1977.

73. Strandell T: Heart volume and its relation to anthropometric data in old men compared with young men. *Acta Med Scand* 176:205–218, 1964.

74. Kane RL, McMahon TA, Wagner RL, Abelmann WH: Ventricular elastic modulus as a function of age in the Syrian golden hamster. *Circ Res* 38:74–80, 1976.

75. Janz RF, Kubert BR, Mirsky I, Korecky B, Taichman GC: Effect of age on passive elastic stiffness of rat heart muscle. *Biophys J* 16:281–290, 1976.

76. Kort AA, Lakatta EG: Calcium-dependent mechanical oscillations occur spontaneously in unstimulated mammalian cardiac tissues. *Circ Res* 54:396–404, 1984.

77. Lakatta EG, Lappe DL: Diastolic scattered light fluctuation, resting force and twitch force in mammalian cardiac muscle. *J Physiol* 315:369–394, 1981.

78. Stern MD, Kort AA, Bhatnager GM, Lakatta EG: Scattered-light intensity fluctuations in diastolic rat cardiac muscle caused by spontaneous Ca^{2+}-dependent cellular mechanical oscillations. *J Gen Physiol* 82:199–153, 1983.

79. Ziman B, Spurgeon HA, Stern MD, Lakatta EG: A Ca^{2+} myofilament interaction modulates resting length of single rat ventricular myocytes (abstr). *Circulation* 82:III214, 1990.

80. Fabiato A, Fabiato F: Contraction induced by a calcium-triggered release of calcium from the sarcoplasmic reticulum of single skinned cardiac cells. *J Physiol* 249:469–495, 1975.

81. Dani AM, Cittadine A, Inesi G: Calcium transport and contractile activity in dissociated mammalian heart cells. *Am J Physiol* 237:C147–C155, 1979.

82. Kort AA, Lakatta EG: Bimodal effect of electrical stimulation on light fluctuations monitoring spontaneous sarcoplasmic reticulum Ca^{2+} release in rat cardiac muscle. *Circ Res* 63: 960–968, 1988.

83. Lappe DL, Lakatta EG: Intensity fluctuation spectroscopy monitors contractile muscle. *Science* 207:1369–1371, 1980.

84. Hano O, Bogdanov KY, Lakatta EG: Enhanced calcium intolerance manifest as aftercontractions and ventricular fibrillation in hearts of aged rat. J Mol Cell Cardiol 22(Suppl 1):S.24, 1990.

85. Kort AA, Capogrossi MC, Lakatta EG: Frequency, amplitude, and propagation velocity of spontaneous Ca^{2+}-dependent contractile waves in intact adult rat cardiac muscle and isolated myocytes. *Circ Res* 57:844–855, 1985.

86. Lakatta EG, Capogrossi MC: Probability of occurrence and frequency distribution of spontaneous contractile waves in unstimulated Ca^{2+} tolerant adult rat myocytes. *Fed Proc* 44:829, 1985.

87. Kort AA, Lakatta EG: Restitution of action potential triggered and spontaneous sarcoplasmic reticulum Ca^{2+} release in rat papillary muscle. *Circulation* 72:Part II, III-328, 1985.

88. Capogrossi MC, Suarez-Isla BA, Lakatta EG: The interaction of electrically stimulated twitches and spontaneous contractile waves in single cardiac myocytes. *J Gen Physiol* 88:615–633, 1986.

89. Jewell RB: A reexamination of the influence of muscle length on myocardial performance. *Circ Res* 40:221–230, 1977.

90. Lakatta EG, Spurgeon HA: Force staircase kinetics in mammalian cardiac muscle; modulation by muscle length. *J Physiol (Lond)* 299:377–352, 1980.

91. Heyliger CE, Prakash AR, McNeill JH: An assessment of phospholipid methylation in sarcolemma and sarcoplasmic reticulum of the aging myocardium. *Biochim Biophys Acta* 960:462–465, 1988.

92. Ruch S, Im W-B, Kennedy RH, Seifen E, Akera T: Aging: Stimulation rate of cardiac intracellular Na^+ activity and developed tension. *Mech Ageing Dev* 60:303–313, 1991.

93. Guarnieri T, Spurgeon H, Froehlich JP, Weisfeldt ML, Lakatta EG: Diminished inotropic response but unaltered toxicity to acetylstrophanthidin in the senescent beagle. *Circulation* 60:1548–1554, 1979.

94. Buxton ILO, Brunton LL: Action of the cardiac α_1-adrenergic receptor. Activation of cyclic AMP degradation. *J Biol Chem* 260:6733–6737, 1985.

95. Lakatta EG: Regulation of cardiac muscle function in the hypertensive heart. In: Cox RH (ed) *Cellular and Molecular Mechanisms of Hypertension*. New York: Plenum, 1991, pp 149–173.

96. Lecarpentier Y, Bugaisky LB, Chemla D, Mercadier JJ, Schwartz K, Whalen RG, Martin JL: Coordinated changes in contractility, energetics, and isomyosins after aortic stenosis. *Am J Physiol* 252:H275–H282, 1987.

97. Swynghedauw B: Remodeling of the heart in response to chronic mechanical overload. *Eur Heart J* 10:935–943, 1989.

98. Yazaki Y, Komuro I: Molecular analysis of cardiac hypertrophy due to overload (abstr). *J Mol Cell Cardiol* 21(Suppl III):S.29, 1989.

99. Schiaffino S, Samuel JL, Sassoon D, Lompre AM, Garner I, Marotte F, Buckingham M, Rappaport L, Schwartz K: Nonsynchronous accumulation of α_1 skeletal actin and β-myosin heavy chain mRNAs during early stages of pressure-overload-induced cardiac hypertrophy demonstrated by in situ hybridization. *Circ Res* 64:937–948, 1989.

100. Anversa P, Hiler B, Ricci R, Guideri G, Olivetti G: Myocyte cell loss and myocyte hypertrophy in the aging rat heart. *J Am Coll Cardiol* 8:1441–1448, 1986.

101. Korecky B: The effects of load, internal environment and age on cardiac mechanics (abstr). *J Mol Cell Cardiol* 11(Suppl 1):33, 1979.

102. Holloszy JO, Booth FW: Biochemical adaptations to endurance exercise in muscle. *Ann Rev Physiol* 38:273–291, 1976.

103. Tomanek RJ, Taunton CA, Liskop KS: Relationship between age, chronic exercise, and connective tissue of the heart. *J Gerontol* 27:33–38, 1972.

104. Gwathmey JK, Slawsky MT, Perreault CL, Briggs GM, Morgan JP, Wei JY: The effect of exercise conditioning on excitation-contraction coupling in aged rats. *J Appl Physiol* 69:1366–1371, 1990.

105. Chesky JA, LaFollette S, Travis M, Fortado C: Effects of physical training on myocardial enzyme activities in aging rats. *J Appl Physiol* 55:1349–1353, 1983.

106. Xiao RP, Lakatta EG: Mechanisms of altered β-adrenergic modulation of the cardiovascular system with aging. *Rev Clin Gerontol* 1:309–322, 1991.

107. Rendlund DG, Gerstenblith G, Rodeheffer RJ, Fleg JL, Lakatta EG: Potency of the Frank Starling reserve in normal man. *J Am Coll Cardiol*(Part 2):514, 1985.

108. Fleg JL, Gerstenblith G, Schulman SP, Becker LC, O'Connor FC, Lakatta EG: Gender differences in exercise hemodynamics of older subjects: Effects of conditioning status. *Circulation* 82:III239, 1990.

109. Rodeheffer RJ, Gerstenblith G, Becker LC, Fleg JL, Weisfeldt ML, Lakatta EG: Exercise cardiac output is maintained with advancing age in healthy human subjects: Cardiac dilation in increased stroke volume compensate for a diminished heart rate. *Circulation* 69:203–213, 1984.

110. Fleg JL, Schulman S, O'Connor F, Gerstenblith G, Clulow JF, Renlund DG, Lakatta EG: Effect of propranolol on age-associated changes in left ventricular performance during exercise. *Circulation* 84:II187, 1991.

111. Schulman SP, Lakatta EG, Fleg JL, Becker LC, Gerstenblith G: Age-related decline in left ventricular filling at rest and exercise: Another manifestation of decreased beta-adrenergic responsiveness in the elderly. *Am J Physiol* 263: 1932–1938, 1992.

112. Conway J, Wheeler R, Sannerstedt R: Sympathetic nervous activity during exercise in relation to age. *Cardiovasc Res* 5:577–581, 1971.

113. Lakatta EG, Gerstenblith G, Angell CS, Shock NW, Weisfeldt ML: Diminished inotropic response of aged myocardium to catecholamine. *Circ Res* 36:262–269, 1975.

114. Guarnieri T, Filburn CR, Zitnik G, Roth GS, Lakatta EG: Contractile and biochemical correlates of β-adrenergic stimulation of the aged heart. *Am J Physiol* 239:H501–H508, 1980.

115. Fleisch JH: Age-related decrease in beta adrenoceptor activity of the cardiovascular system. *Trends Pharma Sci* 2:337–339, 1981.

116. Xiao Rp, Spurgeon HA, Lakatta EG: Diminished norepinephrine augmentation of calcium current cytosolic [Ca^{2+}] and contraction with aging in single rat ventricular cells (abstr). *J Mol Cell Cardiol* 24(Suppl III):S.54, 1992.

117. Danziger RS, Sakai M, Lakatta EG, Hansford RG: Interactive α- and β-adrenergic actions of norepinephrine in rat cardiac myocytes. *J Mol Cell Cardiol* 22:111–123, 1990.

118. Xiao RP, Capogrossi MC, Spurgeon HA, Lakatta EG: Stimulation of δ opioid receptors in single heart cells blocks β-adrenergic receptor mediated increase in calcium and contraction (abstr). *J Mol Cell Cardiol* 23(Suppl III):S83, 1991.

119. Feldman RD, Limbird LE, Nadeau J, Robertson D, Wood AJ: Alterations in leukocyte beta-receptor affinity with aging. A potential explanation for altered beta-adrenergic sensitivity in the elderly. *N Engl J Med* 310:815–819, 1984.

120. Narayanan N, Derby J: Alterations in the properties of beta-adrenergic receptors of myocardial membranes in aging: Impairments of agonist-receptor interactions and guanine nucleotide regulation accompany diminished catecholamine-responsiveness of adenylate cyclase. *Mech Ageing Dev* 19:127–139, 1982.

121. Scarpace PJ: Decreased beta-adrenergic responsiveness during senescence. *Fed Proc* 45:51–54, 1986.

122. Scarpace PJ: Decreased receptor activation with age. Can it be explained by desensitization? *J Am Geriatr Soc* 36: 1067–1071, 1988.

123. Scarpace PJ, Abrass IB: Beta-adrenergic agonist-mediated desensitization in senescent rats. *Mech Ageing Dev* 35: 255–264, 1986.

124. Scarpace PJ: Forskolin activation of adenylate cyclase in rat myocardium with age: Effects of guanine nucleotide analogs. *Mech Ageing Dev* 52:169–178, 1990.

125. Scarpace PJ, Abrass IB: Decreased beta-adrenergic agonist affinity and adenylate cyclase activity in senescent rat lung. *J Gerontol* 38:143–147, 1983.

126. Scarpace PJ, Baresi LA: Increased beta-adrenergic receptors in the light-density membrane fraction in lungs from senescent rats. *J Gerontol* 43:B163–B167, 1988.

127. Doyle V, O'Malley K, Kelly JG: Human lymphocyte beta-adrenoceptor density in relation to age and hypertension. *J Cardiovasc Pharmacol* 4:738–740, 1982.

128. Tsukimoto G, Lee CH, Hoffman BB: Age-related decrease in beta adrenergic receptor-mediated vascular smooth muscle relaxation. *J Pharmacol Exp Ther* 239:411–415, 1986.

129. Chevalier B, Mansier P, Teiger E, Callen-el Amrani F, Swynghedauw B: Alterations in beta adrenergic and muscarinic receptors in aged rat heart. Effects of chronic administration of propranolol and atropine. *Mech Ageing Dev* 60:215–224, 1991.

130. Krall JF, Connelly M, Tuck ML: Evidence for reversibility of age-relate decrease in human lymphocyte adenylate cyclase activity. *Biochem Biophys Res Commun* 99:1028–1034, 1981.

131. Krall JF, Connelly M, Weisbart R, Tuck ML: Age-related elevation of plasma catecholamine concentration and reduced responsiveness of lymphocyte adenylate cyclase. *J Clin Endocrinol Metab* 52:863–867, 1981.

132. O'Connor SW, Scarpace PJ, Abrass IB: Age-associated decrease in the catalytic unit activity of rat myocardial adenylate cyclase. *Mech Ageing Dev* 21:357–363, 1983.

133. O'Connor SW, Scarpace PJ, Abrass IB: Age-associated decrease of adenylate cyclase activity in rat myocardium. *Mech Ageing Dev* 16:91–95, 1981.

134. Sakai M, Danziger RS, Staddon JM, Lakatta EG, Hansford RG: Decrease with senescence in the norepinephrine-induced phosphorylation of myofilament proteins in isolated rat cardiac myocytes. *J Mol Cell Cardiol* 21:1327–1336, 1989.

135. Lefkowitz RJ, Hansdorff WP, Caron MG: Role of phosphorylation in desensitization of the beta-adrenoceptor. *Trends Pharm Sci* 11:190–194, 1990.

136. Levitzki A: Regulation of hormone-sensitive adenylate cyclase. *Trends Pharm Sci* 8:299–303, 1987.

137. Sibley DR, Lefkowitz RJ: Molecular mechanisms of receptor desensitization using the beta-adrenergic receptor-coupled adenylate cyclase system as a model. *Nature* 317: 124–129, 1985.

138. Strasser RH, Sibley DR, Lefkowitz RJ: A novel catecholamine-activated adenosine cyclic 3′,5′-phosphate independent pathway for beta-adrenergic receptor phosphorylation in wild-type and mutant S_{49} lymphoma cells: Mechanisms of homologous desensitization of adenylate cyclase. *Biochemistry* 25:1371–1377, 1986.

139. Frolkis VV, Bezrukov VV, Bogatskaya LN, Verkhratsky NA, Zamostian VP: Catecholamines in the metabolism and

functions regulation in aging. *Gerontologia* 16:129–140, 1979.

140. Frolkis VV, Bezrukov VV, Schevtchuk VG: Hemodynamics and its regulation in old age. *Exp Gerontol* 10:251–271, 1975.
141. Kulchitskii OK: Effect of acetylcholine on the cyclic GMP level in the rat heart at different ages. *Bull Exp Biol Med* 90:1237–1239, 1980.
142. Kennedy RH, Seifen E: Aging: Effects of chronotropic actions of muscarinic agonists in isolated rat atria. *Mech Ageing Dev* 51:81–87, 1990.
143. Kelliher GJ, Conahan J: Changes in vagal activity and response to muscarinic receptor agonists with age. *J Gerontol* 35:842–849, 1980.
144. Verkhratsky NS: Acetylcholine metabolism peculiarities in aging. *Exp Gerontol* 5:49–56, 1970.
145. Abu-Erreish GM, Neely JR, Whitmer JT, Whitman V, Sanadi DR: Fatty acid oxidation by isolated perfused working hearts of aged rats. *Am J Physiol* 232:E258–E262, 1977.
146. Hansford RG: Metabolism and energy production. In: Weisfeldt ML (ed) *Aging: The Aging Heart: Its Function and Response to Stress*, Vol 12. New York: Raven Press, 1980, pp 25–76.
147. Starnes JW, Rumsey WL: Cardiac energetics and performance of exercised and food-restricted rats during aging. *Am J Physiol* 254:H599–H608, 1988.
148. Starnes JW, Beyer RE, Edington DW: Myocardial adapta-

tions to endurance exercise in aged rats. *Am J Physiol* 245:H560–H566, 1983.
149. Chen JC, Warshaw JB, Sanadi DR: Regulation of mitochondrial respiration in senescence. *J Cell Physiol* 80:141–148, 1972.
150. Hansford RG: Lipid oxidation by heart mitochondria from young adult and senescent rats. *Biochem J* 170:285–295, 1978.
151. Du JT, Beryer TA, Lang CA: Protein biosynthesis in aging mouse tissues. *Exp Gerontol* 12:181–191, 1977.
152. Crie JS, Millward DJ, Bates PC, Griffin EE, Wildenthal K: Age-related alterations in cardiac protein turnover. *J Mol Cell Cardiol* 13:589–598, 1981.
153. Florini JR, Saito Y, Manowitz EJ: Effect of age on thyroxine-induced cardiac hypertrophy in mice. *J Gerontol* 28:293–297, 1973.
154. Geary S, Florini JR: Effect of age on rate of protein synthesis in isolated perfused mouse hearts. *J Gerontol* 27:325–332, 1972.
155. Meerson FZ: The myocardium in hyperfunction, hypertrophy and heart failure. *Circ Res* 25(Suppl 2):I163, 1969.
156. Meerson FZ, Javich MP, Lerman MI: Decrease in the rate of RNA and protein synthesis and degradation in the myocardium under long-term compensatory hyperfunction and on aging. *J Mol Cell Cardiol* 10:145–159, 1978.
157. Grimm AG, Kubora R, Whitehorn WV: Ventricular nucleic acid and protein levels with myocardial growth and hypertrophy. *Circ Res* 19:552–558, 1966.

CHAPTER 37

Hormonal Effects on Cardiac Performance

EUGENE MORKIN

INTRODUCTION

Alterations in cardiac function and metabolism have been described in a number of experimental and clinical disorders of the endocrine system. For the most part, however, the mechanisms of these effects are obscure. New insight into the problem has been provided by studying the actions of thyroid hormone, which has marked positive inotropic effects on the heart that can be related to distinct biochemical changes {1}. Since thyroid hormone has many interactions with other components of the neuroendocrine system, the insights gained from these studies may explain some otherwise perplexing changes in cardiac performance in a variety of endocrine disorders.

In ventricular muscle of rat and rabbit, thyroid hormone causes a rapid induction of the high-ATPase activity V_1 myosin isoform and inhibits expression of the low activity V_3 form {2,3}. This switch in myosin isoforms may relate to the increase in cardiac performance resulting from thyroid hormone administration, since the intrinsic speed of muscle contraction has been shown to correlate with myosin ATPase activity {4}. In addition to its effects on myosin isoenzymes, however, there is evidence that thyroid hormone affects cardiac performance by other mechanisms. In particular, the early inotropic actions of thyroid hormone, which have their onset within 12–24 hours, clearly precede significant changes in myosin isoenzyme composition {5,6}. Although the biochemical basis for the initial inotropic actions of thyroid hormone are unclear, a number of effects of the hormone have been described that might be involved, including its ability to increase the number of Na,K-ATPase pump sites, to stimulate calcium uptake by fragmented sarcoplasmic reticulum (SR), and to activate SR Ca^{2+}-ATPase {7}.

The inotropic response to thyroid hormone and the effects on Ca^{2+} homeostasis are similar in all species studied, but the degree to which myosin isoforms switch is variable (see below). This observation suggests that alterations in Ca^{2+} handling may be more important in determining the effects of T_3 on the inotropic state. Changes in myosin isoforms also may be an important part of the adaptive response in those species in which it

occurs. Both of these mechanisms are discussed in more detail below.

PRIMARY MECHANISM OF THYROID HORMONE ACTIONS

Thyroid hormones are thought to enter the cell by a complex, multipath process {8}. Several well-documented effects of the hormones have been demonstrated at the cell surface, including stimulation of glucose transport and membrane Ca^{2+}-ATPase activity, but the biological roles of these actions remain to be elucidated. Within the cell, 3,5,3',5'-tetraiodo-L-thyronine (T_4), the major circulating form of the hormone, is converted by 5'-deiodinases to 3,5,3'-triiodo-L-thyronine (T_3), the active intracellular form of the hormone. T_3 binds to high-affinity nuclear receptors, which regulate the expression of specific genes {9}. In outline, the mechanism of thyroid hormone action resembles that of steroid hormones. The receptors for glucocorticoids, estrogen, and progesterone have been characterized and found to be related to the retroviral oncogene v-erbA. The protein product of the cellular counterpart of this virus, c-erbA, has been found to bind thyroid hormone {10,11}. Several pieces of evidence suggest that the c-erbA protein is the nuclear thyroid hormone receptor, including similarities in molecular weight and binding affinities for T_3 and its analogs.

These new observations should presage significant advances in our understanding of thyroid hormone action. However, at this time it is not clear how a mechanism involving the binding of hormone to receptors located on a fairly small number of genes can explain the diversity of T_3 actions. In particular, this hypothesis would not seem to explain the ability of the hormone to activate a gene in one tissue and cause repression of the same gene in another tissue. An additional piece of evidence that will need to be reconciled with any plausible scheme of thyroid hormone action is the observation that some T_3 effects may be mediated through release of an autocrine factor {12}.

N. Sperelakis (ed.), Physiology and Pathophysiology of the Heart, Third Edition.

THYROID HORMONE AND CARDIAC MYOSIN ISOENZYMES

Myosin structure and function

The thick filaments are comprised of myosin molecules arranged in parallel; the thin filaments are repeating units of globular actin that are arranged like a double strand of pearls on their long axis. Cardiac myosin is a hexameric protein composed of two heavy polypeptide chains of 210 kDa each. The heavy chains coil around each other to form an α-helical *tail* region, which imparts rigidity and length to the molecule, and divide to form two globular *head* regions. Each globular head region has a site for ATP binding and hydrolysis, and a separate but closely related site for actin binding. In addition to its two heavy chains, myosin contains two pairs of light chains; the precise location of the light chains is uncertain, but seem to be near the ATP- and actin-binding sites on the heavy chains. Three troponin components and tropomyosin, proteins involved in the regulation of contraction, lie along a longitudinal groove between the actin monomers.

It is now almost universally accepted that in both cardiac and skeletal muscles contraction involves the sliding of the thick (myosin) filament of the sarcomere past the thin (actin) filament, utilizing energy supplied by hydrolysis of ATP {13}. This process is controlled by variations in the cytosolic concentration of Ca^{2+}, which binds to the troponin complex in the thin filament. As a result, the thin filament undergoes a conformational change that activates myosin molecules in the thick filament. The sliding between the filaments is thought to be caused by a cyclic interaction between crossbridges, which are comprised of the globular head region of myosin molecules and specific sites on the actin filament.

Initially experiments with hybrid myosins, in which light chains derived from fast skeletal muscle are combined with heavy chains from slow skeletal muscle, and vice versa, appeared to show that both myosin ATPase activity, and hence, muscle-shortening velocity, might be determined by the type of myosin light chains. Later hybridization experiments have failed to confirm the effect of myosin light chains on the rate of Ca^{2+}-ATPase activity or actin-stimulated Mg^{2+}-ATPase activity. Furthermore, full ATPase activity of skeletal myosin has been found to be retained in the bare heavy subunits.

To relate the chemistry of actin-myosin interaction to mechanical events during muscle contraction, Lymn and Taylor {14} proposed a four-step reaction mechanism: (a) binding of ATP and rapid dissociation of actomyosin, (b) hydrolysis of ATP on the free myosin head, (c) recombination of actin with the myosin products complex, and (d) release of myosin products. This mechanism was attractive because it could be related easily to the cycling of myosin crossbridges during contraction: (a) dissociation of the myosin head or crossbridge from the filament, (b) movement of the myosin crossbridge, (c) recombination of the myosin crossbridge with actin, and (d) the drive stroke of the cycle.

Subsequently, several refinements of the Lymn and Taylor model have been made {15,16}, which are presented in fig. 37-1. Rather than a single hydrolysis step, as originally proposed, several additional intermediate states in hydrolysis of ATP by the free myosin head have been identified from changes in myosin fluorescence. Other evidence suggests that the reaction products of ATP hydrolysis, adenosine diphosphate (ADP) and inorganic orthophosphate (P_i), are released sequentially from the active site. Furthermore, kinetic studies have revealed that association-dissociation between actin and the myosin-products complex occurs with great rapidity; this reaction is estimated to occur 1000 times more rapidly than hydrolysis of ATP. In terms of the sliding-filament model of contraction, this would imply that crossbridges (myosin heads) cycle on and off the thin filament many times during a single turn of the ATP cleavage cycle. Presumably, only after myosin heads have undergone the conformational changes associated with ATP hydrolysis would the complexes formed with actin contribute to force development. With a mechanochemical mechanism of this type, several myosin isoenzymes could coexist in a single contractile unit (sarcomere) and work together, without the differences in ATPase limiting the speed of contraction.

Cardiac myosin isoenzymes

Ventricular muscle in humans and large mammals consists of a dominant fiber type with properties similar to red skeletal myosin. Despite their uniform histologic appearance, ventricular muscle cells in most species contain varying amounts of three myosin forms, which are designated V_{1-3}, in order of decreasing electrophoretic mobility and ATPase activity {2,3}. These three myosin forms are composed of combinations of two myosin heavy chain (MHC) types, referred to as α- and β-MHC. Each molecule of the V_1 isoenzyme consists of two α-MHC, whereas the V_3 isoenzyme has two β-MHC. V_2 is a heterodimer of α- and β-MHCs. Myosin molecules also contain two pairs of "essential" and "regulatory" light chains, but the light chain types are the same in all three ventricular myosin isoforms. Since myosin plays a central role in the crossbridge cycle, any alterations in the proportion of myosin isoenzymes would be expected to alter the mechanical performance of the ventricle.

The influence of the thyroid status on the composition of ventricular myosin isoenzymes is illustrated schematically in fig. 37-2. In adult rats, thyroid hormone deficiency produced by hypophysectomy or thyroidectomy causes a decline in synthesis of α-MHCs and increases expression of the β-MHCs, resulting in a predominance of the V_3 form {2,3}. By contrast, in adult rabbits thyroid hormone administration stimulates synthesis of the V_1 form and depresses synthesis of the V_3 form. This conclusion has been confirmed by demonstration that thyroid hormone administration stimulates synthesis of mRNA encoding α-MHC and depresses synthesis of the mRNA for β-MHC {17}. Similar effects of thyroid hormone on MHC regulation have been obtained in fetal heart cells grown in chemically defined medium, indicating that these changes represent direct effects of the hormone {18}.

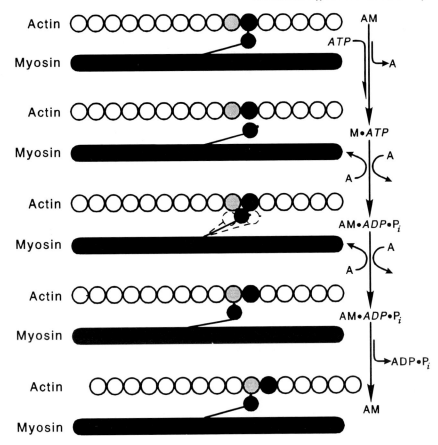

Fig. 37-1. Effects of thyroid status on the distribution of ventricular myosin isoenzymes. In the calf, the faster migrating band in the hyperthyroid state also may contain the V_2 form.

Human ventricular tissue obtained intraoperatively or postmortem shows a strong predominance of the low-activity V_3 isoenzyme {19,20}. Very little is known, however, about the regulation of the human MHC genes. The proximal 600 base pairs of the promoter region of the human and rat genes are closely homologous, suggesting that they be controlled similarly. When the MHC promoter sequences are fused to a marker gene and transfected into fetal rat heart cells, the human and rat constructs are regulated similarly by T_3 {21}. Treatment of a profoundly hypothyroid individual with replacement doses of T_4 has been reported to cause a small increases in α-MHC mRNA content {22}, but the effects of larger amounts of exogenously administered or endogenous hormone have not been quantified.

The effects on myosin isoforms of thyroid hormone treatment have been studied in large mammals, including baboon, dog, and calf {21}. Before treatment α-MHC could not be detected in ventricular muscle from any of these species. After daily treatment with large doses of T_4 for 6 weeks, calf ventricle contained about 40% α-MHCs and the baboon ventricle about 17%. Treatment with T_4 in

the dog did not change the ventricular MHC pattern. Despite these wide differences in the effect of T_4 on α-MHC expression between dog and calf, the hemodynamic responses in these species are very similar. These results provide additional reasons to believe that a switch in MHC isoforms is unlikely to be the major underlying mechanism responsible for the inotropic action of thyroid hormone.

Effects of thyroid status on mechanical performance

THYROTOXICOSIS

The cardiac output is often increased two to three times in thyrotoxic subjects and in animals receiving exogenous thyroid hormone. In the past, these alterations have been attributed mainly to changes in the peripheral circulation mediated by the metabolic effects of thyroid hormone. Also, there are known to be direct chronotropic and inotropic effects on the heart. Experimental evidence and mathematical modeling now suggest, however, that none of these factors are likely to account for an increase in cardiac output of this magnitude, rather the high output

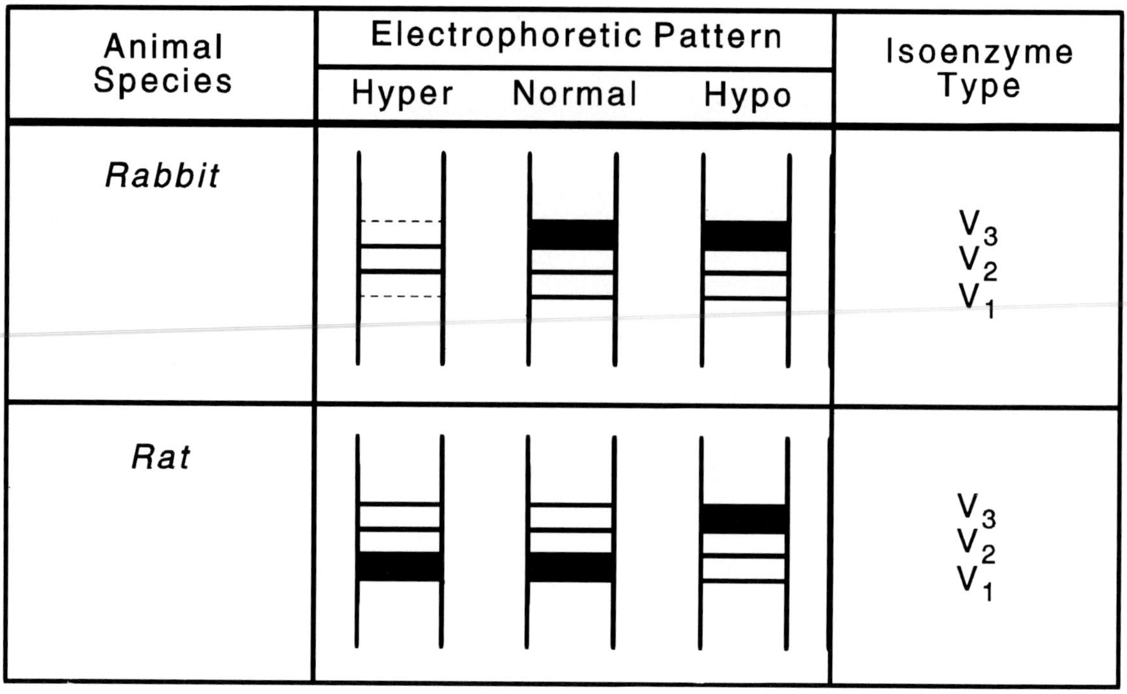

Animal Species	Electrophoretic Pattern			Isoenzyme Type
	Hyper	Normal	Hypo	
Rabbit				V_3 V_2 V_1
Rat				V_3 V_2 V_1

Fig. 37-2. A current model of the relationship between muscle contraction and ATP hydrolysis by actomyosin. Upon binding of ATP to myosin, actin and myosin dissociate, and conformational changes take place in the myosin heads (M*), during which there is rapid attachment and detachment of the myosin heads to actin monomers. The myosin heads or crossbridges contribute to force development only after undergoing conformational changes associated with ATP cleavage.

state probably is caused primarily by changes in the venous circulation that promote venous return {23}. These changes consist of an increase in mean circulatory filling pressure (gradient from peripheral veins to right atrium) and a decrease in venous compliance.

A positive chronotropic effect of thyroid hormone was established nearly 50 years ago by experiments demonstrating that isolated hearts of excised atria from animals treated with thyroid hormone beat at a faster rate than similar control preparations {24,25}. Direct inotropic effects of thyroid hormone were shown by measurements of the mechanical performance of isolated papillary muscles from thyrotoxic cat hearts {26}. In isotonic experiments, muscles from thyrotoxic cats showed a significant increase in the velocity of shortening compared to euthyroid muscles. In isometric experiments, the rate of tension development was increased without much change in maximum active tension. These findings occurred in the presence and absence of intact norepinephrine stores and over a wide range of temperature and contraction frequency. An increase in the rate of isometric tension development also has been found in both intact and glycerinated muscles from thyrotoxic rabbits {27}. Furthermore, the alterations in maximal velocity of shortening correlate closely with myofibrillar ATPase values and are limited to a range of 32–40% of maximal values{28}.

These changes in contractile performance in thyrotoxicosis are accompanied by increases in the resting ca^{2+} concentration and the amplitude of the intracellular Ca^{2+} transient {29}. The thyroid state also profoundly affects the recovery of contractile strength, with much faster recovery in hyperthyroid and slower in hypothyroid muscles {30}.

To gain a clearer description of the effects of the hormone on the intact heart, LV mechanical performance has been assessed in calves with implanted sonomicrometer crystals and pressure transducers {31}. As would be expected, heart rate, LV systolic pressure, and dP/dt increased significantly after treatment. LV internal diameter increased in both systole and diastole, however, fractional shortening was unchanged. The increases in LV end-diastolic diameter and systolic blood pressure combine to increase peak wall stress by about 30%. Despite the increase in afterload, the mean velocity of circumferential fiber shortening (V_{cf}) remains normal. Thus, in the intact heart at rest the direct inotropic effect of thyroid hormone does not produce a greater speed of shortening; speed of shortening remains normal despite a greater afterload.

HYPOTHYROIDISM

The cardiovascular effects of hypothyroidism are generally viewed as the opposite of thyrotoxicosis. Reductions in cardiac output, stroke volume, and heart rate have been reported in hypothyroid subjects and thyroid-deficient animals {32}. Changes in these parameters could reflect alterations in peripheral oxygen demand, rather than direct negative inotropic effects on the myocardium. Experimental studies of open-chested hypothyroid dog preparations or isolated papillary muscles have found depressed myocardial mechanical performance, however. It is perhaps noteworthy that in most studies differences in contractile properties between hypothyroid and control hearts are smaller than between euthyroid and hyperthyroid hearts, and not always statistically significant. Also, the velocity of contraction in isotonically contracting papillary muscles often is underestimated because of the slower activation process in hypothyroidism. Generally, the changes in intracellular Ca^{2+} transients {29} and mechanical restitution {30} are found to be opposite to those in thyrotoxicosis.

These experiments may not be adequate to explain all the evidence of reduced contractile performance in hypothyroid hearts, particularly in human subjects. Pericardial effusions are quite common in hypothyroid subjects, but can be easily recognized by echocardiography. Several other explanations for impaired performance need to be considered, including defects in excitation-contraction coupling, myxedematous infiltration, hypertrophy secondary to hypertension, and severe coronary atherosclerosis.

THYROID HORMONE INTERACTIONS

Changes in ventricular myosin isoform composition resembling mild degrees of hypothyroidism in the rat heart have been noted in several experimental conditions, particularly in pressure/volume load with myocardial dysfunction or frank congestive failure {33,34}. Downregulation of myosin isoforms may occur even though circulating T_4 levels remain normal {35}. Administration of T_4 has been shown to reverse the changes in myosin isoenzymes after aortic coarctation {36}. In the rat postinfarction model of congestive heart failure, in which myosin isoforms are downregulated, short-term use of T_4 improves LV function prior to restoration of the myosin isoform pattern {37}. Administration for longer times returns the myosin isoform distribution toward normal, but the improvement in myocardial performance is not sustained, possibly because of development of hypertrophy or tachycardia {38}. More severe degrees of cardiac dysfunction in humans are accompanied by decreased plasma T_4 and increased rT_3 {39}. The resulting abnormalities in T_4/rT_3 ratios correlate directly with increased mortality. The ability of thyroid hormone to reverse these changes is currently under investigation.

As another example, streptozocin-induced diabetes in the rat causes depression of myocardial performance in association with reduction in myosin ATPase activity and

a switch in myosin isoenzymes from the V_1 to the V_3 form {40,41}. Plasma thyroid hormone concentrations are uniformly reduced, and administration of the hormone returns the myosin isoform pattern toward normal.

These examples suggest that pressure/volume overload or experimental diabetes may cause subtle disturbances in intracellular levels of thyroid hormones, which cause downregulation of myosin isoform patterns and other biochemical abnormalities that may contribute to myocardial dysfunction. On the other hand, some investigators believe that conditions like pressure/volume overload may directly downregulate myosin isoenzymes and produce alterations in intracellular Ca^{2+} homeostasis by mechanism that are independent of changes in thyroid status. According to this view, alterations in circulating thyroid hormone levels are of secondary importance. It should be emphasized, however, that the changes in myosin isoforms reported in experimental animals may have no counterpart in humans.

Use of thyroid analogs to improve cardiovascular performance

The evidence presented above suggests that the performance of the failing heart might be benefitted by administration of a thyroid hormone analog with selective inotropic actions, if myocardial oxygen consumption is not excessively stimulated. Recently, a carboxylic acid analog, 3,5-diiodothyropropanoic acid (DITPA), which has low metabolic activity, has been shown to bind to nuclear T_3 receptors, induce α-MHC expression in heart cell cultures, and improve cardiac performance in hypothyroid rats with significantly less effect on heart rate than T_4 {42}. Since heart rate is a major determinant of myocardial oxygen consumption, DITPA is able to stimulate myocardial performance at lower oxygen costs. When given in combination with captopril (see below), DITPA improves LV performance more than captopril given alone in the rat postinfarction model of heart failure {43}. It remains to be determined whether DITPA or similar cardiotonic thyroid hormone analogs will be useful in the clinical management of congestive failure.

OTHER MECHANISMS FOR THYROID HORMONE ACTIONS ON THE HEART

Catecholamines

In the past, several investigators found support for the hypothesis that excess thyroid hormone enhances or potentiates the cardiovascular actions of catecholamines. Subsequently, a large amount of evidence has accumulated to refute this contention. For example, the positive inotropic and chronotropic response to epinephrine, norepinephrine, and cardiac sympathetic nerve stimulation were compared in T_4-treated and normal dogs {44,45}. Similar results were obtained with catecholamine infusions in thyrotoxic human subjects {46}. The enhanced contractile performance of isolated papillary muscles from thyroxine-treated cats was not influenced by depletion of catecholamine stores with reserpine {26}. No increase was found in myocardial concentration of norepinephrine or epinephrine, or in urinary excretion of catecholamines and their metabolites. Furthermore, low levels of plasma catecholamines and dopamine β-hydroxylase activity have been reported in thyrotoxic subjects.

This evidence indicates that thyrotoxicosis is not associated with increased beta-adrenergic activity or supersensitivity to beta-adrenergic stimulation. There have been suggestions, however, of more subtle interactions between thyroid hormone and catecholamines. For example, thyroid hormone has been found to increase the number of cardiac beta-adrenergic receptors in rat heart. As with may other actions of thyroid hormone, this effect is species specific and is not found in rabbit or calf. In addition, amplification by thyroid hormone of the intracellular system for expression of beta-adrenergic stimulation was suggested by an increase in myocardial phosphorylase *a* activation by catecholamines in rats pretreated with T_4. Despite extensive further study, the mechanism responsible for this observation has not come to light.

Experiments making use of beta-adrenergic antagonists also have failed to reveal a clear role for catecholamines in mediating the effects of thyroid hormone. The effects of beta-adrenergic blockade have been examined in conscious animals {47}, thereby avoiding some of the problems associated with anesthesia or the use of isolated heart preparations. In this study, full beta-adrenergic blocking doses of propanolol had no effect on hemodynamic parameters or LV mechanical performance. The average dose of propanolol required to achieve beta-adrenergic blockade was twice that required in the euthyroid state, however.

Membrane actions

A second site of thyroid hormone action is on the membrane properties of the heart, including effects on heart rate, rhythm, and electrical properties. The most striking electrophysiological abnormalities in experimental hyperthyroidism is a decrease in the duration of the action potential recorded from individual atrial cells {48}. By contrast, the duration of the action potential is prolonged in hypothyroidism. A reduction in action-potential duration increases the electrical excitability of the atrium, as shown by a reduction in the stimulation threshold for a given coupling interval. These effects may explain the tendency of thyrotoxic patients to develop atrial fibrillation.

Several mechanisms have been proposed for the effects of thyroid hormone on myocardial membrane properties, but there is little experimental verification. Because both diastolic depolarization and repolarization of the action potential are related partly to changes in intracellular K^+ conductance, it has been proposed that thyroid hormone may selectively influence these changes {48}. An increase in Na^+ conductance relative to the decrease in K^+ conductance also could explain the changes in diastolic depolarization. In addition, thyroid hormone administration appears to increase sarcolemmal Na,K-ATPase

activity. The number of Na,K-ATPase molecules in the membrane increases without changing the specific activity of the enzyme. Consistent with increased Na,K-ATPase pump activity, there is evidence of a decrease in intracellular Na^+ concentration. Also, thyroid hormone stimulates Ca^{2+} uptake by isolated SR {7}, and both the resting Ca^{2+} concentration and amplitude of the Ca^{2+} transient are reported to be increased in isolated cardiomyocytes {29}.

EFFECTS OF OTHER HORMONES ON CARDIAC PERFORMANCE

Secretions from several endocrine glands, including the anterior pituitary and adrenal cortex, may modulate myocardial contractile performance. Cardiac performance may be impaired in diabetes mellitus, a complex group of disorders characterized by an absolute or relative lack of insulin. There is evidence to suggest that this represents a distinct diabetic cardiomyopathy. Circulating or locally produced angiotensin II may play a role in the development of myocardial hypertrophy in response to pressure/volume overload. Other hormones, such as aldosterone and vasopressin, have important effects on the peripheral circulation, but they do not seem to have major effects on the heart. Atrial natriuretic peptides, although produced in the heart, act primarily to regulate blood pressure and salt and water excretion.

Parathormone

Parathyroid hormone (parathormone) has been reported to have a direct positive inotropic action on the isolated myocardium {49}. Furthermore, removal of the parathyroid glands together with the thyroid results in much more profound depression of cardiac electrical and contractile properties than only removal of the thyroid {50}. Thus the parathyroid glands may be essential for maintenance of normal cardiac performance.

Anterior pituitary hormones

The anterior pituitary gland secretes a number of polypeptide hormones with important actions on the cardiovascular system. Four of these — corticotropin, follicle stimulating hormones, leutinizing hormone, and thyrotropin — produce their biological effects indirectly by altering hormonal secretion from specific target organs (adrenal cortex, gonads, and thyroid). For this reason, the effects of these hormones are the same as those of the hormones secreted by the target gland. There are no known clinical cardiovascular abnormalities of altered secretion of prolactin. Hyperprolactemia induced by prolactin-secretin tumor in rats has been reported to reduce the response to catecholamines {51}. Isolated growth hormone deficiency does not seem to be associated with alterations in cardiac function, but excessive secretion of growth hormone produces a syndrome known as acromegaly, which may be associated with signs and symptoms of cardiac dysfunction. An increase in cardiac mass is usually present, occasionally to an extreme degree {52}. Also, there seems to be an increase in the incidence of hypertension, coronary atherosclerosis, and cardiac dysrhythmias. Because 10–20% of these patients exhibit overt congestive heart failure in the absence of other explanations, the suggestion has been made that a specific acromegalic cardiomyopathy exists. At the time of postmortem, subendocardial fibrosis and septal hypertrophy have been reported in addition to biventricular dilation and hypertrophy {53}.

The incidence of acromegaly with subclinical evidence of cardiac dysfunction is controversial. Jonas et al. {54} reported shortening of the LV ejection time (LVET), prolongation of the preejection phase, and elevation of the PEP/LVET ratio in 7 out of 10 patients. By contrast, Mather et al. {55} found a normal ejection fraction by echocardiography in all but one of 23 patients, and in those with increased LV mass there was no detectable impairment of LV performance by noninvasive techniques. They also pointed out that the abnormal PEP/LVET ratios reported by Jonas et al. {54} were largely the result of a shortened LVET with a relatively normal preejection period, which would not be a typical pattern of subclinical cardiac dysfunction. Possibly, some of the variability noted in these and other studies may be related to the duration of the disease before institution of definitive therapy.

The effects of growth hormone on cardiac growth, ventricular performance, and blood pressure have been studied experimentally {56}. It was found that hypophysectomy prevents the development of cardiac hypertrophy in response to aortic banding. Low blood pressure and cardiac atrophy are observed after banding. The decrease in heart weight relative to body weight in hypophysectomized rats was not corrected by growth hormone, but the weight of the heart increased after aortic constriction to about 12% of the expected weight. Growth hormone treatment did not influence cardiac output and work in hypophysectomized rats, but after aortic constriction these values were higher in hypophysectomized rats treated with growth hormone than in untreated controls. Treatment of hypophysectomized rats with T_4 restored the weight and rate of the heart, the blood pressure, cardiac output, and work to near normal levels. By contrast, after aortic constriction no further increase in the weight of the heart took place. These results indicate that growth hormone is essential to cardiac growth and maintenance of normal cardiac mass, but thyroid hormone is principally responsible for the reduction in cardiac performance after hypophysectomy.

Glucocorticoids

The most common cardiovascular manifestation of adrenal cortical insufficiency (Addison's disease) is arterial hypotension. Orthostatic hypotension and syncope are common, and are thought to be secondary to marked hypovolemia and electrolyte abnormalities. In severe cases, the heart size may be small, perhaps reflecting a reduction in work load. In experimental adrenal insufficiency in the rat, similar changes in blood pressure and heart weight are found. In addition, a decrease occurs in the high-ATPase activity V_1 myosin isoform, which can be reversed by glucocorticoid replacement {57}.

Hypertension is present in 80–90% of patients with glucocorticoid excess (Cushing's syndrome). Hemodynamic, electrocardiographic, and X-ray examination of patients with this condition have revealed no specific cardiac abnormalities except those that are usually associated with either hypertension or electrolyte disturbances.

Hypersecretion of aldosterone (Cohn's syndrome) is associated with arterial hypertension and hypokalemia. Both in the clinical disorder and in a related experimental model (hypertension induced by desoxycorticosterone acetate and salt in the rat), elevations in mineralocorticoids do not seem to directly affect cardiac function.

Angiotensin II

Angiotensin II (Ang II) has important actions on the cardiovascular, endocrine, and central nervous system that are initiated by binding to high-affinity receptors located on the plasma membrane. Although originally perceived as a classic endocrine system in which hormones are secreted into the blood to reach their target organs, recently it has been shown that all components of the system are present locally within the heart and many other tissues {58}. Ang II is formed by a multistep process, beginning with the cleavage of angiotensinogen, a glycoprotein of the α_2-globulin class, by renin, an aspartyl protease, to form the decapeptide angiotensin I (Ang I) and Des-angiotensin I angiotensinogen. Using Ang I as susbtrate, angiotensin converting enzyme (ACE), a dipeptidyl carboxypeptidase, then catalyzes the formation of Ang II. The same enzyme also is responsible for the degradation of bradykinin. Most abundant in the lung, ACE also is present in the heart and other tissues.

The cellular actions of Ang II are initiated when Ang II binds to specific receptors on the external surface of the plasma membrane. Recently, application of two benzylimidazole derivatives, losartan and PD123177, has revealed two Ang II receptor subtypes. The high-affinity, low-capacity receptor subtype (AT_1) is sensitive to losartan, whereas the low-affinity, high-capacity AT_2 subtype is inhibited by PD123177. The AT_1 receptor is the predominant subtype in adrenal cortex, kidney, and liver. The AT_2 receptor is the major subtype in adrenal medulla, uterus, and ovary. The heart contains AT_1 and AT_2 subtypes in approximately equal abundance {59}. Recently, the AT_1 receptor subtype has been cloned {60,61}. Analysis of the predicted amino acid sequence suggests that seven transmembrane domains are present, with 20–30% sequence identity to beta-adrenergic receptors and other G-protein-coupled receptors. In contrast, the AT_2 receptor does not appear to interact directly with the G proteins.

Ang II-bound receptors, probably by activating a G protein, increase the catalytic activity of phospholipase C. This enzyme hydrolyzes phosphatidylinositol 4,5-bisphosphate, a membrane lipid, to form two second messengers, inositol 1,4,5-trisphosphate ($InsP_3$), which mobilizes Ca^{2+} from intracellular stores, and diacylglycerol, which activates protein kinase C. The latter, a family of lipid-dependent enzymes, regulates cell function by catalyzing the phosphorylation of a variety of proteins. The regulatory pathways activated by these two second messengers interact in a number of ways. For example, activation of protein kinase C may depend in part upon Ca^{2+} released in response to $InsP_3$.

Ang II has positive inotropic and chronotropic actions, which are the result of both direct effects and modulation of sympathetic nervous system function. Accumulated evidence suggests that the direct inotropic and chronotropic effects of Ang II are mediated by its effects on Ca^{2+} conductance and homeostasis [62,63]. During the plateau phase of the action potential, Ang II strongly enhances the "slow inward current," which has been closely linked to the contractile properties of cardiac muscle [64]. In addition to enhancing transmembrane Ca^{2+} fluxes, patch-clamp studies suggest that Ang II influences voltage-dependent Na^+ channels [65]. Both effects most likely are mediated by activation of protein kinase C.

In addition to its direct actions, Ang II affects other neurohumoral systems. Facilitation of cardiac sympathetic nervous system activity is probably mediated by promoting the release of norepinephrine from presynaptic vesicles. Ang II also promotes the formation of endoperoxides via the prostaglandin synthesis pathway [66]. These substances, in turn, have a wide variety of effects, including coronary vasodilation and stimulation of adenylate cyclase. The latter may explain their reported effects on heart rate and contractility. Studies in cultured heart cells have provided evidence, however, for a direct positive chronotropic effect that is blocked by specific Ang II antagonists and is not influenced by beta-adrenergic receptor blockade [67,68]. In addition, a centrally mediated inhibition by Ang II of cardiac vagal afferents has been reported [69], which may explain the absence of tachycardia in patients treated with ACE inhibitors.

In addition to its effects on blood pressure and myocardial performance, Ang II may play an important role in promoting the hypertrophic response in both heart and blood vessels. Although the remarkable ability of ACE inhibitors to prevent or reverse hypertensive cardiac hypertrophy has been recognized for some time, this action has not been clearly separated from the concomitant lowering of blood pressure caused by these agents. Recently, treatment with low doses of ACE inhibitors that did not lower blood pressure has been shown to result in prevention or regression of hypertrophy in aortic-banded rats [70,71]. Whatever their precise mechanism of action, ACE inhibitors are effective antihypertensive agents and have been shown to reduce mortality in the rat postinfarction model [72] and patients with congestive heart failure [73]. Losartan, an orally active AT_1 receptor antagonist, also lowers blood pressure in hypertension and improves cardiac function in heart failure [74].

Opioids

The heart has opioid receptors and opioid peptides may affect cardiac function either directly or indirectly by acting synergistically with classical neurotransmitters. Leu-enkephalin has been reported to increase the positive chronotropic response to epinephrine and SR Ca^{2+} uptake in guinea pig heart [75]. Evidence for a direct action of enkephalins has been obtained by use of cultured chick embryo ventricular cells, which are devoid of neural elements [76]. Met-enkephalin, leu-enkephalin, and their nonhydrolyzable analogs increased contractility in a dose-dependent manner that could be antagonized by naloxone. Possibly, enkephalins released from the adrenal medulla together with catecholamines could exert physiological effects on cardiac performance. Cardiac opioid receptors have been shown to be involved in the genesis of arrhythmias during ischemia and reperfusion. Studies using an opioid agonist and antagonist suggest that the cardiac κ-receptors are the most likely receptor-subtype involved [77].

Diabetes mellitus

The incidence of congestive heart failure is increased in diabetes, even when factors such as age, blood pressure, plasma cholesterol, body weight, and coronary artery disease are taken into account [78]. These data, together with postmortem reports [79,80] of cardiomegaly, interstitial fibrosis, and subendocardial thickening of the small coronary arteries in diabetics with clinical evidence of congestive failure, have lead to the proposal that diabetes is associated with a discrete form of cardiomyopathy.

Regan et al. [81] have reported variable degrees of interstitial and perivascular fibrosis in diabetic hearts; significant accumulations of acid-Schiff-positive material were found in the interstitium. The walls of intramural blood vessels were thickened in some cases, usually to a mild extent. There was no evidence that either large or small blood vessel occlusive disease contributed to the pathological alterations in the myocardium.

The study by Regan et al. [81] also included hemodynamic assessment of a small group of diabetic patients without hypertension or angiographically significant coronary artery disease. A consistent reduction in stroke volume and elevation of LV diastolic pressure were found. Increments in afterload significantly increased filling pressure compared to normals without an appropriate response in stroke volume. These changes, which are indicative of reduced ventricular compliance, were interpreted as signifying a preclinical cardiomyopathy. Noninvasive studies [82,83] also have suggested myocardial dysfunction in diabetics; however, the type of abnormalities reported have been variable.

Further support for the concept of a diabetic cardiomyopathy has come from experimental studies of drug-induced diabetes. Studies with chronically diabetic rats, employing both isolated LV papillary muscles and perfused hearts, have shown slowing of relaxation and depression of contractile performance in diabetic hearts [84,85].

Studies in chronically diabetic dogs have indicated that the stiffness of the LV is increased, possibly because of increased collagen content [86]. Regulation of postprandial hyperglycemia with insulin did not reverse these changes {87}. In contrast, in the streptozotocin-treated rat, the pressure-volume relationship of the isolated ventricle is shifted away from the pressure axis, suggesting increased chamber compliance {85}. In neither study was the entire diastolic pressure-volume relation examined, nor was myocardial stiffness measured.

To provide an integrated assessment of changes in ventricular function, conscious hemodynamics and an ex vivo analysis of LV passive-elastic properties was performed in a recent study {88}. After 7 days, diabetic rats exhibited decreases in heart rate and LV systolic function. Overall chamber stiffness was decreased; however, "operating chamber stiffness" calculated at end-diastolic pressure was initially increased and later returned toward normal. After 26 days LV cavity/wall volume and end-diastolic volume were increased, changes suggestive of an early cardiomyopathy. Despite evidence of LV dilation and impaired systolic function in this model, cardiac output is increased or maintained because of the combination of decreased afterload and maintenance of preload {89}. All of these abnormalities were reversed by treatment with insulin.

In the early period after induction of alloxan diabetes in the rat, cardiac function and high-energy phosphate stores were reduced because of impaired glucose utilization {90}. Acute correction of substrate deficiency in the perfused hearts with insulin or high concentrations of glucose restored ATP levels and returned ventricular function toward normal.

Efforts have been made to correlate these mechanical changes to alterations in SR Ca^{2+} {91} uptake and to a change in myosin isoenzymes toward a predominance of the V_3 form {40,41}. These changes are reversible with insulin {92}, but, as pointed out above, thyroid hormone levels are depressed in this model and could be responsible for some of the abnormalities found.

REFERENCES

1. Morkin E, Flink IL, Goldman S: Physiological and biochemical effects of thyroid hormone on cardiac performance. *Prog Cardiovasc Dis* 25:435–464, 1983.
2. Hoh JFY, McGrath PA, Hale PT: Electrophoretic analysis of multiple forms of rat cardiac myosin: Effects of hypophysectomy and thyroid replacement. *J Mol Cell Cardiol* 10:1053–1076, 1978.
3. Hoh JFY, Egerton LJ: Action of triiodothyronine on the synthesis of rat ventricular myosin isozymes. *FEBS Lett* 101:143–148, 1979.
4. Swynghedauw B: Developmental and functional adaptions of contractile proteins in cardiac and skeletal muscles. *Physiol Rev* 66:710–771, 1986.
5. Goodkind M, Damback G, Thyrum P, Luchi R: Effect of thyroxine on ventricular myocardial contractility and ATPase activity in guinea pigs. *Am J Physiol* 226:66–72, 1974.
6. Brooks I, Flynn S, Owen D, Underwood A: Changes in cardiac function following administration of thyroid hormones in thyroidectomized rats: Assessment using the isolated working rat heart preparation. *J Cardiovasc Pharm* 7:290–296, 1985.

7. Dillmann WH: Biochemical basis of thyroid hormone action in the heart. *Am J Med* 88:626–630, 1990.
8. Davis P: Cellular actions of thyroid hormone. In: Braverman. LE, Utiger RD (eds) *Werner and Ingbar's The Thyroid*. New York: J.B. Lippincott, 1991, pp 190–203.
9. Oppenheimer JH: The nuclear receptor-triiodothyronine complex: Relationship to thyroid hormone distribution, metabolism, and biological action. In: Oppenheimer JH, Samuels HH (eds) *Molecular Basis of Thyroid Hormone Action*. New York: Academic Press, 1983, pp 1–34.
10. Sap J, Munoz A, Damm K, Goldberg Y, Ghysdael J, Leutz A, Beug H, Vennstrom B: The c-erbA protein is a high-affinity receptor for thyroid hormone. *Nature* 324:635–640, 1986.
11. Weinberger C, Thompson CC, Ong ES, Lebo R, Gruol DJ, Evans RM: The c-erbA gene encodes a thyroid hormone receptor. *Nature* 324:641–646, 1986.
12. Hinkle PR, Kinsella PA: Thyroid hormone induction of an autocrine growth factor secreted by pituitary tumor cells. *Science* 234:1549–1552, 1986.
13. Eisenberg E, Green LE: The relation of muscle biochemistry to muscle physiology. *Annu Rev Physiol* 42:293–309, 1980.
14. Lymn RW, Taylor EW: Mechanism of adenosine triphosphate hydrolysis by actomyosin. *Biochemistry* 10:4617–4624, 1971.
15. Siemankowski RF, White HD: Kinetics of the interaction between actin, ADP, and cardiac myosin S-1. *J Biol Chem* 259:5045–5053, 1984.
16. Stein LA, Chock PB, Eisenberg E: The rate-limiting step in the actomyosintriphosphtase cycle. *Biochemistry* 23:1555–1563, 1984.
17. Sinha AM, Umeda PK, Kavinsky CJ, Rajamanickam C, Hsu H-J, Jakovcic S, Rabinowitz M: Molecular cloning of mRNA sequences for α- and β-form myosin heavy chains: Expression in ventricles of normal hypothyroid, and thyrotoxic rabbits. *Proc Natl Acad Sci USA* 79:5847–5851, 1982.
18. Gustafson TA, Bahl JJ, Markham BE, Roeske WR, Morkin E: Hormonal regulation of myosin heavy chain and α-actin gene expression cultured fetal rat heart myocytes. *J Biol Chem* 262:13316–13322, 1987.
19. Bouvagnet P, Leger J, Pons F, Deschesne C, Leger JJ: Fiber types and myosin types in human atrial and ventricular myocardium. An anatomical description. *Circ Res* 55:794–804, 1984.
20. Gorza L, Mercadier JJ, Schwartz K, Thornell LE, Sartore S, Schiaffino S: Myosin types in the human heart. An immunofluorescence study of normal and hypertrophied atrial and ventricular myocardium. *Circ Res* 54:694–702, 1984.
21. Morkin E: Regulation of myosin heavy chain genes in the heart. *Circulation* 87:1451–1460, 1993.
22. Ladenson PW, Sherman SI, Baughman KL, Ray PE, Feldman AM: Reversible alterations in myocardial gene expression in a young man with dilated cardiomyopathy. *Proc Natl Acad Sci USA* 89:5251–5255, 1992.
23. Goldman S, Olajos M, Morkin E: Control of cardiac output in thyrotoxic calves. *J Clin Invest* 73:358–365.
24. Priestley JT, Markowitz J, Mann FC: The tachycardia of experimental hyperthyroidism. *Am J Physiol* 98:357–362, 1931.
25. Yater WM: The tachycardia, time factor, survival period and seat of action of thyroxine in the perfused hearts of thyroxinized rabbits. *Am J Physiol* 98:338–343, 1931.
26. Buccino RA, Spann JF, Pool PE, Sonnenblick EH, Braunwald E: Influence of the thyroid state on the intrinsic contractile properties and energy stores of the myocardium. *J Clin Invest* 46:1669–1682, 1967.
27. Skeleton CL, Su JY, Pool E: Influence of hyperthyroidism on

glycerol-extracted cardiac muscle from rabbits. *Cardiovasc Res* 10:380–384.

28. Ebrecht G, Rupp H, Jacob R: Alterations of mechanical parameters in chemically skinned preparation of rat myocardium as a function of isoenzyme pattern of myosin. *Basic Res Cardiol* 77:220–234, 1982.

29. Beekman RE, Hardeveld CV, Simonides WS: Thyroid status and β-agonist effects on cytosolic calcium concentration in single rat cardiac myocytes activated by electrical stimulation or high-K^+ depolarization. *Biochem J* 268:563–569, 1990.

30. Poggesi C, Everts M, Polla B, Tanzi F, Reggiani C: Influence of thyroid state on mechanical restitution of rat myocardium. *Circ Res* 60:142–151, 1987.

31. Goldman S, Olajos M, Friedman H, Roeske WR, Morkin E: Left ventricular performance in conscious thyrotoxic calves. *Am J Physiol* 242 (*Heart Circ Physiol* 11):H113–H121, 1982.

32. Stauer BE, Schulze W: Experimental hypothyroidism: Depression of myocardial contractile function and hemodynamics and their reversibility by substitution with thyroid hormone. *Basic Res Cardiol* 71:624–644, 1976.

33. Rupp H: The adaptive changes in the isoenzyme pattern of myosin from hypertrophied rat myocardium as a result of pressure overload and physical training. *Basic Res Cardiol* 76:79–88, 1981.

34. Mercadier JJ, Lompre AM, Wisenewsky C, Samuel JL, Bercovici J, Swynghedauw B, Schwartz K: Myosin isozyme changes in several models of rat cardiac hypertrophy. *Circ Res* 49:525–532, 1981.

35. Imamura S-I, Matsuoka R, Hiratsuka E, Kimura M, Nakanishi T, Nishikawa T, Furutani Y, Takao A: Adaptational changes of MHC gene expression and isozyme transition in cardiac overloading. *Am J Physiol* (*Heart Circ Physiol* 29) 260:H73–H79, 1991.

36. Izumo S, Lompre AM, Matsuoka R, Koren G, Schwartz K: Myosin heavy chain messenger RNA and protein isoform transitions during cardiac hypertrophy: Interaction between hemodynamic and thyroid hormone-induced signals. *J Clin Invest* 79:970–977, 1988.

37. Gay RG, Gustafson TA, Goldman S, Morkin E: Effects of L-thyroxine in rats with chronic heart failure after healed myocardial infarction. *Am J Physiol* (*Heart Circ Physiol* 22) 253:H341–H346, 1987.

38. Gay RG, Graham S, Aquirre M, Goldman S, Morkin E: Effects of 10- to 12-day treatment with L-thyroxine in rats with myocardial infarction. *Am J Physiol* (*Heart Circ Physiol* 24) 255:H801–H806, 1988.

39. Hamilton MA, Stevenson LW, Luu M, Walden MN: Altered thyroid hormone metabolism in advanced heart failure. *J Am Coll Cardiol* 16:91–95, 1990.

40. Dillman WH: Diabetes mellitus induced changes in cardiac myosin of the rat. *Diabetes* 29:579–582, 1980.

41. Malhotra A, Penpargkul S, Fein F, Sonnenblick EH, Scheuer J: The effects of streptozotocin-induced diabetes in rats on cardiac contractile proteins. *Circ Res* 49:1243–1250, 1981.

42. Pennock GD, Raya TE, Bahl JJ, Goldman S, Morkin E: Cardiac effects of 3,5-diiodothyropropionic acid, a thyroid hormone analog with inotropic selectivity. *J Pharmacol Exp Ther* 263:163–169, 1992.

43. Pennock GD, Raya TE, Bahl JJ, Goldman S, Morkin E: Combination treatment with captopril and the thyroid hormone analog 3,5-diiodothyropropionic acid (DITPA): A new approach to improving left ventricular performance in heart failure. *Circulation* 88:1289–1298, 1993.

44. Margolius HS, Gaffney T: Effect of injected norepinephrine and sympathetic nerve stimulation in hypothyroid and hyperthyroid dogs. *J Pharmacol Exp Ther* 149:329–335, 1965.

45. Van der Shoot JB, Moran NC: An experimental evaluation of the reputed influence of thytoxine on the cardiovascular effects of catecholamines. *J Pharmacol Exp Ther* 149:336–345, 1965.

46. Aoki VS, Wilson WR, Theilen EO: Studies of the reputed augmentation of the cardiovascular effects of catecholamines in patients with spontaneous hyperthyroidism. *J Pharmacol Exp Ther* 181:362–368, 1972.

47. Goldman S, Olajos M, Pieniaszek H, Perrier D, Mayersohn M, Morkin E: Beta-adrenergic blockade with propranolol in conscious euthyroid and thyrotoxic calves: Dosage requirements and effects on heart rate and left ventricular performance. *J Pharmacol Exp Ther* 219:394–399, 1981.

48. Johnson PN, Freedberg AS, Marshall JM: Action of thyroid hormone on the transmembrane potentials from sinoatrial node cells and atrial muscle cells in isolated atria of the rabbit. *Cardiology* 58:273–289, 1973.

49. Katoli Y, Klein D, Kaplan R, Warren G, Kurokanna K: Parathyroid hormone has a positive inotropic action in the rat. *Endocrinology* 111:2252–2254, 1977.

50. Capasso G, Tepper D, Capasso JM, Sonnenblick EH: Effects of hypothyroidism and hypoparathyroidism on rat myocardium: Mechanical and electric alterations. *Am J Med Sci* 29:232–240, 1986.

51. Katovich MJ, Baker SP, Nelson C: Effects of elevated prolactin and its normalization on thyroid hormone, cardiac β-adrenoreceptor number and β-adrenergic responsiveness. *Life Sci* 34:889–898, 1983.

52. Heljtmancik MR, Bradfield JY, Herman GR: Acromegaly and the heart: A clinical and pathologic study. *Ann Intern Med* 34:1445–1456, 1951.

53. Rossi L, Theine G, Caregaro L, Giordano R, Lauro S: Dysrhythmias and sudden death in acromegalic heart disease. A clinicopathological study. *Chest* 72:496–498, 1977.

54. Jonas EA, Aloia JF, Lane JF: Evidence of subclinical heart muscle dysfunction in acromegaly. *Chest* 67:190–194, 1975.

55. Mather HM, Boyd MJ, Jenkins JS: Heart size and function in acromegaly. *Br Med J* 41:697–701, 1979.

56. Beznak M: Effect of growth hormone and thyroxine in cardiovascular system of hypophysectomized rats. *Am J Physiol* 204:279–283, 1963.

57. Sheer D, Morkin E: Effects of thyroid hormone analogs, non-thyroidal hormones, and high carbohydrate diet on cardiac myosin isozyme expression on the rat. *Fed Proc* 42:2212, 1983.

58. Lindpainter K, Ganten D: The cardiac renin-angiotensin system. An appraisal of present experimental and clinical evidence. *Circ Res* 68:905–921, 1990.

59. Sechi LA, Griffin CA, Grady EF, Kalinyak JE, Schambelan M: Characterization of angiotensin II receptor subtypes in heart. *Circulation* 71:1482–1489, 1992.

60. Sasaki K, Yamano Y, Bardhan S, Iwai N, Murray JJ, Hasegawa M, Matsuda Y, Inagami T: Cloning and expression of a complementary DNA encoding a bovine adrenal angiotensin II type-1 receptor. *Nature* 351:230–233, 1991.

61. Murphy TJ, Alexander RW, Griendling KK, Runge MS, Berstein KE: Isolation of a cDNA encoding the vascular type-1 angiotensin II receptor. *Nature* 351:233–236, 1991.

62. Koch-Weser J: Nature of the inotropic action of angiotensin on ventricular myocardium. *Circ Res* 16:230–237, 1965.

63. Freer RJ, Pappano AJ, Peach MJ, Bing KT, McLean MN, Vogel S, Sperelakis N: Mechanism for the positive inotropic effect of angiotensin II on isolated cardiac muscle. *Circ Res* 39:178–183, 1976.

64. Kass RS, Blair ML: Effects of angiotensin II on membrane

current in cardiac Purkinje fibers. *J Mol Cell Cardiol* 13: 797–809, 1981.

65. Moorman JR, Kirsch GE, Lacerda AE, Brown AM: Angiotensin II modulates cardiac Na$^+$ channels in neonatal rat. *Circ Res* 65:1804–1809, 1989.

66. Peach M: Molecular actions of angiotensin. *Biochem Pharmacol* 30:2745–2751, 1981.

67. Allen IS, Cohen NM, Dhallan RS, Gaa ST, Lederer WJ, Rogers TB: Angiotensin II increases spontaneous contractile frequency and stimulates calcium current in cultured neonatal rat heart myocytes: Insight into the underlying biochemical mechanism. *Circ Res* 62:524–534, 1988.

68. Dosemeci A, Dhallan RS, Cohen NM, Lederer WJ, Rogers TB: Phorbol ester increases calcium current and stimulates the effects of angiotensin II on cultured neonatal rat heart myocytes. *Circ Res* 62:347–357, 1988.

69. Lee WB, Ismay MJ, Lumbers ER: Mechanisms by which angiotensin affects the heart rate of the conscious sheep. *Circ Res* 47:286–292, 1980.

70. Baker KM, Chernin MI, Wixson SK, Aceto JF: Renin-angiotensin system involvement in pressure-overload cardiac hypertrophy in rats. *Am J Physiol* 259 (2 Part 2):H324–H332, 1990.

71. Linz W, Schoelkens BA, Ganten D: Converting enzyme inhibition specifically prevents the development and induces the regression of cardiac hypertrophy in rats. *Clin Exp Hypertens* 11:13254–1350, 1989.

72. Pfeffer JM, Pfeffer MA, Braunwald E: Influence of chronic captopril therapy on the infarcted left ventricle of the rat. *Circ Res* 57:84–95, 1985.

73. CONSENSUS Trial Study Group: Effects of enalapril on mortality in severe congestive heart failure: Results of the Cooperative North Scandinavian Enalapril Survival Study (CONSENSUS). *N Engl J Med* 316:1429–1435, 1987.

74. Raya TE, Fonken SJ, Lee RW, Daugherty S, Goldman S, Wong PC, Timmermans PB, Morkin E: Hemodynamic effects of direct angiotensin II blockade compared to converting enzyme inhibition in rat model of heart failure. *Am J Hypertension* 4:334S–340S, 1991.

75. Ruth JA, Cuizon JV, Eiden LE: Leucine-enkephalin increase norepinephrine-stimulated chronotropy and ^{45}Ca^{2+} uptake in guinea-pig atria. *Neuropeptides* 4:185–191, 1984.

76. Laurent S, Marsh JD, Smith TW: Enkephalins have a direct positive inotropic effect on cultured cardiac myocytes. *Proc Natl Acad USA* 82:5930–5934, 1985.

77. Wong TM, Lee AYS, Tai KK: Effects of drugs interacting with opioid receptors during normal perfusion and reperfusion in the isolated rat heart — an attempt to identify cardiac

opioid receptor subtype(s) involved in arrhythmogenesis. *J Mol Cell Cardiol* 22:1167–1175, 1990.

78. Kannel WB, Hjortland M, Castelli WP: Role of diabetes in congestive heart failure: The Framingham study. *Am J Cardiol* 34:29–34, 1974.

79. Rubler S, Diugash J, Yuceoglu YZ, Kumral T, Branwood AW, Grishman A: New type of cardiomegaly associated with diabetic glomerulosclerosis. *Am J Cardiol* 30:595–602, 1972.

80. Hamby RI, Zoneraich S, Sherman L: Diabetic cardiomyopathy. *JAMA* 229:1749–1754, 1974.

81. Regan TJ, Lyons MM, Ahmed SS, Levinson GE, Oldewurtel HA, Ahmad MR, Haider B: Evidence for cardiomyopathy in familial diabetes mellitus. *J Clin Invest* 60:885–899, 1977.

82. Ahmed SS, Jafferi GA, Narang RM, Regan TJ: Preclinical abnormalities of left ventricular function in diabetes mellitus. *Am Heart J* 89:153–158, 1975.

83. Rubler S, Sajadi RM, Araoye MA, Holford FD: Noninvasive estimate of performance in patients with diabetes. *Diabetes* 27:127–134, 1978.

84. Fein FS, Kornstein LB, Strobeck JE, Capasso JM, Sonnenblick EH: Altered myocardial mechanics in diabetic rats. *Circ Res* 47:922–933, 1980.

85. Penpargkul S, Schaible T, Yiptinsoi T, Scheuer J: The effect of diabetes on performance and metabolism of rat heart. *Circ Res* 47:911–921, 1980.

86. Regan TJ, Ettinger PO, Khan MI, Jesranc MV, Lyons MM, Oldewurtel HA, Weber M: Altered myocardial function in chronic diabetes without ischemia in dogs. *Circ Res* 35:222–237, 1974.

87. Regan TJ, Wu CF, Yeh CK, Oldewurtel HA, Haider B: Myocardial composition and function in diabetes. Chronic insulin use. *Circ Res* 49:1268–1277, 1981.

88. Litwin SE, Raya TE, Anderson PG, Daugherty S, Goldman S: Abnormal cardiac function in the streptozotocin-diabetic rat. *J Clin Invest* 86:481–488, 1990.

89. Litwin SE, Raya TE, Daugherty S, Goldman S: Peripheral circulatory control of cardiac output in diabetic rats. *Am J Physiol* 261 (*Heart Circ Physiol* 30):H836–H842, 1991.

90. Miller TB Jr: Cardiac performance in isolated perfused hearts from alloxan diabetic rats. *Am J Physiol* 236:H808–H812, 1979.

91. Penpargkul S, Fein F, Sonnenblick EH, Scheuer J: Depressed cardiac sarcoplasmic reticular function from diabetic rats. *J Mol Cell Cardiol* 13:303–309, 1981.

92. Fein FS, Strobeck JE, Malhotra A, Scheuer J, Sonnenblick EH: Reversibility of diabetic cardiomyopathy with insulin in rats. *Circ Res* 49:1251–1261, 1981.

CHAPTER 38

Cardioplegia Principles and Problems

MARTHA-MARIA GEBHARD, HANS JÜRGEN BRETSCHNEIDER,[†]
& PHILIPP A. SCHNABEL

THE GLOBALLY ISCHEMIC HEART

Suspension of coronary circulation and the shift from aerobic to anaerobic energy metabolism is known to effect a decrease of energy-rich phosphates in the heart muscle cell and is accompanied by insufficiency of contractile function, cellular as well as extracellular accumulation of lactate and hydrogen ions, decrease of cellular as well as subcellular transmembraneous electrolyte gradients, and alteration of the fine structure of the myocardium. With extension of global ischemia and increasing energy deficit in the myocardium, alterations intensify and finally become irreversible.

The different parts in the heart vary in terms of their susceptibility to damage as a result of ischemia. As described by PICK in 1924 {41}, the *primum moriens* of the ischemic heart under physiological conditions is the left ventricular myocardium; the *ultimum moriens* lies in the ventricular parts of the excitation-conduction system. Therefore, if specific preischemic damage to the heart can be excluded, ischemia tolerance of the organ as a whole correlates with the revivability of the left ventricular myocardium.

From the point of view of postischemic functional revivability of the heart, three phases of reversible ischemia can be defined on the basis of characteristic changes in the left ventricular levels of the high-energy phosphates creatine phosphate (CP) and adenosine triphosphate (ATP) (fig. 38-1): (a) the latency period, (b) survival time, and (c) revival time {5,6,39}.

During the first or latency period of ischemia, myocardial function is not yet disturbed. Metabolically, it is characterized by aerobic energy gain as a result of the use of O_2 reserves of myocardial oxymyoglobine, oxyhemoglobine, and physically dissolved oxygen. Under normothermic conditions and depending on the level of O_2

Supported by the Deutsche Forschungsgemeinschaft, Sonderforschungsbereich 89 — Kardiologie — Göttingen.
The authors wish to thank the technical assistants of the Department of Electron Microscopy and of the Department of Physiology and Pathophysiology for their always-skillful support in this work.
[†] Deceased

demand immediately prior to ischemia, these O_2 reserves last for no more than 1–20 ss.

During *survival time*, reperfusion and reoxygenation of the ischemic heart allow immediate resumption of cardiac function. In metabolic terms, survival time includes the aerobic latency period as well as the immediately following first period of anaerobic energy gain and decrease of myocardial CP. It is therefore also called CP time or t-CP. The critical limit of survival time in the dog heart corresponds to a CP concentration of 3 μM/g of wet left ventricular myocardium; depending on the preischemic energy demands of the heart, under normothermic conditions t-CP lasts about 1–3 minutes (fig. 38-1).

Finally, revival time refers to the total duration of reversible global ischemia. In metabolic terms it includes the aerobic latency period, the period of decrease of CP down to about 3 μM/g of left ventricular myocardium, and the immediately ensuing period of ATP breakdown in the left ventricle. Because postischemic recovery latency increases exponentially until reaching full resumption of myocardial function following t-CP and increasing ATP deficit {5,6,16}, a so-called practical limit of revivability of the heart has been distinguished from overall revival time; during this period, the functional recocovery of the heart lasts no more than 20–30 minutes. The practical limit of revivability in the dog heart corresponds to a left ventricular ATP concentration of 4 μM/g and is also called ATP time or t-ATP. The absolute limit of revival time is reached when the left ventricular ATP concentration falls below a minimum of between 1.5 and 2 μM/g {29}. t-ATP in the normothermic dog heart, depending on the preischemic O_2 requirement, lasts no more than 10–15 minutes (fig. 38-1); overall revival time, however, can be as long as 40–60 minutes (fig. 38-1).

These data correspond well with clinical observations on the reversibility of ischemic cardiac arrest and therefore indicate that experimental data on ischemia tolerance in the dog heart can also be applied to the human heart.

PRINCIPLES OF CARDIOPLEGIA

Experimental results involving the untreated globally ischemic heart show that myocardial ultrastructure and

N. Sperelakis (ed.), Physiology and Pathophysiology of the Heart, Third Edition.

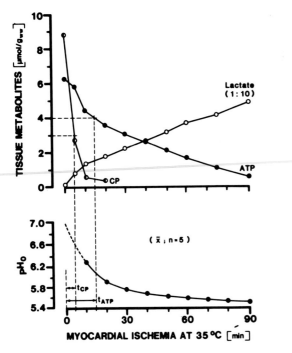

Fig. 38-1. High-energy phosphates, lactate, and interstitial pH during pure global ischemia at 35°C in the left ventricular canine myocardium.

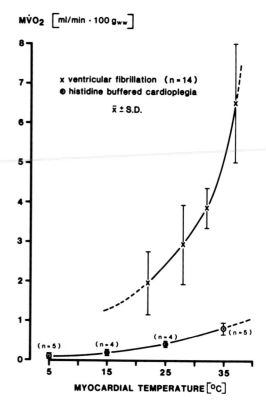

Fig. 38-2. Myocardial temperature and the aerobic energy demand, MVO_2, during ventricular fibrillation {9} or cardioplegic coronary perfusion in the canine heart. The data are even valid in the human heart {44}.

revivability are determined by the energy deficit of the heart defined in relation to normal conditions {5,16,30, 45,47}; it therefore follows that there are three principle ways of artificially prolonging the ischemia tolerance of the heart {6}: (a) through minimization of the cardiac energy demand, (b) through maximization of the energy reserves of the heart muscle, and (c) through amelioration of metabolic energy gain in the myocardium during each of the three phases of ischemia tolerance defined above.

Minimization of cardiac energy demands

The energy demand of any organ is the sum of its basal energy requirement at rest plus that which arises during work. In the heart, the latter is essentially determined by the level of performance of the contractile system {3,7}. Energy demand varies by a factor of approximately 10 if we compare myocardial oxygen consumption (MVO_2) at maximum work with that of the empty beating or fibrillating heart, and by a factor of 100 in relation to the heart arrested in diastole (fig. 38-2). The membraneous ion pumping systems exercise relatively little influence on this relationship, even at very rapid rates {3,7}.

The basal energy requirements of the heart arise from the demands for structural preservation and for metabolic and electrophysiologic readiness for function {6}. The fact that functional reversibility of global ischemia differs during aerobic latency, during t-CP, and after t-CP indicates that the energy consuming systems determining the

work output of the heart can be temporarily switched off without ill effects. However, a reduction of energy turnover below the level of the basal requirement is always accompanied by at least reversible damage to the organ.

Suspension of work output of the heart can be achieved by any type of pharmacologic or electrophysiologic intervention that inacitivates the electrical and mechanical functions of the heart muscle and leads to diastolic cardiac arrest. In its strictest sense, *cardioplegia* means artificial diastolic cardiac arrest. A number of different methods for inducing cardiac arrest are not practicable because they are either irreversibly toxic or because it is difficult to determine the proper dosage. Reduction of myocardial temperature alone is not only difficult to realize homogeneously, it is also insufficiently effective in achieving complete relaxation of the contractile system, as can be deduced from the high-temperature dependency of MVO_2 in the fibrillating heart {9} (fig. 38-2). Pharmacological agents such as tetrodotoxine, acetylcholine, local anesthetics (e.g., procaine), or even calcium antagonists or calcium-complexing agents (e.g., EDTA or citrate) are temperature-sensitive {11}, exhibit a narrow therapeutic range {23}, or can accumulate in the myocardium during cardioplegic coronary perfusion, leading to at least a delay

Table 38-1. The three cardioplegic solutions of Kirklin {23}, of the St. Thomas' hospital {23}, and of Bretschneider {6,18} represent the three essential ionic principles of artificial cardiac arrest

[mmol/l]	Kirklin	St. Thomas' hospital	Bretschneider
Na^+	110	117	15
K^+	30	16	10
Ca^{2+}	0.5	1	—
Mg^{2+}	—	16	4
Substrates	28 Glucose	—	—
Buffering substances	27 HCO_3^-	25 HCO_3^-	180 Histidine 18 His-HCl
Pharmaca	—	1 Procaine-HCl	—
Osmolality	362	318	310

in cardiac recovery upon reperfusion {43}. The cardioplegic methods currently in clinical use are based on essentially three ionic principles of cardiac arrest (table 38-1) and are usually used in combination with hypothermia. The principles involved are

1. An increase of extracellular myocardial potassium concentration $[K]_o$ (e.g., Kirklin's cardioplegia),
2. An increase of extracellular myocardial concentration of ionized magnesium $[Mg^{2+}]_o$ (e.g., St. Thomas's cardioplegia), and
3. A simultaneous reduction of the extracellular myocardial concentration of sodium $[Na]_o$ and ionized calcium $\{Ca^{2+}\}_o$ (Bretschneider's cardioplegia).

The basic principles of action behind these electrolytic concepts are reviewed and discussed in other chapters of this book; certain aspects can be summarized here from the point of view of cardioplegic efficacy.

Increased concentrations of *potassium* in the extracellular compartment of the myocardium effect cardioplegia by deactivating the fast Na and the slow Ca-Na channels in the myocardial sarcolemma. In an otherwise physiological milieu, cardiac arrest based on the use of potassium occurs at concentrations of $[K]_o$ of about 30 mM {34}. However, the slope of the dose-response curve representing the cardioplegic efficacy of $[K]_o$ depends to a considerable degree on such accompanying conditions as temperature and ionic milieu, and it increases under conditions of hypothermia {5}, high $[Mg^{2+}]_o$ {46}, or low $[Ca^{2+}]_o$ {4}. In addition to its effects on the excitability of the heart muscle cell, however, $[K]_o$ also stimulates aerobic and anaerobic energy turnover in the myocardium {34} and causes alterations of volume regulation in myocardial endothelial cells to the point of occlusion of the capillary bed {49}. Cardioplegia with high $[K]_o$ is therefore usually combined with additional plegic measures such as a reduction of $[Ca^{2+}]_o$, an increase of $[Mg^{2+}]_o$, and a lowering of temperature (see table 38-1). Under these more complex conditions, the amount of cardioplegically effective $[K]_o$ is less than 30 mM, but the optimum amount must be determined experimentally in each case.

Magnesium induces diastolic cardiac arrest at extracellular myocardial concentrations of 20–25 mM {42,51}.

The fundamental effects of Mg^{2+} are its inactivation of the fast Na-channel and the competitive inhibition of cellular calcium influx via the slow Ca-Na channel at the sarcolemma {27,42,46,50,51}. Consistent with this is the fact that the slope of the dose-response curve of cardioplegic efficacy with $[Mg^{2+}]_o$ is dependent on $[Na]_o$, $[K]_o$, and $[Ca^{2+}]_o$ and rises if $[Na]_o$ and $[Ca^{2+}]_o$ are decreased in comparison with physiological levels or if $[K]_o$ is enhanced {40,51}. Moreover, especially under low $[Na]_o$, low $[Ca^{2+}]_o$, and high $[K]_o$ conditions, Mg^{2+} is an effective competitive inhibitor of Ca^{2+} at several binding sites of calcium at the outer cell surface, though it provides no substitute for the membrane-stabilizing effects of calcium {12,13,32,40}. Mg^{2+} interferes with Ca^{2+} intracellularly as well as acts Ca-antagonistically by displacing Ca^{2+} from sarcolemmal binding sites {28} and preventing Ca-uptake into the mitochondria {25} while enhancing calcium uptake into the sarcoplasmic reticulum {15,22}. The overall effect of a longer lasting coronary perfusion with perfusate of a high Mg^{2+} concentration is a reduction of myocardial Ca content {51}. In physiological terms, however, the main importance of intracellular magnesium appears to be as an ion essential to numerous phases of cellular metabolism {14,42}. The concentration of free cytoplasmic Mg^{2+} is thought to amount to between 0.3 and 3.0 mM per kg of cell water and varies, in particular, as a consequence of changes in the concentration of cytoplasmic adenine-nucleotide phosphates, up to 90% of which normally exists intracellularly as magnesium complexes {14,55}. Catabolism of cellular ATP as a result of an ischemic impact results in an increase of free cytosolic Mg^{2+}; depending on the concentration gradient, Mg^{2+} leaves the cell and is washed out of the myocardium at the moment of postischemic reperfusion or even during ischemia if there is a residual, noncoronary, collateral blood flow {14,55}.

In light of the above-mentioned considerations, it follows that $[Mg^{2+}]_o$ in cardioplegia should not be lower than the physiological free cytoplasmic concentration of Mg^{2+} in order to prevent myocardial magnesium loss as a result of ischemia, that cardioplegia involving very high doses of $[Mg^{2+}]_o$ may lead to crisis because of its Ca-displacing and membrane-destabilizing effects {18}, but that the optimum level changes as a result of accompanying ionic conditions and therefore must be evaluated in each specific case.

Reduction of *sodium* and *calcium* in the extracellular myocardial compartment to about cytoplasmic concentrations causes cessation of the electrical as well as mechanical activity of the heart muscle cell and induces diastolic cardiac arrest. By contrast, exclusive reduction of $[Na]_o$ causes an increase of myocardial tonus, the degree of which correlates with the quotient $[Ca^{2+}]_o:[Na]_o^2$ or even $[Ca^{2+}]_o:[Na]_o^4$. The reason for this increase of tonus is the increase of intracellular Ca^{2+} concentration, above all via the sarcolemmal Na-Ca exchange system {10,31,36}. In terms of the artificial induction of diastolic cardiac arrest, reduction of $[Na]_o$ to about 1/10 of physiological values, therefore, calls for a reduction of $[Ca^{2+}]_o$ to $1/10^2$ or even $1/10^4$ in order to minimize myocardial energy demand. This is true even though the efficacy of $[Ca^{2+}]_o$ at a given $[Na]_o$ level depends, within certain limits, on the simultaneous concentration of other ions, e.g., $[K]_o$ and especially $[Mg^{2+}]_o$, that interfere with Ca^{2+} {28,40}.

In addition to its role in the activation of the contractile system, calcium plays a decisive part in stabilizing and preserving the structural and functional integrity of myocardial sarcolemmal membranes {12,33}. The critical minimum of $[Ca^{2+}]_o$ in this context is given by various authors as $15–50\,\mu M$ {1,12}. Reduction of $[Ca^{2+}]_o$ below this minimum as a result of a longer-lasting coronary perfusion with calcium-free perfusate or solutions containing Ca-binding (citrate) or Ca-displacing (Mg) additives creates a predisposition to the so-called calcium paradox {37}: irreversible destruction of the organ during reintroduction of calcium after critical minimization of $[Ca^{2+}]_o$. The risk of calcium paradox is significantly lower if, in addition to $[Ca^{2+}]_o$, $[Na]_o$ is also reduced in the coronary perfusate {37}. Binding of calcium at the sarcolemma as well as in the cellular compartment of the myocardium, is enhanced at a $[Na]_o$ level of less than about 25 mM; even longer-lasting coronary perfusion under these conditions does not reduce the calcium concentration per unit of weight of myocardial tissue {4,10,31,40}. Nevertheless, the risk of induction of the calcium paradox is not eliminated.

From the point of view of cardioplegia, the optimal value of $[Ca^{2+}]_o$ has to be sufficiently low to bring about reversible inactivation of Ca-dependent energy consumers in the myocardium, but only so low as to guarantee a definite safety margin against the risk of calcium paradox. The absolute value of $[Ca^{2+}]_o$ is again a function of accompanying $[Na]_o$, $[K]_o$, and especially $[Mg^{2+}]_o$ levels, and has to be experimentally determined.

RESULTS

Under homogeneously aerobic conditions, the energy demand of the heart is revealed by its oxygen consumption, MVO_2.

A comparison of MVO_2 of the fibrillating and the cardioplegically arrested heart (fig. 38-2) makes it evident that (a) each of the cardioplegic solutions discussed above reduces MVO_2 to a similar degree, (b) MVO_2 takes place on a lower order of magnitude under cardioplegic conditions than during ventricular fibrillation, (c) MVO_2 in the fibrillating heart varies to a much higher degree than in the cardioplegically arrested one, and (d) myocardial temperature influences MVO_2 of the fibrillating heart to a distinctively higher degree than MVO_2 of the cardioplegically arrested one. MVO_2 during cardioplegia under normothermia is about 1/8, under hypothermia at 25°C 1/6, and under hypothermia of 15°C 1/5 of MVO_2 during fibrillation at the same temperatures (fig. 38-2).

The anaerobic energy demand of the heart is assumed to be identical with the anaerobic energy turnover, E, of the myocardium. E is the result of the amount of high-energy phosphate bonds ($\triangle\sim P$) supplied, on the one hand, glycolytically by metabolism of glycogen to lactate — around $1.5 \times \triangle$lactate — on the other hand, by metabolism of CP and ATP content of the myocardium:

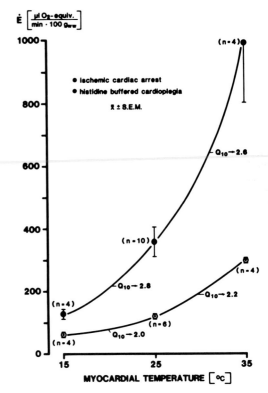

Fig. 38-3. Myocardial temperature and the anaerobic energy turnover E during t-ATP in ischemically and cardioplegically arrested canine hearts.

$$E = (1.5 \,\triangle\text{lactate} + \triangle\sim P): \triangle t.$$

In order to compare this with the preischemic aerobic energy demand of the heart, E can even be expressed in terms of O_2-equivalents per time by correcting the results for a mean ATP/O quotient of 3.0. Comparing the so-calculated E of the ischemically and the cardioplegically arrested heart (fig. 38-3), it can be shown that (a) E under both conditions is significantly lower than preischemic MVO_2; (b) the three cardioplegic solutions discussed above all reduce E to a comparable degree; (c) E in the cardioplegically arrested heart at normothermia as well as under hypothermic conditions is on a lower order of magnitude than in the ischemically arrested one; (d) E in the ischemically arrested heart varies to a clearly higher degree than in the cardioplegically pretreated one; (e) the temperature dependence of E in the untreated ischemic myocardium is much higher than that in the cardioplegically arrested one.

The results discussed above support the hypothesis that myocardial energy demand is above all a function of the activity of the contractile system and consequently that it can be lowered to a comparable degree by fundamentally different methods of inducing diastolic cardiac arrest. In addition, they show that preischemic cardioplegic coronary perfusion is an effective way of equalizing the individually variable levels of preischemic energy demand and therefore of equalizing E during during global ischemia.

Maximization of myocardial energy reserves

From the point of view of ischemia tolerance, the following can be drawn on within certain limits as energy reserves for the ischemic myocardium: (a) the O_2 content, (b) the concentration of high-energy phosphates, and (c) the concentration of glycogen.

Cardiac O_2-*reserves* at the moment of coronary circulatory arrest total about $1.0-1.2\,ml/100\,g$ ventricular tissue; they consist of $0.5-0.6\,ml\;O_2/100\,g$ in the form of oxymyoglobine plus about $0.5\,ml\;O_2/100\,g$ in the form of oxyhemoglobine plus about $0.1\,ml\;O_2/100\,g$ in the form of physically dissolved oxygen; even in the fibrillating or empty beating heart, these reserves are exhausted within $8-12$ seconds (fig. 38-2). Myocardial O_2 reserves can be effectively increased by means of enhancement of the physically dissolved fraction. Nevertheless, these reserves remain of minor importance in relation to the total practically usable revival time, t-ATP, of the ischemic heart, as the following calculations show: Lowering myocardial temperature to 5°C and increasing p_{O_2} to $700\,mmHg$ increases the fraction of physically dissolved O_2 to about $3\,ml/100\,g$ of tissue; if at the same time MVO_2 amounts to ca. $0.1\,ml/min/100\,g$, as in the cardioplegically arrested heart (fig. 38-2), O_2 reserves would at the most allow for an aerobic latency period of about $35-40$ minutes; in relation to the totally usable t-ATP under these conditions (compare fig. 38-4), this would mean a gain of no more than about 5%. Quite apart from these quantitative considerations, it is still unknown what side effects can be expected from high partial pressures of O_2 under conditions of ischemia and minimal MVO_2 in the myocardium {53}.

The *high-energy phosphates* CP and ATP in the myocardium cannot be called on as energy reserves in the strict sense of the word. Within certain limits, levels of these phosphates are lowered by increasing pumping performance of the heart {38}; at the same time preservation of ultrastructure and capacity for functional performance presupposes the concentration found under aerobic conditions {5,6,7,16}. Within the physiological range of variation, however, cardioplegic coronary perfusion and mechanical relief of the heart muscle result in almost complete shift within the high-energy phosphate pool in favor of conservation of energy. Therefore, in hearts arrested by aortic cross clamping, the initial concentrations of CP and ATP are, as a rule, lower than following cardioplegic coronary perfusion (figs. 38-1 and 38-5).

In the nonaltered heart, *reserves of glycogen*, which, with regard to the yield of ATP under unaerobic conditions, is the most favorable substrate for glycolysis, are never the factor limiting t-ATP under the conditions of pure ischemic cardiac arrest or ischemia following cardioplegia by any of the methods currently in clinical use (fig. 38-5, table 38-1; Kirklin's cardioplegic solution is supplemented by glucose). In the case of preischemic chronic hypoxia of the myocardium, the situation could be dif-

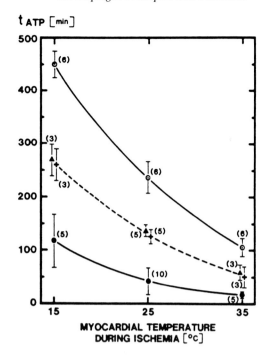

Fig. 38-4. Importance of myocardial temperature and method of cardiac arrest for the length of practically usable revival time, t-ATP, of the globally ischemic canine heart. ● ischemic cardiac arrest; + Kirklin's cardioplegia; ▲ St. Thomas's cardioplegia; ○ Bretschneider's cardioplegia. $\bar{x} \mp SEM$.

ferent {41}; nevertheless, up to now all of the methods applied immediately prior to ischemia in order to increase myocardial glycogen content simultaneously increase the aerobic and anaerobic energy turnover of the heart and thus reduce the otherwise attainable myocardial revival time {29}. It remains to be clarified whether this effect can be delayed by more specific selection of substrate or pharmacological support of metabolic intervention.

Optimization of myocardial energy supply

The efficiency of metabolic energy yield, η, is not a constant under either aerobic or anaerobic conditions and, to a certain extent, is open to influence. η of oxidative energy metabolism is quantified as the ration $\Delta \sim P/\Delta O$; it varies depending on the preferentially metabolized substrate. In keeping with theoretical considerations and in-vitro results, the greatest change in the $\Delta \sim P/\Delta O$ quotient results from the switch from oxidation of free fatty acids to oxydation of glycogen; $\Delta \sim /\Delta O$ under these conditions increases by about 20%, from around 2.7 to 3.2 {2,24}. Although the effect in vivo is necessarily more limited because substrate supply is always more or less mixed, an increase of η during aerobic energy gain is, in principle, one way of extending the aerobic latency period during global myocardial ischemia. From a quantitative point of view, however, extending the aerobic latency period even

TISSUE METABOLITES
$[\mu mol/g_{ww}]$

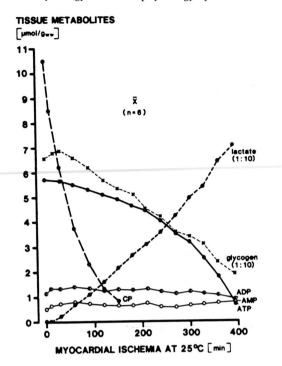

MYOCARDIAL ISCHEMIA AT 25°C $[min]$

Fig. 38-5. Left ventricular canine myocardium during global ischemia at 25°V: High-energy phosphates, glycogen, and lactate following cardioplegia with Bretschneider's solution.

η DURING t_{ATP} [%]

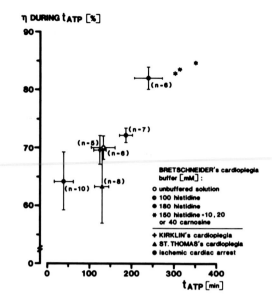

Fig. 38-6. Left ventricular canine myocardium during global ischemia at 25°C: Effect of different methods of artificial cardiac arrest on the mean energetic efficiency, η, of anaerobic glycolysis during t-ATP $\bar{x} \mp$ SD.

by the maximum of 20% is insignificant in terms of the total usable revival time, t-ATP, of the heart.

During anaerobiosis, glycolysis is the only effective pathway of ATP gain. Therefore, under such conditions the efficiency of metabolic energy yield, η, can be given as

$$\eta = 1.5\, \Delta lactate : (1.5\, \Delta lactate + \Delta \sim P).$$

The efficiency of glycolytic energy yield under conditions of pure global ischemia as well as under conditions of global ischemia following preischemic cardioplegia in accordance with Kirklin's or St. Thomas's solution (table 38-1), reaches no more than about 65–70% of anaerobic energy turnover (fig. 38-6), and the adaptation of glycolytic energy supply to anaerobic energy turnover therefore always leaves a deficit of at least 30–35%. The only way to effectively increase η of anaerobic energy metabolism appears to be through an artificial enhancement of myocardial buffering capacity, β, of the globally ischemic heart (fig. 38-6).

The question of an artificial increase of β in the myocardium in order to prevent development of ischemia-caused myocardial acidosis {17} raises two considerations: (a) the need to identify the pH range in need of buffering; and (b) the need to evaluate the quantitative determinants of an increase of β. As can be deduced from the physiological cytoplasmic pH of around 7.0 {17}, the known specific sensitivity of myocardial function to alkalosis {48}, and the marked limitation of the capacity of certain key

enzymes of glycolysis at pH values near 6.0 {29}, the pH range of the globally ischemic heart under consideration for enhancement of buffer capacity lies between 7.0 and 6.0. Thus, from the point of view of β, only buffer substances with a pk of around 6.5 should be appropriate. The potential increase of myocardial buffer capacity is additionally limited by the fact that, for osmotic reasons, only the extracellular compartment of the heart muscle can be used for introducing buffering substances. Buffer substances that can reach the cellular compartment in significant amounts necessarily cause cellular edema because of the accompanying osmotic water shift. Limited to extracellular space, and even under conditions of maximal use of this compartment by means of an optimal equilibration with the buffer solution, the increase of β per unit of weight myocardium reaches only 20–25% of β per unit of weight of buffer solution. Because the non-bicarbonate buffer capacity of the myocardium under physiological conditions amounts to between 20 and 30 mM of H^+ per kilogram of tissue and pH unit {17,48}, it follows that in order to double β of the myocardial tissue between pH 7.0 and 6.0 with a buffer system of pk 6.5 one would need a buffer solution of approximately 100 mM, but that with a buffer system of pk 5.5 one would need a solution well over 200 mM.

Given these quantitative considerations, it follows that an effective preischemic increase of myocardial buffer capacity can be achieved at present only in combination with the cardioplegic principle of reduction of $[Na]_o$ and $[Ca^{2+}]_o$ to about cytoplasmic concentrations (table 38-1), since only such a cardioplegic solution offers the necessary osmotic margin. The buffering system histidine/histidine-hydrochloride (his/his-HCl), presently being used, because of its low pk_2 of about 5.9 at 35°C, 6.1 at 25°C, and 6.3 at 15°C, is far from being an ideal system for buffering the pH range between 7.0 and 6.0; up to now, however, it seems to be the only one which, even in concentrations of more than 150 mM, does not cause any negative side effects, even in the ischemic myocardium.

RESULTS

The main effect of a preischemic increase of myocardial β, as well as quantitative calculations based on the limitations of an artificial increase of β in the myocardium, have been experimentally verified. During global ischemia following preischemic cardioplegic coronary perfusion with a low-sodium, low-calcium solution supplemented by increasing concentrations of the buffering system his/his-HCl, the following changes have been shown to take place in anaerobic energy metabolism parameters: (a) the rate of acidification in the extracellular compartment of the ischemic myocardium, expressed in terms of the time interval during which extracellular pH, pH_O, decreases from preischemic initial values down to 6.0 (t-pH), changes proportionally to the respective β of the cardioplegic solution used (fig. 38-7). Interestingly, however, during untreated global ischemia, as well as during ischemia following cardioplegia according to the Kirklin or St. Thomas's hospital method, t-pH, in keeping with the comparable β of the respective extracellular medium, is about equally long, but in comparison with t-pH after car-

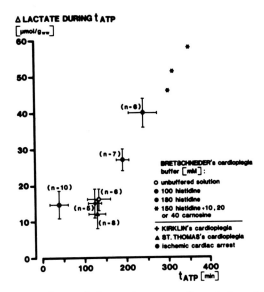

Fig. 38-8. Left ventricular canine myocardium during global ischemia at 25°C: Effect of different methods of artificial cardiac arrest on the formation of lactate during t-ATP. $\bar{x} \mp$ SD.

dioplegia with the histidine-free low-sodium, low-calcium solution is significantly shorter {18}. (b) increasing β of the low-sodium, low-calcium cardioplegic solution is followed by an extension of flux in anaerobic glycolysis and lactate production and by a proportional prolongation of revival time, t-ATP (fig. 38-8). This means that η of anaerobic energy metabolism is increased without a simultaneous increase in the anaerobic energy turnover, E, of the heart (fig. 38-6). Maximal supplementation of the low-sodium, low-calcium cardioplegic solution with histidine effects an increase of the mean value of η during t-ATP by about 20%, in comparison with pure global ischemia as well as with ischemia following Kirklin's or St. Thomas' cardioplegia, or even cardioplegic coronary perfusion with Bretschneider's unbuffered solution. At the same time, t-ATP is nearly doubled (figs. 38-6 and 38-8).

In summary, these results support the hypothesis that the limitation of glycolytic energy gain in the ischemic myocardium could be a manifestation of a specific pH dependence of certain key enzymes involved in anaerobic energy metabolism {29}, thus invalidating the thesis that η of anaerobic energy gain in normally aerobic organs or organisms is a natural constant {29}.

CARDIOPLEGIA: CORRELATIONS BETWEEN ENERGY STATE, ULTRASTRUCTURE, AND POSTISCHEMIC REVIVABILITY OF THE HEART

With the considerable increase in the length of revival time, t-ATP (fig. 38-4), experimental global ischemia at a mean myocardial temperature of 23°C for 210 minutes following Kirklin's or St. Thomas's cardioplegia, or for 300 minutes following Bretscheider's cardioplegia (table 38-1),

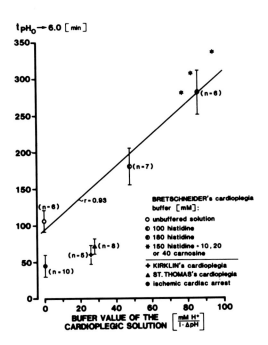

Fig. 38-7. Left ventricular canine myocardium during global ischemia at 25°C: Effect of different methods of artificial cardiac arrest on the rapidity of extracellular acidification, t-pH. $\bar{x} \mp$ SD.

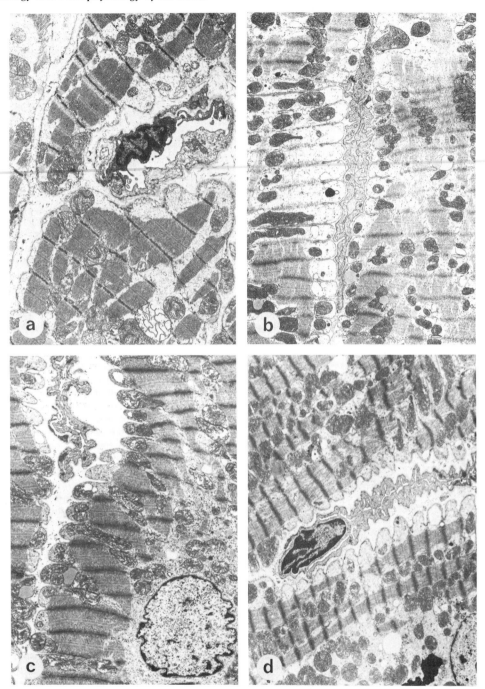

Fig. 38-9. St. Thomas's cardioplegia ultrastructure of left ventricular subendocardium in the canine heart (**a**) after preischemic cardioplegic coronary perfusion and global ischemia that reduced the myocardial ATP concentration to 4 μM/g wet weight; (**b**) after 20 minutes postischemic recovery following preischemic cardioplegic coronary perfusion and 210 minutes global ischemia at 22°C that reduced myocardial ATP to 4 μM/g wet weight; (**c**) after 20 minutes postischemic recovery following multidose cardioplegia by one preischemic and three intraischemic cardioplegic coronary perfusions and in total 210 minutes global ischemia at 13°C that reduced myocardial ATP to 5 μM/g wet weight; (**d**) after 20 minutes postcardioplegic recovery following 60 minutes continuous cardioplegic coronary perfusion at 5°C without ischemia. Original magnification ×7000.

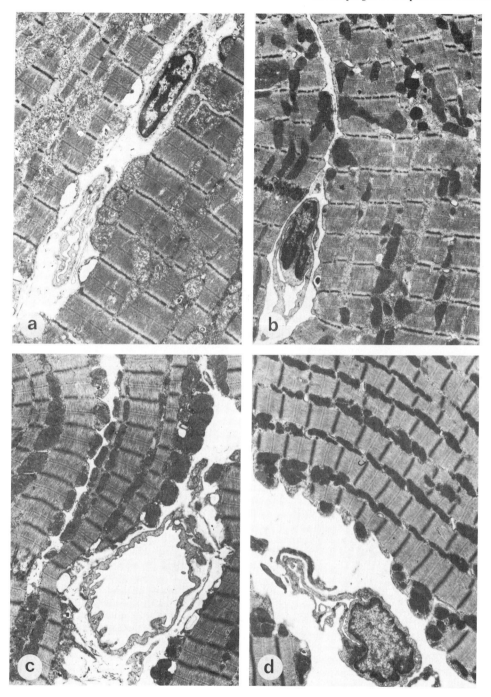

Fig. 38-10. Bretschneider's cardioplegia: Left ventricular subendocardium in the canine heart (**a**) after preischemic cardioplegic coronary perfusion and global ischemia that reduced the myocardial ATP content to 4 μM/g wet weight; (**b**) after 20 minutes post-ischemic recovery following preischemic cardioplegic coronary perfusion and 300 minutes global ischemia at 22°C that reduced myocardial ATP to 4 μM/g wet weight; (**c**) after 20 minutes postischemic recovery following multidose cardioplegia by one preischemic and three intraischemic cardioplegic coronary perfusions and in total 300 minutes global ischemia at 17°C that reduced myocardial ATP to 5 μM/g wet weight; (**d**) after 20 minutes postischemic recovery following 80 minutes continuous cardioplegic coronary perfusion at 10°C without ischemia. Original magnification ×7000.

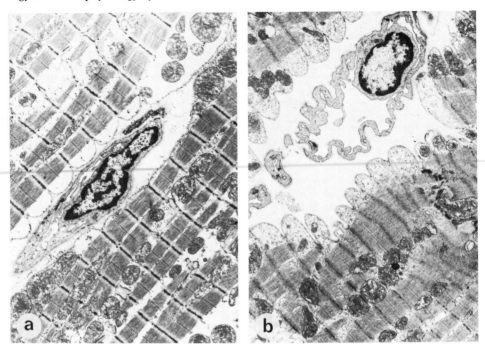

Fig. 38-11. Bretschneider's cardioplegic solution supplemented by 50 μM of Ca^{2+}. Ultrastructure of left ventricular subendocardium in the canine heart (**a**) after preischemic cardioplegic coronary perfusion and global ischemia that reduced the myocardial ATP concentration to 4 μM/g wet weight. (**b**) After 20 minutes postischemic recovery following preischemic cardioplegic coronary perfusion and 300 minutes global ischemia at 22°C that reduced the myocardial ATP concentration to 4 μM/g wet weight. Original magnification ×7000. For details see text.

is spontaneously reversible in dog hearts. However, detailed analysis of the ultrastructure of the left ventricular subendocardium (a) during global ischemia at the critical left ventricular ATP concentration of 4 μM/g wet weight and (b) after 20 minutes of recovery following this critical ischemic stress, reveals greatly differing degrees of alteration and capacity for postischemic regeneration of fine structure, depending on the cardioplegic solution applied prior to ischemia {8,19,20,49,54}. This raises the question of whether the close correlation that has been shown to exist in the untreated globally ischemic heart between energy state and degree of preservation of ultrastructure as well as revivability can be suspended by specific cardioplegic interventions, or whether there are additional factors besides energy state that influence structural preservation and revivability but that, because of the rapidity of damage and the high degree of deviation of all experimental results, cannot reliably be detected in pure global ischemia.

Figures 38-9A, 38-10A, and 38-11A show the state of left ventricular ultrastructure following preischemic cardioplegic coronary perfusion with St. Thomas's solution, Bretschneider's solution, and Bretschneider's solution supplemented by 50 μM of Ca^{2+}, and following an ischemic stress that in all cases reduced the mean ATP concentration of the left ventricular myocardium to 4 μM/g wet

weight; figs. 38-9B, 38-10B, and 38-11B illustrate the respective states of ultrastructure after 20 minutes of recovery from cardioplegia and the critical impact of ischemia: The photographs of myocardial specimens taken during ischemia differ from one another in several respects, but there is a noticeable contrast in the degree of intracellular edema; cellular water content following application of Bretschneider's Ca^{2+}-supplemented cardioplegic solution {20}, and even with St. Thomas's cardioplegia {54}, is significantly higher than in the case of Bretschneider's classical solution. Reperfusion and reoxygenation at this stage of ischemic stress therefore leads to different reactions in myocardial fine structure depending on the cardioplegic solution used: Following cardioplegia by the classic Bretschneider method, the mitochondria again look dark, the contractile system is homogeneously contracted, and there are no signs of cellular edema; by contrast, following Ca^{2+}-supplemented Bretschneider cardioplegia, as well as after cardioplegia according to the St. Thomas's method, mitochondria exhibit restoration deficits, cellular edema shows scarcely any decrease, and the state of the contractile system is very non-homogeneous, with overcontracted and overdistended areas, even after 20 minutes of postischemic recovery.

Supplementing the information gained from these investigations with two further experimental models allows us, within certain limits, to determine whether the very different degrees of preservation and restorability of myocardial ultrastructure at identically reduced mean myocardial ATP concentration are the result of specific characteristics of the preischemically applied cardioplegic solution or whether they are the result of incompatibility reactions, especially of the ischemically altered myocardium, that run counter to certain of the principles assumed in cardioplegia. The first model involves reperfusion of the heart after intermittently repeated application of the respective cardioplegic solution in the course of global ischemia, so-called multidose cardioplegia, as opposed to the single-dose cardioplegia discussed above {18,19}. The second model involves reperfusion after longer-lasting continuous cardioplegic coronary perfusion without ischemia.

Intermittently repeated cardioplegic coronary perfusion, as compared to single-dose cardioplegia with subsequent continuous global ischemia, is accompanied by reduction of ischemic stress, even if the length of ischemia is the same, since the procedure induces a lower mean myocardial temperature during ischemia, on the one hand, and, on the other hand, leads to simultaneous, intermittent aerobiosis and washout of metabolites of anaerobic metabolism such as H^+ and lactate. Figures 38-9C and 38-10C show the effects of the intermittent procedure using St. Thomas's solution and Bretschneider's classic solution, whereas figs. 38-9D and 38-10D illustrate the effects of the same cardioplegic solutions under conditions of continuous application without ischemia. In summary, electron microscopic investigation shows that (a) in the case of the classic Bretschneider cardioplegic solution, multidose cardioplegia not only reduces ischemic stress but further enhances postischemic recovery of myocardial fine structure in comparison with single-dose application and subsequent continuous global ischemia; myocardial mitochondria now exhibit the typical matrix granules of aerobically working heart muscle. Continuous application of this cardioplegic solution for 80 minutes at a mean rate of coronary flow of 150 ml/min/100 g of ventricular weight at 10°C does not bring about ultrastructural alterations in the heart, even after 20 minutes of postcardioplegic reprefusion using a medium of physiological extracellular electrolyte composition, (b) by comparison, intermittent application of St. Thomas's cardioplegic solution, in spite of reduction of ischemic stress, causes intracellular myocardial edema that is, however, less pronounced than following recovery after single-dose application of this same solution; it is, moreover, followed by remarkable alterations of the fine structure of myocardial mitochondria, alterations that are more striking than after single-dose cardioplegia and an identical period of postischemic recovery. The state of contraction of the contractile system is comparably nonhomogeneous following both multidose and single-dose application of the solution. Sixty minutes of continuous coronary perfusion with St. Thomas's cardioplegic solution, again at a mean flow rate of 150 ml/min/100 g of ventricular weight, but at 5°C, and after 20 minutes of postcardioplegic recovery, provides for noticeably better preservation of myocardial fine structure than does single-dose or multidose application and ischemia; nevertheless, even under these experimental conditions, the cardiomyocytes show cellular edema.

In conclusion, the results described must be regarded as indicating: (a) that the principle of cardioplegia by reduction of $[Na]_o$ in combination with an equivalent reduction of $[Ca^{2+}]_o$ and high extracellular buffering by the buffering system his/his-HCl not only substantially extends revival time as defined by left ventricular ATP concentration, but also preserves myocardial fine structure as well as the capacity for postischemic regeneration to a degree that allows us to retain the criterion of minimal left ventricular ATP concentration for revivability of the heart that was determined primarily under conditions of pure global ischemia. The correlation between energy state, structural preservation, and revivability, even under longer-lasting continuous or intermittent application of the cold solution, is not suspended; (b) that supplementing the above-mentioned cardioplegic solution with otherwise critically minimal Ca^{2+} concentration does not affect t-ATP {20}, but during the early stage of a global ischemic impact does alter the volume-regulating mechanisms of the cardiomyocytes to a significant degree, thus detracting from the spontaneous revivability of the heart; (c) that the cardioplegic principle of increase of $[Mg^{2+}]_o$, in combination with a high level of $[K]_o$ and procaine, as realized in the St. Thomas's method, seems to affect the mechanism of cellular volume regulation, even without accompanying global ischemia. The resulting cellular edema, however, increases simultaneously with the ischemic stress of the myocardium. In addition, intermittent application of this cardioplegic solution seems to interfere specifically with myocardial mitochondria, resulting in a markedly delayed, postischemic recovery of oxidative metabolism and energy gain. The cardioplegic principle of increasing $[Mg^{2+}]_o$ and $[K]_o$ supplemented with procaine, as it is realized in the St. Thomas's solution, as well as the Ca^{2+}-supplemented cardioplegic solution of Bretschneider changes the interrelationship between energy state and degree of structural preservation and consequently also the interrelationship between energy state and postischemic revivability of the heart. In comparison with untreated global ischemia, the change is in the direction of a higher critical minimum ATP concentration in the left ventricular myocardium.

CARDIOPLEGIA: UNRESOLVED QUESTIONS AND OUTLOOK

The attempt to interpret the experimental results discussed above leads to the formulation of, on the one hand, unresolved questions with regard to the factors limiting ischemia tolerance in primarily aerobic organs like the heart, and, on the other hand, to the drawing of practical consequences from the surprisingly loose correlation between energy state, ultrastructure, and revivability of the heart, particularly with a view to the fundamental possibilities of further development of organ protection against global ischemia.

First of all, it seems necessary to recognize that the relevancy of energetics for structural and functional integrity of the myocardium is not invalidated as a consequence of an inconstant interrelationship between these factors. The finding indicates only that the actual mean concentration of ATP in the left ventricular myocardium, and consequently even a mean actual energy charge potential from the mean concentrations of adenine nucleotide phosphates in the tissue {2,26}, is not an adequate parameter of myocardial energy state under conditions of global ischemia. The same discrepancy would be found if, on the one hand, specific functions of the heart muscle cell were altered prior to ischemia, or if, on the other hand, the availability of high-energy phosphates for undoubtedly different cellular users of ATP were not guaranteed {16,21,35,38}. It is quite conceivable, for example, that the ATP demand of specific cellular users is dependent on preischemic conditions, i.e., that it differs depending on the type of anesthesia used {52}, hormonal state {6}, or pharmacological pretreatment {43}, or even on the cardioplegic approach adopted prior to ischemia. This could also account for the widely differing results with regard to the factors limiting ischemia tolerance of the heart or the heart muscle cell, even in the normal, healthy state. From the point of view of ischemia tolerance of the whole organ at the cellular level under such conditions, the structural and functional state of the sarcolemma are especially important {5}, because when postischemic reperfusion begins, this cellular structure cannot draw upon latent potential for recovery without placing great demands on all functionally subordinated, subcellular structures and thus placing at risk their postischemic recovery and revivability.

For the present, the practical consequences of these considerations in terms of the examination or development of methods for prolonging ischemia tolerance can be defined as follows {19}:
1. The need for simultaneous analysis of parameters of energy metabolism, fine structure, and function before, during, and following global ischemia, and
2. The need for experimental proof of the principles of cardioplegia under highly standardized but principally different conditions of application. Complex initial conditions, for example, with regard to temperature, premedication, predamage, but even with regard to nonstandardized modes of application of a cardioplegic solution or the supplementation of an experimentally tested solution by further cardioplegic additives, all result in an increase of unintelligibility in the discussion of cardioplegia and increased risk with regard to reversibility in practice.

REFERENCES

1. Alto LE, Dhalla NS: Role of changes in microsomal calcium uptake in the effects of reperfusion of Ca^{2+}-deprived rat hearts. *Circ Res* 48:17–24, 1981.
2. Atkinson DE: *Cellular Energy Metabolism and its Regulation.* New York, San Francisco: Academic Press, 1977.
3. Baller D, Bretschneider HJ, Hellige G: Validity of myocardial oxygen consumption parameters. *Clin Cardiol* 2: 317–327, 1979.
4. Blaustein MP: The interrelationship between sodium and calcium fluxes across cell membranes. *Rev Physiol Biochem Pharmacol* 70:33–82, 1974.
5. Bretschneider HJ: Überlebenszeit und Wiederbelebungszeit des Herzens bei Normo- und Hypothermie. *Verh Dtsch Ges Kreislaufforsch* 30:11–34, 1964.
6. Bretschneider HJ, Gebhard MM, Preusse CJ: Reviewing the pros and cons of myocardial preservation within cardiac surgery. In: Longmore DB (ed) *Towards Safer Cardiac Surgery.* Lancaster: MTP, 1981, pp 21–53.
7. Bretschneider HJ, Hellige G: Pathophysiologie der ventrikelkontraktion — Kontraktilität, Inotropie, Suffizienzgrad und Arbeitsökonomie des Herzens. *Verh Dtsch Ges Kreislaufforsch* 42:14–30, 1976.
8. Bretschneider HJ, Gebhard MM, Gersing E, Presusse CJ, Schnabel PhA: Recent advances for myocardial protection. In: Kaplitt MJ, Borman JB (eds) *Concepts and Controversies in Cardiovascular Surgery.* Norwalk, CT: Appleton-Century-Crofts, 1983, pp 174–185.
9. Buckberg GD, Brazie JR, Nelson RL, Goldstein SM, McConnell DH, Cooper N: Studies on the effects of hypothermia on regional myocardial blood flow and metabolism during cardiopulmonary bypass. I. The adequately perfused beating, fibrillating, and arrested heart. *J Thorac Cardiovasc Surg* 73:87–94, 1977.
10. Chapman RA, Coray A, McGuigan JAS: Sodium-calcium exchange in mamalian heart: The maintenance of low intracellular calcium concentration. In: Drake-Holland AJ, Noble MIM (eds) *Cardiac Metabolism.* Chichester. New York: John Wiley & Sons, 1983, pp 117–149.
11. Clark BJ, Chu D, Aellig WH: Ergot alkaloids and related componds: Action on the heart and circulation. In: *Ergot Alkaloids and Related Compounds. Handbook of Experimental Pharmacology*, Vol 49. Berlin: Springer, 1978, pp 321–420.
12. Crevey BJ, Langer GA, Frank JS: Role of Ca^{2+} in maintenance of rabbit myocardial cell membrane structural and functional integrity. *J Mol Cell Cardiol* 10:1081–1100, 1978.
13. Dawson RMC, Hauser H: Binding of calcium to phospholipids. In: Cuthbert (ed) *Calcium and Cellular Function.* London: Macmillan, 1970, pp 17–41.
14. Ebel H, Günther T: Role of magnesium in cardiac disease. *J Clin Chem Clin Biochem* 16:249–265, 1983.
15. Fabiato A, Fabiato F: Calcium release from the sarcoplasmic reticulum. *Circ Res* 40:119–129, 1977.
16. Fleckenstein A: Die Bedeutung der energiereichen Phosphate für Kontraktilität und Tonus des Myokards. *Verh Dtsch Ges Inn Med* 70:81–99, 1964.
17. Garlick PB, Radda GK, Seeley PJ: Studies of acidosis in the ischaemic heart by phosphorus nuclear magnetic resonance. *Biochem J* 184:547–554, 1979.
18. Gebhard MM: Pathophysiologie der globalen Ischamic des Herzens. *Z Kardiol* 76(Suppl 4):115–129, 1987.
19. Gebhard MM, Bretschneider HJ, Gersing E, Preusse CJ, Schnabel PhA: Bretschneider's histidine-buffered cardioplegic solution: Concept — application — efficiency. In: Roberts A (ed) *Myocardial Protection in Cardiac Surgery.* New York: Marcel Dekker, 1987, pp 95–119.
20. Gebhard MM, Gersing E, Brockhoff CJ, Schnabel PhA, Bretschneider HJ: Impedance spectroscopy: A method for surveillance of ischemia tolerance of the heart. *Thorac Cardiovasc Surg* 35, 1987.
21. Gudbjarnason S, Mathes P, Ravens KG: Functional compartmentation of ATP and creatine phosphate in heart muscle. *J Mol Cell Cardiol* 1:325–330, 1970.
22. Hasselbach W, Fassold E, Migala A, Rauch B: Magnesium

dependence of sarcoplasmic reticulum calcium transport. *Fed Proc* 40:2657–2661, 1981.

23. Hearse DJ, Braimbridge MV, Jynge P: *Protection of the Ischemic Myocardium: Cardioplegia.* New York: Raven Press, 1981.

24. Hütter JF, Schweickhardt C, Piper HM, Spieckermann PG: Inhibition of fatty acid oxidation and decrease of oxygen consumption of working rat heart by 4-bromochrotonic acid. *J Mol Cell Cardiol* 16:105–108, 1984.

25. Jacobus WE, Tiozzo R, Lugli G, Lehninger AL, Carafoli E: Aspects of energy-linked calcium accumulation by rat heart mitochondria. *J Biol Chem* 250:7863–7870, 1975.

26. Kammermeier H, Schmidt P, Jüngling E: Free energy change of ATP-hydrolysis: A causal factor of early hypoxic failure of the myocardium. *J Mol Cell Cardiol* 14:267–277, 1982.

27. Kimelberg KH: Alterations in phospholipid-dependent $(Na^+ + K^+)$-ATPase activity due to lipid fluidity: Effects of cholesterol and Mg^{2+}. *Biochim Biophys Acta* 413:143–156, 1975.

28. Kovacs T, O'Donnell JM: An analysis of calcium-magnesium antagonism in contractility and ionic balance in isolated trabecular muscle of rat ventricle. *Pflügers Arch* 360:267–282, 1970.

29. Kübler W, Spieckermann PG: Regulation of glycolysis in the ischemic and the anoxic myocardium. *J Mol Cell Cardiol* 1:351–377, 1970.

30. Kübler W, Katz A: Mechanism of early "pump" failure of the ischemic heart: Possible role of adenosine triphosphate depletion and inorganic phosphate accumulation. *Am J Cardiol* 40:467–471, 1977.

31. Langer GA: Sodium-calcium exchange in the heart. *Ann Rev Physiol* 44:435–449, 1982.

32. Langer GA: Calcium at the sarcolemma. *J Mol Cell Cardiol* 16:147–153, 1984.

33. Langer GA: The effect of pH on cellular and membrane calcium binding and contraction of myocardium. *Circ Res* 57:374–382, 1985.

34. Lochner W, Arnold G, Müller-Ruchholtz ER: Metabolism of the artificially arrested and of the gas-perfused heart. *Am J Cardiol* 22:299–311, 1968.

35. Müller-Ruchholtz ER, Lochner W: Utilization of glycolytic energy for external heart work. *J Mol Cell Cardiol* 3:15–29, 1971.

36. Mullins LJ: The role of Na-Ca exchange in heart. In: Sperelakis N (ed) *Physiology and Pathophysiology of the Heart.* Boston: Martinus Nijhoff, 1984.

37. Nayler WG, Daly MJ: Calcium and the injured cardiac myocytes. In: Sperelakis N (ed) *Physiology and Pathophysiology of the Heart.* Boston: Martinus Nijhoff, 1984.

38. Opie LH: Substrate and energy metabolism of the heart. In: Sperelakis N (ed) *Physiology and Pathophysiology of the Heart.* Boston: Martinus Nijhoff, 1984.

39. Optiz E, Schneider M: Über die Sauerstoffversorgung des Gehirns und den Mechanismus von Mangelwirkungen. *Ergebn Physiol* 46:126–260, 1956.

40. Pang DC: Influence of cations and agents on sarcolemmal calcium binding. In: Tajuddinm M, Das PK, Tariq M, Dhalla NS (eds) *Advances in Myocardiology*, Vol 1. Baltimore, MD: University Park Press, 1980, pp 43–53.

41. Pick EP: Über das primum und ultimum moriens im Herzen. *Klin Wschr* 16:662–667, 1924.

42. Polimeni PhI, Page E: Magnesium in heart muscle. *Circ Res* 33:367–374, 1973.

43. Preusse CJ, Gebhard MM, Schnabel PhA, Ulbricht LJ, Bretschneider HJ: Post-ischemic myocardial function after pre-ischemic application of propranolol or verapamil. *J Cardiovasc Surg* 25:158–164, 1984.

44. Preusse CH, Winter J, Schulte HD, Bircks W: Energy demand of cardioplegically perfused human hearts. *J Cardiovasc Surg* 26:558–563, 1985.

45. Reimer KA, Jennings RB, Hill ML: Total ischemia in dog hearts in vitro: High energy phosphate depletion and associated defects in energy metabolism, cell volume regulation, and sarcolemmal integrity. *Circ Res* 4:901–911, 1981.

46. Reuter H, Scholz H: A study of the ion selectivity and the kinetic properties of the calcium dependent slow inward current in mammalian cardiac muscle. *J Physiol (Lond)* 264:17–47, 1977.

47. Rona G, Boutet M, Hüttner I: Membrane permeability alterations as manifestation of early cardiac muscle cell injury. In: Fleckenstein A, Rona G (ed) *Recent Advances in Studies on Cardiac Structure and Metabolism, Vol 6: Pathophysiology and Morphology of Myocardial Cell Alteration.* Baltimore, MD: University Park Press, 1975, pp 439–451.

48. Roos A, Boron WF: Intracellular pH: *Physiol Rev* 61:296–434, 1981.

49. Schnabel PhA, Gebhard MM, Pomykaj Th, Schmiedl A, Preusse CJ, Richter J, Bretschneider HJ: Myocardial protection: Left ventricular ultrastructure after different forms of cardiac arrest. *Thorac Cardiovasc Surg* 35:148–156, 1987.

50. Schuurmans Steckhoven F, Bonting SL: Transport adenosine triphosphatases: Properties and functions. *Physiol Rev* 61:1–76, 1981.

51. Shine KI: Myocardial effects of magnesium. *Amer J Physiol* 237:H413–H423, 1979.

52. Spieckermann PG, Kettler D: Effects of anaesthesia on myocardial tolerance to ischemia. *Int Anaesthesiol Clin* 12:51–81, 1974.

53. Vladimirov YA, Olenev VJ, Suslova TB, Cheremisina ZP: Lipid peroxidation in mitochondrial membrane. *Adv Lipid Res* 17:173–249, 1980.

54. Warnecke H, Hetzer R, Franz P, Borst HG: Standardized comparison of cardioplegic methods in the isolated paracorporeal dog heart. *Thorac Cardiovasc Surg* 28:322–328, 1980.

55. Wu ST, Pieper GM, Salhany JM, Eliot RS: Measurement of free magnesium in perfused and ischemically arrested heart muscle. A quantitative phosphorus-31 nuclear magnetic reasonance and multiequilibria analysis. *Biochemistry* 30: 7399–7403, 1981.

CHAPTER 39

Effects of the Volatile Anesthetic Agents on the Heart

MARGARET G. PRATILA & VASILIOS PRATILAS

INTRODUCTION

It took only just over a year after William Morton showed the feasibility of surgical anesthesia to demonstrate the marked effects of volatile anesthetic agents on the heart. On January 28, 1848, Hannah Greener, aged 15, was the first patient to die during chloroform anesthesia (presumably of ventricular fibrillation).

Increasing amounts of research at the cellular level and in intact animals, in addition to clinical studies, have emphasized this effect. The many hundreds of papers that have been written on the cardiac effects of the anesthetic agents and the many millions of dollars spent on monitoring the heart in the perioperative period attest to the importance of the effects of anesthetic agents on the heart.

One of the exciting advances in understanding the effects of anesthetic agents on the heart has been the application of microelectrode techniques of electrophysiology that allow us to study the effects of anesthetic agents on the cell uninfluenced by uncontrolled autonomic nervous system activity. It is to these studies that we shall mainly direct our attention. Anesthetic effects influencing the coronary circulation have also become increasingly important with the advent of coronary bypass surgery.

SINOATRIAL NODE

Hauswirth and Schaer {1} in 1967 described the effects of halothane on action potentials from single rabbit sinoatrial (SA) nodal fibers. They showed a decrease of the maximal diastolic potential (MDP) and a decreased rate of diastolic depolarization. These effects were confirmed by Reynolds and his colleagues {2}. At 1% concentration, halothane had a moderate negative chronotropic action on the SA nodal fibers. This was the result of a reduced rate of diastolic depolarization and an increase in threshold potential. At 2% halothane the rate of diastolic depolarization was further reduced and maximal diastolic potential, overshoot, and amplitude of the action potential were also decreased. At 4% halothane a progressive reduction in maximal diastolic potential, overshoot, and amplitude occurred. Arrest of the fiber followed. The arrest did not follow progressive slowing of rate, but was associated with

a marked loss of maximal diastolic potential, increase in the threshold potential, and ultimate loss of excitability. These fibers were unresponsive to electrical stimulation. The arrest was completely reversed when halothane was washed out. The effects are summarized in fig. 39-1.

Maylie et al. {3} have recently indicated that generation of the pacemaker potential in the SA node is related to the activation of an inward current with high equilibrium potential rather than decreasing potassium ion conductance. Kampine and his colleagues {4} have further examined the SA nodal suppression caused by halothane in the light of the findings of Maylie et al. Halothane has been shown to inhibit inward Ca^{2+} current through the slow ionic channel in myocardium, demonstrated by depression of the maximum rate of rise ($+V_{max}$) of the slow action potential {5}. The negative chronotropic action of halothane and the dose-dependent depression of $+V_{max}$ in phase 4 and phase 0 demonstrated by Kampine et al. are consistent with inhibition of slow calcium channels in the SA node. Introduction of calcium ($2\times$ concentration) produced a parallel shift in the dose-response curve in an upward direction and blunted the overall depression of phases 4 and 0. Introduction of a calcium channel blocker (verapamil) produced a parallel depression of the dose-response curve and potentiated depression of the heart rate and $+V_{max}$ of phase 0. It would appear that halothane interacts with calcium competitively.

Halothane 0.5% and initial exposure to 1% halothane resulted in hyperpolarization of the transmembrane potential in guinea pig and cat SA nodal fibers {6}. Initial exposure to 1.12% and 2.25% enflurane did not produce the same effect. Enflurane 2.25% and 4.50% produced a significant negative chronotropic action, an increase in the duration of phase 4, and a decreased rate of rise in phase 4. The rate of rise of phase 0 was decreased and the duration of the action potential was prolonged at 4.5% enflurane (fig. 39-2). The effects of enflurane are obviously less marked than those of halothane.

The clinical use of methoxyflurane has decreased markedly due to its adverse renal effects and its slow uptake and elimination. However, it is the prototype of the halogenated ethers. Reynolds and his coworkers {2} demonstrated a biphasic effect on the SA node. There is a decrease in rate that is preceded by a brief initial accelera-

HALOTHANE SA NODE

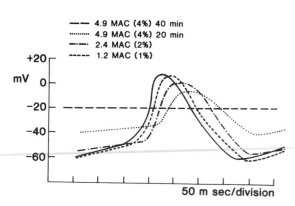

Fig. 39-1. A schematic presentation of the effects of halothane on the SA nodal action potential {1,2}. The effects of concentration and time are shown. MAC values allow comparison between agents.

SA NODE ENFLURANE

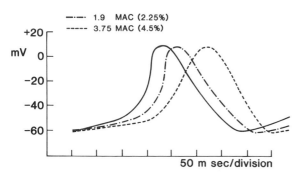

Fig. 39-2. A schematic presentation of the effects of enflurane on the SA nodal action potential {6}.

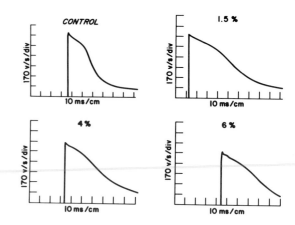

Fig. 39-3. The effects of enflurane on rabbit atrium at 1.5% (1.25 MAC), 4% (3.3 MAC), and 6% (5 MAC).

tion. This acceleration is due chiefly to a slight loss in maximal diastolic potential. It is not reversed by propranolol. The decrease in rate is associated with a further decrease in maximal diastolic potential and an increase in threshold potential. Overshoot is reduced. An arrest of activity invariably occurred at 1% methoxyflurance and frequently occurred at 0.5%. Arrest followed a loss of MDP, an increase in threshold potential, and finally a loss of excitability. As with the other volatile agents, this effect was reversible. When the rate was increased by epinephrine, exposure to methoxyflurane had little effect.

ATRIA

Hauswirth {7} has shown that single rabbit atrial fibers are not very sensitive to even 2% halothane. Although the

overshoot was significantly decreased and repolarization slightly prolonged, there was no marked change in resting potential or amplitude of the action potential, as is seen in the SA node. Similar effects are seen with 1% methoxyflurane {8}. Enflurane {9} also produced a decreased overshoot and prolonged repolarization, but 6% enflurane (a dose far in excess of clinical values) was necessary before a reduction in amplitude occurred. Resting potential was virtually unchanged (fig. 39-3).

Azari et al. {10} used left atrial guinea pig strips to quantitate the relative degree of myocardial depression with sevoflurane, halothane, and isoflurane, and also the degree of beta-adrenergic responsiveness to isoproterenol. They found least inotropic depression with sevoflurane and less blunting of the beta-adrenegic response.

Polic et al. {11} studied the relation between the automaticity of the sinoatrial node and subsidiary atrial pacemakers (SAP) using an isolated perfused canine right atrial preparation. Halothane 1% or 2% did not produce a significant pacemaker shift to the SAP sites. Increasing concentrations of epinephrine or norepinephrine produced shifts to the SAP sites. These shifts were not influenced by exposure to halothane. The authors concluded that epinephrine or norepinephrine augment the automaticity of subsidiary atrial pacemakers more than the SA node with or without halothane; also that ectopic atrial rhythms with halothane require epinephrine or augmented adrenergic tone.

Atrial arrhythmias are common manifestations of digitalis toxicity {12}. Polic et al. {13} found that increasing ouabain concentrations do not sufficiently enhance automaticity of SAP compared to the SA node to account for digitalis-induced atrial tachyarrhythmias. In preparations with borderline toxic ouabain concentrations, halothane favors pacemaker shifts from the SA node to sites of SAP and in some caused atrial electrical quiescence.

Increase in vagal tone protects against catecholamine/halothane-produced ventricular fibrillation in dogs {14}. Volatile anesthetic agents have also been shown to affect muscarinic receptor/G-protein coupling {15}. A major action of acetylcholine is to increase membrane K^+ conductance by muscarinic receptor stimulation {16}. This, in turn, may cause hyperpolarization and a reduced spontaneous pacemaker activity by lowering the slope of phase 4 of the pacemaker action potential. Acetylcholine shortens the effective refractory period of atrial cells {17} and slows impulse conduction in the AV node by a decrease in the inward Ca^{2+} current {18}. Seifen et al. {19} studied the chronotropic and inotropic effects of norepinephrine and acetylcholine alone and in the presence of halothane, enflurane, and isoflurane. They found that in isolated guinea pig atria these three anesthetics do not alter the effects of norepinephrine or acetylcholine, and do not induce arrhythmias.

ATRIOVENTRICULAR NODE

There is no doubt clinically that the presently used volatile anesthetic agents have a marked effect on the atrioventricular (AV) node. It is not uncommon to see P waves unrelated to QRS complexes on the monitoring ECG during anesthesia. With the termination of anesthesia there is termination of the dysrhythmia.

Scherlag et al. {20} and Damato et al. {21} described a method of studying AV nodal conduction in intact dogs by His bundle stimulation and recording. This His bundle electrogram allows subdivision of the PR interval into two components {22,23}. Conduction time between the atrial depolarization potential and the His bundle deflection (AH interval) primarily represents impulse propagation in the region of the AV node. Conduction to the distal bundle of His and Purkinje network (HV interval) is measured from the His deflection to the beginning of the QRS complex.

The effects of the anesthetic agents on AV nodal conduction have mainly been studied by His stimulation and recording. Atlee and Rusy {24}, in their initial studies utilizing catheter electrocardiography, found a concentration-dependent depression of AV conduction by halothane. This depression was most marked proximal to the bundle of His (intraatrial and AV node, AH recording). Since atropine did not significantly alter the effect of halothane, vagal stimulation was not felt to be a factor. Beta blockade with propranolol further slowed conduction, indicating sympathetic enhancement of AV conduction was present even at 2% halothane. Rapid atrial pacing also slowed conduction. The arrival of an impulse during the absolute refractory period with no transmission or during the relative refractory period when decremental conduction occurs was felt to be the probable cause. Prolongation of the refractory period was considered the most likely mechanism of halothane-produced depression of AV conduction.

In a later study {25}, Atlee and Alexander showed that an increased concentration of halothane prolonged AV nodal and His-Purkinje conduction time in spontaneously beating hearts in which heart rate was constant and rate did not influence conduction time. The functional refractory period was prolonged at slow heart rates (120 beats/min), but unaffected at rapid rates (200 beats/min).

Atlee et al. {26} also studied the effects of the antidysrhythmics lidocaine and diphenylhydantoin in the presence of halothane. There was further prolongation of AV conduction to that produced by halothane. AV conduction was more sensitive to drug effect than His-Purkinje or total intraventricular conduction. They believed this might represent potentiation of the normal slowing of conduction through the AV node in response to increases in heart rate (fatigue response). They concluded that the antidysrhythmics failed to reverse the depressant effects of halothane on AV conduction. This may explain their ineffectiveness in the treatment of certain dysrhythmia during halothane anesthesia.

The problem with these early studies is that light anesthesia with halothane was used as a control. In a more recent study, chronically instrumented dogs were used and the true awake-to-anesthetized state was obtained {27}. The results of these studies in producing prolongation of AV nodal conduction is more apparent at light levels of anesthesia (1%–1.5% halothane) and is more a function of changes in autonomic tone than of increasing concentration. Hantler and his colleagues {28} also studied halothane related to an "unanesthetized" control by using total spinal anesthesia. Sympathetic nervous system activity was thereby eliminated. AH interval was prolonged at fast rates following exposure to halothane, but not at slow rates.

In intact unpremedicated dogs, methoxyflurane produced a dose-dependent increase in the effective refractory period of the AV conduction system {29}. This was not influenced by vagotomy, which suggests the effect is independent of parasympathetic control.

Methoxyflurane is one of the few agents on which microelectrode studies are available. Reynolds et al. {8} showed that the activity of the AV node remained normal, even after complete arrest of the SA nodal fiber. This finding correlates well with the frequent development of nodal rhythm during methoxyflurance anesthesia {30}.

His bundle studies in the presence of 1–2 MAC (minimal alveolar concentration) enflurane showed a prolongation of AV nodal, but not His-Purkinje or ventricular conduction times {31}. [Minimum alveolar concentration is that concentration (vol/vol) of an inhalational anesthetic that prevents 50% of subjects from moving in response to a painful stimulus.] AV nodal conduction time increased as heart rate was increased. This rate dependency was enhanced by enflurane. His-Purkinje and ventricular conduction were not affected by rate or enflurane. The atrial effective refractory period, functional refractory period of the AV node, and AV nodal conductivity were depressed by enflurane. Halothane does not prolong the atrial effective refractory period {32}. This may be important in explaining the decreased incidence of supraventricular dysrhythmia during enflurane anesthesia compared to halothane. The effects of enflurane on the His-Purkinje and ventricular conduction system contrast with those the authors report for halothane. Since conduction changes are necessary for ventricular dysrhythmia caused by reentry of excitation, they felt their findings might partially explain the clinical impression of a decreased incidence of ventricular dysrhythmia with enflurane compared to halothane.

Zaidan et al. {33} have shown that 3/4 MAC enflurane did not influence ventricular pacing employed as treatment of third-degree heart block produced by cardioplegic solutions during cardiopulmonary bypass. This is support from a clinical source for the findings of Atlee et al.

Blitt et al. {34} studied the effects of 1.25, 2, and 2.5 MAC isoflurane on AV conduction by His-bundle electrocardiography during atrial pacing in dogs. There were no changes in AH interval. Atrial pacing to 200 beats/min did not influence the AH interval, unlike the effects of halothane. The stability of cardiac rhythm observed clinically with isoflurane may be related to this lack of effect on the AV node.

More recently, Atlee investigated the effects of 1.2, 1.7, and 2.3 MAC enflurane, halothane, and isoflurane on AV conduction times compared with awake (control) dogs that were chronically instrumented for His-bundle studies. Both halothane and enflurane produced increases in AV nodal conduction time (18% and 17%, respectively) compared to the awake state. There was, however, little increase in time with increasing depth of anesthesia. Isoflurane had virtually no effect on AV nodal conduction time {35}.

Wilton et al. {36} studied the effects of equipotent concentrations of halothane, enflurane, and isoflurane on sinus node function (corrected sinus node recovery time), atrial-His and His-ventricular conduction times, and AV refractoriness (assessed by Wenckebach periodicity), and compared them to chloralose, which does not alter AV function {37}, in intact dogs. No evidence of sinus node dysfunction occurred. Enflurane produced a significant prolongation of atrial-His conduction at higher paced rates compared to halothane, isoflurane, and chloralose. AV refractoriness was impaired by enflurane and halothane, but not by isoflurane. His-ventricular conduction was unaltered.

Atlee and Yeager {38} have shown in chronically instrumented dogs that clinically relevant concentrations of enflurane and isoflurane compared with the awake state produced the largest increase in atrial and AV nodal refractoriness. These effects were more pronounced in dogs with intact autonomic function. Halothane had little or no significant effects on atrial or AV nodal refractoriness. This increased refractoriness should oppose reentry of excitation, and enflurane and isoflurane should be more effective against SVT due to atrial or AV nodal reentry.

PURKINJE FIBERS

Reynolds et al. {2} reported that when quiescent canine Purkinje fibers were exposed in vitro to 1% halothane, the resting membrane potential (RMP) was unchanged and the rate of phase 4 depolarization was virtually unaffected. Hauswirth {7}, however, found in sheep Purkinje fibers that RMP was increased, and overshoot and the duration of the action potential were decreased at 1% halothane.

This disparity could be due to species differences. At 2% halothane or above, rate slowed in spontaneously beating fibers as a result of an increase in threshold potential and a decreased rate of rise in phase 4 depolarization. A steep increase in the slope of phase 2 caused almost a complete loss of plateau. Action potential (AP) duration was shortened. In driven fibers the same effect on the plateau was seen. In many fibers, AP duration was not shortened due to a decrease in phase-3 repolarization. Pruett and his coworkers {39} have also shown similar results at equivalent concentrations — a shortened AP duration, decreased overshoot, depressed rate of phase-4 depolarization, and reduced maximum diastolic potential. $+V_{max}$, however, increased and membrane responsiveness was enhanced. Amplitude and $+V_{max}$ were decreased in the slow-response APs of fibers partially depolarized by 20 mM KCL.

Quiescent Purkinje fibers exposed to 1% methoxflurane had a slightly less negative resting potential, but did not develop automatically. In spontaneously beating fibers, 0.5% and 1% methoxyflurane caused marked increases in rate, mainly due to an increase in the slope of phase-4 depolarization. While a sharp increase in phase-2 repolarization occurred, the duration of action potential remained about the same due to a decrease in the terminal part of phase-3 repolarization. $+V_{max}$ in phase 0 was also slightly decreased.

The actions of enflurane are similar to those observed with halothane. In spontaneously active Purkinje fibers, however, enflurane enhances the rate of phase-4 depolarization and significantly reduces MDP (fig. 39-4). Threshold potential also appears to be at a less negative voltage. These findings have also been reported by Pruett and his colleagues {39}. These authors showed enhancement of membrane responsiveness in Purkinje fibers by both halothane and enflurane. Since membrane responsiveness reflects the fast inward current carried by sodium ions, they suggest normalization of membrane responsiveness after exposure to halothane and enflurane might be due to alteration in voltage- and/or time-dependent changes in sodium conductance, similar to that reported by Chen et al. {40} for lidocaine.

Several types of voltage-dependent Ca^{2+} channels exist {41}. Two distinct types of calcium channel currents have been shown to be present in a variety of cell membranes including the sarcolemma. They have been described in sinoatrial, atrial, ventricular, and Purkinje cells {42–45}.

The long-lasting (L-type) channel is activated at more positive membrane potentials and decays slowly. The transient (T-type) channel is activated at more negative membrane potentials and has a rapid decay. The L-type channel current is enhanced by beta-adrenergic agents {42,43} and by calcium channel agonists, e.g., Bay K-8644. It is decreased by calcium channel blockers, for example, nifedipine {42,43,46}.

The T type is not affected by calcium channel agonists or antagonists but is blocked by Ni^{2+} and tetramethrin. The two types are thought to have different functions.

The L type is the main channel for the slow inward current in cardiac ventricular cells, whose main function is contraction {44}. It must therefore provide the major part

Canine Purkinje Fibres (2.35 mM K⁺)

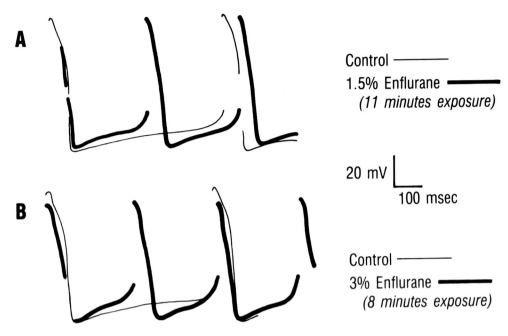

A

Control ——————
1.5% Enflurane ▬▬▬▬
(11 minutes exposure)

20 mV ⌊
    100 msec

B

Control ——————
3% Enflurane ▬▬▬▬
(8 minutes exposure)

Fig. 39-4. The effects of enflurane on spontaneously firing canine Purkinje fibers at 1.5% (**A**; 0.73 MAC) and 3% (**B**; 1.5 MAC).

of the external calcium ions required for excitation-contraction coupling. In the AV node the L-type current is responsible for the slow action potential and its plateau. T-type channels have a greater density in cells that have pacemaker or conduction functions {42,45,46}.

Eskinder et al. {47} have recently studied the effects of halothane, enflurane, and isoflurane on the L- and T-type channels in patch-clamped canine cardiac Purkinje fibers. All three agents produced similar and nonselective depression of L- and T-type calcium currents. Since the L-type channel contributes to the slow diastolic depolarization as well as the plateau and repolarization phases of the cardiac action potential, the authors believe suppression of this inward current may be one of the mechanisms by which these agents alter the action potential in cardiac Purkinje fibers. Similar suppression of the L-type current has been observed in ventricular muscle cells (see below).

We observed that enflurane caused dose-related inhibition of post-overdrive hyperpolarization in canine Purkinje fibers and postulated this could reflect enflurane produced inhibition of the Na⁺-K⁺ exchange pump {48}.

Lazlo et al. {49} reported the effects of halothane, enflurane, and isoflurane on automaticity and recovery following overdrive suppression in Purkinje fibers. All the anesthetics, but especially enflurane, increased the rate of normal automaticity of Purkinje fibers exposed to

epinephrine. Recovery times were shortened by enflurane, to a lesser extent by halothane, and were virtually unaffected by isoflurane.

More recently, they examined the effects of these agents on postdrive membrane hyperpolarization using Purkinje fibers from normal and infarcted hearts {50}. Pacing produced a greater increase in the maximum diastolic potential of the normal compared to the abnormal fibers. Unlike our study, no anesthetic altered the effect of pacing on postdrive hyperpolarization in normal or infarcted hearts. However, our study was at higher concentrations, longer pacing, and higher rates. Inhibition of postdrive hyperpolarization by enflurane could partially explain its greater propensity to increase automaticity in normal Purkinje fibers when compared to halothane or isoflurane.

Polic et al. {51} have shown that halothane, enflurane, and isoflurane have a greater action in decreasing the action potential duration (APD) of Purkinje fibers exhibiting long APDs (proximal fibers) than short APDs (distal fibers). This reduces the normal regional differences of APD. The relative actions on Purkinje fiber repolarization were enflurane > isoflurane > halothane. This differs from their relative anesthetic potencies, halothane > isoflurane > enflurane, and their negative inotropic effects halothane = enflurane > isoflurane. The authors postulate that these actions reduce regional differences of Purkinje fiber APD and might alter the occurrence of dysrhythmias when there is abnormal conduction in the ventricular conduction system and differences in the refractory periods in different regions.

The interaction between anesthetic agents and endogenous or exogenous catecholamine have long been a topic for study. In a recent article, Freeman and Muir {52} studied the effects of halothane on Purkinje fibers from false tendons (provide rapid conduction of impulses to the endocardium) and Purkinje fiber-muscle junctions (PMJs; provide conduction from terminal Purkinje fibers to the endocardial muscle fibers). They confirmed Hauswirth's findings {7} that halothane decreased action potential duration in Purkinje fibers and ventricular muscle. There was also decreased conduction in false tendon Purkinje fibers. The reduction in phase 0 depolarization, AP amplitude, and overshoot with halothane are attributed to a decrease in the peak inward Na^+ current {53}. Halothane also depressed conduction in PM junctions. This may be due to depression of inward Na^+ current combined with alteration in passive membrane properties, leading to a decrease of gap junctional conductance and cell-to-cell coupling {54,55}. The P-M junction is considered a potential site for initiation of cardiac arrhythmias {56}. Depression by halothane of the P-M junction suggests that reduction of intracellular coupling is a possible cause of arrhythmias. Freeman and Muir {57} further studied the effects of alpha-adrenoceptive stimulation in the presence of halothane on impulse propagation in cardiac Purkinje fibers. Halothane decreased the effective refractory period and action potential duration. Alpha-adrenergic stimulation restored both ERP and APD, an effect antagonized by prazosin. There was no additional effect on normal impulse propagation but significant slowing of conduction of premature impulses.

Vodanovic et al. {58} recently studied the effect of alpha- (prazocin) and beta- (metoprolol) adrenergic receptor blockade on the decrease in conduction velocity produced by epinephrine in the presence of halothane or isoflurane in canine left ventricular false tendons. They found epinephrine in the presence of halothane decreased conduction velocity within 2–5 minutes, with a return to baseline by 10 minutes. Metoprolol had no effect but decreased conduction velocity was prevented by prazosin. Phenylephrine produced a greater decrease in conduction velocity when combined with halothane than with isoflurance. The transient negative dromotropic effects of the catecholamine in the presence of volatile anesthetic agents are alpha-adrenergic mediated.

Oshita et al. {59} studied halothane/epinephrine interaction by using the sensitivity of slow Ca^{2+} channels to epinephrine (epinephrine threshold for the development of slow responses) ETSR {60} as an indicator. They studied the effects of halothane, selective alpha$_1$ blockers (prazosin, droperidol), beta$_1$ blockers (metoprolol), and calcium entry blockers (verapamil) alone and in combination with halothane on the ETSR in canine trabeculae. Halothane at 1% had no effect, but at 2% and 4%

significantly increased the ETSR. Alpha$_1$ blockade with prazosin or droperidol had no effect, while beta$_1$ block with metoprolol increased ETSR. Similar findings occurred when prazosin or metoprolol was given with 2% halothane. Verapamil also increased ETSR in a dose-related manner. This suggests halothane decreases the sensitivity of slow Ca^{2+} channels to epinephrine and is related to calcium entry blockade by halothane.

Zuckerman and Wheeler {61} used single rat myocytes to evaluate whether the mechanism of dysrhythmia production by a combination of halothane and catecholamine originates in a single cell. The incidence of spontaneous contractile waves between stimulated beats, early aftercontractions, and late aftercontractions was measured on exposure to isoproterenol, norepinephrine, and phenylephrine with and without halothane. All of the above end points can produce arrhythmias in multicell preparations. The addition of halothane reduced the incidence of these phenomena. This arrhythmicity does not arise in a single cell, and altered impulse propagation and possible reentry is a more probable explanation.

Vodanovic et al. {62} showed that epinephrine in the presence of halothane or isoflurane decreases conduction velocity in canine Purkinje fibers more than epinephrine alone. The decrease with halothane and epinephrine was greater than that with isoflurane and epinephrine.

Halothane and enflurane, but not isoflurane, opposed the induction of triggered rhythmic activity in quiescent but partially depolarized Purkinje fibers from infarcted hearts. This activity is the result of delayed afterdepolarization attributed to intracellular calcium ion overload {63}. This, in turn, produces Na^+-Ca^{2+} exchange, producing the transient inward current {64} that is responsible for delayed afterdepolarization.

VENTRICULAR MUSCLE

Halothane depresses intraventricular conduction, but to a lesser extent than conduction through the AV node {26}. Ventricular automaticity is somewhat depressed by halothane, as shown by studies in isolated cell preparations {2,65} and intact animals {65,66}. At 2% halothane, Hauswirth {7} found in sheep ventricular cells an unchanged resting membrane potential, a decreased overshoot, a reduced duration of the action potential, and shortened effective refractory period. The $\dot{V}_{max}$ of phase-0 depolarization was also decreased. Recent work has confirmed Hauswirth's findings {5}. Up to 2% halothane had little effect on normal APs. At 2% and above, a slight decrease in amplitude and duration occurred so that the plateau was shortened. $\dot{V}_{max}$ of the normal fast AP was not depressed at any concentration of halothane.

Enflurane also has little effect on the resting membrane potential of normal guinea pig APs {67}. Amplitude and $\dot{V}_{max}$ were virtually unaffected by even 6% enflurane. However, loss of plateau and AP duration occurred at higher concentrations (fig. 39-5).

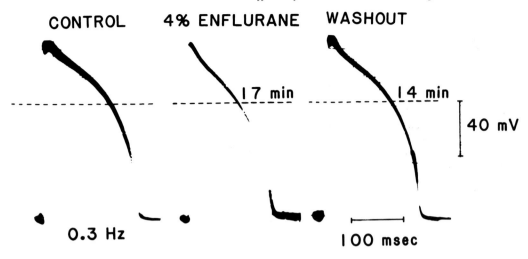

Fig. 39-5. The effect of enflurane 4% (2.35 MAC) on normal guinea pig ventricular muscle action potential, showing some loss of plateau and AP duration.

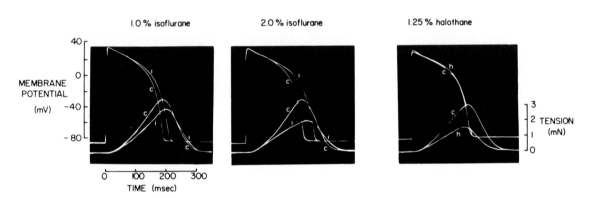

Fig. 39-6. Simultaneously recorded normal action potentials and twitch responses in the same papillary muscle. Control (c), isoflurane (i), and halothane (h). From Lynch C III: Anesthesiology 64:620–631, 1986. Reproduced with permission.

Since the slow inward current is in part responsible for maintaining the plateau of the action potential {68}, the decrease in duration may be attributed to the depression of the slow inward currents by the volatile anesthetic agents that we shall discuss later.

We cannot, however, exclude the possibility that potassium conductance is increased by these agents. This also would shorten the duration of the action potential.

Isoflurane 1%–4% caused no significant change in normal AP amplitude, $\dot{V}_{max}$, or resting membrane potential. AP duration was, however, significantly prolonged {69} (fig. 39-6).

VENTRICULAR CONTRACTION

All volatile anesthetic agents are known to depress myocardial contractility. Nitrous oxide was thought to be innocuous for many years {70}. Clinical {71} and recent laboratory reports have shown a direct negative inotropic effect of N_2O {72,73}. The negative inotropic effect of N_2O is associated with a decrease in intracellular calcium availability without change in myofibrillar Ca^{2+} responsiveness {72}. In further studies in isolated ferret ventricular papillary muscle, 50% N_2O caused a significant reduction in contractility {74}. In the presence of ryanodine 10^{-6} M, which suppresses utilization of Ca^{2+} from the sarcoplasmic reticulum, a further significant reduction in contractile variables occurred. The authors concluded that at least part of the negative inotropic effect of N_2O is due to inhibition of trans-sarcolemmal calcium influx. This depressant effect of the anesthetic agents has been shown both in clinical situations {75–79} and in the laboratory {80–85}.

The mechanism of myocardial depression by the volatile anesthetic agents has been and continues to be the basis for a great number of investigations. It is unlikely that a single factor will provide an adequate explanation.

The volatile agents could influence the cardiac excitation-contraction process in a number of ways:

1. An effect on myocardial contractile proteins
2. An effect on calcium ion release by the sarcoplasmic reticulum
3. An effect on myocardial slow channels

The sites of action of these agents are not easy to differentiate, since a change in influx of Ca^{2+} through the sarcolemma necessarily changes the release or sequestration of Ca^{2+} by the sarcoplasmic reticulum, which then changes the amount of Ca^{2+} available to activate the contractile proteins. It has been suggested that the volatile anesthetic agents interact directly with the myocardial contractile protein by changing its shape, blocking ionic channels, or preventing structural change in the protein. Evidence for this direct action is provided by the work of Seeman {86}, Halsey {87,88}, Woodbury {89}, Metcalfe {90}, and Cheng {91} and their coworkers. Trudell has suggested a change in the fluidity of the phospholipid bilayer at anesthetic concentrations, thus affecting the membrane lipoproteins involved in slow-channel gating {92}. It has been postulated that alterations in fluidity would affect fast- and slow-channel gating equally, and fast sodium-channel gating is unaffected by both halothane {5} and enflurane {67}. However, the work of Rosenberg et al. {93} and of Pang et al. {94} showed that variation in structure of phospholipid molecules, the phospholipid-cholesterol ratio, and anesthetic concentration caused an increase or a decrease in the internal fluidity of the bilayer. These findings may partially explain the differing anesthetic actions on fast- and slow-channel gating.

The sarcoplasmic reticulum (SR) is a membranous system in the cardiac muscle that controls the amount and duration of calcium ion availability for contraction. Lipophilic volatile anesthetics have been shown to accumulate in the SR {95}. It has been suggested that the SR might be an important site at which anesthetic agents act to inhibit contractility {96}. Lain et al. {97} showed decreased uptake of calcium in homogenized and differentially centrifuged muscle. Although they showed a decreased calcium uptake, their halothane concentration was much greater than that which is clinically relevant. The work of Lee and colleagues {98}, which also shows decreased Ca^{2+} uptake, suffers also from an uncertain concentration of halothane.

Su et al. have shown inhibition of Ca^{2+} uptake by the cardiac SR in the presence of a clinically relevant concentration of halothane, enflurane, and isoflurane {99–102}. They used mechanically skinned myocardial fibers, which allows free movement of the perfusing medium through the outer cell membrane. There is depression of Ca^{2+} uptake by the sarcoplasmic reticulum, which con-

tributes to the negative inotropic effect. Halogenated anesthetics also decrease the calcium ion sensitivity of the contractile proteins {100,103}.

Measurements of La^{3+} displaceable calcium ions in dog trabecular muscle indicate that halothane reduces the amount of superfically bound calcium ions {104}. Blanck {105–107} and coworkers have also studied the effects of halothane, enflurane, and isoflurane. All stimulate Ca^{2+} uptake by the SR in vitro. This occurs at low ATP concentrations and clinical ranges of the anesthetic agents. Their data suggest that all three agents increase the affinity of $[Ca^{2+}, Mg^{2+}]$-ATPase for ATP. Since the rate of uptake is not stimulated beyond the maximum velocity of the enzyme, the authors suggest that ATP availability, rather than enzyme alteration, is improved. At higher concentrations of ATP ($>5\,mM$) and higher clinical concentrations of the anesthetic agents, inhibition of Ca^{2+} uptake occurs. However, at normal ATP levels and clinical concentration, all three agents seems to have little effect on Ca^{2+} uptake. Clinical significance, if any, lies in the fact that if ATP declines, as in ischemic heart disease or during ischemic arrest during cardiopulmonary bypass, Ca^{2+} uptake might be depressed.

More recently the inhibitory effects of halothane on two separate binding sites on the voltage-dependent channel have been demonstrated {108}. The authors suggest that halothane produces a significant alteration in the conformation or exposure of the channel, and also that halothane alters the sarcolemmal lipid environment, rather than producing a direct effect on the voltage-dependent calcium channel itself.

Komai and Rusy concluded from their work on the effects of halothane in rested-state and potential-state contractions in rabbit papillary muscle that trans-sarcolemmal calcium influx and stored calcium are equally influenced, resulting in a negative inotropic action. Halothane reduced the amount of stored calcium by inhibiting uptake and accelerating the loss of the cation during rest {109}.

More recently, these authors found that halothane and isoflurane depressed Ca^{2+} influx across the sarcolemma {110,111}. They also suggest halothane has a direct effect on the sarcoplasmic reticulum, making it pervious to calcium ions and reducing the amount of calcium stored. Isoflurane does not have this effect and may in fact make the sarcoplasmic reticulum less pervious. Halothane may further reduce the myofibrillar response to activated Ca^{2+} when the muscle fiber length is shortened.

Wilde et al. {112} have studied the effects of halothane, enflurane, and isoflurane in isolated single rat ventricular cells. All reduce the availability of Ca^{2+} for myocyte shortening. The mechanisms by which these agents cause their effect differ. Halothane is the most potent in inhibiting the increase in cytosolic Ca^{2+} that results from direct action of the sarcoplasmic reticulum calcium release channel (caffeine stimulation) or indirect release following sarcoplasmic reticulum stimulated calcium release, while enflurane appears to have no effect. Both isoflurane and enflurane appear to alter the L-type Ca^{2+} channels in the sarcolemma.

Hirota et al. {113} have studied the effects of halothane

on the Ca^{2+} channel using both electrophysiologic and biochemical techniques. Their work with single ventricular myocytes confirms the work cited above. Their results also demonstrate that halothane does not produce use-dependent inhibition of I_{Ca}. This inhibition appears to require blockade of activated channels in the hydrophilic phase {114}. Halothane is both hydrophobic and lipid soluble. Halothane directly decreased cAMP content of single ventricular myocytes. The authors suggest that the decrease of I_{Ca} by halothane is in part due to the inactivation of the cAMP-induced phosphorylation of the Ca^{2+} channels as a result of this decrease. The decrease in I_{Ca} was greater with halothane than has been shown with cAMP inhibition alone {115}. Additional mechanisms, not involving the phosphorylation-dependent gate, must be involved.

During phase 2 or the plateau of the action potential, an inward movement of calcium ions occurs through the kinetically slow ion-transport system {116}. If this system is blocked by verapamil, a marked negative inotropism occurs in the presence of virtually normal action potentials {117}. The calcium entering the cell through these channels contributes to the contractile process {118}. Early workers {7,119} showed halothane produced this negative inotropism with little effect on cardiac action potentials. Electromechanical dissociation is not uncommon clinically and is manifested as severe hypotension with a virtually normal electrocardiogram.

The effects of halothane {5}, enflurane {67} (fig. 39-7), and methoxyflurane {120} (fig. 39-8) on the slow channels have been studied by simultaneous measurements of action potentials and contractions in guinea pig papillary muscles. All three agents produce a depression of the inward calcium current that enters the myocardial cells through the voltage-dependent slow channels. Slow-channel action potentials were obtained by depolarization to $-40\,mV$ with 26 mM K^+, thus inactivating fast sodium channels {121}. Cells at this level of depolarization are inexcitable due to lack of inward current {122}. Slow-channel current can be increased by elevating the intracellular cyclic AMP level {123-125}. The $\dot{V}_{max}$ of the slow action potential reflects the rate of depolarizing current flow {126}.

The depressant effects of halothane on $\dot{V}_{max}$ are more marked than those of enflurane. Additionally, halothane is slightly more depressant than enflurane on tension produced by the muscle during the slow AP. These findings appear to support investigators who have found halothane to be more depressant {77,78,82} rather than those who have suggested that enflurane was more or equally depressant {79,83-85}. At lower concentrations, halothane 0.5% (0.65 MAC) {5} and enflurane 1% (0.6 MAC) {67} both produced a negative inotropic effect without an effect on the slow AP. Obviously a mechanism other than slow-channel depression is involved in this early cardiac depression.

Lynch recently compared the effects of isoflurane and halothane on guinea pig papillary muscle {69}. With normal APs, isoflurane (1.3% and 2.5%) depressed peak tension significantly less at high frequencies of stimulation than did equivalent does of halothane (0.75% or 1.5%).

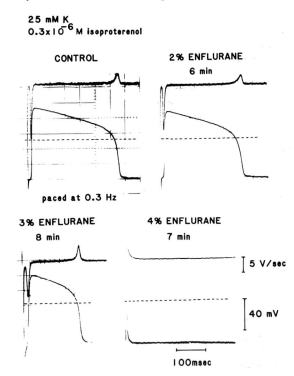

Fig. 39-7. Effect of enflurane on slow cardiac action potentials from guinea pig ventricular muscle at 2% (1.2 MAC), 3% (1.8 MAC), and 4% (2.35 MAC). Note marked effects on slow AP at 4% compared to fig. 39-5, the fast AP.

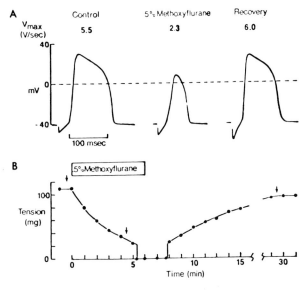

Fig. 39-8. Effect of 5% methoxyflurane on (A) the slow action potentials of guinea pig papillary muscle and (B) tension developed.

At all frequencies, dT/dt was depressed less by isoflurane than by halothane. For this to occur, either duration of tension development must be decreased, or the pattern and rate of tension development altered, by the anesthetic during contraction.

Isoflurane (1.3% and 2.5%) and enflurane (1.7% or 3.5%) markedly depressed the late-peaking slow AP contraction observed with low-frequency stimulation. Halothane (0.75% or 1.5%) caused a similar contractile depression at all frequencies. At frequencies above 1 Hz, however, isoflurane depressed early-peaking slow AP tension and dT/dt max significantly less than halothane or enflurane. At 0.3 Hz, isoflurane caused depression of the $\dot{V}_{max}$ of slow APs. Isoflurane altered the pattern of tension development in a manner different from that of halothane, suggesting differing mechanisms of myocardial depression.

Like halothane and enflurane, isoflurane depressed the $\dot{V}_{max}$ of the slow APs, but this depression is small when compared with the depression of late peak tension. Lynch felt that this suggested that Ca^{2+} entry contributed little to the contractile depression produced by isoflurane and that an alteration in myocardial SR uptake and/or release was involved {69}.

We discussed the types of Ca^{2+} channels in the section on Purkinje fibers. In ventricular muscle the L-type predominates while the T-type contributes little to the total inward Ca^{2+} current during the action potential. Bosnjak et al. {127}, using patch-clamp techniques, have shown that halothane, enflurane, and isoflurane produce similar depression of peak inward calcium current at equivalent anesthetic concentrations without a shift in the current-voltage relationship for channel activation. Bosnjak has proposed that since halothane and enflurane depress myocardial contractility more than isoflurane {128}, their effects are most likely due to differential actions at other cellular sites {129}.

Frazer and Lynch {130} recently reported that both halothane and isoflurane decrease Ca^{2+} uptake, enhance Ca^{2+} efflux, and increase ATPase activity. This latter effect may be largely explained by the enhanced efflux that prevents accumulation of Ca^{2+} from causing feedback inhibition of the ATPase. Casella et al. {131} previously reported that the volatile anesthetic agents did not depress initial Ca^{2+} uptake by cardiac SR vesicles but did depress their ability to retain Ca^{2+}.

Frazer and Lynch {132} also presented a molecular basis for the different actions of halothane and isoflurane on myocardial function. They studied the effects of halothane and isoflurane in a Ca release channel rich fraction of homogenized centrifuged canine ventricular muscle in the presence of ryanodine. Ryanodine binds to open Ca release channels. The increased binding in the presence of halothane compared to isoflurane corresponds to an increased number of open Ca release channels. Increase in open channels enhances Ca^{2+} release from the sarcoplasmic reticulum, and results in less accumulation of Ca for release to activate ventricular contraction. In addition, Ca^{2+} that leaks from the SR is eliminated by exchange for Na^+ as long as a Na^+ gradient is present. In ischemic ATP-depleted myocardium with intracellular Na^+ accumulation, this effect of halothane may lead to sustained diastolic Ca^{2+} levels and enhanced cell damage.

Miao et al. {133} studied the effects of halothane, enflurane, and isoflurane on the homogenized, centifuged canine ventricular membrane vesicle fraction with little Ca release capability. Enflurane enhanced Ca^{2+} uptake and free phosphate production, which is consistent with an increase rate of turnover of Ca-ATPase. Isoflurane had no effect. Halothane decreased Ca^{2+} uptake while increasing free phosphate production, which would occur with increased Ca^{2+} leak from the SR vesicles.

Halothane has been shown to depress myocardial function in normal and hypertrophied muscle {134}. Rooke and Su compared the effects of halothane on normal and hypertrophied skinned rabbit left ventricular fibers {135}. Halothane depressed contractile protein responsiveness to calcium equally in normal and hypertrophied muscle. There was decreased calcium storage in the sarcoplasmic reticulum with halothane but less so in hypertrophied muscle than in normal. Thus hypertropied muscle is not more sensitive to halothane.

Baum {136} studied the effects of the calcium channel agonist BAY K8644 on the impairment of I_{Ca} by halothane in single guinea pig ventricular myocytes. He found there was no specific antagonism. Although BAY K8644 resulted in increased calcium current at baseline, during exposure to 1% halothane, and during recovery compared to non-BAY K8644 exposed cells, the depression of current as a percentage of baseline current was identical.

Desflurane (difluoromethyl-1-fluro-2,2,2,-trifluoroethyl ether) is a new volatile anesthetic that has recently completed clinical trials. It is a structural analogue of isoflurane. Boban et al. {137} have compared the effects of isoflurane and desflurane in isolated guinea pig hearts. Heart rate was similarly decreased and AV conduction time prolonged with both agents. Desflurane produced a significantly greater depression of left ventricular pressure at 1 and 2 MAC than isoflurane.

Sevoflurane, a newly introduced inhalational anesthetic, was studied by Nakao et al. {138} by the whole-cell patch-clamp technique in collagenase-digested single ventricular bullfrog cells and compared to halothane. This tissue has little sarcoplasmic reticulum and, therefore, calcium current can be measured without the effect of SR-mediated calcium mobilization. Both sevoflurane and halothane suppress Ca^{2+} current in a concentration-dependent manner with equal depression at equal MAC concentrations.

CLINICAL IMPLICATIONS

Halothane, like many antidysrhythmic drugs, produces depression of phase-4 depolarization. It has been shown to moderate the cardiotoxic effects of digitalis {139,140} and even to have therapeutic value in ouabain-induced ventricular tachycardia {141}. Ectopic pacemaker cells in digitalis-induced ventricular tachycardia are situated either in the left bundle branch or more distal Purkinje fibers, with retrograde activation of the bundle of His {142}. Logic and Morrow {143} have shown that halothane can suppress glycoside enhancement of these ectopic pacemakers. Digitalis inhibits the ATP-dependent Na^+-K^+ pump {144}. The resultant increase in intracellular sodium ionic concentration stimulates the sodium-calcium transport system {145}. Intracellular calcium concentration increases and myocardial contractility improves. Cardiotoxicity of digitalis is a result of a greater inhibition of the pump. Halothane antagonizes the increased rate of phase-4 depolarization and may therefore prevent the increased automaticity in ectopic pacemaker cells. The enhanced membrane responsiveness reported by Pruett and Gramling {146} may also contribute to the prevention of reentrant dysrhythmias, not only of digitalis toxicity but also those produced by ischemia. Finally, the competitive action of halothane with calcium on the slow channel may also be a factor {4}.

Diethyl ether, methoxyflurane, enflurane, and isoflurane also increase tolerance to digitalis toxicity when administered prior to ouabain infusion and restore sinus rhythm when administered acutely during ouabain-induced ventricular tachycardia {147}. Methoxyflurane and enflurane both increase the rate of phase-4 depolarization in the SA node. This would tend to produce nodal rhythm, which is frequently seen during anesthesia with these agents. Enflurane has also been shown to increase membrane responsiveness {39}, so this may in part explain their action in moderating digitalis-induced dysrhythmias. While their effect on the AV node remains somewhat unclear, they certainly do not antagonize the AV nodal depression of digitalis. As is true with digitalis, effective refractory periods of the ventricles are shortened. The sympathetic nervous system is thought to be involved in the genesis of digitalis-induced ventricular dysrhythmias {148}. Halothane {149}, enflurane {150}, and isoflurane {151} are thought to decrease sympathetic nervous activity and thus confer increased tolerance to digitalis.

Gallagher and McClernan {152} investigated the effects of halothane on ventricular tachycardia (VT) produced by different electrophysiologic mechanisms in intact dogs: (1) Abnormal automaticity, (2) Reentry, (3) Delayed afterdepolarization-induced triggered activity (DAD), and (4) Early afterdepolarization triggered activity (EAD) were studied. In groups 1 and 2 VT was achieved by left anterior descending coronary artery ligation and infarction. Halothane reduced the frequency of ventricular beats in group 1 and abolished reentry in 50% of group 2 dogs. Halothane restored sinus rhythm in 80% of dogs in group 3, but had no effect on EADs in group 4. A recent study {153} suggests a role for the L-type Ca^{2+} channel in EADs since they could be induced with the Ca^{2+} current agonist BAY K8644 in voltage-clamped sheep Purkinje fibers. However an inward Na^+ current such as the Na^+ window current could also be involved {154}.

Deutsch et al. {155} produced ventricular tachycardia by programmed stimulation 4–6 days after creating myocardial infarction in dogs. Halothane and enflurane suppressed the induction of VT. Both drugs prolonged refractory periods in normal and infarcted myocardium, while isoflurane was only effective in normal myocardium.

While we have discussed the antidysrhythmic effects of the volatile anesthetic agents, in clinical situations dysrhythmias are not infrequent. This is particularly true in the presence of catecholamines. Initially there was discussion as to whether the underlying mechanism was that of increased automaticity or reentry {156–158}. All evidence now points to reentry. In Zink's work there were critical levels for both blood pressure and atrial rate. A rise in intraventricular systolic pressure causes stretch of Purkinje fibers. This, in turn, slows conduction velocity and increases the rate of diastolic depolarization, both of which favor reentry {157}. The bigeminal beat is thought to be a fusion beat of a reentrant impulse that has its origins in the upper interventricular septum, with the next normal beat conducted through the AV node. The findings of Reynolds and Chiz support this work {160}. Epinephrine, in concentrations without effect on velocity of impulse conduction in Purkinje fibers, markedly potentiated a modest slowing of conduction produced by halothane. This effect was antagonized by alpha blockade, but not by beta blockade.

Clinically we term these findings *sensitization of the myocardium by halothane*, i.e., the dose of intravenous exogenous epinephrine needed to produce ventricular premature contractions (VPCs) is lower in the presence of halothane anesthesia than in the awake state. In comparing the presently used volatile agents, Joas and Stevens {161} have shown that in dogs during epinephrine injection, the stability of heart rhythm is greatest with isoflurane, then with enflurane, and is least with halothane. Both Johnston et al. {163} for halothane, and Horrigan et al. {162} for enflurane, have shown larger doses of epinephrine are required when the vehicle of injection is lidocaine. This contradicts the often-quoted adage that lidocaine should not be given during halothane-induced dysrhythmias because it depresses an already depressed (by halothane) AV conduction.

Verapamil, a slow-calcium-channel inhibitor, is known to inhibit myocardial contractility, depress the SA and AV nodes, and decrease vascular smooth muscle tone {164}. Dysrhythmias occurring during anesthesia have been successfuly treated with verapamil {165}. Verapamil also produces blockade of the fast sodium channels {165}, which contributes to its depression of cardiac output {167}.

The effects of verapamil during halothane {168}, enflurane {169}, and isoflurane {170,171} anesthesia have been studied. Verapamil produced a rise in the epinephrine dysrhythmogenic threshold and epinephrine-induced ventricular dysrhythmia in the intact dog during 1 MAC halothane anesthesia {168}. There was a further depression in mean arterial pressure and cardiac function compared to halothane alone. Cardiac output, however, varied. After a uniform initial rise, cardiac output remained high in some dogs or fell in others. This may represent an additive effect of halothane on the balance of the two cardiovascular effects of verapamil, i.e., beneficial afterload reduction versus deleterious direct myocardial depression {172}.

Verapamil in the presence of enflurane anethesia decreased mean arterial pressure, cardiac output, and heart rate, and left ventricular dP/dt decreased. Enflurane caused hemodynamic depression below control at 25% of the verapamil dosage {169}. Animals receiving 1 MAC isoflurane compared to those receiving 1 MAC enflurane had a greater sympathetic tone and tolerated higher plasma levels of verapamil. There was also less reflex increase in epinephrine {170}. These findings may indicate isoflurane as the inhalational agent of choice in patients taking verapamil. Kates et al. {171} confirmed the additive myocardial depressant effects of isoflurane and verapamil. They also showed only partial reversal by calcium, which might indicate depression of the slow channels, is not the sole mechanism in the cardiac depression.

The effects of the phosphodiesterase inhibitors amrinone, milrinone, and 3-isobutyl-1-methylxanthine (IBMX) were studied in halothane and isoflurane depressed guinea pig hearts {173}. Under control conditions, contractile force and heart rate were increased most with IBMX and least with amrinone. In isoflurane-treated hearts, the phoshodiesterase inhibitors increased contractile force to a greater degree, while heart rate increased, as in the control group. In halothane-treated hearts, amrinone and milrinone were less effective, while IBMX gave the same increase in contraction as in the isoflurane group.

Takada et al. {174} recently compared the antiarrhythmic action of Na^+, K^+, and Ca^{2+} channel blockers on halothane- and epinephrine-induced ventricular dysrhythmias in rats. The K^+ channel blockers amiodarone and E-4031 were far more effective than either the Na^+ channel blockers (lidocaine and flecainide) or the Ca^{2+} channel blocker, verapamil. They suggest that the K^+ channel may have a role in the genesis of halothane-epinephrine dysrhythmias.

CORONARY CIRCULATION

Ischemic heart disease has become increasingly important to the anesthesiologist for several reasons. These include an aging population, the increased incidence of coronary artery bypass surgery, and the acceptance of patients for noncardiac surgery who would previously have been considered too great a risk. The following is a highly simplified outline of myocardial oxygenation so that we may discuss the effects of the volatile anesthetic agents.

Myocardial oxygen supply is mainly dependent on blood flow through the coronary arteries and the oxygen-carrying capacity of the blood. Coronary blood flow is greatest in early diastole. The pressure gradient across the coronary vessels is influenced by the aortic diastolic pressure (LVEDP). Heart rate also influences coronary flow because of its effects on the length of diastole. If diastolic pressure or LVEDP are changed, coronary flow changes unless coronary vascular resistance also changes. In the ischemic heart, atheromatous changes preclude this decrease in coronary vascular resistance and coronary flow depends upon pressure and diastolic time.

Anemia, acid-base balance and adequate ventilation are more important than the anesthetic agents per se on the oxygen-carrying capacity of the blood. Factors influencing myocardial oxygen consumption have been well reviewed {175}. The most important are heart rate, the myocardial contractile state, and myocardial wall tension. Increased heart rate means increased myocardial work. N. Ty Smith {176} has listed 58 indicators in assessing the myocardial contractile state. This itself indicates a lack of agreement on both method of evaluation and definition of contractility. $LV_{dP/dt}$ has been considered a reasonable index {177–180}. Increases are associated with increased myocardial oxygen consumption, while decreases have the opposite effect. The rate-pressure product (heart rate × systolic blood pressure) also has an adequate correlation with myocardial oxygen consumption under clinical conditions {181,182}. A rate-pressure product of >11,000 occurred in patients who developed ischemic changes during surgery {183}. Myocardial wall tension is determined by ventricular pressure, intraventricular volume, and myocardial mass. Increases in intraventricular pressure or volume increase wall tension and thus myocardial work.

The effects of the inhalational agents on myocardial contractility have been discussed in the previous section on ventricular contraction and also have been reviewed by Smith {176} and Sonntag {184}. Suffice it to say that halothane, enflurane, and isoflurane all caused myocardial depression and therefore decreased myocardial work.

The restriction of coronary blood flow during systole is greatest at the endocardium and least at the epicardium {185}. The endocardium is therefore more vulnerable to ischemic changes {186}. Another important facet of the coronary circulation is the division into the larger conductance vessels on the epicardial surface and the smaller precapillary resistance vessels within the myocardium {187}. The larger vessels do not play a part in overall coronary resistance until neurogenic stimulation occurs {188}. This factor may be of importance in view of the effects of volatile anesthetic agents on autonomic control of the circulation {189}.

Early work performed in anesthetized animals with open chests showed only slight effects on stimulation of adrenergic nerves {190,191}. Later investigations in chronically instrumented animals have shown that adrenergic stimulation or blockade has profound effects on coronary blood flow {192,193}. Alpha- and beta-receptors have been demonstrated in the coronary vascular bed {194}. Klocke et al. {195} have reviewed sympathetic influences on the coronary circulation. As yet they are incompletely understood.

The effects of the volatile anesthetics on coronary circulation have been investigated in animal studies and in humans.

ANIMAL STUDIES

Eberlein {196}, Saito et al. {197}, and Weaver {198}, utilizing flow meters, have shown that halothane and methoxyflurane decreased coronary artery flow, while diethyl ether increased flow, in dogs. Other experiments using washout of ^{85}Kr from the coronary vein as an estimate of myocardial blood flow have shown decreases in ventricular function and oxygen consumption accompanied by equivalent decreases in myocardial blood flow {199}. Since the heart of *Sus scrofa* more nearly resembles that of humans {200}, Merin et al. studied the effect of halothane in pigs {201}. Dose-related depression in left ventricular function by halothane was again accompanied by equivalent decreases in coronary blood flow and oxygen consumption.

Decrease in coronary blood flow with halothane and increase with diethyl ether are most likely due to alterations in cardiac oxygen requirements {202}. However, Domenech et al. {203} studied the circumflex diastolic coronary vascular resistance in the working heart and total mean coronary resistance in the isolated nonworking heart of the dog during 100% oxygen and 2–3% halothane in oxygen. They concluded that the decreased resistance they observed was due to a direct action of halothane on coronary vessels. This action was not modified by beta-adrenergic block.

Sawyer et al. {204} were able to contrast local and systemic effects of halothane on the vascular bed supplied by the right coronary artery by using an extracorporeal circuit containing an isolated donor lung. Local administration of halothane caused marked coronary vasodilation without an effect on $R_{dP/dt}$ or systemic pressure. Systemic halothane caused marked reduction of systemic pressure and $RV_{dP/dt}$, and was without effect on coronary resistance. They concluded that while the direct local effect is to produce dilation, reflex baroreceptor stimulation and decreased cardiac metabolism during halothane antagonize local effects. This was supported by the finding that systemic halothane during alpha blockade produced a significant decrease in coronary resistance. They also compared the effects of halothane and enflurane on the right coronary circulation in the pig {205}. Halothane and enflurane both cause coronary vasodilation as a direct effect. Systemically, halothane and enflurane both cause coronary vasodilation as a direct effect. Halothane and enflurane also cause decreases in systemic pressure without a change in coronary resistance, local effects being effectively antagonized by indirect effects.

Verrier and his colleagues {206} measured myocardial blood flow as an indicator of oxygen supply during autoregulation and maximal vasodilation at various coronary arterial perfusion pressures at stable oxygen demand. The relationship between pressure and blood flow provided an index of coronary vascular reserve. Pressure-flow relations in the left circumflex coronary artery were compared during halothane (approx. 1 MAC) and nitrous oxide anesthesia. Myocardial oxygen demand and blood flow decreased during halothane anesthesia. The interesting point was that the pressure-flow relationship during maximal vasodilation shifted to the left. This reflects the lower coronary arterial perfusion pressure at which flow becomes zero. The authors aptly explain this by the vascular waterfall theory. This shift also reflects the lower coronary arterial perfusion at which subendocardial ischemia occurs during autoregulation of blood flow. Greater coronary vascular reserve is present during halothane anesthesia than with nitrous oxide.

The use of lightly anesthetized animals as controls may produce erroneous results {189,207}. Vatner and Smith, using chronically instrumented dogs, showed that halothane produced a dose-related decrease in ventricular function at 1% and 2% {208}, but coronary flow did not decrease with increased concentration. Merin et al. {80} found a dose-related decrease in myocardial blood flow. The latter group felt that the presence of tachycardia, with its effect on oxygen demand, was a factor in the conflicting findings. These authors also studied the effects of enflurane {84}. Dose-dependent depression of ventricular function was accompanied by depression of myocardial blood flow and oxygenation. Comparison with halothane in the same dog showed dose-dependent negative inotropic effects accompanied by equivalent decreases in cardiac oxygen demand.

Kenny et al. {209} studied the direct and temporal effects of halothane and isoflurane on coronary hemodynamics in chronically instrumented dogs. Induction of anesthesia with halothane caused a significant increase in coronary blood flow, which was secondary to increases in heart rate, blood pressure, and pressure work index. When autonomic nervous reflexes were eliminated, halothane did not cause an alteration in coronary blood flow. Isoflurane produced a larger increase in coronary blood flow, and when autonomic reflexes were eliminated isoflurane continued to produce an increase in coronary flow. Peak flow occurred at 2.1 ± 0.4 minutes and declined to control levels by 6 minutes, despite the continued presence of isoflurane. Halothane thus produces an increase in coronary flow only in relation to increased oxygen demand. Isoflurane produces a small but transient increase in flow when increased oxygen demand is prevented. Moore et al. {210} compared the effects of halothane and isoflurane in open chest dogs anesthetized with fentanyl, in whom acute ischemia was induced by occlusion of the left anterior descending coronary artery. They found that isoflurane produced an increase in blood flow in contiguous myocardium, blood flow through collaterals to ischemic myocardium was well maintained, and transmural steal was not increased. Lactate production from ischemic myocardium confirmed that no worsening of ischemia occurred. Halothane caused a dose-dependent reduction in myocardial flow to normally perfused myocardium. Ischemia did not become worse in the presence of halothane.

Bernard et al. {211} compared the effects of sevoflurane in chronically instrumented dogs. They found sevoflurane to be virtually identical to isoflurane in its effects on systemic and coronary hemodynamics. A decrease in coronary vascular resistance occurred. Manohar and Parks {212} previously reported a dose-dependent decrease in coronary blood flow with sevoflurane. The reason for the difference in results is unclear.

Pagel et al. {213} have compared the effects of desflurane, isoflurane, halothane, and enflurane in chronically instrumented dogs. Desflurane, like isoflurane, increased diastolic coronary blood flow velocity and decreased diastolic coronary vascular resistance in the presence of a functional autonomic nervous system. This may be due to direct coronary vasodilation. Following autonomic blockade, desflurane produces relatively little coronary vasodilation. This is in contrast to isoflurane, which produced an increase in coronary diastolic flow velocity in the presence of autonomic block.

The mechanism of the vasodilatation produced by the volatile anesthetic agents has been intensively studied over the past few years {214}. Endothelial cells control the state of vascular smooth muscle tone, not only by metabolism of vasoactive substances but also by secretion of vasodilators [endothelium-derived relaxing factor (EDRF) {215} and prostacyclin] and vasoconstrictors [endothelium-derived constricting factor (EDCF) and endothelin {216}]. EDRF is an endogenous vasodilator produced by endothelial cells. Production can be stimulated by substances such as acetylcholine, adenosine triphosphate, bradykinin, and calcium ionophore {217}, and also by vasoconstrictors such as phenylephrine, norepinephrine, and serotonin {218,219}. These cause an increase in endothelial cell cytosolic calcium, which together with the cofactors NADPH and calmodulin activates EDRF synthase, which, in turn, metabolizes L-arginine to citrulline and EDRF. EDRF causes relaxation of vascular smooth muscle through activation of guanylate cyclase and an increase in vascular smooth muscle cyclic GMP {220}.

Palmer et al. {221} established the chemical identity of EDRF as nitric oxide (NO), and Amezcua et al. {222} have shown that acetylcholine-induced vasodilation is due to release of nitric oxide. Other EDRFs have been described more recently {223}, including a hyperpolarizing factor {224} that produces relaxation by interaction with the voltage-operated calcium channel.

Blaise et al. {225} have shown that isoflurane is able to prevent smooth muscle contraction in canine coronary artery rings in response to 5-hydroxytryptamine only in the presence of intact endothelium. Muldoon et al. {226} studied the effect of halothane on the relaxation produced by acetylcholine and bradykinin in norepinephrine-contracted canine carotid and femoral artery rings and rabbit thoracic aortic rings. Relaxation was attenuated by 2% halothane in the acetylcholine/bradykinin group but not in the group where relaxation was produced by nitroglycerine (an endothelium-independent mechanism). They suggested halothane may interfere with the synthesis, release, or transport of EDRF. Halothane caused decreases in tension in canine carotid and rabbit aortic rings produced by nonepinephrine but increased tension in femoral artery rings. These results were unaffected by mechanical removal of the endothelium, which suggests a direct action on vascular smooth muscle.

Stone and Johns {227} studied the effects of halothane, enflurane, and isoflurane in rat thoracic aortic rings precontracted with phenylephrine. Endothelial intact rings showed vasoconstriction at low concentrations of enflurane and isoflurane with vasodilatation at higher concentrations. Although halothane produced vasoconstriction in some rings, its overall effect differed little from control. Rebound vasoconstriction occurred with discontinuance of all three agents. Vasoconstriction was potentiated with indomethacin addition. This suggests enflurane and isoflurane in low concentrations cause vasoconstriction

through inhibition of EDRF and/or stimulation of EDCF. At higher concentrations direct vasodilation occurs. Eskinder et al. {228} studied the effects of 2% and 3% halothane on cGMP levels and guanylate cyclase enzyme activity in rings of canine middle cerebral arteries that were preconstricted with 5-hydroxytryptamine. They compared halothane to sodium nitroprusside. Halothane produced increases in cGMP levels that were dose dependent. Nitroprusside also increased cGMP levels. Nitroprusside but not halothane modulated the activity of soluble guanylate cyclase enzyme. Halothane stimulated particulate guanylate cyclase enzyme activity. The authors suggest that halothane-induced vasodilation of cerebral blood vessels is partly mediated by an increase in tissue cGMP levels.

Halothane is an antagonist of the voltage-operated calcium channel in endothelial cells {229}. Luckhoff and Busse {230} have suggested that formation and/or activation of EDRF may be controlled by membrane potential. The effects of halothane on hyperpolarization and calcium-sensitive potassium channels is tissue dependent {231, 232}. The effect of halothane on endothelium Ca^{2+}-dependent K^+ channels is unknown.

Brendel and Johns {233} have created a model for differentiating EDRF-dependent relaxation from direct vascular smooth muscle relaxation by denuding rat thoracic aortic rings of endothelium and using L-NAME (a specific inhibitor of EDRF synthase). Isoflurane at 1%, 2%, and 3% produced dose-dependent vasodilation of endothelium-intact, endothelium-denuded, and L-NAME-treated vascular rings preconstricted with phenylephrine or KCl. The authors conclude that isoflurane vasodilation is not mediated by EDRF and does not involve the production of cyclic GMP. Greenblatt et al. {234} attempted to resolve the differing results obtained by the above investigators by studying intact animals rather than isolated tissues. Using radiolabeled microspheres, systemic and regional hemodynamics were measured in the cerebrum, cerebellum, heart, kidney, gastrointestinal tract, spleen, liver, skeletal muscle, skin, ear, and white and brown fat of rats. L-NMMA (an EDRF inhibitor) caused significantly greater increases in blood pressure in isoflurane-anesthetized rats than in the halothane group. Vascular resistance in heart, kidney, GI tract, hepatic artery, and skin was also greater in the isoflurane group than in the halothane group. These data indicate that EDRF plays a significant role in vascular control in both groups but that EDRF vasorelaxation is greater in coronary, renal, hepatic, splanchnic, and cutaneous circulations with isoflurane.

Bollen et al. in 1987 {235} published their work showing halothane relaxes previously constricted isolated porcine coronary artery segments more than isoflurane. They recently {236} repeated this work in human coronary arteries obtained from cardiac transplantation recipients. Underlying pathology was ischemic cardiomyopathy, viral cardiomyopathy, and AV malformation with pulmonary hypertension. Responses to the anesthetic agents were as previously reported for porcine coronary arteries and did not vary between groups. They also studied the effects of halothane and isoflurane on small and medium preconstricted porcine artery segments {237}. As with the larger epicardial arteries, halothane relaxes these arteries more than isoflurane. They also compared the ability of halothane and isoflurane to inhibit calcium channel activation by BAY K8644. Although halothane produced partial relaxation in potassium-constricted arteries, an additional mechanism for halothane relaxation must be in place. As Nugent {238} has pointed out, neither halothane nor isoflurane has an effect on the basal tensions of these isolated arteries or rings. They modify the tension only in contracted rings, unlike nitroglycerine.

Yoshida and Okabe {239} in a recent article suggest that sevoflurane selectively impairs endothelium-dependent relaxation of canine mesenteric arterial rings and not endothelium-independent relaxation via inactivation of EDRF. They also sugest this action is mediated by generation of a superoxide anion radical and/or other oxygen free radicals, possibly $-OH$. The mechanism of this generation is unknown.

HUMAN STUDIES

Sonntag et al. {240} found that 0.7% and 1.54% halothane caused a decrease in myocardial function in healthy patients in a dose-related manner without a change in heart rate. Myocardial blood flow and oxygen consumption also showed a dose-related decrease. Myocardial oxygenation was adequate, as evidenced by decreased oxygen extraction and unchanged lactate levels. The rate-pressure product correlated poorly with myocardial oxygen consumption, although there was a dose-related decrease during halothane anesthesia. Changes in arterial blood pressure and contractile function of the heart were more closely related to myocardial oxygen consumption but still not ideal. As they felt then, an ideal clinical correlate of myocardial oxygen demand is still unavailable.

ISCHEMIC HEART DISEASE

In ischemic heart disease there is an imbalance between myocardial oxygen supply and myocardial oxygen consumption. Experimentally produced ischemia by ligation of coronary arteries has been studied in the dog under halothane {241,242} and epidural anesthesia {243} with improvement in myocardial perfusion and oxygenation. Merin {244} has, however, has made the point that the control state was hyperdynamic with rapid heart rates. Anesthesia reduced heart rate and blood pressure. These, together with a depression of cardiac contractility, might depress myocardial oxygen demand more than a decreased coronary perfusion pressure decreased myocardial oxygen supply. Work in chronically instrumented animals {245} does not show a beneficial effect of halothane on the ischemic heart, and halothane $\frac{1}{2}$ and 1 MAC did not protect ventricular function following global myocardial ischemia {246}. Gerson et al. {247} used elevation of the ST segment on epicardial electrograms in response to temporary occlusion of the left descending coronary artery

as an index of ischemia. They compared 1% halothane to nitroprusside-propranolol and found the reduction of the ST segment to be significantly greater with halothane.

Later investigations utilized narrowed, rather than completely occluded, vessels in an attempt to provide conditions nearer to those present in clinical situations. Lowenstein and his coworkers {248} studied the effect of halothane between 0.5% and 2% on left ventricular myocardium supplied by a critically narrowed coronary artery (left anterior descending) and a normal coronary artery (left circumflex). An inspired halothane concentration well tolerated by myocardium supplied by the normal coronary artery produced dysfunction and paradox (i.e., ischemia) in the myocardium supplied by the narrowed coronary artery, despite normal global left ventricular function. The authors proposed that clinically unsuspected intraanesthetic compromise of such an area may be an important cause of perioperative myocardial infarction, despite the absence of an ischemic episode or hemodynamic instability. They felt a local decrease in perfusion pressure was the cause of the dysfunction.

This is supported by the work of Behrenbeck et al. {249}, which showed no difference in regional myocardial function in ischemic or nonischemic areas with increasing concentrations of halothane as long as perfusion was maintained. The former group also produced critical constriction of the left circumflex coronary artery {250}. Critical constriction of a coronary artery supplying a large area of the myocardium may cause a severe loss of regional myocardial perfusion, which is accompanied by an equally severe loss of global perfusion. The effects of enflurane in the presence of critical constriction of the left anterior descending coronary artery were to produce marked reduction in segmental wall function with matching global dysfunction {251}. Critical constriction produced slightly greater depression of left anterior descending segmental function, compared with the left circumflex segment, and significantly more depression of global function.

Hickey et al. {252} saw virtually no effect on hemodynamics, metabolism, or ECG findings at 40% decrease in left anterior descending coronary flow as a result of stenosis at 1.2 MAC halothane anesthesia. Low arterial pressure and 2.1 MAC produced evidence of ischemia. Merin et al. {253} produced a 60% reduction in flow to the left anterior descending coronary artery in swine, which resulted in ischemia of the cardiac muscle supplied by that vessel. Their object was to compare the effects of halothane with fentanyl-supplemented nitrous oxide anesthesia. Neither protected against ischemia or the degree of ischemia, and depression of ventricular function was not different. They concluded a decrease in oxygen supply due to coronary stenosis was no more deleterious to metabolic function when oxygen supply/demand was high, as with fentanyl, or when it was low, as with halothane. Lowenstein et al. {254}, however, using values from Merin et al. {253}, Waters et al. {255}, and Verrier et al. {206}, calculated that with the degree of narrowing reported by Merin and the hemodynamic state, a low-demand–low-pressure anesthetic (halothane) will be better tolerated than a high-demand–high-pressure anesthetic (fentanyl).

There are inherent problems in these studies. Coronary stenosis is imposed upon a preexisting stable anesthetic state, unlike the clinical situation, in which anesthesia is imposed upon severe narrowing of one or more coronary arteries {254}. Also such localized constrictions are unlikely clinically. More widespread coronary artery involvement might produce more evidence of global ischemia with hemodynamic correlates.

CLINICAL INVESTIGATIONS

Lieberman et al. {256} studied the effect of halothane in patients undergoing coronary artery bypass grafting by monitoring a V5 surface EKG. A total of 73% of their patients had evidence of left ventricular dysfunction prior to surgery. No evidence of new ischemic changes occurred prior to coronary artery bypass. Slogoff et al. {257} showed a 26% incidence of ischemia in patients given a morphine-based anesthetic, with a markedly higher incidence when beta blockade was withheld. Kistner et al. {258} also compared halothane and morphine in patients undergoing coronary artery bypass and found in a well-monitored situation that halothane was superior in avoiding ischemic and adverse hemodynamic changes. Delaney et al. {75} compared halothane and enflurane $\frac{3}{4}$ MAC in patients with coronary artery disease. Halothane decreases the contractile state, heart rate, and afterload, and therefore presumably myocardial oxygen consumption, while slightly increasing preload. Enflurane reduced afterload only. Similar findings have been described for isoflurane {259}, which reduces systemic vascular resistance to a greater extent than enflurane, while stroke volume and cardiac output are less impaired {260}. Isoflurane causes significantly less impairment of myocardial contractile performance compared to halothane and enflurane, despite the fact that its effects on contractile proteins and their enzyme systems are similar {261}.

Inhalational anesthetics are used in addition to high-dose opiates for coronary artery bypass procedures (CABG) to produce a smoother hemodynamic course {262}. The use of isoflurane has remained controversial, since Reiz et al. showed both electrocardiographic and metabolic evidence of myocardial oxygen imbalance during isoflurane anesthesia in patients with coronary artery disease {263}. This was attributed to decreased perfusion and redistribution of flow (coronary steal) as a result of vasodilation. Subsequent studies have also indicated ischemic changes as a result of this steal effect {264,265}. A retrospective study by Slogoff et al. {266} in patients with steal-prone anatomy undergoing CABG, however, failed to show an increased incidence of ischemic ECG changes with isoflurane.

Pulley et al. {267} have recently published a prospective study in which heart rate and arterial pressure were kept constant. Myocardial ischemia was monitored by ECG changes, regional wall changes on echocardiography, and myocardial lactate production. Anesthesia was with high-dose fentanyl supplemented with isoflurane or halothane. Their findings do not support coronary steal as a cause of

myocardial ischemia, and neither isoflurane or halothane is a likely cause of myocardial ischemia by this mechanism. Thompson et al. {268} compared desflurane and isoflurane in patients undergoing CABG. Both agents were used as primary agents in patients who had ejection fractions greater than 0.34. There were no differences between the two groups on the incidence of myocardial ischemia (ECG changes), perioperative myocardial infarction, or perioperative mortality.

In conclusion, we have summarized the effects of the volatile anesthetics in clinical use on the electrophysiology of the heart and their effects on the heart and coronary circulation with particular reference to ischemic heart disease, the major coincidental pathologic process faced by an anesthesiologist today. As we mentioned, above, high-dose opiate anesthesia with fentanyl or sufentanil supplemented with the inhalational anesthetic agents is the choice of the majority of anesthesiologists for this type of surgery. There is no single anesthetic agent that provides ideal conditions for surgery in patients with coronary artery disease. A judicious combination of various pharmacologic agents and careful monitoring is the "best" anesthesia.

REFERENCES

1. Hauswirth O, Schaer H: Effects of halothane on the sinoatrial node. *J Pharmacol Exp Ther* 158:36–39, 1967.
2. Reynolds AK, Chiz JF, Pasquet AF: Halothane and methoxflurane: A comparison of their effects on cardiac pacemaker fibers. *Anesthesiology* 33:602–610, 1970.
3. Maylie J, Morad M, Weiss J: A study of pacemaker potential in rabbit sino-atrial node: Measurement of potassium activity under voltage-clamp conditions. *J Physiol* 311:161–178, 1981.
4. Kampine JP, Bosnjak ZJ, Turner LA: Effects of halothane on SA node: Role of calcium. *Anesthesiology* 55:A58, 1981.
5. Lynch C, Vogel S, Sperelakis N: Halothane depression of myocardial slow action potentials. *Anesthesiology* 55:360–368, 1981.
6. Merlos JR, Bosnjak ZJ, Purlock RV, Turner LA, Kampine JR: Halothane and enflurane effects on SA node cells. *Anesthesiology* 53:S143, 1980.
7. Hauswirth O: Effects of halothane on single atrial, ventricular, and Purkinje fibers. *Circ Res* 24:745–750, 1969.
8. Reynolds AK, Chiz JF, Pasquet AF: Pacemaker migration and sinus node arrest with methoxyflurane and halothane. *Can Anaesth Soc J* 18:137–144, 1971.
9. Pratila MG, Vogel S, Sperelakis N: Effects of enflurane on rabbit atrium. Unpublished data.
10. Azari DM, Cork RC, Conzen P, Vollmar B, Kramer TH: Inotropic effects of sevoflurane compared to isoflurane and halothane. *Anesthesiology* 77:A628, 1992.
11. Polic S, Atlee JL III, Laszlo A, Kampine JP, Bosnjak ZJ: Anesthetics and automaticity in latent pacemaker fibers. II. Effects of halothane and epinephine or norepinephrine on automaticity of dominant and subsidiary atrial pacemakers in the canine heart. *Anesthesiology* 75:298–304, 1991.
12. Hoffman BF, Bigger JT Jr: Digitalis and the allied cardiac glycosides. In: Culman AG, Goodman LS, Rall TW, Murad F (eds) *The Pharmacological Basis of Therapeutics*, 7th ed. New York: Macmillan, 1985, pp 716–747.

13. Polic S, Atlee JL III, Laszlo A, Kampine JP, Bosnjak ZJ: Anesthetics and automaticity in latent pacemaker fibers. III. Effects of halothane and ouabain on automaticity of the SA node and subsidiary atrial pacemakers in the canine heart. *Anesthesioloy* 75:305–312, 1991.

14. Waxman MB, Sharma AD, Asta J, Cameron DA, Wald RW: The protective effect of vagus nerve stimulation on catecholamine-halothane-induced ventricular fibrillation in dogs. *Can J Physiol Pharmacol* 67:801–809, 1989.

15. Anthony BL, Dennison RL, Aronstam RS: Disruption of muscarinic receptor-AG protein coupling is a general property of liquid volatile anesthetics. *Neurosci Lett* 99: 191–196, 1989.

16. Szabo A, Otero AB: A-protein mediated regulation of K^+ channels in heart. *Ann Rev Physiol* 52:293–305, 1990.

17. Zipes DP, Mihalick MJ, Robbins AT: Effects of selective vagal and stellate ganglion stimulation on atrial refractoriness. *Cardiovasc Res* 8:647–655, 1974.

18. Sperelakis N, Josephson I: The slow action potential and properties of the myocardial slow Ca channels. In: Sperelakis N (ed) *Physiology and Pathophysiology of the Heart*, 2nd ed. Boston: Kluwer Academic Publishers, 1989, pp 195–225.

19. Seifen AB, Kennedy RH, Serifen E: Effects of volatile anesthetics on response to norepinephrine and acetylcholine in guinea pig atria. *Anesth Analg* 73:304–309, 1991.

20. Scherlag BJ, Helfant RH, Damato AN: A catheterization technique for His-bundle stimulation and recording in intact dog. *J Appl Physiol* 25:425–428, 1968.

21. Damato AN, Lau SH, Bobb GA, Wit AL: Recording of AV nodal activity in the intact dog heart. *Am Heart J* 80: 353–366, 1970.

22. Narula OS, Scherlag BJ, Samet P, Javier RP: Atrial ventricular block: Localization and classification by His-bundle recordings. *Am J Med* 50:146–165, 1971.

23. Kastor JA: Atrioventricular block. *N Engl J Med* 292: 462–465, 572–574, 1975.

24. Atlee JL, Rusy BF: Halothane depression of A-V conduction studied by electrograms of the bundle His in dogs. *Anesthesiology* 36:112–118, 1972.

25. Atlee JL, Alexander SC: Halothane effects on conductivity of the AV node and His Purkinje system in the dog. *Anesth Analg* 56:378–386, 1977.

26. Atlee JL, Homer LD, Tober RE: Diphenylhydantoin and lidocaine modification of AV conduction in halothane anesthetized dogs. *Anesthesiology* 43:49–60, 1975.

27. Atlee JL III, Houge JC, Malkinson CE: Halothane and AV conduction: Awake vs. anesthesia. *Anesthesiology* 55:A53, 1981.

28. Hantler CB, Kroll DA, Tait AR, Knight PR: Cardiac effects of halothane with spinal anesthesia. *Anesthesiology* 55:A4, 1981.

29. Morrow DH, Haley JV, Logic JR: Anesthesia and digitalis. VII. The effect of pentobarbital, halothane and methoxyflurane on the AV conduction and inotropic responses to ouabain. *Anesth Analg* 51:430–438, 1972.

30. Jacques A, Hudon F: Effect of epinephrine on the human heart during methoxyflurane anesthesia. *Can Anaesth Soc J* 10:53, 1963.

31. Atlee JR III, Rusy BF: Atrioventricular conduction times and atrioventricular nodal conductivity during enflurane anesthesia in dogs. *Anesthesiology* 47:498–503, 1977.

32. Atlee JR, Rusy BF, Kruel JF: Supraventricular excitability in dogs during anesthesia with halothane and enflurane. *Anesthesiology* 49:407–413, 1978.

33. Zaidan JR, Curling PE, Kaplan JA: Effect of enflurane on pacing threshold. *Anesthesiology* 55:A59, 1981.

34. Blitt CD, Raessler KL, Wightman MA, Groves BM, Wall CL, Geha DG: Atrioventricular conduction in dogs during anesthesia with isoflurane. *Anesthesiology* 50:210–212, 1979.

35. Atlee JL III, Brownlee SW, Burstrom RE: Conscious-state comparisons of the effects of inhalation anesthetics on specialized atrioventricular conduction times in dogs. *Anesthesiology* 64:703–710, 1986.

36. Wilton NCT, Hantler CB, Landau SN, Larsen LO, Knight PR: Effects of volatile anesthetic agents on sinus node function and atrioventricular conduction in dogs: A comparison with chloralose anesthesia. *J Cardiothorac Vasc Anesth* 2:188–193, 1988.

37. Duchene-Maruliaz P, Fabry-Delaigue R, Gueorguiev G, Kantelip JP, Marullaz PD, Delargue RF, Gueorguiev A, et al.: Influence of chloralose and pentobarbitane anesthesia on atrioventricular conduction in dogs. *Br J Pharmacol* 77: 309–317, 1982.

38. Atlee JR III, Yeager TS: Electrophysiologic assessment of the effects of enflurane, halothane and isoflurane on properties affecting supraventricular re-entry in chronically instrumented dogs. *Anesthesiology* 71:914–952, 1989.

39. Pruett JK, Mote PS, Grover TE, Augeri JM: Enflurane and halothane effects on cardiac Purkinje fibers. *Anesthesiology* 55:A65, 1981.

40. Chen C, Gettes LS, Katzung BG: Effect of lidocaine and quinidine on steady-state characteristics and recovery kinetics of $(dV/dt)_{max}$ in guinea pig ventricular myocardium. *Circ Res* 37:20–29, 1975.

41. McCleskey EW, Fox AP, Feldman D, Tsien RW: Different types of calcium channels. *J Exp Biol* 124:177–190, 1986.

42. Hagiwara N, Irisawa H, Kameyama M: Contribution of two types of calcium currents to the pacemaker potentials of rabbit sino-atrial node cells. *J Physiol* 395:233–253, 1988.

43. Bean BP: Two kinds of calcium channels in canine atrial cells. *J Gen Physiol* 87:1–30, 1985.

44. Nilius B, Hess P, Lansman JB, Tsien RW: A novel type of calcium channel in ventricular cells. *Nature* 316:443–446, 1985.

45. Tseng GN, Boyden PA: Multiple types of Ca^{2+} currents in single canine Purkinje cells. *Circ Res* 65:1735–1750, 1989.

46. Hirano Y, Fozzard HA, January CT: Characteristics of L and T type Ca^{2+} currents in canine cardiac Purkinje cells. *Am J Physiol* 256:H1478–H1492, 1989.

47. Eskinder H, Rusch NJ, Supan FD, Kampine JP, Bosnjak ZJ: The effects of volatile anesthetics on L- and T-type calcium channel currents in canine cardiac Purkinje cells. *Anesthesiology* 74:919–926, 1991.

48. Pratila M, Vogel S, Sperelakis N: Inhibition by enflurane and methoxyflurane of postdrive hyperpolarization in canine Purkinje fibers. *J Pharmacol Exp Ther* 229:603–607, 1984.

49. Laszlo A, Polic S, Atlee JR III, Kampine JP, Bosnjak ZJ: Anesthetics and automaticity in latent pacemaker fibers: 1) Effects of halothane, enflurane and isoflurane on automaticity and recovery of automaticity from overdrive suppression in Purkinje fibers derived from canine hearts. *Anesthesiology* 75:98–105, 1991.

50. Laszlo A, Polic S, Kampine JP, Turner LA, Atlee JL III, Bosnjak ZJ: Halothane, enflurane and isoflurane on abnormal automaticity and triggered rhythmic activity of Purkinje fibers from 24-hour-old infarcted canine hearts. *Anesthesiology* 75:847–853, 1991.

51. Polic S, Bosnjak ZJ, Marijik J, Hoffman RG, Kampine JP, Turner LA: Actions of halothane, isoflurane and enflurane on the regional action potential characteristics of canine Purkinje fibers. *Anesth Analg* 73:603–611, 1991.

52. Freeman LC, Muir WW III: Effects of halothane on impulse propagation in Purkinje fibers and at Purkinje-muscle junctions: Relationship of V_{max} to conduction velocity. *Anesth Analg* 72:5–10, 1991.

53. Ikemoto Y, Yatani A, Imoto Y, Arimurah H: Reduction in the myocardial sodium current by halothane and thiamyl. *Jpn J Physiol* 36:107–121, 1986.

54. Terrar DA, Victory JGG: Influence of halothane on electrical coupling in cell pairs isolated from guinea-pig ventricle. *Br J Pharmacol* 95:509–514, 1988.

55. Burt JM, Spray DC: Volatile anesthetics block intercellular communication between neonatal rat myocardial cells. *Circulation Res* 65:829–837, 1989.

56. Sasyniuk BI, Mendez C: A mechanism for re-entry in canine ventricular tissue. *Circ Res* 28:3–15, 1971.

57. Freeman AC, Muir WW III: Alpha-adrenoceptor stimulation in the presence of halothane: Effects on impulse propagation in cardiac Purkinje fibers. *Anesth Analg* 72:11–17, 1991.

58. Vodanovic S, Turner LA, Kampine JP, Bosnjak ZJ: Alpha-adrenergic receptors mediate the negative dromotropic effect of catecholamines in the presence of volatile anesthetics. *Anesthesiology* 77:A3–A594, 1992.

59. Oshita S, Oka H, Hiraoka I, Takeshita H: Halothane increases epinephrine threshold for the development of slow responses in isolated canine trabeculae. *Anesth Analg* 73:449–454, 1991.

60. Ehara T, Hasegawa J, Mitsuige T: Depolarization produced by cathecholamines in guinea-pig ventricular muscle cells exposed to potassium-rich media and its dependence on temperature. *J Mol Cell Cardiol* 15:555–564, 1983.

61. Zuckerman RL, Wheeler DM: Effect of halothane on arrhythmogenic responses induced by sympathetic agents in single rat heart cells. *Anesth Analg* 72:596–603, 1991.

62. Vodanovic S, Turner LA, Marijic J, Kampine JP, Bosnjak ZJ: Effects of epinephrine and volatile anesthetics on conduction velocity in canine Purkinje fibers. *Anesthesiology* 75:A569, 1991.

63. Wit AL, Rosen MR: Afterdepolarizations and triggered activity. In: Fozzard HA, Haber E, Jennings RB, Katz AM, Morgan HE (eds) *The Heart and Cardiovascular System*. New York: Raven Press, 1986, pp 1449–1490.

64. Orchard CH, Eisner DA, Allen DA: Oscillation of intracellular Ca^{2+} in mammalian cardiac muscle. *Nature* 304:735–738, 1983.

65. Hashimoto K, Endoh M, Kimura T: Effects of halothane on automaticity and contractile force of isolated blood-perfused canine ventricular tissue. *Anesthesiology* 42:15–25, 1975.

66. Logic JR, Morrow DH: The effect of halothane on ventricular automaticity. *Anesthesiology* 36:107–118, 1972.

67. Lynch C, Vogel S, Pratila MG, Sperelakis N: Enflurane depression of myocardial slow action potentials. *J Pharmacol Exp Ther* 222:405–409, 1982.

68. Vassalle M: Electrogenesis of the plateau and pacemaker potential. *Am Rev Physiol* 41:425–440, 1979.

69. Lynch C III: Differential depression of myocardial contractility by halothane and isoflurane in vitro. *Anesthesiology* 64:631–650, 1986.

70. Goldberg AH, Sohn YZ, Phear WPC: Direct myocardial effects of nitrous oxide. *Anesthesiology* 37:373–380, 1972.

71. Lappas DC, Buckley MJ, Laver MB, Daggett WM, Lowenstein E: Left ventricular performance and pulmonary circulation following addition of nitrous oxide to morphine during coronary-artery surgery. *Anesthesiology* 43:61–69, 1975.

72. Carton EG, Waner LA, Housmans PR: Effects of nitrous oxide on contractility, relaxation and the intracellular calcium transient of isolated mammalian ventricular myocardium. *J Pharmacol Exp Ther* 257:843–849, 1991.

73. Lawson D, Frazer MJ, Lynch C III: Nitrous oxide effects on isolated mycardium: A re-examination in vitro. *Anesthesiology* 73:930–943, 1990.

74. Carton EG, Housmans PR: Role of transsarcolemmal Ca^{2+} entry in the negative inotropic effect of nitrous oxide in isolated ferret myocardium. *Anesth Analg* 74:575–579, 1992.

75. Delaney TJ, Kistner JR, Lake CL, Miller ED Jr: Myocardial function during halothane and enflurane anesthesia in patients with coronary artery disease. *Anesth Analg* 59:240–244, 1980.

76. Stevens WC, Cromwell TH, Halsey MJ, Eger EI II, Shakespeare TF, Bahlman SH: The cardiovascular effects of a new inhalational anesthetic, Forane, in human volunteers at constant arterial carbon dioxide tension. *Anesthesiology* 35:8–16, 1971.

77. Rathod R, Jacobs HK, Kramer NE, Rao TLK, Salem MR, Towne WD: Echocardiograhic assessment of ventricular performance following induction with two anesthetics. *Anesthesiology* 49:86–90, 1978.

78. Kaplan JA, Miller ED, Bailey DR: A comparative study of enflurane and halothane using systolic time intervals. *Anesth Analg* 55:263–268, 1976.

79. Smith NT, Calverley RK, Prys-Roberts C, Eger EI II, Jones CW: Impact of nitrous oxide on the circulation during enflurane anesthesia in man. *Anesthesiology* 48:345–349, 1978.

80. Merin RG, Kumazawa T, Luka NL: Myocardial function and metabolism in the conscious dog and during halothane anesthesia. *Anesthesiology* 44:402–514, 1976.

81. Kemmotsu O, Hashimoto Y, Shimosato S: Inotropic effects of isoflurane on mechanics of contraction in isolated cat papillary muscles from normal and failing hearts. *Anesthesiology* 39:470–477, 1973.

82. Kemmotsu O, Hashimoto Y, Shimosato S: The effects of fluroxene and enflurane on contractile performance of isolated papillary muscles from failing hearts. *Anesthesiology* 40:252–260, 1974.

83. Ritzman RJ, Erickson HH, Miller ED: Cardiovascular effects of enflurane and halothane in the rhesus monkey. *Anesth Analg* 55:85–91, 1976.

84. Merin RG, Kumazawa T, Luka NL: Enflurane depresses myocardial function perfusion and metabolism in the dog. *Anesthesiology* 45:501–507, 1976.

85. Brown BR, Crout JR: A comparative study of the effects of five general anesthetics on myocardial contractility. *Anesthesiology* 34:236–245, 1971.

86. Seeman P: The membrane expansion theory of anesthesia. In: Fink BR (ed) *Molecular Mechanisms of Anesthesia. Progress in Anesthesiology*, Vol 1. New York: Raven Press, 1975, pp 243–252.

87. Halsey MJ: Structure-activity relationships of inhalational anesthetics. In: Halsey MJ, Millar RA, Sutton JA (eds) *Molecular Mechanisms in General Anesthesia*. Edinburgh: Churchill Livingstone, 1974, pp 3–16.

88. Halsey MJ, Brown FF, Richards RE: Perturbations of model protein systems as a basis for the central and peripheral mechanisms of general anaesthesia. *Molecular Interactions and Activity in Proteins. Ciba Foundation Symposium 60*. Amsterdam: Excerpta Medica, 1978.

89. Woodbury JW, d'Arrigo JS, Eyring H: Molecular mechanism of general anesthesia lipoprotein conformation change theory. In: Fink BR (ed) *Molecular Mechanisms of An-*

esthesia. *Progress in Anesthesiology*, Vol 1. New York: Raven Press, 1975, pp 253–276.

90. Metcalfe JC, Hoult JRS, Colley CM: The molecular implications of a unitary hypothesis of anesthetic action. In: Halsey MJ, Millar RA, Sutton JA (eds) *Molecular Mechanisms in General Anaesthesia*. Edinburgh: Churchill Livingstone, 1974, pp 145–163.

91. Cheng SC, Brunner EA: Is anesthesia caused by excess GABA? In: Fink BR (ed) *Molecular Mechanisms of Anesthesia. Progress in Anesthesiology*, Vol 2. New York: Raven Press, 1980, pp 137–144.

92. Trudell JR: A unitary theory of anesthesia based on lateral phase separations in nerve membranes. *Anesthesiology* 46:5–10, 1977.

93. Rosenberg PH, Eibl H, Stier A: Biphasic effects of halothane on phospholipid and synaptic plasma membranes: A spin label study. *Mol Pharmacol* 11:879–882, 1975.

94. Pang KY, Chang TL, Miller KW: On the coupling between anesthetic induced membrane fluidization and cation permeability in lipid vesicles. *Mol Pharmacol* 15:729–738, 1979.

95. Mastrangelo CJ, Trudell JR, Edmunds HN, Cohen EN: Effect of clinical concentrations of halothane on phospholipid membrane fluidity. *Mol Pharmacol* 14:463–467, 1978.

96. Menn RG: Inhalational anesthetics and myocardial metabolism: Possible mechanism of functional effects. *Anesthesiology* 34:236–245, 1971.

97. Lain RF, Hess ML, Gertz EW, Briggs FN: Calcium uptake activity of canine myocardial sarcoplasmic reticulum in the presence of anesthetic agents. *Circ Res* 23:597–604, 1968.

98. Lee SL, Alto LE, Dhalla NS: Subcellular effects of some anesthetic agents on rat myocardium. *Can J Physiol Pharmacol* 57:65–70, 1974.

99. Su JY, Kerrick WGL: Effects of halothane on Ca^{2+} activated tension development in mechanically disrupted rabbit myocardial fibers. *Pflügers Arch* 375:111–117, 1978.

100. Su JY, Kerrick WGL: Effects of halothane on caffeine-induced tension transients in functionally skinned myocardial fibers. *Pflügers Arch* 380:29–34, 1979.

101. Su JY, Kerrick WGL: Effects of enflurane on functionally skinned myocardial fibers from rabbits. *Anesthesiology* 52:385–389, 1980.

102. Su JY, Bell JG: Effects of isoflurane on functionally skinned myocardial fibers from rabbits. *Anesthesiology* 57:A11, 1982.

103. Murat I, Ventura-Clapier R, Vassort G: Halothane enflurane and isoflurane decrease calcium sensitivity and maximum force in detergent-treated rat cardiac fibers. *Anesthesiology* 69:892–899, 1988.

104. Ohnishi ST, DiCamillo CA, Singer M, Price HL: Correlation between halothane-induced myocardial depression and decreases in La^{3+}-displaceable Ca^{2+} in cardiac muscle cells. *J Cardiovasc Pharmacol* 2:67–75, 1980.

105. Blanck TJJ, Thompson M: Calcium transport by cardiac sarcoplasmic reticulum: Modulation of halothane action by substrate concentration and pH. *Anesth Analg* 60:390–394, 1981.

106. Conahan TJ, Blanck TJJ: Sarcoplasmic reticulum: Enflurane effect on Ca^{2+} dynamics. *Anesthesiology* 51:S146, 1979.

107. Blanck TJJ, Thompson M: Enflurane and isoflurane stimulate calcium transport by cardiac sarcoplasmic reticulum. *Anesth Analg* 61:142–145, 1982.

108. Drenger B, Runge SR, Hoehner P, Quigg M, Blanck TJJ: Halothane inhibits binding of calcium channel blockers to cardiac sarcolemma. In: Blanck TJJ, Wheeler DM (eds) *Mechanisms of Anesthetic Action in Skeletal, Cardiac and Smooth Muscle*. New York: Plenum Press, 1991, pp 109–123

109. Komai H, Rusy BF: Effect of halothane on rested state and potentiated-state contractions in rabbit papillary muscle: Relationship to negative inotropic actions. *Anesth Analg* 61:403–409, 1982.

110. Komai H, Rusy BF: Direct effect of halothane and isoflurane on the function of the sarcoplasmic reticulum in intact rabbit atria. *Anesthesiology* 72:694–698, 1990.

111. Komai H, Rusy BF: Contribution of the known subcellular effects of anesthetics to their negative inotropic effect in intact myocardium. In: Blanck TJJ, Wheeler DM (eds) *Mechanisms of Anesthetic Action in Skeletal, Cardiac and Smooth Muscle*. New York: Plenum Press, 1991, pp 115–123.

112. Wilde DW, Gutta R, Haney MF, Knight PR: Effects of volatile anesthetics on the intracellular Ca^{2+} concentration in cardiac muscle cells. In: Blanck TJJ, Wheeler DM (eds) *Mechanisms of Anesthetic Action in Skeletal, Cardiac and Smooth Muscle*. New York: Plenum Press, 1991, pp 125–141.

113. Hirota K, Ito Y, Kuze S, Momose Y: Effects of halothane on electrophysiologic properties and cyclic adenosine 3',5'-monophosphate content in isolated guinea pig hearts. *Anesth Analg* 74:564–567, 1992.

114. Hille B: Local anesthetics: Hydrophilic and hydrophobic pathways for the drug-receptor reaction. *J Gen Physiol* 69:487–515, 1977.

115. Kameyama M: Hescheler J, Hofmann F, Trautwein W: Modulation of Ca current during phosphorylation cycle in the guinea pig heart. *Pflügers Arch* 407:123–128, 1986.

116. Weidmann S: Heart: Electrophysiology. *Ann Rev Physiol* 36:155–169, 1974.

117. Shigenobu K, Schneider JA, Sperelakis N: Blockade of slow Na$^+$ and Ca^{2+} currents in myocardial cells by verapamil. *J Pharmacol Exp Ther* 190:280–288, 1974.

118. Fabiato A, Fabiato F: Calcium and cardiac excitation-contraction coupling. *Ann Rev Physiol* 41:473–484, 1979.

119. Awalt CH, Frederickson EL: The contractile and cell membrane effects of halothane. *Anesthesiology* 25:90, 1964.

120. Lynch C, Vogel S, Pratila MG, Sperelakis N: Methoxy-flurane depression of myocardial slow action potentials. Unpublished findings.

121. Shigenobu K, Sperelakis N: Calcium current channels induced by catecholamines in chick embryonic hearts whose fast Na$^+$ channels are blocked by TTX or elevated K$^+$. *Circ Res* 31:932–952, 1972.

122. Reuter H, Scholz H: A study of the ion selectivity and kinetic properties of the calcium-dependent slow inward current in cardiac muscle. *J Physiol (Lond)* 264:17–47, 1977.

123. Watanabe AM, Besch HR Jr: Cyclic adenosine monophosphate modulation of slow Ca^{2+} influx channels in guinea pig hearts. *Circ Res* 35:316–324, 1974.

124. Sperelakis N, Schneider JA: A metabolic control mechanism for calcium ion influx that may protect the ventricular myocardial cell. *Am J Cardiol* 37:1079–1085, 1976.

125. Reuter H, Scholz H: The regulation of the calcium conductance of cardiac muscle by adrenalin. *J Physiol (Lond)* 264:49–62, 1977.

126. Kass RS, Siegelbaum SA, Tsien RW: Three microelectrode voltage clamp experiments in calf Purkinje fibers: Is slow inward current adequately measured? *J Physiol (Lond)* 290:201–225, 1979.

127. Bosnjak ZJ, Supan FD, Rusch NJ: The effects of halothane, enflurane and isoflurane on calcium current in isolated canine ventricular cells. *Anesthesiology* 74:340–345, 1991.

128. Housmans PR, Murat I: Comparative effects of halothane, enflurane and isoflurane at equipotent anesthetic concentrations on isolated ventricular myocardium of the ferret. 1

Contractility. *Anesthesiology* 69:451–463, 1988.

129. Bosnjak ZJ, Aggarwal A, Turner LA, Kampine JM, Kampine JP: Differential effects of halothane, enflurane, and isoflurane on Ca^{2+} transient and papillary muscle tension in guinea pigs. *Anesthesiology* 76:123–131, 1992.

130. Frazer MJ, Lynch C III: Halothane and isoflurane effects on Ca^{2+} fluxes of isolated myocardial sarcoplasmic reticulum. *Anesthesiology* 77:316–323, 1992.

131. Casella ES, Suite DA, Fisher YI, Blanck TJJ: The effect of volatile anesthetics on the pH dependence of calcium uptake by cardiac sarcoplasmic reticulum. *Anesthesiology* 67:386–390, 1987.

132. Frazer MJ, Lynch C III: Ca release channels of cardiac sarcoplasmic reticulum are activated by halothane, but not by isoflurane. *Anesthesiology* 77:A630, 1992.

133. Miao N, Frazer MJ, Lynch C III: Volatile anesthetic actions on cardiac sarcoplasmic reticulum Ca-ATPase. *Anesthesiology* 77:A631, 1992.

134. Shimosato S, Yasuda I, Kemmotsu O, Shanks C, Gamble C: Effect of halothane on altered contractility of isolated heart muscle obtained from cats with experimentally produced ventricular hypertrophy and failure. *Br J Anaesth* 45:2–9, 1973.

135. Rooke GA, Su JY: Left ventricular hypertrophy in rabbits does not exaggerate the effects of halothane on the intracellular components of cardiac contraction. *Anesthesiology* 77:513–521, 1992.

136. Baum VC: Will the calcium channel against BAY K 8644 inhibit halothane-induced impairment of calcium current? *Anesth Analg* 74:865–869, 1992.

137. Boban M, Stowe DF, Buljubasic N, Kampine Jr, Bosnjak ZJ: Direct comparative effects of isoflurane and desflurane in isolated guinea pig hearts. *Anesthesiology* 76:775–780, 1992.

138. Nakao M, Hiraiwa K, Maehara Y, Yoge O: Seroflurane as well as halothane depress calcium current of single ventricular myocyte. *Anesthesiology* 77:A624, 1992.

139. Morrow DH, Townley NT: Anesthesia and digitalis toxicity: An experimental study. *Anesth Analg* 43:510–519, 1964.

140. Reynolds AK, Horne ML: Studies on the cardiotoxicity of ouabain. *Can J Physiol Pharmacol* 47:165–170, 1969.

141. Morrow DH, Knapp DE, Logic JR: Anesthesia and digitalis toxicity. V. Effect of the vagus on ouabain-induced ventricular automaticity during halothane. *Anesth Analg* 49:23–27, 1970.

142. Damato AN, Lau SH, Bobb GA: Digitalis-induced bundle-branch ventricular tachycardia studied by electrode catheter recordings of the specialized conducting tissues of the dog. *Circ Res* 28:16–22, 1971.

143. Logic JR, Morrow DH: The effect of halothane on ventricular automaticity. *Anesthesiology* 36:107–118, 1972.

144. Matsui H, Schwartz A: Mechanism of cardiac glycoside inhibition of the $(Na^+\text{-}K^+)$-dependent ATPase from cardiac tissue. *Biochim Biophys Acta* 151:655–663, 1968.

145. Baker PF, Blaustein MP, Hodgkin AL, Steinhardt RA: The influence of calcium on sodium efflux in squid axons. *J Physiol (Lond)* 200:431–458, 1969.

146. Pruett JK, Gramling ZW: Halothane enhanced membrane responsiveness in canine Purkinje fibers. *Fed Proc* 38:589, 1979.

147. Ivankovich AD, Miletich DJ, Grossman RK, Albrecht RF, El-Etr AA, Cairoli VJ: The effect of enflurane, isoflurane, fluroxene, methoxyflurane and diethyl ether anesthesia on ouabain tolerance in the dog. *Anesth Analg* 55:360–365, 1976.

148. Pearle DL, Gillis RA: Effect of digitalis on response of the

149. Skovsted P, Price ML, Price HL: The effects of carbon dioxide on preganglionic sympathetic activity during halothane, methoxyflurane and cyclopropane anesthesia. *Anesthesiology* 37:70–75, 1972.

150. Brown FF III, Owens WD, Felts JA, Spitznagel EL Jr, Cryer PE: Plasma epinephrine and norepinephrine levels during anesthesia: Enflurane-N_2O-O_2 compound with fentanyl-N_2O-O_2. *Anesth Analg* 61:366–370, 1982.

151. Skovsted P, Sapthavichaikul S: The effects of isoflurane on arterial pressure, pulse rate, autonomic nervous activity and barostatic reflexes. *Can Anaesth Soc J* 24:304–314, 1977.

152. Gallagher JD, McClernan CA: The effects of halothane on ventricular tachycardia in intact dogs. *Anesthesiology* 75:866–875, 1991.

153. January CT, Riddle JM: Early afterdepolarizations: Mechanism of induction and block. *Circ Res* 64:977–990, 1989.

154. Colombe A, Coraboeuf E, Malecot C, Deroubaix E: Role of the "Na^+ window" current and other ionic currents in triggering early afterdepolarizations and resulting re-excitations in Purkinje fibers. In: Zipes DP, Jalife J (eds) *Cardiac Electrophysiology and Arrhythmias*. Orlando: Grune and Stratton, 1985, pp 43–49.

155. Deutsch N, Hantler CB, Tait AR, Uprichard A, Schork MA, Knight PR: Suppression of ventricular arrhythmias by volatile anesthetics in a canine model of chronic myocardial infarction. *Anesthesiology* 72:10212–1021, 1990.

156. Hashimoto K, Hashimoto K: The mechanism of sensitization of the ventricle to epinephrine by halothane. *Am Heart J* 83:652–658, 1972.

157. Hashimoto K, Endoh M, Kimura T: Effects of halothane on automaticity and contracile force of isolated blood-perfused canine ventricular tissue. *Anesthesiology* 42:15–25, 1975.

158. Zink J, Sasyniuk BI, Dresel PE: Halothane-epinephrine induced cardiac arrhythmias and the role of heart rate. *Anesthesiology* 43:548–555, 1975.

159. Singer DH, Lazzara R, Hoffman BF: Electrophysiological effects of canine peripheral A-V conducting system. *Circ Res* 26:361–378, 1970.

160. Reynolds AK, Chiz JF: Epinephrine-potentiated slowing of conduction in Purkinje fibers. *Res Commun Chem Pathol Pharmacol* 9:633–642, 1974.

161. Joas TA, Stevens WC: Comparison of the arrhythmic doses of epinephrine during Forane, halothane and fluroxene anesthesia in dogs. *Anesthesiology* 35:48–53, 1971.

162. Horrigan RW, Eger EI II, Wilson C: Epinephrine-induced arrhythmias during enflurane anesthesia in man: A nonlinear dose-response relationship and dose-dependent protection from lidocaine. *Anesth Analg* 57:547–550, 1970.

163. Johnston RR, Eger EI II, Wilson C: A comparative interaction of epinephrine with enflurane, isoflurane and halothane in man. *Anesth Analg* 55:709–712, 1976.

164. Singh BN, Ellrodt G, Peter GT: Verapamil: A review of its pharmacological properties and therapeutic use. *Drugs* 15:169–197, 1978.

165. Brichard G, Zimmerman PE: Verapamil in cardiac dysrhythmias during anesthesia. *Br J Anaesth* 42:1005–1012, 1970.

166. Bayer R, Kalusche D, Kaufmann R, Mannhold R: Inotropic and electrophysiological actions of verapamil and D-600 in myocardium. III. Effects of the optical isomers on transmembrane action potentials. *Naunyn-Schmiedebergs Arch Pharmacol* 290:81–97, 1975.

167. Merin RG: Slow channel inhibitors, anesthetics and cardio-

vascular function. *Anesthesiology* 55:198–200, 1981.

168. Kapur PA, Flacke WE: Epinephrine-induced arrhythmias and cardiovascular function after verapamil during halothane anesthesia in the dog. *Anesthesiology* 55:218–225, 1981.

169. Kapur PA, Flacke WE, Olewine SK, Van Etten PA: Cardiovascular and catecholamine responses to verapamil during enflurane anesthesia. *Anesthesiology* 55:A14, 1981.

170. Kapur PA, Flacke WE, Olewine SK: Comparison of effects of isoflurane versus enflurane on cardiovascular and catecholamine responses to verapamil in dogs. *Anesth Analg* 61:193–194, 1982.

171. Kates RA, Kaplan JA, Hug CC, Guyton R, Dorsey LM: Hemodynamic interactions of verapamil and isoflurane in dogs. *Anesth Analg* 61:194–195, 1982.

172. Ellrodt GK, Chew CYC, Singh BN: Therapeutic implications of slow-channel blockade in cardio-cirlatory disorders. *Circulation* 62:669–679, 1980.

173. Himmel HM, Schappert T, Ravens U: Combined effects of volatile anesthetics and phosphodiesterase inhibitors on contractile performance in guinea pig hearts. *Anesth Analg* 73:76–82, 1991.

174. Takada K, Sumikawa K, Kamibuyashi T, Hayashi Y, Yamatodans A, Yoshiya I: Comparative efficacy of cation-channel blockers to prevent halothane-epinephrine arrhythmias in rats. *Anesthesiology* 77:3A A592, 1992.

175. Braunwald E: Control of myocardial oxygen consumption. *Am J Cardiol* 27:416–432, 1971.

176. Smith NT: Myocardial function and anaesthesia. In: Prys-Roberts C (ed) *The Circulation of Anaesthesia.* Oxford: Blackwell Scientific, 1980, pp 59–60.

177. Shimosato S: Isovolumic intraventricular pressure change: An index of myocardial contractility during anesthesia. *Anesthesiology* 31:327–333, 1969.

178. Pollack GH: Isovolumic intraventricular pressure. *Anesthesiology* 32:381–383, 1970.

179. Mason DT, Braunwald E, Covell JW, Sonnenblick EH, Ros J Jr: Assessment of cardiac contractility: The relation between the rate of pressure rise and ventricular pressure during isovolumic systole. *Circulation* 44:47–58, 1971.

180. Prys-Roberts C, Gersh RJ, Baker AB, Reuben SR: The effects of halothane on the interactions between myocardial contractility, aortic impedance and left ventricular performance. I. Theoretical considerations and results. *Br J Anaesth* 44:634–639, 1972.

181. Nelson RR, Gobel FL, Jorgensen CR, Wang K, Wang Y, Taylor HL: Hemodynamic predictors of myocardial oxygen consumption during static and dynamic exercise. *Circulation* 50:1179–1189, 1974.

182. Gobel FL, Nordstrom LA, Nelson RR, Jorgensen CR, Wang Y: Rate-pressure product as an index of myocardial oxygen consumption during exercise in patients with angina pectoris. *Circulation* 57:549–556, 1978.

183. Roy WL, Edelist G, Gilbert B: Myocardial ischemia during noncardiac surgical procedures in patients with coronary-artery disease. *Anesthesiology* 51:393–397, 1979.

184. Sonntag H: Actions of anesthetics on the coronary circulation in normal subjects and patients with ischemic heart disease. *Int Anesthesiol Clin* 18:111–135, 1980.

185. Brandi G, McGregor M: Intramural pressure in the left ventricle of the dog. *Cardiovasc Res* 3:472–475, 1969.

186. Hoffman JIE: Determinants and prediction of transmural myocardial perfusion. *Circulation* 58:381–391, 1978.

187. Cohen MV, Kirk ES: Differential response of large and small coronary arteries to nitroglycerin and angiotensin: Autoregulation and tachyphylaxis. *Circ Res* 33:445–453, 1973.

188. Braunwald E, Ross J Jr, Sonnenblick EH: Regulation of coronary blood flow. In: *Mechanisms of Contraction of the Normal and Failing Heart,* 2nd ed. Boston: Little Brown, 1976, pp 200–231.

189. Vatner SF, Franklin D, Braunwald E: Effects of anesthesia and sleep on circulatory response to carotid sinus nerve stimulation. *Am J Physiol* 220:1249–1255, 1971.

190. Berne RM: Effect of epinephrine and nor-epinephrine on coronary circulation. *Circ Res* 6:644–655, 1958.

191. Hardin RA, Scott JB, Haddy FJ: Effect of epinephrine and norepinephrine on coronary vascular resistance in dogs. *Am J Physiol* 201:276–280.

192. Hackett JG, Abboud FM, Mark AL, Schmid PG, Heistad DD: Coronary vascular responses to stimulation of chemoreceptors and baroreceptors: Evidence for reflex activation of vagal cholinergic innervation. *Circ Res* 31:8–17, 1972.

193. Vatner SF, Higgins CB, Braunwald E: Effects of norepinephrine on coronary circulation and left ventricular dynamics in the conscious dog. *Circ Res* 34:812–823, 1974.

194. Pitt B, Elliot EC, Gregg DE: Adrenergic receptor activity in the coronary arteries of the unanesthetized dog. *Circ Res* 21:75–84, 1967.

195. Klocke FJ, Ellis AK, Orlick AE: Sympathetic influences on coronary perfusion and evolving concepts of driving pressure, resistance and transmural flow regulation. *Anesthesiology* 52:1–5, 1980.

196. Eberlein HJ: Der einfluss von anasthetika autdas koronargefasssystem. *Wien Z Inn Med* 46:400–403, 1965.

197. Saito T, Wakisaka K, Yudate T: Coronary and systemic circulation during (inhalation) anesthesia in dogs. *Far East J Anesth* 5:105–111, 1966.

198. Weaver PC: Study of the cardiovascular effects of halothane. *Ann R Coll Surg Engl* 49:114–136, 1971.

199. Kumazawa T, Merin RG: Effects of inhalation anesthetics on cardiac function and metabolism in the intact dog. *Recent Adv Cardiac Struct Metab* 10:71–79, 1975.

200. Douglas WR: Of pigs and men and research: A review of applications and analogies of the pig, *Sus scrofa,* in human medical research. *Space Life Sci* 3:226–234, 1972.

201. Merin RG, Verdouw PD, DeJong JW: Dose-dependent depression of cardiac function and metabolism by halothane in swine (*Sus scrofa*). *Anesthesiology* 46:417–423, 1977.

202. Wolff G, Claudi B, Rist M, Wardak MR, Niederer W, Graedel E: Regulation of coronary blood flow during ether and halothane anaesthesia. *Br J Anaesth* 44:1139–1149, 1972.

203. Domenech RJ, Macho P, Valdes J, Penna M: Coronary vascular resistance during halothane anesthesia. *Anesthesiology* 46:236–240, 1977.

204. Sawyer DC, Ely SW, Korthuis RJ, Scott JB: Effects of halothane in right coronary circulation in the dog. *Anesth Analg* 59:559, 1980.

205. Sawyer DC, Ely SW, Scott JB: Halothane and enflurane effects on the coronary circulation. *Anesthesiology* 53:S129, 1980.

206. Verrier ED, Edelist G, Consigny PM, Robinson S, Hoffman JIE: Greater coronary vascular reserve in dogs anesthetized with halothane. *Anesthesiology* 53:445–459, 1980.

207. Muggenburg BA, Mauderly JL: Cardiopulmonary function of awake, sedated and anesthetized beagle dogs. *J Appl Physiol* 37:152–157, 1974.

208. Vatner SP, Smith NT: Effects of halothane on left ventricular function and distribution of regional blood flow in dogs and primates. *Circ Res* 34:155–167, 1974.

209. Kenny D, Proctor LT, Schmeling WT, Kampine JP, Warther DC: Isoflurane causes only minimal increases in coronary

blood flow independent of oxygen demand. *Anesthesiology* 75:640–649, 1991.

210. Moore PG, Kien ND, Reitan JA, White DA, Safwat AM: No evidence for blood flow redistribution with isoflurane or halothane during acute coronary artery occlusion in fentanyl-anesthetized dogs. *Anesthesiology* 75:854–865, 1991.

211. Bernard JW, Wouters PF, Doursout MF, Florence B, Chelly JE, Merin RG: Effects of seroflurane and isoflurane on cardiac and coronary dynamics in chronically instrumented dogs. *Anesthesiology* 72:659–662, 1992.

212. Manohar M, Parks CM: Porane systemic and regional organ blood flow during 1 and 1–5 minimal alveolar concentrations of seroflurane anesthesia without and with 50% nitrous oxide. *J Pharmacol Exp Ther* 231:640–648, 1984.

213. Pagel PS, Kampine JR, Schmeling WT, Warltier DC: Comparison of the systemic and coronary hemodynamic actions of resflurane, isoflurane, halothane and enflurane in the chronically instrumented dog. *Anesthesiology* 74:539–551, 1991.

214. Vanhoutte PM: The endothelium-modulator of vascular smooth muscle tone. *N Engl J Med* 319:512–513, 1988.

215. Furchgott RF, Zawadzki JV: The obligatory role of endothelial cells in the relaxation of arterial smooth muscle by acetylcholine. *Nature* 288:373–376, 1980.

216. Masaki T, Kimura S, Yanagisawa M, Goto K: Molecular and cellular mechanism of endothelin regulation: Implications for vascular function. *Circulation* 84:1457–1468, 1991.

217. Johns RA: Endothelium-derived relaxing factor: Basic review and clinical implications. *J Cardiothor Anesth* 5:69–79, 1991.

218. Cohen RA, Shepherd JT, Vanhoulte PM: 5-hydroxytryptamine can mediate endothelium-dependent relaxation of coronary arteries. *Am J Physiol* 245:H1077–1080, 1983.

219. Martin W, Furchgott RF, Villani GM, Jothianandan D: Depression of contractile responses in rat aorta by spontaneously released endothelium-derived relaxing factor. *J Pharmacol Exp Ther* 237:529–538, 1986.

220. Holzmann S: Endothelium-induced relaxation by acetylcholine associated with larger rises in cyclic GMP in coronary arterial straps. *J Cyclic Nucleotide Res* 8:409–419, 1982.

221. Palmer RMJ, Ferrige AG, Mocada S: Nitric oxide release accounts for the biological activity of endothelium-derived relaxing factor. *Nature* 327:524–526, 1987.

222. Amezcua JL, Dusting GJ, Palmer RMJ, Moncada S: Acetylcholine includes vasodilation in the rabbit isolated heart through the release of nitric oxide, the endogenous nitro vasodilator. *Br J Pharmacol* 95:830–834, 1988.

223. Hoeffner U, Feletou M, Flavahan NA, Vanhoutte PM: Canine arteries release two different endothelium derived relaxing factors.

224. Feletou M, Vanhoutte PM: Endothelium-dependent hyperpolarization of canine coronary smooth muscle. *Br J Pharmacol* 93:515–524, 1988.

225. Blaise A, Sill JC, Nugent M, Van Dyke RA, Vanhoutte PM: Isoflurane causes endothelium-dependent inhibition of contractile responses of canine coronary arteries. *Anesthesiology* 67:513–517, 1987.

226. Muldoon SM, Hart JL, Bowen KA, Freas W: Attenuation of endothelium-mediated vasodilation by halothane. *Anesthesiology* 68:31–37, 1988.

227. Stone DJ, Johns RA: Endothelium-dependent effects of halothane, enflurane and isoflurane on isolated rat aortic vascular rings. *Anesthesiology* 71:126–132, 1989.

228. Eskinder H, Hillard CJ, Flynn MB, Bosnjak ZJ, Kampine JP: Role of guanylate cyclase-cAMP systems in halothane-induced vasodilation in canine cerebral arteries. *Anesthesiology* 77:482–487, 1992.

229. Blaise A, Hughes J, Sill JC, Buluran J, Caille A: Attenuation of contraction of isolated canine coronary arteries by enflurane and halothane. *Can J Anaesth* 38:111–115, 1990.

230. Luckhoff A, Busse R: Calcium enflux into endothelial cells and formation of endothelium-derived relaxing factor 15 controlled by the membrane potential. *Pflügers Arch* 416:305–311, 1990.

231. Scharff O, Foder B: Halothane inhibits hyper-polarization and potassium channels in human red blood cells. *Eur J Pharmacol* 159:165–173, 1989.

232. Nicoll RA, Madison DV: General anesthetics hyperpolarize neurons in the vertebrate central nervous system. *Science* 217:1055–1057, 1982.

233. Brendel JK, Johns RA: Isoflurane does not vasodilate rat-thoracic aortic rings by endothelium-derived relaxing factor or other cyclic GMP-mediated mechanisms. *Anesthesiology* 77:126–131, 1992.

234. Greenblatt EP, Loeb AL, Longnecher DE: Endothelium-dependent circulatory control — a mechanism for the differing peripheral vascular effects of isoflurane versus halothane. *Anesthesiology* 77:1178–1185, 1992.

235. Bollen BA, Tinker JH, Hermsmeyer K: Halothane relaxes previously constricted isolated porcine coronary artery segments more than isoflurane. *Anesthesiology* 66:748–752, 1987.

236. Bollen BA, McKlveen RE, Stevenson JA: Halothane relaxes previously constricted human epicardial coronary artery segments more than isoflurane. *Anesth Analg* 75:4–8, 1992.

237. Bollen BA, McKlveen RE, Stevenson JA: Halothane relaxes pre-constricted small and medium isolated porcine coronary artery segments more than isoflurane. *Anesth Analg* 75:9–17, 1992.

238. Nugent M: Anesthesia and myocardial ischemia: The gains of the past have largely come from control of myocardial oxygen demand; the breakthroughs of the future will involve optimizing myocardial oxygen supply. *Anesth Analg* 75:1–3, 1992.

239. Yoshida K, Okabe E: Selective impairment of endothelium-dependent relaxation by seroflurane: Oxygen free radical participation. *Anesthesiology* 76:440–447, 1992.

240. Sonntag H, Merin RG, Donath U, Radke J, Schenk HD: Myocardial metabolism and oxgenation in man awake and during halothane anesthesia. *Anesthesiology* 51:204–210, 1979.

241. Bland JHL, Lowenstein EL: Halothane-induced decrease in experimental myocardial ischemia in the non-failing canine heart. *Anesthesiology* 45:287–293, 1976.

242. Smith G, Rogers K, Thorburn J: Halothane improves the balance of oxygen supply to demand in acute experimental myocardial ischemia. *Br J Anaesth* 52:577–583, 1980.

243. Klassen GA, Bramwell RS, Bromage PR: Effect of acute sympathectomy by epidural anesthesia on the canine coronary circulation. *Anesthesiology* 52:8–15, 1980.

244. Merin RC: Is anesthesia beneficial for the ischemic heart? *Anesthesiology* 53:439–440, 1980.

245. Prys-Roberts C, Roberts JG, Foex P, Clarke TNS, Bennett MJ, Ryder WA: Interaction of anesthesia, beta receptor blockade and blood loss in dogs with induced myocardial infarction. *Anesthesiology* 45:326–339, 1976.

246. Nugent M, Walls JT, Tinker JH, Harrison CE: Post-ischemic myocardial function. No anesthetic protection. *Anesthesiology* 53:S108, 1980.

247. Gerson JL, Hickey RF, Bainton CR: Treatment of myocardial ischemia with halothane or nitroprusside-

propranolol. *Anesth Analg* 62:10–14, 1982.

248. Lowenstein E, Foex P, Francis CM, Davis WL, Yusuf S, Ryder WA: Regional ischemic ventricular dysfunction in myocardium supplied by a narrowed coronary artery with increasing halothane concentration in the dog. *Anesthesiology* 55:349–359, 1981.

249. Behrenbeck T, Nugent M, Quasha A, Hoffman E, Ritman E, Tinker JH: Halothane and ischemic regional myocardial wall dynamics. *Anesthesiology* 53:S140, 1980.

250. Francis CM, Glazebrook C, Lowenstein E, Davies WL, Foex P, Ryder WA: Effect of halothane on the performance of the heart in the case of critical constriction of the left circumflex coronary artery. *Br J Anaesth* 52:953P, 1980.

251. Cutfield GR, Francis CM, Foex P, Lowenstein E, Davies WL, Ryder WA: Myocardial function and critical constriction of the left anterior descending coronary artery: Effects of enflurane. *Br J Anaesth* 52:953P, 1980.

252. Hickey RF, Verrier ED, Baer RW, Vlahakes GJ, Hoffman JIE: Does deliberate hypotension produce myocardial ischemia when the coronary artery is stenotic? *Anesthesiology* 53:S89, 1980.

253. Merin RG, Verdouw PD, De Jong JW: Myocardial functional and metabolic responses to ischemia in swine during halothane and fentanyl anesthesia. *Anesthesiology* 56:84–92, 1982.

254. Lowenstein E, Hill RD, Rajogopalan B, Schneider RC: Winnie the Pooh revisited, or, the more recent adventures of Piglet. *Anesthesiology* 56:81–83, 1982.

255. Waters DD, Daluz P, Wyatt HL, Swan JHC, Forrester JS: Early changes in regional and global left ventricular function induced by graded reductions in regional coronary perfusion. *Am J Cardiol* 39:537–543, 1977.

256. Lieberman RW, Jobes DR, Schwartz AJ, Andrews RW: Incidence of ischemia during CABG using halothane. *Anesthesiology* 51:S90, 1979.

257. Slogoff S, Keats AS, Oh E: Preoperative propranolol therapy and aorto-coronary bypass operation. *JAMA* 240:1487–1490, 1978.

258. Kistner JR, Miller ED, Lake CL, Ross WT Jr: Indices of myocardial oxygenation during coronary artery revascularization in man with morphine versus halothane anesthesia. *Anesthesiology* 50:324–330, 1979.

259. Caverly RK, Smith NT, Jones CW, Prys-Roberts C, Eger EI

II: Ventilatory and cardiovascular effects of enflurane anesthesia during spontaneous ventilation in man. *Anesth Analg* 57:610–618, 1978.

260. Tarnow J, Eberlein HJ, Oser G, Patschke D, Schneider E, Schweichel E, Wilde J: Influence of modern inhalational anesthetics on hemodynamics, myocardial contractility, LV volumes and myocardial oxygen supply. *Anesthetist* 26:220–230, 1977.

261. Pask GT, England PJ, Prys-Roberts C: Effects of volatile inhalational anesthetics on isolated bovine cardiac myofibrillar ATPase. *J Mol Cell Cardiol* 13:293–301, 1981.

262. Sahlman L, Milocco I, Appelgren L, William-Olsson G, Ricksten S: Control of intraoperative hypertension with isoflurane in patients with coronary artery disease. Effects on regional myocardial blood flow and metabolism. *Anesth Analg* 68:105–111, 1989.

263. Reiz S, Balfors E, Sorensen MB, Anola S, Friedman A, Truedsson H: Isoflurane: A powerful coronary dilator in patients with coronary artery disease. *Anesthesiology* 59:91–97, 1983.

264. Khambatta HJ, Sonntag H, Larsen R, Stephan H, Stone JG, Kettler D: Global and regional myocardial blood flow and metabolism during equipotent halothane and isoflurane anesthesia in patients with coronary artery disease. *Anesth Analg* 67:936–942, 1988.

265. Buffington CW, Romson JL, Levine A, Duttlinger NC, Huang AH: Isoflurane induces coronary steal in a canine model of chronic coronary occlusion. *Anesthesiology* 66:280–292, 1987.

266. Slogoff S, Keats AS, Dear WE, Abadia A, Lawyer JT, Moulds JP, Williams TM: Steal prone coronary anatomy and myocardial ischemia associated with four primary anesthetic agents in humans. *Anesth Analg* 72:22–27, 1991.

267. Pulley DD, Kirvassilis GV, Kelermenos N, Kater K, Barzilai B, Genton RE, Efstathiou C, Lappas DG: Regional and global myocardial circulatory and metabolic effects of isoflurane and halothane in patients with steal-prone coronary anatomy. *Anesthesiology* 75:756–766, 1991.

268. Thompson IR, Bowering JB, Hudson RJ, Frais MA, Rosenbloom M: A comparison of desflurane and isoflurane in patients undergoing coronary artery surgery. *Anesthesiology* 75:776–781, 1991.

CHAPTER 40

Effects of Toxic Substances on the Heart

VICTOR J. FERRANS

INTRODUCTION

The reactions of the heart to toxic injury can be classified according to whether they are caused by (a) a direct toxic effect of the agent; (b) an exaggeration of the pharmacologic effect of the agent, either on the myocardium itself or on the coronary or systemic circulation; or (c) an allergic or hypersensitivity phenomena. Most cardiotoxic drugs produce the feature of either an acute toxic or an acute allergic reaction, and these usually develop shortly after administration of single or multiple doses of a particular drug. These lesions demonstrate an unequivocal cause-and-effect relationship, whether they result from an overdose, a side effect, or a hypersensitivity reaction. The clinical features of these reactions usually include electrocardiographic ischemic changes, arrhythmias, acute cardiac failure, and sudden death. From the morphologic standpoint, drug-induced myocardial lesions usually consist of multifocal areas of myocardial degeneration, necrosis, inflammation, or fibrosis; however, large, confluent areas of necrosis and fibrosis resembling myocardial infarcts develop in certain toxic reactions. Some agents, such as digitalis and quinidine, can cause rapidly fatal changes in cardiovascular function (particularly arrhythmias) without accompanying morphologic alterations; cardiomegaly in these circumstances is attributable to preexisting heart disease. Less frequently, drugs or chemicals may produce long-term cardiac alterations with clinical and morphological manifestations of a chronic cardiomyopathy. In this review, the morphologic reactions of the heart to toxic injury are described under the following categories: (a) cardiac hypertrophy; (b) cardiomyopathies; (c) cardiac necrosis, including infarctlike myocardial necrosis, hypersensitivity (allergic) myocarditis, and toxic myocarditis; (d) pericarditis; and (e) vascular changes, including hypersensitivity vasculitis, toxic vasculitis, fibromuscular hyperplasia, and thromboembolism. Cardiovascular developmental abnormalities also may be produced by drugs or chemicals. Consideration of these effects is outside the scope of this chapter.

CARDIAC HYPERTROPHY

Cardiac hypertrophy is defined as an increase in the mass of the heart muscle beyond the limits of normal for age, sex, and body weight {1}. This increase in mass usually develops as a compensatory response to an increase in the workload of the heart. Such an increase may result from congenital lesions, acquired valvular dysfunction, pulmonary disease (cor pulmonale), systemic hypertension, variously mediated drug effects, or unknown causes, as in the cardiomyopathies.

In most types of heart disease, the degree of hypertrophy is similar in the various regions of a given cardiac chamber (symmetric hypertrophy). The exception to this is hypertrophic cardiomyopathy, in which the ventricular septum becomes thickened to a much greater extent (asymmetric hypertrophy) than the free walls of both ventricles. Most of the increment in muscle mass that occurs in hypertrophy is mediated through increases in mitochondria and myofibrils. However, the quantitative relations between these two components vary considerably according to the cause and stage of the hypertrophy.

Very considerable degrees of cardiac hypertrophy can be induced in experimental animals by the administration of growth hormone {2}, thyroid hormone {3}, triiodothyroacetic acid (TRIAC) {4}, norepinephrine {5}, isoproterenol {6}, and carbon monoxide {7}. Norepinephrine and isoproterenol induce hypertrophy at dose levels lower than those that produce cardiac necroses. In fact, long-term infusion of norepinephrine produces cardiac hypertrophy at doses that do not result in elevation of systemic arterial pressure {5}. The hypertrophy produced in newborn animals by administration of TRIAC to their mothers during pregnancy is of special interest in that it resembles, in some respects, the hypertrophy that occurs in hypertrophic cardiomyopathy {4}.

CARDIOMYOPATHIES

The cardiomyopathies (heart muscle diseases) can be classified into (a) hypertrophic, (b) ventricular-dilated or congestive, and (c) restrictive/obliterative {8}.

N. Sperelakis (ed.), Physiology and Pathophysiology of the Heart, Third Edition.

769

Hypertrophic cardiomyopathy

In most patients, hypertrophic cardiomyopathy is familial; however, in a few instances it is associated with other diseases, such as Friedreich's ataxia, Fabry's disease, hyperthyroidism, and lentiginosis {8}. It also occurs in cats, pigs, and dogs, but a suitable model strain of these animals has not been developed yet {9}. The genetic defect is heterogeneous and consists of mutations in the synthesis of the heavy chain of cardiac myosin {10}.

The disease is of great pharmacologic interest because of the many complex ways in which its clinical manifestations can be drastically altered by beta-adrenergic blockers, various inotropic agents, and substances that modify calcium transport.

Dilated cardiomyopathies

The terms *ventricular-dilated* or *congestive cardiomyopathy* describe a heterogeneous group of heart muscle diseases (in which congenital, hypertensive, valvular, and pulmonary heart disease are excluded as etiologic factors) that have congestive heart failure (systolic pump failure) and dilatation of both ventricular chambers as common features (fig. 40-1). Mural thrombi and focal endocardial thickening are common, as are small foci of myocytolysis and myocardial fibrosis {8}.

The etiology of the disorder remains unknown in many patients with dilated cardiomyopathy (idiopathic dilated cardiomyopathy); in other patients, the cardiomyopathy is associated with chronic alcoholism (alcoholic cardiomyopathy), with sequelae of viral infection, or with toxic agents. Ethyl alcohol, antineoplastic agents of the anthracycline family, cobalt, and furazolidone have been identified as toxic agents capable of inducing syndromes of chronic cardiomyopathy.

Alcoholic cardiomyopathy

Ethyl alcohol has several detrimental effects on myocardial metabolism, including depression of mitochondrial functions, decrease in the uptake of calcium by sarcoplasmic reticulum, accumulation of lipid, and indirect effects mediated by acetaldehyde (which can inhibit protein synthesis and promote release of catecholamines), by acetate, and by thiamine. Nevertheless, the pathogenetic mechanism of alcoholic cardiomyopathy remains uncertain {8,11,12}.

Cardiomyopathy develops only in a small percentage of alcoholic patients, although many alcoholic individuals have less obvious cardiac anatomic and functional abnormalities. The complete clinical picture of alcoholic cardiomyopathy seen in humans has not been reproduced in experimental animals by ethanol feeding, even though various morphologic and functional changes have been observed in such animals. It appears likely that the toxic effects of ethanol on myocardium are modified by other factors and that the "alcoholic" cardiomyopathy observed clinically in human patients is a multifactorial disease {8,11}.

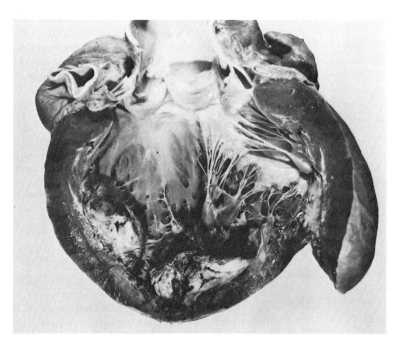

Fig. 40-1. Gross photograph of dilated heart of patient with cardiomyopathy and history of chronic alcoholism. Mural thrombi fill the apical region of the left ventricle.

Histologic and ultrastructural studies have been useful in the recognition of some of the diseases leading to the nonspecific picture of progressive cardiac dilatation and failure seen in dilated cardiomyopathy {13}. Nevertheless, the anatomic findings in dilated cardiomyopathy do not differ significantly in patients with and without a history of chronic alcoholism. Myocardial biopsies in both groups of patients have revealed a wide variety of nonspecific degenerative changes, which tend to reflect the duration and severity of the heart disease. Alcoholic patients often show accumulations of lipid droplets in cardiac muscle cells; however, this is a nonspecific change.

Alcoholic cardiomyopathy may be complicated by concomitant deficiency of thiamine or other nutrients, or by other toxic materials ingested with the ethanol. The most striking example of this was the epidemic of severe, acute cardiomyopathy, often associated with pericardial effusion and lactic acidosis, that developed in chronically malnourished, alcoholic patients who had ingested large amounts of beer to which cobalt salts had been added during the manufacturing process to improve the quality of the foam. Structural findings in these patients with "cobalt-beer cardiomyopathy" included prominent vacuolization, myofibrillar lysis, glycogen accumulation, and edema of the muscle cells. Experiments in animals showed that protein malnutrition is an important factor modulating the absorption of cobalt from the gastrointestinal tract and that cobalt-beer cardiomyopathy differs in some respects from the acute toxic cardiomyopathy produced by large doses of cobalt alone {11}.

Anthracycline cardiomyopathy

Although anthracycline antibiotics also can produce acute (ventricular arrhythmias and depression of contractility) and subacute (pericarditis and myocarditis) cardiac toxicity, these agents are well known for the distinctive type of chronic congestive cardiomyopathy that they produce in humans and experimental animals {14–16}. This complication generally is dose dependent (usually at least >400 mg/mm^2 total cumulative dose). Mechanisms for this toxicity are incompletely understood, and include drug binding by intercalation into the DNA in cardiac myocytes, inhibition of several enzyme systems, and promotion of peroxidative damage (mediated by oxygen free radicals) to cell membranes, mitochondrial membranes, DNA, enzymes, and membranes of sarcoplasmic reticulum {14,15}.

In addition to the three types of cardiotoxicity just described, recent observations have demonstrated that doxorubicin causes very late, delayed ventricular dysfunction in young adults who underwent antineoplastic therapy successfully during childhood and survived for 10 years or longer. Cardiac morphologic findings in these patients have not been consistent, and the exact mechanisms mediating this greatly delayed cardiotoxicity remain to be determined. It has been suggested that previous therapy with doxorubicin prevents proper growth of the heart during adolescence. It is thought that the selective cardiotoxicity of anthracyclines is due to the fact that the heart,

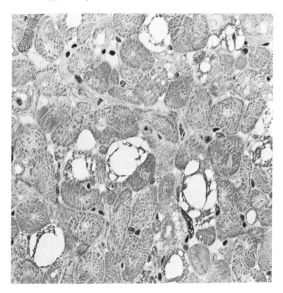

Fig. 40-2. Severe cytoplasmic vacuolization of cardiac myocytes is the characteristic finding in anthracycline cardiotoxicity. Plastic-embedded tissue, alkaline toluidine blue stain, ×400.

unlike other organs such as the liver, has very limited defenses (i.e., low levels of superoxide dismutase, catalase, and glutathione peroxidase) against peroxidative damage {15}.

The drug toxicity leads to two major cardiac morphological lesions, which are ventricular dilatation and myocardial cellular degeneration. The latter is manifested microscopically by myofibrillar loss and a distinctive type of cytoplasmic vacuolization (fig. 40-2). The vacuolization is a prominent but focal finding that involves individual cells rather than large, confluent areas of myocardium, and is caused by massive dilatation of tubules of sarcoplasmic reticulum. These changes also can involve the conduction system of the heart. Doxorubicin has been shown to inhibit the expression of several muscle-specific proteins {17}, and it seems likely that this inhibition contributes to the decrease in myofibrillar content of the affected myocytes. Nucleolar segregation develops transiently in cardiac myocytes and other cell types after administration of large doses of anthracyclines {18}, but is not a feature of the chronic cardiomyopathy induced by these agents.

The immune effector cells of the heart, including interstitial dendritic cells (antigen-preventing cells), macrophages, and CD4$^+$ T-helper lymphocytes, increase considerably in number after doxorubicin treatment {19}. These observations are interpreted as indicating that release of components from damage cardiac myocytes elicits immune reactions mediated by these cells {19}. The severity of the cardiac morphologic changes induced by anthracyclines has been evaluated by myocardial biopsies, which are useful in determining whether or not patients at risk of developing anthracycline cardiomyopathy can receive additional amounts of the drug {20}. Previous radiation to the heart is a significant risk factor in the development of anthracycline cardiomyopathy.

Considerable efforts have been made to diminish the cardiotoxicity of anthracyclines without compromising their therapeutic effectiveness {15}. The most successful results in this regard have been obtained with ICRF-187, a compound that appears to act by chelating iron, which is needed to catalyze the formation of oxygen free radicals with cytotoxic properties. When given concomitantly with doxorubicin, ICRF-187 reduces markedly the severity of the cardiomyopathy in animals {15} as well as in patients undergoing treatment for metastatic carcinoma of the breast {21}. In dogs, the administration of ICRF-187 has allowed the dose of doxorubicin to be increased four-fold without producing significant degrees of chronic cardiomyopathy {15}. Compounds that act as free radical scavengers (vitamin E, N-acetylcysteine) have been considerably less successful than ICRF-187 in blocking the cardiotoxic effects of doxorubicin {15}. New, less cardiotoxic antibiotics of the anthracycline family are becoming available for clinical use. Reduced cardiotoxicity also has been obtained by modified dose scheduling, in which prolonged (up to 96 hours) rather than rapid infusions of doxorubicin are used {15}.

Antineoplastic agents other than the anthracyclines also are capable, but usually only rarely, of producing cardiac damage. Among these are cyclophosphamide, busulfan, mitomycin C, mitoxanthrone, anthracenedione, cisplatinum, 5-fluorouracil, vincristine, VP-16, m-AMSA, the anthrapyrazoles, and taxol {22–28}. Cyclophosphamide is cardiotoxic only when administered in massive doses {22–24}, as in patients being prepared for bone marrow transplantation, in whom cyclophosphamide has

been reported to precipitate an acute cardiomyopathy, characterized by hemorrhagic myocardial necrosis and pericardial effusion (figs. 40-3 and 40-4). Busulfan has caused endocardial fibrosis; mitomycin C has caused myocardial fibrosis. Myocardial infarction and development or exacerbation of symptoms of ischemic heart disease have followed the administration of vincristine, vinblastine, 5-fluorouracil, and VP-16.

The pathogenesis of these abnormalities is not understood. Various ECG changes have been reported after cisplatinum therapy, and severe arrhythmias have followed treatment with m-AMSA {24,27}. Drugs of the anthrapyrazole group have antineoplastic properties that in several respects resemble those of the anthracyclines {28}. However, the clinical use of some anthrapyrazoles has been associated in some instances with the sudden onset of congestive heart failure and acute cardiac dilatation, particularly in patients who had been previously treated with anthracyclines (unpublished observations). Cardiac morphologic changes in such patients have not been defined in detail. Taxol, a naturally occurring agent found in the bark of the yew tree, is extremely effective in the treatment of carcinoma of the ovary. In a few patients, bradycardia and some degree of depression of cardiovascular function have followed very short-term use of this agent. Taxol is known to exert marked effects on the microtubules of various cell types, but the relationship between these effects and the antineoplastic and cardiotoxic properties of this agent remains uncertain {26}.

Furazolidone cardiomyopathy

Furazolidone, an antibiotic of the nitrofuran group, produces dilated cardiomyopathy in ducks, chickens, and

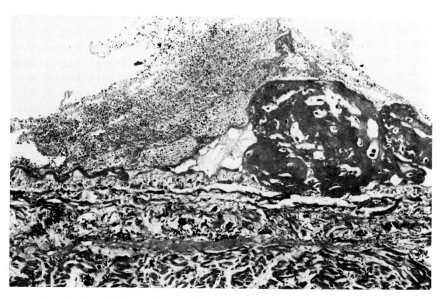

Fig. 40-3. Fibrinous pericarditis and epicardial hemorrhage in heart of patient with acute cardiomyopathy due to administration of large amounts of cyclophosphamide in preparation for bone marrow transplantation. H & E stain, ×40.

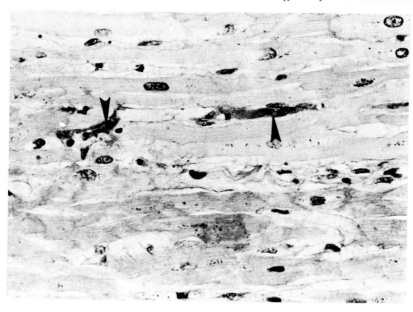

Fig. 40-4. Same heart as in fig. 40-3, showing microthrombi (arrowheads) in left ventricular capillaries. Periodic acid-Schiff stain, ×400.

turkeys {29–32}. When administered to the young of these avian species, it causes, in a dose-dependent manner, severe ventricular dilatation without hypertrophy, necrosis, or fibrosis. The principal alteration in cardiac muscle cells is diffuse myofibrillar lysis {31}. The sarcoplasm of affected myocytes contains scattered masses of free thick and thin myofilaments, clumps of Z-band material, and accumulations of cytoskeletal filaments. Supplements of selenium, vitamin E, and taurine do not protect against furazolidone-induced cardiomyopathy {32}; however, propranolol has been reported to be protective {33}. It appears that furazolidone does not induce cardiomyopathy in mammals. The biochemical mechanisms mediating this cardiomyopathy remain unknown.

Other agents that induce toxic cardiomyopathies

In addition to the agents mentioned above, which cause well-defined syndromes of dilated cardiomyopathy, other drugs can induce depression of myocardial contractility, with or without associated bradyarrhythmias or tachyarrhythmias, and with or without the morphologic changes of toxic myocarditis (see below). Important among these are tricyclic antidepressants, phenothiazines, lithium carbonate, emetine, chloroquine, amiodarone, quinidine, calcium blockers, and radiographic contrast agents, zidovudin (AZT) and FIAC {12,34–41}.

Amitriptyline has been responsible for most of the cardiovascular reactions attributed to tricyclic antidepressants. The cardiotoxic actions of these agents usually occur only with preexisting ischemic heart disease or after drug overdosage, and are manifested by arrhythmias and direct depression of myocardial function. Phenothiazines also

are prone to producing hypotension, by virtue of their alpha-adrenergic blockading effect and inhibition of central pressor reflexes; in addition, patients on phenothiazines show a tendency toward prolongation of the QT interval, a change that facilitates the development of arrhythmias. It has been suggested that myocardial changes induced by tricyclic antidepressants and phenothiazines persist after withdrawal of these drugs; however, no controlled studies have been made of these problems.

Emetine, an alkaloid used in the treatment of amebiasis and schistosomiasis, frequently produces electrocardiographic changes. These may persist for several months after termination of treatment. Rarely, emetine causes depression of cardiovascular function and death from cardiac failure or arrhythmias {34–36}.

Electrocardiographic alterations are frequent in patients receiving lithium carbonate. T-wave changes are common; tachyarrhythmias, atrioventricular conduction disturbances, and left bundle branch block occur at toxic serum lithium concentrations. These effects are reversible in the majority of patients; however, a few patients receiving lithium carbonate develop dilated cardiomyopathy, which does not improve after the drug is discontinued {34–36}.

Chloroquine occasionally produces electrocardiographic changes, usually bundle branch block; dilated cardiomyopathy also may develop, in association with deposits of electron-dense lamellae and "curvilinear bodies" within lysosomes of cardiac myocytes. These structures contain phospholipids and glycolipids, which accumulate because of chloroquine-induced inhibition of lysosomal acid hydrolases {39}.

Radiographic contrast agents often produce electro-

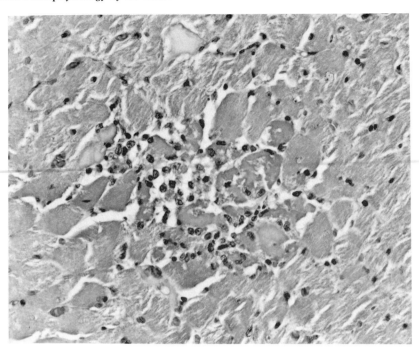

Fig. 40-5. Myocardial necrosis in rat sacrificed 24 hours after the administration of 5 ml/kg of diatrizoate meglumine sodium, used as radiographic contrast material. Hematoxylin-eosin stain, ×400.

cardiographic changes and depression of myocardial function, particularly when used for ventriculography or coronary arteriography. This effect seems to be mediated by a calcium-chelating action rather than by changes in osmolarity. Tissue damage (fig. 40-5) also can be produced by these agents. Significant depression of myocardial function also can result from the use of other agents that interfere with the movement of calcium ions, i.e., verapamil and quinidine {34–36}. Accumulations of irregularly arranged, concentric, electron-dense lamellae in the cytoplasm of cardiac myocytes and endothelial cells have been found in certain patients receiving prolonged treatment with amiodarone, a powerful antiarrhythmic agent. These lamellae represent intralysosomal deposits of phospholipids and glycolipids {40}. Similar deposits have been observed in cornea and in pulmonary alveolar macrophages of patients receiving amiodarone {40}.

Zidovudine [azidothymidine (AZT)] inhibits the replication of human immunodeficiency virus (HIV), prolongs survival, and delays the progression of acquired immune deficiency syndrome (AIDS) {37}. Ultrastructural and biochemical studies of the hearts of rats treated with AZT revealed marked and widespread mitochondrial swelling with disrupted cristae after 35 days of therapy with doses of 1 mg/ml of drinking water. Other cardiac structures appeared to be unaffected. After a 14-day recovery, these ultrastructural changes did not reverse. Mitochondrial cytochrome b mRNA expression was depressed in AZT-treated rat hearts. Expression of mRNA for several cardiac contractile and other mitochondrial proteins was unchanged. Nevertheless the AZT-treated rats showed no clinical or necropsy evidence of cardiac dysfunction. In contrast to this, however, other investigators have presented clinical evidence strongly implicating AZT therapy in the pathogenesis of dilated cardiomyopathy in some patients with AIDS {38}.

It must be pointed out that dilated cardiomyopathy develops in 11–22% of adult patients with AIDS, that the exact causes of this cardiomyopathy have not been established, and that AZT therapy is only one of the factors to be considered in this regard. In some of these patients the cardiomyopathy was associated with other evidence of toxicity of AZT, including myositis and necrosis of skeletal muscle cells (changes that clearly differ from those reported in rat heart). Myocardial ultrastructural changes in the hearts of patients with possible AZT-related cardiomyopathy are yet to be defined. Lewis et al. concluded that the cardiotoxic effect of AZT is due to inhibition of replication of mitochondrial DNA {37}.

Among other antiviral agents, FIAC [1-(2-deoxy-2-fluoro-β-D arabinofuranosyl)-5-iodocytosine] has been found to have some cardiotoxic effects when given in large doses to rats {41}. These effects consist of myofibrillar loss, necrosis (fragmentation and hypereosinophilia involving small groups of myocytes in both ventricles), inflammation (primarily lymphocytes and histiocytes), and fibrosis. Early ultrastructural changes consisted of dilatation of the sarcoplasmic reticulum of the myocyte and swelling of the capillary endothelial cells. The mechanism mediating these changes is not known.

Obliterative and restrictive cardiomyopathies

Obliterative cardiomyopathies are characterized by endocardial fibrous thickening and endocardial mural thrombosis, changes that lead to partial obliteration of the ventricular cavities. Löffler's syndrome and endomyocardial fibrosis are the most important entities in this group. Restrictive cardiomyopathies are those in which infiltrative processes (for example, amyloidosis) or diffuse accumulation of fibrous tissue in the ventricular walls reduce myocardial compliance and interfere with ventricular filling {8}.

Löffler's syndrome (fibroplastic parietal endocarditis) is a disorder of unknown etiology in which hypereosinophilia in blood and heart (and often also in other tissues) is accompanied by marked endocardial fibrous thickening and mural thrombosis {42}. These processes also can involve the cardiac valves. The eosinophilia can be transient, and it is thought that Löffler's syndrome and endomyocardial fibrosis (in which eosinophilia is lacking at the time when heart disease becomes clinically evident) represent two parts of the spectrum of endomyocardial disease associated with eosinophilia. Eosinophils can release products capable of inducing endocardial damage by mechanisms that involve the release of several cytotoxic proteins from the specific granules of these cells.

Endocardial mural thickening of mild degree can occur in association with toxic or ischemic lesions that cause myocardial necrosis {13}; however, fibrous thickening of mural and valvular endocardium also can be produced by methysergide and ergotamine tartrate {43–46}. The cardiac valves most frequently involved are the mitral and aortic, which become thickened and distorted by a layer of dense fibrous tissue that is devoid of elastic fibers and resembles that found in the lesions of carcinoid heart disease {47}. In the atrioventricular valves, the fibrosis may lead to thickening and fusion of the chordae tendineae. These lesions can lead to valvular stenosis and regurgitation. Mural endocardial thickening also occurs in the late stages of allylamine cardiotoxicity {48} and in radiation-induced myocardial fibrosis. Calcification of mural endocardium can occur in domestic animals as the result of the ingestion of toxic plants {25}.

CARDIAC NECROSIS AND MYOCARDITIS

Cardiac necrosis

Although much of the research on the mechanisms of cardiac muscle cell necrosis has centered on ischemic injury and its modification by pharmacologic agents, many of the principles derived from these studies are applicable to toxic myocardial injury. Two basic forms of cardiac muscle cell necrosis are recognizable: coagulation necrosis and necrosis with contraction bands (myofibrillar damage leading to myocytolysis) {13}.

Coagulation necrosis

Ischemia of less than 20 minutes duration produces reversible damage, characterized by glycogen depletion, mitochondrial swelling, mild intracellular edema, and relaxation of sarcomeres (reflecting loss of contractility). Irreversible injury with the features of coagulation necrosis develops when the period of ischemia exceeds 20 minutes. The percentage of irreversibly damaged cells increases as the period of ischemia is prolonged up to 60 minutes, at which time most of the cells in the ischemic areas become irreversibly injured. In addition to the changes mentioned above, coagulation necrosis is characterized by (a) intramitochondrial flocculent precipitates (amorphous densities), which are thought to be derived from mitochondrial lipids; (b) margination of nuclear chromatin, which is regarded as evidence of irreversible nuclear damage; (c) small holes in the plasma membrane, signifying loss of its permeability barrier function, and (d) various degrees of dissociation of intercellular junctions, leading to electrical uncoupling of cells. These changes progress to fully developed coagulation necrosis, in which the muscle cells have relaxed sarcomeres with indistinct myofilaments. Coagulation necrosis is characteristically limited to central areas of myocardial infarcts, in which reflow does not occur after ischemic damage develops.

Necrosis with contraction bands

In contrast to coagulation necrosis, peripheral areas of infarcts show a different type of necrosis, known as necrosis with contraction bands, which is characterized by (a) hypercontraction of sarcomeres, (b) intramitochondrial electron-dense calcific deposits, and (c) progression to myocytolysis. The distinctive features of this type of necrosis are related to the entry of large amounts of calcium ions, which originate from partial perfusion of peripheral areas of ischemic lesions, into cells that are damaged by ischemia. Additional damage is caused by the generation of oxygen free radicals, particularly during the reperfusion period {49}. The passage of calcium through damaged, abnormally permeable plasma membranes is responsible for the hypercontraction; this passage occurs either when severely but temporarily ischemic tissue is reperfused with arterial blood or when necrosis develops because of other factors not related to a reduction in coronary blood flow. Thus necrosis with contraction bands is seen in many forms of cardiac toxic injury, including the lesions caused by catecholamines and vasodilating antihypertensive agents {13} (fig. 40-6). Progression of necrosis with contraction bands to myocytolysis is mediated through lysis of the myofilaments, a change that follows a variable time course and results in an empty appearance of the cells. In infarcted myocytes this lysis is retarded by therapy with corticosteroids, under which circumstances the cells appear "mummified" {50}.

Flow through the ischemic area often cannot be reestablished when attempts are made to reperfuse tissue that has been ischemic for a long time (in excess of 90 minutes). Under these circumstances, the microcirculation in the ischemic area may suffer irreversible damage (i.e., endothelial cell swelling, occlusion by microthrombi or platelet aggregates), giving rise to the "no reflow" phenomenon {13}.

Inflammation

Inflammation basically is a protective response by which injured tissue is restored to its normal state. However, inflammation also can be the cause of additional tissue damage, and modification of myocardial inflammatory responses constitutes an important aspect of cardiac pharmacology.

Acute inflammation

Acute inflammation is manifested by vascular dilatation, tissue edema, and infiltration by leukocytes. These manifestations result from the release of vasopermeability factors (kinins, vasoactive amines, leukokines, anaphylatoxins from complement, prostaglandins, and cytokines) and leukotactic factors (these vary in their ability to attract different types of inflammatory cells in areas of cellular injury or necrosis). The diagnosis of acute myocarditis is dependent on the finding of myocyte damage and acute inflammatory cells, which have the capacity to neutralize offending chemical and infective agents, and to destroy remnants of injured cells and extracellular components of connective tissue {13}.

Polymorphonuclear neutrophilic leukocytes, which are strongly phagocytic cells, constitute the most prominent feature of acute inflammation in the heart, where they first become marginated (i.e., adherent to the luminal surfaces of capillaries and postcapillary venules) before passing into the extravascular compartment. Neutrophils contain powerful proteases, including elastase, as well as oxidases, all of which can cause considerable tissue damage. They are also capable of producing large amounts of oxygen free radicals. Monocytes and lymphocytes invade tissues at somewhat later stages of acute inflammation. As they leave the vascular compartment, blood monocytes undergo a gradual transformation into macrophages, which play a most important role in phagocytic and hydrolytic processes. Lymphocytes have the capacity of mediating responses involving specific humoral (B lymphocytes) or cell-mediated (T lymphocytes) immune responses. The interstitial dendritic cells of the heart {51} participate in inflammatory processes by presenting antigens to T lymphocytes and macrophages; in this respect, they play an important role in the activation of these two types of cells to function as immune effector cells.

Mast cells, which are abundant in myocardium, also participate in acute inflammatory and hypersensitivity reactions by serving as mediator cells capable of releasing histamine, together with other components of mast cell granules, either on direct contact of the cell with a chemical or through the interaction of antigens with IgE bound to the mast cell surface. Many of the properties of mast cells in tissues are shared by basophilic leukocytes in blood.

Eosinophilic leukocytes, which also are phagocytic and capable of releasing toxic products (major basic protein), also can participate in acute inflammation as well as in chronic inflammation. These cells are important components of the inflammatory reaction in allergic and parasitic disorders, including allergic myocarditis; however, their specific role in these processes is not well understood. They also occur in other, unrelated cardiac disorders, such as Löffler's syndrome of hypereosinophilia and endomyocardial fibrosis {52}.

Subacute inflammation

Subacute inflammation is a delayed phase of acute inflammation, and is characterized by the accumulation of monocytes and lymphocytes, and by the formation of granulation tissue. The latter is composed of rapidly proliferating fibroblasts, pericytes, and capillary endothelial cells in a matrix of developing connective tissue. The synthesis of connective tissue proteins by these cells mediates the fibrous tissue deposition by which healing occurs. Modulation of the proliferation and protein synthetic activity of connective tissue cells in the heart by fibronectin {53} and by various growth factors {54} is a subject of considerable interest.

Chronic inflammation

Chronic inflammation is characterized by the continuing presence of lymphocytes, monocytes (or monocyte-derived cells such as macrophages and epithelioid cells), and plasma cells in the tissues. It usually results from the persistence of material that elicits an immunologic reaction, and it causes continuing tissue damage, either because of immunologic injury or because of excessive deposition of collagen. Chronic inflammation can be granulomatous, in which the macrophages and epithelioid cells are associated with multinucleated giant cells and form nodular masses {55}.

Cardiac cellular damage produced by toxic agents

It is obvious that many highly specific biochemical and pharmacological mechanisms can mediate the cardiac cellular damage produced by toxic drugs and chemical agents. It is difficult to establish structural-functional correlations with respect to such lesions; even highly specific, localized disturbances of the delicate equilibrium of cell functions can lead rapidly to a picture of generalized cell damage or cell necrosis. Examples of toxic agents producing specific damage to various subcellular organelles of cardiac muscle cells include (a) compounds that interfere with mitochondrial enzymes (cyanide {56}, thyroid hormone {3}), uncouple oxidative phosphorylation (dinitrophenol {57}), or bind to mitochondrial DNA (acriflavine {58}) and produce a number of alterations in mitochondrial morphology; (b) compounds that induce intracellular calcification, usually localized within mitochondria (dihydrotachysterol {59}, sodium phosphate {60}); (c) compounds that primarily cause myofibrillar lesions (sympathomimetic amines {61–63}, plasmocid {64,65}, diuretics or other agents leading to potassium deficiency {66}); (d)

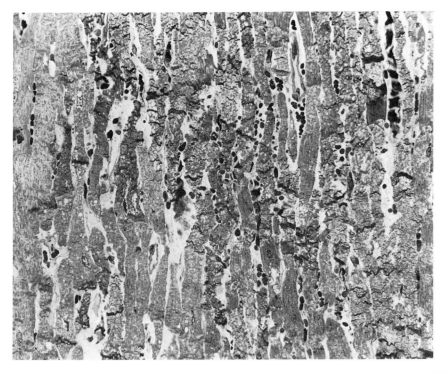

Fig. 40-6. Necrosis with contraction bands in left ventricular papillary muscle of dog given overdose of minoxidil. Plastic-embedded tissue, alkaline toluidine blue stain, ×250.

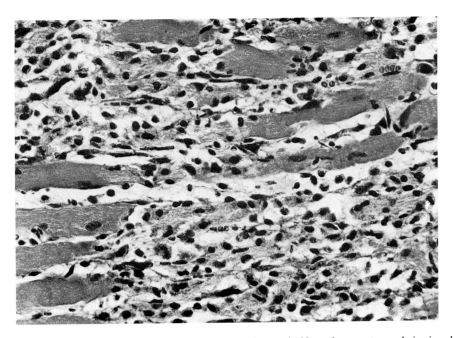

Fig. 40-7. Left ventricular myocardium of rat with hydralazine-induced necrosis. Necrotic myocytes are being invaded by inflammatory cells. H & E stain, ×400.

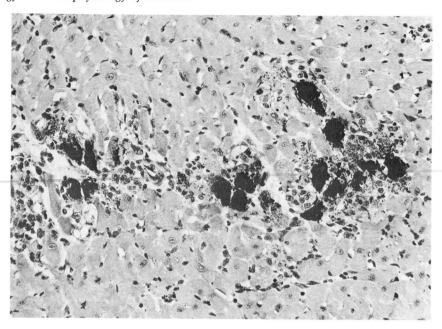

Fig. 40-8. Heavily calcified, necrotic myocytes are surrounded by moderate inflammatory infiltrate in heart of rat given large dose of dihydrotachysterol. Von Kossa stain, ×250.

compounds that cause accumulations of electron-dense lamellae (chloroquine {39}, amiodarone {40}); (e) compounds that produce nuclear or nucleolar lesions (anthracyclines {18}); and (f) compounds that promote the formation of free radicals and produce massive dilatation of the sarcoplasmic reticulum (anthracyclines {14–16}) (figs. 40-6 to 40-8).

Although the changes just cited seldom are specific, they can provide valuable clues as to the mode of action of a given agent. Many of the changes in the contractile apparatus, nucleus, or membrane systems (plasma membrane/T tubules and sarcoplasmic reticulum) are associated with complex alterations in the overall concentrations of Ca, Mg, Na, and K, as well as with changes in the intracellular compartmentalization of these ions {67}. Furthermore, these ionic alterations and changes in intracellular pH can be associated with activation and release of lysosomal hydrolytic enzymes, including cathepsin D and other proteases and phospholipases {68,69}. These variously interrelated changes, together with alterations in the permeability of plasma membranes, act as determinants of whether or not cellular injury progresses to necrosis {13}.

On the basis of the pathogenesis and morphology of the resulting lesions, acute toxic cardiac damage can be classified into the following categories: (a) myocardial infarcts and infarctlike lesions; (b) hypersensitivity myocarditis; and (c) toxic myocarditis.

Myocardial infarction associated with toxic reactions

Grossly evident myocardial infarction may occur when the coronary arteries are involved by drug-induced arteritis (as from amphetamines), fibromuscular intimal proliferation (oral contraceptives), embolization from infective endocarditis (associated with intravenous drug abuse), or, in patients with normal coronary arteries, following exposure to toxic levels of carbon monoxide, nitrates, thyroid preparations, methysergide or ergot derivatives, and certain antineoplastic agents {35}. Large, infarctlike areas of necrosis, not related to obstruction of large, extramural coronary arteries, have been produced in experimental animals by the administration of toxic doses of isoproterenol {61,63}. It was originally thought that this necrosis resulted from isoproterenol-induced increases in cardiac rate, contractility, and oxidative metabolism to an extent beyond the limits of the oxygen supply system. More recently, however, it has become evident that isoproterenol also produces other highly complex effects, including a marked increase in calcium uptake, stimulation of the adenyl cyclase system, aggregation of platelets, and induction of the formation of free radicals capable of causing peroxidative damage {12,70}. Other sympathomimetic amines, including epinephrine, norepinephrine, dopamine, and dobutamine, are capable of inducing myocardial necroses, which are small, patchy and multifocal, and usually are localized in left ventricular subendocardium {38,61–63,71}. These lesions are associated with epicardial and endocardial hemorrhage; in addition, the small intramural coronary arteries may show segmental medial necrosis {71}.

Other toxic effects of catecholamines are of practical importance. Cardiac lesions produced by release of large amounts of catecholamines occur in patients with pheochromocytomas, tetanus, acutely stressful situations, subarachnoid hemorrhage, and other CNS lesions {12,72}. Ischemic cardiac damage can be aggravated by high circulating levels of catecholamines in patients with acute myocardial infarction {12}. The ingestion of certain foods containing tyramine can produce severe hypertensive crises in patients undergoing therapy with monoamine oxidase inhibitors {73}. Therapy with beta-adrenergic blockers and exposure to chloroform and other halogenated hydrocarbons, including a number of fluorinated compounds and halogen-containing anesthetic and refrigerating agents, can sensitize the myocardium to the effects of sympathomimetic amines {34}.

Hypersensitivity myocarditis

Hypersensitivity myocarditis associated with drug therapy is characterized by infiltration of the heart muscle with numerous eosinophils, mixed with mononuclear cells, predominantly lymphocytes and plasma cells {35,36}. The cellular infiltrate may be focal or diffuse, and is associated with foci of myocytolysis. Fibrotic changes are absent, and all lesions are similar in age and appearance. True granulomatous lesions are not present, although giant cells of myogenic origin may be found. Vascular involvement is frequent and consists of a bland-appearing vasculitis affecting small arteries, arterioles, and venules. The inflammatory reaction also may involve the pericardium, but characteristically spares the cardiac valves. The absence of extensive myocardial necrosis or fibrosis distinguishes drug-related hypersensitivity myocarditis from other forms of myocarditis in which eosinophils are prominent. Endocardial fibrosis is not a feature of hypersensitivity myocarditis. Hypersensitivity myocarditis represents the most common form of drug-induced heart disease. The clinical criteria for the diagnosis of this disorder are (a) previous use of the drug without incident; (b) the hypersensitivity reaction bears no relationship to the magnitude of the dose of the drug; (c) the reaction is characterized by classic allergic symptoms, symptoms of serum sickness, or syndromes suggesting infectious disease; (d) immunologic confirmation; and (e) persistence of symptoms until the drug is discontinued. Drugs known to be associated with hypersensitivity myocarditis include methyldopa, hydrochlorothiazide, sulfadiazine, sulfisoxazole, sulfonylureas, chloramphenicol, p-aminosalicylic acid (PAS), amitriptyline, carbamazepine, indomethacin, penicillin, phenindione, phenylbutazone, oxyphenbutazone, tetracycline, diphenylhydantoin, acetazolamide, ampicillin, chlorthalidone, spironolactone, and streptomycin. Many of these drugs also have been associated with hypersensitivity vasculitis. The pathogenesis of drug-induced hypersensitivity myocarditis remains unclear, but appears to be immunologically mediated, perhaps as a delayed hypersensitivity reaction in which the drug or one of its meta-bolites act as a hapten and combines with an endogenous macromolecule; it is this combination that is antigenic. Hypersensitivity myocarditis also has developed after injection of horse serum, tetanus toxoid, and smallpox vaccine.

Toxic myocarditis

Drugs can cause myocardial injury not only by producing hypersensitivity myocarditis but also by direct toxic effects, which result in cell damage and cell death. This type of drug toxicity is dose related. Depending upon its rate of progression, it can cause either acute toxic myocarditis or a more chronic picture of drug-induced cardiomyopathy. In acute toxic myocarditis there is interstitial edema, multifocal areas of cardiac muscle cell necrosis with contraction bands, and an inflammatory cell infiltrate consisting of lymphocytes, plasma cells, and polymorphonuclear leukocytes. The areas of necrosis show different stages of progression. Eosinophils may be present, but seldom are prominent. There is endothelial cell damage, but not a true vasculitis. Microthrombi have been reported after administration of adenosine diphosphate, cyclophosphamide, catecholamines, and thromboxane A {13}. The paucity of eosinophils and the presence of various stages of cell death and healing by fibrosis serve to differentiate toxic myocarditis from hypersensitivity myocarditis.

Among the drugs and chemicals known to cause toxic myocarditis are daunorubicin, doxorubicin, 5-fluorouracil, emetine, antimony compounds, amphetamines, cyclophosphamide, catecholamines, lithium carbonate, phenothiazines, plasmocid, paraquat, and mitomycin C {35,36}. It should be remembered that a cellular inflammatory reaction may be poorly developed or totally absent in toxic myocarditis due to antineoplastic or immunosuppressive agents. Other agents capable of inducing focal myocardial necrosis and fibrosis are histamine; methylxanthines; a large variety of poisonous plants, some of which have fluoroacetate, an inhibitor of the Krebs cycle, as their toxic factor; gossypol, which is found in cottonseed meal, used to feed swine {25}; monensin, a polyether antibiotic that acts as a Na-selective carboxylic ionophore {74}; rapeseed oil, the most important ingredient of which is erucic acid {75}; brominated vegetable oils; arsenicals, which also can cause peripheral vascular disease (black leg) {35,36}; and allylamine, a highly toxic aliphatic amine used in industry {48,76}.

Corticosteroids produce degenerative lesions in the hearts of animals and, to a lesser extent, in those of humans {35,77}. Cobalt, copper, tellurium, cadmium, and zinc, when given in toxic doses, can precipitate systemic lesions, often with cardiac and skeletal muscle involvement, that resemble those resulting from deficiency of selenium and vitamin E, and that can be at least partially prevented by dietary supplements of selenium and vitamin E {78,79}. Other metallic salts capable of inducing cardiac toxicity include those of lead, nickel, barium, vanadium, lanthanum, and manganese {25}. Oral hypoglycemic agents have been associated with adverse cardiovascular effects, the mechanisms of which have not been elucidated {12}.

Other agents that recently have become of considerable interest as causes of toxic myocarditis, with or without concomitant involvement of coronary vessels, include vasodilating and inotropic drugs {71}, various cytokines {80–84}, and the substances responsible for the toxic oil syndrome {85} and the eosinophilia-myalgia syndrome (contaminated tryptophan) {85–88}.

A peculiar type of chronic myocarditis associated with vasculitis, hemorrhage, and fibrosis (figs. 40-5, 40-9, and 40-10) has been observed in atrial myocardium of dogs and pigs treated with minoxidil, a vasodilating antihypertensive agent that also can produce foci of left ventricular papillary muscle necrosis {71,89–93}. The papillary muscle necrosis (fig. 40-6) is thought to be a consequence of the tachycardia, hypotension, and hypoperfusion that occur when large doses of minoxidil are given. The vascular lesions consist of (a) bland arteritis involving small coronary arteries, which on ultrastructural study show foci of endothelial cell loss, medial smooth cell necrosis and intramural accumulations of red blood cells, inflammatory cells, and large numbers of platelets {92}.

Atrial and ventricular lesions similar to those just described have been induced by minoxidil in old (24-month) rats, but not in young rats {93}. In dogs, the atrial lesions are localized to the right atrium; in rats and pigs, to the left atrium {92}. The exact mechanism of these lesions and their selective localization remain to be elucidated. Lesions similar to those produced by minoxidil have been observed after administration of large doses of theobromine, digoxin, epinephrine, norepinephrine, diazoxide, and hydralazine to dogs {71,92}.

Recent investigations {see 71 for review} have demonstrated that various combinations of these atrial and ventricular lesions are also produced in dogs by a large variety of compounds that have very diverse chemical structures but possess vasodilating and/or inotropic properties. Included among these compounds are SKF 94120, SKF 95654, CI-914, CI-930, UD-CG 115BS, BTS 43993, and UK61.260. It has been concluded from these studies that the dog is much more sensitive than other species of animals to the induction of these lesions and that caution is necessary in extrapolating these results to the clinical use of these agents in human patients. The study in rats has important implications in terms of the relationships of drug toxicity to the aging process.

The development of cytokines as DNA recombinant products has led to a number of clinical uses for these agents, and several important manifestations of cardiovascular toxicity have become evident after their therapeutic use. The most frequently recognized cardiovascular complication of cancer immunotherapy with interleukin-2 (IL-2) is the vascular leak syndrome (VLS), which is thought to result, at least in part, from the interaction between IL-2-activated lymphocytes (lymphokine activated killer cells or LAK cells) and endothelial cells {80,81}. VLS is characterized by an increase in vascular permeability, with fluid retention, peripheral edema, ascites, pleural effusion, and pulmonary edema. IL-2 therapy also can result in myocardial toxicity. Cardiac arrhythmias have been reported in 14–21% of patients undergoing IL-2 therapy. Other major cardiotoxic effects reported include myocardial infarction, myocarditis, and cardiomyopathy.

Myocardial infarction has occurred in up to 4% of patients treated with IL-2. At necropsy, only some of

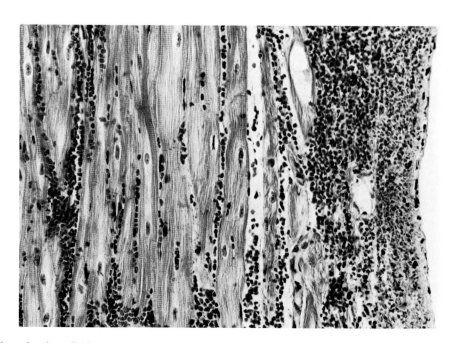

Fig. 40-9. Extensive subendocardial hemorrhage in left ventricle of dog given toxic dose of minoxidil. H & E stain, ×100.

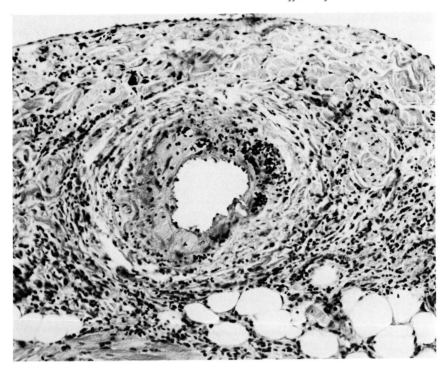

Fig. 40-10. Inflammatory reaction surrounds area of medial necrosis and intramural hemorrhage in small artery in right atrial epicardium of dog receiving toxic dose of minoxidil. H & E stain, ×80.

these patients have had anatomic evidence of preexisting atherosclerotic coronary artery disease. To investigate this cardiotoxicity, immunohistochemical and ultrastructural studies were made of the hearts of rats treated with several large doses of IL-2. Cardiac changes consisted of focal lymphocytic and eosinophilic infiltration, myocyte vacuolization, myofibrillar loss and necrosis, and microcirculatory damage and plugging of capillaries by massess of lymphocytes (fig. 40-11). It was concluded that two factors were responsible for the myocardial necrosis: (a) Cytotoxic damage mediated by contact with lymphocytes (fig. 40-12) and (b) ischemia secondary to microvascular damage {81}.

The potential for cardiotoxicity of IL-1 is suggested by a recent study {82} showing that IL-1 decreases the contractile response of cultured myocytes to beta-adrenergic agonists. Another study {83} using rat cremaster muscle as a model system demonstrated that the combination of IL-1 and tumor necrosis factor (TNF) causes a vascular leak syndrome that is dependent upon the adherence of lymphocytes and neutrophils to the endothelium of capillaries and venules, and results in capillary damage, aggregation of platelets, and extravasation of fluid and plasma proteins.

In clinical practice, administration of interferons (IFN) causes an appreciable degree of discomfort, but life-threatening complications are infrequent. In rare instances patients exhibit severe chest pain, suffer myocardial infarctions, and experience other cardiovascular disorders, e.g., arrhythmias, hypotension, and hypertension {see 84

for review}. Nevertheless, administration of large doses of interferon-α to rats failed to produce consistent cardiac morphorlogic changes, although arrthymias and ischemic changes were noted on electrocardiographic study {84}.

PERICARDITIS

Pericarditis with or without effusion has been reported to occur in patients with drug-induced systemic lupus erythematosus. In the majority of these patients, the pericarditis is only one of the many manifestations of the lupus-like syndrome. A relatively large number of drugs has been implicated in the induction of lupus-like syndromes. Among these agents are hydralazine, procainamide, isoniazid, p-aminosalicylic acid, diphenylhydantoin, methylphenylethylhydantoin, mephenytoin, primidone, trimethadione, ethosuximide, methsuximide, trimethadione, penicillin, penicillamine, sulfonamides, tetracycline, propylthiouracil, methyldopa, barbiturates, griseofulvin, streptomycin, quinidine, phenylbutazone, chlorpromazine, methotrimeprazine, perphenazine, promazine, and reserpine. In many of the reports of the agents just mentioned, the evidence linking drug usage to the lupus-like syndrome is highly circumstantial. Drug-induced lupus has been most clearly documented in the case of hydralazine and procainamide {35}.

Drugs that cause toxic myocarditis, hypersensitivity myocarditis, or large areas of myocardial necrosis often

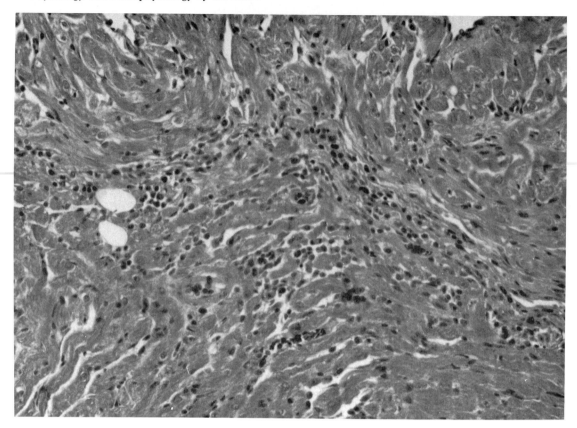

Fig. 40-11. Lymphocytic myocarditis in rat sacrificed after being treated for 3 days with multiple doses of interleukin-2 {81}. Hematoxylin-eosin stain, ×100.

also cause pericarditis by extension of the inflammation to the pericardium, particularly the visceral pericardium. Pericardial hemorrhage (fig. 40-3) can occur as a result of cyclophosphamide toxicity {22,23} and therapy with anticoagulants. The latter problem is encountered in some patients with uremia who are given heparin during the course of hemodialysis {35}.

VASCULAR CHANGES

Morphologic changes of considerable practical importance are induced by drugs or chemicals that modify the lesions of atherosclerosis, either through changes in plasma lipids and lipoproteins, or through more direct effects on vascular walls. Other toxic chemicals exert their effects on blood vessels by inducing connective tissue changes leading to the formation of nonatherosclerotic aneurysms in the aorta and other large arteries. These effects usually are mediated through biochemical inhibition of specific steps in the synthesis of connective tissue proteins, as in the case of penicillamine and β-aminopropionitrile {94}.

Hypersensitivity vasculitis

The anatomic features of hypersensitivity vasculitis may be summarized as follows: (a) Only small vessels, primarily arterioles, capillaries, and venules, are involved; (b) muscular and elastic arteries and large veins are spared; (c) aneurysms are not found; (d) all lesions appear to be of about the same age; (e) fibrinoid necrosis is not present; and (f) eosinophils and mononuclear cells are the predominant components of the inflammatory reaction and are present in all three layers of the involved vessel and in adjacent areas of interstitial connective tissue {35}. Drugs reported to induce hypersensitivity vasculitis include allopurinol, ampicillin, bromide, carbamazepine, chloramphenicol, chlortetracycline, chlorpropamide, chlorthalidone, chromolyn sodium, colchicine, dextran, diazepam, diphenylhydantoin, diphenhydramine, griseofulvin, indocin, isoniazid, levamisole, methylthiouracil, oxyphenbutazone, phenylbutazone, potassium iodide, procainamide, propylthiouracil, quinidine, spironolactone, sulfonamides, tetracycline, and trimethadione {35}.

In contrast to drug-induced vasculitis, the lesions of periarteritis nodose, a collagen-vascular disease of unknown origin, are characterized by (a) involvement of

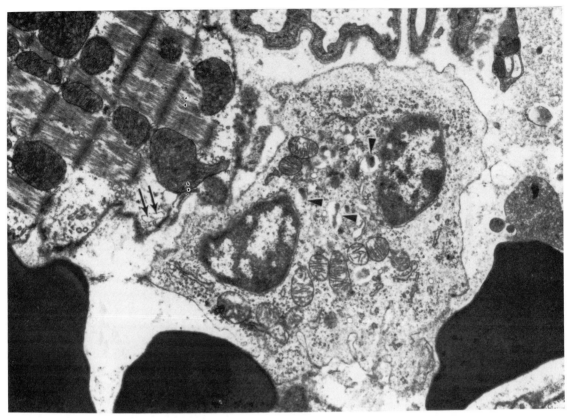

Fig. 40-12. Electron micrographs of myocardium of rat treated as described in fig. 40-11. Area of close contact between a granular lymphocyte and a cardiac myocyte. Such contacts mediate the cytotoxicity of these lymphocytes through the release of perforin and other toxic substances from the cytoplasmic granules of the lymphocytes. ×10,000.

muscular arteries; (b) fibrinoid necrosis of the vascular walls; (c) frequent occlusion of the vascular lumina by thrombus or granulation tissue; and (d) weakening of the media, with formation of aneurysms. Vascular lesions in other collagen-vascular diseases have nonspecific features and occasionally may resemble those in periarteritis nodose. The exception is Wegener's granulomatosis, in which the lesions affect small arteries, arterioles, and venules (pulmonary vessels often are involved), forming granulomas with acute and chronic inflammatory cells and multinucleated giant cells. Nevertheless, granulomatous lesions are not diagnostic of Wegener's granulomatosis, and fibrinoid necrosis is not diagnostic of collagen-vascular diseases {35}.

Toxic vasculitis

Toxic vasculitis is usually necrotizing, with morphologic features similar to those of periarteritis nodose. Medium-sized and small arteries are most often affected; however, smaller vessels also may be involved. The lesions tend to be segmental and to be heavily infiltrated by polymorphonuclear leukocytes. Fibrinoid necrosis, superimposed thrombi, and aneurysm formation are usually found in various stages of evolution. These lesions are most frequently associated with the use of penicillin or sulfonamides; less commonly, with organic arsenicals, gold salts, mercurials, bismuth, amphetamine, methamphetamine, DDT, heterologous serum, and sulfonamides. The pathogenesis of drug-induced toxic vasculitis remains incompletely understood {35,36}.

Vascular lesions associated with oral contraceptives

Vascular proliferative lesions, not related to atherosclerosis, have been found in women taking oral contraceptives (fig. 40-13), in pregnant and immediately postpartal women, and in a few men with severe liver disease (the implication in the latter patients being that of inadequate inactivation of certain steroids). These lesions may be associated with thrombosis and may occur in the systemic, portal, or pulmonary circulation. The lesions consist of fibromuscular intimal thickenings containing smooth muscle cells, collagen, and proteoglycans; inflammatory cells and vascular necrosis usually are not present {95}.

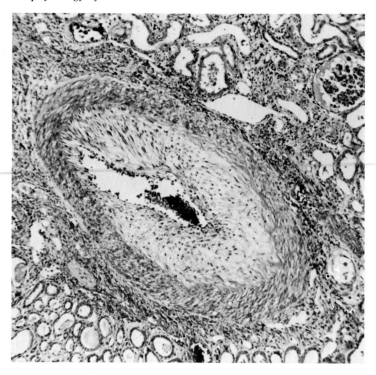

Fig. 40-13. Fibromuscular intimal proliferation, presumed to be due to oral contraceptives, has caused considerable luminal narrowing in small renal artery. Movat pentachrome stain, ×80.

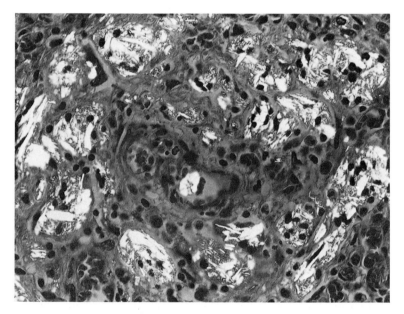

Fig. 40-14. Micrograph taken with partially polarized light to demonstrate numerous talc deposits around small pulmonary blood vessel of patient who had history of intravenous drug abuse. H & E stain, ×100.

Other drug-induced vascular lesions

Other drug-induced arterial lesions include those induced by (a) ergotamine (intimal proliferation, medial hypertrophy, and hyalinization, with or without superimposed thrombosis and gangrene); (b) methysergide maleate (intimal proliferation, often leading to vascular occlusion), a compound that, as mentioned previously, also can aggravate symptoms of coronary artery disease and produce retroperitoneal, endocardial, and mediastinal fibrosis; (c) vitamin D (calcification of arterial elastic lamina {25,36}); and (d) the lesions, already mentioned, produced by digoxin, theobromine, catecholamines, minoxidil, and other vasodilating/inotropic agents {71,89–93}. In addition, disseminated arterial lesions similar to those in periarteritis nodosa are found in patients using amphetamines intravenously; pulmonary arteriolar granulomatous lesions (fig. 40-14) occur in patients who inject themselves intravenously with suspensions of drug tablets containing talc or other silicates {96}, and drug-related infective vasculitis can develop in patients receiving intravenously administered drugs. In the latter patients, the infection may be only a localized phlebitis or may progress to infective arteritis or endocarditis. Drug-induced thrombophlebitis not related to infection also is a common complication of intravenous therapy.

Two new syndromes of combined vascular and cardioneural involvement have been described recently as resulting from the ingestion of contaminated oil (Spanish toxic oil syndrome) and L-tryptophan. Early in the course of studies of the Spanish toxic oil syndrome (caused by ingestation of vegetable oil that had been adulterated by the addition of rapeseed oil and oleoanilides), it was recognized that vascular lesions were a major problem, attributable to endothelial damage by the toxic oil. However, most clinical attention has been directed to the pulmonary complications of this syndrome and its evolution into a sclerodermalike illness. In a study of 11 patients who died of the toxic oil syndrome, James et al. {85} observed evidence of major injury to the coronary arteries, neural structures, and the conduction system of the heart. Obliterative fibrosis of the sinus node in four cases resembled that found in fatal scleroderma heart disease, and in eight patients the cardiac lesions resembled those of lupus erythematosus. The more impressive pathologic features involved the coronary arteries and neural structures, which were abnormal in every heart. The arterial disease included widespread focal fibromuscular dysplasia, but there was also an unusual myointimal proliferative degeneration of both small and large coronary arteries in five patients, four of whom were young women. Coronary arteritis was rarely found. Inflammatory and noninflammatory degeneration of cardiac nerves was widespread. Fatty infiltration, fibrosis, and degeneration were present in the coronary chemoreceptors. In most respects these cardiac abnormalities resemble those described in the eosinophilia-myalgia syndrome.

In 1989, an epidemic outbreak of a new disorder, which became known as the eosinophilia-myalgia syndrome, was observed among individuals who had been taking dietary supplements of L-tryptophan for various health reasons {86–88}. The tryptophan responsible for this disorder was produced by a single manufacturer, using a newly developed process. It is now thought that this syndrome represents a toxic reaction to a yet not fully identified contaminant of this tryptophan. The syndrome was characterized by hypereosinophilia, severe pulmonary disease, fasciitis, peripheral nerve disease, and eventual evolution into a scleroderma-like disease. In three necropsy patients with the eosinophilia-myalgia syndrome, James et al. {87,88} observed fibrosis of the sinus node and other components of the conduction system, cardioneuropathy of widespread distribution, fibromuscular intimal hyperplasia of small coronary arteries, and inflammatory arteritis; however, endocardial fibrosis was not evident. The exact mechanism responsible for these changes is not known. James et al. {87,88} concluded that this combination of cardiac pathologic changes was likely to cause or aggravate electrical instability of the heart and to contribute to the sudden death that has been reported in some patients with the eosinophilia-myalgia syndrome.

REFERENCES

1. Ferrans VJ: Cardiac hypertrophy: Morphological aspects. In: Zak R (ed) *Growth of the Heart in Health and Disease*. New York: Raven Press, 1984, pp 187–239.
2. Rubin SA, Buttrick P, Malhotra A, Melmed S, Fishbein MC: Cardiac physiology, biochemistry and morphology in response to excess growth hormone in the rat. *J Mol Cell Cardiol* 4:429–438, 1990.
3. Gerdes AM, Kriseman J, Bishop SP: Changes in myocardial cell size and number during development and reversal of hyperthyroidism in neonatal rats. *Lab Invest* 48:598–602, 1983.
4. Hawkey CM, Olsen EGJ, Symons C: Production of cardiac muscle abnormalities in offspring of rats receiving triiodothyroacetic acid (triac) and the effect of beta adrenergic blockade. *Cardiovasc Res* 15:196–205, 1981.
5. Laks MM, Morady F: Norepinephrine — The myocardial hypertrophy hormone? *Am Heart J* 91:674–675, 1976.
6. Bartolome JV, Trepanier PA, Chait EA, Slotkin TA: Role of polyamines in isoproterenol-induced cardiac hypertrophy: Effects of α-difluoromethylornithine, an irreversible inhibitor of ornithine decarboxylase. *J Mol Cell Cardiol* 14:461–466, 1982.
7. Clubb FJ Jr, Penney DG, Baylerian MS, Bishop SP: Cardiomegaly due to myocyte hyperplasia in perinatal rats exposed to 200 ppm carbon monoxide. *J Mol Cell Cardiol* 18:477–486, 1986.
8. Ferrans VJ, Rodriguez ER: The pathology of the cardiomyopathies. In: Giles TD, Sander GE (eds) *Cardiomyopathy*. New York: PSG Publishing, 1988, pp 15–54.
9. Liu SK: Cardiac disease in the dog and cat. In: Roberts HR, Dodds WJ (eds) *Pig Model for Biomedical Research*. Taipei: Pig Research Institute, 1982, pp 110–133.
10. Watkins H, Rosenzweig A, Hwang DS, Levi T, McKenna W, Seidman C, Seidman JG: Characteristics and prognostic implications of myosin missense mutations in familial hypertrophic cardiomyopathy. *N Engl J Med* 1108–1114, 1992.
11. Ferrans VJ, Buja LM, Roberts WC: Cardiac morphologic changes produced by ethanol. In: Rothschild MA, Oratz M, Schreiber S (eds) *Alcohol and Abnormal Protein Biosynthesis*. New York: Pergamon Press, 1974, pp 139–185.

12. Opie LH: Metabolic and drug-induced injury to the myocardium. In: Bristow MR (ed) *Drug-Induced Heart Disease.* Amsterdam: Elsevier/North Holland Biomedical Press, 1980, pp 81–102.

13. Ferrans VJ, Butany JW: Ultrastructural pathology of the heart. In: Trump BF, Jones RT (eds) *Diagnostic Electron Microscopy*, Vol 4. New York: John Wiley & Sons, 1983, pp 319–473.

14. Ferrans VJ, Sanchez JA, Herman EH: Pathologic anatomy of animal models of anthracycline-induced cardiotoxicity. In: Muggia F, Speyer J (eds) *Cancer and the Heart.* Johns Hopkins University Press, 1992, pp 89–113.

15. Herman EH, Ferrans VJ, Sanchez JA: Methods of reducing anthracycline cardiac toxicity. In: Muggia F, Speyer J (eds) *Cancer and The Heart.* Johns Hopkins University Press, 1992, pp 114–169.

16. Ferrans VJ, Sanchez JA, Herman EH: Role of myocardial biopsy in the diagnosis of anthracycline toxicity. In: Muggia F, Speyer J (eds) *Cancer and The Heart.* Johns Hopkins University Press, 1992, pp 198–216.

17. Ito H, Miller SC, Billingham ME, Akimoto H, Torti SV, Wade R, Gahlmann R, Lyons G, Kedes L, Torti FM: Doxorubicin selectively inhibits muscle gene expression in cardiac muscle cells in vivo and in vitro. *Proc Natl Acad Sci USA* 87:4275–4279, 1990.

18. Mirski A, Daskal I, Busch H: Effects of adriamycin on ultrastructure of nucleoli in the heart and liver cells of the rat. *Cancer Res* 36:1580–1584, 1976.

19. Zhang J, Herman EH, Ferrans VJ: Dendritic cells in the hearts of spontaneously hypertensive rats treated with doxorubicin with or without ICRF-187. *Am J Pathol* 1993, in press.

20. Billingham ME: Role of endomyocardial biopsy in diagnosis and treatment of heart disease. In: Silver MD (ed) *Cardiovascular Pathology*, 2nd ed. New York: Churchill Livingstone, 1991, pp 1465–1486.

21. Speyer JL, Green MD, Kramer E, Rey M, Sanger J, Ward C, Dubin N, Ferrans VJ, Stecy P, Zeleniuch-Jacquotte A, Wernz J, Feit F, Slater W, Blum R, Muggia F: Protective effect of the bispiperazinedione ICRF-187 against doxorubicin-induced cardiac toxicity in women with advanced breast cancer. *N Engl J Med* 319:745–752, 1988.

22. Applebaum FR, Strauchen JA, McGraw RG Jr, Savage DD, Kent KM, Ferrans VJ, Herzig GP: Acute lethal carditis caused by high-dose combination chemotherapy. A unique clinical and pathological entity. *Lancet* 1:58–62, 1976.

23. Gottdiener JS, Applebaum FR, Ferrans VJ, Deisseroth A, Ziegler J: Cardiotoxicity associated with high-dose cyclophosphamide therapy. *Arch Intern Med* 141:758–763, 1981.

24. Von Hoff DD, Rozencweig M, Piccart M: The cardiotoxicity of anti-cancer agents. *Sem Oncol* 9:23–33, 1982.

25. Van Vleet JF, Ferrans VJ: Myocardial diseases of animals. *Am J Pathol* 124:98–178, 1986.

26. Rowinsky EK, Onetto N, Canetta RM, Arbuck SG: Taxol. The first of the taxanes, an important new class of anti-tumor agents. *Sem Oncol* 19:646–662, 1992.

27. Torti FM, Lum BL: Cardiac toxicity. In: de Vita VT Jr, Hellman S, Rosenberg SA (eds) *Cancer: Principles and Practice of Oncology*, 2nd ed. Vol 2. Philadelphia: JB Lippincott, 1989, pp 2153–2162.

28. Fry DW: Biochemical pharmacology of anthracenediones and anthrapyrazoles. *Pharmac Ther* 55:109–125, 1991.

29. Van Vleet JF, Ferrans VJ: Congestive cardiomyopathy induced in ducklings fed graded amounts of furazolidone. *Am J Vet Res* 44:76–85, 1983.

30. Van Vleet JF, Ferrans VJ: Furazolidone-induced congestive cardiomyopathy in ducklings: Regression of cardiac lesions after cessation of furazolidone ingestion. *Am J Vet Res* 44:1007–1013, 1983.

31. Van Vleet JF, Ferrans VJ: Furazolidone-induced congestive cardiomyopathy in ducklings: Myocardial ultrastructural alterations. *Am J Vet Res* 44:1014–1023, 1983.

32. Van Vleet JF, Ferrans VJ: Furazolidone-induced congestive cardiomyopathy in ducklings: Lack of protection from selenium, vitamin E, and taurine supplements. *Am J Vet Res* 44:1143–1148, 1983.

33. Gwathmey J, Hamllin RL: Protection of turkeys against furazolidone-induced cardiomyopathy. *Am J Cardiol* 52:626–628, 1983.

34. Horowitz JD: Drugs that induce heart problems. Which agents? What effects? *Cardiovasc Med* 8:308–315, 1983.

35. McAllister HA Jr, Mullick FG: The cardiovascular system. In: Riddell R (ed) *Pathology of Drug-Induced and Toxic Diseases.* New York: Churchill-Livingstone, 1982, pp 201–228.

36. Fenoglio JJ Jr, Silver MD: The effects of drugs on the cardiovascular system. In: Silver MD (ed) *Cardiovascular Pathology*, 2nd ed. New York: Churchill-Livingstone, 1991, pp 1205–1229.

37. Lewis W, Papoian T, Gonzalez B, Louie H, Kelly DP, Payne RM, Grody WW: Mitochondrial ultrastructural and molecular changes induced by zidovudine in rat hearts. *Lab Invest* 65:228–236, 1991.

38. Herskowitz A, Willoughby SB, Baughman KL, Schulman SP, Bartlett JD: Cardiomyopathy associated with antiretroviral therapy in patients with HIV infection: A report of six cases. *Ann Intern Med* 116:311–313, 1992.

39. McAllister HA Jr, Ferrans VJ, Hall RJ, Strickman NE, Bossart MI: Chloroquine cardiomyopathy. *Arch Pathol Lab Med* 111:953–956, 1987.

40. Arbustini E, Grasso M, Salerno JA, Gavazzi A, Pucci A, Bramerio M, Calligaro A, Ferrans VJ: Endomyocardial biopsy finding in two patients with idiopathic dilated cardiomyopathy receiving long-term treatment with amiodarone. *Am J Cardiol* 67:661–662, 1991.

41. Herman EH, Zhang J, Chadwick DP, Ferrans VJ, Green MD: The antiviral drug FIAC causes myocardial alterations in rats. *FASEB J*, 1993, in press.

42. Fauci AS, Harley JB, Roberts WC, Ferrans VJ, Gralnick HR, Bjornson BH: The idiopathic hypereosinophilic syndrome. Clinical, pathophysiologic and therapeutic considerations. *Ann Intern Med* 97:78–92, 1982.

43. Graham JR: Cardiac and pulmonary fibrosis during methysergide therapy for headache. *Am J Med Sci* 254:1–12, 1967.

44. Kunkel RS: Fibrotic syndromes with chronic use of methysergide. *Headache* 11:1–5, 1971.

45. Bana DS, McNeal PS, LeCompte PM, Shah Y, Graham JR: Cardiac murmurs and endocardial fibrosis associated with methysergide therapy. *Am Heart J* 88:640–655, 1975.

46. Mason JW, Billingham ME, Friedman JP: Methysergide-induced heart disease. A case of multivalvular and myocardial fibrosis. *Circulation* 56:889–890, 1977.

47. Ferrans VJ, Roberts WC: The carcinoid endocardial plaque. An ultrastructural study. *Hum Pathol* 7:387–409, 1976.

48. Boor PJ, Ferrans VJ: Ultrastructural alterations in allylamine cardiovascular toxicity. Late myocardial and vascular lesions. *Am J Pathol* 121:39–54, 1985.

49. Ferrari R, Ceconi C, Curello S, Guarnieri C, Caldarera CM, Albertini A, Visioli O: Oxygen-mediated myocardial damage during ischemia and reperfusion: Role of the cellular defenses against oxygen toxicity. *J Mol Cell Cardiol* 17:937–946, 1985.

50. Kloner RA, Fishbein MC, Lew H, Maroko PR, Braunwald

E: Mummification of the infarcted myocardium by high dose corticosteroids. *Circulation* 57:56–63, 1978.

51. Zhang J, Yu Z-X, Fujita S, Ferrans VJ, Yamaguchi ML: Interstitial dendritic cells of the rat heart. Quantitative and ultrastructure changes in experimental myocardial infarction. *Circulation* 1993, Vol. 87, No. 3:909–920.

52. McAllister HA Jr, Ferrans VJ: Eosinophilic and granulomatous inflammation of the heart. In: Kapoor AS (ed) *Cancer and the Heart.* New York: Springer-Verlag, 1986, pp 246–263.

53. Casscells W, Kimura H, Sanchez JA, Yu Z-X, Ferrans VJ: Immunohistochemical study of fibronectin in experimental myocardial infarction. *Am J Pathol* 137:801–810, 1990.

54. Casscells W, Ferrans VJ: Growth factors in the heart. In: Oberpriller JO, Oberpriller JC (eds) *The Development and Regenerative Potential of Cardiac Muscle.* New York: Harwood Academic, 1991, pp 399–414.

55. McAllister HA Jr, Ferrans VJ: Granulomas of the heart and major blood vessels. In: Ioachim HL (ed) *Pathology of Granulomas.* New York: Raven Press, 1983, pp 75–123.

56. Suzuki T: Ultrastructural changes of heart muscle in cyanide poisoning. *Tohoku J Exp Med* 95:271–287, 1968.

57. Poche R: Uber den Einfluss von Dinitrophenol und Thyroxin auf die Ultrastruktur des Herzmuskels bei der Ratte. *Virchows Arch Pathol Anat* 335:282–297, 1962.

58. Laguens R, Meckert PC, Segal A: Effect of acriflavine on the fine structure of the heart cell mitochondria of normal and exercised rats. *J Mol Cell Cardiol* 4:185–193, 1972.

59. Raute-Kreinsen U, Berlet H, Buhler F, Rixner P: Elektronenmikroskopische Befunde am Herzmuskel der Ratte bei experimentell induzierten Elektrolyt-veranderungen. *Virchows Arch Pathol Anat* 375:331–344, 1977.

60. Nienhaus H, Poche R, Reimold E: Elektrolytverschiebungen, histologische Veranderungen der Organe and Ultrastruktur des Herzmuskels nach Belastung mit Cortisol, Aldosteron und primaren Natriumphosphat bei der Ratte. *Virchows Arch Pathol Anat* 337:245–269, 1963.

61. Ferrans VJ, Hibbs RG, Weily HS, Weilbaecher DG, Walsh JJ, Burch GE: A histochemical and electron microscopic study of epinephrine-induced myocardial necrosis. *J Mol Cell Cardiol* 1:11–22, 1970.

62. Ferrans VJ, Hibbs RG, Cipriano PR, Buja LM: Histochemical and electron microscopic studies of norepinephrine-induced myocardial necrosis in rats. *Recent Adv Stud Card Struct Metab* 1:495–525, 1972.

63. Rona G, Huttner I, Boutet M: Microcirculatory changes in myocardium with particular reference to catecholamine-induced cardiac muscle cell injury. In: Meesen H (ed) *Handbuch der allgemeinen Pathologie, Vol III, part 7, Mikrozirkulation/Microcirculation.* Berlin: Springer-Verlag, 1977, pp 791–888.

64. Berger JM, Bencosme SA: Divergence in patterns of atrial and ventricular cardiocyte degeneration: Studies with plasmocid. *J Mol Cell Cardiol* 2:41–49, 1971.

65. Ferrans VJ, Saito K: Selective loss of actin filaments from cardiac myocytes. *Pathol Res Pract* 181:489–644, 1986.

66. Sarkar R, Levine DZ: Repair of the myocardial lesion during potassium repletion in kaliopenic rats: An ultrastructural study. *J Mol Cell Cardiol* 11:1165–1172, 1979.

67. Trump BF, Berezesky IR, Laiho KU, Osornio AR, Mergner WJ, Smith MW: The role of calcium in cell injury. A review. In: *Scanning Electron Microscopy II.* AMF O'Hare, III: SEM Inc, 1980, pp 437–462.

68. Decker RS, Wildenthal K: Lysosomal abnormalities in hypoxic and reoxygenated hearts. I. Ultrastructural and cytochemical changes. *Am J Pathol* 98:425–444, 1980.

69. Decker RS, Poole AR, Crie JS, Dingle JT, Wildenthal R: Lysosomal alterations in hypoxia and reoxygenated hearts. II. Immunohistochemical and biochemical changes in cathepsin D. *Am J Pathol* 98:445–455, 1980.

70. Singal PK, Beamish RE, Dhalla NS: Potential oxidative pathways of catecholamines in the formation of lipid peroxides and genesis of heart disease. In: Spitzer JJ (ed) *Myocardial Injury.* New York: Plenum Press, 1982, pp 391–401.

71. Dogterom P, Zbinden G: Cardiotoxicity of vasodilators and positive inotropic/vasodilating drugs in dogs. An overview. *Crit Rev Toxicol* 22:203–241, 1992.

72. Ferrans VJ, Van Vleet JF: Morphological aspects of myocardial lesions associated with stress. In: Beamish RE, Singal PK, Dhalla NS (eds) *Stress and Heart Disease.* Boston: Martinus Nijhoff, 1985, pp 211–227.

73. Blackwell B, Marley E, Price J, Taylor D: Hypertensive interactions between monoamine oxidase inhibitors and food stuffs. *Br J Psychiat* 113:349–365, 1967.

74. Van Vleet JF, Amstutz HE, Weirich WE, Rebar AH, Ferrans VJ: Clinical, clinicopathologic, and pathologic alterations in monensin toxicosis in cattle. *Am J Vet Res* 44:2133–2144, 1983.

75. Bhatnagar MK, Yamashiro S: Ultrastructural alterations of the myocardium of rats fed rapeseed oils. *Res Vet Sci* 26:183–188, 1979.

76. Boor PJ, Ferrans VJ: Ultrastructural alterations in allylamine-induced cardiomyopathy. Early lesions. *Lab Invest* 47:76–86, 1982.

77. Clark AF, Tandler B, Vignos PJ: Glucocorticoid-induced alterations in the rabbit heart. *Lab Invest* 47:603–610, 1982.

78. Van Vleet JF, Boon GD, Ferrans VJ: Induction of lesions of selenium-vitamin E deficiency in weanling swine fed silver, cobalt, tellurium, zinc, cadmium, and vanadium. *Am J Vet Res* 42:789–799, 1981.

79. Van Vleet JF, Boon GD, Ferrans VJ: Induction of lesions of selenium-vitamin E deficiency in ducklings fed silver, cobalt, cadmium, copper, tellurium or zinc and protection by selenium or vitamin E supplements. *Am J Vet Res* 42:1206–1217, 1981.

80. Fujita S, Puri RK, Yu Z-X, Travis WD, Ferrans VJ: An ultrastructural study of in vivo interactions between lymphocytes and endothelial cells in the pathogenesis of the vascular leak syndrome induced by interleukin-2. *Cancer* 68:2169–2174, 1991.

81. Zhang J, Yu Z-X, Hilbert SL, Yamaguchi M, Chadwick DP, Herman EH, Ferrans VJ: Cardiotoxicity of human recombinant interleukin-2 in rats: A morphological study. *Circulation* 1993, ol. 87, No. 4:1340–1353.

82. Gulick T, Chung MK, Pieper SJ, Lange LG, Schreiner GF: Interleukin-1 and tumor necrosis factor inhibit cardiac myocyte β-adrenergic responsiveness. *Proc Natl Acad Sci USA* 86:6753, 1989.

83. Yi ES, Ulich TR: Endotoxin, interleukin-1, and tumor necrosis factor cause neutrophil-dependent microvascular leakage in postcapillary venules. *Am J Pathol* 140:656–663, 1992.

84. Zbinden G: Effects of recombinant human alpha-interferon in a rodent cardiotoxicity model. *Toxicol Lett* 50:25–35, 1990.

85. James TN, Gomez-Sanchez MA, Martinez-Tello FJ, Posada-De La Paz M, Abaitua-Borda I, Soldevilla LB: Cardiac abnormalities in the toxic oil syndrome, with comparative observations on the eosinophilia-myalgia syndrome. *J Am Coll Cardiol* 18:1367–1379, 1991.

86. Silver RM, Heyes MP, Maize JC, Quearry B, Vionnet-Fuasset M, Sternberg EM: Scleroderma, fascitis, and eosino-

philia associated with the ingestion of tryptophan. *N Engl J Med* 322:874–881, 1990.

87. James TN: Abnormalities of the coronary arteries, neural structures and conduction system of the heart observed postmortem in the eosinophilia-myalgia syndrome, with a discussion of comparative findings from the toxic oil syndrome. *Trans Am Clin Climatol Assoc* 102:52–83, 1990.

88. James TN, Kamb ML, Sandberg GA, Silver RM, Kilbourne EM: Postmortem studies of the heart in three fatal cases of the eosinophilia-myalgia syndrome. *Ann Intern Med* 115:102–110, 1991.

89. Herman EH, Ferrans VJ, Balazs T: Minoxidil and cardiac lesions. *Circulation* 64:1299–1300, 1981.

90. Van Vleet JF, Herman EH, Ferrans VJ: Cardiac morphologic alterations in acute minoxidil cardiotoxicity in miniature swine. *Exp Mol Pathol J* 41:10–25, 1984.

91. Jett GK, Herman EH, Jones M, Ferrans VJ, Clark RJ: Influence of minoxidil on regional blood flow and morphology

in beagle dogs. *Cardiovasc Drugs Ther* 1:687–694, 1988.

92. Herman EH, Ferrans VJ, Young RSK, Balazs T: A comparative study of minoxidil-induced myocardial lesions in beagle dogs and miniature swine. *Toxicol Pathol* 17:182–192, 1989.

93. Herman E, Chadwick D, Zhang J, Ferrans V: Minoxidil-induced cardiac lesions in rats of different ages. *FASEB J* 1993, in press.

94. Pinnell SR: Disorders of collagen. In: Stanbury JB, Wyngaarden JB, Fredrickson DS (eds) *The Metabolic Basis of Inherited Disease*. New York: McGraw-Hill, 1978, pp 1366–1394.

95. Irey NS, Norris HJ: Intimal lesions associated with female reproductive steroids. *Arch Pathol* 96:227–234, 1973.

96. Arnett EN, Battle WE, Russo JV, Roberts WC: Intravenous injection of talc-containing drugs intended for oral use: A cause of pulmonary granulomatosis and pulmonary hypertension. *Am J Med* 60:711–718, 1976.

CHAPTER 41

Adenosine and Adenine Nucleotide Action on Cardiac Cellular Excitation

YOSHIHISA KURACHI

INTRODUCTION

A variety of evidence indicates that adenosine and adenine nucleotides act as endogenous modulators of cellular activity in various physiological responses. The cardiovascular action of these substances has been known for over 60 years, as in 1929 Drury and Szent-Györgyi {1} examined the effects of various adenine compounds on the heart. The molecular mechanisms responsible for the effects of these substances, however, have been clarified only in the last decade. The clinical relevance of adenosine and ATP, especially in treating supraventricular tachycardia, has also been recently recognized {2}. In this chapter, recent progress in the understanding of molecular mechanisms underlying the effects of purinergic receptor activation on cardiac cellular electrical activity are reviewed.

DIRECT OR CYCLIC AMP-INDEPENDENT ACTION OF ADENOSINE

Adenosine-induced K^+ channel activation and termination of paroxysmal supraventricular tachycardia

It is well known that excitation of vagal nerves can terminate paroxysmal supraventricular tachycardia (PSVT), which include the atrioventricular node in the circuit. Adenosine was shown to have the same effects on PSVT as acetylcholine (ACh). Recently venous injection of adenosine or ATP has been used as an effective therapy to terminate PSVT {2,3}. ATP is supposed to act on the heart after being degraded to adenosine.

Figure 41-1 shows an example of adenosine-induced termination of PSVT. The patient was a 68-year-old man who suffered from PSVT because of a concealed Wolff-Parkinson-White syndrome. The excitation antegrade-conducted the atrioventricular node, retrograde-conducted an accessory pathway, and caused reentrant tachycardia. Ten seconds after adenosine (5 mg) was injected intravenously, the tachycardia was terminated by a transient A-H block and the sinus rhythm recovered. The characteristics of adenosine-injection therapy for PSVT are as follows: (a) The effect appears rapidly and consistently

(>90% of patients), (b) the effect is transient and short lived, and (c) no serious side effects occur. The relative contraindications are (a) extreme old age, (b) ischemic heart disease, (c) asthma, and (d) use of dipyridamole.

As shown in fig. 41-2, we examined the dose dependency of the effect of adenosine on cardiac excitation and the effects of aminophylline and dipyridamole on the adenosine effect. The patient was a 60-year-old woman who had suffered from recurrent PSVT based on a James bundle. In the sinus rhythm, adenosine (4 mg) was injected intravenously. At 15 seconds after the injection, the A-H interval was prolonged to twice the control level, an effect that disappeared after 30 seconds. Adenosine (1 mg) did not affect the cardiac excitation. The effect of adenosine on the A-H interval was not affected by atropine, was enhanced prominently by dipyridamole, and was blocked by aminophylline. In other cases, adenosine caused sinus bradycardia, in addition to prolongation of the A-H interval, which was also augmented by dipyridamole and blocked by aminophylline. Since dipyridamole inhibits the transport of adenosine into the cells and aminophylline is an inhibitor of P_1-purinergic receptors {4}, the prolongation of the sinus cycle and the A-H interval observed after adenosine injection appears to be caused by the binding of adenosine to cardiac P_1 purinoceptors.

The following sections will show what mechanisms underlie this direct effect of adenosine on sinus cycle and atrioventricular conduction. In brief, adenosine activates the muscarinic K^+ (K_{ACh}) channels in sinoatrio and atrioventricular nodal cells, atrial cells, and Purkinje fibers, but not in ventriclular cells. Activation of the K_{ACh} channel by adenosine decreases the resting membrane resistance of these tissues, which may be responsible for the adenosine-induced slowing of the sinus rate and the atrioventricular conduction. In the cardiac cell membrane, a pertussis toxin-sensitive G protein (G_K) couples m_2-muscarinic and P_1-purinergic receptors with the K_{ACh} channel.

N. Sperelakis (ed.), Physiology and Pathophysiology of the Heart, Third Edition.

789

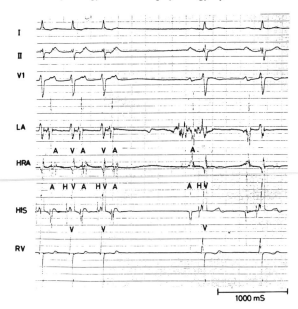

Fig. 41-1. Termination of PSVT by adenosine. Concealed WPW syndrome in a 68-year-old male. LA = esophageal lead; HRA = high right atrium; HIS = His bundle; RV = right ventricle; A = atrial ECG; B = His ECG; V = ventricular ECG.

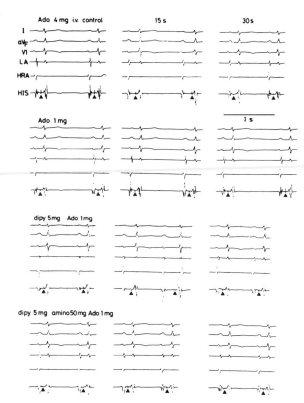

Fig. 41-2. Effects of dipyridamole and aminophylline on adenosine-induced atrioventricular condition disturbance. Arrows indicate His ECG. See text for details.

Molecular mechanisms underlying adenosine activation of muscarinic K⁺ channel

ADENOSINE AND ACETYLCHOLINE ACTIVATE THE MUSCARINIC K⁺ CHANNEL VIA GTP-BINDING PROTEINS IN CARDIAC ATRIAL CELLS

The similarity of the effects of adenosine on cardiac membrane potential to those of ACh has been known since the early studies in the 1950s. Figure 41-3 shows the properties of adenosine- and ACh-activated K⁺ channel currents {53}: The K⁺ channels activated by adenosine and ACh have the same conductance and kinetic properties; i.e., the unitary channel conductance is 40–50 pS with symmetrical 150 mM K⁺ and displays prominent inward rectification at potentials more positive than E_K. The open-time histogram of the channel can be fitted by a single exponential curve with a time constant of about 1 ms. The channel does not open at random intervals but in bursts. Adenosine and ACh increase the frequency of bursts. The effects of adenosine and ACh are selectively antagonized by theophylline and atropine added to the pipette solution, respectively. We interpret these results to indicate that adenosine and ACh regulate the same K⁺ channel, i.e., the muscarinic K⁺ channel (K_{ACh}), in cardiac atrial cells, but do so by activating different membrane receptors (P_1, more specifically A_1-purinergic receptors in the case of adenosine and m_2-muscarinic cholinergic receptors in the case of ACh).

In the inside-out patch configuration, in the presence of ACh or adenosine in the extracellular side of the membrane, K_{ACh} channels are activated by intracellular GTP (fig. 41-4A). This GTP-induced activation is blocked by the A promoter of pertussis toxin (PTX; or islet-activating protein, IAP) with nicotinamide adenine dinucleotide (fig. 41-4B). Since PTX specifically ADP ribosylates and inhibits the functions of a family of G proteins, these observations strongly indicate that m_2-muscarinic and P_1-purinergic receptors link with the K_{ACh} channels via PTX-sensitive G proteins *in the cell membrane* without a mandatory involvement of intracellular second messengers (fig. 41-5) {5}. Consistent with this model, in the absence of agonists (adenosine or ACh), GTP failed to activate the channel, but GTP-γS and GppNHp, nonhydrolyzable GTP analogues, gradually increased the frequency of K_{ACh} channel openings. AlF₄⁻, an activator of G proteins, also activates the channel in the absence of agonists {6}.

A SIMPLIFIED MODEL FOR THE G_K ACTIVATION OF THE K_{ACh} CHANNEL

Using the inside-out patch clamp technique, it is easy to control the intracellular and extracellular ionic conditions

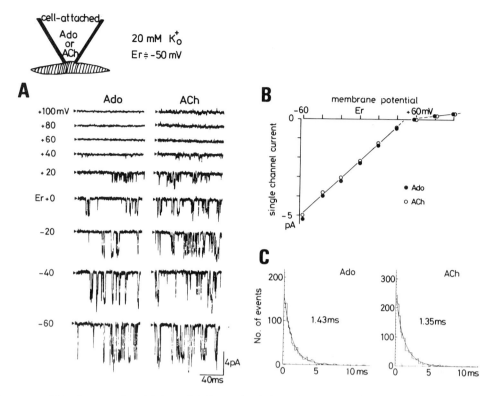

Fig. 41-3. Conductance and kinetic properties of Ado- and ACh-regulated channel currents. **A:** Examples of Ado- and ACh-regulated channel currents recorded from guinea pig atrial myocytes at various membrane potentials in the cell-attached form. The current-recording pipettes contained Ado ($10\,\mu M$) or ACh ($5.5\,\mu M$) in these experiments. All records were low-pass filtered at $1\,kHz$ ($-3\,dB$). The closed arrow at each trace represents the zero current level. **B:** Current-voltage relations of Ado- (closed circles) and ACh- (open circles) regulated channels. The slope conductance of the unitary current was $46\,pS$ in this example. **C:** Open-time histograms of Ado- and ACh-regulated channels at Er. Both distributions were fitted by a single exponential curve with the time constants indicated in each graph. Reproduced from Kurachi et al. {5}, with permission.

as well as metabolites. Thus, it is possible to further examine the molecular mechanisms underlying the muscarinic regulation of the K_{ACh} channel. We first examined the effects of intracellular Mg^{2+} on the regulation of K_{ACh} channel {7}.

Mg^{2+} free-EDTA internal solution was perfused in the inside-out patches (adenosine or ACh in the pipettes). Under this condition, channel opening did not resume when GTP was applied to the intracellular side of the membrane. When Mg^{2+} was also added, the channels started to open. In the absence of intracellular Mg^{2+}, the K_{ACh} channels did not open, even when GTP-γS was used in place of GTP. Once the channels started to open with GTP-γS, the openings persisted after removal of GTP-γS and Mg^{2+}. These observations indicate that (a) intracellular Mg^{2+} is essential for GTP activation of the K_{ACh} channel, and (b) for deactivation of the channel openings, it is necessary that GTP, bound to the α subunit of G_K, is hydrolyzed to GDP.

Based on these results, a simplified model was proposed for the molecular mechanism underlying G_K activation of the K_{ACh} channel using the analogy of G protein regulation of adenylyl cyclase (fig. 41-6): In the absence of agonists, G_K remains in a trimeric complex composed of $G_{K\alpha}$ and $G_{K\beta\gamma}$, and the K_{ACh} channel is closed (state 1). In this state, GDP may be bound to $G_{K\alpha}$. When an agonist (either ACh or adenosine) binds to the membrane receptor, some signal is transmitted to G_K (state 2). If Mg^{2+} is present on the intracellular side of the membrane, GTP binds to $G_{K\alpha}$, probably in exchange for GDP, and activates G_K (state 3). During activation G_K may be dissociated into its subunits ($G_{\alpha-GTP}$ and $G_{\beta\gamma}$), and potentially either subunit may activate the K_{ACh} channel. When GTP, which is bound to $G_{K\alpha}$, is hydrolyzed to GDP, G_K is deactivated and goes back to state 1 or 2. Since GTPγS and GppNHp are not hydrolyzed to GDP, G_K, when activated by GTPγS or GppNHp, may stay in state 3 and the openings of the K_{ACh} channel are continuously stimulated. GTP-dependent channel activation, as well as AlF$_4^-$-dependent activation, requires Mg^{2+}, whereas G protein subunit activation of the channel does not require intracellular Mg^{2+}. These observations are consistent with the notion that dissociation of the trimer into G_α and $G_{\beta\gamma}$ is Mg^{2+} dependent.

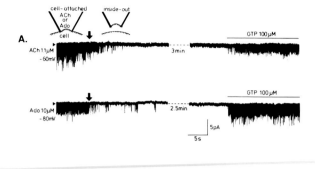

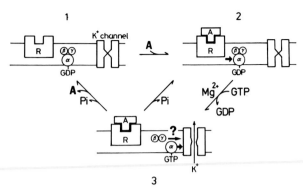

3

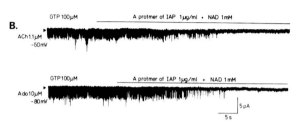

Fig. 41-6. Simplified scheme of activation of a K^+ channel regulated by GTP-binding protein in the atrial cell membrane. R is a membrane receptor (m-ACh or Ado receptor); A is an agonist (ACh or ADo); α, β, and γ are the subunits of the GTP-binding protein. This scheme does not represent any quantitative relations and does not exclude the possibility of several other steps between each component. Reproduced from Kurachi et al. {7}, with permission.

Fig. 41-4. Activation of a K^+ channel by Ado and ACh requires intracellular GTP and is blocked by PTX (or IAP). **A:** The cells were bathed in the internal solution. The concentration of agonists and the patch membrane potential are indicated at each current trace. At the arrow in each trace, the patch was excised from the cell, yielding an "inside-out" patch. Activation of the channel was blocked in the inside-out patches. During the period shown by the bar above each trace, the internal solution containing GTP (100 μM) was perfused. Activation of the channel resumed abruptly by adding GTP to the bath. **B:** The patches are the same as those in A. With GTP present in the intracellular side of the membrane, the channels remained activated. The A (active) promoter of PTX (or IAP) with NAD 1 mM was added to the internal solution containing GTP during the period indicated by the bar above each trace. Channel activation was gradually blocked by IAP within 1–3 minutes. When the A promoter was perfused in the absence of NAD, the activation of the channel was not blocked. Reproduced from Kurachi et al. {5}, with permission.

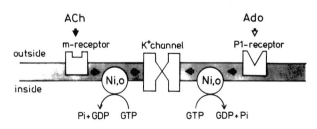

Fig. 41-5. Simplified scheme of purinergic and muscarinic activation of a K^+ channel in atrial cell membrane. In cardiac atrial cell membrane, two different membrane receptors (P1-purinergic and muscarinic ACh receptors) link with a K^+ channel via GTP-binding proteins N_i (G_i) and/or N_o (G_o). This scheme does not represent any quantitative relations between the components. Reproduced from Kurachi et al. {5}, with permission.

G PROTEIN SUBUNIT ACTIVATION OF THE K_{ACh} CHANNEL

Experiments designed to identify which G protein subunit activates the K_{ACh} channel have been performed using G protein subunits purified from brain and erythrocytes or recombinant subunits. Logothetis et al. {8} reported that nanomolar concentrations of $G_{\beta\gamma}$ activated the K_{ACh} channel. In contrast, Yatani et al. {9} and Codina et al. {10} reported that only $G_{i\alpha\text{-}GTP\gamma S}$ (picomolar range) activated the channel. They also reported that $G_{\alpha40}$ from human erythrocytes (probably $G_{i3\alpha}$) is much more potent than $G_{i1\text{ or }2\alpha}$ and $G_{o\alpha}$. Yatani et al. {11} also reported that recombinant $G_{i\alpha}S$ ($G_{i1\text{-}\alpha}$, $G_{i2\text{-}\alpha}$, and $G_{i3\alpha}$) are equally potent in activating the K_{ACh} channel.

Codina et al. {10} and Kirsh et al. {12} proposed that the effects of $G_{\beta\gamma}$ on the K_{ACh} channel are either due to contaminating $G_{\alpha\text{-}GTP\gamma S}$ in the $G_{\beta\gamma}$ preparation or to the effects of a detergent, CHAPS, which was used to suspend the $G_{\beta\gamma}$ preparation. Kim et al. {13} proposed that $G_{\beta\gamma}$ activation of the K_{ACh} channel was indirectly caused by arachidonic acid metabolites that were released by $G_{\beta\gamma}$ activation of PLA_2 and that the physiological functional arm of G_K to the K_{ACh} channel was $G_{K\alpha}$. However, these possibilities were shown to be unlikely, and it was strongly indicated that the activating effect of $G_{\beta\gamma}$ on the K_{ACh} channel is attributable to the function of $G_{\beta\gamma}$ protein itself (fig. 41-7) {14–17}. By comparing the effects of G protein subunits on the ATP-sensitive K (K_{ATP}) and the K_{ACh} channels, we concluded that $G_{K\beta\gamma}$ is the physiological functional arm of G_K responsible for activation of the K_{ACh} channel {17,18}.

Logothetis et al. {19} showed that exogenous $G_{\alpha41\text{-}GDP}$ blocked exogenous $G_{\beta\gamma}$-activation of the K_{ACh} channel. They also showed that $G_{\alpha41\text{-}GDP}$ blocked GTP-γS-induced activation of the K_{ACh} channel. We recently found that the

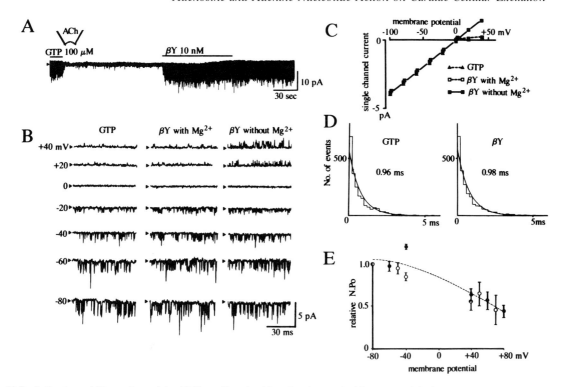

Fig. 41-7. Activation of K_{ACh} channel by GTP or $G_{\beta\gamma}$. **A:** After forming an inside-out patch in internal solution containing 2 mM $MgCl_2$, 100 μM GTP activated the K_{ACh} channel with 0.3 μM ACh in the pipette solution. After washing out GTP, channel activity disappeared. Subsequent application of Gd2f94b$_g$ activated the K_{ACh} channel irreversibly. Bars above the tracing indicate perfusing protocol. The patch was held at −80 mV. **B:** Expanded recordings of the K_{ACh} channel at various holding potentials induced by GTP, $G_{\beta\gamma}$ with 2 mM Mg^{2+}, or without Mg^{2+} (indicated above each column). **C:** Current-voltage (I/V) relationship of the K_{ACh} channel. Filled triangles, open squares, and filled squares represent I/V relationship induced by GTP with Mg^{2+} (2 mM), $G_{\beta\gamma}$ with Mg^{2+} (2 mM), and $G_{\beta\gamma}$ without Mg^{2+}, respectively. Strong inward rectification was noted using GTP with Mg^{2+} and $G_{\beta\gamma}$ with Mg^{2+}. **D:** Open-time histograms of the K_{ACh} channel currents induced by GTP and $G_{\beta\gamma}$ at −80 mV. **E:** Voltage-dependent channel activity in the absence of Mg^{2+} induced by $G_{\beta\gamma}$ (filled circles) and by GppNHp (open circles). The relative $N \cdot P_o$ was obtained in reference to the $N \cdot P_o$ induced by 10 nM $G_{\beta\gamma}$ or GppNHp (10 μM) at −80 mV. The results were expressed as mean ± SD (n = 3 each). Reproduced from Ito et al. {17}, with permission.

GDP-bound form of the transducin α subunit inhibited the agonist-mediated/GTP-induced or GTP-γS-induced K_{ACh} channel activity irreversibly {18}. This inhibition was only restored by $T_{\beta\gamma}$ or $G_{\beta\gamma}$. These results again strongly support the notion that $G_{K\beta\gamma}$ is the physiological functional arm of G_K to activate the K_{ACh} channel.

The present questions concerning G_K subunit activation of K_{ACh} channels are as follows: (a) Which PTX-sensitive G protein is G_K? (b) How does $G_{\beta\gamma}$ interact with the K_{ACh} channel? (c) How is the specificity of signaling from the receptor to the K_{ACh} channel preserved?

ADENOSINE ACTIVATION OF THE ATP-SENSITIVE K⁺ CHANNEL

Since the initial reports that G proteins might be involved in the regulation of the K_{ATP} channel in the pancreatic β cell {20} and skeletal muscle cell {21}, G protein has

also been found to activate the K_{ATP} channel in cardiac myocytes {17,22,23}. We found that GTP-γS-bound $G_{i1\,or\,2\alpha}$ of PTX-sensitive G proteins purified from bovine brain activated the K_{ATP} channel in the guinea pig ventricular cell membrane (figs. 41-8A and 41-8B). $G_{\beta\gamma}$ inhibited the adenosine-dependent/GTP-induced activation of K_{ATP} channels (fig. 41-8C). These results indicate that α subunits of the PTX-sensitive G proteins activate the K_{ATP} channel in ventricular cell membrane.

In fig. 41-9A, we compared the effects of $G_{i1\alpha\text{-GTP}\gamma S}$ and $G_{\beta\gamma}$ on the K_{ATP} and K_{ACh} channels in the atrial cell membrane where both channels are expressed. In the cell-attached form, the K_{ACh} channel was activated vigorously by ACh (1 μM) in the pipette. In the inside-out patch condition, the openings of the K_{ACh} channel decreased to a minimal background level. The internal solution contained 100 μM ATP to keep the K_{ATP} channel in the phosphorylated condition. When $G_{i1\alpha\text{-GTP}\gamma S}$ (300 pM) was applied to the internal side of the membrane, bursting K⁺

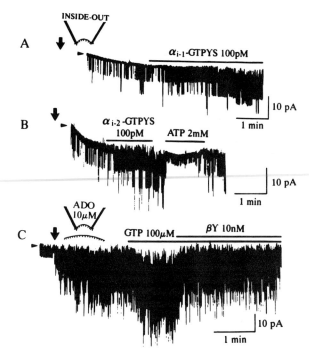

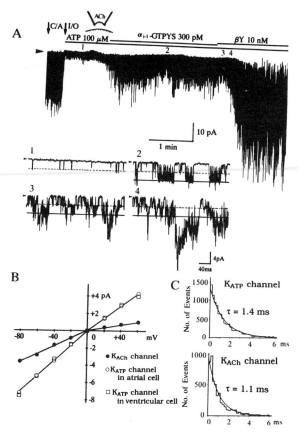

Fig. 41-8. Activation of the K$_{ATP}$ channel by G$_{i1-2\alpha-GTP\gamma S}$ in ventricular myocytes. The inside-out patch from ventricular myocytes was formed in internal solution containing 100 µM ATP and 0.5 mM MgCl$_2$. When G$_{i-1,2\alpha-GTP\gamma S}$ was added to the internal solution, burstlike openings of a K$^+$ channel with large conductance (~90 pS) appeared (**A,B**), which could be suppressed by 2 mM ATP (**B**). Arrows above each trace indicate where the inside-out patch was formed. No agonist in the pipette solution in A and B. **C:** 10 µM adenosine (ADO). Arrowheads indicate the zero current level. The holding potential was −80 mV. The protocol for perfusing GTP, ATP, GTP-γS-bound G$_{i-1,2\alpha}$, and G$_{\beta\gamma}$ are indicated by the bars above each current trace. Reproduced from Ito et al. {17}, with permission.

channel openings with a conductance of ~90 pS were induced. On the other hand, the background openings of the K$_{ACh}$ channel were not affected significantly (fig. 41-9A, 2). Openings of the 90-pS K$^+$ channel were blocked by 1 µM glibenclamide, indicating that this was indeed the K$_{ATP}$ channel. Subsequent application of G$_{\beta\gamma}$ (10 nM) to the patch dramatically increased openings of the 40–45 pS K$_{ACh}$ channel in the same patch membrane (fig. 41-9A, 3 and 4). The G$_{\beta\gamma}$-induced openings of the K$_{ACh}$ channel were not affected by glibenclamide.

From these results, we proposed that upon stimulation of P$_1$-purinergic or m$_2$-muscarinic receptors, PTX-sensitive G proteins are dissociated into G$_{\alpha-GTP}$ and G$_{\beta\gamma}$. G$_{\alpha-GTP}$ activates the K$_{ATP}$ channel and G$_{\beta\gamma}$ activates the K$_{ACh}$ channel (fig. 41-10), although we do not know whether the G protein coupled to the K$_{ACh}$ channels is identical to that coupled to the K$_{ATP}$ channels. The former mechanism exists in both ventricular and atrial cells, while the latter may exist in atrial cells but not in ventricular cells. These results also further support the activating effects of G$_{\beta\gamma}$ on the K$_{ACh}$ channel.

Fig. 41-9. Effects of G$_{i-1\alpha-GTP\gamma S}$* and G$_{\beta\gamma}$ on the K$_{ATP}$ and K$_{ACh}$ channels in the atrial cell membrane. **A:** The pipette solution contained 1 µM ACh. The inside-out patch was formed at the arrow above the current trace in the internal solution containing 100 µM ATP and 0.5 mM MgCl$_2$. G$_{i-1\alpha-GTP\gamma S}$ (300 pM) was first applied to the internal side of the patch, which clearly induced opening of the K$_{ATP}$ channel (~90 pS) (A-2) without affecting background activity of the K$_{ACh}$ channel. Subsequently, G$_{\beta\gamma}$ (10 nM) was applied to the patch, which caused a dramatic increase of 45 pS K$_{ACh}$ channel openings in the same patch (A-3,4). Numbers above the current trace indicate the location of each expanded current trace below. In the expanded current trace, the dotted line is the first level of the K$_{ACh}$ channel and the continuous line is that of the K$_{ATP}$ channel. The arrowhead at each trace is the zero current level. **B:** The current-voltage relation of G$_{i-1\alpha-GTP\gamma S}$-induced K$_{ATP}$ channel in the ventricular (open squares) and the atrial (open circles) cell membrane, and G$_{\beta\gamma}$-induced K$_{ACh}$ channel in the atrial cell membrane (closed circles). **C:** The open-time histograms of G$_{i-1\alpha-G0TP\gamma S}$-induced K$_{ATP}$ channel (in ventricle) and G$_{\beta\gamma}$-induced K$_{ACh}$ channel (in atrium) at −80 mV. Reproduced from Ito et al. {17}, with permission.

Since cardiac myocytes contain millimolar concentrations of ATP, adenosine activation of the K$_{ATP}$ channel may not be operative under physiological condition. However, this mechanism may play an important role in protection of cardiac mycoytes during ischemia (Gross G.J., Wisconsin Medical School, personnal communication).

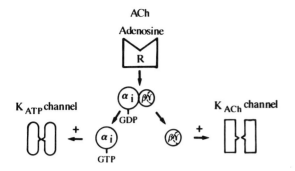

Fig. 41-10. Proposed mechanism of the PTX-sensitive G protein subunit — activation of the K_{ATP} and K_{ACh} channels in cardiac cell membrane. Upon stimulation of the receptors by adenosine or ACh, PTX-sensitive G proteins may be functionally dissociated into $G_{\alpha\text{-}GTP}$ and $G_{\beta\gamma}$. $G_{\alpha\text{-}GTP}$ may activate the K_{ATP} channel, while $G_{\beta\gamma}$ activates the K_{ACh} channel. This scheme does not represent any quantitative relationship between each component and does not take into account possible intermediate steps between components. The former mechanism exists in both ventricular and atrial cells, while the later may exist in atrial but not in ventricular cells. Since cardiac myocytes contain millimolar concentrations of intracellular ATP, the G protein activation of the K_{ATP} channel system may not be operative under physiological conditions. However, the system might play significant role in the ischemia-induced shortening of the cardiac action potential. Although we cannot completely exclude the possibility that $G_{i\alpha\text{-}GTP}$ pathway may partly contribute to the G_K activation of the K_{ACh} channel, the pathway cannot be the major regulatory mechanism for the K_{ACh} channel. Reproduced from Ito et al. {17}, with permission.

INDIRECT OR CYCLIC AMP-DEPENDENT ACTION OF ADENOSINE

Subcellular mechanism for indirect action of adenosine

Adenosine antagonizes the electrophysiological and biochemical effects of beta-adrenergic agonists on the heart, which is related to the regulation of intracellular cyclic AMP and is observed only when the heart is pretreated with beta-adrenergic agonists {24–27}. The antagonistic effect of adenosine on beta-agonist action can be explained by the dual control of adenylyl cyclase acivity by stimulatory and inhibitory G proteins {28}.

The molecular mechanism responsible for the antagonistic effect of adenosine against beta-adrenergic agonist action on the L-type Ca channel current was electrophysiologically shown by Isenberg and Belardinelli {25}, Cerbai et al. {26}, and Kato et al. {27}. The mechanism appears to be identical to the muscarinic antagonism of beta agonists {29}.

Adenosine does not affect the ventricular action potential or the Ca^{2+} current in the absence of beta agonists. When the action potential or the Ca^{2+} current is augmented by isoproterenol, adenosine reduces the action potential or the current to the control value (fig. 41-11). This phenomenon is explained by the dual control mechanism of adenylyl cyclase activity by G proteins (fig. 41-12); that is, the A_1-purinergic receptors couple to cardiac adenylyl cyclase via the inhibitory G proteins (G_i, probably G_{i2}). The beta-adrenergic receptors couple to the adenylyl cyclase via the stimulatory G proteins (G_s). Under beta-

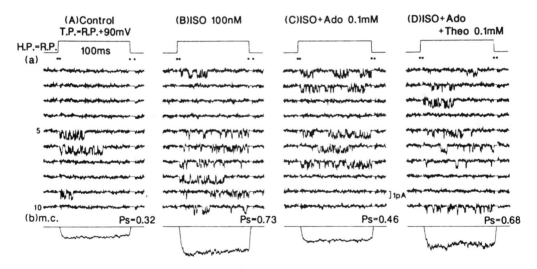

Fig. 41-11. Effect of isoproterenol (ISO), adnosine (Ado), and theophylline (Theo) on singel-channel Ca^{2+} current. **A:** Control. **B:** 100 nM ISO. **C:** 0.1 mM Ado and ISO. **D:** ISO, Ado, and 0.1 mM Theo. Traces labeled as (a) are 10 consecutive sweeps in order of depolarization sequence. Artifacts produced by capacitive transients were erased at the intervals indicated by the two dots. Traces labeled (b) are mean currents (m.c.) from all traces, including blanks. Mean currents were obtained by averaging the idealized openings and are shown on a constant arbitrary scale. About 1000 depolarization steps (100 ms in duration) from the resting potential (R.P.) to R.P. +9 mV were applied repetitively at 2 Hz in each solution. The pipette solution contained 100 mM Ba^{2+}. T.P. = test potential; H.P. = holding potential; Ps = ratio of the number of channel currents containing sweeps to total number of sweeps. Reproduced from Kato et al. {27}, with permission.

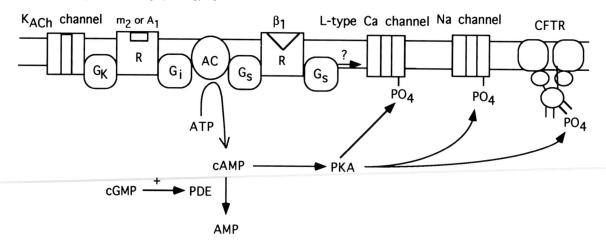

Fig. 41-12. Signaling mechanisms responsible for direct and indirect effects of adenosine in cardiac myocytes. See text for details.

adenergic stimulation, activated G_s stimulates the adenylyl cyclase activity, resulting in formation of cyclic AMP. Cyclic AMP activates the specific protein kinase (A-kinase), which phosphorylates the Ca^{2+} channel. Thus, the cardiac Ca^{2+} current is augmented by beta-stimulation {29}. Under this condition, activation of G_i by adenosine inhibits the G_s-stimulated adenylyl cyclase activity, resulting in the decrease of cyclic AMP to control. The Ca^{2+} channel cannot be maintained phosphorylated without continuous generation of cyclic AMP, and its activity decreases to control levels. In the absence of beta stimulation, intracellular cyclic AMP in the cardiac myocytes may be minimal. Thus, even when the adenylyl cyclase activity is suppressed by activation of G_i with adenosine, the intracellular cyclic AMP level or the Ca^{2+} current is not affected by adenosine. Since the cardiac Na^+ channel and the delayed outward K^+ channel are also regulated by intracellular cyclic AMP-dependent protein kinase {30–32}, similar antagonistic regulation by adenosine also may exist on these channels.

Although regulation of adenylyl cyclases by G protein subunits was shown to be more complicated than previously proposed {33}, adenylyl cyclases expressed in the heart (type V and type VI) seemed not to be affected by $G_{\beta\gamma}$ when preactivated by $G_{s\alpha\text{-GTP}\gamma S}$ {34}. The precise mechanism underlying antagonistic interaction of subunits of G_s and G_i has not yet been determined.

Adenosine may also suppress the adenylyl cyclase activity via the P site by increasing intracellular AMP {34,35}. However, the contribution of this pathway to the antagonism of adenosine against beta-adrenergic stimulation is not clear electrophysiologically.

Clinical relevance

In addition to teminating PSVT due to the direct action of adenosine on the K_{ACh} channel, this substance was used to differentiate the subcellular mechanism underlying ventricular tachycardia {36}. As shown in fig. 41-13, adenosine is an useful diagnostic tool for detecting cardiac tachyarrhythmias {3}.

EFFECTS OF ATP ON CARDIAC CELLULAR EXCITATION

In addition to P_1-purinergic receptors, cardiac myocytes possess purinergic receptors mainly responding to ATP. Although the purinergic receptors responding to ATP are usually classified as P_2 {4}, an unidentified class of ATP receptors, in addition to various subtypes of P_2 purinoceptors, may exist in cardiac myocytes {37}. Thus, in this chapter we may call those receptors ATP receptors. The cardiac ATP receptors exhibit a variety of effects on cardiac excitation by activating a specific nonselective cation channel, the L-type Ca^{2+} current, PI turnover, and by stimulating various transporter systems, such as Na^+-H^+ exchanger and the bicarbonate-dependent regulatory mechanism of intracellular pH.

Effects of ATP in the whole heart

ATP EFFECT ON THE SINUS PACEMAKER ACTIVITY

Figure 41-14 shows the effects of ATP on the sinus rhythm of isolated rabbit hearts under Langendorff perfusion {38}. ATP initially accelerated and then slowed the heart rate. The sinus slowing caused by ATP was blocked by theophylline and disappeared in hearts pretreated with PTX (or IAP), indicating that activation of P_1 purinoceptor either by ATP itself or by adenosine being degradated from ATP may be responsible for the sinus slowing. In contrast, the ATP-induced sinus acceleration was not affected by either theophylline or PTX. In the PTX-

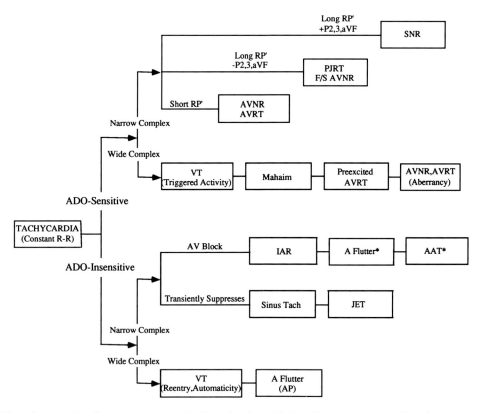

Fig. 41-13. Flow diagram identifying potential mechanism of tachycardia based on response to adenosine and morphology of the arrhythmia. AAT = automatic atrial tachycardia; AP = accessory pathway; AVNR = atrioventricular nodal reentry; AVRT = atrioventricular reciprocating tachycardia; F/S = fast/slow; IAR = intraatrial reentry; JET = junctional ectopic tachycardia; PJRT = permanent form of junctional reciprocating tachycardia; SNR = sinus node reentry; VT = ventricular tachycardia. *Infrequent termination of these forms of arrhythmia to adenosine have been reported. Reproduced from Belardinelli and Lerman {3}, with permission.

treated hearts, ATP persistently accelerated the sinus rate, which was blocked by apamin, suggesting that P_2 purinoceptors are involved. Further subtypes of P_2 purinoceptors involved in this action were not examined. The ATP-induced sinus acceleration was blocked partially by indomethacin and aspirin (cyclooxygenase inhibitors), and completely by neomycin (a phospholipase C inhibitor). Therefore, it was suggested that cardiac P_2 receptors may be coupled, at least in part, to prostaglandin synthesis and possibly to PI turnover via a PTX-insensitive stimulation of phospholipase C.

ATP EFFECT ON CARDIAC INOTROPY

Studies of the effect of ATP on contractility in intact mammalian hearts or heart tissues have produced variable results, probably due to activation of the P_1 purinoceptor by adenosine produced from ATP, in addition to activation of ATP receptors. In single cell preparations, extracellular ATP was shown to consistently cause positive inotropy by increasing $[Ca^{2+}]_i$ {39}. Recently, a variety of

ionic or subcellular mechanisms responsible for the ATP-induced positive inotropy have been proposed (fig. 41-15).

Subcellular mechanisms of ATP action on heart

ATP EFFECT ON NONSELECTIVE CATION CHANNELS AND L-TYPE Ca^{2+} CHANNEL

In various cardiac cells it was shown that extracellular ATP activates a nonselective cation channel {40–42}. The cation channel was activated and desensitized quickly. This channel activation causes depolarization of the membrane {41}. It was also shown that extracellular ATP enhances the L-type Ca^{2+} channel current in rat ventricular myocytes without cyclic AMP production {43}. Thus initial depolarization due to activation of the cation channel and stimulation of the Ca^{2+} channel itself may facilitate Ca^{2+} influx across the cardiac cell membrane, which may be mainly responsible for the increase of $[Ca^{2+}]_i$ induced by extracellular ATP {39,44}.

In bovine and frog atrial cells, it was also shown that

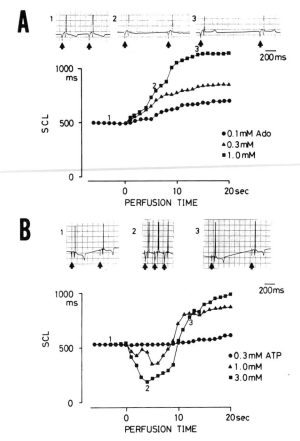

ATP activates an inward-rectifying K_{ACh} channel {40,45}. In these cells, adenosine has no effect on the K_{ACh} channel. The membrane receptors to ATP in these cells cannot be classified as a classical P_2 purinoceptor, since the receptors are not antagonized by [α,β-methylene]ATP. Subclassification of this ATP receptor coupled to the K_{ACh} channel has not yet been performed.

ATP EFFECTS ON MEMBRANE TRANSPORT SYSTEMS

Extracellular ATP, in the presence of Mg^{2+}, induces transient acidification followed by sustained alkalinization. The acidifying effect of ATP has been ascribed to the stimulation of Cl^-/HCO_3^- exchange {46}, whereas the alkalinization has been attributed to activation of the Na^+/H^+ antiport {47}. In addition, in the presence of Na/H antiport inhibitors, ATP can accelerate the recovery of intracellular pH (pH_i) following acidification induced by NH_4Cl through stimulation of a bicarbonate-dependent alkalinizing transporter {48}. Since a change in pH_i has profound effects on cardiac excitation-contraction coupling {49,50}, ATP can be expected to improve the ability of cardiac myocytes to maintain their pH_i, and thus, normal function. Sustained alkalinization may in part be responsible for the ATP-induced positive inotropy, as has been suggested for $α_1$-adrenergic agonists {48,51}. The ATP-induced transient acidification may cause a transient increase of $[Ca^{2+}]_i$ by mobilizing Ca^{2+} from storage sites {52}.

PI TURNOVER INDUCED BY EXTRACELLULAR ATP

It was shown that extracellular ATP enhances the formation of inositol 1,4,5-trisphospate as well as inositol monophosphate and bisphosphate formation in rat ventricular myocytes {53} and in fetal mice ventricular myocytes {54}. However, the role of IP_3 formation in the ATP-induced positive inotropy is not clear. In fetal mice ventricular myocytes, it was also shown that extracellular ATP inhibits isoproterenol-induced accumulation of cyclic AMP. The formation of IP_3 was PTX insensitive, while inhibition of cyclic AMP accumulation was PTX sensitive.

Fig. 41-14. Effects of adenosine and ATP on the sinus pacemaker rhythm of rabbit heart. **A:** Slowing of the sinus pacemaker induced by adenosine (Ado). **B:** Transient acceleration and subsequent slowing of the sinus pacemaker induced by high concentrations of ATP. A,B: The upper panels show examples of electrocardiograms recorded from each heart. Arrows are the P waves. Numbers in the lower graph indicate the examples in the upper panels. Tyrode solution containing various concentrations of drugs reached the heart at time 0. Before application of drugs, control Tyrode solution was perfused for at least 15 minutes in all experiments. Reproduced from Takikawa et al. {38}, with permission.

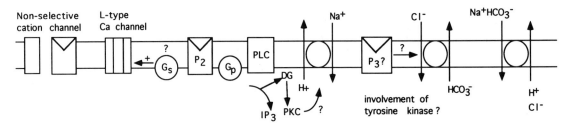

Fig. 41-15. Subcellular signaling mechanisms for cardiac ATP receptors. P_2-purinergic receptors activate a nonselective cation channel and PLC and PI turnover via pertussis-toxin insensitive G proteins (G_p), and stimulate the L-type Ca^{2+} channel, possibly via G_s without involvement of cyclic AMP. Putative P_3-purinergic receptors stimulate the Cl^-/HCO_3^- exchanger via an unknown mechanism, resulting in intracellular acidification. It is suggested that tyrosine kinase might be involved in P_3 stimulation of the Cl^-/HCO_3^- exchanger. Intracellular acidification may cause an increase of intracellular Ca^{2+}. Extracellular ATP also stimulates the Na/H antiport and the amiloride-insensitive intracellular alkalinization mechanism via unknown mechanisms.

CONCLUSIONS

Cardiac myocytes have P_1 (more specifically A_1) purinergic receptors and ATP receptors. P_1 purinoceptors are most effectively activated by adenosine. The action of P_1 purinoceptors on the heart can be classified into direct (cyclic AMP independent) and indirect (cyclic AMP dependent) actions, like m_2-muscarinic cholinergic action {55}. The effects of extracellular ATP on cardiac function are usually attributed to cardiac P_2 purinoceptors. However, characterization of ATP receptors has not been satisfactorily done so far. Subclassification of P_2 purinoceptors and the effects of each subclass on cardiac excitation should be examined. A novel class of ATP receptors in cardiac myocytes is also suggested {37}.

Adenosine applied to the heart decelerates the heart beat and atrioventricular conduction and decreases atrial contraction {35}. This direct acton is characteristic of supraventricular tissues and is mainly related to the P_1-purinoceptor activation of cardiac K_{ACh} channels via PTX-sensitive G proteins {5}. As an indirect action, adenosine antagonizes the electrophysiological and biochemical effects of beta-adrenergic agonists on the heart, which is related to regulation of intracellular cyclic AMP and is observed only when the heart is pretreated with beta-adrenergic agonists {24,25,27}. The antagonistic effect of adenosine on beta agonists can be demonstrated in all cardiac cells and is explained by dual control of adenylyl cyclase activity by stimulatory and inhibitory G proteins {28}. Recently, the P_1 purinoceptor was also found to couple to the K_{ATP} channels via PTX-sensitive G proteins in cardiac myocytes {17,22,23}, which may not have physiological significance in cardiac tissues but may play an important role in protection of cardiac myocytes during ischemia.

ATP receptors are, on the other hand, coupled to activation of a nonselective cation channel {41,42}, the L-type Ca^{2+} channel {43}, PI turnover {53,54}, Ca^{2+} mobilization {39,41,56}, several transporter systems {46–48}, and possibly to prostaglandin synthesis {38} in the heart. Characterization of cardiac ATP receptors has not yet been completed.

REFERENCES

1. Drury AN, Szent-Györgyi A: The physiological activity of adenine compounds with especial reference to their action upon the mammalian heart. *J Physiol (Lond)* 68:213–237, 1929.
2. Kurachi Y: Molecular regulation of muscarinic receptor-gated K^+ channel in mammalian hearts. *Asian Med J* 32:179–190, 1989.
3. Belardinelli L, Lerman BB: Adenosine: Cardiac electrophysiology. *PACE* 14:1672–1680, 1991.
4. Burnstock G, Brown CM: An introduction tp purinergic receptors. In: Burnstock G (ed) *Purinergic Receptors*. London: Chapman and Hall, 1981, pp 1–45.
5. Kurachi Y, Nakajima T, Sugimoto T: On the mechanism of activation of muscarinic K^+ channels by adenosine in isolated atrial cells: Involvement of GTP-binding proteins. *Pflügers Arch* 407:264–274, 1986.
6. Kurachi Y, Nakajima T, Ito H: Intracellular fluoride activation of muscarinic K channel in atrial cell membrane. *Circulation* 76:IV105, 1987.
7. Kurachi Y, Nakajima T, Sugimoto T: Role of intracellular Mg^{2+} in the activation of muscarinic K^+ channel in cardiac atrial cell membrane. *Pflügers Arch* 407:572–574, 1986.
8. Logothetis DE, Kurachi Y, Galper J, Neer EJ, Clapham DE: The $\beta\gamma$ subunits of GTP-binding proteins activate the muscarinic K^+ channel in heart. *Nature* 325:321–326, 1987.
9. Yatani A, Codina J, Brown AM, Birnbaumer L: Direct activation of mammalian atrial muscarinic potassium channels by GTP regulatory protein G_K. *Science* 235:207–211, 1987.
10. Codina J, Yatani A, Grenet D, Brown AM, Birnbaumer L: The α subunit of G_K opens atrial potassium channels. *Science* 236:442–445, 1987.
11. Yatani A, Mattera R, Codina J, Graf R, Okabe K, Padrell E, Iyenger R, Brown AM, Birnbaumer L: The G protein-gated atrial K^+ channel is stimulated by three distinct $G_{i\alpha}$-subunits. *Nature* 336:680–689, 1988.
12. Kirsh GE, Yatani A, Codina J, Birnbaumer L, Brown AM: α-subunit of G_K activates K^+ channels of chick, rat and guinea pig. *Am J Physiol* 254:H1200–H1205, 1988.
13. Kim D, Lewis DL, Graziadel L, Neer EJ, Bar-Sagi D, Clapham DE: G-protein $\beta\gamma$-subunits activate the cardiac muscarinic K^+ channel via phospholipase A_2. *Nature* 337:557–560, 1989.
14. Kurachi Y, Ito H, Sugimoto T, Katada T, Ui M: Activation of atrial muscarinic K^+ channels by low concentrations of $\beta\gamma$ subunits of rat brain G protein. *Pflu gers Arch* 413:325–327, 1989.
15. Kurachi Y, Ito H, Sugimoto T, Shimizu T, Miki I, Ui M: Arachidonic acid metabolites as intracellular modulators of the G protein-gated cardiac K^+ channel. *Nature* 337:555–557, 1989.
16. Nakajima T, Sugimoto T, Kurachi Y: Platelet-activating factor activates cardiac G_K via arachidonic acid metabolites. *FEBS Lett* 289:239–243, 1991.
17. Ito H, Tung RT, Sugimoto T, Kobayashi I, Takahashi K, Katada T, Ui M, Kurachi Y: On the mechanism of G protein $\beta\gamma$ subunit activation of the muscrinic K^+ channel in guinea pig atrial cell membrane: Comparison with the ATP-sensitive K^+ channel. *J Gen Physiol* 99:961–983, 1992.
18. Yamada M, Ho Y-K, Katada T, Kurachi Y: Activation of cardiac muscarinic K^+ channels by transducin $\beta\gamma$ subunits. *Biophy J* 64:A388, 1993.
19. Logothetis DE, Kim D, Northup JK, Neer EJ, Clapham DE: Specificity of action of guanine nucleotide-binding regulatory protein subunits on the cardiac muscarinic K^+ channel. *Proc Natl Acad Sci USA* 85:5814–5818, 1988.
20. Dunne MJ, Bullett MJ, Li G, Wollheim CB, Petersen OH: Galanin activates nucleotide-dependent K^+ channels in insulin-secreting cells via a pertussis toxin-sensitive G-protein. *EMBO J* 8:413–420, 1989.
21. Parent L, Coronado R: Reconstitution of the ATP-sensitive potassium channel of skeletal muscle: Activation by a G protein-dependent process. *J Gen Physiol* 94:445–463, 1989.
22. Kirsch GE, Codina J, Birnbaumer L, Brown AM: Coupling of ATP-sensitive K^+ channels to A1 receptors by G proteins in rat ventricular myocytes. *Am J Physiol* 259:H820–H826, 1990.
23. Tung RT, Kurachi Y: G protein activation of cardiac ATP-sensitive K^+ channel. *Circulation* 82:III462, 1990.
24. Belardinelli L, Isenberg G: Actions of adenosine and isoproterenol on isolated mammalian ventricular myocytes. *Circ Res* 53:287–297, 1983.
25. Isenberg G, Belardinelli L: Ionic basis for the antagonism between adenosine and isoproterenol on isolated mammalian ventricular myocytes. *Circ Res* 55:309–325, 1984,

26. Cerbai E, Klöckner U, Isenberg G: Ca-antagonistic effects of adenosine in guinea pig atrial cells. *Am J Physiol* 255: H872–H878, 1988.
27. Kato M, Yamaguchi H, Ochi R: Mechanism of adenosine-induced inhibition of calcium current in guinea pig ventricular cells. *Circ Res* 67:1134–1141, 1990.
28. Gilman AG: G proteins: Transducers of receptor-generated signals. *Ann Rev Biochem* 56:615–649, 1987.
29. Trautwein W, Heshceler J: Regulation of cardiac L-type calcium current by phosphorylation and G proteins. *Ann Rev Physiol* 52:257–274, 1990.
30. Ono K, Kiyosue T, Arita M: Isoproterenol, DBcAMP, and forskolin inhibit cardiac sodium current. *Am J Physiol* 256:C1131–C1137, 1989.
31. Yazawa K, Kameyama M: Mechanism of receptor-mediated modulation of the delayed outward potassium current in guinea-pig ventricular myocytes. *J Physiol (Lond)* 421: 135–150, 1990.
32. Nagel G, Hwang T-C, Nastiuk KL, Nairn AC, Gadsby DC: The protein kinase A-regulated cardiac Cl$^-$ channel resembles the systic fibrosis transmembrane conductance regulator. *Nature* 360:81–84, 1992.
33. Tang W-J, Gilman AG: Type-specific regulation of adenylyl cyclase by G protein βγ subunits. *Science* 254:1500–1503, 1991.
34. Tang W-J, Gilman AG: Adenylyl cyclases. *Cell* 70:869–872, 1992.
35. Schrader J: Sites of action and production of adenosine in the heart. In: Burnstock (ed) *Purinergic Receptors*. London: Chapman and Hall, 1981, pp 119–162.
36. Lerman BB, Belardinelli L, West GA, Berne RM, DiMarco JP: Adenosine-sensitive ventricular tachycardia: Role of endogenous adenosine. *Circulation* 76:21–31, 1986.
37. Vassort G, Scamps F, Pucéat M, Clément O: Multiple site effects of extracellular ATP in cardiac tissues. *NIPS* 7:212–215, 1992.
38. Takikawa R, Kurachi Y, Mashima S, Sugimoto T: Adenosine-5'-triphosphate-induced sinus tachycardia mediated by prostaglandin synthesis via phospholipase C in the rabbit heart. *Pflügers Arch* 417:13–20, 1990.
39. Danziger RS, Raffaeli S, Moreno-Sanchez R, Sakai M, Capogrossi MC, Spurgeon HA, Hansford RG, Lakatta EG: Extracellular ATP has a potent effect to enhance cytosolic calcium and contractility in single ventricular myocytes. *Cell Calcium* 9:193–199, 1989.
40. Friel DD, Bean BP: Two ATP-activated conductances in bullfrog atrial cells. *J Gen Physiol* 91:1–27, 1988.
41. Hirano Y, Abe S, Sawanobori T, Hiraoka M: External ATP-induced changes in [Ca^{2+}]$_i$ and membrane currents in mammalian atrial myocytes. *Am J Physiol* 260:C673–C680, 1991.
42. Bean BP: Pharmacology and electrophysiology of ATP-activated ion channels. *Trends Pharm Sci* 13:87–90, 1992.
43. Scamps F, Rybin V, Puceat M, Tkachuk V, Vassort G: A G$_s$ protein couples P$_2$-purinergic stimulation to cardiac Ca channels without cyclic AMP production. *J Gen Physiol* 100:675–701, 1992.
44. De Young MB, Scarpa A: ATP receptor-induced Ca^{2+} transients in cardiac myocytes: Source of mobilized Ca^{2+}. *Am J Physiol* 257:C750–C758, 1989.
45. Friel DD, Bean BP: Dual control by ATP and acetylcholine of inwardly rectifying K$^+$ channels in bovine atrial cells. *Pflügers Arch* 415:651–657, 1990.
46. Pucéat M, Clément O, Vassort G: Extracellular MgATP activates the Cl$^-$/HCO$_3^-$ exchanger in single cardiac cells. *J Physiol (Lond)* 444:241–256, 1991.
47. Pucéat M, Clément O, Terzic A, Vassort G: α$_1$-adrenoceptor and purinoceptor agonists modulate the Na/H antiport in single cardiac cells. *Am J Physiol* 1993, in press.
48. Terzic A, Pucéat M, Clément-Clomienne O, Vassort G: Phenylephrine and ATP enhance an amiloride insensitive bicarbonate-dependent alkalinizing mechanism in rat single cardiomyocytes. *Naunyn-Schmiedbergs Arch Pharmacol* 346:597–600, 1992.
49. Kurachi Y: The effects of intracellular protons on the electroreical activity of single ventricular cells. *Pflügers Arch* 394:264–270, 1982.
50. Orchard CH, Kentish JC: Effects of changes of pH on the contractile function of cardiac muscle. *Am J Physiol* 258: C967–C981, 1990.
51. Pucéat M, Terzic A, Clément O, Samps F, Vogel SM, Vassort G: Cardiac α$_1$-adrenoceptors mediate a positive inotropic effect via myofibrillar Ca-sensitization. *Trends Pharmacol Sci* 13:263–265, 1992.
52. Pucéat M, Clément O, Scamps F, Vassort G: Extracellular ATP-induced acidification leads to cytosolic calcium transient rise in single rat cardiac myocytes. *Biochem J* 274:55–62, 1991.
53. Leggssyer A, Poggioli J, Renard D, Vassort G: ATP and other adenine compounds increase mechanical activity and inositol triphosphate production in rat heart. *J Physiol (Lond)* 401:185–199, 1988.
54. Yamada M, Hammamori Y, Akita H, Yokoyama M: P$_2$-purinoceptor activation stimulates phosphoinositide hydrolysis and inhibits accumulation of cAMP in cultured ventricular myocytes. *Circ Res* 70:477–485, 1992.

II VASCULAR SMOOTH MUSCLE AND CORONARY CIRCULATION

CHAPTER 42

Vascular Smooth Muscle Cells and Other Periendothelial Cells of Mammalian Heart

MICHAEL S. FORBES

INTRODUCTION

The mammalian heart is characterized by a vascular supply that is truly prodigious. It is curious that, of the many studies addressed to the heart, few have been directly concerned with the ultrastructure of the *medial* or *periendothelial* cells of myocardial blood vessels. The term *vascular smooth muscle cells* comes most readily to mind when one is describing such cells, but it has become apparent that less highly developed cells occupy the walls of the heart's microvessels. Such cells, which include entities known as *primitive smooth muscle cells* and *pericytes*, are the positional and, perhaps, the functional equivalents of the definitive smooth muscle cells of the larger myocardial blood vessels. This chapter describes the structure of true vascular smooth muscle cells (VSMC) and considers, in addition, the spectrum of periendothelial cells within the vasculature of the heart.

DEFINITIVE VASCULAR SMOOTH MUSCLE CELLS

General features

The packing and orientation of smooth muscle cells of the major arteries and veins of the heart may vary considerably according to the species under examination, the particular vessel being investigated, and perhaps even the individual selected for study. Though the conventional picture of arteries is one in which the muscle cells wind in circles or spirals about the endothelial cylinder (figs. 42-1, 42-2, and 42-4), it is not unusual to find longitudinally running bundles of cells at the outermost level of the tunica media, for example, in the anterior descending {1} and right coronary arteries {2} of the dog, and the right coronary artery of shrew {2}. It is intriguing, furthermore, to consider the orientation of smooth muscle cells in the right coronary artery of the vervet (*Cercopithecus aethiops*); in some planes of section an inner longitudinal, a central circular, and an outer longitudinal muscle layer can be detected (fig. 42-6). Further observation along lengths of this artery indicate that only the central layer intrinsically forms a complete covering of the vessel. The inner and

outer "layers" appear to be spiral bundles of cells whose longitudinal axes are aligned at an extremely steep pitch with respect to the vessel axis. The cells of the central layer themselves are canted, forming an angle of ca. 30° with respect to true circular orientation (fig. 42-4).

It should be recalled that the physiologic state of the blood vessel at the time of fixation will be a major factor in the orientation of smooth muscle cells as observed with the microscope {e.g., 3}. Thus the morphologic study of the blood vessel wall requires thorough appreciation of the conditions under which a vessel has been preserved and benefits from the use of techniques that effectively reconstruct the three-dimensional architecture (or allow its visualization in toto, as with scanning electron microscopy of enzymatically digested vessels {e.g., 2,4-6}.

The tunica media of coronary arteries and their branches is usually an unbroken covering composed primarily of vascular smooth muscle cells (VSMC). The other broad categories of myocardial blood vessels (veins, venules, arterioles, and capillaries) frequently are characterized by large gaps in the tunica media. The muscular arteries of the heart do not contain distinct strata of VSMC, delimited by sheets of elastin, as is the case in larger "elastic" arteries. Thus to speak of the relative numbers of "layers" in myocardial blood vessels is inexact at best. Still the general conclusion can be drawn that as the size of the mammal (and its heart) increases, so do the overall diameters and wall thicknesses of comparably located arterial segments. For example, the coronary arteries of a mouse seldom achieve medial thicknesses of more than 6–7 mm and contain a maximum of only 3–4 layers of VSMC; in comparison, the medial layer of dog right coronary artery is massive, possessing 12–15 layers of muscle cells (fig. 42-5).

In overall form, arterial VSMC are flattened, tapered, straplike cells (figs. 42-1, 42-3, and 42-4). In many instances, the cells from arteries of larger mammalian hearts do not taper to rounded ends, but instead exhibit distinct indentations that may originate from nearly any point on the sarcolemma (figs. 42-1, 42-3, 42-4, and 42-8). In such cases, the tips of the cells are particularly elaborate (fig. 42-8). The VSMC of smaller vessels (and this is true for most of the vessels from smaller mammals) tend to be less complex in their surface contours (e.g., fig. 42-7). Such

N. Sperelakis (ed.), Physiology and Pathophysiology of the Heart, Third Edition.

803

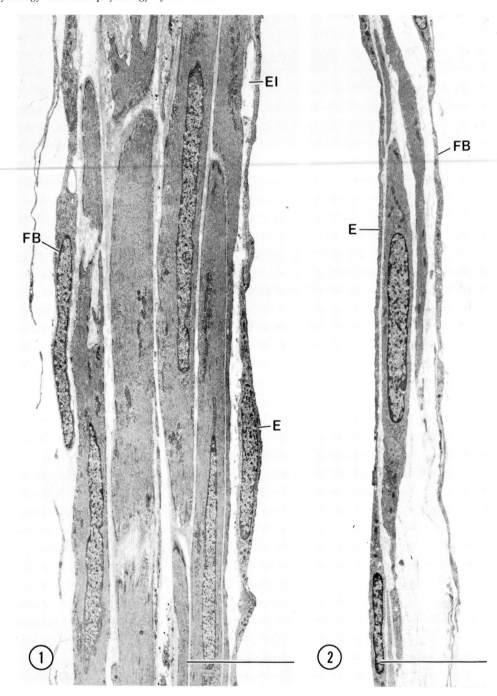

Fig. 42-1. Myocardial blood vessel of squirrel monkey (*Saimiri sciureus*). Survey micrograph of wall of anterior descending coronary artery, the vessel viewed here in transverse thin section. Approximately four layers of vascular smooth muscle cells form the tunica media of the artery along its largest segments. The medial layer is bordered on its adluminal side by the tunica intima, the complex of a layer of endothelial cells (E) and the elastica interna (EI), and on its abluminal surface by connective tissue elements, including collagen and fibroblasts (FB), which together with occasional examples of nerve tissue comprise the tunica adventitia. Scale bar represents 5 μm.

Fig. 42-2. Myocardial blood vessel of squirrel monkey. The accompanying vein of the artery shown in fig. 42-1. Micrograph equivalent in magnification and orientation, which serves to demonstrate the profound contrast in wall structure that exists between the two divisions of the myocardial circulatory system. The three tunicae are extant, the tunica adventitia perhaps constituting the greatest portion of the vessel wall. Labels as in fig. 42-1. Scale bar represents 5 μm.

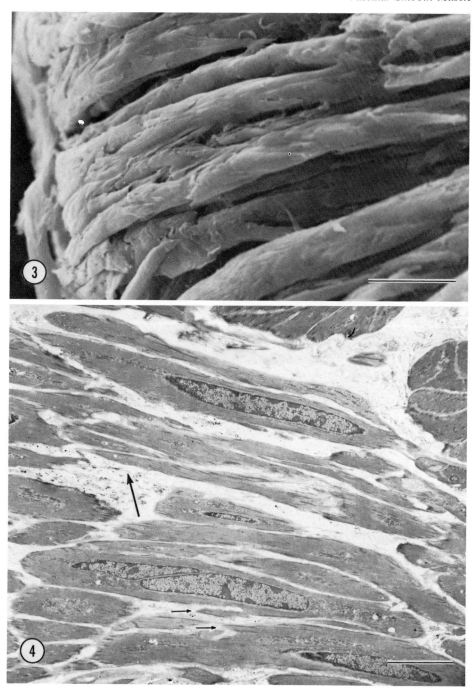

Fig. 42-3. Scanning electron micrograph of smooth muscle cells of a dog right coronary artery from which the adventitial material has been removed by sequential exposure to hydrochloric acid and collagenase, coupled with mechanical dissection. At this point on the vessel's circumference, all the smooth muscle cells wind about the vessel axis in circumferential orientation (cf. fig. 42-5, however, for a more complete appreciation of the medial architecture of this vessel). The overall fusiform shape of the cells is evident, but their topography is noticeably irregular, marked by various excrescences and indentations. Scale bar represents 10 μm.

Fig. 42-4. Low-power transmission electron micrograph of right coronary artery of vervet monkey (*Cercopithecus aethiops*). At the upper regions of the field there appear bundles of spirally oriented smooth muscle cells (cf. fig. 42-26). The major component of the wall is invested in cells that are sectioned en face, but are obliquely oriented with respect to the vessel axis (large arrow). Note fusiform nuclei and minor cytoplasmic projections (small arrows). Scale bar represents 10 μm.

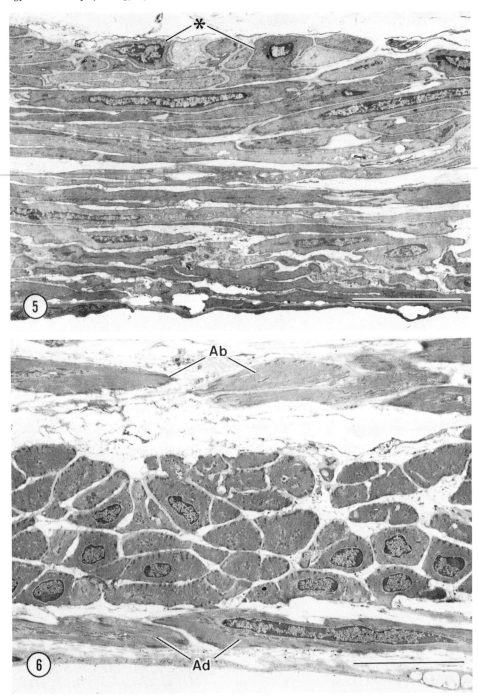

Fig. 42-5. Right coronary artery of dog; vessel viewed in transverse section. The bulk of the medial layer is composed of smooth muscle cells that are arranged circularly about the vessel and therefore are caught in longititudinal section (cf. figs. 42-1 and 42-3). The outermost abluminal layers of smooth muscle, however, are seen in cross section (*), which indicates that they are longitudinally oriented along the outer surface of the vessel wall. Scale bar represents 10 μm.

Fig. 42-6. Right coronary artery of vervet monkey; longitudinal section. Three distinct strata of smooth muscle cells constitute the tunica media of this vessel. The immediately adluminal cells (Ad) run parallel to the vessel axis, while a central stratum of approximately circularly oriented cells forms the major protion of the medial layer. It is the latter cells that are equivalent to the cells seen en face in fig. 42-4; the spirally oriented cells in fig. 42-4 may correspond to either the adluminal band or the abluminal (Ab) layer, which is separated from the medial wall by a large gap. Scale bar represents 10 μm.

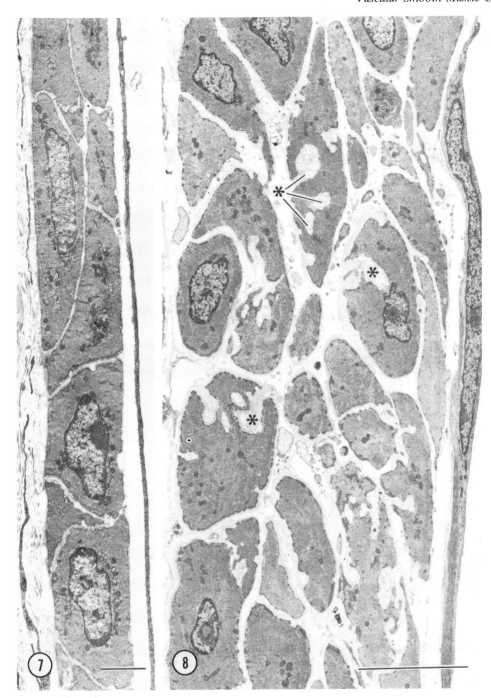

Fig. 42-7. Longitudinal section of mouse anterior descending coronary artery; the circularly applied smooth muscle cells thus appear in transverse section, and in this orientation display profiles closely fitted to one another. Accordingly, there is a minimum of intervening connective tissue. Scale bar represents 2 μm.

Fig. 42-8. Squirrel monkey right coronary artery, viewed at the same magnification and similar orientation to that of the mouse artery shown in fig. 42-7. In contrast to that vessel, the VSMC here are strikingly pleiomorphic in profile, and are characterized by involved sarcolemmal indentations and cavities (*). The cells are separated by large spaces, which are occupied by the thick surface coats of the cells and by connective tissue elements. Scale bar represents 5 μm.

cells are more tightly fitted together within the medial layer, perhaps in part because of the lower incidence there of elements of connective tissue.

Arterial VSMC are individually noteworthy by dint of the extreme degree of polarity observed by their cytoplasmic components, including nuclei (see *The nucleus ...*), cytoskeletal and contractile fibrils (see *Fibrillar elements ...*), and various other organelles (see *"Miscellaneous" organelles*). The bipolar form is not necessarily retained in the smallest myocardial vessels, however, and secondary ("circumferential") projections are prominent features of pericytes on venules and capillaries (see *Cytoskeletal elements* and figs. 42-28 to 42-33), and venous VSMC as well may be branched {3} (see *Comparison of arterial/arteriolar ...*).

Organelles and cell systems

As pointed out above, a striking characteristic of the muscle cells in coronary arteries is their marked bipolar conformation. Not only is this embodied in the overall shape of these cells (figs. 42-1, 42-3, and 42-4), but it is also evident in their internal construction, which in each cell is developed around the nucleus and the associated cytoplasm, which extends from each of its poles. These and other constituents are described below in greater detail.

NUCLEUS, ASSOCIATED ORGANELLES AND THE CENTRAL SARCOPLASMIC CORE

Most VSMC in the cardiac circulatory system appear to be mononucleate. The nucleus in each muscle cell is distinctly fusiform, its tips aimed directly at the cell ends (figs. 42-1 and 42-4). Though infoldings of the nuclear membrane can be found (fig. 42-4), these are rather infrequent, and the profile that the nucleus presents in thin sections usually is unremarkable, save for its occasional great length (up to ca. 25 μm).

Golgi saccules and centrioles are generally located near the nucleus (fig. 42-9). The Golgi apparatus seldom displays a memorable morphology, though in other vessels this organellar system has been shown to react noticeably to the administration of ionophoric agents {7}. As many as four centrioles may be encountered; given the rarity of multiple nuclear profiles in VSMC, the significance of this observation is unclear.

There is a distinct association between each smooth muscle nucleus and the sharply delimited cylinders or cones of cytoplasm that extend from its apices out toward the cell ends (fig. 42-9). There results a compartmentation of the cell contents, such that certain organelles (Golgi saccules, centrioles, microtubules, intermediate filaments, mitochondria, and lysosomes) are lodged primarily within the *central sarcoplasmic core* (figs. 42-9 to 42-11), whereas the remaining voluminous cortical region of the cell is virtually completely filled with myofilaments (see below). The central sarcoplasmic core can be envisioned as an entity that forms a medullary zone within the muscle cell and surrounds the nucleus; its major portion is fusiform, but a retinue of thin digitlike ramifications also extends

into the peripheral regions of the cell (fig. 42-10). This internal compartment provides both enclosure and transcellular distribution of the cytoskeleton (see below) and the mitochondrial complement (see *"Miscellaneous" organelles*) of the smooth muscle cell.

FIBRILLAR ELEMENTS (CYTOSKELETAL AND CONTRACTILE)

The cytoskeleton and contractile apparatus of coronary arterial VSMC are largely isolated from one another, as discussed in the preceding section. The cytoskeleton is composed of longitudinally oriented microtubules and intermediate filaments (figs. 42-10 to 42-12). In many sections that pass through the central sarcoplasmic core, intermediate filaments ("10-nm" filaments, "skeletin" filaments {8}) appear as the predominant fibril (figs. 42-10 and 42-11), but their overall incidence may very considerably between adjacent cells in the blood vessel wall. Microtubules accompany, or are accompanied by, intermediate filaments in the various recesses of the sarcoplasmic core system (figs. 42-10 to 42-12); they observe the same longitudinal disposition, and frequently appear surrounded by a "halo," 10 nm or so in width, which emphasizes their presence (figs. 42-10 and 42-11). The orientation of microtubules may in fact be a dictating force for the similar alignment observed for intermediate filaments {9,10}. In visceral smooth muscle cells, intermediate filaments have been implicated {11,12} as forming segmental frameworks that interact via their anchorage in intracellular dense bodies (see the following section). This sort of system seems largely absent from cardiac vessels {2}. Rather, there exists a system of cytoskeletal supports, consisting solely of filaments and tubules that are distributed, albeit thinly at some points, throughout the smooth muscle cell, without the intercalation of prominent stationary points of attachment.

The collection of myofilaments that characterizes the peripheral myoplasm appears to consist largely of 5- to 8-nm-diameter actin filaments (figs. 42-10 and 42-12). The occurrence of myosin filaments is often sporadic in specimens of myocardial vessels. When these 15- to 19-nm "thick" filaments are preserved, they usually appear in the majority of VSMC in the particular vessel, and yet may be absent from certain of its cells; no particular distribution of "haves" and "have-nots" is evident within the vessel wall, however.

The consensus among investigators concerned with the mechanics of smooth muscle is that arterial and venous VSMC are dependent for their contractile activity upon the presence of filamentous myosin (for reviews, see Murphy {13} and Somlyo {14}). It therefore seems likely that a total lack of thick filaments bespeaks inadequate fixation of the specimen under examination. Still, a failproof fixation regimen, that which consistently produces thick filaments, has not yet been offered, nor has the mosaic occurrence of thick filaments among adjacent VSMC been investigated.

The propensity of myofilaments to be grouped into bundles is most evident in longitudinal sections of myo-

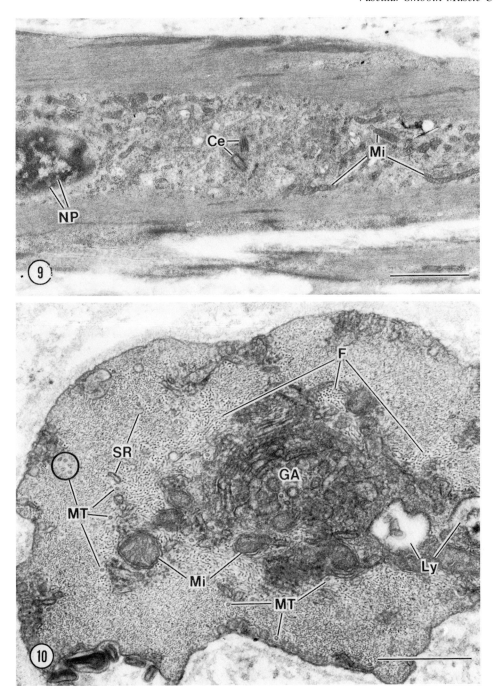

Fig. 42-9. Longitudinal thin section through the center of a VSMC from vervet right coronary artery; the relationship between the nucleus (NP, nuclear pores) and the central sarcoplasmic core is demonstrated. A pair of centrioles (Ce) is located in the core, as is the nucleus; other organelles indigenous to the core include mitochondria (Mi) and ribosomes. The peripheral regions of the cells are filled for the most part with myofilaments. Scale bar represents 2 μm.

Fig. 42-10. Squirrel monkey right coronary artery. Transverse section through VSMC at point distal to the nucleus. The central sarcoplasmic core here is dominated by saccules and tubules of the Golgi apparatus, and is characterized as well by numerous intermediate filaments (F) and microtubules (MT), all cut as well in transverse section. Profiles of mitochondria (Mi) and sarcoplasmic reticulum (SR) also occupy the core, as do lysosomes (Ly), here represented by multivesicular bodies. Thin, peripheral extensions of the core are represented by microtubule profiles, typically surrounded by electron-lucent halos. Scale bar represents 0.5 μm.

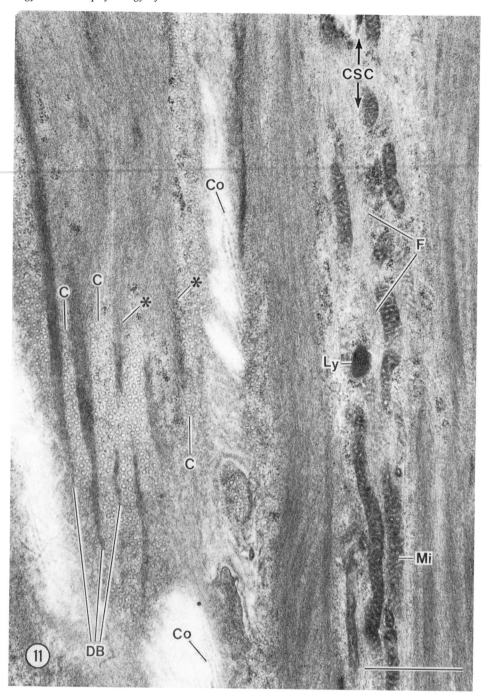

Fig. 42-11. Vervet right coronary artery. In this section, the smooth muscle cells are cut longitudinally. The surface of one cell (at the left) is exposed en face, and in the cell at the right the central sarcoplasmic core (CSC) is evident as a relatively clear zone that contains longitudinally oriented mitochondria (Mi), numerous intermediate filaments (F), and a lysosome (Ly). Microtubules also observe preferential location in this region (cf. fig. 42-10), but their lower numbers render them less obvious in longitudinal sections. The myofilaments of these smooth muscle cells tend to group in large bundles, which lead, at their extremities, into dense subsarcolemmal adhesion plaques (dense bodies: DB); transitions between myofilament bundles and dense bodies are indicated by asterisks. Alternating with the subsarcolemmal stripes formed by dense bodies are rows of sarcolemma decorated with numerous surface-connected caveolae (C). Collagen fibrils (Co) are closely associated with the surfaces of the muscle cells. Scale bar represents 1 µm.

Vascular Smooth Muscle Cells   811

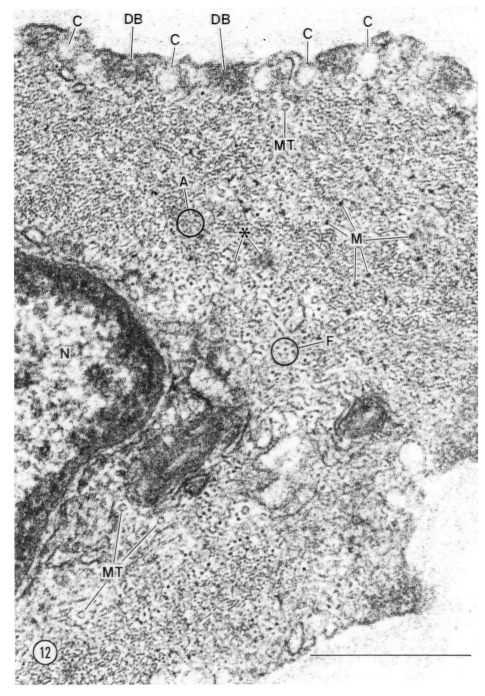

Fig. 42-12. Transverse section of VSMC from right coronary artery of squirrel monkey. All the categories of fibrils are visible in this field, including actin (A) and myosin (M) filaments, which are the basis of the cell's contractile apparatus and occupy the cortical portion of the myoplasm. The alternation of caveolae (C) with subsarcolemmal dense bodies (DB) is evident (cf. fig. 42-11). Small internal dense bodies (*) appear in limited numbers. Punctate actin profiles can be discerned within the subsarcolemmal dense bodies, indicating their probable termination there. The cytoskeletal fibrils — microtubules (MT) and intermediate filaments (F) — are far less numerous at this level of the cell, though they specifically populate the central sarcoplasmic core (figs. 42-10 and 42-11) and its ramifications. N = nucleus. Scale bar represents 0.5 µm.

cardial VSMC (fig. 42-11). Many such bundles terminate in the opaque subsarcolemmal substance of the *dense bodies* (fig. 42-11; see below). Stereoscopic images have served to demonstrate this association, in VSMC, of myofilaments with dense bodies {2,14}, and profiles of actin filaments frequently can be discerned in thin transverse sections of dense bodies (fig. 42-12).

SURFACE COAT, SARCOLEMMA, DENSE BODIES, AND CAVEOLAE

The outermost covering of VSMC is composed of lightly opaque, amorphous material. This material is likely constituted in the main by glycoproteinaceous moieties; the most general (and least chemically committal) term for the material seen by electron microscopy is the *surface coat*. Surface coats can display a wide array of appearances in different mammals and in vessels of different sizes. Specifically, where VSMC are closely packed (fig. 42-7) the surface coat is a consistently thin layer, the most opaque portion of which is at most 50 nm thick and often separated from the sarcolemma proper by a relatively lucent space, 30–50 nm in width {2}. In contrast, where the VSMC are widely separated (e.g., in monkey coronary arteries), the surface coats (figs. 42-8 and 42-13) are thick and thrown into irregular profiles, and form elaborate whorls and filigrees, particularly within the recesses that characterize the muscle cell tips in such vessels {2} (figs. 42-8 and 42-16).

Much of the sarcolemma of arterial VSMC is segmented into a series of lengthwise divisions by the alternation of stripelike dense bodies and bands of caveolae (fig. 42-11). Relatively few isolated, intracellular dense bodies (fig. 42-12) are found in coronary VSMC, in contrast to VSMC of larger vessels such as carotid artery (unpublished observations) and PAMV {14}, for which the terminologic distinction has been made between the intracellular, "free-floating" densities and the longitudinal, subsarcolemmal striations; the former have been denoted as *dense bodies* and the latter as *surface patches* {14}. There has also been drawn an analogy between the Z discs of striated muscle and dense bodies of VSMC, both of which serve as regions in which actin filaments anchor {14}. Similarly, the subsarcolemmal dense bodies of VSMC are analogous to the fasciae adherentes of heart, those portions of the intercalated discs in which the thin filaments belonging to the myofibrils terminate {15,16}. A partial substitute for internal dense bodies in coronary VSMC may reside in smearings of the opaque material that extend away from subsarcolemmal locations to points deep in the myoplasm.

Sarcolemmal inpocketings (*caveolae*, lit. "small caves") are a substantial component of muscle cells. Such flask-shaped invaginations add considerable surface area to certain myocardial cells {17-19}, and it is likely that this is the case for VSMC as well. Caveolae appear to be permanently connected to the sarcolemma, with their lumina open to the extracellular fluid space. This stands in contrast to the mobile "micropinocytotic" vesicles of vascular endothelial cells. The caveolae of smooth muscle are not limited to single invaginations, but may participate in extensive structures, so-called beaded tubules (figs. 42-14 and 42-17) of varying lengths {2,20}. These complexes bear close resemblance to the forming elements of the system of transverse tubules of skeletal and cardiac muscle {2,16,21}, and for this reason smooth muscle caveolae collectively may be considered to represent the equivalent of T tubules, in both the analogous and homologous senses {2,20}.

Most surfaces of arterial VSMC — abluminal, adluminal, and lateral — are decorated with caveolae (e.g., figs. 42-10 to 42-12). Farther down the vascular tree, the VSMC of arterioles become thinner and presumably less voluminous, and frequently lack caveolae on their adluminal surfaces, as do pericytes on the smallest vessels (figs. 42-30 and 42-31; see *Cytoskeletal elements*).

SARCOPLASMIC RETICULUM

A variety of smooth-surfaced tubules and saccules are present in smooth muscle cells. Some are concentrated in the Golgi apparatus (see *The nucleus . . .* and fig. 42-10), but the majority of these profiles — primarily located in the central sarcoplasmic core and its ramifications, or close beneath the sarcolemma — are known collectively as the *sarcoplasmic reticulum* (SR). This collection of intracellular membranous structures is considered functionally equivalent to the more structured SR networks in striated and cardiac muscle {22–25}. In large vessels, the division of SR into *peripheral*, *deep*, and *central* categories has been made {26}. The relatively small volumes of coronary artery VSMC usually allow a more limited distinction, that between the peripheral and central SR (figs. 42-10 and 42-13). The alternation of dense bodies and caveolae creates a subtle subsarcolemmal compartmentation that exists in addition to the more noticeable overall cortical and medullary arrangement of cell components (see *The nucleus . . .* and *Fibrillar elements . . .*). Thus much of the sarcoplasmic reticulum is specifically located beneath the ribbons of sarcolemma that bear caveolae. The more notable component of the peripheral SR division is *junctional* SR (J-SR), those segments that are juxtaposed to the inner surface of the sarcolemma (figs. 42-13 to 42-15). The J-SR winds as multibranched tubules among the sarcolemmal invaginations formed by caveolae (figs. 42-13 to 42-15), and appears to make connection with both surface sarcolemma and caveolae through the interposition of so-called junctional processes. One form taken by the processes is that of thin profiles ("pillars" {27,28}), which resemble unit membranes and whose opaque limiting substance frequently can be seen to fuse with the apposed membrane leaflets of the J-SR and sarcolemma/caveola (figs. 42-13 to 42-15) {2,28}. As has been discussed {2,20}, the T tubules of smooth muscle are likely to be represented by caveolae; the complexes constituted by appositions of caveolae with J-SR are therefore the equivalent of the "internal couplings" typical of other muscle types {e.g., 16,21}, while the J-SR-sarcolemma complexes clearly are the homologues of peripheral couplings {2,20}.

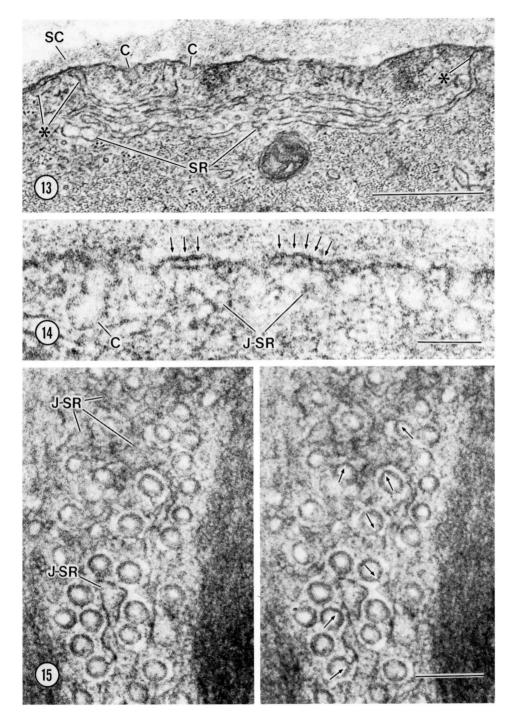

Fig. 42-13. Squirrel monkey anterior descending coronary artery; smooth muscle cell in transverse section. Layered profiles of sarcoplasmic reticulum (SR) are present, tubular extensions of which are closely apposed (*) to the sarcolemma. C = caveolae. Note the varying thickness of the muscle cell's surface coat (SC). Scale bar represents 0.5 μm.

Fig. 42-14. Same vessel as in fig. 42-13. Subsarcolemmal couplings formed between the sarcolemma and saccules of junctional sarcoplasmic reticulum (J-SR). Distinct linear structures ("pillars": arrows) connect the apposed membranes. The J-SR profiles are interspersed with caveolae, two of which (at C) are fused to form a short "beaded tubule." Scale bar represents 0.1 μm.

Fig. 42-15. Squirrel monkey anterior descending artery. Stereo micrograph pair (10° separation) showing the marked interdigitation of junctional SR (J-SR) and surface-connected caveolae, and demonstrating the pillarlike structures (arrows) that connect the two. Scale bar represents 0.2 μm.

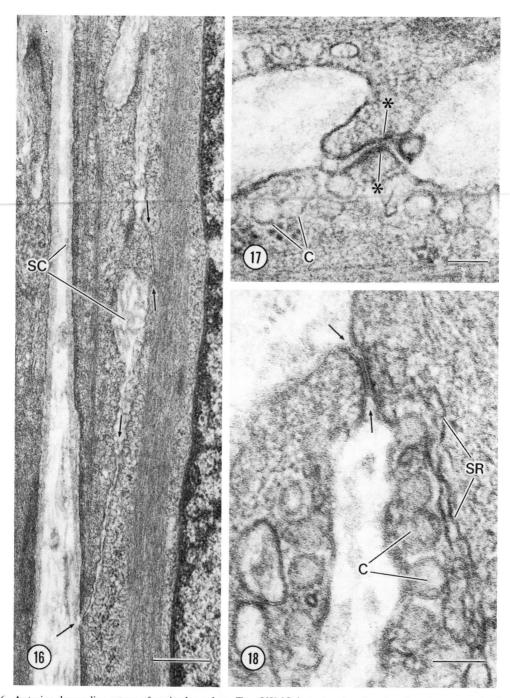

Fig. 42-16. Anterior descending artery of squirrel monkey. Two VSMC form two junctional regions known as simple appositions (between arrows). Although the apposed sarcolemmata run parallel for rather great distances, no intracellular or extracellular densities can be discerned, nor does the structured surface coat (SC) appear to enter the intercellular gaps at these points. Scale bar represents 0.5 μm.

Fig. 42-17. Right coronary artery of dog heart. The upper muscle cell has formed a small digital protrusion that approaches the lower cell, forming an "intermediate" contact, characterized primarily by accumulations of electron-opaque material (*) immediately beneath the apposed sarcolemmal regions. In the adjacent sarcolemmata numerous caveolae appear, some of which (C) are fused to form a beaded caveolar chain. Scale bar represents 0.1 μm.

Fig. 42-18. Squirrel monkey right coronary artery. Gap junction (between arrows), ca. 6 nm in length, formed between a slender process of one smooth muscle cell with the main body of another. Homocellular gap junctions are frequently found in coronary arteries, but most are of a limited size, such as the one shown here. Note the close association of caveolae (C) with tubules of sarcoplasmic reticulum (SR). Scale bar represents 0.1 μm.

JUNCTIONS (HOMOCELLULAR AND HETEROCELLULAR)

A multitude of intermembranous connections are demonstrable in the walls of myocardial blood vessels {2}. *Homocellular* junctions form both between individual medial cells and also within them (i.e., they are *intracellular*, developing at points of juxtaposition of sarcolemmal regions belonging to the same cell). *Heterocellular* junctions are those that join the adluminal VSMC with the underlying endothelium {2}.

A wide variety of VSMC homocellular junctions has already been described in coronary arteries {2}. These include *simple appositions*, in which sarcolemmal surfaces are poised in parallel array with one another, separated by a space of ca. 17-20 nm (fig. 42-16), which usually does not admit the electron-opaque substance of the cell coat. *Intermediate* junctions (fig. 42-17) display a spectrum of morphologies, which range from a short pair of intracellular densities that face one another across an empty-appearing, 17- to 20-nm gap to *quasi*-desmosomal complexes, which are characterized by structured extracellular material. *Desmosomes* themselves appear between VSMC of cat coronary arteries {2}. Short *gap junctions* are present in coronary arterial VSMC of mouse, guinea pig, dog, and squirrel monkey {2} (fig. 42-18), and these may be located either *inter*cellularly or *intra*cellularly.

The heterocellular junctions of myocardial arteries are less varied in morphology than the homocellular connections. Most often seen between smooth muscle and endothelium are simple appositions, which usually incorporate an endothelial extrusion that extends abluminally to approach the overlying smooth muscle cell. No discernible intracellular structures are present in either of the cells that participate in a simple myoendothelial junction. On the other hand, there is occasionally encountered a heterocellular junction of the intermediate category (fig. 42-19), which is marked by intracellular accumulations of opaque substance similar to those of homocellular counterparts.

A third category of heterocellular junctions, myoendothelial gap junctions, has been clearly identified in arteries and arterioles of the mouse heart {2} (fig. 42–20), but examples have not yet been found in equivalent vessels of other species. Myoendothelial gap junctions are frequently characterized by an abluminal endothelial protrusion or an adluminal VSMC protrusion. The frequent presence of such junctions in these thin-walled vessels of mouse heart may be indicative of a function of adhesion and structural stabilization, rather than necessarily one of electrical continuity {2}.

Heterocellular junctions (including gaplike junctions; fig. 42-21) are frequently encountered in veins, venules, and capillaries. In veins, in particular, unusual junctional profiles are found (fig. 42-22) that do not clearly correspond in form to the junctional categories already described.

"MISCELLANEOUS" ORGANELLES

In a review of this kind, there inevitably accumulate categories of cell structures that are lumped together and accounted for, both for the purposes of completeness and, primarily, because relatively little research has been devoted to them. Such is the case, to greater or lesser degrees, with the mitochondria, rough endoplasmic reticulum, ribosomes, glycogen particles, and lysosomes of vascular smooth muscle cells, all of which are considered below. The Golgi apparatus and centrioles have already been dealt with earlier in this chapter.

As noted earlier, mitochondria of myocardial VSMC are in large part restricted in their occurrence to the central sarcoplasmic core and its extensions, these last including subsarcolemmal cavities in which mitochondria may contact the SR and caveolae {20}. Such complexing may be related to the intracellular transfer of Ca^{2+} ion within the smooth muscle cell {14}. Mitochondria of coronary artery VSMC are small and elongate, and usually are aligned with the longitudinal axis of the cell (e.g., fig. 42-11).

Ribosome-decorated tubules — "rough" endoplasmic reticulum — and alpha-rosettes of glycogen are much in evidence in VSMC of the neonatal animal, but disappear for the most part from mature cells, though occasional examples of rough ER may persist in the central sarcoplasmic core (fig. 42-19), along with free ribosomes and scattered glycogen particles.

Lysosomes of myocardial VSMC assume a number of forms {2}, including uniformly opaque membrane-bounded spheroids (fig. 42-11), variegate bodies with light and dark components (probably secondary lysosomes), and multivesicular structures (fig. 42-10). The occurrence, in the extracellular spaces of the rat coronary artery media, of collections of multisized vesicles has suggested the hypothesis that VSMC waste products are liberated from the cell via exocytosis of lysosomes {29}.

COMPARISON OF ARTERIAL/ARTERIOLAR VS. VENOUS/VENULAR SMOOTH MUSCLE CELLS

The two major blood vessel categories of the heart can be readily distinguished from one another on the basis of the thick muscular walls of arteries, and the thin walls and large lumina of veins (figs. 42-1 and 42-2). Arterioles (fig. 42-26) and venules usually exhibit characteristics similar to those of the respective "parent" vessels. Some vessel segments, however, offer highly equivocal profiles whose periendothelial components are, to more or less degrees, intermediate in structure between smooth muscle cells and pericytes (fig. 42-27); these transitional forms are considered further in the following section.

A good deal more information is available on the structure of the arterial side of the heart's circulatory system than is the case for its venous complement. Veins in general are frequently described as bearing longitudinally oriented smooth muscle cells, but in fact the shape and orientation of these cells can vary tremendously

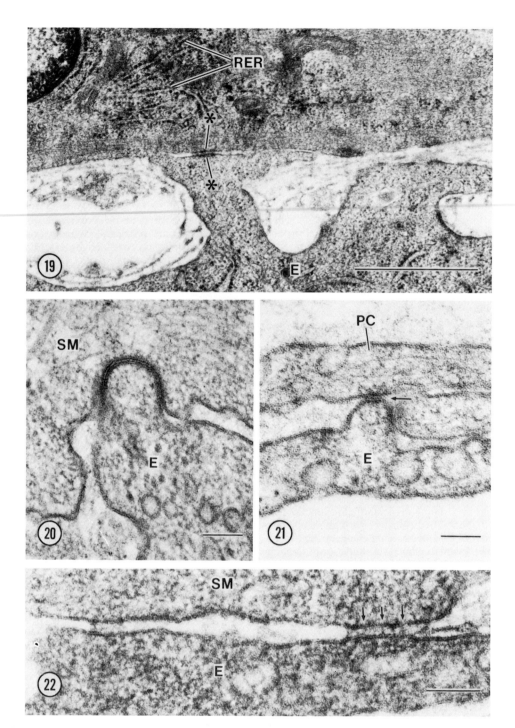

Fig. 42-19. Myointimal region of a large artery in rhesus monkey right papillary. Two hummocks of an endothelial cell (E) approach the adluminal surface of the subjacent smooth muscle cell. The left-hand endothelial protrusion comes into close contact with the smooth muscle sarcolemma, and part of the apposition is composed of a heterocellular intermediate contact, identifiable by its thin opaque plaques (asterisk; cf. fig. 42-17). RER = rough endoplasmic reticulum. Scale bar represents 1 μm.

Fig. 42-20. Myoendothelial gap junction in mouse right coronary artery. This example is formed by a domelike endothelial process (E) that fits into a closely correspondent invagination of the overlying smooth muscle cell (SM). Scale bar represents 0.1 μm.

Fig. 42-21. Wall of a venule from rhesus monkey right papillary muscle. The endothelium (E) juts up to abut the process of a pericyte (PC), there forming a short, close apposition (arrow), which resembles the myoendothelial gap junction seen in fig. 42-20. Scale bar represents 0.1 μm.

Fig. 42-22. Transverse section through anterior coronary vein of squirrel monkey. The limiting membranes of the smooth muscle (SM) and endothelial cell (E) run in approximately parallel array, and along this length two regions appear, which are notable because of the presence in the intercellular gap of strands of material, some of which is collected into linear bodies (arrows) that extend to contact both apposed membranes. Scale bar represents 0.1 μm.

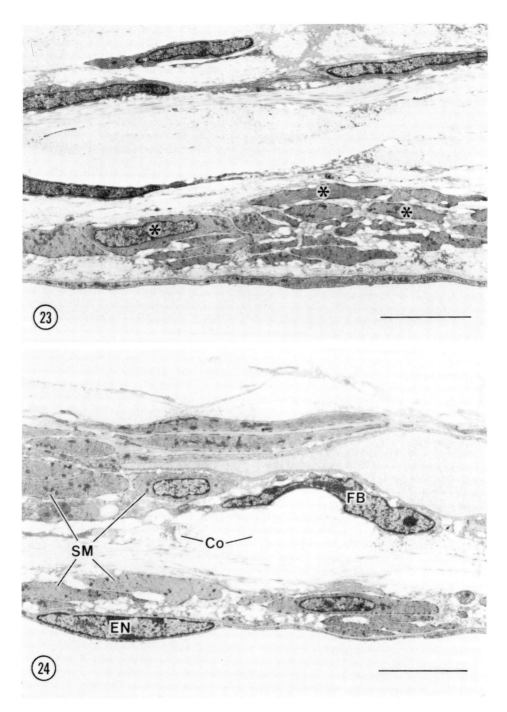

Fig. 42-23. Anterior vein of rhesus monkey; vessel cut in transverse section. At this point on the circumference of the vein, the smooth muscle cells occupy positions equivalent to the tunica media of arteries. The orientations of these cells are varied, however, there being an admixture of circumferentially (*) and longitudinally aligned cells. Scale bar represents 5 μm.

Fig. 42-24. Same vein as in fig. 42-23 at another point on its circumference. Smooth muscle cells (SM) are located both in subendothelial positions (EN = endothelial cell nucleus) and in "adventitial" regions [note the fibroblast (FB) and bands of collagen (Co), which are interposed between the two groups of V̇SMC]. Scale bar represents 5 μm.

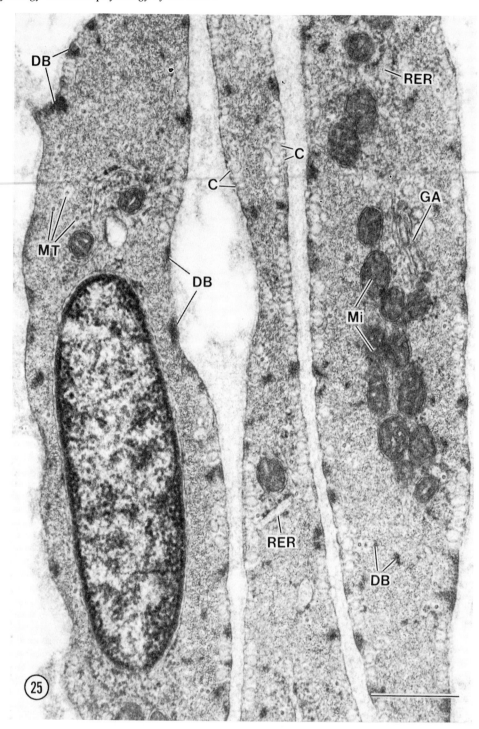

Fig. 42-25. VSMC in transversely sectioned anterior vein of rhesus monkey heart. Such cells are characterized by thin, flattened profiles. Present in this field are a number of organelles and structures that are found in arterial VSMC as well. These include mitochondria (Mi), Golgi saccules (GA), and cisternae of rough endoplasmic reticulum (RER); in venous VSMC, these last appear more prominent than in arterial VSMC. In these transversely sectioned profiles, fibrillar elements such as microtubules (MT) and myofilaments also are caught in transverse section (thus indicating that the cell bodies and processes are aligned along the length of the vessel). Dense bodies (DB) are present free in the myoplasm, as well as apposed to the sarcolemma, where they are interspersed with groups of caveolae (C). Scale bar represents 0.5 μm.

with the vein type, the particular segment, the point on the vessel circumference, etc. {3,30}. In fact it may be difficult to discern clearly delineated tunics in veins, since VSMC may appear within levels of the vessel wall which, in arteries, would rightly belong to the tunica intima or tunica adventitia {3} (fig. 42-24). The great variation in incidence and orientation of VSMC in a collection of human veins studied by Kügelgen (data summarized by Rhodin {3}) is tacit promotion for evaluation, on an individual basis, of any particular segment of any particular vein, of any particular species. Therefore the descriptions of myocardial veins given here may be anecdotal, in view of the relatively few observations thus far made on such vessels. At its widest points, the anterior vein of rhesus monkey (which accompanies the right coronary artery) display 4–5 "layers" of VSMC bodies and processes at some points around its circumference (fig. 42-23), and at others none at all. Fibroblasts and bands of collagen may abut the endothelium while VSMC are located farther abluminally; in certain regions, connective tissue is the major vessel wall component. Additional variations are found in the VSMC orientation (as judged by the alignment of myofilaments); abluminal longitudinal VSMC profiles are intermingled with more adluminal, concentric elements, and vice versa (fig. 42-23). "Stellate" VSMC have been reported as well {3}. This suggests that some venous VSMC possess both longitudinal and circumferential processes, thus resembling the pericytes of venules and capillaries {31}, and this would account in part for the heterogeneity of VSMC orientation in veins.

There is probably only a single generality that can be made concerning the structure of the VSMC of myocardial veins; they present notably thinner profiles than those of VSMC in corresponding arteries (figs. 42-1 and 42-23 to 42-25). Examples of the organelles and cell systems described in the preceding sections can be found in venous VSMC (fig. 42-25), though some specific complexes, such as homocellular gap junctions, have not yet been encountered. It is interesting to note that in the same vein thick (myosin) filaments may appear in some VSMC, but not in others, as is the case in arteries (see *Fibrillar elements* . . .). Certainly the possibility of branching complicates the concept of the *central sarcoplasmic core* (see *The nucleus* . . .) in venous VSMC, as does their relative thinness. A great deal of study, specifically addressed to cardiac vein ultrastructure, will be required before further generalities can be established.

COMPARATIVE STRUCTURAL ASPECTS OF VASCULAR SMOOTH MUSCLE CELLS AND OTHER PERIENDOTHELIAL CELLS

Pericytes are classically recognized as those cells of periendothelial location that partially envelop the endothelial profiles of microvessels, such as capillaries and postcapillary venules, and in addition, bear surface coat material ("basal lamina") that is continuous with that intrinsic to the endothelial cells (figs. 42-28 and 42-30). The *Rouget cells*, periendothelial cells of amphibian microcirculation,

have clearly visible contractile abilities {32}. On the other hand, belief in the contractile abilities of their phylogenetic counterparts, the pericytes, has repeatedly waxed and waned since the time of Rouget's observations. During the 1920s, Zimmerman {33}, Vimtrup {34}, and Krogh {35} supported the contractile role, whereas later — perhaps coincidental with the advent of transmission electron microscopy — the function of pericytes was deemed less clear, and their contractile ability, in some cases, came to be denied outright (see Majno {36} and Zweifach {37}). The concept did not die out, however, and supporting evidence has resurfaced in force recently {6,30,38–44}.

In microvascular networks, there is seen a gradual transition between capillaries and venules (and sometimes between arterioles and capillaries) with respect to luminal diameter and types, and numbers of periendothelial cells {33,36,45}. The ultrastructure of periendothelial cells also changes gradually from that exemplified by features typical of smooth muscle cells. Thus in many vessels there can be found intermediate forms (*primitive smooth muscle cells*; fig. 42-27). In several studies of mouse heart it has been documented that many basic ultrastructural features are mutually comparable for smooth muscle cells, primitive smooth muscle cells, and pericytes {20,31,38}. These features fall into five categories:
1. Cytoskeletal elements
2. Excitation-contraction coupling system (SR and "T system")
3. Contractile (force-generating) apparatus
4. Force-transmitting devices (heterocellular junctions)
5. Effector system (efferent innervation)

Cytoskeletal elements

Microtubules and intermediate filaments form an organized skeletal network within periendothelial cells such as pericytes. A structural study of mouse heart microcirculation {31} showed that these fibrils are likely responsible for the configuration and maintenance of the pericyte's numerous cytoplasmic processes; this seems likely to be the case in primate heart as well (figs. 42-30 and 42-31). Microtubules are especially prominent within the longitudinal stems of pericytes (figs. 42-30 and 42-31), and intermingle in both longitudinal stems and circumferential processes with varying numbers of intermediate filaments (fig. 42-33; also see Forbes et al. {31}).

The cytoskeletal fibrils of pericytes are notable in that they are restricted to the abluminal cytoplasmic region, whereas microfilaments are massed next to the adluminal surfaces (figs. 42-30 and 42-33). A bilayered internal segmentation is therefore typical of pericytes; this sort of cytoplasmic compartmentation compares favorably with the arrangement characteristic of the definitive VSMC of the myocardial vascular supply: a myofilament-filled cortex about a central core that is free of contractile elements.

Excitation-contraction coupling system

Smooth-surfaced saccules and tubules, the structural analogues of sarcoplasmic reticulum in VSMC (see *Sarco-*

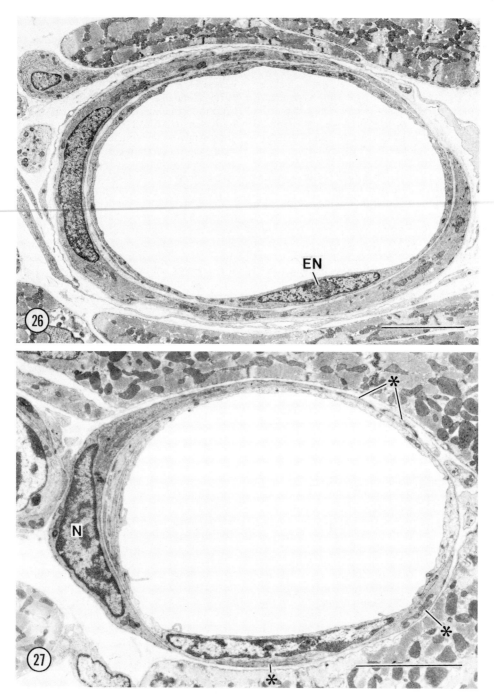

Fig. 42-26. Transverse section through "typical" arteriole in right ventricular wall of squirrel monkey (*Saimiri sciureus*). At most points of the circumference of this vessel, a single layer of smooth muscle is present, almost completely enveloping the endothelial cylinder. The VSMC component is in its essence identical to that of coronary arteries in its organellar content, though the individual cells appear less voluminous. EN = endothelial cell nucleus. Scale bar represents 5 μm.

Fig. 42-27. Blood vessel in mouse left ventricular wall. Although this vessel is of a diameter (ca. 14 μm, lesser axis) characteristic of arterioles or venules (cf. fig. 42-26), its medial layer consists of a "primitive smooth muscle cell," which displays features intermediate between those of pericytes and smooth muscle cells; these features include a protruding nuclear profile (N) and extensive cytoplasmic processes (*), which appear as isolated profiles in this micrograph, but were found, in succeeding sections, to be confluent with the nucleated portion of the cell. In such cells, surface caveolae appear at both the abluminal and adluminal surfaces, in contrast to pericytes, which form the periendothelial layer of small vessels (cf. figs. 42-30 and 42-31). Scale bar represents 5 μm.

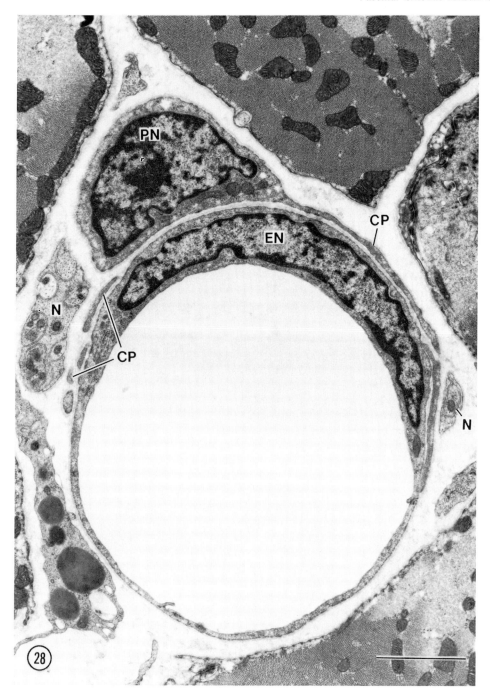

Fig. 42-28. Transverse section of small vessel (luminal diameter ca. 7.9 μm: probably a venous capillary) of rhesus monkey papillary muscle. The cell body of the pericyte is characterized by a protrusive nucleus (PN); profiles of its circumferential process (CP) appear at various points about the endothelial cylinder (EN = nucleus of endothelial cell). The vessel is hemmed in by cardiac muscle cells, and elements of nervous tissue (N) are closely associated with the vessel's abluminal surface. Scale bar represents 2 μm.

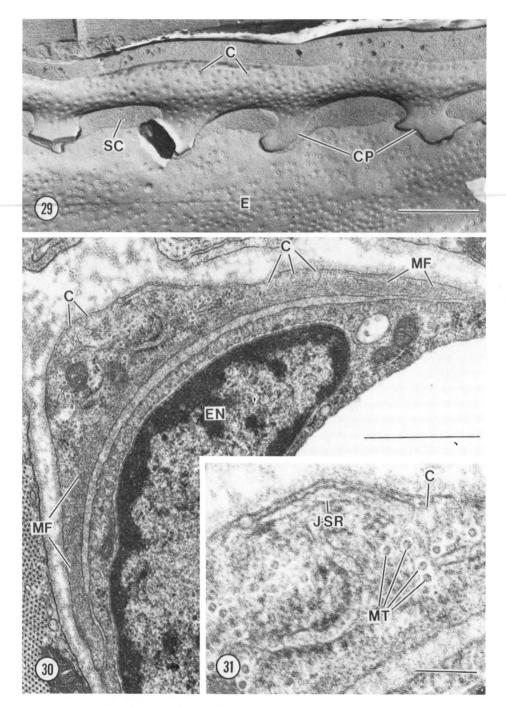

Fig. 42-29. Freeze-fracture replica of a small blood vessel (fractured longitudinally) from right papillary of rhesus monkey. Reproduced in the field are the contours of a pericyte that overlies the vessel's endothelial wall (E). The circumferential processes of the pericyte (CP) lack caveolar openings at their thinnest portions; this image corresponds favorably to the appearance of these processes in thin sections (fig. 42-30). SC = replica of surface coat material between pericyte and endothelium. Scale bar represents 1 μm.

Fig. 42-30. Transverse section through capillary (5.4 μm luminal diameter) from rhesus right papillary muscle. A profile of pericyte cytoplasm is closely applied to the endothelium (EN = endothelial nucleus). Caveolae (C) are restricted in occurrence to the upper (abluminal) plasmalemma of the pericyte, and they appear only within the thicker portions. The attenuated tips of the processes are completely filled with microfilaments (MF), which elsewhere are massed subjacent to the adluminal plasmalemma. Microtubules are located only in the abluminal cytoplasm, and thus are segregated from the more basal microfilaments. Both tips of the pericyte come into close apposition with the endothelium. Scale bar represents 1 μm.

Fig. 42-31. Detail of fig. 42-30, showing subplasmalemmal saccule (J-SR) equivalent to junctional SR of vascular smooth muscle. The orientation of microtubules (MT) is predominantly along the longitudinal stem of the pericyte. C = caveola. Scale bar represents 0.2 μm.

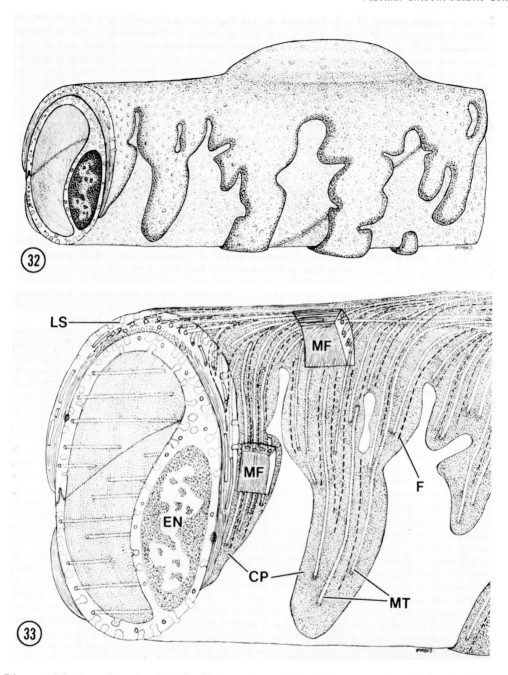

Fig. 42-32. Diagram of the three-dimensional relationship borne by a pericyte to its accompanying cylinder of capillary endothelium (drawn on the basis of observations made on mouse heart). The pericyte's nucleus typically is protrusive (cf. fig. 42-28), and its cytoplasm forms two major longitudinal stems and numerous, less extensive circumferential processes, the latter of which may branch from either the main cell body or the longitudinal stems (see fig. 42-33). The outer (abluminal) surfaces of the pericyte are characterized by caveolar indentations. From Forbes et al. {31}, courtesy of Alan R. Liss, Inc.

Fig. 42-33. Drawing based on the diagram shown in fig. 42-32, demonstrating by surface projection and cutaway views the intracytoplasmic organization of pericyte fibrils. Microfilaments (MF), presumably composed of actin, are restricted to the adluminal cytoplasm, whereas the cytoskeletal fibrils, microtubules (MT), and intermediate filaments (F) occupy the more abluminal cytoplasmic regions. Note that numbers of all three categories of fibrils are diverted from the longitudinal stem (LS) into the circumferential processes (CP), so that the same stratification of fibrils is maintained in all branches of the pericyte. EN = endothelial nucleus. From Forbes et al. {31}, courtesy of Alan R. Liss, Inc.

plasmic reticulum), in pericytes are primarily present as subplasmalemmal profiles (figs. 42-30 and 42-31). The subsarcolemmal endoplasmic reticulum of pericytes frequently generates bridging structures that contact the inner plasmalemmal leaflet and strongly resemble the junctional processes of VSMC couplings (see *Sarcoplasmic reticulum*).

Caveolae, which are abundant on all surfaces of the thicker VSMC, generally occupy only abluminal plasmalemmal positions in pericytes; limited numbers of adluminal caveolae are found in the primitive smooth muscle cells of larger microvessels and the VSMC of arterioles. Examples of caveolar tubules, consisting of two to three vesicular elements fused end to end, can be found both in pericytes and in the transitional forms of periendothelial cells; these are not so extensive as the "beaded tubules" of mouse coronary arterial VSMC {20}, yet demonstrate the propensity of the limiting membrane to form significant invaginations in periendothelial cells of all vessel categories.

Contractile apparatus

A major identifying feature of most myocardial pericytes is the collection of 7- to 8-nm-diameter *microfilaments* that populate the adluminal cytoplasm of the cell, the portion that is closest to the underlying endothelium (figs. 42-30 and 42-33). In the microvascular beds of brain {46} and retina {42}, these microfilaments have been shown, by means of decoration with heavy meromyosin, to be chemically equivalent to the F-actin of muscle cells. Immunological studies have confirmed the presence of both muscle and nonmuscle actin in pericytes {47}. In myocardial pericytes, the microfilaments are aligned along the longitudinal axes of the various processes; this, together with their juxtaendothelial location, places them in an ideal position to exert contractile influence, particularly in the numerous circumferential processes, which may in some instances nearly surround the endothelial cylinder {31}. A major problem in the promotion of the concept of pericyte contractility is the general absence of thick, myosinlike filaments; under certain conditions, however, tactoidal bodies reminiscent of myosin aggregates have been detected in the cytoplasm of brain pericytes {46}, and tropomyosin of the smooth muscle variety has been demonstrated by immunological means in pericytes of a number of circulatory beds, including that of the heart {48,49}. Furthermore, mechanisms have been proposed for smooth muscle contraction that do not require the palpable presence of thick filaments per se {50}; I have already noted the capricious occurrence of myosin filaments in definitive VSMC of myocardial vessels (see *Fibrillar elements . . .*) {2}. Added to these circumstances is the relative difficulty that attends the capture of transverse sections of pericyte processes, in which authoritative identification of discrete myosin filaments, if present, could best be made.

Force-transmitting devices

The arteries and veins of mammalian heart incorporate numerous appositions between the medial and intimal tunics (see *Junctions . . .*). A variety of heterocellular junctions are present in microvessels as well, including simple appositions (fig. 42-30), intermediate contacts {31}, and gap junctions (fig. 42-21). Pericytes vary in their encompassment of individual myocardial vessels, and may in fact be inferior in this parameter in comparison to their counterparts in the skeletal muscle microcirculation {40,41}. Still, the presence of numerous traction points between myocardial pericytes and the accompanying endothelium may provide sites for transfer of contractile force to the vessel lining, thereby providing graded amounts of deformation to the luminal contour of capillaries and venules.

Effector system

Both efferent and afferent axon terminals are known to accompany myocardial vessels at all levels of the circulatory bed {38}. The chemical nature of the efferent nerves associated with pericytes on capillaries and postcapillary venules varies between species. In the mouse, the majority of terminals appear to be cholinergic (as judged in animals treated by administration of 5- or 6-hydroxydopamine, which labels adrenergic terminals {38}). On the other hand, cat myocardium, which is profusely supplied with adrenergic nerves {51}, contains a system of blood vessels that at all its levels is similarly supplied with terminals filled with numerous small dense-cored vesicles (unpublished observations).

The gap between axon terminal and abluminal vessel surface is smallest in microvessels (in mouse averaging ca. 170 nm, with a minimum distance of 46 nm {38}); this is perhaps related in some instances to the progressive narrowing of the perivascular space that accompanies the diminution of vessel bore. The pertinent observation is that a substantial structural relationship exists between terminal axons and pericytes in mammalian heart, such that the pericyte surfaces are within reasonable diffusion distances of neurotransmitter substances. It has been demonstrated {41} that skeletal pericytes contract in response to intravascularly administered norepinephrine, angiotensin, or vasopressin, and that myocardial pericytes are unaffected by such treatment. The pericytes of skeletal muscle differ from myocardial pericytes in that they generally are not associated with efferent axon terminals {40}. It remains to be seen what effects would result in heart from extravascular application of vasoactive agents or induced release of neurotransmitter from the terminal axons themselves.

It should be noted that over the years a number of different functions have been proposed for pericytes in various vascular beds, including the provision of a source of stem cells for definitive VSMC, regulation of blood vessel growth during wound healing, maintenance of structural stability in the blood vessel wall, participation in the blood-brain barrier, etc. An extensive review on pericytes in general is given by Sims {52}. Strong evidence of pericyte contractility, however, has come from the study in vitro of retinal pericytes, which can visibly deform an underlying silicone rubber matrix, forming wrinkles in the matrix at right angles to the bundles of F-actin in the pericytes {43,44}. Furthermore, the contractile responses of pericytes are altered in pericyte-endothelial cocultures, suggesting an interaction similar to that seen between endothelium and definitive vascular smooth muscle cells {44}.

CONCLUSIONS AND SUMMARY

The walls of myocardial blood vessels in mammals are occupied by a spectrum of muscle and musclelike cells, various forms of which are collectively known by numerous appellations: smooth muscle cells, primitive smooth muscle cells, transitional cells, medial cells, mural cells, perivascular cells, pericapillary cells, Rouget cells, etc. A reasonable unifying term that at once encompasses this spectrum of vascular components is, simply, *periendothelial cells*, for this term aptly describes their positioning, yet does not relegate them to strict residence within a medial tunic (consider, for example, the far-flung VSMC that appear in veins: See *Comparison of arterial/arteriolar . . .* and fig. 42-24). The use of *periendothelial cells* furthermore sidesteps the debate as to whether three distinct tunics can be identified in microvessels such as capillaries. [Incidentally, for capillaries of mammalian myocardium, the answer is clear to this reviewer: The *tunica intima* is of course represented by the endothelial cylinder, the *t. media* by pericyte bodies and processes, and the *t. adventitia* by the fibroblasts and the numerous elements of neural tissue (including Schwann cells) that appear in the perivascular space.]

The spectrum of fine structure attributes possessed by periendothelial cells is not restricted solely to the stretches of "microvessels" that connect arteries and veins in the individual heart, but can also exist interspecifically, such as is demonstrated in the numerous instances when anatomically equivalent vessels display strikingly different profiles and distributions of VSMC (e.g., figs. 42-7 and 42-8). With the application of more effective regimens of preservation, it has become apparent that VSMC are far more complex than was indicated by early electron micrographs. This has been shown to be the case as well with "minor" periendothelial cells such as myocardial pericytes, which in well-fixed tissue display obvious complements of microfilaments, which are likely the basis of a contractile apparatus. Taken together with recent physiological observations, then, there must remain the possibility, which would be of great functional significance, that modulation of vessel bore occurs, to one or another degree, at all levels of the circulatory system of the heart.

ACKNOWLEDGMENTS

The research that contributed to this work as reported was carried out at the University of Maryland (PHS grants NS-06779 and NS-08261) and at the University of Virginia (grants-in-aid from the American Heart Association {78–753} and its Virginia affiliate {A81–737}, as well as PHS grant HL-28329, all the Virginia-based support to M.S. Forbes) and PHS grant HL-19242. Dr. Forbes was also recipient of Research Career Development Award 5-K04 HL00550 from the National Institutes of Health during part of the course of the research that contributed to this chapter.

The contributions made during the course of this research by Drs. Erland R. Nelson, Marshall L. Rennels, and S. David Gertz, and especially by Miss Barbara A. Plantholt, are acknowledged, as is the able technical assistance of Messrs. Rafa Rubio and Lawrence A. Hawkey. Primate heart material was generously contributed by Drs. S.K. Jirge and K.R. Brizzee of the Tulane University Delta Regional Primate Research Center (Covington, LA: Dr. Peter Gerone, Director).

REFERENCES

1. Boucek RJ, Takashita R, Fojaco R: Relation between microanatomy and functional properties of the coronary arteries (dog). *Anat Rec* 147:199–207, 1963.
2. Forbes MS: Ultrastructure of vascular smooth-muscle cells in mammalian heart. In: Kalsner S (ed) *The Coronary Artery*. London: Croom-Helm, 1982, pp 3–58.
3. Rhodin JAG: Architecture of the vessel wall. In: Bohr DF, Somlyo AP, Sparks HV Jr (eds) *Handbook of Physiology. Sect 2: The Cardiovascular System. Vol 2: Vascular Smooth Muscle*. Bethesda, MD: American Physiological Society, 1980, pp 1–32.
4. Uehara Y, Suyama K: Visualization of the adventitial aspect of the vascular smooth muscle cells under the scanning electron microscope. *J Electr Microsc* 27:157–159, 1978.
5. Murakami M, Sugita A, Shimada T, Nakamura K: Surface view of pericytes on the retinal capillary in rabbits revealed by scanning electron microscopy. *Arch Histol Jpn* 42:287–303, 1979.
6. Mazanet R, Franzini-Armstrong C: Scanning electron microscopy of pericytes in rat red muscle. *Microvasc Res* 23:361–369, 1982.
7. Somlyo AP, Garfield RE, Chacko S, Somlyo AV: Golgi organelle response to the antibiotic X537A. *J Cell Biol* 66:425–443, 1975.
8. Eriksson A, Thornell L-E: Intermediate (skeletin) filaments in heart Purkinje fibers: A correlative morphological and biochemical identification with evidence of a cytoskeleton function. *J Cell Biol* 80:231–247, 1979.
9. Goldman RD: The role of three cytoplasmic fibers in BHK-21 cell motility. I. Microtubules and the effects of colchicine. *J Cell Biol* 51:752–762, 1971.
10. Forbes MS, Dent JN: Filaments and microtubules in the gonadotrophic cell of the lizard, *Anolis carolinensis*. *J Morphol* 143:409–434, 1974.
11. Cooke P: A filamentous cytoskeleton in vertebrate smooth muscle fibers. *J Cell Biol* 68:539–556, 1976.
12. Tsukita S, Tsukita S, Ishikawa H: Association of actin and 10 nm filaments with the dense body in smooth muscle cells of the chicken gizzard. *Cell Tissue Res* 229:233–242, 1983.
13. Murphy RA: Mechanics of vascular smooth muscle. In: Bohr DF, Somlyo AP, Sparks HV Jr (eds) *Handbook of Physiology. Sect 2: The Cardiovascular System. Vol 2: Vascular Smooth Muscle*. Bethesda, MD: American Physiological Society, 1980, pp 325–352.
14. Somlyo AV: Ultrastructure of vascular smooth muscle. In: Bohr DF, Somlyo AP, Sparks HV Jr (eds) *Handbook*

of Physiology. Sect 2: The Cardiovascular System. Vol 2: Vascular Smooth Muscle. Bethesda, MD: American Physiological Society, 1980, pp 33–68.

15. Forbes MS, Sperelakis N: Structures located at the level of the Z bands in mouse ventricular myocardial cells. *Tissue Cell* 12:467–489, 1980.

16. Forbes MS, Sperelakis N: Ultrastructure of mammalian cardiac muscle. In: Sperelakis N (ed) *Physiology and Pathophysiology of the Heart*. Boston: Martinus Nijhoff, 1994, pp 1–35.

17. Gabella G: Inpocketings of the cell membrane (caveolae) in the rat myocardium. *J Ultrastruct Res* 65:135–147, 1978.

18. Masson-Pévet M, Gros D, Besselsen E: The caveolae in rabbit sinus node and atrium. *Cell Tissue Res* 208:183–196, 1980.

19. Levin KR, Page E: Quantitative studies on plasmalemmal folds and caveolae of rabbit ventricular myocardial cells. *Circ Res* 46:244–255, 1980.

20. Forbes MS, Rennels ML, Nelson E: Caveolar systems and sarcoplasmic reticulum in coronary smooth muscle cells of the mouse. *J Ultrastruct Res* 67:325–339, 1979.

21. Forbes MS, Sperelakis N: The membrane systems and cytoskeletal elements of mammalian myocardial cells. In: Shay JW, Dowben RM (eds) *Cell and Muscle Motility*, Vol 3. New York: Plenum Press, 1983, pp 89–155.

22. Somlyo AP, Devine CE, Somlyo AV, North SR: Sarcoplasmic reticulum and the temperature-dependent contraction of smooth muscle in calcium-free solutions. *J Cell Biol* 51:722–741, 1971.

23. Somlyo AV, Somlyo AP: Strontium accumulation by sarcoplasmic reticulum and mitochondria in vascular smooth muscle. *Science* 174:955–958, 1971.

24. Somlyo AP, Devine CE, Somlyo AV: Sarcoplasmic reticulum, mitochondria and filament organization in vascular smooth muscle. In: Betz E (ed) *Vascular Smooth Muscle*. Berlin: Springer, 1979, pp 119–121.

25. Devine CE, Somlyo AV, Somlyo AP: Sarcoplasmic reticulum and mitochondria as cation accumulation sites in smooth muscle. *Philos Trans R Soc Lond [B]* 265:17–23, 1973.

26. Popescu LM, Diculescu I: Calcium in smooth muscle sarcoplasmic reticulum in situ: Conventional and X-ray analytical electron microscopy. *J Cell Biol* 32:911–919, 1975.

27. Forbes MS, Sperelakis N: Bridging junctional processes in couplings of skeletal, cardiac, and smooth muscle. *Muscle Nerve* 5:674–681, 1982.

28. Somlyo AV: Bridging structures spanning the junctional gap at the triad of skeletal muscle. *J Cell Biol* 80:743–750, 1979.

29. Joris I, Majno G: Cellular breakdown within the arterial wall: An ultrastructural study of the coronary artery in young and aging rats. *Virchows Arch [Pathol Anat]* 364:111–127, 1974.

30. Franklin KJ: The physiology and pharmacology of veins. *Physiol Rev* 8:346–364, 1928.

31. Forbes MS, Rennels ML, Nelson E: Ultrastructure of pericytes in mouse heart. *Am J Anat* 149:71–92, 1977.

32. Rouget C: Mémoire sur le dévelopment, la structure et les propriétiés physiologiques des capillaires sanguins et lymphatiques. *Arch Physiol Norm Pathol* 5:603–663, 1873.

33. Zimmerman KW: Der feinere Bau der Blutcapillaren. *Z Anat Entwicklungsgesch* 68:3–109, 1923.

34. Vimtrup BJ: Beiträge zur Anatomie der Kapillaren. I. Ueber kontraktile Elemente in der Gafässwand der Blutkapillaren. *Z Gesamte Anat* 65:150–182, 1922.

35. Krogh A: *The Anatomy and Physiology of Capillaries*. New Haven, CT: Yale University Press, 1929.

36. Majno G: The ultrastructure of the vascular membrane. In: Hamilton WF, Dow P (eds) *Handbook of Physiology. Circulation*. Washington, DC: American Physiological Society, 1965, pp 2293–2375.

37. Zweifach BW: Microcirculation. *Annu Rev Physiol* 35:117–150, 1973.

38. Forbes MS, Rennels ML, Nelson E: Innervation of myocardial microcirculation: Terminal autonomic axons associated with capillaries and postcapillary venules in mouse heart. *Am J Anat* 149:71–92, 1977.

39. Rennels ML, Nelson E: Capillary innervation in the mammalian central nervous system: An electron microscopic demonstration. *Am J Anat* 144:233–241, 1975.

40. Tilton RG, Kilo C, Williamson JR: Pericyte-endothelial relationships in cardiac and skeletal muscle capillaries. *Microvasc Res* 18:325–335, 1979.

41. Tilton RG, Kilo C, Williamson JR, Murch DW: Differences in pericyte contractile function in rat cardiac and skeletal muscle microvasculatures. *Microvasc Res* 18:336–352, 1979.

42. Wallow IH, Burnside B: Actin filaments in retinal pericytes and endothelial cells. *Invest Ophthal Vis Sci* 19:1433–1441, 1980.

43. Kelley C, D'Amore P, Hechtman HB, Shepro D: Microvascular pericyte contractility in vitro: Comparison with other cells of the vascular wall. *J Cell Biol* 104:483–490, 1987.

44. Dodge AB, Hechtman HB, Shepro D: Microvascular endothelial-derived autacoids regulate pericyte contractility. *Cell Motil Cytoskel* 18:180–188, 1991.

45. Rhodin JAG: Ultrastructure of mammalian venous capillaries, venules, and small collecting veins. *J Ultrastruct Res* 25:452–500, 1968.

46. Le Beux YJ, Willemot J: Actin- and myosin-like filaments in rat brain pericytes. *Anat Rec* 190:811–826, 1978.

47. Herman IM, D'Amore PA: Microvascular pericytes contain muscle and nonmuscle actins. *J Cell Biol* 101:43–52, 1985.

48. Joyce NC, Haire MF, Palade GE: Contractile proteins in pericytes. I. Immunoperoxidase localization of tropomyosin. *J Cell Biol* 100:1379–1386, 1985.

49. Joyce NC, Haire MF, Palade GE: Contractile proteins in pericytes. II. Immunocytochemical evidence for the presence of two isomyosins in graded concentrations. *J Cell Biol* 100:1387–1395, 1985.

50. Panner BJ, Honig CR: Filament ultrastructure and organization in vertebrate smooth muscle. *J Cell Biol* 35:303–321, 1967.

51. Yamauchi A: Ultrastructure of the innervation of the mammalian heart. In: Challice CE, Viràgh S (eds) *Ultrastructure of the Mammalian Heart*. New York: Academic Press, 1973, pp 127–178.

52. Sims DE: The pericyte — a review. *Tissue Cell* 18:153–174, 1986.

CHAPTER 43

Pathogenesis of Coronary Atherosclerosis

S. DAVID GERTZ, ADI KURGAN, & SHMUEL BANAI

INTRODUCTION

The purported increase in the incidence of ischemic heart disease in civilized communities during the first two thirds of this century has been attributed variously to the decline and/or extinction of infectious disease, to a "less than optimal adaptation to changing patterns of lifestyle," and to advances in diagnostic techniques. In the United States between 1974 and 1977, 52% of all causes of death were attributed to cardiovascular diseases {1}. By 1981 and 1982 this figure declined slightly to 49%, and by 1986 and 1987 to 41% and 40%, respectively. Since 1974 ischemic heart diseases have accounted for approximately 65% of all cardiovascular diseases and were responsible for every third death in the United States during this period. The mortality rate for coronary artery disease in the United States has declined significantly during the last third of this century — to 21% in 1987 {1–4}, and further reduction is being witnessed since the middle 1980s due in large part to the widespread use of thrombolytic agents during evolving acute myocardial infarction {5–9}. Nevertheless, the incidence of coronary artery disease has not declined, more than half a million Americans still die of coronary artery disease each year, and this entity remains the cause of more deaths in the United States than any other disease.

Atherosclerotic stenosis of the coronary arteries has been considered to be the underlying causative factor in ischemic heart disease in as many as 99% of the cases. The arteritides such as syphilitic, rheumatic, temporal, or periarteritis; congenital anomalies of the coronary vessels; and spasm with "normal" coronary arteries, when considered together, account for a very small percentage of the etiologic factors. Progress in our understanding of the pathogenesis of atherosclerosis has been inhibited in part because of its insidious onset and its usually protracted period of asymptomatic development. Unfortunately, in the majority of cases "asymptomatic" coronary atherosclerosis is usually detected only when death occurs from other causes or when coronary vessels are visualized by angiography. It was not until studies of American males who died in the Korean War that the higher prevalence of this disease within the second decade of life was documented. Since then, considerable effort has been directed toward increasing our understanding of the pathogenesis

of atherosclerosis, which is essential if it is our goal to prolong man's active lifespan.

In this chapter we review current concepts concerning the normal coronary arterial wall; pathologic changes in atherosclerosis; the distribution of coronary atherosclerosis and plaque composition; the major theories of the pathogenesis of atherosclerosis, with emphasis on lipids and atherosclerosis and the response-to-injury theory; hemodynamic factors in atherogenesis; vasoconstriction, vasospasm, and atherogenesis; plaque rupture and the pathogenesis of acute coronary syndromes; and the accelerated atherosclerotic syndromes.

NORMAL CORONARY ARTERIAL WALL

The coronary artery wall, like that of all muscular arteries, consists of three distinct layers or tunicae: intima, media, and adventitia.

Intima

The intima, the innermost layer, is bounded on its luminal side by a usually single, continuous, interdigitated layer of endothelial cells that are attached to one another by a series of junctional complexes of varying types depending on location and vessel caliber. These cells are arranged to permit marginal overlap which provides for a degree of cellular reserve, and hence maintenance of continuity, when the vessel is subjected to excessive dilatation or other mechanical stresses associated with normal pulsatile flow. The endothelial junctions are partially responsible for the regulation of transport from the lumen to the remainder of the arterial wall, including the limitation of intercellular passage of macromolecules as evidenced by the nonpenetration of horseradish peroxidase in the intact endothelium. Small macromolecules of the size of the low-density lipoproteins may be transported across the endothelium in vesicular chains {10}; disruption of this transport system is considered by some to contribute to the accumulation of these lipids within the arterial wall.

The intima is limited on its external side by the internal elastic lamina — a perforated, circular sheet of elastic tissue. The internal elastic membrane in the fetus is es-

N. Sperelakis (ed.), Physiology and Pathophysiology of the Heart, Third Edition.

827

sentially a continuous tube of elastic tissue with localized splitting occurring only a few days after birth prior to the more advanced development of the media {11}. The 2–7 micron wide fenestrations in the internal elastic lamina appear to restrict the migration of cells from the media to the subendothelial space to only limited passage. This is supported by numerous studies which have confirmed the morphologic association between intimal fibromuscular hyperplasia characteristic of atherosclerosis and disruption of the internal elastic lamina.

Between the endothelium and internal elastic lamina are a variety of loose connective tissue components including an often ill-defined connective tissue meshwork, the basement membrane, which consists primarily of proteoglycans and collagen type IV. The endothelium is tenuously attached to this lamina by half-desmosomes. In the fetus and newborn, the endothelium is closely apposed to the internal elastic lamina; however, shortly after birth the subendothelial space becomes widened by the influx of cells and connective tissue such that, in the epicardial coronary arteries of the adult, the intima represents approximately one sixth of the total wall thickness. In general, only an occasional smooth muscle cell can be found between the two limiting layers of the intima. With increasing age, however, and at sites of intimal cusions (usually found at branch points), the number of intimal smooth muscle cells increases.

The endothelium performs a wide variety of functions that serve to maintain the integrity of the vascular system and hence the tissues supplied. The nonthrombogenicity of the endothelial surface has been related to the secretion of a thin layer of complex carbohydrate found on the luminal surface of the endothelial lining. This glycocalyx has a particular affinity for ruthenium red staining and has been shown to be thinner in areas of the arterial tree prone to atherosclerosis {12}. Endothelial cell-derived molecules, which contribute to the maintenance of arterial patency, include prostacyclin (PGI-2), a potent inhibitor of platelet aggregation and a vasodilator; antifactor VIII, which interferes with intrinsic coagulation; plasminogen activators, which participate in fibrinolysis; and a variety of other vasodilator molecules, including bradykinin and endothelial cell-derived relaxing factor. Molecules that can be thought of as participating in the hemostatic functions of endothlelial cells include Von Willebrand factor for facilitating platelet adhesion to subendothelium in the initial stages of thrombogenesis and endothelin, which has been shown to have powerful vasoconstrictive properties {for recent reviews see {13–15}.

Other functions of the endothelium include its regenerative and proliferative role in response to vascular injury, controlled exchange of fluids and metabolic substances of various molecular sizes between blood and surrounding tissues, and the metabolism of lipoproteins through interactions with lipoprotein lipase and specialized surface receptors {16–20} (see also *Lipids and atherogenesis*).

Media

The media consists primarily of smooth muscle cells arranged in multiple concentric spiral lamellar units. (One lamellar unit consists of two smooth muscle cell layers divided by one layer of elastic membrane containing variable amounts of collagen, elastin, and proteoglycans.) The collagen and elastic fibers (as well as proteoglycans) which surround the smooth muscle cells are presumably elaborated by the smooth muscle cells themselves {21–23}. The smooth muscle cell is considered to be a multipotential cell whose capabilities of migration, proliferation, and synthesis are manifest in the intimal thickening of atherosclerosis {24,25} (see *Pathologic changes . . .*).

The smooth muscle cells of the contractile phenotype contain large amounts of myofilaments and minimal rough endoplasmic reticulum. Smooth muscle cells respond to vasoactive substances like angiotensin and alpha-adrenergic agonists by vasoconstriction, and to nitrous oxide and prostacyclin by relaxation and vasodilatation. Smooth muscle cells of the synthetic phenotype appear to have lost most of their myofilament content and develop extensive rough endoplasmic reticulum and Golgi complex. Synthetically active cells appear to express numerous growth factor receptors on the cell surface and respond to mitogens such as PDGF by proliferation, migration, and secretion of macromolecules which form the connective tissue matrix of the vascular wall. Activated smooth muscle cells can synthesize and secrete growth factors which can bind to their own receptors resulting in self-stimulation to further mitosis (autocrine stimulation) or bind to receptors on adjacent smooth muscle cells (paracrine stimulation) {for review see 26}.

On the external, abluminal aspect of the media is the less continuous, and not always present, external elastic lamina. The fenestrated lamellae of elastic tissue are essential for the mechanical adaptation of the arterial wall in response to the increased wall tension that occurs with systole and for elastic recoil in diastole. This lamellar structure is therefore largely responsible for the maintenance of arterial tone to ensure proper distal propulsion of blood and to permit gradual dampening of the pulsatile aspects of flow toward the smaller vessels.

Adventitia

The adventia is the outermost supporting layer of the coronary vessels consisting of dense and loose connective tissue including bundles of collagen and elastic fibers with a mixture of loosely arranged smooth muscle cells and fibroblasts. The latter represents the predominant cell type in this layer. Vasa vasora are found in this layer, extending, according to Wolinsky and Glagov, as far luminally as the approximately 29th lamellar unit in the case of the aortic media {27}. Although arteries of up to 29 lamellar units are thought to be capable of being sustained from the lumen, the area of supply of the vasa vasora has been shown in some vessels to extend far enough inward so that only the innermost layers of the media are supplied exclusively from the lumen. The presence and significance of perivascular nerves and their terminals, often found in the outer media and adventitia of coronary vessels, and even abutting on pericytes at the capillary level, are discussed in Chapter 42.

PATHOLOGIC CHANGES IN THE ARTERIAL WALL IN ATHEROSCLEROSIS

Atherosclerosis is the form of arteriosclerosis that involves generally the larger and medium-size muscular arteries, and is the entity that forms the pathogenetic basis underlying most forms of ischemic heart disease. Atherosclerosis has been referred to primarily as a disease of the intima. However, changes are also found in the media which include medial thinning, calcific deposits, the phenotypic changes of the smooth muscle cells referred to above, and even foam cell accumulation which may depend on the degree of vascular injury, age of the lesion, and lipoprotein levels in the blood. The adventitia is also involved with changes including increased fibrous tissue deposition, inflammatory cell infiltrates (primarily lymphocytic), and increased vascularization {28}. The pathological substrate of this disease is intimal fibromuscular hyperplasia, associated with a variable degree of lipid and calcific deposits, which may result either in encroachment on the lumen or aneurysmal dilatation {29}.

Atherosclerotic lesions have been classified into three types: fatty streak, fibrous plaque, and complicated lesion {for reviews see 4,11–13,28,30–43}.

Fatty streak

The fatty streak has been considered to be the earliest of these three lesion types and can generally be found in all persons by age 10 {13,44} Fatty streaks increase in frequency up to the third decade and in absolute surface area involved during all decades {32}. This is a nonobstructive lesion characterized by focal accumulation within the intima of relatively small numbers of smooth muscle cells, foam cells, and T lymphocytes.

The degree of luminal protrusion of fatty streaks ranges from slightly raised to not at all. The yellow color seen upon gross inspection of these lesions is associated with the lipid deposition (cholesterol esters and free cholesterol) within these intimal cells as well as extracellularly. Fatty streaks are distributed throughout the arterial tree, but display a predilection for arterial curvatures and branch orifices {45}.

It remains a matter of controversy as to whether the foam cells, which increase in number with increased lipid deposition, have their origin from smooth muscle cells or from macrophages of monocytic origin. This question arose initially because of the fact that foam cells exhibit phagocytic properties, often show ultrastructural features resembling leukocytes, particularly monocytes, and have the ability to produce acid hydrolases and catalases. On the other hand, it has been shown that smooth muscle in tissue culture can be transformed into foam cells following lipid imbibition. Recent immunohistochemical studies employing monoclonal antibodies to antigens thought to be specific to monocyte/macrophage antigens, and antibodies to smooth muscle cell α-actin, have shown that, in all likelihood, these cells have their origin from both monocytes and from smooth muscle cells, with the distribution within the wall of these two antigenic types varying with the experimental model studied {38,41,42,46}.

Among the many functions attributed to the macrophage foam cells (see *Foam cells*) are the ability to secrete chemotactic and mitogenic factors. Growth factors secreted by the macrophages are mitogenic to various cell types and cause proliferation of endothelial cells, smooth muscle cells, and fibroblasts. These growth factors include platelet-derived growth factor (PDGF), fibroblast growth factor (FGF), interleukin-1 (IL-1), epidermal growth factor (EGF), and transforming growth factor-β (TGF-β) {47–49}. Foam cells have also been shown to secrete collagenase and elastase which are of particular significance in view of the fact that disruption of the internal and other elastic laminae of the arterial wall are considered to be among the very early steps in atherogenesis leading to luminal compromise and/or aneurysmal dilatation {29,50–53}.

Fibrous plaque

Fibrous plaques are generally considered to be the characteristic lesion of well-developed atherosclerosis. Lesions in the coronary vessels occur generally later than in the aorta, and occur earlier as a rule in men than in women. Macroscopically, fibrous plaques are white in appearance and protrude to varying degrees into the vascular lumen, accounting for the term *raised lesions*. The fibrous plaque, as its name implies, consists primarily of fibrous tissue (see *Distribution of . . . plaque composition*) with substantial numbers of smooth muscle cells, fewer foam cells than the fatty streak, and a highly variable degree of intracellular as well as extracellular lipid (see *Lipids and atherogenesis*). The smooth muscle cells are intertwined with variable amounts of collagen, elastic fibers, and several proteoglycans {54} such that the contribution of the smooth muscle cell to intimal thickening is not only by virtue of its proliferation and migration, but also because of the products it synthesizes. It has been suggested that the proteoglycans, possibly in combination with these other connective tissue components, participate in the accumulation of extracellular lipids within the plaque and within the media {55}. In well-advanced plaques, the accumulated smooth muscle cells, macrophage foam cells, and intercellular substances within the intima take the form of a dome-shaped fibrous cap covering a deeper central core of necrotic cellular debris mixed with cholesterol-ester-rich extracellular lipid {25,56}. In many cases, the fatty streak and fibrous plaque occupy the same anatomic position in the coronary arteries {57} with the former occurring generally earlier. However, this is not always the case, since some fatty streaks, particularly those in the non-branchpoint areas, actually may regress, and thus, the suggestion that the fatty streak represents the unequivocal precursor to the fibrous plaque remains unconfirmed.

Complicated lesion

Complicated lesions are fibrous plaques that have been altered by increased cellular necrosis, hemorrhage, calcific deposits, or desquamation of the overlying endothelial surface (or deeper wall injury) and thrombus formation.

The calcific deposits in the intima of advanced lesions, in addition to the possibility of a luminal origin, have also been considered to be derived from precipitation of this ion during injury, from necrosis of intimal smooth muscle cells, or from deterioration of attached platelets thought to have internal calcium-transport systems very similar to those of the smooth muscle cells {51}. Calcific deposits can also be found in early stages of atherogenesis. Elastic tissue has been shown to have an extremely high affinity for calcium {58,59}, and studies of experimental arterial aneurysm involving light microscopic assessment of sections stained with von Kossa's stain or alizarin red with energy-dispersive x-ray microanalysis and transmission electron microscopic studies using pyroantimonate staining have identified the preferential localization of calcium to the internal elastic lamina and elastic lamellar network of the media {29}.

The complicated lesion can result in the compromise of coronary perfusion as a result of partial or total arterial occlusion due to the marked luminal protrusion of the lesion itself (>75% *reduction in luminal cross-sectional area by atherosclerotic plaque*) or because of the superimposition of thrombus, which may also result in the occlusion of smaller coronary vessels distally following platelet shower or embolization. Progression of central necrosis within the plaque and accumulation of its "gruel" is often associated with weakening of the arterial wall, which may result in dissection within the wall, aneurysm, hemorrhage, or plaque rupture, followed by thrombus formation and/or embolization of fragments of the plaque to the distal arterial tree (see *Plaque rupture*).

DISTRIBUTION OF CORONARY ATHEROSCLEROSIS AND PLAQUE QOMPOSITION

The extent of the atherosclerotic process in patients with symptomatic or fatal coronary artery disease has only relatively recently been appreciated due to the extensive studies of Roberts and associates in which the four major epicardial coronary arteries (right, left anterior descending, left circumflex, and left main) have been examined by sectioning of these arteries at 5-mm intervals. In one study of 889 patients with fatal coronary artery disease {60}, it has been shown that all patients had at least 1 of the 4 major epicardial coronary arteries narrowed more than 75% in luminal cross-sectional area at some point by atherosclerotic plaque, and three or four arteries were so narrowed in 57%. Multivessel disease (more than one coronary artery narrowed 75% or more) was present in over 80% of the patients, and none of the arteries was totally devoid of atherosclerotic plaque. This emphasizes the diffuse nature of the distribution of atherosclerosis in these patients.

Among the three major acute coronary syndromes — sudden coronary death, acute myocardial infarction, and unstable angina pectoris — the degree of luminal cross-sectional area narrowing by plaque was found to be greatest among those with unstable angina {61–63}. Necropsy studies of patients considered to have died of sudden cardiac death have shown that more extensive luminal cross-sectional area narrowing occurs in the proximal compared to the distal halves of the epicardial coronary arteries, but the number of arteries narrowed >75% at some point is not significantly different from those with acute myocardial infarction {64}.

Several recent necropsy studies have addressed the question of the composition of the atherosclerotic plaque in the major subtypes of symptomatic or fatal coronary artery disease and over the various age groups. Kragel et al. {63} reported that the frequency of plaque rupture, plaque hemorrhage, and luminal thrombus was significantly greater among patients with first fatal acute myocardial infarction than in those with sudden cardiac death or unstable angina which were not associated with myocardial necrosis. However, the percent of 5-mm long segments of the four major arteries containing multiluminal vascular channels, considered by many to result from the recanalization of organizing thrombus, was greatest in the group with unstable angina.

These differences in frequency of acute lesions in the three patient populations have been related to differences in plaque composition. By quantitative computerized planimetry, fibrous tissue is the principal component of the atherosclerotic plaque in all three patient populations {65–68}. In all three clinical subtypes, the mean percents of plaque area occupied by dense fibrous tissue, calcific deposits, and pultaceous debris increase with increasing degrees of luminal narrowing, and the mean percent of cellular fibrous tissue decreases {65–67}. However, when restricting the analysis to arterial segments narrowed greater than 75% in cross-sectional area, patients with acute myocardial infarction had significantly more lipid-rich pultaceous debris, and significantly less cellular fibrous tissue and calcific deposits, than similarly narrowed segments of patients with "uncomplicated" unstable angina or sudden coronary death.

The characteristic necropsy finding in patients with first fatal acute myocardial infarction {68–69} is an occlusive thrombus found almost exclusively at sites of rupture of plaques with a high percentage of lipid-rich pultaceous debris. The coronary arteries of patients with sudden coronary death (without myocardial necrosis) are also severely narrowed, but the frequencies of plaque rupture and occlusive thrombus are lower. In patients with unstable angina uncomplicated by subsequent acute myocardial infarction, the lumen is significantly more narrowed than the other two populations with more extensive distribution of multiluminal channels with or without small nonocclusive thrombi (see *Plaque rupture* and *Pathogenesis of acute coronary syndromes*).

Comparisons, using the same technique of computerized planimetry at 5-mm intervals, between the composition of plaques in the four major coronary arteries of elderly patients with myocardial infarcts at necropsy (90 years and over) with that of two populations of younger patients with infarcts (53–68 years and 33–38 years) showed that fibrous tissue was the dominant component in all three patient populations {67}. Restricting the analysis to severely narrowed sections (>75% in cross-sectional area) has shown that while the percentage of plaque occupied by acellular fibrous tissue increases with increasing age, the percentages of cellular fibrous tissue and foam cells were significantly higher in the youngest subjects {66–67}. This is supported by several recent immunohistochemical studies {38–42}. Katsuda et al. {42} described the cell composition of 27 fixed, paraffin-embedded atherosclerotic lesions in the aorta of young adults ranging in age from 15 to 34 years. In the latter study, fibrofatty lesions (advanced fatty streaks) were found to consist of substantial numbers of foam cells, approximately two thirds of which (those found in the deeper layers of the lesions and being contiguous with the underlying media) were HHF35-positive (smooth muscle) and one third (those closer to the lumen) of which were HAM56-positive (monocyte-macrophage derived). In a recent immunohistochemical study of the response of normal iliac arteries to acute retrograde balloon pullback injury in rabbits, Stadius et al. {43} showed that as the intima increased in area, macrophage-type (RAM-11-positive) cells predominated along the internal elastic lamina (abluminal) aspect of the intimal lesion, while smooth-muscle cell antigen-postitive (HHF-35-positive) cells occupied the portion of the intima adjacent to the lumen.

THEORIES OF ATHEROGENESIS

Introduction

Scarpa (1804) and Lobstein (1833) are credited with providing the first pathologic descriptions of arteriosclerosis and its association with ischemic heart disease {70}. Since that time, numerous theoories of the etiology and pathogenesis of atherosclerosis have been presented. Each of these theories attempts to identify the mechanism(s) responsible for one or all of the pathologic alterations that characterize atherosclerosis, namely, smooth muscle proliferation, connective tissue formation, variable degrees of lipid deposition, and foam cell accumulation. It is the purpose of this section to present the major theories that have been entertained and that have not been totally excluded by scientific investigation. It should be emphasized that the question of which of the presented mechanisms represents the most likely remains unanswered. Moreover, the available evidence indicates that atherogenesis may be initiated by a wide variety of pathogenetic factors, singly or in combination. Current concepts concerning the pathogenesis of atherosclerosis continue to be influenced by the two major theories advanced in the middle of the last century — the thrombogenic theory and the insudation theory. A brief review of two other, less substantiated theories will be presented first.

Degeneration and clonal senescence theories

The *degeneration theory* is considered to have been advanced initially by Thoma in 1833 {71}, who suggested that the components of the atherosclerotic plaque have their origin as products of fatty and hyaline degeneration

of connective tissue components of the arterial wall. Evidence of degenerative processes in the arterial wall exists particularly in the late stages of plaque development {72,73}, and, indeed, aging is an undisputed risk factor. On the other hand, it is known that atherosclerotic lesions occur in the young and in the absence of other signs of tissue degeneration.

A related hypothesis is that often referred to as the *clonal senescence theory*. Martin and Sprague {74} suggested that atherogenesis is a function of declining stem cell activity. According to this theory, intimal smooth muscle cell proliferation is normally controlled by reciprocal feedback by way of *chalones*, which are considered to be endocrine substances that inhibit mitosis and that possibly are secreted by smooth muscle cells themselves {73}. With age, these smooth muscle cells are not adequately replaced, which results in a failure of this inhibitory control system, thus permitting uncontrolled smooth muscle cell proliferation.

Monoclonal theory

Benditt and Benditt {75} suggested that individual atherosclerotic lesions are clones from single smooth muscle cells that serve as progenitors for all subsequent cells. This was based on their observations that most individual atherosclerotic lesions from subjects with glucose-6-phosphate dehydrogenase deficiency (G-6-PD) contained either one or the other of the two isoenzymes of G-6-PD, whereas most tissues from control subjects contained both isoenzymes. According to this theory, each atherosclerotic lesion represents a benign neoplasm derived from a cell that has been subjected to mutation by a noxious substance such as a chemical or viral agent {76}. Although support for this theory is not widespread, it has yet to be completely disproven. Arguments against this theory of smooth muscle cell proliferation include the observation that the finding of a single-enzyme phenotype consistently throughout a lesion does not necessarily imply a clonal origin, since a single lesion could arise from more than one cell that contained the same isoenzyme {77}.

Thrombogenic or encrustation theory

This, the oldest theory, was first initiated by von Rokitansky {78} and later revised by Duguid {79,80}. This theory suggests that atherogenesis is preceded by deposition of thrombi (platelets, fibrin, and leukocytes) on the intimal surface that are later incorporated into the arterial wall by overgrowth of endothelium. The lipid content of the atherosclerotic plaque was considered to be derived from breakdown products of the platelets and leukocytes that form these thrombi. At this early stage, the importance of intimal smooth-muscle-cell proliferation had not been appreciated.

Insudation-inflammation theory

This theory, advanced by Virchow {81,82}, holds that atherosclerosis is initiated by local (mechanical) intimal injury, which is followed by the increased passage (imbibition or insudation) and accumulation of blood constituents (fluid and cellular) from the arterial lumen into the intima. Virchow suggested that this insudation results in an inflammatory process with edema, fatty degeneration of the intimal cells, and connective tissue proliferation in reaction to the degenerative mucoid pool. It was not intended by Virchow to imply that the inflammation was initiated by lipid insudation — as many investigators often misinterpret; rather, that the intimal injury occurred first, thus predisposing the arterial wall to increased permeability followed by a secondary inflammatory process.

At this stage, the insudation theory did not define the precise form in which lipid is transported to the atheroma. Anitschkow {83,84} showed that the addition of cholesterol to the diet of rabbits resulted in hypercholesterolemia followed by the deposition of cholesterol and its esters within atherosclerotic plaques in the aorta. He thus modified the theory of Virchow by suggesting that hypercholesterolemia is the inciting cause of the intimal changes typical of atherosclerosis. Other factors, such as mechanical or pharmacologic ones, were considered to be of secondary importance. Because of these obervations, it was the general consensus for years that conquering the problem of atherosclerosis was dependent solely upon clarifying and reversing the biochemical alterations of plasma lipids.

Lipids and atherosclerosis

Since the observation of the presence of cholesterol (free and esterified) in arterial lesions {83–85}, hypercholesterolemia has been suggested to be an important risk factor for the development of atherosclerosis. It is known that in persons with homozygous (and probably heterozygous), familial hypercholesterolemia, cholesterol accumulates more rapidly in the arterial wall, and clinical manifestations of cardiovascular pathology appear earlier in life {86,87}. A variety of epidemiologic studies have provided evidence for a high degree of correlation between dietary-induced hypercholesterolemia and increased prevalence of coronary disease {88}. It has been suggested that the higher the total and LDL cholesterol levels, the greater the chance of an atherosclerotic event, and lowering of the serum cholesterol in patients with hypercholesterolemia may result in a reduced overall mortality from coronary artery disease and regression of the atherosclerotic lesions {89–97}. A negative correlation has also been reported between plasma high-density lipoproteins (HDL-C) and coronary artery disease {98}. It has been suggested that HDL may exert an antiatherogenic effect by way of "reverse cholesterol transport" {99} by prevention of the deposition or removal of cholesterol deposits out of cells and toward the liver for catabolism and excretion {100–102}. Rubin et al. have shown that overexpression of apolipoprotein A-I gene in transgenic mice results in an increase in plasma HDL associated with the inhibition of early atherogenesis {103}.

In order to understand current hypotheses concerning the role of lipids (particularly LDL) in the genesis of the atherosclerotic plaque, a brief review of basic concepts of LDL-cell interaction is in order {104}: (a) Cells bind LDL to specialized, high-affinity, membrane-bound receptors. (b) LDL is internalized, probably by endocytosis, and fuses with primary lysosomes. (c) LDL is broken down into protein and cholesterol ester. (d) Protein is broken down into free amino acids that leave the cell. (e) Cholesterol ester is hydrolyzed into free cholesterol which is released from the lysosome into the cell. (f) The cholesterol then suppresses endogenous cholesterol synthesis, stimulates esterification as stored cholesterol, and suppresses synthesis of new LDL receptors, reducing LDL-cell interaction. Patients with familial hypercholesterolemia (phenotype II-a) have a deficiency in LDL receptors which presumably accounts for the markedly elevated LDL levels in these patients.

The source, nature, and fate of the lipids that accumulate in atherosclerotic lesions have been the subject of considerable investigation. It has been suggested variously that the extracellular lipids are themselves capable of contributing to the initiation of the atherogenic process or, alternatively, that these lipids represent byproducts of this process. It has generally been accepted that most lipids that are found in the vascular wall arrive there by crossing the endothelial "barrier" in the form of lipoproteins, although there is some evidence for a smooth muscle cell origin for some of the arterial lipids.

Many theories have been advanced concerning the role of lipids, particularly LDL, in the genesis of the atherosclerotic lesion. Among the most widely entertained theories concerning factors responsible for lipid accumulation in large vessel walls are as follows: a defect in membrane LDL receptor function, altered transcellular (endocytotic) transport of lipoproteins, impaired lysosomal degradation of lipoproteins, and altered endothelial permeability. Studies by Stein et al. {56} have suggested a possible role for a carrier protein, cholesterol ester transfer protein (CETP), in the regulation of this flux.

The major component of the lipids in atheromatous lesions is derived from circulating cholesterol in the form of LDL. Triglycerides and phospholipids, which also enter the arterial wall as components of LDL or VLDL, and which are also actively synthesized and metabolized by the arterial wall, represent a relatively minor component of the lipid composition of most atheromatous lesions {105}. Nonetheless, a number of studies have suggested a correlation between hypertriglyceridemia and coronary heart disease {85}, and apoprotein characteristics of very-low-density lipoproteins (VLDL) have been found in human atherosclerotic lesions {106,107}.

The possibility that chylomicrons (containing exogenous cholesterol and triglycerides) might be atherogenic has been discussed by Zilversmit, who hypothesized that the interaction of triglyceride-rich lipoprotein with arterial lipoprotein lipase constitutes an atherogenic process {108}. According to this hypothesis, chylomicrons may bind to subendothelial tissues exposed following endothelial cell loss. Triglycerides would then be hydrolyzed by lipoprotein lipase, followed by internalization of cholesterol-rich chylomicron remnants by arterial smooth muscle cells.

Ross and Harker {109} suggested that hyperlipidemia may initiate atherogenesis by itself causing endothelial damage. This was supported by the studies of Jackson and Gotto {110}, who suggested that chronically elevated levels of LDL may result in the increase in the relative proportion of cholesterol to phospholipid within the plasma membranes of the endothelium, thereby causing a decrease in the maleability of these cell surfaces, leading to a lowering of their yield threshold, which would be of particular importance at sites of increased wall shear such as the arterial curvature or branch points {111–113}.

In accordance with the reaction-to-injury hypothesis, another possible explanation for the more severe and widespread atherogenesis in animals fed a hyperlipidemic diet may be found in the reported effect of hypercholesterolemia on platelet aggregation. Carvalho et al. {114} reported a 25-fold increase in platelet aggregation by epinephrine in patients with type-II hyperlipoproteinemia. In another study, a significant increase in ADP-induced platelet aggregation was reported following oral administration of cholesterol {115}, and a significant decrease in collagen- and thrombin-induced platelet aggregation was found in human subjects fed a low-fat, low-cholesterol diet {116}. Accumulation of lipid at sites of endothelial injury in animals fed a high-cholesterol diet is well known. On the other hand, Moore and colleagues {117–119} found a variety of atherosclerotic lesions following repeated catheter injury in normolipemic animals, including fatty streaks, edematous plaques, fibrous (lipid-free) plaques, and raised lesions, with intracellular as well as extracellular lipid deposition covered partially or totally with thrombus formation. Cholesterol clefts were also seen in such lesions as early as 2 weeks. Thus, evidence exists that lipid accumulation in atherosclerotic lesions is not dependent upon hypercholesterolemia; it may occur in animals fed normal diets, provided this is associated with repeated insult to the endothelial lining {118}.

It has been suggested that focal hemodynamic stress, such as that which occurs at arterial curvatures or branch points, may enhance the local accumulation of LDL within the arterial wall by increasing LDL endocytosis {28,120} or by enchancing the binding of LDL to its specific receptor sites. This enhanced LDL-receptor binding has been found to be due to an increase in the number of receptors, suggesting that increased shear forces can result in an enhanced expression of LDL receptors {28}.

Although the precise mechanisms by which lipids become entrapped within the arterial wall remain uncertain, accumulation of lipid within macrophages resulting in foam cell formation has been identified as an important event in the early stages of atherogenesis. Macrophages are not thought to accumulate native plasma low-density lipoproteins under normal circumstances. In recent years, several lipoprotein modifications have been identified that provide new insights concerning the significance of lipids in atherogenesis {28,121}. The oxidized form of LDL (Ox-LDL) has been reported to increase the accumulation of foam cells within the plaque by its chemoattractant properties for blood monocytes.

This Ox-LDL is taken up within these foam cells after its recognition by non-downregulating scavenger receptors and may cause endothelial and smooth muscle cell injury because of its cytotoxic properties {12,28,122}. Furthermore, studies of the effect of the antioxidant probucol in Watanabe Heritable Hyperlipidemic rabbits have demonstrated a marked reduction in the frequency and size of atherosclerotic lesions {124,125}.

Lipoprotein (a) has been proposed as a factor contributing to acute coronary occlusion, particularly in patients with familial hypercholesterolemia {126–128}. This lipoprotein modification contains apolipoprotein (a), which is a glycosylated protein whose structure is very similar to plasminogen {129,130}. It has been suggested, therefore, that this glycosylated sequence may compete with plasminogen, thus reducing its capacity for fibrinolysis and increasing the likelihood of thrombosis {131}.

In summary, the most widely entertained theories concerning factors responsible for lipid accumulation in large vessel walls include: (a) a defect in membrane LDL receptor function, (b) altered transcellular (endocytototic) transport of lipoproteins, (c) impaired lysosomal degradation of lipoproteins, and (d) altered endothelial permeability {132}. Although accumulation of lipid is an undisputed, major component of the atherosclerotic plaque, and indeed, the lipid-insudation hypothesis has virtually dominated atherosclerotic research for most of this century, a number of serious questions have arisen. These include inconsistencies in the ability to demonstrate the known complications of human atherosclerosis, including plaque ulceration and thrombosis, in dietary-induced lesions and the fact that lipid accumulation may be detected in a variety of species including humans, even without elevated levels of serum lipids {104,133}. In addition, although evidence has been presented suggesting a causative relationship between lipid insudation and smooth muscle cell proliferation, this theory has not adequately explained this cellular proliferation, which forms a major, if not the principal, component of the atherosclerotic plaque.

Response-to-injury theory

This theory, as advocated most recently by Ross and colleagues {30,37,134,135}, represents a synthesis of ideas from a number of other theories and is predicated upon the concept that atherogenesis is preceded by damage to the endothelial lining. Indeed, prior damage to the arterial intima is a presupposition for both the lipid imbibition theory of Virchow and the thrombosis encrustation theory of Rokitansky (see above).

According to this theory, injury to the endothelial lining, whether continual or repetitive, structural or functional, might be so subtle as to result in alteration of the permeability characteristics of the endothelial lining without obvious morphologic changes, or severe enough to result in extensive endothelial damage in the form of cellular fragmentation or desquamation. Damage to the endothelial lining could result in the loss of the antithrombogenic properties of these cells, loss of the relaxing factors synthesized by these cells (see above), or enhancement of secretion of vasoconstrictor molecules such as endothlelin-1. Exposure of the arterial wall to increased concentrations of plasma constituents, including various lipoprotein fractions and modifications, is followed by the adherence of platelets to exposed subendothelial connective tissue and the attraction of a variety of cellular elements of the blood, including monocytes.

The discharge of products of the platelet-release reaction is associated with further platelet aggregation and thrombus formation. The release of platelet-derived growth factors (PDGF) from α-granules of platelets stimulates smooth muscle cell proliferation {117,136} and migration from the media into the intima through normal or pathologic fenestrations in the internal elastic lamina. The attraction and adhesion of monocytes to the sites of arterial injury can result in their migration to the subendothelial position, and they too may secrete a variety of chemoattractant and proliferation-stimulating growth factors for smooth muscle cells, such as "platelet derived" growth factors and fibroblast growth factors. These cells also can convert to macrophages, which take up modified (e.g., oxidized) or unmodified lipoproteins, resulting in foam cell formation. Release of modified, toxic lipoproteins or other toxic anions from these cells can result in further endothelial and/or connective tissue damage, followed by further stimulation of the release of growth factors from endothelial cells, platelets, monocytes, and even smooth muscle cells themselves. This proliferation, accompanied by increased formation of connective matrix primarily by smooth muscle cells, constitutes intimal fibromuscular hyperplasia pathognomonic of arteriosclerosis.

Support for the proliferative role of discharge products of the platelet-release reaction with respect to smooth muscle cells is also derived from studies by Moore et al. {117,118} in which rabbits were made thrombocytopenic with antiplatelet antibodies. Following endothelial damage, such animals showed a virtual absence of smooth muscle cell proliferation, with consequent inhibition of atherosclerotic lesions and fibrous plaques. Studies of swine that were homozygous for Von Willebrand disease, in which platelet adhesion to the subendothelium is impaired, have shown the absence of atherosclerotic lesions in spite of dietary-induced hypercholesterolemia {137}. The hypercholesterolemic, non-Von-Willebrand swine showed extreme atherosclerosis. On the other hand, other studies on the susceptibiliy to atherosclerosis of coronary arteries of swine with Von Willebrand disease following balloon-catheter injury and administration of an atherdogenic diet did not appear to show any appreciable differences between affected and nonaffected animals {138}. Platelets also release thromboxane A_2, one of the many prostaglandin derivatives of arachidonic acid. Thromboxane A_2 is a potent vasoconstrictor and stimulant of platelet aggregation. The precursor of thromboxane A_2, however, can be converted in the endothelial cells to another derivative, prostacyclin (PGI_2), which favors vasodilation and inhibits platelet aggrega-

tion, presumably by increasing platelet cyclic AMP {139, 140}.

It has been shown that smooth muscle cell proliferation in rats occurs only in those areas that require more than 7 days for endothelial regeneration {141}. Thus the possibility of the existence of a critical lesion size has been suggested in which a critical amount of endothelium must be desquamated before smooth muscle cell proliferation can be initiated. This is supported by studies suggesting that small areas of denudation, up to approximately 20 cells in width, do not result in smooth muscle cell proliferation {142,143}. This raises another question of whether the mitogenicity of the growth factors, including those derived from the platelet-release reaction, from monocytes or from endothelial cells is immediate, or whether an accumulation of mitogenic substance(s) may be required over a long time period {141}.

The studies of Reidy and Schwartz {143} have also shown that after endothelial injury, those areas of the intima that are recovered first have the least extensive intimal hyperplasia. Of interest, recent studies by Banai et al. {144} have shown that increasing the extracellular concentration of magnesium in vitro beyond the normal serum concentration (up to 2.4 mM Mg) results in a dose-dependent increase in endothelial cell migration. Further studies are therefore necessary to test whether compounds that accelerate endothelial cell regrowth may limit the extent of intimal hyperplasia in vivo.

Hemodynamic factors in atherogenesis

Considerable additional support for the reaction-to-injury hypothesis is obtained from information that has accumulated regarding the effects of hemodynamic forces on the arterial wall. That hemodynamic factors might contribute to the initiation of atherosclerosis has been suggested by the well-known predilection of this process for arterial curvatures and branch orifices. These areas have been shown to display increased intimal permeability, as evidenced by increased accumulation of Evans blue dye in the intima and adjacent medial layers {145,146}. This altered permeability has been shown to correspond to the pattern of intimal lipid deposition, as shown by increased sudanophilia, seen in coronary arteries of animals subjected to an atherogenic diet {45}. Such areas represent frequent sites of atherosclerotic plaque formation {145}. Endothelial cell turnover is reported to be greater at branch orifices {146,147}, and the sensitivity of these cells to changing flow patterns is manifested by distinct variability in their axis of orientation at these sites. At branch orifices, damage to endothelial cells in nontreated control animals has been detected with the aid of scanning electron microscopy. This damage has been found to range from craterlike and balloonlike vesicular defects to focal areas of cellular desquamation {145,148–150}. These sites have also been shown to be favored sites for the accumulation of platelet aggregates {151} and deposition of leukocytes, particularly monocytes {152}.

Hemodynamic forces are considered to act on the arterial wall by two principal mechanisms: (a) Shear stress acts parallel to the axis of the blood vessel and represents the drag force that the adjacent blood exerts on the endothelial lining. (b) Lateral pressure force acts perpendicular to the axis of flow; this force is thought to facilitate the interaction of fluid and cellular elements of the blood with the vascular wall.

SHEAR FORCES

This force represents the drag or friction force of the blood on the luminal surface that is independent of turbulence. It is proportional to the blood viscosity and rate of flow, and inversely proportional to the luminal radius. That such forces might damage the vascular wall is suggested by several reports of functional and structural changes in the endothelial lining associated with areas such as arterial curvatures and branch orifices {45,145, 147,149}. This is supported by the classic studies of Fry, in which an intravascular grooved plug was used to acutely narrow the arterial lumen {111}. He reported that when the shear force of the blood approached $379 \pm 85 \, \text{dyn/cm}^2$, the "acute yield stress of the endothelial surface," rapid cellular deterioration occurred, resulting in focal or widespread endothelial desquamation. That shear forces of this magnitude (at or exceeding the yield stress of the endothelial lining) might exist in vivo has been suggested previously {113,145}. This is particularly true in highly pulsatile arterial systems, such as the coronary arteries, which are notorious for their numerous anatomic curvatures and rapid tapering, and which are frequently subjected to abrupt, rapid, and wide fluctuations in velocity and demand for flow {153}.

Shear stress is also expected to be high in areas of arterial constriction, such as coarctation, atherosclerotic stenosis, or arterial spasm. On the other hand, it has been suggested that plaques tend to develop in those parts of the branch orifice where shear forces are relatively low, implying that increased shear forces may exert a protective effect for the development of atherosclerotic lesions {154}. In a scanning electron microscopic study combined with blood flow analyses, endothelial damage was found at the site of partial (50%) coronary artery constriction {113}. This damage ranged from vesicular defects (craters and balloons) to endothelial desquamation and was found to be more extensive on the proximal slope of the constriction where shear forces are expected to be greatest. Extensive platelet deposition and thrombus formation was found on exposed subendothelium at sites of focal constriction, even though, and probably particularly because, the reduction in transluminal diameter was insufficient to alter the rate of distal arterial flow.

LATERAL PRESSURE FORCES

Increased lateral intravascular pressure that occurs in association with hypertension is thought to contribute to vascular injury in two major ways. First, it is known that endothelial cells are involved in the transport of plasma lipoproteins, mediated in part by lipoprotein lipase, thought to be located on the endothelial surface. In-

creased lateral pressure might alter lipid transport in a direct fashion by pressure damage to the endothelial barrier or indirectly through minimal cellular damage, which interferes with normal metabolic processes. Studies of experimental hypertension have shown that elevated arterial pressure increased the permeability of the vessel wall to lipids, particularly in animals with experimental atherosclerosis {155–157}, and lesion formation in these animals is greater than in control, nonhypertensive animals {157–159}.

A variety of studies have been concerned with pathologic changes in blood vessels associated with animal (spontaneous and experimental) and human hypertension. In studies of spontaneously hypertensive rats, increased intimal thickening, hyalinization, and fibrosis have been reported, with medial hyperplasia and hypertropy, resulting in overall thickening of the wall and, in some instances, total luminal obstruction {160}. Haudenschild et al. {161} demonstrated intimal changes in a combined scanning and transmission electron microscopic study of deoxycorticosterone-salt-treated rats and spontaneously hypertensive rats. Distortion of endothelial shape was reported with subintimal thickening due to accumulation of extracellular material such as precipitated plasma proteins, reticulated basement membrane and collagen fibers, and fragments of elastin that appeared to show a blood as well as a vessel wall origin. Of interest, withdrawal of the hypertensive stimulus (DOC-salt) and normalization of blood pressure, even when combined with a prolonged period of low-salt diet, did not result in a discernible regression of these intimal changes suggesting that vascular injury, once induced, may not completely reverse, and that areas of prior damage might serve as foci for subsequent more-advanced damage to the vascular wall. It has also been shown that permeability is increased in elastic and muscular arteries in hypertension as evidenced by enhancement of vesicular transport and by increased protein passage through endothelial junctions and discontinuities {162–165}.

Thus it is generally accepted that increased arterial pressure can alter intimal permeability by (a) increasing filtration pressure, (b) stretching the endothelial surface and increasing its permeability, and (c) direct mechanical damage to the endothelial surface resulting in exposure of subendothelial layers. Microscopic studies have provided evidence for most, if not all, of the known histopathologic alterations in vascular intima and media associated with hypertension that are common to atherogenesis. Moreover, it has repeatedly been confirmed that the risk of hypertension for atherosclerosis, particularly in ischemic heart disease and cerebrovascular disease, increases progressively with increasing blood pressure, and conversely, the risk for atherosclerosis appears diminished by therapeutic reduction in blood pressure {166}.

Vasoconstriction, vasospasm, and atherogenesis

The observations of the effect of hemodynamic forces on the integrity of the vascular wall have provided greater insight into the relationship between episodes of arterial constriction, such as atherosclerotic stenosis and coronary vasospasm, and the pathogenesis of ischemic heart disease. Considerable evidence has accumulated implicating coronary vasospasm as a major, if not the principal, causative factor in Prinzmetal's variant angina {167–169} and as a contributory factor to classic angina pectoris and acute myocardial infarction {170–175}. It has been assumed that the threat posed by such episodes for the initiation of myocardial ischemia depends on the degree to which the reduction in luminal diameter results in the interference with distal coronary blood flow. However, the results of several studies suggest a modification to this assumption {113, 145,173,176}.

Coronary vasospasm, like atherosclerotic stenosis, may result in myocardial ischemia and/or infarction, not only as a result of a critical vascular constriction, when coronary flow would be dangerously reduced, but also as a result of marked endothelial damage, which may occur even, and perhaps particularly, when the reduction in luminal diameter is not sufficient to alter the rate of distal coronary flow. Such endothelial damage may result in thrombus formation at the site of spasm (or constriction), followed by partial or total arterial occlusion at that site (especially if spasm is superimposed upon preexisting arteriosclerosis), or occlusion of smaller coronary vessels distally after platelet shower or embolization. Turitto and Baumgartner {177} determined that the rate and extent of formation of platelet microthrombi on exposed subendothelium actually increase with increasing shear rate up to the highest shear rate tested of $10,000\,\mathrm{s}^{-1}$. It is not certain whether shear rates in excess of this would continue to favor an increased rate and extent of thrombus formation or at what point such increased shear forces might favor embolization. Nonetheless, the latter report further supports the suggestion that areas of focal partial arterial constriction, such as spasm or atherosclerotic stenosis, are a much-favored site for marked endothelial damage, platelet deposition, and thrombus formation, even, and possibly particularly, when the reduction in luminal diameter is insufficient to alter the rate of flow.

The possibility that coronary arterial spasm might itself contribute to the initiation of atherogenesis has been suggested on the basis of observations of endothelial damage and platelet attachment at these sites in experimental systems {113,178}. As per the response-to-injury hypothesis, the endothelial damage at sites of spasm (whether from mechanical effects of shear forces or endothelial compression associated with the vascular contriction) would be followed by platelet attachment to exposed subendothelial tissues, infiltration of lipoprotein molecules and scavenging macrophages, and proliferation and intimal migration of arterial smooth muscle cells. Support for this hypothesis is also obtained from the work of Gutstein et al. {179} who showed that rats whose aortae were subjected to repetitive vasoconstriction manifest fibrocalcific lesions as well as many of the intermittent stages associated with atherogenesis, and by the report of Betz and Scholte {180} who showed arteriosclerotic lesions following vasoconstriction induced by electrical stimulation. Although the prevalence of coronary spasm in the total spectrum of ischemic heart diseases has classically been considered to be minimal,

a variety of experimental and clinical studies have emphasized that this entity may be far more prevalent than previously thought {14,15,170–175,181–187}. The suggested relationship between vasospasm and coronary atherosclerosis greatly expands the role of spasm by its inclusion not only in the progression of acute coronary syndromes (see below), but also in their pathogenesis.

PLAQUE RUPTURE: THEORIES AND PATHOPHYSIOLOGY

Classification of vascular injury

As emphasized by the response to injury hypothesis, damage to the arterial wall is a key factor in the initiation of atherogenesis. Vascular injury is also responsible for the further progression of atherosclerosis and is thus a key factor in the pathogenesis of acute coronary syndromes. Fuster et al. {14,15} have classified vascular injury into three types. Type I represents functional impairment of the endothelium without obvious morphologic changes that may lead to the accumulation of lipids and monocytes. Such impairment may occur at sites of arterial curvatures or branch points where the hemodynamic shear may be sufficient to affect endothelial function but below the yield stress that causes endothelial desquamation. Type II includes structural damage to the endothelial lining and subendothelial portions of the intima but with intact internal elastic lamina. Such damage may result from a wide variety of injurious stimuli (see *Response to injury hypothesis*) followed by platelet attachment to exposed subendothelial tissues, release of chemotactic and mitogenic factors, and migration and proliferation of smooth muscle cells into the intima. Type III lesions include those with damage to endothelium, intima, and media. These are thought to be the most thrombogenic lesions, and the most rapidly progressing, particularly when at sites of large lipid pools. From the studies of Fuster and associates and others, it has become apparent that the severity of the injury is an important determinant of the course of development of the acute coronary syndromes (see below).

Theories on the pathogenesis of plaque rupture

Angiographic and necropsy studies have suggested a direct pathogenetic relationship between rupture of a coronary arterial atherosclerotic plaque, coronary thrombus formation, and acute myocardial infarction (AMI) {188–198}. Suggestions concerning the local pathophysiologic factor(s) responsible for the initiation of plaque rupture have included hemorrhage into a plaque following injury to the vasa vasora, mechanical compression associated with coronary spasm, increased intraluminal arterial pressure, circumferential tensile stress on the "fibrous cap" of the plaque, and hemodynamic shear forces {199}.

Injury to vasa vasora

Damage to small vascular channels within atherosclerotic plaques has been suggested as a source of plaque hemorrhage {200–203}, but it has not been shown how this might result in plaque rupture. Extravasation of erythrocytes from injury to intraplaque vascular channels is known to occur in large plaques, but this must be distinguished from hemorrhage associated with plaque rupture. The former is not associated with fibrin and platelets {204}. Moreover, Constantinides {205}, in a detailed analysis of serial sections of 17 cases of fatal coronary thrombosis, showed that the associated plaque hemorrhage could always be traced to an entry of blood from the lumen through the same crack in the plaque. Thus, although intraplaque vascular channels are seen often, there is no evidence that such channels are associated with plaque hemorrhage which accompanies rupture of a coronary atherosclerotic plaque.

Mechanical compression by vasospasm

A variety of studies have suggested an association between vasomotion and the consequences of coronary artery disease {206,207}, and vasoconstriction or spasm has been proposed as a cause of rupture of an atherosclerotic plaque {207–209}. The dominant histopathologic component of coronary atherosclerotic plaques is fibrous tissue, and when the luminal narrowing is severe, the underlying media is often severely attenuated {68,69}. Nevertheless, a variety of studies, including those involving provocative testing with ergonovine maleate, have identified spasm in coronary arteries at, and in close proximity to, sites of severe luminal narrowing {168–170, 210,211}. Recent experimental studies have suggested that sites of atherosclerotic narrowing may be hypercontractile because of possible loss of endothelial-dependent arterial relaxation associated with structural or functional damage to these cells {212,213}. Joris and Majno {141} reported endothelial desquamation following experimental vasospasm induced by periarterial application of L-epinephrine, and Kurgan et al. {187} demonstrated endothelial damage associated with spasm after periarterial application of calcium chloride. Thus, it appears that vasospasm may occur at sites of atherosclerotic stenosis, and vasospasm may be associated with damage to the arterial intima. However, that vasospasm may cause arterial injury sufficient to cause plaque rupture remains an important but still unanswered question.

Circumferential tensile stress

Plaque rupture involves plaques heavily laden with extracellular lipid material (pultaceous debris) covered by a thin residuum of fibrous tissue (cap) adjacent to the lumen {204,214,215}. Computerized histomorphometric analysis of Movat-stained sections of 101 sites of plaque rupture in the infarct-related arteries of 37 patients with a fatal first acute myocardial infarction {68} showed that the atherosclerotic plaques at sites of rupture consisted of about 32% pultaceous debris, whereas plaques unassociated with rupture contained approximately 5% pultaceous debris {199}.

The eccentric extracellular lipid "pools" within the atherosclerotic plaque are thought to be associated with increased circumferential tensile stress on the thin residuum of fibrous tissue adjacent to the lumen, and variations in mechanical strength of the plaque cap, such as that which may result from infiltration of foam cells, might further contribute to the likelihood of rupture at such sites {216}. This hypothesis is based on a computerized reconstruction of the distribution of tensile stress within the arterial wall in response to theoretical elevation of intraluminal pressure. Values for tensile strengths of the various components of the atherosclerotic plaque were obtained by micromechanical testing of samples of intima and media obtained from the coronary arteries of human cadavers. Although the applicability of this model to the biophysical forces generated in vivo in the highly pulsatile coronary arterial system may be questioned, the studies of Richardson et al. {215} provide valuable information concerning the potential for components of the atherosclerotic plaque to yield in response to increased lateral pressure forces. In a recent study by Loree et al. {217} in which the biomechanical properties of normal and diseased vessels were incorporated into a model of atherosclerotic vessels, it was concluded that the thickness of the fibrous cap is more important in the distribution of circumferential stress in the plaque than the degree of luminal narrowing. This, therefore, emphasized the importance of the physical properties of the various components of the plaque.

Hemodynamic shear force

Plaque rupture occurs at sites of marked luminal narrowing, but the degree is often insufficient to reduce the rate of distal coronary blood flow (fig. 43-1). Morphometric analysis of the sites of plaque rupture in the infarct-related arteries of the 37 patients with first fatal acute myocardial infarction (see above) showed that the mean percent reduction in luminal cross-sectional area by atherosclerotic plaque alone was $81 \pm 9\%$. Although the latter is significantly greater than the mean percent cross-sectional narrowing of all segments of the infarct-related arteries that did not have plaque rupture ($68 \pm 9\%$, $p = 0.002$), this "severe" degree of cross-sectional narrowing corresponds to approximately 56% reduction in transluminal diameter, which is insufficient, by itself, to substantially reduce the rate of distal coronary flow. This observation is supported by the necropsy studies of Falk {192} which show that of 103 sites of plaque rupture, the lumen was narrowed by less than 75% in cross-sectional area in 39 (38%), by 75–94% in 69 (67%), and >94% in 12 (12%). From quantitative high-resolution angiographic studies, the "critical stenosis" beyond which coronary flow is sufficiently reduced to be symptomatic has been determined to range between 70% and 80% reduction in luminal diameter which corresponds approximately to 90–95% reduction in cross-sectional area {218}. Thus, even moderately narrowed atherosclerotic plaques may rupture, and infarcts frequently develop in association with coronary arteries that previously were not severely narrowed {219,220}.

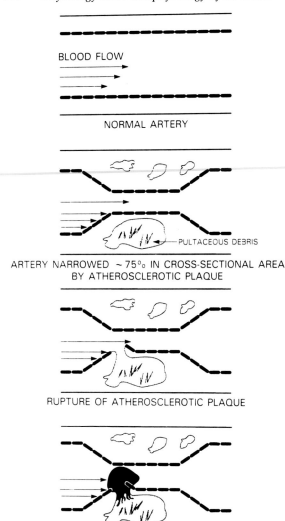

BLOOD FLOW

NORMAL ARTERY

——————— PULTACEOUS DEBRIS

ARTERY NARROWED ~75% IN CROSS-SECTIONAL AREA
BY ATHEROSCLEROTIC PLAQUE

RUPTURE OF ATHEROSCLEROTIC PLAQUE

OCCLUSIVE THROMBUS AT SITE OF PLAQUE RUPTURE

Fig. 43-1. Hemodynamic shear force as a factor in rupture of the atherosclerotic plaque. Reprinted withd permission from Gertz SD, Roberts WC: Hemodynamic shear force in rupture of coronary arterial atherosclerotic plaques. *Am J Cardiol* 66: 1368–1372, 1990.

Hemodynamic wall shear at sites of "subcritical" arterial narrowing has been calculated to be sufficiently strong to cause marked endothelial damage followed by platelet deposition and thrombus formation on exposed subendothelial tissues (see *Hemodynamic factors in atherogenesis*, above). Correlative scanning electron microscopic and blood flow studies of the coronary arteries of dogs, and the common carotid artery of rabbits, have shown that marked endothelial damage, with extensive platelet deposition and thrombus formation on exposed subendothelial tissues, may occur at the site of a partial arterial constriction (40–60% reduction in trans-

luminal diameter) even, and perhaps particularly, when the reduction in luminal diameter is insufficient to alter substantially the rate of distal coronary blood flow {113, 141}. That shear forces of the magnitude sufficient to exceed the yield stress of the endothelial lining (see *Hemodynamic factors in atherogenesis*, above) might be possible at sites of plaque rupture in humans can be estimated as follows {199}: By applying Poiseuille's Law, shear stress may be expressed as

$$t = 4Qn/\pi r^3,$$

where t = shear force in dynes/cm², Q = coronary blood flow distal to the site of constriction in ml/s, n = viscosity of the blood in Poise, and r = luminal radius at site of constriction in cm. Assuming the average luminal diameter of a "normal" coronary artery to be 3.0 mm, the luminal radius of such a coronary artery at the site of a 50% diameter reduction would be 0.075 cm. The viscosity of the blood, assuming normal hematocrit, is approximately 0.047 Poise, and coronary blood flow, e.g., in the left anterior descending coronary artery distal to the site of a 50% subcritical stenosis, can be assumed to remain at 150 ml/min with maintenance of normal arterial pressure, although flow may increase more than threefold during exercise. The shear force under these conditions is calculated to be more than 350 dynes/cm², which is well within the range of shear forces hypothesized by Fry {145} to be capable of inducing endothelial damage. These calculations assume steady, laminar flow. In circumstances of pulsatile flow, a much greater velocity gradient would be expected at the arterial wall, especially at sites of arterial constriction, that could result in more than a fivefold increase in shear stress over that in steady flow {221,222}. The shear force might increase even further during exercise, but this increase may be offset partially by autoregulatory mechanisms.

It may be argued that just because shear force can cause marked endothelial damage, this does not prove that it is capable of causing plaque rupture. Indeed, further multidisciplinary studies are necessary to confirm this hypothesis. Nonetheless, intimal damage so produced, even if initially of minimal mural depth, may increase the likelihood of rupture at such sites, particularly when occurring in segments with extensive amounts of pultaceous debris and a correspondingly thinner residuum of fibrous tissue between the lipid pool and the arterial lumen. Exposure of thrombogenic stimuli, such as collagen fibrils and pultaceous debris, may result in partial or total arterial occlusion at such sites by platelet adhesion and thrombus formation, or facilitation of such occlusion by spasm consequent to the release of vasoactive compounds from platelets at these.

Vasoconstriction at sites of endothelial desquamation also might increase the likelihood of plaque rupture by the mechanical effects of the constriction itself on the arterial wall, or by further increasing the intensity of the hemodynamic shear on the already damaged intima if the constriction remains below the "critical stenosis." Intimal damage associated with hemodynamic shear might also be expected to facilitate the sequence proposed by

Richardson et al. {215} by decreasing the circumferential tensile force necessary to rupture the plaque at sites of extensive pultaceous debris and an attenuated fibrous tissue residuum.

Thus, it appears likely that coronary atherosclerotic plaques may rupture even when, and perhaps particularly because, the reduction in luminal cross-sectional area is insufficient to reduce distal coronary flow (fig. 43-1). Increased shear force associated with the acutely narrowed arterial segments may, by itself, cause intimal damage sufficiently severe to cause plaque rupture, or it may participate with intramural circumferential stress and mechanical forces associated with active vasoconstriction, as one component of a multifactorial pathogenesis of plaque rupture.

PATHOGENETIC PROGRESSION OF ACUTE CORONARY SYNDROMES

A variety of angiographic and necropsy studies have shown that thrombus formation, superimposed upon plaque fissure or rupture, is the underlying pathogenetic precursor to the acute coronary syndromes {for recent reviews see 4,14,15,219,220,223–226}.

Acute myocardial infarction

In patients with acute myocardial infarction, plaque rupture is usually severe (severe type II or type III lesion), it usually occurs at sites of extensive lipid-rich pultaceous debris, and collateral coronary circulation to the supplied myocardium is usually poor. Plaque rupture is itself responsible for total or near-total obstruction of the infarct-related artery in only a small minority of cases {68}, and luminal obstruction is due in most cases to total thrombotic occlusion of an artery whose luminal narrowing by atherosclerotic plaque alone is insufficient to result in a significant reduction in the rate of distal arterial flow {199}.

Sudden coronary death

In sudden coronary death without evidence of left ventricular necrosis, the coronary arteries are less severely narrowed, and collateral circulation is likely to be poorer than in patients with unstable angina. The percent of plaque occupied by pultaceous debris is significantly less in sudden death than in acute myocardial infarction. This may explain the lower frequencies of severe plaque rupture and occlusive thrombus observed in patients with sudden coronary death {63}. It has been suggested, therefore, that sudden coronary death may be associated with dynamic coronary obstruction at the site of nonocclusive thrombus due to superimposed spasm in the presence of poor collateral circulation or to extensive platelet shower from the site of a relatively small plaque fissure. Under such circumstances, ischemia of large areas of the myocardium might occur without necrosis but with fatal disturbances of conduction.

Unstable angina pectoris

Patients with unstable angina experience transient reductions in myocardial perfusion. Necropsy studies have shown that the degree of luminal narrowing is more severe in patients with unstable angina than in those with acute myocardial infarction (see above, *Distribution coronary atherosclerosis and plaque composition*) and the extent of collateral circulation is thought to be greater. The plaques in patients with unstable angina (compared to patients with acute myocardial infarction) have a greater percentage of fibrous tissue, less pultaceous debris, a higher frequency of multiluminal vascular channels, smaller nonocclusive thrombi, and a lower observed frequency of plaque rupture {63}. In view of the studies of Richardson et al. {215} and Loree et al. {217}, the lower percentage of plaque occupied by pultaceous debris, and the correspondingly higher percentage of fibrous tissue, may explain, at least in part, the suggestion that patients with unstable angina have plaque fissure that is less severe than that usually found in acute myocardial infarction. On the background of arteries severely narrowed by atherosclerotic plaque, thrombus formation in these patients may be either nonocclusive but sufficient to result in reduced supply relative to demand, nonocclusive but made transiently occlusive by superimposed vasospasm, or occlusive but rapidly dissolved by the fibrinolytic system.

ACCELERATED ATHEROSCLEROTIC SYNDROMES

Injury to the endothelium and vessel wall represents a pivotal initiating event in the pathogenesis of atherosclerosis, both in its chronic and accelerated forms (fig. 43-2). Vascular smooth muscle cell (SMC) proliferation, and elaboration by these cells of abundant extracellular matrix, is the characteristic response of the arterial wall to various types of injury. The accelerated form of this proliferative response is the cause of premature coronary occlusion and of morbidity and mortality in patients undergoing *heart transplantation*, *coronary artery bypass grafting*, and *percutaneous transluminal coronary angioplasty* {227–229}. In the following section we confine our remarks to the first two accelerated syndromes.

Accelerated arteriosclerosis in heart transplantation

Hemodynamically significant coronary artery narrowing is a major long-term problem in the transplanted heart where the incidence of arteriosclerotic occlusion is 20–50% at 5 years {230–233}. Arrhythmias, congestive heart failure, silent myocardial infarction, and sudden death are often the first clinical manifestations of accelerated coronary arteriosclerosis in transplant recipients, since these patients do not experience anginal pain. The pathogenesis of this accelerated vascular disease is poorly understood, but it may result from a chronic immunologic injury directed against the arteries of the donor. The

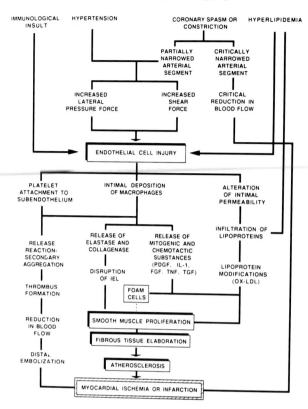

Fig. 43-2. Diagram depicting the role of four of the many risk factors in the pathogenesis of atherosclerosis and ischemic heart disease.

concept of ongoing immune-mediated vascular injury as the cause of this syndrome is suggested by the demonstration of both humoral and cellular immune components associated with the vascular damage. The arterial narrowing tends to be diffuse and concentric, and once this highly diffuse graft arteriosclerosis develops to the point of clinical manifestation, retransplantation is usually the only recourse.

Accelerated arteriosclerosis in coronary bypass vein grafts

Occlusion of vein grafts contributes significantly to morbidity and mortality after coronary artery bypass graft surgery and is responsible, in the majority of cases, for the recurrence of myocardial ischemia, infarction, and compromised ventricular function. Early occlusion (prior to hospital discharge) occurs in 8–12% of vein grafts, and by 1 year 12–20% of vein grafts become occluded. Histological studies of vein grafts occluded within 1 year show marked intimal hyperplasia with superimposed thrombus {234}. This accelerated process of intimal hyperplasia is believed to be initiated by endothelial damage in venous bypass grafts subjected to arterial pressure.

The principal pathophysiologic substrate in both cases (as in restenosis after balloon angioplasty) is *proliferation of activated vascular smooth muscle cells.* Endothelial cell injury, e.g., that caused by high shear stress or by immune mechanisms, leads to platelet deposition and liberation of growth-promoting factors (e.g., fibroblast growth factors, platelet-derived growth factor, epidermal growth factor, transforming growth factor-α, and insulin-like growth factor) from endothelial cells, smooth muscle cells, platelets, and probably macrophages. This results in activation of medial smooth muscle cells, which change their characteristic quiescent, contractile phenotype to become more rounded, synthetic cells. Activated smooth muscle cells proliferate and migrate into the intima and elaborate abundant matrix proteins, resulting in encroachment on the arterial lumen {235–237}. These changes are accompanied by an increase in the expression of numerous genes with upregulation of several growth factors, and expression of their receptors, which further perpetuates the smooth muscle cell proliferation.

A variety of agents have been found to be effective inhibitors of smooth muscle proliferation in vitro, and several animal studies have reported favorable reductions in the extent of the intimal proliferative response to vascular injury. However, clinical studies have failed to identify any single agent effective enough to inhibit this process. Recent in vitro studies by Epstein et al. {238} focused on the use of recombinant DNA to facilitate the development of highly specific targeted therapy. This strategy is based on the observation that rapidly proliferating smooth muscle cells, like cancer cells, often express high levels of surface receptors that are either absent, or present in low density, in normally proliferating cells. Epstein et al. demonstrated that activated SMC can be selectively targeted and killed using the chimeric toxin transforming growth factor-α, pseudomonas exotoxin-40 (TGFα-PE40). This type of molecule is cytotoxic to cells displaying the ligand-specific growth factor receptor because the cell-killing domain of Pseudomonas toxin enters the cell only when the ligand portion of the fusion-protein binds to its receptor. Such studies involving specific targeting of proliferating cells by use of chimeric toxins, and the development of specific antisense gene sequences to prevent the proliferating capability of these cells {239}, are two promising new approaches designed to interfere with smooth muscle cell proliferation, which is recognized to be the principal pathogenetic substrate of the arteriosclerotic process underlying both acute and accelerated coronary syndromes (fig. 43-2).

REFERENCES

1. World Health Statistics Annual. Vol 1: Vital Statistics and Causes of Death. Geneva: World Health Organization, 1977, pp 272–279; 1978, pp 218–225; 1979, pp 134–141; 1980, pp 108–115; 1985, pp 154–165; 1986, pp 256–261; 1987, pp 174–177; 1988, pp 192–199; 1989, pp 216–219.
2. Cooper R, Stamler L, Dyer A, Garside D: The decline in mortality from coronary heart disease, USA, 1968–1975. *J Chronic Dis* 31:709–720, 1978.
3. Stern MP: The recent decline in ischemic heart disease mortality. *Ann Intern Med* 91:630–640, 1979.
4. Clark LT: Atherogenesis and thrombosis: Mechanisms,

pathogenesis, and therapeutic implications. *Am Heart J* 123:1106–1109, 1992.

5. Chesebro JH, Knatterud G, Roberts R, Borer J, Cohen LS, Dalen J, Dodge HT, Francis CK, Hillis D, Ludbrook P, Markis JE, Mueller H, Passamani ER, Powers ER, Rao AK, Robertson T, Ross A, Ryan TJ, Sobel BE, Willerson J, Williams DO, Zaret BL, Braunwald E: Thrombolysis in myocardial infarction (TIMI) trial, phase I: A comparison between intravenous tissue plasminogen activator and intravenous streptokinase: Clinical findings through hospital discharge. *Circulation* 76:142–154, 1987.

6. Serruys PW, Simoons ML, Suryapranata H, Vermeer F, Wijns W, van den Brand M, Bar F, Zwaan C, Hanno Krauss X, Remme WJ, Res J, Verheugt FWA, van Domburg R, Lubsen J, Hugenholtz PG: Preservation of global and regional left ventricular function after early thrombolysis in acute myocardial infarction. *J Am Coll Cardiol* 7:729–742, 1986.

7. White HD, Norris RM, Brown MA, Takayama M, Maslowski A, Bass NM, Ormiston JA, Whitlock T: Effect of intravenous streptokinase on left ventricular function and early survival after acute myocardial infarction. *N Engl J Med* 317:850–855, 1987.

8. O'Rourke M, Baron D, Keogh A, Kelly R, Nelson G, Barnes C, Raftos J, Graham K, Hillman K, Newman H, Healey J, Woolridge J, Rivers J, White H. Whitlock R, Norris R: Limitation of myocardial infarction by early infusion of recombinant tissue-type plasminogen activator. *Circulation* 77:1311–1315, 1988.

9. Gruppo Italiano Per Lo Studio Della Streptochinasi Nell'infarto Miocardico (GISSI): Effectiveness of intravenous thrombolytic treatment in acute myocardial infarction. *Lancet* 1:397–401, 1986.

10. Stein O, Stein Y, Eisenberg S: Radioautographic study of the transport of ^{125}iodine-labeled serum lipoproteins in rat aorta. *Z Zellforsch Mikrosk Anat* 138:223–237, 1973.

11. Vlodaver Z, Edwards JE: Pathology of coronary atherosclerosis. *Prog Cardiovasc Dis* 14:256–274, 1971.

12. Wissler RW: Principles of the pathogenesis of atherosclerosis. In: Braunwald E (ed) *Heart Disease: A Text Book of Cardiovascular Medicine*. Philadelphia: WB Saunders, 1980, pp 1221–1245.

13. Stary HC, Blankenhorn DH, Chandler AB, Glagov S, Insull W Jr, Richardson M, Rosenfeld ME, Schaffer SA, Schwartz CJ, Wagner WD, Wissler RW: A definition of the intima of human arteries and of its atherosclerosis-prone regions: A report from the Committee on Vascular Lesions of the Council on Arteriosclerosis, American Heart Association. *Arterioscler Thromb* 12:120–134, 1992.

14. Fuster V, Badimon L, Badimon JJ, Chesebro JH: The pathogenesis of coronary artery disease and the acute coronary syndromes (first of two parts). *N Engl J Med* 326:242–250, 1992.

15. Fuster V, Badimon L, Badimon JJ, Chesebro JH: The pathogenesis of coronary artery disease and the acute coronary syndromes (second of two parts). *N Engl J Med* 326:310–318, 1992.

16. Wall RT, Harker LA: The endothelium and thrombosis. *Annu Rev Med* 31:361–371, 1980.

17. Hoak JC, Czervionke RL, Fry GL, Haycraft DL, Brotherton AA: Role of the vascular endothelium. *Philos Trans Roc Lond B* 294:331–338, 1981.

18. Nawroth PP, Stern DM: A pathway of coagulation on endothelial cells. *J Cell Biochem* 28:253–264, 1985.

19. Reidy MA, Schwartz SM: Arterial endothelium — assessment of in vivo injury. *Exp Mol Pathol* 41:419–434, 1984.

20. Reidy MA: Biology of disease. A reassessment of endothelial injury and arterial lesion formation. *Lab Invest* 53:513–520, 1985.

21. Ross R, Klebanoff SJ: The smooth muscle cell. I. In vivo synthesis of connective tissue proteins. *J Cell Biol* 50:159, 1971.

22. Wight TN, Ross R: Proteoglycans in primate arteries. II. Synthesis and secretion of glycosaminoglycans by arterial smooth muscle cells in culture. *J Cell Biol* 67:675–686, 1975.

23. Narayanan S, Sanberg LB, Ross R, Layman D: The smooth muscle cell. III. Elastin synthesis in arterial smooth muscle cell culture. *J Cell Biol* 68:411–419, 1976.

24. Campbell GR, Campbell JH: Smooth muscle phenotypic changes in arterial wall homeostasis: Implications for the pathogenesis for the pathogenesis of atherosclerosis. *Exp Mol Pathol* 42:139–162, 1985.

25. Wissler RW: The cellular pathobiology of atherosclerosis in 1983. *Adv Exp Med Biol* 183:1–16, 1985.

26. Casscells W: Migration of smooth muscle and endothelial cells: Critical events in restenosis. *Circulation* 86:723–729, 1992.

27. Wolinsky H, Glagov S: Comparison of abdominal and thoracic aortic medial structure in mammals: Deviation of man from the usual pattern. *Circ Res* 25:677–686, 1969.

28. Schwartz CJ, Kelley JL, Nerem RM, Sprague EA, Rozek MM, Valente AJ, Edwards EH, Prasad ARS, Kerbacher JJ, Logan SA: Pathophysiology of the atherogenic process. *Am J Cardiol* 64:23G–30G, 1989.

29. Gertz SD, Kurgan A, Eisenberg D: Aneurysm of the rabbit common carotid artery induced by periarterial application of calcium chloride in vivo. *J Clin Invest* 81:649–656, 1988.

30. Ross R: The arterial wall and atherosclerosis. *Ann Rev Med* 30:1–15, 1979.

31. Stemerman MB: Hemostasis, thrombosis and atherogenesis. *Atheroscl Rev* 6:105–146, 1979.

32. Oeser J, Fehr R, Brinkmann B: Aortic and coronary atherosclerosis in a Hamburg autopsy series. Virch Arch *[Pathol Anat]* 384:131–148, 1979.

33. Velican C, Velican D: Coronary intimal necrosis occurring as an early stage of atherosclerotic involvement. *Atherosclerosis* 39:479–496, 1981.

34. Constantinides P: Atherosclerosis — a general survey and synthesis. *Surv Synth Path Res* 3:477-498, 1984.

35. Altman RFA, Ramos de Souza AS: Mechanism of progression and regression of atherosclerosis. *World Rev Nutrit Diet* 46:219–251, 1985.

36. Jokinen MP, Clarkson TB, Prichard RW: Animal models in atherosclerosis research. *Exp Mol Pathol* 42:1–28, 1985.

37. Ross R: The pathogenesis of atherosclerosis. In: Braunwald E (ed) *Heart Disease: A Textbook of Cardiovascular Medicine*, 4th ed. Philadelphia: WB Saunders, 1992, pp 1106–1124.

38. Watanabe T, Hirata M, Yoshikawa Y, Nagafuchi Y, Toyoshima H, Watanabe T: Role of macrophages in atherosclerosis: Sequential observations of cholesterol-induced rabbit aortic lesion by the immunoperoxidase technique using monoclonal antimacrophage antibody. *Lab Invest* 53:80–90, 1985.

39. Gown AM, Toyohiro T, Ross R: Human atherosclerosis: II. Immunocytochemical analysis of the cellular composition of human theroscleotic lesions. *Am J Pathol* 125:191–207, 1986.

40. Tsukada T, Tippens D, Gordon D, Ross R, Gown AM: HHF35, A muscle-actin-specific monoclonal antibody: I. Immunocytochemical and biochemical characterization. *Am J Pathol* 126:51–60, 1987.

41. Munro JM, van der Walt JD, Munro CS, Chalmers JAC, Cox EL: An immunohistochemical analysis of human aortic fatty streaks. *Hum Pathol* 18:375–380, 1987.

42. Katsuda S, Boyd HC, Fligner C, Ross R, Gown AM: Human atherosclerosis: III. Immunocytochemical analysis of the cell composition of lesions of young adults. *Am J Pathol* 140:907–14, 1992.

43. Stadius ML, Rowan R, Fleischhauer, JF, Kernoff R, Billingham M, Gown AM: Time course and cellular characteristic of the iliac artery response to acute balloon injury: An angiographic, morphometric, and immunocytochemical analysis in the cholesterol-fed New Zealand white rabbit. *Arterioscler Thromb* 12:1267–1273, 1992.

44. Stary HC: Evolution of atherosclerotic plaques in the coronary arteries of young adults. *Arteriosclerosis* 3:471a, 1983.

45. Flaherty JT, Ferrans VJ, Pierce JE, Carew TE, Fry DL: Localizing factors in experimental atherosclerosis. In: Likoff W, Segal BL, Insull W, Mayer JH (eds) *Atherosclerosis and Coronary Heart Disease*. New York: Grune and Stratton, 1972, pp 40–84.

46. Fowler S, Shiu H, Haley NJ: Characterization of lipid-laden aortic cells from cholesterol-fed rabbits. *Lab Invest* 41:372–378, 1979.

47. Ross R, Masuda J, Raines EW: Cellular interactions, growth factors, and smooth muscle proliferation in atherogenesis. *Ann NY Acad Sci* 589:102–111, 1990.

48. Libby P, Hansson GK: Involvement of the immune system in human atherogenesis. *Lab Invest* 64:5–15, 1991.

49. Higashiyama S, Abraham JA, Miller J, Fiddes JC, Klagsbrun M: A heparin-binding growth factor secreted by macrophage-like cells that is related to EGF. *Science* 251:936–939, 1990.

50. Werb Z, Gordon S: Elastase secretion by stimulated macrophages. *J Exp Med* 142:361–377, 1975.

51. Mendlowitz M: Arterial calcium metabolism, hypertension and arteriosclerosis. *Cardiology* 67:81–89, 1981.

52. Anidjar S, Dobrin PB, Eichorst M, Graham GP, Chejfec G: Correlation of inflammatory infiltrate with the enlargement of experimental aortic aneurysms. *J Vasc Surg* 16:139–147, 1992.

53. Nakashima Y, Sueishi K: Alteration of elastic architecture in the lathyritic rat aorta implies the pathogenesis of aortic dissecting aneurysm. *Am J Pathol* 140:959–969, 1992.

54. Wight TN: Proteoglycans in pathological conditions: Atherosclerosis. *Fed Proc* 44:381–385, 1985.

55. Smith EB, Smith RH: Early changes in the aortic intima. *Atheroscl Rev* 3:119–136, 1976.

56. Stein O, Halperin G, Stein Y: Cholesterylester efflux from extracellular and cellular elements of the arterial wall. Model systems in culture with cholesteryl linoleyl ether. *Arteriosclerosis* 6:70–78, 1986.

57. McGill HC Jr: Persistent problems in the pathogenesis of atherosclerosis. *Arteriosclerosis* 4:443–451, 1984.

58. Hall DA: Elastic tissue alterations in vascular disease. In: Blumenthal HT (ed) *Cowdrys Arteriosclerosis*, 2nd ed. Springfield, IL: Charles C. Thomas, 1967, pp 121–140.

59. Yu SY: Elastic tissue and arterial calcification. In: Blumenthal HT (ed) *Cowdry's Arteriosclerosis*, 2nd ed. Springfield, IL: Charlesar C. Thomas, 1967, pp 170–192.

60. Roberts WC, Potkin BN, Solus DE, Reddy SG: Mode of death, frequency of healed and acute myocardial infarction, number of major epicardial coronary arteries severely narrowed by atherosclerotic plaque, and heart weight in fatal atherosclerotic coronary artery disease: Analysis of 889 patients studied at necropsy. *J Am Coll Cardiol* 15:196–203, 1990.

61. Roberts WC, Virmani R: Quantification of coronary arterial narrowing in clinically-isolated unstable angina pectoris: An analysis of 22 necropsy patients. *Am J Med* 67:792–799, 1979.

62. Roberts WC: Pathology of coronary atherosclerosis. In: Sabiston DC Jr, Spencer FC (eds) *Surgery of the Chest*, 5th ed. Philadelphia: WB Saunders, 1990, pp 1654–1661.

63. Kragel AH, Gertz SD, Roberts WC: Morphologic comparison of frequency and types of acute lesions in the major epicardial coronary arteries in unstable angina pectoris, sudden coronary death and acute myocardial infarction. *J Am Coll Cardiol* 18:801–808, 1991.

64. Roberts WC: Sudden cardiac death: A diversity of causes with focus on atherosclerotic coronary artery disease. *Am J Cardiol* 65:13B–19B, 1990.

65. Kragel AH, Reddy SG, Wittes JT, Roberts WC: Morphometric analysis of the composition of coronary arterial plaques in isolated unstable angina pectoris with pain at rest. *Am J Cardiol* 66:893–895, 1990.

66. Dollar AL, Kragel AH, Fernicola DJ, Waclawiw MA, Roberts WC: Composition of atherosclerotic plaques in coronary arteries in women <40 years of age with fatal coronary artery disease and implications for plaque reversibility. *Am J Cardiol* 67:1223–1227, 1991.

67. Gertz SD, Malekzadeh S, Dollar AL, Kragel AH, Roberts WC: Composition of atherosclerotic plaques in the four major epicardial coronary arteries in patients >90 years of age. *Am J Cardiol* 67:1228–331, 1991.

68. Gertz SD, Kragel AH, Kalan JM, Braunwald E, Roberts WC: The Thrombolysis in Myocardial Infarction (TIMI) Investigators: Comparison of coronary and myocardial morphologic findings in patients with and without thrombolytic therapy during first fatal acute myocardial infarction. *Am J Cardiol* 66:904–909, 1990.

69. Kragel AH, Reddy SG, Wittes JT, Roberts WC: Morphometric analysis of the composition of atherosclerotic plaques in the four major epicardial coronary arteries in acute myocardial infarction and in sudden coronary death. *Circulation* 80:1747–1756, 1989.

70. Leibowitz JO: The History of Coronary Heart Disease. Berkeley, CA: University of California, 1970.

71. Thoma R: Uber die Abhangigkeit der Hindegewebsneubildung in der Arterienintima von den mechanischen Bendigungen des Blutumlaufes. *Virchows Arch (Pathol Anat)* 93:443–505, 1883.

72. Blumenthal HT, Lansing AL, Wheeler PA: Calcification of the media of the human aorta and its relation to intimal arteriosclerosis, aging and disease. *Am J Pathol* 20:665–679, 1944.

73. Walton KW: Pathogenetic mechanisms in atherosclerosis. *Am J Cardiol* 35:542–558, 1975.

74. Martin GM, Sprague CA: Symposium on in vitro studies related to atherogenesis: Life histories of hyperplastoid cell lines from aorta and skin. *Exp Mol Pathol* 18:125–141, 1973.

75. Benditt EP, Benditt JM: Evidence for a monoclonal origin of human atherosclerotic plaques. *Proc Natl Acad Sci USA* 70:1753–1756, 1973.

76. Benditt EP: The monoclonal theory of atherogenesis. *Atheroscl Rev* 3:77–85, 1978.

77. Failkow PJ: The origin and development of human tumors studies with cell markers. *N Engl J Med* 291:26–35, 1974.

78. Von Rokitansky C: A Manual of Pathological Anatomy (trans GE Day). London: New Sydenham Society, 1852.

79. Duguid JB: Thrombosis as a factor in the pathogenesis of aortic atherosclerosis. *J Pathol Bacteriol* 60:57–61, 1948.

80. Duguid JB: Mural thrombosis in arteries. *Br Med Bull* 2:36–38, 1955.
81. *Virchow R: Phlogose und Thrombose im Gefasssystem. In: Gesammelte Abhandlungen zur wissenschaftlichen Medizin.* Frankfurt-am-Main: Meidinger, 1856.
82. Virchow R: Gesammelte Abhandlungen zur wissenschaftlichen Medizin: Phlogose und Thrombose im Gefasssystem. Berlin: Max Hirsch, 1862.
83. Anitschkow NN: Uber Veranderungen der Kaninchenaorta bei experimentelle Cholesterinsteatose. *Beitr Pathol Anat* 56:379–404, 1913.
84. Anitschkow NN: A history of experimentation on arterial atherosclerosis in animals. In: Blumenthal HT (ed) *Cowdrys Arteriosclerosis*, 2nd ed. Springfield, IL: Charles C. Thomas, 1967, pp 21–44.
85. Dolder MA, Oliver MF: Myocardial infarction in young men: Study of risk factors in nine countries. *Br Heart J* 37:493–503, 1975.
86. Castelli WP, Doyle JT, Gordon T, Hames CG, Hjortland MC, Hulley SB, Kagan A, Zukel WJ: HDL, cholesterol and other lipids in coronary heart disease: The co-operative lipoprotein phenotyping study. *Circulation* 55:767–72, 1977.
87. Fredrickson DS, Goldstein JL, Brown MS: The familial hyperlipoproteinemias. In: Stanbury JB, Wyngaarden JB, Fredrickson DS (eds) *The Metabolic Basis of Inherited Disease*, 4th ed. New york: McGraw-Hill, 1978, pp 604–655.
88. Stamler J: Life styles, major risk factors, proof and public policy. *Circulation* 58:3–19, 1978.
89. The Lipid Research Clinics Coronary Primary Prevention Trial results: I. Reduction in incidence of coronary heart disease. *JAMA* 251:351–364, 1984.
90. Canner PL, Berge KG, Wenger NK, Stamler J, Friedman L, Prineas RJ, Friedenwald W for the Coronary Drug Project Research Group: Fifteen year mortality in Coronary Drug Project patients: Long-term benefit with niacin. *J Am Coll Cardiol* 8:1245–1255, 1986.
91. Brown G, Albers JJ, Fisher LD, Schaefer SM, Lin JT, Kaplan C, Zhao XQ, Bisson BD, Fitzpatrick VT, Dodge HT: Regression of coronary artery disease as a result of intensive lipid-lowering therapy in men with high levels of apolipoprotein B. *N Engl J Med* 323:1289–1298, 1990.
92. Buchwald H, Varco RL, Matts JP, Long JM, Fitch LL, Campbell GS, Pearce MB, Yellin AE, Edmiston WA, Smink RD Jr, Sawin HS, Campos CT, Hansen BJ, Tuna N, Karnegis JN, Sanmarco ME, Amplatz K, Caataneda-Zuniga WR, Hunter DW, Bissett JK, Weber FJ, Stevenson JW, Leon AS, Chalmers TC and the POSCH Group: Effect of partial ileal bypass surgery on mortality and morbidity from coronary heart disease in patients with hypercholesterolemia: Report of the Program on the Surgical Control of the Hyperlipidmias (POSCH). *N Engl J Med* 323:946–955, 1990.
93. Blankenhorn DH, Nessim SA, Johnson RL, Sanmarco ME, Azen SP, Cashen-Hemphill L: Beneficial effects of combined colestipol-miacin therapy on coronary atherosclerosis and coronary venous bypass grafts. *JAMA* 257:3233–3240, 1987.
94. Blankenhorn DH, Johnson RL, Mack WJ, el Zein HA, Vailas LI: The influence of diet on the appearance of new lesions in human coronary arteries. *JAMA* 263:1646–1652, 1990.
95. Ornish D, Brown SE, Scherwitz LW, Billings JH, Armstrong WT, Ports TA, McLanahan SM, Kirkeeide RL, Brand RJ, Gould KL: Can lifestyle changes reverse coronary heart disease? The Lifestyle Heart Trial. *Lancet* 336:129–133, 1990.
96. Kane JP, Malloy MKJ, Ports TA, Phillips NR, Diehl JC, Havel RJ: Regression of coronary atherosclerosis during treatment of familial hypercholesterolemia with combined drug regimens. *JAMA* 264:3007–3012, 1990.
97. Roberts WC: Lipid-lowering therapy after an atherosclerotic event. *Am J Cardiol* 65:16F–18F, 1990.
98. Gwynne JT: HDL and atherosclerosis: An update. *Clin Cardiol* 14:I17–I24, 1991.
99. Reichl D, Miller NE: Pathophysiology of reverse cholesterol transport: Insights from inherited disorders of lipoprotein metabolism. *Arteriosclerosis* 9:785–797, 1989.
100. Badimon JJ, Badimon L, Galvez A, Dische R, Fuster V: High density lipoprotein plasma fractions inhibit aortic fatty streaks in cholesterol-fed rabbits. *Lab Invest* 60:455–461, 1989.
101. Badimon JJ, Badimon L, Fuster V: Regreesion of atherosclerotic lesions by high density lipoprotein plasma fraction in the cholesterol-fed rabbit. *J Clin Invest* 85:1234–1241, 1990.
102 Miller GJ: High density lipoproteins and atherosclerosis. *Annu Rev Med* 31:97–108, 1980.
103. Rubin EM, Krauss RM, Spangler EA, Verstuyft JG, Clift SM: Inhibition of early atherogenesis in transgenic mice by human apolipoprotein AI. *Nature* 353:265–267, 1991.
104. Steinberg D: Underlying mechanisms in atherosclerosis. *J Pathol* 133:75–87, 1981.
105. Haimovici H: Antherogenesis: Recent biological concepts and clinical implications. *Am J Surg* 134:174–178, 1977.
106. Hoff HF, Heideman CL, Jackson RL, Bayardo RJ, Kim H, Gotto AM Jr: Localization patterns of plasma apolipoproteins in human atherosclerotic lesions. *Circ Res* 37:72–79, 1975.
107. Onitini AC, Lewis B, Bentall H, Jamieson C, Wisheart J, Faris I: Lipoprotein concentrations in serum and in biopsy samples of arterial intima: A quantitative comparison. *Atherosclerosis* 23:513–519, 1976.
108. Zilversmit DB: Atherogenesis: A postprandial phenomenon. *Circulation* 60:473–485, 1979.
109. Ross R, Harker L: Hyperlipidemia and atherosclerosis. *Science* 193:1094–1100, 1976.
110. Jackson RL, Gotto AM Jr: Hypothesis concerning membrane structure, cholesterol, and atherosclerosis. In: Paoletti R, Gotto AM Jr (eds) *Atherosclerosis Reviews*, Vol 1. New York: Raven Press, 1976, p 1.
111. Fry DL: Acute vascular endothelial changes associated with increased blood velocity gradients. *Circ Res* 22:165–197, 1968.
112. Fry DL, Haupt MW, Pap JM: Effect of endothelial integrity, transmural pressure, and time on the intimal-medial uptake of serum ^{125}I-albumin and ^{125}I-LDL in an in vitro porcine arterial organ-support system. Arterioscler Thromb 12: 1313–1328, 1992.
113. Gertz SD, Uretzky G, Wajnberg RS, Navot N, Gotsman MS: Endothelial cell damage and thrombus formation following partial arterial constriction: Relevance to the role of coronary artery spasm in the pathogenesis of myocardial infarction. *Circulation* 63:476–486, 1981.
114 Carvalho ACA, Colman RW, Lees RS: Platelet function in hyperlipoproteinemia. *N Engl J Med* 290:434–438, 1974.
115. Yamazaki H, Sano T, Kobayashi I, Takahashi T, Shimamoto T: Enhancement of ADP-induced platelet aggregation by adrenaline and cholesterol in vivo and its prevention. In: Shimamoto T, Numano F (eds) *Atherogenesis II.* Amsterdam: Excerpta Medica, 1973, pp 177–194.
116. Iacono JM, Binder RA, Marshall MW, Shoene NW, Jencks JA, Mackin JF: Decreased susceptibility to thrombin and

collagen platelet aggregation in man fed low fat diet. *Haemostasis* 3:306–318, 1975.

117. Moore S: Pathogenesis of atherosclerosis. *Metabolism* 34(Suppl 1):13–16, 1985.

118. Moore S, Freidman RJ, Singal DP, Gauldie J, Blajchman MA, Roberts RS: Inhibition of injury induced thromboatherosclerotic lesions by antiplatelet serum in rabbits. *Thromb Haemost* 35:70–81, 1976.

119. Moore S: Endothelial injury and atherosclerosis. *Exp Mol Pathol* 31:182–190, 1979.

120. Sprague EA, Steinbach BL, Nerem RM, Schwartz CJ: Influence of a laminar steady state fluid-imposed wall shear stress on the binding, internalization and degradation of low density lipoproteins (LDL) by cultured arterial endothelim. *Circulation* 76:648–657, 1987.

121. Steinbrecher UP, Lougheed M: Scavenger receptor-independent stimulation of cholesterol esterification in macrophages by low density lipoprotein extracted from human aortic intima. *Arterioscler Thromb* 12:608–625, 1992.

122. Steinberg D: Modified forms of LDL and their pathophysiologic significance. 8th International Symposium on Atherosclerosis. Rome: CIC Edizioni Internazional, 1988, pp 1–7.

123. Hessler JR, Morel DW, Lewis LJ, Chisholm GM: Lipoprotein oxidation and lipoprotein-induced cytotoxicity. *Arteriosclerosis* 3:215–222, 1983.

124. Carew T, Schwenke DC, Steinberg D: Antiatherogenic effect of probucol unrelated to its hypocholesterolemic effect: Evidence that the antioxidants in vivo can selectively inhibit low density lipoprotein degradation in macrophage-rich fatty streaks and slow the progression of atherosclerosis in the Watanabe heritable hyperlipidemic (WHHL) rabbit. *Proc Natl Acad Sci USA* 84:7725–7729, 1987.

125. Kita T, Nagano Y, Yokode M, Ishii K, Kume N, Ooshima A, Yoshida H, Kawai C: Probucol prevents the progression of atherosclerosis in Watanabe heritable hyperlipidemic rabbit, an animal model for familial hypercholestrolemia. *Proc Natl Acad Sci USA* 84:5928–5931, 1987.

126. Rosengren A, Wilhelmensen L, Eriksson E, Risberg B, Wedel H: Lipoprotein (a) and coronary heart disease: A prospective case-control study in a general population sample of middle aged men. *Br Med J* 301:1248–1251, 1990.

127. Dahlen GH, Guiyton JR, Attar M, Farmer JA, Kautz JA, Gotto AM Jr: Associations of levels of lipoproteinLp(a), plasma lipids, and other lipoproteins with coronary artery disease documented by angiography. *Circulation* 74:758–765, 1986.

128. Seed M, Hoppichler F, Reaveley D, McCarthy S, Thompson GR, Boerwinkle E, Utermann G: Relation of serum lipoprotein(a) concentration and apolipoprotein(a) phenotype to coronary heart disease patients with familial hypercholesterolemia. *N Engl J Med* 332:1494–1499, 1990.

129. McLean JW, Tomlinson JE, Kuang WJ, Eaton DL, Chen EY, Fless GM, Scanu AM, Lawn RM: cDNA sequence of human apolipoprotein(a) is homologous to plasminogen. *Nature* 330:132–137, 1987.

130. Frank SL, Klisak I, Sparkes RS, Mohandas T, Tomlinson JE, McLean JW, Lawn RM, Lusis AJ: The apoprotein(a) gene resides on human chromosome 6q26–27 in close proximity to the homologous gene for plasminogen. *Hum Genet* 79:352–356, 1988.

131. Karadi I, Kostner GM, Gries A, Nimpf J, Romics L, Malle E: Lipoprotein(a) and plasminogen are immunochemically related. *Biochim Biophys Acta* 960:91–97, 1988.

132. Wolinsky H: A proposal linking clearance of circulating lipoproteins to tissue metabolic activity as a basis for understanding atherogenesis. *Circ Res* 47:301–311, 1980.

133. Stehbens WE: The role of lipid in the pathogenesis of atherosclerosis. *Lancet* 1:724–726, 1975.

134. Ross R, Bowen-Pope DF, Raines EW: Platelet derived growth factor: Its potential roles in wound healing, atherosclerosis, neoplasia, and growth and development. *Ciba Found Symp* 116:98–112, 1985.

135. Ross R: Mechanisms of atherosclerosis — a review. *Adv Nephrol* 19:79–86, 1990.

136. Grotendorst GR, Seppa HEJ, Kleinman HK, Martin GR: Attachment of smooth muscle cells to collagen and their migration toward platelet-derived growth factor. *Proc Natl Acad Sci USA* 78:3669–3672, 1981.

137. Fuster V, Bowie EJW, Lewis JC, Fass DN, Owen CA Jr, Brown AL: Resistance to arteriosclerosis in pigs with von Willebrand's disease. *J Clin Invest* 61:722–730, 1978.

138. Griggs TR, Reddick RL, Sultzer D, Brinkhous KM: Susceptibility of atherosclerosis in aortas and coronary arteries of swine with von Willebrand's disease. *Am J Pathol* 102:137–145, 1981.

139. Moncada S, Gryglewski R, Bunting SL, Vane JR: An enzyme isolated from arteries transforms prostaglandin endoperoxides to an unstable substance that inhibits platelet aggregation. *Nature* 163:663–665, 1976.

140. Mustard JF, Kinlough-Rathbone RL, Packham MA: Prostaglandins and platelets. *Ann Rev Med* 31:89–96, 1980.

141. Joris I, Majno G: Endothelial changes induced by arterial spasm. *Am J Pathol* 102:346–358, 1981.

142. Hirsch EZ, Robertson AL: Selective acute arterial endothelial injury and repair. I. Methodology and surface characteristics. *Atherosclerosis* 28:271–287, 1977.

143. Reidy MA, Schwartz SM: Endothelial regenerating. III. Time course of intimal changes after small defined injury to rat aortic endothelium. *Lab Invest* 44:301–308, 1981.

144. Banai S, Haggroth L, Epstein SE, Casscells W: Influence of extracellular magnesium on capillary endothelial cell proliferation and migration. *Circ Res* 67:645–650, 1990.

145. Fry DL: Hemodynamic forces in atherogenesis. In: Scheinberg P (ed) *Cerebrovascular Diseases*. New York: Raven Press, 1976, pp 77–95.

146. Caplan BA, Schwartz CJ: Increased endothelial cell turnover in areas of in vivo Evans blue up-take in the pig aorta. *Atherosclerosis* 17:401–417, 1973.

147. Wright HP: Endothelial turnover. *Thromb Diath Heamorrh* 40(Suppl):79–85, 1970.

148. Gertz SD, Forbes MS, Sunaga T, Kawamura J, Rennels ML, Shimamoto T, Nelson E: Ischemic carotid endothelium: Transmission electron microscopic studies. *Arch Pathol Lab Med* 100:522–526, 1976.

149. Nelson E, Gertz SD, Forbes MS, Rennels ML, Heald FD, Khan MA, Farber TM, Miller E, Husain MM, Earl FL: Endothelial lesions in the aorta of egg yolk-fed miniature swine: A study by scanning and transmission electron microscopy. *Exp Mol Pathol* 25:208–220, 1976.

150. Lewis JC, Kottke BA: Endothelial damage and thrombocyte adhesion in pigeon atherosclerosis. *Science* 196:1007–1009, 1977.

151. Geissinger HD, Mustard JF, Rowsell HC: The occurrence of microthrombi on the aortic endothelium of swine. *Can Med Assoc J* 87:405–408, 1962.

152. Gerrity RG, Naito HK, Richardson M, Schwartz CJ: Dietary induced atherogenesis in swine: Morphology of the intima in prelesion stage. *Am J Pathol* 95:775–786, 1979.

153. Texon M: *Hemodynamic Basis of Atherosclerosis*. New York: McGraw-Hill, 1970.

154. Ku DN, Giddens DP, Zarins CK, Glagov S: Pulsatile flow and atherosclerosis in the human carotid bifurcation. Posi-

tive correlation between plaque location and low and oscillating shear stress. *Arteriosclerosis* 5:293–302, 1985.

155. Veress B, Balint A, Kocze A, Nazy Z, Jellinek H: Increasing aortic permeability by atherogenic diet. *Atherosclerosis* 11:369–371, 1970.

156. Bretherton KN, Day AJ, Skinner SL: Effect of hypertension on the entry of ^{125}I-labeled low density lipoprotein into
the aortic intima in normal-fed rabbits. *Atherosclerosis* 24:99–106, 1976.

157. Schwartz SM: Hypertension, endothelial injury and atherosclerosis. *Cardiovasc Med* 2:991–1002, 1977.

158. Heistad DD, Lopez JAG, Baumbach GJ: Hemodynamic determinants of vascular changes in hypertension and atherosclerosis. *Hypertension* 17(Suppl III):III7–III11, 1991.

159. Bondjers G, Glukhova M, Hansson GK, Postnov YV, Reidy MA, Schwartz SM: Hypertension and atherosclerosis: Cause and effect, or two effects with one unknown cause? *Circulation* 84(Suppl VI):VI2–VI16, 1991.

160. Wexler BC, Iams SG, Judd JT: Arterial lesions in repeatedly bred spontaneously hypertensive rats. *Circ Res* 38:494–501, 1976.

161. Haudenschild CC, Prescott MF, Chobanian AV: Effects of hypertension and its reversal on aortic intima lesions of rat. *Hypertension* 2:33–44, 1980.

162. Giacomelli F, Weiner J, Spiro D: The cellular pathology of experimental hypertension. V. Increased permeability of cerebral arterial vessels. *Am J Pathol* 59:133–160, 1970.

163. Huttner I, Boutet M, More RH: Studies on protein passage through arterial endothelium. III. Effect of blood pressure levels on the passage of fine structural protein tracers through rat arterial endothelium. *Lab Invest* 29:536–546, 1973.

164. Bevan RD: An autoradiographic and pathological study of cellular proliferation in rabbit arteries correlated with an increase in arterial pressure. *Blood Vessels* 13:100–128, 1976.

165. Fry DL: Steady-state macromolecular transport across a multilayered arterial wall. *Math Model* 6:353–368, 1985.

166. Spence JD: Hemodynamic effects of antihypertensive drugs. Possible implications for the prevention of atherosclerosis. *Hypertension* 6(Suppl III):III163–III168, 1984.

167. Dhurandhar RW, Watt DL, Silver MD, Trimble AS, Adelman AG: Prinzmetal's variant form of angina with arteriographic evidence of coronary spasm. *Am J Cardiol* 30:902–905, 1972.

168. Chahine RA, Luchi RJ: Coronary arterial spasm: Culprit or bystander? *Am J Cardiol* 37:936–937, 1976.

169. Meller J, Pichard A, Dack S: Coronary arterial spasm in Prinzmetal's variant angina: A proved hypothesis. *Am J Cardiol* 37:938–940, 1976.

170. Maseri A, L'Abbate A, Baroldi G, Chierchia S, Marzilli M, Ballestra AM, Severi S, Parodi O, Biagini A, Distance A, Pesola A: Coronary vasospasm as a possible cause of myocardial infarction. *N Eng J Med* 299:1271–1277, 1978.

171. Braunwald E: Coronary artery spasm as a cause of myocardial ischemia. *J Lab Clin Med* 97:299–312, 1981.

172. Hellstrom HR: The injury-spasm and vascular autoregulatory hypothesis of ischemic disease. *Am J Cardiol* 49:802–810, 1982.

173. Epstein SE, Cannon RO, Watson RM, Leon MB, Bonow RO, Rosing DR: Dynamic coronary obstruction as a cause of angina pectoris: Implications regarding therapy. *Am J Cardiol* 55:61B–68B, 1985.

174. Conti CR: Myocardial infarction: Thoughts about patho-

genesis and the role of coronary artery spasm. *Am Heart J* 110:187–193, 1985.

175. Maseri A, Chierchia S, Koski JC: Mixed angina pectoris. *Am J Cardiol* 56:30E–33E, 1985.

176. Folts JD, Crowell EB, Rowe GG: Platelet aggregation in partially obstructed vessels and its elimination with aspirin. *Circulation* 54:365–370, 1976.

177. Turitto VT, Baumgartner HR: Platelet interaction with subendothelium in flowing rabbit blood: Effect of blood shear rate. *Microvasc Res* 17:38–4, 1979.

178. Gertz SD, Wajnberg RS, Kurgan A, Uretzky G: Effect of magnesium sulfate on thrombus formation following partial arterial constriction: Implications for coronary vasospasm. *Magnesium* 6:225–235, 1987.

179. Gutstein WH, Lataillade JN, Lewis L: Role of vasoconstriction in experimental arteriosclerosis. *Circ Res* 10:925–932, 1962.

180. Betz E, Schlote W: Responses of vessel walls to chronically applied electrical stimuli. *Basic Res Cardiol* 74:10–20, 1979.

181. Lown B, De Silva RA: Is coronary arterial spasm a risk factor for coronary atherosclerosis? *Am J Cardiol* 45:901–903, 1980.

182. Marzilli M, Goldstein S, Trivella MG, Palumbo C, Maseri A: Some clinical considerations regarding the relation of coronary vasospasm to coronary atherosclerosis: A hypothetical pathogenesis. *Am J Cardiol* 45:882–886, 1980.

183. Dalen JE, Ochene IS, Alpert JS: Coronary spasm, coronary thrombosis and myocardial infarction: A hypothesis concerning the pathophysiology of acute myocardial infarction. *Am Heart J* 104:1119–1124, 1982.

184. Gutstein WH: Coronary spasm and coronary atherosclerosis. *Am J Cardiol* 48:389–390, 1981.

185. Luchi RJ, Chahine RA: Coronary artery spasm, coronary artery thrombosis, and myocardial infarction. *Ann Intern Med* 95:502–505, 1981.

186. Braunwald E: A symposium: Experimental and clinical aspects of coronary vasoconstriction. *Am J Cardiol* 56:1E–29E, 1985.

187. Kurgan A, Gertz SD, Wajnberg RS: Intimal changes associated with arterial spasm induced by periarterial application of calcium chloride. *Exp Mol Pathol* 39:176–193, 1983.

188. Chapman I: Morphogenesis of occluding artery thrombosis. *Arch Pathol Lab Med* 80:256–261, 1965.

189. Friedman M, Van Den Bovenkamp GJ: The pathogenesis of a coronary thrombus. *Am J Pathol* 48:19–31, 1966.

190. Ridolfi RL, Hutchins GM: The relationship between coronary artery lesions and myocardial infarcts: Ulceration of atherosclerotic plaques precipitating coronary thrombosis. *Am Heart J* 93:468–486, 1977.

191. Horie T, Sekiguchi M, Hirosawa K: Coronary thrombosis in pathogenesis of acute myocardial infarction: Histopathological study of coronary arteries in 108 necropsied cases using serial section. *Br Heart J* 40:153–161, 1978.

192. Falk E: Plaque rupture with severe pre-existing stenosis precipitating coronary thrombosis: Characteristics of coronary atherosclerotic plaques underlying fatal occlusive thrombi. *Br Heart J* 50:127–134, 1983.

193. Ambrose JA, Winters SL, Stern A, Eng A, Teichholz LE, Gorlin R, Fuster V: Angiographic morphology and the pathogenesis of unstable angina pectoris. *J Am Coll Cardiol* 5:609–616, 1985.

194. Fuster V, Badimon L, Cohen M, Ambrose JA, Badimon JJ, Chesebro J: Insights into the pathogenesis of acute ischemic syndromes. *Circulation* 77:1213–1220, 1988.

195. Davies MJ: Successful and unsuccessful coronary thrombolysis. *Br Heart J* 61:381–384, 1989.

196. Falk E: Morphologic features of unstable atherothrombotic plaques underlying acute coronary syndromes. *Am J Cardiol* 63:114E–120E, 1989.

197. Muller JE, Tofler GH, Stone PH: Circadian variation and triggers of onset of acute cardiovascular disease. *Circulation* 79:733–743, 1989.

198. Alpert JS: The pathophysiology of acute myocardial infarction. *Cardiology* 76:85–95, 1989.

199. Gertz SD, Roberts WC: Hemodynamic shear force in rupture of coronary arterial atherosclerotic plaques. *Am J Cardiol* 66:1368–1372, 1990.

200. Paterson JC: Vascularization and hemorrhage of the intima of arteriosclerotic coronary arteries. *Arch Pathol* 22: 313–324, 1936.

201. Paterson JC: Capillary rupture with intimal hemorrhage as a causative factor in coronary thrombosis. *Arch Pathol* 25: 474–487, 1938.

202. Barger AC, Beeuwkes R, Lainey LL, Silverman KJ: Hypothesis: Vasa vasorum and neovascularization of human coronary arteries. A possible role in the pathophysiology of atherosclerosis. *N Engl J Med* 310:175–177, 1984.

203. Baroldi G, Mariani F, Silver MD, Giuliano G: Correlation of morphologic variables in the coronary atherosclerotic plaque with clinical patterns of ischemic heart disease. *Am J Cardiovasc Pathol* 2:159–172, 1988.

204. Davies MJ, Thomas AC: Plaque fissuring — the cause of acute myocardial infarction, sudden ischaemic death, and crescendo angina. *Br Heart J* 53:363–373, 1985.

205. Constantinides P: Plaque fissures in human coronary thrombosis. *J Atheroscler Res* 6:1–17, 1966.

206. Wilson RF: An artery has many masters. *Circulation* 81: 1147–1150, 1990.

207. Santamore WP, Yelton BW Jr, Ogilby JD: Dynamics of coronary occlusion in the pathogenesis of myocardial infarction. *J Am Coll Cardiol* 18:1397–1405, 1991.

208. Hellstrom HR: Evidence in favor of the vasospastic cause of coronary artery thrombosis. *Am Heart J* 97:449–452, 1979.

209. Alpert JS: Coronary vasomotion, coronary thrombosis, myocardial infarction and the camel's back. *J Am Coll Cardiol* 5:617–8, 1985.

210. Maseri A, Pesola A, Marzilli M, Severi S, Paroldi O, L'Abbate A, Ballestra AM, Maltinti G, De Nes DM, Biagini A: Coronary vasospasm in angina pectoris. *Lancet* 2:713–717, 1977.

211. Gensini GG: Coronary artery spasm and angina pectoris. *Chest* 68:709–713, 1975.

212. Ganz P, Alexander RW: New insights into the cellular mechanisms of vasospasm. *Am J Cardiol* 56:11E–15E, 1985.

213. Hoak JC: The endothelium, platelets, and coronary vasospasm. *Adv Intern Med* 34:353–375, 1989.

214. Tracy RE, Devaney K, Kissling G: Characteristics of the plaque under a coronary thrombus. *Virchows Arch (Pathol Anat)* 405:411–427, 1985.

215. Richardson PD, Davies MJ, Born GVR: Influence of plaque configuration and stress distribution on fissuring of coronary atherosclerotic plaques. *Lancet* 2:941–944, 1989.

216. Constantinides P, Lawder J: Experimental thrombosis and hemorrhage in atherosclerotic arteries. *Fed Proc* 22: 251–259, 1963.

217. Loree HM, Kamm RD, Stringfellow RG, Lee RT: Effects of fibrous cap thickness on peak circumferential stress in model atherosclerotic vessels. *Circ Res* 71:850–858, 1992.

218. McMahon MM, Brown BG, Cukingnan R, Rolett EL, Bolson E, Frimer M, Dodge HT: Quantitative coronary angiography: Measurement of the "critical" stenosis in patients with unstable angina and single-vessel disease without collaterals. *Circulation* 60:106–113, 1979.

219. Little WC, Constantinescu M, Applegate RJ, Kutcher MA, Burrows MT, Kahl FR, Santamore WP: Can angiography predict the site of a subsequent myocardial infarction in patients with mild-to-moderate coronary artery disease? *Circulation* 78:1157–1166, 1988.

220. Ambrose JA, Tannenbaum MA, Alexopoulos D, Hjemdahl-Monsen CE, Leavy J, Weiss M, Barrico S, Gorlin R, Fuster V: Angiographic progression of coronary artery disease and the development of myocardial infarction. *J Am Coll Cardiol* 12:56–62, 1988.

221. Blaumanis OR, Grady PA, Nelson E: Hemodynamic and morphological aspects of cerebral vasospasm. In: Price TR, Nelson E (eds) *Cerebrovascular Diseases.* New York: Raven Press, 1979, pp 283–294.

222. McDonald DA: *Blood Flow in Arteries.* Baltimore, MD: Williams and Wilkins, 1974.

223. Cohen M, Fuster V: Insights into the pathogenetic mechanisms of unstable angina. *Haemostasis* 20(Suppl 1): 102–112, 1990.

224. Fuster V, Stein B, Ambrose JA, Badimon L, Badimon JJ, Chesebro JH: Atherosclerotic plaque rupture and thrombosis: Evolving concepts. *Circulation* 82(Suppl II):II47–II59, 1990.

225. Shah PK, Forrester JS: Pathophysiology of acute coronary syndromes. *Am J Cardiol* 68:16C–23C, 1991.

226. Little WC, Downes TR, Applegate RJ: The underlying coronary lesion in myocardial infarction: Implications for coronary angiography. *Clin Cardiol* 14:868–874, 1991.

227. Barnhart GR, Pascoe EA, Mills AS, Szentpetery S, Eich DM, Mohanakumar T, Hastillo A, Thompson JA, Hess ML, Lower RR. Accelerated coronary arteriosclerosis in cardiac transplant recipients. *Transplant Rev* 1:31–46, 1987.

228. Fuster VF, Chesebro JH: Role of platelets and platelet inhibitors in aortocoronary artery vein-graft disease. *Circulation* 73:227–232, 1986.

229. McBride W, Lange RA, Hillis DL. Restenosis after successful coronary angioplasty: Pathophysiology and prevention. *N Engl J Med* 318:1734–1737, 1988.

230. Billingham ME: Cardiac transplant atherosclerosis. *Transplant Proc* 19(Suppl 5):19–25, 1987.

231. Hess ML, Hastillo JA, Thompson DJ, Sansonetti S, Szentpetery GB, Lower RR: Lipid mediators in organ transplantation: Does cyclosporin accelerate coronary atherosclerosis? *Transplant Proc* 19(Suppl 5):71–73, 1987.

232. Uretsky BF, Murali S, Reddy PS, Rabin B, Lee A, Griffith BP, Hardesty RL, Tento A, Bahnson HT: Development of coronary artery disease in cardiac transplant patients receiving immunosuppressive therapy with cyclosporin and prednisone. *Circulation* 76:827–834, 1987.

233. Nitkin RS, Schroeder JS: Accelerated coronary artery disease risk in heart transplant patients. *J Am Coll Cardiol* 5:535, 1985.

234. Vlodaver Z, Edwards JE: Pathologic changes in aortic-coronary arterial saphenous vein grafts. *Circulation* 44:719–728, 1971.

235. Clowes AW, Schwartz SM: Significance of quiescent smooth muscle migration in the injured rat carotid artery. *Circ Res* 56:139–145, 1985.

236. Clowes AW, Clowes MM, Reidy MA: Kinetics of cellular proliferation after arterial injury: III. Endothelial and smooth muscle growth in chronically denuded vessels. *Lab Invest* 54:295–303, 1986.

237. Ip JH, Fuster V, Badimon L, Badimon J, Taubman MB, Chesebro JH: Syndromes of accelerated atherosclerosis: Role of vascular injury and smooth muscle cell proliferation. *J Am Coll Cardiol* 15:1667–1687, 1990.

238. Epstein SE, Siegall CB, Sadatoshi Biro Fu YM, FitzGerald

D, Pastan I: Cytotoxic effects of recombinant chimeric toxin on rapidly proliferating vascular smooth muscle cells. *Circulation* 84:778–787, 1991.

239. Simons M, Edelman ER, DeKeyser JL, Langer R, Rosenberg RD: Antisense c-myb oligonucleotides inhibit intimal arterial smooth muscle cell accumulation in vivo. *Nature* 359:67–70, 1992.

CHAPTER 44

Endothelial Control of Vascular Smooth Muscle:
Importance of Nitric Oxide

CATHERINE M. VENTURINI & UNA S. RYAN

INTRODUCTION

One hundred and twenty-five years ago, Virchow saw the endothelium as "... a membrane as simple as any that is met in the body"; today this is far from our view of vascular biology. The endothelial lining of blood vessels possesses functional properties of great intricacy. It provides (a) a nonthrombogenic surface; (b) mediates the passage of solutes, nutrients, lipids, and hormones to the interstitium; (c) maintains a patent lumen; and (d) regulates vascular tone. The regulation of smooth muscle is a dynamic process that is under fine control by the endothelium. This chapter reviews the morphology of the myoendothelial junction, the role of endothelium-derived relaxing factors in the control of vascular tone, and endothelial control of smooth muscle proliferation.

MORPHOLOGY OF THE MYOENDOTHELIAL JUNCTION

Intima

Blood vessels, historically, are divided into three distinct morphological areas: intima, media, and adventitia. The internal elastic lamina denotes the border between intima and media. The intimal layer is defined as {1} the "region of the arterial wall from, and including, the endothelial surface at the lumen, to the luminal margin of the media." The media consists mostly of layers of smooth muscle cells and makes up the bulk of the vessel. The adventitia is comprised of connective tissue, fibroblasts, nerves, and vasa vasorum.

A clear definition of intima comprising endothelium and media as smooth muscle is not strictly held in all species. Thomas {2} and Koo {3} described focal clusters of smooth muscle cells in the intima of vessels of healthy, untreated pigs. Blood vessels from infants and children under the age of five were examined by Stary as an indicator of the state of healthy human blood vessels. Smooth muscle cells were observed in the intima of each of 63 children studied {4}.

There appears to be a population of resident intimal smooth muscle cells in the "normal" blood vessel of hu-

mans (fig. 44-1) but this is not true in some other animals, even several species of nonhuman primate {5}. These cells may be the source of plaque smooth muscle and the site from which atherosclerotic lesions grow {for review see 6,7}. It is important to consider these differences in vascular morphology when developing animal models of atherosclerosis.

Myoendothelial interactions

The majority of smooth muscle cells are located in the media of normal blood vessels and are separated from the endothelium by the internal elastic lamina. Still, the endothelium and smooth muscle are in close communication, both in the intima and across the intimal-medial barrier.

Serial thin sections demonstrate extensions of smooth muscle cells through the internal elastic lamina that physically contact the abluminal surface of the endothelial lining {8}. Myoendothelial contacts have been seen as cytoplasmic projections passing through the fenestrae in the lamina of human renal biopsies {9}. The contacts are numerous and in small pulmonary arteries 150 such interactions were visualized in one thin section {10}.

Endothelial cell-smooth muscle cell interactions are primarily via gap junctions where cytoplasmic bridges of smooth muscle cells extend through fenestrations in the internal elastic lamina to contact the endothelium {11}. Gap junctions provide a pathway for the transportation of ions and small molecules {12} and could provide a route of entry of mediators from endothelium to smooth muscle and vice versa. In addition, some endothelium-derived factors are freely diffusible and penetrate smooth muscle cells directly, independent of gap junctions. Others bind to receptors on the surface of the smooth muscle cell and elicit responses through second messengers.

The endothelium and smooth muscle cells form an integrated alliance through membrane interaction. The close association of these two cell types allows for the efficacy of the most influential of the endothelium-derived vasomodulating factors, endothelium-derived relaxing factor (EDRF), and demonstrates the transducing role of the endothelium. Thus a blood-borne agonist, interacting with receptors on the endothelial cells, leads to release of a mediator that modulates smooth muscle relaxation.

N. Sperelakis (ed.), Physiology and Pathophysiology of the Heart, Third Edition.

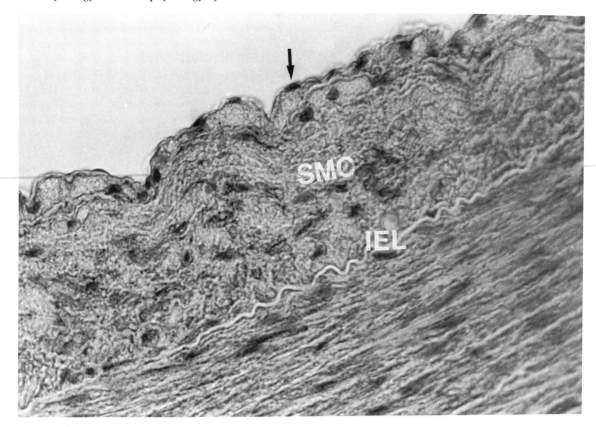

Fig. 44-1. Light micrograph of a rabbit aorta, showing smooth muscle cells (SMC) stained with antibodies to α-actin (HHF35) within the intima. IEL = internal elastic lamina; endothelium is indicated by the arrow. Counterstained with hematoxylin. Original magnification 40×.

ENDOTHELIUM-DEPENDENT RELAXATION

One of the most important functions of the endothelium is the regulation of vascular tone. Many humoral regulators of blood pressure exert their effects by binding cell surface receptors on the endothelium and eliciting a second messenger response. In the past 15 years, a new mode of cellular communication has come to light that does not require cell surface receptor binding.

The best defined mediator of this type is nitric oxide (NO). This mediator accounts for the vasodilatory effect of many endothelial receptor agonists. A labile free radical gas, it activates guanylate cyclase and exerts its effects through its redox potential. The general physiology and pathophysiology of NO, and its role in the central nervous system and inflammatory disease, have been comprehensively reviewed recently {13}.

Endothelium-derived relaxing factor

Furchgott and Zawadski demonstrated that endothelial cells control acetylcholine-induced vasodilation in preconstricted aortic rings {14}. The humoral nature and short half-life of this endothelium-derived substance (coined EDRF) were demonstrated in pharmacological preparations in which this substance is transferred from a superfused "donor" vessel segment to a detector strip of smooth muscle {15}.

Early recognition of pharmacological properties of this factor assisted in the delineation of its function. The factor is inhibited by hemoglobin and methylene blue {16}. It elicits an increase in cGMP in the target smooth muscle cells {17}. Its effects are potentiated by superoxide dismutase {18}.

Based on the similarities of the action of EDRF and acidified nitrite, Furchgott {19} suggested that EDRF may be nitric oxide (NO). The biological actions of EDRF and authentic NO were demonstrated to be similar in vascular strip preparations {21} and on platelets {22}. These studies demonstrated that NO, like EDRF, has a short half-life under physiological conditions and activates guanylate cyclase.

There is a degree of controversy over the chemical identity of EDRF. However, pharmacological, biochemical, and chemical evidence suggest that EDRF is NO or a labile nitroso precursor {20}, and it is celar that NO, or a closely related species, activates guanylate cyclase in many target cells. EDRF/NO is responsible for a wide variety of effects throughout the body, not just in vasomotor control.

Endothelium-derived nitric oxide

In the atmosphere, it takes thunder and lightning to generate NO, but a wide variety of cells can make it, with the proper stimulus {23}. The enzyme responsible for the generation of NO is nitric oxide synthase (NOS; EC 1.14.13.39). Endothelial NOS has been characterized {24} and cloned {25}.

NOS reacts with the guanidino nitrogen of L-arginine {26} and incorporates molecular oxygen into its products: NO and citrulline {27}. There is a requirement for a unique cadre of cofactors: FAD, FMN, tetrahydrobiopterin, and NADPH {for review see 28}. Endothelial NOS is closely controlled by calcium in the 100–500 nM range, regulating the reversible binding of calmodulin {29,30}. There is some evidence that the enzyme can localize to the cell membrane {31}.

Endothelium-dependent relaxation occurs basally, perhaps as a function of sheer stress or flow {32}. A wide variety of agonists increase the production of NO: acetylcholine, bradykinin, substance P, thrombin, adenine nucleotides, and calcium ionophore. NO release explains the mechanism of action of these vasodilators. It seems that calcium is the rate-limiting cofactor in the generation of NO from NOS in endothelium. Increases in endothelial intracellular calcium may be the mechanism of NO generation by most of these agonists {33}.

NO formed by endothelial cells will quickly diffuse across membranes to nearby smooth muscle cells because it is a gas. It is not limited, as are other larger signaling molecules, by the ability of the producing cell to release it or the target cell to bind or recognize it.

There is some evidence that NO can exist as an adduct of free thiols that have a longer half-life than NO. S-nitrosothiols have been identified in human plasma, primarily as S-nitrosoalbumin {34}. Nitric oxide may react reversibly with free thiol containing proteins to form S-nitrosoproteins under physiologic conditions {35}. These S-nitroso compounds may represent a mechanism for the transfer of a stable form of nitric oxide through the blood. However, it is not clear whether these reactions of NO with protein are important in the transfer of NO abluminally from endothelium to smooth muscle or whether they play a role in intracellular storage of NO.

Luminally released NO binds rapidly with oxyhemoglobin, which is abundant in the red blood cells and is converted to inactive nitrite:

$$NO + O_2Hb \rightarrow NO_3^- + Hb^+;$$

and on the venous side, NO reacts with deoxyhemoglobin {36}:

$$NO + Hb \rightarrow NOHb$$

In this manner NO is effectively removed by the blood, preventing its action on cells downstream.

Another important mechanism of clearing NO is superoxide (O_2^-):

$$NO+ \rightarrow ONOO^- \rightarrow NO_3^-$$

This explains early observations with superfused arterial segments that superoxide dismutase potentiates while O_2^--generating compounds inhibit the bioactivity of EDRF.

The importance of NO in the physiological control of blood flow, vessel tone, and blood pressure has been clearly demonstrated by the use of inhibitors of its production. Administration of an altered form of arginine, L-N^G-monomethyl-L-arginine (L-NMMA), into the isolated brachial artery of humans causes direct vasoconstriction and inhibits vasodilation to acetylcholine or bradykinin {37}. Blood pressure increases approximately 30% in animals after an infusion of L-NMMA {38}. The smooth muscle of arterial vessels appears to be under a constant, basal vasodilatory stimulus, due to the production of NO from the vascular endothelium.

One of the ways that endothelial cells communicate with the underlying smooth muscle is by NO release (fig. 44-2). The smooth muscle cells respond when NO binds the soluble guanylate cyclase in the cytosol of the cells. The heme group of guanylate cyclase is obligatory for activation by NO {39}. Vascular relaxation is mediated by the resulting increase in cyclic GMP (cGMP) {for review see 40}.

Induction of NO synthase in the blood vessel

We have so far discussed only the constitutive nitric oxide synthase that is present in endothelial cells and is responsible for the basal and agonist-induced production of NO. Normally, smooth muscle cells do not generate NO. However, inducible NOS (iNOS) is expressed in both endothelial cells and smooth muscle cells in response to inflammatory stimuli.

NO generation is dramatically increased in response to cytokines in vascular endothelial cells in culture. Low levels of NOS activity, from constitutive NOS, can be detected in untreated endothelial cells in culture. When cells are exposed to LPS and interferon-γ, there is a sharp increase in NOS activity and NO generation {43}. The activity of this induced enzyme is calcium independent {44}, unlike the calcium-regulated constitutive enzyme.

The production of NO can be induced in vascular smooth muscle cells as well as endothelial cells. iNOS activity in cultured smooth muscle cells was demonstrated after stimulation with TNF and IFN-γ {43} or IL-1 {44}. Induction increases smooth muscle cGMP {45}.

The induction of NOS takes place spontaneously in deendothelialized aortic rings preconstricted with phenylephrine over a period of 8 hours. The relaxation is potentiated by L-arginine, accompanied by an increase in smooth muscle cGMP, and is inhibited by L-NMMA, indicating the production of NO directly from vascular smooth muscle. This spontaneous relaxation is inhibited by cycloheximide, an inhibitor of protein synthesis, indicating iNOS is synthesized de novo during the induction period {46}.

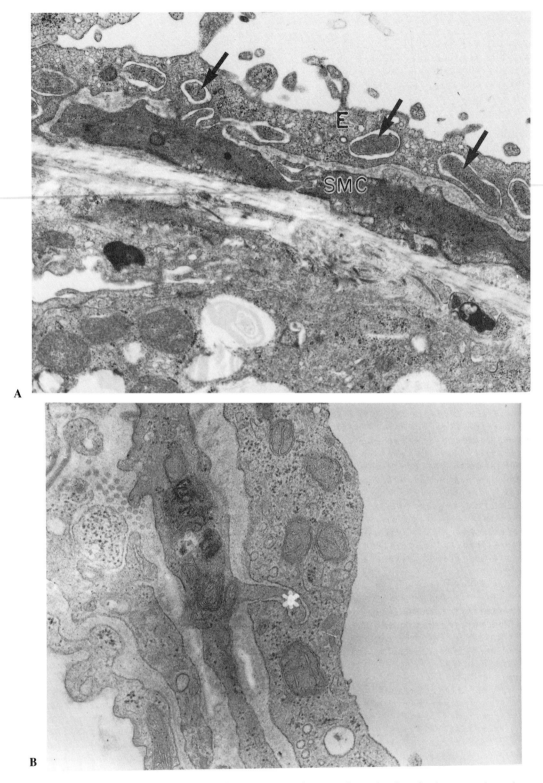

Fig. 44-2. **A:** Electron micrograph of a small pulmonary artery in a rat lung showing the large number of myoendothelial interdigitations (arrows) between smooth muscle cells (SMC) and endothelium (E). Original magnification. **B:** Higher magnification of a myoendothelial interaction (*) in a rat pulmonary arteriole. Original magnification.

In vivo LPS also triggers the expression of iNOS in blood vessels. In rats that were injected with endotoxin {47}, calcium-independent NOS activity is seen in the aorta and a significant decrease in blood pressure results. In fact, the expression of iNOS after endotoxin treatment is widespread, including the heart, spleen, liver, and gut {23}.

The induction of NOS in the blood vessel has important relevance to severe hypotension seen in septic shock. The cardiovascular damage of septic shock is largely due to endotoxin in the blood. Endotoxin has been shown to stimulate the synthesis of cytokines, and overproduction of NO may be a mechanism accounting for the breakdown of vascular tone regulation in these patients.

Endotoxin-mediated hypotension is reversed in dogs treated with an inhibitor of NOS {48}. However, in endotoxin-treated rabbits, a higher dose of L-NMMA caused a precipitous decline in blood pressure and death {49}. These higher doses of L-NMMA may have caused a total blockade of NO synthesis, causing severe ischemia. In patients with severe septic shock, L-NMMA caused a rapid dose-dependent increase in mean arterial pressure {50}. NO synthase inhibitors may be useful in the treatment of septic shock if complete inhibition of NO production is avoided {51}.

The constitutive and inducible NOS enzymes have many characteristics in common. They are regulated by similar cofactors (FAD, FMN, NADPH, BH4), use the same substrate (L-arginine), and are of a similar molecular weight. However, they produce nitric oxide at a different rate and are differentially inhibited by competitive analogues of arginine {for summary see 13}.

One of the most important functional differences between the constitutive and inducible enzymes is the calcium dependency. Much of the work on the inducible enzyme has been conducted in the macrophage, which is induced in a manner similar to the smooth muscle cell. In the macrophage, inducible NOS activity is independent of added calcium, and is not inhibited by agents that interfere with the functioning of calmodulin {52}. An interesting observation from the characterization of murine macrophage iNOS is that calmodulin copurifies with the enzyme so tightly that it can be considered a subunit of the enzyme {53}. It is very unusual that calmodulin binding is not dependent on calcium concentration. So it seems that the tight affinity of calmodulin to the protein is a sharp distinction between the two types of NOS {for review see 28}.

The role of NO in the regulation of smooth muscle tone is multifaceted. In the simplest state, endothelial cells produce NO from L-arginine via the constitutive NOS. This is probably calcium regulated and NO diffuses to the surrounding tissue, stimulates smooth muscle cell guanylate cyclase, and the vessel relaxes, providing a patent system of tubes through which blood can flow. In response to several vasodilatory agonists, the endothelial cell generates an additional burst of NO and the vessels relax transiently. However in some pathological states where cytokines and endotoxin are present, both endothelial cells and smooth muscle cells are induced to express the

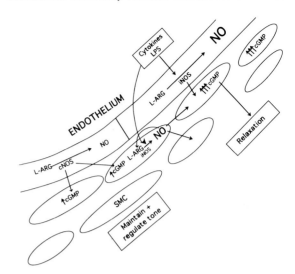

Fig. 44-3. L-Arg:NO pathway in regulation of vascular tone (left), and induction of NOS leading to hypotension (right).

protein iNOS, which is not regulated by calcium, and a large sustained generation of NO follows. This can lead to systemic hypotension, as in states of septic shock. Endothelial control of smooth muscle cell function is lost in this induced state, and a marked lowering of blood pressure results (fig. 44-3).

REGULATION OF SMOOTH MUSCLE CELL PROLIFERATION

The endothelium also regulates smooth muscle cell proliferation. Mechanical {54} and air-induced {55} endothelial denudation stimulate medial outgrowth. The regeneration of the endothelial lining coincides with a decrease in smooth muscle cell proliferation {56}. Further, endothelial desquamation leads to an increase in DNA synthesis {57} and early protooncogene expression {58}, similar to that of cultured human atherosclerotic plaque cells {59}.

Cultured endothelial cells produce a heparinlike factor, which inhibits smooth muscle cell proliferation in vitro {60}. Regenerating endothelium accumulates more heparan sulfate containing glycosaminoglycans {61}. This glycosaminoglycan is less prevalent in atherosclerotic tissue {62}.

Another mechanism by which the endothelium may control proliferation of smooth muscle is by the antiproliferative function of NO. Nitric oxide generating vasodilators and 8-bromo cyclic GMP, a cell-permeable analog of the second messenger of NO {63,64}, and authentic NO {65} inhibit cultured smooth muscle cell serum-induced DNA synthesis. Inhibition of proliferation was limited in the presence of hemoglobin and augmented with superoxide dismutase. Atrial natriuretic factor, which also increases cGMP, inhibits smooth muscle cell proliferation {66}.

This effect of NO may be specific for smooth muscle cells in the synthetic phenotype. 8-bromo cyclic GMP did not inhibit DNA synthesis in rabbit aortic smooth muscle cells from explants {67}. However, when these cell were passaged and differentiated into a synthetic phenotype, both 8-bromo cGMP and SIN-1, an NO donor, inhibited DNA synthesis {68}. Nitric oxide may act as an antiproliferative agent in cells differentiated into a synthetic phenotype, such as those found in atherosclerotic plaque.

Further evidence that NO inhibits smooth muscle cell proliferation involves induction of NOS in smooth muscle cells in culture. Stimulation of ^{3}H-thymidine incorporation by growth factors was reduced when NO synthase was induced by IL-1β {69} or IFN-γ {70}. This is reversed by treatment with NOS inhibitors. Further, impairment of NO production was observed after treatment with the mitogen, PDGF, indicating that growth factors may repress NO induction {69}. Advanced glycosylation endproducts, which accumulate on basement membrane proteins of diabetic patients, chemically inactivate NO {71} and block the antiproliferative effect of NO on smooth muscle and renal mesangial cells {72}.

One of the first alterations following hypercholesterolemia is loss of endothelium-dependent relaxation. There is a wealth of evidence, in vitro and in vivo in several animal models, indicating that diet-induced experimental atherosclerosis leads to impaired endothelium-dependent vasodilation early in the disease process {for review see 71}. This occurs before the appearance of morphological changes in the artery and endothelium-independent relaxations remain intact {74–80}. Impaired responses have been demonstrated in nonhuman primates {81,82} and patients in the early stages of coronary atherosclerosis {83}. Low density lipoproteins are inhibitors of NO {84,85} and inhibit arteriolar relaxation {86}.

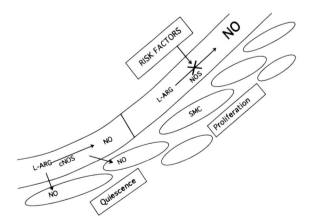

Fig. 44-4. Cardiovascular risk factors, such as hypertension, hypoxia, and hypercholesterolemia, may lead to SMC prolification via loss of NO.

There are several mechanisms proposed for the loss of endothelium-dependent relaxation after hypercholesterolemia (fig. 44-4). L-arginine supplementation does not augment endothelium-dependent vasorelaxation in normal vessels {87}, and plasma L-arginine levels are normal in patients with hypercholesterolemia {88}. However, L-arginine augments endothelium-dependent vasodilation in cholesterol-fed rabbit vessels from various beds {89,90,91}. Infusion of L-arginine had a similar effect in the forearm {92} and coronary microcirculation {93} of hypercholesterolemic humans. This suggests that an L-arginine deficiency may be responsible for a decreased synthesis of NO. Further, reduction in NO synthesis could contribute to the smooth muscle cell proliferation seen in early atherogenesis.

Chronic oral administration of L-arginine in the drinking water of rabbits also receiving moderate cholesterol supplementation decreased the surface area and intimal thickness of atherosclerotic lesions in the thoracic aorta {94}. There was an associated improvement in the loss of endothelium-dependent relaxation.

Alternatively, loss of NO-induced relaxation could result from increased destruction of NO, for example, by superoxide anion or through insufficient regulation of superoxide anion levels by SOD {95}. Although the relationship between NO and smooth muscle cell proliferation is far from delineated, it seems clear that states that lead to intimal thickening also involve the loss of NO bioactivity. Further, elevation of cGMP in the smooth muscle prevents its proliferation. Overall, there seems to be a link between the loss of endothelium-dependent relaxation and smooth muscle cell outgrowth.

Endothelin-derived constrictor substances

Although not a main focus of this chapter, it is interesting to consider the role of constrictor substances on vascular tone and remodeling as well as their interrelationships with vasodilators such as NO. Vasoconstrictor substances such as angiotensin II, neutropeptide Y, and endothelin are potent hypertensive agents, acting both on smooth muscle cells and in the central nervous system. These vasoconstrictors tend to be mitogenic for a variety of cell types, including smooth muscle cells, and tend to worsen intimal hyperplasia. On the other hand, vasodilators, such as atrial natriuretic peptide, bradykinin, and related neurokinins, substance P, calcitonin gene related peptide, prostacyclin, and NO, presumably act to balance vasoconstrictor molecules in maintaining homeostatic mechanisms.

The role of one of the endothelium-derived vasoconstrictors, endothelin, and its regulation by one of the endothelium-derived vasorelaxing substances, NO, serves to illustrate this point. Endothelin-1 (ET-1) is a potent vasoconstrictor with long-lasting pressor effects {96}, and it has also been shown to be an endothelial mitogen {97}. Endothelin gene expression has been shown to be upregulated by thrombin, TGF-β, epinephrine, vasopressin, phorbol esters, and the calcium ionophone A23187, as well as increased shear stress. It has been shown that not only the endogenous preproendothelin-1 gene, but also a supernumerany gene transfected into endothelial cells using gene therapy methodology are upregulated by thrombin and downregulated by NO {98}. These regulatory mechanisms have also been demonstrated in vivo: Thrombin and A23187 enhance ET-1 release, while NO inhibits its production {99}. Furthermore, in an animal model of restenosis following angioplasty ET-1 administration clearly worsens intimal hyperplasic {100}.

Understanding the control of ET-1 secretion and its interrelationship with NO is likely to prove fruitful in developing therapeutic approaches both to regulating vascular tone and hyperplastic responses to injury.

SUMMARY

While the blood vessel wall is morphologically delineated into distinct layers, the functional interactions between the endothelium and smooth muscle cells indicate a complex collaboration important for the maintenance of vascular tone and which, when out of balance, can lead to such pathophysiological conditions as loss of vasoregulatory control and intimal hyperplasia.

Integral components of the complex collaboration between the endothelial and smooth muscle layers are small molecular weight mediators, such as NO and CO, which can easily traverse between the two cell types, perhaps via myoendothelial contacts, and interact directly, without the requirement for receptor occupancy, to mediate constrictor and relaxation responses.

The collaboration between endothelial cells and smooth muscle cells may reach well beyond vasoregulation. As a generalization, constrictor substances tend to be promotors of vascular smooth muscle cell growth, while relaxing substances tend to inhibit smooth muscle cell growth. Thus through understanding of endothelial-smooth muscle cell interactions, it may be possible to link the mechanisms responsible for vascular remodelling in hypertension, hypercholesterolemia, and atherosclerosis.

ACKNOWLEDGMENTS

This work was supported by NIH grants HL-52608 and HL-46029.

REFERENCES

1. Stary HC (Chairman), et al.: A definition of the intima of human arteries and of its atherosclerosis-prone regions. *Circulation* 85:391–405, 1992.
2. Thomas WA, Lee KT, Kim DN: Cell population kinetics in atherogenesis: Cell births and losses in intimal cell mass-derived lesions in the abdominal aortas of swine. *Ann NY Acad Sci* 454:305–315, 1985.
3. Koo EWY, Gotlieb AI: Neointimal formation in the porcine aortic organ culture: I. Cellular dynamics over 1 month. *Lab Invest* 64:743–753, 1991.
4. Stary HC: Macrophages, macrophage foam cells and eccentric intimal thickening in the coronary arteries of young children. *Atherosclerosis* 64:91–108, 1987.
5. Stary HC: Ultrastructure of experimental coronary artery atherosclerosis in cynomolgus macaques: A comparison with the lesions of other primates. *Atherosclerosis* 43:151–175, 1982.
6. Schwarz SM, Heimark RL, Majesky MW: Developmental mechanisms underlying pathology of arteries. *Phys Rev* 70:1177–1209, 1990.
7. Benditt EP, Gown AM: Atheroma: The artery wall and the environment. *Int Rev Exp Pathol* 21:55–118, 1980.
8. Rhodin JAG: The ultrastructure of mammalian arterioles and precapillary sphincters. *J Ultrastruct Res* 18:181–223, 1967.
9. Sosa-Melgarejo JA, Berry CL: Myoendothelial contacts in arteriosclerosis. *J Pathol* 167:235–239, 1992.
10. Ryan US, Ryan JW: Vital functions and activities of endothelial cells. In: Nossel HL, Vogel HJ (eds) *The Biology of the Endothelial Cell*. New York: Academic Press, 1982, pp 301–309.
11. Davies PF: Current concepts of vascular endothelial and smooth muscle cell communication. *Surv Synth Pathol Res* 4:357–373, 1985.
12. Lowenstein WR: Junctional intercellular communication and the control of growth. *Biochim Biophys Acta* 560:1–65, 1979.
13. Moncada S, Palmer RMJ, Higgs EA: Nitric oxide: Physiology, pathophysiology, and pharmacology. *Physiol Rev* 43:109–142, 1991.
14. Furchgott RW, Zawadski JV: The obligatory role of endothelial cells in the relaxation of arterial smooth muscle by acetylcholine. *Nature* 288:373–376, 1980.
15. Rubanyi GM, Lorenz RR, Vanhoutte PM: Bioassay of endothelium-derived relaxing factor(s): Inactivation by catacholamines. *Am J Physiol* 249:H95–H101, 1985.
16. Martin W, Villani GM, Jothianandan D, Furchgott RW: Selective blockade of endothelium-dependent and glyceryl trinitrite-induced relaxation by hemoglobin and methylene blue in the rabbit aorta. *J Pharm Exp Ther* 232:708–716, 1985.
17. Rappaport RM, Murad F: Agonist induced endothelium-dependent relaxation in the rat thoracic aorta may be mediated through cyclic GMP. *Circ Res* 52:352–357, 1983.
18. Greglewski RJ, Palmer RMJ, Moncada S: Superoxide anion is involved in the breakdown of endothelium-derived relaxing factor. *Br J Pharmacol* 87:685–694, 1986.
19. Furchgott RW: Studies on relaxation of rabbit aorta by sodium nitrite: The basis for the proposal that the acid-activatable inhibitory factor from retractor penis is inorganic nitrite and the endothelium-derived relaxing factor is nitric oxide. In: Rubanyi GM, Vanhoutte PM (eds) *Vasodilation: Vascular Smooth Muscle, Peptides, Autonomic Nerves and Endothelium*. New York: Raven Press, 1988, pp 40–414.
20. Ignarro LJ: Pharmacological, biochemical, and chemical evidence that EDRF is NO or a labile nitroso precursor. In: Ryan US, Rubanyi GM (eds) *Endothelial Regulation of Vascular Tone*. New York: Marcel Dekker, 1992, pp 37–49.
21. Palmer RMJ, Ferringe AG, Moncada S: Nitric oxide release accounts for the biological activity of endothelium-derived relaxing factor. *Nature* 327:524–526, 1987.
22. Radomski MW, Palmer RMJ, Moncada S: Comparative pharmacology of endothelium-derived relaxing factor, nitric oxide and prostacyclin in platelets. *Br J Pharmacol* 92:181–187, 1987.
23. Salter M, Knowles M, Moncada S: Widespread distribution and changes in activity if Ca^{2+}-dependent and Ca^{2+}-independent nitric oxide synthases. *FEBS Lett* 291:145–149, 1991.
24. Palmer RMJ, Ashton DS, Moncada S: Vascular endothelial

cells synthesize nitric oxide from L-arginine. *Nature* 333: 664–666, 1988.

25. Lamas S, Marsden PA, Li GK, Tempst P, Michel T: Endothelial nitric oxide synthase: Molecular cloning and characterization of a distinct constitutive enzyme isoform. *Proc Natl Acad Sci USA* 89:14519–14522, 1992.

26. Palmer RMJ, Moncada S: A novel citrulline producing enzyme implicated in the formation of nitric oxide by Vascular endothelial cells. *Biochem Biophys Res Commun* 158:348–352, 1989.

27. Leone A, Palmer RMJ, Knowles RG, Francis PL, Ashton DS, Moncada S: Constitutive and inducible nitric oxide synthases incorporate molecular oxygen into both nitric oxide and citrulline. *J Biol Chem* 35:22790–23795, 1991.

28. Nathan C: Nitric oxide as a secretory product of mammalian cells. *FASEB J* 6:3051–3064, 1992.

29. Bredt DS, Snyder SH: Isolation of nitric oxide synthetase, a calmodulin-requiring enzyme. *Proc Natl Acad Sci USA* 87:682–685, 1990.

30. Busse R, Mulsch A: Calcium-dependent nitric oxide synthesis in endothelial cytosol is mediated by calmodulin. *FEBS Lett* 265:133–136, 1990.

31. Pollock JS, Fostermann U, Mitchell JA, Warner TD, Schmidt HHHW, Nakane M, Murad F: Purification and characterization of particulate endothelium-derived relaxing factor synthase from cultured and native bovine aortic endothelial cells. *Proc Natl Acad Sci USA* 88:10480–10484, 1991.

32. Lamontagne D, Pohl U, Busse R: Mechanical deformation of vessel wall and shear stress determine the basal release of endothelium-derived relaxing factor in the intact rabbit coronary vascular bed. *Circ Res* 70:123–130, 1992.

33. Ryan US, Avdonin P, Hayes B, Broschat KO: Signal transduction in endothelial cells. In: Ryan US, Rubanyi GM (eds) *Endothelial Regulation of Vascular Tone.* New York: Marcel Dekker, 1992, pp 73–90.

34. Stamler JS, Jaraki O, Osbourne J, Simon DI, Keaney J, Vita J, Singel, D, Valeri CR, Loscalzo J: Nitric oxide circulates in mammalian plasma primarly as an S-nitroso adduct of serum albumin. *Proc Natl Acad Sci USA* 89: 7674–7677, 1992.

35. Stamler JS, Simon DI, Osbourne JA, Mullins ME, Jaraki O, Michel T, Singel DJ, Loscalzo J: S-nitrosylation of tissue-type plasminogen activator confers vasodilatory and antiplatelet properties on the enzyme. *Proc Natl Acad Sci USA* 89:8087–8091, 1992.

36. Wennmalm A, Benthin G, Petersson AS: Dependence of the metabolism of nitric oxide in healthy human whole blood on the oxygenation of its red cell haemoglobin. *Br J Pharmacol* 106:507–508, 1992.

37. Vallance P, Collier J, Moncada S: Effects of endothelium-derived nitric oxide on the peripheral arteriolar tone in man. *Lancet* 2:997–1000, 1989.

38. Rees DD, Palmer RMJ, Schulz R, Hodson HF, Moncada S: Characterization of three inhibitors of endothelial nitric oxide synthase in vivo and in vitro. *Br J Pharmacol* 101: 746–752, 1990.

39. Ignarro LJ, Adams JB, Horwitz PM, Wood KS: Activation of soluble guanylate cyclase by NO-hemoproteins involves NO-heme exchange. Comparison of heme-containing and heme deficient enzyme forms. *J Biol Chem* 261:4997–5002, 1986.

40. Ignarro LJ, Kadowitz PJ: The pharmacological and physiological role of cyclic GMP in vascular smooth muscle relaxation. *Ann Rev Pharm Tox* 25:171–191, 1985.

41. Radomski MW, Palmer RMJ, Moncada S: Glucocorticoids inhibit the expression of an inducible, but not the constitutive, nitric oxide synthase in vascular endothelial cells. *Proc*

Natl Acad Sci USA 87:10043–10047, 1990.

42. Gross SS, Jaffe EA, Levi R, Kilbourne RG: Cytokine-activated endothelial cells express an isotype of nitric oxide synthase which is tetrahydrobiopterin-dependent, calmodulin-dependent, and inhibited by arginine analogs with a rank order of potency characteristic of activated macrophages. *Biochem Biophys Res Commun* 178:823–829, 1991.

43. Busse R, Mulsch A: Induction of nitric oxide synthase by cytokines in vascular smooth muscle. *FEBS Lett* 275:87–90, 1990.

44. Beeley D, Schwarz JH, Brenner BM: Interleukin-1 induces prolonged L-arginine dependent cyclic guanosine monophosphate and nitrite production in rat vascular smooth muscle cells. *J Clin Invest* 87:6002–608, 1991.

45. Mollace V, Salvamini D, Angaard E, Vane J: Nitric oxide from vascular smooth muscle cells: Regulation of platelet reactivity and smooth muscle cell guanylate cyclase. *Br J Pharmacol* 104:633–638, 1991.

46. Rees DD, Cellak S, Palmer RMJ, Moncada S: Dexamethasone prevents the induction by endotoxin of a nitrix oxide synthase and the associated effects on vascular tone: An insight into endotoxin shock. *Biochem Biophys Res Commun* 173:541–547.

47. Knowles RG, Salter M, Brooks SL, Moncada S: Anti-inflammatory glucocorticoids inhibit the induction by endotoxin of nitric oxide synthase in the lung, liver, and aorta of the rat. *Biochem Biophys Res Commun* 172:1990.

48. Kilbourne RG, Jurbran A, Gross SS, Griffith OW, Levi R, Adams J, Lodato RF: Reversal of endotoxin-mediated shock by N^G-monomethyl-L-arginine, an inhibitor of nitric oxide synthase. *Biochem Biophys Res Commun* 172:1132–1138, 1990.

49. Wright CE, Rees DD, Moncada S: Protective and pathological role of nitric oxide in endotoxin shock. *Cardiovasc Res* 26:48–57, 1992.

50. Petros A, Bennett D, Vallance P: Effect of nitric oxide synthase inhibitors on hypotension in patients with septic shock. *Lancet* 338:1557–1558, 1991.

51. Nava E, Palmer RMJ, Moncada S: Inhibition of nitric oxide synthesis in septic shock: How much is beneficial? *Lancet* 338:1555–1557, 1991.

52. Steur DJ, Cho HJ, Kwon NS, Wiese M, Nathan C: Purification and characterization of the cytokine induced macrophage nitric oxide synthase: An FAD and FMN containing flavoprotein. *Proc Natl Acad Sci USA* 88:7773–7777, 1991.

53. Cho HJ, Xie QW, Calaycay J, Mumford RA, Swierdeck KM, Lee TD, Nathan C: Calmodulin as a tightly bound subunit of calcium-, calmodulin-independent nitric oxide synthase. *J Exp Med* 176:599–604, 1992.

54. Helin P, Lorenson I, Garbarasch C: Atherosclerosis in rabbit aorta induced by mechanical dilation: Biochemical and morphological studies. *Atherosclerosis* 13:1319–1331, 1971.

55. Fishman JA, Ryan GB, Karnovsky MJ: Endothelial regeneration in the carotid artery and the significance of endothelial denudation in the pathogenesis of myointimal thickening. *Lab Invest* 32:339–345, 1975.

56. Clowes AW, Reidy MA, Clowes MM: Kinetics of cellular proliferation after arterial injury: 1. Smooth muscle growth in the absence of endothelium. *Lab Invest* 49:327–333, 1983.

57. De May JGR, Dijkstra EH, Vrijdag MJJF: Endothelium reduces DNA synthesis in isolated arteries. *Am J Physiol* 260:H1128–H1134, 1991.

58. Miano JM, Tota RR, Vlasic NN, Danishefsky KJ, Stemmerman MB: Early proto-oncogene expression in rat

aortic smooth muscle cells following endothelial removal. *Am J Pathol* 137:761–765, 1990.

59. Parkes JL, Cardell RR, Hubbard FC, Hubbard D, Meltzer A, Penn A: Cultured human atherosclerotic plaque smooth muscle cells retain transforming potential and display enhanced expression of the *myc* proto-oncogene. *Am J Pathol* 138:765–775, 1991.

60. Castellot JJ Jr, Addinizio ML, Rosenberg R, Karnovsky MJ: Cultured endothelial cells produce a heparin-like inhibitor of smooth muscle cell growth. *J Cell Biol* 90:372–377, 1981.

61. Richardson M, Ihnatowycz I, Moore S: Glycosaminoglycan distribution in rabbit aortic wall following balloon catheter de-endothelialization: An ultrastructural study. *Lab Invest* 43:509–516, 1980.

62. Hollman J, Schmidt A, von Bassewitz DB, Buddecke E: Relationship of sulfated glycosaminoglycans and cholesterol content in normal and atherosclerotic human aorta. *Arteriosclerosis* 9:154–158, 1989.

63. Garg UC, Hassid A: Nitric oxide generating vasodilators and 8-bromo cGMP inhibit mitogenesis and proliferation of cultured vascular smooth muscle cells. *J Clin Invest* 83:1774–1777, 1989.

64. Kariya K, Kwawhara Y, Araki S, Fukuzaki H, Takai Y: Antiproliferative action of cyclic GMP-elevating vasodilators in cultured rabbit aortic smooth muscle cells. *Atherosclerosis* 80:143–147, 1989.

65. Nakaki T, Nakayama, Kato R: Inhibition by nitrix oxide and nitric oxide producing vasodilators of DNA synthesis in vascular smooth muscle cells. *Eur J Pharm* 189:347–353, 1990.

66. Abell TJ, Richards AM, Ikrahm H, Espiner EA, Yandle T: Atrial naturetic factor inhibits the proliferation of vascular smooth muscle cell stimulated by PDGF. *Biochem Biophys Res Commun* 160:1392–1396, 1989.

67. Southgate K, Newby AC: Serum-induced proliferation of rabbit aortic smooth muscle cells from the contractile state is inhibited by *-bromo-cAMP, but not 8-bromo cGMP. *Atherosclerosis* 82:113–123, 1990.

68. Assander JW, Southgate KM, Newby AC: Does nitric oxide inhibit smooth muscle proliferation? *J Cardiovasc Pharmacol* 17(Suppl 3):S104–S107, 1991.

69. Scott-Burden T, Schini VB, Elizondo E, Junquero DC, Vanhoutte P: Platelet-derived growth factor suppresses and fibroblast growth factor enhances cytokine-induced production of nitric oxide by cultured smooth muscle cells: Effects on proliferation. *Circ Res* 71:1088–1100, 1992.

70. Nunokawa Y, Tanaka S: Interferon-γ inhibits proliferation of rat vascular smooth muscle cells by nitric oxide generation. *Biochem Biophys Res Commun* 188:409–415, 1992.

71. Bucala R, Tracey KJ, Cerami A: Advanced glycosylation products quench nitric oxide and mediate defective endothelium-dependent vasodilation in experimental diabetes. *J Clin Invest* 87:432–438, 1991.

72. Hogan M, Cerami A, Bucala R: Advanced glycosylation endproducts block the antiproliferative effect of nitric oxide. *J Clin Invest* 90:1110–1115, 1992.

73. Flavahan NA: Atherosclerosis or lipoprotein-induced endothelial dysfunction: Potential mechanisms underlying reduction in EDRF/NO activity. *Circulation* 85:1927–1938, 1992.

74. Verbeuren TJ, Jordaens FH, Zonnekeyn LL, Van Hove CE, Coene M-C, Hermann AG: Effect of hypercholesterolemia on vascular reactivity in the rabbit: I. Endothelium-dependent and endothelium-independent contractions in isolated arteries of control and hypercholesterolemic rabbits. *Circ Res* 58:552–564, 1986.

75. Bossaller C, Habib GB, Yamamoto H, Williams C, Wells S, Henry, PD: Impaired muscarinic endothelium-dependent relaxation and cyclic guanosine 5′-monophosphate formation in atherosclerotic tissue. *J Clin Invest* 79:170–174, 1987.

76. Cohen RA, Zitnay KM, Haudenschild CC, Cunningham LD: Loss of selective endothelial cell vasoactive functions caused by hypercholesterolemia in pig coronary arteries. *Circ Res* 63:903–910, 1988.

77. Shimokawa H, Vanhoutte PM: Impaired endothelium-dependent relaxation to aggregating platelets and related vasoactive substances in porcine coronary arteries in hypercholesterolemia and atherosclerosis. *Circ Res* 64:900–914, 1989.

78. Kolodgie FD, Virmani R, Rice HE, Mergner WJ: Vascular reactivity during the progression of atherosclerotic plaque: A study in Watanabe Heritable Hyperlipidemic rabbits. *Circ Res* 66:1112–1126, 1990.

79. Merkel LA, Rivera LM, Bilder GE, Perrone MH: Differential alteration of vascular reactivity in rabbit aorta with modest elevation of serum cholesterol. *Circ Res* 67:550–555, 1990.

80. Tagawa H, Tomoike H, Nakamura M: Putative mechanisms of the impairment of endothelium-dependent relaxation of the aorta with atheromatous plaque in heritable hyperlipidemic rabbits. *Circ Res* 68:330–337, 1991.

81. Quillen JE, Selke FW, Armstrong ML, Harrison DG: Long-term cholesterol feeding alters the reactivity of primate coronary microvessels to platelet products. *Arterioscler Thromb* 11:639–644, 1991.

82. McLenachan JM, Williams JK, Fish RD, Ganz P, Selwyn AP: Loss of flow mediated endothelium dependent dilation occurs early in the development of atherosclerosis. *Circulation* 84:1273–1278, 1991.

83. Zieher AN, Drexler H, Wollschlager H, Just H: Modulation of coronary vasomotor tone in humans: Progressive endothelial dysfunction with different early stages of coronary atherosclerosis. *Circulation* 83:391–401, 1991.

84. Takahashi M, Yui Y, Yasumoto H, Aoyama T, Morishita H, Hattori R, Kawai C: Lipoproteins are inhibitors of endothelium-dependent relaxation of rabbit aorta. *Am J Physiol* 258:H1–H8, 1990.

85. Galle J, Mulsch A, Bassange E: Effects of native and oxidized low density lipoproteins on formation and inactivation of endothelium-derived relaxing factor. *Arterioscler Thromb* 11:198–203, 1991.

86. Tanner FC, Noll G, Boulanger CM, Luscher TF: Oxidized low density lipoproteins inhibit relaxations of porcine coronary arteries: Role of scavenger receptor and endothelium-derived nitric oxide. *Circulation* 83:2012–2020, 1991.

87. Rees DD, Palmer RMJ, Moncada S: Role of endothelium derived nitric oxide in the regulation of blood pressure. *Proc Natl Acad Sci USA* 86:3375–3378, 1989.

88. Pasini FL, Frigerio C, De Giorgi L, Blardi P, Di Perri T: L-arginine plasma concentrations in hypercholesterolemia. *Lancet* 340:549, 1992.

89. Girerd XJ, Hirsch AT, Cooke JP, Dzau VJ, Creager M: L-arginine augments endothelium-dependent vasodilation in cholesterol fed rabbits. *Circ Res* 67:1301–1308, 1990.

90. Cooke JP, Andon NA, Gireard ZJ, Hirsch AT, Creager MA: Arginine restores cholinergic relaxation of hypercholesterolemic rabbit thoracic aorta. *Circulation* 83:1057–1062, 1991.

91. Rossitch E, Alexander E, Black PM, Cooke JP: L-arginine normalizes endothelial function in cerebral vessels from hypercholesterolemic rabbits. *J Clin Invest* 87:1295–1299, 1991.

92. Creager MA, Gallagher SJ, Gireard XJ, Coleman S, Dzau VJ, Cooke JP: L-arginine improves endothelium-dependent vasodilation in hypercholesterolemic humans. *J Clin Invest* 90:1248–1253, 1992.

93. Drexler H, Zeiher AM, Meinzer K, Just H: Correction of endothelial dysfunction in coronary microcirculation of hypercholesterolemic patients by L-arginine. *Lancet* 338: 1546–1550, 1991.

94. Cooke JP, Singer AH, Tsao P, Zera P, Rowan RA, Billingham ME: Antiatherogenic effects of L-arginine in the hypercholesterolemic rabbit. *J Clin Invest* 90:1168–1172, 1992.

95. Minor RL, Myers PR, Guerra RJ, Bates JN, Harrison DG: Diet-induced atherosclerosis increases the release of nitrogen oxides from rabbit aorta. *J Clin Invest* 86:2109–2116, 1990.

96. Yanagisawa M, Masaki T: Endothelin, a novel endothelium-derived peptide. Pharmacological activities, regulation and possible roles in cardiovascular control. *Biochem Pharmacol* 38:1877–1883, 1989.

97. Hirata Y, Takagi Y, Fukuda Y, Marumo F: Endothelin is a potent mitogen for rat vascular smooth muscle cells. *Atherosclerosis* 78:225–228, 1989.

98. Ryan US, Zhong R, Hayes BA, Rapp NS, Sauther ML: Regulation of endothelin-1 expression in normal and transfected endothelial cells. *J Cardiovasc Pharmacol*, in press.

99. Boulanger C, Luscher TF: Release of endothelin from the porcine aorta. Inhibition by endothelium-derived nitric oxide. *J Clin Invest* 85:587–590, 1990.

100. Trachtenberg JD, Sun S, Rapp NS, Choi ET, Callow AD, Ryan US: The effect of ET-1 infusion on the development of intimal hyperplasia following balloon catheter injury. *J Cardiovasc Pharmacol*, in press.

CHAPTER 45

Electrophysiology of Vascular Smooth Muscle

NICHOLAS SPERELAKIS & YUSUKE OHYA

INTRODUCTION

This chapter provides an overview of the electrophysiology of vascular smooth muscle and of how the actions of some vasoactive substances are mediated by changes in electrical properties of the cell membrane. Emphasis is given to the role of the Ca^{2+} ion and to the action of inhibitor drugs.

Compared to skeletal muscle or cardiac muscle, less is known about the electrical properties of vascular smooth muscle (VSM) because of the difficulty of making satisfactory electrical recordings from the very small smooth muscle cells with the tough connective tissue that is often present. However, considerable progress has been made during the past few years. For the sake of convenience, this article will draw heavily upon the work done in our laboratory, even though many of the facts and principles concerning VSM resulted from the efforts of numerous other investigators. To attempt to give proper credit to all these published studies would make this chapter unwieldy.

Vascular smooth muscle consists of an assembly of short (e.g., 200 μm in length) and thin (e.g., 5 μm in diameter) cells (Somlyo and Somlyo, 1968a). Contiguous cells often come into close contact, forming various types of specialized junctions. The degree of low-resistance electrical coupling between the VSM cells is uncertain and controversial. Some investigators who conclude that low-resistance connections exist in one vessel conclude that they may not exist in another vessel (Mekata, 1980). Motor nerves of the autonomic nervous system innervate the muscle cells and exercise some control over their state of contraction. The neurons release neurotransmitters, such as norepinephrine, acetylcholine, ATP, etc., at periodic neuron varicosities distributed along the length of the blood vessels. The nerve fibers are generally confined to the border between the outer adventitia layer and the media (muscle) layer. Thus many VSM cells become influenced by neurotransmitter secreted at a relatively distant point, i.e., there usually are no close neuromuscular junctions, as found in skeletal muscle.

The neurotransmitters, some vasoactive hormones and autacoids, and some vasoactive drugs appear to exert their primary effect on the electrical properties of the cell membrane of the VSM cells. Changes in the level of the resting membrane potential control the level of contraction

of the VSM cells, depolarization increasing the state of contraction and hyperpolarization diminishing the state of contraction (i.e., producing relaxation). Changes in the conductance of the cell membrane for certain ions, e.g., Ca^{2+}, have profound effects on the degree of contraction.

The Ca^{2+} necessary for raising the myoplasmic Ca^{2+} to activate the contractile myofilaments (e.g., elevating free $[Ca]_i$ from $<10^{-7}M$ to $>10^{-5}M$) may come from two sources: (a) Ca^{2+} influx across the surface membrane and (b) Ca^{2+} release from some internal store, such as the sarcoplasmic reticulum (SR), brought about by the Ca^{2+} influx (Ca^{2+}-induced-release mechanism), a change in potential across the SR membrane, and/or production of inositol triphosphate. Some vasoactive substances may exert a primary or seondary effect to facilitate or depress Ca^{2+} release from the SR. Some vasoactive agents produce contraction without an associated change in membrane potential, termed *pharmacomechanical coupling*, but often changes in membrane conductance can be detected (Droogmans et al., 1977; Kuriyama et al., 1982).

It is often mentioned that there are two general categories of VSM: those that generate action potentials in vitro (spiking VSM) and those that normally do not fire action potentials in vitro (nonspiking VSM; Somlyo and Somlyo, 1968b; Somlyo et al., 1969; Johansson, 1971; Kuriyama et al., 1982). The spikes, when they occur, bring about contraction or increase the state of contraction. An example of spiking VSM is the rat portal vein, while examples of nonspiking muscle are some of the large arteries in rabbit (Somlyo and Somlyo, 1968b; Johansson, 1978). However, some of the nonspiking VSM in vitro (and electrically inexcitable) may actually fire spikes in situ in response to summated excitatory junction potentials (EJPs; Zelcer and Sperelakis, 1981a). In addition, the nonspiking VSM can be made to spike in vitro by lowering the K^+ conductance with Ba^{2+} or tetraethylammonium (TEA^+; Droogmans et al., 1977; Harder and Sperelakis, 1979).[1] This means that the membrane possesses a full

---

[1] Ba^{2+} ion is now believed to be not only a K^+ channel blocker (especially the Ca^{2+}-dependent K^+ channel), but also a charge carrier through voltage-dependent Ca^{2+} channels (Benham et al., 1985; Inoue et al., 1985). As Ba^{2+} ion by itself does not induce inactivation of Ca^{2+} channels and has a high affinity for binding

N. Sperelakis (ed.), Physiology and Pathophysiology of the Heart, Third Edition.
© *1995 Kluwer Academic Publishers. ISBN 0-7923-2612-1. All rights reserved.*

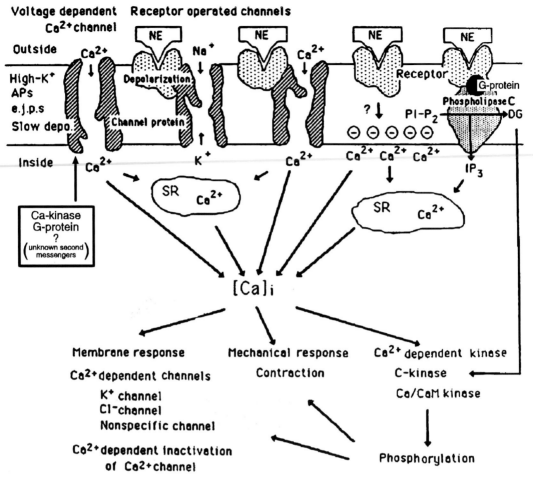

Fig. 45-1. Diagrammatic representation of the various sources of Ca^{2+} for contraction of vascular smooth muscle. Several major sources are depicted: (1) a voltage-dependent Ca^{2+} channel; that is, the channel responsible for the rising phase of the action potential and for the high K^+ contraction, which is the site of action of Ca^{2+} antagonists; (2) a receptor-operated postsynaptic channel that is nonspecific, allowing Na^+, K^+, and Ca^{2+} to pass; this channel is responsible for the excitatory postsynaptic potentials (EPSP or e.j.p.); (3) a receptor-operated Ca^{2+} channel that is specific for Ca^{2+} ion; (4) a variant of (3), receptor-operated release of Ca^{2+} ion bound to fixed negative charges at the inner surface of the cell membrane; (5) Ca^{2+} release from the intracellular store site, possibly sarcoplasmic reticulum (SR), by inositol triphosphate (IP_3); binding of agonist to the receptor activates phosphatidyl bis-phosphate (P_1-P_2) turnover. The key enzyme of this reaction is phospholipase C, and this activity is regulated by a GTP-binding protein on the regulatory subunit. The main metabolites of this turnover are IP_3 and diacylglycerol (DG). DG is used for the activation of C kinase together with Ca^{2+}. The receptors involved in mechanisms (2)–(5) are depicted as alpha-adrenergic receptors and norepinephrine (NE) as the neurotransmitter. The major intracellular sources of Ca^{2+} ions are the SR and, perhaps, Ca^{2+} bound to the inner surface of the cell membrane. Ca^{2+} release from the SR may be brought about by a rise in intracellular Ca^{2+} and by a potential change across the SR membrane, as well as IP_3. High K^+ depolarizes and thereby leads to activation of the voltage-dependent Ca^{2+} channel [mechanism (1)], causing a contraction. Exogenous NE activates the alpha receptor (alpha 1), which in turn (a) depolarizes by activating the receptor-operated channels [mechanism (2)], thereby activating the voltage-dependent Ca channel [mechanism (1)]; or directly stimulating the voltage-dependent Ca channel (mechanism 1); (b) causes a direct rise in intracellular Ca^{2+} by mechanism (3) or (4); and (c) produces an intracellular second messenger, IP_3, which triggers Ca^{2+} release from the SR.

complement of voltage-dependent Ca^{2+} channels for inward current and is capable of regenerative excitation.

VSM cells have relatively low resting potentials

sites in the Ca^{2+} channel, Ba^{2+} ion can pass through the Ca^{2+} channel easier than Ca^{2+} ion (Ohya et al., 1988).

($-40\,mV$ to $\sim70\,mV$), due to a low K^+ permeability (P_K), although in some vessels the resting potentials are often greater than $-70\,mV$. The VSM cells are capable of exhibiting automaticity, at least under certain experimental conditions. An inward slow current (I_{si}), carried almost exclusively by Ca^{2+} ion in many types of VSM cells, is responsible for the depolarizing phase of the spikes. There appear to be no functional fast Na^+ channels and inward fast Na^+ current. Therefore, agents like tetrodotoxin (TTX) that block fast Na^+ channels have no effect on the VSM spikes, whereas agents like verapamil that block Ca^{2+} channels depress and block the VSM spikes.

For a detailed description of the electrical properties of VSM and electromechanical and pharmacomechanical coupling, the reader is referred to a number of reviews, including those by Johansson (1971), Bolton (1979), Johansson and Somlyo (1980), Kuriyama et al. (1982), and Ohya and Sperelakis (1991).

SOURCES OF Ca^{2+} FOR CONTRACTION

The Ca^{2+} ions for activation of the contractile proteins come from two major sources: (a) Ca^{2+} influx from the interstitial fluid bathing the cells and (b) release of Ca^{2+} from the sarcoplasmic reticulum (SR) stores. These various possible sources of Ca^{2+} for contraction are diagrammatically depicted in fig. 45-1.

The Ca^{2+} influx across the sarcolemma is down an electrochemical gradient and through the voltage-dependent and time-dependent Ca^{2+} channels, one major focus of this chapter. This Ca^{2+} inward current is responsible for the rising phase of the AP in most VSM cells. It is these Ca^{2+} channels that are blocked by various Ca^{2+} antagonists like verapamil, bepridil, nifedipine, diltiazem, Mn^{2+}, Cd^{2+}, and La^{3+}, as indicated in fig. 45-1.

The Ca^{2+} influx acts to directly elevate $[Ca]_i$ and, in addition, it might cause the release of more Ca^{2+} from the SR by the Ca-triggered, Ca-release mechanism of Fabiato and Fabiato (1979). It is also possible that Ca^{2+} release from the SR may be controlled by depolarization of the sarcolemma, which could lead to depolarization of the SR by somehow being reflected across the diadic junctions formed between sarcolemma and SR[2] (junctional SR is continuous with the network SR surrounding bundles of myofilaments). The level of $[Ca]_i$ in a noncontracting cell is estimated to be about $10^{-7} M$, and the $[Ca]_i$ necessary for peak contraction is about $10^{-5} M$, as estimated in the studies using skinned muscle preparations (Itoh et al., 1981) and using Ca^{2+}-sensitive dyes (Williams et al., 1986).

Contractions initiated by action potentials or by elevated $[K]_o$ presumably occur by means of activation of the voltage-dependent Ca^{2+} channels to allow Ca^{2+} influx down its electrochemical gradient (fig. 45-1). Ca^{2+} release from the SR may also contribute. High $[K]_o$ depolarizes by reducing E_K, as calculated from the Nernst equation ($E_K = -61 \, mV \log[K]_i/[K]_o$). Most Ca^{2+} antagonists (Ca^{2+} channel blockers) selectively block Ca^{2+} influx through the voltage-dependent Ca^{2+} channel. Therefore, these drugs inhibit this type of contraction to a greater extent than those induced by agonists.

Contractions initiated by norepinephrine (NE) may be brought about by somewhat different mechanism(s) (Bolton, 1979; Kuriyama et al., 1982; fig. 45-1):
1. NE binding to alpha-adrenergic receptors on the VSM cell (postsynaptic) membrane increase conductance for Na^+ (and perhaps Ca^{2+}), thereby producing the equivalent of a large excitatory postsynaptic potential [EPSP; and/or excitatory junctional potential (EJP)]. This EPSP depolarization should activate the voltage-dependent Ca^{2+} channels and cause a large Ca^{2+} influx.
2. NE directly stimulates opening of voltage-dependent Ca^{2+} channels. NE also shifts the threshold potential of the Ca^{2+} channels to the negative direction (Nelson et al., 1990).
3. The receptor-operated channel, if analogous to the ion channels in the postsynaptic membrane at the vertebrate skeletal neuromuscular junction activated by ACh (nicotinic receptor), is nonspecific so that a number of cations, including Na^+, Ca^{2+}, and K^+, can pass through. If so, then some Ca^{2+} influx would occur through these voltage-independent synaptic channels. Casteels (1980) has shown that NE increases the permeability for Na^+, Ca^{2+}, K^+, and Cl^- ions. There is no evidence that Ca^{2+} antagonists block Ca^{2+} influx through the postsynaptic channels (similar to the lack of effect of tetrodotoxin [TTX] on Na^+ influx through the ACh-operated postsynaptic channels).
4. It has been postulated (see reviews by Bolton, 1979; Johansson and Somlyo, 1980; Casteels, 1980; and Van Breemen et al., 1979) that there is a separate set of alpha-receptor-operated channels that allows only Ca^{2+} ions to pass through. Major evidence for this view comes from the fact that addition of exogenous NE to VSM completely depolarized by elevated $[K]_o$ and in contracture produces a considerably greater force of contraction. However, it is difficult to distinguish between mechanisms (1) and (2). Even if Na^+ influx is increased upon addition of NE to K^+-depolarized VSM cells, this would not rule out the possibility of this type of receptor-operated Ca^{2+} channel. The most compelling argument for this type of channel is Casteels' finding that low concentrations of NE bring about some contraction without an accompanying depolarization (higher doses produced depolarization and greater contraction).
5. A variation of the third mechanism is that, instead of a protein channel embedded in the lipid bilayer membrane and coupled to the alpha receptor, activation of the alpha receptor could instead somehow cause the release of Ca^{2+} bound to negative charges at the inner surface of the cell membrane (see fig. 45-1). It may be presumed that Ca^{2+} antagonists do not greatly affect Ca^{2+} influx through this receptor-operated mechanism.
6. Activation of the alpha receptor could also cause the release of Ca^{2+} from the SR via a second messenger that is produced intracellularly. NE is known to increase the turnover of phosphatidylinositol (PI) in VSM, and one of the metabolites formed (inositol 1,4,5-triphosphate, IP_3; for review see Berridge, 1984) has recently been demonstrated to cause Ca^{2+} release and tension development in skinned arterial VSM cells (Suematsu et al., 1984; Somlyo et al., 1985). Similarly, angiotensin II increases PI turnover (Smith et al., 1984). Thus IP_3 may be a common intracellular messenger mediating agonist-induced Ca^{2+} release from

the SR in smooth muscle cells. Diacylglycerol (DG), another metabolite of PI turnover, may also play an important role in the regulation of vascular tone via protein phosphorylation related to activation of C kinase (for review see Nishizuka, 1984; Itoh et al., 1986).

In summary, NE produces contraction via several mechanisms: (a) the voltage-dependent Ca^{2+} channel (activated by EPSP, depolarization, and/or receptor activation), (b) the receptor-operated channel of the nonspecific postsynaptic type or the postulated specific Ca^{2+} type, and (c) Ca^{2+} release from the intracellular Ca^{2+} store sites.

ELECTRICAL PROPERTIES OF VASCULAR SMOOTH MUSCLES

Resting membrane potentials

In general, the basic electrical properties of VSM cells, such as resting potentials and action potential (AP) characteristics, are similar to those in other types of smooth muscle, for example, intestinal muscle. The resting membrane potential of vascular smooth muscles (VSM) is reported to be about −40 mV to ∼−70 mV (Johansson and Somlyo, 1980; Jones, 1980; Kuriyama et al., 1982). Such variation is considered to be due to differences in the experimental approaches of each investigator, and in the species and regions of the experimental animals. For example, Harder and Sperelakis (1978) found a mean resting potential (E_m) in guinea pig superior mesenteric artery of −54 ± 0.6 mV (table 45-1A). The mean resting

potential for the small coronary arteries of the dog was −54 ± 1.0 mV and that for the large coronary arteries was −56 ± 2 mV (table 45-1B; Belardinelli et al., 1979; Harder et al., 1979).

There is a small contribution of the electrogenic pump potential to the resting E_m in VSM cells. For example, Harder and Sperelakis (1978) found a contribution of about 8 mV in guinea pig superior mesenteric artery; that is, the resting E_m rapidly decreased from a control value of −54 mV to −46 mV when ouabain (10^{-5} M) was added to inhibit the Na,K-ATPase and thus stop the Na-K pump (table 45-1A). Thus −46 mV represents the net diffusion potential (E_{diff}) that reflects the ionic distributions and the relative ionic conductances (see Sperelakis, 1979a). The electrogenic pump potential (V_p) is in parallel with E_{diff} so that removal of V_p (i.e., −54 mV) permits the measurement of E_{diff} (namely, −46 mV; see fig. 45-23).

The P_{Na}/P_K ratio can be calculated from E_{diff} using the Goldman constant-field equation, adopting values for $[Na]_i$ (15 mM) and $[K]_i$ (160 mM) and assuming that Cl^- is passively distributed

$$E_{diff} = \frac{RT}{F} \ln \frac{P_{Na}[Na]_o + P_K[K]_o + P_{Cl}[Cl]_i}{P_{Na}[Na]_i + P_K[K]_i + P_{Cl}[Cl]_o}.$$

The value of $[K]_i$ can be estimated by running a complete curve of E_m versus $\log[K]_o$ and extrapolating to zero potential (fig. 45-2). By this method, a value of 160 mM was obtained for $[K]_i$ in guinea pig superior mesenteric artery and a P_{Na}/P_K ratio of 0.17 was calculated (in 4 mM $[K]_o$; Harder and Sperelakis, 1978). This ratio is considerably higher than that found for skeletal muscle or cardiac

Table 45-1. Summary of some electrical properties of the resting membrane in arterial smooth muscle

Condition	Resting E_m (mV)	Input resistance r_{in} (MΩ)	P_{Na}/P_K ratio
A. Guinea pig superior mesenteric artery			
Control	−54 ± 0.6	8.5 ± 0.3	—
Ouabain (10^{-5} M)[1]	−46 ± 1.0[a]	—	0.17
Cl^--free solution	−55 ± 0.6	8.5 ± 0.4	—
Ba^{2+} (1.0 mM)	−24 ± 0.8[a]	24.0 ± 1.8*	0.42
Low Na^+ solution	−66 ± 1.3[a]	—	—
B. Dog coronary arteries	−56 ± 2	9.0 ± 0.4	—
Large diameter	−53 ± 2	10.0 ± 1.0	—
Small diameter	−55 ± 1.0	—	—
Small diameter	−54 ± 1.3	—	—

Values given are the mean ± 1 SE.
[a] Significantly different from control value at $p < 0.05$.
The small coronary arteries were intramural and less than 0.5 mm in diameter; the large coronary arteries were extramural and more than 1.0 mm in diameter. Measurements of E_m were made after only 1–5 minutes exposure to ouabain so that depolarization due to ion shifts (i.e., rundown of the ionic gradients) did not occur. The value listed is for a $[K]_o$ of 4.0 mM. Data taken from Harder and Sperelakis (1978), Harder et al. (1979), Belardinelli et al. (1979), Harder and Sperelakis (1979), and Mras and Sperelakis (1981).

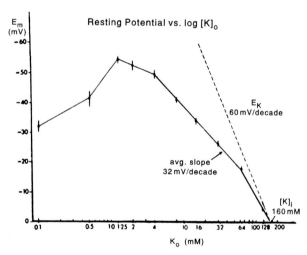

Fig. 45-2. Resting potential (E_m) as a function of external K^+ concentration, $[K]_o$ (log scale) for vascular smooth muscle of guinea pig superior mesenteric artery. The vertical bars represent the mean ± 1 SEM for 10–23 impalements in 4–6 muscles. The curve extrapolated to zero potential gives an estimated internal K^+ concentration, $[K]_i$, of 160 mM. The broken line gives the K^+ equilibrium potential (E_K) as calculated from the Nernst equation and has a slope of 60 mV/10-fold change in $[K]_o$. From Harder and Sperelakis, 1987, with permission.

muscle. The ratio is high because of a low P_K and not because of a high P_{Na}.

In guinea pig superior mesenteric artery, Cl^- ions appear to be passively distributed, i.e., Cl^- distributes itself in accordance with the average membrane potential (Harder and Sperelakis, 1978). This means that, for a membrane at rest for a long period, the Cl^- equilibrium potential (E_{Cl}), calculated from the Nernst equation, equals the resting E_m. The evidence for passive Cl^- distribution is based on the fact that the resting E_m upon equilibration in Cl^--free Ringer solution was nearly exactly equal to that in Ringer solution in the presence of Cl^- (table 45-1A); that is, following a transient depolarization that is expected to occur during Cl^- washout from the cells, the potential returns to the original value within 10 minutes. If $[Cl]_i$ was higher than that predicted from the resting E_m (due to an inwardly directed Cl^- pump), then hyperpolarization should have been observed after equilibration in Cl^--free solution. The fact that the input resistance (r_{in}) in Cl^--free solution was about the same as that in the presence of Cl^- (table 45-1A) suggests that Cl^- conductance (g_{Cl}) is relatively low in this muscle. This conclusion is also supported by the fact that Ba^{2+} ion (1 mM), a depressant of K^+ conductance (g_K),[2] rapidly produced a large depolarization in normal Cl^--containing Ringer solution (table 45-1A). When g_{Cl} is high, Ba^{2+} has relatively little effect (Sperelakis et al., 1967). Hence, there is no evidence for a Cl^- pump in this tissue.

In low-Na^+ solution, the membrane should become hyperpolarized, as expected because of the removal of much of the depolaring Na^+ influx. Under such conditions, guinea pig superior mesenteric artery cells become hyperpolarized by about 12 mV, from the control value of -54 mV to a value of -66 mV in low Na^+ solution (table 45-1A).

The input resistance (r_{in}), that is, the resistance that the impaled microelectrode "looks into," may be calculated from the slope of the steady-state voltage-current curve through the origin (i.e., at infinitesimally small applied current). Depolarizing and hyperpolarizing current pulses are applied through the voltage-recording microelectrode by means of a balanced bridge circuit (Sperelakis and Lehmkuhl, 1964) or by a second independent voltage-recording microelectrode impaled very close to the current-injecting microelectrode in the same cell. r_{in} generally ranges between 5 and 15 MΩ for VSM. For example, the average value was 8.5 MΩ in guinea pig superior mesenteric artery (table 45-1A), and 9 and 10 MΩ, respectively, in large and small coronary artery of the dog (table 45-1B). Assuming a cell length (L) of 200 μm and a radius (a) of 2.5 μm, and assuming no low-resistance coupling between cells, an r_{in} of 9 MΩ gives a membrane resistivity (R_m) of 283 Ωcm^2 ($R_m = r_{in} \times \pi 2aL$). This value would be underestimated if the cells are connected by low-resistance pathways. Addition of Ba^{2+} ion (0.5 or 1.0 mM), a blocker

of K^+ conductance, greatly increases r_{in}. It was reported by Harder (1980) that the slope of the curve of E_m versus log $[K]_o$ was much higher (58 mV/decade) in the middle cerebral artery of the cat than that in the cat mesenteric artery (36 mV/decade) or guinea pig superior mesenteric artery (32 mV/decade; fig. 45-2); that is, the VSM cell membrane in the cerebral artery was more K^+ selective (lower P_{Na}/P_K ratio). This property would make the membrane potential more sensitive to changes in $[K]_o$. In general, regional differences of the resting membrane potential are attributed to the different value in P_{Na}/P_K ratio.

The degree of low-resistance coupling between VSM cells is not really known, and the interpretations are controversial. The structure that accounts for this low-resistance pathway is called the nexus, or gap junction, and is the region of close apposition between adjacent cells. Since much of the basic data obtained in electrical coupling studies in smooth muscle are similar to those in cardiac muscle, the reader is referred to a review article by Sperelakis (1979b) that summarized many of the facts and arguments for cardiac muscle. Mekata (1980) reported that r_{in} (measured from polarizing current pulses of 0.5 nA or less injected through the voltage-recording microelectrode by means of a bridge circuit) of the circumflex coronary artery of the dog varied over a wide range of 10–400 MΩ (mean of 181 MΩ). Since he could not measure any electrotonic potential beyond 0.4 mm, when external polarizing current pulses were applied by a partitioned-chamber method of Abe and Tomita (1968), Mekata concluded that low-resistance coupling between VSM cells must be poor in this vessel. In contrast, Mekata concluded that the cells in the anterior descending coronary artery were well coupled (length constant of 2.44 mm).

Depolarization produced in low $[K]_o$ (<1.25 mM; fig. 45-2) may be due to two factors: (a) inhibition of the electrogenic Na-K pump and (b) a reduction in g_K (and P_K). After a period in low $[K]_o$ (or K^+-free solution), elevation of $[K]_o$ back to the normal level (e.g., 4 mM) causes a pronounced hyperpolarization that overshoots the normal resting E_m; this is thought to be due to great stimulation of the electrogenic pump due to the preceding Na^+ loading (i.e., increase in $[Na]_i$; Bonaccorsi et al., 1977; Haddy, 1978). This K^+-induced hyperpolarization is associated with relaxation of the VSM. Webb and Bohr (1978, 1979) reported that the K^+-induced relaxation was greater in VSM from spontaneously hypertensive rats (SHR) than in normotensive rats. This finding was consistent with the results of Bonacorsi et al. (1977), who found that the contribution of the electrogenic pump potential to the resting E_m was greater in the SHR animals.

Development of tension in VSM is closely associated with changes in E_m; for example, this is well known for K^+ contractures. In addition, the amplitude of the norepinephrine-induced contraction is altered by changes in the resting E_m level, e.g., depolarization by a few millivolts greatly increases tension development (Casteels et al., 1977; Haeusler, 1978). Hyperpolarization has the opposite effect, decreasing the contractile response to norepinephrine (Haeusler, 1978); nitroprusside-induced hyperpolarization reduces the tension developed by K^+

---

[2] Forbes and Sperelakis (1982) have shown that there are junctional processes and pillars that connect the sarcolemma and surface caveolae with the membrane of the junctional SR, which may be involved in the transfer of excitation from the sarcolemma to the SR.

and by norepinephrine (Ito et al., 1978). In some experiments, the NE-induced contractions occurred without depolarization at low doses (10^{-9} to 10^{-7}M) and with depolarization at high doses (10^{-6} to 10^{-5}M; Mekata and Niu, 1972; Casteels et al., 1977; Droogmans et al., 1977; Kuriyama and Suzuki, 1978), but in other cases 10^{-8}M norepinephrine (10^{-9}M in SHR animals) produced significant depolarization with the contraction in rat pulmonary artery. However, NE brings about additional tension in arteries that are already maximally depolarized by K^+ (Somlyo and Somlyo, 1968a,b; Haeusler, 1978), perhaps by releasing Ca^{2+} sequestered in the SR.

Excited membrane properties

INEXCITABILITY OF SOME VSM PREPARATIONS IN VITRO

The VSM cells in some isolated arterial strip preparations are often inexcitable by electrical stimulation for unknown reasons (Somlyo and Somlyo, 1968b; Somlyo et al., 1969; Johansson, 1971; Kuriyama et al., 1982). There are some exceptions to this, including cultured rat aortic VSM cells (see below). Venous VSM cells are usually excitable in isolated preparations and may even be spontaneously active (Somlyo and Somlyo, 1968b; Somlyo et al., 1969; Johansson, 1971; Kuriyama et al., 1982). Mesenteric arteries of guinea pig also can exhibit spontaneous electrical activity under appropriate conditions of temperature and pressure (Zelcer and Sperelakis, 1982). The arterial VSM cells that are electrically inexcitable in vitro probably fire action potentials in situ, in response to summated EJPs following neurotransmitter release.

INDUCTION OF EXCITABILITY BY TEA OR Ba^{2+} ION

Exposure of the isolated arterial VSM to agents that depress K^+ conductance (g_K) at rest and during excitation, such as Ba^{2+} ion (fig. 45-3A,B) and tetraethylammonium (TEA; fig. 45-3C,D), induce electrical excitability. These agents allow large overshooting APs to be elicited by electrical stimulation (fig. 45-3D), and sometimes spontaneous discharge also occurs (fig. 45-3B). Inhibition of g_K suppresses the outward K^+ current, which should permit a greater net inward current and thus facilitate regenerative excitation; that is, for a given amount of inward current (through voltage-dependent slow channels) a decrease in

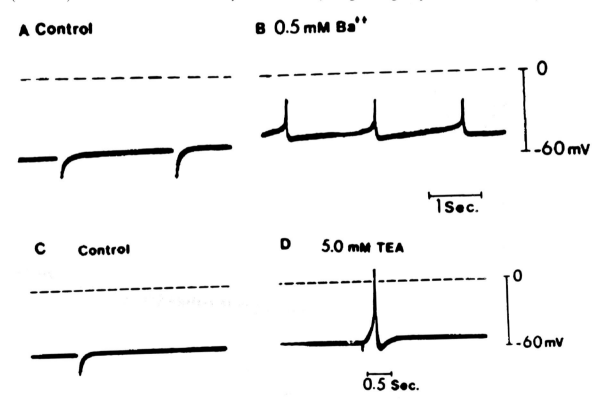

Fig. 45-3. Induction of excitability by Ba^{2+} (A and B) and tetraethylammonium ion (TEA^+) in guinea pig superior mesenteric artery muscle. **A:** Control showing a large resting potential of about -55 mV and lack of spontaneous action potentials (APs) or responses to external electrical stimulation (two shock artifacts shown). **B:** Record taken from same cell 5 minutes after the addition of 0.5 mM Ba^{2+}, illustrating the partial depolarization and production of spontaneous APs. **C:** Control showing a large resting potential of about -58 mV and lack of spontaneous APs or responses to intense external electrical stimulation (one shock artifact depicted). **D:** Record taken from the same cell 5 minutes after the addition of 5 mM TEA^+, illustrating a large overshooting AP produced in response to electrical stimulation. Modified from Harder and Sperelakis (1979), with permission.

the simultaneous K^+ outward current gives a greater net inward current. A minimum net inward current is required before a regenerative AP can occur. Ba^{2+} and TEA not only depress the resting g_K but also slow the kinetics of g_K turn-on during depolarization, thus allowing the inward slow current (I_{si}) to predominate. The lack of electrical excitability in vitro in normal Ringer solution may be due to one or more factors, such as (a) too early a turn-on of g_K, (b) lack of anomalous rectification (i.e., instantaneous decrease in g_K with depolarization), (c) inactivation of some of the slow channels causing insufficient I_{si}, or (d) an increase in g_{Cl} (which tends to clamp or hold the E_m at E_{Cl}).

TEA has been shown to induce spikes in common carotid artery of the rabbit (Mekata, 1971) and the rabbit saphenous artery (Holman and Surprenant, 1979), and low doses of TEA allow NE to induce spike activity (Harder, 1981). Droogmans et al. (1977) showed that the spontaneous APs induced by TEA in rabbit-ear artery were Ca^{2+} dependent. Hence, the TEA-induced APs in arterial smooth muscle provide a useful assay system for the effect of various vasoactive substances on the inward Ca^{2+} current (Ca^{2+} influx) of VSM cells.

When APs are induced by agents like TEA, their maximal rate of rise (max dV/dt) varies from 2 to 12 V/s. For example, in guinea pig superior mesenteric artery (Harder and Sperelakis, 1979), the average max dV/dt (in 1.8 mM Ca^{2+}) was 6 + 0.7 V/s (table 45-2). Those of small and large coronary artery of dog were 6 ± 1 V/s and 5 ± 1 V/s, respectively. The AP duration (measured at 50% repolarization) was 50–75 ms. The average amplitude of these spikes was 59 mV, i.e., there usually was a small overshoot of about 5 mV (table 45-2). However, in some conditions the APs undershoot to various degrees, i.e., their peak does not reach the zero potential level. This may be due to a premature increase in g_K.

The max dV/dt increases only slightly with hyperpolarization (produced by injected hyperpolarizing current pulses), whereas max dV/dt decreases greatly with depo-

larization (Harder and Sperelakis, 1979). Decrease of max dV/dt to 50% of its maximal value (half-inactivation of the Ca^{2+} channels) occurs by -47 mV, and complete inactivation (max dV/dt = 0) occurs at -22 mV. This behavior is consistent with the behavior of slow channels in visceral smooth muscle and cardiac muscle. The curve of max dV/dt versus E_m is more or less typical of Ca^{2+} channel APs.

The specific blocker of fast Na^{2+} channels, TTX, has no effect on the rate of rise or overshoot of the APs of VSM cells (or of visceral smooth muscle). This was shown, for example, in guinea pig superior mesenteric artery (Harder and Sperelakis, 1979). This indicates that an inward fast Na^+ current does not contribute to the depolarizing phase of the AP and that fast Na^+ channels are either absent or nonfunctional (silent).

The max dV/dt and overshoot of the APs of most types of VSM are increased greatly by elevation of $[Ca]_o$ and decreased by lowering of $[Ca]_o$. This was shown, for example, in guinea pig superior mesenteric artery (Harder and Sperelakis, 1979; fig. 45-4) and in dog coronary arteries (Harder et al., 1979). In both arteries, a plot of AP amplitude (proportional to overshoot) against $\log[Ca]_o$ gave a straight line with a slope of about 30 mV/decade (table 45-2). Since this is about the same as the theoretical slope of 30.5 mV/decade calculated from the Nernst equation for a divalent cation, the results indicate that the inward current during the APs in these two types of arteries is carried almost exclusively by Ca^{2+} ion; that is, Na^+ ion carries little or no inward current. This conclusion is further supported by the results of experiments in which $[Na]_o$ was varied (and $[Ca]_o$ held constant). Variation in $[Na]_o$ over a wide range (0–150 mM) had little or no effect on the amplitude orr max dV/dt of the APs (Harder and Sperelakis, 1979). In addition, a plot of max dV/dt versus $\log[Ca]_o$ (between 1.0 and 5.0 mM) gave a straight line.

The results of Ca^{2+}-antagonistic agents, such as verapamil and bepridil, are consistent with the conclusion that the inward current during the APs is carried entirely by Ca^{2+} channels, i.e., fast Na^+ channels do not participate. In guinea pig superior mesenteric artery (Harder and Sperelakis, 1979; fig. 45-5A,B) and dog coronary arteries (Belardinelli et al., 1979; Harder et al., 1979), it was demonstrated that verapamil and bepridil depress and block the Ca^{2+}-dependent APs. If a significant participation of fast Na^+ channels occurred in VSM, then one could expect that verapamil and bepridil would not completely block the APs. Mn^{2+}, an inorganic Ca^{2+} antagonist, also blocked the APs (fig. 45-5C,D). A number of other calcium antagonists, including mesudipine, nifedipine, and diltiazem, were also shown to block the K^+ contracture of both arterial and venous smooth muscles (Sperelakis and Mras, 1983).

Because of the complete Ca^{2+} dependence of the APs, the TEA-induced APs should make a good assay system for determining the effects of vasoactive substances on the Ca^{2+} influx and on other membrane properties of the VSM cells, as will be shown below. The rate of rise of the AP is proportional to the inward current (for a constant membrane capacitance, C_m), and the inward current

Table 45-2. Summary of the properties of the TEA-induced action potentials in arterial smooth muscles

Parameter	Small diameter (<0.5 mm)	Large diameter (>1.0 mm)	Guinea-pig superior mesenteric artery[a]
Resting E_m (mV)	-53 ± 2	-56 ± 2	-54 ± 1.3
Amplitude of TEA-induced action potential (mV)	54 ± 1	56 ± 1	59 ± 1
Max dV/dt (V/s)	6 ± 1	5 ± 1	6 ± 0.7
Ca^{2+} dependency (mV/decade)	31	30	29

The data are given as the mean ± SE.
[a] The duration (at 50% repolarization) of the spikes in the guinea pig was 50–75 ms. From Harder et al. (1979) and Harder and Sperelakis (1979), with permission.

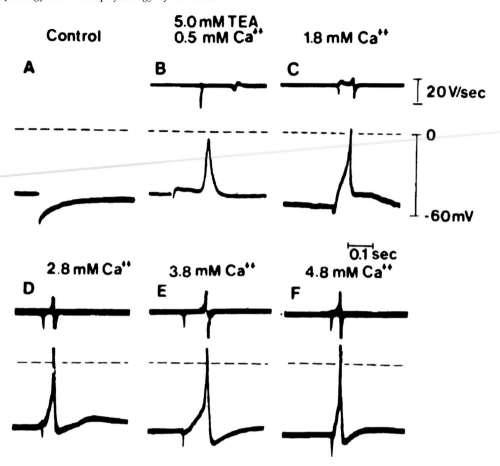

Fig. 45-4. Ca^{2+} dependency of stimulated action potentials in the presence of TEA^+ in normally inexcitable vascular smooth muscle from guinea pig superior mesenteric artery. All records were taken from one impalement. **A:** Control record showing a large resting potential of -58 mV and lack of spontaneous action potentials or responses to intense external electrical stimulation (one shock artifact depicted). **B–F:** Production of APs (in response to electrical stimulation) after addition of 5 mM TEA, illustrating an increase in amplitude and the maximal rate of rise dV/dt max or APs as $[Ca]_o$ is increased from 0.5 mM (B) to 1.8 mM (C), 2.8 mM (D), 3.8 mM (E), and 4.8 mM (F). The upper trace in B–F gives dV/dt, the maximal deflection of which is proportional to dV/dt max. The horizontal broken line gives the zero potential level. Taken from Harder and Sperelakis (1979), with permission.

(assuming the electrochemical driving force is unchanged) is proportional to the number of activated slow channels. Thus if a drug depresses the max dV/dt by 50%, this corresponds to a block of half of the slow channels (assuming the conductance per channel is unaffected). This analysis also assumes that the drug did not affect other membrane properties such as g_K. As we have seen above, changes in g_K can have profound effects on the max dV/dt of the AP, because the rate of rise is proportional to the net inward current and not the absolute inward slow current.

Effects of vasoactive substances on electrical properties

The electrical activity of VSM cells is greatly influenced by a number of substances. Here we introduce several substances that affect electrical and mechanical properties of VSM tissues, especially the coronary artery. For comparison, we also refer the reader to the results from other VSM tissues (for review see Somlyo and Somlyo, 1968b; Kuriyama et al., 1982; Bulbring and Tomita, 1987).

AUTONOMIC NEUROTRANSMITTERS

NE

In general, application of NE depolarizes the membrane and contracts the tissues. Such depolarization is accompanied by an increase or a decrease in the membrane resistance (Kuriyama et al., 1982; Itoh et al., 1983; Bolton et al., 1984). A decrease in the membrane resistance is considered to be caused mainly by an increase in Na^+ influx (also K^+, Ca^{2+}). The increase in the resistance is

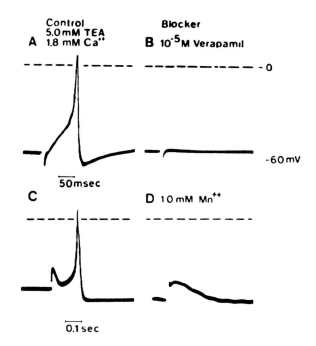

Control
5.0 mM TEA
A 1.8 mM Ca⁺⁺

Blocker
B 10^{-5}M Verapamil

50msec

C

D 10 mM Mn⁺⁺

0.1 sec

Fig. 45-5. Blockade of TEA-induced action potential by slow channel blockers in isolated vascular smooth muscle from guinea pig mesenteric arteries. **A:** Control record illustrating large overshooting AP induced by 5 mM TEA upon electrical stimulation. **B:** Record taken from the same cell, illustrating complete blockade of AP within 5 minutes after the addition of 10^{-5}M verapamil (shock artifact only visible). **C:** Another control record depicting the large overshooting AP induced by 5 mM TEA upon electrical stimulation. **D:** Record taken from same cell showing complete blockade of action potential within 30 seconds after the addition of 1.0 mM Mn^{2+} (shock artifact only visible). Taken from Sperelakis (1982), with permission.

considered to be caused by inhibition of the K^+ channel (Takata, 1980). Activation of receptor-operated Ca^{2+} channels is also supposed to be present; however, little about this is known. Following a low dose of NE, VSM tissues contract without a change in the membrane potential (pharmacomechanical coupling; Somlyo and Somlyo, 1968b; Somlyo et al., 1969; Droogmans et al., 1977; Van Breeman et al., 1979; Casteels, 1980). This excitatory action by NE is mediated by an activation of alpha adrenoceptor. In most arteries, the receptor subtype for this alpha action is α_1 and is blocked by prazosin, an α_1-selective blocker (Itoh et al., 1983; Kuriyama and Makaita, 1983). On the contrary, activation of beta adrenoceptors relaxes the tissues with or without hyperpolarization of the membrane potential (Mulvany et al., 1982; Bulbring and Tomita, 1987).

In some arteries, application of NE also produces rhythmic potential changes, which are suppressed in Na^+-free solution (Itoh et al., 1983). NE also induces spontaneous spike (Ca^{2+}-dependent) activity (Harder, 1981).

ACh

ACh, the muscarinic transmitter, has various effects on electrical and mechanical activity of VSM cells, and the interpretation of these effects is complicated (Kuriyama et al., 1982). ACh has been considered to have an inhibitory effect on VSM cells. ACh relaxes the tissue with or without hyperpolarization of the membrane, in some tissues (Kuriyama and Suzuki, 1978; Takata, 1980; Bolton et al., 1984). However, after the discovery of an endothelium-dependent relaxing factor (EDRF; Furchgott and Zawadzki, 1980), which is released from endothelium by ACh, such responses are mainly attributed to the effect of EDRF (Bolton et al., 1984; for review see Furchgott, 1984; Vanhoutte et al., 1986). Hyperpolarization is also induced by the unknown substance, endothelium-derived hyperpolarizing factor (EDHF), released from edothelium (Bolton et al., 1984; Bolton and Clapp, 1986; Komori and Suzuki, 1987). Actually, after the endothelial denudation, ACh itself sometimes contracts the VSM cell (with or without membrane depolarization) in such arteries (for example, rabbit mesenteric artery; Kuriyama and Suzuki, 1978; Itoh et al., 1983). However, some arteries are relaxed by ACh, even without the endothelium (guinea pig mesenteric artery; Bolton and Clapp, 1986). ACh depolarizes the membrane and contracts the portal vein as intestinal tissues (Takata, 1980). In pig coronary artery, ACh contracts the cell without a change in membrane activity (Ito et al., 1979). In guinea pig coronary artery, ACh contracts the tissue with membrane hyperpolarization (Kitamura and Kuriyama, 1979), which is considered to be partly due to activation of Ca^{2+}-dependent K^+ channels (Meech and Standen, 1975). On the contrary, still another coronary artery, the canine coronary artery, is relaxed by ACh without a change in the membrane potential (Ito et al., 1980).

HISTAMINE

Histamine also has various actions on VSM tissues. Both contraction and relaxation are observed in different animals and/or regions. Harder (1980) demonstrated that histamine (10^{-7} to 10^{-5}M) enhanced the TEA-induced APs in dog coronary arteries (<0.5 mm o.d.) and that this effect was blocked by the H_1-receptor antagonist, pyrilamine maleate. In quiescent preparations in the absence of TEA, histamine (10^{-6}M) hyperpolarized by 9 mV (from −55 to −64 mV) and reduced r_{in} to about half of the control value, consistent with an increase in g_K. Because the histamine-induced hyperpolarization was prevented by 1 mM Mn^{2+}, it was suggested that this increase in g_K was mediated by an increased Ca^{2+} influx and elevated $[Ca]_i$ due to the Meech–Gardos effect (Ca^{2+}-dependent K^+ channel; Meech and Standen, 1975). Casteels and Suzuki (1980) reported, in rabbit-ear artery, that histamine activates both H_1 receptors (blocked by mepyramine) and H_2 receptors (blocked by cimetidine), H_1 activation tending to depolarize and increase force development, and H_2 activation tending to hyperpolarize and decrease force development. Since K^+-free medium prevented the hyperpolarizing effect of H_2 activation, it appears that stimulation of the electrogenic pump is responsible for the hyperpolarization. Because they found that the effects of histamine on force were independent of changes in E_m, they concluded that H_1 activation induces release of Ca^{2+} from intracellular stores and that H_2 activation inhibits this release.

The presence of H_1 receptors on the endothelium has been reported, and this activation triggers EDRF release and relaxes the tissues (Toda, 1986).

ANGIOTENSIN II

Angiotensin II (AII) is a potent vasoconstrictor for maintaining the blood pressure. It contracts the VSM cell via membrane responses and/or hydrolysis of PIP_2 (Smith et al., 1984; Satoh et al., 1987). In rat portal vein, AII depolarizes the membrane and increases the spike activity (Takata and Kuriyama, 1979). AII (10^{-6} M), given as a bolus, rapidly depolarized cultured rat aortic VSM cells by about 10–30 mV (Zelcer and Sperelakis, 1981b). Sometimes the AII-induced depolarization triggered APs (with spike and plateau components). The AII-induced depolarization disappeared in Na^+-free solution, suggesting that the depolarization may be due to an increase in Na^+ conductance. In further studies on AII by Johns and Sperelakis (1982), continuous exposure of the cultured rat

aortic VSM cells to AII (rather than bolus injection) also produced an AII-induced peak depolarization of about 20 mV, which triggered an action potential consisting of a spike plus plateau (ca. 20-second duration; fig. 45-6). Membrane resistance was also lowered significantly, consistent with an AII-induced increase in conductance for an inward-depolarizing current.

These experiments demonstrate that AII has a direct effect on VSM cells to depolarize them and that this may be one important mechanism whereby angiotensin increases the degree of contraction of VSM cells. The results also demonstrate that functional angiotensin receptors are present in the cultured cells.

ENDOTHELIUM-DEPENDENT RELAXING FACTOR AND CONSTRICTING FACTOR (EDRF AND EDCF)

Various factors are released from the endothelium (for review see Furchgott, 1984; Vanhoutte et al., 1986). EDRF is one of them, which relaxes VSM tissues with increases in intracellular cyclic-GMP levels (Rapoport and Murad, 1983). After the first report by Furchgott and Zawadzki (1980), experiments have been intensively performed on this substance. Now EDRF is thought to be nitric oxide (Ignarro et al., 1987). There appear to be one or more other factors released from endothelium that hyperpolarize and relax VSM tissues (Bolton et al., 1984;

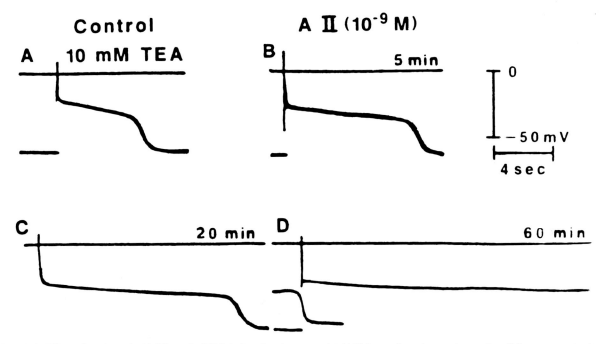

Fig. 45-6. Effect of angiotensin (A II) on the TEA-induced action potential (AP) in a cultured smooth muscle cell from rat aorta. **A:** Control AP induced by electrical stimulation in the presence of 10 mM TEA. **B–D:** Addition of 10^{-9} M A II (continuous exposure) progressively increased the AP duration at 5 minutes (B), 20 minutes (C), and 60 minutes (D). All records were from the same impalement. Taken from Johns and Sperelakis (1982), with permission.

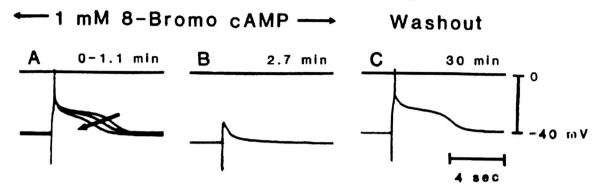

Fig. 45-7. Depression and abolition of TEA-induced action potentials in cultured rat aortic cells by 8-bromo-cAMP (A-C). **A:** Superimposed traces of a control action potential (in 15 mM TEA) and depression of the action potential within 1.1 minutes after addition of 1 mM 8-bromo-cAMP. **B:** Abolition of the action potential after 2.7 minutes. **C:** Recovery of the action potential upon washout for 30 minutes. (Records A–C were from the same cell.) The stimulation frequency was 0.04 Hz in both experiments. The time and voltage calibrations apply to all records. Adapted from Ousterhout and Sperelakis (1987), with permission.

Bolton and Clapp, 1986; Komori and Suzuki, 1987). The mechanism of this hyperpolarization is proposed to be an activation of the K^+ conductance or the Na-K pump (Komori and Suzuki, 1987; Vanhoutte, 1987).

Another factor released from the endothelium is EDCF, which contracts the VSM tissues (Hickey et al., 1985; Lugcher and Vanhoutte, 1986). One of them was identified as endothelin. Endothelin depolarized the membrane and also enhanced the Ca channel activity (Yanagisawa et al., 1988; Inoue et al., 1990; Klockner and Isenberg, 1991). Harder and Madden (1987) and Nagao and Suzuki (1987) reported that some factor is triggered from the endothelium by electrical stimulation that depolarizes the membrane and contracts the tissues. Some prostaglandins are also released from endothelium to contract VSM cells (Altiere et al., 1986).

EFFECTS OF SECOND MESSENGERS (CYCLIC AMP AND CYCLIC GMP) AND RELEASED AGENTS

The effects of cyclic nucleotide analogs and related agents on the TEA-induced APs in the cultured aortic reaggregates were examined (Ousterhout and Sperelakis, 1987). Superfusion with analogs of cyclic AMP (dibutyryl or 8-bromocyclic AMP, 1 mM; fig. 45-7) or agents that activate adenylate cyclase, such as isoproterenol (1–10 mM) and forskolin (1–10 mM), depressed or abolished the TEA-induced APs. Abolition of the APs by these agents was reversible and was accompanied by some hyperpolarization of the membrane. Superfusion with 8-bromo cyclic GMP (0.1–1 mM) also depressed or abolished the TEA-induced APs, whereas dibutyryl cyclic GMP (1 mM) and sodium nitroprusside (10 mM) had little effect (table 45-3; Sperelakis and Ousterhout, 1987). Synthetic atrial natriuretic factor (ANF, 0.01–0.1 mM), which activates the particulate form of guanylate cyclase (Fujii et al., 1986), had inhibitory effects in a few experiments (Sperelakis and Ousterhout, 1987). These results are consistent with the hypothesis that cyclic AMP, and possibly cyclic GMP, may

Table 45-3. Summary of the effects of cyclic nucleotides and related agents on the TEA-induced action potentials of cultured rat aortic cells

Compound	Effect of APs
8-bromo cyclic AMP (10^{-3} M)	Abolished
Dibutyryl cyclic AMP (10^{-3} M)	Abolished
Isoproterenol (10^{-6} M)	Abolished or depressed
Forskolin (10^{-6} M)	Abolished
8-bromo cGMP (10^{-4}–10^{-3} M)	Abolished or depressed
Dibutyryl cGMP (10^{-3} M)	No effect
Nitroprusside (10^{-6}–10^{-5} M)	Depressed slightly
Atrial natriuretic factor (10^{-8}–10^{-7} M)	Abolished or depressed

Taken from Ousterhout and Sperelakis (1987), with permission.

decrease the inward Ca^{2+} current, or increase an outward K^+ current, in the cultured aortic cells. Depression of membrane excitability may therefore be a contributing factor in the relaxation of aortic smooth muscle produced by some agents that increase intracellular levels of cyclic nucleotides.

Effects of some drugs on coronary artery

The mechanisms of action of certain vasoactive substances on coronary artery has been investigated (namely, the vasodilators: adenosine, nitroglycerin, and verapamil; and the vasoconstrictor: cardiac glycoside). Patients under treatment with cardiac glycosides sometimes develop coronary constriction, and Fleckenstein et al. (1975) suggested that this effect is mediated by an increase in Ca influx. Schnaar and Sparks (1972) found that the contractile responses of small coronary arteries were relaxed by adenosine but not by nitroglycerine, whereas the great vessels were relaxed by nitroglycerin but not by adenosine. They suggest that these effects were mediated by inhibition of Ca^{2+} influx. Ca^{2+} antagonists are now used clinically to prevent an attack of angina pectoris. These drugs especially have potent effects on variant angina, which is induced by coronary vasospasm. The primary target of those drugs is the coronary artery. These drugs also reduce preload and afterload of the heart, and consequently protect the heart from angina pectoris and possibly heart failure. Many Ca^{2+} antagonists are being developed and are currently used (for reviews see Fleckenstein, 1977; Godfraind et al., 1986; Ohya et al., 1986).

BLOCKADE BY Ca^{2+} ANTAGONISTIC AGENTS

Verapamil was first shown by Kohlhardt et al. (1972) to produce a decrease in contraction of cardiac muscle by inhibition of the Ca^{2+} influx from the extracellular fluid. The methoxy derivative of verapamil, D-600, had the same effect but was somewhat more potent. Another Ca^{2+}-antagonistic agent, nifedipine, was also shown to block the inward slow current in cardiac muscle (Kohlhardt and Flekenstein, 1977). Verapamil is not specific for Ca^{2+} influx, but also depressed Na^+ influx through myocardial slow channels, i.e., verapamil is a nonspecific blocker of slow channels (McLean et al., 1974). Similar findings were made by Labrid et al. (1979). In smooth muscle, verapamil inhibits Ca^{2+} influx in VSM cells (Peiper et al., 1971; Haeusler, 1972; Massingham, 1973; Bilek et al., 1974). The Ca^{2+} antagonistic drugs have vasodilatory effects, including on the coronary arteries. Bepridil also was shown to have coronary vasodilatory effects (Cosnier et al., 1977; Michelin et al., 1977) and an antianginal effect (Jouve et al., 1978).

Verapamil (10^{-5}M) rapidly depressed and abolished the TEA-induced APs in both small and large dog coronary arteries (table 45-4). The verapamil blockade is consistent with the Ca^{2+} dependency of the AP. As expected, the inhibitory effect of verapamil could be reversed by elevation of $[Ca^{2+}]_o$. Bepridil also rapidly depressed (10^{-6}M) and abolished (10^{-5}M) the TEA-induced APs (table 45-4; Harder and Sperelakis, 1981). Thus these results can explain the antianginal action of depridil, namely, inhibiting Ca^{2+} influx into the VSM cells of the coronary arteries and thereby exerting a relaxing effect on the VSM cells. $MnCl_2$ (1 mM), a relatively specific blocker of slow channels, exerted effects similar to those of verapamil and bepridil, namely, depression and block of the TEA-induced APs in both small and large coronary arteries (Sperelakis, 1982; table 45-4).

EFFECTS OF ADENOSINE

Adenosine (10^{-5}M) suppressed the TEA-induced Ca^{2+}-dependent action potentials in canine small coronary arteries within 1 minute (table 45-4; Harder et al., 1979). When the VSM cells blocked by adenosine were superfused with adenosine deaminase to destroy the adenosine, there was nearly complete recovery of the APs within 2 minutes. The depression of the max dV/dt by adenosine reflects an inhibition of the inward Ca^{2+} current. Adenosine had no significant effect on the resting potential (E_m) or input resistance (r_{in}). In contrast, adenosine (10^{-5}M) had no

effect on the amplitude or max dV/dt of the TEA-induced Ca^{2+}-dependent APs in the large coronary arteries (table 45-4; Harder et al., 1979).

EFFECTS OF NITROGLYCERIN

Nitroglycerin (10^{-5}M) abolished the TEA-induced Ca^{2+}-dependent APs in the large dog coronary arteries within 5 minutes (table 45-4; Harder et al., 1979). Fifty percent depression of both parameters was produced by about 5×10^{-6}M nitroglycerin, and 10^{-7}M nitroglycerin had a slght effect. The depression of max dV/dt by nitroglycerin corresponds to a depression of the inward Ca^{2+} current. Elevation of $[Ca]_o$ by 3 mM restored the APs depressed by nitroglycerin, indicating that the inhibitory effects of the drug are antagonized by Ca^{2+} ion. Nitroglycerin had no significant effect on the resting E_m or r_{in}. However, nitroglycerin (10^{-5}M) had no effect on either the amplitude or max dV/dt of the Ca^{2+}-dependent APs in the small coronary arteries (table 45-4; Harder et al., 1979). Ito et al. (1980) reported that high doses of nitroglycerin slightly hyperpolarized the membrane potential in dog coronary artery.

CARDIAC GLYCOSIDE POTENTIATION OF Ca^{2+} INWARD CURRENT

The effects of the cardiac glycosides, ouabain and digoxin, known to produce coronary vasoconstriction, were studied on the electrical activity of isolated small (0.5 mm o.d.) coronary arteries of the dog (Belardinelli et al., 1979). The cardiac glycosides (4×10^{-9} to 1×10^{-7}M) increased the amplitude and maximal rate of rise (dV/dt) of the TEA-induced Ca^{2+}-dependent APs in a dose-dependent manner (fig. 45-8A,B and table 45-4). In most experiments, a submaximal dose of TEA (usually 5 mM) was used so that the potentiating effects of the cardiac glycosides could be readily discerned. Significant enhancement by digoxin occurred at 4×10^{-9}M, and maximal potentiation occurred at 1×10^{-7}M. Increase in digoxin concentration to 10^{-6}M

Table 45-4. Summary of the effects of some vasoactive substances on the TEA-induced action potentials of small and large coronary arteries of the dog heart

Substance	Small diameter (<0.5 mm)	Large diameter (>1.0 mm)
Verapamil (1.5×10^{-6}M)	Blocked	Blocked
Bepridil (1×10^{-5}M)	Blocked[a]	—
Mn^{2+} (10^{-3}M)	Blocked	Blocked
Adenosine (10^{-5}M)	Blocked	No effect
Nitroglycerin (10^{-5}M)	No effect	Blocked
Cardiac glycosides (10^{-8}–10^{-6}M)	Potentiated	—

[a]Tested on intermediate-sized arteries (0.5–1.0 mm diameter). Data taken from Harder and Sperelakis (1979), Harder and Sperelakis (1978), Harder et al. (1979), Belardinelli et al. (1979), and Sperelakis (1982).

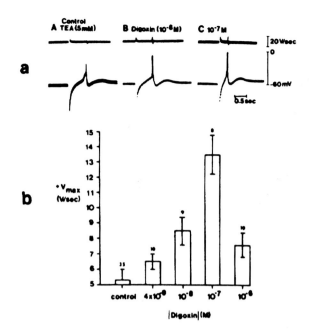

Fig. 45-8. **a:** Illustration of potentiating effect of digoxin on the amplitude and maximal rate of rise of the action potential. A: Elicitation of an undershooting action potential by electrical stimulation in the presence of TEA (5 mM). B,C: Records from same cell as in A taken within 2 minutes after the addition of 10^{-8} M (B) and 10^{-7} M (C) digoxin, showing a marked increase in the amplitude and maximal rate of rise of the action potentials. Upper trace gives dV/dt. **b:** Summary of data demonstrating the dose dependency of digoxin on the maximal rate of rise of the action potential. The tissue was bathed in 5 mM TEA to allow the elicitation of action potentials. Each bar gives the mean ± SE for the number of cells impaled (indicated by the number over the bars) in three to six coronary arteries. Significant increases in both maximal rate of rise and amplitude occurred at 10^{-8} M, and the peak effect occurred at 10^{-7} M. At higher doses of digoxin (10^{-6} M) there was a significant decrease in the maximal rate of rise and amplitude. Taken from Belardinelli et al. (1979), with permission.

produced a smaller potentiation than did 10^{-7} M, consistent with a blocking effect of high concentrations of cardiac glycosides on the slow channels (Vanhoutte et al., 1981; Sperelakis, 1982) and with some depolarization.

The cardiac glycosides also rapidly (e.g., 3–10 minutes) produced spontaneous APs in the presence of subthreshold doses of TEA (e.g., 5 mM) and increased the frequency of the spontaneous APs produced by 10 or 15 mM TEA (Belinardinelli et al., 1979). A small elevation in [Ca]$_o$ (e.g., by 1 mM) caused a marked increase in frequency, amplitude, and rate of rise of the APs, i.e., the effects of the glycosides were greatly enhanced in elevated [Ca]$_o$, consistent with the effect of the glycosides being mediated by an increase in Ca^{2+} conductance, hence Ca^{2+} influx. Verapamil (5×10^{-6} M) abolished all APs produced by the glycosides. Phentolamine (5×10^{-6} M), an alpha-adrenergic antagonist, did not prevent the effects of the

glycosides, and phenylephrine (5×10^{-6} M), an alpha-adrenergic agonist, had no significant effect on the resting potential or action potentials (Belinardinelli et al., 1979). These results suggest that the effects of the glycosides were not mediated by release of catecholamines from sympathetic nerve terminals or by activation of the alpha-adrenergic receptors. The effects of the cardiac glycosides occurred before any significant depolarization was evident (Belinardinelli et al., 1979). Significant depolarization was observed only after relatively long periods (e.g., 15 minutes) in high doses of glycoside, 10^{-6} M for digoxin and 10^{-7} M for ouabain. At 10^{-6} M, ouabain depolarized by 12 mV (from the control value of -54 mV to -42 mV) within 15 minutes. In summary, the data indicate that the low concentrations of cardiac glycosides ($<10^{-7}$ M) increase inward Ca^{2+} current in VSM by a mechanism that is independent of membrane depolarization, i.e., independent of the well-known action of the glycosides to inhibit the Na,K-ATPase and hence the Na-K cation pump. This Ca^{2+}-influx potentiating action of cardiac glycosides can account for their coronary vasoconstrictor effect and may be important in digitalis toxicity.

The effects of various substances on electrical and mechanical properties of dog coronary artery are summarized and listed in table 45-5.

NERVE-MUSCULAR INTERACTION

Almost all blood vessels are innervated by postganglionic sympathetic nerves. The transmitter release from these perivascular nerve terminals is initiated by the APs generated in the ganglionic cell body. Under experimental conditions transmitter release can be evoked by electrical stimulation in isolated blood vessels. The neuroeffector transmission between the adrenergic nerve terminals and vascular smooth muscle (VSM) can be regulated or modulated by a number of factors that act locally on the nerve terminals (prejunctional site; for review, see Langer, 1981; Vanhoutte et al., 1981; Kuriyama et al., 1982; Neild and Zelcer, 1982).

Production of EJPs, facilitation, and initiation of APs

Perivascular nerve stimulation with brief impulses evokes excitatory junction potentials (EJPs) in VSM cells. The amplitude of the EJP is thought to reflect the amount of transmitter released, and norepinephrine (NE) and ATP are believed to be the coneurotransmitters released from the sympathetic nerves (Hirst and Neild, 1978; Hirst and Neild, 1983).

The EJP rises quickly, reflecting the maximum synaptic current, and decays more slowly, as a passive exponential decay, reflecting the R_M C_M (time constant τ_M) properties of the VSM cell membrane. The duration of the EJP at 50% amplitude (EJP$_{50}$) is about 500 ms. The EJPs became successively larger in amplitude upon repetitive nerve stimulation, i.e., there is facilitation of neurotransmitter release. This phenomenon is illustrated in figs. 45-9 to 45-12. Facilitation of EJP amplitude does not occur in

Table 45-5. Effects of various agents on the electrical and mechanical activities of VSM tissues

	Membrane potential	APs	Contraction (C) relaxation (R)	Second messenger
NE (α_1)	$\uparrow \rightarrow$	$\uparrow \rightarrow$	C	PI-P_2 (+)
NE (α_2)	$\uparrow$		C	c-AMP (−)
Isop (β)	$\downarrow \rightarrow$	$\downarrow \rightarrow$	R	c-AMP (+)
ACh	$\uparrow \rightarrow \downarrow$		C,R	PI-P_2 (+), c-GMP (+)
Histamine	$\uparrow \rightarrow \downarrow$	$\uparrow \rightarrow$	C,R	PI-P_2 (+)
TxA_2	$\uparrow \rightarrow$		C	PI-P_2 (+)
AII	$\uparrow \rightarrow$	$\uparrow$	C	PI-P_2 (+)
ANP	$\rightarrow$	$\rightarrow$	R	c-GMP (+), PI-P_2 (−)
EDRF (NO)	$\rightarrow$	?	R	c-GMP (+)
EDHF	$\downarrow$	$\downarrow$	R	?
NG	$\downarrow \rightarrow$	$\downarrow \rightarrow$	R	c-GMP (+)
Adenosine	$\downarrow \rightarrow$	$\downarrow \rightarrow$	R	?
Cardiac glycoside	$\uparrow \rightarrow$	$\uparrow \rightarrow$	C	?
Endothelin	$\uparrow \rightarrow$	?	C	?

NR, norepinephrine; Isop, isoprenaline; ACh, acetylcholine; TxA_2, thromboxane A_2; AII, angiotensin II; ANP, atrial natriuretic factor; EDRF, endotheliun-dependent relaxing factor; NO, nitric oxide; NG, nitroglycerine; EDCF, endothelium-dependent constricting factor; $\uparrow$, enhance; $\rightarrow$ no change, $\downarrow$, decrease; PI-P_2, turnover of phosphatidylinositol biphosphate. EDHF, endothelium-dependent hyperpolarizing factor.

the renal artery of the guinea pig, but rather fatigue occurs, i.e., depression of EJP amplitude upon repetitive stimulation.

Repetitive nerve stimulation at a higher frequency produces temporal summation of the EJPs, which can reach the threshold voltage for action potential generation and subsequent contraction of the vascular smooth muscle. This is illustrated in figs. 45-9 and 45-10.

Release of transmitter is controlled by the level of excitation at the nerve terminals. In guinea pig mesenteric artery, EJPs were found to be dependent on external Na^+ and Ca^{2+} ions, and spikes were dependent on external Ca^{2+} ions (Zelcer and Sperelakis, 1982; fig. 45-10). Lowering $[Na]_o$ decreased EJP amplitude, but had no significant effect on spike max dV/dt. In contrast, lowering $[Ca]_o$ produced a significant decrease in both EJP amplitude and spike max dV/dt. Raising $[Ca]_o$ increased both parameters. These results suggest that transmitter release and EJP generation require external Ca^{2+} and Na^+. Intracellular Ca^{2+} may also be important.

It has been demonstrated that ω-conotoxin (ω-CTX) irreversibly blocked the EJPs in guinea pig vas deferens at 10–100 nM (Brock et al., 1989) and inhibited the EJPs in rat small mesenteric arteries at 0.1–3 nM (Pruneau and Angus, 1990). This effect was thought to be due to inhibition of excitation-secretion coupling, possibly mediated by the block of N-type Ca^{2+} channels.

Modulation of neurotransmitter release

Various vasoactive substances produce their effects on vascular tissues, in part by modulating neurotransmission.

Adrenergic α_2, cholinergic, and purinergic stimulation, and several prostaglandins attenuate transmitter release, presumably by acting through receptors on the nerve terminal. Beta-adrenergic stimulation, in contrast, enhances transmitter release.

ADRENERGIC FEEDBACK

Norepinephrine

In guinea pig mesenteric artery, norepinephrine decreases the amplitude of the EJPs (fig. 45-11). This phenomenon was previously reported to be mediated via presynaptic α_2-adrenoceptors that reduce the amount of neurotransmitter release (Kuriyama and Makita, 1983).

Isoproterenol

Isoproterenol acts on the beta-adrenoceptors and increases the intracellular cyclic AMP level. Figure 45-12 shows that application of 0.1 µM isoproterenol increased the amplitudes of the first EJP and the mean (11 pulses) EJP. These parameters were increased to 147 ± 12% and 117 ± 4% of the control values, respectively (table 45-6). The facilitatory action of isoproterenol on EJP amplitude was abolished by 0.3 µM propranolol (fig. 45-12). Isoproterenol had no effect on the resting potential or on the current/voltage relationship assessed by the electrotonic potentials in guinea pig mesenteric arteries.

Electrical responses induced by nerve stimulation

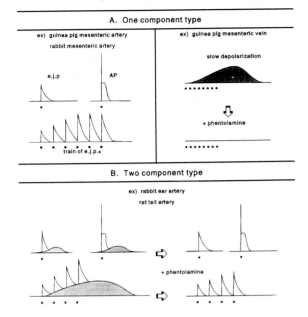

Fig. 45-9. Diagrammatic illustrations of the electrical responses induced by nerve stimulation. **A:** Electrical responses of one-component type. Left column: Fast EJP. Single electrical subthreshold intensity induced fast EJP only; when the stimulation is strong enough, action potential is produced following EJP. Train of stimulations induced train of EJPs and these EJPs show facilitation. Right column: Slow depolarization type. This depolarization was abolished by phentolaminc (alpha blocker), indicating that this response is mediated by NE released from the nerve terminal. **B:** Two-component type. In some vascular smooth muscle (e.g., rabbit ear artery), fast EJPs and following slow depolarization can be seen. Only slow depolarization is abolished by phentolamine. It is well known that these fast EJPs were produced by ATP, a cotransmitter that is released with NE from the nerve terminal.

HISTAMINE

A novel type of histamine receptor (H₃) was found on the perivascular adrenergic nerve terminals of guinea pig mesenteric artery (Ishikawa and Sperelakis, 1987; fig. 45-13). Histamine depresses EJP amplitude. Neither 2-methyl-histamine, an H₁ agonist, nor dimaprit, an H₂ agonist, decreased EJP amplitude, but N-α-methylhista-mine, a nonselective histamine derivative and H₃ agonist, mimicked the histamine depression with 10-fold higher potency than histamine itself. These results suggest that an H₃ receptor exists at the adrenergic nerve terminals. This novel class of histamine receptor is pharmacologically distinct from H₁- and H₂-histaminergic receptors. This H₃ receptor on nerve terminals is much more sensitive to histamine than are H₂ receptors on the VSM membrane, so that they may play an important function in the physiological control of the circulation. Stimulation of H₃ receptors may produce vasodilation by inhibiting the sympathetic

tone, i.e., they reduce the contractile influence of the sympathetic nerves on VSM.

CYCLIC NUCLEOTIDES

Second messenger systems are involved in signal transduction at the adrenergic nerve terminals in guinea pig mesenteric artery (Ishikawa and Sperelakis, 1989). Isoproterenol enhanced the EJP amplitude without modifying the passive membrane properties of the VSM cells. Forskolin (1–10 μM) markedly potentiated the isoproterenol-induced stimulation of EJP amplitude (table 45-6). Furthermore, 8-bromo cAMP, a permeable analog of cAMP, enhanced EJP amplitude without changing the resting potential (table 45-6; fig. 45-14), thus mimicking the effects of isoproterenol and forskolin. 8-bromo cGMP also augmented the EJP amplitude (table 45-6), but hyperpolarized the VSM cell membrane by approximately 4 mV (fig. 45-14) and decreased the input resistance, presumably by increasing the K⁺ conductance.

PROTEIN KINASE C

The effects of phorbol esters, direct activators of protein kinase C (PK-C), were examined to investigate the possible involvement of PK-C on the nerve terminal (Sperelakis et al., 1991). Phorbol-12-myristate-13-acetate (PMA) was applied in normal Krebs solution. After an incubation time of about 60 minutes, PMA (30, 100, and 300 nM) consistently enhanced the EJP amplitude evoked by nerve stimulation in a concentration-dependent manner (fig. 45-15). These facilitatory effects of PMA on EJP amplitude were significant for the first EJP as well as for the averaged EJP amplitude (table 45-6). PMA had no effect on the resting potential of the VSM cell.

From these results with the cyclic nucleotides and phorbol ester (table 45-6), three different protein kinase-dependent phosphorylation systems (cAMP/PK-A, cGMP/PK-G, and DAG/PK-C) could be involved in regulating neurotransmitter release from the perivascular nerve terminals.

PERTUSSIS TOXIN AND CHOLERA TOXIN

Pertussis toxin

The possible involvement of GTP-binding protein (G-protein) in neuromuscular transmission at the adrenergic nerve terminal of guinea pig mesenteric artery was investigated by pretreatment of blood vessels with pertussis toxin (PT), a bacterial exotoxin that catalyzes ADP ribosylation of G proteins (Nozaki and Sperelakis, 1989). PT was used to abolish the effect of G proteins (Gᵢ or Gᵢ-like protein).

In control conditions, EJP amplitude was suppressed by NE in a dose-dependent manner. In VSM preincubated with PT, the inhibition of EJP amplitude by NE was greatly attenuated. These effects of PT pretreatment were time and temperature dependent. Similar results were obtained with histamine. Since PT pretreatment had no obvious effect on the postsynaptic membrane (resting

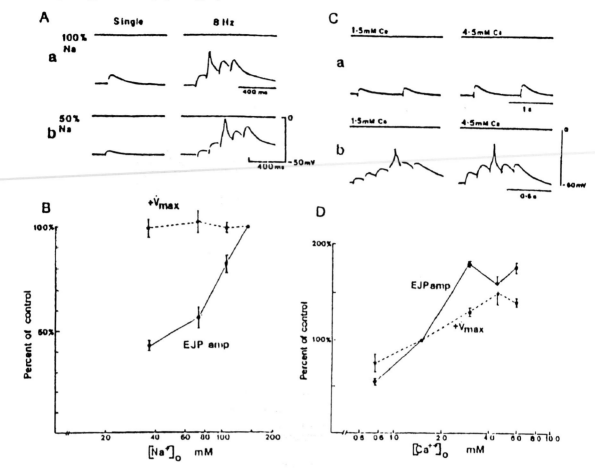

Fig. 45-10. Effects of [Na]$_o$ and [Ca]$_o$ on EJPs and action potentials. **A:** The effects of decreasing external Na$^+$ (replacement with choline $+10^6$ g/ml atropline) are shown using data from a single impalement. (a) Control responses to single and 8 Hz stimuli. (b) After 12 minutes in 50% [Na]$_o$. **B:** The relationship between the external Na concentration (log scale) and EJP amplitude (solid line) and spike max dV/dt (dashed line). **C:** The effects of changing external Ca^{2+} (a and b) from a single cell. **D:** Graph showing the relationship between the external Ca^{2+} concentration (log scale) and EJP amplitude (solid line) and spike max dV/dt (dashed line). Numbers in parentheses are numbers of cells impaled and numbers of preparations. Each point represents the mean $\pm$ SEM for paired data. Data were normalized relative to the amplitude of EJPs in each cell, in the normal Na$^+$ or Ca^{2+} solution. Taken from Zelcer and Sperelakis (1982), with permission.

potentials, depolarization by NE and ATP, and input resistance), these results suggest that PT pretreatment has mainly a presynaptic effect. Therefore, the NE and histamine effects on EJP amplitude may be mediated by PT-sensitive G proteins in the presynaptic nerve terminals.

Cholera toxin

The effects of cholera toxin (CTX) on the electrical properties of VSM cells of guinea pig mesenteric artery were also investigated (Nozaki and Sperelakis, 1991). CTX is a bacterial exotoxin that ribosylates subunits of the stimulatory G protein (G$_S$). EJP amplitude was markedly enhanced by treating isolated blood vessels with CTX (10 µg/ml for 1 hr). The VSM cells also became hyperpo-

larized (control: -68 ± 2.8 mV; CTX: -74.6 ± 2.1 mV), and their input resistances were significantly reduced (control: 12 ± 0.5 MΩ; CTX: 8.2 ± 0.5 MΩ). These effects persisted after washout for 35 minutes. The enhancement of EJP amplitude by CTX could not be abolished by injecting currents to depolarize the VSM membrane by 5 mV (to counter the hyperpolarization). CTX also abolished the effects of isoproterenol and 8-br-cAMP on the EJPs. These results suggest that CTX elevates cAMP levels in the nerve terminals and in the VSM cells.

SUMMARY MODEL

The model for modulation of neurotransmitter release is depicted in fig. 45-16. EJP amplitude (initial one and mean

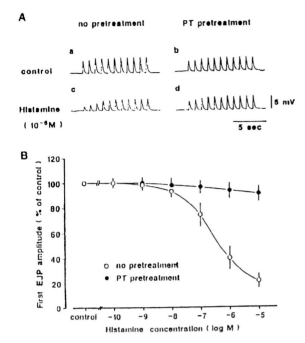

A

no pretreatment   PT pretreatment

control   a   b

Histamine   c   d | 5 mV

(10⁻⁶ M)   5 sec

B

Fig. 45-11. Effect of norepinephrine (NE) on excitatory junction potentials (EJPs) in guinea pig mesenteric artery preincubated with pertussis toxin (PT) or without PT. **A:** Actual traces of EJPs recorded before and after addition of NE (10^{-6} M) to tissues with PT pretreatment (b and d) or without pretreatment (a and c). Repetitive nerve stimulation was $30\,\mu s$ in duration, $30\,V$ in intensity, at $1\,Hz$ for a total of 11 pulses. **B:** Concentration-response curves showing effects of various concentrations of NE on EJP amplitude. Amplitude of first EJP in a train of stimuli was expressed as a fraction of that in control (NE free). EJPs were recorded 5–10 minutes after the application of each concentration of NE. Guinea pig mesenteric arteries were either pretreated for 24 hours at 21°C with 2×10^{-7} g/ml PT (●) or incubated under identical conditions without PT (○). Vertical bars indicate mean ± SE (n = 3–7). Taken from Nozaki and Sperelakis (1989), with permission.

of 11 EJPs) was used as the index of neurotransmitter released, because most of the agents tested had no significant effect on the electrical properties of the postsynaptic VSM cells, including resting potential and input resistance. The cotransmitters released at the nerve terminals in guinea pig mesenteric artery are ATP and NE. ATP is responsible for the fast component of the EJP and NE is responsible for the slow component (fig. 45-9). There is negative feedback regulation of the neurotransmitter release via receptors on the presynaptic membrane. NE acts on an α_2 receptor and G_i coupling protein (evidenced by the pertussis toxin data) to inhibit neurotransmitter release, as depicted in fig. 45-16. ATP acts on a P_2 receptor to inhibit release. Histamine acts on an H_3 receptor and G_i coupling protein to inhibit release.

Beta-adrenoceptor agonists, such as NE and isoproterenol, act on the beta-adrenoceptors and G_S coupling

protein (evidenced by the cholera toxin data) to stimulate transmitter release. This effect is presumably mediated by cAMP elevation. Addition of 8-Br-cAMP and 8-Br-cGMP produced marked stimulation of EJP amplitude due to stimulated transmitter release; 8-Br-cGMP also produced a small hyperpolarization of the postsynaptic VSM cell. Forskolin, a direct activator of adenylate cyclase, also potentiated transmitter release. Activation of protein kinase-C by phorbol esters also greatly potentiated neurotransmitter release, and therefore the amplitude of the EJPs. Therefore, phosphorylation of some proteins, perhaps in or near the presynaptic membrane, by PK-C, PK-A, and PK-G potentiate transmitter release.

In conclusion, there is regulation of neurotransmitter release at the adrenergic nerve terminals in vascular smooth muscle, via specific receptors for agonists on the presynaptic membrane. Such regulation includes negative feedback inhibition by the neurotransmitters themselves, including NE (via α_2 receptor), ATP (via P_2 receptor), and histamine (via H_3 receptor). These receptors are functionally connected to G_i coupling proteins for exerting their effects A positive feedback component occurs with NE activation of β_2 receptors presynaptically, which stimulate cAMP production via a coupling protein. Any agonist that stimulates phosphohpase-C (PL-C), and thereby IP_3 and DAG production, would activate PK-C and thereby potentiate transmitter release.

MEMBRANE CURRENTS AND IONIC CHANNELS OF VSM CELLS

In the past, the voltage-clamp method has not been successfully applied to many smooth muscle tissues because of the rapid decrement of potential due to the two-or three-dimensional spread of the current. Recent advances in techniques of dispersing single cells (Hermsmeyer, 1979; Inoue et al., 1985; Klockner and Isenberg, 1985) and a voltage clamp (patch clamp) using a suction pipette (Hamill et al., 1981) have greatly facilitated our understanding of the electrical phenomena observed in VSM tissues. Figure 45-17 shows a schematic drawing of various channels on VSM cells. This chapter mainly reviews the different and unique features of the VSM ion channels from other excitable tissues.

Voltage-dependent Ca²⁺ channels

The voltage-dependent Ca^{2+} channel is one of the important pathways of Ca^{2+} ion entry from the extracellular space into the cytosol (Somlyo and Somlyo, 1968b; Bolton, 1979; Johansson and Somlyo, 1980; Kuriyama et al., 1982). In most VSM cells, the AP is considered to be due to an activation of the voltage-dependent Ca^{2+} channels, not fast Na^+ channels, as suggested by studies using conventional intracellular voltage recording. Contraction induced by applying high-K^+ solution (high-K^+ contraction) is also considered to be induced by activation of voltage-dependent Ca^{2+} channels, because such contraction is inhibited by application of Ca^{2+} antagonists and by a

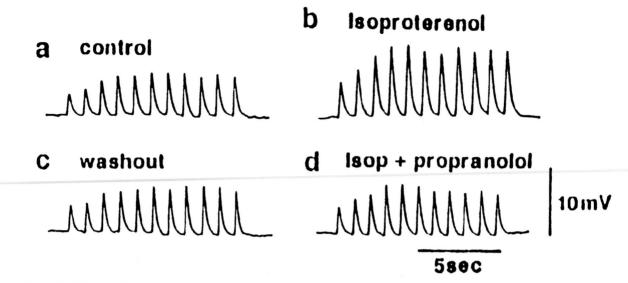

Fig. 45-12. Effects of isoproterenol on EJP amplitude and input resistance of the muscle cells of guinea pig mesenteric arteries. Repetitive nerve stimulation was 30 μs in duration, 30 V in intensity, at 1 Hz for a total of 11 pulses. **A:** EJPs were recorded from the same cell before (**a**) and 8 minutes after application of 0.1 μM isoproterenol (**b**). EJPs were also recorded before (**c**) and 10 minutes after the combined application of isoproterenol (0.1 μM) and propranolol (0.5 μM) (**d**). Note that propranolol blocked the isoproterenol potentiation of EJP amplitude. Taken from Ishikawa and Sperelakis (1989), with permission.

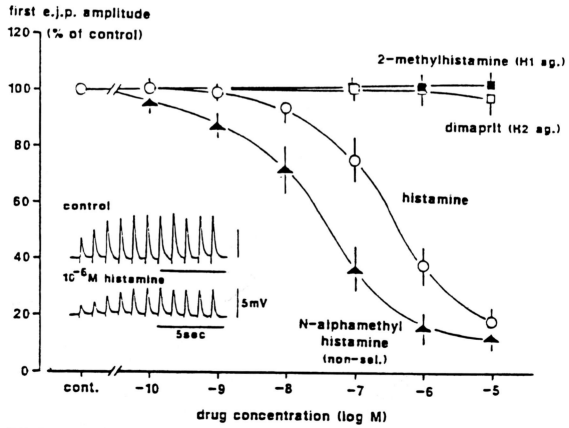

Fig. 45-13. Concentration-response curves for the effects of four histamine receptor agonists on neurotransmission in the guinea pig mesenteric artery. The amplitude of the first EJP in a train of stimuli was expressed as a fraction of that in the control. The EJPs were recorded 5–10 minutes after application of each agonist. The **inset** shows the inhibitory effect of histamine on the EJPs. The histamine-induced depression of EJP amplitude was not mimicked by 2-methylhistamine or dimaprit. A nonselective histamine derivative, N-α-methylhistamine mimicked the histamine depression with 10-fold higher potency than histamine itself. Taken from Ishikawa and Sperelakis (1987), with permission.

Table 45-6. Summary of effects of cyclic nucleotides, agents that affect cyclic AMP level, and phorbol ester on EJP amplitude in guinea pig mesenteric artery

	Relative EJP amplitude (%)	
	First EJP	Mean EJP
Isoproterenol (0.1 µM)	147 ± 12	117 ± 4
Forskolin (30 µM)	274 ± 7	139 ± 3
8-Br-cAMP		
0.1 mM	289 ± 23	143 ± 12
1.0 mM	592 ± 20	183 ± 19
8-Br-cGMP (1 mM)	266 ± 27	155 ± 8
Phorbol ester		
30 nM	132 ± 2[a]	99 ± 1
100 nM	194 ± 12[a]	113 ± 1.5[a]
300 nM	391 ± 12[a]	178 ± 10[a]

The values given are the mean ± SEM. The exposure time to PMA was >40–60 minutes.
[a] $p < 0.05$.
Data taken from Nozaki and Sperelakis (1991).

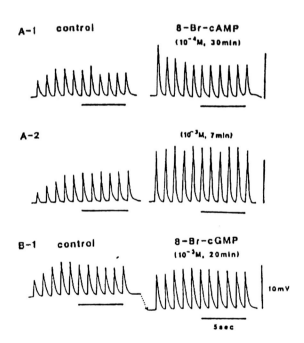

Fig. 45-14. Enhancement of the EJP amplitude by cyclic nucleotide analogs in guinea pig mesenteric arteries. **A:** Control EJPs were elicited by stimulation of the perivascular nerves at 1 Hz. After addition of 8-bromo cyclic AMP (8-Br-cAMP), the amplitude of the EJPs was increased (A1: 10^{-4} M, 30 minutes; A2: 10^{-3} M, 7 minutes). B1: Addition of 8-Br-cGMP (10^{-3} M, 20 minutes) hyperpolarized the membrane and increased the EJP amplitude. Both traces in each row were obtained from the same cell. Taken from Ishikawa and Sperelakis (1989), with permission.

reduction in the extracellular Ca^{2+} concentration. Previously the method for the estimation of the function of voltage-dependent Ca^{2+} channels in VSM cells was mainly the recording of APs or contractions. After the establishment of the patch-clamp method, the properties of Ca^{2+} channels of VSM cells could be examined directly, as has been done with other excitable tissues.

REGIONAL DIFFERENCES

Venous cells (e.g., portal vein), which have spontaneous activity, have a relatively high density of Ca^{2+} channels, as estimated by the maximum amplitude of inward Ca^{2+} currents under physiological conditions (150–300 pA/cell, cell capacitance of 15–30 pF), even with the presence of outward currents (Ohya et al., 1988A; fig. 45-18). However, in most arterial cells, which are usually quiescent in vitro, without suppression of the outward currents (K^+ channel) a net inward current cannot be seen (Tsien, 1983; Bean et al., 1986; Okabe et al., 1987; Matsuda et al., 1990). After elimination of the outward current, a small Ca^{2+} current is recorded from aortic cells (including A10 cell line; Friedman et al., 1986), pulmonary arterial cells (Okabe et al., 1987), and rabbit coronary artery (Matsuda et al., 1990; 50–100 pA/cell, cell capacitance of 10–25 pF). From rat and guinea pig mesenteric artery and rabbit ear artery, which are considered to be resistance vessels, a Ca^{2+} channel current of about 100 pA/cell is recorded, even with isotonic Ba^{2+} (100 mM) in the bath (Bean et al., 1986; Ohya and Sperelakis, 1989A; fig. 45-18). The above observations, together with the different distribution of K^+ channels, may partly account for the different behavior of each vascular tissue.

REGULATION OF THE Ca^{2+} CHANNEL

Control of the Ca^{2+} channel has been thoroughly investigated in neurons and heart cells (for review see Reuter, 1983; Tsien, 1983; Sperelakis et al., 1985). Many features of the Ca^{2+} channels are the same among these cell types, including VSM cells. However, several differences between VSM cells and cardiac cells must be considered. For example, in cardiac cells β stimulation enhances electrical and mechanical activity. Such phenomena are explained mainly by an enhancement of Ca^{2+} current induced by cyclic AMP-dependent phosphorylation of the Ca^{2+} channel. On the contrary, in VSM cells β stimulation relaxes the cell with or without suppression of the electrical activity (Bulbring and Tomita, 1987). Intracellular application of cyclic AMP and extracellular application of dibutyryl cyclic AMP have no effect on the Ca^{2+} current of intestinal and portal venous cells (Ohya et al., 1987A; Ohya and Sperelakis, 1988). However, intracellular ATP is essential for the activation of Ca^{2+} channels of VSM cells (Ohya and Sperelakis, 1989a,b). Therefore, in smooth-muscle cells, cyclic AMP-dependent phosphorylation does not play an important role in the regulation of Ca^{2+} channels. Other phosphorylation mechanisms are probably present. It was recently reported, using cloned Ca channels, that lack of cAMP stimulation of Ca^{2+}

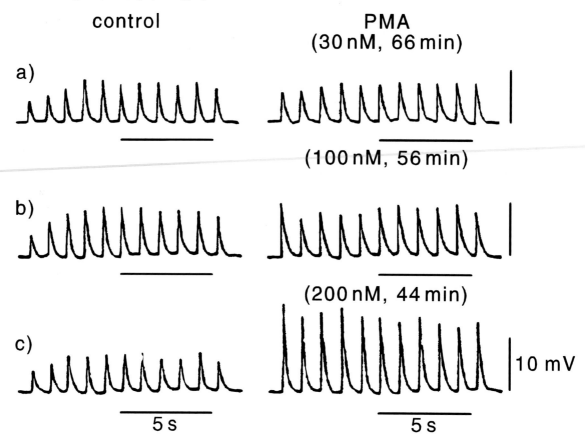

control

**PMA
(30 nM, 66 min)**

a)

(100 nM, 56 min)

b)

(200 nM, 44 min)

c)

10 mV

5 s   5 s

Fig. 45-15. Effects of phorbol-12-myristate-12-acetate (PMA) on the EJPs in guinea pig mesenteric artery. Perivascular nerves were stimulated by a train of *rectangular* current pulses (25 μs duration, 30 V intensity, 1 Hz frequency, and total of 11 pulses). Each record was obtained from a different cell. EJPs were recorded before (control) and after application of PMA: (a) 30 nM, 65 minutes; (b) 100 nM, 56 minutes; and (c) 300 nM, 44 minutes. Note the marked potentiation of the EJP amplitude (first, and total of the 11) produced by the protein kinase-C activator. From Ishikawa and Sperelakis (1989), with permission.

channel activity of VSM cells is mainly attributed to the difference in the β-subunit of the Ca^{2+} channel between cardiac muscle and smooth muscle, and not in the α_1-subunit (Klockner et al., 1992).

Inactivation mechanisms for I_{Ca} in smooth muscle cells are important for regulation of the cytosolic Ca^{2+} concentration. Voltage-dependent and Ca^{2+}-dependent mechanisms are considered to be the main inactivation mechanisms in VSM cells. An increase in the intracellular concentration of Ca^{2+} induced either by applying a conditioning pulse, which evokes Ca^{2+} current, or by the intracellular perfusion technique, suppressed the Ca^{2+} current (Ohya et al., 1988a; fig. 45-19). Together with the evidence that Ba^{2+} current through the Ca^{2+} channel decays more slowly than Ca^{2+} current, and an increase in the intracellular EGTA concentration also slows the decay of the Ca^{2+} current, the above inhibitory effects produced by intracellular Ca^{2+} indicate the presence of Ca^{2+}-dependent inactivation mechanisms for the Ca^{2+} channel. Voltage-dependent inactivation mechanisms are also present,

because application of the conditioning pulse at a low potential, which does not evoke Ca^{2+} current, inhibits the Ca^{2+} current, and because Ba^{2+} current does decay without the presence of Ca^{2+}. Both mechanisms may also be present in cardiac cells (Tsien, 1983; Josephson et al., 1984; Lee et al., 1985). In VSM cells, about 50% of the Ca channels are not available for opening with the resting $[Ca]_i$ (0.1 μM), and increase in $[Ca]_i$ to the level for inducing contraction greatly decreases the availability because of the Ca^{2+}-induced inactivation mechanism (fig. 45-19).

TWO TYPES OF Ca^{2+} CHANNELS

As in other excitable membranes, VSM cells have two types of Ca^{2+} channels, i.e., fast and slow types (Bean et al., 1986; Friedman et al., 1986; Aaronson et al., 1986; Yatani et al., 1987; Rusch and Hermsmeyer, 1988; fig. 45-20). These two channels are distinguished by differences in their voltage dependency of activation and inactivation,

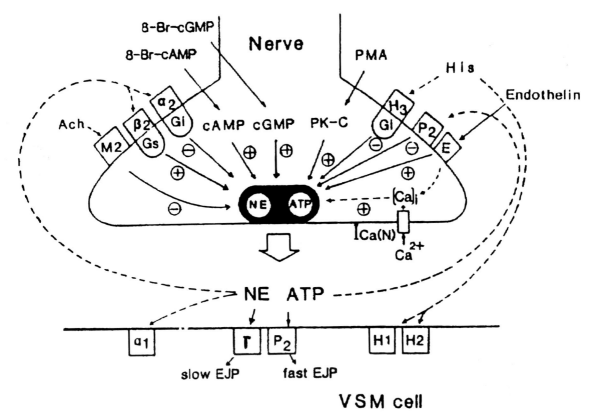

Fig. 45-16. Model for modulation of neurotransmitter release at adrenergic nerve terminals in guinea pig mesenteric artery. As depicted, norepinephrine (NE) and ATP are cotransmitters released simultaneously. A number of feedback mechanisms are depicted, as well as stimulation of neurotransmitter release by cAMP, cGMP, and phorbol esters (PK-C).

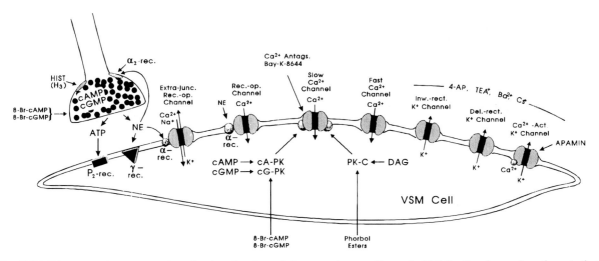

Fig. 45-17. Diagrammatic representation of various ion channels in a vascular smooth muscle (VSM) cell and a number of agents that may either activate or inhibit these channels. Depicted are three different types of Ca^{2+} channels (fast, slow, and receptor operated) and a nonselective ion channel (extrajunctional, receptor operated), which allows Ca^{2+}, Na^{2+}, and K^+ to pass through. The voltage-dependent Ca^{2+} slow channels are blocked by Ca^{2+} antagonists and enhanced by Ca^{2+} agonists (Bay-K-8644). The three different K^+ channels (inward rectifier, delayed rectifier, and Ca^{2+} activated) are blocked by TEA^+, Ba^{2+}, and Cs^+. Also shown is an adrenergic nerve terminal from which norepinephrine (NE) and ATP are released to activate α or γ receptors and purinergic (P_2) receptors, respectively, on the postsynaptic membrane. Release of neurotransmitters may be modulated by substances such as NE, histamine, and cyclic nucleotides. Other vasoactive substances, such as angiotensin II, may also affect ion channels in the membrane.

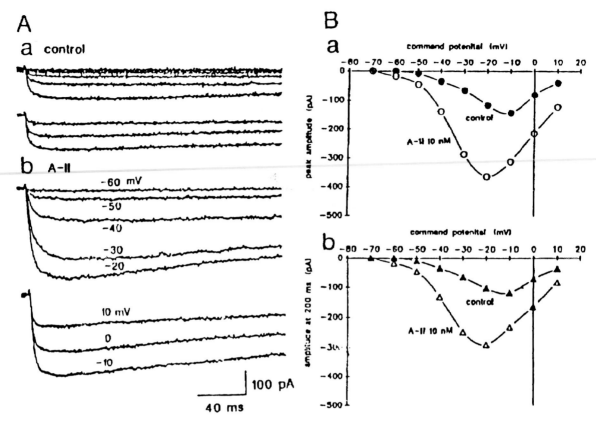

Fig. 45-18. Effects of angiotensin-II (A-II) on the Ca^{2+} channel current recorded from single smooth muscle cells isolated from guinea pig portal vein. **A:** Ba^{2+} current recorded before (a) and 3 minutes after (b) application of 10 nM A II. Step command pulses were applied over the voltage range of -60 mV to 10 mV from a holding potential (HP) of -90 mV. **B:** Peak current amplitude (a; circles) and amplitude measured at 200 ms (b; triangles) before (filled symbols) and after (unfilled symbols) A II application, were plotted against the command potentials. Data in A and B were collected from the same cell. Bath solution contained 2 mM Ba^{2+} as the charge carrier. Pipette solution contained high Cs^+, with 5 mM ATP and 0.1 mM GTP. Taken from Ohya and Sperelakis (1991), with permission.

sensitivity to dihydropyridine derivatives (Ca^{2+} channel antagonists and agonists), single-channel conductance, permeability to various divalent cations, etc. (table 45-7). However, the amount of fast type compared to slow type reported is variable in each cell, in each region, and in each species. In arterial smooth muscle cells, the distribution of fast T-type current is small (Ohya and Sperelakis, 1989). It was reported that only few or no fast T-type current is seen in the rabbit coronary artery (Matsuda et al., 1990), but that both types are present in guinea pig coronary artery (Gamitkevidr and Isenberg, 1990). In pathological conditions, changes of distribution of slow-type channels were reported. Rusch and Hermsmeyer showed, using cultured azygous vein cells from neontal SHR and WKY, that a higher density of distribution of slow L-type Ca^{2+} channels occurred in SHR than in WKY (Rusch and Hermsmeyer, 1988). It was reported that incubation of the cells with cholesterol increases the slow L-type current in cultured arterial cells (Sen et al., 1992).

This observation may be important in considerations of the mechanisms of vasospasm and atherosclerosis.

Ca^{2+} ANTAGONISTS

A Ca^{2+} antagonist is a compound that blocks the Ca^{2+} channel, mainly the voltage-dependent Ca^{2+} channel. Both inorganic (Co, Mn, Ni, La) and organic (nifedipine, nicardipine, diltiazem, verapamil, etc.) Ca antagonists block the Ca^{2+} channel currents. Organic compounds are considered to possess a higher affinity (sensitivity) for vascular tissues than for other excitable tissues such as cardiac cells (Fleckenstein, 1977; Godfraind et al., 1986; Ohya et al., 1986). The possible explanations considered for this high sensitivity are the following: (a) The nature of the Ca^{2+} channel is different. Recent advances in molecular biology show that the α_1 subunit of the Ca^{2+} channel, which is the receptor site for the Ca^{2+} antagonists, differs between tissues. (b) VSM cells have relatively low mem-

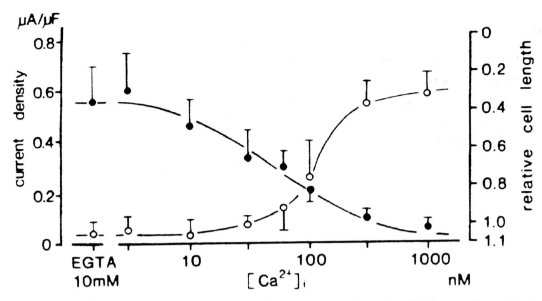

Fig. 45-19. Effects of $[Ca^{2+}]_i$ on the amplitude of I_{Ca} and the shortening of smooth muscle cells. To normalize amplitudes of I_{Ca} recorded in individual cells, the amplitude of I_{Ca} was expressed as a current density. The shortening of the single smooth was expressed as a relative cell length after exposure to the pipette solution. Individual records were obtained in the test pipette solution in the absence (EGTA 10 mM without addition of $CaCl_2$, the control) or presence of various $[Ca^{2+}]_i$ (3–1000 nM). Current density (closed circles) and relative length of smooth muscle cells (open circles) were plotted against the $[Ca^{2+}]_i$. Each point indicates mean ± SD (n = 7–20). Values obtained above 30 nM $[Ca^{2+}]_i$ for the shortening are statistically significant. Continuous curve of the I_{Ca} was drawn by the best least-squares fit to the equation described in the text, and the relation line for changes in the cell length was drawn by eye.

brane potentials, which increases the amount of channels in an inactivated state. Ca^{2+} antagonists bind to the inactivated Ca^{2+} channel with higher affinity, according to the modulated receptor hypothesis (Bean et al., 1983; Bean, 1984). (c) The distribution of fast and slow Ca^{2+} channels is different.

(d) Differences in the methods for estimation of K_d the value; i.e., in cardiac cells, voltage clamp or APs are used, while in smooth muscle cells, isometric tension recording (high K^+ simulation, agonist stimulation) is mainly used. Bean et al. (1986) reported in rat mesenteric artery, the K_d value for the high-affinity binding site of nitrendipine was almost the same as in cardiac cells (0.46 nM in VSM cells, 0.1–1 nM in cardiac cells). However, a half-blocking concentration of this drug in VSM cells was lower than in cardiac cells (100–300 nM vs. 700 nM). They suggested that this is because the resting state of the channel binds nitrendipine more tightly in vascular muscle than in cardiac muscle. Further experiments are needed to clarify this point. (e) Differences in accessibility of the drug to the Ca^{2+} channel. Ca^{2+} antagonist access to the channel is at the outer surface, at the intracellular surface, or within the plasma membrane. The accessibility may be affected by charge or composition of the membrane lipid. For example, methoxy-verapamil has been shown to block the Ca^{2+} channels by acting on the inner surface of the cell membrane in cardiac muscles (Hescheler et al., 1982). However, from a similar study in smooth muscle cells, Ohya et al. (1989) concluded that Ca^{2+} antagonists bound

to the outside of the membrane, not to the inside. It was demonstrated that ^3H-bepridil and ^3H-verapamil readily enter VSM cells (rabbit aorta) (Mras and Sperelakis, 1982; Pang and Sperelakis, 1983). In smooth muscle and cardiac muscle, the order of uptake observed was bepridil > verapamil ≫ nifedipine > diltiazem (Pang and Sperelakis, 1983). This order of uptake was in the same order as their lipid solubilities (Pang and Sperelakis, 1984). Possible secondary intracellular effects, in addition to block of the voltage-dependent Ca^{2+} channels, are not fully understood yet and should be clarified for VSM cells.

Actions of these drugs on the single Ca^{2+} channels in VSM cells have not been clarified in detail. Those actions in the case of cardiac cells are reviewed elsewhere (Hess et al., 1984). Ca^{2+} agonists are derivatives of dihydropyridines (Bay-K-8644, CGP28392, etc), which enhance the voltage-dependent Ca^{2+} current (slow-type) in VSM cells (Bean et al., 1986; Caffrey et al., 1986; Yatani et al., 1987A). In single-channel recording, a prolongation of the mean open time was observed (Caffrey et al., 1986; Benham et al., 1987A). Such effects are the same as those observed in other excitable cells (Hess et al., 1984).

Modulation of Ca^{2+} channels by agonists

Agonists may modify the voltage-dependent Ca^{2+} channels of vascular smooth muscle cells, as occurs in cardiac cells by beta-adrenergic agonists. However, one group (Aaronson et al., 1986) has reported that NE enhances the

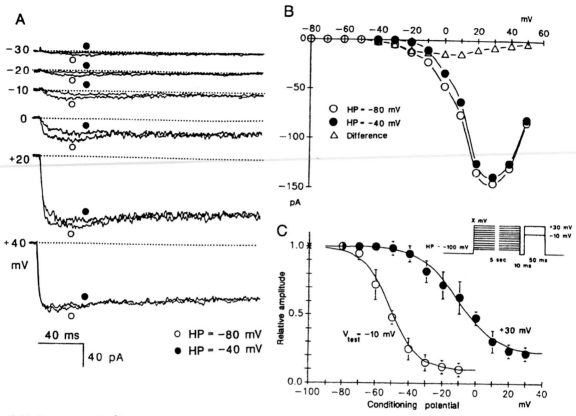

Fig. 45-20. Two types of Ca^{2+} channel currents recorded from single smooth muscle cell of guinea pig small mesenteric artery. **A:** Traces of the Ca^{2+} channel currents recorded at six different command potentials from holding potentials (HPs) of $-80\,mV$ ($\bigcirc$) and $-40\,mV$ ($\bullet$). Dotted lines indicate the zero current level. **B:** I/V curves of the peak current amplitudes obtained from the holding potentials (HPs) of $-80\,mV$ ($\bigcirc$) and $-40\,mV$ ($\bullet$) for the same cell as in A. The difference curve between these two currents is also plotted ($\triangle$). **C:** Steady-state inactivation curves for the fast current ($\bigcirc$) and slow currents ($\bullet$). Various levels of conditioning pulses (5 seconds) were applied before application of the test pulse (to $-10\,mV$ for the fast current and to $+30\,mV$ for the slow current); 10-ms intervals were used between the conditioning pulse and the test pulse. HP was kept at $-100\,mV$. Data are shown as mean $\pm$ SD (n = 3–5). Continuous curves were drawn by fitting the data to a Boltzmann distribution (for the fast current, k = 8.3 mV, V_h = -51.3 mV, s = 0.1; for the slow current, k = 11.0 mV, V_h = -11.2 mV, s = 0.23). The pipette contained high Cs^+ and 5 mM ATP, and the bath contained isotonic Ba^{2+} solution. Taken from Ohya and Sperelakis (1989), with permission.

Table 45-7. Differences between two types of Ca^{2+} channels in VSM cells

	Fast (T type)	Slow (L Type)
Threshold	Low ($-60 \sim -40\,mV$)	High ($-20 \sim -30\,mV$)
Current decay	Fast	Slow
Voltage for half inhibition	$-60 \sim -40\,mV$	Over $-20\,mV$
Ca^{2+}-dependent inactivation	$- \sim \pm$	$+$
Permeation of divalent cation	Ba = Ca	Ba > Ca
Single-channel conductance	7 pS	26 pS
(isotonic Ba^{2+} in the pipette)	8 pS	24 pS
Cell-free recording	Possible	Rundown
Dihydropyridine sensitivity	$\pm \sim +$	$++$
Regulated by phosphorylation		

Ca^{2+} channel current in rabbit ear artery, whereas another group (Droogmans et al., 1987) has reported that it is inhibited. It was reported that NE enhanced the fast-type Ca^{2+} channels in cultured rat portal vein cells (Pacaud et al., 1987). Others observed no significant changes in rat mesenteric artery and dog saphenous vein (Bean et al., 1986; Yatani et al., 1987A). ACh enhanced the Ca^{2+} channel current of rabbit coronary artery (Matsuda et al., 1990). Some of the variability in these findings may be due to the use of different protocols and experimental conditions. However, it is likely that agonists affect the ion channel activity via a number of different mechanisms. Furthermore, there might be some factor that regulates the response to agonists, which is lost from the cell by perfusion under whole-cell voltage-clamp configuration. Ca^{2+}-induced Ca^{2+} channel inactivation also may modify agonist action on the Ca^{2+} channels. It was reported that this mechanism was present in vascular muscles, as in cardiac muscles and neurons, and that the threshold concentration of intracellular Ca^{2+} required to inactivate the Ca^{2+} channels was lower than in cardiac muscle (Ohya et al., 1988). Agonists trigger Ca^{2+} release from the store sites, and this released Ca^{2+} may inhibit the Ca^{2+} channel activation. The Ca^{2+}-induced Ca^{2+} inactivation mechanism, along with possible unknown factors, makes agonist action on Ca^{2+} channels complicated.

Ang-II enhanced the Ca^{2+} channel current in guinea pig portal venous cells (Ohya and Sperelakis, 1991). To ensure consistent results, the conditions were as follows: (a) Ba^{2+} ion was used as a charge carrier to record the Ca^{2+}-channel currents, and the single cells were stored in the Ca^{2+}-free solution before experimentation, to avoid Ca^{2+} loading of the store sites. (b) The pipettes used had a relatively small tip diameter to avoid losing unknown intracellular factors. (c) Ang-II was applied in the bath solution after the same preincubation time for stabilizing the intracellular content by the pipette solution (after making whole-cell configuration). Ang-II enhanced the Ca^{2+}-channel currents in about 90% of the cells used. The threshold concentration of Ang-II to enhance the current was about 10^{-10} M. Half-enhancement of the maximal response was observed at about 10^{-8} M.

Besides enhancement of the amplitude, Ang-II also shifted the current/voltage relationship in the negative direction by 5–15 mV. With 2 mM Ba^{2+}, the threshold was between −60 mV and −50 mV, and maximum amplitude was observed around −10 mM; with 2 mM Ca^{2+}, threshold was about −40 mV, and maximum amplitude was at about 0 mV. If simple extrapolation is applied, in the physiological condition (2 mM Ca^{2+}) the threshold potential should be shifted to be between −55 and −45 mV. This value is similar to the resting potential reported for this tissue. This could explain why Ang-II enhanced spike activity without depolarization (Takata and Kuriyama, 1979; Johns and Sperelakis, 1982). Furthermore, the shift of the threshold potential by agonists may contract the vascular smooth muscle, even without membrane depolarization.

A secondary effect of Ang-II on the Ca^{2+} channels was also observed, namely, an inhibitory effect. After the Ca^{2+} channels were stimulated, the current decreased gradually. This phenomenon was most evident with high concentrations of Ang-II. This is not due to the Ca^{2+}-induced Ca^{2+} channel inactivation, because Ba^{2+} ion was used (instead of Ca^{2+}) in the bath solution as the charge carrier.

Possible involvement of GTP-binding protein (G protein) in Ang-II action

Involvement of G protein in the regulation of Ca^{2+} channels by Ang-II in vascular smooth muscle cells was investigated by the whole-cell voltage-clamp method (Ohya and Sperelakis, 1991). The analogues of GTP, GDP-βS and GTP-γS, are considered to be good tools to examine the involvement of G protein in the receptor coupling to various effectors (Gilman, 1987). Single cells from guinea pig portal vein were used. Either GTP (0.1 mM), GDP-βS (0.3 mM or 1 mM), or GTP-γS (0.3 mM or 1 mM) was contained in the pipette solution for diffusion into the cell interior. GTP-γS is considered to (a) substitute for endogenous GTP in the binding site of the G protein; (b) be a poor substrate for the GTPase, causing its effect to be persisten; and (c) cause slowly increasing activation of G protein in the absence of agonist stimulation (Gilman, 1987). In electrophysiological studies, persisting and strong effects of GTP-γS in the activation of the G_K channel in atrial cells and in the inhibition of the Ca^{2+} currents of neuronal cells and cardiac cells were observed (Hescheler et al., 1987; Yatani et al., 1987; Ikeda and Schofield, 1989).

In experiments of guinea pig portal vein, GTP-γS (0.3 mM and 1 mM) produced a slowly progressive increase in the basal current amplitude and inhibited the subsequent Ang-II action, perhaps due, at least in part, to substitution for endogenous GTP in the G protein and to the increased basal level. The slow increase in the basal amplitude might be due to a slow increase in degree of activation of G protein.

GDP-βS is a competitive inhibitor of GTP binding to the G proteins (Gilman, 1987). There are several reports with electrophysiological studies showing that intracellular GDP-βS blocks the agonist-dependent responses (Holz et al., 1986; Dolphin and Scott, 1987; Hescheler et al., 1987; Ikeda and Schofield, 1989). In our observations, GDP-β-S suppressed the effect of Ang-II dose dependently and time dependently (fig. 45-21). Therefore, this result, together with those of GTP-γS, provides positive evidence of the involvement of G protein.

Pertussis toxin (PTX) is the bacterial toxin that ribosylates the subunit of G_i or G_i-like protein, and consequently inhibits the action of this G protein (Dolphin and Scott, 1987). Preincubation of muscle tissues with pertussis toxin (PTX; 10^{-6} g/ml; for up to 6 hr at 36°C) or intracellular application of preactivated PTX (10^{-6} g/ml) with NAD (10^{-3} M) did not inhibit the Ang-II action. In biochemical studies and voltage-clamp studies, these procedures were demonstrated to be effective in ribosylating the G protein in cardiac tissues (Kurachi et al., 1986; Inoue and Isenberg, 1990) and vascular tissues (Ito et al., 1978; Suematsu et al., 1984). To confirm these results, the muscle tissues

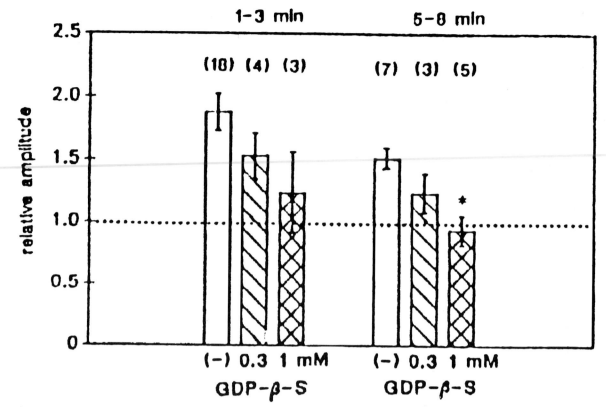

Fig. 45-21. Relative amplitudes of the Ba^{2+} current affected by 10 nM angiotensin II (A-II) with and without the presence of GDP-β-S. The basal current amplitude before application of A-II was normalized to 1.0 (horizontal dotted line). Pipette solution contained either 0.1 mM GTP as control (--) or GDP-β-S at 0.3 or 1 mM. Incubation with the pipette solution was either short (1–3 minutes) or long (5–8 minutes). The number of cells for each condition is indicated in parentheses. *Statistical significance compared with control.

were treated by PTX (10^{-6} M) for 24 hours at 36°C, and the mechanical force produced by high K^+ and Ang-II was measured. There was no significant difference between control tissue (incubation without PT) and PT-pretreated tissue in the contraction induced by 10 nM Ang-II (Y. Ohya, unpublished observations).

Another important toxin for investigation of the involvement of GTP-binding protein in the agonist response is cholera toxin (CTX). CTX ribosylates G_S protein (Gilman, 1987; Inoue and Isenberg, 1990). In vascular smooth muscle, CTX was reported to inhibit agonist-induced contraction, probably due to increasing cytosol cAMP level (Ousterhout and Steinsland, 1981; Asano et al., 1988). In our experiments, CTX did not change the Ang-II response, suggesting that G_S does not have an important role in this system. These results suggest that Ang-II-induced stimulation of Ca^{2+} channels in vascular smooth muscle cells may be mediated by a G protein that is not PTX sensitive or CTX sensitive. Because of variability of G protein as well as receptors, receptor coupling of G-protein in other vascular tissues and in other receptors may not be the same.

Possible mechanisms underlying agonist modulation of Ca^{2+} channels

REGULATION BY C KINASE

Neurotransmitters and hormones promote the breakdown of membrane phospholipids and the formation of two putative second messengers, inositol-1,4,5-triphosphate (IP_3) and 1,2-diacylglycerol (DAG), by activating phospholipase C (reviewed in Nishizuka, 1984). Phospholipase C is known to be modified by G protein. Therefore, products from this phospholipid breakdown may be the candidates to explain the G-protein-mediated Ang-II action. IP_3 is known to release Ca^{2+} from intracellular stores (reviewed in Berridge and Irvine, 1984), including the SR of vascular smooth muscle (Somlyo et al., 1985). Recent studies also suggest an important role of IP_4 in regulating Ca^{2+} influx (Irvine and Moor, 1986). We have previously reported that neither IP_3 or IP_4, perfused into the cell, modify the Ca^{2+} channel current directly, suggesting that these two phospholipid metabolites were not candidates for modifying the Ca^{2+} channels in vascular smooth muscles (Ohya et al., 1988).

Activation of protein kinase C has been suggested (Rasmussen et al., 1987) to be involved in agonist-induced Ca^{2+} influx, responsible for the tonic phase of smooth muscle contraction. Phorbol esters, which activate protein kinase C (PK-C), produce a slowly developing sustained contracture of vascular muscle that is dependent at least partially on $[Ca]_o$ (Danthuluri and Deth, 1986; Gleason and Flaim, 1986; Itoh and Lederis, 1987). To examine a possible role of PK-C in modulation of electrical activity of VSM cells, the effects of phobol 12,13-diacetate (PDA) were determined on the membrane potential and APs in cultured aortic reaggregates (Ousterhout and Sperelakis, unpublished observations). Superfusion with PDA produced a gradual depolarization and, in most cases, also allowed the appearance of an active AP (plateau-type) in response to electrical stimulation. This AP response was abolished by verapamil. When APs were elicited in the presence of TEA, PDA also depolarized and, at first, prolonged the AP duration. After prolonged exposure to PDA (20–30 minutes), the APs became depressed or abolished. Therefore, phorbol esters had several effects on membrane excitability, including depolarization accompanied by induction or enhancement of Ca^{2+}-dependent APs, followed by depression of the APs.

The depolarization produced by the phorbol esters could be due to inhibition of K^+ channels, and the induction of APs could result from the depression of a K^+ conductance and/or the activation of a Ca^{2+} conductance. For example, in cultured aortic cells (A7r5 cell line; Fish et al., 1988) and neonatal rat cardic myocytes, phorbol esters increased the slow (sustained) Ca^{2+} channel current (Dosemeci et al., 1988). The subsequent depression of the APs could be due, in part, to depolarization-induced inactivation of the Ca^{2+} channels, or to a more direct inhibition of the Ca^{2+} channels. Such dual actions of phorbol esters on the Ca^{2+} channels were reported in cultured neurons and cardiac myocytes (Wertz and MacDonald, 1987; Lederer et al., 1988). Thus, C kinase might be involved in the agonist actions on Ca^{2+} channels. However, since several reports suggested that C kinase did not have stimulatory effects, further study is required to clarify the action of C kinase.

DIRECT REGULATION BY G PROTEIN

Direct regulation of ionic channels by G protein has been reported in several tissues (reviewed in Rosenthaul et al., 1988). In some neurons G protein (G_o) mediates the inhibition of Ca^{2+} channels produced by receptor activation by agonists (Casteels, 1980). In cardiac cells, G protein (G_S) was reported to directly enhance the activity of Ca^{2+} channels (Yatani et al., 1987B).

Effects of GTP-γS, which activates the G protein directly, on single Ca^{2+} channels were examined in single cells isolated from guinea pig portal vein (Ohya and Sperelakis, 1988). The activity of single Ca^{2+} channels (conductance of 18–22 pS) was recorded in cell-attached patch configuration with 100 mM Ba^{2+} and Bay-K-8644 in

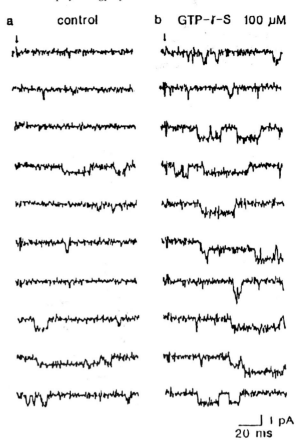

a control   **b** GTP-ϒ-S 100 µM

$\underline{\hspace{1cm}}$ | 1 pA
20 ms

Fig. 45-22. Effects of GTP-γ-S on the Ca^{2+} channel activity in a single cell isolated from guinea pig portal vein, using the open-cell-attached configuration in the presence of 1 mM Bay-K-8644. After one end of the cell was disrupted in the cell-attached configuration, control recordings were obtained (a). Bath application of 0.1 mM GTP-γ-S (access into the cell interior) enhanced the channel openings (b). Taken from Ohya and Sperelakis (1991), with permission.

the pipette and high K^+ solution in the bath. One end of the cell was disrupted mechanically by another electrode during the single-channel recording in the cell-attached configuration, so that the cell interior communicated with the bath solution (open-cell-attached configuration; see Ohya and Sperelakis, 1991). In this configuration, chemicals applied to the bath solution can diffuse into the cell. Conversely, intracellular factors may diffuse out of the cell. Rundown of the single Ca^{2+} channel activity was prevented by using 1 µM Bay-K-8644. After obtaining the control records, 0.1 mM GTP-γS was applied inside the cell. GTP-γS, which activates the G protein without agonist stimulation, enhanced the Ca^{2+} channel activity in about 30% of the cells. Figure 45-22 shows results obtained from such an experiment. As can be seen, the single-channel activity of the Ca^{2+} channels was stimulated. Single-channel current amplitude was not affected. These results are consistent with the possibility that a G protein may directly regulate Ca^{2+} channels in vascular smooth muscle cells. However, the failure in about 70% of the cells may also suggest that the regulation of voltage-dependent Ca^{2+} channels in VSM involves multiple factors.

Receptor-associated channels

Several mechanisms can explain agonist-induced contraction: (a) agonist-induced depolarization, with increasing or decreasing membrane resistance; (b) directly stimulating voltage-dependent Ca^{2+} channels; (c) opening of receptor-operated Ca^{2+} channels and release of Ca^{2+} from store sites by several mechanisms (see *Sources of Ca^{2+} for contraction*).

RECEPTOR-OPERATED CHANNELS

Depolarization induced by agonists with a decrease in resistance is considered to be due mainly to Na^{2+} influx (Kuriyama et al., 1982; Bolton et al., 1984). Application of an agonist to VSM cells may activate several types of channels. One is an inward current channel that predominantly carries Na^{2+} but is also nearly nonspecific for other cations, such as K^+, Ca^{2+}, etc. (Bolton et al., 1984). However, although the presence of this channel has been reported, little is known, especially about its Ca^{2+} dependency. Various agonists release Ca_{2+} from the store sites, and this released Ca^{2+} may activate the Ca^{2+}-dependent channels (K^+ channel, Cl^- channel, and nonspecific channel), as observed in other cells (for example, lacrimal grand; Marry et al., 1984).

RECEPTOR-OPERATED Ca^{2+} CHANNEL

To explain pharmacomechanical coupling, the presence of receptor-operated Ca^{2+} channels has been postulated. Benham and Tsien (1987) reported that extracellular application of ATP evoked Ca^{2+}-permeable channel activation in rabbit-ear artery (selectivity for Ca^{2+} over Na^+ was 3:1 under physiological conditions). That study is the first direct demonstration of receptor-operated Ca^{2+} channels in VSM cells.

Ca^{2+}-DEPENDENT CHANNELS

Increased Ca^{2+} in the cytosol may activate K^+ channels, Cl^- channels, and nonselective channels (Marry et al., 1984). Such channels may modify the membrane responses to agonists.

K^+ channels

The K^+ channels are important for controlling membrane excitability, because application of a K^+-channel blocker depolarizes the membrane and produces a condition in which Ca^{2+}-dependent spikes are easily evoked. However, the background K^+ current that is important for setting of the resting membrane potential has not yet been determined.

Ca^{2+}-ACTIVATED K^+ CHANNEL

In smooth muscle cells, there is a large distribution of Ca^{2+}-activated K^+ channels (Benham et al., 1985; Inoue et al., 1985; Singer and Walsh, 1987). Several types of Ca^{2+}-activated K^+ channels have been reported in VSM cells. These have a different single-channel conductance, different Ca^{2+} sensitivity, and different drug sensitivity. The large-conductance type (BK channel) is the same one as commonly observed in various types of cells. The single-channel conductance is about 200–270 pS in the symmetrical high-K^+ condition and is activated by over 10^{-7} M Ca^{2+} from inside the membrane (Benham et al., 1985; Inoue et al., 1985; Singer and Walsh, 1987). Low concentrations of TEA ($K_d = 0.1$–0.3 mM) from **outside** the membrane and charybdotoxin bath block this channel (Inoue et al., 1985). In the whole-cell clamp, activation of this channel is observed as a transient outward and an oscillatory outward current (spontaneously appearing) in smooth muscle cells (Benham and Bolton, 1986; Ohya et al., 1987B). Triggered Ca^{2+} release from store sites is important in the regulation of these currents (Ohya et al., 1987B). The transient outward current always follows Ca^{2+} current, and it is considered that Ca^{2+} influx is also important for this current (Ca^{2+} influx may trigger Ca^{2+} from the store site by the mechanism of Ca^{2+}-induced Ca^{2+} release from the store site). Applications of voltage steps, agonists, or caffeine induce the appearance of the oscillatory outward current. Intracellular application of IP_3, which is believed to be a second messenger for the agonist-induced contraction, also activated this current (Ohya et al., submitted).

Another class of Ca-dependent K channel that has medium conductance (~90 pS in symmetrical K condition) was also recorded in rabbit portal vein (Inoue et al., 1985). This channel is less sensitive to TEA. In A7r5 cells and rat portal vein cells, Ca-dependent K channels with a small conductance (30–40 pS symmetrical K^+ condition) were recorded (Kajioka et al., 1990; van Renterghem and Lazdunski, 1992). This channel is inhibited by charybdotoxin and 4AP. Another Ca^{2+}-dependent K channel is a unique channel that is activated by Ca^{2+} from outside the membrane (Inoue et al., 1985, 1986). This channel was observed in rabbit portal venous cells and porcine coronary arterial cells. Single-channel conductance is about 180 pS (in symmetrial K condition). Although the function of these channels is not known, they may be involved in setting the resting membrane potential or in repolarizing the membrane after each Ca^{2+}-dependent APs.

Drugs or agonists may modify these Ca^{2+}-dependent channels. Agonists that increase intracellular Ca also activate Ca^{2+}-dependent K channels. It was reported that beta stimulation or intracellular cAMP directly activate BK channels in rat aortic cells (Sadeshima et al., 1988). Stimulation of G kinase (by nitroglycerin) also activates this channel (Fujino et al., 1991). cAMP- and cGMP-dependent phosphorylation thus may modify channel activity.

Ca^{2+}-INSENSITIVE OUTWARD CURRENT (DELAYED OUTWARD CURRENT)

Classification of outward currents in smooth muscle cells is still controversial. There are at least two types of Ca^{2+}-insensitive outward current. One is TEA sensitive (K_d = 2–5 mM; vs. K_d = 0.1–0.3 mM for the Ca^{2+}-activated K^+ channel; Ohya et al., 1987B), and the other is 4-aminopyridine sensitive (K_d = 0.3 mM; Okabe et al., 1987). The TEA-sensitive current is commonly observed in VSM and visceral smooth muscle cells. A large amount of 4-aminopyridine-sensitive channels is found in most arterial cells (rabbit pulmonary artery, rabbit coronary artery; Okabe et al., 1987). The threshold of this channel is about −40 mV and, due to the presence of this channel, no net inward current is observed in these cells.

ATP-DEPENDENT K CHANNELS

One class of K channel that is activated with decreased concentration of intracellular ATP has been reported in various tissues, such as skeletal muscle, cardiac muscle, pancreatic β cell, and smooth muscle cells. This channel is considered to be a target of K channel openers (lemakalim, cromakalim, pinacidil, etc.; Standen et al., 1989; Cook and Quast, 1990; Kajioka et al., 1992; Miyoshi et al., 1992). This channel is inhibited by glibenclamide. It was recently reported that opening of ATP-sensitive K channel was facilitated in the presence of GDP (Kajioka et al., 1992). Single-channel conductance values for this channel reported varied between researchers. It was postulated that during ischemia this channel will activate, hyperpolarize the membrane, and thereby relax the arteries (coronary artery, mesenteric artery; Silbergerg and van Breeman, 1992).

Na^+ channels

In smooth muscle cells, the Na^+ channel has been considered to be absent or nonfunctional. Recently Sturek and Hermsmeyer (1986) reported the presence of a large Na^+ current in cultured VSM cells that was insensitive to TTX. Okabe et al. (in press) reported the presence of a TTX-sensitive Na^+ current in rabbit pulmonary artery. Fast Na^+ currents, very sensitive to TTX, were also observed in rat and rabbit portal vein cells (Xiong et al.,

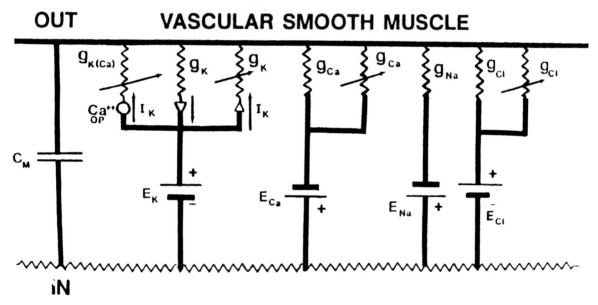

Fig. 45-23. Electrical equivalent circuit for the cell membrane of arterial vascular smooth muscle cells. The conductance pathways (channels) are shown both for the resting membrane (g_K, g_{Na}, g_{Ca}, and g_{Cl}) and for the excited membrane (g'_{Ca}, g'_K, and $g_{K(Ca)}$). The arrow through the resistances (for the excited membrane) represents the fact that the resistance (conductance) varies with the membrane potential and time, i.e., these are voltage-dependent conductances. $g_{K(Ca)}$ is intracellular Ca^{2+} dependent and voltage dependent, but not time dependent. The equilibrium potentials for the four major ions of concern (E_K, E_{Na}, E_{Ca}, and E_{Cl}), as calculated from the Nernst equation for the known ion distributions, are depicted as batteries of differing polarities and magnitudes, as indicated. The resistance channels are presumably due to protein molecules in the phospholipid bilayer matrix of the membrane, and the parallel capacitance (C_m) component is due to the lipid bilayer. Ca^{2+} antagonists block the Ca^{2+} channels, whereas TEA^+ and Ba^{2+} block the resting K^+ channels (depress g_K) and depress the kinetics of activation of g'_K. There may be several types of voltage-dependent K^+ channel (Ca^{2+} insensitive), that allow K^+ to pass more readily outward (outwardly directed rectification or delayed rectification). The AP rising velocity and overshoot is determined by the inward Ca^{2+} current carried through the Ca^{2+} channels. The repolarization of the AP is brought about by a sharp increase in g'_K and $g_{K(Ca)}$, which are activated by the depolarization and intracellular Ca^{2+}. Inexcitability may be produced when ($g_K + g'_K + g_{K(Ca)}$) is too high.

unpublished observations). The function of these channels is not known.

Cl⁻ channels

The presence of Ca^{2+}-dependent and Ca^{2+}-independent Cl^- channels has been reported in arterial smooth muscle cells. Ca^{2+}-dependent Cl^- channels are activated during agonist stimulation, and they may produce depolarization (because E_{Cl} is less negative than resting E_m; Byrne and Large, 1988; Amedee et al., 1990; Droogmans et al., 1991; Klockner and Isenberg, 1991). Ca^{2+}-independent Cl current was recorded in A7r5 cells that are voltage dependent (Soejima and Kokubun, 1988).

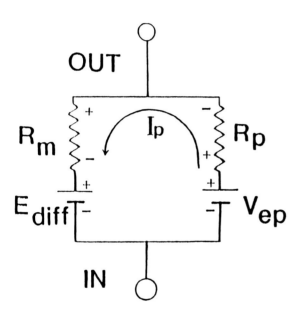

Fig. 45-24. Hypothetical electrical equivalent circuit for an electrogenic sodium pump in vascular smooth muscle cells. The model consists of a pump pathway (R_p) in parallel with the membrane resistance (R_m) pathway and the membrane capacitance (C_m). The pump protein Na,K-ATPase and the ion-channel conductance proteins are floating in the lipid bilayer membrane as parallel elements. The net diffusion potential (E_{diff}; determined by the ion equilibrium potentials and relative ion conductances) is depicted in series with R_m. The electrogenic Na^+ pump potential (V_{ep}; determined by the rate of the pump turnover and the Na^+-K^+ coupling ratio) is depicted in series with the pump resistance (R_p). R_p is assumed to have a constant value close to R_m, but to be independent of changes in R_m when the pump is operating at a constant rate; R_p is assumed to become infinite when the pump is stopped. (Alternatively, the internal resistance of V_{ep} can be considered as becoming infinite when the pump is stopped.) Membrane potential (E_m) is modified by electrogenic sodium pump by following equation:

$$E_m = \left(\frac{R_m}{R_m + R_p}\right) V_{ep} + \left(\frac{R_p}{R_m + R_p}\right) E_{diff}.$$

Other channels

Leak channels that conduct Ca^{2+} (Benham and Tsien, 1987) and stretch-dependent cation channels (Kirber et al., 1987; Davis et al., 1992) have been reported in VSM cells. However, little is known about them at present. They may be important for VSM because vascular tissue always has a basal tension or tone.

CONCLUSIONS

It is concluded that the electrical-equivalent circuit of the cell membrane of arterial VSM cells is as depicted in fig. 45-23. There are two types of voltage-dependent channels: One is the slow channel, which is specific for Ca^{2+} ion and blocked by the Ca^{2+}-channel blockers, such as verapamil, bepridil, nifedipine, diltiazem, and Mn^{2+}. The other type is a fast type, which is resistant to the slow L-type Ca channel blockers, but blocked by a low concentration of Ni^{2+} (e.g., $30\,\mu M$) and by tetramethrine. There are probably one or more types of voltage-dependent K^+ channels, including the outward delayed-rectifier channel, which is responsible for repolarization of the AP. Ca^{2+}-activated K channels contribute to the repolarization phase. Agents like Ba^{2+} and TEA^+ may affect all types of K^+ channels, namely, the resting g_K, the delayed-rectifier channel, and the Ca_{2+}-dependent K^+ channel. The resting potential, more correctly E_{diff}, is determined by the resting values for the K^+ and Na^+ conductances (g_{Na}/g_K ratios) and the magnitude of E_K and E_{Na}. At this moment, K channel that is responsible for g_C is not known. The electrogenic pump potential (V_{ep}) contribution to the resting potential is illustrated in fig. 45-24.

ACKNOWLEDGMENTS
The work of the authors and their associates summarized in this chapter was supported by NIH grant HL-19242 and by grants from Wallace Laboratories and from Smith, Kline and French Laboratories. The authors would like to acknowledge their assoicates who were involved in these studies: M.J. McLean, MD, PhD; D. Harder, PhD; E. Zelcer, PhD; S. Mras, PhD; P.-A. Molyvdas, MD; D. Jones, MD; D. Johns, MD; D. Pang, PhD; S. Ishikawa, MD, PhD; J. Ousterhout, PhD. They also thank R. Hentz for typing the manuscript.

REFERENCES

Aaronson PI, Benham CD, Bolton TB, Hess P, Lang RJ, Tsien RW: Two types of single-channel and whole-cell calcium or barium currents in single smooth muscle cells of rabbit ear artery and the effects of noradrenaline. *J Physiol* 377:36, 1986.

Abe Y, Tomita T: Cable properties of smooth muscle. *J Physiol (Lond)* 196:87–100, 1968.

Altiere RJ, Kiritsy-Roy JA, Catravas JD: Acetylcholine-induced contractions in isolated rabbit pulmonary arteries: Role of thromboxane A_2. *J Pharmacol Exp Ther* 236:535–541, 1986.

Amedee T, Benham CD, Bolton TB, Byrne NG, Large WA: Potassium, chloride and nonselective cation conductances opened by noradrenaline in rabbit ear artery cells. *J Physiol* 423:551–568, 1990.

Asano M, Masuzawa K, Matsuda T: Role of stimulatory GTP-binding protein (G_s) in reduced β-adrenoceptor coupling in the femoral artery of spontaneously hypertensive rats. *Br J Pharmacol* 95:241–251, 1988.

Bean BP, Sturek M, Puga A, Hermsmeyer K: Calcium channels in muscle cells isolated from rat mesenteric arteries: Modulation by dihydropyridine drugs. *Circ Res* 59:229–235, 1986.

Bean BP, Cohen CJ, Tsien RW: Lidocaine block of cardiac sodium channels. *J Gen Physiol* 81:613–642, 1983.

Bean BP: Nitrendipine block of cardiac calcium channels: High-affinity binding to the inactivated state. *Proc Natl Acad Sci USA* 81:6388–6392, 1984.

Belardinelli L, Harder D, Sperelakis N, Rubio R, Berne RM: Cardiac glycoside stimulation of inward Ca^{2+} current in vascular smooth muscle of canine coronary artery. *J Pharmacol Exp Ther* 209:62–66, 1979.

Benham CD, Hess P, Tsien RW: Two types of calcium channels in single smooth muscle cells from rabbit ear artery studied with whole-cell and single channel recordings. *Circ Res* 61(Suppl I):110–116, 1987a.

Benham CD, Bolton TB, Bryne NG, Large WA: Action of extracellular adenosine triphosphate in single smooth muscle cells dispersed from the rabbit ear artery. *J Physiol* 387:473–488, 1987b.

Benham CD, Bolton TB, Byrne NG, Large WA: Action of externally applied adenosine triphosphate on smooth muscle cells dispersed from rabbit ear artery. 387:473–488, 1987.

Benham CD, Tsien RW: A novel receptor-operated Ca^{2+}-permeable channel activated by ATP in smooth muscle. *Nature* 328:275–278, 1987.

Benham CD, Bolton TB, Lang RJ, Takewaki T: The mechanism of action of Ba^{2+} and TEA on single Ca^{2+}-activated K^+-channels in arterial and intestinal smooth muscle cell membrane. *Pflügers Arch* 403:120–127, 1985.

Benham CD, Bolton TB: Spontaneous transient outward currents in single visceral and vascular smooth muscle cells of the rabbit. *J Physiol* 381:385–406, 1986.

Berridge MJ, Irvine RF: Inositol trisphosphate, a novel second messenger in cellular signal transduction. *Nature* 312:315–321, 1984.

Berridge MJ: Inositol triphosphate and diacylglycerol as second messengers. *Biochem J* 220:345–360, 1984.

Bilek I, Laven R, Peiper R, Regnat K: The effect of verapamil on the response to noradrenaline or to potassium-depolarization in isolated vascular strips. *Microvasc Res* 7:181–189, 1974.

Bolton TB, Lang RJ, Takewaki T: Mechanism of action of noradrenaline and carbachol on smooth muscle of guinea-pig anterior mesenteric artery. *J Physiol* 351:549–572, 1984.

Bolton TB, Clapp LH: Endothelial-dependent relaxant actions of carbachol and substance P in arterial smooth muscle. *Br J Pharmacol* 87:713–733, 1986.

Bolton TB: Mechanisms of action of transmitters and other substances on smooth muscle. *Physiol Rev* 59:606–718, 1979.

Bonaccorsi A, Hermsmeyer K, Aprigliano O, Smith CP, Bohr DF: Mechanism of potassium relaxation of arterial muscle. *Blood Vessels* 14:261–276, 1977.

Brock JS, Cunnane TC, Evans RJ, Ziogas J: Inhibition of transmitter release from sympathetic nerve ending by ω-conooxin. *Clin Exp Pharmacol Physiol* 16:333–339, 1989.

Brown AM, Birnbaumer L: Direct G protein gating of ion channels. *Am J Physiol* 254:H401–H410, 1988.

Bulbring E, Tomita T: Catecholamine action on smooth muscle. *Pharmacol Rev* 39:49–96, 1987.

Byrne NG, Large WA: Membrane ionic mechanisms activated by noradrenaline in cells isolated from the rabbit portal vein. *J Physiol* 404:557–573, 1988.

Caffrey JM, Josephson IR, Brown AM: Calcium channels of amphibian stomach and mammalian aorta smooth muscle cells. *Biophys J* 49:1237–1242, 1986.

Casteels R, Kitamura K, Kuriyama H, Suzuki H: The membrane properties of the smooth muscle cells of rabbit pulmonary artery. *J Physiol* 271:41–61, 1977.

Casteels R, Suzuki H: The effect of histamine on the smooth muscle cells of the ear artery of the rabbit. *Pflügers Arch* 387:17–25, 1980.

Casteels R: Electro and pharmacomechanical coupling in vascular smooth muscle. *Chest* 78(Suppl):150–156, 1980.

Cook NS, Quast U: Potassium channel pharmacology. In: Cook NS (ed) *Potassium Channels*. 1990, pp 181–225.

Cosnier D, Duchenne-Marullaz P, Rispat G, Streichenberger G: Cardiovascular pharmacology of bepridil (1[3 isobutoxy 2 benzylphenyl amino] propyl pyrrolidine hydrochloride) a new potential anti-anginal compound. *Arch Int Pharmacodyn Ther* 225:133–151, 1977.

Danthuluri NR, Deth RC: Acute desensitization to angiotensin II: Evidence for a requirement of agonist-induced diacylglycerol production during tonic contraction of rat aorta. *Eur J Pharmacol* 125:1103–1107, 1986.

Davis MJ, Donovitz JA, Hood JD: Stretch-activated single-channel and whole cell currents in vascular smooth muscle cells. *Am J Physiol* 262:C1083–C1088, 1992.

Dolphin AC, Scott RH: Calcium channel currents and their inhibition by (−)-bacrophen in rat sensory neurones: Modulation by guanine nucleotides. *J Physiol* 86:1–17, 1987.

Dosemeci A, Dhalla RS, Cohen NM, Lederer WJ, Roger TB: Phorbol ester increases calcium current and stimulates the effects of angiotensin II on cultured neonatal rat heart myocytes. *Circ Res* 62:347–355 1988.

Droogmans G, Raeymaekers L, Casteels R: Electro and pharmacomechanical coupling in the smooth muscle cells of the rabbit ear artery. *J Gen Physiol* 70:129–148, 1977.

Droogmans G, Declerck I, Casteel R: Effect of adrenergic agonists on Ca^{2+}-channel currents in single ventricular smooth muscle cells. *Pflügers Archiv* 409:7–12, 1987.

Droogmans G, Callewaert G, Declerck I, Casteels R: ATP-induced Ca^{2+}-release and Cl^- current in cultured smooth muscle cells from pig aorta. *J Physiol* 440:623–634, 1991.

Fabiato A, Fabiato F: Calcium and cardiac excitation-contraction coupling. *Ann Rev Physiol* 41:473–484, 1979.

Fish RD, Sperti G, Colucci WS, Clapham DE: Phorbol ester increases the dihydropyridine-sensitive calcium conductance in a vascular smooth muscle cell line. *Circ Res* 62:1049–1052, 1988.

Fleckenstein A, Nakayama K, Fleckenstein-Grun G, Byon YK: Interactions of vasoactive ions and drugs with Ca-dependent excitation-contraction coupling of vascular smooth muscle. In: Carafoli E (ed) *Calcium Transport in Contraction and Secretion*. Amsterdam: North Holland, 1975, pp 555–564.

Fleckenstein A: Specific pharmacology of calcium in myocardium, cardiac pacemaker and vascular smooth musecl. *Ann Rev Pharmacol Toxicol* 17:149–166, 1977.

Forbes MS, Sperelakis N: Bridging junctional processes in couplings of skeletal, cardiac, and smooth muscle. *Muscle Nerve* 5:674–681, 1982.

Friedmann E, Suarez-Kurtz G, Kaczorowski GJ, Katz GM, Reuben JP: Two calcium currents in a smooth muscle cell line. *Am J Physiol* 250:H699–H703, 1986.

Fujii K, Ishimatsu T, Kuriyama H: Mechanisms of vasodilation induced by α-human atrial natriuretic polypeptide in rabbit and guinea-pig renal arteries. *J Physiol* 377:315–332, 1986.

Fujino K, Nakaya S, Wakatsuki T, Myoshi Y, Nakaya Y, Mori H, Inoue I: Effects of nitroglycerin on ATP-induced Ca^{2+}-mobilization, Ca^{2+}-activated K channels and contraction of cultured smooth muscle cells of porcine coronary artery. *J Pharmacol Exp Ther* 256:371–377, 1991.

Furchgott RF, Zawadzki JV: The obligatory role of the endothelial cells in the relaxation of arterial vascular smooth muscle by acetylcholine. *Nature* 288:373–376, 1980.

Furchgott RF: The role of endothelium in the responses of vascular smooth muscle to drugs. *Ann Rev Pharmacol Toxicol* 24:175–197, 1984.

Gamitkevidr VY, Isenberg G: Contribution of two types of calcium channels to membrane conductance by single myocytes from guinea-pig coronary artery. *J Physiol* 426:19–42, 1990.

Gilman AG: G protein: Transducers of receptor-generated signals. *Ann Rev Biochem* 56:615–649, 1987.

Gleason MM, Flaim SF: Phorbol ester contracts rabbit thoracic aorta by increasing intracellular calcium and by activating calcium influx. *Biochem Biophys Res Commun* 138:1362–1365, 1986.

Godfraind T, Miller R, Wibo M: Calcium antagonism and calcium entry blockade. *Pharmacol Rev* 38:321–416, 1986.

Haddy FJ: The mechanism of potassium vasodilation. In: Vanhoutte PM, Leusen I (eds) *Mechanisms of Vasodilation*. Basel: Karger, 1978, pp 200–205.

Haeusler G: Differential effect of verapamil on excitation-contraction coupling in smooth muscle and on excitation-secretion coupling in adrenergic nerve terminals. *J Pharmacol Exp Ther* 180:672–682, 1972.

Haeusler G: Relationship between noradrenaline-induced depolarization and contraction in vascular smooth muscle. *Blood Vessels* 15:46–54, 1978.

Hamill OP, Marty A, Neher E, Sackmann B, Sigworth FJ: Improved patch-clamp technique for high resolution current recording from cells and cell-free membrane patches. *Pflügers Arch* 391:85–100, 1981.

Harder D, Sperelakis N: Membrane electrical properties of vascular smooth muscle from guinea pig superior meseoteric artery. *Pflügers Arch* 378:11–119, 1978.

Harder D, Belardinelli L, Sperelakis N, Rubio R, Berne RM: Differential effects of adenosine and nitroglycerin on the action potentials of large and small coronary arteries. *Circ Res* 44:176–182, 1979.

Harder DR, Sperelakis N: Action potentials induced in guinea pig arterial smooth muscle by tetraethylammonium. *Am J Physiol* 237:C75–86, 1979.

Harder DR, Madden JA: Electrical stimulation by the endothelial surface of pressurized cat middle cerebral artery results in TTX-sensitive vasoconstriction. *Circ Res* 60:831–836, 1987.

Harder DR: Membrane electrical activation of arterial smooth muscle. In: Crass C, Barnes CD (eds) *Research Topics in Physiology: Vascular Smooth Muscle*. New York: Academic Press, 1981, pp 71–97.

Harder DR: Membrane electrical effects of histamine on vascular smooth muscle of canine coronary artery. *Circ Res* 46:372–377, 1980.

Hartshorne DJ, Siemankowski RF: Regulation of smooth muscle actomyosin. *Ann Rev Physiol* 43:519–530, 1981.

Hermsmeyer K: High shortening velocity of isolated single arterial muscle cells. *Experientia* 35:1599–1602, 1979.

Hescheler J, Pelzer D, Trube G, Trautwein W: Does the organic calcium channel blocker D-600 act from inside or outside on the cardiac cell membrane? *Pflügers Arch* 393:287–291, 1982.

Hescheler J, Rosenthal W, Trautwein W, Schultz G: The GTP-binding protein, G_o, regulates neuronal calcium channels. *Nature* 325:445–447, 1987.

Hess P, Lansman JB, Tsien RW: Different modes of Ca^{2+} channel gating behavior favored by dihydropyridine Ca^{2+} agonists and antagonists. *Nature* 311:538–544, 1984.

Hickey KA, Rubanyi G, Paul RJ, Highsmith RF: Characterization of a coronary vasoconstrictor produced by cultured endothelial cells. *Am J Physiol* 248:C550–C556, 1985.

Hirst GD, Neild TO: An analysis of excitatory junctional potentials recorded from arterioles. *J Physiol* 280:87–104, 1978.

Hirst GDS, Neild TD: Localization specialized noradrenaline receptors at neuromuscular junctions on aterioles of the guinea-pig. *J Physiol* 313:343–350, 1983.

Holman ME, Surprenant AM: Some properties of the excitatory junction potentials recorded from saphenous arteries of rabbits. *J Physiol* 287:337–351, 1979.

Holz IV GG, Rane SG, Dunlap K: GTP-binding proteins mediate transmitter inhibition of voltage-dependent calcium channels. *Nature* 319:670–672, 1986.

Ignarro LJ, Buga GM, Wood KS, Byrns RE, Chaudhuri G: Endothelium-derived relaxing factor produced and released from artery and vein is nitric oxide. *Proc Natl Acad Sci USA* 84:9265–9269, 1987.

Ikeda SR, Schofield GG: Somatostatin blocks a calcium current in rat sympathetic ganglion neurones. *J Physiol* 409:221–240, 1989.

Inoue R, Kitamura K, Kuriyama H: Two Ca^{2+} dependent K^+ channels classified by the application of tetraethylammonium distributed to smooth muscle membranes of the rabbit portal portal vein. *Pflügers Arch* 405:173–179, 1985.

Inoue R, Okabe K, Kitamure K, Kuriyama H: A newly identified Ca^{2+} dependent K^+ channel in the smooth muscle membrane of single cells dispersed from the rabbit portal vein. *Pflügers Arch* 406:138–143, 1986.

Inoue R, Isenberg G: Acetylcholine activates nonselective cation channels in guinea pig ileum through a G protein. *Am J Physiol* 258:C1173–C1178, 1990.

Inoue Y, Oike K, Nakao K, Kitamura K, Kuriyama H: Endothelin augments unitary calcium channel currents on the smooth muscle cell membrane of guinea-pig portal vein. *J Physiol* 423:171–191, 1990.

Irvine RF, Moor RM: Micro-injection of inositol 1,3,4,5-tetrakis-phosphate activates sea urchin eggs by a mechanism dependent on external Ca^{2+}. *Biochem J* 240:917–920, 1986.

Ishikawa S, Sperelakis N: Cyclic nucleotide regulation of neurotransmission in guinea-pig mesenteric artery. *J Cardiovasc Pharm* 13:836–845, 1989.

Ishikawa S, Sperelakis N: A novel class (H_3) of histamine receptors on perivascular nerve terminals. *Nature* 327:158–160, 1987.

Ito Y, Suzuki H, Kuriyama H: Effects of sodium nitroprusside on smooth muscle cells of rabbit pulmonary artery and portal vein. *J Pharmacol Exp Ther* 207:1022–1031, 1978.

Ito Y, Kitamura K, Kuriyama H: Effects of acetylcholine and catecholamine on the smooth muscle cell of the porcine coronary artery. *J Physiol* 294:595–611, 1979.

Ito Y, Kitamura K, Kuriyama H: Nitroglycerine and catecholamine actions on smooth muscle cells by the canine coronary artery. *J Physiol* 309:171–183, 1980.

Itoh T, Kuriyama H, Suzuki H: Excitation-contraction coupling in smooth muscle cell of the guinea-pig mesenteric artery. *J Physiol (Lond)* 321:513–551, 1981.

Itoh H, Lederis K: Contraction of rat thoracic aorta strips induced by phorbol 12-myristate 13-acetate. *Am J Physiol* 252:C244–C249, 1987.

Itoh T, Kanmura Y, Kuriyama H, Sumimoto K: A phorbol ester has dual actions on the mechanical response in the rabbit mesenteric and porcine coronary artery. *J Physiol (Lond)* 375:515–534, 1986.

Itoh T, Kuriyama H, Suzuki H: Differences and similarities in the noradrenaline- and caffeine-induced mechanical responses in the rabbit mesenteric artery. *J Physiol* 337:609–629, 1983.

Johansson B, Somlyo AP: Electrophysiology and excitation-contraction coupling. In: Bohr DF, Somlyo AP, Sparks HV (eds) *Handbook of Physiology. Sect 2: The Cardiovascular System. Vol 2: Vascular Smooth Muscle.* Bethesda, MD: American Physiological Society, 1980, pp 301–323.

Johansson B: Electromechanical and mechanoelectrical coupling in vascular smooth muscle. *Angiologia* 8:129–143, 1971.

Johansson B: Processes involved in vascular smooth muscle contraction and relaxation. *Circ Res* 43:14–20, 1978.

Johns DW, Sperelakis N: Angiotensin-II depolarization of cultured vascular smooth muscle cells (abstr 815). *Circulation* 66(Suppl 2):II204, 1982.

Jones AW: Content and fluxes of electrolytes. In: Bohr DF, Somlyo AP, Sparks HV (eds) *Handbook of Physiology. Sect 2: The Cardiovascular System. Vol 2: Vascular Smooth Muscle.* Bethesda, MD: American Physiological Society, 1980, pp 253–299.

Josephson IR, Sanchez-Chapula J, Brown AM: A comparison of calcium currents in rat and guinea pig single ventricular cells. *Circ Res* 54:144–156, 1984.

Jouve A, Sommer A, Romano JP, Heuillet G, Lavaurs G: Painful manifestations of coronary heart disease: Angina pectoris. *Arch Mala Coeur* 65:533–542, 1972.

Kajioka S, Oike M, Kitamura K: Nicorahdil opens a calcium-dependent potassium channel in smooth muscle cells of the rat portal vein. *J Pharmacol Exp Ther* 254:905–913, 1990.

Kajioka S, Kitamura K, Kuriyama H: Guanosine diphosphate activates an adenosine 5'-triphosphate-sensitive K+ channel in the rabbit portal vein. *J Physiol (Lond)* 444:397–418, 1992.

Kirber MT, Singer JJ, Walsh JV: Stretch-activated channels in freshly dissociated smooth muscle cells. *Biophys J* 51:252, 1987.

Kitamura K, Kuriyama H: Effects of acetylcholine on the smooth muscle cell of isolated main coronary artery of the guinea pig. *J Physiol* 239:119–133, 1979.

Klockner U, Isenberg G: Action potentials and net membrane currents of isolated smooth muscle cells (urinary bladder of the guinea-pig). *Pflügers Arch* 405:329–339, 1985.

Klockner U, Isenberg G: Endothelin depolarizes myocytes from porcine coronary and human mesenteric arteries through a Ca-activated chloride current. *Pflügers Arch* 418:168–175, 1991.

Klockner V, Itagaki K, Bodi I, Schwartz A: β-subunit expression is required for cAMP-dependent increase of cloned cardiac and vascular calcium channel. *Pflügers Arch* 420:413–415, 1992.

Kohlhardt M, Bauer B, Krause H, Fleckenstein A: Differentiation of the transmembrane Na and Ca channels in mammalian cardiac fibers by the use of specific inhibitors. *Pflügers Arch* 335:309–322, 1972.

Kohlhardt M, Fleckenstein A: Inhibition of the slow inward current by nifedipine in mammalian ventricular myocardium. *Naunyn-Schmiedebergs Arch Pharmacol* 298:267–272, 1977.

Komori K, Suzuki H: Electrical responses of smooth muscle cells during cholinergic vasodilation in the rabbit saphenous artery. *Circ Res* 61:586–593, 1987.

Kurachi Y, Nakajima T, Sugimoto T: On the mechanism of activation of muscarinic K+ channels by adenosine in isolated atrial cells: Involvement of GTP-binding proteins. *Pflügers Arch* 407:264–274, 1986.

Kuriyama H, Ito Y, Suzuki H, Kitamura K, Itoh T: Factors modifying contraction-relaxation cycle in vascular smooth muscle. *Am J Physiol* 243:H641–H662, 1982.

Kuriyama H, Makita Y: Modulation of noradrenergic transmis-

sion in the guinea-pig mesenteric artery: An electrophysiological study. *J Physiol* 335:609–627, 1983.

Kuriyama H, Suzuki H: The effects of acetylcholine on the membrane and contractile properties of smooth muscle cells of the rabbit superior mesenteric artery. *Br J Pharmacol* 64:493–501, 1978.

Labrid C, Grosset A, Dureng G, Mironneau J, Duchene-Marullaz P: Some membrane interactions with bepridil, a new antianginal agent. *J Pharmacol Exp Ther* 211:546–554, 1979.

Langer SZ: Presynaptic regulation of the release of catecholamines. *Pharmacol Rev* 32:337–362, 1981.

Lee KS, Marban E, Tsien RW: Inactivation by calcium channel in mammalian heart cells: Joint dependence on membrane potential and intracellular calcium. *J Physiol* 364:395–411, 1985.

Luscher TF, Vanhoutte PM: Endothelium-dependent contractions to acetylcholine in the aorta of the spontaneously hypertensive rat. *Hypertension* 8:344–348, 1986.

Marry A, Tan YP, Trautmann A: Three types of calcium-dependent channels in rat lacrimal glands. *J Physiol* 357:293–325, 1984.

Massingham R: A study of compounds which inhibit vascular smooth muscle contraction. *Eur J Pharmacol* 22:75–82, 1973.

Matsuda JJ, Volkka ●, Shibaza BF: Calcium currents in isolated rabbit coronary arterial smooth muscle myocytes. *J Physiol* 429:657–680, 1990.

McLean MJ, Shigenobu K, Sperelakis N: Two pharmacological types of cardiac slow Na+ channels as distinguished by verapamil. *Eur J Pharmacol* 26:379–382, 1974.

Meech RIF, Standen NB: Potassium activation in *Helix aspersa* neurones under voltage clamp: A component mediated by calcium influx. *J Physiol* 249:211–239, 1975.

Mekata F, Niu H: Biophysical effects of adrenaline on the smooth muscle of the rabbit common carotid artery. *J Gen Physiol* 59:92–102, 1972.

Mekata F: Electrophysiological properties of the smooth muscle cell membrane of the dog coronary artery. *J Physiol* 298:205–212, 1980.

Mekata F: Electrophysiological studies of the smooth muscle cell membrane of rabbit common cartotid artery. *J Gen Physiol* 57:738–751, 1971.

Michelin MT, Cheucle M, Duchene-Marullaz P: Comparison of the effects of bepridil, dipyridamole, and propranolol on the cardiac activity and the coronary venous debt in anesthetized dogs. *Therapie* 32:485–499, 1977.

Miyoshi Y, Nakaya Y, Wakatsuki T, Nakaya S, Fujino K, Saito K, Inoue I: Endothelin blocks ATP-sensitive K+ channels and depolarizes smooth muscle cells of porcine coronary artery. *Circ Res* 70:612–616, 1992.

Mras S, Sperelakis N: Comparison of ³H-bepridil and ³H-verapamil uptake into rabbit aortic rings. *J Cardiovasc Pharmacol* 4:777–783, 1982.

Mulvany MJ, Nilsson H, Flatman JA: Role of membrane potential in the response of rat small mesenteric arteries to exogenous noradrenaline stimulation. *J Physiol* 332:363–373, 1982.

Nagao T, Suzuki H: Non-neural electrical responses of smooth muscle cells of the rabbit basilar artery to electrical field stimulation. *Jpn J Physiol* 37:497–513, 1987.

Neild TO, Zelcer E: Noraderengic neuromuscular transmission with special reference to arterial smooth muscle. *Prog Neurobiol* 19:141–158, 1982.

Nelson MT, Patlak JB, Worley JF, Standen NB: Calcium channels, potassium channels, and voltage dependence of arterial smooth muscle tone. *Am J Physiol* 259:C3–C18, 1990.

Nishizuka Y: The role of protein kinase C in cell surface signal transduction and tumor promotion. *Nature* 308:693–698, 1984.

Nozaki M, Sperelakis N: Pertussis toxin effects on transmitter release from perivascular nerve terminals. *Am J Physiol* 256: H455–H459, 1989.

Nozaki M, Sperelakis N: Cholera toxin and G_s protein modulation of signal transduction in guinea pig mesenteric artery. *Eur J Pharmacol* 197:57–62, 1991.

Ohya Y, Terada K, Satoh S, Fujiwara T, Nagao T, Komori K, Nozaki M, Kuriyama H: Action of calcium antagonists on smooth muscle cells of vascular tissues. Current knowledge on actions of Ca antagonist. In: Aoki K (ed) *Essential Hypertension — Calcium Mechanisms and Treatment.* Heidelberg: Springer-Verlag, 1986, pp 81–94.

Ohya Y, Kitamura K, Kuriyama H: Regulations of calcium current by intracellular calcium in smooth muscle cells of rabbit portal vein. *Circ Res* 62:375–383, 1988a.

Ohya Y, Kitamura K, Kuriyama H: Modulation of ionic current in smooth muscle balls of the rabbit intestine by intracellular perfused ATP and cAMP. *Pflügers Arch* 408:465–473, 1987a.

Ohya Y, Kitamura K, Kuriyama H: Cellular calcium regulates outward currents in rabbit intestinal smooth muscle cell. *Am J Physiol* 252:C401–C410, 1987b.

Ohya Y, Terada K, Yamaguchi K, Inoue R, Okabe K, Kitamura K, Hiraza M, Kuriyama H: Effects of inositol phosphates on the membrane activity of smooth muscle cells of the rabbit portal vein — electrophysiological evidences. Submitted.

Ohya Y, Terada K, Kitamura K, Kuriyama H: D-600 blocks the Ca^{2+} channel from the outer surface of smooth muscle cell membrane of rabbit intestine and portal vein. *Pflügers Arch* 408:80–82, 1987c.

Ohya Y, Sperelakis N: ATP regulation of the slow calcium channels in vascular smooth muscle cells of guinea-pig mesenteric artery. *Circ Res* 64:145–154, 1989a.

Ohya Y, Sperelakis N: Involvement of a GTP-binding protein in stimulating action on calcium channels in vascular smooth muscle. *Circ Res* 68:763–771, 1991.

Ohya Y, Sperelakis N: Modulation of single slow (L-type) calcium channels by intracellular ATP in vascular smooth muscle cells. *Pflügers Arch* 414:257–264, 1989b.

Ohya Y, Terada K, Yamaguchi K, Inoue B, Okabe K, Kitamura K, Hirata M, Kuriyama H: Effects of inositol phosphates on the membrane activity of smooth muscle cells of the rabbit portal vein. *Pflügers Arch* 412:382–389, 1988b.

Ohya Y, Sperelakis N: *Physiologist* 31:A88, 1988.

Okabe K, Kitamura K, Kuriyama H: Features of 4-aminopyridine sensitive outward current observed in single smooth muscle cells from the rabbit pulmonary artery. *Pflügers Arch* 409: 561–568, 1987.

Okabe Y, Kitamura K, Kuriyama H: Direct evidence for the existence of a tetrodotoxin sensitive Na channel in freshly dispersed single smooth muscle cell of the rabbit main pulmonary artery. *Pflügers Arch,* in press.

Ousterhout J, Sperelakis N: Cyclic nucleotides depress action potentials in cultured aortic smooth muscle cells. *Eur J Pharmacol* 144:7–14, 1987.

Ousterhout JK, Steinsland OS: Effects of cholera toxin on vasoconstriction and cyclic AMP content of the isolated rabbit ear artery. *Life Sci* 28:2687–2695, 1981.

Pacaud P, Lorrand G, Mironneau C, Mironneau J: Opposing effects of noradrenaline on the two classes of voltage-dependent calcium channels of single vascular smooth muscle cells in short-term primary cultures. *Plfügers Arch* 410:557–559, 1987.

Pang DC, Sperelakis N: Nifedipine, diltiazem, bepridil and verapamil uptakes into cardiac and smooth muscles. *Eur J Pharmacol* 87:199–207, 1983.

Pang DC, Sperelakis N: Uptakes of calcium antagonists into muscles as related to their lipid solubilities. *Biochem Pharmacol* 33:821–826, 1984.

Peiper U, Griebel L, Wende W: Activation of vascular smooth muscle of rat aorta by noradrenaline and depolarization: Two different mechanisms. *Pflügers Arch* 330:74–89, 1971.

Pruneau D, Angus JA: ω-conotoxin GVIA is a potent inhibitor of sympathetic neurogenic response in rat small mesenteric arteries. *Br J Pharmacol* 100:180–184, 1990.

Rapoport RM, Murad F: Agonist-induced endothelium-dependent relaxation in rat thoracic aorta may be mediated through cGMP. *Circ Res* 52:351–357, 1983.

Rasmussen H, Takuwa Y, Parks S: Protein kinase C in the regulation of smooth muscle contraction. *FASEB J* 1:177–180, 1985.

Reuter H: Calcium channel modulation by neurotransmitters, enzymes and drugs. *Nature* 301:569–574, 1983.

Rosenthal W, Hescheler J, Trautwein W, Schultz G: Control of voltage-dependent Ca^{2+} channels by G protein-coupled receptors. *FASEB J* 2:2784–2790, 1988.

Rusch NJ, Hermsmeyer K: Calcium currents are altered in the vascular muscle cell membrane of spontaneously hypertensive rats. *Circ Res* 63:999–1002, 1988.

Sadoshima J, Akaike N, Kanaide H, Nakamura M: Cyclic AMP modulates Ca-activated K channel in cultured smooth muscle cells of rat aortas. *Am J Physiol* 255:H754–H759, 1988.

Satoh S, Itoh T, Kuriyama H: Actions of angiotensin II and noradrenaline on smooth muscle cells of the canine mesenteric artery. *Pflügers Arch* 410:132–138, 1987.

Schnaar RC, Sparks HV: Response of large and small coronary arteries in nitroglycerin, $NaNO_2$ and adenosine. *Am J Physiol* 223:223–228, 1972.

Sen L, Bialecki RA, Smith T, Smith TW, Colucci WS: Cholesterol increases the L-type voltage-sensitive calcium channel current in arterial smooth muscle cells. *Circ Res* 71:1008–1014, 1992.

Silberberg SD, van Breemen C: A potassium current activated by lemakalim and metabolic inhibition in rabbit mesenteric artery. *Pflügers Arch* 420:118–120, 1992.

Singer JJ, Walsh JV: Characterization of calcium-activated potassium channels in single smooth muscle cells using the patch-clamp technique. *Pflügers Arch* 408:98–111, 1987.

Smith JB, Smith L, Brown EP, Barnes D, Sabir MA, Davis JS, Farese RO: Angiotensin II rapidly increases phosphatidase-phosphoinositide synthesis and phosphoinositide hydrolysis and mobilizes intracellular calcium in cultured arterial muscle cells. *Proc Natl Acad Sci USA* 81:7812–7816, 1984.

Soejima M, Kokubun S: Single anion-selective channel and its ion selectivity in the vascular smooth muscle cell. *Pflügers Arch* 411:304–311, 1988.

Somlyo AP, Somlyo AV: Vascular smooth muscle. I Normal structure, pathology, biochemistry and biophysics. *Pharmacol Rev* 20:197–272, 1968a.

Somlyo AV, Somlyo AP: Electromechanical and pharmacomechanical coupling in vascular smooth muscle. *J Pharmacol Exp Ther* 159:129–145, 1968b.

Somlyo AV, Vinall P, Somlyo AP: Excitation-contraction coupling and electrical events in two types of vascular smooth muscle. *Microvasc Res* 1:354–373, 1969.

Somlyo AV, Bond M, Somlyo AP, Scapra A: Inositol triphosphate-induced calcium release and contraction in vascular smooth muscle. *Proc Natl Acad Sci USA* 82:5231–5235, 1985.

Sperelakis N, Inoue Y, Nozaki M, Ishikawa S: Neuromuscular transmission at adrenergic nerve terminals with vascular smooth muscle in guinea-pig mesenteric artery. In: Sperelakis N, Kuriyama H (eds) *Electrophysiology and Ion Channels of Vascular Smooth Muscle and Endothelial Cells.* Elsevier Publishers, 1989, pp 3–15.

Sperelakis N, Schneider MF, Harris EJ: Decreased K^+ conductance produced by Ba^{2+} in frog sartorius fibers. *J Gen Physiol* 50:1565–1583, 1967.

Sperelakis N, Lehmkuhl D: Effect of current on transmembrane potential in cultured chick heart cells. *J Gen Physiol* 47:895–927, 1964.

Sperelakis N, Mras S: Depression of contractions of rabbit aorta and guinea pig vena cava by mesudipine and slow channel blockers. *Blood Vessels* 20:172–183, 1983.

Sperelakis N, Ousterhout J: Smooth muscle electrophysiology: Role of calcium and effects of specific inhibitors. In: Singh BN (ed) *Calcium Channel Blockade in Cardiovascular Therapeutics.* Littleton, MA: PSG, in press.

Sperelakis N, Wahler GM, Bkaily G: Properties of myocardial calcium slow channels and mechanisms of action of calcium antagonistic drugs. In: Shamoo AE (ed) *Current Topics in Membranes and Transport,* Vol 25. New York: Academic Press, 1985, pp 4376.

Sperelakis N: Electrophysiology of vascular smooth muscle of coronary artery. In: Kalsner S (ed) *The Coronary Artery.* London: Croom Helm, 1982, pp 118–167.

Sperelakis N: Origin of the cardiac resting potential. In: Berne RM, Sperelakis N (eds) *Handbook of Physiology. Sect 2: The Cardiovascular System. Vol 1: The Heart.* Bethesda, MD: American Physiological Society, 1979A, pp 187–267.

Sperelakis N: Propagation mechanisms in heart. *Ann Rev Physiol* 41:441–457, 1979B.

Standen NB, Quayle JM, Davies NW, Brayden JE, Huang Y, Nelson MT: Hyperpolarizing vasodilators activate ATP-sensitive K^+ channels in arterial smooth muscle. *Science* 245:177–180, 1989.

Sturek M, Hermsmeyer K: Calcium and sodium channels in spontaneously contracting vascular muscle cells. *Science* 233:475–478, 1986.

Suematsu E, Hirata M, Hashimoto T, Kuriyama H: Inositol 1,4′,5-triphosphate releases Ca^{2+} from intracellular store sites in skinned cells of porcine coronary artery. *Biochem Biophys Res Commun* 120:481–485, 1984.

Takata Y, Kuriyama H: Effects of angiotensin II and 1-Sar, 8-Isoleu angiotensin II on electrical and mechanical properties of the portal vein from rats of different ages. *Jpn J Pharmacol* 29:639–651, 1979.

Takata Y: Regional differences in electrical mechanical properties of guinea-pig mesenteric vessels. *Jpn J Physiol* 30:709–728, 1980.

Toda N: Mechanism of histamine induced relaxation in isolated monkey and dog coronary artery. *J Pharmacol Exp Ther* 239:529–535, 1986.

Tsien RW: Calcium channels in excitable cell membranes. *Ann Rev Physiol* 45:341–358, 1983.

Van Breemen C, Aaronson T, Loutzenhifer R: Sodium-calcium interactions in mammalian smooth muscle. *Pharmacol Rev* 30:167–208, 1979.

Van Renterghem C, Lazdunski M: A small-conductance carybdotoxin-sensitive, apamin-resistant Ca^{2+}-activated K^+ channel in aortic smooth muscle cels. (A7r5 line and primary culture). *Pflügers Arch* 420:417–423, 1992.

Vanhoutte PM, Rubanyi GM, Miller VM, Houston DS: Modulation of vascular smooth muscle contraction by the endothelium. *Ann Rev Physiol* 48:317–320, 1986.

Vanhoutte PM, Verbeuran TJ, Webb RC: Local modulation of the adrenergic neuroeffector interaction in the blood vessel wall. *Physiol Rev* 61:151–247, 1981.

Vanhoutte PM: The end of the quest? *Nature* 327:459–460, 1987.

Webb RC, Bohr DF: Potassium-induced relaxation as an indicator of Na^+-K^+ ATPase activity in vascular smooth muscle. *Blood Vessels* 15:198–207, 1978.

Webb RC, Bohr DF: Potassium relaxation of vascular smooth muscle from spontaneously hypertensive rats. *Blood Vessels* 16:71–79, 1979.

Wertz MA, MacDonald RL: *J Neurosci* 7:1639–1647, 1987.

Williams DA, Fogarty KE, Tsien RW, Fay FS: Calcium gradients in single smooth muscle cells revealed by the digital imaging microscope using Fura-2. *Nature* 318:558–561, 1986.

Yanagisawa M, Kurihara H, Kimura S, Tomobe Y, Kobayashi M, Mitsui M, Yazaki Y, Goto K, Masaki T: A novel potent vasoconstrictor peptide produced by vascular endothelial cells. *Nature* 332:411–415, 1988.

Yatani A, Seidel CL, Allen J, Brown AM: Whole-cell and single-channel calcium currents of isolated smooth muscle cells from saphenous vein. *Circ Res* 60:523–533, 1987.

Yatani A, Cardina J, Imoto JP, Reves L, Birnbaumer L, Brown AM: A G protein directly regulates mammalian cardiac calcium channels. *Science* 238L:1288–1292, 1987.

Zelcer E, Sperelakis N: Ionic dependence of electrical activity in small mesenteric arteries of guinea-pig. *Pflügers Arch* 392:72–78, 1981.

Zelcer E, Sperelakis N: Spontaneous electrical activity in pressurized small mesenteric hypertensive rats. *Blood Vessels* 19:301–310, 1982.

Zelcer E, Sperelakis N: Angiotensin induction of active responses in cultured reaggregates of rat aortic smooth muscle cells. *Blood Vessels* 18:263–279, 1981B.

CHAPTER 46

Electromechanical and Pharmacomechanical Coupling in Vascular Smooth Muscle Cells

GUY DROOGMANS & LUDWIG MISSIAEN

INTRODUCTION

The contractile response of smooth-muscle cells is triggered by an increase of the free cytoplasmic calcium concentration ($[Ca^{2+}]_i$). This change in $[Ca^{2+}]_i$ can be brought about by an increased influx of Ca^{2+} ions from the extracellular medium or by a mobilization of Ca^{2+} ions from intracellular pools.

Excitatory agonists induce a contractile response that is poorly correlated with the concomitant changes in membrane potential. This has led to the introduction of the term *pharmacomechanical coupling*, as opposed to *electromechanical coupling* (caused by depolarization of the cell membrane), and to a subdivision of Ca^{2+} entry into voltage-gated and receptor-mediated mechanisms {1}. Both entry mechanisms and the agonist-induced Ca^{2+} release will be reviewed in this chapter.

Ca^{2+}-ENTRY MECHANISMS

Voltage-operated Ca^{2+} entry

GENERAL CHARACTERISTICS OF VOLTAGE-GATED Ca^{2+} CHANNELS

Single-channel studies have revealed multiple types of Ca^{2+} channels with different unitary conductances in smooth muscle cells {2–7}. We will mainly focus on the L-type Ca^{2+} channels, which are responsible for the upstroke of the action potential and for the Ca^{2+} influx activated by membrane depolarization. These channels show a threshold for activation around −40 mV and are fully activated around 0 mV.

Inactivation of these currents is clearly voltage dependent, but also shows a component dependent on intracellular Ca^{2+}. This latter component might be important during agonist stimulation: The rise in $[Ca^{2+}]_i$ due to Ca^{2+} release from internal stores might downregulate the channels {8,9}. Recently, a positive feedback of intracellular Ca^{2+} has been described that results in an enhanced Ca^{2+} current via a Ca^{2+}-dependent activation of calmodulin-dependent protein kinase II {10}.

The voltage ranges for steady-state activation and in-

activation overlap in a region between −30 and −20 mV {11}. The window current at these potentials may account for the tonic component of Ca^{2+} influx and contraction during a sustained depolarization of the cell membrane, e.g., during K^+ depolarization.

These L-type Ca^{2+} channels are voltage dependently blocked by dihydropyridines (DHP). The block is less pronounced if the channels are activated from a more hyperpolarized potential, which suggests a much higher affinity of DHP for the inactivated state of the channel {3,12–14}.

Intracellular ATP dose dependently enhanced the L-type Ca^{2+} current without altering its voltage-dependent features {15,16}. Unlike in cardiac cells, cAMP had no effect on the L-type Ca^{2+} current in smooth-muscle cells {15}. It has been proposed that beta agonists increase the L-type Ca^{2+} current by a direct coupling of the receptor to the channel via a G-protein {17}. It has recently been shown that the vasodilating action of PTH was correlated with the inhibition of voltage-gated Ca^{2+} channels {18}, and that this effect was mediated by a cAMP-dependent mechanism {19}.

MODULATION OF VOLTAGE-GATED Ca^{2+} CHANNELS BY AGONISTS

The modulation of L-type Ca^{2+} channels by excitatory agonists is a puzzling and controversial issue. In some tissues the Ca^{2+} current (i_{Ca}) is enhanced, while in others the current is decreased by the agonist. Even in the same tissue and under comparable experimental conditions, it has been reported that noradrenaline either enhances {20} or inhibits L-type Ca^{2+} channels {21}. The latter effect occurred through activation of α_1-adrenergic receptors, while the former was not related to either α or β stimulation. Table 46-1 gives an overview of the modulating effects of various agonists on i_{Ca} in different smooth muscle tissues. This modulation consists in most tissues of a change of the peak amplitude of i_{Ca} while the voltage-dependent characteristics of the channels are not significantly modified. A shift in the voltage dependence of activation has been observed occasionally {22}.

Most of the reported effects are probably mediated via the stimulation of phospholipase C and activation via DG

N. Sperelakis (ed.), Physiology and Pathophysiology of the Heart, Third Edition.
© 1995 Kluwer Academic Publishers. ISBN 0-7923-2612-1. All rights reserved.

Table 46-1. Receptor-mediated modulation of Ca^{2+} channels

Tissue	Agonist	i_{Ca}	Ref.
Rabbit ear artery	Noradrenaline	↑	20
Rabbit ear artery	Noradrenaline	↓	21, 32
Rat portal vein	Noradrenaline	↓	33
Rat portal vein	Noradrenaline	↑	34
Rabbit mesenteric artery	Noradrenaline	↑	22
Rabbit aorta	Noradrenaline	↓	35
Guinea pig portal vein	Angiotensin II	↑	26
Rabbit aorta	Angiotensin II	↑	36
Rabbit saphenous artery	Histamine	↑	27
Toad stomach	Acetylcholine	↑	25, 37
Toad stomach	Substance P	↑	38
Porcine coronary artery	Endothelin	↑	31
Rat aorta (A7r5 cells)	Vasopressin	↓	23, 39
Guinea pig vas deferens	Noradrenaline	↓	40
Rabbit basilar artery	Serotonin	↑	41
Colonic smooth muscle	Substance P	↑	42
Guinea pig urinary bladder	Vasopressin	↑	43
Rabbit coronary artery	Acetylcholine	↑	44
Rabbit portal vein	ATP	↓	45
Porcine coronary artery	Beta agonists	↑	46

of a Ca^{2+}-activated protein kinase C (PKC), which is thought to phosphorylate a number of endogenous proteins, including ion channels. A variety of DG analogues mimic this PKC-activating action of DG, and have been used as a tool to delineate the role of PKC activation in agonist-mediated responses. The inhibitory effect of the peptides vasopressin and bombesin on i_{Ca} in aortic smooth muscle (cell line A7r5) could be mimicked by DG and phorbol esters {23}. However, it has also been reported that in the same cells i_{Ca} is increased by TPA {24}. The stimulating effect of acetylcholine on i_{Ca} in smooth muscle cells of toad stomach could be mimicked by analogues of DG that are able to activate PKC {25}. The reduction of i_{Ca} induced by noradrenaline in rabbit ear artery becomes irreversible if the GTP-binding proteins, which link receptor occupation to the stimulation of phospholipase C, are permanently activated by GTP-γ-S {21}. The stimulation of i_{Ca} by angiotensin II in guinea pig portal vein {26}, and by histamine in rabbit saphenous artery {27}, are also mediated by GTP-binding proteins. It is puzzling that the effect of histamine in the latter tissue becomes inhibitory if the cells are internally perfused with a non-hydrolyzable GTP analogue.

Arachidonic acid causes a gradual depression of the Ca^{2+} current in rabbit ileum, which could not be prevented by the PKC-inhibitor staurosporine and which could not be mimicked by phorbol esters {28}. Since Ca^{2+} activates phospholipase A_2, it is possible that the inhibition of the Ca^{2+} current in response to Ca^{2+}-mobilizing agonists is mediated by arachidonic acid.

It is interesting to note that phosphatase inhibitors reduce i_{Ca} in gastric and colonic smooth muscle [29] but enhance it in guinea pig taenia coli [30], suggesting that phosphorylation may either inhibit or stimulate L-type Ca^{2+} channels.

It has also been shown that endothelin augments the current through L-type Ca^{2+} channels without modifying the voltage-dependent parameters of the current {31}. It is not clear whether this is a direct action on the channels or whether it is mediated via second messengers.

INDIRECT MODULATION

Besides these direct modulating effects, several mechanisms have been described whereby receptor activation may control the flow of Ca^{2+} through voltage-operated channels by its effect on the membrane potential. The inhibition of a K^+ current (M current) in nonmammalian visceral smooth muscle by acetylcholine {47} induces depolarization and activation of the tissue. On the other hand, stimulation of this M current by beta-adrenergic agonists will hyperpolarize the cell and induce relaxation {48}. Stimulation or suppression of a Ca^{2+}-dependent K^+ channel {49–53} will affect the membrane potential, and thereby modulate the influx of calcium via voltage-gated pathways.

Similarly, activation of a nonselective cation channel either directly gated by the agonist {9,54–58} or indirectly via agonist-induced Ca^{2+} release {59–63} and the concomitant rise in $[Ca^{2+}]_i$ will not only cause a Ca^{2+} influx through these channels, but will also depolarize the cell membrane and thereby activate Ca^{2+} channels. The ATP-activated nonselective cation channel {64} shows some selectivity for Ca^{2+} over Na^+ (3–4:1), and may therefore gate a Ca^{2+} influx during activation. Influx of Ca^{2+} through the ATP-gated channels increments $[Ca^{2+}]_i$ and inactivates L-type Ca^{2+} channels in guinea pig urinary bladder {9}. These effects were observed in voltage-clamped cells and are probably less pronounced under normal physiological conditions, where activation of these channels will presumably lead to a depolarization of the cell membrane and the concomitant activation of voltage-gated Ca^{2+} channels.

Activation of a Ca^{2+}-activated Cl^- current due to release of internal calcium by agonists {34,65–71} might also depolarize the cell membrane, and activate voltage-gated Ca^{2+} channels, thereby leading to an influx of extracellular calcium.

Receptor-mediated Ca^{2+} entry

This Ca^{2+} influx may occur independently of a change of the membrane potential through Ca^{2+}-selective as well as through nonselective cation channels in response to occupation of cell surface receptors by specific agonists. We will mainly focus on the influx that is promoted by the agonist-induced discharge of internal Ca^{2+} pools. This mechanism, which assumes a close interaction between internal stores and the plasma membrane, originated partly as a result of studies in smooth muscle {72,73} and evolved into a variety of models to explain agonist-induced Ca^{2+}

entry in excitable and nonexcitable cells. Until now no convincing electrophysiological evidence has been presented for the existence of such a channel in smooth muscle cells. The channel activated by ATP is directly gated by the agonist, while the other nonselective cation channels are activated by intracellular Ca^{2+}. Recently a channel has been described in mast cells that is activated by store depletion and inactivated by intracellular calcium {74}.

At least four different pathways for reloading empty stores have been proposed.
1. Through a direct link between the store and the extracellular space {73}. This connection may be controlled by GTP {75} and is stimulated by store depletion.
2. Ca^{2+} will accumulate in a narrow space between the store and the plasma membrane, from which it will then be transferred into the store by means of the endoplasmic reticulum Ca^{2+} pump {76}. An empty store stimulates this Ca^{2+} transfer.
3. Ca^{2+} will first enter into the bulk of the cytosol before being accumulated into the pool. A messenger is needed to signal the state of filling of the store to the plasma membrane {77}. It has been proposed that the luminal $[Ca^{2+}]$ in the endoplasmic reticulum store activates a tyrosine phosphatase that shifts a 130-kDa protein towards a tyr-dephosphorylated state. Ca^{2+} depletion of the store would favor phosphorylation of the 130-kDa protein, which then gates a Ca^{2+}-permeable membrane channel {78}. Alternative possibilities are that the luminal Ca^{2+} content is signalled to the plasma membrane via a cytochrome P450-dependent mechanism {79,80} or via a cyclic GMP-mediated signaling system {81}.
4. Ca^{2+} will enter the cytoplasm through the $Ins(1,3,4,5)P_4$ receptor, which is supposed to be a Ca^{2+} channel. The $Ins(1,3,4,5)P_4$ receptor makes direct contact with the $Ins(1,4,5)P_3$ receptor {82}. Since the $Ins(1,4,5)P_3$ receptor senses luminal Ca^{2+} {83–85}, this protein can be part of the mechanism by which the state of filling of the store is signaled to the plasma membrane. A slight variant is a direct activation of a Ca^{2+}-permeable plasma-membrane channel by $Ins(1,3,4,5)P_4$ that is produced by a Ca^{2+}-mediated (by the released Ca^{2+}) activation of the $Ins(1,4,5)P_3$-3-kinase converting $Ins(1,4,5)P_3$ to $Ins(1,3,4,5)P_4$ {86}.

Various reviews have covered the issue of Ca^{2+} entry in nonexcitable cells {87,88}. In this review we will focus on the information obtained in smooth muscle. All models except model 3 presume a close contact between the endoplasmic reticulum and the plasma membrane, for which there is both morphological {89} and functional evidence {90,91} in smooth muscle.

The emptying of the agonist-sensitive Ca^{2+} store is a sufficient stimulus to activate Ca^{2+} entry into the cell to replenish the store {73,92}. It was observed in rabbit ear artery that the rate of filling and the maximum degree of filling depend on the external $[Ca^{2+}]$. Since the rapid filling is not accompanied by a contractile response, it was assumed that cytosolic $[Ca^{2+}]$ does not reach the threshold for contraction during the reloading. The organic Ca^{2+}-

channel antagonist D600 does not affect the refilling, excluding the involvement of voltage-operated Ca^{2+} channels. Based on these observations, a model was proposed in which the internal Ca^{2+} pool is refilled *directly* from the extracellular medium. The permeability of this pathway for Ca^{2+} is controlled by the extent of filling of the agonist-sensitive store.

A7r5 vascular smooth muscle cells represent a suitable model to further study receptor-mediated Ca^{2+} entry {93}. These cells, which only express $Ins(1,4,5)P_3$-sensitive Ca^{2+} stores, exhibit an increased rate of $^{45}Ca^{2+}$ uptake if their stores are initially depleted by pretreating them with vasopressin. This increased rate of Ca^{2+} entry is not blocked by the Ca^{2+} channel blocker verapamil. Mn^{2+} can be used as a surrogate of Ca^{2+} to study the entry pathway. Mn^{2+} entry in A7r5 cells is also increased when the pools are depleted. In order to investigate whether Mn^{2+} is accumulated in a store, we have exposed intact cells to $^{54}Mn^{2+}$, then permeabilized the cells and observed whether $^{54}Mn^{2+}$ is released by application of A23187. Mn^{2+}, which, at least in micromolar concentrations, is a poor substrate for the Ca^{2+} pump, is found to accumulate in the store. The conclusion from these experiments is that Mn^{2+} (and therefore Ca^{2+}) enters the cell through a direct pathway into the store. An alternative explanation would be that Ca^{2+} accumulates in a narrow space between the plasma membrane and the endoplasmic reticulum, where it reaches high concentrations and from where it will then be pumped into the store.

An alternative approach to establish the nature of the Ca^{2+}-entry pathway is to study the effect of Ca^{2+}-pump inhibitors on the process of Ca^{2+} entry. The rationale of these experiments is to study whether or not a Ca^{2+} pump is involved in the refilling process. AlF_4^-, cyclopiazonic acid, and thapsigargin have been used for that purpose. Low $[AlF_4^-]$ reversibly blocks the endoplasmic reticulum Ca^{2+} pump by interacting with the phosphate-binding site of the ATPase {94,95}. AlF_4^- is also effective when applied to intact cells {96,97}. The effect of AlF_4^- on the reloading of the store has been observed by measuring force development as an estimate of the free $[Ca^{2+}]_i$. Blocking the endoplasmic reticulum Ca^{2+} pump in the rabbit ear artery with AlF_4^- is unable to prevent the reloading of an empty norepinephrine-sensitive Ca^{2+} store, suggesting that no Ca^{2+} pump is involved in the reloading process in that tissue {96}. The same effect is not observed in rat myometrium. The use of Ca^{2+} pump inhibitors, therefore, points to differences in Ca^{2+} entry between various smooth muscle tissues.

The use of Ca^{2+} pump inhibitors has also pointed to the existence of different refilling mechanisms in the same smooth muscle tissue. Only part of the Ca^{2+}-entry pathway is blocked by cyclopiazonic acid in dog mesenteric artery, while another component of it is unaffected {98}. Thapsigargin, another drug that specifically blocks internal Ca^{2+} pumps in smooth muscle {99–102}, is unable to completely prevent repletion of the store in rat aorta and dog mesenteric artery {103}. Recently evidence was presented for the coexistence of two refilling pathways in canine mesenteric artery {98}. Phenylephrine induces a biphasic contraction and therefore presumably a biphasic Ca^{2+} release in Ca^{2+}-free solution. The first component is due to Ca^{2+} release from a store that is refilled via a Ca^{2+} pump. A second more slow component of the contraction represents Ca^{2+} release from a store that can reload in the absence of Ca^{2+} pumping. The refilling of that store is blocked by the Ca^{2+}-channel blocker nifedipine and enhanced by the Ca^{2+}-channel activator Bay K 8644. The authors propose that the store is linked to the plasma membrane by a voltage-sensitive connection. Such a voltage-sensitive connection has also been proposed for dog trachea {104}. The proposed connection, therefore, differs from the one in A7r5 cells {93} and rabbit ear artery {73}, which are both assumed to be voltage independent.

van Breemen and coworkers envisage a special organization of the endoplasmic reticulum close to the plasma membrane (the *superficial buffer barrier*). They assume that a fenestrated superficial endoplasmic reticulum is separated from the cell membrane by a narrow restricted cytoplasmic space {72,105}. According to the model, enhanced Ca^{2+} entry would be partially buffered by Ca^{2+} uptake into the superficial endoplasmic reticulum. Since Ca^{2+} uptake into the superficial endoplasmic reticulum is mediated by a Ca^{2+} pump, which is a saturable transporter, it could be bypassed by a very high rate of Ca^{2+} entry. Ca^{2+} entering at slower rates could be effectively removed from the cytoplasm before exiting through the fenestrations into the deeper myoplasm.

Clearly, the issue of how emptying the pools stimulates Ca^{2+} entry in smooth muscle is far from resolved. Much more refined techniques (e.g., electrophysiology) are needed to further address the issue. It is, however, also possible that the rather divergent results obtained from various tissues could represent the existence of different mechanisms of Ca^{2+} entry.

Ca^{2+} RELEASE FROM INTERNAL STORES

Mitochondria probably do not make a significant contribution to the regulation of cytoplasmic Ca^{2+} in smooth muscle {106}, because they have only a low affinity for Ca^{2+}. The apparent K_m for Ca^{2+} ($10–20\,\mu M$) is higher than the level of free cytoplasmic Ca^{2+} reached during a maximal contraction. The mitochondrial Ca^{2+} content does neither significantly increase during a maximal physiological increase in $[Ca^{2+}]_i$ {107,108}. Pathological calcification of mitochondria, with as much as a 1000-fold increase in mitochondrial Ca^{2+} content, can occur when the cytoplasmic $[Ca^{2+}]_i$ rises to abnormally high levels. The ability of mitochondria to serve as high-capacity, low-affinity Ca^{2+} buffers could protect cells from Ca^{2+} proteases during periods of pathological Ca^{2+} overload {106}.

The endoplasmic reticulum or a part thereof seems to be the physiologically important Ca^{2+} reservoir in smooth muscle. The endoplasmic reticulum occupies about 1.5% of the cell volume in some smooth muscles {89} but much more in others like aorta {109}. The luminal $[Ca^{2+}]$ in the endoplasmic reticulum could be as high as $15\,mM/l$ {110,111}, although most of it may be bound to Ca^{2+}-binding proteins. The internal stores in smooth muscle may release their Ca^{2+} through two types of Ca^{2+}-release channels: the $Ins(1,4,5)P_3$ receptor and the ryanodine receptor, which will be discussed below.

$Ins(1,4,5)P_3$ receptor

SMOOTH-MUSCLE $Ins(1,4,5)P_3$ RECEPTOR

The general principles of the signal-transducing pathway in smooth muscle are well known: Agonist binding to cell surface receptors stimulates inositol-lipid breakdown, thereby producing $Ins(1,4,5)P_3$, which then releases Ca^{2+} from intracellular stores. $Ins(1,4,5)P_3$ mobilizes Ca^{2+} from nonmitochondrial Ca^{2+} pools by interacting with a specific receptor in the membrane of these internal stores {112}.

$Ins(1,4,5)P_3$ seems to be the major physiological messenger for the Ca^{2+}-release component of pharmacomechanical coupling {113}. Indeed, the ability of $Ins(1,4,5)P_3$ to mobilize Ca^{2+} has now been demonstrated in many different types of smooth muscle. In addition, the time course of the tension development upon flashing the photolabile inactive precursor of $Ins(1,4,5)P_3$ [caged $Ins(1,4,5)P_3$] was comparable to the tension rise in intact muscle after agonist stimulation {114}.

The $Ins(1,4,5)P_3$ receptor has been isolated from smooth muscle of bovine aorta {115} and rat vas deferens {116}. The latter tissue expresses a high density of $Ins(1,4,5)P_3$ receptors, about 25% of that in cerebellum, which is the richest source of $Ins(1,4,5)P_3$ receptors so far.

The smooth-muscle $Ins(1,4,5)P_3$ receptor consists of 4 single subunits with a M_r of 224,000 {115} and 260,000 {116} as determined by SDS/PAGE. Its ability to bind to wheat germ agglutinin suggests that the receptor is a glycoprotein. The purified receptor of aorta consists of large structures with surface dimensions of $25 \times 25\,nm^2$. It has a pinwheel appearance with fourfold symmetry and four radial arms radiating from a central humb, suggesting that four subunits form the channel. $Ins(1,4,5)P_3$ binds to the receptor with a K_d of $2.4\,nM$ (aorta) and $10\,nM$ (vas deferens). Only a single population of binding sites seems to occur in smooth muscle. Channel activity of the purified receptor from aorta has been reported {117}.

Gene diversity and alternative splicing result in the existence of several subtypes of the $Ins(1,4,5)P_3$ receptor {118–122}. Quantitative differences have been reported in the expression of these subtypes between uterus, cerebellum, and other tissues {119}. The genes encoding the gastrointestinal smooth muscle receptor and that from brain might be different {121}, and both receptors might therefore exhibit different functional properties. It has been reported that the purified $Ins(1,4,5)P_3$ receptor from adult cerebellum and vas deferens have different K_m values for phosphorylation by cyclic AMP-dependent protein kinase {118}.

KINETICS OF THE RELEASE

The Ins(1,4,5)P$_3$-induced Ca^{2+} release presents a fast and a slow release component in nonmuscle cells {123–125}. Photoreleasing a high concentration of Ins(1,4,5)P$_3$ in guinea pig portal vein smooth muscle results in a [Ca^{2+}]$_i$ rise within approximately 10 ms {126}, which points to the existence of a fast release component. ^{45}Ca^{2+}-flux experiments in permeabilized A7r5 smooth muscle cells in addition revealed a slow component {127}. This slow release was not related to Ins(1,4,5)P$_3$ metabolism, and also not to a slow dissociation of Ca^{2+} from binding proteins. The slow release neither represents a slow diffusion of Ca^{2+} from uptake compartments to structurally different release sites {128,129}, nor a spontaneous inactivation of the Ins(1,4,5)P$_3$ receptor. The slow-release component might represent a partially open state of the Ins(1,4,5)P$_3$ receptor occurring when the luminal free Ca^{2+} concentration is low {127}.

CONTROL BY CYTOSOLIC Ca^{2+}

A biphasic effect of Ca^{2+} on the Ins(1,4,5)P$_3$ receptor was first observed in smooth muscle {130,131}. This biphasic Ca^{2+} dependence occurs in other tissues as well {122,132,133}. Increasing the [Ca^{2+}] to 300 nM augments the effectiveness of Ins(1,4,5)P$_3$ in releasing Ca^{2+} {130}. The Ins(1,4,5)P$_3$ receptor can therefore be considered as a *Ca^{2+}-induced Ca^{2+}-release channel*. This positive feedback exerted by Ca^{2+} could be very important and would lead to a very rapid release from internal stores. The stimulatory effect of cytosolic Ca^{2+} on the smooth muscle Ins(1,4,5)P$_3$ receptor can be more easily demonstrated when the pools contain less Ca^{2+} {134}.

The Ins(1,4,5)P$_3$ receptor consists of an amino-terminal Ins(1,4,5)P$_3$-binding domain, a carboxy-terminal Ca^{2+} channel, and a coupling domain between this binding site and the channel {135}. The sequence of the coupling domain may contain a Ca^{2+}-binding site, and it is possible that there are further Ca^{2+}-binding sites at other regions of the molecule, in particular in the transmembrane spanning regions {136}.

High [Ca^{2+}] inhibit the release in smooth muscle {130, 134,137}. This inhibition by Ca^{2+} presents a negative feedback on the release. Negative feedback could underlie the ceiling to agonist-induced [Ca^{2+}]$_i$ rises in single smooth muscle cells {138}.

CONTROL BY LUMINAL Ca^{2+}

Luminal Ca^{2+} controls the Ins(1,4,5)P$_3$ receptor in rat hepatocytes {83–85}. The Ca^{2+} content of the store also seems to control the release process in A7r5 smooth muscle cells {127}. Store depletion shifts the dose-response relationship for Ins(1,4,5)P$_3$-induced Ca^{2+} mobilization to the right (fig. 46-1). Luminal Ca^{2+} may directly interact with the channel or via some associated protein. The latter seems to occur with the ryanodine receptor, where [Ca^{2+}]-dependent conformational changes of calsequestrin affect the Ca^{2+}-channel function {139}. It was recently suggested

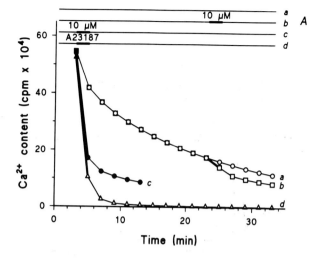

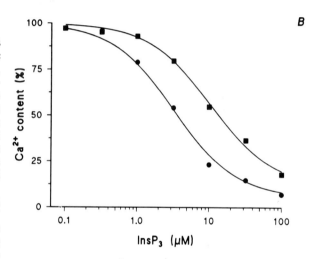

Fig. 46-1. Luminal Ca^{2+} interferes with the InsP$_3$-induced Ca^{2+} release process. The nonmitochondrial Ca^{2+} stores in permeabilized A7r5 smooth muscle cells were loaded to steady state. The stores in **A** are challenged for 2 minutes with 10 μM InsP$_3$ after 3 minutes (c) or 23 minutes (b) of efflux. **B** illustrates the percentage Ca^{2+} remaining in the stores after a 2 minutes application of the indicated [InsP$_3$] after 3 minutes (●) or 23 minutes of efflux (■). Each curve is typical for three experiments. Methods: ^{45}Ca^{2+} fluxes were performed on monolayers of saponin-permeabilized A7r5 cells (3 × 10^5 cells/4 cm^2 well) at 25°C. The stores were loaded for 10 minutes in a medium containing 120 mM KCl, 30 mM imidazole (pH 6.8), 5 mM MgCl$_2$, 5 mM ATP, 0.44 mM EGTA, 10 mM NaN$_3$, and 150 nM free Ca^{2+} (23 μCi/ml). The wells were then washed three times in an efflux medium containing 120 mM KCl, 30 mM imidazole (pH 6.8), 2 mM MgCl$_2$, 1 mM ATP, 1 mM EGTA, 5 mM NaN$_3$, and 2 μM thapsigargin. One milliliter of this medium was then added to the monolayers and replaced every 2 minutes. The time course of the ^{45}Ca^{2+} washout was calculated by summing in retrograde order the amount of ^{45}Ca^{2+} remaining in the cells at the end of the efflux and the amounts of ^{45}Ca^{2+} collected during the successive time intervals. Reprinted with permission from Nature 357:599–602, Copyright 1992 Macmillan Magazines Limited.

{131} that the "loading dependence" of the Ins(1,4,5)P$_3$-dependent Ca^{2+} release could represent the stimulatory effect of cytosolic Ca^{2+}. The feedback control will be less effective if the Ca^{2+} store is only partly loaded with Ca^{2+}.

PARTIAL Ca^{2+} RELEASE

Even a prolonged stimulation with a submaximal dose of Ins(1,4,5)P$_3$ is unable to release all the Ca^{2+} accumulated in the Ins(1,4,5)P$_3$-sensitive store {124–126,133,140–142}. It is therefore said that low doses of Ins(1,4,5)P$_3$ only induce a *partial release*, implying that the release in response to a submaximal Ins(1,4,5)P$_3$ stimulus suddenly stops despite the fact that there is still a large amount of Ca^{2+} left in the Ins(1,4,5)P$_3$-sensitive store. One hypothesis to explain this partial release is that individual stores present a heterogeneous Ins(1,4,5)P$_3$ sensitivity and that low [Ins(1,4,5)P$_3$] completely discharge only the most sensitive stores, while leaving the less sensitive pools more or less untouched (an *all-or-none release*) {125,140,142}. The other hypothesis is that a low [Ins(1,4,5)P$_3$] releases Ca^{2+} from the whole population of stores and that the release mechanism somehow inactivates (a *steady-state mechanism*) {82,88,143}.

We have presented experimental evidence that the partial release in A7r5 smooth muscle cells probably does not represent the manifestation of an all-or-none emptying of the most sensitive stores, but instead represents a partial emptying of all the stores through a process that is activated by luminal Ca^{2+} and that therefore slows down as the pools become depleted {127}.

A steady-state model can, however, explain a more complete release if there is a time delay between the decrease of the luminal [Ca^{2+}] below the threshold for channel activation and the actual closure of the channel or if cytosolic Ca^{2+} is allowed to exert its positive feedback on the Ins(1,4,5)P$_3$ receptor {130–133}. Since the rate of Ca^{2+} release will depend on the density of the release channels and on the initial Ca^{2+} content of the stores, it is possible that the pattern of Ca^{2+} release (steady state or all-or-none) not only depends on intrinsic properties of the Ins(1,4,5)P$_3$ receptor, but also on the density of Ins(1,4,5)P$_3$ receptors, Ca^{2+} pumps, luminal Ca^{2+}-binding proteins, passive Ca^{2+} leaks, etc., all of which might differ amongst various cell types.

EFFECT OF NUCLEOTIDES

The Ins(1,4,5)P$_3$-induced Ca^{2+} release in permeabilized smooth muscle cells requires ATP {144}. Ins(1,4,5)P$_3$ seems, however, also to release Ca^{2+} in the absence of adenine nucleotides {130,145,146}, although the release is much smaller than in the presence of ATP {126}. ATP increases the open probability of the channel twofold, but only in the presence of Ins(1,4,5)P$_3$ {117,146}. Phosphorylation of the receptor is not involved, because the poorly hydrolyzable ATP analogue AMP-PNP is also effective {126,146}.

Low concentrations of adenine nucleotides stimulate the release, but higher concentrations inhibit it {147}. The Ins(1,4,5)P$_3$ receptor may therefore have two adenine nucleotide binding sites, one coupled to stimulation of the release, the other to inhibition of the release. The latter inhibitory site could be the Ins(1,4,5)P$_3$-binding site itself {147}, since ATP competitively inhibits the Ca^{2+} release {148,149}. However, the inhibitory site and the Ins(1,4,5)P$_3$-binding site could be different in cerebellum {150}.

The intracellular [ATP] in smooth muscle is 1–2 mM, and remains constant even during maximal agonist stimulation {151}. It is therefore unlikely that ATP would regulate the Ins(1,4,5)P$_3$ receptor under normal physiological conditions.

Guanine nucleotides have little effect on the Ins(1,4,5)P$_3$ receptor {147,150}, although they may enlarge the capacity of the Ins(1,4,5)P$_3$-sensitive Ca^{2+} stores by connecting them with Ins(1,4,5)P$_3$-insensitive Ca^{2+} stores {75}. This is consistent with the fact that purified Ins(1,4,5)P$_3$ receptors alone can induce a flux of Ca^{2+} {152}. There are some claims that a GTP-binding protein might regulate the Ins(1,4,5)P$_3$-mediated Ca^{2+} release in smooth muscle {153–155}.

EFFECT OF THE SULPHYDRYL REAGENT THIMEROSAL

The sulphydryl reagent thimerosal has the potential of becoming a valuable tool for further probing the Ins(1,4,5)P$_3$ signaling pathway. This topically used antibacterial and antifungal agent also releases Ca^{2+} from internal stores in mammalian cells {156,157}. Thimerosal has more recently been shown to induce Ca^{2+} oscillations in oocytes {158–161}, HeLa cells {162}, endothelial cells {163}, and pancreatic acinar cells {164}. Thimerosal does not induce a rise in intracellular Ins(1,4,5)P$_3$ concentration {162}.

Low concentrations of thimerosal (<10 μM) sensitize the smooth-muscle Ins(1,4,5)P$_3$ receptor {165}. At higher concentrations, an inhibitory effect becomes also apparent. The stimulation of the Ins(1,4,5)P$_3$ receptor occurs at lower doses than those required to inhibit the endoplasmic reticulum Ca^{2+} pump. Still higher doses aspecifically increase the passive Ca^{2+} leak. Thimerosal is therefore a pharmacological tool that, at least at low concentrations, can rather specifically activate the smooth muscle Ins(1,4,5)P$_3$ receptor.

Ryanodine receptor

RYANODINE RECEPTOR IN SMOOTH MUSCLE

The ryanodine receptor becomes activated when the cytosolic [Ca^{2+}] rises to produce the phenomenon of Ca^{2+}-induced Ca^{2+} release. The channel in smooth muscle is sensitive to Ca^{2+}, adenine nucleotides, Mg^{2+}, caffeine, pH, and ryanodine, and therefore resembles the channel in skeletal muscle {166,167}. Skeletal-muscle ryanodine receptors form junctional feet spanning the gap between the T-tubule and the sarcoplasmic reticulum {168}. In smooth muscle, similar bridging structures have been identified between the surface membrane and the superficial endoplasmic reticulum, although they are less well developed than skeletal-muscle junctional feet {89}.

These bridges might represent the ryanodine receptors in smooth muscle {166}.

The plant alkaloid ryanodine has been successfully applied to smooth muscle fibres to open the channel and hence to deplete the intracellular stores. The generally used concentration to induce a gradual depletion of the intracellular stores in smooth muscle is $10\,\mu M$ {169–172}. Very high concentrations (greater than $500\,\mu M$) of ryanodine are needed to transfer the channel into a permanently closed state {167}. The smooth muscle ryanodine receptor therefore seems to be less sensitive to ryanodine than the receptor of other tissues.

The ryanodine receptor has been purified from vascular smooth muscle and incorporated in bilayers {167}. The channel conducts Ca^{2+} and monovalent cations. It is activated by Ca^{2+} and caffeine, and inhibited by ruthenium red. The channel shares many common features with the skeletal and cardiac ryanodine receptors. The identical sedimentation coefficients and the observation of four subconductance levels may also indicate a similar structure composed of four subunits. There are, however, some functional differences between the ryanodine receptor in smooth muscle and that in cardiac and skeletal muscle, e.g., subconducting states are not observed in the purified smooth muscle ryanodine receptor.

Some smooth muscle cells, such as the myometrium {173–175} and A7r5 vascular smooth muscle cells {93}, do not respond to caffeine and ryanodine, and therefore probably do not express a ryanodine receptor. The presence or absence of a ryanodine receptor is influenced by cell growth and differentiation in cultured rat aorta cells {176}. Proliferation of these cells is accompanied by a loss of sensitivity to caffeine.

Recently, a novel type of ryanodine receptor was described that is not activated by caffeine and therefore seems to be distinct from the known receptors {177,178}. The receptor is also present in smooth muscle.

FUNCTION OF THE SMOOTH-MUSCLE RYANODINE RECEPTOR

Ryanodine receptors in smooth muscle could be involved in the following phenomena: (a) amplifying the agonist-induced Ca^{2+} signal, (b) setting up cytosolic Ca^{2+} oscillations, and (c) inducing Ca^{2+} waves.

Amplifying the agonist-induced Ca^{2+} signal

Ryanodine receptors in cardiac muscle exhibit Ca^{2+}-induced Ca^{2+} release in the physiological range of $[Ca^{2+}]$. It has been proposed {179} for smooth muscle that agonists trigger a release of Ca^{2+} from a small store near the receptor in the plasma membrane, which then triggers further release of Ca^{2+} through the ryanodine receptor. It has also been proposed {180} that Ca^{2+} influx via voltage-dependent Ca^{2+} channels can trigger subsequent Ca^{2+}-induced Ca^{2+} release contributing to the contraction.

Ca^{2+}-induced Ca^{2+} release in guinea pig taenia caeci is only activated when the $[Ca^{2+}]$ has risen above $1\,\mu M$. The threshold for contraction development in that smooth muscle is $100\,nM$ and a maximal contraction is reached at $3–10\,\mu M$. The ryanodine receptor could therefore not play an important role in triggering a physiological contraction. It is, however, possible that the ryanodine receptor could fulfill a more important role in the intact cell, because the $[Ca^{2+}]$ in the vicinity of a release channel can become much higher than the bulk $[Ca^{2+}]$ in the cytoplasm {181}. It is also possible that some soluble component of the cytosol, which might be lost after saponin treatment, enhances the Ca^{2+} sensitivity of the Ca^{2+}-induced Ca^{2+}-release mechanism in the intact cell.

Setting up cytosolic Ca^{2+} oscillations

The use of systems that can record the intracellular $[Ca^{2+}]$ in single cells has revealed that the intracellular $[Ca^{2+}]$ often oscillates, especially after modest agonist stimulation. The oscillator is called cytosolic if the individual spikes are due to the periodic release of internally stored Ca^{2+} {182}. Cytosolic Ca^{2+} oscillations occur in many smooth muscles, e.g., vascular smooth muscle {8,183–186}, intestinal smooth muscle {187}, and tracheal smooth muscle {188}.

Various models have been proposed to explain these oscillations {182,189}. One of them (the "two pool" model) assumes that agonists induce a gradual influx of external Ca^{2+} into the cell. This Ca^{2+} then accumulates in the intracellular store until these pools become overloaded, at which time Ca^{2+} will be released through the process of Ca^{2+}-induced Ca^{2+} release. The $Ins(1,4,5)P_3$ receptor is activated by a rise in cytosolic $[Ca^{2+}]$. This protein therefore fulfills the necessary criteria to act as a Ca^{2+}-induced Ca^{2+}-release channel {130–133} and could therefore be involved in the setting up of Ca^{2+} oscillations {83,127}. Also the ryanodine receptor is a Ca^{2+}-induced Ca^{2+}-release channel. The caffeine-sensitive store could therefore also be involved in setting up cytosolic Ca^{2+} oscillations in smooth muscle. The finding that $1\,mM$ caffeine induces a small increase in frequency and amplitude of the Ca^{2+} oscillator in rabbit jejunal cells, while higher caffeine concentrations induce a rapid burst of transient outward currents followed by a prolonged quiet period with no transient currents, is compatible with the involvement of a ryanodine receptor {183}. Similar responses are observed in rabbit ear-artery cells {183}, rabbit portal vein {8}, and rabbit small intestine {172}. High concentrations of caffeine {10–20 mM} also inhibit the oscillations in rat aortic smooth muscle {184} and rabbit portal vein {186}. Although inhibitory effects of caffeine would be compatible with the involvement of the ryanodine receptor for generating oscillations, they do not exclude the involvement of $Ins(1,4,5)P_3$-sensitive stores, because of the known inhibitory effects of caffeine on the $Ins(1,4,5)P_3$ receptor {84,190,191}. The stimulatory effect of low caffeine concentrations on the oscillator {8,172,183} can be explained by oscillation models that rely on Ca^{2+}-induced Ca^{2+} release from overloaded caffeine-sensitive stores. Caffeine would lower the threshold for Ca^{2+}-induced Ca^{2+} release and thereby increase the oscillation frequency. This enhancing effect of caffeine can, however, also be explained by oscillation models in which Ca^{2+} is periodically released from an overloaded $Ins(1,4,5)P_3$-sensitive store. The enhancing effect of low caffeine concentrations would then be explained by this oscillator in the $Ins(1,4,5)P_3$-sensitive store receiving an increased supply of Ca^{2+}, due to the inability of the caffeine-sensitive pool to accumulate Ca^{2+} {84}.

Ca^{2+} waves

The initial $[Ca^{2+}]_i$ rise upon agonist stimulation often starts in a specific region of the cell and then spreads through the rest of the cell as a Ca^{2+} wave {155,185,192–194}. One model to explain Ca^{2+} waves assumes that Ca^{2+} waves represent the slow diffusion of $Ins(1,4,5)P_3$ {195}. The other assumes that Ca^{2+} diffuses in the cell and triggers further release through Ca^{2+}-induced Ca^{2+} release {112,196}. The ryanodine receptor could be involved in inducing the Ca^{2+}-induced Ca^{2+} release, which is necessary for wave propagation. However, also the smooth muscle $Ins(1,4,5)P_3$ receptor fulfills the necessary criteria to act as a Ca^{2+}-induced Ca^{2+} release channel {130,131,134}.

REFERENCES

1. Somlyo AV, Somlyo AP: Electromechanical and pharmacomechanical coupling in vascular smooth muscle. *J Pharmacol Exp Ther* 159:129–145, 1968.
2. Friedman ME, Suarez Kurtz G, Kaczorowski GJ, Katz GM, Reuben JP: Two calcium currents in a smooth muscle cell line. *Am J Physiol* 250:H699–H703, 1986.
3. Benham CD, Hess P, Tsien RW: Two types of calcium channels in single smooth muscle cells from rabbit ear artery studied with whole-cell and single-channel recordings. *Circ Res* 61:I10–I16, 1987.
4. Yoshino M, Someya T, Nishio A, Yabu H: Whole-cell and Ca channel currents in mamalian intestinal smooth muscle cells: Evidence for the existence of two types of Ca channels. *Pflügers Arch* 411:229–231, 1988.
5. Loirand G, Mironneau C, Mironneau J, Pacaud P: Two types of calcium currents in single smooth muscle cells from rat portal vein. *J Physiol (Lond)* 412:333–349, 1989.
6. Wang R, Karpinski E, Pang PKT: Two types of calcium channels in isolated smooth muscle cells from rat tail artery. *Am J Physiol* 256:H1361–H1368, 1989.
7. Simard JM: Calcium channel currents in isolated smooth muscle cells from the basilar artery of the guinea pig. *Pflügers Arch* 417:528–536, 1991.
8. Komori S, Bolton T: Calcium release induced by inositol 1,4,5-trisphosphate in single rabbit intestinal smooth muscle cells. *J Physiol (Lond)* 433:495–517, 1991.
9. Schneider P, Hopp HH, Isenberg G: Ca^{2+} influx through ATP-gated channels increments $[Ca^{2+}]_i$ and inactivates I_{Ca} in myocytes from guinea-pig urinary bladder. *J Physiol (Lond)* 440:479–496, 1991.
10. McCarron JG, McGeown JG, Reardon S, Ikebe M, Fay FS, Walsh JV Jr: Calcium-dependent enhancement of calcium current in smooth muscle by calmodulin-dependent protein kinase II. *Nature* 357:74–77, 1992.
11. Droogmans G, Callewaert G: Ca-channel current and its modification by the dihydropyridine agonist BAY K 8644 in

12. Bean BP: Nitrendipine block of cardiac calcium channels: High affinity binding to inactivated state. *Proc Natl Acad Sci USA* 81:6388–6392, 1984.
13. Bean BP, Sturek M, Puga A, Hermsmeyer K: Calcium channels in muscle cells isolated from rat mesenteric arteries: Modulation by dihydropyridine drugs. *Circ Res* 59:229–235, 1986.
14. Yatani A, Seidel CL, Allen J, Brown AM: Whole-cell and single-channel calcium currents of isolated smooth muscle cells from saphenous vein. *Circ Res* 60:523–533, 1987.
15. Ohya Y, Kitamura K, Kuriyama H: Modulation of ionic currents in smooth muscle balls of the rabbit intestine by intracellularly perfused ATP and cyclic AMP. *Pflügers Arch* 408:465–473, 1987.
16. Ohya Y, Sperelakis N: ATP regulation of the slow calcium channels in vascular smooth muscle cells of guinea pig mesenteric artery. *Circ Res* 64:145–154, 1989.
17. Welling A, Felbel J, Peper K, Hofmann F: Beta-adrenergic receptor stimulates L-type calcium current in adult smooth muscle cells. *Blood Vessels* 28:154–158, 1991.
18. Wang R, Karpinski E, Pang PKT: Parathyroid hormone selectively inhibits L-type calcium channels in single vascular smooth muscle cells of the rat. *J Physiol (Lond)* 441:325–346, 1991.
19. Wang R, Wu LY, Karpinski E, Pang PK: The effects of parathyroid hormone on L-type voltage-dependent calcium channel current in vascular smooth muscle cells and ventricular myocytes are mediated by a cyclic AMP dependent mechanism. *FEBS Lett* 282:331–334, 1991.
20. Benham CD, Tsien RW: Noradrenaline modulation of calcium channels in single smooth muscle cells from rabbit ear artery. *J Physiol (Lond)* 404:767–784, 1988.
21. Droogmans G, Declerck I, Casteels R: Effect of adrenergic agonists on Ca-channel currents in single vascular smooth muscle cells. *Pflügers Arch* 409:7–12, 1987.
22. Nelson MT, Standen NB, Brayden JE, Worley JF: Noradrenaline contracts arteries by activating voltage-dependent calcium channels. *Nature* 336:382–385, 1988.
23. Galizzi JP, Qar J, Fosset M, Van Renterghem C, Lazdunski M: Regulation of calcium channels in aortic muscle cells by protein kinase C activators (diacylglycerol and phorbol esters) and by peptides (vasopressin and bombesin) that stimulate phosphoinositide breakdown. *J Biol Chem* 262:6947–6950, 1987.
24. Fish RD, Sperti G, Colucci WS, Clapham DE: Phorbol ester increases the dihydropyridine-sensitive calcium conductance in a vascular smooth muscle cell line. *Circ Res* 62:1049–1054, 1988.
25. Vivaudou MB, Clapp LH, Walsh JV, Singer JJ: Regulation of one type of Ca current in smooth muscle cells by diacylglycerol and acetylcholine. *FASEB J* 2:2497–2504, 1988.
26. Ohya Y, Sperelakis N: Involvement of a GTP-binding protein in stimulating action of angiotensin-II on calcium channels in vascular smooth muscle cells. *Circ Res* 68:763–771, 1991.
27. Oike Y, Kitamura K, Kuriyama H: Histamine H_3-receptor activation augments voltage-dependent Ca^{2+} current via GTP hydrolysis in rabbit saphenous artery. *J Physiol (Lond)* 448:133–152, 1992.
28. Shimada T, Somlyo AP: Modulation of voltage-dependent Ca channel current by arachidonic acid and other long-chain fatty acids in rabbit intestinal smooth muscle. *J Gen Physiol* 100:27–44, 1992.
29. Ward SM, Vogalis F, Blondfield DP, Ozaki H, Fusetani N,

Uemura D, Publicover NG, Sanders KM: Inhibition of electrical slow waves and Ca^{2+} currents of gastric and colonic smooth muscle by phosphatase inhibitors. *Am J Physiol* 261:C64–C70, 1991.

30. Usuki T, Obara K, Someya T, Ozaki H, Karaki H, Fusetani N, Yabu H: Calyculin-A increases voltage-dependent inward current in smooth muscle cells isolated from guinea pig taenia coli. *Experientia* 47:939–941, 1991.

31. Goto K, Kasuya Y, Matsuki N, Takuwa Y, Kurihara H, Ishikawa T, Kimura S, Yanagisawa M, Masaki T: Endothelin activates the dihydropyridine-sensitive, voltage-dependent Ca^{2+} channel in vascular smooth muscle. *Proc Natl Acad Sci USA* 86:3915–3918, 1989.

32. Declerck I, Himpens B, Droogmans G, Casteels R: The α_1-agonist phenylephrine inhibits voltage-gated Ca^{2+}-channels in vascular smooth muscle cells of rabbit ear artery. *Pflügers Arch* 417:117–119, 1990.

33. Pacaud P, Loirand G, Mironneau C, Mironneau J: Opposing effects of noradrenaline on the two classes of voltage-dependent calcium channels of single vascular smooth muscle cells in short-term primary culture. *Pflügers Arch* 410:557–559, 1987.

34. Pacaud P, Loirand G, Mironneau C, Mironneau J: Noradrenaline activates a calcium-activated chloride conductance and increases the voltage-dependent calcium current in cultured single cells of rat portal vein. *Br J Pharmacol* 97:139–146, 1989.

35. Tomita T: Ionic channels in smooth muscle studied with patch-clamp methods. *Jpn J Physiol* 38:1–18, 1988.

36. Bkaily G, Peyrow M, Sculptoreanu A, Jacques D, Chahine M, Regoli D, Sperelakis N: Angiotension II increases I_{si} and blocks I_K in single aortic cell of rabbit. *Pflügers Arch* 412:448–450, 1988.

37. Clapp LH, Vivaudou MB, Walsh JV, Singer JJ: Acetylcholine increases voltage-activated Ca current in freshly dissociated smooth muscle cells. *Proc Natl Acad Sci USA* 84:2092–2096, 1987.

38. Clapp LH, Vivaudou MB, Singer JJ, Walsh JV: Substance P, like acetylcholine, augments one type of Ca current in isolated smooth muscle cells. *Pflügers Arch* 413:565–567, 1989.

39. Van Renterghem C, Romey G, Lazdunski M: Vasopressin modulates the spontaneous electrical activity in aortic cells (line A7r5) by acting on three different types of ionic channels. *Proc Natl Acad Sci USA* 85:9365–9369, 1988.

40. Imaizumi Y, Takeda M, Muraki K, Watanabe M: Mechanisms of NE-induced reduction of Ca current in single smooth muscle cells from guinea pig vas deferens. *Am J Physiol* 260:C17–C25, 1991.

41. Worley JF, Kotlikoff MI: Dihydropyridine-sensitive single calcium channels in airway smooth muscle cells. *Am J Physiol* 259:L468–L480, 1990.

42. Mayer EA, Loo, DDF, Snape WJ, Sachs G: The activation of calcium and calcium-activated potassium channels in mammalian colonic smooth muscle by substance-P. *J Physiol (Lond)* 420:47–71, 1990.

43. Bonev A, Isenberg G: Arginine-vasopressin induces mode-2 gating in L-type Ca^{2+} channels (smooth muscle cells of the urinary bladder of the guinea-pig). *Pflügers Arch* 420:219–222, 1992.

44. Matsuda JJ, Volk KA, Shibata EF: Calcium currents in isolated rabbit coronary arterial smooth muscle myocytes. *J Physiol (Lond)* 427:657–680, 1990.

45. Xiong ZL, Kitamura K, Kuriyama H: ATP activates cationic currents and modulates the calcium current through GTP-binding protein in rabbit portal vein. *J Physiol (Lond)* 440:143–165, 1991.

46. Fukumitsu T, Hayashi H, Tokuno H, Tomita T: Increase in calcium channel current by β-adrenoceptor agonists in single smooth muscle cells isolated from porcine coronary artery. *Br J Pharmacol* 100:593–599, 1990.

47. Sims SM, Singer JJ, Walsh JV: Cholinergic agonists suppress a potassium current in freshly dissociated smooth muscle cells of the toad. *J Physiol (Lond)* 367:503–529, 1985.

48. Sims SM, Clapp LH, Walsh JV, Singer JJ: Dual regulation of M current in gastric smooth muscle cells — beta-adrenergic-muscarinic antagonism. *Pflügers Arch* 417:291–302, 1990.

49. Cole WC, Carl A, Sanders KM: Muscarinic suppression of Ca^{2+}-dependent K-current in colonic smooth muscle. *Am J Physiol* 257:C481–C487, 1989.

50. Cole WC, Sanders KM: G-proteins mediate suppression of Ca^{2+}-activated K-current by acetylcholine in smooth muscle cells. *Am J Physiol* 257:C596–C600, 1989.

51. Gelband CH, Silberberg SD, Groschner K, van Breemen C: ATP inhibits smooth muscle Ca^{2+}-activated K^+ channels. *Proc R Soc (Lond) B* 242:23–28, 1990.

52. Groschner K, Silberberg SD, Gelband CH, van Breemen C: Ca^{2+}-activated K^+ channels in airway smooth muscle are inhibited by cytoplasmic adenosine triphosphate. *Pflügers Arch* 417:517–522, 1991.

53. Kume H, Kotlikoff MI: Muscarinic inhibition of single K_{Ca} channels in smooth muscle cells by a pertussis-sensitive G-protein. *Am J Physiol* 261:C1204–C1209, 1991.

54. Benham CD, Tsien RW: A novel receptor-operated Ca-permeable channel activated by ATP in smooth muscle. *Nature* 328:275–278, 1987.

55. Nakazawa K, Matsuki N: Adenosine triphosphate-activated inward current in isolated smooth muscle cells from rat vas deferens. *Pflügers Arch* 409:644–646, 1987.

56. Benham CD, Bolton TB, Byrne NG, Large WA: Action of externally applied adenosine triphosphate on single smooth muscle cells dispersed from rabbit ear artery. *J Physiol (Lond)* 387:473–488, 1987.

57. Friel DD: An ATP-sensitive conductance in single smooth muscle cells from the rat vas deferens. *J Physiol (Lond)* 401:361–380, 1988.

58. Declerck I, Droogmans G, Casteels R: Excitatory agonists and Ca-permeable channels in arterial smooth muscle cells. In: Aoki K (ed) *Essential Hypertension 2*. Berlin: Springer Verlag, 1989, pp 45–56.

59. Sims SM: Cholinergic activation of a non-selective cation current in canine gastric smooth muscle cells is associated with contraction. *J Physiol (Lond)* 449:377–398, 1992.

60. Komori S, Bolton TB: Actions of guanine nucleotides and cyclic nucleotides on calcium stores in single patch-clamped smooth muscle cells from rabbit portal vein. *Br J Pharmacol* 97:973–982, 1989.

61. Amedee T, Benham CD, Bolton TB, Byrne NG, Large WA: Potassium, chloride and non-selective cation conductances opened by noradrenaline in rabbit ear artery cells. *J Physiol (Lond)* 423:551–568, 1990.

62. Loirand G, Pacaud P, Baron A, Mironneau C, Mironneau J: Large conductance calcium-activated non-selective cation channels in smooth muscle cells isolated from rat portal vein. *J Physiol (Lond)* 437:461–475, 1991.

63. Pacaud P, Bolton TB: Relation between muscarinic receptor cationic current and internal calcium in guinea-pig jejunal smooth muscle cells. *J Physiol (Lond)* 441:477–499, 1991.

64. Benham CD: ATP-activated channels gate calcium entry in

single smooth muscle cells dissociated from rabbit ear artery. *J Physiol (Lond)* 419:689–701, 1989.

65. Byrne NG, Large WA: Membrane mechanism associated with muscarinic receptor activation in single cells freshly dispersed from the rat anococcygeus muscle. *Br J Pharmacol* 92:371–379, 1987.

66. Byrne NG, Large WA: Action of noradrenaline on single smooth muscle cells freshly dispersed from the rat anococcygeus muscle. *J Physiol (Lond)* 389:513–525, 1988.

67. Pacaud P, Loirand G, Baron A, Mironneau C, Mironneau J: Ca^{2+} channel activation and membrane depolarization mediated by Cl-channels in response to noradrenaline in vascular myocytes. *Br J Pharmacol* 104:1000–1006, 1991.

67. Sun XP, Supplisson S, Torres R, Sachs G, Mayer E: Characterization of large-conductance chloride channels in rabbit colonic smooth muscle. *J Physiol (Lond)* 448:355–382, 1992.

68. Pacaud P, Loirand G, Lavie JL, Mironneau C, Mironneau J: Calcium-activated chloride current in rat vascular smooth muscle cells in short-term primary culture. *Pflügers Arch* 413:629–636, 1989.

69. Droogmans G, Callewaert G, Declerck I, Casteels R: ATP-induced Ca^{2+} release and Cl^- current in cultured smooth muscle cells from pig aorta. *J Physiol (Lond)* 440:623–634, 1991.

70. Soejima M, Kokubun S: Single anion-selective channel and its ion selectivity in the vascular smooth muscle cell. *Pflügers Arch* 411:304–311, 1988.

71. Van Helden DF: An α-adrenoceptor-mediated chloride conductance in mesenteric veins of the guinea-pig. *J Physiol (Lond)* 401:489–501, 1988.

72. van Breemen C: Ca^{2+} requirement for activation of intact aortic smooth muscle. *J Physiol (Lond)* 272:317–329, 1977.

73. Casteels R, Droogmans G: Exchange characteristics of the noradrenaline-sensitive calcium store in vascular smooth muscle cells of rabbit ear artery. *J Physiol (Lond)* 317:263–279, 1981.

74. Hoth M, Penner R: Depletion of intracellular calcium stores activates a calcium current in mast cells. *Nature* 355:353–356, 1992.

75. Ghosh TK, Mullaney JM, Tarazi FI, Gill DL: GTP-activated communication between distinct inositol 1,4,5-trisphosphate-sensitive and -insensitive calcium pools. *Nature* 340:236–239, 1989.

76. Putney JW Jr: A model for receptor-regulated Ca^{2+} entry. *Cell Calcium* 7:1–12, 1986.

77. Takemura H, Hughes AR, Thastrup O, Putney JW Jr: Activation of calcium entry by tumor promotor thapsigargin in parotid acinar cells. Evidence that an intracellular calcium pool, and not an inositol phosphate, regulates calcium fluxes at the plasma membrane. *J Biol Chem* 264:12266–12271, 1989.

78. Vostal JG, Jackson WL, Shulman NR: Cytosolic and stored calcium antagonistically control tyrosine phosphorylation of specific platelet proteins. *J Biol Chem* 266:16911–16916, 1991.

79. Alvarez J, Montero M, Garcia-Sancho J: Cytochrome P-450 may link intracellular Ca^{2+} stores with plasma membrane Ca^{2+} influx. *Biochem J* 274:193–197, 1991.

80. Alvarez J, Montero M, Garcia-Sancho J: Cytochrome P450 may regulate plasma membrane Ca^{2+} permeability according to the filling state of the intracellular Ca^{2+} stores. *FASEB J* 6:786–792, 1992.

81. Pandol SJ, Schoeffield-Payne MS: Cyclic GMP mediates the agonist-stimulated increase in plasma-membrane calcium entry in the pancreatic acinar cell. *J Biol Chem* 265:12846–12853, 1990.

82. Irvine RF: "Quantal" Ca^{2+} release and the control of Ca^{2+} entry by inositol phosphates — a possible mechanism. *FEBS Lett* 263:5–9, 1990.

83. Missiaen L, Taylor CW, Berridge MJ: Spontaneous calcium release from inositol trisphosphate-sensitive calcium stores. *Nature* 352:241–244, 1991.

84. Missiaen L, Taylor CW, Berridge MJ: Luminal Ca^{2+} promoting spontaneous Ca^{2+} release from inositol trisphosphate-sensitive stores in rat hepatocytes. *J Physiol (Lond)* 455:623–640, 1992.

85. Nunn DL, Taylor CW: Luminal Ca^{2+} increases the sensitivity of Ca^{2+} stores to inositol 1,4,5-trisphosphate. *Mol Pharmacol* 41:115–119, 1992.

86. Lückhoff A, Clapham DE: Inositol 1,3,4,5-tetrakisphosphate activates an endothelial Ca^{2+}-permeable channel. *Nature* 355:356–358, 1992.

87. Putney JW Jr: Capacitative Ca^{2+} entry revisited. *Cell Calcium* 11:611–624, 1990.

88. Irvine RF: Inositol tetrakisphosphate as a second messenger: confusions, contradictions, and a potential resolution. *BioEssays* 13:419–427, 1991.

89. Devine CE, Somlyo AV, Somlyo AP: Sarcoplasmic reticulum and excitation-contraction coupling in mammalian smooth muscles. *J Cell Biol* 52:690–718, 1972.

90. van Breemen C, Saida K: Cellular mechanisms regulating $[Ca^{2+}]_i$ smooth muscle. *Ann Rev Physiol* 51:315–329, 1989.

91. Stehno-Bittel L, Sturek M: Spontaneous sarcoplasmic reticulum calcium release and extrusion from bovine, not porcine, coronary artery smooth muscle. *J Physiol (Lond)* 451:49–78, 1992.

92. Casteels R, Droogmans G, Missiaen L: Agonist-induced entry of Ca^{2+} in smooth muscle cells. *Neurochem Int* 17:297–302, 1990.

93. Missiaen L, Declerck I, Droogmans G, Plessers L, De Smedt H, Raeymaekers L, Casteels R: Agonist-dependent Ca^{2+} and Mn^{2+} entry dependent on state of filling of Ca^{2+} stores in aortic smooth muscle cells of the rat. *J Physiol (Lond)* 427:171–186, 1990.

94. Missiaen L, Wuytack F, De Smedt H, Vrolix M, Casteels R: AlF_4^- reversibly inhibits "P"-type cation-transport ATPases, possibly by interacting with the phosphate-binding site of the ATPase. *Biochem J* 253:827–833, 1988.

95. Missiaen L, Wuytack F, De Smedt H, Amant F, Casteels R: AlF_4^--induced inhibition of the ATPase activity, the Ca^{2+}-transport activity and the phosphoprotein-intermediate formation of plasma-membrane and endo(sarco)plasmic-reticulum Ca^{2+}-transport ATPases in different tissues. Evidence for a tissue-dependent functional difference. *Biochem J* 261:655–660, 1989.

96. Missiaen L, Kanmura Y, Wuytack F, Raeymaekers L, Declerck I, Droogmans G, Casteels R: AlF_4^- inhibits the accumulation of Ca in the endoplasmic reticulum in intact myometrial strips, but not in the rabbit ear artery. *Pflügers Arch* 414:423–429, 1989.

97. Himpens B, Missiaen L, Droogmans G, Casteels R: AlF_4^- induces Ca^{2+} oscillations in guinea-pig ileal smooth muscle. *Pflügers Arch* 417:645–650, 1991.

98. Low AM, Kwan CY, Daniel EE: Evidence for two types of internal Ca^{2+} stores in canine mesenteric artery with different refilling mechanisms. *Am J Physiol* 262:H31–H37, 1992.

99. Ghosh TK, Bian J, Short AD, Rybak SL, Gill DL: Persistent intracellular calcium pool depletion by thapsigargin and its influence on cell growth. *J Biol Chem* 266:24690–24697, 1991.

100. Baro I, Eisner DA: The effects of thapsigargin on $[Ca^{2+}]_i$ in

isolated rat mesenteric artery vascular smooth muscle cells. *Pflügers Arch* 420:115–117, 1992.

101. Xuan Y-T, Wang O-L, Whorton AR: Thapsigargin stimulates Ca^{2+} entry in vascular smooth muscle cells: Nicardipine-sensitive and -insensitive pathways. *Am J Physiol* 262:C1258–C1265, 1992.

102. Verboomen H, Wuytack F, De Smedt H, Himpens B, Casteels R: Functional difference between SERCA2a and SERCA2b Ca^{2+} pumps and their modulation by phospholamban. *Biochem J* 286:591–596, 1992.

103. Low AM, Gaspar V, Kwan CY, Darby PJ, Bourreau JP, Daniel E: Thapsigargin inhibits repletion of phenylephrine-sensitive intracellular Ca^{2+} pool in vascular smooth muscles. *J Pharm Exp Ther* 258:1105–1113, 1991.

104. Bourreau JP, Abela AP, Kwan CY, Daniel EE: Acetylcholine Ca^{2+} stores refilling directly involves a dihydropyridine-sensitive channel in dog trachea. *Am J Physiol* 261: C497–C505, 1991.

105. Chen Q, Cannell M, van Breemen C: The superficial buffer barrier in vascular smooth muscle. *Can J Physiol Pharmacol* 70:509–514, 1992.

106. Somlyo AP, Himpens B: Cell calcium and its regulation in smooth muscle. *FASEB J* 3:2266–2276, 1989.

107. Somlyo AP, Somlyo AV, Shuman H: Electron probe analysis of vascular smooth muscle: Composition of mitochondria, nuclei and cytoplasm. *J Cell Biol* 81:316–344, 1979.

108. Bond M, Shuman H, Somlyo AP, Smolyo AV: Total cytoplasmic calcium in relaxed and maximally contracted rabbit portal vein smooth muscle. *J Physiol (Lond)* 357:185–201, 1984.

109. Somlyo AP: Excitation-contraction coupling and the ultrastructure of smooth muscle. *Circ Res* 57:497–508, 1985.

110. Bond M, Kitazawa T, Somlyo AV, Somlyo AP: Release and recycling of calcium by the sarcoplasmic reticulum in guinea-pig portal vein smooth muscle. *J Physiol (Lond)* 355: 677–695, 1984.

111. Iino M: Calcium release mechanisms in smooth muscle. *Jpn J Pharmacol* 54:345–354, 1990.

112. Berridge MJ, Irvine RF: Inositol phosphates and cell signalling. *Nature* 341:197–205, 1989.

113. Kobayashi S, Kitazawa T, Somlyo AV, Somlyo AP: Cytosolic heparin inhibits muscarinic and α-adrenergic Ca^{2+} release in smooth muscle. Physiological role of inositol 1,4,5-trisphosphate in pharmacomechanical coupling. *J Biol Chem* 264:17997–18004, 1989.

114. Walker JW, Somlyo AV, Goldman YE, Somlyo AP, Trentham DR: Kinetics of smooth muscle and skeletal muscle activation by laser pulse photolysis of caged inositol-1,4,5-trisphosphate. *Nature* 327:249–252, 1987.

115. Chadwick CC, Saito A, Fleischer S: Isolation and characterization of the inositol trisphosphate receptor from smooth muscle. *Proc Natl Acad Sci USA* 87:2132–2136, 1990.

116. Mourey RJ, Verma A, Supattapone S, Snyder SH: Purification and characterization of the inositol 1,4,5-trisphosphate receptor protein from rat vas deferens. *Biochem J* 272:383–389, 1990.

117. Mayrleitner M, Chadwick CC, Timmerman AP, Fleischer S, Schindler H: Purified IP_3 receptor from smooth muscle forms an IP_3 gated and heparin sensitive Ca^{2+} channel in planar bilayers. *Cell Calcium* 12:505–514, 1991.

118. Danoff SK, Ferris CD, Donath C, Fischer GA, Munemitsu S, Ullrich A, Snyder SH, Ross CA: Inositol 1,4,5-trisphosphate receptors: Distinct neuronal and non-neuronal forms derived by alternative splicing differ in phosphorylation. *Proc Natl Acad Sci USA* 88:2951–2955, 1991.

119. Nakagawa T, Okano H, Furuichi T, Aruga J, Mikoshiba K: The subtypes of the mouse inositol 1,4,5-trisphosphate receptor are expressed in a tissue-specific and developmentally specific manner. *Proc Natl Acad Sci USA* 88:6244–6248, 1991.

120. Südhof TC, Newton CL, Archer BT III, Ushkaryov YA, Mignery GA: Structure of a novel $InsP_3$ receptor. *EMBO J* 10:3199–3206, 1991.

121. Ross CA, Danoff SK, Schell MJ, Snyder SH, Ullrich A: Three additional inositol 1,4,5-trisphosphate receptors: Molecular cloning and differential localization in brain and peripheral tissues. *Proc Natl Acad Sci USA* 89:4265–4269, 1992.

122. Parys JB, Sernett SW, Delisle S, Snyder PM, Welsh MJ, Campbell KP: Isolation, characterization and localization of the inositol 1,4,5-trisphosphate receptor protein in *Xenopus laevis* oocytes. *J Biol Chem* 267:18776–18782, 1992.

123. Champeil P, Combettes L, Berthon B, Doucet E, Orlowski S, Claret M: Fast kinetics of calcium release induced by *myo*-inositol trisphosphate in permeabilized rat hepatocytes. *J Biol Chem* 264:17665–17673, 1989.

124. Meyer T, Stryer L: Transient calcium release induced by successive increments of inositol 1,4,5-trisphosphate. *Proc Natl Acad Sci USA* 87:3841–3845, 1990.

125. Ferris CD, Cameron AM, Huganir RL, Snyder SH: Quantal calcium release by purified reconstituted inositol 1,4,5-trisphosphate receptors. *Nature* 356:350–352, 1992.

126. Somlyo AV, Horiuti K, Trentham DR, Kitazawa T, Somlyo AP: Kinetics of Ca^{2+} release and contraction induced by photolysis of caged D-*myo*-inositol 1,4,5-trisphosphate in smooth muscle. The effects of heparin, procaine and adenine nucleotides. *J Biol Chem* 267:22316–22322, 1992.

127. Missiaen L, De Smedt H, Droogmans G, Casteels R: Ca^{2+} release induced by inositol 1,4,5-trisphosphate is a steady-state phenomenon controlled by luminal Ca^{2+} in permeabilized cells. *Nature* 357:599–602, 1992.

128. Satoh T, Ross CA, Villa A, Supattapone S, Pozzan T, Snyder SH, Meldolesi J: The inositol 1,4,5-trisphosphate receptor in cerebellar Purkinje cells: Quantitative immunogold labelling reveals concentration in an ER subcompartment. *J Cell Biol* 111:615–624, 1990.

129. Menniti FS, Bird G St J, Takemura H, Thastrup O, Potter BVL, Putney JW Jr: Mobilization of calcium by inositol trisphosphates from permeabilized rat parotid acinar cells. Evidence for translocation of calcium from uptake to release sites within the inositol 1,4,5-trisphosphate- and thapsigargin-sensitive calcium pool. *J Biol Chem* 266:13646–13653, 1991.

130. Iino M: Biphasic Ca^{2+} dependence of inositol 1,4,5-trisphosphate-induced Ca release in smooth muscle cells of the guinea pig taenia caeci. *J Gen Physiol* 95:1103–1122, 1990.

131. Iino M, Endo M: Calcium-dependent immediate feedback control of inositol 1,4,5-trisphosphate-induced Ca^{2+} release. *Nature* 360:76–78, 1992.

132. Bezprozvanny I, Watras J, Ehrlich BE: Bell-shaped calcium-response curves of $Ins(1,4,5)P_3$- and calcium-gated channels from endoplasmic reticulum of cerebellum. *Nature* 351: 751–754, 1991.

133. Finch EA, Turner TJ, Goldin SM: Calcium as a coagonist of inositol 1,4,5-trisphosphate-induced calcium release. *Science* 252:443–446, 1991.

134. Missiaen L, De Smedt H, Droogmans G, Casteels R: Luminal Ca^{2+} controls the activation of the $Ins(1,4,5)P_3$ receptor by cytosolic Ca^{2+}. *J Biol Chem* 267:22961–22966, 1992.

135. Mignery GA, Südhof TC: The ligand binding site and transduction mechanism in the inositol-1,4,5-trisphosphate receptor. *EMBO J* 9:3893–3898, 1990.

136. Mignery GA, Johnston PA, Südhof TC: Mechanism of Ca^{2+} inhibition of inositol 1,4,5-trisphosphate ($InsP_3$) binding to

the cerebellar InsP$_3$ receptor. *J Biol Chem* 267:7450–7455, 1992.

137. Suematsu E, Hirata M, Hashimoto T, Kuriyama H: Inositol 1,4,5-trisphosphate releases Ca^{2+} from intracellular store sites in skinned single cells of porcine coronary artery. *Biochem Biophys Res Commun* 120:481–485, 1984.

138. Williams DA, Becker PL, Fay FS: Regional changes in calcium underlying contraction of single smooth muscle cells. *Science* 235:1644–1648, 1987.

139. Ikemoto N, Ronjat M, Meszaros LG, Koshita M: Postulated role of calsequestrin in the regulation of calcium release from sarcoplasmic reticulum. *Biochemistry* 28:6764–6771, 1989.

140. Muallem S, Pandol SJ, Beeker TG: Hormone-evoked calcium release from intracellular stores is a quantal process. *J Biol Chem* 264:205–212, 1989.

141. Taylor CW, Potter BVL: The size of inositol 1,4,5-trisphosphate-sensitive Ca^{2+} stores depends on inositol, 1,4,5-trisphosphate concentration. *Biochem J* 266:189–194, 1990.

142. Oldershaw KA, Nunn DL, Taylor CW: Quantal Ca^{2+} mobilization stimulated by inositol 1,4,5-trisphosphate in permeabilized hepatocytes. *Biochem J* 278:705–708, 1991.

143. Tregear R, Dawson AP, Irvine RF: Quantal release of Ca^{2+} from intracellular stores by InsP$_3$: Tests of the concept of control of Ca^{2+} release by intraluminal Ca^{2+}. *Proc R Soc Lond B* 243:263–268, 1991.

144. Smith T, Smith L, Higgins B: Temperature and nucleotide dependence of calcium release by *myo*-inositol 1,4,5-trisphosphate in cultured vascular smooth-muscle cells. *J Biol Chem* 260:14413–14416, 1985.

145. Iino M: Calcium-dependent inositol trisphosphate-induced calcium release in the guinea-pig taenia caeci. *Biochem Biophys Res Commun* 142:47–52, 1987.

146. Ehrlich BE, Watras J: Inositol 1,4,5-trisphosphate activates a channel from smooth muscle sarcoplasmic reticulum. *Nature* 336:583–586, 1988.

147. Iino M: Effect of adenine nucleotides on inositol 1,4,5-trisphosphate-induced calcium release in vascular smooth muscle cells. *J Gen Physiol* 98:681–698, 1991.

148. Guillemette G, Balla T, Baukal AJ, Catt KJ: Inositol 1,4,5-trisphosphate binds to a specific receptor and releases microsomal calcium in the anterior pituitary gland. *Proc Natl Acad Sci USA* 84:8195–8199, 1987.

149. Maeda N, Kawasaki T, Nakade S, Yokota N, Taguchi T, Kasai M, Mikoshiba K: Structural and functional characterization of inositol 1,4,5-trisphosphate receptor channel from mouse cerebellum. *J Biol Chem* 266:1109–1116, 1991.

150. Ferris CD, Huganir RL, Snyder SH: Calcium flux mediated by purified inositol 1,4,5-trisphosphate receptor in reconstituted lipid vesicles is allosterically regulated by adenine nucleotides. *Proc Natl Acad Sci USA* 87:2147–2151, 1990.

151. Kushmerick MJ, Dillon PF, Meyer RA, Brown TR, Krisanda JM, Sweeney HL: ^{31}P NMR spectroscopy, chemical analysis, and free Mg^{2+} of rabbit bladder and uterine smooth muscle. *J Biol Chem* 261:14420–14429, 1986.

152. Ferris CD, Huganir RL, Supattapone S, Snyder SH: Purified inositol 1,4,5-trisphosphate receptor mediates calcium flux in reconstituted lipid vesicles. *Nature* 342:87–89, 1989.

153. Saida K, van Breemen C: GTP requirement for inositol-1,4,5-trisphosphate induced Ca^{2+} release from sarcoplasmic reticulum in smooth muscle. *Biochem Biophys Res Commun* 144:1313–1316, 1987.

154. Saida K, Twort C, van Breemen C: The specific GTP requirement for inositol 1,4,5-trisphosphate-induced Ca^{2+} release from skinned vascular smooth muscle. *J Cardiovasc Pharmac* 12(Suppl 5):47–50, 1988.

155. Neylon CB, Nickashin A, Little PJ, Tkachuk VA, Bobik A: Thrombin-induced Ca^{2+} mobilization in vascular smooth muscle utilizes a slowly ribosylating pertussin toxin-sensitive G protein. Evidence for the involvement of a G protein in inositol trisphosphate-dependent Ca^{2+} release. *J Biol Chem* 267:7295–7302, 1992.

156. Hecker M, Brune B, Decker K, Ullrich V: The sulphydryl reagent thimerosal elicits human platelet aggregation by mobilization of intracellular calcium and secondary prostaglandin endoperoxide formation. *Bioch Biophys Res Commun* 159:961–968, 1989.

157. Hatzelmann A, Haurand M, Ullrich V: Involvement of calcium in the thimerosal-stimulated formation of leukotriene by fMLP in human polymorphonuclear leucocytes. *Bioch Pharmacol* 39:559–567, 1990.

158. Swann K: Thimerosal causes calcium oscillations and sensitizes calcium-induced calcium release in unfertilized hamster eggs. *FEBS Lett* 278:175–178, 1991.

159. Swann K: Different triggers for calcium oscillations in mouse eggs involve a ryanodine-sensitive calcium store. *Biochem J* 287:79–84, 1992.

160. Carroll J, Swann K: Spontaneous cytosolic calcium oscillations driven by inositol trisphosphate occur during *in vitro* maturation of mouse oocytes. *J Biol Chem* 267:11196–11201, 1992.

161. Miyazaki S-I, Shirakawa H, Nakada K, Honda Y, Yuzaki M, Nakade S, Mikoshiba K: Antibody to the inositol trisphosphate receptor blocks thimerosal-enhanced Ca^{2+}-induced Ca^{2+} release and Ca^{2+} oscillations in hamster eggs. *FEBS Lett* 309:180–184, 1992.

162. Bootman MD, Taylor CW, Berridge MJ: The thiol reagent, thimerosal, evokes Ca^{2+} spikes in HeLa cells by sensitizing the inositol 1,4,5-trisphosphate receptor. *J Biol Chem*, 267:25113–25119, 1992.

163. Gericke M, Droogmans G, Nilius B: Thimerosal induced changes of intracellular calcium in human endothelial cells. *Cell Calcium*, 14:201–207, 1993.

164. Thorn P, Brady P, Llopis J, Gallacher DV, Petersen OH: Cytosolic Ca^{2+} spikes evoked by the thiol reagent thimerosal in both intact and internally perfused single pancreatic acinar cells. *Pflügers Arch* 422:173–178, 1992.

165. Parys JB, Missiaen L, De Smedt H, Droogmans G, Casteels R: Bellshaped activation of unositol-1,4,5-trisphosphate-induced Ca^{2+} release by thimerosal in permeabilized A7r5 smooth-muscle cells. *Pflügers Arch* 424:516–522, 1993.

166. Iino M: Calcium-induced calcium release mechanism in guinea pig taenia caeci. *J Gen Physiol* 94:363–383, 1989.

167. Herrmann-Frank A, Darling E, Meissner G: Functional characterization of the Ca^{2+}-gated Ca^{2+} release channel of vascular smooth muscle sarcoplasmic reticulum. *Pflügers Arch* 418:353–359, 1991.

168. Lai FA, Erickson HP, Rousseau E, Liu Q-Y, Meissner G: Purification and reconstitution of the calcium release channel from skeletal muscle. *Nature* 331:315–319, 1988.

169. Hwang KS, van Breemen C: Ryanodine modulation of ^{45}Ca efflux and tension in rabbit aortic smooth muscle. *Pflügers Arch* 408:343–350, 1987.

170. Hisayama T, Takayanagi I: Ryanodine: Its possible mechanism of action in the caffeine-sensitive calcium store of smooth muscle. *Pflüger Arch* 412:376–381, 1988.

171. Kanmura Y, Missiaen L, Raeymaekers L, Casteels R: Ryanodine reduces the amount of calcium in intracellular stores of smooth-muscle cells of the rabbit ear artery. *Pflügers Arch* 413:153–159, 1988.

172. Bolton TB, Lim SP: Properties of calcium stores and transient outward currents in single smooth muscle cells of rabbit intestine. *J Physiol (Lond)* 409:385–401, 1989.

173. Ashoori F, Takai A, Tomita T: The response of non-

pregnant rat myometrium to oxytocin in Ca-free solution. *Br J Pharmacol* 84:175–183, 1985.

174. Kanmura Y, Missiaen L, Casteels R: Properties of intracellular calcium stores in pregnant rat myometrium. *Br J Pharmacol* 95:284–290, 1988.

175. Savineau JP: Caffeine does not contract skinned uterine fibers with a functional Ca store. *Eur J Pharmacol* 149:187–190, 1988.

176. Masuo M, Toyo-oka T, Shin WS, Sugimoto T: Growth-dependent alterations of intracellular Ca^{2+}-handling mechanisms of vascular smooth muscle cells. *Circ Res* 69:1327–1339, 1991.

177. Giannini G, Clementi E, Ceci R, Marziali G, Sorrentino V: Expression of a ryanodine receptor-Ca^{2+} channel that is regulated by TGF-β. *Science* 257:91–94, 1992.

178. Hakamata Y, Nakai J, Takeshima H, Imoto K: Primary structure and distribution of a novel ryanodine receptor/calcium release channel from rabbit brain. *FEBS Lett* 312:229–235, 1992.

179. Saida K, van Breemen C: A possible Ca^{2+}-induced Ca^{2+} release mechanism mediated by norepinephrine in vascular smooth muscle. *Pflügers Arch* 397:166–167, 1983.

180. Ito K, Ikemoto T, Takakura S: Involvement of Ca^{2+} influx-induced Ca^{2+} release in contractions of intact vascular smooth muscles. *Am J Physiol* 261:H1464–H1470, 1991.

181. Stern MD: Buffering of calcium in the vicinity of a channel pore. *Cell Calcium* 13:183–192, 1992.

182. Berridge MJ, Galione A: Cytosolic calcium oscillators. *FASEB J* 2:3074–3082, 1988.

183. Benham CD, Bolton TB: Spontaneous transient outward currents in single visceral and vascular smooth muscle cells of the rabbit. *J Physiol (Lond)* 381:385–406, 1986.

184. Weissberg PL, Little PJ, Bobik A: Spontaneous oscillations in cytoplasmic calcium concentration in vascular smooth muscle. *Am J Physiol* 256:C951–C957, 1989.

185. Johnson EM, Theler J-M, Capponi AM, Vallotton MB: Characterization of oscillations in cytosolic free Ca^{2+} concentration and measurement of cytosolic Na^+ concentration

changes evoked by angiotensin II and vasopressin in individual rat aortic smooth muscle cells. Use of microfluorometry and digital imaging. *J Biol Chem* 266:12618–12626, 1991.

186. Wang Q, Hogg RC, Large WA: Properties of spontaneous inward currents recorded in smooth muscle cells isolated from the rabbit portal vein. *J Physiol (Lond)* 451:525–537, 1992.

187. Sims SM, Vivaudou MB, Hillemeier C, Biancani P, Walsh JV Jr, Singer JJ: Membrane currents and cholinergic regulation of K^+ current in esophageal smooth muscle of the dog trachea. *Am J Physiol* 258:G794–G802, 1990.

188. Janssen LJ, Sims SM: Acetylcholine activates non-selective cation and chloride conductances in canine and guinea-pig tracheal myocytes. *J Physiol (Lond)* 453:197–218, 1992.

189. Berridge MJ: Calcium oscillations. *J Biol Chem* 265:9583–9586, 1990.

190. Parker I, Ivorra I: Caffeine inhibits inositol trisphosphate-mediated liberation of intracellular calcium in *Xenopus* oocytes. *J Physiol (Lond)* 433:229–240, 1991.

191. Brown GR, Sayers LG, Kirk CJ, Michell RH, Michelangeli F: The opening of the inositol 1,4,5-trisphosphate-sensitive Ca^{2+} channel in rat cerebellum is inhibited by caffeine. *Biochem J* 282:309–312, 1992.

192. Wier WG, Blatter LA: Ca^{2+}-oscillations and Ca^{2+}-waves in mammalian cardiac and vascular smooth muscle cells. *Cell Calcium* 12:241–254, 1991.

193. Mayer EA, Kodner A, Sun XP, Wilkes J, Scott D, Sachs G: Spatial and temporal patterns of intracellular calcium in colonic smooth muscle. *J Memb Biol* 125, 107–118, 1992.

194. Blatter LA, Wier WG: Agonist-induced $[Ca^{2+}]_i$ waves and Ca^{2+}-induced Ca^{2+} release in mammalian vascular smooth muscle cells. *Am J Physiol* 263:H576–H586, 1992.

195. Meyer T: Cell signaling by second messenger waves. *Cell* 64:675–678, 1991.

196. Kargacin G, Fay FS: Ca^{2+} movement in smooth muscle cells studied with one- and two-dimensional diffusion models. *Biophys J* 60:1088–1100, 1991.

CHAPTER 47

Regulation of Calcium and Chloride Channels in Vascular Smooth Muscle Cells by Norepinephrine

JEAN G. MIRONNEAU

INTRODUCTION

Agonists such as norepinephrine (NE) or angiotensin II increase cytoplasmic Ca^{2+} concentration in vascular smooth muscle through several mechanisms, including (a) stimulation of Ca^{2+} influx through receptor-operated channels; (b) activation of voltage-dependent Ca^{2+} channels, opened in response to membrane depolarization evoked by increases in membrane conductances for various ions; and (c) release of Ca^{2+} from intracellular store sites [1–3].

In strips of rat portal vein, low concentrations of NE (10^{-7}M) augmented the frequency and amplitude of spontaneous contractions with a small increase in the basal tone. Higher concentrations of NE (10^{-6}M or more) also induced an oscillatory response, in which oscillations of augmented frequency, but of smaller amplitude, were superimposed on a large tone variation. In contrast, vascular smooth muscles having no spontaneous activity (i.e., vena cava) responded to NE application by a sustained tone. These observations suggest that the membrane mechanisms involved in NE stimulation could be dependent on the ion channel types, transduction pathways, and adrenoceptors subtypes that are present in a given vascular tissue.

ION CHANNELS RESPONSIBLE FOR DEPOLARIZATION

It is well known that most agonists depolarize the smooth muscle membrane, modulate action potentials and slow waves in their frequency and pattern. Two different mechanisms, Cl^- channels and nonspecific cation channels, have been proposed to account for agonist-induced depolarization. Although these mechanisms appear to be nonadditive, they may coexist in different structures. As will be described later, activation of Cl^- channels is sufficient to support NE-induced depolarization in portal vein smooth muscle.

Direct evidence that NE activated a depolarizing current was obtained with the patch-clamp technique by microejecting 10 μM NE on single cells held at −70 mV. A similar response was obtained with phenylephrine, but not with clonidine. With depolarizations, the NA-evoked current decreased in amplitude, was null near 0 mV, and reversed at positive membrane potentials (fig. 47-1A). The NE-activated current was selectively blocked by prazosin (1 μM) and phentolamine (1 μM), whereas it remained unaffected in the presence of yohimbine (1 μM) and propranolol (10 μM). In this experiment, the external Cl^- concentration ($[Cl]_o$) was 146 mM and the internal Cl^- concentration ($[Cl]_i$) was 130 mM, so that the equilibrium potential for Cl^- ions was estimated to be −3 mM. In addition, CsCl was used instead of KCl in both external and internal solutions in order to block K^+ currents [4].

The current/voltage relationship obtained by plotting the peak current induced by NE against membrane potential was linear, and the reversal potential was obtained at 0 mV, close to the calculated E_{Cl}.

In order to confirm the chloride nature of the NE-induced current, the reversal potential was determined with various Cl^- concentrations in the bath and pipette solutions. The mean potentials obtained in four different Cl^- solutions were plotted on the ordinate against the calculated equilibrium potential for Cl^- ions (E_{Cl}) on the abscissa (fig. 47-1B). The experimental points are closely distributed along a straight line with a slope of 1.0, as expected for a pure Cl^- current. The absence of any change in the reversal potential by replacing internal Cs^+ with Na^+ ions suggests that it is unlikely that NE opens a cation channel in smooth muscle cells of rat portal vein.

It has to be noted that, in vascular smooth muscle $[Cl]_i$ is estimated to be about 60 mM, so that the reversal potential for the Cl^- current is around −20 mV. Therefore, depolarizing Cl^- current can be activated by NE at the resting membrane potential (−60 mV).

The role of Ca^{2+} ions in activating Cl^- channel was examined first by comparing the NE-induced response in the presence of Ba^{2+} and Ca^{2+} ions. No responses were observed when the cells were perfused for at least 20 minutes in 5 mM Ba^{2+} solution. After replacement of Ba^{2+} with Ca^{2+}, inward currents were evoked within 5 minutes by NE applications. Similarly, when the pipette solution contained 10 mM EGTA in order to reduce $[Ca]_i$ into the nanomolar concentration range, the responses to NE were never observed, even in the presence of 5 mM $[Ca]_o$. In contrast, the NE-induced current was not affected

N. Sperelakis (ed.), *Physiology and Pathophysiology of the Heart, Third Edition.*

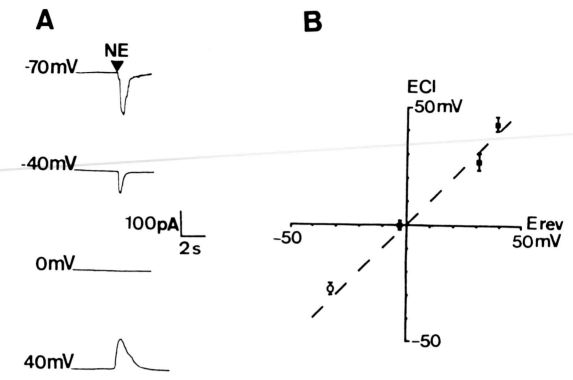

Fig. 47-1. Cl⁻ currents in response to norepinephrine (NE, 10 µM) in isolated cells of rat portal vein. **A:** Membrane currents to ejections of NE (▼) at different holding potentials (noted near the current traces). The external Cl⁻ concentration was 146 mM and the pipette concentration was 130 mM. **B:** Reversal potential (E_{rev}) of the NE-induced current as a function of the equilibrium potential (E_{Cl}), for reference Cl⁻ (146 mM:130 mM) gradient (●), low external Cl⁻ (■), and low pipette Cl⁻ concentrations (○). The dashed line predicts the reversal potential for pure Cl⁻ conductance. Each point represents the mean of 3–15 cells, with SEM shown by vertical lines. CsCl was used instead of KCl in both external and pipette solutions. NE (▼) was ejected for 100–500 ms at a distance of about 100 µm from the cell. From Pacaud et al. {4}, with permission.

in the presence of 3 mM Co²⁺ applied externally to block the voltage-dependent Ca²⁺ channels. Caffeine (10 mM) applied to the bathing solution also induced a transient increase in Cl⁻ current, as caffeine is known to release Ca²⁺ from the intracellular store. Interestingly, the NE-induced response was lost after caffeine application, as expected if the intracellular store was completely emptied. These results suggest that the Cl⁻ current is activated by a release of Ca²⁺ from the intracellular store in response to α₁-adrenoceptor activation.

Activation of Ca²⁺-dependent Cl⁻ current supports the NE-induced depolarization as E_{Cl} in physiological conditions is clearly different from the resting potential. In K⁺-containing solutions, but in the presence of 2.5 mM Co²⁺ to inhibit Ca²⁺ channels, applications of NE produced a large depolarization, reaching 30–40 mV when the cell was held initially at −60 mV (fig. 47-2A). At depolarized membrane potential (e.g., −45 mV), the NE-induced response was composed of an early hyperpolarization, corresponding to activation of Ca²⁺-dependent K⁺ channels, followed by a depolarization that reached the threshold for activation of voltage-dependent Ca²⁺

channels. The delay between NE application and the onset of Cl⁻ current was about 1–2 seconds. In cells showing spontaneous spikes, the first spike appeared 3–4 seconds after NE application, and the increase in spike amplitude was observed only after 5–10 seconds (fig. 47-2B). These observations indicate that activation of Cl⁻ channels clearly precedes stimulation of Ca²⁺ channels.

Cl⁻ channel blocking agents have been classified in different categories according to their binding kinetics {5}. Recently, a high-affinity ligand (IAA 94, a derivative of indanyloxyacetic acid) has been used in epithelia to purify different proteins corresponding to the Cl⁻ channels {6}. Compounds known as Cl⁻ channel blockers produced inhibitory effects on the Ca²⁺-activated Cl⁻ current in response to NE or caffeine. As illustrated in fig. 47-3, DIDS, DPC, and 9-AC produced a concentration-dependent inhibition of Cl⁻ current. The antagonist concentrations required to produce half-maximal inhibition were 16.5 µM DIDS, 117 µM 9-AC, and 300 µM DPC. The decreasing rank order of potency was, therefore, DIDS > 9-AC > DPC. In contrast, IAA and picrotoxin were ineffective on Ca²⁺-activated Cl⁻ current of portal vein myocytes. These

A

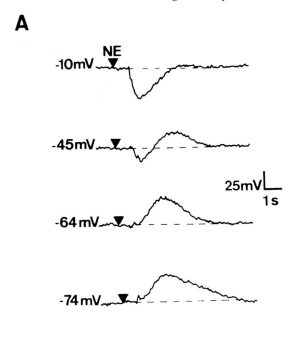

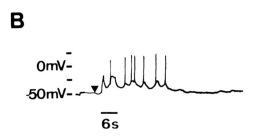

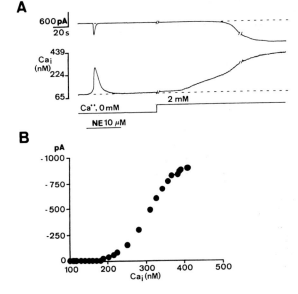

Fig. 47-3. Concentration-response curves for the effects of different compounds on Cl^- current activated by Ca^{2+} influx or internal Ca^{2+} release. DPC (■), 9-AC (●), and DIDS (△) were added for 9 minutes, and the effects were measured at steady state. Cl^- currents are expressed as a fraction of control current in the absence of inhibitory compounds. Modified from Baron et al. {7}, with permission.

B

Fig. 47-2. Membrane responses to NE (10 μM) in isolated cells of rat portal vein. **A:** Depolarization and hyperpolarization in response to ejections of NE (▼) recorded using current-clamp at different initial potentials in K^+-containing solution. **B:** Burst of action potentials superimposed on the NE-induced depolarization in K^+-containing solution. From Pacaud et al. {4}, with permission.

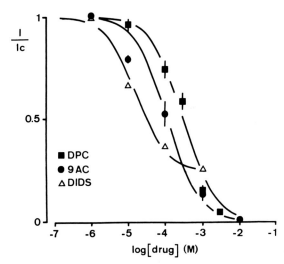

Fig. 47-4. Amplitude of the Ca^{2+}-activated Cl^- current as a function of $[Ca]_i$. Addition of external Ca^{2+} (lower trace) gradually increased $[Ca]_i$ (middle trace) and activated an inward current at a holding potential of -50 mV (top trace). Application of NE (10 μM) in Ca^{2+}-free solution induced a transient rise in $[Ca]_i$ by releasing intracellularly stored Ca^{2+}. This rise in $[Ca]_i$ activated a transient Cl^- current. This cell was pretreated for 30 minutes with 3 mM amytal and 5 μM CCCP to deplete the intracellular ATP pool. Broken lines represent the current level and the $[Ca]_i$ obtained at a holding potential of -50 mV in Ca^{2+}-free solution. From Pacaud et al. {8}, with permission.

observations suggest that different subtypes of Cl^- channels may be identified on the basis of their pharmacological properties {7}.

Sensitivity of Cl^- channels to $[Ca]_i$ was studied by combining the patch-clamp technique and microspectrofluorimetry (indo-1). In conditions in which the intracellular ATP concentration was greatly reduced by pretreatment with amytal and CCCP, the $[Ca]_i$ range for Cl^- current activation was between 180 and 500 nM, thus spanning a factor of threefold (fig. 47-4). Such a variation is steeper than that predicted by a simple binding isotherm and indicates that the Ca^{2+} regulation mechanism most probably involves simultaneous binding of several Ca^{2+} ions. Interestingly, the amplitude of the Cl^- current reached during the transient rise induced by NE through the action of inositol phosphates on Ca^{2+} stores was similar to that produced by a same level of $[Ca]_i$ in the absence of NE. This observation was true for all the $[Ca]_i$ values, including the threshold concentration, so that the dose-response curve was not shifted by NE. This suggests that the gating of Ca^{2+}-dependent Cl^- channels was mainly controlled by the $[Ca]_i$ level independently of the rate of increase in $[Ca]_i$ {8}. Moreover, the Cl^- current remained activated as long as the $[Ca]_i$ was above the threshold concentration, suggesting that the Cl^- channels had no intrinsic inactivation.

STIMULATION OF VOLTAGE-DEPENDENT Ca^{2+} CHANNELS BY NE

In portal vein smooth muscle, two types of Ca^{2+} channels have been separated {9,10}, which resemble the T-type and L-type Ca^{2+} channels described in other excitable cells. When the holding potential was held at $-70\,mV$, single-channel currents, typified by brief openings of about $-1\,pA$ in amplitude, were recorded in 90 mM Ba^{2+} solution. At more depolarized test potentials, a second type of channel activity was seen with long-lasting openings of $-1.5\,pA$ in amplitude. The slope conductances of the two channels types were 8 pS and 17 pS, respectively.

Single-channel current recordings provide the most direct approach for the identification of the NE-sensitive Ca^{2+} channel and for characterizing the modulatory effect. Ca^{2+} influx is proportional to $N_T.P_f.P_o.i$, where N_T is the total number of Ca^{2+} channels per cell, P_f is the probability that the channel is functional (i.e., that it responds to depolarization), P_o is the probability of a functional channel being open for a given time at a given membrane potential, and i is the amplitude of the single-channel current. Figure 47-5 shows records of large-conductance channel activity in the cell-attached mode at $+10\,mV$ (from a holding potential of $-70\,mV$) in the absence and presence of 10 µM NE (without a dihydropyridine agonist, Bay K 8644 in the bath solution). NE did not change single-channel current amplitude. By contrast, there was a marked change in the probability of the large-conductance Ca^{2+} channel being open. This is seen as an increase of P_f from 0.12 ± 0.03 (control) to 0.22 ± 0.04, and P_o from a mean value of 0.085 ± 0.004 (control) to 0.287 ± 0.011 in 10 µM NE. Similarly, NE increased the small-conductance Ca^{2+} channel activity recorded at $+10\,mV$ (from a holding potential of $-70\,mV$). The probability of the channel being open was enhanced by NE, which acted by increasing P_f from 0.25 ± 0.02 (control) to 0.44 ± 0.04, and P_o from a value of 0.026 ± 0.005 (control) to 0.044 ± 0.009 in 10 µM NE.

These increases in the probability of the Ca^{2+} channels being open induced by NE could result from a shift in the activation curve, as proposed in arterial smooth muscle {11}, or from an increase in the maximal open probability. In the absence of Bay K 8644, in cells where Ca^{2+} channel activity was recorded during depolarizing pulses, no evidence of Ca^{2+} channel activity was observed when the

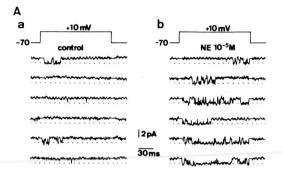

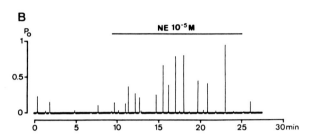

Fig. 47-5. Effect of NE on the large-conductance Ca^{2+} channel. **A:** Activity of the Ca^{2+} channel was recorded in the cell-attached configuration from a holding potential of $-70\,mV$ to $+10\,mV$, in the absence of Bay K 8644, before (a) and during bath application of 10 µM NE (b). Dashed lines indicate the mean single-channel current level obtained from amplitude histograms. **B:** Channel open probability for individual sweeps plotted against time. The open-state probability P_o was determined by dividing the time that the channel spends in the open state during a depolarization by the total time of the depolarization. Sweeps with no detectable openings were assigned a P_o value of zero. P_f corresponds to the ratio of the number of sweeps with at least one opening over the total number of sweeps in the ensemble. The NE effect is shown as an increase in P_o and P_f. From Pacaud et al. {12}, with permission.

membrane patch potential was held steady at -50 and $-30\,mV$ (without voltage steps) in the absence and presence of 10 µM NE {12}. Moreover, when 1 mM heparin was added to the pipette solution, upon applying NE (10 µM) both the rise in $[Ca]_i$ and the Ca^{2+}-activated Cl^- current were completely inhibited. Under these conditions, the amplitude of the Ca^{2+} current and the corresponding $[Ca]_i$ transient evoked by repetitive depolarizations were increased during NE applications. This result indicates that NE does not produce a detectable Ca^{2+} entry through voltage-dependent Ca^{2+} channels at a holding potential of $-50\,mV$.

The sequence of events induced by activation of α_1-adrenoceptors in rat portal vein can be summarized as follows: (a) NE releases intracellular Ca^{2+} stores through $InsP_3$ production; (b) the Ca^{2+} released opens Cl^- channels, thus producing inward current and membrane depolarization; (c) this depolarization produces Ca^{2+} entry through voltage-dependent Ca^{2+} channels; (d) the open probability of Ca^{2+} channels is enhanced by NE.

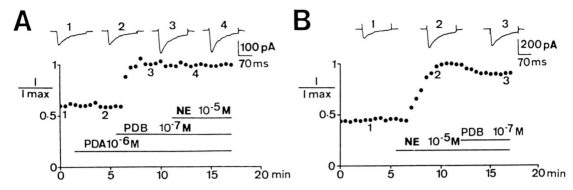

Fig. 47-6. Effect of externally applied phorbol esters and NE on Ca^{2+} channel currents evoked by depolarizations to 0 mV from a holding potential of −60 mV. **A:** Time course of the peak Ba^{2+} current during cumulative applications of phorbol 13,20-diacetate (PDA, 1 μM), phorbol 12,13-dibutyrate (PDB, 0.1 μM), and NE (10 μM). PDB induced a sustained increase in Ba^{2+} current, while PDA and NE were ineffective. **B:** Time course of the peak Ba^{2+} current during cumulative applications of NE and PDB. NE induced an increase in inward current, while PDB reduced the current by about 10–20%. Currents are expressed as a fraction of their maximal values. **Inset:** Current traces corresponding to numbers on the curves. External solution contained 5 mM Ba^{2+}. From Loirand et al. {14}, with permission.

ELECTROPHYSIOLOGICAL STUDY OF THE TRANSDUCTION MECHANISM

One of the most common transduction pathways between α_1-adrenoceptors and ion channels involves phosphatidylinositol hydrolysis by phospholipase C (PLC), leading to the generation of two second messengers: 1,4,5-inositol trisphosphate ($InsP_3$) and diacylglycerol (DAG) {13}. This transduction coupling has been explored by studying (a) the effects of substances that replicate the action of DAG on Ca^{2+} channels, for example, phorbol esters activating protein kinase C (PKC); (b) the effects of substances stimulating or inhibiting G-protein activity on both Cl^- channels and Ca^{2+} channels; (c) the nature of phospholipids that are hydrolyzed by PLC activity.

External application of 0.1 μM phorbol dibutyrate approximately doubled the Ca^{2+} channel current, but addition of 10 μM NE was ineffective (fig. 47-6A). Similarly, when the Ca^{2+} channel current was stimulated by a maximal dose of NE, phorbol dibutyrate was ineffective or produced a slight inhibition of current (fig. 47-6B). The latter effect is compatible with the existence of regulatory sites, which are presumably phosphorylated by PKC. These results support the idea that Ca^{2+} channels are stimulated by NE and phorbol ester through a transduction pathway that involves activation of PKC {14}.

Effects of guanine nucleotides were studied on the stimulatory effect of NE on Cl^- channels. With intracellular application of GDP-β S (1 mM), a stable analog of GDP, NE was unable to induce a noticeable Cl^- current. In contrast, GTP-γ S (1 mM), a stable analog of GTP, induced a transient and a sustained Cl^- current. Under these conditions, NE failed to enhance the Cl^- current, suggesting that the G protein was fully activated. Incubation of the cells in the presence of 10 μg/ml pertussis toxin for 6 hours had no effect on the NE-induced activation of Cl^- channels. Moreover, internal application of a monoclonal antibody raised against the C-terminal branch of the α_q subunit completely suppressed the stimulatory effect of NE, thus indicating that this G protein was of the G_q family (Leprêtre and Mironneau, unpublished data). Similar regulatory effects of guanine nucleotides were obtained on the NE-induced stimulation of Ca^{2+} channels.

In order to identify the membrane phospholipids that are hydrolyzed by PLC, autoantibodies directed against phosphatidylinositides have been used {15}. The NE-induced activation of Cl^- channels was dose dependently inhibited by increasing the concentration of antibodies from 0.0004 to 0.012 mg IgG/ml. Intracellular applications of either purified IgG from healthly patients or purified IgG from breast cancer serum (preincubated with a 1 nM solution of phosphatidylinositol) had no effect on the activation of Cl^- channels induced by NE (fig. 47-7). Therefore, inhibition of the NE-induced Cl^- current by these autoantibodies suggests that phosphatidylinositol is involved in the transduction process activated by occupancy of α_1-adrenoceptors.

PHARMACOLOGICAL STUDY OF THE TRANSDUCTION MECHANISM

It is established that specific binding sites for different Ca^{2+} channel antagonists are localized on the α_1 subunit of the Ca^{2+} channel protein {16,17}. The binding site for $(+)[^3H]$isradipine in intact strips of portal vein had a high affinity (about 0.1 nM) and was modulated by the membrane potential. Depolarization increased the affinity of dihydropyridine to the specific binding site, without alterations of the maximal binding capacity {18}. This property has been demonstrated in intact strips of several veins or in cell suspensions that are depolarized during preincubation in high K^+ solutions {19,20}. The binding site for $(−)[^3H]$desmethoxyverapamil (D888) in intact strips of rat portal vein had a high affinity (about 0.3 nM) and was modulated

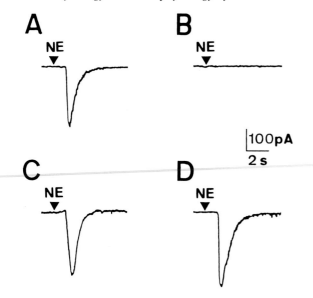

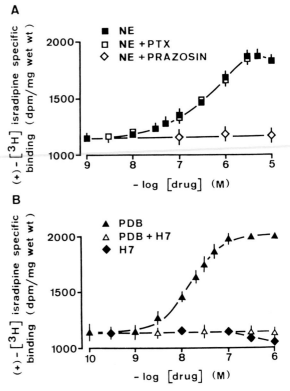

Fig. 47-7. Effect of auto-antiphosphatidylinositol antibodies on Ca^{2+}-activated Cl^- current in response to application of NE. Cl^- current was recorded at a holding potential of $-60\,mV$ and NE ($10\,\mu M$, ▼) was applied in control (**A**), in the presence of $0.012\,\mu g/ml$ IgG from breast cancer serum (**B**), and from healthy patients (**C**) in the pipette solution, and when $0.012\,mg/ml$ IgG from breast cancer serum preincubated with a $1\,nM$ solution of phosphatidylinositol (**D**) was added to the pipette solution. From Loirand et al. {15}, with permission.

by membrane potential. Both membrane depolarization and hyperpolarization produced a gradual decrease in D888 binding capacity. These observations support the idea that membrane potential variation changes the conformational state of Ca^{2+} channels in such a way that there is less access of D888 to the binding site {21}.

[^{3}H]isradipine binding sites

Isradipine-specific binding in intact venous strips was increased in a concentration-dependent manner by NE (fig. 47-8A). The maximal effect was obtained with $3-10\,\mu M$ NE and corresponded to an increase of about 80% of isradipine binding. A similar enhancement was produced by $1\,\mu M$ phorbol dibutyrate (fig. 47-8B). The stimulatory effect of NE was suppressed by incubation in the presence of $1\,\mu M$ prazosin, but remained unaffected after pretreatment with $10\,\mu g/ml$ pertussis toxin (PTX) for 6 hours. The effect of phorbol dibutyrate was prevented by the addition of PKC inhibitors ($1-10\,\mu M$ H7). There is evidence that modulation of isradipine binding may depend on a phosphorylation process. Using isolated membranes of portal vein, the phorbol dibutyrate-induced increase in isradipine binding was obtained only when the membranes were incubated in the presence of $10\,\mu M$ ATP and $5\,mM$ Mg^{2+} (fig. 47-9A). These results suggest that isradipine binding is modulated by a phosphorylation-dependent mechanism through activation of PKC.

Fig. 47-8. Effect of NE and phorbol esters on $(+)[^3H]$isradipine binding to intact strips of rat portal vein. **A:** Binding studies were performed with $0.15\,nM$ $(+)[^3H]$isradipine in the presence of increasing concentrations of NE (■), NE + $10\,\mu M$ prazosin (◇), and in strips pretreated with pertussis toxin ($10\,mg/ml$) for 6 hours (□). **B:** Isradipine binding in the presence of PDB (▲), H7 (◆), and PDB + $10\,\mu M$ H7 (△). The specific binding in the absence of drugs was $1150 \pm 50\,dpm/mg$ wet weight (n = 4). Nonspecific binding was not changed in the presence of the different compounds. Data shown are means $\pm$ SEM of 3–6 experiments. From Mironneau et al. {20}, with permission.

Equilibrium binding studies in the presence of $1\,\mu M$ phorbol dibutyrate or $10\,\mu M$ NE indicated that the linear pattern of the Scatchard plot was not affected, but the apparent K_D value was decreased from $0.14\,nM$ to $0.05\,nM$ (fig. 47-9B). Thus, the effects of $10\,\mu M$ NE were comparable to those produced by $135\,mM$ external KCl (membrane potential close to zero mV), indicating that they could not be due only to the depolarization produced by NE ($20-25\,mV$). When portal vein strips were incubated in the presence of cromakalim, the membrane potential was hyperpolarized by about $25-30\,mV$ {22}. Addition of $10\,\mu M$ NE in the presence of cromakalim depolarized the membrane potential close to resting value. Under these conditions, $10\,\mu M$ NE or a combination of $10\,\mu M$ $AlCl_3$ and $10\,mM$ NaF significantly decreased the apparent K_D value. Finally, to confirm that the effects of NE on isradipine binding involved activation of PKC, specific binding of $(+)[^3H]$isradipine was determined after treatment with PKC inhibitors. In the presence of $10\,\mu M$ H7,

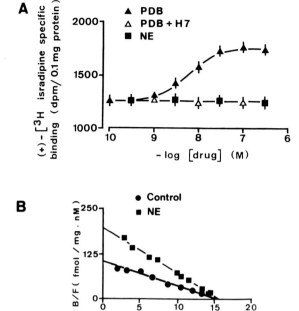

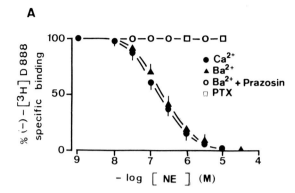

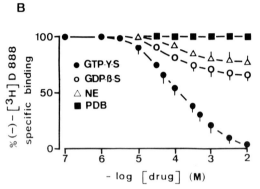

Fig. 47-9. Effect of phorbol esters and NE on $(+)[^3H]$isradipine binding to equine portal vein smooth muscle membranes. **A:** Binding studies were performed with 0.15 nM $(+)[^3H]$isradipine in the presence of increasing concentrations PDB (▲), NE (■), and PDB + 10 μM H7 (△). The incubation medium contained 10 μM ATP and 5 mM Mg^{2+}. The specific binding in the absence of drugs was 1250 ± 60 dpm/0.1 mg protein (n = 4). Data shown are means ± SEM of four experiments. **B:** Scatchard analysis of specific binding in control and in the presence of 10 μM NE, showing an increase in affinity without variations of the maximal binding capacity. Similar observations were obtained from five separate experiments. From Mironneau et al. {20}, with permission.

Fig. 47-10. Effect of NE and guanine nucleotides on $(-)[^3H]$D888 binding to intact strips of rat portal vein. **A:** Specific binding of $(-)$D888 (0.35 nM) in the presence of increasing concentrations of NE in solutions containing 2 mM Ca^{2+} (●), 2 mM Ba^{2+} (▲), and 2 mM Ba^{2+} + 1 μM prazosin (○), and in strips incubated in the presence of PTX (10 μg/ml) for 6 hours (□). **B:** Specific binding of $(-)$D888 in the presence of increasing concentrations of GTP-γ S (●), GDP-β S (○), NE (△), and PDB (■). Results are expressed as a percentage of specific binding obtained in the absence of substances and are means ± SEM of 4–8 experiments. From Rakotoarisoa et al. {24}, with permission.

the decrease in apparent K_D induced by NE was completely removed. These results differ from those obtained in rat aorta, which suggest that the increase in affinity of isradipine by NE in arterial smooth muscle would be only dependent on membrane depolarization {23}.

[^3H]Desmethoxyverapamil binding sites

In intact strips of portal vein, increasing concentrations of NE produced a concentration-dependent inhibition of desmethoxyverapamil (D888) specific binding (fig. 47-10A). The inhibitory effect of NE was completely suppressed in the presence of 1 μM prazosin, but also after preteatment with 10 μg/ml pertussis toxin for 6 hours. Interestingly, increasing concentrations of phorbol dibutyrate were ineffective on D888 specific binding. These results suggest the existence of a second transduction pathway involving a pertussis toxin-sensitive G protein {24}.

In isolated membranes, phorbol dibutyrate remained

without effect on $(-)[^3H]$D888 binding, even in the presence of 10 μM ATP and 5 mM Mg^{2+}. Activation of the G protein by GTP-γ S produced a concentration-dependent inhibition of D888 binding (fig. 47-10B). Equilibrium binding studies in the presence of 0.3 mM GTP-γ S indicated an increase of the K_D value and a decrease of the B_{max} value. As GTP-γ S accelerated the kinetics of the $(-)[^3H]$D888-receptor complex, this observation suggests that GTP-γ S might transform high-affinity D888 binding sites into low-affinity D888 sites and might account for the apparent decrease in B_{max} value.

Although contractile experiments have shown that removal of the pertussis toxin-sensitive transduction pathway increases D888 affinity for its binding sites, electrophysiological experiments are needed for definitive establishment of this second transduction process in vascular smooth muscle.

ADRENOCEPTOR SUBTYPES

Three different subtypes of α_1-adrenergic receptors have been defined on the basis of both binding and functional experiments, and molecular biological approach. The α_{1A} subtype has a high affinity for prazosin, WB4101, 5-methylurapidil, phentolamine, and (+)niguldipine, and is not activated by the alkylating agent, chloroethylchlonidine (CEC). The α_{1B} subtype shows a lower affinity for the competitive antagonists mentioned above and is potently inactivated by CEC {25–28}. Both α_{1A} and α_{1B} subtypes have similar high affinity for prazosin {29}. The bovine α_{1C} subtype is sensitive to CEC, albeit its high affinity for prazosin and WB4101 {28}. On the other hand, another subclassification is proposed, in which the α_1 adrenoceptors are separated into three subtypes (α_{1H}, α_{1L}, α_{1N}). Prazosin has a higher affinity for the α_{1H} subtype than for the α_{1L} and α_{1N} subtypes. In addition, the α_{1N} subtype has a higher affinity for HV723 than the other α_1 subtypes {30}.

According to these criteria, it has been shown that the α_1-adrenoceptor sites of rat portal vein smooth muscle correspond to α_{1H} and α_{1L} subtypes, as [³H]prazosin binds to two distinct populations of binding sites with high and low affinities. The fact that the high-affinity binding sites for prazosin were inactivated in a concentration-dependent manner by pretreatment with CEC in membrane preparations as well as in intact strips of rat portal vein suggests that the α_{1H} subtype may correspond to the α_{1B} subtype. The six α-adrenoceptor antagonists used (prazosin, HV723, WB4101, 5-methylurapidil, phentolamine, yohimbine) showed competitive inhibition of both high- and low-affinity binding sites for [³H]prazosin and, therefore, were not considered as useful probes for further α_1-adrenoceptor subclassification in portal vein smooth muscle (Sayet, Neuilly, Rakotoarisoa, Mironneau, and Mironneau, unpublished data).

Selective inhibition of the $\alpha_1{}^B$ subtype by CEC pretreatment had little or no effect on the NE-induced contraction, suggesting that the contractile response was predominantly mediated through the α_{1A} or α_{1N} subtypes. In CEC-pretreated strips, NE-induced contractions were inhibited by high concentrations of prazosin, WB4101, and HV723.

It has been previously proposed that the diversity of α_1-adrenoceptor-induced responses may be, in part, related to the distinct subtypes of receptors that may activate different emchanisms of signal transduction {27}. Responses to the α_{1A} subtype reportedly require Ca^{2+} influx through voltage-dependent channels, whereas responses to the α_{1B} subtype seem to involve mobilization of intracellular Ca^{2+} stores by an inositol phosphate mechanism {26}. In portal vein smooth muscle, activation of the α_{1A} subtype was responsible for mobilization of intracellular Ca^{2+} stores, as shown by measuring cytoplasmic Ca^{2+} with fura-2 and inositol phosphates. The transient Ca^{2+} peak and inositol phosphate production induced by $10\,\mu M$ NE were concentration-dependently inhibited by prazosin WB4101 and HV723 (Leprêtre, Arnaudeau, Sayet, and Mironneau, unpublished data). Furthermore, supramaximal concentrations of antagonists ($1\,\mu M$) did not affect the NE-induced stimulation of Ca^{2+} channels, suggesting that other α adrenoceptors were involved in Ca^{2+} channel modulation. This is the first observation that in vascular smooth muscle cells NE modulates voltage-dependent Ca^{2+} channels independently of phosphatidylinositol hydrolysis. More experiments are needed to clarify the different transduction pathways that can modulate Ca^{2+} channels in response to activation of the different α adrenoceptors.

CONCLUSIONS

In this report the ionic mechanisms involved in the NE-induced contractions have been explored in portal vein smooth muscle by means of both electrophysiological and pharmacological techniques. The main transduction process between α_1 adrenoceptors and ion channels involves activation of phospholipase C and production of

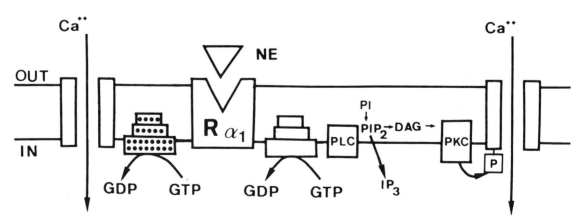

Fig. 47-11. Diagram depicting two transduction pathways between α_1-adrenoceptors and voltage-dependent Ca^{2+} channels in portal vein myocytes. One coupling involves activation of PLC through a PTX-insensitive Gq-protein. Hydrolysis of phosphatidylinositol bisphosphate (PIP2) leads to generation of $InsP_3$ and DAG. Another coupling involves a direct interaction of a PTX-sensitive G protein with the Ca^{2+} channel.

both InsP$_3$ and DAG (fig. 47-11). The α_{1A}-adrenoceptor subtype is coupled to phospholipase C through activation of a G$_q$ protein, which is insensitive to pertussis toxin. Both production of inositol phosphates and release of Ca^{2+} from intracellular stores are concentration dependently inhibited by prazosin with a high affinity (nanomolar range). InsP$_3$ produces a release of Ca^{2+} from intracellular stores. When [Ca]$_i$ is higher than 180 nM, Cl$^-$ channels are activated and produce a depolarization. This depolarization is large enough to reach the threshold potential for activation of voltage-dependent Ca^{2+} channels, leading to Ca^{2+} influx and contraction.

It is possible that this mechanism of a required depolarization might represent a common mechanism involved in many agonist-mediated contractions of smooth muscle. However, the nature of the channels responsible for the depolarization could differ from one tissue to another. In vascular smooth muscle, Ca^{2+}-activated Cl$^-$ channels seem to play the major role: in the portal and mesenteric veins in response to NE {4,31,32}, and in the coronary and mesenteric arteries in response to endothelin {33}. However, in visceral smooth muscle Ca^{2+}-activated cation channels seem to be more important: in the ileum and jejunum in response to acetylcholine {34–36}. In addition, NE increases the open-state probability of both types (T and L) of Ca^{2+} channel. For the large-conductance Ca^{2+} channel, the change in the open-state probability seems to be induced through a PKC-dependent pathway. For the small-conductance Ca^{2+} channel, the intracellular mechanism involved in the increase of the open-state probability by NE is not known and may use the same or a different pathway. (+)[^{3}H]isradipine binding to Ca^{2+} channels in intact strips of rat portal vein is increased by NE through a PKC-dependent pathway, involving a phosphorylation process. PKC-dependent phosphorylation of Ca^{2+} channels increases the affinity of dihydropyridine without affecting the number of dihydropyridine binding sites.

These results are in good agreement with the single Ca^{2+} channel recordings showing no modification of the number of functional channels in the presence of NE. The transduction coupling between the α adrenoceptor subtypes and Ca^{2+} channels is not completely understood, as it might involve hydrolysis of phospholipids other than phosphatidylinositol or a direct coupling through a G protein (Leprêtre, Arnaudeau, Sayet, and Mironneau, unpublished data). Pharmacological data show that (−)[^{3}H]D888 binding to Ca^{2+} channels is modulated by GTP analogs in a way that suggests that a pertussis toxin-sensitive G protein interacts directly with Ca^{2+} channels in response to activation of α adrenoceptors. Taken together, these results suggest that several transduction pathways between α adrenoceptors and Ca^{2+} channels are involved in the contractile effect of NE in vascular smooth muscle.

ACKNOWLEDGMENTS

This work was supported by grants from CNRS, INSERM, Région Aquitaine, and Ministère de la Recherche et de l'Espace, France. We thank Ms. Biendon for her excellent assistance.

REFERENCES

1. Bolton TB: Mechanisms of action of transmitters and other substances on smooth muscle. *Physiol Rev* 59:606–718, 1979.
2. Kuriyama H, Ito Y, Suzuki H, Kitamura K, Itoh T: Factors modifying contraction-relaxation cycle in vascular smooth muscle. *Am J Physiol* 243:H641–H662, 1982.
3. Mironneau J: Noradrenaline modulation of ionic channels in vascular smooth muscle cells. In: Sperelakis N, Kuriyama H (eds) *Electrophysiology and Ion Channels of Vascular Smooth Muscle Cells and Endothelial Cells.* New York: Elsevier, 1991, pp 47–54.
4. Pacaud P, Loirand G, Mironneau C, Mironneau J: Noradrenaline activates a calcium-activated Cl conductance and increases the voltage-dependent calcium current in cultured single cells of rat portal vein. *Br J Pharmacol* 97:139–146, 1989.
5. Gögelein H: Cl channels in epithelia. *Biochem Biophys Acta* 947:521–547, 1988.
6. Landry DW, Akabas MH, Redhead C, Edelman A, Cragoe EJ, Al Awqati Q: Purification and reconstitution of Cl channels from kidney and trachea. *Science* 244:1469–1472, 1989.
7. Baron A, Pacaud P, Loirand G, Mironneau C, Mironneau J: Pharmacological block of Ca^{2+}-activated Cl$^-$ current in rat vascular smooth muscle cells in short-term primary culture. *Pflügers Arch* 419:553–558, 1991.
8. Pacaud P, Loirand G, Grégoire G, Mironneau C, Mironneau J: Calcium-dependence of the calcium-activated chloride current in smooth muscle cells of rat portal vein. *Pflügers Arch* 421:125–130, 1992.
9. Loirand G, Pacaud P, Mironneau C, Mironneau J: Evidence for two distinct calcium channels in rat vascular smooth muscle cells in short-term primary culture. *Pflügers Arch* 407:566–568, 1986.
10. Loirand G, Pacaud P, Mironneau C, Mironneau J: Two types of calcium currents in single smooth muscle cells from rat portal vein. *J Physiol (Lond)* 412:333–349, 1989.
11. Nelson MT, Patlak JB, Worley JF, Standen NB: Calcium channels, potassium channels, and voltage-dependence of arterial smooth muscle tone. *Am J Physiol* 259:C3–C18, 1990.
12. Pacaud P, Loirand G, Baron A, Mironneau C, Mironneau J: Ca^{2+} channel activation and membrane depolarization mediated by Cl$^-$ channels in response to noradrenaline in vascular myocytes. *Br J Pharmacol* 104:1000–1006, 1991.
13. Berridge MJ, Irvine RF: Inositol trisphosphate, a novel second messenger in cellular signal transduction. *Nature* 312:315–320, 1984.
14. Loirand G, Pacaud P, Mironneau C, Mironneau J: GTP-binding proteins mediate noradrenaline effects on calcium and chloride currents in cultured rat portal vein myocytes. *J Physiol (Lond)* 428:517–529, 1990.
15. Loirand G, Faiderbe S, Baron A, Geffard M, Mironneau J: Autoantiphosphatidylinositol antibodies specifically inhibit noradrenaline effects on Ca^{2+} and Cl$^-$ channels in rat portal vein myocytes. *J Biol Chem* 267:4312–4316, 1992.
16. Catterall WA: Structure and function of voltage-sensitive ion channels. *Science* 242:50–61, 1988.
17. Hosey MM, Lazdunski M: Calcium channels: Molecular pharmacology, structure and regulation. *J Membr Biol* 104:81–105, 1988.
18. Dacquet C, Loirand G, Rakotoarisoa L, Mironneau C, Mironneau J: (+)[^{3}H]PN 200-110 binding to microsomes and intact strips of portal vein smooth muscle: Characterization and modulation by membrane potential and divalent cations. *Br J Pharmacol* 97:256–262, 1989.

19. Morel N, Godfraind T: Prolonged depolarization increases the pharmacological effect of dihydropyridines and their binding affinity for calcium channels of vascular smooth muscle. *J Pharmacol Exp Ther* 234:711–715, 1987.

20. Mironneau C, Rakotoarisoa L, Sayet I, Mironneau J: Modulation of [³H]dihydropyridine binding by activation of protein kinase C in rat vascular smooth muscle. *Eur J Pharmacol* 208:223–230, 1991.

21. Rakotoarisoa L, Sayet I, Mironneau C, Mironneau J: Selective modulation by membrane potential of desmethoxyverapamil binding to calcium channels in rat portal vein. *J Pharmacol Exp Ther* 255:942–947, 1990.

22. Weir AW, Weston AH: The effects of BRL 34915 and nicorandil on electrical and mechanical activity and on ⁸⁶Rb efflux in rat blood vessels. *Br J Pharmacol* 88:121–128, 1986.

23. Morel N, Godfraind T: Characterization in rat aorta of the binding sites responsible for blockade of noradrenaline-evoked calcium entry by nisoldipine. *Br J Pharmacol* 102:467–477, 1991.

24. Rakotoarisoa L, Mironneau C, Sayet I, Mironneau J: Guanine nucleotide-binding proteins modulate desmethoxyverapamil binding to calcium channels in vascular smooth muscle. *J Pharmacol Exp Ther* 259:164–168, 1991.

25. Morrow AL, Creese I: Characterization of α_1-adrenergic receptor subtypes in rat brain: A reevaluation of [³H]WB4101 and [³H]prazosin binding. *Mol Pharmacol* 29:321–330, 1986.

26. Han C, Abel PW, Minneman KP: α_1-adrenoceptor subtypes linked to different mechanisms for increasing intracellular Ca^{2+} in smooth muscle. *Nature* 329:333–335, 1987.

27. Minneman KP: α_1-adrenergic receptor subtypes, inositol phosphates, and sources of cell Ca^{2+}. *Pharmacol Rev* 40:87–119, 1988.

28. Lomasney JW, Cotecchia S, Lefkowitz RJ, Caron MG: Molecular biology of α-adrenergic receptors: Implications for receptor classification and for structure-function relationships. *Biochim Biophys Acta* 1095:127–139, 1991.

29. Hanft G, Gross G: Subclassification of α_1-adrenoceptor recognition sites by urapidil derivatives and other selective antagonists. *Br J Pharmacol* 97:691–700, 1989.

30. Muramatsu I, Ohmura T, Kigoshi S, Hashimoto S, Oshita M: Pharmacological subclassification of α_1-adrenoceptors in vascular smooth muscle. *Br J Pharmacol* 99:197–201, 1990.

31. Byrne NG, Large WA: Membrane ionic mechanisms activated by noradrenaline in cells isolated from the rabbit portal vein. *J Physiol (Lond)* 404:557–573, 1988.

32. Van Helden DF: Electrophysiology of neuromuscular transmission in guinea pig mesenteric veins. *J Physiol (Lond)* 401:469–488, 1988.

33. Klöckner U, Isenberg G: Endothelin depolarizes myocytes from porcine coronary and human mesenteric arteries through a Ca-activated chloride current. *Pflügers Arch* 418:168–175, 1991.

34. Inoue R, Isenberg G: Effect of membrane potential on acetylcholine-induced inward current in guinea pig ileum. *J Physiol (Lond)* 424:57–72, 1990.

35. Inoue R, Isenberg G: Intracellular calcium ions modulate acetylcholine-induced inward current in guinea pig ileum. *J Physiol (Lond)* 424:73–92, 1990.

36. Pacaud P, Bolton TB: Relation between muscarinic receptor cationic current and internal calcium in guinea pig jejunal smooth muscle cells. *J Physiol (Lond)* 441:477–499, 1991.

CHAPTER 48

Calcium-Activated K$^+$ Channels from Coronary Smooth Muscle: Mechanisms of Modulation and Role in Cardiac Function

L. TORO

INTRODUCTION

Coronary blood flow is determinant for the normal function of the heart. In fact, localized spasm of the coronary arteries largely contributes to the development of myocardial ischemia, angina, infarction, and sudden death. Coronary vasospasm occurs when coronary smooth muscle is exposed to circulating or to in situ produced vasoconstrictors. Thus a fundamental problem is to determine which molecules at the plasma membrane of coronary smooth muscle cells are the targets of vasoactive substances and to understand the mechanisms of their response. In this regard, increasing evidence supports the idea that the large conductance ("maxi") calcium-activated K (K$_{Ca}$) channels play an important role in determining vascular tone and the resting membrane potential of smooth muscle cells {8,67,78,81,90,100}. Special characteristics of this type of channels in smooth muscle make them good candidates for this physiological role, i.e., their high density per cell (>15,000/cell), their large conductance, and their responsiveness to both vasoconstrictors and vasorelaxants {for recent reviews see 83,97,98}. The mechanisms of K$_{Ca}$ channel regulation by vasoactive substances in coronary smooth muscle are beginning to be understood. We and others have found that the binding of intracellular Ca^{2+} to the channel protein is not the sole mechanism of K$_{Ca}$ channel activation, but other mechanisms are likely to be involved, which may themselves change the channel affinity for Ca^{2+}. Among the mechanisms responsible for the modification in K$_{Ca}$ channel activity of coronary smooth muscle after a stimulus are (a) ligand modulation, (b) phosphorylation, and (c) G-protein gating. These mechanisms of K$_{Ca}$ channel regulation will be discussed in this review, with special emphasis on K$_{Ca}$ channels from coronary smooth muscle (table 48-1).

POTASSIUM CHANNELS AND CONTRACTILITY OF CORONARY SMOOTH MUSCLE

The coronary artery is a nonregenerative type of smooth muscle {89} that can be induced to contract vigorously by substances that block K$^+$ channels {101}. We and others have observed that coronary smooth muscle possesses predominant K$_{Ca}$ channels at both the macroscopic and single-channel level {26,36,88,99,106}; in addition, this type of K channels is diverse and is present as several isoforms that differ in conductance and mode of gating {99}.

The abundance and diversity of K$_{Ca}$ channels in coronary smooth muscle may warrant their importance in coronary function. Several findings support this hypothesis: (a) cromakalim, traditionally known as a K$_{ATP}$ channel opener {22} and recently as an activator of K$_{Ca}$ channels from coronary and other smooth muscles {28,29}, has spasmolytic effects on coronary smooth muscle {20,60}; (b) arachidonic acid relaxes coronary vessels {110} and activates K$_{Ca}$ channels from coronary {83}, pulmonary {70} and aortic smooth muscles {38}; (c) strong vasoconstrictors, such as angiotensin II (Ag-II) {93}, thromboxane A$_2$ (TXA$_2$) {86}, and endothelin {36}, inhibit coronary K$_{Ca}$ channel activity; (d) the bradycardic agent tedisamil blocks K$_{Ca}$ channels from portal vein {76}, and (e) calcium-dependent K currents are enhanced in aortic smooth muscle cells exposed to high blood pressure, probably as a compensatory mechanism to limit pressure-induced vasoconstriction {79}. Thus vasoconstriction is related to K$_{Ca}$ channel inhibition, which would depolarize the cell membrane and promote Ca^{2+} entry, causing the activation of the contractile machinery; while vasodilation is related to the activation of K$_{Ca}$ channels, which would hyperpolarize the cell membrane and avoid a rise of [Ca^{2+}]$_i$ through voltage-dependent Ca^{2+} channels causing relaxation. Despite these experimental findings, it is important to keep in mind that coronary smooth muscle also possesses other types of K channels, like delayed rectifier {103}, ATP sensitive {71,104}, and inward rectifier (our unpublished observations) K channels, which could also be involved in the response to vasoactive substances. In this regard it has been recently shown that vasopressin, endothelin, and Ag-II can also inhibit K$_{ATP}$ channels {62,63,104} from coronary smooth muscle grown from explants. Which type of channels have a major role in controlling the contraction of coronary smooth muscle cells, and under which circumstances? This question awaits more experimental endeavors.

N. Sperelakis (ed.), Physiology and Pathophysiology of the Heart, Third Edition.

Table 48-1. Regulatory properties of "maxi" Ca-activated K channels

Cell type or tissue	Regulatory agent	Effect	Mechanism proposed	Ref.
CSM	AA	(+)	Ligand modulation	83
	ACh	(+)	$[Ca^{2+}]_i$	27
	Adrenergic agents	(+)	Phosphorylation and G-protein gating	85
	Ag-II	(−)	Ligand modulation	93
	cGMP	(+)	Ligand modulation?	26
	Endothelin	(+,−)	$[Ca^{2+}]_i$	36,42
	Nitroglycerin	(+)	cGMP-dependent phosphorylation?	26
	TXA_2	(−)	Ligand modulation	86
	Vasopressin	(+)	$[Ca^{2+}]_i$	104
SM	AA	(+)	Ligand modulation	41
	ACh	(−)	G-protein gating?	14,15,45
		(+)	$[Ca^{2+}]_i$	64
	Adrenergic agents	(+)	Phosphorylation	80
		(+)	G-protein gating	44,95
	Adenosine, ANF	(+)	GMP mediated	107
	ATP	(+)	Phosphorylation	78
	GMP, cGMP, GDP, GTP	(+)	Ligand modulation?	107
	$[H^+]$	(−)	Ligand modulation	46
	Substance P	(+)	$[Ca^{2+}]_i$	57,58
		(−)	?	57
Brain	ATP	(+)	Phosphorylation	13
Chromaffin	ACh	(−)	Direct?	30
Epithelia	$[H^+]$	(−)	Ligand modulation	12,18
Kidney	Antidiuretic hormone	(+)	Phosphorylation	34
	AA	(+)	$[Ca^{2+}]_i$	54
	Prostaglandin E_2	(+)	$[Ca^{2+}]_i$	54
Pancreatic B cells	$[H^+]$	(−)	Ligand modulation	17
Pancreatic duct cells	Secretin	(+)	Phosphorylation	32
Pituitary tumor cells	Somatostatin	(+)	Dephosphorylation	105
	Thyrotropin releasing hormone	(+)	?	52
Skeletal muscle	$[H^+]$	(−)	Ligand modulation	51

CSM, coronary smooth muscle; SM, smooth muscle; AA, arachidonic acid; ACh, acethylcholine; Ag-II, angiotensin II; TXA_2, thromboxane A_2; (+), activation; (−), inhibition; ?, not known.

GENERAL PROPERTIES OF CORONARY SMOOTH MUSCLE K_{Ca} CHANNELS

Large-conductance K_{Ca} channels are present in a broad spectrum of tissues, including smooth muscle, brain, skeletal muscle, epithelia, and secretory glands. Because of their large conductance ($\approx 150-300\,pS$) they have been called "maxi" or "big" K_{Ca} channels {16,50,59}. As mentioned before, in smooth muscle they are particularly abundant {92} and in coronary smooth muscle they are present as several isoforms {99}.

The electrical activity of K_{Ca} channels from coronary smooth muscle has been studied in isolated cells using the patch-clamp technique or in artificial membranes after reconstitution of isolated plasmalemmal membranes. In isolated cells robust K_{Ca} currents have been observed. Wilde and Lee {106} described two types of K_{Ca} currents sensitive to internal Ca ($[Ca^{2+}]_i$) in dog coronary arteries, and noticed that these types of K currents were the predominant currents in these cells. We have made similar observations using isolated cells from porcine coronary artery {96}, and recently Volk et al. {103} have shown

that K_{Ca} currents represent an important component of the outward current in rabbit coronary smooth muscle. Consistent with these results is our finding that "maxi" K_{Ca} channels are abundant and have functional "isoforms" in isolated plasmalemmal membranes from porcine coronary smooth muscle (245 and 295 pS in 50/250 mM KCl gradient) {99}, and the finding of other investigators that patches of the corresponding cells contain primarily K_{Ca} channels (148 pS in 5.4/140 mM K gradient; 216 pS and 300 pS in 140/140 mM K) {26,36,88}.

K_{Ca} channels from coronary smooth muscle are voltage and Ca sensitive, similar to the ones described in other tissues {50}. An interesting feature, however, is that in isolated cells from coronary artery K_{Ca} channels may be active at $[Ca^{2+}]_i$ as low as $10^{-8}\,M$ {36}, supporting the hypothesis that they participate in the control of the resting membrane potential of the cell.

The pharmacology of K_{Ca} channels from coronary smooth muscle has not been extensively studied. We have demonstrated at the single-channel level that externally applied tetraethylammonium (TEA) inhibits coronary smooth muscle K_{Ca} channel activity in a dual manner

A

Putative topology of a "maxi" K_{Ca} channel

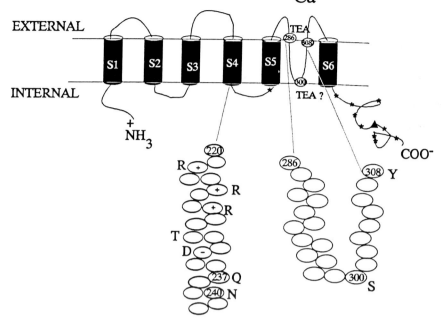

B

Sequence alignement of the "pore" region of a "maxi" K_{Ca} channel and a *Shaker* B K channel

Slo: L S Y W T C V Y F L I V T M $\boxed{S}$ T V G Y G D V $\boxed{Y}$ 308

Sh: D A F W - - - - W A V V T M $\boxed{T}$ T V G Y G D M $\boxed{T}$ 449

Fig. 48-1. Molecular characteristics of a "maxi" K_{Ca} channel. **A:** Putative topology of a K channel subunit {for a recent review see 9}. S4 domain (putative "voltage sensing" domain) and putative "pore" region are enlarged. Tyrosine (Y) at position 308 seems to be responsible for the high *external* TEA sensitivity (Ki ≈ 200 μM) of this channel. Serine (S) at position 300 seems not to confer a low internal TEA sensitivity (Ki ≈ 50 mM for coronary K_{Ca} channels). * marks putative PKC-dependent phosphorylation sites; ▲ marks putative PKA-dependent phosphorylation sites. Numbers correspond to the amino acid position in the primary sequence of the *slowpoke* K_{Ca} channel {2}. **B:** Comparison of the primary sequences of two voltage-dependent K channels: *Slo* (slowpoke K_{Ca} channel) and *Sh* (*Shaker* B K channel). Boxes mark sites found to confer K channels their TEA sensitivities {for review see 55}. In the *Sh*B K channel, when T at position 441 is mutated for an S (as present in *slo* K channel which has a high internal Ki), the Ki for internal TEA becomes larger (Ki$_{wild}$ type = 0.7 vs. Ki$_{mutant}$ = 7.4 mM); substituting T at position 449 for a Y (as present in the *slo* K_{Ca} channel, which has a low external Ki of ≈200 μM) shifts Ki for external TEA from 30 mM in the wild type to 650 μM in the mutant. Accordingly, when Y at position 308 in the *slo* K_{Ca} channel is mutated to T, the K_{Ca} channel acquires the TEA sensitivity of the *Sh*B K channel, that is, its phenotype changes from low to high Ki for external TEA (2).

{99}. TEA is a "fast" blocker of this channel, as manifested in the reduction of current amplitude {109}, but can also cause a reduction in open probability (K½ ≈ 150–380 μM). The mechanism of this reduction in open time is not known yet. The mechanism of "fast" blockade induced by TEA and the K_d value of this process (100–300 μM at 0 mV) are common to all studied K_{Ca} channels, including a K_{Ca} channel (*slowpoke*) cloned from the *Drosophila melanogoster slo* locus {2,69}. On the contrary, the change in gating produced by micromolar concentrations of external TEA has only been observed in K_{Ca} channels from coronary smooth muscle {99}. These features suggest that K_{Ca} channels comprise a family of channels with common external domains for at least one binding site for TEA. This common binding site for external TEA is thought to be located in the external "mouth" of the "pore" or conduction pathway of the channel protein (fig. 48-1). Adelman et al. {2} demonstrated that a tyrosine residue at position 308 of the *slowpoke* K_{Ca} channel provides a high-affinity binding site for TEA responsible for the "fast" blockade, since its mutation with a valine promoted the expression of a K_{Ca} channel with much less TEA affinity. It is important to point out that molecular biology studies on other voltage-dependent K channels revealed that a tyrosine in the corresponding position confers these channels a high sensitivity to external TEA {39,40,55,56}. These findings indicate that K_{Ca} channels not only share structural characteristics within members of the same family, but also with other K channels.

Another K_{Ca} channel blocker of coronary smooth muscle is charybdotoxin, whose mechanism of blockade is "slow," producing long-lived closed events {61}. K_{Ca} channels isoforms from coronary smooth muscle are all blocked by CTX {99}, indicating that they share common "pore" domains and that their main structural and functional differences might be related to regions other than the conduction pathway. These assumptions will only be proven when cloned K_{Ca} channels from coronary smooth muscle are available to perform structure-function studies at the molecular level.

Recently we have demonstrated that maxi K_{Ca} channels from coronary smooth muscle can be "opened" by externally applied niflumic acid, a nonsteroidal antiinflammatory agent {94} (fig. 48-2). This property of maxi K_{Ca} channels is shared with other K_{Ca} channels from other tissues (uterine smooth muscle, skeletal muscle, and *Drosophila melanogaster*), suggesting that K_{Ca} channels possess a common binding domain for this drug. It would be interesting to determine if this drug affects K_{ATP} channels, which are also present in coronary smooth muscle {71,104}. The relevance of this finding resides in that niflumic acid could serve as a prototype of "maxi" K_{Ca} channels activators in the design of therapeutic drugs useful to relax the coronary vessel.

MODULATION OF CORONARY SMOOTH MUSCLE BY VASOACTIVE METABOLITES

Acetylcholine

The role of acetylcholine on the modulation of K_{Ca} channels from coronary smooth muscle has been addressed at the single cell level {27}. K_{Ca} channel activity was studied at the macroscopic level by measuring STOCs and "spikelike hyperpolarizations" (SLHs), while single-channel activity was studied in cell-attached patches. Perfusion with $10\,\mu M$ ACh caused an increase of SLHs, leading to hyperpolarization of the membrane, an increase

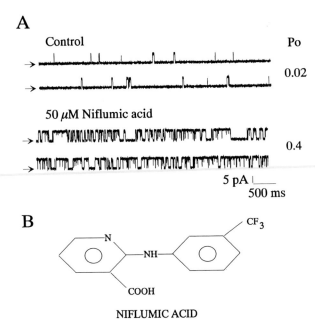

Fig. 48-2. Niflumic acid "opens" K_{Ca} channels from coronary smooth muscle. **A:** Externally applied niflumic acid ($50\,\mu M$) increases channel open probability by increasing the mean open time and diminishing the duration of the closed states {94}. K_{Ca} channels were reconstituted into lipid bilayers; 250 KCl internal/5 KCl, 245 NaCl external; holding potential, $V_H = 0\,mV$. **B:** Chemical structure of niflumic acid. Po, open probability. In this and the following figures, arrows mark the closed state of the channel.

of the STOCs, and an enhancement of single K_{Ca} channel activity. In agreement with a role of K_{Ca} channels on ACh-induced SLHs and STOCs, these events disappeared after dialysis of the internal solution with $10\,mM$ EGTA. The fact that activation of K_{Ca} channels was observed in cell-attached patches when ACh was present in the bath suggested to the authors that activation occurred via a cytosolic messenger. This messenger seems to be Ca^{2+} released from intracellular stores, since heparin, which inhibits IP_3-induced calcium release, suppressed the ACh-increased STOCs but not the basal STOCs. In addition, the ACh-induced STOCs were reversibly blocked by atropine, suggesting a muscarinic receptor associated mechanism. In tracheal smooth muscle a similar mechanism (rise in $[Ca^{2+}]_i$) for ACh-induced activation of K_{Ca} channel has been recently proposed {64}.

It is interesting to note that in colonic and tracheal smooth muscle ACh can also produce inhibition of K_{Ca} channels. This inhibition is probably due to a direct effect of a pertussis toxin-sensitive G protein on K_{Ca} channels {14,15,45}, and not due to a change in $[Ca^{2+}]_i$. Therefore, it would be interesting to determine if ACh can modulate K_{Ca} channels from coronary smooth muscle by alternative mechanisms (e.g., ligand modulation, phosphorylation, G-protein gating). Studies in cell-attached patches with ACh in the pipette, in outside-out patches with ACh in the bath, and in lipid bilayers may give light to other modulatory mechanisms of ACh.

Adrenergic agents

Beta-adrenergic agents relax smooth muscle and consequently are important dilators of the coronary circulation {110}. Consistent with the hypothesis that K_{Ca} channels have a physiological role as modulators of coronary smooth muscle contractility, we have recently observed that isoproterenol activates "maxi" K_{Ca} channels from coronary smooth muscle in the presence of GTP + Mg^{2+}, and that this effect is reversed by the beta-antagonist propranolol. Because these experiments were performed after fusion of membrane vesicles with a lipid bilayer, it is very likely that the receptor, the channel, and a coupling G protein are intimately associated in a macromolecular complex and do not diffuse away in the lipid bilayer. In view of the functional characteristics of the reconstituted protein complex, and the fact that the bilayer system permits a better experimental control of the channel environment (increasing evidence suggests that this is almost impossible to achieve using excised patches), we decided to explore with this technique the possible mechanisms underlying beta-adrenergic stimulation. As will be discussed later, we have recently shown that K_{Ca} channels not only can be activated by PKA-dependent phosphorylation as expected for a beta-receptor mediated G_s activation of the adenylyl cyclase pathway, but can also be activated by $G_{\alpha s}$ or GTPγS when phosphorylation is inhibited. Therefore, at least *two independent mechanisms* may explain how beta-adrenergic stimulation increases K_{Ca} channel activity in the coronary smooth muscle: (a) PKA-dependent phosphorylation and (b) direct G-protein stimulation by $G_{\alpha s}$ protein {84,85}.

Angiotensin II (Ag-II)

Angiotensin II is one of the most potent vasoconstrictors of the coronary vessels. Plasma membrane receptors for Ag-II have been detected in a number of vascular smooth muscles, and its action on cell metabolism has been widely studied {33}. Binding of Ag-II to its receptor activates the formation of IP_3 and diacylglycerol through a G-protein-mediated activation of phospholipase C. Consequently, there is an increase in intracellular Ca that is caused by IP_3-induced Ca release from internal stores. Besides these actions, Ag-II may also produce an increase of Ca currents, blockade of K currents {7,68}, and depolarization of the plasma membrane {37}.

We have reported that Ag-II may inhibit coronary K_{Ca} channels incorporated into lipid bilayers {93}. The inhibition produced by Ag-II was dose dependent with a K½ of 58 nM. Ag-II affected both the open and closed states of K_{Ca} channels. Since the experiments were performed in the absence of GTP, Mg^{2+}, or ATP, it was difficult to postulate an inhibition mediated by an endogenous G protein or an endogenous protein kinase. A more suitable explanation was a direct effect of Ag-II on K_{Ca} channels or

a closely coupled protein. This does not mean, however, that in the intact tissue parallel pathways of regulation do not take place, leading to the same final response: depolarization and contraction of coronary arteries. Therefore, it is of interest to determine the site of modulatory binding of Ag-II. Some possibilities are (a) a receptor that belongs to the family of Ag-II receptors functionally coupled to the K_{Ca} channel, (b) the channel protein itself, or (c) an unknown closely associated protein (e.g., regulatory subunit). The involvement of a specific receptor may be tested with the peptide antagonist [Sar¹, Ala⁸]-angiotensin II (saralasin), or non-peptide antagonists like DuP753 (to Ag-II-1 type receptor) and PD123177 (to Ag-II-2 type receptor). Testing DuP753 would be especially interesting, since it has antihypertensive properties {108}.

Arachidonic acid (AA)

Arachidonic acid relaxes coronary vessels {82}. We have observed that externally applied arachidonic acid (10–50 μM) to reconstituted coronary K_{Ca} channels increases channel activity in a dose-dependent manner {83}. Thus the increase in K_{Ca} channel activity may contribute to the hyperpolarization and relaxation of the coronary vessel. A role for arachidonic acid in the regulation of K_{Ca} channels from pulmonary artery {41,70} and aorta {38} has also been suggested. However, the specificity of this effect in coronary smooth muscle has to be determined in order to correlate this effect with a physiological role of this lipid. Besides the role of arachidonic acid and its metabolites as external vasoactive substances, the possibility also exists that these compounds are synthesized in the smooth muscle itself and that they act as intracellular modulators of channel activity. This type of action has been demonstrated in cardiac cells where lipoxygenase metabolites of arachidonic acid (derived after phospholipase A2 cleavage of membrane phospholipids) modulate the muscarinic K channel (48). The question remains open whether this lipid itself modulates channel activity or if one or more of its metabolites exert a regulatory action on coronary smooth muscle K_{Ca} channels in vivo.

Endothelin

Endothelin was isolated from the supernatant of cultured endothelial cells {108}. This vasoactive peptide has been shown to produce either contraction or relaxation of the coronary vessels {25,43}. Relaxation has been explained as mediated by the release of endothelium-derived relaxing factor (EDRF) and prostacyclin from endothelial cells {19}. On the other hand, contraction is thought to occur by several mechanisms that raise $[Ca^{2+}]_i$, including the activation of Ca^{2+} channels and induction of phosphoinositide breakdown after stimulation of phospholipase C {31,102}.

Recently Hu et al. {36} have demonstrated in coronary smooth muscle that endothelin may modulate K_{Ca} channel activity in a dual manner (inhibition and activation), depending on the peptide concentration. This evidence provides an alternate explanation for endothelin opposing effects on coronary smooth muscle. Endothelin at concentrations between 0.1 and 1 nM increased channel activity in cell-attached patches of isolated coronary smooth muscle cells. On the contrary, when endothelin concentration was raised to 10–100 nM, K_{Ca} channel activity diminished. Klöckner and Isenberg {42}, however, found that 100 nM endothelin increased the frequency of spontaneous transient outward currents (STOCs), thought to be the result of simultaneous activation of K_{Ca} channels {5}. This discrepancy seems not to be related to differences in species, since both investigations were carried out using porcine coronary smooth muscle cells. The main reason for these differences using high endothelin concentrations could be that the inhibitory effect was observed at the single-channel level in cell-attached experiments, while the activation was seen using the whole-cell configuration. It is possible that in the whole-cell experiments an important intermediate of the endothelin-induced inhibition of K_{Ca} channel activity is lost due to diffusion into the patch pipette. Another explanation could be that since enzymatic treatment may modify the structure of membrane proteins (receptors and channels), different cell dissociation procedures give rise to the discrepancies in the results. Nevertheless, both groups propose that endothelin regulates K_{Ca} channel activity through changes in the internal Ca concentration.

Many questions remain open: Can endothelin regulate K_{Ca} channels directly? Is modulation by endothelin through a metabolite of the phosphoinositide cascade? Are phosphorylation and/or dephosphorylation of the channel protein involved?

Nitroglycerin and cGMP

The chemical identity of endothelial relaxing factor (EDRF) is thought to be nitrogen oxide (NO) {72}, although more recent data suggest that EDRF is not solely or mainly composed of NO {65}. NO-containing compounds, such as nitroglycerin, are important as pharmacologic and therapeutic agents due to their vasorelaxing properties. These agents activate the soluble form of guanylate cyclase (GC), leading to increased levels of cGMP followed by relaxation. In addition, NO causes hyperpolarization of coronary smooth muscle at rest {91}, suggesting that it may activate K conductances. In accordance, Fujino et al. {26} have recently reported that 4-aminopyridine-sensitive K_{Ca} channels from coronary smooth muscle cells, grown in explants, are stimulated by nitroglycerin (10 μM). These authors also tested the effect of cGMP on K_{Ca} channel activity. The permeant analog Br-cGMP (300 μM) was used in cell-attached patches, while cGMP (300 μM) was added to the intracellular side of inside-out patches. As expected for a NO-related relaxing effect, cGMP or its permeant analog induced the activation of K_{Ca} channels. Thus activation of K_{Ca} channels by NO compounds via cGMP may account in part for the relaxation of coronary smooth muscle. On the other hand, the role of cGMP in smooth muscle relaxation has been attributed to the activation of cGMP-dependent protein

kinase (PKG), which leads to a decrease in internal $[Ca^{2+}]$ {53}. Thus it would be interesting to establish if activation of PKG is also involved in the increase of K_{Ca} channel activity (via phosphorylation) and/or if cGMP may by itself enhance channel activity. Since Fujino et al. {26} reported that cGMP could increase channel activity in inside-out patches where soluble PKG may be lost, it is plausible that this cyclic nucleotide may act directly on the gating of K_{Ca} channels.

Thromboxane A_2 (TXA$_2$)

One of the events during platelet aggregation at the site of coronary artery damage (where smooth muscle is exposed) is the activation of the arachidonic acid metabolic pathway. Arachidonic acid from the plasma membrane of platelets is metabolized by the enzyme cyclooxygenase to produce cyclic endoperoxides. These compounds are subsequently metabolized to TXA$_2$ (primarily) and prostaglandins (fig. 48-3). Thromboxane A_2 reaches the smooth muscle at the coronary lesion, causing vasoconstriction {82}. The mechanism of activation of TXA$_2$ on the coronary smooth muscle is not well understood. However, in astrocytoma cells it has been shown that it may activate phospholipase C via a pertussis toxin-insensitive G protein {66}.

We have recently found that the TXA$_2$ mimetic U-46619 inhibits K_{Ca} channels from coronary smooth muscle incorporated into lipid bilayers (fig. 48-4). We used the stable analog U46619, since TXA$_2$ is chemically unstable (half life = 30 seconds at 37°C) {73}. U46619 (50–150 nM) reduced channel activity between 15% and 60% of the control open probability. The inhibitory effect of the TXA$_2$ agonist modified both the open and closed states of the channel, and the inhibition could be reversed by internal Ca^{2+}. This inhibition is specific since it takes place only when U46619 is added to the external side of the channel. Moreover, the inactive hydrolysis derivative TXB$_2$ (1 μM) had no effect on channel activity, and the TXA$_2$ receptor antagonist SQ29,548 prevented or reversed the action of U46619 {86}. These findings are in agreement with the vasoconstrictor action of TXA$_2$, since inhibition of K channels would lead to depolarization and contraction of coronary smooth muscle.

Since our experimental protocol did not include GTP, Mg, or ATP in the solution facing the internal side of the channel, a mechanism involving the activation of an endogenous G protein or an endogenous protein kinase seems to be unlikely. Therefore it is possible that the channel itself has a site for the TXA$_2$ action or that a TXA$_2$ receptor protein is closely associated with the channel. This mechanism of inhibition of K_{Ca} channels by TXA$_2$ may be parallel to the activation of phospholipase C in the intact cell. It would be interesting to test in single cells if TXA$_2$ inhibits K_{Ca} channels through the activation of phospholipase C according to the following metabolic cascade: (a) interaction of TXA$_2$ with its receptor; (b) activation of a G protein after TXA$_2$ receptor occupancy; (c) activation of phospholipase C, or in addition, inhibition of K_{Ca} channels, by the activated G protein; (d) phospholipase C mediated formation of inositol-1,4,5-

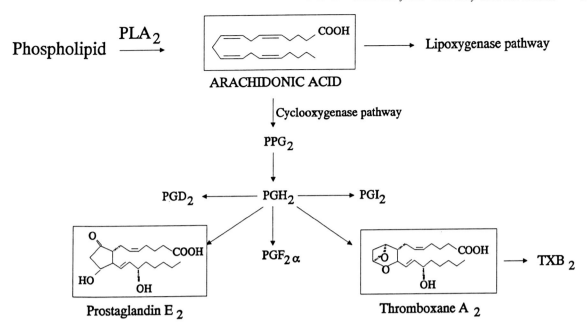

Fig. 48-3. Metabolic pathway of arachidonic acid metabolism. Arachidonic acid and thromboxane A_2 can modulate K_{Ca} channel activity of coronary smooth muscle. Prostaglandin E_2 and arachidonic acid modulate K_{Ca} channels from kidney. PG, prostaglandin; TXB_2, thromboxane B_2 (inactive analog of thromboxane A_2); PLA_2, phospholipase A_2.

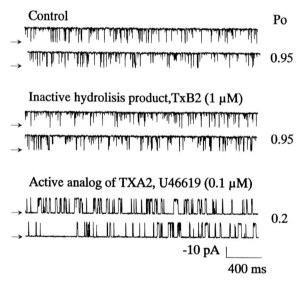

Fig. 48-4. Thromboxane A_2 activates K_{Ca} channels from coronary smooth muscle. Channel records show that thromboxane B_2 (TXB_2), the inactive analog of thromboxane A_2 (TXA_2), does not produce any effect on reconstituted K_{Ca} channels from coronary smooth muscle. On the contrary, externally applied U46619 (active analog of TXA_2) has a strong inhibitory action on K_{Ca} channel activity {86}. This inhibition may explain in part the vasoconstrictor effect of TXA_2, since inhibition of K_{Ca} channel gating would lead to depolarization, raise $[Ca^{2+}]_i$, and consequently, contract the coronary artery. $V_H = -40\,mV$; 250/250 KCl.

trisphosphate, IP3, and diacylglycerol; (e) activation of protein kinase C by diacylglycerol; and (f) protein kinase C mediated phosphorylation of K_{Ca} channels or of a closely related molecule that inhibits channel activity. Also the possibility that IP3 or diacylglycerol may by themselves regulate channel activity has to be explored.

Vasopressin

Vasopressin is a peptidic hormone released by the pituitary gland. Besides its action as an antidiuretic hormone, it is also known as a potent vasoconstrictor. Vasopressin increases the levels of diacylglycerol and IP_3, with a concomitant increase in $[Ca^{2+}]_i$. Recently, Wakatsuki et al. {104} demonstrated that vasopressin (100–200 nM) increases the activity of K_{Ca} channels and decreases that of K_{ATP} channels in coronary smooth muscle cells grown from explants. Thus in this case it appears that the constrictor action of vasopressin is related to its ability to block K_{ATP} channels and not to its modulation of K_{Ca} channels. However, to what extent do smooth muscle cells in tissue culture correspond to the cells in the intact tissue? The study of this problem using several experimental approaches may answer this question.

The mechanism of activation of K_{Ca} channels by vasopressin seemed to be through the increase in intracellular Ca^{2+} and not due to a direct effect on the channel protein. The latter mechanism was discarded due to the fact that in outside-out patches vasopressin did not activate K_{Ca} channels; in cell-attached patches, when internal calcium was chelated with fura-2/AM, vasopressin also failed to increase K_{Ca} channel activity. The role of $[Ca^{2+}]_i$ in increasing K_{Ca} channel activity should be addressed to determine if, for example, the increase in $[Ca^{2+}]_i$ causes an increase of Ca-calmodulin-dependent phosphorylation of the channel protein.

MODULATION OF K_{Ca} CHANNELS FROM OTHER TISSUES

The regulatory properties of K_{Ca} channels seem to be a common characteristic of this type of membrane proteins. We have recently reviewed their regulation by neurotransmitters, hormones, nucleotides, lipids, and intracellular pH {83,97}, and their mechanisms of action {98}. In this review, other and recent contributions to this field will be discussed. For a general overview see table 48-1.

Acetylcholine and substance P (SP)

Muraki et al. {64}, using β-escin permeabilized cells, have shown that ACh and SP may activate K_{Ca} channels from trachea and urinary bladder smooth muscle in the presence of GTP. Because ACh and SP were applied to the bath and their action was prevented by heparin (an inhibitor of IP_3-induced Ca^{2+} release from internal stores), the authors concluded that the mechanism of activation of K_{Ca} channels was most likely via a rise of $[Ca^{2+}]_i$. On the contrary, Kume and Kotlikoff {45} provided evidence in the same smooth muscle (tracheal myocytes) for an inhibitory modulation of K_{Ca} channels by ACh via a pertussis-sensitive G protein. An explanation to this apparent discrepancy is that Kume and Kotlikoff {45} studied the modulation of K_{Ca} channels by ACh that occurs in an area contiguous to the channel protein. Several questions arise: Which is the physiological relevance of these two opposite mechanisms? Do they occur within a different time frame? Are any of these opposite mechanisms modulated by other factors?

Eicosanoids

Recently Ling et al. {54} proposed that AA and prostaglandin (PG) E_2 (fig. 48-3) activate K_{Ca} channels via the release of $[Ca^{2+}]_i$ from intracellular stores. The authors showed that 50 μM AA and 500 nM PGE_2 increased K_{Ca} channel activity in cultured principal cells of kidney cortical collecting tubule. The installation of the activation had a lag time, and PGE_2 did not activate K_{Ca} channels in cell-free patches, suggesting that AA and PGE_2 do not activate directly K_{Ca} channels, but a secondary messenger is involved. A mechanism of Ca activation of the K_{Ca} channels was proposed on the basis that thapsigargin (250 nM; known to deplete Ca^{2+} stores) prevented the action of both AA and PGE_2. Previous studies, however, have shown that AA may exert its stimulatory action without the necessity of $[Ca^{2+}]_i$ to increase {41}. It is obvious from these studies that AA action on K_{Ca} channels occurs via distinct mechanisms depending on the cell source. How are these differences related to the physio-logy of each cell type? This is a question that needs further investigation.

Thyrotropin-releasing hormone (TRH)

Thyrotropin-releasing hormone is a neuropeptide that stimulates phosphatidyl turnover and Ca^{2+} release from internal stores. In perforated patches {52} and cell-attached patches {21}, but not outside-out patches, TRH was able to induce an increase in K_{Ca} channel open probability, suggesting that an intracellular signal-transduction mechanism is involved in this response. Whether the simple increase of $[Ca^{2+}]_i$ or other mechanisms such as G-protein gating or phosphorylation are responsible for activation of K_{Ca} channels after TRH stimulation is still unclear.

MECHANISMS OF REGULATION OF MAXI-K_{Ca} CHANNELS

Table 48-1 compiles the actions of various metabolites capable of producing a change in K_{Ca} channel activity in channels from coronary smooth muscle and other tissues and indicates the possible mechanisms involved in the modulatory process: (a) changes in intracellular calcium, $[Ca^{2+}]_i$; (b) ligand modulation (direct action on the channel or a closely associated molecule); (c) phosphorylation/dephosphorylation; and/or (d) G-protein gating {for a recent review see 98}. It is important to stress that the physiological response of K_{Ca} channels to a stimulus may involve more than one mechanism that can be either activatory or inhibitory.

Ligand modulation

The mechanism of ligand modulation implies that the protein constituting the "maxi" K_{Ca} channel possesses a receptor site for its modulator or else that the binding of the agonist to a closely associated receptor molecule (e.g., a regulatory subunit, associated receptor) can cause a modification in channel gating (fig. 48-6A). The existence of this type of mechanism has been experimentally supported not only using excised patches, but with a more stringent control of the solutes in the microenvironment of the channel by using reconstituted channels in lipid bilayers. Metabolites found to modulate K_{Ca} channels in this fashion are (a) in coronary smooth muscle, angiotensin II {93}, thromboxane A_2 {86}, and (b) in other tissues, nucleotides {107}, arachidonic acid {41}, and protons {12,17,18,46,51}.

As discussed in the previous section, K_{Ca} channels from coronary smooth muscle, incorporated into lipid bilayers, are inhibited by the vasoconstrictors Ag-II {93} and TXA_2 {86} (fig. 48-4), and activated by AA {83} without a requirement of added nucleotides or protein kinases, suggesting a "direct" action of these vasoactive substances on K_{Ca} channels or a closely associated protein (regulatory subunit?).

A typical example of "direct" modulation of K_{Ca} channels in other systems is AA. Kirber et al. {41} and Katz et

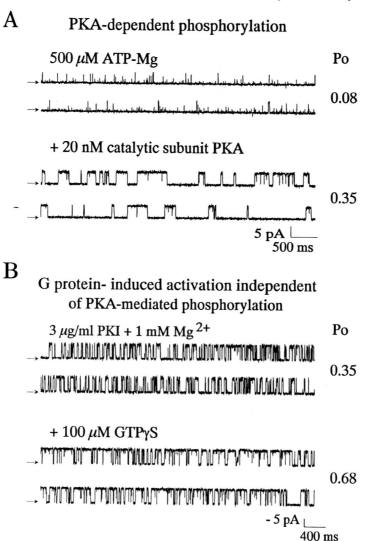

A   PKA-dependent phosphorylation

500 μM ATP-Mg   Po

0.08

+ 20 nM catalytic subunit PKA

0.35

5 pA |___
     500 ms

B   G protein- induced activation independent
     of PKA-mediated phosphorylation

3 μg/ml PKI + 1 mM Mg^{2+} Po

0.35

+ 100 μM GTPγS

0.68

- 5 pA |___
       400 ms

Fig. 48-5. Phosphorylation and G-protein-mediated activation of K_{Ca} channels are two independent processes. **A:** Phosphorylation of K_{Ca} channels from coronary smooth muscle by PKA causes activation. **B:** Activation of K_{Ca} channels by a G protein (with GTP-γS) in the presence of a PKA inhibitor (PKI). The G-protein-mediated activation of channel activity did not require a PKA-phosphorylating process; thus K_{Ca} channels (or a closely associated molecule) from coronary smooth muscle can be activated by both a direct G-protein gating mechanism and by PKA-dependent phosphorylation in an independent manner {84,85}. 250/250 KCl; V_H = 20 mV (A); V_H = −40 mV (B).

al. {38} demonstrated that K_{Ca} channels from vascular smooth muscle can be activated by AA at concentrations ranging from 50 nM to 20 μM. Because this effect could be reproduced by fatty acids that are not substrates of the cyclooxygenase nor of the lipoxygenase metabolic pathways, and occurred in inside-out patches in the "absence" of nucleotides and calcium (5 mM EGTA), it was suggested that AA may directly modulate K_{Ca} channel activity {41}. This type of mechanism has also been postulated for the activation of a small conductance K+ channel ($\approx$30 pS) from smooth muscle of the toad *Bufo marinus* {70}. These results are consistent with the idea that AA may modulate the channel or a closely associated molecule, and that this effect cannot be explained by changes in calcium, transduction pathways leading to phosphorylation, or G proteins. However, it is possible that in the complex cellular machinery AA also serves as a second messenger stimulating a G protein {1}, which in turn triggers a metabolic cascade or activates the channel in a direct "membrane delimited" way.

A   **Ligand modulation**

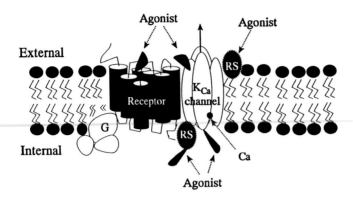

B

**Phosphorylation and G-protein gating
may occur as independent mechanisms**

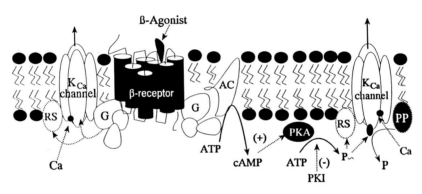

G protein gating   PKA-mediated phosphorylation

Fig. 48-6. Schemes proposing possible routes or mechanisms of ligand modulation, phosphorylation, and G-protein gating of K_{Ca} channels from coronary smooth muscle. **A:** Ligand modulation. The extracellular or intracellular interaction of the agonist (e.g., arachidonic acid) with a receptor, the channel, or a closely related molecule (e.g., regulatory subunit, RS) modulates K_{Ca} channel activity. **B:** Possible pathways of modulation explaining beta-adrenergic stimulation of K_{Ca} channels from coronary smooth muscle. After binding of the β-agonist to its receptor, at least two independent mechanisms may occur: (1) G-protein gating (left) and (2) PKA-mediated phosphorylation (right) {85}. G_S, G_S protein; PKI, protein kinase inhibitor; RS, regulatory subunit; PP, phosphatase; (+) activation; (−) inhibition.

Phosphorylation/dephosphorylation

PKA-DEPENDENT PHOSPHORYLATION

The first direct evidence that a calcium-activated K^+ channel may be activated by PKA-mediated phosphorylation was put forward by Ewald et al. {23}, who demonstrated that an intermediate-K_{Ca} channel (40–60 pS) from neurons of *Helix aspersa* could be activated by the kinase in isolated membrane patches and in bilayers. Since then

several laboratories have searched for agonists that trigger the metabolic cascade leading to modulation of K_{Ca} channels via PKA-dependent phosphorylation. Up to the present, agonists that have been shown to induce PKA-dependent phosphorylation are beta-adrenergic agents, in aorta and trachea smooth muscle {47,80}, and secretin in pancreatic duct cells {32}. The general transduction scheme for PKA-dependent phosphorylation would be (a) binding of the agonist to its receptor, (b) activation of a coupled G protein (G_s), (c) activation of adenylyl cyclase and increase in cAMP levels, (d) activation of cAMP-dependent protein kinase (PKA), and (e) ATP-dependent phosphorylation of the effector (e.g., K_{Ca} channel) or a closely related molecule (e.g., regulatory subunit or G-protein?) (fig. 48-6B).

In coronary smooth muscle, phosphorylation of K_{Ca} channels by PKA has received little attention. As mentioned before, in studies in which we explored the mechanisms of regulation of K_{Ca} channels after beta-adrenergic stimulation, we found that they can be activated by both PKA-dependent phosphorylation (fig. 48-5A) and G-protein activation in an independent manner {85} (fig. 48-5B).

PKA may induce both an increase in channel open probability or an inhibition of channel activity in K_{Ca} channels from several sources. For example, K_{Ca} channels from gonadotrophs of ovine pituitary {87}, a "type 2" K_{Ca} channel from brain vesicles {77}, and K_{Ca} channels from human nonpregnant myometrium {75} are inhibited by PKA-dependent phosphorylation. On the other hand, activation of K_{Ca} channels has been shown in a variety of tissues, including aortic, tracheal, and colonic myocytes {11,47,80}, pancreatic duct cells {32}, brain {13,77}, and our own observations in coronary {85} and pregnant uterine smooth muscle {74}. The activation of K_{Ca} channels by phosphorylation increases the affinity of the channels for Ca^{2+} without a modification of the Hill coefficient of the process {77}. Because the change in channel gating produced by phosphorylation is comparable with the one observed after Ca^{2+} activation, it is possible that phosphorylation modulates the Ca^{2+} sensor of K_{Ca} channels. Therefore, phosphorylation or dephosphorylation of different sites in K_{Ca} channels may contribute to the variety in Ca^{2+} affinities found in K_{Ca} channels of the same class.

The dual regulation by phosphorylation of the same class of channels may be explained by the existence of several isoforms of K_{Ca} channels with different relevant phosphorylation sites, or else by the assumption that the regulatory proteins or subunits associated with the channel-forming protein differ according to the tissue. In fact, several isoforms of K_{Ca} channels have been observed in coronary smooth muscle {99} and at least two types in brain {24,77}. Moreover, molecular studies of *slowpoke* (cloned K_{Ca} channel from *Drosophila*) transcripts indicate that a large number of K_{Ca} channels isoforms may exist {49}.

PHOSPHORYLATION BY OTHER PROTEIN KINASES

To our knowledge the actions of other protein kinases, such as calmodulin-dependent protein kinase, cGMP-protein kinase, and protein kinase C, on K_{Ca} channels have not been reported yet. Even though phosphorylation of K_{Ca} channels from coronary smooth muscle by protein kinase C (PKC) has not been demonstrated directly, modulation of K_{Ca} channels by PKC-dependent phosphorylation is likely to occur, since several agonists, such as angiotensin II, thromboxane A_2, bradykinin, and histamine, known to increase lipid turnover via phospholi-

pase C (PLC), control K_{Ca} channel activity {6,97} (table 48-1). Moreover, the K_{Ca} channel (*slowpoke*) cloned from *Drosophila* has more consensus sites for PKC- than for PKA-dependent phosphorylation {2,4}. The modulation of K_{Ca} channel activity by these agonists could occur through the following scheme: agonist → receptor → G_{plc}-*protein* → PLC → *IP₃ + diacylglycerol*; [IP₃ → release Ca^{2+}]; [diacylglycerol → activation of PKC → PKC-mediated phosphorylation]. In this sequence of reactions modulation of K_{Ca} channels by PKC-mediated phosphorylation would be the final step; however, it is obvious that other ways of regulation are possible as well. We have italicized modulatory candidates other than Ca^{2+} and phosphorylation that need to be explored: G_{plc}-protein, IP₃, and diacylglycerol.

PHOSPHORYLATION/DEPHOSPHORYLATION

K_{Ca} channels, similar to other proteins regulated by phosphorylation, can also be dephosphorylated. A balance between these two chemical modifications on the channel protein or a closely associated molecule (G protein?, channel subunit?) may be relevant to control cellular excitability and function.

Modulation of K_{Ca} channels by phosphorylation/dephosphorylation cycles has been suggested from experiments in intact cells from colonic smooth muscle and pituitary tumor {11,105} and in K_{Ca} channels from brain after incorporation into lipid bilayers 13}, for review see 98. It is interesting that both types of experiments point to the conclusion that endogenous phosphatases may be in close association with K_{Ca} channels {11,13}. Moreover, the experiments in lipid bilayers support the idea that K_{Ca} channels form stable complexes with modulatory proteins, in this case PK and phosphatases, that remain functionally coupled after incorporation into the lipid bilayer {13}, as was previously proposed for the complex receptor/G-protein/K_{Ca} channel {95}.

G-protein gating

G-protein gating type of modulation was first proposed for the muscarinic K^+ channel from atrial cells {6,10}. This mechanism requires that after the agonist is bound to its receptor, a coupled G protein is activated, followed by the direct interaction of the activated G protein, with the channel protein modifying its gating properties. Recent evidence in coronary {84,85}, myometrial {95}, tracheal {44,45}, and colonic {14,15} smooth muscles has put forward the hypothesis that K_{Ca} channels might be coupled and be substrates of G-protein modulation.

In coronary smooth muscle, direct evidence that supports this hypothesis involves studies in lipid bilayers in which we have demonstrated that K_{Ca} channels from coronary smooth muscle may be modulated by both endogenous G proteins (GTP- or GTPγS-mediated stimulation) or exogenous purified G proteins under conditions in which PKA-dependent phosphorylation is inhibited {84,85} (fig. 48-5B). The receptor involved in this activation seems to be beta-adrenergic, since isoproterenol could activate K_{Ca} channels incorporated into lipid bilayers solely in the presence of GTP and Mg^{2+}, which are necessary to activate the endogenous G protein. In other tissues, the agonists that have produced activation of K_{Ca} channels by G proteins are acetylcholine and beta-adrenergic agents.

ADRENERGIC STIMULATION

Beta-adrenergic stimulation causes an increase in K_{Ca} channel activity in smooth muscle from coronary arteries {85}, aorta {80}, trachea {44}, and uterus {3,95}. Because these channels are abundant in smooth muscle and their activation would lead to hyperpolarization of the cell membrane, it is very plausible that they play a major role during beta-adrenergic induced relaxation. In tracheal smooth muscle isoprenalin causes 10 times more relaxation than forskolin (which activates adenylyl cyclase) {35}, indicating that mechanism(s) other than PKA-dependent phosphorylation (of K_{Ca} channels?) may be involved after beta-adrenergic stimulation. In fact in cell-attached patches from the same tissue, isoprenaline in the bath increased the open probability of K_{Ca} channels about seven times, while PKA-dependent phosphorylation in inside-out patches only caused a fourfold increase in channel activity {47}. In this type of experiment it has been assumed that if the agonist is not required in the pipette to activate the channel, then the most likely mechanism to occur is one that involves a second messenger, such as cAMP, and the subsequent activation of K_{Ca} channels via PKA-dependent phosphorylation. Even though phosphorylation may partially explain these results, how can one explain that beta-adrenergic stimulation is more potent in stimulating K_{Ca} channel activity than the sole PKA-mediated phosphorylation? One can speculate that although the agonist was present in the bath and not in the pipette (close to the channel), it is possible that the tip of the pipette does not make an absolute barrier and that a receptor (near the pipette tip) is able to activate a G protein coupled to the channel inducing its activation. Thus a G-protein-gated mechanism may be parallel to PKA-dependent phosphorylation of K_{Ca} channels after beta-adrenergic stimulation.

Can a G protein directly modulate K_{Ca} channels?

We have tested the hypothesis that beta-adrenergic stimulation of K_{Ca} channels may involve a G-protein gating mechanism aside from the G-protein mediated activation of the adenylyl cyclase pathway, which leads to phosphorylation. To this end, we have used reconstituted membrane vesicles in lipid bilayers; in this system, most likely, the exchange of the vesicle content with the experimental solution is much more efficient than in isolated patches in which the solution exchange may be substantially limited by the geometry and attached components (e.g., microfilaments) of the membrane patch. We found that K_{Ca} channels from coronary smooth muscle in lipid bilayers (in the absence of added phosphorylating agents) were activated by GTP or GTPγS solely in the presence of

Mg^{2+} from the "intracellular" side {84}, as previously shown for myometrium smooth muscle {95}. In addition, experiments in the presence of inhibitors of PKA-dependent phosphorylation, such as AMP-PNP (adenylyl-imidodiphosphate, a nonphosphorylating analog of ATP), PKI, or IP20, gave similar results (fig. 48-5B), indicating that activation of K_{Ca} channels by GTP or GTP-γS was not due to phosphorylation via "contaminant" or "endogenous" ATP, cAMP, or protein kinase A. In agreement with a G-protein gating mechanism triggered by beta-adrenergic stimulation, K_{Ca} channel activity was potentiated by "extracellular" application of the beta agonist isoproterenol in the presence of GTP and Mg^{2+}, and inhibited by external application of the beta antagonist, propranolol {85}. These results taken together strongly suggested to us that K_{Ca} channels can be activated through a coupled GTP-dependent protein and that this mechanism may participate in the beta-adrenergic stimulation of K_{Ca} channels. Furthermore, they stressed the fact that the beta receptor, the stimulatory G protein, and the K_{Ca} channel were coupled and formed a stable association that was not disrupted after incorporation into the lipid bilayer.

Which is the nature of the G protein that gates K_{Ca} channels, and how are K_{Ca} channels gated?

Experiments performed on K_{Ca} channels from coronary smooth muscle, in lipid bilayers, indicate that the stimulatory G protein may be G_s {85}. Stimulation of K_{Ca} channels by the activated $G\alpha_s$ subunit (α_s^*) resembles the increase in channel activity observed with GTP-γS, strongly suggesting that the endogenous G protein is G_s. Both GTP-γS and α_s^* caused a shift in the voltage-activation curve towards more negative potentials, making the channel behave as if its affinity for Ca^{2+} was higher {84}, and induced a change in kinetics that fundamentally consisted of a decrease in the time the channel remained in the long closed states. Furthermore, the potentiation of K_{Ca} channels with α_s^* was persistent in the presence of the PKA inhibitor, PKI, indicating that PKA-mediated phosphorylation was not the cause of channel activation. Consistent with these results in coronary smooth muscle, Kume et al. {44} have recently shown that the α subunit of G_S may activate K_{Ca} channels in tracheal myocytes.

In summary, two independent mechanisms for beta-adrenergic stimulation of K_{Ca} channels may be proposed: (a) direct G-protein gating and (b) phosphorylation via PKA. Certainly it is possible that other parallel mechanisms may occur.

MUSCARINIC REGULATION

K_{Ca} channels from coronary {27}, colonic {14,15}, and tracheal smooth muscle {45} are modulated by muscarinic agents. K_{Ca} channels from coronary {27} and tracheal {64} smooth muscle are activated, probably due to a rise in $[Ca^{2+}]_i$; while those from tracheal {45} and colonic {14,15} myocytes are inhibited, most likely via a G-protein action.

Cole et al. {14} observed that acetylcholine (ACh,

$10 \mu M$) diminished K_{Ca} channel activity when present in the bath and pipette solutions. This inhibition was absent in inside-out patches with ACh in the pipette or when ACh was only applied to the bath but not to the pipette in the cell-attached mode. Furthermore, the inhibition of whole-cell currents required GTP or nonhydrolyzable GTP analogs (GTP-γS or 5'-guanylylimidodiphosphate) in the pipette {15}. These results indicated that (a) in inside-out patches essential internal components were lost (GTP?), preventing muscarinic inhibition to take place, (b) in cell-attached patches the coupling molecule (G-protein?) between the muscarinic receptor and the channel was functional only if they were in "close" proximity, and (c) a GTP-dependent protein coupled the receptor occupancy with channel inhibition.

Similarly, Kume and Kotlikoff {45} demonstrated that K_{Ca} channels are inhibited by extracellular metacholine ($50 \mu M$) in outside-out patches. An interesting observation was that the inhibition could take place in the absence of added GTP in the pipette. However, this "basal" inhibition was larger and more consistent when GTP or GTP-γS was included in the pipette and was abolished in the presence of GDP-βS. These results favored the idea that metacholine induced inhibition of K_{Ca} channels through a GTP-dependent mechanism (G protein). This idea implies that in outside-out patches the intracellular milieu is not completely exchanged with the pipette content, as was traditionally thought, but that a sufficient amount of nucleotides remain in the microenvironment of the G protein and channel, permitting the activation of the former and the inhibition of the latter.

The role of a G protein in the muscarinic-induced inhibition of K_{Ca} channels was confirmed by its inhibition with pertussis toxin. Intracellular dialysis or incubation of the cells with pertussis toxin suppressed the muscarinic-mediated inhibition of K_{Ca} whole-cell {15} and single-channel currents {44,45}. These experiments taken together with those previously described are consistent with a role of a pertussis toxin-sensitive G protein in the muscarinic inhibition of K_{Ca} channels. In this context, the fact that ACh could not inhibit K_{Ca} channels in inside-out patches when it was only present in the pipette may be explained by the absence of GTP in the external solution necessary to activate the proximal G protein. On the other hand, the requirement of ACh in the pipette in cell-attached experiments supports the idea that (a) after ACh binds to its receptor, a closely related G protein is activated, gating the channel in a direct mode, and (b) a diffusible second messenger produced after the G-protein activation was not involved in the inhibition of K_{Ca} channels. In conclusion, it is very like that muscarinic inhibition of K_{Ca} channels involves a protein-protein interaction between the G protein and the K_{Ca} channel protein (G-protein gating). The identity of this G protein is still an enigma; neither $G\alpha_{i-2}$, $G\alpha_{i-3}$, nor $G\alpha_{o-1}$ were able to mimic the muscarinic response of K_{Ca} channels from tracheal myocytes {44}.

CONCLUSIONS

Study of the coronary smooth muscle physiology at the molecular level utilizing single cells and reconstituted membrane vesicles gives light to our understanding of how coronary arteries behave in physiological or pathophysiological situations. The complexity of the mechanisms of action of vasoactive substances that lead to spasm or counteract constriction makes necessary the use of various experimental approaches to discern which mechanisms are involved and when they occur. In this context, reconstitution experiments have been valuable to better control the microenvironment of the channel under study, which is difficult or uncertain when excised membrane patches are used. The studies summarized and discussed in this review converge to the same conclusion: K_{Ca} channels from coronary smooth muscle cells are modulated by vasoactive substances and may play an important role in coronary physiology and consequently in cardiac function.

ACKNOWLEDGMENTS

Supported by Grant-in-Aid 900963 from the American Heart Association and NIH grant HL47382.

REFERENCES

1. Abramson SB, Leszczynska-Piziak J, Weissmann G: Arachidonic acid as a second messenger: Interactions with a GTP-binding protein of human neutrophils. *J Immunol* 147: 231–236, 1991.
2. Adelman JP, Shen K-Z, Kavanaugh MP, Warren RA, Wu Y-N, Lagrutta A, Bond CT, North RA: Calcium-activated potassium channels expressed from cloned complementary DNAs. *Neuron* 9:209–216, 1992.
3. Anwer K, Toro L, Oberti C, Stefani E, Sanborn BM: Ca^{2+}-activated K$^+$ channels in pregnant rat myometrium: Modulation by a β-adrenergic agent. *Am J Physiol* 263:C1049–C1056, 1992.
4. Atkinson NS, Robertson GA, Ganetzky B: A component of calcium-activated potassium channels encoded by the *Drosophila slo* locus. *Science* 253:551–555, 1991.
5. Benham CD, Bolton TB: Spontaneous transient outward currents in single visceral and vascular smooth muscle cells of the rabbit. *J Physiol* 381:385–406, 1986.
6. Birnbaumer L, vanDongen AMJ, Codina J, Yatani A, Mattera R, Graf R, Brown AM: Identification of G protein-gated and G protein-modulated ionic channels. Molecular basis for G protein action. In: Armstrong CM, Oxford GS (eds) *Secretion and its control*. New York: Rockefeller University Press 1989, pp 18–54.
7. Bkaily G, Peyrow M, Sculptoreanu A, Jacques D, Chahine M, Regoli D, Sperelakis N: Angiotensin II increases I_{si} and blocks I_{kappa} in single aortic cell of rabbit. *Pflügers Arch* 412:448–450, 1988.
8. Brayden JE, Nelson MT: Regulation of arterial tone by activation of calcium-dependent potassium channels. *Science* 532:535, 1992.
9. Brown AM, Functional bases for interpreting amino acid sequences of voltage-dependent K$^+$ channels. *Annu Rev Biophys Biomol Struct* 22:173–198, 1993.

10. Brown AM, Birnbaumer L: Ionic channels and their regulation by G protein subunits. *Annu Rev Physiol* 52:197–213, 1990.

11. Carl A, Kenyon JL, Uemura D, Fusetani N, Sanders KM: Regulation of Ca^{2+}-activated K^+ channels by protein kinase A and phosphatase inhibitors. *Am J Physiol Cell Physiol* 261:C387–C392, 1991.

12. Christensen O, Zeuthen T: Maxi K^+ channels in leaky epithelia are regulated by intracellular Ca^{2+}, pH and membrane potential. *Pflügers Arch* 408:249–259, 1987.

13. Chung S, Reinhart PH, Martin BL, Brautigan D, Levitan IB: Protein kinase activity closely associated with a reconstituted calcium-activated potassium channel. *Science* 253:560–562, 1991.

14. Cole WC, Carl A, Sanders KM: Muscarinic suppression of Ca^{2+}-dependent K current in colonic smooth muscle. *Am J Physiol* 257:C481–C487, 1989.

15. Cole WC, Sanders KM: G proteins mediate suppression of Ca^{2+}-activated K current by acetylcholine in smooth muscle cells. *Am J Physiol* 257:C596–C600, 1989.

16. Cook DI, Young JA: Ca^+ ion channels and secretion. In: Young, Wong (eds) Epithelial secretion of water and electrolytes. Berlin: Springer-Verlag, 1990, pp 15–38.

17. Cook DL, Ikeuchi M, Fujimoto WY: Lowering of pH_i inhibits Ca^{2+}-activated K^+ channels in pancreatic B-cells. *Nature* 311:269–271, 1984.

18. Copello J, Segal Y, Reuss L: Cytosolic pH regulates maxi K^+ channels in *Necturus* gall-bladder epithelial cells. *J Physiol (Lond)* 434:577–590, 1991.

19. D'Orleans-Juste P, De Nucci G, Vane JR: Endothelin-1 contracts isolated vessels independently of dihydropyridine-sensitive Ca^{2+} channel activation. *Eur J Pharmacol* 165:289–295, 1989.

20. Daut J, Maier-Rudolph W, Von Beckerath N, Mehrke G, Günther K, Goedel-Meinen L: Hypoxic dilation of coronary arteries is mediated by ATP-sensitive potassium channels. *Science* 247:1341–1344, 1990.

21. Dubinsky JM, Oxford GS: Dual modulation of K channels by thyrotropin-releasing hormone in clonal pituitary cells. *Proc Natl Acad Sci USA* 82:4282–4286, 1985.

22. Escande D, Thuringer D, Leguern S, Cavero I: The potassium channel opener cromakalim (BRL 34915) activates ATP-dependent K^+ channels in isolated cardiac myocytes. *Biochem Biophys Res Commun* 154:620–625, 1988.

23. Ewald DA, Williams A, Levitan IB: Modulation of single Ca^{2+}-dependent K^+-channel activity by protein phosphorylation. *Nature* 315:503–506, 1985.

24. Farley J, Rudy B: Multiple types of voltage-dependent Ca^{2+}-activated K^+ channels of large conductance in rat brain synaptosomal membranes. *Biophys J* 53:919–934, 1988.

25. Folta A, Joshua IG, Webb RC: Dilator actions of endothelin in coronary resistance vessels and the abdominal aorta of the guinea pig. *Life Sci* 45:2627–2635, 1989.

26. Fujino K, Nakaya S, Wakatsuki T, Miyoshi Y, Nakaya Y, Mori H, Inoue I: Effects of nitroglycerin on ATP-induced Ca^{2+}-mobilization, Ca^{2+}-activated K channels and contraction of cultured smooth muscle cells of porcine coronary artery. *J Pharmacol Exp Ther* 256:371–377, 1991.

27. Ganitkevich V, Isenberg G: Isolated guinea pig coronary smooth muscle cells: Acetylcholine induces hyperpolarization due to sarcoplasmic reticulum calcium release activating potassium channels. *Circ Res* 67:525–528, 1990.

28. Gelband CH, Carl A, Post JM, Bowen SM, Ishikawa T, Keef KD, Sanders KM, Hume JR: Effect of cromakalim and lemakalim on whole-cell and single-channel K^+ currents in canine colonic, renal and coronary smooth muscle cells. In: Speralakis N, Kuriyama H (eds) *Ion Channels of Vascular*

Smooth Muscle Cells and Endothelial Cells. New York: Elsevier Science, 1991, pp 125–138.

29. Gelband CH, Lodge NJ, Van Breemen C: A Ca^{2+}-activated K^+ channel from rabbit aorta: Modulation by cromakalim. *Eur J Pharmacol* 167:201–210, 1989.

30. Glavinovic MI: Effect of acetylcholine on single Ca^{2+}-activated K^+ channels in bovine chromaffin cells. *Neuroscience* 39:815–822, 1990.

31. Goto K, Kasuya Y, Matsuki N, Takuwa Y, Kurihara H, Ishikawa T, Kimura S, Yanagisawa M, Masaki T: Endothelin activates the dihydropyridine-sensitive, voltage-dependent Ca^{2+} channel in vascular smooth muscle. *Proc Natl Acad Sci USA* 86:3915–3918, 1989.

32. Gray MA, Greenwell JR, Garton AJ, Argent BE: Regulation of maxi-K^+ channels on pancreatic duct cells by cyclic AMP-dependent phosphorylation. *J Membr Biol* 115:203–215, 1990.

33. Griendling KK, Tsuda T, Berk BC, Alexander RW: Angiotensin II stimulation of vascular smooth muscle. *J Cardiovasc Pharmacol* 14(Suppl 6):S27–S33, 1989.

34. Guggino SE, Suarez-Isla BA, Guggino WB, Sacktor B: Forskolin and antidiuretic hormone stimulate a Ca^{2+}-activated K^+ channel in cultured kidney cells. *Am J Physiol* 249:F448–F455, 1985.

35. Honda K, Satake T, Takagi K, Tomita T: Effects of relaxants on electrical and mechanical activities in the guinea-pig tracheal muscle. *Br J Pharmac* 87:665–671, 1986.

36. Hu S, Kim HS, Jeng AY: Dual action of endothelin-1 on the Ca^{2+}-activated K^+ channel in smooth muscle cells of porcine coronary artery. *Eur J Pharmacoly* 194:31–36, 1991.

37. Johns DW, Sperelakis N: Angiotensin stimulates Ca^{2+}-dependent action potentials in cultured smooth muscle cells. *Eur J Pharmacol* 187:183–191, 1990.

38. Katz G, Roy-Contancin L, Bale T, Reuben JP: Arachidonic, linoleic, and other unsaturated fatty acids enhance K^+ and depress Na^+ and Ca^{2+} channel activity. *Biophys J* 57:506, 1990.

39. Kavanaugh MP, Hurst RS, Yakel J, Varnum MD, Adelman JP, North RA: Multiple subunits of a voltage-dependent potassium channel contribute to the binding site for tetraethylammonium. *Neuron* 8:493–497, 1992.

40. Kavanaugh MP, Varnum MD, Osborne PB, Christie MJ, Busch AE, Adelman JP, North RA: Interaction between tetraethylammonium and amino acid residues in the pore of cloned voltage-dependent potassium channels. *J Biol Chem* 266:7583–7587, 1991.

41. Kirber MT, Ordway RW, Clapp LH, Walsh JV Jr, Singer JJ: Both membrane stretch and fatty acids directly activate large conductance Ca^{2+}-activated K^+ channels in vascular smooth muscle cells. *FEBS Lett* 297:24–28, 1992.

42. Klöckner U, Isenberg G: Endothelin depolarizes myocytes from porcine coronary and human mesenteric arteries through a Ca-activated chloride current. *Pflügers Arch* 418:168–175, 1991.

43. Kodama M, Kanaide H, Abe S, Hirano K, Kai H, Nakamura M: Endothelin-induced Ca-independent contraction of the porcine coronary artery. *Biochem Biophys Res Commun* 160:1302–1308, 1989.

44. Kume H, Graziano MP, Kotlikoff MI: Stimulatory and inhibitory regulation of calcium-activated potassium channels by guanine nucleotide-binding proteins. *Proc Natl Acad Sci USA* 89:11051–11055, 1992.

45. Kume H, Kotlikoff MI: Muscarinic inhibition of single K_{Ca} channels in smooth muscle cells by a pertussis-sensitive G protein. *Am J Physiol Cell Physiol* 261:C1204–C1209, 1991.

46. Kume H, Takagi K, Satake T, Tokuno H, Tomita T: Effects of intracellular pH on calcium-activated potassium channels

in rabbit tracheal smooth muscle. *J Physiol (Lond)* 424: 445–457, 1990.

47. Kume H, Takai A, Tokuno H, Tomita T: Regulation of Ca^{2+}-dependent K^+-channel activity in tracheal myocytes by phosphorylation. *Nature* 341:152–154, 1989.

48. Kurachi Y, Ito H, Sugimoto T, Shimizu T, Miki I, Ui M: Arachidonic acid metabolites as intracellular modulators of the G protein-gated cardiac K^+ channel. *Nature* 337: 555–557, 1989.

49. Lagrutta A, Bond CT, Warren RA, North RA, Adelman JP: Diversity of slowpoke potassium channel transcripts. *Biophys J* 61:A377, 1992.

50. Latorre R, Oberhauser A, Labarca P, Alvarez O: Varieties of calcium-activated potassium channels. *Annu Rev Physiol* 51:385–399, 1989.

51. Laurido C, Candia S, Wolff D, Latorre R: Proton modulation of a Ca^{2+}-activated K^+ channel from rat skeletal muscle incorporated into planar bilayers. *J Gen Physiol* 98:1025–1043, 1991.

52. Levitan ES, Kramer RH: Neuropeptide modulation of single calcium and potassium channels detected with a new patch clamp configuration. *Nature* 348:545–547, 1990.

53. Lincoln TM, Cornwell TL: Towards an understanding of the mechanism of action of cyclic AMP and cyclic GMP in smooth muscle relaxation. *Blood Vessels* 28:129–137, 1991.

54. Ling BN, Webster CL, Eaton DC: Eicosanoids modulate apical Ca^{2+}-dependent K^+ channels in cultured rabbit principal cells. *Am J Physiol Renal Fluid Electro Physiol* 263: F116–F126, 1992.

55. MacKinnon, R: Using mutagenesis to study potassium channel mechanisms. *J Bioenerg Biomembr* 23:647–663, 1991.

56. MacKinnon R, Yellen G: Mutations affecting TEA blockade and ion permeation in voltage-activated K^+ channels. *Science* 250:276–279, 1990.

57. Mayer EA, Loo DDF, Kodner A, Reddy SN: Differential modulation of Ca^{2+}-activated K^+ channels by substance P. *Am J Physiol* 257:G887–G897, 1989.

58. Mayer EA, Loo DDF, Snape WJ Jr, Sachs G: The activation of calcium and calcium-activated potassium channels in mammalian colonic smooth muscle by substance P. *J Physiol (Lond)* 420:47–71, 1990.

59. McManus OB: Calcium-activated potassium channels: Regulation by calcium. *J Bioenerg Biomembr* 23:537–560, 1991.

60. McPherson GA, Keily SG, Angus JA: Spasmolytic effect of cromakalim in dog coronary artery in vitro. *Naunyn-Schmiedebergs Arch Pharmacol* 343:519–524, 1991.

61. Miller C, Moczydlowski E, Latorre R, Phillips M: Carybdotoxin, a protein inhibitor of single Ca^{2+}-activated K^+ channels from mammalian skeletal muscle. *Nature* 313:316–318, 1985.

62. Miyoshi Y, Nakaya Y: Angiotensin II blocks ATP-sensitive K^+ channels in porcine coronary artery smooth muscle cells. *Biochem Biophys Res Commun* 181:700–706, 1991.

63. Miyoshi Y, Nakaya Y, Wakatsuki T, Nakaya S, Fujino K, Saito K, Inoue I: Endothelin blocks ATP-sensitive K^+ channels and depolarizes smooth muscle cells of porcine coronary artery. *Circ Res* 70:612–616, 1992.

64. Muraki K, Imaizumi Y, Watanabe M: Ca-dependent K channels in smooth muscle cells permeabilized by β-escin recorded using the cell-attached patch-clamp technique. *Pflügers Arch* 420:461–469, 1992.

65. Myers PR, Guerra R Jr, Harrison DG: Release of NO and EDRF from cultured bovine aortic endothelial cells. *Am J Physiol* 256:H1030–H1037, 1989.

66. Nakahata N, Matsuoka I, Ono T, Nakanishi H: Thromboxane A2 activates phospholipase C in astrocytoma cells via pertussis toxin-insensitive G-protein. *Eur J Pharmacol* 162:407–417, 1989.

67. Oberti C, Anwer K, Sanborn BM, Stefani E, Toro L: Calcium-activated K channels as modulators of human myometrial contractility. *Biophys J* 64:A199, 1993.

68. Ohya Y, Sperelakis N: Involvement of a GTP-binding protein in stimulating action of angiotensin II on calcium channels in vascular smooth muscle cells. *Circ Res* 68:763–771, 1991.

69. Olcese R, Toro L, Perez G, Kavanaugh MP, North RA, Adelman JP, Stefani E: Macroscopic (cut-open oocyte) and reconstituted (bilayer) single channel currents of slowpoke Ca-activated K channels. *Biophys J* 64:A200, 1993.

70. Ordway RW, Walsh JV Jr, Singer JJ: Arachidonic acid and other fatty acids directly activate potassium channels in smooth muscle cells. *Science* 244:1176–1179, 1989.

71. Ottolia M, Toro L: ATP-sensitive potassium channels from coronary smooth muscle reconstituted in lipid bilayers. *Biophys J* 64:A311, 1993.

72. Palmer RMJ, Ferrige AG, Moncada S: Nitric oxide release accounts for the biological activity of endothelium-derived relaxing factor. *Nature* 327:524–526, 1987.

73. Patscheke H: Current concepts for a drug-induced inhibition of formation and action of thromboxane A2. *Blut* 60: 261–268, 1990.

74. Perez G, Stefani E, Toro L: Dual hormonal regulation of PKA-dependent phosphorylation in K(Ca) channels from uterine smooth muscle. *Biophys J* 64:A386, 1993.

75. Perez G, Toro L, Stefani E: Protein kinase A (PKA) modulates calcium activated potassium channel (KCa) from human myometrium. *Biophys J* 61:A255, 1992.

76. Pfründer D, Kreye VAW: Tedisamil blocks single large-conductance Ca^{2+}-activated K^+ channels in membrane patches from smooth muscle cells of the guinea-pig portal vein. *Pflügers Arch* 418:308–312, 1991.

77. Reinhart PH, Chung S, Martin BL, Brautigan DL, Levitan IB: Modulation of calcium-activated potassium channels from rat brain by protein kinase A and phosphatase 2A. *J Neurosci* 11:1627–1635, 1991.

78. Robertson BE, Corry PR, Nye PCG, Kozlowski RZ: Ca^{2+} and Mg-ATP activated potassium channels from rat pulmonary artery. *Pflügers Arch* 421:94–96, 1992.

79. Rusch NJ, De Lucena RG, Wooldridge TA, England SK, Cowley JAW: A Ca^{2+}-dependent K^+ current is enhanced in arterial membranes of hypertensive rats. *Hypertension* 19:301–307, 1992.

80. Sadoshima J-I, Akaike N, Kanaide H, Nakamura M: Cyclic AMP modulates Ca-activated K channel in cultured smooth muscle cells of rat aortas. *Am J physiol* 255:H754–H759, 1988.

81. Savaria D, Lanoue C, Cadieux A, Rousseau E: Large conducting potassium channel reconstituted from airway smooth muscle. *Am J Physiol* 262:L327–L336, 1992.

82. Schrader BJ, Berk SI: Antiplatelet agents in coronary artery disease. *Clin Pharm* 9:118–124, 1990.

83. Scornik F, Toro L: Modulation of Ca-activated K channels from coronary smooth muscle. In: Sperelakis N, Kuriyama H (eds) *Ion Channels of Vascular Smooth Muscle Cells and Endothelial Cells.* Sperelakis New York: Elsevier Science, 1991, pp 111–124.

84. Scornik FS, Codina J, Birnbaumer L, Stefani E, Toro L: Activation of calcium activated potassium K(Ca) channels from pig coronary artery by GTP gammaS may involve a G protein. *Biophys J* 61:A254, 1992.

85. Scornik FS, Codina J, Birnbaumer L, Toro L: Modulation of coronary smooth muscle Kca channels by $G_s\alpha$ independent of phosphorylation by protein kinase A. *Am J Physiol* 265: H1460–H1465, 1993.

86. Scornik FS, Toro L: U46619, a thromboxane A_2 agonist, inhibits KCa channel activity from pig coronary artery. *Am J*

Physiol 262:C708–C713, 1992.

87. Sikdar SK, McIntosh RP, Mason WT: Differential modulation of Ca^{2+}-activated K^+ channels in ovine pituitary gonadotrophs by GnRH, Ca^{2+} and cyclic AMP. *Brain Res* 496: 113–123, 1989.

88. Silberberg SD, Van Breemen C: An ATP, calcium and voltage sensitive potassium channel in porcine coronary artery smooth muscle cells. *Biochem Biophys Res Commun* 172:517–522, 1990.

89. Sperelakis N: Electrophysiology of vascular smooth muscle of coronary artery. In: Kalsner S (ed) *The Coronary Artery.* New York: Oxford University, 1982, pp 118–167.

90. Suarez-Kurtz G, Garcia ML, Kaczorowski GJ: Effects of charybdotoxin and iberiotoxin on the spontaneous motility and tonus of different guinea pig smooth muscle tissues. *J Pharmacol Exp Ther* 259:439–443, 1991.

91. Tare M, Parkington HC, Coleman HA, Neild TO, Dusting GJ: Hyperpolarization and relaxation of arterial smooth muscle caused by nitric oxide derived from the endothelium. *Nature* 346:69–71, 1990.

92. Tomita T: Ionic channels in smooth muscle studied with patch-clamp methods. *Jpn J Physiol* 38:1–18, 1988.

93. Toro L, Amador M, Stefani E: Ang II inhibits calcium-activated potassium channels from coronary smooth muscle in lipid bilayers. *Am J Physiol* 258:H912–H915, 1990.

94. Toro L, Ottolia M, Olcese R, Stefani E: Niflumic acid activates large conductance K(Ca) channels. *Biophys J* 64:A2, 1993.

95. Toro L, Ramos-Franco J, Stefani E: GTP-dependent regulation of myometrial KCa channels incorporated into lipid bilayers. *J Gen Physiol* 96:373–394, 1990.

96. Toro L, Silberberg SD, Brown AM, Stefani E: K^+ and Ca^{2+} currents from coronary smooth muscle cells. *Biophys J* 55:543, 1989.

97. Toro L, Stefani E: Calcium-activated K^+ channels: Metabolic regulation. *J Bioenerg Biomembr* 23:561–576, 1991.

98. Toro L, Stefani E: Modulation of maxi calcium-activated K channels. Role of ligands, phosphorylation and G-proteins. In: Dickey B, Birnbaumer L (eds) *Handbook of Experimental Pharmacology, Vol 108. GTPases in Biology.* New York: Springer-Verlag, 1993, pp 561–579.

99. Toro L, Vaca L, Stefani E: Calcium-activated potassium channels from coronary smooth muscle reconstituted in lipid bilayers. *Am J Physiol Heart Circ Physiol* 260:H1779–H1789, 1991.

100. Trieschmann U, Isenberg G: Ca^{2+}-activated K^+ channels contribute to the resting potential of vascular myocytes. Ca^{2+}-sensitivity is increased by intracellular Mg^{2+} ions. *Pflügers Arch* 414:S183–S184, 1989.

101. Uchida Y, Nakamura F, Tomaru T, Sumino S, Kato A, Sugimoto T: Phasic contractions of canine and human coronary arteries induced by potassium channel blockers. *Jpn Heart J* 27:727–740, 1986.

102. Van Renterghem C, Vigne P, Barhaini J, Schmid-Alliana A, Frelin C, Lazdunski M: Molecular mechanisms of action of the vasoconstrictor peptide endothelin. *Biochem Biophys Res Commun* 157:977–985, 1988.

103. Volk KA, Matsuda JJ, Shibata EF: A voltage-dependent potassium current in rabbit coronary artery smooth muscle cells. *J Physiol (Lond)* 439:751–768, 1991.

104. Wakatsuki T, Nakaya Y, Inoue I: Vasopressin modulates K^+-channel activities of cultured smooth muscle cells from porcine coronary artery. *Am J Physiol Heart Circ Physiol* 263:H491–H496, 1992.

105. White RE, Schonbrunn A, Armstrong DL: Somatostatin stimulates Ca^{2+}-activated K^+ channels through protein dephosphorylation. *Nature* 351:570–573, 1991.

106. Wilde DW, Lee KS: Outward potassium currents in freshly isolated smooth muscle cell of dog coronary arteries. *Circ Res* 65:1718–1734, 1989.

107. Williams DLJ Jr, Katz GM, Roy-Contancin L, Reuben JP: Guanosine 5′-monophosphate modulates gating of high-conductance Ca^{2+}-activated K^+ channels in vascular smooth muscle cells. *Proc Natl Acad Sci USA* 85:9360–9364, 1988.

108. Yanagizawa M, Kurihara H, Kimura S, Tomobe Y, Kobayashi M, Mitsui Y, Yazaki Y, Goto K: A novel potent vasoconstrictor peptide produced by vascular endothelial cells. *Nature* 332:411–415, 1988.

109. Yellen G: Ionic permeation and blockade in Ca-activated K-channels of bovine chromaffin cells. *J Gen Physiol* 84:157–186, 1984.

110. Young MA, Vatner SF: Regulation of large coronary arteries. *Circ Res* 59:579–596, 1986.

CHAPTER 49

ATP-Sensitive Potassium Channels: Properties, Distribution, and Role in Cardiovascular Regulation

JOSEPH E. BRAYDEN

INTRODUCTION

Potassium channels play an important role in both the inhibitory and excitatory activity of many tissues. The degree of membrane permeability to potassium is a key regulator of membrane potential, and hence an important determinant of the level of activation of most excitable tissues {1}. In vascular smooth muscle the resting membrane potential is determined by membrane conductance to several ions, including potassium, sodium, and chloride, and in part by sodium/potassium pump activity {2}. Blockade of potassium conductances results in substantial membrane depolarization, with the onset of regenerative electrical activity in some normally quiescent vascular preparations. Conversely, activation of potassium channels results in pronounced hyperpolarization and inhibition of force in vascular smooth muscle.

Numerous potassium channels with different pharmacological and biophysical properties have been identified. Chief among these in vascular smooth muscle are calcium-activated potassium channels, delayed rectifier potassium channels, inward rectifier potassium channels, and ATP-sensitive potassium (K_{ATP}) channels {2,6}. The relative importance of each of these channels is both species and tissue specific. However, recent evidence has indicated the general significance of the K_{ATP} channel as a mediator of vasodilation induced by numerous means. The purpose of this chapter is to provide a brief historical overview of the significance of K_{ATP} channels in the cardiovascular system and then to provide evidence for involvement of K_{ATP} channels in the regulation of coronary artery function. A number of excellent reviews of the biophysics and physiology of the ATP-sensitive potassium channel have been published and should be consulted for more detail on these topics {4–9}.

GENERAL PROPERTIES OF K_{ATP} CHANNELS

K_{ATP} channels were first identified in cardiac myocytes by Noma in 1983 {10} and since then have been described in pancreatic beta cells {11,12}, skeletal muscle {13}, certain neurons {14,15}, and most recently in vascular {16} and nonvascular smooth muscle {17}. The primary dis-

tinguishing feature of this channel is that it is inhibited by exposure of the intracellular face of the cell membrane to ATP (Ki: 50–500 µM). This particular characteristic provides the possibility for regulation of channel activity, and therefore electrical excitability, by cellular metabolism. K_{ATP} channels are highly selective for potassium and are also specifically inhibited by sulfonylurea compounds, such as glibenclamide and tolbutamide {18,19}, which have been used as antidiabetic agents for many years. Using the patch-clamp technique, investigators have found the single-channel conductance of K_{ATP} channels in cardiac cells to be in the range of 50–70 pS in symmetrical K^+ solutions, i.e., when the intracellular and extracellular sides of the membrane are exposed to the same $[K^+]$, usually 140 mM K^+. However, this single-channel conductance value can vary considerably from tissue to tissue, or depending on the conditions of study (see below). Unlike other K^+ channels, such as the inward rectifier, delayed rectifier, and calcium-activated potassium channels, K_{ATP} channels show only a weak voltage dependence in their level of activity (i.e., their open-state probability is only slightly affected by changes in membrane potential) {3}.

REGULATORS OF K_{ATP} CHANNELS

ATP/ADP ratio and pH_i

Significant inhibition of K_{ATP} channels by ATP occurs at concentrations of the nucleotide that are far below physiological levels in cells. This would suggest that metabolic regulation of the channel might be likely to occur only under extreme conditions where formation of ATP is severely limited. However, various factors can alter the sensitivity of the channel to inhibition by ATP. For instance, in cardiac muscle the ratio of ATP to ADP may be particularly important, with a decrease in this ratio associated with an increase in channel activity {20,21}. Thus conditions resulting in altered metabolism of ADP as well as ATP could influence K_{ATP} channel activity. Another condition that affects inhibition by ATP is intracellular pH. This has been particularly well documented in skeletal

N. Sperelakis (ed.), *Physiology and Pathophysiology of the Heart, Third Edition.*

muscle cells {22}. As intracellular pH falls, the inhibitory effect of ATP decreases.

Inhibition by sulfonylureas

As indicated above, another key distinguishing feature of K_{ATP} channels is the inhibition of channel activity by sulfonylurea agents. This effect is highly selective for K_{ATP} channels, although there are apparently some tissue-specific differences in affinity of these drugs for the channel. For instance, the Ki for glibenclamide inhibition of K_{ATP} channels in pancreatic beta cells is in the range of 4–50 nM {12,23}, whereas in cardiac and smooth muscle it is in the range of 5–20 μM {7,16}.

Other regulators

Other substances, such as guanine nucleotides, MgATP (in cardiac and smooth muscle), or cyclic AMP (in cardiac and beta cells), are either required to sustain channel activity or may participate in mechanisms of activation of the channel. In the absence of MgATP, K_{ATP} channel activity in membrane patches isolated from cardiac myocytes declines ("runs down") with time. MgATP can prevent or reverse this loss of channel activity, suggesting that some phosphorylation event is important in maintaining full channel activity {24,25}. Similarly, G proteins may help to maintain K_{ATP} channel activity {26} and may be involved in the mechanisms of coupling of receptor activation and K_{ATP} channel activity {27}. In pancreatic beta cells, cyclic AMP and the catalytic subunit of protein kinase A enhance the activity of K_{ATP} channels {28}.

K^+ channel openers

K_{ATP} channels can be activated by a number of substances, chief among these are the so-called potassium channel openers {23}. Agents such as cromakalim, pinacidil, RP49356, and nicorandil activate K_{ATP} channels in cardiac muscle cells {29–31}; diazoxide and cromakalim activate K_{ATP} channels in insulin-secreting cells {32}. In cardiac myocytes, potassium channel openers decrease the sensitivity of K_{ATP} channels to ATP and thereby can activate these channels in the face of a constant level of ATP {29,33}.

PHYSIOLOGICAL SIGNIFICANCE OF K_{ATP} CHANNELS IN NON-SMOOTH MUSCLE TISSUES

Cardiac muscle

In cardiac muscle under normal conditions, the K_{ATP} channel may play little role in the electrophysiological behavior and excitability of this tissue. However, K_{ATP} channels may be particularly important in relation to the response of cardiac muscle to ischemic or hypoxic insult. During global ischemia the K_{ATP} channel is activated as a result of a reduction in the formation of ATP {34}. Activation of K_{ATP} channels will shorten the cardiac action

potential. This may result in a reduction of calcium influx and a depression of contractility of the cardiac cells, and may account in part for the negative inotropic, perhaps cardioprotective, effect in the ischemic myocardium. Others have postulated that activation of K_{ATP} channels during conditions of *regional* ischemia may have proarrhythmic effects due to an enhanced rate of repolarization {35}. Thus, depending on the nature and severity of ischemic insult, the effect of activation of K_{ATP} channels may be either beneficial or detrimental.

Possible role in skeletal muscle fatigue

In skeletal muscle, K_{ATP} channels may be particularly relevant physiologically in relation to the response of muscle to fatigue. It has been proposed that as intracellular levels of ATP and intracellular pH fall during exercise, K_{ATP} channels are activated, and this leads to hyperpolarization and entry of some muscle cells in a given motor unit into a rest state {9}. Concomitant accumulation of potassium ions outside cells may also induce local vasodilation within the skeletal muscle to enhance blood flow and oxygen delivery to the working muscle.

Role in mechanism of insulin release

One of the best-defined physiological roles for K_{ATP} channels relates to the mechanism of insulin release from pancreatic beta cells {36}. When plasma levels of glucose are low, the intracellular concentration of ATP or the ATP/ADP ratio is such that K_{ATP} channels are tonically activated and the beta cell membrane is hyperpolarized. As plasma glucose is elevated, glucose enters the beta cell and glycolysis is increased. The ATP thus generated is sufficient to inhibit a large percentage of K_{ATP} channels and the beta cell depolarizes. Calcium influx is then increased and this triggers the release of insulin. Blockade of K_{ATP} channels by sulfonylureas has effects similar to those caused by enhanced synthesis of ATP in the beta cell, and eventually leads to depolarization, increased calcium entry, and enhanced release of insulin, accounting for the efficacy of these agents in non-insulin-dependent diabetes.

Possible role in neurons

Little is known about the function of K_{ATP} channels in neurones, although a role in regulation of the release of neurotransmitters has been suggested. Amoroso et al. {37} have proposed that increased or decreased delivery of glucose to cells in the substantia nigra, either in various diabetic states or during periods of ischemia or hypoxia, can change the level of activity of K_{ATP} channels in these cells. Subsequent changes in membrane potential may modulate release of GABA, an inhibitory neurotransmitter. This may, in turn, lead to alterations in locomotor activity. The significance of K_{ATP} channels in other parts of the nervous system remains to be elucidated.

K$_{ATP}$ CHANNELS IN VASCULAR SMOOTH MUSCLE

The level of vascular smooth muscle tone at any moment is determined by a balance of excitatory and inhibitory inputs. It is clear that regulation of activity along these pathways involves multiple mechanisms that ultimately determine the concentration of free calcium within the muscle cells. Voltage-dependent calcium channels in the vascular smooth muscle cell membrane are important determinants of the degree of calcium entry, and the level of membrane potential will play a critical role in such calcium channel activity {6}. Because activation of potassium channels in vascular smooth muscle will have significant effects on membrane potential and, therefore, calcium channel activity, potassium channels represent an important control point in regulation of vascular tone. Among the various potassium channels, K$_{ATP}$ channels are now thought to play an important role as mediators of the response of vascular smooth muscle to a variety of pharmacological and endogenous vasodilators as well as to changes in metabolic activity, which can directly influence blood flow in various tissues.

Discovery and distribution of K$_{ATP}$ channels in vascular smooth muscle

The presence of K$_{ATP}$ channels in vascular smooth muscle was suggested by pharmacological evidence, namely, that sulfonylureas had inhibitory effects on the vasodilator actions of substances such as cromakalim, minoxidil, and diazoxide {38,39,40,41}.

K$_{ATP}$ channels were first definitively identified in vascular smooth muscle only recently by Standen et al. {16} using the patch-clamp technique. Based on these studies, it is now clear that potassium-selective ion channels that are inhibited by ATP (1 mM) applied to the intracellular face of the membrane are present in patches of membranes from smooth muscle cells isolated from rat and rabbit mesenteric arteries. The concentration of ATP required to inhibit channel activity by 50% is about 50 μM. Single-channel activity returns after removal of ATP and is

greatly reduced by glibenclamide. These channels are not inhibited by blockers of calcium-activated potassium channels, such as tetraethylammonium chloride (1 mM) or charybdotoxin (100 nM), but are inhibited by other sulphonylureas, such as tolbutamide, and by concentrations of barium (50–100 μM), which have been shown to inhibit K$_{ATP}$ channels in skeletal muscle {42}. The slope conductance of these channels is large, about 130 pS in the presence of 60 mM K$_o$/120 mM K$_i$, but is about 30 pS in physiological concentrations of potassium {43}. Single K$_{ATP}$ channels from these arteries are also activated by K$^+$-channel openers, such as cromakalim and pinacidil, as well as at least one endogenous vasodilator, calcitonin gene-related peptide (see below).

K$_{ATP}$ channels have been identified in several different vascular tissues. Kajioka and colleagues have observed K$_{ATP}$ channels in smooth muscle cells isolated from the portal vein of rabbits {44} and rats {45}. These channels are of lower conductance than in arterial smooth muscle cells (10–15 pS in physiological K$^+$ solutions, 50 pS in symmetrical 140 mM K$^+$ solutions). The channels are inhibited by ATP and glibenclamide, and are activated by potassium channel openers such as pinacidil. Inoue et al. {46,47} have observed a potassium channel in cultured smooth muscle cells from porcine coronary arteries that is inhibited by ATP and glibenclamide, and activated by the K$^+$-channel opener nicorandil. The single-channel conductance is about 30 pS in physiological K$^+$ solutions. This channel has the interesting property of being activated by physiological levels of calcium (>0.1 mM Ca^{+2}) in the *extracellular* medium and, probably because of this characteristic, is tonically active at physiological membrane potentials. These high levels of channel activity at physiological membrane potentials suggest an important role for K$_{ATP}$ channels in regulation of resting membrane potential of coronary arteries.

K$_{ATP}$ channels with large single-channel conductance (260 pS in symmetrical 150 mM K$^+$) have also been observed in renal afferent arterioles from the rabbit {48}. These channels are inhibited by ATP and glibenclamide, and are activated by diazoxide. K$_{ATP}$ channels from canine aortic smooth muscle have been incorporated into planar

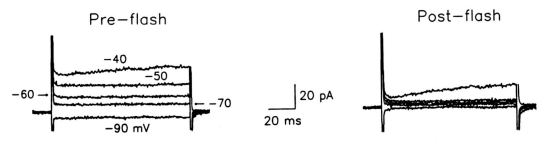

Fig. 49-1. Release of "caged" ATP blocks ATP-sensitive K$^+$ current in pulmonary arterial smooth muscle cells. Whole cell currents were recorded before (Pre-flash) and after (Post-flash) exposing a cell loaded with caged ATP to two brief flashes of light from a xenon lamp, which releases ATP within the cell. Currents were elicited by command pulses to the potentials indicated from a holding potential of −80 mV. The instantaneous (time-independent) currents in the "Pre-flash" example were shown in other cells to be glibenclamide and ATP sensitive. From Clapp and Gurney {50}, with permission.

lipid bilayers {49}, and these large-conductance, potassium-selective channels are also inhibited by ATP and gliben-clamide, and are activated by cromakalim.

The presence of K_{ATP} channels in other vascular smooth muscle preparations has been confirmed by several investigators using the whole-cell current recording technique. Clapp and Gurney {50} found a glibenclamide-sensitive potassium current in vascular smooth muscle cells isolated from rabbit pulmonary artery. These investigators also found that release of ATP by flash photolysis of caged ATP within ATP-depleted cells caused a rapid (within 1 second) block of this potassium current (see fig. 49-1). These experiments clearly indicate the substantial capability of ATP to modulate membrane potential by inhibition of K^+ currents in vascular smooth muscle. Whole-cell potassium currents that are inhibited by glibenclamide and activated by K^+-channel openers (BRL 38227, lemakalim) have also been observed in smooth muscle cells isolated from human mesenteric artery and from rabbit portal vein {51}.

Role of K_{ATP} channels in regulation of vascular smooth muscle

RESPONSE TO PHARMACOLOGICAL VASODILATORS

As mentioned above, a group of chemically distinct substances, including agents such as cromakalim, pinacidil, diazoxide, minoxidil, and nicorandil, have been classified as potassium channel openers. A key feature that these substances have in common is their ability to increase potassium conductance in vascular smooth muscle and thereby hyperpolarize the smooth muscle cell membrane and inhibit tone {4}. A common target of these agents by which they hyperpolarize vascular smooth muscle is the K_{ATP} channel.

The ability of K^+ channel openers to activate K_{ATP} channels in vascular smooth muscle has been demonstrated most comprehensively for cromakalim {16}. As shown in fig. 49-2, single K_{ATP} channels in patches of membrane from rabbit arterial smooth muscle cells are activated by cromakalim. The open-state probability of K_{ATP} channels can be enhanced by 10- to 100-fold by cromakalim, depending on the concentration of ATP to which the cells are exposed. In the presence of cromakalim, glibenclamide dramatically decreases the open-state probability of K_{ATP} channels.

Several investigators have found that K^+ channel openers increase the efflux of labeled K^+ or rubidium and that this effect is inhibited by K_{ATP} channel blockers {52,53}. As would be predicted, the K^+-channel openers can also induce hyperpolarization of vascular smooth muscle cells, either in the intact tissue {23,54} (fig. 49-2) or in isolated cells {50}. This response is inhibited or abolished by glibenclamide or other K_{ATP} channel blockers, but not by blockers of other K^+ channels, such as charybdotoxin, apamin, or low concentrations of TEA^+.

In the presence of tone, isolated arteries are relaxed by the K^+ channel openers (fig. 49-2), and this response can

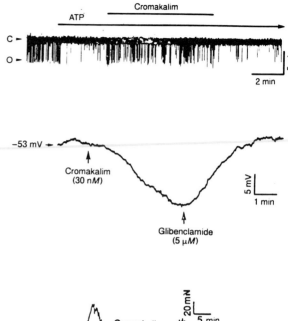

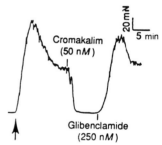

Fig. 49-2. K_{ATP} channels in vascular smooth muscle are activated by K^+ channel openers and inhibited by sulfonylureas. The recording in the top panel shows the inhibitory effect of ATP (1 mM) and the excitatory action of cromakalim (1 μM) on single potassium channels in an inside-out patch of membrane from a rabbit mesenteric arterial smooth muscle cell. The membrane was voltage clamped to −60 mV. C and O correspond to the open and closed levels of the channel. The recording in the middle panel demonstrates the hyperpolarizing effects of cromakalim and block of that effect by glibenclamide in an isolated, intact segment of rabbit middle cerebral artery. (Top and middle records from Brayden et al. {54}, with permission. The lower trace shows the vasodilator effect of cromakalim and reversal of the dilation by glibenclamide in a segment of rabbit mesenteric artery. Active tone was induced using norepinephrine (10 μM) added at the time indicated by the arrow. From Standen et al. {16}, with permission.

be reversed by application of glibenclamide or barium chloride {38–40}. Thus data from a variety of approaches, from single-channel and membrane-potential studies to ion-flux and force measurements, uniformly suggest that K^+ channel openers can activate K_{ATP} channels and that, for many of these agents, this represents the primary and perhaps sole mechanism of vasodilation.

It should be noted that K^+ channel openers can activate other types of potassium channels {4}. High concentrations of cromakalim, diazoxide, or pinacidil can increase the opening of large-conductance calcium-activated potassium channels in vascular smooth muscle. However, the effects of K^+ channel openers on potassium efflux and vascular tone are in general unaffected by blockers of K_{Ca} channels, such as charybdotoxin or low concentrations of TEA^+. Therefore it seems unlikely that the physiological effects of K^+ channel openers are mediated by activation of K_{Ca} channels. Any role of other K^+ channels in this response remains to be determined, but the evidence to date most strongly implicates the K_{ATP} channel as a key mediator of the vascular response to K^+ channel openers.

There is some regional heterogeneity with respect to the apparent distribution of K_{ATP} channels or the distribution of receptors for K^+ channel openers in some vascular beds. For instance, although large diameter arteries in the cerebral circulation relax and hyperpolarize in response to cromakalim {54}, arteries from more distal sites in the same vascular bed are unresponsive to cromakalim {55,56}. This observation may be specific to the cerebral circulation, as large and small arteries from other vascular beds respond well to K^+ channel openers.

RESPONSES TO ENDOGENOUS VASODILATORS

Evidence is also available to suggest that activation of K_{ATP} channels is an important mechanism of action of endogenous vasodilators, such as neurotransmitters, cellular metabolites, and endothelial factors.

Neuropeptides

Calcitonin gene-related peptide (CGRP) is a potent endogenous vasodilator found in perivascular nerves in many tissues {57}. CGRP activates K_{ATP} channels in smooth muscle cells isolated from rabbit mesenteric arteries {43} (fig. 49-3). CGRP also hyperpolarizes the smooth muscle cells in intact mesenteric arteries, and this action is abolished by glibenclamide but is not affected by inhibitors of calcium-activated potassium channels. However, in contrast to the actions of cromakalim, CGRP-induced vasodilation is only partially inhibited by glibenclamide (fig. 49-3). Thus, for this, as well as some other endogenous dilators (see below), membrane hyperpolarization due to activation of K_{ATP} channels may account for only part of the overall mechanism of dilation.

Vasoactive intestinal polypeptide (VIP) is another potent vasodilator that is found in perivascular nerves throughout the cardiovascular system. The effects of K_{ATP} channel blockers on the hyperpolarizing and vasodilator actions of this peptide are comparable to those indicated above for CGRP, suggesting a similar mechanism of action for VIP in some vascular beds {16}.

Endothelium-dependent vasodilators

Another endogenous substance that may activate K_{ATP} channels is the so-called endothelium-derived hyperpolarizing factor {58}. This still unidentified factor is probably distinct from the well-known and intensely studied EDRF/

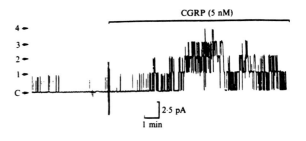

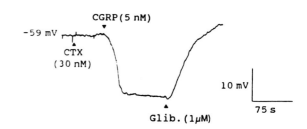

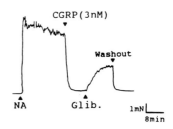

Fig. 49-3. Neuropeptides activate K_{ATP} channels in vascular smooth muscle. In the **top panel** the excitatory effect of calcitonin gene-related peptide (CGRP) on K_{ATP} channels in a smooth muscle cell isolated from the rabbit mesenteric artery is clearly demonstrated. CGRP also hyperpolarizes smooth muscle cells in the intact mesenteric artery, and this effect is reversed by glibenclamide (**middle panel**). CGRP is a potent inhibitor of force, but in contrast to K^+ channel opener-induced vasodilation, only part of the dilator response is reversed by glibenclamide (**lower panel**). From Nelson et al. {43}, with permission.

nitric oxide {59,60}. At least in the rabbit, EDHF seems to activate K_{ATP} channels but, as for other endogenous vasodilators, only part of the dilation to endothelium-dependent vasodilators is due to the membrane hyperpolarization (fig. 49-4) {61,62}. In arteries from other species EDHF is present, but probably does not activate K_{ATP} channels {63}.

Endotoxins and septic shock

Profound hypotension and shock that are unresponsive to vasopressor agents are often associated with endotoxemia. This pathological vascular response to endotoxemia may

Mesenteric Resistance Artery

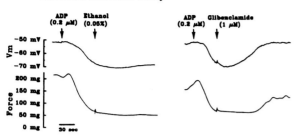

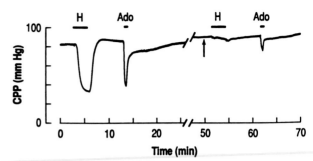

Fig. 49-4. Effects of glibenclamide on adenosine diphosphate-induced hyperpolarization and vasodilation of a mesenteric resistance artery isolated from the rabbit. Force and membrane potential were recorded simultaneously. ADP causes a substantial hyperpolarization and relaxation of tone (**left panel**). The hyperpolarization is abolished by glibenclamide; glibenclamide inhibits the relaxation by about 50%. From Brayden {56}, with permission.

Fig. 49-5. Coronary vasodilation induced by hypoxia or adenosine is inhibited by glibenclamide. Hypoxia (H) for 3 minutes or 1 μM adenosine (ado) induced a substantial fall in coronary perfusion pressure (CPP) in an isolated guinea pig heart perfused at a constant rate. Following a recovery period, glibenclamide (2 μM) was added to the perfusate at the time indicated by the arrow. In the presence of glibenclamide, the response to hypoxia was abolished and the response to adenosine was greatly attenuated. From Daut et al. {73}, with permission.

in part be due to activation of K_{ATP} channels {64}. In a canine model of endotoxemia, glibenclamide was able to cause vasoconstriction and restore blood pressure to normal levels. It should be noted, however, that enhanced release of EDRF/NO may also play a role in this disease process {65}.

ROLE OF K_{ATP} CHANNELS IN CONTROL OF CORONARY CIRCULATION

Response to vasoconstrictors

As indicated previously, K_{ATP} channels have been identified in coronary artery smooth muscle. These channels have been further characterized as targets of the actions of modulators of coronary artery vascular tone. Endothelin {47}, vasopressin {66}, and angiotensin II {67} *inhibit* activity of this channel in cardiac smooth muscle cells. In light of evidence suggesting that K_{ATP} channels are tonically active in coronary artery smooth muscle cells {46,67}, inhibition of these channels could represent an important mechanism of depolarization and constriction by a variety of agents in the coronary circulation.

K_{ATP} channels and regulation of resting coronary smooth muscle tone

Further evidence to support the concept that in coronary arteries K_{ATP} are active under resting conditions and contribute to maintenance of basal coronary vascular tone comes from studies of blood flow in canine hearts in vivo and in isolated perfused rabbit hearts {68}. Infusion of glibenclamide in these preparations causes large increases in coronary vascular resistance that are reversed upon removal of the K_{ATP} channel blocker.

Adenosine

Adenosine has long been implicated as an important endogenous vasodilator in the coronary circulation {69}. Studies by several groups using canine {70–72}, guinea pig {73, 74}, and porcine {75} models of coronary artery blood flow have concluded that activation of K_{ATP} channels plays a significant role in the coronary vasodilator response to adenosine. This suggestion is based primarily on the inhibitory effect of glibenclamide on adenosine-induced vasodilation of the intact coronary vascular bed (fig. 49-5).

Adenosine hyperpolarizes the vascular smooth muscle cells in isolated bovine {76} and rabbit (Brayden, unpublished) coronary arteries, and this response is glibenclamide sensitive. Although excitatory actions of adenosine on single K_{ATP} channels in vascular smooth muscle have not yet been reported, adenosine can activate K_{ATP} channels in cardiac muscle cells {27}. Thus the profile of effects of adenosine strongly suggests that this nucleoside acts, at least in part, by mechanisms that are similar to those described for other endogenous vasodilators.

K_{ATP} channels and coronary pathophysiology

HYPOXIA

Coronary arteries dilate in response to hypoxia. The underlying mechanism of hypoxia-induced vasodilation appears to involve K_{ATP} channels. Daut and colleagues {73} found that hypoxia induced a pronounced vasodilation in isolated, intact guinea pig hearts and that this response was blocked by glibenclamide (fig. 49-5). Metabolic inhibitors, such as dinitrophenol, cyanide {73}, or 2-deoxyglucose {74}, also induce a glibenclamide-sensitive vasodilation in this preparation. Thus it seems likely that interventions that alter cellular metabolism, and therefore production of ATP, may be sufficient to activate K_{ATP}

channels in coronary vascular smooth muscle cells and cause vasodilation. In these studies, adenosine did not appear to be a mediator of the hypoxic vasodilation, as 8-phenyltheophylline, an adenosine receptor antagonist, inhibited the response to exogenous adenosine but had little or no effect on the dilator response to hypoxia.

ISCHEMIA/REPERFUSION

Reactive hyperemia in the coronary circulation, which occurs following a brief period of ischemia, may involve activation of K_{ATP} channels {72,77}. Whether this is related to release of adenosine during the period of reperfusion or to other mechanisms whereby arterial K_{ATP} channels are activated remains to be elucidated. The autoregulatory vasodilator response of small ($<100\,\mu m$) epicardial arteries that occurs during mild or severe coronary stenosis or during coronary artery occlusion in vivo may also involve activation of K_{ATP} channels {78}.

FUTURE PERSPECTIVES

Identification of the precise mechanisms by which various agents activate K_{ATP} channels in vascular smooth muscle, including the type and extent of involvement of second messenger systems such as G proteins, cyclic nucleotides, and protein kinases, will be the next important step in the development of this field. Preliminary reports of success in cloning the K_{ATP} channel are just beginning to emerge {79}, and this development should open several new avenues for dissecting the signal transduction pathways involved in activation of this channel. The development of even more selective activators of the K_{ATP} channel may provide new drugs for treatment of cardiovascular diseases, such as hypertension, ischemia, and vasospasm. Further understanding of the precise distribution of K_{ATP} channels within the cardiovascular system will help determine the potential for selective modulation of blood flow within different tissues using K^+ channel openers.

SUMMARY

K_{ATP} channels represent a population of potassium channels with distinct biophysical and pharmacological properties. Important fingerprints of this channel include the inhibitory actions of intracellular ATP and of sulfonylurea compounds, and the excitatory actions of K^+ channel openers on these channels. K_{ATP} channels are likely to play an important regulatory role under normal and pathophysiological conditions in the cardiovascular system. The evidence presented in this chapter indicates that activation of K_{ATP} channels by pharmacological and endogenous vasodilators represents a powerful, general mechanism of vasodilation. By virtue of their regulation by cellular metabolism, K_{ATP} channels are also likely to play an important role in the alterations in cellular function that occur during pathophysiological stresses such as hypoxia, ischemia, and septic shock. In the coronary circulation, in

distinction to most other vascular beds, smooth muscle K_{ATP} channels appear to be active tonically. Thus K_{ATP} channels are in position to participate in the regulation of coronary blood flow as a result of either an increase or a decrease in channel activity, which may occur in response to chemically diverse substances, including K^+ channel openers, neuropeptides, adenosine, as well as potent vasoconstrictors such as vasopressin or endothelin.

ACKNOWLEDGMENTS

I would like to acknowledge Dr. M.T. Nelson for his comments on this chapter. I am also thankful to other colleagues, including Nick Standen, Noel Davies, John Quayle, Jurgen Hescheler, Huang Yu, Jurgen Daut, and Mark Nelson, who have made major contributions to the advancement of our understanding of K_{ATP} channels in the cardiovascular system. Work by the author reported in this chapter was supported by NIH grant HL-35911 and an Established Investigator award from the American Heart Association.

REFERENCES

1. Hille B: Potassium channels and chloride channels. In: Hille B (ed) *Ionic Channels of Excitable Membranes.* Sunderland, MA: Sinauer Associates, 1992, pp 115–139.
2. Hirst GDS, Edwards FR: Sympathetic neuroeffector transmission in arteries and arterioles. *Physiol Rev* 69:546–604, 1989.
3. Ashcroft FM: Adenosine 5′-triphosphate-sensitive potassium channels. *Ann Rev Neuroscience* 11:97–118, 1988.
4. Quast U, Cook NS: Moving together: K^+ channel openers and ATP-sensitive K^+ channels. *Trends Pharm Sci* 10:431–435, 1989.
5. Ashcroft SJH, Ashcroft FM: Properties and functions of ATP-sensitive K-channels. *Cellu Signali* 2:197–214, 1990.
6. Nelson MT, Patlak JB, Worley JF, Standen NB: Calcium channels, potassium channels and the voltage-dependence of arterial tone. *Am J Physiol* 259:C3–C18, 1990.
7. Nichols CG, Lederer W: Adenosine triphosphate-sensitive potassium channels in the cardiovascular system. *Am J Physiol* 261:H1675–H1686, 1991.
8. Rorsman P, Trube G: Biophysics and physiology of ATP-regulated K^+-channels (K_{ATP}). In: Cook NS (ed) *Potassium Channels: Structure, Classification and Therapeutic Potential.* Chichester, UK: Horwood, 1990, pp 96–116.
9. Standen NB: Potassium channels, metabolism and muscle. *Exp Physiol* 77:1–25, 1992.
10. Noma A: ATP-regulated K^+ channels in cardiac muscle. Nature 305:147–148, 1983.
11. Cook DL, Hales CN: Intracellular ATP directly blocks K^+ channels in pancreatic beta cells. Nature 311:271–273, 1984.
12. DeWeille JR, Schmid-Antomarchi H, Fosset M, Lazdunski M: ATP-sensitive K^+ channels that are blocked by hypoglycemia-inducing sulphonylureas in insulin secreting cells are activated by galanin, a hyperglycemia-inducing hormone. *Proc Natl Acad Sci USA* 85:1312–1316, 1988.
13. Spruce AE, Standen NB, Stanfield PR: Voltage-dependent, ATP-sensitive potassium channels of skeletal muscle membrane. *Nature* 316:736–738, 1985.
14. Ashford MLJ, Sturgess NC, Trout NJ, Gardner NJ, Hales CN: Adenosine 5′-triphosphate-sensitive ion channels in

neonatal rat cultured central neurones. *Pflügers Arch* 412: 297–304, 1988.

15. De Weille JR, Fosset M, Mourre C, Schmid-Antomarchi H, Bernardi H, Lazdunski M: Pharmacology and regulation of ATP-sensitive K$^+$ channels. *Pflügers Arch* 414(Suppl 1): S80–S87, 1989.

16. Standen NB, Quayle JM, Davies NW, Brayden JE, Huang Y, Nelson MT: Hyperpolarizing vasodilators activate ATP-sensitive K$^+$ channels in arterial smooth muscle. *Science* 245:177–180, 1989.

17. Bonev A, Nelson MT: ATP-sensitive potassium channels in smooth muscle cells from guinea pig urinary bladder. *Am J Physiol*, 264:C1190–C1200, 1993.

18. Schmid-Antomarchi H, DeWeille J, Fosset M, Lazdunski M: The receptor for antidiabetic sulfonylureas controls the activity of the ATP-modulated K$^+$ channel in insulin-secreting cells. J Biol Chem 262:15840–15844, 1987.

19. Sturgess NC, Ashford MLJ, Cook DL, Hales CN: The sulfonylurea receptor may be an ATP-sensitive potassium channel. *Lancet* 8453:474–475, 1985.

20. Findlay I: ATP^{4-} and ATP.Mg inhibit the ATP-sensitive K$^+$ channel of rat ventricular myocytes. *Pflügers Arch* 412:37–41, 1988.

21. Lederer WJ, Nichols CG: Nucleotide modulation of the activity of rat heart ATP-sensitive K$^+$ channels in isolated membrane patches. J Physiol 419:193–211, 1989.

22. Davies NW: Modulation of ATP-sensitive K$^+$ channels in skeletal muscle by intracellular protons. Nature 343:375–377, 1990.

23. Cook NS, Quast U: Potassium channel pharmacology. In: Cook NS (ed) *Potassium Channels: Structure, Classification and Therapeutic Potential*. Chichester, UK: Horwood, 1990, pp 181–255.

24. Findlay I, Dunne MJ: ATP maintains ATP-inhibited channels in an operational state. *Pflügers Arch* 407:238–240, 1986.

25. Ohno-Shosaku T, Zunkler BJ, Trube G: Dual effects of ATP on K$^+$ currents of mouse pancreatic beta-cells. *Pflügers Arch* 408:133–138, 1987.

26. Dunne MJ, Peterson OH: GTP and GDP activation of K$^+$ channels that can be inhibited by ATP. *Pflügers Archiv* 407:564–565, 1988.

27. Kirsch GE, Codina J, Birnbaumer L, Brown AM: Coupling of ATP-sensitive K$^+$ channels to A$_1$ receptors by G proteins in rat ventricular myocytes. *Am J Physiol* 259:H820–H826, 1990.

28. Ribalet B, Ciani S, Eddlestone GT: ATP mediates both activation and inhibition of K(ATP) channel activity via cAMP-dependent protein kinase in insulin-secreting cell lines. *J Gen Physiol* 94:693–717, 1989.

29. Thuringer D, Escande D: Apparent competition between ATP and the potassium channel opener RP 49356 on ATP-sensitive K$^+$ channels of cardiac myocytes. *Mol Pharm* 36: 897–902, 1989.

30. Escande D, Thuringer D, Leguern S, Cavero I: The potassium channel opener cromakalim (BRL 34915) activates ATP-dependent K$^+$ channels in isolated cardiac myocytes. *Biochem Biophys Res Commun* 154:620–625, 1988.

31. Escande D, Thuringer D, Leguern S, Courteix J, Laville M, Cavero I: Potassium channel openers act through an activation of ATP-sensitive K$^+$ channels in guinea-pig cardiac myocytes. *Pflügers Arch* 414:669–675, 1989.

32. Zunkler BK, Lenzen S, Manner K, Panten U, Trube G: Concentration-dependent effects of tolbutamide, meglitinide, glipizide, glibenclamide and diazoxide on ATP-regulated K$^+$ currents in pancreatic beta cells. *Naunyn-Schmeidebergs Arch Pharm* 337:225–230, 1988.

33. Fan Z, Nakayama K, Hiraoka M: Multiple actions of pinacidil on adenosine triphosphate-sensitive potassium channels in guinea-pig ventricular myocytes. *J Physiol* 430:273–295, 1990.

34. Gasser RNA, Vaughan-Jones RD: Mechanism of potassium efflux and action potential shortening during ischaemia in isolated mammalian cardiac muscle. *J Physiol (Lond)* 431: 713–741, 1990.

35. Wolleben CD, Sanguinetti MC, Siegl PKS: Influence of ATP-sensitive potassium channel modulators on ischemia-induced fibrillation in isolated rat hearts. *J Mol Cell Cardiol* 21: 783–788, 1989.

36. Rorsman P, Berggren P, Bokvist K, Efendic S: ATP-regulated K$^+$ channels and diabetes mellitus. *News Physiol Sci* 5: 143–147, 1990.

37. Amoroso S, Schmid-Antomarchi H, Fosset M, Lazdunski M: Glucose, sulfonylureas, and neurotransmitter release: Role of ATP-sensitive K$^+$ channels. *Science* 247:852–854, 1990.

38. Winquist RJ, Heaney LA, Wallace AA, Baskin EP, Stein RB, Garcia ML, Kaczarowski GJ: Glyburide blocks the relaxation response to BRL 34915 (cromakalim), minoxidil sulfate and diazoxide in vascular smooth muscle. *J Pharmacol Exp Ther* 248:149–156, 1989.

39. Wilson C: Inhibition by sulphonylureas of vasorelaxation induced by K$^+$ channel activators in vitro. *J Auton Pharmacol* 9:71–78, 1989.

40. Cavero I, Mondot S, Mestre M: Vasorelaxant effects of cromakalim in rats are mediated by glibenclamide-sensitive potassium channels. *J Pharmacol Exp Ther* 248:1261–1268, 1989.

41. Grover GJ, McCullough JR, Henry DE, Conder ML, Sleph PG: The anti-ischemic effects of the potassium channel activators pinacidil and cromakalim and the reversal of these effects with the potassium channel blocker glyburide. *J Pharmacol Exp Ther* 251:98–110, 1989.

42. Quayle JM, Standen NB, Stanfield PR: The voltage-dependent block of ATP-sensitive potassium channels of frog skeletal muscle by caesium and barium ions. *J Physiol (Lond)* 405:677–697, 1988.

43. Nelson MT, Huang Y, Brayden JE, Hescheler J, Standen NB: Arterial dilations to calcitonin gene-related peptide involve activation of K$^+$ channels. *Nature* 344:770–773, 1990.

44. Kajioka S, Kitamura K, Kuriyama H: Guanosine diphosphate activates an adenosine 5'-triphosphate-sensitive K$^+$ channel in the rabbit portal vein. *J Physiol* 444:397–418, 1991.

45. Kajioka S, Oike M, Kitamura K: Nicorandil opens a calcium-dependent potassium channel in smooth muscle cells of the rat portal vein. J Pharm Exp Ther 254:905–913, 1990.

46. Inoue I, Nakaya Y, Nakaya S, Mori H: Extracellular Ca^{2+}-activated K channel in coronary artery smooth muscle cells and its role in vasodilation. *FEBS Lett* 255:281–284, 1989.

47. Miyoshi Y, Nakaya Y, Wakalsuki T, Nakaya S, Fujino K, Saito K, Inoue I: Endothelin blocks ATP-sensitive K$^+$ channels and depolarizes smooth muscle cells of porcine coronary artery. *Circ Res* 70:612–616, 1992.

48. Lorenz JN, Schnermann J, Brosius FC, Briggs JP, Furspan PE: Intracellular ATP can regulate afferent arteriolar tone via ATP-sensitive K$^+$ channels in the rabbit. *J Clin Invest* 90:733–740, 1992.

49. Kovacs RJ, Nelson MT: ATP-sensitive K$^+$ channels from aortic smooth muscle incorporated into planar lipid bilayers. *Am J Physiol* 261:H604–H609, 1991.

50. Clapp LH, Gurney AM: ATP-sensitive K$^+$ channels regulate resting potential of pulmonary arterial smooth muscle cells. *Am J Physiol* 262:H916–H920, 1992.

51. Russel SN, Smirnov SV, Aaronson PI: Effects of BRL 38227 on potassium currents in smooth muscle cells isolated from rabbit portal vein and human mesenteric artery. *Br J Pharmacol* 105:549–556, 1992.

52. Post JM, Jones AW: Stimulation of arterial ^{42}K efflux by ATP depletion and cromakalim is antagonized by glyburide. *Am J Physiol* 260:H848–H854, 1991.

53. Quast U, Cook NS: In vitro and in vivo comparisons of two K$^+$ channel openers, diazoxide and cromakalim, and their inhibition by glibenclamide. *J Pharmacol Exp Ther* 250: 261–271, 1989.

54. Brayden JE, Quayle JM, Standen NB, Nelson MT: Role of potassium channels in the vascular response to endogenous and pharmacological vasodilators. *Blood Vessels* 28:147–153, 1991.

55. McCarron JG, Quayle JM, Halpern W, Nelson MT: Cromakalim and pinacidil dilate small mesenteric arteries but not small cerebral arteries. *Am J Physiol* 261:H287–H291.

56. Brayden JE: Hyperpolarization and relaxation of resistance arteries in response to adenosine diphosphate: Distribution and mechanism of action. *Circ Res* 69:1415–1420, 1991.

57. Mulderry PK, Ghatei MA, Rodrigo J, Allen JM, Rosenfeld MG, Polak JM, Bloom JR: Calcitonin gene-related peptide in cardiovascular tissues of the rat. *Neuroscience* 14:947–954, 1985.

58. Taylor SG, Weston AH: Endothelium-derived hyperpolarizing factor: A new endogenous inhibitor from the vascular endothelium. *Trends Pharm Sci* 9:272–274, 1988.

59. Furchgott RF: Role of endothelium in responses of vascular smooth muscle. *Circ Res* 53:557–573, 1983.

60. Palmer RMJ, Ferrige AG, Moncada S: Nitric oxide release accounts for the biological activity of endothelium-derived relaxing factor. *Nature* 327:524–526, 1987.

61. Brayden JE: Membrane hyperpolarization is a mechanism of endothelium-dependent cerebral vasodilation. *Am J Physiol* 259:H668–H673, 1990.

62. Jiang CW, Poole-Wilson PA, Collins P: Comparison of rabbit coronary arterial relaxation induced by acetylcholine and lemakalim: Activation of ATP-sensitive potassium channels. *Cardiovasc Res* 25:930–935, 1991.

63. Eckman DM, Frankovich JD, Keef KD: Comparison of the actions of acetylcholine and BRL 38227 in the guinea-pig coronary artery. *Br J Pharmacol* 106:9–16, 1992.

64. Landry DW, Oliver JA: The ATP-sensitive K$^+$ channel mediates hypotension in endotoxemia and hypoxic lactic acidosis in dog. *J Clin Invest* 89:2071–2074, 1992.

65. Kilbourn RG, Gross SS, Jubran A, Adams J, Griffith OW, Levi R, Lodata RF: N^G-methyl-L-arginine inhibits tumor necrosis factor-induced hypotension: Implications for the involvement of nitric oxide. *Proc Natl Acad Sci USA* 87: 3629–3632, 1990.

66. Wakatsuki T, Nakya Y, Inoue I: Vasopressin modulates K$^+$-channel activities of cultured smooth muscle cells from porcine coronary artery. *Am J Physiol* 263:H491–H496, 1992.

67. Myoshi Y, Nakaya Y: Antiotensin II blocks ATP-sensitive K$^+$ channels in porcine coronary artery smooth muscle cells. *Biochem Biophys Res Commun* 181:700–706, 1991.

68. Samaha FF, Heineman FW, Ince C, Fleming J, Balaban RS: ATP-sensitive potassium channel is essential to maintain basal coronary vascular tone in vivo. *Am J Physiol* 262: C1220–C1227, 1992.

69. Berne RM: The role of adenosine in regulation of coronary blood flow. *Circ Res* 47:807–813, 1980.

70. Belloni FL, Hintze TM: Glibenchamide attenuates adenosine-induced bradycardia and coronary vasodilation. *Am J Physiol* 261:H720–H727, 1991.

71. Yoneyama F, Yamada H, Satoh K, Taira N: Vasodepressor mechanisms of 2-(1-octynyl)-adenosine (YT-146), a selective adenosine A2 receptor agonist, involve the opening of glibenclamide-sensitive K$^+$ channels. *Eur J Pharmacol* 213: 199–204, 1992.

72. Clayton FC, Hess TA, Smith MA, Grover GJ: Coronary reactive hyperemia and adenosine-induced vasodilation are mediated partially by a glyburide-sensitive mechanism. *Pharmacology* 44:92–100, 1992.

73. Daut J, Maier-Rudolph W, von Beckerath N, Mehrke G, Gunther K, Goedel-Meinen L: Hypoxic dilation of coronary arteries is mediated by ATP-sensitive potassium channels. *Science* 247:1341–1344, 1990.

74. von Beckerath N, Cyrys S, Dischner A, Daut J: Hypoxic vasodilation in isolated, perfused guinea-pig heart: An analysis of the underlying mechanisms. *J Physiol (Lond)* 442: 297–319, 1991.

75. Merkel LA, Lappe RW, Rivera LM, Cox BF, Perrone MH: Demonstration of vasorelaxant activity with an A1-selective adenosine agonist in porcine coronary artery: Involvement of potassium channels. *J Pharm Exp Ther* 260:437–443, 1991.

76. Sabouni MH, Hargittai PT, Lieberman EM, Mustafa SJ: Evidence for adenosine receptor-mediated hyperpolarization in coronary smooth muscle. *Am J Physiol* 257:H1750–H1752, 1989.

77. Kanatsuka H, Sekiguchi N, Satao K, Akai K, Wang Y, Komaru T, Ashikawa K, Takishima T: Microvascular sites and mechanisms responsible for reactive hyperemia in the coronary circulation of the beating canine heart. *Circ Res* 71:912–922, 1992.

78. Komaru T, Lamping KG, Eastham CL, Dellsperger KC: Role of ATP-sensitive potassium channels in coronary microvascular autoregulatory responses. *Circ Res* 69:1146–1151, 1991.

79. Ho K, Vassilev PM, Kanazirska MV, Lytton J, Hebert SC: The primary structure and functional expression of a mammalian ATP-sensitive potassium channel (abstr). *J Am Soc Nephrol* 3:808, 1992.

CHAPTER 50

Mechanisms of Action of K^+ Channel Openers and Closers in Smooth Muscle Cells

KENJI KITAMURA, MASAHIRO KAMOUCHI, & HIROSI KURIYAMA

INTRODUCTION

Chronic vasoconstriction of resistant vessels for various etiologic reasons induces regional and systemic hypertension. The etiology of the hypertension is not fully understood, but clinical treatment with antihypertensive agents shows Ca^{2+} regulation on the membrane and in the cytosol are closely related to the pathologic change of the blood vessels. At present, various kinds of drugs are used as antihypertensive and antianginal agents, for example, alpha-adrenoceptor blockers, beta-adrenoceptor blockers, nitroso compounds, angiotensin converting enzyme (ACE) inhibitors, Ca^{2+} channel blockers, and diuretic agents. Among these, alpha-adrenoceptor blockers and ACE inhibitors reduce blood pressure by preventing binding of noradrenaline to the adrenoceptors and reducing the active form of angiotensin II, respectively; nitro compounds are thought to activate mainly the Ca^{2+} extrusion system through cyclic guanosine 3':5'-monophosphate (cGMP); and Ca^{2+} channel blockers are known to block selectively the voltage-dependent Ca^{2+} channel. Mechanisms of vasodilation or antihypertensive actions of beta-adrenoceptor blockers and diuretic agents are not yet fully understood. Antihypertensive actions of beta-adrenoceptor blockers are thought not to be related to the beta-adrenoceptor blocking action but to the membrane-stabilizing action or local anesthetic action. It is commonly believed that such actions are in part closely related to the nonspecific blocking actions of ion channels. A diuretic agent, cicletanine, is reported to modify the voltage-dependent Ca^{2+} channel in the ventricular cells by enhancing the cAMP concentration or facilitation of the channel phosphorylation {1}, suggesting enhancement of Ca^{2+} extrusion from the vascular smooth muscle cells. Therefore, control of the cytosolic Ca^{2+} concentration at the membrane is one of the most common mechanisms of action of various antihypertensive agents.

The contraction of the smooth muscle cells is mainly regulated by intracellular Ca^{2+} concentration ($[Ca^{2+}]_i$), which is regulated by influx and efflux across the cell membrane and release and uptake through the membrane of the sarcoplasmic reticulum. In various smooth muscle cells producing spontaneous action potentials (for example, stomach, small intestine, urinary bladder, myo-

metrium, ureter, portal vein, etc.), automatic membrane depolarization by pacemaking activity opens the voltage-dependent Ca^{2+} channel, followed by activation of the voltage- and Ca^{2+}-dependent K^+ channels, to form the rising and falling phases of the action potential. Other smooth muscle cells, such as arterial smooth muscle cells, do not produce an action potential spontaneously, but several agonists produce membrane depolarization and trigger the action potential in some cases.

Hyperpolarization of the membrane impedes the opening of the voltage-dependent Ca^{2+} channel of the smooth muscle cells so that muscle contraction is prevented. For example, in visceral smooth muscle cells, stimulation of beta-adrenoceptors hyperpolarizes the membrane as well as activating adenylate cyclase to stimulate Ca^{2+} efflux through production of cyclic adenosine 3':5'-monophosphate (cAMP). As a consequence, the frequency of the action potential generation decreases during membrane hyperpolarization or is completely inhibited, depending upon the degree of membrane hyperpolarization. On the other hand, K^+ channel blockers, such as tetraethylammonium (TEA) and 4-aminopyridine (4-AP), produce membrane depolarization and evoke the action potential {2,3}. Because of the asymmetrical distribution of ions, movement of K^+ across the membrane always makes the membrane more hyperpolarized. Furthermore, the membrane depolarization and hyperpolarization have been reported to increase and reduce, respectively, the synthesis of inositol 1,4,5-trisphosphate ($InsP_3$) in smooth muscle cells {4,5}. Therefore, control of K^+ channel activity is also very important for regulation of $[Ca^{2+}]_i$ and smooth muscle contraction.

K CHANNELS IN SMOOTH MUSCLE CELLS

In visceral smooth muscle cells, it is known that noradrenaline and isoprenaline produce membrane hyperpolarization through activation of alpha- and beta-adrenoceptors, respectively. In Ca-free solution, the hyperpolarization induced by catecholamines is abolished and apamin, a bee venom, is a selective blocker of this hyperpolarization. Nicorandil contains NO_2 in the structure. Therefore, this drug was expected to produce vasodilation through a

N. Sperelakis (ed.), *Physiology and Pathophysiology of the Heart, Third Edition.*

similar mechanism to that for other nitroso compounds, such as nitroglycerin and sodium nitrite. Later, nicorandil was proven to synthesize cGMP and was thought to activate Ca pumping out into the sarcolemma and sarcoplasmic reticulum via activation of the cGMP-dependent protein kinase. Nicorandil was found to produce a large hyperpolarization of the vascular smooth muscle cell membranes and to inhibit action potential generation {6,7}. The hyperpolarization induced by nicorandil was not inhibited by removal of $[Ca^{2+}]_o$, and K^+ channel blockers are relatively insensitive to the nicorandil-induced hyperpolarization {8}. From these experiments, mainly done with microelectrode and sucrose gap methods, one could classify the hyperpolarization into Ca-dependent and Ca-resistant components, as well as K channel blocker sensitive and resistant components. The basis of the hyperpolarization in the smooth muscle cells was unclear until introduction of the patch-clamp technique to the smooth muscle cells. However, such pharmacological properties are still important for identification of K^+ channels recorded by voltage-clamp experiments.

At present, various K^+ channels have been found by whole-cell voltage-clamp and single-channel current recording experiments with the patch-clamp method in smooth muscle cells. So far K^+ currents can be classified into two classes from the macroscopic current recording, i.e., voltage-dependent and -independent K^+ channels. The former is subclassified into voltage-gated and Ca^{2+}-dependent K^+ channels, and the latter into receptor-operated and ATP-sensitive K^+ channels. In table 50-1, K^+ channels identified in a variety of smooth muscle cells are listed.

Voltage-dependent K^+ currents are easily induced by membrane depolarization from a holding potential near the resting membrane potential ($-60\,mV$). Sufficient depolarization of the membrane to produce an inward Ca^{2+} current evokes a transient outward current following the Ca^{2+} current {9–12}. In Ca^{2+}-free solution, the transient outward current ceased as well as the inward Ca^{2+} current.

Perfusion of high concentrations of EGTA ($\geq 1\,mM$) also abolished the transient outward current, suggesting a Ca^{2+}-dependent current. The current was inhibited by submillimolar concentrations of TEA in the bath, but not by millimolar concentrations of 4-AP. Charybdotoxin (ChTX), but not apamin, also blocked the current. From these pharmacological profiles, the Ca^{2+}-dependent component of the transient outward current $[I_{TO(Ca)}]$ is closely related to the large-conductance Ca^{2+}-dependent K^+ channel (maxi-K^+ channel), which is commonly distributed in various smooth muscle cells.

It was found from the pharmacological profiles that activation of the same K^+ (maxi-K^+) channel also produced a current oscillation during the membrane depolarization (oscillatory outward current, I_{OO} {9,13}; spontaneously transient outward current, STOC {14}). Recently, Xiong et al. {13} directly proved that the sporadic and simultaneous opening of dozens of maxi-K^+ channels was modulated by either heparin or caffeine using an inside-out patch membrane. There is no difference between the pharmacological properties of $I_{TO(Ca)}$ and I_{OO}. However, in Ca^{2+}-free solution, I_{OO} appeared for more than 10 minutes, whereas $I_{TO(Ca)}$ was immediately abolished. One of the interesting profiles of $I_{TO(Ca)}$ and I_{OO} is that both currents are modulated by several agents that act on the intracellular Ca^{2+} store site. Caffeine ($\geq 1\,mM$) transiently augmented these currents then inhibited current generation, while procaine gradually inhibited it. Ryanodine, an open-channel locker of the store site Ca^{2+} channel, abolished both currents. Perfusion of $InsP_3$ augmented and heparin inhibited the frequency of I_{OO} generation {9,14–17}. On the other hand, $InsP_3$ and heparin did not act on the transient outward current. Therefore, both Ca^{2+}-dependent outward currents are speculated to be regulated by Ca^{2+} release from the store site. Generation of I_{OO} is closely related to both caffeine and $InsP_3$-sensitive store sites through Ca^{2+}-induced and $InsP_3$-induced Ca^{2+} release mechanisms, but $I_{TO(Ca)}$ is likely to be related to the Ca^{2+}-induced Ca^{2+} release

Table 50-1. K channel in smooth muscle cells (classification by macroscopic currents)

	Blockers	Openers	Tissues
Voltage-dependent K^+ current			
Voltage-gated K^+ current			
a. Transient outward current (A-like current)	4AP		Guinea pig ureter
b. Delayed outward current			
a) TEA-sensitive K^+ current	TEA		Rabbit portal vein
b) TEA-insensitive K^+ current	4AP		Rabbit pulmonary artery
Ca^{2+}-activated K^+ current			
a. Transient outward current	TEA; ChTX; IbTX	$[Ca]_i$; cAMP; GMP;	Rabbit ear artery & portal vein
b. Oscillatory outward current	TEA; ChTX; IbTX	$[Ca]_i$; cAMP; GMP;	
Voltage-independent K^+ current			
Receptor-operated K^+ current	Apamin	Norad; ATP; Isop	Visceral tissues
ATP-sensitive K^+ current			
a. Ca^{2+}-insensitive K^+ current	Glibenclamide	K^+ channel openers	Rabbit mesenteric artery & portal vein
b. Ca^{2+}-sensitive K^+ current	Glibenclamide	K^+ channel openers	Rat portal vein & pig coronary artery
M current	ACh; SP	cAMP; Isop	Toad stomach

mechanism. I_{OO} has also been modulated by protein kinase C indirectly by regulating Ca^{2+} mobilization at the store site {18}.

In addition to the Ca^{2+}-dependent component, a depolarization of the membrane from a lower holding potential (-80 mV) evoked another transient outward current, which did not disappear in the Ca^{2+}-free solution {19–21}. Elevation of the holding potential to -50 mV or application of 4-aminopyridine (4-AP) inhibited the Ca^{2+}-independent component of the transient outward current, suggesting this current is classified as an A current. The unitary conductance of the A current was 14 pS, similar to that in the dorsal root ganglion (DRG) cell from the guinea pig (20 pS), and the channel was rapidly inactivated following transient opening during the membrane depolarization {19,22}.

Delayed K^+ current was also evoked by membrane depolarization in Ca^{2+}-free solution. The current reached the maximum amplitude within 100 ms and inactivated very slowly. The delayed K^+ current, in the rabbit pulmonary and mesenteric arteries, portal vein, and dog trachea, was inhibited by millimolar concentrations of 4-AP {11,12,23,24}. On the other hand, inhibitory effects of TEA on the delayed K^+ current were inconsistent between preparations. In the rabbit small intestine and rat portal vein, the delayed K^+ current was inhibited by millimolar concentrations of TEA {9,25}, whereas the delayed K^+ current in dog trachea and rabbit portal vein cells was inhibited only when more than 10 mM of TEA was present {11,12,23}. The delayed K^+ current recorded in the rabbit pulmonary and mesenteric arteries was resistant to TEA. Even when Na^+ was replaced with TEA in the bath, half of the current amplitude was not inhibited {24}. The unitary conductance of the delayed K^+ current in the rabbit portal vein was estimated to be 5 pS {23}.

At least four Ca^{2+}-dependent K^+ channels have been classified in various smooth muscle cells by unitary conductance. The large-conductance Ca^{2+}-dependent K^+ channels (maxi-K^+ channel; B-K^+ channel) are widely and densely distributed in many smooth muscle cells {26–34}. The unitary conductance of the maxi-K^+ channel is in the range 200–300 pS in the symmetrical high-K^+ condition. Submicromolar concentrations of $[Ca^{2+}]_i$ open the channel, but millimolar concentration of $[Ca^{2+}]_o$ do not change channel activity. $[Ba^{2+}]_i$ is a good substitute to inhibit of the maxi-K^+ channel {27}. TEA, applied from the extracellular side at submillimolar concentrations, effectively blocks the maxi-K^+ channel. However, the same concentration of TEA added to the intracellular side does not inhibit the channel {28}. Apamin and 4-AP had no action on the maxi-K^+ channel. Quinidine, a blocker of the Ca^{2+}-dependent K^+ channel, also inhibited the maxi-K^+ channel in toad stomach cells {35}. Isoprenaline and cAMP are thought to activate the maxi-K^+ channel through protein kinase A {33}. Furthermore, cGMP is also reported to augment maxi-K^+ channel activity via protein kinase G {31,36}.

The small conductance Ca^{2+}-dependent K^+ channel (92 pS in symmetrical high K^+ solutions), found in the rabbit portal vein, is insensitive to 1 mM TEA {28}. The $[Ca^{2+}]_i$ sensitivity of this K^+ channel was nearly the same as that of the maxi-K^+ channel, and $[Ca^{2+}]_o$ did not affect the channel activity. The small-conductance Ca^{2+}-dependent K^+ channel in skeletal muscle (12 pS) was blocked by apamin {37}, but those in *Aplysia* neurons (35 pS) {38}, red blood cells (40 pS) {39}, and rabbit portal vein (92 pS) {28} were not sensitive to apamin.

A different type of small-conductance $[Ca^{2+}]_i$-dependent K^+ channel (10 pS) was found in rat portal vein, which was sensitive to high concentrations of TEA and 4-AP {25,40}. This channel was insensitive to ChTX and apamin, but sensitive to glibenclamide, a blocker of ATP-sensitive K^+ channels. This current did not show voltage-dependent activation.

In rabbit portal vein and pig coronary artery, novel Ca^{2+}-dependent K^+ channels were also found {41,42}. K^+ channels in both cells are activated by $[Ca^{2+}]_o$ at a physiological range and are less voltage dependent. However, the two $[Ca^{2+}]_o$-dependent K^+ channels are different, because the unitary conductance and pharmacological properties are distinct. The $[Ca^{2+}]_o$-dependent K^+ channel in the rabbit portal vein was inhibited by millimolar concentrations of TEA inside, but not outside. On the other hand, the K^+ channel in the pig coronary artery was blocked by glibenclamide {43}.

The ATP-sensitive K^+ channel, first found in cardiac cells {44}, has now been confirmed in skeletal muscle, pancreatic β cells, and smooth muscle cells {45–47}. The ATP-sensitive K^+ channel is inhibited by submillimolar concentrations of intracellular ATP. However, for continuous activation a small amount of ATP or other nucleotide is required. Removal of Ca^{2+} on both sides of the membrane does not affect the channel activity. Unitary conductance of the ATP-sensitive K^+ channel is in the range 30–135 pS in high K^+ conditions. Glibenclamide inhibited all ATP-sensitive K^+ channels observed in various cells. As mentioned above, several Ca^{2+}-dependent K^+ channels found in smooth muscle cells are also classified into the ATP-sensitive K^+ channel, since those are inhibited by glibenclamide and intracellular ATP $[ATP]_i$.

GATING MECHANISMS OF THE ATP-SENSITIVE K^+ CHANNEL

In the first paper on the ATP-sensitive K^+ channel in the guinea pig and rabbit ventricular cells, Noma {44} demonstrated that this channel has an inward rectifying property. As the ATP-sensitive K^+ channel shows high selectivity to K^+, other impermeable cations in the cell, such as Na^+ or Mg^{2+}, plug the channel from the inside and obstruct unidirectional K^+ permeation {48}. However, Nichols and Lederer {49} speculate that another intracellular factor also contributes to the inward rectifying property of the channel, because inward rectification was observed in the permeabilized cells but not in the inside-out membrane.

The activity of the ATP-sensitive K^+ channel was rapidly reduced after excision of the membrane in ATP-free solution (rundown) {46,50–54}. The rundown probably occurs due to channel dephosphorylation by depletion of ATP inside the membrane, since readministration of low concentrations of ATP or withdrawal of high concentrations of ATP activate the ATP-sensitive K$^+$ channel in various cells {51–53,55,56}. Ribalet et al. {55} reported that cAMP-dependent protein kinase or cAMP also enhanced the channel activity, and a specific inhibitor of the cAMP-dependent protein kinase inhibited the activity. Therefore, we may conclude that channel phosphorylation by cAMP-dependent protein kinase is one of the activation pathways of the ATP-sensitive K$^+$ channel at low concentrations of ATP. Reactivation of the channel by ATP requires Mg^{2+} {57}, and nonhydrolyzable ATP analogues, such as AMP-PNP, AMP-PCP, ATPγS, and ADPβS, have little or no effect on the channel reactivation {53,58,59}.

Other mechanisms are also involved in reactivation of the ATP-sensitive K$^+$ channel. In insulin-secreting cells, GTP and its analogues (GTP-γS, GDP, and GDP-βS) have been reported to activate the channel when Mg^{2+} is simultaneously present {60}. Tung and Kurachi {61} also reported that in guinea pig ventricular cells various nucleoside diphosphates could activate the ATP-sensitive K$^+$ channel in the dephosphorylated condition. However, they did not see any action of triphosphate and monophosphate forms of nucleotide on the K$^+$ channel. Similarly, Kajioka et al. {54} demonstrated that in the smooth muscle cells of rabbit portal vein, K$^+$ channel openers only opened the ATP-sensitive K$^+$ channel when GDP or GTP was present in the cell. On the other hand, GTP-γS had no action on the channel activity but GDP-βS reduced it. GTP binding protein was not involved in channel reactivation, since GTP-γS did not mimic the GTP action in the smooth muscle cells nor did GDP-βS antagonize the GTP action in the insulin-secreting cells. Mg^{2+} is essential for reactivation of the channel by nucleoside diphosphate in cardiac cells, but not in smooth muscle cells {54,61}. Although there are several discrepancies in the reactivating mechanisms by nucleoside diphosphate between cardiac, smooth muscle, and pancreatic β cells, they may all bind on to the ATP-sensitive K$^+$ channel, then open the activation gate of the dephosphorylated channel. ATP may independently open the activation gate by shifting the channel state from dephosphorylation to phosphorylation.

From an analysis of the unitary current, the ATP-sensitive K$^+$ channel has one open and three closed states in guinea pig ventricular cells, and one open and two closed states in rabbit portal vein {54,62}. The ATP-sensitive K$^+$ channel in the rabbit portal vein has a longer mean open time than in ventricular cells. The apparently longer mean open time and the lack of a very fast closed state in rabbit portal vein are probably due to the use of a lower cut-off filter for noise reduction. Opening of the ATP-sensitive K$^+$ channel in insulin secreting cells and guinea pig ventricular cells occurred in bursts with a very brief closed time (0.3–0.4 ms) {55,62}, whereas those in smooth muscle cells were not interrupted by such brief closure {25,46,54,63}. [ATP]$_i$ did not modify the mean open and closed times, but reduced the burst duration and increased the longer closed time in guinea pig ventricular cells {62}, while reducing the mean open time mainly by

chopping up the long duration of the channel opening and increasing the longer closed time {54}. Thus, micromolar to millimolar concentrations of [ATP]$_i$ reduced the open probability of the ATP-sensitive K$^+$ channel. The simplest kinetics model of the ATP-sensitive K$^+$ channel in cardiac and smooth muscle cells is

$$C_1 - C_2 - O_{burst},$$

and [ATP]$_i$ shifts the states to the left. The ATP-sensitive K$^+$ channel in frog skeletal muscle has two open and four closed states {64}.

The inhibitory actions of ATP on the ATP-sensitive K$^+$ channel are also mimicked by AMP-PNP, AMP-PCP, or ATP-γS and other nucleoside triphosphates, such as GTP, UTP, and CTP, suggesting the presence of high-affinity binding sites for these nucleoside triphosphates {52,53,65–69}. Reduction in pH decreased the ATP sensitivity of the channel in cardiac and skeletal muscle cells, but increased the apparent ATP inhibition in pancreatic β cells {52,64, 69}. In the case of skeletal muscle, since reduction in pH shifted the ATP-dependent inhibition curve for the channel activity in parallel, Davies et al. {64} proposed a simple proton binding model for prevention of ATP binding to the channel. However, the same model is not applicable to the cardiac and pancreatic ATP-sensitive K$^+$ channel. In cardiac cells, a low pH (6.25) reduced the ATP sensitivity of the channel with increase in the Hill coefficient for ATP binding {69}, suggesting modulation of the ATP binding site by protons.

Extracellular Na$^+$ also modulates the ATP sensitivity of the channel in ventromedial hypothalamic neurons, but not in the insulin-secreting cells, by unknown mechanisms {70}.

MECHANISMS OF K$^+$ CHANNEL ACTIVATION BY VARIOUS AGENTS

Receptor agonists

Hyperpolarization induced by isoprenaline and other catecholamines is prevented by treatment with either propranolol or phentolamine, suggesting adrenoceptor-mediated hyperpolarization. Yamaguchi et al. {71} demonstrated a hyperpolarization induced by isoprenaline using an isolated single-cell preparation of the toad stomach. Ouabain, an inhibitor of the Na$^+$-K$^+$ pump, abolished the hyperpolarization induced by isoprenaline, but they did not think that electrogenic Na$^+$ transport was the main contributor to the hyperpolarization, because even in the presence of ouabain changes in the membrane resistance were still seen without membrane hyperpolarization. They speculated that inhibition of the isoprenaline-mediated hyperpolarization induced by ouabain occurs due to a shift of the K$^+$ equilibrium potential. Yamanaka and Kitamura {72} reported that histamine via activation of the H$_2$ receptor also produced hyperpolarization in the guinea pig ileum circular muscle cells. Receptors for these agents (isoprenaline and histamine) are known to link with adenylate cyclase via GTP-binding protein to produce cAMP. Therefore, we can speculate that a simple causal relation occurs between hyperpolarization and cAMP-dependent activation of the maxi-K$^+$ channel. Indeed, application of dibutyryl cAMP and theophylline hyperpolarized the smooth muscle membrane of the rabbit pulmonary artery. Forskolin, an activator of adenylate cyclase, also produced membrane hyperpolarization in cultured rabbit aortic smooth muscle cells {73}. In tracheal myocytes, Kume et al. {33} and Savarie et al. {74} reported cAMP with protein kinase A activated the maxi-K$^+$ channel. As ChTX attenuated the relaxation induced by noradrenaline of tracheal tissue, which was precontracted by carbachol, it was speculated that synthesis of cAMP by isoprenaline or other agents was closely related to the generation of hyperpolarization {74}. All these findings may lead us to the conclusion that beta-adrenoceptor or H$_2$ receptor stimulation produces hyperpolarization by the maxi-K$^+$ channel via cAMP synthesis. There is no evidence that ChTX inhibits hyperpolarization induced by isoprenaline or histamine, although ChTX could inhibit the relaxant action induced by isoprenaline, salbutamol, or theophylline in guinea pig trachealis {75–77}. Contrary to the above speculation, the relaxant action of noradrenaline and the efflux of ^{86}Rb$^+$ stimulated by ATP or noradrenaline in various smooth muscle cells were inhibited by apamin, which does not block the maxi-K$^+$ channel {77–80}. To solve these inconsistencies, we need further information about the hyperpolarization induced by noradrenaline and isoprenaline.

ATP is known to activate a nonselective cation channel in various smooth muscle cells (ear artery {81}, vas deferens {82}, uterus {83}, portal vein {84}), whereas ATP hyperpolarizes the membrane in guinea pig small intestine and dog kidney cells {85,86}. The hyperpolarization induced by ATP was sensitive to [Ca^{2+}]$_o$ and was inhibited by apamin in guinea pig small intestine and by ChTX in dog kidney cells. Unfortunately, as an apamin-sensitive K channel has not been found in smooth muscle cells, the mechanism of channel activation by ATP is obscure. The slow component of the neurotensin-induced hyperpolarization was [Ca^{2+}]$_o$ dependent and was blocked by apamin, suggesting the existence of a common pathway for the apamin-sensitive K$^+$ channel for the hyperpolarization induced by ATP and neurotensin {85,87}.

Nitric oxide

It is known that a neurotransmitter from the nonadrenergic, noncholinergic (NANC) nerve in the enterogastric tract produces an apamin-sensitive hyperpolarization or relaxation {78,85,88–92}. To identify an unknown neurotransmitter of the NANC nerve, analogues of L-arginine were applied, since such analogues were known to inhibit nitric oxide synthase {93}. Several experiments showed that arginine analogues and oxyhemoglobin reduced the amplitude of the IJP or muscle relaxation induced by electrical field stimulation in canine gut {94–97}, suggesting that a neurotransmitter of the NANC neuron in these tissues is nitric oxide or a nitric oxide releasing compound. Furthermore, in opossum esophagus the hyperpolarization

induced by nitroprusside and the IJP were inhibited by methylene blue, a blocker of soluble guanylate cyclase {98}. Recently, Ward et al. {99} confirmed that nitric oxide produced membrane hyperpolarization and cGMP synthesis, and a membrane-permeable cGMP, 8 bromo cGMP, mimicked the membrane hyperpolarization in the dog colon. These may indicate that nitric oxide released from a nerve terminal permeates the membrane and activates soluble guanylate cyclase to produce cGMP, which activates a certain K$^+$ channel, possibly by channel phosphorylation with protein kinase G. However, in dog colon hyperpolarization induced by nitric oxide was not inhibited by methylene blue and the IJP was not inhibited by arginine analogues, suggesting that several mechanisms are involved in the membrane hyperpolarization induced by a neurotransmitter from NANC neurons in various tissues.

Nitric oxide is also known as endothelium-derived relaxing factor in vascular tissues {93}. Although nitric oxide could produce hyperpolarization in vascular smooth muscle cells, this substance is not the endothelium-dependent hyperpolarizing factor {100–102}. The hyperpolarization induced by acetylcholine was not blocked by glibenclamide, but that induced by nitric oxide gas or sodium nitrite was blocked by glibenclamide {102–104}. On the other hand, Nelson et al. {73} reported that in rabbit mesenteric artery the hyperpolarization induced by acetylcholine was blocked by glibenclamide. As Parkington et al. {69} noted that acetylcholine produced transient and prolonged hyperpolarization, and the latter component was inhibited by either nitro arginine methyl ester or indomethacin, more than two substances may be released from the endothelial cells as the endothelium-dependent hyperpolarizing factor. Although no specific blocker for the hyperpolarization induced by endothelium-derived factor has been found, calmidazolium, a calmodulin inhibitor, has been reported to block the endothelium-dependent hyperpolarization and relaxation resistant to nitro-L-arginine in canine coronary artery {105,106}. However, this inhibitory effect of calmidazolium is not an action on the K$^+$ channel, but on the synthetic process of the endothelium-derived hyperpolarizing factor or on the smooth muscle membrane.

K$^+$ channel openers

In cardiac and pancreatic beta-cells, chemicals classified as K$^+$ channel openers activate the ATP-sensitive K$^+$ channel {44,62,107–112}. However, in smooth muscle cells several results indicate that K$^+$ channel openers open different K$^+$ channels. In guinea pig mesenteric vein, the hyperpolarization induced by nicorandil and cromakalim was classified into fast and slow components by their Ca^{2+} sensitivity {113}. A glibenclamide-sensitive outward current induced by pinacidil and LP 805 was classified into a Ca^{2+}-independent current in rabbit portal vein, since the amplitude of the outward current induced by K$^+$ channel openers was not attenuated by removal of [Ca^{2+}]$_o$ or addition of a high concentration of EGTA in the cell {114}. On the other hand, in the rat portal vein a glibenclamide-sensitive outward current produced by nicorandil or cromakalim was sensitive to $[Ca^{2+}]_o$ {40}.

Single-channel current recording also revealed that K^+ channel openers activate several different types of K^+ channel in smooth muscle cells. In 1987, Kusano et al. {115} first reported that cromakalim opens a large-conductance Ca^{2+}-dependent K^+ channel in cultured cells of bovine and rabbit aorta (200 pS with symmetrical high K^+ solution). High concentrations of TEA could block this K^+ channel current. Gelband et al. {116} demonstrated that cromakalim increased the open probability of the maxi-K^+ channel by reducing the closed time of the slow component in the rabbit thoracic aorta. Recently, Gelband et al. {117} reported that cromakalim and lemakalim, an active isomer of cromakalim, increased the open probability of the large conductance Ca^{2+}-dependent K^+ channel (maxi-K^+ channel), which was very sensitive to the external application of low concentrations of TEA, in the canine colon and renal and coronary arteries. They also reported that glibenclamide reduced the open probability of the maxi-K^+ channel induced by K^+ channel openers in the inside-out membrane patch. Similarly, Hermsmeyer {118} demonstrated that ChTX could partly inhibit the outward current induced by pinacidil, but he also noted that an ATP-sensitive K^+ channel was distributed in the same rat azygos veins, with unitary conductance of 50 pS. It is interesting that lemakalim had no action on the maxi-K^+ channel pretreated by TEA {117}. It is speculated that a binding site for TEA on the maxi-K^+ channel is situated at the outer mouth of the channel (see later section), whereas lemakalim probably binds to the channel via a hydrophobic pathway. The gating mechanism of the maxi-K^+ channel is modulated by cAMP and cGMP or other metabolic processes, but activation of the maxi-K^+ channel by cromakalim is not related to such metabolic pathways, as lemakalim is reported to increase neither cAMP nor cGMP content {119}. Therefore, we may expect that lemakalim activates the channel in a direct way rather than by a known second messenger system and that binding of TEA in the channel leads to a kinetic change of the open gate regulated by K^+ channel openers in the maxi-K^+ channel.

Standen et al. {46} first reported that a similar ATP-sensitive K^+ channel to those in cardiac and pancreatic β cells is presented in smooth muscle cells of the rabbit mesenteric artery. The unitary conductance of this ATP-sensitive K^+ channel is larger than those in cardiac and β cells but relatively the same as the maxi-K^+ channel (135 pS). However, pharmacological properties of the ATP-sensitive K^+ channel in the mesenteric artery resemble those in cardiac and pancreatic β cells in being Ca^{2+} insensitive, ChTX insensitive, TEA resistant, and glibenclamide sensitive. In rabbit portal vein, an ATP-sensitive K^+ channel with smaller unitary conductance than in the rabbit mesenteric artery was reported to be present, but the pharmacological properties of the channel are much the same {54}. In rat portal vein, a different type of ATP-sensitive K^+ channel was activated by K^+ channel openers {25,40}. The outward current induced by cromakalim or nicorandil was attenuated by removal of

$[Ca^{2+}]_o$, and the unitary current (10 pS in asymmetrical K^+ concentrations) was sensitive to $[ATP]_i$, $[Ca^{2+}]_i$ and glibenclamide, but not to apamin and ChTX. Noack et al. {120} also estimated that in the same cells (rat portal vein) lemakalim opened a small-conductance K^+ channel (17 pS), which was sensitive to glibenclamide but insensitive to $[Ca^{2+}]_o$. They speculated that the difference in sensitivity to $[Ca^{2+}]$ may be due to interference of the channel with Mn^{2+}, as this Japanese group always use Mn^{2+} as a Ca^{2+} substitute. Another possible explanation for the discrepancy is that these researchers saw different channels, since K^+ channel openers produce hyperpolarization with transient Ca^{2+}-resistant and slow Ca^{2+}-sensitive components {113}. Indeed, Okabe et al. {40} demonstrated that cromakalim still produced an outward current, even in the presence of Mn^{2+}, although a major part of the outward current was inhibited by removal of Ca^{2+}. Another Ca^{2+}-dependent K^+ channel, which was sensitive to $[ATP]_i$ and glibenclamide, was reported to be present in the pig coronary artery {43}. The unitary conductance of this channel was 30 pS and it was inhibited by 5 mM 4-AP.

Most of the K^+ channel openers are hydrophobic agents and the rate of channel activation is slower than other channel modulators, such as ATP or GDP. Using a concentration jump technique, Takano and Noma {56} reported that nicorandil, a water-soluble agent, activated the channel with a time constant of about 1 second, whereas the opening rate of the channel on removal of ATP was about 100 ms. Pinacidil and cromakalim, applied from either side, activated the ATP-sensitive K^+ channel in rat portal vein and pig coronary artery {25,43,54}. Although a high concentration was required to activate the channel, nicorandil also activated the channel from the intracellular membrane side {121}. In rabbit portal vein, Kajioka et al. {54} reported that pinacidil and cromakalim activated the ATP-sensitive K^+ channel in the cell-attached condition when drugs were applied in the bath. This indicates that K^+-channel openers have to penetrate the membrane first, then reach the binding site. Thuringer and Escande {122} showed a competitive antagonism of ATP on the RP 49356- (a K^+ channel opener) induced channel activation and a prolongation of onset of blocking action of ATP by RP 49356. They speculate that K^+ channel openers bind to a site where the drug competes with ATP or an ATP binding protein. Takano and Noma {56} also speculated that a target of nicorandil is an ATP-sensitive gating mechanism, because nicorandil reduced the apparent binding rate of ATP but did not change the unbinding rate. However, Takano and Noma also proposed another unknown mechanism for the nicorandil-induced channel activation in ATP-free condition, because the ATP-regulated channel gate should open fully in ATP free condition {66,123}. From all of these findings, we can speculate that the binding sites for K^+ channel openers are located at the intracellular face of the channel or in the membrane where the drug can easily interact with the ATP-regulating gate.

Fan et al. {62} demonstrated that pinacidil did not modify the mean open and fast-closed times, but increased the mean burst duration and reduced the long closed time in guinea pig ventricular cells. ATP did not modify the mean burst duration, but increased the fast and slow closing times, suggesting that pinacidil modulates an ATP-dependent regulating mechanism of the channel, possibly by binding to a different site from the inhibitory ATP-binding site. In rabbit portal vein, on the other hand, Kajioka et al. {54} reported that pinacidil increased the mean open time and reduced the mean closed time, whereas ATP reduced the mean open time by chopping up the long opening of the channel. These indicate that K⁺ channel openers and ATP do not compete for the same site. As a very high rate of channel transition was not seen in the rabbit portal vein due to the use of a low-frequency cut-off filter, the burst channel opening was not seen in the smooth muscle cells.

The rundown phenomenon is well documented as a result of channel dephosphorylation due to depletion of ATP, because readministration of ATP could reactivate the channel {51,53,124}. Pinacidil did not activate the dephosphorylated channel but activated the phosphorylated channel in ventricular cells {61}. However, when the channel was activated by nucleoside diphosphates, pinacidil could open the channel. Similarly, in the smooth muscle cells of the rabbit portal vein, pinacidil lost the ability to activate the ATP-sensitive K⁺ channel after rundown of the channel but possessed the ability with the coexistence of GDP {54}. It is interesting that in inside-out membrane patches of the rabbit portal vein, activity of the ATP-sensitive K⁺ channel was not seen in the absence of pinacidil or other K⁺ channel openers, even in the presence of GDP. This indicates that K⁺ channel openers open the ATP-sensitive K⁺ channel only in the operative state (either phosphorylated by ATP or activated by nucleoside diphosphates).

MECHANISMS OF K⁺ CHANNEL INHIBITION BY VARIOUS AGENTS

TEA

TEA is the first K⁺ channel blocker that has been demonstrated to have an inhibitory action on the large-conductance Ca^{2+}-dependent K⁺ channel (maxi-K⁺ channel) in various cells by single-channel current analysis (pituitary neuron {125}, skeletal muscle {126}, chromaffin cells {127}, smooth muscle cells {27,28}). The mode of channel inhibition by TEA differs, depending on the side of the membrane TEA to which is applied {28}. Submillimolar concentrations of TEA, applied from the outside of the channel, effectively block the maxi-K⁺ channel (K_i = 0.2–0.3 mM), whereas higher concentrations of intracellular TEA (K_i = 10–30 mM) are required to block the channel {27,28,125–128}. Inhibition by TEA occurs with reduction in the apparent amplitude of the unitary current without change in the mean open time but with an increase in the long closed interval. There is little voltage dependency for the blocking actions of TEA at either side {28,128}. Using a noise reduction filter with a cut-off

frequency of more than 3 kHz, current noise amplitude is augmented while the channel is open, suggesting plug-in block by the TEA molecule. As inhibition appears to be voltage independent, binding sites of TEA are located separately near the pore opening on either side of the membrane {129}. The distance to the TEA binding site on either side of the membrane from the channel mouth is estimated to be 0.1–0.26 of the electric field {126–128}, and this value is close to those in other K⁺ channels {129,130}.

Other K⁺ channels are also blocked by high concentrations of TEA (1–10 mM) on either side of the membrane, such as the voltage-dependent (delayed) K⁺ channel in squid giant axon and visceral smooth muscle cells, the ATP-sensitive K⁺ channel, delayed rectifier K⁺ channel in skeletal muscle cells, and the transient K⁺ current in human T lymphocytes {9,129–132}. However, in rabbit pulmonary artery and possibly other arterial smooth muscle cells, the voltage-dependent (delayed) K⁺ channel seems to be insensitive to 10 mM TEA {24}. In the delayed K⁺ channel in frog skeletal muscle, TEA did not change the mean open time. Therefore, channel block by TEA is independent of the gating mechanism {133}. However, a cloned K⁺ channel, the RCK2 channel (a *Shaker*-type delayed rectifier K⁺ channel), was blocked by intracellular TEA with a slow blocking rate. Thus the apparent unitary current amplitude did not decrease {130}. It has been reported that external TEA prevents the close of the inactivation gate of the transient K⁺ channel in human T lymphocytes {132} and prolongs the open time of the transient K⁺ channel with reduction in the apparent amplitude of the unitary current in the rat olfactory receptor neurons {134}.

Recently, an aromatic amino acid, such as phenylalanine or tyrosine, in the pore-forming region of the *Shaker* K⁺ channel (position 449), was found to be essential for forming the high-affinity site for external TEA binding {135–137}, and substitution of the amino acid at the 449 position by a hydrophobic amino acid (isoleucine or valine) formed a K⁺ channel pore with very low TEA sensitivity {137}. Furthermore, they found that external TEA sensitivity of the *Shaker* K⁺ channel was determined by the number of tyrosine-containing subunits at the 449 position. Yellen et al. {138} also reported that intracellular TEA binding to the *Shaker* K⁺ channel was strongly affected by threonine at the 372 position. On the other hand, Kirsch et al. {139} reported that nine amino acids between the 368 and 388 positions markedly interfered in both the internal and external TEA sensitivity of the Kv2.1 channel. As both the Kv2.1 host channel and its mutated channel have tyrosine at the 380 position, they concluded that the aromatic amino acid in this position did not affect the TEA sensitivity, although substitution of threonine by tyrosine at the 380 position of the *Shaker* K⁺ channel increased TEA sensitivity {139}.

4-AP

4-AP blocks A channels, transient K⁺ channels, delayed rectifier K⁺ channels, and ATP-sensitive K⁺ channels in various cells {25,40,134,140–143}. The block induced by 4-AP occurs in a voltage-dependent manner {24,142, 144,145}. Yeh et al. {142,144} and Okabe et al. {24} reported that 4-AP strongly blocked the K^+ currents evoked by lower depolarizing pulses than larger depolarizing pulses in the squid axon membrane and the smooth muscle cells of the rabbit pulmonary artery. Simurda et al. {146} also reported that the transient K^+ current in dog ventricular cells, blocked by 4-AP, was partly relieved by repetitive membrane depolarization. The block produced by 4-AP applied externally showed strong dependence on extracellular pH {24,147,148}. On superfusion with alkaline solution in the bath, the current inhibition induced by external 4-AP was more pronounced than that in acidic solution, whereas changes in the external pH did not affect external 4-AP-induced inhibition of the K^+ channel {24,148}. As 4-AP has a large pKa value (9.17), the ionized form of 4-AP has no or little action on the K^+ channel and 4-AP must permeate the membrane, probably through a hydrophobic pathway, before acting on the channel. Therefore it is speculated that the binding site of the 4-AP molecule is on the inside of the membrane. Kasai et al. {22} and Davies et al. {143} showed that $[4-AP]_i$ blocked the ATP-sensitive K^+ channel with reduction in the unitary current amplitude, similar to the blocking action of TEA on various K^+ channels, but external 4-AP did not reduce the unitary current amplitude. As the internal 4-AP-induced block increased with membrane depolarization, they estimated that ionized 4-AP bound just over half of the membrane electric field of the ATP-sensitive K^+ channel, which was being opened with 1:1 stoichiometry {143}. On the other hand, the fast-inactivating transient K^+ current in rat melanotrophs and the voltage-dependent K^+ current in the rabbit pulmonary arterial cells were speculated to be blocked by 4-AP in the resting state {24,149}. In this case, 4-AP was time-dependently dissociated from the binding site in the channel, which was activated by a strong depolarization. Kasai et al. {22} demonstrated that 4-AP also reduced the mean open time as well as reducing the unitary conductance in DRG neurons of the guinea pig. In rat portal vein, 4-AP did not reduce the unitary conductance of the ATP-sensitive K^+ channel, but reduced the open probability of the channel (probably with reduction in the mean open time) {25}. The channel block by 4-AP with fast and slow kinetics indicates that there are two different pathways or mechanisms for inhibition. It is well known that local anesthetics block the voltage-dependent Na^+ channel through hydrophobic and hydrophilic pathways, and the former modifies the gating mechanism of the channel and the latter produces a plug-in block of the channel at the open state {150}. Fast and slow blocking kinetics and two different dissociation constant for reduction in the peak ensemble average current (1 mM) and the unitary conductance (12 mM) indicate the presence of two different mechanisms of action of the A current of DRG neurons {22}. 4-AP probably acts on the K^+ channel via hydrophobic and hydrophilic pathways, similar to the action of local anesthetics on the voltage-dependent Na^+ channel.

Glibenclamide

Glibenclamide and other sulfonylurea derivatives are thought to be specific channel blockers of the ATP-sensitive K^+ channel in various cells (pancreatic cells {151–154}, cardiac cells {109,155}, smooth muscle cells {25,54,63}). However, glibenclamide has also been reported to inhibit other K^+ channels. In the human neuroblastoma cell line (SH-SY5Y) glibenclamide (1–20 μM) produces a voltage-independent but time-dependent inhibition of the K^+ channel, which is insensitive to $[ATP]_i$ and $[Ca^{2+}]_o$ {156}. Glibenclamide also inhibits the maxi-K^+ channel in smooth muscle cells recorded in the cell-attached condition {117}. However, Xiong et al. {13} reported that glibenclamide had no effect on the maxi-K^+ channel of the rabbit portal vein in the cell-free condition. As glibenclamide inhibited I_{OO}, actions of glibenclamide observed in the cell-attached condition are possibly due to an indirect action on the maxi-K^+ channel through modulation of Ca^{2+}-induced Ca^{2+} release mechanisms {157}.

Glibenclamide inhibited the ATP-sensitive K^+ channel with a Hill coefficient of 1.26 in guinea pig ventricular cells {158}. From a radioligand binding experiment, there are high- and low-affinity binding sites in brain, β cells, and cardiac and smooth muscle cells {159–161}. K^+ channel openers (cromakalim, lemakalim, pinacidil, minoxidil, and nicorandil, but not diazoxide) did not interact with the glyburide binding site, suggesting a different binding site for K^+ channel openers and sulfonylurea {161}.

Glibenclamide is a very hydrophobic agent with a pKa value of 6.3. As inhibitory effects of glibenclamide on the ATP-sensitive K^+ channel were enhanced by perfusion of an acidic solution over the extracellular surface but not in the intracellular space, the un-ionized form of glibenclamide is probably responsible for inhibition of the ATP-sensitive K^+ channel in guinea pig ventricular cells {162}. Findlay {162} also demonstrated that tolbutamide, a less hydrophobic sulfonylurea than glibenclamide, also inhibited the ATP-sensitive K^+ channel in the same way as glibenclamide. However, tolbutamide showed faster recovery from the inhibition than glibenclamide. Therefore, Findlay {158,162} concluded that the sulphonylurea receptor is located in the lipid phase of the membrane.

Quinidine

Quinine and quinidine were found to be specific blockers of the Ca^{2+}-dependent K^+ channel, which is not sensitive to apamin, in erythrocytes {163,164}. However, quinine and quinidine have been reported to block various K^+ channels in various preparations, such as A current, delayed K^+ current, Ca^{2+}-dependent K^+ current, Ca^{2+} inward current, and Na^+ inward current {10,35,165–169}. Quinidine blocked the maxi-K^+ channel in toad stomach cells with reduction in the amplitude of the unitary conductance, but at a slower rate than TEA {35}. Wong {35} also demonstrated that quinidine only acted internally and was knocked off by inward movement of K^+, producing inward rectification. On the other hand, quinine acts from the external surface of the maxi-K$^+$ channel of bovine chromaffin cells without change in the mean closed time, and the blocking action was augmented by membrane hyperpolarization {170}. The reason for this difference has not yet been solved. Recently, Snyders et al. {166} has reported that quinidine blocks a cloned human cardiac K$^+$ channel (HK2) with 1:1 stoichiometry at the open state and that it is unbound before channel closing. Quinidine blocks the channel by binding at the internal mouth (0.19 of the electric field from the inner surface). Quinidine has a relatively large pKa value of 8.9, indicating that at a pH 7.2–7.4 quinidine is present predominantly in the ionized form. Therefore external quinidine in the neutral form should permeate the membrane and be ionized before reaching the binding site (inner mouth of the channel).

Charybdotoxin

ChTX is a 37 amino acid protein from the venom of the scorpion *Leiurus quinquestriatus* var. hebraeus and is thought to be a specific blocker of the maxi-K$^+$ channel {171}. ChTX also selectively blocks the maxi-K$^+$ channel in smooth muscle cells {46,54,114}. In molluscan neurons ChTX was reported to block the small-conductance Ca^{2+}-dependent K$^+$ channel (35 pS) as well as the maxi-K$^+$ channel {38}. ChTX inhibited the apamin-sensitive afterhyperpolarizing potential in bullfrog sympathetic ganglion cells, but not the apamin-insensitive afterhyperpolarizing potential in rat hippocampal CA1 cells {172,173}. The Ca^{2+}-insensitive and voltage-dependent K$^+$ channel in rat DRG neurons and human and murine T lymphocytes was also shown to be blocked by ChTX {174,175}. Recently, ChTX has been reported to block all K$^+$ channels distributed in the human T lymphocytes (one voltage-dependent and three Ca^{2+}-dependent K$^+$ channels) {176}.

Mechanisms of inhibitory actions of charybdotoxin have been well investigated in the skeletal muscle maxi-K$^+$ channel incorporated into the planar membrane {171, 177–179}. ChTX inhibits the Ca^{2+}-dependent K$^+$ channel with 1:1 stoichiometry, and the binding site is estimated to be located on the outer mouth of the channel {177}, because ChTX does not block the maxi-K$^+$ channel from the intracellular side and shares a common binding site with [TEA]$_o$ {178}. MacKinnon and Miller {179} showed that internal K$^+$ and another permeable ion, [Rb$^+$]$_i$, enhanced the [ChTX]$_o$ dissociation rate, but the impermeable ions [Na$^+$]$_i$, [Li$^+$]$_i$, and [Cs$^+$]$_i$ did not accelerate the dissociation. ChTX, which blocks both open and closed channels, probably plugs the channel physically at the external mouth. Increase in the ChTX concentration, membrane depolarization, and binding to the open channel accelerated the association rate, but did not change the dissociation rate {177}.

The binding site of ChTX is located on the external loop between the S5 and S6 transmembrane structures of the *Shaker* K$^+$ channel, because point mutations at the 422 glutamate, 427 lysine, and 452 glycine alter the toxin inhibition by an electrostatic mechanism, but mutations in the external loop between S1 and S2, or S3 and S4, do not alter the ChTX inhibition {180,181}.

Iberiotoxin

So far, iberiotoxin (IbTX) is thought to be a selective blocker of the maxi-K$^+$ channel {182–184}. IbTX is also a 37 amino acid peptide that is purified from the venom of the scorpion *Buthus tamulus* and has 68% homology with ChTX. Blocking of the maxi-K$^+$ channel by IbTX is very similar to that by ChTX. However, IbTX induces a long silent period between the normal burst channel opening and reduces the mean open time, indicating that IbTX more tightly binds to the channel than ChTX {182,184}. As only external IbTX inhibits the maxi-K$^+$ channel and the IbTX binding is relieved by TEA, this toxin also binds to the outer mouth of the channel {184}. IbTX produces concentration-dependent inhibition of ^{125}I-ChTX binding, but does not replace 10–20% of bound ChTX in the bovine aortic muscle {182}. On the other hand, IbTX neither affected ChTX binding in the A-type K$^+$ channel in rat brain nor blocked the fast-inactivating transient K$^+$ channel in T lymphocytes and *Shaker* K$^+$ channels of *Drosophila* {182}. From studies of hybrid IbTX and ChTX, the 21–24 amino acid residues of IbTX have been reported to be crucial for IbTX binding {183,185}.

Apamin and leiurotoxin

Apamin is an 18 amino acid peptide purified from honeybee venom (*Apis mellifera*). Apamin, applied from the external membrane side, inhibits the small conductance Ca^{2+}-dependent K$^+$ channel (12 pS) but has no effect on the maxi-K$^+$ channel in rat skeletal muscle {37}. Apamin also has no effect on the maxi-K$^+$ channel in various smooth muscle cells, and an apamin-sensitive K$^+$ channel has not yet been identified in smooth muscle cells.

Leiurotoxin, purified from the scorpion venom of *Leiurus quinquestriatus* var. hebraeus, is a 31 amino acid peptide and has been reported to inhibit apamin binding, although leiurotoxin has no structural homology to apamin {186}. Leiurotoxin blocks the apamin-sensitive K$^+$ channel in guinea pig hepatocytes and bullfrog sympathetic ganglion cells {173,186,187}. On the other hand, a small-conductance Ca^{2+}-dependent K$^+$ channel, which was responsible for the afterhyperpolarization in rat hippocampal CA1 neurons, was not inhibited by leiurotoxin {173}.

Dendrotoxins

α-dendrotoxin is a 59 amino acid peptide purified from the Green Mamba (*Dendroaspis angusticeps*), which has a similar amino acid sequence to dendrotoxin I from Black Mamba (*Dendroaspis polylepsis*). Dendrotoxin selectively blocks the 4-AP-sensitive K$^+$ current in the frog motor nerve fiber, guinea pig DRG, and rat ganglion cells {188–191}. On the other hand, dendrotoxin does not bind to the membrane of human T lymphocytes {192}, which have a voltage-dependent K$^+$ channel sensitive to ChTX {174}, and in rat brain membrane ChTX inhibited dendrotoxin binding, due to a nonselective channel blocking action of ChTX {175}. Some of the cloned voltage-dependent K$^+$ channels from rat and mouse were inhibited by dendrotoxin (RCK1, RCK5, MK1, and MK2) {192,193}. Dendrotoxin binding was modified by β-bungarotoxin (21 kDa), a purified snake venom from *Bungarus multicinctus*, and mast cell degranulating peptide (MCD) purified from the bee venom of *Apis mellifera* {194–197}.

Noxiustoxin

Noxiustoxin is a 39 amino acid peptide purified from the scorpion venom of *Centruroides noxius*. Noxiustoxin did not interact with ChTX binding to the bovine aortic preparations, but inhibited the ChTX binding in rat brain synaptic membrane and the maxi-K$^+$ channel activity in skeletal muscle cells {198–200}. In rat synaptosomes noxiustoxin blocked both Ca^{2+}-independent and -dependent ^{86}Rb efflux, and the former was more than 10 times more sensitive to the toxin than the latter {201}. Sands et al. {174} and Leonard et al. {176} also reported that noxiustoxin blocked a voltage-dependent K$^+$ channel, which was blocked by ChTX, but not Ca^{2+}-dependent, ChTX-sensitive K$^+$ channels in human and murine T lymphocytes. Garcia et al. {183} considered that noxiustoxin blocked the ChTX-sensitive, voltage-dependent K$^+$ channel, but neither the delayed rectifier nor the maxi-K$^+$ channels.

CONCLUSIONS

Due to the voltage-dependent properties of the dihydropyridine-sensitive Ca^{2+} channel, the opening and blocking of K$^+$ channels was believed to control [Ca^{2+}]$_i$ indirectly via regulation of the Ca^{2+} channel. However, recent evidence from arterial cells has shown that the membrane potential (depolarization and hyperpolarization) directly modulates the InsP$_3$ synthetic system, the main [Ca]$_i$ mobilizing system for receptor-mediated contraction in smooth muscle cells. Therefore, we are required to have a higher estimate for roles of the K$^+$ channel on smooth muscle function than before. There are many K$^+$ channels with a wide variety of properties in smooth muscle cells, and the activity of each channel is affected by different K$^+$ channel modulators in different ways. Although we do not have any specific K$^+$ channel modulator at present, control of the K$^+$ channel activity may become important for the treatment of disease.

ACKNOWLEDGMENTS

The authors are grateful to Dr. K.E. Creed, Murdoch University, Australia, for her English editing. This work was supported by Grants-in-Aid for Scientific Research from the Ministry of Education, Science and Culture, Japan.

REFERENCES

1. Gisbert MP, Mery PF, Fishmeister R: A patch-clamp study of the effects of cicletanine on whole-cell calcium current in ventricular myocytes. *Drugs Exp Clin Res* 14:109–115, 1988.
2. Casteels R, Kitamura K, Kuriyama H, Suzuki H: The membrane properties of the smooth muscle cells of the rabbit main pulmonary artery. *J Physiol* 271:41–61, 1977.
3. Hara Y, Kitamura K, Kuriyama H: Actions of 4-aminopyridine on vascular smooth muscle tissues of the guinea-pig. *Br J Pharmacol* 68:99–106, 1980.
4. Sasaguri T, Watson SP: Protein kinase C regulates the tonic but not the phasic component of contraction in guinea-pig ileum. *Br J Pharmacol* 98:791–798, 1989.
5. Itoh T, Seki N, Suzuki S, Ito S, Kajikuri J, Kuriyama H: Membrane hyperpolarization inhibits agonist-induced synthesis of inositol 1,4,5-trisphosphate in rabbit mesenteric artery. *J Physiol* 451:307–328, 1991.
6. Sumimoto K, Domae M, Yamanaka K, Nakao K, Hashimoto T, Kitamura K, Kuriyama H: Actions of nicorandil on vascular smooth muscles. *J Cardiovasc Pharmacol* 10(Suppl. 8):S66–S75, 1987.
7. Furukawa K, Itoh T, Kajiwara M, Kitamura K, Suzuki H, Ito Y, Kuriyama H: Vasodilating actions of 2-nicotinamidoethyl nitrate on porcine and guinea-pig coronary arteries. *J Pharmacol Exp Ther* 218:248–259, 1981.
8. Inoue T, Ito Y, Takeda K: The effects of 2-nicotinamidoethyl nitrate on smooth muscle cells of the dog mesenteric artery and trachea. *Br J Pharmacol* 80:459–470, 1983.
9. Ohya Y, Kitamura K, Kuriyama H: Cellular calcium regulates outward currents in rabbit intestinal smooth muscle cell. *Am J Physiol* 251:C335–346, 1987.
10. Nakao K, Inoue R, Yamanaka K, Kitamura K: Actions of quinidine and apamin on after-hyperpolarization of the spike in circular smooth muscle cells of the guinea-pig ileum. *Naunyn-Schmiedebergs Arch Pharmacol* 334:508–513, 1986.
11. Hume JR, Leblanc N: Macroscopic K$^+$ currents in single smooth muscle cells of the rabbit portal vein. *J Physiol* 413:49–73, 1989.
12. Muraki K, Imaizumi Y, Kojima T, Kawai T, Watanabe M: Effects of tetraethylammonium and 4-aminopyridine on outward currents and excitability in canine tracheal smooth muscle cells. *Br J Pharmacol* 100:507–515, 1990.
13. Xiong Z, Kitamura K, Kuriyama H: Evidence for contribution of Ca^{2+} storage sites on unitary K$^+$ channel currents in inside-out membrane of rabbit portal vein. *Pflügers Arch* 420:112–114, 1992.
14. Benham CD, Bolton TB: Spontaneous transient outward currents in single visceral and vascular smooth muscle cells of the rabbit. *J Physiol* 381:385–406, 1986.
15. Ohya Y, Terada K, Yamaguchi K, Inoue R, Okabe K, Kitamura K, Hirata M, Kuriyama H: Effects of inositol phosphates on the membrane activity of smooth muscle cells of the rabbit portal vein. *Pflügers Arch* 412:382–389, 1988.
16. Sakai T, Terada K, Kitamura K, Kuriyama H: Ryanodine inhibits the Ca-dependent K current after depletion of Ca stored in smooth muscle cells of the rabbit ileal longitudinal muscle. *Br J Pharmacol* 95:1089–1100, 1988.
17. Bolton TB, Lim SP: Properties of calcium stores and transient outward currents in single smooth muscle cells of rabbit intestine. *J Physiol* 409:385–401, 1989.
18. Kitamura K, Xiong Z, Teramoto N, Kuriyama H: Roles of inositol trisphosphate and protein kinase C in the spontaneous outward current modulated by calcium release in rabbit portal vein. *Pflügers Arch* 421:539–551, 1992.

19. Beech DJ, Bolton TB: A voltage-dependent outward current with fast kinetics in single smooth muscle cells isolated from the rabbit portal vein. *J Physiol* 412:397–414, 1989.

20. Lang RJ: Identification of the major membrane currents in freshly dispersed single smooth muscle cells of guinea-pig ureter. *J Physiol* 412:375–395, 1989.

21. Imaizumi Y, Muraki K, Watanabe M: Characteristics of transient outward currents in single smooth muscle cells from the ureter of the guinea-pig. *J Physiol* 427:301–324, 1989.

22. Kasai H, Kameyama M, Yamaguchi K, Fukuda J: Single transient K channels in mammalian sensory neurons. *Biophys J* 49:1243–1247, 1986.

23. Beech DJ, Bolton TB: Two components of potassium current activated by depolarization of single smooth muscle cells from the rabbit portal vein. *J Physiol* 418:293–309, 1989.

24. Okabe K, Kitamura K, Kuriyama H: Features of 4-aminopyridine sensitive outward current in single smooth muscle cells from the rabbit main pulmonary artery. *Pflügers Arch* 409:561–568, 1987.

25. Kajioka S, Oike M, Kitamura K: Nicorandil opens a calcium-dependent potassium channel in smooth muscle cells of the rat portal vein. *J Pharmacol Exp Ther* 254:905–913, 1990.

26. Berger W, Grygorcyk R, Shwarz W: Single K$^+$ channels in membrane evaginations of smooth muscle cells. *Pflügers Arch* 402:18–23, 1984.

27. Benham CD, Bolton TB, Lang RJ, Tekewaki T: The mechanism of action of Ba^{2+} and TEA on single Ca^{2+}-activated K$^+$-channels in arterial and intestinal smooth muscle cell membranes. *Pflügers Arch* 403:120–127, 1985.

28. Inoue R, Kitamura K, Kuriyama H: Two Ca-dependent K-channels classified by the application of tetraethylammonium distribute to smooth muscle membranes of the rabbit portal vein. *Pflügers Arch* 405:173–179, 1985.

29. McCann JD, Welsh MJ: Calcium-activated potassium channels in canine airway smooth muscle. *J Physiol* 372:113–127, 1986.

30. Singer JJ, Walsh JV Jr: Characterization of calcium-activated potassium channels in single smooth muscle cells using the patch-clamp technique. *Pflügers Arch* 408:98–111, 1987.

31. Williams DL, Katz GM, Roy-Contancin L, Reuben JP: Guanosine 5'-monophosphate modulates gating of high-conductance Ca^{2+}-activated K$^+$ channels in vascular smooth muscle cells. *Proc Natl Acad Sci USA* 85:9360–9364, 1988.

32. Bregestovski PD, Printseva OY, Serebryakov V, Stinnakre J, Turmin A, Zamoyski V: Comparison of Ca^{2+}-dependent K$^+$ channels in the membrane of smooth muscle cells isolated from adult and foetal human aorta. *Pflügers Arch* 413:8–13, 1988.

33. Kume H, Takagi K, Satake T, Tokuno H, Tomita T: Effects of intracellular pH on calcium-activated potassium channels in rabbit tracheal smooth muscle. *J Physiol* 424:445–457, 1990.

34. Kihara M, Matsuzawa K, Tokuno H, Tomita T: Effects of calmodulin antagonists on calcium-activated potassium channels in pregnant rat myometrium. *Br J Pharmacol* 100:353–359, 1990.

35. Wong BS: Quinidine blockade of calcium-activated potassium channels in dissociated gastric smooth muscle cells. *Pflügers Arch* 414:416–422, 1989.

36. Taniguchi J, Furukawa KI, Shigekawa M: Maxi K$^+$ channel activity stimulated by G kinase in the canine coronary arterial smooth muscle. *Jpn J Pharmacol* 58(Suppl II):397p, 1992.

37. Blatz AL, Magleby KL: Single apamin-blocked Ca-activated K$^+$ channels of small conductance in rat cultured skeletal muscle. *Nature* 323:718–720, 1986.

38. Hermann A, Erxleben C: Charybdotoxin selectively blocks small Ca-activated K channels in *Aplysia* neurons. *J Gen Physiol* 90:27–47, 1987.

39. Wolff D, Cecchi X, Spalvins A, Canessa M: Charybdotoxin blocks with high affinity the Ca-activated K$^+$ channel of Hb A and Hb S red cells: Individual differences in the number of channels. *J Memb Biol* 106:243–252, 1988.

40. Okabe K, Kajioka S, Nakao K, Kitamura K, Kuriyama H, Weston AH: Actions of cromakalim on ionic currents recorded from single smooth muscle cells of the rat portal vein. *J Pharmacol Exp Ther* 250:832–839, 1990.

41. Inoue R, Okabe K, Kitamura K, Kuriyama H: A newly identified Ca^{2+} dependent K$^+$ channel in the smooth muscle membrane of single cells dispersed from the rabbit portal vein. *Pflügers Arch* 406:138–143, 1986.

42. Inoue I, Nakaya Y, Nakaya S, Mori H: Extracellular Ca^{2+}-activated K$^+$ channel in coronary artery smooth muscle cells and its role in vasodilation. *FEBS Lett* 255:281–284, 1989.

43. Inoue I, Nakaya S, Nakaya Y: An ATP-sensitive K$^+$ channel activated by extracellular Ca^{2+} and Mg^{2+} in primary cultured arterial smooth muscle cells. *J Physiol* 430:132P, 1990.

44. Noma A: ATP-regulated K$^+$ channels in cardiac cells. *Nature* 305:147–148, 1983.

45. Ashcroft FM: Adenosine 5'-triphosphate-sensitive potassium channels. *Ann Rev Neurosci* 11:97–118, 1988.

46. Standen NB, Quayle JM, Davies NW, Brayden JE, Huang Y, Nelson MT: Hyperpolarizing vasodilators activate ATP-sensitive K$^+$ channels in arterial smooth muscle. *Science* 245:177–180, 1989.

47. de Weille JR, Lazdunski M: Regulation of the ATP-sensitive potassium channel In: Narahashi T (ed) *Ion Channels*, Vol II. New York: Plenum Press, 1990, pp 205–222.

48. Horie M, Irisawa H, Noma A: Voltage-dependent magnesium block of adenosine-triphosphate-sensitive potassium channel in guinea-pig ventricular cells. *J Physiol* 387:251–272, 1987.

49. Nichols CG, Lederer WJ: The regulation of ATP-sensitive K$^+$ channel activity in intact and permeabilized rat ventricular myocytes. *J Physiol* 423:91–110, 1990.

50. Trube G, Hescheler J: Inward-rectifying channels in isolated patches of the heart cell membrane: ATP-dependence and comparison with cell-attached patches. *Pflügers Arch* 401:178–184, 1984.

51. Findlay I, Dunne MJ: ATP maintains ATP-inhibited K$^+$ channels in an operational state. *Pflügers Arch* 407:238–240, 1986.

52. Misler S, Falke LC, Gillkis KD, McDaniell ML: A metabolite-regulated potassium channel in rat pancreatic B-cells. *Proc Natl Acad Sci USA* 83:7119–7123, 1986.

53. Ohno-Shosaku T, Zünkler BJ, Trube G: Dual effects of ATP on K$^+$ currents of mouse pancreatic β-cells. *Pflügers Arch* 408:133–138, 1987.

54. Kajioka S, Kitamura K, Kuriyama H: Guanosine diphosphate activates an adenosine-5'-triphosphate-sensitive K$^+$ channel in the rabbit portal vein. *J Physiol* 444:397–418, 1991.

55. Ribalet B, Ciani S, Eddlestone GT: ATP mediates both activation and inhibition of K(ATP) channel activity via cAMP-dependent protein kinase in insulin-secreting cell lines. *J Gen Physiol* 94:693–717, 1989.

56. Takano M, Noma A: Selective modulation of the ATP-sensitive K$^+$ channel by nicorandil in guinea-pig cardiac cell membrane. *Naunyn-Schmiedebergs Arch Pharmacol* 342:592–597, 1990.

57. Findlay I: The effects of magnesium upon adenosine triphosphate-sensitive potassium channels in a rat insulin-secreting cell line. *J Physiol* 391:611–629, 1987.

58. Dunne MJ, Petersen OH: Intracellular ADP activates K^+ channels that are inhibited by ATP in an insulin-secreting cell line. *FEBS Lett* 208:59–62, 1986.

59. Takano M, Qin D, Noma A: ATP-dependent decay and recovery of K^+ channels in guinea-pig cardiac myocytes. *Am J Physiol* 258:H45–50, 1990.

60. Dunne MJ, Petersen OH: GTP and GDP activation of K^+ channels that can be inhibited by ATP. *Pflügers Arch* 407: 564–565, 1986.

61. Tung RT, Kurachi Y: On the mechanism of nucleotide diphosphate activation of the ATP-sensitive K^+ channel in ventricular cell of guinea-pig. *J Physiol* 1991.

62. Fan Z, Nakayama K, Hiraoka M: Pinacidil activates the ATP-sensitive K^+ channel in inside-out and cell-attached patch membranes of guinea-pig ventricular myocytes. *Pflügers Arch* 415:387–394, 1990.

63. Nelson MT, Huang Y, Brayden JE, Hesceler J, Standen NB: Arterial dilations in response to calcitonin gene-related peptide involve activation of K^+ channels. *Nature* 344: 770–773, 1990.

64. Davies NW, Standen NB, Stanfield PR: The effect of intracellular pH on ATP-dependent potassium channels of frog skeletal muscle. *J Physiol* 445:549–568, 1992.

65. Cook DL, Hales CN: Intracellular ATP directly blocks K^+ channels in pancreatic B-cells. *Nature* 311:271–273, 1984.

66. Kakei M, Noma A, Shibasaki T: Properties of adenosine-triphosphate-regulated potassium channels in guinea-pig ventricular cells. *J Physiol* 363:441–462, 1985.

67. Spruce AE, Standen NB, Stanfield PR: Voltage-dependent ATP-sensitive potassium channels of skeletal muscle membrane. *Nature* 316:736–738, 1985.

68. Noma A, Shibasaki T: Intracellular ATP and cardiac membrane currents. In: Narahashi T (ed) *Ion Channels*, Vol I. New York: Plenum Press, 1988, pp 183–212.

69. Lederer WJ, Nichols CG: Nucleotide modulation of the activity of rat heart ATP-sensitive-K^+ channels in isolated membrane patches. *J Physiol* 419:193–211, 1989.

70. Treherne JM, Ashford MLJ: Extracellular cations modulate the ATP sensitivity of ATP-K^+ channels in rat ventromedial hypothalamic neurons. *Proc R Soc Lond B* 247:121–124, 1992.

71. Yamaguchi H, Honeyman TW, Fay FS: β-Adrenergic actions on membrane electrical properties of dissociated smooth muscle cells. *Am J Physiol* 254:C423–C431, 1988.

72. Yamanaka K, Kitamura K: Electrophysiological and mechanical characteristics of histamine receptors in smooth muscle cells of the guinea-pig ileum. *Eur J Pharmacol* 144: 29–37, 1987.

73. Pavenstädt H, Lindeman V, Lindeman S, Kunzelmann K, Späth M, Greger R: Effect of depolarizing and hyperpolarizing agents on the membrane potential difference of primary cultures of rabbit aorta vascular smooth muscle cells. *Pflügers Arch* 419:69–75, 1991.

74. Savarie D, Lanoue C, Cadieux A, Rousseau E: Large conducting potassium channel reconstituted from airway smooth muscle. *Am J Physiol* 262:L327–L336, 1992.

75. Jones TR, Charette L, Garcia ML, Kaczorowski GJ: Selective inhibition of relaxation of guinea-pig trachea by charybdotoxin, a potent Ca^{2+}-activated K^+-channel inhibitor. *J Pharmacol Exp Ther* 255:697–706, 1990.

76. Murry MA, Berry JL, Cook SJ, Foster RW, Green KA, Small RC: Guinea-pig isolated trachealis: The effects of charybdotoxin on mechanical activity, membrane potential changes and the activity of plasmalemmal K^+-channels. *Br J Pharmacol* 103:1814–1818, 1991.

77. Berry JL, Small RC, Hughes SJ, Smith RD, Miller AJ, Hollingworth M, Edwards G, Weston AH: Inhibition by adrenergic neurone blocking agents of the relaxation induced by BRL 38227 in vascular, intestinal and uterine smooth muscle. *Br J Pharmacol* 107:288–295, 1992.

78. Maas AJJ, Den Hertog A: The effects of apamin on the smooth muscle cells of the guinea-pig taenia coli. *Eur J Pharmacol* 58:151–156, 1979.

79. Allen SL, Beech DJ, Foster RW, Morgan GP, Small RC: Electrophysiological and other aspects of the relaxant action of isoprenaline in guinea-pig isolated trachealis. *Br J Pharmacol* 86:843–854, 1985.

80. Weir SW, Weston AH: Effects of apamin on responses to BRL 34915, nicorandil and other relaxants in the guinea-pig taenia caeci. *Br J Pharmacol* 88:113–120, 1986.

81. Benham CD, Tsien RW: A novel receptor-operated Ca^{2+}-permeable channel activated by ATP in smooth muscle. *Nature* 328:275–278, 1987.

82. Nakazawa K, Matsuki N: Adenosine triphosphate-activated inward current in isolated smooth muscle cells from rat vas deferens. *Pflügers Arch* 409:644–646, 1987.

83. Honoré E, Martin C, Mironneau C, Mironneau J: An ATP-sensitive conductance in cultured smooth muscle cells from pregnant rat myometrium. *Am J Physiol* 257:C297–C305, 1989.

84. Xiong Z, Kitamura K, Kuriyama H: ATP activates cationic currents and modulates the calcium current through GTP-binding protein in rabbit portal vein. *J Physiol* 440:143–165, 1991.

85. Yamanaka K, Furukawa K, Kitamura K: The different mechanisms of action of nicorandil and adenosine triphosphate on potassium channels of circular smooth muscle of the guinea-pig small intestine. Naunyn-Schmiedebergs Arch. *Pharmacol* 331:96–103, 1985.

86. Tauc M, Gastineau M, Poujeol P: Toxin pharmacology of the ATP-induced hyperpolarization in Madin-Darby canine kidney cells. *Biochim Biophys Acta* 1105:155–160, 1992.

87. Yamanaka K, Kitamura K, Kuriyama H: Effects of neurotensin on electrical and mechanical properties of smooth muscle in longitudinal and circular layers of the guinea-pig ileum. *Pflügers Arch* 408:10–17, 1987.

88. Vladimilova A, Shuba MF: Strychnine, hydrastine and apamin effects on synaptic transmission in smooth muscle cells. *Neurofyziologiya* 10:296–299, 1978.

89. Banks BEC, Brown C, Burgess GM, Burnstock G, Claret M, Cocks TM, Jenkinson DH: Apamin blocks certain neurotransmitter-induced increases in potassium permeability. *Nature* 282:415–417, 1977.

90. Maas AJJ: The effects of apamin on responses evoked by field stimulation on guinea-pig taenia coli. *Eur J Pharmacol* 73:1–9, 1981.

91. Bauer V, Kuriyama H: The nature of non-cholinergic, non-adrenergic transmission in longitudinal and circular muscles of the guinea-pig ileum. *J Physiol* 332:375–391, 1982.

92. Komori, K, Suzuki H: Distribution and properties of excitatory and inhibitory junction potentials in circular muscle of the guinea-pig stomach. *J Physiol* 370:339–355, 1986.

93. Moncada S, Palmer MJ, Higgs EA: Nitric oxide: Physiology, pathophysiology and pharmacology. *Pharmacol Rev* 43: 109–142, 1991.

94. Toda N, Baba H, Okamura T: Role of nitric oxide in non-adrenergic, non-cholinergic nerve-mediated relaxation in dog duodenal longitudinal muscle strips. *Jpn J Pharmacol* 53:281–284, 1990.

95. Bult H, Boeckxstaens GE, Pelckmans PA, Jordaens FH, Van Maercke YM, Herman AG: Nitric oxide as an inhibitory non-adrenergic, non-cholinergic neurotransmitter. *Nature* 345:346–347, 1990.

96. Dalziel HH, Thornbury KD, Ward SM, Sanders KM: Involvement of nitric oxide synthetic pathway in inhibitory junction potentials in canine proximal colon. *Am J Physiol* 260:G789–G792, 1991.

97. Ward SM, McKeen E, Sanders KM: Role of nitric oxide in non-adrenergic, non-cholinergic inhibitory junction potentials in canine ileocolonic sphincter. *Br J Pharmacol* 105:776–782, 1992.

98. Du C, Conklin JL: Cyclic GMP; possible mediator of inhibitory junction potentials in opossum esophageal circular smooth muscle. *Am J Physiol* 1992, in press.

99. Ward SM, Dalziel HH, Bradley ME, Buxton ILO, Keef K, Westfall DP, Sanders KM: Involvement of cyclic GMP in non-adrenergic, non-cholinergic inhibitory neurotransmission in dog proximal colon. *Br J Pharmacol* 1992, in press.

100. Suzuki H, Chen G, Yamamoto Y, Miwa K: Nitroarginine-sensitive and insensitive components of the endothelium-dependent relaxation in the guinea-pig carotid artery. *Jpn J Physiol* 42:335–347, 1992.

101. Parkington HC, Tonta MA, Tare M, Coleman H: Complex endothelium-dependent hyperpolarisation in coronary arterial smooth muscle. *Jpn J Pharmacol* 58(Suppl II):388P, 1992.

102. Garland CJ, McPherson GA: Evidence that nitric oxide does not mediate the hyperpolarization and relaxation to acetylcholine in the rat small mesenteric artery. *Br J Pharmacol* 105:429–435, 1992.

103. McPherson GA, Angus JA: Evidence that acetylcholine-mediated hyperpolarization of the rat small mesenteric artery does not involve the K^+ channel opened by cromakalim. *Br J Pharmacol* 103:1184–1190, 1991.

104. Fujii K, Tominaga M, Ohmori S, Kobayashi K, Koga T, Takata Y, Fujishima M: Decreased endothelium-dependent hyperpolarization to acetylcholine in smooth muscle of the mesenteric artery of spontaneously hypertensive rats. *Circ Res* 70:660–669, 1992.

105. Nagao T, Illiano S, Vanhoutte PM: Calmodulin antagonists inhibit endothelium-dependent hyperpolarization in the canine coronary artery. *Br J Pharmacol* 107:382–386, 1992.

106. Illiano S, Nagao T, Vanhoutte PM: Calmidazolium, a calmodulin inhibitor, inhibits endothelium-dependent relaxations resistant to nitro-L-arginine in the canine coronary artery. *Br J Pharmacol* 107:387–392, 1992.

107. Escande D, Thuringer D, Le Guern S, Cavero I: The potassium channel opener cromakalim (BRL 34915) activates ATP-dependent K^+ channels in isolated cardiac myocytes. *Biochem Biophys Res Commun* 154:620–625, 1988.

108. Escande D, Thuringer D, Le Guern S, Courteix J, Laville M, Cavero I: Potassium channel openers act through an activation of ATP-sensitive K^+ channels in guinea-pig cardiac myocytes. *Pflügers Arch* 414:669–675, 1989.

109. Sanguinetti MC, Scott AL, Zingaro GJ, Siegel PK: BRL 34915 (cromakalim) activates ATP-sensitive K^+ current in cardiac muscle. *Proc Natl Acad Sci USA* 85:8360–8364, 1988.

110. Arena JP, Kass RS: Activation of ATP-sensitive K channels in heart cells by pinacidil. *Am J Physiol* 257:H2092–H2096, 1989.

111. Hiraoka M, Fan Z: Activation of the ATP-sensitive K^+ channel by nicorandil (2-nicotinamidoethyl nitrate) in isolated ventricular myocytes. *J Pharmacol Exp Ther* 250:278–285, 1989.

112. Nakayama K, Fan Z, Marumo F, Hiraoka M: Interrelation between pinacidil and intracellular ATP concentrations on activation of the ATP-sensitive K^+ current in guinea pig ventricular myocytes. *Circ Res* 67:1124–1133, 1990.

113. Nakao K, Okabe K, Kitamura K, Kuriyama H, Weston AH: Characteristics of cromakalim-induced relaxations in the smooth muscle cells of guinea-pig mesenteric artery and vein. *Br J Pharmacol* 95:795–804, 1988.

114. Kamouchi M, Kajioka S, Sakai T, Kitamura K, Kuriyama H: A target K^+ channel for the LP-805-induced hyperpolarization in smooth muscle cells of the rabbit portal vein. *Naunyn-Schmiedebergs Arch Pharmacol* 1993, in press.

115. Kusano K, Barros F, Katz GM, Roy-Contancin L, Reuben JP: Modulation of K channel activity in aortic smooth muscle by BRL 34915 and scorpion toxin. *Biophys J* 51:55a, 1987.

116. Gelband CH, Lodge NJ, Van Breemen C: A Ca^{2+}-activated K^+ channel from rabbit aorta: Modulation by cromakalim. *Eur J Pharmacol* 167:201–210, 1989.

117. Gelband CH, Carl A, Post JM, Bowen SM, Ishikawa T, Keef KD, Sanders KM, Hume JR: Effects of cromakalim and lemakalim on whole-cell and single-channel K^+ currents in canine colonic, renal and coronary smooth muscle cells. In: Sperelakis N, Kuriyama H (eds) *Ion Channels of Vascular Smooth Muscle Cells and Endothelial Cells.* New York: Elsevier, 1991, pp 125–138.

118. Hermsmeyer K: Potassium channel currents of vascular muscle. In: Sperelakis N, Kuriyama H (eds) *Ion Channels of Vascular Smooth Muscle Cells and Endothelial Cells.* New York: Elsevier, 1991, pp 107–110.

119. Coldwell MC, Howlett DR: Specificity of action of the novel antihypertensive agent, BRL 34915, as a potassium channel activator. Comparison with nicorandil. *Biochem Pharmacol* 36:3663–3669, 1987.

120. Noack T, Deitmer P, Edwards G, Weston AH: Characterization of potassium currents modulated by BRL 38227 in rat portal vein. *Br J Pharmacol* 106:717–726, 1992.

121. Shen WK, Tung RT, Machulda MM, Kurachi Y: Essential role of nucleotide diphosphates in nicorandil-mediated activation of cardiac ATP-sensitive K^+ channel: A comparison with pinacidil and lemakalim. *Circ Res* 69:1152–1158, 1991.

122. Thuringer D, Escande D: Apparent competition between ATP and the potassium channel opener RP 49356 on ATP-sensitive K^+ channels of cardiac myocytes. *Mol Pharmacol* 36:897–902, 1989.

123. Qin D, Takano M, Noma A: Kinetics of ATP-sensitive K^+ channels revealed with oil-gate concentration jump method. *Am J Physiol* 257:H1624–H1633, 1989.

124. Findlay I: ATP-sensitive K^+ channels in rat ventricular myocytes are blocked and inactivated by internal divalent cations. *Pflügers Arch* 410:313–320, 1987.

125. Wong BS, Lecar H, Adler M: Single calcium-dependent potassium channels in clonal anterior pituitary cells. *Biophys J* 39:313–317, 1984.

126. Blatz AL, Magleby KL: Ion conductance and selectivity of single calcium-activated potassium channels in cultured rat muscle. *J Gen Physiol* 84:1–23, 1984.

127. Yellen G: Ionic permeation and blockade in Ca^{2+}-activated K^+-channels of bovine chromaffin cells. *J Gen Physiol* 84:157–186, 1984.

128. Hu SL, Yamamoto Y, Kao CY: Permeation, selectivity, and blockade of the Ca^{2+}-activated potassium channel of the guinea pig taenia coli myocyte. *J Gen Physiol* 94:849–862, 1989.

129. Armstrong CM, Hille B: The inner quaternary ammonium

ion receptor in potassium channels of the node of Ranvier. *J Gen Physiol* 59:388–400, 1972.

130. Kirsch GE, Taglialatela M, Brown AM: Internal and external TEA block in single cloned K$^+$ channels. *Am J Physiol* 261:C583–C590, 1991.

131. Spruce AE, Standen NB, Stanfield PR: The action of external tetraethyl-ammonium ions on unitary delayed rectifier potassium channels of frog skeletal muscle. *J Physiol* 393:467–478, 1987.

132. Grissmer S, Caharlan M: TEA prevents inactivation while blocking open K$^+$ channels in human T lymphocytes. *Biophys J* 55:203–206, 1989.

133. Stanfield PR: Tetraethylammonium ions and the potassium permeability of excitable cells. *Rev Physiol Biochem Pharmacol* 97:1–67, 1983.

134. Lynch JW, Barry PH: Properties of transient K$^+$ currents and underlying single K$^+$ channels in rat olfactory receptor neurons. *J Gen Physiol* 97:1043–1072, 1991.

135. MacKinnon R, Yellen G: Mutations affecting TEA blockade and ion permeation in voltage-activated K$^+$ channels. *Science* 250:276–279, 1990.

136. Kavanaugh MP, Varnum MD, Osborne PB, Christie MJ, Busch AE, Adelman JP, North RA: Interaction between tetraethylammonium and amino acid residues in the pore of cloned voltage-dependent potassium channels. *J Biol Chem* 266:7583–7587, 1991.

137. Heginbotham L, MacKinnon R: The aromatic binding site for tetraethylammonium ion on potassium channels. *Neuron* 8:483–491, 1992.

138. Yellen G, Jurman M, Abramson T, MacKinnon R: Mutations affecting internal TEA blockade identify the probable pore-forming region of a K$^+$ channel. *Science* 251:939–942, 1991.

139. Kirsch GE, Drewe JA, Hartmenn HA, Taglialatela M, DeBiasi M, Brown AM, Joho RH: Differences between the deep pores of K$^+$ channels determined by an interacting pair of nonpolar amino acid. *Neuron* 8:499–505, 1992.

140. Thompson SH: Aminopyridine block of transient potassium current. *J Gen Physiol* 80:1–18, 1982.

141. Meves H, Pichon Y: The effect of internal and external 4-aminopyridine on the potassium currents in intracellularly perfused squid giant axons. *J Physiol* 268:511–532, 1975.

142. Yeh JZ, Oxford GS, Wu CH, Narahashi T: Dynamics of aminopyridine block of potassium channels in squid axon membrane. *J Gen Physiol* 68:519–535, 1976.

143. Davies NW, Pettit AI, Agarwal R, Standen NB: The flickery block of ATP-dependent potassium channels of skeletal muscle by internal 4-aminopyridine. *Pflügers Arch* 419:25–31, 1991.

144. Yeh JZ, Oxford GS, Wu CH, Narahashi T: Interactions of aminopyridines with potassium channels of squid axon membranes. *Biophys J* 16:77–82, 1976.

145. Hermann A, Gorman ALF: Effects of 4-aminopyridine on potassium currents in a molluscan neuron. *J Gen Physiol* 78:63–86, 1981.

146. Simurda J, Simurdova M, Cupera P: 4-Aminopyridine sensitive transient outward current in dog ventricular fibres. *Pflügers Arch* 411:442–449, 1988.

147. Molgó J, Lundh H, Thesleff S: Potency of 3,4-diaminopyridine and 4-aminopyridine on mammalian neurotransmission and the effects of pH changes. *Eur J Pharmacol* 61:25–34, 1980.

148. Plant TD, Standen NB: The action of 4-aminopyridine (4-AP) on the early outward current (I$_A$) in *Helix aspersa* neurones. *J Physiol* 332:18P–19P, 1982.

149. Kehl SJ: 4-aminopyridine causes a voltage-dependent block of the transient outward K$^+$ current in rat melanotrophs. *J Physiol* 431:515–528, 1990.

150. Hille B: Local anesthetics: Hydrophilic and hydrophobic pathways for the drug-receptor reaction. *J Gen Physiol* 69:497–515, 1977.

151. Sturgess NC, Kozlowski RZ, Carrington CA, Hales CN, Ashford MLJ: Effects of sulfonylureas and diazoxide on insulin secretion and nucleotide-sensitive channels in an insulin secreting cell line. *Br J Pharmacol* 95:83–94, 1988.

152. Trube G, Rorsmann P, Ohno-Shosaku T: Opposite effects of tolbutamide and diazoxide on the ATP-dependent K$^+$ channel in mouse pancreatic β-cells. *Pflügers Arch* 407:493–499, 1986.

153. Dunne MJ, Ilott MC, Petersen OH: Interaction of diazoxide, tolbutamide and ATP^{4-} on nucleotide-dependent K$^+$ channels in an insulin-secreting cell line. *J Memb Biol* 99:215–224, 1987.

154. de Weille JR, Fosset M, Mourre C, Schmid-Antomarchi H, Bernardi H, Lazdunski M: Pharmacology and regulation of ATP-sensitive K$^+$ channels. *Pflügers Arch* 414(Suppl 1): S80–87, 1989.

155. Ciampolillo F, Tung DE, Cameron JS: Effects of diazoxide and glyburide on ATP-sensitive K$^+$ channels from hypertrophied ventricular myocytes. *J Pharmacol Exp Ther* 260:254–260, 1992.

156. Reeve HL, Vaughan PFT, Peers C: Glibenclamide inhibits a voltage-gated K$^+$ current in the human neuroblastoma cell line SH-SY5Y. *Neurosci Lett* 135:37–40, 1992.

157. Xiong Z, Kajioka S, Sakai T, Kitamura K, Kuriyama H: Pinacidil inhibits the ryanodine-sensitive outward current and glibenclamide antagonizes its action in cells from the rabbit portal vein. *Br J Pharmacol* 102:788–790, 1991.

158. Findlay I: Inhibition of ATP-sensitive K$^+$ channels in cardiac muscle by the sulphonylurea drug glibenclamide. *J Pharmacol Exp Ther* 261:540–545, 1992.

159. Geisen K, Hetzel V, Ökomomopoulos R, Pünter J, Weyer R, Summ HD: Inhibition of [^{3}H]glibenclamide binding to sulfonylurea receptors by oral antidiabetics. *Arzneim Forsch* 35:707–712, 1985.

160. Niki I, Kelly RP, Ashcroft SJH, Ashcroft FM: ATP-sensitive K-channels in HIT T15b cells studied by patch clamp methods, ^{86}Rb$^+$ efflux and glibenclamide binding. *Pflügers Arch* 415:47–55, 1989.

161. Gopalakrishnan M, Johnson DE, Janis RA, Triggle DJ: Characterization of binding of the ATP-sensitive potassium channel ligand, [^{3}H]glyburide, to neuronal and muscle preparations. *J Pharmacol Exp Ther* 257:1162–1171, 1991.

162. Findlay I: Effects of pH upon the inhibition by sulphonylurea drugs of ATP-sensitive K$^+$ channels in cardiac muscle. *J Pharmacol Exp Ther* 262:71–79, 1992.

163. Armondo-Hardy M, Ellory JC, Ferreira HG, Fleminger S, Lew VL: Inhibition of the calcium-induced increase in the potassium permeability of human red blood cells by quinine. *J Physiol* 250:32P–33P, 1975.

164. Burgess GM, Claret M, Jenkinson DH: Effects of quinine and apamin on the calcium-dependent potassium permeability of mammalian hepatocytes and red blood cells. *J Physiol* 317:67–90, 1981.

165. Walden J, Speckmann EJ: Effects of quinine on membrane potential and membrane currents in identified neurons of *Helix pomatia*. *Neurosci Lett* 27:139–143, 1981.

166. Snyders DJ, Knoth KM, Roberds SL, Tamkun MM: Time-, voltage-, and state-dependent block by quinidine of a cloned human cardiac potassium channel. *Mol Pharmacol* 41:322–330, 1992.

167. Hermann A, Gorman ALF: Action of quinidine on ionic currents of molluscan pacemaker neurons. *J Gen Physiol* 83:919–940, 1984.

168. Iwatsuki N, Petersen OH: Inhibition of Ca^{2+}-activated K$^+$ channels in pig pancreatic acinar cells by Ba^{2+}, Ca^{2+},

quinine, and quinidine. *Biochem Biophys Acta* 819:249–257, 1985.

169. Snyders DJ, Hondeghem LM: Effects of quinidine on the sodium current of ventricular guinea-pig myocytes. *Circ Res* 66:565–579, 1990.

170. Glavinovic MI, Trifaró JM: Quinine blockade of currents through Ca²⁺-activated K⁺ channels in bovine chromaffin cells. *J Physiol* 399:139–152, 1988.

171. Miller C, Moczydlowski E, Latorre R, Phillips M: Charybdotoxin, a protein inhibitor of single Ca²⁺-activated K⁺ channels from skeletal muscle. *Nature* 313:316–318, 1985.

172. Goh JW, Pennefather PS: Pharmacological and physiological properties of the afterhyperpolarization current of bullfrog ganglion neurons. *J Physiol* 394:315–330, 1987.

173. Goh JW, Kelly MEM, Pennefather PS, Chicchi GG, Cascieri MA, Garcia ML, Kaczorowski GJ: Effect of charybdotoxin and leiurotoxin I on potassium currents in bullfrog sympathetic ganglion and hippocampal neurons. *Brain Res* 591: 165–170, 1992.

174. Sands SB, Lewis RS, Caharan MD: Charybdotoxin blocks voltage-gated K⁺ channels in human and murine T lymphocytes. *J Gen Physiol* 93:1061–1074, 1989.

175. Schweitz H, Stanfield CE, Bidard JN, Fagni L, Maes P, Lazdunski M: Charybdotoxin blocks dendrotoxin-sensitive voltage-activated K⁺ channels. *FEBS Lett* 250:519–522, 1989.

176. Leonard RJ, Garcia ML, Slaughter RS, Reuben JP: Selective blockers of voltage-gated K⁺ channels depolarize human T lymphocytes: Mechanism of the antiproliferative effect of charybdotoxin. *Proc Natl Acad Sci USA* 89:10094–10098, 1992.

177. Anderson CS, MacKinnon R, Smith C, Miller C: Charybdotoxin block of single Ca²⁺-activated K⁺ channels. *J Gen Physiol* 91:317–333, 1988.

178. Miller C: Competition for block of a Ca²⁺-activated K⁺ channel by charybdotoxin and tetraethylammonium. *Neuron* 1:1003–1008, 1988.

179. MacKinnon R, Miller C: Mechanism of charybdotoxin block of the high-conductance, Ca²⁺-activated K⁺ channel. *J Gen Physiol* 91:335–349, 1988.

180. MacKinnon R, Miller C: Mutant potassium channels with altered binding of charybdotoxin, a pore-blocking peptide inhibitor. *Science* 245:1382–1385, 1989.

181. MacKinnon R, Heginbotham L, Abramson T: Mapping the receptor site for charybdotoxin, a pore-blocking potassium channel inhibitor. *Neuron* 5:767–771, 1990.

182. Galvez A, Gimenez-Gallego G, Reuben JP, Roy-Contancin L, Feiogenbaum P, Kaczorowski GJ, Garcia ML: Purification and characterization of a unique potent, peptidyl probe for the high conductance calcium-activated potassium channel from venom of the scorpion *Buthus tamulus*. *J Biol Chem* 265:11083–11090, 1990.

183. Garcia ML, Galvez A, Garcia-Carvo M, King VF, Vazquez J, Kaczorowski GJ: Use of toxins to study potassium channels. *J Bioenerg Biomemb* 23:615–646, 1991.

184. Candia S, Garcia ML, Latorre R: Mode of action of iberiotoxin, a potent blocker of the large conductance Ca²⁺-activated K⁺ channel. *Biophys J* 63:583–590, 1992.

185. Sugg EE, Garcia ML, Johnson BA, Kaczorowski GJ, Patchett AA, Reuben JP: In: Rivier JE, Marshall GR (eds) *Peptide: Chemistry, Structure and Biology*. Leiden: Escom Science, 1990, pp 1069–1070.

186. Castle NA, Strong PN: Identification of two toxins from scorpion (*Leiurus quinquestriatus*) venom which block

187. Abia A, Lobaton CD, Moreno A, Garcia-Sancho J: *Leiurus quinquestriatus* venom inhibits different kinds of Ca²⁺-dependent K⁺ channels. *Biochim Biophys Acta* 856:403–407, 1986.

188. Weller U, Bernhardt U, Siemen D, Dreyer F, Vogel W, Habermann E: Electrophysiological and neurobiochemical evidence for the blockade of a potassium channel by dendrotoxin. *Naunyn-Schmiedebergs Arch. Pharmacol* 330:77–83, 1985.

189. Benoit E, Dubois JM: Toxin I from the snake *Dendroaspis polylepis*: A highly selective blocker of the type of K⁺ channel in myelinated nerve fiber. *Brain Res* 377:374–377, 1986.

190. Petersen M, Penner R, Pierau FK, Dreyer F: β-Bungarotoxin inhibits a non-inactivating K⁺ current in guinea pig dorsal root ganglion neurones. *Neurosci Lett* 68:141–145, 1986.

191. Stanfield C, Marsh S, Halliwell J, Brown D: 4-Aminopyridine and dendrotoxin induce repetitive firing in rat visceral neurons by blocking a slowly inactivating outward current. *Neurosci Lett* 64:299–304, 1986.

192. Rhem H, Temple BL: Voltage-gated K⁺ channels of the mammlian brain. *FASEB J* 5:164–170, 1991.

193. Stühmer W, Ruppersberg J, Schröter K, Sakmann B, Stocker M, Giese K, Perschke A, Baumann A, Pongs O: Molecular basis of functional diversity of voltage-gated K⁺ channels in mammalian brain. *EMBO J* 8:3235–3244, 1989.

194. Rehm H, Lazdunski M: Purification and subunit structure of a putative K⁺ channel protein identified by its binding properties for dendrotoxin I. *Proc Natl Acad Sci USA* 85: 4919–4923, 1988.

195. Rehm H, Lazdunski M: Existence of different populations of the dendrotoxin I binding protein associated with neuronal K⁺ channels. *Biochem Biophys Res Commun* 153:231–240, 1988.

196. Bidard JN, Mourre C, Lazdunski M: Two potent central convulsant peptides: A bee venom toxin, the MCD peptide and snake venom toxin dendrotoxin I known to block K⁺ channels have interacting receptor sites. *Biochem Biophys Res Commun* 143:383–389, 1987.

197. Rehn H, Bidard JN, Schweitz H, Lazdunski M: The receptor site for the bee venom mast cell degranulating peptide: Affinity labelling and evidence for a common molecular target for mast cell degranulating peptide and dendrotoxin I, a snake toxin active on K⁺ channels. *Biochemistry* 27:1827–1832, 1988.

198. Valdevia HH, Smith JH, Martin BM, Coronado R, Possani LD: Charybdotoxin and noxiustoxin, two homologous peptide inhibitors of the K⁺(Ca²⁺) channel. *FEBS Lett* 226:280–284, 1988.

199. Vázquez J, Feigenbaum P, King VF, Kaczorowski GJ, Garcia ML: Characterization of high affinity binding sites for charybdotoxin in synaptic plasma membrane from rat brain. *J Biol Chem* 265:15564–15571, 1990.

200. Vázquez J, Feigenbaum P, Katz G, King VF, Reuben JP, Roy-Contancin L, Slaughter RS, Kaczorowski GJ, Garcia ML: Characterization of high affinity binding sites for charybdotoxin in sarcolemmal membranes from bovine aortic smooth muscle. *J Biol Chem* 264:20902–20909, 1989.

201. Blaustein MP, Rogowski RS, Schneider MJ, Krueger BK: Polypeptide toxins from the venoms of Old World and New World scorpions preferentially block different potassium channels. *Mol Pharmacol* 40:932–942, 1991.

CHAPTER 51

Ion Channels of Endothelial Cells

BERND NILIUS & GUY DROOGMANS

INTRODUCTION

The total mass of endothelial cells is presumably one of the largest complex functional organs in the body, with complex interactions in terms of signaling between various cell types. The interaction between the different cells is either by humoral factors or by a direct cell-to-cell coupling and, moreover, signal transduction can be integrated at the cell surface of endothelial cells. A great variety of completely different functions are coordinated by these cell interactions as control of vasomotor activity of vascular smooth muscle cells, cell proliferation, migration of blood cells through the vessel wall regulated by different chemotactic signals, immunological responses, control of the thrombogenic as well as the thrombolytic activity within the blood vessel, and control of the coagulation potential in the blood.

Endothelial cells (EC) are positioned at the boundary between intravascular and interstitial compartments, and are thereby exposed to biochemical mediators in the blood and to physical factors acting at the vascular wall, such as stretch, shear stress, and pressure. They also receive signals from the abluminal site of the blood vessel, e.g., histamine released from mast cells, neurotransmitters from nerve varicosities, cytokines from macrophages, and other migratory cells. Endothelial cells respond to all these stimuli by synthesizing and releasing various messengers that interact with neighboring cell types (humoral communication), but, in addition, endothelial cells can also communicate via physical contacts with neighboring cells (contact-mediated communication).

Humoral compounds that are released by endothelial cells are proteins, e.g., platelet-derived growth factor (PDGF) and interleukins; peptides, e.g., endothelins; as well as smaller products, e.g., prostaglandins, and, especially, endothelium-derived relaxation factor (EDRF), which is believed to play a key role in the regulation of vascular tone. Other secreted vasoactive compounds (endothelium-derived contracting factors different from endothelins, endothelium-derived hyperpolarization factor) are not yet chemically characterized.

In all of these complex signal functions, ion channels are involved. Their significance in triggering or modulation of endothelial cell functions will be reviewed in this chapter.

IMPORTANCE OF INTRACELLULAR Ca^{2+} FOR ENDOTHELIAL CELL FUNCTION

The control of intracellular Ca^{2+} plays the key role in most of the functions of endothelial cells. The first endothelium-derived factor found was prostacyclin (PGI_2). PGI_2 is released by agonists such as bradykinin, histamine, serotonin (5-HT), thrombin, lipoproteins (HDL), fibrin, interleukin-1 (IL-1), interferon, epidermal growth factor (EGF), transforming growth factor α (TGFα), and tumor necrosis factor (TNF). Also hypoxia and mechanical factors such as flow (shear stress) increase the release of PGI_2. The very trigger is an increase of the intracellular Ca^{2+} concentration, $[Ca^{2+}]_i$. PGI_2 activates an adenyl cyclase in neighboring cells (mainly platelets) that induces an increase to a variable extent in cAMP.

The most powerful vasorelaxing mediator has been termed *endothelium-derived relaxing factor* (EDRF). This substance also has widespread importance for many other mechanisms. EDRF is released by shear stress (flow), calcium ionophores such as A23187, autacoids, bradykinin, histamine, norepinephrine, substance P, vasopressin, acetylcholine, thrombin, and platelet-derived products such as ATP and ADP. EDRF has been identified as endogenous nitric oxide. It is produced by a Ca^{2+}-calmodulin-NADPH dependent synthase that catalyzes oxidation of the N-guanidine terminal of L-arginine and is released as the easily diffusable NO or bound to cysteine (S-nitroso-cysteine). An increase in intraendothelial Ca^{2+} by release from Ca^{2+} stores and by sustained Ca^{2+} influx via membrane channels is the trigger event for activation of the NO synthase and the release of EDRF {1; for reviews see 2–4}. EDRF activates a soluble guanylate cyclase in neighboring cells that leads to an increase in cGMP. By this mechanism EDRF induces relaxation of smooth muscle cells. NO has now been determined to be a general messenger not only in the vascular system, but also as a central and peripheral neuronal messenger involved in synaptic modulation and perhaps even in long-term potentiation.

961

All these properties make endothelial cells one of the body's largest endocrine glands. EDRF production depends on a sustained increase in Ca^{2+} in the cell. Another example of the importance of $[Ca^{2+}]_i$ is the Ca^{2+}-dependent activation of the enzyme lyso-PAF-acetyl transferase that triggers the synthesis of platelet-activating factor (PAF) in endothelial cells {2}.

The most important tigger in all these cell functions is an increase in the intracellular Ca^{2+} activity. There is now a large body of evidence that Ca^{2+} influx into vascular endothelial cells and the intracellular Ca^{2+} pattern is regulated by different voltage- and agonist-gated ion channels {for a review see 3 and 4}. After stimulation of endothelial cells by various vasoactive agonists, the functionally important sustained elevation of intracellular Ca^{2+} depends on extracellular Ca^{2+} and is supposedly mediated by a transmembrane Ca^{2+} influx. The concerted action of several ion channels in relation to the control of intracellular Ca^{2+} is the main subject of this article.

POTASSIUM CHANNELS IN ENDOTHELIAL CELLS

Potassium channels are widely distributed in endothelial cells. The existence of inwardly rectifying potassium chan-

nels in endothelial cells that pass inward currents at hyperpolarized membrane potentials more readily than outward currents at depolarized potentials is well documented {5,6}. In most excitable and nonexcitable cells, these channels are responsible for stabilization of the resting membrane potential near the K^+ equilibrium potential, E_K. Inward currents can be measured at potentials negative to E_K; positive to E_K outward currents are almost blocked. Unlike the cardiac inward rectifier, however, it is questionable whether this block depends on intracellular Mg^{2+}. Figure 51-1 shows an experiment in which the inwardly rectifying K^+ channel has been measured in the whole-cell configuration of the patch-clamp technique and also as single-channel currents from a cell-attached patch. Whole-cell currents, after subtraction of leakage currents, show a small outward component near the reversal potential towards positive potentials. In the single-channel recordings an almost complete rectification can be observed. The inwardly rectifying K^+ channel has a conductance of approximately 30 pS in 140 mM/l symmetrical K^+ concentrations on either side of the membrane for the inward movement of K^+.

In capillary endothelial cells, and also in larger vessels, the inward rectifier is blocked by vasoactive agonists, such as angiotensin II, vasopressin, and histamine. Figure 51-

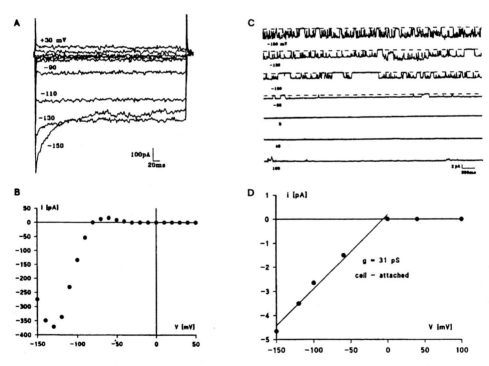

Fig. 51-1. Inwardly rectifying K^+ channels in endothelial cells. **A:** Whole-cell measurement of an K^+-inward rectifier in endothelial cells from human umbilcal veins. From a holding potential of 0 mV, 400 ms voltage steps were applied to the indicated test potential. **B:** After subtraction of the linear leak currents obtained from currents between -50 and $+20$ mV, the current-voltage relationship of the inward rectifier current was obtained. Note the small outward component between -80 and -40 mV. **C:** Single-channel measurements of the inwardly rectifying K^+ current in endothelial cells from umbilical vein at different holding potentials. **D:** Single-channel IV curve for the 30 pS inwardly rectifying K^+ channel. (From Nilins et al. {63}, modified, with permission.)

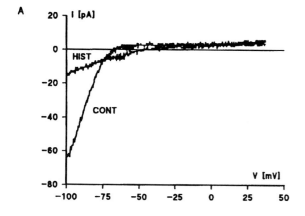

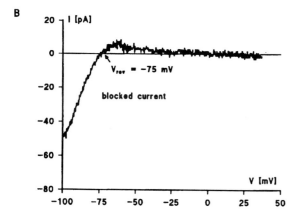

Fig. 51-2. Histamine-induced block of the endothelial K^+-inward rectifier currents. **A:** Current-voltage (IV) relationships obtained from human endothelial cells by linear voltage ramps (umbilical vein in the whole-cell patch-clamp configuration). The IV curve of the nonstimulated cell crosses the voltage axis at approximately -70 mV, indicating a rather negative membrane potential. Application of $100 \mu M$ histamine reduces the inward component of the K^+ current. The zero current can now be obtained at approximately -35 mV, indicating an agonist-mediated depolarization of the cell. The intracellular Ca^{2+} concentration is buffered at 10^{-7} M. Thus the block is not Ca^{2+} mediated. **B:** The current blocked by histamine matches completely the current-voltage relationship of the inwardly rectifying K^+ channel. Histamine blocks the inward rectifier. (From Nilins et al. {63} with permission.)

2A shows such an agonist-induced block of the inward rectifier in an isolated endothelial cell from human umbilical veins. The endothelial cell was stimulated with histamine. Before and during stimulation linear voltage ramps were applied to measure the instantaneous current-voltage relationships (IV curves). The blocked current has the typical IV curve of the inward rectifier (fig. 51-2B, compare with fig. 51-1). An inward rectifier block would depolarize the cell (see also the shift of the zero current potential from -70 to -35 mV; fig. 51-2A). This shift towards more positive potentials decreases the driving force for in-

wardly transported Ca^{2+}, e.g., via CRAC or other Ca^{2+}-permeable nonselective channels (see below). The block appears independently from the intracellular Ca^{2+} concentration, develops extremely quickly within 2–5 seconds, and can be mimicked by GTPS, thus a G-protein-mediated mechanism seems to be involved {7,8,63}. The mechanism of this block is still to be elucidated. It could provide a negative feedback via the driving force for Ca^{2+} entry. It is worthwhile to mention that supposedly not all endothelial cells have an inward rectifier potassium channel {8,9,63}. Even within the same cell population, an inward rectifier cannot be found in all cells.

An inwardly rectifying K^+ channel has also been described in cultured bovine aortic endothelial cells and in human endothelial cells from umbilical veins {10–12}. This channel has a conductance of approximately 30 pS in the inward direction but only of 10 pS in the outward direction. It is activated by intracellular calcium with an apparent $K_{0.5}$ value of approximately 720 nM $[Ca^{2+}]_i$. Thus this channel is not identical with the above-described inward rectifier. The channel is also activated via G-protein-dependent mechanism. GTP sensitizes the channel to Ca^{2+}, e.g., shifts the Ca^{2+}-activation curve to lower concentrations (apparent $K_{0.5}$ is approx. 230 nM). GTPS activated the channel irreversibly. This channel is supposedly identical to a Ca^{2+}-activated K^+ channel that appears after stimulation of endothelial cells with ATP {12}. It is well established that vasoactive agonists, such as bradykinin, ATP, histamine, thrombin, and acetylcholine, release intracellular calcium. Therefore, under physiological conditions the channel could be activated by these agonists and hyperpolarization would result {13–15}. Assuming a low intracellular Cl^- concentration in endothelial cells, a similar mechanism could also be mediated by activation of chloride-selective ion channels {16,17} (see below).

In addition to these small-conductance Ca^{2+}-activated K^+ channels, high-conductance Ca^{2+}-activated K^+ channels have also been described in both cultured and native endothelial cells {8,13,14}. These channels show a half-maximal activation at approximately $1 \mu M$ $[Ca^{2+}]_i$ at $+20$ mV and have single-channel conductances between 150 and 220 pS. They are blocked by charybdotoxin in the nanomolar range and also by tetraethylammonium chloride (TEA) or tetrabutylammonium chloride (TBA). These high-conductance Ca^{2+}-activated K^+ channels are also activated by the application of vasoactive agonists.

It is now known that Ca^{2+}-activated K^+ channels are involved in the modulation of NO synthesis (see below) by the following mechanism: Ca^{2+}-activated K^+ channels are activated by an intracellular increase in $[Ca^{2+}]_i$ and play a substantial supportive role for Ca^{2+} influx into endothelial cells by hyperpolarizing the cells and thereby increasing the driving force for Ca^{2+} {15,20,21}. Such hyperpolarization would become significant if the normal polarization of an endothelial cell is really in a rather positive range. The values reported for resting potentials in cultured endothelial cells are, however, sometimes far from the potassium equilibrium potential and scatter substantially (between -85 and -20 mV). In coronary endothelial cells, for example, membrane potentials between -20 and $-30\,mV$ have been measured. They are shifted towards the expected potassium equilibrium potential after application of various vasoactive agonists such as ATP or bradykinin {20}. This shift in the resting membrane potential increases the driving force for calcium. However, there is some question as to whether technical problems during measurement of resting potentials in the extremely flat EC could alter membrane potential. By use of nystatin-perforated patches, the membrane potential measured in endothelial cells is always between -70 and $-80\,mV$.

The inward rectifier K^+ channel could generate N-shaped IV curves and therefore a bistable resting potential. Such a bistable resting potential could be observed in cultured bovine and guinea pig coronary endothelium {15}. In these cells one population of cells shows a resting potential around $-25\,mV$, and a second population has resting potentials close to $-85\,mV$. Any increase in intracellular Ca^{2+} stabilizes the more negative potential and therefore results in an increased driving force for Ca^{2+}. Different types of Ca^{2+}-activated or agonist-activated K^+ channels could be responsible for hyperpolarization of endothelial cells.

Until now, several outward ion currents activated by different agonists, such as bradykinin, thrombin, platelet-activating factor (PAF), ATP, histamine, and acetyl-choline, have been described at the level of whole-cell measurements and will not be reviewed in this context. Intracellular Ca^{2+} release might be the activator in all these earlier described experiments {see 6,9,18 for reviews}. Voltage-gated A-type K^+ channels will be reviewed under *Voltage-dependent ion channels in endothelial cells.*

Cl⁻ CHANNELS IN ENDOTHELIUM

Until now, cation-permeable channels attracted the most interest in endothelial cells. Not very much is known of anion channels. It seems possible that morphological changes in endothelial cells are connected to changes in the normally very low Cl^- conductance {16}. A high-conductance Cl^- channel is normally almost silent in intact cells or in cell-attached patches. This channel becomes active after excision of the patches. Single-channel conductance between 350 and $400\,pS$ has been reported in symmetrical Cl^- solutions. Channel openings seem to be voltage dependent: The open probability increases at more positive potentials. A prolonged increase in intracellular Ca^{2+} seems to activate the channel; in addition, inhibition of a Ca^{2+}-phospholipid activated protein kinase (PKC) increased the incidence of the appearance of the channel in cell-attached patches. Zn^{2+} blocks the channel from

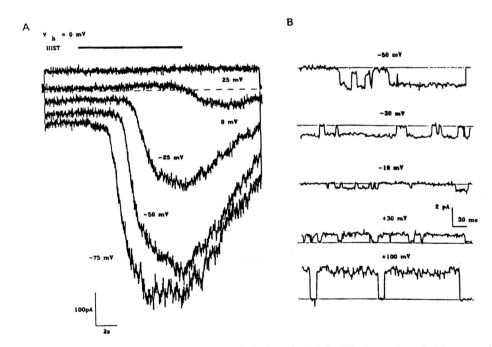

Fig. 51-3. Histamine induces a nonselective cation current. **A:** A single endothelial cell is clamped at a holding potential of $0\,mV$. A 20-second step to different holding potentials (starting at $-75\,mV$, $25\,mV$ spaced) is applied. After 2 seconds, $100\,\mu M$ histamine are applied to the surface of the cell through a multibarreled fast perfusion pipette. Development of an inward current can be seen that appears in dependence on the membrane potential. The size of the current is $650\,pA$ at $-75\,mV$. The reversal potential is approximately $+20\,mV$. This current is not a chloride current that would reverse near $-40\,mV$ (whole-cell patch-clamp mode, fast sampling with $2\,ms$ interval). **B:** Single-channel recordings after application of histamine to the bath (cell-attached patch, bath solution in the pipette, 1-kHz sampling). The single-channel conductance in this experiment was $26\,pS$. The reversal potential is $0\,mV$.

both sides of the membrane. However, any physiological role in intact cells is uncertain {17,18 for a review, 19}.

AGONIST-GATED ION CHANNELS

Vasoactive compounds, hormones, and neurotransmitters, such as acetylcholine, bradykinin, histamine, serotonin, angiotensin, thrombin, and ATP, are all activators of endothelial ion channels. In most cases ion channels are activated by an increase in intracellular Ca^{2+} concentration. In whole-cell measurements, K^+ currents have been described that are activated by muscarinic effects of acetylcholine. These currents are blocked by atropine and are inwardly rectifying and Ca^{2+} independent {20} or non-rectifying {21}. All other yet described agonist-activated K^+ channels are Ca^{2+} activated and have already been described.

Of special interest are nonselective cation channels activated by various agonists. In endothelial cells, histamine activates a nonselective cation channel in human endothelial from umbilical veins that is also permeable to Ca^{2+}, Ba^{2+}, and Mn^{2+}. Figure 51-3 shows patch-clamp measurements of this channel. In fig. 51-3A whole-cell ion currents activated by histamine are depicted. A single endothelial cell was clamped at different potentials. At the time indicated, 100 μM histamine was applied. After a latency of some seconds a current appears that reverses near 20 mV. This current cannot be carried by Cl^- because the expected reversal potential would be close to -40 mV (100 mM aspartate and 40 mM Cl^- in the pipette, but 140 mM Cl^- in the bath). This current can amount to a substantial size, in the range of even nanoamperes. Surprisingly, in measurements from membrane patches perforated with nystatine, these whole-cell currents are much smaller. Single-channel recordings are characterized by long openings after activation (fig. 51-3B).

The size of the unitary currents depends on the membrane potential, e.g., the driving force for the permeating cations. Although asymmetrical ion compositions have been used at both sides of the membrane, the potential at which the current reverses its directions is still close to 0 mV. Thus the channel cannot discriminate between Na^+ and K^+. From the almost linear current-voltage relationship, a single-channel conductance of 26 pS can be calculated. The permeation ratio of this channel is $P_{Na}:P_K:P_{Ca} = 1:0.9:0.2$. The single-channel conductance is approximately 25 pS for Na^+ and K^+ and 4 pS for Ca^{2+}. From a quantitative analysis of single-channel current-voltage relationships, affinities of 35 mM, 40 mM, and 17 mM for Na^+, K^+, and Ca^{2+}, respectively, were estimated for binding the permeable cations at a site within the channel. Current is decreased by elevation of extracellular Ca^{2+} because of the higher Ca^{2+} affinity of the channel but the much smaller conductance for Ca^{2+}. The channel can be downregulated by phorbol esters such as PMA and TPA, which activate PKC. The small conductance for Ca^{2+} and the low extracellular Ca^{2+} concentration (Ca_e^{2+}) only permit a small Ca^{2+} influx via this nonselective cation channel. This influx could be in the range of 5–10 pA,

which is still enough to explain the Ca_e^{2+}-dependent plateau of the Ca_i^{2+} signal after application of histamine.

This channel in human endothelial cells is less Ca^{2+} permeable than in another report on the histamine-activated cation channel in native endothelial cells from rat intrapulmonary artery {23}. In this report, an approximately 25 pS, histamine-activated, cation-selective channel could be observed that is not dependent on intracellular Ca^{2+}. This channel is about 15 times more permeable for Ca^{2+} than for K^+ and Na^+, is independent of GTPS, and is not activated by acetylcholine.

In endothelial cells from bovine pulmonary arteries, bradykinin and also thrombin-activated nonselective cation channels {9 for a review; 24,25,26}. These channels have conductances of 35–40 pS for Cs^+, but 15–20 pS for Ba^{2+}.

An agonist-gated small-conductance ion channel has been recently described with single-channel measurements in cultured endothelial cells from bovine aortae, which is very selective for Mn^{2+} and supposedly also Ca^{2+} {27}. This channel can be activated by the vasoactive agonists ATP, bradykinin, and inositol. It has a single-channel conductance of 2.5 pS for Mn^{2+}, and its probability of opening is increased by $Ins(1,3,4,5)P_4$ but not $Ins(1,4,5)P_3$. The channel is dependent on $[Ca^{2+}]_i$. At 1 μM $[Ca^{2+}]_i$ the open probability of this small-conductance channel is approximately 50% of that at 1 mM $[Ca^{2+}]_i$. A possible relation to Ca^{2+}-release-activated Ca^{2+} channels (CRAC) will be discussed later.

Another supposedly agonist-activated small-conductance channel has been discussed on the basis of whole-cell measurements in bovine aortic endothelial cells {28}. Bradykinin activated a current that amounts to only 5–25 pA/cell at -60 mV, is nonselective for cations, and is obviously Ca^{2+} permeable. In the presence of Ca^{2+} as the main charge carrier, this current inactivates in approximately 3 minutes, but is stable, with Na^+ being the main charge carrier. Both Na^+ and Ca^{2+} currents are blocked by lanthanum. These findings will also be discussed later in relation to the CRAC mechanism.

MECHANICALLY GATED ION CHANNELS IN ENDOTHELIAL CELLS

It is well documented that endothelial cells respond to blood flow, e.g., to mechanical signals {see 18,29,30 for reviews}. Endothelium is subjected to flow-related forces such as pressure (stretch, perpendicular to the surface) and shear stress (a force tangential to the surface of the endothelial cells that is generated by the friction between blood and the endothelial surface). Many effects of endothelial cells are related to blood flow: secretion of prostacyclin (PGI_2), EDRF, tissue plasminogen activator (TPA), cytoskeletal rearrangement, cell cycle entry, and others. Ion channels could be significantly involved in modulation of these responses and would provide mechanosensing properties to endothelial cells. The functional link between mechanical stimuli and biological responses could be channel-mediated Ca^{2+} entry.

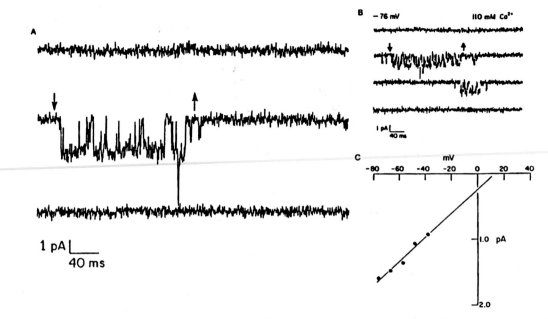

Fig. 51-4. Stretch-activated ion channels in cultured endothelial cells from neonatal pig aorta. **A:** Opening of a nonselective cation channel in an inside-out patch by application of suction pulses (between the arrows) of $1.3–2.7 \, \text{dyn/cm}^2$ through the pipette. The pipette contains $150 \, \text{mM} \, Na^+$, the bath solution $150 \, \text{mM} \, K^+$. Under these asymmetrical conditions the single-channel conductance is approximately $40 \, \text{pS}$. **B:** The stretch-activated channel is permeable for calcium. Between the arrows a suction pulse is applied and opens a channel with isotonic ($110 \, \text{mM}$) calcium in the pipette. **C:** The stretch-activated channel has an ohmic current-voltage relationship. Single-channel conductance is $19 \, \text{pS}$. From Lansman et al. {31}, with kind permission of Nature.

Stretch as a stimulus to open membrane channels in endothelial cells has already been described {31}. Figure 51-4A shows opening of an ion channel induced by application of $10–20 \, \text{mmHg}$ negative pressure. Channel activation disappears when the suction is removed. In this example the current is carried by sodium ions. If the pipette solution is changed to $110 \, \text{mM} \, Ca^{2+}$ (fig. 51-4B), stretch-induced channel opening can also be recorded: Currents are now carried by calcium ions. Thus the stretch-activated channel is permeable to Ca^{2+}. The current-voltage relationship is ohmic, reflecting a single-channel conductance of $19 \, \text{pS}$ in isotonic calcium solutions (fig. 51-4C). Single-channel conductance in isotonic potassium solutions is $56 \, \text{pS}$, and the conductance when sodium is the charge carrier is $40 \, \text{pS}$. The channel is about six times more permeable to calcium than sodium ions (permeation ratio of Ca^{2+} to Na^+, $P_{Ca}:P_{Na}$, is $1.2–8.4$ {31}). Stretch-activated nonselective cation channels have been also described in endothelial cells from porcine cerebral capillaries {32}. These channels may contribute to regulation of cerebrospinal salt and water content. Single-channel conductance is between 24 and $37 \, \text{pS}$ for monovalent cations and $16–19 \, \text{pS}$ for Ca^{2+} and Ba^{2+}.

Most of the mechanosensitive ion channels are blocked by amiloride. It can be speculated that an amiloride-blocked cationic channel in brain microvessels {33} has some relation to this stretch-activated channel. This amiloride-sensitive channel has a permeation ratio of

$P_{Na}:P_K = 1.5:1$ with approximately $23 \, \text{pS}$ conductance for Na^+. Modulation of stretch-activated ion channels is now being studied in several laboratories and seems to depend on changes in the cytoskeleton that focus membrane distorsion from a large area on the site of a single ion channel.

The functionally more significant mechanical signal for endothelial cells seems to be shear stress rather than stretch per se. A potassium-selective ion channel could act as a mechanosensor mediating a hyperpolarizing response due to shear stress, even in the physiological range of $0.5–25 \, \text{dyn/cm}^2$ {34}. Opening this channel is believed to induce non-EDRF-dependent vasorelaxation via electrical coupling of endothelial cells with the neighboring vascular smooth muscle cells {30,35}.

Hyperpolarization of endothelial cells spreads to smooth muscle cells, which are coupled with the endothelium by low-resistance gap junction pathways. This hyperpolarization of smooth muscle cells would cause relaxation. On the other hand, activation of K^+ channels and subsequent hyperpolarization of endothelial cells increases the driving force for Ca^{2+}, which could lead to an increase of $[Ca^{2+}]_i$ followed by activation of NO synthase and EDRF release.

Another transmembrane current induced by shear stress appears to be associated with opening of a nonselective ion channel and induced intracellular Ca^{2+} transients that disappear in Ca^{2+}-free solutions. Obviously, Ca^{2+}

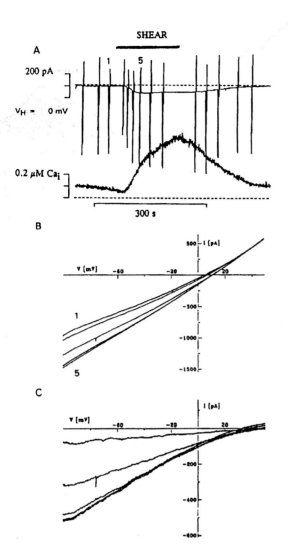

A

SHEAR

200 pA

$V_H = 0$ mV

0.2 μM Ca$_i$

300 s

B

500 — I (pA)

V (mV) −60 −20 20

−500

−1000

1 5 −1500

C

V (mV) −60 −20 20

I (pA)

−200

−400

−600

Fig. 51-5. Shear stress induces Ca^{2+} transients and inward currents in human vascular endothelial cells at 10 mM extracellular calcium. **A:** Simultaneous measurement of intracellular calcium and membrane currents. The bar indicates the application of shear stress on the surface of a single endothelial cell (approximately 10 dyne/cm^2). A holding potential of 0 mV was applied throughout the experiment (slow sampling rate of 3 Hz). **B:** Application of linear voltage ramps from −100 to 50 mV (500 ms, sampling rate 5 kHz). **C:** Shear stress induced currents were obtained by subtracting an averaged ramp current before application of shear stress from currents 2–6 during shear stress. The reversal potential obtained is close to 30 mV. From Schwarz et al. {37}, with permission of Pflügers Archiv.

permeates through shear stress activated channels. Figure 51-5 shows such an experiment in which a single isolated endothelial cell is stimulated by shear stress. A Ca^{2+} signal develops together with an inward current (fig. 51-5A). Application of voltage ramps allows measurement of the shear stress induced current (fig. 51-5B; currents evoked

by linear voltage ramps are shown as fast blips in panel A and are depicted with a fast time resolution in panel B as instantaneous IV curves). Shear stress activated currents can be directly obtained by subtracting the IV curves before application of shear stress from the IV curves obtained during this mechanical activation (fig. 51-5C). The shear stress-evoked current has a reversal potential near +35 mV. It can be concluded that shear stress opens a nonselective cation channel that is, however, approximately 12 times more permeable to Ca^{2+} than to Na$^+$ or Cs$^+$. This pathway is insensitive to activators of protein kinase C; is permeable to Ni^{2+}, Ba^{2+}, and Co^{2+}; but is reversibly blocked by La^{3+} and nonsteroid-inflammatory inhibitors, such as mefenamic acid. It can be discriminated from the agonist-induced nonselective channel. Incubation of endothelial cells with cytochalasin B as a modulator of the cytoskeleton increases the sensitivity of the endothelial cells to respond to shear stress {36,37; for a review including shear stress responses, see 29,30,38,39}.

This now directly demonstrated increase in intracellular Ca^{2+} by shear stress might be the link that couples mechanical stimulation to increased synthesis of NO by Ca^{2+}-dependent activation of NO synthase. Interestingly, regions with reduced shear stress (e.g., bifurcations of vessels) are favored sites for the appearance of atherosclerotic plaques.

Ca^{2+} ENTRY VIA Ca^{2+}-RELEASE-ACTIVATED Ca^{2+}-CHANNEL ENTRY (CRAC)

Intracellular Ca^{2+} ions play a fundamental role in linking the information of receptor stimulation at the level of the plasma membrane to various distinct functions in nonexcitable cells, such as enzyme secretion, synthesis of various compounds, control of cell proliferation, and cell differentiation. The initial rise in intracellular Ca^{2+} concentration ([Ca^{2+}]$_i$) upon receptor stimulation originates from release of Ca^{2+} ions from intracellular stores sensitive to Ins(1,4,5)P$_3$. The activator Ca^{2+} responsible for the more long-lasting effects on the different cell functions comes from the extracellular medium. Nonexcitable cell types lack voltage-operated Ca^{2+} channels but have supposedly developed a special Ca^{2+}-entry mechanism, Ca^{2+}-release-activated Ca^{2+}-permeable channels (CRAC), which appear to be coupled to the state of filling of the internal stores with Ca^{2+}: The mere emptying of these intracellular stores (e.g., by extracellular agonists, intracellular messengers, etc.) seems to increase Ca^{2+} permeability at the plasma membrane {40–42}.

Figure 51-6 summarizes some of the key experiments that provide evidence for the existence of a CRAC mechanism in endothelial cells. Ca^{2+} stores in the endoplasmic reticulum of endothelial cells ("calciosomes") possess Ins(1,4,5)P$_3$-receptor Ca^{2+}-release channels, Ca^{2+} pumps of the isoforms Serca2a,b and supposedly also Serca3 for refilling, and also have Ca^{2+} leaks. Between these stores and a Ca^{2+}-permeable entry channel (CRAC), functional crosstalk is expected (fig. 51-6A). The long-lasting Ca^{2+} plateau after stimulation with an agonist (e.g., histamine)

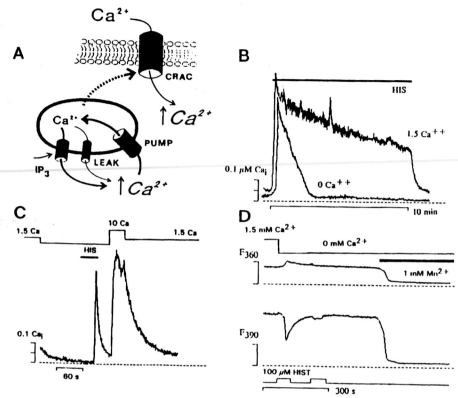

Fig. 51-6. Concept and evidence for Ca^{2+}-release activated channels: CRAC. **A:** Receptor stimulation of a cell by various agonists induces the production of Ins(1,4,5)P$_3$ via activation of a phospholipase C. Ins(1,4,5)P$_3$ opens a Ca^{2+}-release channel in Ca^{2+} stores of the endoplasmic reticulum. Discharge of the store signals a membrane Ca^{2+}-permeable channel to open. The signal pathway is still unknown. Refilling of the store by a Ca^{2+} pump closes CRAC again. **B:** Long-lasting Ca^{2+} signals depend on extracellular Ca^{2+}. The Ca^{2+} plateau disappears in Ca^{2+}-free media. The Ca^{2+} peak is due to IP$_3$-mediated Ca^{2+} release. Ca^{2+} influx from the extracellular space is necessary. (Nilius, unpublished results, endothelial cells from human umbilical vein.) **C:** After depletion of the intracellular Ca^{2+} stores and prevention of refilling (Ca^{2+}-free solution outside) reapplication of Ca^{2+} induces Ca^{2+} signals that disappear after refilling the stores. (Nilius, unpublished results, endothelial cells, human umbilical vein.) **D:** Evidence for existance of CRAC in an endothelial cell loaded with Fura-2/AM. Similar to panel C, stores are discharged by histamine in Ca^{2+}-free solutions. A second application of histamine with no effect proves that the stores are empty. Refilling is prevented by incubation in Ca^{2+}-free (decrease by increase in [Ca^{2+}]$_i$), respectively. Thus, Mn^{2+} must have entered the cell (Nilius, unpublished results, human umbilical vein, endothelium). This kind of experiment performed in many nonexcitable cells provides the most clear evidence for the existence of CRAC.

in the presence of extracellular Ca^{2+} disappears in Ca^{2+}-free solutions (fig. 51-6B). Calcium, which maintains the long-lasting plateau, enters the endothelial cell from the extracellular medium. The Ca^{2+} plateau maintained, however, is inevitably necessary for biological effects such as NO synthesis or synthesis of prostacyclin, which also disappear in Ca^{2+}-free extracellular media. Further evidence is given in fig. 51-6C that after stimulation with an agonist in nonexcitable cells, Ca^{2+} entry is related to discharge of Ca^{2+} stores. A single endothelial cell is exposed to Ca^{2+}-free extracellular medium. Application of histamine in Ca^{2+}-free medium induced only a fast and now transient Ca^{2+} peak without a Ca^{2+} plateau. Refilling of the store is prevented in Ca^{2+}-free solution {41}. Reapplication of Ca^{2+} without an agonist increases [Ca^{2+}]$_i$, again transiently, indicating that a transmembrane pathway is

still open for Ca^{2+} to enter the cell. This entry is controlled by the driving force for Ca^{2+}. A similar approach is represented in fig. 51-6D. Ca^{2+} stores were depleted by histamine. Refilling is prevented in Ca^{2+}-free extracellular solutions, as shown by a second histamine stimulus. Reapplication of Mn^{2+} as a substitute for Ca^{2+} induces quenching of both the Ca^{2+}-independent fura-2 fluorescence signal at 360 nm and the Ca^{2+}-dependent 390-nm signal. This indicates that Mn^{2+} can enter the endothelial cell through a still open transmembrane pathway. Entry is always inactivated by refilling the stores. These kinds of experiments have provided clear evidence for the existence of a CRAC mechanism in endothelial cells.

Figure 51-7A shows the first direct measurement of this important mechanism in mast cells {43}. An isolated single mast cell was loaded via a patch pipette with a high

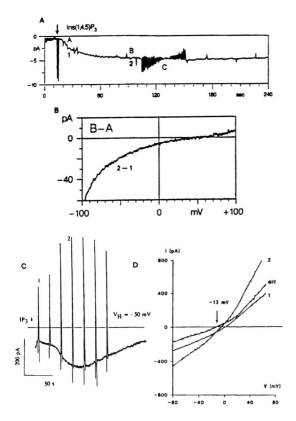

Fig. 51-7. Examples of direct measurements of CRAC in mast cells and endothelial cells. **A:** The cells are loaded via a patch pipette with Ins(1,4,5)P_3. At the arrow, the cell membrane has been perforated under the patch pipette and the cell is then loaded by diffusion from the pipette with IP_3. In A–C voltage ramps from -100 to $+100$ mV or steps are applied to measure current-voltage relationships for the current activated by Ins(1,4,5)P_3. The holding potential is 0 mV throughout the measurement. Store depletion gates a highly Ca^{2+}-selective, low-conductance channel and generates an inward current, even at 0 mV. From Hoth and Penner {43} with the kind permission of Nature. **B:** Current-voltage relationship of the Ca^{2+}-release-activated current. This IV curve was obtained by subtracting ramp A (panel A, before development of the inward current) from ramp B (panel A, at the maximal inward current). From Hoth and Penner {43} with the kind permission of Nature. **C:** The same experimental protocol but in a human endothelial cell (umbilical vein). The cell is loaded with 30 μM Ins(1,4,5)P_3 via the patch pipette. An inward current developed at a holding potential of -40 mV. **D:** The Ins(1,4,5)P_3-induced current was obtained by subtracting the ramp current 1 from 2 (panel C). The reversal potential is -13 mV (E_{Cl} is -40 mV in this experiment). The Ins(1,4,5)P_3-induced current is a nonselective cation current. (Experiments in C,D: Nilius, Droogmans, unpublished results on human endothelial cells, umbilical vein.)

concentration of Ins(1,4,5)P_3, which was used to deplete intracellular Ca^{2+} stores. Even at holding potentials of 0 mV, an inward current is activated (fig. 51-7A). By application of linear voltage ramps, a current could be dissected that reversed at very positive potentials and

seems thus to be highly selective for Ca^{2+} (fig. 51-7B). Activation of this current was shown to be strikingly coupled to depletion of intracellular Ca^{2+} stores {44}.

A similar experiment done in endothelial cells also evoked an inward current by intracellular loading of the cell with Ins(1,4,5)P_3 via a patch pipette (fig. 51-7C). However, this current reversed near 0 mV and seems to be mediated by activation of more nonselective cation currents rather than highly selective Ca^{2+} channels (fig. 51-7D). Also in different protocols in which measurements of a CRAC-like current component was tried, the supposedly Ca^{2+}-release-activated channels seem to be less Ca^{2+} selective than in mast cells.

Figure 51-8 shows two of these different protocols. After application of bradykinin (BK), a small inward current is activated that shows inactivation during administration of the agonist (fig. 51-8A, see also *Agonist-gated ion channels*). All possibly masking K^+ currents have been blocked. This inward current reflects activation of a transmembrane Ca^{2+} pathway {25}. IV curves recorded before and during BK stimulation are shown in panel B and were used to construct the agonist-activated current. The reversal potential of the BK-activated current was close to 0 mV, indicating that this current might be mediated through a rather nonselective cation channel. The current is tiny: At -60 mV only approximately 15 pA/cell are activated.

Another piece of evidence for the existence of such a CRAC mechanism in endothelial cells comes from experiments shown in fig. 51-8D: Ca^{2+} stores are refilled by the action of a Ca^{2+}-ATPase that can be selectively blocked by a tumor-promoting agent, the sesquiterpene lactone thapsigargin, extracted from the umbelliferous plant *Thapsia garcanica* {44}.

Thapsigargin increases $[Ca^{2+}]_i$ by preventing refilling of normally leaky Ca^{2+} stores in endothelial cells (see also fig. 51-6A). In these experiments, depletion of the stores can be directly monitored by application of agonists such as histamine that, after application of thapsigargin, are unable to further increase $[Ca^{2+}]_i$ by Ca^{2+} release. Using the perforated patch whole-cell configuration, thapsigargin-induced inward currents could be recorded (fig. 51-8D) {45}. The onset of the thapsigargin-induced current seemed to match the time course of intracellular $[Ca^{2+}]_i$ changes induced by thapsigargin. The thapsigargin-induced inward current lags behind the changes in $[Ca^{2+}]_i$ and reverses near 0 mV. Thus thapsigargin activates a supposedly nonselective transmembrane pathway in endothelial cells, rather than a highly Ca^{2+}-selective channel.

These Ca^{2+}-release and CRAC processes are also of a more general interest because they are related to the biologically important role of luminal Ca^{2+} inside the Ca^{2+} store in the regulation of many cell functions, such as intracellular protein traffic, secretion of mature processed proteins from the endoplasmic reticulum (ER), retention of the partially processed ones, and control of cell proliferation. The mechanism of signal transduction between the intraluminal Ca^{2+} in a store and the opening of a Ca^{2+}-permeable channel in the plasma membrane is now the subject of intense studies. Summing up all data obtained

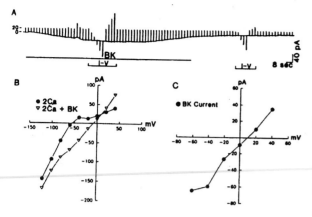

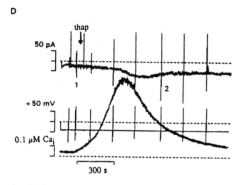

Fig. 51-8. Agonist-induced and thapsigargin-induced currents in endothelial cells that might be related to CRAC. **A:** Application of bradykinin (BK) induced an inward current at −60 mV holding potential in bovine aortic endothelial cells. The small blips indicate ramp currents obtained at 500-ms voltage ramps from −120 to +60 mV. The IV curves so recorded are depicted in panel B and C. **B:** IV curves in the absence (closed circle) and presence (open triangles) of BK. All K$^+$ currents are blocked by 140 mM tetraethylammonium chloride and buffering of $[Ca^{2+}]_i$ to 10^{-8} M. Only 2 mM Ca^{2+}, 5.4 mM K$^+$, and 1 mM Mg^{2+} are the extracellular cations. **C:** BK-activated membrane currents from subtraction of both IV curves shown in panel B. This current reflects Ca^{2+} entry through a not very Ca^{2+}-selective pathway (reversal potential near 0 mV) {28}. **D:** Simultaneous measurement of the effects of 2 μM thapsigargin on $[Ca^{2+}]_i$ and on the transmembrane currents. The top panel shows the transmembrane current measured at a holding potential of −40 mV. The artifacts in this recording are due to currents induced by repetitive application of short voltage ramps. After application of thapsigargin an inward current is activated. Analysis of the voltage ramps (not shown) reveals a reversal potential of the currents activated by thapsigargin near 0 mV (a perforated patch-clamp technique with the pore-forming nystatine was applied). This thapsigargin-activated current is again supposedly through a nonselective pathway. From Gerick et al. {45} with permission of Pflügers Archiv.

from various types of nonexcitable cells, the mechanism of signaling between the intracellular Ca^{2+} store and the membrane channel could include:
1. A cytosolic 130-kDa signal protein that is dephosphorylated at a tyrosine residue, depending on a phos-

phatase that is activated by the intraluminal (store) Ca^{2+}. The protein is phosphorylated by a tyr-kinase activated by cytosolic Ca^{2+}. CRAC might be gated by the phosphorylated protein {46}.
2. cGMP is involved. The intracellular cGMP content is increased in endothelial cells after stimulation with agonists {47}. cGMP is supposed to gate a Ca^{2+}-permeable membrane channel {48,49}.
3. Ins(1,3,4,5)P$_4$ gates CRAC: The predicted channel is activated by Ins(1,3,4,5)P$_4$ {50}. In this respect, the highly Mn^{2+}-, Ca^{2+}-selective channel, activated by Ins(1,3,4,5)P$_4$ {27}, could be a candidate for CRAC.
4. CRAC is controlled via cytochrome P450 {51}.
5. Direct activation of CRAC by an increase in $[Ca^{2+}]_i$ {1–127} (see *Agonist-gated ion channels*).
6. Ins(1,4,5)P$_3$-receptors that provide Ca^{2+} permeability after Ins(1,4,5)P$_3$ binding and are sensitized by Ca^{2+} may be located in the plasma membrane and may act as modified Ca^{2+}-entry channels by binding Ins(1,4,5)P$_3$ at the cytosolic side of the cell membrane {52}.

Other different mechanisms are still under discussion. Although there is already much progress in elucidating this important Ca^{2+}-entry pathway, most of the mechanisms discussed are still largely speculative.

VOLTAGE-DEPENDENT ION CHANNELS IN ENDOTHELIAL CELLS

In any tissue it is always very intriguing to look for the existence of calcium channels because of their special functional significance. In most of the studies published on endothelium, there are statements on the absence of voltage-gated Ca^{2+} channels {see 9 for review}. In capillary endothelial cells dissociated from bovine adrenal glands, however, voltage-gated Ca^{2+} channels exist and share some similarities with the classical L- and T-type calcium channels known in excitable tissues such as myocardium {53,54}. In these cells, Ca^{2+} channels similar to T-type channels have a conductance of approximately 8 pS. Ca^{2+} transients could be evoked in these cells by short pulses of high potassium concentrations and were found to be sensitive to cadmium and amiloride, which suggest a role of T-type Ca^{2+} channels in the control of $[Ca^{2+}]_i$ because amiloride is known to be an efficient blocker of T-type Ca channels. It is, however, difficult to imagine a functional role of the latter channels at the low resting membrane potential in most endothelial cells.

Calcium channels similar to the L type have a single-channel conductance of approximately 20 pS and are sensitive to dihydropyridine calcium agonists. Another Ca^{2+} channel has a tiny conductance of 2.8 pS in 110 mM Ba^{2+}. This channel appears sensitive to the Ca^{2+} agonist BayK 8644 but not to the Ca^{2+} antagonist nicardipine. It is present at more hyperpolarized potentials than the other Ca^{2+} channels, shows very long openings, and could be involved in low-threshold (around −40 mV) Ca^{2+} entry {54}.

Other voltage-gated ion channels are less well characterized. In some endothelial cells, transient A-type potassium channels can be activated by depolarizing voltage steps {55}. These currents are blocked by externally applied 4-aminopyridine and show inactivation at depolarized holding potentials. There is, however, some evidence that this current may arise from K^+ depletion and accumulation in restricted paracellular spaces {26}.

CELL-CELL COMMUNICATION IN ENDOTHELIAL CELLS AND ADJACENT CELLS

Endothelial cells are connected to each other via gap junction channels. These channels are clearly resolvable in electron microscopy. The channels are about 30 Å in diameter and have a molecular weight of approximately 1 kDa. Endothelial cells are electrically coupled via these high-conductance channels. In addition to these structures, similar connections have been described between endothelail cells and smooth muscle cells. Experimental evidence in cocultures of endothelium with smooth muscle cells have indicated that there is gap-junctional transfer of [³H]-uridine phosphate between endothelial and smooth muscle cells. Furthermore, regions have been described in which the overall thickness of cell-cell contacts between the endothelium and the smooth muscle layer is in the range of 150 Å, typical for cell-cell contacts via gap junction channels. In these regions ordered domains of connexons can be seen {56,57}.

These direct connections between endothelial cells and smooth muscle cells via gap junctional channels could be of functional significance: hyperpolarization of an endothelial cell by activation of agonist-gated, Ca^{2+}-activated, or shear-stress-dependent K^+ channels could spread via the low-resistance gap junction channel towards smooth muscle cells, thereby inducing hyperpolarization-mediated relaxation and vasodilation {see 35 for a review}.

LEAK CURRENTS, DRIVING FORCE, AND [Ca²⁺]ᵢ

It has been already discussed in detail that regulation of Ca^{2+} influx in endothelial cells may be at least partially controlled by the driving force for Ca^{2+}. It has been shown that depolarization of endothelial cells with increased extracellular K^+ concentrations and preincubation with K^+-channel blockers (TEA) does not disturb the release component of the Ca^{2+} signal (initial Ca^{2+} peak after stimulation with ATP or bradykinin) but decreases the Ca^{2+} plateau. Release of EDRF was also decreased when the Ca^{2+} plateau was diminished by both mechanisms {58}. It has been concluded that activation of K^+ channels would hyperpolarize endothelial cells, thereby supporting Ca^{2+} influx. However, for such an intriguing mechanism a pathway for Ca^{2+} must be available. Possible candidates could be (a) CRAC channels that are always open due to the existence of a population of empty stores, (b) the existence of a "leaky Ca^{2+} channel" that is permeable to Ca^{2+}. We have tried to test this hypothesis on the existence of a "leaky" Ca^{2+}-entry pathway directly by using the method of simultaneous voltage clamp and intracellular

Ca^{2+} measurements. To avoid Ca^{2+} entry through a high-resistance pathway between the rim of the pipette and the cell surface, we have used the perforated patch-clamp technique. Pores formed by nystatin are impermeable to Ca^{2+} {59,60}. Therefore, changes in intracellular Ca^{2+} by variation of the membrane potential must be mediated by a transmembrane pathway. In a nonstimulated endothelial cell, application of a voltage ramps or voltage steps to more negative membrane potentials induced small inward currents simultaneously with an increase in [Ca²⁺]ᵢ. A significant correlation could be obtained between [Ca²⁺]ᵢ and the driving force for Ca^{2+}. Nickel ions (5 mM) completely and reversibly blocked the Ca^{2+} transients and currents. Thus the Ca^{2+} influx pathway should be considered to be a passive leak. Until now we do not know the nature of this leak pathway. However, this leak could be a candidate for providing increased Ca^{2+} influx by cell hyperpolarization. It is intriguing to speculate whether already depleted stores in endothelial cells are responsible for generating a sustained leak through which Ca^{2+} could permeate, controlled only by the electrochemical driving force. Block of this pathway by nickel — which also inhibits CRAC-induced Ca^{2+} entry — may hint of such a possibility {41,61}.

CONCLUSIONS

Ion channels are involved in various functions of endothelial cells. Their functional significance obviously arises from the multiple effects of modulating or even maintaining intracellular Ca^{2+} signals. Ion channels are involved in the control of Ca^{2+} signaling in almost every cell. In the endothelium, however, we still have little information on the existence, properties, modulation, and functional impact of ion channels. Another problem arises from the possibly very different pattern of ion channels present in different types of endothelial cells. Until now, there is still no clear picture of which channels really belong as "standard tools" for the functioning of an endothelial cell.

Not much is known of electrogenic transporters in endothelial cells. Currents related to activation of Na^+,K^+-ATPase have recently been measured and reflect a high density of pump sites in endothelial cells {62}. Until now, it is not clear whether the Na^+-Ca^{2+} antiporter contributes to Ca^{2+} signaling in the endothelium. Any increase in intraendothelial Ca^{2+} can release vasorelaxing factors, such as NO and PGI_2, as well as vasoconstricting factors, such as endothelins. The consequences of a common pathway for different signals has still to be assessed. It is not at all clear how a common signaling pathway can be bifurcated into functionally opposite effects.

At least four different mechanisms that include ion transport through not very selective pathways have to be considered. Mechanically gated ion channels may provide a Ca^{2+} entry pathway that is not highly selective for Ca^{2+} but seems to be more permeable for divalents than for monovalents. Until now, no details are available to further characterize these important mechanosensing properties

of endothelial cells. Nonselective ion channels gated by
agonists that bind to surface receptors seem to be — at
least when activated by histamine — permeable to Ca^{2+}.
These channels may provide a Ca^{2+}-entry route after
stimulation of endothelial cells by agonists. G-protein
activation might be involved in gating of these channels.
Downregulation by protein kinase C provides a negative
feedback mechanism for Ca^{2+} signaling. An intriguing
mechanism proposes gating of Ca^{2+}-permeable ion channels by Ca^{2+} release from Ca^{2+} stores in the endoplasmic
reticulum via binding of $Ins(1,4,5)P_3$ to the $Ins(1,4,5)P_3$-
receptor Ca^{2+}-release channel in the membranes of the
endoplasmic reticulum (ER). By an unknown mechanism,
the ER store signals to a Ca^{2+}-permeable membrane
channel in the plasma membrane to open (Ca^{2+}-release
activated Ca^{2+} permeable channels, CRAC). We have
some indication that in endothelial cells this pathway
involves a nonselective cation channel.

Ca^{2+} influx can be modulated by the action of various
K^+ channels. Hyperpolarization of endothelial cells always
reacts in an increase in $[Ca^{2+}]_i$ accompanied by increased
synthesis of EDRF. Ca^{2+} influx sensitive to the driving
force could be mediated by a transmembrane pathway
blocked by nickel or a nonspecific leak that allows Ca^{2+}
ions to enter an endothelial cell following the driving
force. It is intriguing to speculate whether the agonist and
leak pathways are related to CRAC mechanisms.

REFERENCES

1. Mayer B, Schmidt K, Humbert P, Böhme E: Biosynthesis of endothelium-derived relaxing factor: A cytosolic enzyme in porcine aortic endothelial cells Ca^{2+}-dependently converts L-arginine into an activator of soluble guanylcyclase. *Biochem Biophys Res Commun* 164:678–685, 1989.
2. Knowles RG, Moncada S: Nitric oxide as a signal in blood vessels. *Topics Biol Sci* 17:399–402, 1992.
3. Nathan C: Nitric oxide as a secretory product of mammalian cells. *FASEB J* 6:3051–3064, 1992.
4. Moncada S: The L-arginine: nitric oxide pathway. *Acta Physiol Scand* 145:201–227, 1992.
5. Takeda K, Schini V, Stoeckel H: Voltage-activated potassium but not calcium currents in cultured bovine aortic endothelial cells. *Pflügers Arch* 410:385–393, 1987.
6. Bregestovski PD, Ryan US: Voltage-gated and receptor-mediated ionic currents in the membrane of endothelial cells. *J Mol Cell Cardiol* 21(Suppl 1):103–108, 1989.
7. Hoyer J, Popp R, Meyer J, Gall H-J, Gögelein H: Angiotensin II, vasopressin and GTPcS inhibit inward-rectifying K^+ channels in porcine cerebral capillary endothelial cells. *J Membr Biol* 123:55–62, 1991.
8. Nilius B, Riemann D: Ion channels in human endothelial cells. *Gen Physiol Biophys* 9:89–112, 1990.
9. Takeda K, Klepper M: Voltage-dependent and agonist-activated ionic currents in vascular endothelial cells: A review. *Blood Vessels* 27:169–183, 1990.
10. Vaca L, Schilling WP, Kunze DL: G-protein-mediated regulation of a Ca^{2+}-dependent K^+-channel in cultured vascular endothelial cells. *Pflügers Arch* 422:66–74, 1992.
11. Sauve R, Chahine M, Tremblay J, Hamet P: Single-channel analysis of the electrical response of bovine aortic endothelial cells to bradykinin stimulation: Contribution of a Ca^{2+}-

dependent K^+-channel. *J Hypertension* 8(Suppl 7):193–201, 1990.
12. Sauve R, Parent L, Simoneau C, Roy G: External ATP triggers a biphasic activation process of a calcium-activated K^+ channel in cultured bovine aortic endothelial cells. *Pflügers Arch* 412:469–481, 1988.
13. Rusko J, Tanzi F, Van Breemen C, Adams DJ: Calcium-activated potassium channels in native endothelial cells from rabbit aorta: Conductance, Ca^{2+} sensitivity and block. *J Physiol (Lond)* 455:601–621, 1992.
14. Fichtner H, Fröbe U, Kohlhardt M: Single non-selective cation channels and Ca^{2+}-activated-K^+ channels in aortic endothelial cells. *J Membr Biol* 98:125–133, 1987.
15. Mehrke G, Pohl U, Daut J: Effects of vasoactive agonists on the membrane potentials of cultured bovine aortic and guinea-pig coronary endothelium. *J Physiol (Lond)* 439:277–299, 1991.
16. Ueda S, Lee S-L, Fanburg BL: Chloride efflux in cyclic AMP-induced configurational change of bovine pulmonary artery endothelial cells. *Circ Res* 66:957–967, 1990.
17. Groschner K, Kukovetz WR: Voltage-sensitive chloride channels of large conductance in the membrane of pig aortic endothelial cells. *Pflügers Arch* 421:209–217, 1992.
18. Revest PA, Abbott NL: Membrane ion channels of endothelial cells. *Top Pharm Sci* 13:404–407, 1992.
19. MacGregor GG, Kemp PJ: A large conductance anion channel in cultured bovine endothelial cells. *J Physiol (Lond)*, New Castle Meeting 1992, P37.
20. Oleson S-P, Davies PF, Clapham DE: Muscarinic-activated K^+ current in bovine aortic endothelial cells. *Circ Res* 62:1059–1064, 1988.
21. Busse R, Fichtner H, Lückhoff A, Kohlhardt M: Hyperpolarization and increased free calcium in acetylcholine-stimulated endothelial cells. *Am J Physiol* 255:H965–H969, 1988.
22. Nilius B: Permeation properties of a non-selective cation channel in human vascular endothelial cells. *Pflügers Arch* 416:609–611, 1990.
23. Yamamoto Y, Chen G, Miwa K, Suzuki H: Permeability and Mg^{2+} blockade of histamine-operated cation channel in endothelial cells from rat intrapulmonary artery. *J Physiol (Lond)* 450:395–408, 1992.
24. Johns A, Lategan TW, Lodge NJ, Ryan US, van Breemen C, Adams DJ: Calcium entry through receptor-operated channels in bovine pulmonary artery endothelial cells. *Tissue Cell* 19:733–745, 1987.
25. Lodge NC, Ryan US, van Breemen C, Adams DJ: Bradykinin and thrombin-activated cation channels in cultured endothelial cells from bovine pulmonary artery. *Biophys J* 53:265, 1988.
26. Adams DJ, Barakeh J, Laskey R, van Breemen C: Ion channel regulation of intracellular calcium in vascular endothelial cells. *FASEB J* 3:2389–2400, 1989.
27. Lückhoff A, Clapham DE: Inositol 1,3,4,5-tetrakisphosphate activates an endothelial Ca^{2+}-permeable channel. *Nature* 355:356–358, 1992.
28. Mendelowitz D, Bacal K, Kunze DL: Bradykinin-activated calcium influx pathway in bovine aortic endothelial cells. *Am J Physiol* 262:H942–H948, 1992.
29. Nollert MU, Diamond SL, McIntire LV: Hydrodynamic shear stress and mass transport modulation of endothelial cell metabolism. *Biotechnol Bioengin* 38:588–602, 1991.
30. Davies PF: How do vascular endothelial cells respond to flow? *News Physiol Sci* 4:22–25, 1989.
31. Lansman JB, Hallam TJ, Rink TJ: Single stretch-activated ion channels in vascular endothelial cells as mechanotransducers? *Nature* 235:811–813, 1987.

32. Popp R, Hoyer J, Meyer J, Galla H-J, Gögelein H: Stretch-activated non-selective cation channels in the antiluminal membrane of porcine cerebral capillaries. *J Physiol (Lond)* 454:435–449, 1992.

33. Vigne P, Champigny R, Marsault R, Barbry P, Frelin C, Lazdunski M: A new type of amiloride-sensitive cationic chanel in endothelial cells of brain microvessels. *J Biol Chem* 264:7663–7668, 1989.

34. Oleson S-O, Clapham DE, Davies PF: Haemodynamic shear stress activates a K^+ current in vascular endothelial cells. *Nature* 331:168–170, 1988.

35. Davies PF, Oleson S-P, Clapham DE, Morrel EM, Schoen FJ: Endothelial communication. *Hypertension* 11:563–572, 1988.

36. Schwarz G, Droogmans G, Callewaert G, Nilius B: Shear stress induced calcium transients in human endothelial cells from umbilical cord veins. *J Physiol (Lond)* 458:527–538, 1992.

37. Schwarz G, Droogmans G, Nilius B: Shear stress induced membrane currents in human vascular endothelial cells. *Pflügers Arch* 421:394–396, 1992.

38. Nilius B: Ion channels and regulation of transmembrane Ca^{2+} influx in endothelium. In: Sperelakis N, Kuriyama H (eds) *Electrophysiology and Ion Channels of Vascular Smooth Muscle and Endothelial Cells.* New York: Elsevier, 1991, pp 317–325.

39. Nilius B: Regulation of transmembrane calcium fluxes in endothelium. *News Physiol Sci* 6:110–114, 1991.

40. Putney JW Jr: Capacitative calcium entry revisited. *Cell Calcium* 11:611–624, 1990.

41. Jacob R: Agonist-stimulated divalent cation entry into single cultured human umbilical vein endothelial cells. *J Physiol (Lond)* 421:55–77, 1990.

42. Meldolesi J, Clementi E, Fasolato C, Zacchetti D, Pozzan T: Ca^{2+} influx following receptor activation. *Trends Pharmacol Sci* 12:289–292, 1991.

43. Hoth M, Penner R: Depletion of intracellular calcium stores activates a calcium current in mast cells. *Nature* 355:353–356, 1992.

44. Thastrup O, Cullen PJ, Drobak BK, Hanley MR, Dawson AP: Thapsigargin, a tumor promotor, discharges intracellular Ca^{2+} stores by specific inhibition of the endoplasmic reticulum Ca^{2+}-ATPase. *Proc Natl Acad Sci USA* 87:2466–2470, 1991.

45. Gericke M, Droogmans G, Nilius B: Thapsigargin induces transmembrane currents and discharges intracellular calcium stores in human endothelial cells. *Pflügers Arch*, 422:552–557, 1993.

46. Vostalt JG, Jackson WL, Shulman NR: Cytosolic and stored calcium antagonistically control tyrosine phosphorylation of specific platelet proteins. *J Biol Chem* 266:16911–16916, 1991.

47. Wiemer G, Wirth K: Production of cGMP via activation of B_1 and B_2 kinin receptors in cultured bovine aortic endothelial cells. *J Pharmacol Exp Ther* 262:729–733, 1992.

48. Pandol SJ, Schoeffield-Payne: Cyclic GMP mediates the agonist-stimulated increase in plasma membrane calcium entry in the pancreatic acinar cell. *J Biol Chem* 265:12846–12853, 1990.

49. Pandol SJ, Schoeffield-Payne: Cyclic GMP regulates free cytosolic calcium in the pancreatic acinar cells. *Cell Calcium* 11:477–486, 1990.

50. Irvine RF: Inositol phosphates and Ca^{2+} entry toward a proliferation or simplification. *FASEB J* 6:3085–3091, 1992.

51. Alvarez J, Montero M, Garcia-Sancho J: Cytochrome P450 may regulate plasma membrane Ca^{2+} permeability according to the filling state of the intracellular Ca^{2+}-stores. *FASEB J* 6:786–792, 1992.

52. Khan AA, Steiner JP, Klein MG, Schneider MF, Snyder SH: IP_3 receptor: Localization to plasma membrane of T cells and cocapping with the T cell receptor. *Science* 257:813–818, 1992.

53. Bossu JF, Feltz A, Rodeau JL, Tanzi F: Voltage-dependent calcium currents in freshly dissociated capillary endothelial cells. *FEBS Lett* 255:377–380, 1989.

54. Bossu JL, Elhamdani A, Feltz A, Tanzi F, Aunis D, Thierse D: Voltage-gated Ca entry in isolated bovine capillary endothelial cells: Evidence of a new type of Bay K 8644-sensitive channel. *Pflügers Arch* 420:200–207, 1992.

55. Takeda K, Schini V, Stoeckel H: Voltage-activated potassium, but not calcium currents in cultured bovine aortic endothelial cells. *Pflügers Arch* 410:385–393, 1987.

56. Larson DM, Sheridan JD: Junctional transfer in cultured vascular endothelium: I. Dye and nucleotide transfer. *J Membr Biol* 83:157–168, 1985.

57. Davies PF, Ganz P, Diehl PS: Methods in laboratory investigation: Reversible microcarrier-mediated junctional communication between endothelial and smooth muscle cell monolayers: An in vitro model of vascular interactions. *Lab Invest* 53:710–718, 1985.

58. Lückhoff A, Busse R: Calcium influx into endothelial cells and formation of endothelium-derived relaxing factor is controlled by the membrane potential. *Pflügers Arch* 416:305–311, 1990.

59. Horn R, Marty A: Muscarinic activation of ionic currents measured by a new whole cell recording method. *J Gen Physiol* 92:145–159, 1988.

60. Korn SJ, Horn R: Influence of sodium-calcium exchange on calcium current rundown and the duration of calcium-dependent chloride currents in pituitary cells, studied with whole cell and perforated patch recording. *J Gen Physiol* 94:789–812, 1989.

61. Nilius B, Droogmans G, Gericke M, Schwarz G: Nonselective ion pathways in human endothelial cells. In: Siemen W, Hescheler J (eds) *Nonselective Cation Channels* — Birkhänser Verlag, Basel Switzerland 269–280, 1993.

62. Oike M, Droogmnas G, Nilius B: Electrogenic Na^+/K^+-transport in human endothelial cells. *Pflügers Arch* 424: 301–307, 1993.

63. Nilins B, Schwarz G, Droogmans G: Modulation by histamine of an inwardly rectifying potassium channel in human endothelial cells. *J Physiol (Lond)* 472:359–371, 1993.

CHAPTER 52

Cyclic Nucleotides and Protein Phosphorylation in Vascular Smooth Muscle Relaxation

BRIAN M. BENNETT & SCOTT A. WALDMAN

INTRODUCTION

Vascular smooth muscle contractility is regulated by a complex balance between a variety of antagonistic and synergistic signal transduction pathways and intracellular second messenger molecules. Contraction is initiated by increases in the concentration of intracellular activator calcium ($[Ca^{2+}]_i$), which is regulated by the interplay of a variety of systems, including receptor- and voltage-operated Ca^{2+} channels, other ion channels, and receptor-mediated increases in the metabolism of signal-transducing phospholipids. Calcium interacts with a number of receptor proteins, particularly calmodulin, which alters the activity of other enzymes, ultimately resulting in increases in the activity of actin-activated myosin ATPase and smooth muscle contraction. Relaxation of vascular smooth muscle involves reducing $[Ca^{2+}]_i$ by increasing the efflux of this cation out of the cell, decreasing its influx, or increasing its intracellular sequestration. Additionally, the sensitivity of the contractile apparatus to Ca^{2+} may be decreased, so that there is a decreased contractile response at any given intracellular concentration of Ca^{2+}.

Smooth muscle relaxation is mediated by the intracellular second messengers cyclic AMP and cyclic GMP. The production and metabolism of these cyclic nucleotides and the regulation of intracellular concentrations of Ca^{2+} are highly interdependent. Experimental evidence suggests that each of these messenger molecules exerts regulatory influences on the intracellular concentration of the others. However, which of the several possible interacting mechanisms predominates in mediating vascular smooth muscle relaxation in a variety of physiological or pathophysiological conditions remains to be defined.

This chapter concentrates on defining the mechanisms by which cyclic AMP and cyclic GMP regulate vascular tone. These mechanisms are defined by available experimental evidence, focusing on their relationships to the regulation of $[Ca^{2+}]_i$ and on the Ca^{2+} sensitivity of the contractile apparatus. Although vascular smooth muscle function is the focus of this chapter, evidence obtained with other types of smooth muscle, and in some cases, with tissues other than smooth muscle, is evaluated. It is hoped that the review presented herein allows the reader to appreciate the complexity of vascular smooth muscle function at the molecular level and the gaps in understanding that remain to be filled.

CYCLIC GMP

Low levels of cyclic GMP in biological systems slowed progress in understanding the biochemistry and physiology of this cyclic nucleotide. The observations that cyclic AMP accumulation was associated with vascular relaxation stimulated by catecholamines and that cholinergic-mediated vasoconstriction was associated with cyclic GMP accumulation misled many to suggest that cyclic AMP was responsible for relaxation while cyclic GMP mediated smooth muscle contraction [1,2]. This hypothesis was challenged when increases in cyclic GMP stimulated by cholinergic agents were detected only after the onset of smooth muscle contraction [3]. The proposal that cyclic GMP was involved in the regulation of smooth muscle relaxation followed the observation of increased cyclic GMP levels associated with relaxation of ductus deferens, tracheal, and vascular smooth muscle to glyceryl trinitrate (GTN) and sodium nitroprusside (SNP) [4–6].

In the ensuing years, the involvement of cyclic GMP in vascular smooth muscle relaxation has been firmly established. It is generally accepted that the vasodilator effects of a number of compounds and therapeutic agents, in addition to endogenous substances such as endothelium-derived relaxing factor (EDRF) and atrial natriuretic peptides (ANPs), are mediated by increased intracellular accumulation of this cyclic nucleotide.

Guanylyl cyclase, which catalyzes the formation of cyclic GMP from GTP, exists in both a cytosolic and particulate or membrane-bound form in most tissues examined [7]. These isoenzymes differ in their kinetic, physicochemical, and antigenic properties. Furthermore, these isoenzyme forms are regulated by different agents: The soluble enzyme is activated by the nitrovasodilators, EDRF, protoporphyrin IX, and arachidonate, while particulate guanylyl cyclase is activated by the heat-stable enterotoxin produced by *E. coli*, atrial natriuretic peptides, and hemin [8].

N. Sperelakis (ed.), Physiology and Pathophysiology of the Heart, Third Edition.

975

SOLUBLE GUANYLYL CYCLASE

Soluble guanylyl cyclase has been purified to apparent homogeneity from a variety of tissues {8}. This protein can be purified in association with heme as an apparent prosthetic group {9,10}, and this heme is required for enzyme activation by nitric oxide (NO). The immunopurified enzyme from rat lung exists as a heterodimer of 82-kDa (α_1) and 70-kDa (β_1) subunits (SDS gels) {11}, while that of bovine lung consists of α_1 and β_1 subunits of 73 kDa and 70 kDa {12}. Both α_1 and β_1 subunits have been cloned and sequenced {13–16}, and have deduced molecular weights of 77.5 and 70 kDa, respectively. Sequence analysis of the α_1 subunits from rat and bovine lung indicates that they are the same. A second β subunit (β_2) has been isolated from rat kidney {17} and has substantial sequence homology with the β_1 subunit from lung. The β_2 subunit contains an additional 86 amino acids at the carboxyl terminal, which end with the consensus recognition sequence for isoprenylation/carboxy-methylation, suggesting that it may associate with the plasma membrane. The carboxyl terminal regions of the α and β subunits possess a high degree of sequence homology with each other, and have partial sequence homology with the putative catalytic domains of particulate guanylyl cyclase {18} and of adenylyl cyclase {19}. Expression of either subunit alone in COS-7 or L- cells did not result in guanylyl cyclase activity, whereas coexpression of the two subunits yielded catalytically active enzyme. That could be stimulated by SNP {14,20,21}. Thus while each subunit appears to contain a catalytic domain, the presence of both subunits is required for both basal and stimulated enzyme activity.

Early studies of the kinetic properties of guanylyl cyclase utilized GTPase inhibitors to maintain constant substrate concentrations. One of these inhibitors, sodium azide, was a potent activator of soluble guanylyl cyclase {22}. It was by this fortuitous observation that a relationship between nitrovasodilators and cyclic GMP was discovered. In addition to azide, other agents, such as SNP, organic nitrates, sodium nitrite, hydroxylamine, phenylhydrazine, nitrosoamines, nitrosoureas, amyl nitrite, nicorandil, and molsidomine, also activate the enzyme.

Nitrovasodilators activate soluble guanylyl cyclase in broken cell preparations from numerous tissues. It has been suggested that these agents require either enzymatic or nonenzymatic conversion to NO {23} or S-nitrosothiols {24} prior to activation of guanylyl cyclase. Thus NO has been proposed as the proximal activator of guanylyl cyclase by these agents, and its formation may represent the final common pathway by which the nitrovasodilators influence enzyme activity and vascular motility. Nitric oxide activates soluble guanylyl cyclase from all tissues tested. Maximum activation by NO is similar to that with other nitrovasodilators and is not additive with those agents.

In 1980, Furchgott and Zawadzki described a class of vasodilators that required intact endothelium to express their vasorelaxant effects {25}. In these studies with rabbit aorta, relaxation stimulated by acetylcholine was dependent on the interaction of acetylcholine with endothelial cells. Indeed, many other agents have been shown to require endothelial cells to promote relaxation, including histamine, bradykinin, the calcium ionophore A23187, ATP, and thrombin {26}. The data suggested that these agents stimulated the release of a factor or factors from endothelial cells (EDRF) that subsequently acted on the smooth muscle cells to induce relaxation. Soon after these observations, Rapoport and Murad demonstrated that the endothelium-dependent vasodilators, acetylcholine, A23187, and histamine, elevated cyclic GMP in rat thoracic aorta {27}.

Subsequent to these and many other studies, NO was identified as the molecule that accounted for the biological properties of EDRF {28}, and the enzyme (NO synthase) that catalyzes the formation of NO from L-arginine has been purified from endothelial cells {29} and cloned {30}. Whereas it appears that NO is the sole nitrogen oxide-containing species generated by NO synthase {31}, discrepancies in some of the properties of EDRF and NO have led to the proposal that NO is released from endothelial cells in a stabilized form such as S-nitrosothiol {32} or a nitrosyl-iron complex with thiol ligands {33}. Regardless of the chemical nature of the released form of EDRF, it is generally accepted that NO is the proximal activator of vascular smooth muscle guanylyl cyclase by the endothelium-dependent vasodilators.

It is now apparent that endothelial cells respond to stimuli such as shear stress and pulsatile flow {34–36} and that EDRF release is an important determinant of vascular tone under normal physiological conditions. In addition, vascular responsiveness in pathophysiological conditions such as hypertension and atherosclerosis may involve a reduction in EDRF-mediated vasodilator tone {36}, while induction of NO synthase in vascular smooth muscle and endothelial cells is likely a major determinant of the pathological vasodilation seen in endotoxic shock.

Whereas the enzymatic basis for endogenous NO formation by endothelial cells is now established, the mechanism of metabolic activation of therapeutic nitrovasodilator agents such as the organic nitrates is not. The biotransformation of organic nitrates (e.g., GTN) to either inorganic nitrite alone or to nitrite and NO can occur by a variety of enzymatic and nonenzymatic pathways, e.g., glutathione *S*-transferases {37}, cytochromes P-450 {38,39}, hemoproteins such as hemoglobin and myoglobin {40}, and various thiol compounds {41}. Biotransformation of GTN by vascular glutathione *S*-transferases {42} and cytochrome P-450 {43} has been demonstrated, and both enzyme systems have been implicated in mediating, at least in part, the vasodilator effects of GTN {44–47}.

In the latter study, the cytochrome P-450 substrate, 7-ethoxyresorufin, had a marked inhibitory effect on GTN-induced relaxation of isolated rat aorta (fig. 52-1), concomitant with inhibition of both cyclic GMP accumulation and vascular biotransformation of GTN {47}. This suggested a significant role of the cytochrome P-450–cytochrome P-450 reductase system in mediating the conversion of GTN to an activator (presumably NO) of guanylyl cyclase. In addition, incubation of rat hepatic

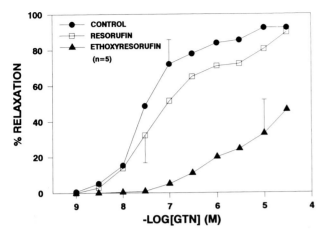

Fig. 52-1. Effect of resorufin and 7-ethoxyresorufin on GTN-induced relaxation of isolated rat aorta. Aortic strips were pre-contracted with $10\,\mu M$ phenylephrine and treated with diluent (control) (●), $1\,\mu M$ resorufin (□), or $1\,\mu M$ 7-ethoxyresorufin (▲) and GTN concentration-response curves were obtained. The EC_{50} value for 7-ethoxyresorufin-treated tissues was significantly different from that of control or resorufin-treated tissues. From Bennett et al. {47}, with permission.

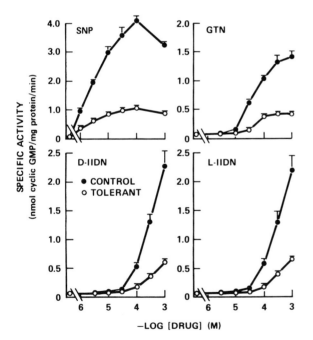

Fig. 52-2. Effect of GTN tolerance on activation of crude soluble guanylyl cyclase by SNP, GTN, D-isoidide dinitrate (D-IIDN), and L-isoidide dinitrate (L-IIDN). Rat aortas were divided in half and treated with either diluent (control) or 0.5 mM GTN for 1 hour, washed for 1 hour, and then homogenized. The $105,000\times g$ supernatant fraction was used for determination of guanylyl cyclase activity. Reproduced from Bennett et al. {52}, with permission; copyright 1988, American Heart Association.

microsomes with GTN results in the formation of an activator of rat aortic guanylyl cyclase {48}. The relaxant effect of SNP was inhibited by 7-ethoxyresorufin, suggesting that cytochrome P-450 can facilitate NO release from SNP in addition to NO released spontaneously from SNP.

Tolerance to the vasodilator effects of organic nitrates following prolonged exposure to these agents is associated with both decreased vascular biotransformation and decreased cyclic GMP accumulation {49}. Although desensitization of guanylyl cyclase to activation by SNP, GTN, and NO is observed in broken cell preparations from GTN-tolerant blood vessels (fig. 52-2) {50–53}, vasodilation by SNP and endothelium-dependent vasodilators is only modestly affected compared to the loss of vasodilator activity of GTN {52–56}. On the other hand, biotransformation of GTN is decreased in tolerant issues {57}, and in cells allowed to recover from GTN tolerance, GTN biotransformation and cyclic GMP responses returned towards control values {58}. Thus the metabolic activation system for organic nitrates in vascular smooth muscle appears to be the primary target for the tolerance-inducing effects of these drugs. Agents that generate NO by other mechanisms appear capable of activating guanylyl cyclase to a degree sufficient to permit vasodilation, even though a substantial portion of vascular guanylyl cyclase has been inactivated during GTN tolerance development.

PARTICULATE GUANYLYL CYCLASE

The particulate guanylyl cyclases are a family of membrane-spanning proteins. They contain an extracellular domain that confers ligand specificity, while the cytoplasmic portion of the enzyme contains putative protein tyrosine kinase and cyclase catalytic domains {59,60}. Three mammalian isoforms (designated GC-A, GC-B, and GC-C) have been identified and sequenced {18,61–64}. They have deduced molecular weights of 114–121 kDa and M_r values of 120–180 kDa on SDS gels. The GC-A and GC-B isoforms exhibit considerable sequence homology, especially within the carboxyl terminal cytosolic region. The GC-A isoform binds and is activated by ANP and brain natriuretic peptide (BNP), with a higher affinity for ANP. The GC-B isoform is activated by low concentrations of C-type natriuretic peptide {65} and by rather higher concentrations of ANP and BNP {62,63,65}. The GC-C isoform has considerably less sequence homology with GC-A and GC-B, especially across the extracellular domain. This isoform binds and is activated by the heat-stable enterotoxin produced by *E. coli* {64}.

Evidence supporting a role for particulate guanylyl cyclase in mediating vascular smooth muscle relaxation emerged from studies using ANP and related peptides. The vascular relaxant properties of these peptides in vitro were similar to those of SNP in that relaxation was endothelium independent and occurred in the absence of extracellular Ca^{2+} {66,67}. ANP-induced vascular relaxation was preceded by cyclic GMP accumulation and cyclic GMP-dependent protein kinase activation {68}. In contrast to the nitrovasodilators, ANP specifically activated particulate guanylyl cyclase in tissues and cultured cells from blood vessels, kidney, and adrenal gland {69–71}. Furthermore, incubation of lung fibroblasts with both ANP and SNP resulted in cyclic GMP levels that were additive {71}. Other studies have examined the effects of ANP on protein phosphorylation and Ca^{2+} dynamics in vascular smooth muscle (see below) and are, for the most part, consistent with a role for cyclic GMP in mediating the relaxant effects of ANP. However, the plasma levels of ANP required for vasodilation following bolus or intravenous infusion are typically much higher than the circulating level of ANP {72}. Thus the physiological relevance of circulating ANP in the regulation of vascular tone is uncertain.

CYCLIC AMP

There is substantial evidence that elevations of intracellular cyclic AMP concentrations are associated with relaxation of vascular smooth muscle. Thus hormones and autacoids that interact with specific receptors, such as beta-adrenoceptor agonists, adenosine, prostaglandins, vasoactive intestinal peptide, and glucagon, induce smooth muscle relaxation by increasing intracellular cyclic AMP {73–76}. Similarly, agents that directly activate adenylyl cyclase and increase the synthesis of intracellular cyclic AMP, such as forskolin, relax vascular smooth muscle {77,78}. Furthermore, the cell-permeant dibutyryl cyclic AMP directly relaxes precontracted smooth muscle.

ADENYLYL CYCLASE

Adenylyl cyclase is a membrane-bound protein in mammalian vascular smooth muscle cells. The protein has been purified and cloned, and consists of a short intracellular amino terminal, two 40-kDa cytoplasmic loop domains, and two intensely hydrophobic domains separating the cytoplasmic loops and hypothesized to contain six transmembrane helices {19}. The cytoplasmic loops are highly homologous amongst the six adenylyl cyclases cloned from mammalian cells and also amongst particulate guanylyl cyclases {19,59,60,76}. Catalytic activity requires the two intracellular loops, since point mutations in or expression of either loop alone results in a protein with significantly inhibited catalytic function {76,79}. Interestingly, the nucleotide-binding domain is presumed to be in the cytoplasmic loops, yet these loops do not share homology with other nucleotide-binding proteins, except guanylyl cyclase {76}.

Receptors are coupled to the activation of adenylyl cyclase and increases in intracellular cyclic AMP through a complex cascade of reactions mediated by guanine nucleotide-binding (G) proteins {75}. These represent a family of regulatory proteins that amplify extracellular signals and produce second messenger responses in a variety transmembrane signaling cascades, including adenylyl cyclase, phosphatidyl inositol metabolism, and

calcium and potassium channel function. G proteins are heterotrimeric, composed of alpha, beta, and gamma subunits. The alpha subunit possesses a guanine nucleotide binding site that has intrinsic GTP-phosphohydrolase activity. Heterotrimeric G proteins complex specifically with unoccupied receptors in the plasma membrane when there is no guanine nucleotide occupying the alpha subunit. This complex converts a low-affinity receptor into one of high affinity. Hormones that increase intracellular concentrations of cyclic AMP bind to these high-affinity receptors, inducing GTP to bind to the alpha subunit and activate the G protein.

Activation results in the dissociation of the heterotrimeric structure into a free beta-gamma complex and an activated alpha subunit associated with receptor. Alpha subunits with GTP bound have decreased affinity for receptors and this complex dissociates, returning the receptor to its original low-affinity state. Free alpha subunit bound to GTP activates the catalytic domain of adenylyl cyclase, increasing the production of cyclic AMP. Enzyme activation is terminated by the intrinsic GTP phosphohydrolase activity of the alpha subunit, which catalyzes the conversion of GTP to GDP. Occupancy of the guanine nucleotide binding site of the free alpha subunit by GDP decreases the affinity of this subunit for adenylyl cyclase and increases its affinity for the beta-gamma complex, which reforms the original heterotrimeric complex. Once GDP dissociates from the heterotrimer, this complex again associates with a receptor, converting it from low to high affinity and starting the cascade again.

Critical features of this regulatory mechanism are the three integrated molecular cycles, including the G-protein heterotrimer association-dissociation, the shuttling of receptor affinity from low to high, and the enzymatic hydrolysis of GTP to GDP. This mechanism permits significant amplification of the original hormonal signal, since each ligand-receptor complex can activate multiple G proteins, each of which can activate a molecule of adenylyl cyclase. Furthermore, this cascade provides an automatic "off switch" for signal generation and amplification in the form of the GTP phosphohydrolase activity intrinsic to alpha subunits of G proteins. It is by this mechanism involving receptors, G proteins, and adenylyl cyclase that autacoids and hormones increase intracellular concentrations of cyclic AMP.

CYCLIC NUCLEOTIDE PHOSPHODIESTERASES

Regulation of the concentrations of cyclic AMP and cyclic GMP in cells is a dynamic process, reflecting the relative activities of the synthetic enzymes, adenylyl and guanylyl cyclase, respectively, and the metabolic enzymes, phosphodiesterases. Phosphodiesterases are a family of enzymes that degrade cyclic nucleotides to their respective 5′-nucleotide monophosphates. Over the past several years, multiple forms of phosphodiesterases have been identified in many tissues. Originally these enzymes were categorized by their chromatographic characteristics on DEAE-cellulose. More recently, phosphodiesterases have been subdivided into five different classes (type I–V) on the basis of their protein structure, nucleotide sequence, substrate specificity and affinity, endogenous regulators, and sensitivities to specific inhibitors {80–82}.

Type I phosphodiesterase catalyzes the metabolism of cyclic AMP and cyclic GMP, and is specifically regulated by interaction with Ca^{2+} calmodulin {83,84}. It is not sensitive to either inhibition or activation by cyclic GMP and is selectively inhibited by calmodulin antagonists such as trifluperazine. Type I phosphodiesterase is found in vascular smooth muscle, including aorta and pulmonary artery, primarily in the cytosolic compartment {85}. This form of phosphodiesterase is activated by increases in $[Ca^{2+}]_i$ and complexing with Ca^{2+} calmodulin. Thus type I phosphodiesterase potentiates the action of contractile agents that raise $[Ca^{2+}]_i$ by coordinately decreasing cyclic nucleotide concentrations. Indeed, changes in $[Ca^{2+}]_i$ have been demonstrated to alter the Ca^{2+}-calmodulin-sensitive phosphodiesterase activity in vascular smooth muscle {86}. Interestingly, type I phosphodiesterase in brain is a substrate for phosphorylation by Ca^{2+}-calmodulin kinase and cyclic AMP-dependent protein kinase (A-kinase), resulting in a decrease in the affinity of this protein for Ca^{2+} calmodulin and, therefore, decreased activity {87,88}. Moreover, this enzyme is resistant to phosphorylation by these kinases when Ca^{2+} calmodulin is bound.

These data suggest that in the presence of contractile agents that elevate $[Ca^{2+}]_i$, type I phosphodiesterase activity may be a balance between occupancy and stimulation by Ca^{2+} calmodulin, and phosphorylation and inactivation by Ca^{2+}-calmodulin kinase. In contrast, agents that induce relaxation by lowering the concentration of $[Ca^{2+}]_i$ and/or increasing the concentration of cyclic AMP may inhibit this phosphodiesterase because of reduced concentrations of Ca^{2+} calmodulin and phosphorylation of the enzyme by A kinase. Whether these different modes of regulation are active under physiological conditions in vascular smooth muscle remains to be determined.

Type II phosphodiesterase metabolizes cyclic AMP and cyclic GMP with equal affinity. However, it is insensitive to regulation by Ca^{2+} calmodulin and is activated by cyclic GMP, which regulates this enzyme at a site other than the catalytic nucleotide-binding domain {89}. The type II phosphodiesterase is located primarily in the cytoplasm and has been identified in aorta and pulmonary artery vascular smooth muscle {83,84}. It is specifically inhibited by agents such as dipyridamole. The role of this phosphodiesterase and its unique allosteric activation by cyclic GMP have been studied primarily in the heart. It has been suggested that in this organ type II phosphodiesterase may mediate the inhibition by cyclic GMP of the cyclic AMP-induced slow inward Ca^{2+} current {90}. Furthermore, it has been suggested that this enzyme mediates the inhibition by muscarinic agonists, which increase intracellular concentrations of cyclic GMP, of beta-adrenoceptor agonist-induced inotropy in the heart {91}. The role of this phosphodiesterase in vascular smooth muscle function remains unclear.

Type III phosphodiesterase has been identified in the cytoplasm and membrane compartments of vascular

smooth muscle {85,92,93}. This enzyme is unique in that it specifically catalyzes the hydrolysis of cyclic AMP but is inhibited in a competitive fashion by cyclic GMP. Type III phosphodiesterase is insensitive to Ca^{2+} calmodulin and is specifically inhibited by the bipyridine inodilators amrinone, enoximone, and milrinone. A role for this phosphodiesterase in regulating the cyclic nucleotide concentration and contractility of vascular smooth muscle has been suggested. Thus specific inhibitors of type III phosphodiesterase relaxed precontracted rat aorta in a concentration-dependent fashion {92,94}. Relaxation produced by these compounds was endothelium independent and unaffected by agents inhibiting the production of EDRF. Interestingly, agents that inhibit soluble guanylyl cyclase activity in smooth muscle, such as methylene blue, also prevent the relaxation induced by inhibitors of type III phosphodiesterase {92}. These data suggest that although type III phosphodiesterase selectively metabolizes cyclic AMP, the net result of its activity may be an increase in intracellular concentrations of both cyclic AMP and cyclic GMP {92,94}. Indeed, this may reflect the ability of type III phosphodiesterase to utilize cyclic GMP as substrate, albeit at only 10% of the maximum rate of catalysis as cyclic AMP {81}.

Furthermore, this phosphodiesterase may mediate the synergy between cyclic AMP and cyclic GMP in vascular smooth muscle, since type III phosphodiesterase is inhibited by cyclic GMP. Thus agents that increase intracellular cyclic GMP concentrations, such as SNP, also enhance isoproterenol-induced increases in cyclic AMP in rat aorta, presumably by inhibiting the metabolism of cyclic AMP by type III phosphodiesterase {95}. Thus this phosphodiesterase is an important regulator of cyclic nucleotide concentrations and represents one focus of crosstalk between the two cyclic nucleotide systems in vascular smooth muscle.

Type IV phosphodiesterase also specifically metabolizes cyclic AMP compared to cyclic GMP. It is localized in the cytoplasm and membranes in vascular smooth muscle, including aorta and pulmonary artery {83,84}. This phosphodiesterase is insensitive to cyclic GMP and Ca^{2+} calmodulin, and is specifically inhibited by denbufylline and rolipram. In contrast to inhibitors of type III phosphodiesterase, which are also cyclic AMP selective, inhibitors of the type IV form of the enzyme relax vascular smooth muscle in an endothelium-dependent fashion. Thus rolipram and denbufylline induced relaxation in bovine aorta only in the presence of intact and functional endothelium. Also, agents that inhibit the production of EDRF and cyclic GMP, such as N^G-monomethyl-L-arginine (L-NMMA), inhibited the ability of rolipram or denbufylline to relax aorta {92}. L-NMMA inhibition of relaxation induced by rolipram could be overcome by L-arginine, a substrate for the production of EDRF. Similarly, methylene blue prevented rolipram or denbufylline from inducing relaxation in bovine aorta. The above data may reflect the interactions of cyclic AMP and cyclic GMP on the activities of type III and IV phosphodiesterases in smooth muscle. Thus increases in cyclic GMP concentration in smooth muscle induced by EDRF may inhibit type III phosphodiesterase sufficiently to permit the inhibition of type IV phosphodiesterase by agents such as rolipram to increase cyclic AMP to concentrations sufficient to induce relaxation. This model predicts that inhibitors of type III and IV phosphodiesterases and agents that increase intracellular cyclic GMP would be synergistic in their ability to relax vascular smooth muscle and, indeed, this has been observed {92}.

Type V phosphodiesterase specifically metabolizes cyclic GMP compared to cyclic AMP {96}. It is localized in the cytoplasm of vascular smooth muscle cells {85,96}. Type V phosphodiesterase is insensitive to regulation by Ca^{2+} calmodulin or cyclic nucleotides but is selectively inhibited by zaprinast (M&B 22,948). Indeed, zaprinast increased intracellular concentrations of cyclic GMP in intact aorta at drug concentrations that specifically inhibit type V phosphodiesterase activity {96}. Interestingly, vascular smooth muscle relaxation by zaprinast was endothelium dependent and was inhibited by L-NMMA {92}. In addition, zaprinast potentiated vascular smooth muscle relaxation by ANP {83}. Thus, as observed for the type IV phosphodiesterase, inhibitors of type V phosphodiesterase require the production of cyclic GMP in order to manifest their vasorelaxant activity. These data suggest a role for type V phosphodiesterase in the metabolism of cyclic GMP and regulation of contractility in vascular smooth muscle.

CYCLIC NUCLEOTIDE-DEPENDENT PROTEIN KINASES

Most, if not all, of the effects of cyclic nucleotides in vascular smooth muscle are thought to be mediated by cyclic nucleotide-dependent protein kinases. These homologous proteins bind cyclic AMP or cyclic GMP with relative selectivity, which activates a catalytic function involving the transfer of phosphate groups from ATP to serine or threonine residues on target proteins. Both kinases demonstrate specificity for the proteins and their domains to which they will donate a phosphate group, although there is significant overlap in this substrate specificity. Recent data suggest that the effects of cyclic AMP and GMP in vascular smooth muscle may be mediated predominantly by cyclic GMP-dependent protein kinase {97}. This will be discussed in more detail in a later section of this review.

CYCLIC GMP-DEPENDENT PROTEIN KINASE

Agents that elevate cyclic GMP, including nitrovasodilators, endothelium-dependent vasodilators, and ANP, activate cyclic GMP-dependent protein kinase (G kinase) {98,99}. This activation and subsequent phosphorylation of key proteins has been suggested as the mechanism underlying regulation of vascular smooth muscle tone by these agents. In contrast to the broad distribution of cyclic AMP-dependent protein kinase (A kinase) in mammalian tissues, the distribution of G kinase is more limited, with

appreciable amounts of the enzyme occurring in smooth muscle, cerebellum, heart, lung, and platelets {100}. Approximately three quarters of the total G-kinase activity of rabbit aorta is found in the soluble fraction {101}. The enzyme has been purified from bovine lung {102,103} and sequenced {104}.

The native enzyme is a dimer comprised of two identical subunits of 76.3 kDa, each of which possesses a catalytic domain in the carboxyl-terminal region. The amino-terminal region contains the subunit dimerization site, autophosphorylation sites (thought to be involved in inhibition of the catalytic domain), a hinge region, and two binding sites for cyclic GMP. The two sites differ in their kinetics and cyclic nucleotide analog selectivities, and binding of cyclic GMP at both sites is required for full activation of the enzyme. The enzyme can be activated by cyclic AMP, but requires at least 10-fold higher concentrations of this cyclic nucleotide {103,105–108}.

Two isoforms of G kinase, designated type Iα and type Iβ, have been purified from bovine aorta {107,108}, porcine coronary artery {109}, and bovine tracheal smooth muscle {110} and are also present in human aorta {109}. The two isoforms are present in approximately equal amounts in these tissues. The type Iα isoform appears to be the same as the bovine lung G kinase, while the type Iβ isoform differs from type Iα only in the amino-terminal region of the protein {108,111}. It is not known whether the two isoforms are products of two homologous genes or arise from alternative splicing of mRNA from one gene. The two isoforms differ with respect to autophosphorylation sites, dissociation kinetics of cyclic GMP, and the concentration of cyclic GMP required for half-maximal activation. This is presumably due to the differences in the amino-terminal sequence {108}. In a recent study {109}, the potency of various cyclic GMP analogs for the activation of the type Iα isoform correlated with the potency for relaxation of porcine coronary artery. This suggests that the type Iα isoform may be the relevant isoform for mediating the relaxant effects of cyclic GMP.

A variety of studies have been performed to elucidate the endogenous protein substrates of G kinase in vascular smooth muscle and to correlate phosphorylation of these proteins with the functional changes known to occur following increases in cyclic GMP accumulation. Early studies focused on endogenous phosphorylation in broken cell preparations of rabbit aorta and cultured rabbit vascular smooth muscle cells exposed to cyclic GMP. Endogenous protein phosphorylation could only be demonstrated in the particulate fraction {112}.

Three proteins of 250, 130, and 85 kDa (designated G_0, G_1, and G_2) demonstrated increased phosphorylation {112}, with G_1 being the major G-kinase substrate. The G_2 protein is thought to be a degradation product of G_1 {113}. The similar molecular sizes of G_1 and the plasma membrane Ca^{2+}-pumping ATPase suggested that the Ca^{2+}-pumping ATPase might be a substrate for G kinase. Using a Ca^{2+}-pumping ATPase preparation purified from bovine aortic smooth muscle by calmodulin affinity chromatography and reconstituted into phospholipid liposomes, exogenous G kinase was found to phosphorylate a 135-kDa protein of identical mobility to that of the Ca^{2+}-pumping ATPase {114}. Furthermore, G kinase was found to stimulate Ca^{2+} uptake into these proteoliposomes. The authors suggested that cyclic GMP regulation of the plasma membrane Ca^{2+} pump involved phosphorylation of the pump itself. The results of a number of other studies argue against the plasma membrane Ca^{2+}-pumping ATPase being a substrate for G kinase {115–119}. Vrolix et al. {115} utilized a Ca^{2+}-pumping ATPase preparation from pig stomach smooth muscle purified by calmodulin affinity chromatography. However, the membranes from which the ATPase was solubilized were first extracted with 0.6 M KCl rather than the 1.2 M KCl used by Furakawa and Nakamura {114}. This resulted in extraction of a 130-kDa G-kinase substrate (presumably G_1) from the crude membrane fraction concomitant with less ^{32}P-labelling of the 130-kDa protein in the Ca^{2+}-pumping ATPase preparation {115}. The authors concluded that the 130-kDa protein in the ATPase preparation was not the ATPase itself, but a contaminant protein that comigrated with the ATPase. They suggested that this 130-kDa protein was myosin light chain kinase (MLCK), based upon crossreactivity with antibodies to chicken gizzard MLCK.

In other studies, however, MLCK and the G_1 protein from porcine {117} or rat {120} aortic smooth muscle differed in molecular mass by 13–20 kDa and had quite different solubility properties. Purification of the Ca^{2+}-pumping ATPase from porcine aortic smooth muscle by Yoshida et al. {119} also utilized calmodulin affinity chromatography. These authors found that a high salt wash of the affinity gel prior to elution of the ATPase resulted in the removal of all G-kinase substrates from the Ca^{2+}-pumping ATPase preparation, thus providing further evidence that the Ca^{2+}-pumping ATPase is not a G-kinase substrate.

The studies of Baltensperger et al. {116,117} utilized an enriched plasma membrane fraction from porcine aorta that contained endogenous G-kinase activity and that demonstrated ATP-dependent Ca^{2+} uptake. Electrophoretic analysis on an acidic gel system demonstrated that the G_1 phosphoprotein and the acyl phosphate intermediate of the Ca^{2+}-pumping ATPase had different M_r values. Furthermore, overlay experiments using ^{125}I-calmodulin demonstrated interaction with the Ca^{2+}-pumping ATPase, but not with the G_1 protein {115}. The Ca^{2+} uptake properties of the plasma membrane vesicles were found to be independent of the phosphorylation level of G_1, suggesting that the pumping activity of the ATPase was not regulated by G_1 phosphorylation. In a subsequent study {117}, it was found that the G_1 phosphoprotein could be oxidatively crosslinked to plasma membrane-bound actin. It was proposed that the G_1 protein might act as a membrane attachment protein for actin and could therefore play a regulatory role in cytoskeletal reorganization, leading to vascular smooth muscle relaxation. Taken together, the balance of evidence suggests that the G_1 protein is not the Ca^{2+}-pumping ATPase and that the Ca^{2+}-pumping ATPase is not a G-kinase substrate.

A role for the 240-kDa G-kinase substrate (G_0) in the regulation of the plasma membrane Ca^{2+}-pumping ATPase has been described recently {121}. In this study, a purified Ca^{2+}-pumping ATPase preparation from porcine aorta that contained G_0 was activated by G kinase in a concentration-dependent manner concomitant with a concentration-dependent phosphorylation of G_0 by the G kinase. No activation of the Ca^{2+}-pumping ATPase was observed in enzyme preparations devoid of G_0.

In addition to the plasma membrane G-kinase substrates G_0, G_1, and G_2, a number of investigators have demonstrated the G-kinase-dependent phosphorylation of vascular smooth muscle phospholamban {122–125}. In sarcoplasmic reticulum membrane fractions of bovine pulmonary artery, phosphorylation of phospholamban after addition of exogenous G kinase was observed {122}, and this was associated with an increase in Ca^{2+} uptake by the membrane fraction {126}. In another study, phosphorylation of phospholamban was observed in microsomal fractions of cultured rat aortic smooth muscle cells after stimulation of endogenous G kinase with cyclic GMP or ANP, or after the addition of purified G kinase {124}.

Huggins et al. {123} demonstrated the phosphorylation of phospholamban in microsomes from sheep pulmonary artery after exposure to exogenous G kinase. However, in intact rabbit aorta, ^{32}P-labeling of phospholamban could not be demonstrated in tissues after a 10-minute exposure to a relatively high concentration of SNP (150 nM). The authors concluded that there is a functional separation between increases in cyclic GMP and phospholamban phosphorylation, possibly due to inaccessibility of G kinase to phospholamban in the intact cell, or to the action of phospholamban phosphatase or phosphodiesterase in close proximity to phospholamban {123}.

In contrast to the above study, phosphorylation of phospholamban in intact cultured rat aortic smooth muscle cells was observed after exposure to 100 nM SNP or ANP, with maximal phosphorylation occurring after 1 minute {125}. The increase in phospholamban phosphorylation was associated with an increase in Ca^{2+}-activated ATPase activity in membranes isolated from stimulated cells. Furthermore, studies using confocal laser scanning microscopy indicated that G kinase and phospholamban were localized to the same cellular regions {125}. These results suggest that G kinase may indeed be located in close proximity to phospholamban in situ and that phosphorylation of phospholamban by G kinase with subsequent activation of the sarcoplasmic reticulum Ca^{2+}-pumping ATPase may be one mechanism by which cyclic GMP mediates a reduction in $[Ca^{2+}]_i$.

Relatively few other studies, in addition to that noted above, have been performed using intact cells. Rapoport et al. {127,128} examined GMP-dependent protein phosphorylation in rat aortic strips. A variety of agents were tested, including SNP, 8-bromo-cyclic GMP, and the endothelium-dependent vasodilator, acetylcholine. All of these agents produced a qualitatively similar pattern of protein phosphorylation. The pattern of phosphorylation observed with acetylcholine could be abolished if the endothelium was removed from the vessel prior to exposure to the relaxant. In these studies, phosphorylation of proteins was observed in both the soluble and particulate compartments. Altered phosphorylation of nine proteins was observed. While most proteins had increased phosphorylation, two were decreased in their phosphorylation. The molecular sizes of those proteins demonstrating increased phosphorylation ranged from 49 kDa to 21 kDa. The proteins demonstrating decreased phosphorylation had molecular sizes of 22 kDa and were later identified as the phosphorylatable light chains of myosin {129}.

In summary, progress has been in the identification of some of the protein substrates of G kinase in vascular smooth muscle. Activation of Ca^{2+}-pumping ATPases in the plasma membrane and sarcoplasmic reticulum via G-kinase-dependent phosphorylation of G_0 and phospholamban would provide explanations for the effects of cyclic GMP on Ca^{2+} efflux and sequestration (see below), while a role of G_1 as a membrane attachment protein for actin might at least partially explain relaxant effects of cyclic GMP that are independent of changes in $[Ca^{2+}]_i$. What is still lacking is knowledge of the relative role of the identified G-kinase substrates in mediating relaxation and the identity and function of other G-kinase substrates.

CYCLIC AMP-DEPENDENT PROTEIN KINASE

Two forms of cyclic AMP-dependent protein kinase (A kinase) that differ in the characteristics of their regulatory subunits have been described. Type I and type II kinase are composed of two regulatory and two catalytic subunits {130,131}. These kinases are tightly regulated, and the catalytic subunits are maintained in the inactive conformation by the regulatory subunits in the absence of cyclic AMP. Each regulatory subunit binds two molecules of cyclic AMP, which induces conformational changes in that subunit, stabilizing a structure that has a lower affinity for the catalytic subunits. Binding of four cyclic AMP molecules results in the dissociation of the tetrameric kinase into a regulatory subunit dimer and two active catalytic monomeric subunits {130–132}. Monomeric catalytic subunits are active and participate in the regulation of intracellular processes by phosphorylating target proteins {133,134}. Isoenzymes of A kinase, corresponding to type I and type II kinase, have been identified in bovine coronary and carotid arteries {135,136}. About 60–70% of the total A kinase is found in the cytosol, composed of equal amounts of the type I and type II isoforms {135–138}.

A role for A kinase in mediating vascular smooth muscle relaxation has been suggested by correlating increased enzyme activity with physiological responses. Thus relaxation of bovine coronary arteries by isoproterenol was associated with increases in type II kinase activity {136}. Activation of type II kinase and relaxation was inhibited by the beta-adrenoceptor antagonist propranolol. Similarly, isoproterenol and forskolin increased intracellular concentrations of cyclic AMP, activated A kinase, and induced relaxation in bovine coronary arteries precontracted with KCl {138}. Furthermore, adenosine produced a time- and concentration-dependent increase in A-kinase activity and relaxation in bovine circumflex arteries {139}.

Identification of the proteins phosphorylated by A kinase has led to attempts to correlate changes in phosphorylation of proteins with alterations in intracellular Ca^{2+} concentrations. Membrane proteins ranging in size from 11 to 256 kDa have been identified in various blood vessels as undergoing alterations in phosphorylation as a result of cyclic AMP accumulation or A-kinase activation {140–144}. More recently, identification of some of these proteins has been achieved. Phospholamban is a regulatory protein that inhibits the activity of the 100-kDa Ca^{2+}-pumping ATPase responsible for sequestration of intracellular Ca^{2+} in sarcoplasmic reticulum. This protein has been identified in vascular smooth muscle from a variety of sources and has been shown to be a substrate for A kinase {141,145,146}.

These data suggest that one mechanism by which cyclic AMP may induce vascular smooth muscle relaxation involves activating A kinase, resulting in the phosphorylation of phospholamban, which subsequently dissociates from the Ca^{2+}-pumping ATPase. This dissociation removes the inhibition mediated by phospholamban, activating the transporter, increasing the sequestration of Ca^{2+} into the sarcoplasmic reticulum, and lowering $[Ca^{2+}]_i$. It is noteworthy that the data supporting this model involving A kinase was obtained in studies of cell-free systems. Interestingly, studies on intact cells in vitro suggest that agents that increase intracellular cyclic AMP concentrations in vascular smooth muscle result in the activation of G kinase, which phosphorylates phospholamban on the same serine residues as A kinase, resulting in relaxation {97}. Thus, regardless of the kinase involved, cyclic AMP and GMP both appear to regulate vascular smooth muscle relaxation by a convergent mechanism involving phospholamban and increased Ca^{2+} sequestration into sarcoplasmic reticulum.

Cyclic AMP has also been reported to increase the activity of a sarcolemmal Ca^{2+}-pumping ATPase, which results in the extrusion of Ca^{2+}, lowering the intracellular concentration of this cation, and relaxation. Activation of the sarcolemmal Ca^{2+}-pumping ATPase by cyclic AMP or A kinase has been reported in microsomes purified from rat mesenteric arteries and porcine aorta {142,147}. Interestingly, A kinase phosphorylates the 130-kDa plasma membrane Ca^{2+}-pumping ATPase in erythrocytes, decreasing the Km and increasing the Vmax of this enzyme {148}. These data suggest that another mechanism by which A kinase mediates vascular smooth muscle relaxation is by phosphorylating the sarcolemmal Ca^{2+}-pumping ATPase and increased extrusion of Ca^{2+}. However, more recent studies demonstrated that cyclic AMP or forskolin were unable to increase the activity of the Ca^{2+}-pumping ATPase in vascular smooth muscle cells in vitro {149}. Also, cyclic AMP and A kinase were unable to phosphorylate the Ca^{2+} pump protein purified from bovine aortic smooth muscle {149}. Although these studies suggest that the sarcolemmal Ca^{2+}-pumping ATPase is not likely to be one of the primary protein substrates for A-kinase phosphorylation in vascular smooth muscle cells; nevertheless, the predominant Ca^{2+}-pumping ATPase isoform found in vascular and nonvascular smooth muscle

(PMCA1b isoform) {150,151} contains the consensus sequence for phosphorylation by A kinase.

Another target for phosphorylation by cyclic AMP and A kinase is myosin light chain kinase (MLCK). A kinase phosphorylates MLCK, reducing the affinity of this enzyme for Ca^{2+} calmodulin and its ability to phosphorylate myosin, resulting in relaxation {152–154}. Thus phosphorylation of MLCK by A kinase mediates vascular smooth muscle relaxation by reducing the Ca^{2+} sensitivity of the contractile apparatus. This mechanism is discussed in greater detail in a later section of this review.

MECHANISMS OF VASCULAR RELAXATION

Vascular smooth muscle contraction

Discussions concerning the molecular mechanisms underlying vascular smooth muscle relaxation are predicated on an understanding of those mechanisms mediating contraction. Since the primary focus of this chapter is smooth muscle relaxation, this brief review of contraction will serve only to highlight those mechanisms in order to put into context mechanisms mediating relaxation. The reader is referred to other chapters for a more complete discussion of the mechanisms underlying vascular smooth muscle contraction.

Smooth muscle contractility and relaxation are intimately dependent upon the concentration of intracellular activator calcium ($[Ca^{2+}]_i$). Thus contraction is dependent upon an increase in $[Ca^{2+}]_i$, increased sensitivity of the contractile apparatus to $[Ca^{2+}]_i$, or both. In contrast, relaxation is dependent upon a decrease in $[Ca^{2+}]_i$, a decreased sensitivity of the contractile apparatus to $[Ca^{2+}]_i$, or both. In addition, relaxation can be mediated by uncoupling of myosin light chain phosphorylation from force generation {155}. Intracellular concentrations of Ca^{2+} can be increased by two major mechanisms, electromechanical and pharmacomechanical coupling {156}. In electromechanical coupling, $[Ca^{2+}]_i$ is regulated by depolarization of smooth muscle cells. Depolarization activates L-type Ca^{2+} channels, which mediate the influx of Ca^{2+}, increase $[Ca^{2+}]_i$, and induce contraction. Pharmacomechanical coupling refers to increases in $[Ca^{2+}]_i$ mediated by ligand-receptor interaction at the extracellular surface of the sarcolemma and the stimulation of transmembrane signaling mechanisms. Generally, the predominate mechanism by which contraction is initiated in blood vessels is pharmacomechanical coupling.

Several mechanisms have been suggested that might participate in pharmacomechanical coupling. Thus contractile agonists, such as norepinephrine, bind to their receptors and activate a sarcolemmal phospholipase C, increasing the metabolism of membrane phosphatidyl inositides {157}. This increase in metabolism results in the production of 1,4,5-inositol triphosphate (IP_3) and diacylglycerol (DAG). Increases in IP_3 result in the release of Ca^{2+} from the sarcoplasmic reticulum, increases in $[Ca^{2+}]_i$, and contraction {158}. Contractile agonists may also increase the influx of Ca^{2+} by activating L-type Ca^{2+} channels or nonspecific ion channels in the sarcolemma {159–161}.

As indicated above, contraction also can be mediated by increasing the sensitivity of the contractile apparatus to Ca^{2+}. One mechanism by which this might occur involves the activation of protein kinase C. Thus phorbol esters, which are potent activators of protein kinase C, induce sustained contractions of blood vessels associated with low or only small increases in $[Ca^{2+}]_i$ {162–166}. Although phorbol esters are not naturally occurring in vascular smooth muscle, IP_3 and DAG are produced in response to contractile agents, as pointed out above. IP_3 increases $[Ca^{2+}]_i$ by releasing this cation from the sarcoplasmic reticulum, and protein kinase C is a Ca^{2+}-dependent enzyme. DAG increases the sensitivity of protein kinase C to activation by Ca^{2+} such that the Ca^{2+} requirement of protein kinase C may be satisfied by resting $[Ca^{2+}]_i$ {167}. Thus, activation of phosphatidyl inositide metabolism by contractile agents could increase contraction in the absence of large increases in $[Ca^{2+}]_i$ through a protein kinase C-mediated mechanism. In addition, DAG is the product of other lipid metabolic enzymes, including phospholipase D and phospholipases C, which utilize phospholipids other than those containing inositol {168, 169}. Activation of these enzymes could increase DAG in the absence of IP_3, activate protein kinase C, and induce contraction in the absence of increases in $[Ca^{2+}]_i$ {170}. Indeed, this may be the mechanism by which prostaglandin $F_{2\alpha}$ induces vascular smooth muscle contraction {171}. The specific target proteins phosphorylated by protein kinase C that increase the sensitivity of the contractile apparatus to Ca^{2+} remain unclear, but candidates include the thin filament proteins caldesmon and calponin, cytoskeletal proteins, or myosin light chain phosphatase.

Evidence that agonist-coupled G proteins may mediate the increased sensitivity of the myofilaments to Ca^{2+} has emerged through the use of plasma membrane-permeabilizing agents such as staphylococcal α-toxin, which allow clamping of $[Ca^{2+}]_i$ while maintaining intact receptor and signal transduction systems {172–176}. In these and other studies {177}, agonists such as norepinephrine, or the nonhydrolyzable GTP analogue GTP-γS, increased the Ca^{2+} sensitivity of the myofilaments (i.e., shifted the pCa^{2+}-tension curve to the left) and increased the level of myosin light chain phosphorylation at constant $[Ca^{2+}]_i$. Both Kitazawa et al. {176} and Kobota et al. {178} have presented evidence that this effect is mediated by inhibition of myosin light chain phosphatase(s). Although a role of protein kinase C in myosin light chain phosphatase inhibition has not been established, Gong et al. {179} have proposed that arachidonic acid may be the downstream mediator of this phosphatase inhibition, subsequent to agonist-coupled G-protein activation.

Increased $[Ca^{2+}]_i$, resulting from electromechanical or pharmacomechanical coupling, binds to and activates calmodulin in vascular smooth muscle cells. The Ca^{2+}-calmodulin complex binds to myosin light chain kinase (MLCK), decreasing the autoinhibition characteristic of this enzyme {180–182}. Activated MLCK phosphorylates the 20-kDa light chain of myosin on serine 19, increasing the actin-activated myosin ATPase activity {183}. This promotes crossbridge cycling between thick and thin filaments, force generation, and smooth muscle contraction.

Although force development in vascular smooth muscle is accompanied by an increase in the level of myosin phosphorylation, it has been demonstrated that the maintenance of isometric tension can be preserved despite a reduction in the level of myosin light chain phosphorylation and $[Ca^{2+}]_i$. These data are consistent with the suggestion that Ca^{2+}-dependent phosphorylation of myosin light chain initiates an initial rapid cycling of crossbridges and development of force. In contrast, as the muscle approaches the sustained phase of isometric contraction, $[Ca^{2+}]_i$ and myosin light chain phosphorylation decrease, and rapid cycling crossbridges give way to stable latchbridges. These latchbridges are dependent on adequate $[Ca^{2+}]_i$, although with a greater sensitivity to that ion than is found during the transient phase of force generation {184}. Since both force development and force maintenance are subject to regulation by $[Ca^{2+}]_i$, both processes are expected to be altered by cyclic nucleotide-induced changes in $[Ca^{2+}]_i$.

EFFECTS OF CYCLIC NUCLEOTIDES ON MYOSIN LIGHT CHAIN KINASE PHOSPHORYLATION AND ON ALTERATIONS IN THE SENSITIVITY OF THE CONTRACTILE APPARATUS TO $[Ca^{2+}]_i$

Previous studies suggested that alterations in the phosphorylation state of MLCK might be a major site of regulation of vascular smooth muscle relaxation. Both A kinase and G kinase phosphorylate MLCK in cell-free preparations {152,154}. Phosphorylation of MLCK by A kinase decreased the affinity of this enzyme for the Ca^{2+}-calmodulin complex, the ability of this enzyme to phosphorylate myosin, and consequently, its ability to induce actin-activated myosin ATPase activity {153}. Phosphorylation of MLCK by A kinase and resultant alterations in enzyme activity were dependent on the concentration of Ca^{2+}. Thus, in the presence of high Ca^{2+} concentration, A kinase phosphorylated MLCK without altering its activity {140,185–187}. In contrast, at lower Ca^{2+} concentration, A-kinase phosphorylation of MLCK inhibited the enzyme. Although G kinase phosphorylated MLCK, this modification was without effect on the MLCK activity {154,187}.

These data suggested a model for regulation of vascular smooth muscle contractility in which increases in $[Ca^{2+}]_i$ result in binding of the Ca^{2+}-calmodulin complex to MLCK, altering the sensitivity of MLCK to inhibition by A-kinase-mediated phosphorylation. Thus, in the absence of elevated $[Ca^{2+}]_i$ and binding of Ca^{2+}-calmodulin, A kinase phosphorylates MLCK at a site that reduces the affinity of this protein for Ca^{2+} calmodulin, decreases the sensitivity of MLCK to increases in $[Ca^{2+}]_i$, and inhibits contraction. In the presence of elevated $[Ca^{2+}]_i$ and binding of Ca^{2+} calmodulin, A kinase phosphorylates MLCK at a different site, which does not alter its sensitivity to increases in $[Ca^{2+}]_i$ or its ability to mediate contraction. Presumably, G kinase phosphorylates MLCK at a site similar to that phosphorylated by A kinase in the presence of Ca^{2+} calmodulin, since G kinase does not alter the sensitivity of MLCK to increases in $[Ca^{2+}]_i$.

More recently, data have become available that significantly alter earlier hypotheses. It has been demonstrated that MLCK possesses six phosphorylation sites (peptides A–F), defined by proteolytic mapping {188}. Interestingly, only phosphorylation on peptide A decreased the sensitivity of MLCK to increases in $[Ca^{2+}]_i$. Phosphorylation of peptides B–F did not alter the affinity of MLCK for Ca^{2+} calmodulin or its ability to phosphorylate myosin light chains {188}. Furthermore, peptide A was phosphorylated by Ca^{2+}-calmodulin-dependent protein kinase II and A kinase {188,189}. These data suggest that large increases in $[Ca^{2+}]_i$ activate Ca^{2+}-calmodulin kinase II, which phosphorylates MLCK at the peptide A site, decreasing the sensitivity of MLCK to increases in $[Ca^{2+}]_i$. Similarly, increases in cyclic AMP activate A kinase, which phosphorylates MLCK at the peptide A site, decreasing the sensitivity of MLCK to increases in $[Ca^{2+}]_i$. Presumably increases in cyclic GMP and activation of G kinase result in the phosphorylation of MLCK on peptides other than peptide A, and therefore do not alter the sensitivity of MLCK to increases in $[Ca^{2+}]_i$ or its ability to phosphorylate myosin.

Data supporting this hypothesis have been obtained with bovine trachealis muscle {188}. In these experiments, the trachealis was contracted with carbachol or by depolarization with KCl. These treatments increased the phosphorylation of MLCK and markedly decreased the Ca^{2+} sensitivity of MLCK. Indeed, there was a significant correlation of phosphorylation of MLCK on peptide A and decreased sensitivity of MLCK to Ca^{2+}. Similarly, arterial smooth muscle contracted with KCl demonstrated a decreased sensitivity of myosin phosphorylation to increases in $[Ca^{2+}]_i$ when compared with tissue contracted with histamine or unstimulated tissue {190}. Furthermore, MLCK extracted from tissue contracted with KCl demonstrated a decreased sensitivity to Ca^{2+} calmodulin compared to that extracted from histamine-contracted or unstimulated tissue {190}. These data demonstrate that the decreased sensitivity of MLCK activity to increases in $[Ca^{2+}]_i$ in intact cells correlates with alterations in the activity of MLCK in biochemical assays. Presumably in these different experiments contraction with KCl produces large increases in $[Ca^{2+}]_i$, which activate Ca^{2+}-calmodulin kinase II, resulting in the phosphorylation of MLCK on peptide A and decreased sensitivity of that enzyme to intracellular Ca^{2+}.

The above data suggest that different contractile agents produce their biological effects by altering $[Ca^{2+}]_i$ and/or the phosphorylation state of MLCK. Regulation of the sensitivity of MLCK to $[Ca^{2+}]_i$ may play an important role in the response of vascular smooth muscle to relaxing agents that increase intracellular concentrations of cyclic AMP. As with be discussed below, it appears that the major mechanism by which cyclic GMP and G kinase relax blood vessels is by decreasing $[Ca^{2+}]_i$ without altering MLCK. In addition, cyclic AMP appears to regulate vascular smooth muscle relaxation predominantly by activating G kinase and decreasing $[Ca^{2+}]_i$, as discussed below. However, A kinase is found in vascular smooth muscle cells and agents that induce vascular smooth muscle relaxation by increasing intracellular cyclic AMP presumably activate A kinase. Increases in cyclic AMP and activation of A kinase could therefore potentially mediate vascular smooth muscle relaxation by two different mechanisms. As pointed out above, A kinase phosphorylates MLCK on peptide A, decreasing the sensitivity of this enzyme to intracellular Ca^{2+} and reducing the phosphorylation of myosin, resulting in relaxation. Interestingly, A kinase also increases $[Ca^{2+}]_i$ by phosphorylating L-type Ca^{2+} channels and increasing the influx of this cation {191, 192}. Increases in $[Ca^{2+}]_i$ could activate Ca^{2+}-calmodulin kinase II, which phosphorylates MLCK on peptide A, decreasing the sensitivity of this protein to intracellular Ca^{2+} and decreasing myosin phosphorylation and relaxation.

Evidence for this mechanism comes from studies with arterial smooth muscle. In vessels precontracted using histamine or phenylephrine, low-dose forskolin (an activator of adenylyl cyclase) produced small increases in intracellular concentrations of cyclic AMP and decreased $[Ca^{2+}]_i$, myosin phosphorylation, and force generation {193}. Relaxation was presumably mediated in these experiments by cyclic AMP activating G kinase and decreasing $[Ca^{2+}]_i$ without altering the sensitivity of MLCK to $[Ca^{2+}]_i$. In contrast, vessels precontracted by electromechanical coupling using KCl required high doses of forskolin to induce relaxation. High-dose forskolin produced large increases in intracellular concentrations of cyclic AMP and decreased myosin phosphorylation and force generation without altering $[Ca^{2+}]_i$ {193}. In this case, relaxation was mediated by a decrease in the sensitivity of MLCK to intracellular Ca^{2+}, presumably due to phosphorylation of MLCK by A kinase or Ca^{2+}-calmodulin kinase II. These data suggest that large increases in intracellular cyclic AMP relax vessels primarily by decreasing the sensitivity of MLCK to intracellular Ca^{2+}, without producing significant alterations in $[Ca^{2+}]_i$.

Mechanisms in addition to regulation of MLCK activity may be involved in the alteration of the Ca^{2+} sensitivity of myofibrils by cyclic nucleotides. As discussed above, cyclic GMP does not appear to affect MLCK activity. However, in α-toxin-permeabilized rat mesenteric artery in which $[Ca^{2+}]_i$ was controlled and intracellular Ca^{2+} stores were depleted, both cyclic AMP and cyclic GMP shifted the pCa^{2+}-tension curve to the right (fig. 52-3) {194}. In histamine-contracted porcine carotid arteries, McDaniel et al. {155} found that GTN and SNP, in addition to lowering $[Ca^{2+}]_i$, uncoupled stress from myosin light chain phosphorylation in that significant relaxation of the arteries occurred in the absence of sustained reductions of $[Ca^{2+}]_i$ or myosin light chain phosphorylation. Similarly, Abe et al. {195} reported that GTN-induced relaxation of porcine coronary artery was greater than expected from the reduction in $[Ca^{2+}]_i$ elicited by GTN.

EFFECTS OF CYCLIC NUCLEOTIDES ON THE CONCENTRATION OF INTRACELLULAR CALCIUM

Evidence suggests that cyclic nucleotides induce vascular smooth muscle relaxation, in part by decreasing $[Ca^{2+}]_i$.

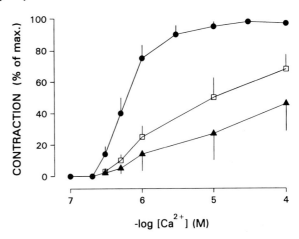

Fig. 52-3. Effect of cyclic nucleotides on the Ca^{2+}-force relationship in α-toxin permeabilized rat superior mesenteric artery. Ca^{2+}-force curves were formed in the absence (●) or presence of 30 μM cyclic AMP (▲) or 30 μM cyclic GMP (□). Experiments were performed in the presence of 2 μM ionomycin in order to deplete sarcoplasmic reticulum Ca^{2+} stores. Modified from Nishimura and Van Breemen {194}, with permission.

Early work demonstrated an antagonistic relationship between agents that increased contraction and $[Ca^{2+}]_i$ and those that induced relaxation and decreased $[Ca^{2+}]_i$. Thus there is a dose-dependent relationship between norepinephrine concentration, contraction, and $[Ca^{2+}]_i$ in rat aorta {196}. Agents that increased intracellular concentrations of cyclic GMP, such as SNP, were more effective at inducing relaxation at low norepinephrine concentrations. Presumably, this reflects the increased efficacy of cyclic GMP to decrease $[Ca^{2+}]_i$ when the concentrations of this cation are low. In contrast, when high concentrations of agonist are employed, $[Ca^{2+}]_i$ is high and agents that increase the concentration of cyclic GMP are ineffective at reducing $[Ca^{2+}]_i$ below that required for relaxation. Similar results were obtained using agents that induce contraction by electromechanical coupling, such as depolarization by KCl {196}. Relaxation by cyclic GMP under these conditions was greatly reduced and was thought to reflect the ability of L-type Ca^{2+} channels to elevate $[Ca^{2+}]_i$ above the level that can be reduced by cyclic GMP.

There are a variety of mechanisms by which cyclic nucleotides could decrease $[Ca^{2+}]_i$ and induce relaxation (table 52-1; fig. 52-4). Increased efflux of Ca^{2+} out of the cell may be mediated directly by a sarcolemmal Ca^{2+}-pumping ATPase or indirectly by activation of a Na, K-ATPase, which decreases intracellular Na^+, activating a sarcolemmal Na^+-Ca^{2+} exchanger. Membrane hyperpolarization by activation of K^+ channels would also serve to increase Ca^{2+} efflux by Na^+-Ca^{2+} exchange. Also Ca^{2+} may be depleted from the cytoplasm by sequestration by a Ca^{2+}-pumping ATPase in the sarcoplasmic reticulum. In addition, relaxing agents may decrease the influx of Ca^{2+} by regulating L-type Ca^{2+} channels. Finally, relaxing agents may alter the production of second messengers that

Table 52-1. Mechanisms by which cyclic nucleotides may mediate vascular smooth muscle relaxation

1. Decreased $[Ca^{2+}]_i$
   A. Decreased influx of Ca^{2+}
      1. Activation of K_{Ca} channels or Na^+/K^+ ATPase → hyperpolarization → decreased Ca^{2+} influx via potential-dependent Ca^{2+} channels
      2. Uncoupling of agonist-induced phosphatidyl inositide turnover → decreased Ca^{2+} influx via receptor-operated Ca^{2+} channels
   B. Increased efflux of Ca^{2+}
      1. Increased activity of plasma membrane Ca^{2+}-pumping ATPase
      2. Activation of K_{Ca} channels or Na^+/K^+ ATPase → hyperpolarization → increased activity of Na^+/Ca^{2+} exchanger
      3. Activation of Na^+/K^+ ATPase → decreased intracellular Na^+ → increased activity of Na^+/Ca^{2+} exchanger
   C. Increased sequestration of Ca^{2+}
      1. Increased activity of sarcoplasmic reticulum Ca^{2+}-pumping ATPase
   D. Decreased mobilization of Ca^{2+}
      1. Uncoupling of agonist-induced phosphatidyl inositide turnover → decreased IP_3 formation
2. Decreased sensitivity of the contractile apparatus to Ca^{2+}
   A. Decreased affinity of myosin light chain kinase for Ca^{2+}-calmodulin → decreased phosphorylation of myosin light chain
   B. Increased Ca^{2+} sensitivity of myofibrils
   C. Altered actin-plasma membrane interaction → cytoskeletal reorganization

are critical for elevations of $[Ca^{2+}]_i$ induced by contractile agents and required for vascular smooth muscle contraction. Evidence has been obtained for the involvement of cyclic nucleotide in most of these mechanisms of lowering $[Ca^{2+}]_i$.

It is noteworthy that there is significant convergence of the mechanisms by which cyclic AMP and cyclic GMP mediate vascular smooth muscle relaxation. The major mechanisms by which cyclic nucleotides alter cellular physiology is through protein phosphorylation on serine and threonine residues mediated by cyclic nucleotide-dependent protein kinases. Indeed, as pointed out above, there are kinases that are specifically activated by cyclic AMP or cyclic GMP. Furthermore, these cyclic nucleotide-selective kinases appear to phosphorylate specific, although overlapping, protein substrates within target cells. Finally, both cyclic AMP and cyclic GMP-specific protein kinases are present in vascular smooth muscle and could potentially mediate relaxation. Although these enzymes are selective for cyclic nucleotides, each can be activated by either cyclic AMP or cyclic GMP. Indeed, G kinase can be activated by cyclic AMP, although at least a 10-fold higher concentration of cyclic AMP compared to cyclic GMP is required for this activation. Similarly, A kinase can be activated by cyclic GMP, although a 10-fold higher concentration of cyclic GMP compared to cyclic AMP is required. It is significant that in vascular smooth muscle,

the concentration of cyclic AMP is about 10-fold greater than cyclic GMP. Thus, elevations in cyclic AMP could activate both A and G kinase, while cyclic GMP may activate only G-kinase.

Data to support this hypothesis come from studies of vascular smooth muscle cells in culture {97,197,198}. Primary cultures of rat aortic smooth muscle cells exhibited increases in $[Ca^{2+}]_i$ when treated with agents that induce contraction by electromechanical (KCl) or pharmacomechanical (arginine vasopressin) coupling. Pretreatment of these cells with agents that increase cyclic GMP concentrations, such as ANP or 8-bromo-cyclic GMP, inhibited the increase in $[Ca^{2+}]_i$ induced by KCl or vasopressin. These data suggest that agents that increase intracellular cyclic GMP induce relaxation by decreasing $[Ca^{2+}]_i$, presumably by activating G kinase. Interestingly, rat aortic smooth muscle cells passaged several times in culture lost their ability to respond to natriuretic peptides and 8-bromo-cyclic GMP with a decrease in $[Ca^{2+}]_i$. This resulted from a loss of G kinase in the passaged cells as demonstrated by Western blot analysis using affinity-purified polyclonal antibodies to this protein. These data demonstrated that the effects of cyclic GMP in decreasing $[Ca^{2+}]_i$ were mediated by G kinase. Of significance, however, was the observation that in passaged cells the response to agents that increase cyclic AMP was an increase in $[Ca^{2+}]_i$ rather than a decrease. Thus, in primary cultures but not passaged cells, forskolin pretreatment of cells increased intracellular cyclic AMP and prevented the increase in $[Ca^{2+}]_i$ induced by vasopressin or KCl. However, both primary cultures and passaged cells contain the same amount of A kinase, suggesting that the loss of response to cyclic AMP in passaged cells resulted from the loss of G kinase. When G kinase was restored to deficient passaged cells, these cells regained their ability to respond to agents that increase intracellular cyclic AMP with a decrease in $[Ca^{2+}]_i$ (fig. 52-5). These data demonstrate that in vascular smooth muscle cells, agents that elevate cyclic AMP activate both G and A kinases. Activation of G kinase may result in the decrease in $[Ca^{2+}]_i$ induced by agents that increase cyclic AMP concentrations. In contrast, activation of A kinase may decrease the Ca^{2+} sensitivity of the contractile apparatus by increasing $[Ca^{2+}]_i$, activating Ca^{2+}-calmodulin kinase II, and phosphorylating MLCK on peptide A, resulting in relaxation. Therefore, in the ensuing discussions relaxation mechanisms induced by increases in cyclic GMP and activation of G kinase may also be induced by agents that increase cyclic AMP in these tissues.

Regulation of calcium influx

As described above, electromechanical coupling involves depolarization of vascular smooth muscle cells and activation of voltage-dependent L-type Ca^{2+} channels, with a resultant increased influx of Ca^{2+} and elevations of $[Ca^{2+}]_i$. One mechanism by which cyclic nucleotides could induce relaxation is to alter the influx of Ca^{2+} through these channels. Thus exposure of rabbit coronary arteries to isoproterenol during Ca^{2+} loading in the presence of KCl

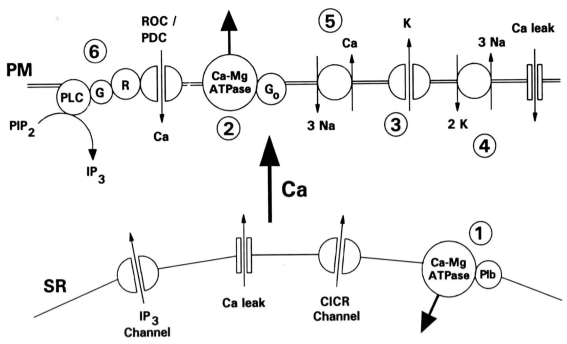

Fig. 52-4. Some of the proposed mechanisms by which cyclic nucleotides may lower $[Ca^{2+}]_i$, leading to vascular smooth muscle relaxation. It is assumed that under resting conditions or conditions of low stimulation, there is vectoral transport of Ca^{2+} from the superficial sarcoplasmic reticulum (SR) towards the plasma membrane (PM), where Ca^{2+} is extruded by the Ca^{2+}-pumping ATPase (②) and the Na^+-Ca^{2+} exchanger (⑤) (superficial buffer barrier hypothesis; for details see Chen and Van Breeman {158}. Ca^{2+} release from the SR is mediated by IP_3-sensitive Ca^{2+} channels, Ca^{2+}-induced Ca^{2+} release channels (CICR), and passive Ca^{2+} leak. **(a)**: Phosphorylation of phospholamban (Plb) by A or G kinase would result in stimulation of the SR Ca^{2+}-pumping ATPase (①), increasing Ca^{2+} sequestration and providing additional Ca^{2+} for vectoral Ca^{2+} transport. **(b)** Phosphorylation of the G-kinase substrate G_o may result in stimulation of the PM Ca^{2+}-pumping ATPase (②), leading to increased Ca^{2+} extrusion. **(c)** Phosphorylation of Ca^{2+}-activated K^+ channels (③) by A kinase and possibly G kinase may result in increased channel open probability. The resulting membrane hyperpolarization would serve to decrease Ca^{2+} entry by potential-dependent Ca^{2+} channels (PDC) and to increase Ca^{2+} extrusion by the Na^+/Ca^{2+} exchanger (⑤). **(d)** Activation of the Na^+/K^+ ATPase (④) by A or G kinase would result in membrane hyperpolarization and decreased intracellular Na^+, both of which would serve to increase Ca^{2+} extrusion by the Na^+-Ca^{2+} exchanger. **(e)** Inhibition of agonist-induced phosphatidyl inositide turnover by cyclic GMP may involve uncoupling of receptor (R) G-protein (G) phospholipase C (PLC) interaction (⑥), resulting in decreased IP_3 formation and decreased Ca^{2+} mobilization from the SR via IP_3-sensitive Ca^{2+} channels. This uncoupling may also inhibit Ca^{2+} entry via receptor-operated Ca^{2+} channels (ROC).

resulted in the inhibition of contraction subsequently induced by histamine {199}. These data suggest that isoproterenol, an agent that increases intracellular cyclic AMP, decreased $[Ca^{2+}]_i$ by inhibiting the influx of this cation through potential-operated Ca^{2+} channels. Similarly, isoproterenol inhibited $^{45}Ca^{2+}$ influx into rabbit aortic smooth muscle depolarized by incubation in high K^+ (145 mM), low Na^+ (0 mM) buffer, and this effect paralleled increases in cyclic AMP and relaxation in this tissue {200–202}. Furthermore, dibutyryl cyclic AMP and forskolin directly relaxed this tissue and decreased the influx of Ca^{2+} {200}.

Although these physiological data suggest a role for cyclic AMP in inhibiting the influx of Ca^{2+} through L-type Ca^{2+} channels, biochemical studies suggest otherwise. L-type Ca^{2+} channels have been characterized in a variety of tissues, including heart, skeletal muscle, and smooth muscle {203,204}. The alpha subunit of this protein, which

is the site of binding for the Ca^{2+}-entry blockers, is an excellent substrate for phosphorylation of A kinase in vitro, predominantly on serine residues. The beta subunit is also a substrate for phosphorylation by A kinase. It is significant that L-type Ca^{2+} channels are activated by phosphorylation by A kinase, permitting an increased influx of Ca^{2+} into muscle cells {191,192,205,206}. Indeed, 8-bromo-cyclic AMP and forskolin produced increases in the influx of Ca^{2+} into guinea pig ventricular myocytes, which could be blocked by inhibitors of A kinase. These data suggest that phosphorylation by L-type Ca^{2+} channels may result in increased influx of Ca^{2+} into some smooth muscle cells with a concomitant increase in $[Ca^{2+}]_i$. The mechanisms whereby increases in $[Ca^{2+}]_i$ mediated by cyclic AMP and A kinase induce vascular smooth muscle relaxation most likely involve a reduction of the Ca^{2+} sensitivity of the contractile apparatus, as described above {181,182}.

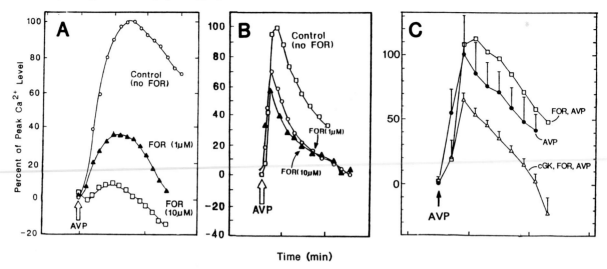

Fig. 52-5. Effect of forskolin on $[Ca^{2+}]_i$ in cultured rat aortic smooth muscle cells. Cells were loaded with fura-2/AM and incubated with forskolin (FOR) or diluent (0.95% ethanol) for 5 minutes before the addition of 50 nM arginine vasopressin (AVP). **a:** Cells in primary culture. **b,c:** Cells in passage 20–23. In panels a and b, cells were treated with diluent (○), 1 μM forskolin (▲), or 10 μM forskolin (□). In panel c, treatments were diluent (●), 10 μM forskolin (□), or 10 μM forskolin in cells in which G kinase (cGK) had been repleted (△). Time courses of experiments were 2 minutes in panels a and c, and 4 minutes in panel b. From Lincoln and Cornwell {97}, with permission, S. Karger AG, Basel.

With respect to cyclic GMP, many studies have reported inhibition of Ca^{2+} influx into vascular smooth muscle, both in blood vessels contracted with agonists or K^+ and using SNP, EDRF, or atrial peptides to induce increases in cyclic GMP {100,207–211}. In studies in which inhibition of Ca^{2+} influx using agonist or K^+-contracted tissues was compared, a greater effect on inhibition of agonist-induced Ca^{2+} influx has been observed, suggesting that cyclic GMP is better able to modulate Ca^{2+} influx when changes in the membrane potential are minimal {209–212}. In experiments using patch-clamped rabbit pulmonary artery, SNP was found to decrease Ca^{2+} influx through L-type Ca^{2+} channels {213}, and in biochemical studies exogenous G kinase was found to inhibit Ca^{2+} uptake in pig aortic microsomes via putative receptor-operated Ca^{2+} channels {214}. While these reports suggest that inhibition of Ca^{2+} influx by cyclic GMP could be mediated by a direct inhibitory effect on Ca^{2+} channels, other studies suggest that reduced Ca^{2+} influx by cyclic nucleotides may be secondary to hyperpolarization mediated by opening of K^+ channels.

Three types of K^+ channels have been described in vascular smooth muscle, including the ATP-sensitive, delayed rectifier, and Ca^{2+}-activated K^+ channels (K_{Ca}) {160}. Although the effects of cyclic nucleotides on the first two types is unclear, a role for cyclic AMP in directly regulating K_{Ca} channels has been suggested {215}. Previous studies demonstrated that beta-adrenoceptors mediated the hyperpolarization of vascular smooth muscle cells, suggesting that these receptors were coupled to the activity of a K^+ channel {216}. The Ca^{2+} dependence of this channel was suggested by studies demonstrating a

requirement for Ca^{2+} or an inhibition by lanthanum of the hyperpolarization induced by isoproterenol {217}. In studies of cultured rat aortic smooth muscle using the patch-clamp technique with whole cells and single channels, isoproterenol increased the probability that K_{Ca} channels were open {215}. These effects of isoproterenol were precisely reproduced by incorporating cyclic AMP and purified A kinase into incubations. Furthermore, the concentration dependence of activation of the K^+ channels by Ca^{2+} was shifted to the left upon cyclic AMP-mediated phosphorylation, suggesting an increased sensitivity of these channels to activation by low $[Ca^{2+}]_i$.

These studies suggest that agents that elevate cyclic AMP concentrations in vascular smooth muscle cells increase the sensitivity of K_{Ca} channels to low $[Ca^{2+}]_i$, increasing their probability of being opened with only small changes in $[Ca^{2+}]_i$. Opening of these channels hyperpolarizes vascular smooth muscle cells, which would result in decreased influx of Ca^{2+} through L-type Ca^{2+} channels, decreased $[Ca^{2+}]_i$, and relaxation. These data further emphasize the multifunctional role of cyclic AMP in regulating smooth muscle relaxation by alterations in Ca^{2+} influx. Thus cyclic AMP may initially produce increases in $[Ca^{2+}]_i$ by directly activating L-type Ca^{2+} channels, which decreases the sensitivity of the contractile apparatus to $[Ca^{2+}]_i$, promoting relaxation. In addition, this cyclic nucleotide activates the K_{Ca} channel both by small increases in $[Ca^{2+}]_i$ and by direct phosphorylation, resulting in hyperpolarization, decreased Ca^{2+} influx, and relaxation.

Regulation of K_{Ca} channels by cyclic GMP has also been investigated. Hyperpolarization of the membrane of several vascular tissues by nitrovasodilators has been reported {218–221}. In a recent study, GTN was found to activate large conductance K_{Ca} channels in cultured porcine coronary artery smooth muscle cells {222}. Williams et al. {223} reported that SNP and ANP enhanced the activity of large-conductance K_{Ca} channels of bovine aortic smooth muscle cells. When various guanine nucleotides were tested for their effect on K_{Ca} channel activity in excised membrane patches, only 5'-GMP consistently enhanced channel activity at low nucleotide concentrations. This suggested that increased cyclic GMP accumulating in response to SNP and ANP does not directly affect channel activity. However, an effect of cyclic GMP on K_{Ca} activity mediated by G kinase was not ruled out.

In summary, there is evidence that both cyclic AMP and cyclic GMP can modulate K_{Ca} channel activity in vascular smooth muscle. The hyperpolarization that would result from K_{Ca} channel opening would limit Ca^{2+} influx through plasma membrane Ca^{2+} channels. An action of cyclic nucleotides on K_{Ca} channels would explain some of the differences observed in agonist and K^+-contracted tissues, since Ca^{2+} entry through L-type Ca^{2+} channels in depolarized cells would not be expected to be sensitive to small changes in the membrane potential resulting from K_{Ca} channel activation.

Regulation of calcium efflux

Calcium efflux appears to be mediated by two different mechanisms in vascular smooth muscle cells. One mechanism involves active transport of Ca^{2+} out of cells by a plasma membrane Ca^{2+}-pumping ATPase. The other mechanism by which Ca^{2+} is extruded from smooth muscle cells is a sarcolemmal Na^+-Ca^{2+} exchanger, which may be coupled to other Na,K-ATPase or K^+ channel activity. Thus activation of Na,K-ATPase would decrease $[Na^+]_i$, which in turn would increase the driving force for Ca^{2+} extrusion by the Na^+-Ca^{2+} exchanger. The Na^+-Ca^{2+} exchanger in vascular smooth muscle appears to be electrogenic and sensitive to changes in membrane potential {224–226}. Membrane hyperpolarization either by K^+ channel activation or increase Na,K-ATPase activity would therefore also serve to increase Ca^{2+} extrusion by this exchanger.

The quantitative contribution of these different mechanisms to the regulation of Ca^{2+} efflux from vascular smooth muscle cells has not been completely defined. Studies in a variety of systems, including giant squid axons and vascular smooth muscle cells, suggest that the Ca^{2+}-pumping ATPase has a higher affinity but lower capacity for Ca^{2+} and probably contributes significantly to maintenance of $[Ca^{2+}]_i$ at low resting levels of this cation. In contrast, the Na^+-Ca^{2+} exchanger appears to have a lower affinity but higher capacity for Ca^{2+} and probably contributes significantly to the extrusion of this cation at the high $[Ca^{2+}]_i$ generated during contraction {149,226,227}. However, according to the superficial buffer barrier hypothesis, under resting conditions vectoral transport of Ca^{2+} from the sarcoplasmic reticulum into the narrow cytoplasmic space between the sarcoplasmic reticulum and the plasma membrane could elevate the local Ca^{2+} concentration to a level that would be amenable to Na^+-Ca^{2+} exchange {158}.

Earlier data suggested a role for cyclic AMP in regulating the activity of the Ca^{2+}-pumping ATPase and relaxation in vascular smooth muscle. Thus incubation of inside-out plasma membrane vesicles purified from rat mesenteric arteries or porcine aorta with A kinase purified from the same tissue stimulated uptake of Ca^{2+} into these vesicles {142,147}. However, more recent studies have demonstrated that neither forskolin nor cyclic AMP analogs evoke significant increases in the efflux of Ca^{2+} by the Ca^{2+}-pumping ATPase from cultured rat aortic smooth muscle cells {149}. Furthermore, there was no significant phosphorylation of the Ca^{2+}-pumping ATPase purified from bovine aortic smooth muscle when this protein was incubated in the presence of ATP and the catalytic subunit of A kinase {149}. These data suggest that cyclic AMP and A kinase do not play significant roles in regulating $[Ca^{2+}]_i$ by altering the activity of the Ca^{2+}-pumping ATPase. In contrast, there is considerable evidence to suggest that cyclic GMP regulates Ca^{2+} efflux by activation of the plasma membrane Ca^{2+}-pumping ATPase {114,115,118, 119,142,149,210,228}. Although a number of biochemical studies have shown that the Ca^{2+}-pumping ATPase itself is not a substrate for G kinase (see above), phosphorylation of G_0 by G kinase appears to mediate the activation of the Ca^{2+}-pumping ATPase {119}.

In the intact rat aorta, the norepinephrine-induced increase in $^{45}Ca^{2+}$ efflux (which reflects release of stored Ca^{2+} followed by membrane transport) was enhanced by low concentrations of SNP, suggesting cyclic GMP-mediated stimulation of the plasma membrane Ca^{2+}-pumping ATPase {210}. In cultured rat aortic smooth muscle cells, SNP, ANP, and 8-bromo-cyclic GMP all increased the component of $^{45}Ca^{2+}$ efflux that was independent of extracellular Na^+ (i.e., efflux mediated by the Ca^{2+}-pumping ATPase rather than the Na^+-Ca^{2+} exchanger) {149}. Furthermore, this effect on Ca^{2+} efflux was especially evident at lower $[Ca^{2+}]_i$ (0.1 μM), suggesting that cyclic GMP regulation of the Ca^{2+}-pumping ATPase could have a significant effect on vascular smooth muscle tone at the $[Ca^{2+}]_i$ associated with force maintenance (i.e., the lower levels of $[Ca^{2+}]_i$ seen in the "latch" state).

The membrane hyperpolarization resulting from cyclic nucleotide-mediated activation of K_{Ca} channels (see above) would be expected to increase Ca^{2+} efflux by Na^+-Ca^{2+} exchange. A stimulatory effect of cyclic nucleotides on the plasma membrane Na,K-ATPase would also serve to increase Ca^{2+} extrusion by the exchanger, since this would decrease $[Na^+]_i$ and hyperpolarize the plasma membrane, both of which would increase the driving force of Na^+ entry. A kinase increased Na,K-ATPase activity and Ca^{2+} uptake in inside-out plasma membrane vesicles prepared from rat aorta {141}. Uptake of Ca^{2+} was blocked by ouabain, an inhibitor of Na,K-ATPase, suggesting that the Na^+-Ca^{2+} exchange mechanism coupled to the ATPase was mediating Ca^{2+} uptake. Similarly, cyclic AMP analogs and isoproterenol hyperpolarized rabbit pulmonary artery, and this effect was inhibited by ouabain {229}. In addition, these agents induced relaxation and activated Na,K-ATPase, and these effects were inhibited by ouabain in tail arteries from a variety of species {230}. More recently, analogs of cyclic AMP were demonstrated to activate the Na,K-ATPase in smooth muscle membranes and to decrease the $[Na^+]_i$ in vascular smooth muscle cells {149,231}. The above-mentioned reports of stimulation of Na,K-ATPase by cyclic AMP are, however, difficult to reconcile with the reported inhibition of Na,K-ATPase activity following phosphorylation of the catalytic subunit of the pump by A kinase {232}.

With respect to cyclic GMP-mediated activation of the Na,K-ATPase, exposure of rat aortic strips to ouabain or K^+-free media inhibited the relaxation induced by SNP, EDRF, or 8-bromo-cyclic GMP {233,234}. However, in cultured primary rat aortic smooth muscle cells, 8-bromo-cyclic GMP had no effect on $[Na^+]_i$, in contrast to the 30% reduction in $[Na^+]_i$ caused by dibutyryl or 8-bromo-cyclic AMP {149}. In a subsequent study {235}, these investigators obtained evidence suggesting that ANP or 8-bromo-cyclic GMP stimulated the Na^+-Ca^{2+} exchanger independent of an effect on membrane potential or Na,K-ATPase activity. Na^+-Ca^{2+} exchange activity was assessed by the $[Na^+]_o$-dependent $^{45}Ca^{2+}$ efflux from cells under conditions where the Ca^{2+}-pumping ATPase was inhibited (pH 8.8 and 20 mM Mg^{2+}). This $^{45}Ca^{2+}$ efflux was augmented by exposure of cells to ANP or 8-bromo-cyclic GMP. Furthermore, 8-bromo-cyclic GMP had no effect on $[Na^+]_i$, intracellular pH, or the membrane potential, suggesting that the observed effect on the Na^+-Ca^{2+} exchanger was not secondary to alteration of these parameters.

The above data suggest that at low $[Ca^{2+}]_i$, the main sarcolemmal extrusion mechanism for maintaining Ca^{2+} is the high-affinity, low-capacity Ca^{2+}-pumping ATPase selectively regulated by cyclic GMP. At higher concentrations of $[Ca^{2+}]_i$, for example, those produced by contractile stimuli, the Na^+-Ca^{2+} exchanger makes a significantly greater contribution to Ca^{2+} extrusion and can be regulated by both cyclic GMP and cyclic AMP.

Regulation of calcium sequestration

Cyclic nucleotides can decrease $[Ca^{2+}]_i$ by sequestering this ion in intracellular storage sites. One mechanism by which this occurs is the increased transport of Ca^{2+} into the sarcoplasmic reticulum. A role for cyclic AMP in this process was suggested by studies of the amount of Ca^{2+} stored in intracellular sites in rabbit ear and coronary arteries and guinea-pig mesenteric arteries {199,236}. Calcium-depleted vessels were loaded with this cation by exposure to KCl, and the amount incorporated into intracellular sites was quantified by assessing the amplitude of contraction induced by histamine. Exposure of vessels to isoproterenol during Ca^{2+} loading increased the amplitude of contraction produced by histamine. These data suggested that isoproterenol increased the sequestration of Ca^{2+} into intracellular sites during the loading process. Similar conclusions were reached in studies of the effect of dibutyryl-cyclic AMP on net ^{45}Ca uptake during Ca^{2+}

loading {201}. Although these data suggest that cyclic AMP increases intracellular sequestration of Ca^{2+}, promoting relaxation, this effect appears to be mediated by G kinase rather than A kinase, as discussed in detail above {97,198}.

Studies utilizing both intact and skinned blood vessel preparations have provided evidence for Ca^{2+} sequestration by agents that increase cyclic GMP. Uptake of ^{45}Ca into saponin-skinned primary rat aortic smooth muscle cells in culture was increased by cyclic GMP {237}. In intact blood vessels or vascular smooth muscle cells, evidence for cyclic GMP-mediated increases in Ca^{2+} sequestration have been obtained using SNP {209}, 8-bromo-cyclic GMP {238,239}, and ANP {240}, although it is difficult to dissociate increased sequestration into the sarcoplasmic reticulum from inhibition of Ca^{2+} mobilization. It is noteworthy that IP_3- or caffeine-induced release of Ca^{2+} from fully loaded intracellular Ca^{2+} stores was not affected by cyclic GMP {237}.

The cyclic GMP-mediated increases in Ca^{2+} sequestration appear to be due to G-kinase-dependent phosphorylation of phospholamban, as discussed in detail above. The abundance of phospholamban in vascular smooth muscle varies with the source of vascular tissue, with significant amounts found in dog, rabbit, and rat aorta, and in bovine pulmonary artery, and low amounts in porcine aorta and coronary artery. Thus the relative importance of phospholamban phosphorylation by G kinase in the lowering of $[Ca^{2+}]_i$ would also be expected to vary between vascular tissues, and this appears to be the case. For example, contrast the lack of effect of G kinase on Ca^{2+} uptake into sarcoplasmic reticulum-enriched fractions of porcine aorta {142} with stimulation of Ca^{2+} uptake by G kinase in those from bovine pulmonary artery {126}.

Regulation of calcium mobilization

In addition to the effects of cyclic nucleotides on the lowering of $[Ca^{2+}]_i$, there is substantial evidence that cyclic nucleotides exert inhibitory effects on Ca^{2+} mobilization. Agonist-induced increases in $[Ca^{2+}]_i$ mediated by release of Ca^{2+} from intracellular stores are attenuated by a number of agents that increase cyclic GMP. Thus, norepinephrine-, histamine-, angiotensin II-, or arginine vasopressin-induced Ca^{2+} transients were decreased by SNP {209,210}, GTN {195,241}, ANP {197,240,242,243}, EDRF {207}, and 8-bromo-cyclic GMP {197,238,243}.

The mechanism by which this occurs could be by either decreasing the amount of IP_3 formed during agonist stimulation or by inhibition of the effects of IP_3 on Ca^{2+} release from the sarcoplasmic reticulum. Inhibition of IP_3-induced Ca^{2+} release may not be the primary site of attenuated Ca^{2+} mobilization, since Ca^{2+} release from fully loaded Ca^{2+} stores in skinned vascular smooth muscle cells by IP_3 is not altered by cyclic GMP {237}. On the other hand, several investigators have reported inhibitory effects of cyclic GMP on phosphatidyl inositide turnover. Thus, SNP, EDRF, and 8-bromo-cyclic GMP {244,245}, GTN {246}, and ANP {247} inhibited the agonist-induced increases in phosphatidyl inositide turnover. In a subsequent study, the norepinephrine-induced increase in IP_3 content of rat aorta was attenuated by SNP or 8-bromo-cyclic GMP {248}.

The mechanism of attenuated phosphatidyl inositide hydrolysis was addressed by Hirata et al. {245}, who found that cyclic GMP inhibited both arginine vasopressin-induced GTPase activation and GTP-γS-induced formation of inositol phosphates in homogenates of bovine aortic smooth muscle cells. They proposed that the action of cyclic GMP involved inhibition of agonist-induced G-protein activation and of coupling between the G protein and phospholipase C. In another study, however, pertussis toxin-sensitive and -insensitive G proteins were not found to be substrates for G kinase in vitro {249}, and ANP did not significantly affect angiotensin II-induced increases in inositol phosphates {249}. If one of the actions of cyclic GMP in intact cells is to inhibit agonist-induced G-protein activation, then one might expect that, in addition to inhibitory effects on Ca^{2+} mobilization, an inhibitory effect on the increased sensitivity of the myofibrils to Ca^{2+} may occur, since this is also associated with agonist-induced G-protein activation.

CONCLUSIONS

Data presented herein suggest that cyclic nucleotides can mediate vascular smooth muscle relaxation by a variety of mechanisms involving alterations in intracellular concentrations of Ca^{2+} or the sensitivity of the contractile apparatus to that cation. Which of these mechanisms predominates varies with the experimental conditions, the type of blood vessel studied, and the source of blood vessels. Thus it is difficult to determine which of these mechanisms participate, and which predominates, in vascular smooth muscle relaxation in vivo. However, it is clear from the data presented that there is a complex relationship between the regulation of intracellular concentrations of cyclic nucleotides and Ca^{2+} and vascular smooth muscle contractility. This complexity is reflected in the precision with which the contractile tone of vascular smooth muscle regulates total peripheral resistance and regional blood flow to meet physiological requirements. The relative roles of these mechanisms in maintaining vascular tone and their contributions to vascular relaxation under various physiological and pathophysiological conditions will be elucidated as further investigations in this important area are conducted.

ACKNOWLEDGMENTS

This work was supported by research grants from the Medical Research Council of Canada and the Heart and Stroke Foundation of Ontario (BMB) and from the W.W. Smith Charitable Trust (SAW). BMB was the recipient of a Heart and Stroke Foundation of Canada Scholarship, and SAW was the recipient of a PMA Faculty Development Award in Pharmacology and Toxicology. The authors wish to thank Mrs. Janet LeSarge for her assistance in the preparation of this manuscript.

REFERENCES

1. Lee TP, Kuo JF, Greengard P: Role of muscarinic cholinergic receptors in regulation of guanosine 3',5'-monophosphate content in mammalian brain, heart muscle and intestinal smooth muscle. *Proc Natl Acad Sci USA* 69: 3287–3291, 1972.
2. Dunham EW, Haddox MK, Goldberg ND: Alteration of vein cyclic 3',5'-nucleotide concentrations during changes in contractility. *Proc Natl Acad Sci USA* 71:815–819, 1974.
3. Schultz G, Schultz K, Hardman JG: Effects of norepinephrine on cyclic nucleotide levels in the ductus deferens of the rat. *Metabolism* 24:429–437, 1975.
4. Schultz K-D, Schultz K, Schultz G: Sodium nitroprusside and other smooth muscle relaxants increase cyclic GMP levels in rat ductus deferens. *Nature* 265:750–751, 1977.
5. Katsuki S, Arnold WP, Murad F: Effects of sodium nitroprusside, nitroglycerin, and sodium azide on levels of cyclic nucleotides and mechanical activity of various tissues. *J Cyclic Nucleotide Res* 3:239–247, 1977.
6. Diamond J, Blisard KS: Effects of stimulant and relaxant drugs on tension and cyclic nucleotide levels in canine femoral artery. *Mol Pharmacol* 12:688–692, 1976.
7. Mittal CK, Murad F: Guanylate cyclase: Regulation of cyclic GMP metabolism. In: Nathanson JA, Kebabian JW (eds) *Handbook of Experimental Pharmacology*, Vol 58/1, *Cyclic Nucleotide Biochemistry*. Berlin: Springer-Verlag, 1982, pp 225–260.
8. Waldman SA, Murad F: Cyclic GMP synthesis and function. *Pharmacol Rev* 39:163–196, 1987.
9. Gerzer R, Bohme E, Hoffman F, Schultz G: Soluble guanylate cyclase purified from bovine lung contains heme and copper. *FEBS Lett* 132:71–74, 1981.
10. Ignarro LJ, Degnan JN, Baricos WH, Kadowitz PJ, Wolin MS: Activation of purified guanylate cyclase by nitric oxide requires heme. Comparison of heme-deficient, heme-reconstituted and heme-containing forms of soluble enzyme from bovine lung. *Biochem Biophys Acta* 718:49–59, 1982.
11. Kamisaki Y, Saheki S, Nakane M, Palmieri JA, Kuno T, Chang BY, Waldman SA, Murad F: Soluble guanylate cyclase from rat lung exists as a heterodimer. *J Biol Chem* 261:7236–7241, 1986.
12. Humbert P, Niroomand F, Fischer G, Mayer B, Koesling D, Hinsch K-H, Gausephol H, Frank R, Schultz G, Böhme E: Purification of soluble guanylate cyclase from bovine lung by a new immunoaffinity chromatographic method. *Eur J Biochem* 190:273–278, 1990.
13. Nakane M, Saheki S, Kuno T, Ishii K, Murad F: Molecular cloning of a cDNA coding for 70 kilodalton subunit of soluble guanylate cyclase from rat lung. *Biochem Biophys Res Commun* 158:1139–1147, 1988.
14. Nakane M, Arai K, Saheki S, Kuno T, Buechler W, Murad F: Molecular cloning and expression of cDNAs coding for soluble guanylate cyclase from rat lung. *J Biol Chem* 265: 16841–16845, 1990.
15. Koesling D, Herz J, Gausepohl H, Niroomand F, Hinsch K-D, Mülsch H, Böhme E, Schultz G, Frank R: The primary structure of the 70 kDa subunit of bovine soluble guanylate cyclase. *FEBS Lett* 239:23–34, 1988.
16. Koesling D, Harteneck C, Humbert P, Bosserhoff A, Frank R, Schultz G, Böhme E: The primary structure of the larger subunit of soluble guanylyl cyclase from bovine lung. *FEBS Lett* 266:128–132, 1990.
17. Yuen PST, Potter LR, Garbers DL: A new form of guanylyl cyclase is preferentially expressed in rat kidney. *Biochemistry* 29:10872–10878, 1990.
18. Chinkers M, Garbers DL, Chang M-S, Lowe DG, Chin H,

Goeddel DV, Schulz S: A membrane form of guanylate cyclase is an atrial natriuretic peptide receptor. *Nature* 338: 78–83, 1989.

19. Krupinski J, Coussens F, Bakalyar HA, Tang W-J, Feinstein PG, Orth K, Slaughter C, Reed RR, Gilman AG: Adenylyl cyclase amino acid sequence: Possible channel- or transporter-like structure. *Science* 244:1558–1564, 1989.

20. Harteneck C, Koesling D, Söling A, Schultz G, Böhme E: Expression of soluble guanylyl cyclase. *FEBS Lett* 272: 221–223, 1990.

21. Buechler WA, Nakane M, Murad F: Expression of soluble guanylyl cyclase activity requires both enzyme subunits. *Biochem Biophys Res Commun* 174:351–357, 1991.

22. Kimura H, Mittal CK, Murad F: Activation of guanylate cyclase from rat liver and other tissues by sodium azide. *J Biol Chem* 250:8016–8022, 1975.

23. Mittal CK, Murad F: Properties and oxidative regulation of guanylate cyclase. *J Cyclic Nucleotide Res* 3:381–391, 1977.

24. Ignarro LJ, Lippton H, Edwards JC, Baricos WH, Hyman AL, Kadowitz PJ, Gruetter CA: Mechanisms of vascular smooth muscle relaxation by organic nitrates, nitrites, nitroprusside and nitric oxide: Evidence for the involvement of S-nitrosothiols as active intermediates. *J Pharmacol Exp Ther* 218:739–749, 1981.

25. Furchgott RF, Zawadzki JV: The obligatory role of endothelial cells in the relaxation of arterial smooth muscle by acetylcholine. *Nature* 288:373–376, 1980.

26. Furchgott RF: Role of endothelium in responses of vascular smooth muscle. *Circ Res* 53:557–573, 1983.

27. Rapoport RM, Murad F: Agonist-induced endothelium-dependent relaxation in rat thoracic aorta may be mediated through cyclic GMP. *Circ Res* 52:352–357, 1983.

28. Palmer RMJ, Ferrige AG, Moncada S: Nitric oxide release accounts for the biological activity of endothelium-derived relaxing factor. *Nature* 327:524–526, 1987.

29. Pollock JS, Förstermann U, Mitchell JA, Warner TD, Schmidt HHHW, Nakane M, Murad F: Purification and characterization of particulate endothelium-derived relaxing factor synthase from cultured and native bovine aortic endothelial cells. *Proc Natl Acad Sci USA* 88:10480–10484, 1991.

30. Lamas S, Marsden PA, Li GK, Tempst P, Michel T: Endothelial nitric oxide synthase: Molecular cloning and characterization of a distinct constitutive enzyme isoform. *Proc Natl Acad Sci USA* 89:6348–6352, 1991.

31. Mülsch A, Vanin A, Mordvintcev P, Hauschildt S, Busse R: NO accounts completely for the oxygenated nitrogen species generated by enzyme L-arginine oxygenation. *Biochem J* 288:597–603, 1992.

32. Myers PR, Minor RL Jr, Guerra R Jr, Bates JN, Harrison DG: Vasorelaxant properties of the endothelium-derived relaxing factor more closely resemble S-nitrosocysteine than nitric oxide. *Nature* 345:161–163, 1990.

33. Mülsch A, Mordvintcev P, Vanin AF, Busse R: The potent vasodilating and guanylyl cyclase activating dinitrosyl-iron (II) complex is stored in a protein-bound form in vascular tissue and is released by thiols. *FEBS Lett* 294:252–256, 1991.

34. Pohl U, Busse R, Kuon E, Bassenge E: Pulsatile perfusion stimulates the release of endothelial autacoids. *J Appl Cardiol* 1:215–235, 1986.

35. Rubanyi GM, Romero JC, Vanhoutte PM: Flow-induced release of endothelium-derived relaxing factor. *Am J Physiol* 250:H1145–H1149, 1986.

36. Moncada S, Palmer RMJ, Higgs EA: Nitric oxide: Physiology, pathophysiology and pharmacology. *Pharmacol Rev* 43:109–142, 1991.

37. Keen JH, Habig WH, Jakoby WB: Mechanism for the several activities of the glutathione S-transferases. *J Biol Chem* 251:6183–6188, 1976.

38. Servent D, Delaforge M, Ducrocq C, Mansuy D, Lenfant M: Nitric oxide formation during microsomal hepatic denitration of glyceryl trinitrate: Involvement of cytochrome P-450. *Biochem Biophys Res Commun* 163:1210–1216, 1989.

39. McDonald BJ, Bennett BM: Cytochrome P-450 mediated biotransformation of organic nitrates. *Can J Physiol Pharmacol* 68:1552–1557, 1990.

40. Bennett BM, Kobus SM, Brien JF, Nakatsu K, Marks GS: Requirement for reduced, unliganded hemoprotein for the hemoglobin- and myoglobin- mediated biotransformation of glyceryl trinitrate. *J Pharmacol Exp Ther* 237:629–635, 1986.

41. Feelisch M, Noack E: Nitric oxide (NO) formation from nitro-vasodilators occurs independently of hemoglobin or non-heme iron. *Eur J Pharmacol* 142:465–469, 1987.

42. Tsuchida S, Maki T, Sato K: Purification and characterization of glutathione transferases with an activity towards nitroglycerin from human aorta and heart. Multiplicity of the human class mu forms. *J Biol Chem* 265:7150–7157, 1990.

43. McDonald BJ, Bennett BM: Biotransformation of glyceryl trinitrate by rat aortic cytochrome P450. *Biochem Pharmacol* 45:268–270, 1993.

44. Yeates RA, Schmid M, Leitold M: Antagonism of glycerol trinitrate activity by an inhibitor of glutathione S-transferase. *Biochem Pharmacol* 38:1749–1753, 1989.

45. Lau DT-W, Benet LZ: Effects of sulfobromophthalein and ethacrynic acid on glyceryl trinitrate relaxation. *Biochem Pharmacol* 43:2247–2254, 1992.

46. Nigam R, Whiting T, Bennett BM: Effects of inhibitors of glutathione S-transferase on glyceryl trinitrate activity in isolated rat aorta. *Can J Physiol Pharmacol* 71:179–184, 1993.

47. Bennett BM, McDonald BJ, Nigam R, Long PG, Simon WC: Inhibition of nitrovasodilator- and acetylcholine-induced relaxation and cyclic GMP accumulation by the cytochrome P-450 substrate, 7-ethoxyresorufin. *Can J Physiol Pharmacol* 70:1297–1303, 1992.

48. Bennett BM, McDonald BJ, St James MJ: Hepatic cytochrome P-450-mediated activation of rat aortic guanylyl cyclase by glyceryl trinitrate. *J Pharmacol Exp Ther* 261: 716–723, 1992.

49. Ahlner J, Andersson RGG, Torfgård K, Axelsson KL: Organic nitrate esters: Clinical use and mechanisms of action. *Pharmacol Rev* 43:351–418, 1991.

50. Axelsson K, Andersson RGG: Tolerance towards nitroglycerin, induced in vivo, is correlated to a reduced cyclic GMP response and an alteration in cyclic GMP turnover. *Eur J Pharmacol* 88:71–79, 1983.

51. Waldman SA, Rapoport RM, Ginsberg R, Murad F: Desensitization to nitroglycerin in vascular smooth muscle from rat and human. *Biochem Pharmacol* 35:3525–3531, 1986.

52. Bennett BM, Schröder H, Hayward DL, Waldman SA, Murad F: Effect of in vitro organic nitrate tolerance on relaxation, cyclic GMP accumulation, and guanylate cyclase activation by glyceryl trinitrate and the enantiomers of isoidide dinitrate. *Circ Res* 63:693–701, 1988.

53. Mülsch A, Busse R, Bassenge E: Desensitization of guanylate cyclase in nitrate tolerance does not impair endothelium-dependent responses. *Eur J Pharmacol* 158: 191–198, 1988.

54. Keith RA, Burkman AM, Sokoloski TD, Fertel RH: Vascular tolerance to nitroglycerin and cyclic GMP generation

in rat aortic smooth muscle. *J Pharmacol Exp Ther* 221: 525–531, 1982.

55. Molina CR, Andresen JW, Rapoport RM, Waldman S, Murad F: The effect of in vivo nitroglycerin therapy on endothelium-dependent and -independent vascular relaxation and cyclic GMP accumulation in rat aorta. *J Cardiovasc Pharmacol* 10:371–378, 1987.

56. Rapoport RM, Waldman SA, Ginsberg R, Molina CR, Murad F: Effects of glyceryl trinitrate on endothelium-dependent and -independent relaxation and cyclic GMP levels in rat aorta and human coronary artery. *J Cardiovasc Pharmacol* 10:82–89, 1987.

57. Brien JF, McLaughlin BE, Breedon TH, Bennett BM, Nakatsu K, Marks GS: Biotransformation of glyceryl trinitrate occurs concurrently with relaxation of rabbit aorta. *J Pharmacol Exp Ther* 237:608–614, 1986.

58. Bennett BM, Leitman DC, Schröder H, Kawamoto JH, Nakatsu K, Murad F: Relationship between biotransformation of glyceryl trinitrate and cyclic GMP accumulation in various cultured cell lines. *J Pharmacol Exp Ther* 250: 316–323, 1989.

59. Koesling D, Böhme E, Schultz G: Guanylyl cyclases, a growing family of signal-transducing enzymes. *FASEB J* 5:2785–2791, 1991.

60. Schulz S, Yuen PST, Garbers DL: The expanding family of guanylyl cyclases. *Trends Pharmacol Sci* 12:116–120, 1992.

61. Lowe DG, Chang M-S, Hellmiss R, Chen E, Singh S, Garbers DL, Goeddel DV: Human atrial natriuretic peptide receptor defines a new paradigm for second messenger signal transduction. *EMBO J* 8:1377–1384, 1989.

62. Schulz S, Singh S, Bellett RA, Singh G, Tubb DJ, Chin H, Garbers DL: The primary structure of a plasma membrane guanylate cyclase demonstrates diversity within this receptor family. *Cell* 58:1155–1162, 1989.

63. Chang M-S, Lowe DG, Lewis M, Hellmiss R, Chen E, Goeddel DV: Differential activation by atrial and brain natriuretic peptides of two different receptor guanylate cyclases. *Nature* 341:68–72, 1989.

64. Schulz S, Green CK, Yuen PST, Garbers DL: Guanylate cyclase is a heat stable enterotoxin receptor. *Cell* 63: 941–948, 1990.

65. Koller KJ, Lowe DG, Bennett GL, Minamino N, Kangawa K, Matsuo H, Goeddel DV: Selective activation of the B natriuretic peptide receptor by C-type natriuretic peptide (CNP). *Science* 252:120–123, 1991.

66. Winquist RJ, Faison EP, Waldman SA, Schwartz K, Murad F, Rapoport RF: Atrial natriuretic factor elicits an endothelium-independent relaxation and activates particulate guanylate cyclase in vascular smooth muscle. *Proc Natl Acad Sci USA* 81:7661–7664, 1984.

67. Rapoport RM, Waldman SA, Schwartz K, Winquist RJ, Murad F: Effects of atrial natriuretic factor, sodium nitroprusside, and acetylcholine on cyclic GMP levels and relaxation in rat aorta. *Eur J Pharmacol* 115:219–229, 1985.

68. Fiscus RR, Rapoport RM, Waldman SA, Murad F: Atriopeptin II elevates cyclic GMP, activates cyclic GMP-dependent protein kinase and causes relaxation in rat thoracic aorta. *Biochim Biophys Acta* 846:179–184, 1985.

69. Waldman SA, Rapoport RM, Murad F: Atrial natriuretic factor selectively activates particulate guanylate cyclase and elevates cyclic GMP in rat tissues. *J Biol Chem* 250: 14332–14334, 1984.

70. Leitman DC, Andresen JW, Catalano RM, Waldman SA, Tuan JJ, Murad F: Atrial natriuretic peptide binding, cross-linking, and stimulation of cyclic GMP accumulation and particulate guanylate cyclase activity in cultured cells. *J Biol Chem* 263:3720–3728, 1988.

71. Leitman DC, Agnost VL, Tuan J, Andresen JW, Murad F: Atrial natriuretic factor and sodium nitroprusside increase cyclic GMP in cultured rat lung fibroblasts by activating different forms of guanylate cyclase. *Biochem J* 224:69–74, 1987.

72. Winquist RJ, Hintze TH: Mechanisms of atrial natriuretic factor-induced vasodilation. *Pharmacol Ther* 48:417–426, 1990.

73. Kramer GL, Hardman JG: Cyclic nucleotides and blood vessel contraction. In: Bohr DF, Somlyo AP, Sparks HV Jr (eds) *Handbook of Physiology. The Cardiovascular System*, Vol 2, *Vascular Smooth Muscle*. Bethesda, MD: American Physiological Society, 1980, pp 179–199.

74. Hardman JG: Cyclic nucleotides and smooth muscle contraction: Some conceptual and experimental considerations. In: Bulbring E, Bradding A, Jones AW, Tomita T (eds) *Smooth Muscle: An Assessment of Current Knowledge*. London: Edward Arnold, 1981, pp 249–262.

75. Birnbaumer L, Abramowitz J, Brown AM: Receptor-effector coupling by G-proteins. *Biochim Biophys Acta* 1031:163–224, 1990.

76. Tang W-J, Gilman A: Adenylyl cyclases. *Cell* 70:869–872, 1992.

77. Seamon KB, Daly JW: Forskolin: Its biological and chemical properties. *Adv Cycl Nucleot Prot Phosphoryl Res* 20:1–150, 1986.

78. Abe A, Karaki H: Effect of forskolin on cytosolic Ca^{2+} level and contraction in vascular smooth muscle. *Am J Physiol* 254: H840–H854, 1989.

79. Tang W-J, Krupinski J, Gilman A: Expression and characterization of calmodulin-activated (Type I) adenylyl cyclase. *J Biol Chem* 266:8595–8603, 1991.

80. Pang DC: Cyclic AMP and cyclic GMP phosphodiesterases: Target for drug development. *Drug Dev Res* 12:85–92, 1988.

81. Beavo JA: Multiple isozymes of cyclic nucleotide phosphodiesterase. *Adv Second Messenger Phosphoprotein Res* 22:1–35, 1988.

82. Beavo J, Reifsnyder DH: Primary sequence of cyclic nucleotide phosphodiesterase isozymes and the design of selective inhibitors. *Trends Pharmacol Sci* 11:150–155, 1990.

83. Weishaar RE, Kobylarz-Singer D, Keiser JA, Haleen SJ, Major TC, Rapundalo S, Peterson JT, Panek R: Subclasses of cyclic GMP phosphodiesterase and their role in regulating the vascular and renal effects of atrial natriuretic peptide. *Hypertension* 15:528–540, 1990.

84. Weishaar RE, Kobylarz-Singer D, Keiser JA, Wright CD, Cornicelli J, Panek R: Cyclic nucleotide phosphodiesterases in the circulatory system: Biochemical, pharmacological, and functional characteristics. *Adv Second Messenger Phosphoprotein Res* 25:249–269, 1992.

85. Ivorra MD, Le Bec A, Lugnier C: Characterization of membrane-bound cyclic nucleotide phosphodiesterases from bovine aortic smooth muscle. *J Cardiovascular Pharm* 19: 532–540, 1992.

86. Saitoh Y, Hardman JG, Wells JN: Differences in the association of calmodulin with cyclic nucleotide phosphodiesterase in relaxed and contracted arterial strips. *Biochemistry* 24:1613–1618, 1985.

87. Sharma RK, Wang JH: Differential regulation of bovine brain calmodulin-dependent cyclic nucleotide phosphodiesterase isozymes by cyclic AMP-dependent protein kinase and calmodulin-dependent phosphatase. *Proc Natl Acad Sci USA* 82:2603–2607, 1985.

88. Sharma RK, Wang JH: Calmodulin and Ca^{2+}-dependent phosphorylation and dephosphorylation of 63 kDa subunit-

containing bovine brain calmodulin-stimulated cyclic nucleotide phosphodiesterase isozyme. *J Biol Chem* 261: 1322–1328, 1986.

89. Macphee CH, Harrison SA, Beavo JA: Immunological identification of the major platelet low-Km cAMP phosphodiesterase: Probable target for anti-thrombotic agents. *Proc Nat Acad Sci USA* 83:6660–6663, 1986.

90. Hartzell HC, Fischmeister R: Opposite effects of cyclic GMP and cyclic AMP on Ca^{2+} current in single heart cells. *Nature* 323:273–275, 1986.

91. Fischmeister R, Hartzell C: Mechanism of action of acetylcholine on calcium current in single cells from frog ventricle. *J Physiol (Lond)* 376:183–202, 1986.

92. Komas N, Lugnier C, Stoclet J-C: Endothelium-dependent and independent relaxation of the rat aorta by cyclic nucleotide phosphodiesterase inhibitors. *Br J Pharmacol* 104: 495–503, 1991.

93. Rascon A, Lindgren S, Stavenow L, Belfrage P, Andersson K-E, Manganiello VC, Degerman E: Purification and properties of the cGMP-inhibited cAMP phosphodiesterase from bovine aortic smooth muscle. *Biochim Biophys Acta* 1134:149–156, 1992.

94. Kauffman RF, Shenck KM, Utterback BG, Crowe VG, Cohen MC: In vitro vascular relaxation by new inotropic agents. Relationship to phosphodiesterase inhibition and cyclic nucleotides. *J Pharmacol Exp Ther* 242:864–872, 1987.

95. Maurice DH, Haslam RJ: Nitroprusside enhances isoprenaline-induced increases in cAMP in rat aortic smooth muscle. *Eur J Pharmacol* 191:471–475, 1990.

96. Lugnier C, Schoeffter P, Le Bec A, Strouthou E, Stoclet JC: Selective inhibition of cyclic nucleotide phosphodiesteras of human, bovine and rat aorta. *Biochem Pharmacol* 35: 1743–1751, 1986.

97. Lincoln TM, Cornwell TL: Towards an understanding of the mechanism of action of cyclic AMP and cyclic GMP in smooth muscle relaxation. *Blood Vessels* 28:129–137, 1991.

98. Fiscus RR, Rapoport RM, Murad F: Endothelium-dependent and nitrovasodilator-induced activation of cyclic GMP-dependent protein kinase in rat aorta. *J Cycl Nucleotide Prot Phosphoryl Res* 9:415–425, 1983.

99. Fiscus RR, Rapoport RM, Waldman SA, Murad F: Atriopeptin II elevates cyclic GMP, activates cyclic GMP-dependent protein kinase and causes relaxation in rat thoracic aorta. *Biochim Biophys Acta* 846:179–184, 1985.

100. Lincoln TM: Cyclic GMP and mechanisms of vasodilation. *Pharmacol Ther* 41:479–502, 1989.

101. Ives HE, Casnellie JE, Greengard P, Jamieson JD: Subcellular localization of cyclic GMP-dependent protein kinase and its substrates in vascular smooth muscle. *J Biol Chem* 255:3777–3785, 1980.

102. Gill GN, Holdy KE, Walton GM, Kanstein CB: Purification and characterization of 3′:5′-cyclic GMP-dependent protein kinase. *Proc Natl Acad Sci USA* 73:3918–3922, 1976.

103. Lincoln TM, Dills WL, Corbin JD: Purification and subunit composition of guanosine 3′:5′-monophosphate-dependent protein kinase from bovine lung. *J Biol Chem* 252: 4269–4275, 1977.

104. Takio K, Wade RD, Smith SB, Krebs EG, Walsh KA, Titani K: Guanosine cyclic 3′,5′-phosphate-dependent protein kinase, a chimeric protein homologous with two separate protein families. *Biochemistry* 23:4207–4218, 1984.

105. Landgraf W, Hullin R, Gobel C, Hoffman F: Phosphorylation of cGMP-dependent protein kinase increases the affinity for cAMP. *Eur J Biochem* 154:113–117, 1986.

106. Foster JL, Guttmann J, Rosen OM: Autophosphorylation

of cGMP-dependent protein kinase. *J Biol Chem* 256: 5029–5036, 1981.

107. Lincoln TM, Thompson M, Cornwell TL: Purification and characterization of two forms of cyclic GMP-dependent protein kinase from bovine aorta. *J Biol Chem* 263: 17632–17637, 1988.

108. Wolfe L, Corbin JD, Francis SH: Characterization of a novel isozyme of cGMP-dependent protein kinase from bovine aorta. *J Biol Chem* 264:7734–7741, 1989.

109. Sekhar KR, Hatchett RJ, Shabb JB, Wolfe L, Francis SH, Wells JN, Jastorff B, Butt E, Chakinala MM, Corbin JD: Relaxation of pig coronary arteries by new and potent cGMP analogs that selectively activates type 1α, compared with type 1β, cGMP-dependent protein kinase. *Mol Pharmacol* 42:103–108, 1992.

110. Keilbach A, Landgraf W, Hofmann F: Two immunologically different isoforms of cGMP-dependent protein kinase are localized in mammalian smooth muscle. *Biol Chem Hoppe Seyler* 371:742, 1990.

111. Wernet W, Flockerzi V, Hofmann F: The cDNA of the two isoforms of bovine cGMP-dependent protein kinase. *FEBS Lett* 251:191–196, 1989.

112. Casnellie JE, Ives HE, Jamieson JD, Greengard P: Cyclic GMP-dependent protein phosphorylation in intact medial tissue and isolated cells from vascular smooth muscle. *J Biol Chem* 255:3770–3776, 1980.

113. Parks TP, Nairn AC, Greengard P, Jamieson JD: The cyclic nucleotide-dependent phosphorylation of aortic smooth muscle membrane proteins. *Arch Biochem Biophys* 255: 361–371, 1987.

114. Furukawa K, Nakamura H: Cyclic GMP regulation of the plasma membrane $(Ca^{2+} - Mg^{2+})$ ATPase in vascular smooth muscle. *J Biochem* 101:287–290, 1987.

115. Vrolix M, Raeymaekers L, Wuytack F, Hofmann F, Casteels R: Cyclic GMP-dependent protein kinase stimulates the plasmalemmal Ca^{2+} pump of smooth muscle via phosphorylation of phosphatidylinositol. *Biochem J* 255:855–863, 1988.

116. Baltensperger K, Carafoli E, Chiesi M: The Ca^{2+}-pumping ATPase and the major substrates of the cGMP-dependent protein kinase in smooth muscle sarcolemma are distinct entities. *Eur J Biochem* 172:7–16, 1988.

117. Baltensperger K, Chiesi M, Carafoli E: Substrates of cGMP kinase in vascular smooth muscle and their role in the relaxation process. *Biochemistry* 29:9753–9760, 1990.

118. Imai S, Yoshida Y, Sun HT: Sarcolemmal $(Ca^{2+} + Mg^{2+})$-ATPase of vascular smooth muscle and the effects of protein kinases thereupon. *J Biochem* 107:755–761, 1990.

119. Yoshida Y, Cai J-Q, Imai S: Plasma membrane Ca^{2+}-pump ATPase is not a substrate for cGMP-dependent protein kinase. *J Biochem* 111:559–562, 1992.

120. Sarcevic B, Robinson PJ, Pearson RB, Kemp BE: The smooth muscle 132 kDa cyclic GMP-dependent protein kinase substrate is not myosin light chain kinase or caldesmon. *Biochem J* 271:493–499, 1990.

121. Yoshida Y, Sun H-T, Cai J-Q, Imai S: Cyclic GMP-dependent protein kinase stimulates the plasma membrane Ca^{2+} pump ATPase of vascular smooth muscle via phosphorylation of a 240 kDa protein. *J Biol Chem* 266:19819–19825, 1991.

122. Raeymaekers L, Hofmann F, Casteels R: Cyclic GMP-dependent protein kinase phosphorylates phospholamban in isolated sarcoplasmic reticulum from cardiac and smooth muscle. *Biochem J* 252:269–273, 1988.

123. Huggins JP, Cook EA, Piggott JR, Mattinsley TJ, England PJ: Phospholamban is a good substrate for cyclic GMP-

dependent protein kinase in vitro, but not in intact cardiac or smooth muscle. *Biochem J* 260:829–835, 1989.

124. Sarcevic B, Brookes V, Martin TJ, Kemp BE, Robinson PJ: Atrial natriuretic peptide-dependent phosphorylation of smooth muscle cell particulate fraction proteins is mediated by cGMP-dependent protein kinase. *J Biol Chem* 264:20648–20654, 1989.

125. Cornwell TL, Pryzwansky KB, Wyatt TA, Lincoln TM: Regulation of sarcoplasmic reticulum protein phosphorylation by localized cyclic GMP-dependent protein kinase in vascular smooth muscle cells. *Mol Pharmacol* 40:923–931, 1991.

126. Raeymaekers L, Eggermont JA, Wuytack F, Casteels R: Effects of cyclic nucleotide dependent protein kinases on the endoplasmic reticulum Ca^{2+} pump of bovine pulmonary artery. *Cell Calcium* 11:261–268, 1990.

127. Rapoport RM, Draznin MB, Murad M: Sodium nitroprusside-induced protein phosphorylation in intact rat aorta is mimicked by 8-bromo cyclic GMP. *Proc Natl Acad Sci USA* 79:6470–6474, 1982.

128. Rapoport RM, Draznin MB, Murad F: Endothelium-dependent relaxation in rat thoracic aorta may be mediated through cyclic GMP-dependent protein phosphorylation. *Nature* 306:174–176, 1983.

129. Draznin MB, Rapoport RM, Murad F: Myosin light chain phosphorylation in contraction and relaxation of intact rat thoracic aorta. *Int J Biochem* 18:917–928, 1986.

130. Hanks SK, Quinn AM, Hunter T: Protein kinase family: Conserved features and deduced phylogeny of the catalytic domains. *Science* 241:42–52, 1988.

131. Taylor SS, Buechler JA, Slice LW, Knighton DK, Durgerian S, Ringheim GE, Neitzel JJ, Yonemoto WM, Sowadski JM, Dospmann W: cAMP-dependent protein kinase: A framework for a diverse family of enzymes. *Cold Springs Harbor Symp* 53:121–130, 1988.

132. Corbin JD, Sugden PH, West L, Flockhart DA, Lincoln TM, McCarthy D: Studies on the properties and mode of action of the purified regulatory subunit of bovine heart adenosine 3′:5′-monophosphate-dependent protein kinase. *J Biol Chem* 253:3997–4003, 1978.

133. Krebs EG, Beavo JA: Phosphorylation-dephosphorylation of enzymes. *Annu Rev Biochem* 48:923–959, 1979.

134. Bramson HN, Thomas N, Matsueda R, Nelso NC, Taylor SS, Kaiser ET: Modification of the catalytic subunit of bovine heart cAMP-dependent protein kinase with affinity labels related to peptide substrates. *J Biol Chem* 257:10575–10581, 1983.

135. Singh D: Distribution and localization of adenosine 3′,5′-monophosphate-dependent protein kinase in mammalian artery. *Blood Vessels* 17:312–323, 1980.

136. Silver PJ, Schmidt-Silver C, DiSalvo J: Beta-adrenergic relaxation and cAMP kinase activation in coronary areterial smooth muscle. *Am J Physiol* 242:H177–H184, 1982.

137. Singh D: Adenosine 3′,5′-monophosphate-dependent protein kinase from mammalian artery: Isolation and properties of the isoenzymes. *Cell Mol Biol* 27:419–428, 1981.

138. Vegesna RVK, Diamond J: Effects of isoproterenol and forskolin on tension, cyclic AMP levels, and cyclic AMP-dependent protein kinase activity in bovine coronary artery. *Can J Physiol Pharmacol* 62:1116–1123, 1984.

139. Silver PJ, Walus K, DiSalvo J: Adenosine-mediated relaxation and activation of cyclic AMP-dependent protein kinase in coronary arterial smooth muscle. *J Pharmacol Exp Ther* 228:342–347, 1984.

140. Bhalla RC, Sharma RV, Gupta RC: Isolation of two myosin light-chain kinases from bovine carotid artery and their

regulation by phosphorylation mediated by cyclic AMP-dependent protein kinase. *Biochem J* 203:583–592, 1982.

141. Brockbank KJ, England PJ: A rapid method for the preparation of sarcolemmal vesicles from rat aorta, and the stimulation of calcium uptake into the vesicles by cyclic AMP-dependent protein kinase. *FEBS Lett* 122:67–71, 1980.

142. Suematsu E, Hirata M, Kuriyama H: Effects of cAMP- and cGMP-dependent protein kinases, and calmodulin on Ca uptake by highly purified sarcolemmal vesicles of vascular smooth muscle. *Biochim Biophys Acta* 773:83–90, 1984.

143. Chiesi M, Gasser J, Carafoli E: Properties of the Ca-pumping ATPase of sarcoplasmic reticulum from vascular smooth muscle. *Biochem Biophys Res Commun* 124:797–806, 1984.

144. Boulanger-Saunier C, Kattenburg DM, Stoclet J-C: Cyclic AMP-dependent phosphorylation of a 16kd protein of rat aortic myocytes. *FEBS Lett* 193:283–288, 1985.

145. Raeymaekers L, Jones LR: Evidence for the presence of phospholamban in the endoplasmic reticulum of smooth muscle. *Biochim Biophys Acta* 882:258–265, 1986.

146. Watras J: Regulation of calcium uptake in bovine aortic sarcoplasmic reticulum by cyclic AMP-dependent protein kinase. *J Mol Cell Cardiol* 20:711–723, 1988.

147. Kattenberg DM, Daniel EE: Effects of endogeneous cyclic AMP-dependent protein kinase catalytic subunit on Ca-uptake by plasma membrane vesicles from rat mesenteric artery. *Blood Vessels* 21:257–266, 1984.

148. James PH, Pruschy M, Vorherr TE, Penniston JT, Carafoli E: Primary structure of the cAMP-dependent phosphorylation site of the plasma membrane calcium pump. *Biochemistry* 28:4253–4258, 1989.

149. Furukawa K, Tawada Y, Shigekawa M: Regulation of the plasma membrane Ca^{2+} pump by cyclic nucleotides in cultured vascular smooth muscle cells. *J Biol Chem* 263:8058–8065, 1988.

150. De Jaegere S, Wuytack F, Eggermont JA, Verboomen H, Casteels R: Molecular cloning and sequencing of the plasma-membrane Ca^{2+} pump of pig smooth muscle. *Biochem J* 271:655–660, 1990.

151. Khan I, Grover AK: Expression of cyclic-nucleotide-sensitive and -insensitive isoforms of the plasma membrane Ca^{2+} pump in smooth muscle and other tissues. *Biochem J* 277:345–349, 1991.

152. Adelstein RS, Conti MA, Hathaway DR: Phosphorylation of smooth muscle myosin light chain kinase by the catalytic subunit of adenosine 3′,5′-monophosphate-dependent protein kinase. *J Biol Chem* 253:8347–8350, 1978.

153. Silver PJ, DiSalvo J: Adenosine 3′,5′-monophosphate-mediated inhibition of myosin light chain phosphorylation in bovine aortic actomyosin. *J Biol Chem* 254:9950–9954, 1979.

154. Nishikawa M, De Lanerolle P, Lincoln TM, Adelstein RS: Phosphorylation of mammalian myosin light chain kinase by the catalytic subunit of cyclic AMP-dependent protein kinase and by cyclic GMP-dependent protein kinase. *J Biol Chem* 259:8429–8439, 1984.

155. McDaniel NL, Chen X-L, Singer HA, Murphy RA, Rembold CM: Nitrovasodilators relax arterial smooth muscle by decreasing $[Ca^{2+}]_i$ and uncoupling stress from myosin phosphorylation. *Am J Physiol* 263:C461–C467, 1992.

156. Somlyo AV, Somlyo AP: Electromechanical and pharmacomechanical coupling in vascular smooth muscle. *J Pharmacol Exp Ther* 159:129–145, 1968.

157. Berridge MJ: Inositol triphosphate and diacylglycerol as

second messengers. *Biochem J* 220:345–360, 1984.

158. Chen Q, Van Breeman C: Function of smooth muscle sarcoplasmic reticulum. *Adv Second Messenger Phosphoprotein Res* 26:335–350, 1992.

159. Benham CD, Tsien RW: A novel receptor-operated Ca^{2+}-permeable channel activated by ATP in smooth muscle. *Nature* 328:275–278, 1987.

160. Nelson MT, Patlak JB, Worley JF, Standen NB: Calcium channels, potassium channels, and voltage dependence of arterial smooth muscle tone. *Am J Physiol* 259:C3–C18, 1990.

161. Ohya Y, Speralakis N: Involvement of a GTP-binding protein in stimulating action of angiotensin II on calcium channels in vascular smooth muscle cells. *Circ Res* 68:763–771, 1991.

162. Rasmussen H, Forder J, Kofima I, Scriabine A: TPA-induced contraction of isolated rabbit vascular smooth muscle. *Biochem Biophys Res Commun* 122:776–784, 1984.

163. Danthuluri NR, Deth RC: Phorbol-ester-induced contraction of arterial smooth muscle and inhibition of alpha-adrenergic response. *Biochem Biophys Res Commun* 125:1103–1109, 1984.

164. Chatterjee M, Tejada M: Phorbol ester induced contraction in chemically-skinned vascular smooth muscle. *Am J Physiol* 251:C1–C6, 1986.

165. Miller JR, Hawkins DJ, Wells JN: Phorbol diesters alter the contractile responses of porcine coronary artery. *J Pharmacol Exp Ther* 239:38–42, 1986.

166. Jiang MJ, Morgan KG: Intracellular calcium levels in phorbol ester-induced contractions of vascular smooth muscle. *Am J Physiol* 253:H1365–H1371, 1987.

167. Nishizuka Y: Studies and perspectives of protein kinase C. *Science* 233:305–312, 1986.

168. Martinson EA, Goldstein D, Brown JH: Muscarinic receptor activation of phosphatidylcholine hydrolysis. *J Biol Chem* 264:14748–14754, 1989.

169. Matozaki T, Williams JT: Multiple sources of 1,2-diacylglycerol in isolated rat pancreatic acini stimulated by cholecystokinin. *J Biol Chem* 264:14729–14734, 1989.

170. Morgan KG: The role of calcium in the control of vascular tone. *Cardiovasc Drugs Ther* 4:1355–1362, 1990.

171. Bradley AB, Morgan KG: Alteration in cytoplasmic calcium sensitivity during porcine coronary artery contractions as detected by aequorin. *J Physiol (Lond)* 385:437–448, 1987.

172. Nishimura J, Kolber M, Van Breemen C: Norepinephrine and GTPγ-S increase myofilament Ca^{2+} sensitivity in α-toxin permeabilized arterial smooth muscle. *Biochem Biophys Res Commun* 157:677–683, 1988.

173. Kitazawa T, Kobayashi S, Horiuchi K, Somlyo AV, Somlyo AP: Receptor coupled, permeabilized smooth muscle: Role of the phosphatidylinositol cascade, G-proteins and modulation of the contractile response to Ca^{2+}. *J Biol Chem* 264:5339–5342, 1989.

174. Nishimura J, Khalil RA, Drenth JP, Van Breemen C: Evidence for increased myofilament Ca^{2+} sensitivity in norepinephrine-activated vascular smooth muscle. *Am J Physiol* 259:H2–H8, 1990.

175. Kitazawa T, Gaylinn BD, Denney HG, Somlyo AP: G-protein-mediated Ca^{2+} sensitization of smooth muscle contraction through myosin light chain phosphorylation. *J Biol Chem* 266:1708–1715, 1991.

176. Kitazawa T, Masuo M, Somlyo AP: G-protein-mediated inhibition of myosin light-chain phosphatase in vascular smooth muscle. *Proc Natl Acad Sci USA* 88:9307–9310, 1991.

177. Fujiwara T, Itoh T, Kubota Y, Kuriyama H: Effect of guanosine nucleotides on skinned smooth muscle tissue of the rabbit mesenteric artery. *J Physiol (Lond)* 408:535–547, 1989.

178. Kubota Y, Nomura M, Kamm KE, Mumby MC, Stull JT: GTPγS-dependent regulation of smooth muscle contractile elements. *Am J Physiol* 262:C405–C410, 1992.

179. Gong MC, Fuglsand A, Alessi D, Kobayashi S, Cohen P, Somlyo AV, Somlyo AP: Arachidonic acid inhibits myosin light chain phosphatase and sensitizes smooth muscle to calcium. *J Biol Chem* 267:21492–21498, 1992.

180. Means AR, VanBerkum MFA, Bagchi I, Lu KP, Rasmussen CD: Regulatory functions of calmodulin. *Pharmacol Ther* 50:255–270, 1991.

181. Stull JT, Gallagher PJ, Herring BP, Kamm KE: Vascular smooth muscle contractile elements. Cellular regulation. *Hypertension* 17:723–732, 1991.

182. Rembold CM: Regulation of contraction and relaxation in arterial smooth muscle. *Hypertension* 20:129–137, 1992.

183. Ikebe M, Koretz, J, Hartshorne DJ: Effects of phosphorylation of light chain residues threonine 18 and serine 19 on the properties and conformation of smooth muscle myosin. *J Biol Chem* 263:6432–6437, 1988.

184. Hai C-M, Murphy RA: Ca^{2+}, crossbridge phosphorylation, and contraction. *Annu Rev Physiol* 51:285–298, 1989.

185. Conti MA, Adelstein RS: The relationship between calmodulin binding and phosphorylation of smooth myosin kinase by the catalytic subunit of 3′,5′ cAMP-dependent protein kinase. *J Biol Chem* 256:3178–3181, 1981.

186. Vallet B, Molla A, Demaille JG: Cyclic adenosine 3′,5′-monophosphate-dependent regulation of purified bovine aortic calcium/calmodulin-dependent myosin light chain kinase. *Biochim Biophys Acta* 674:256–264, 1981.

187. Hathaway DR, Konick MV, Codican SA: Phosphorylation of myosin light chain kinases. *J Mol Cell Cardiol* 17:841–850, 1985.

188. Stull JT, Hsu L-C, Tansey MG, Kamm KE: Myosin light chain kinase phosphorylation in tracheal smooth muscle. *J Biol Chem* 265:16683–16690, 1990.

189. Ikebe M, Reardon S: Phosphorylation of smooth myosin light chain kinase by smooth muscle Ca^{2+}/calmodulin-dependent multifunctional protein kinase. *J Biol Chem* 265:8975–8978, 1990.

190. Gilbert EK, Weaver BA, Rembold CM: Depolarization decreases the $[Ca^{2+}]_i$-sensitivity of myosin light chain kinase in arterial smooth muscle: A comparison of aequorin and fura 2 $[Ca^{2+}]$ estimates. *FASEB J* 5:2593–2599, 1991.

191. Reuter H: Calcium channel modulation by neurotransmitters, enzymes, and drugs. *Nature* 301:569–574, 1983.

192. Brown AM, Yatani A, Imoto Y, Codina J, Mattera R, Birnbaumer L: Direct G-protein regulation of Ca^{2+} channels. *Ann NY Acad Sci* 560:373–386, 1989.

193. McDaniel NL, Rembold CM, Richard HL, Murphy RA: cAMP relaxes arterial smooth muscle predominantly by decreasing cell $[Ca^{2+}]$. *J Physiol (Lond)* 439:147–160, 1991.

194. Nishimura J, Van Breemen C: Direct regulation of smooth muscle contractile elements by second messengers. *Biochem Biophys Res Commun* 163:929–935, 1989.

195. Abe S, Kanaide H, Nakamura M: Front-surface fluorometry with fura-2 and effects of nitroglycerin on cytosolic calcium concentrations and on tension in the coronary artery of the pig. *Br J Pharmacol* 101:545–552, 1990.

196. Lincoln TM, Johnson RM: Possible role of cyclic GMP-dependent protein kinase in vascular smooth muscle function. *Adv Cyclic Nucleotide Prot Phosphoryl Res* 17:285–296, 1984.

197. Cornwell TL, Lincoln TM: Regulation of intracellular Ca^{2+} levels in cultured vascular smooth muscle cells. Reduction of Ca^{2+} by atriopeptin and 8-bromo-cyclic GMP is mediated by

cyclic GMP-dependent protein kinase. *J Biol Chem* 264: 1146–1155, 1989.

198. Lincoln TM, Cornwell TL, Taylor AE: cGMP-dependent protein kinase mediates the reduction of Ca^{2+} by cAMP in vascular smooth muscle cells. *Am J Physiol* 258:C399–C407, 1990.

199. Van Eldere J, Raeymaekers L, Casteels R: Effects of isoprenaline on intracellular Ca uptake and on Ca influx in arterial smooth muscle. *Pflügers Arch* 395:81–83, 1982.

200. Meisheri KD, Van Breeman C: Effects of beta-adrenergic stimulation on calcium movements in rabbit aortic smooth muscle: Relationship with cyclic AMP. *J Physiol (Lond)* 331:429–441, 1982.

201. Hwang KS, Van Breemen C: Effect of dB-c-AMP and forskolin on the ^{45}Ca influx, net Ca uptake and tension in rabbit aortic smooth muscle. *Eur J Pharmacol* 134:155–162, 1987.

202. Abe A, Karaki H: Inhibitory effects of forskolin on vascular smooth muscle of rabbit aorta. *Jpn J Pharmacol* 46: 293–301, 1988.

203. Bahanin J, Borsotto M, Coppola T, Fosset M, Hosey MM, Moure C, Pouron D, Qar J, Romey G, Schmid A, Varedaele S, Van Renterghen C, Lazdunski M: Biochemistry, molecular pharmacology, and functional control of Ca^{2+} channels. *Ann NY Acad Sci* 560:15–26, 1989.

204. Hosey MM, Chang FC, O'Callahan CM, Ptasienski J: L-type calcium channels in cardiac and skeletal muscle. *Ann NY Acad Sci* 560:27–36, 1989.

205. Kameyama M, Hescheler J, Trautwein W, Hofmann F: Modulation of Ca current during the phosphorylation cycle in the guinea pig heart. *Pflügers Arch* 407:123–128, 1986.

206. Rosenberg RL, Hess P, Reeves JP, Smilovitz H, Tsien RW: Calcium channels in planar lipid bilayers: Insights into mechanisms of ion permeation and gating. *Science* 231: 1564–1566, 1986.

207. Collins P, Griffith TM, Henderson AH, Lewis MJ: Endothelium-derived relaxing factor alters calcium fluxes in rabbit aorta: A cyclic guanosine monophosphate-mediated effect. *J Physiol (Lond)* 381:427–437, 1986.

208. Taylor CJ, Meisheri RD: Inhibitory effects of a synthetic atrial peptide on contractions and ^{45}Ca fluxes in vascular smooth muscle. *J Pharmacol Exp Ther* 237:803–808, 1986.

209. Karaki H, Sato K, Ozaki H, Murakami K: Effects of sodium nitroprusside on cytosolic calcium level in vascular smooth muscle. *Eur J Pharmacol* 156:259–266, 1988.

210. Magliola L, Jones AW: Sodium nitroprusside alters Ca^{2+} flux components and Ca^{2+}-dependent fluxes of K^+ and Cl^- in rat aorta. *J Physiol (Lond)* 421:411–424, 1990.

211. Chen X-L, Rembold CM: Cyclic nucleotide-dependent regulation of Mn^{2+} influx, $[Ca^{2+}]_i$, and arterial smooth muscle relaxation. *Am J Physiol* 263:C468–C473, 1992.

212. Godfraind T: EDRF and cyclic GMP control gating of receptor-operated calcium channels in vascular smooth muscle. *Eur J Pharmacol* 126:341–343, 1986.

213. Clapp LH, Gurney AM: Modulation of calcium movements by nitroprusside in isolated vascular smooth muscle cells. *Pflügers Arch* 418:462–470, 1991.

214. Blayney LM, Gapper PW, Newby AC: Inhibition of a receptor-operated calcium channel in pig aortic microsomes by cyclic GMP-dependent protein kinase. *Biochem J* 273: 803–806, 1991.

215. Sandoshima J-I, Akaike N, Kanaide H, Nakamura M: Cyclic AMP modulates Ca-activated K channel in cultured smooth muscle cells of rat aortas. *Am J Physiol* 255: H754–H759, 1988.

216. Ito Y, Kitamura K, Kuriyama H: Effects of acetylcholine and catecholamine on the smooth muscle cell of the porcine coronary artery. *J Physiol (Lond)* 294:595–611, 1979.

217. Bolton TB: Mechanisms of action of transmitters and other substances on smooth muscle. *Physiol Rev* 59:606–718, 1979.

218. Haeusler, G: The effects of sodium nitroprusside (SNP) on vascular smooth muscle. *Experientia* 31:729, 1975.

219. Ito Y, Kitamura K, Kuriyama H: Actions of nitroglycerin on the membrane and mechanical properties of smooth muscles of the coronary artery of the pig. *Br J Pharmacol* 70:197–204, 1980.

220. Karashima S: Actions of nitroglycerin on smooth muscles of the guinea-pig and rat portal veins. *Br J Pharmacol* 71:489–497, 1980.

221. Cheung DW, MacKay MJ: The effects of sodium nitroprusside and 8-bromo-cyclic GMP on electrical and mechanical activities of the rat tail artery. *Br J Pharmacol* 86:117–124, 1985.

222. Fujino K, Nakaya S, Wakatsuki T, Miyoshi Y, Nakaya Y, Mori H, Inoue I: Effects of nitroglycerin on ATP-induced Ca^{2+}-mobilization, Ca^{2+}-activated K channels and contraction of cultured smooth muscle cells of porcine coronary artery. *J Pharmacol Exp Ther* 256:371–377, 1991.

223. Williams DL, Katz GM, Roy-Contancin L, Reuben JP: Guanosine 5'-monophosphate modulates gating of high-conductance Ca^{2+}-activated K^+ channels in vascular smooth muscle cells. *Proc Natl Acad Sci USA* 85:9360–9364, 1988.

224. Ashida T, Blaustein MP: Regulation of cell calcium and contractility in mammalian arterial smooth muscle: The role of sodium-calcium exchange. *J Physiol (Lond)* 392:617–635, 1987.

225. Kahn AM, Allen JC, Shelat H: Na^+-Ca^{2+} exchange in sarcolemmal vesicles from bovine superior mesenteric artery. *Am J Physiol* 254:C441–C449, 1988.

226. Slaughter RS, Shevell JL, Felix FP, Garcia ML, Kaczorowski GJ: High levels of sodium-calcium exchange in vascular smooth muscle sarcolemmal membrane vesicles. *Biochemistry* 28:3995–4002, 1989.

227. Baker PF, Dipolo R: Axonal calcium and magnesium homeostasis. *Curr Top Membr Transp* 22:195–247, 1984.

228. Popescu LM, Panoiu C, Hinescu M, Nutu O: The mechanism of cGMP-induced relaxation in vascular smooth muscle. *Eur J Pharmacol* 107:393–394, 1985.

229. Somlyo AV, Somlyo AP, Smiesko V: Cyclic AMP and vascular smooth muscle. *Adv Cyclic Nucleotide Res* 1:175–194, 1972.

230. Webb RC, Bohr DF: Relaxation of vascular smooth muscle by isoproterenol, dibutyryl-cyclic AMP and theophylline. *J Pharmacol Exp Ther* 217:26–35, 1981.

231. Sheid CR, Fay FS: Beta-adrenergic effects on transmembrane ^{45}Ca fluxes in isolated smooth muscle cells. *Am J Physiol* 246:C431–C438, 1984.

232. Bertorello AM, Aperia A, Walaas SI, Nairn AC, Greengard P: Phosphorylation of the catalytic subunit of Na^+,K^+-ATPase inhibits the activity of the enzyme. *Proc Natl Acad Sci USA* 88:11359–11362, 1991.

233. Rapoport RM, Murad R: Effect of ouabain and alterations in potassium concentration on relaxation induced by sodium nitroprusside. *Blood Vessels* 20:255–264, 1983.

234. Rapoport RM, Schwartz K, Murad F: Effects of Na^+,K^+-pump inhibitors and membrane depolarization agents on acetylcholine-induced endothelium-dependent relaxation and cyclic GMP accumulation in rat aorta. *Eur J Pharmacol* 110:203–209, 1985.

235. Furukawa K-I, Ohshima N, Tawade-Iwata Y, Shigekawa M: Cyclic GMP stimulates Na^+/Ca^{2+} exchange in vascular smooth muscle cells in primary culture. *J Biol Chem* 266: 12337–12341, 1991.

236. Itoh T, Izumi H, Kuriyama H: Mechanisms of relaxation induced by activation of β-adrenoceptors in smooth muscle cells of the guinea pig mesenteric artery. *J Physiol (Lond)* 326:475–493, 1982.

237. Twort CHC, Van Breeman C: Cyclic guanosine monophosphate-enhanced sequestration of Ca^{2+} by sarcoplasmic reticulum in vascular smooth muscle. *Circ Res* 62:961–964, 1988.

238. Chiu PJS, Tetzloff G, Ahn H-S, Sybertz EJ: Comparative effects of vinpocetine and 8-Br-cyclic GMP on the contraction and ^{45}Ca-fluxes in the rabbit aorta. *Am J Hypertens* 1:262–268, 1988.

239. Komori S, Bolton TB: Actions of guanine nucleotides and cyclic nucleotides on calcium stores in single patch-clamped smooth muscle cells from rabbit portal vein. *Br J Pharmacol* 97:973–982, 1989.

240. Hassid A, Yu Y-M: Mechanism of atriopeptin-induced decrease of cytosolic free Ca in rat vascular smooth muscle cells: Evidence for an intracellular locus of action. *J Cardiovasc Pharmacol* 14(Suppl 6):S34–S38, 1989.

241. Kai H, Kanaide H, Nakamura M: Effects of nicorandil on cytosolic calcium concentrations in quin2-loaded rat aortic vascular smooth muscle cells in primary culture. *J Pharmacol Exp Ther* 251:1174–1180, 1990.

242. Meisheri KD, Taylor CJ, Saneii H: Synthetic atrial peptide inhibits intracellular calcium release in smooth muscle. *Am J Physiol* 250:C171–C174, 1986.

243. Meyer-Lehnert H, Caramelo C, Tsai P, Schrier RW: Interaction of atriopeptin III and vasopressin on calcium kinetics and contraction of aortic smooth muscle cells. *J Clin Invest* 82:1407–1414, 1988.

244. Rapoport RM: Cyclic guanosine monophosphate inhibition of contraction may be mediated through inhibition of phosphatidylinositol hydrolysis in rat aorta. *Circ Res* 58:407–409, 1986.

245. Hirata M, Kohse KP, Chang C-H, Ikebe T, Murad F: Mechanism of cyclic GMP inhibition of inositol phosphate formation in rat aorta segments and cultured bovine aortic smooth muscle cells. *J Biol Chem* 265:1268–1273, 1990.

246. Ahlner J, Axelsson KL, Karlson J-OG, Andersson RGG: Glyceryl trinitrate inhibits phosphatidylinositol hydrolysis and protein kinase C activity in bovine mesenteric artery. *Life Sci* 43:1241–1248, 1988.

247. Fujii K, Ishimatsu T, Kuriyama H: Mechanism of vasodilation induced by α-human atrial natriuretic polypeptide in rabbit and guinea-pig renal arteries. *J Physiol (Lond)* 377:315–322, 1986.

248. Langlands JM, Diamond J: The effect of phenylephrine on inositol 1,4,5-trisphosphate levels in vascular smooth muscle using a protein binding assay system. *Biochem Biophys Res Commun* 173:1258–1265, 1990.

249. Lincoln TM: Pertussis toxin-sensitive and insensitive guanine nucleotide binding proteins (G-proteins) are not phosphorylated by cyclic GMP-dependent protein kinase. *Second Messenger Phosphoprotein* 13:99–109, 1991.

CHAPTER 53

Vascular Muscle Membrane Properties in Hypertension

NANCY J. RUSCH, SARAH K. ENGLAND & KENT HERMSMEYER

INTRODUCTION

The direct effect of high blood pressure on the molecular composition and function of coronary arterial membranes is largely unknown. Thus it is difficult to correlate vascular muscle membrane alterations in hypertension to coronary blood flow changes in this disease. However, elevated peripheral vascular resistance, which is a hallmark of hypertension, is a major predisposing factor to cardiac pathology, suggesting that understanding the vascular mechanisms of high blood pressure may be one avenue to reducing myocardial disorders. Hypertension is the most common cause of left ventricular hypertrophy and a frequent precursor of congestive heart failure {1}. Even in borderline hypertensive children, there is significant cardiac hypertrophy and perhaps early stages of cardiac problems {2}. Thus humans may suffer from a loss of cardiac function, possibly beginning in the very initial stages of hypertension, if blood pressure is not normalized. The true impact of hypertension on cardiac pathology is revealed by statistics showing that 25% of Americans (approximately 63 million people) have some form of hypertension, which will predispose them to heart disease {3}.

In light of this, the present chapter will outline vascular muscle membrane changes in hypertension, which may culminate in cardiac disease. This text will focus on the observation that despite the multifaceted etiology of hypertension, arterial muscle membranes exposed to high blood pressure invariably show an enhanced ionic permeability to Na^+, Ca^{2+}, K^+, and Cl^- ions {4–10}. In particular, laboratory and clinical studies have implicated augmented Ca^{2+} influx in vascular smooth muscle cells as a contributing factor to the enhanced arterial tone in hypertension {11}. To counteract this enhanced Ca^{2+} influx, the vascular muscle cell may activate hyperpolarizing K^+ currents and membrane ion transport mechanisms to buffer further rises in cell excitability {12–14}. Figure 53-1 depicts some ion channel and ion transport mechanisms, which may be altered in the vascular muscle membrane in hypertension. Ultimately, changes in ion channel regulation and ion exchange mechanisms, combined with structural alteration of the arterial wall {15}, will determine the final level of peripheral vascular re-

sistance and cardiac afterload. Figure 53-2 shows how altered ionic mechanisms in the vascular muscle membrane might influence arterial reactivity and blood pressure levels in the intact system, thus leading to cardiac pathology in patients with hypertension.

ARTERIAL MUSCLE MEMBRANE MECHANISMS

Arterial sarcolemma shows increased ionic permeability in hypertension

Arterial muscle membranes from hypertensive animals show a generalized increase in membrane permeability to Na^+, K^+, and Cl^- ions. Using radioisotope and ion exchange methods, several laboratories have consistently shown an increased turnover of these ions in aortic, femoral, and caudal arteries of genetic, renal, and salt-sensitive rat models of hypertension {4–10}. The common finding of increased arterial membrane permeability in animals with different genetic and endocrine profiles, but the same unifying presence of high blood pressure, has led to the theory that arterial membrane alterations may represent a "universal defect" of hypertension {16}. It is unclear if altered arterial membrane permeability precedes or is a consequence of high blood pressure, since most studies to date have measured ion exchange in arterial tissues from rats in the established phase of hypertension. However, the persistence of enhanced ionic turnover in arteries at temperatures as low as 2°C implies that "passive" ion flux through ion channels in the arterial plasma membrane, rather than ion exchange by more temperature-sensitive active transport mechanisms, likely is one pathway for increased ion turnover in hypertension {7}.

Voltage-dependent ion channels critically regulate the level of excitation-contraction coupling in arterial muscle cells {17}, and thus recent attention has focused particularly on the regulation of ion currents through these channels in the plasma membrane of arterial muscle in hypertension. Calcium influx through voltage-dependent calcium channels (VDCCs) in arteriolar muscle cells provides activator Ca^{2+} for arterial contraction and replenishes intracellular Ca^{2+} stores {18}. Thus an enhanced

N. Sperelakis (ed.), Physiology and Pathophysiology of the Heart, Third Edition.
© *1995 Kluwer Academic Publishers. ISBN 0-7923-2612-1. All rights reserved.*

VASCULAR MEMBRANE MECHANISMS OF HYPERTENSION?

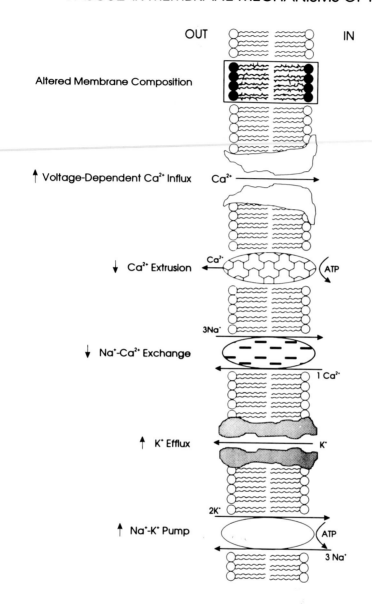

ARTERIAL MUSCLE PLASMA MEMBRANE

Fig. 53-1. Diagrammatic representation of vascular membrane mechanisms associated with hypertension. Ion channel and ion transport mechanisms that may be altered in the vascular muscle membrane include (from top to bottom): (1) membrane composition, (2) voltage-dependent Ca^{2+} channels, (3) Ca^{2+} pump, (4) Na^+-Ca^{2+} exchanger, (5) K^+ channels, and (6) Na^+-K^+ pump.

Ca^{2+} influx through arterial VDCCs in hypertension may increase the level of vascular muscle contraction, potentially elevating peripheral vascular resistance and systemic blood pressure {11}. Activation of arterial K^+ channels and the resulting K^+ efflux would hyperpolarize the vascular muscle membrane, resulting in less voltage-dependent Ca^{2+} influx {17}. Therefore, an increased vascular membrane permeability to K^+ ions would tend to reduce arterial excitability in hypertension by acting as a vascular compensatory mechanism to counteract arterial

REGULATION OF ARTERIAL TONE IN HYPERTENSION
BY VASCULAR MEMBRANE MECHANISMS

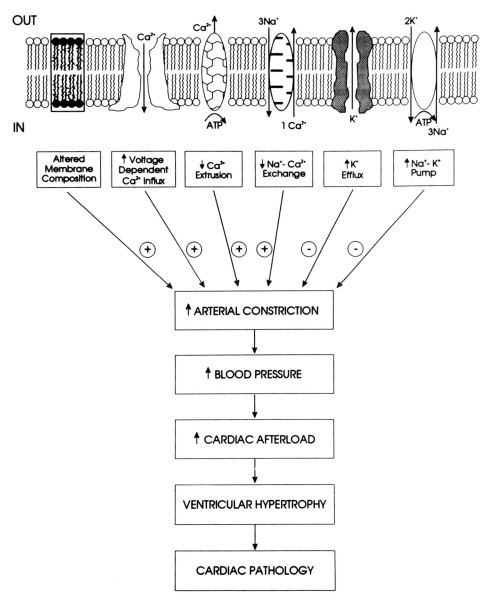

Fig. 53-2. Diagrammatic representation of the effect of vascular membrane mechanisms on regulation of arterial tone in hypertension. As depicted in the figure, the balance between positive and negative modulators of membrane excitation leads to an increased arterial constriction in hypertension. The resultant elevated peripheral resistance may be a predisposing factor of cardiac pathology.

contraction {12–14}. Notwithstanding the less-understood modulatory roles of Na^+ and Cl^- flux on arterial reactivity, the counterbalance between voltage-dependent Ca^{2+} influx and K^+ efflux will help to determine the level of arterial contraction in hypertension.

Are arterial muscle membrane components altered in hypertension?

The molecular basis of the enhanced movement of Na^+, K^+, Ca^{2+}, and Cl^- ions through arterial muscle membranes in hypertension is unknown {14,25}. However, ion channels and their immediate environment must be suspected. Along this reasoning, an altered phospholipid composition of the vascular muscle plasma membrane has been proposed as a primary mechanism by which membrane stability and fluidity may be reduced in hypertension {19–23}.

Remodeling of the membrane structure in hypertension with incorporation of less anionic phospholipid molecules may reduce membrane surface negative charge, providing less binding sites for stabilizing divalent cations and predisposing the arterial cell to excitation by lowering the threshold to physiological stimuli. This hypothesis is supported by measurements showing fewer Ca^{2+} binding sites in arterial muscle membranes in hypertension {19}, and reports that increases in levels of external Ca^{2+} normalize the enhanced ionic flux and vascular reactivity abnormalities in arteries from genetic and renal hypertensive rats {20–23}. A decreased binding of Ca^{2+} in erythrocyte membranes also has been reported in hypertensive patients, and in normotensive patients with family histories of hypertension {24}. Furthermore, decreased membrane fluidity is correlated with an augmented Ca^{2+} influx in arterial muscle cells, suggesting that changes in vascular membrane phospholipid composition in hypertension favor Ca^{2+} influx and activation of arterial smooth muscle {25–27}.

The enhanced ionic permeability of arterial muscle membranes in hypertension also could be attributed to changes in ion channel molecules or regulation {14}. These mechanisms will be discussed as they appear in the text of this chapter, but are briefly listed here for initial consideration. First, a higher density of membrane channels (more ion channels per given membrane surface area) could increase arterial membrane permeability in hypertension. Second, the channel molecular pore structure per se may be altered, with channel types characterized by higher unitary conductances or open state probabilities permitting more ionic flux across arterial membranes. Third, the regulation of ion channels by membrane voltage or cytosolic mediators of channel activity may be altered, promoting an enhanced open state of existing membrane pathways.

Does enhanced calcium influx activate arterial muscle in hypertension?

There is growing experimental evidence that Ca^{2+} influx across that arterial sarcolemma is increased in hypertension, providing a higher level of activator Ca^{2+} for arterial muscle contraction. In particular, the enhanced arterial reactivity in hypertension appears to depend on Ca^{2+} influx through "L-type", voltage-dependent Ca^{2+} channels (VDCCs) in the arterial plasma membrane {11}. L-type VDCCs, named for their conductance of a "long-lasting" Ca^{2+} current in patch-clamp studies {28,29}, provide activator Ca^{2+} for excitation-contraction coupling {12} and refilling of intracellular Ca^{2+} stores in arterial muscle cells {18}. Notably, L-type channels appear to be the predominant VDCC type in most arterial muscle mem-

branes, including those from smaller resistance vessels {30–39}. These Ca^{2+} channels are blocked by the clinically available, organic calcium channel blockers, such as nifedipine, verapamil, and diltiazem {29,40–43}.

In rat models of hypertension, tension-recording studies have implicated an enhanced Ca^{2+} influx through L-type VDCCs as a mechanism for augmented vascular reactivity. In the absence of vasoactive stimuli, aortic and carotid arteries from spontaneously hypertensive rats (SHR) develop a Ca^{2+}-dependent active tone after application of passive stretch. This activation is reversed by Ca^{2+}-free solution or chelation of external Ca^{2+} by ethylene glycol-tetraacetic acid (EGTA) {44–46}. Similar results have been reported in femoral arteries from younger, 6-week-old SHR {47}. In this preparation, passive stretch also evoked a Ca^{2+}-dependent active tone, which was reversed by nifedipine-induced block of L-type VDCCs. This apparent increase in nifedipine-sensitive Ca^{2+} influx in arterial muscle from young SHR suggests that enhanced Ca^{2+} current through L-type VDCCs may be an early vascular change in the development of hypertension. However, it is unclear from the latter study if the augmented Ca^{2+} permeability of SHR arterial membranes preceded or was a consequence of high blood pressure, since mean arterial pressure in the 6-week-old SHR was elevated by 20 mmHg compared to age-matched WKY rats.

Functional studies also indicate that L-type Ca^{2+} current may be amplified during activation of SHR arterial muscle. Femoral, caudal, and carotid arteries from SHR contract with greater sensitivity to depolarizing agonists than WKY arteries, suggesting that the same depolarizing stimulus results in augmented Ca^{2+} influx through VDCCs in SHR membranes {44–53}. For example, the KCl concentrations for half-maximal contraction (ED_{50}) of SHR carotid arteries were 25 mM compared to 37 mM in WKY {44}. Similarly, in isolated rat caudal arterial cells, the ED_{50} values for KCl-induced contraction were 30 mM in SHR and 38 mM in WKY {51}. However, this may not be a universal finding, since although large SHR mesenteric arteries also show an enhanced contractile sensitivity to KCl {49}, KCl dose-response curves reportedly are comparable between WKY and SHR small (100–200 μm) mesenteric resistance vessels {54}. Thus, while there is functional evidence for abnormal Ca^{2+} influx in vascular muscle in hypertension, determining the time course and distribution of abnormalities will require further study in a variety of blood vessels.

A more depolarized membrane potential sometimes is cited as a cause of augmented voltage-dependent Ca^{2+} influx in arteries obtained from hypertensive animals {55,56}. However, comparison of membrane potential values between isolated arterial muscle cells and unpressurized vascular segments from normotensive and hypertensive animals does not support this contention {11, 57–63}. Resting membrane potentials in isolated arterial segments and cells from SHR, Dahl, and DOCA rat models of hypertension range between −50 and −56 mV, comparable to membrane potentials in similar in vitro preparations from age-matched control rats {57–63}. This is not to imply, however, that membrane potentials are the same between in situ arteries exposed to different blood pressure levels in the intact cardiovascular system {61,64–66}. Rather, recent microelectrode measurements in intact vascular beds suggest that a combination of enhanced sympathetic neural output and intraluminal pressurization reduces transmembrane potentials of in situ arteries, and the arterial membrane depolarization is more pronounced in hypertension. For example, resting membrane potential of in situ mesenteric arteries is $-43\,mV$ in WKY compared to $-38\,mV$ in SHR, showing a more depolarized membrane potential in arteries of the hypertensive strain {61,64,65}. Similarly, small cremaster arteries of hypertensive reduced renal mass (RRM) rats exposed to in vivo endogenous physical, humoral, and neurogenic influences show a membrane potential of $-40\,mV$ compared to $-44\,mV$ in intact control vessels {66}.

Thus in the hypertensive animal heightened depolarization of in situ arterial muscle may further activate L-type VDCCs and accentuate Ca^{2+} influx into vascular muscle cells. It could be argued that the final consequence in the integrated system would be an enhanced voltage-dependent Ca^{2+} influx into arterial muscle cells and an increased peripheral vascular resistance. In this context, it is interesting to note that the diameters of resistance vessels in the SHR renal vasculature are 18–35% smaller than in WKY, and that this difference is eliminated by a low-calcium media {67}. This observation suggests that elevated Ca^{2+}-dependent vascular tone, rather than structural changes, may account for smaller microvascular diameters in SHR. Similarly, the L-type VDCC blocker verapamil, but not the nonspecific vasodilator nitroprusside, dilates the forearm vasculature of hypertensive subjects more than normotensive controls {68,69}. In the integrated system, blockers of L-type VDCCs decrease blood pressure to a greater extent in SHR, renal, and salt-sensitive rat models of hypertension than in normotensive animals {69–75}. Clinically approved, L-type VDCC blockers also reduce blood pressure more in hypertensive than normotensive human subjects {76–82}. Together, these data provide compelling evidence that abnormal Ca^{2+} influx across arterial muscle membranes is correlated with the increased vascular tone observed in animal and human hypertension.

Despite functional indications that Ca^{2+} influx through L-type VDCCs augments arterial responsiveness in hypertension {42}, few patch-clamp studies have compared L-type Ca^{2+} current between cardiovascular membranes from normotensive and hypertensive animals. However, an initial study in azygos vein cells from 1- to 3-day-old WKY and SHR has provided evidence that the amplitude of whole-cell, L-type Ca^{2+} current is greater in SHR than WKY vascular membranes {83}. Since the vascular muscle cells for this study were obtained from the low-pressure venous side of the circulation in neonatal rats, this implied that the augmented L-type Ca^{2+} current was genetically determined rather than induced by neural factors or elevated blood pressure. Similar to this finding in vascular muscle, an increased Ca^{2+} current density also has been

reported in cardiac myocytes from rats with renovascular hypertension {84}. However, the single-channel mechanisms contributing to augmented, macroscopic Ca^{2+} current have not been explored, and further studies are needed to determine the molecular nature of L-type VDCC alterations in hypertension.

Are Ca^{2+} transporters in the arterial sarcolemma altered in hypertension?

In addition to Ca^{2+} influx across the plasma membrane, multiple other Ca^{2+} regulatory mechanisms may influence levels of cytosolic free Ca^{2+} concentration ($[Ca]_i$) and arterial contraction {85}. Of these, several reports indicate that the ATP-regulated Ca^{2+} pump of the plasma membrane, which ejects Ca^{2+} from the cell to buffer changes in $[Ca]_i$, may show a reduced activity in hypertension. Early studies have shown that isolated arterial membrane fractions from genetic and salt-sensitive SHR show decreased ATP-dependent membrane transport of Ca^{2+}, compared to membranes from normotensive control animals {86–89}. This apparent reduction in Ca^{2+} extrusion may be related to the slower relaxation rate of arterial muscle from hypertensive animals, although more recent evidence proposes that the thicker smooth muscle cell layer in vascular preparations exposed to a high pressure load may account in part for the delayed vascular muscle relaxation in hypertension {90,91}. In other studies, a compromised calmodulin-stimulated Ca^{2+}-ATPase activity has been reported in erythrocytes from SHR and Milan genetically hypertensive rats {92–94} and in platelets of patients with essential hypertension {95}. The finding of a reduced Ca^{2+} pump activity in 3-week-old SHR suggests that Ca^{2+} pump alterations could stem from an intrinsic membrane defect in genetic hypertension. If this reduced Ca^{2+} pump activity in erythrocytes also was found to pertain to arterial muscle cells from the same 3-week-old SHR, it could be viewed as a potential etiological factor in the pathogenesis of high blood pressure. Similar to alterations reported in other membrane transport pathways in hypertension, it is unclear if altered Ca^{2+} pump function is inherent to the pump molecule or secondary to an altered membrane composition, since Ca^{2+} pump activity is sensitive to its phospholipid environment {96}. The recent purification of this pump and identification of some of its functional domains may provide the opportunity to examine possible molecular alterations in hypertension {96}.

A second possible mechanism of altered Ca^{2+} movement across the vascular muscle plasma membrane in hypertension is the Na^+-Ca^{2+} countertransport system. This passive but electrogenic membrane transport system likely exchanges at least three extracellular Na^+ ions for one intracellular Ca^{2+} ion in cardiac myocytes and other cell types {60}. The effectiveness of the Na^+-Ca^{2+} countertransporter is proportional to the transmembrane Na^+ gradient, and thus under physiological conditions of low intracellular free Na^+ concentration ($[Na]_i$), this countertransport mechanism transfers Ca^{2+} out of the cell with the greatest effectiveness. However, under conditions in which $[Na]_i$ is increased, reduced Na^+-Ca^{2+} counter-transport would lead to a buildup of $[Ca]_i$ to promote vascular muscle contraction. It is hypothesized that Na^+-Ca^{2+} countertransporter activity is compromised by rises in arterial $[Na]_i$ in hypertension, which in the absence of other regulatory mechanisms would increase $[Ca]_i$ and concurrently induce membrane hyperpolarization. The functional impact of these changes on arterial reactivity has been difficult to assess, however, since the capacity of the Na^+-Ca^{2+} countertransporter is small in vascular muscle compared to other muscle cell types {97}. Although there are reports that impaired Ca^{2+} extrusion by this mechanism may maintain arterial contraction in hypertension {98,99}, it is unclear if such a mechanism has physiological importance in the smaller resistance arteries {97,100,104}.

Despite the emphasis on arterial Ca^{2+} regulatory mechanisms in hypertension, the relationship between $[Ca]_i$ and the increased arterial reactivity of hypertension has not been clarified. Small increases in $[Ca]_i$ have been reported at 37°C in aortic muscle cells exposed to high blood pressure in SHR {102} and aortic-coarcted Sprague-Dawley rats {103}. Also, an elevated membrane permeability to Ca^{2+} has been implicated in SHR arterial membranes which may promote at least localized rises in $[Ca]_i$ {104}. However, another study has detected no difference in $[Ca]_i$ between WKY and SHR arteriole muscle cells {105}. Measurements of localized Ca^{2+} in vascular muscle cells may be required to resolve whether possible alterations in $[Ca]_i$ occur in hypertension {11}. Also, although membrane ion channel and transport mechanisms are notable controllers of $[Ca]_i$, the final level of arterial muscle tone in hypertension involves a more complicated network of events. Smooth muscle contraction is not only dependent on the level of $[Ca]_i$ {106}, but also on other cellular pathways that may be affected by the hypertensive disease state. For example, receptor-initiated contraction enabled by the inositol triphosphate (IP_3) signaling pathway is reportedly enhanced in hypertension, implying alterations in intracellular Ca^{2+} mobilization independent of membrane ionic events {107–110}. At the level of the contractile apparatus, an enhanced sensitivity of arterial contractile proteins to $[Ca]_i$ has been reported in some {111,112}, but not all {113,114}, animal models of hypertension, suggesting that biochemical events distal to membrane ion transport may further modulate the degree of arterial contraction. Thus even at the level of the single arterial cell, there are multiple endogenous modulators of Ca^{2+}-dependent contraction that will interact to determine the final level of vasoconstriction in hypertension.

Does augmented K^+ efflux buffer arterial excitability in hypertension?

Potassium efflux through K^+ channels in the arterial sarcolemma causes membrane hyperpolarization, which limits voltage-dependent Ca^{2+} influx and buffers the arterial contractile response to membrane excitation {12–14,17,115,116}. A diversity of K^+ channel types contribute to this attenuation of electrical excitability in vascular muscle cells {117,118}, including Ca^{2+}-dependent K^+ channels {119–126}, delayed rectifier K^+ channels {124, 127,128}, fast transient K^+ channels {124,127}, inward rectifier K^+ channels {129,130}, and ATP-sensitive K^+ channels {12,131–133}. Of these K^+ channel types, the large-conductance Ca^{2+}-dependent K^+ channel [$I_{K(Ca)}$ channel] may primarily control arterial excitability during hypertension {12–14}. The $I_{K(Ca)}$ channel appears to be ubiquitous to most smooth muscle membranes {121,125, 134–138}, and is activated by membrane depolarization and/or rises in $[Ca]_i$ within the physiological range {14, 121,122,137}. The role of this channel is to regulate the tonic contractile tone of arterial smooth muscle by buffering membrane depolarization and the influx of activator Ca^{2+}.

Recent evidence suggests that the membrane mechanism for enhanced arterial K^+ permeability in hypertension is increased K^+ efflux through $I_{K(Ca)}$ channels {12–14}. First, in some vascular muscle cells, patch-clamp studies show that K^+ efflux through single $I_{K(Ca)}$ channels is the predominant pathway for transmembrane K^+ flux at resting membrane potential {120–122,135}. Second, nifedipine normalizes K^+ turnover in arteries of hypertensive rats, implicating a Ca^{2+}-dependent pathway as the route for augmented K^+ efflux {139}. Third, recent patch-clamp studies provide direct evidence that $I_{K(Ca)}$ channels are activated by acute and chronic blood pressure rises, suggesting that this ion channel may act to buffer the increased arterial tone of hypertension {12–14}.

The physiological potential of the $I_{K(Ca)}$ channel to regulate arterial reactivity has been documented in perfused, pressurized arteries. In pressurized rabbit cerebral and rat skeletal muscle arteries, pharmacological block of $I_{K(Ca)}$ channels results in profound arterial constriction, demonstrating the strong buffering power of the $I_{K(Ca)}$ channel in controlling arterial tone {12,13}. The mechanism for $I_{K(Ca)}$ channel activation in intact arteries is likely membrane depolarization and increases in $[Ca]_i$ during pressurization, which increase the open-state probability of this voltage and Ca^{2+}-sensitive K^+ channel in the arterial plasma membrane. The resulting K^+ efflux would counteract pressure-induced constriction of small arteries, providing a compensatory mechanism at the vascular muscle cell level to control local arterial tone {12,13}.

Other studies suggest that the $I_{K(Ca)}$ channel also regulates arterial excitation in chronic hypertension {53, 140}. For example, rat aortas exposed to high pressure after inter-renal aortic coarctation show dose-dependent contractions in response to $I_{K(Ca)}$ channel blockers, whereas aortic segments exposed to normal blood pressure do not {53}. Carotid and aortic arteries obtained from adult SHR, but not from WKY, also constrict after $I_{K(Ca)}$ channel block, suggesting that K^+ efflux through this membrane pathway is required for maintaining vascular relaxation in the face of a chronically increased blood pressure {53,140}. Findings from patch-clamp studies concur with activation of arterial $I_{K(Ca)}$ channels in response to chronic hypertension. For example, aortic muscle membranes exposed to chronically high in situ blood pressure in SHR or aortic-coarcted rats have a higher whole-cell membrane $I_{K(Ca)}$ current density than arterial membranes exposed to normal blood pressure {53}. An enhanced Ca^{2+}-dependent K^+ current also has been demonstrated at the single-channel level in cell-attached patches of SHR aortic muscle membranes. In this preparation, where the $I_{K(Ca)}$ channels were exposed to normal cytosolic mediators at resting membrane potential, $I_{K(Ca)}$ channels showed a fivefold higher open-state probability in SHR than WKY vascular muscle.

The mechanism for this enhanced $I_{K(Ca)}$ channel open state in arterial membranes in hypertension was explored recently in inside-out membrane patches of SHR and WKY aorta {14}. Single-channel conductance and pharmacological sensitivity of the $I_{K(Ca)}$ channel were the same between SHR and WKY aortic muscle membranes, suggesting that at least some functional domains of the $I_{K(Ca)}$ channel were unaltered in hypertension. However, $I_{K(Ca)}$ channels showed an increased Ca^{2+} sensitivity in SHR arteries, suggesting that at the same membrane potential and $[Ca]_i$ level, SHR $I_{K(Ca)}$ channels show a higher open state probability and permit more K^+ efflux than similar K^+ channels in WKY. Thus altered calcium regulation of the arterial $I_{K(Ca)}$ channel, possibly mediated by an altered membrane phospholipid environment in hypertension, may account for the enhanced K^+ efflux reported by earlier investigators using radioisotope methods {4–10}. Further studies will help to pinpoint whether membrane $I_{K(Ca)}$ alterations extend to the small-resistance vessels in hypertension, and if other K^+ channel types are implicated in the modulation of arterial tone during high blood pressure.

Does the electrogenic Na^+-K^+ pump counteract arterial muscle depolarization in hypertension?

The level of resting membrane potential in arterial muscle is determined primarily by the open-state probability of membrane K^+ channels and the activity of the ATP-dependent, Na^+-K^+ pump. This Na^+-K^+ pump transports $2 K^+$ ions into the cell in electrogenic exchange for $3 Na^+$ ions {141}, thus contributing between 1 and $20\,mV$ of voltage to resting membrane potential in different vascular muscle cell types {60}. The hyperpolarizing current produced by the Na^+-K^+ pump may be less than that generated by K^+ efflux across the arterial sarcolemma, but its contribution to resting membrane potential likely still modulates vascular tone, at least in some circumstances. For example, pharmacological block of the Na^+-K^+ pump by cardiac glycosides increases peripheral vascular resistance in intact vascular beds, implying that active Na^+-K^+ exchange counteracts vascular smooth muscle depolarization and contraction in pressurized blood vessels {142,143}.

Two contradictory theories have been advanced to explain how the Na^+-K^+ pump is implicated in hypertension. First, as reviewed elsewhere {144}, an endogenous, circulating inhibitor of the Na^+-K^+ pump may be expressed in hypertension. This circulating inhibitor would act on the renal tubules to reduce reabsorption of Na^+, and thus counteract hypertension by lowering circulating plasma volume. However, inhibition of Na^+-K^+ exchange concurrently would promote arterial constriction and increased vascular tone in hypertension by causing arterial depolar-

ization and voltage-dependent Ca^{2+} influx and permitting $[Ca]_i$ to rise {143,145}.

In contradiction to this perspective of the Na^+-K^+ pump as an etiological factor in hypertension, there is substantial evidence that the arterial muscle Na^+-K^+ pump is activated during hypertension to compensate for the increased inward leak of Na^+ {146}. Caudal arteries from SHR show an increased ouabain-sensitive ^{86}Rb uptake compared to arteries from WKY, indicative of a greater Na^+-K^+ pump capacity in arterial muscle membranes in genetic hypertension {147}. Microelectrode studies also suggest that the Na^+-K^+ pump makes a larger contribution to resting membrane potential in SHR than in WKY caudal and cerebral arteries, as demonstrated by a greater depolarization of SHR resting membrane potential during Na^+-K^+ pump inhibition by low temperature, K^+-free solution, or ouabain {148,149}. Using potassium-induced relaxation of arterial muscle as a functional marker of Na^+-K^+ pump activity, several investigators also have reported enhanced Na^+-K^+ pump electrogenesis in SHR arteries. In these experiments, the Na^+-K^+ pump initially was blocked by exposure to K^+-free solution, and then acutely activated by reintroducing potassium to the incubation medium. The magnitude of the resulting K^+-induced relaxation was considered as an index of Na^+-K^+ pump activity, although this index may not be applicable to all arterial muscle types {150,151}. However, in caudal artery of SHR and in arteries and veins of renal hypertensive rats, where Na^+-K^+ pump activity has been correlated with K^+-induced relaxation {152}, an enhanced K^+-induced relaxation has been reported {153,154}. Since estimation of Na^+-K^+ pump sites using ^{3}H-ouabain binding has shown no difference in pump site density between arterial muscle membranes of SHR and WKY {155,156}, it appears that an altered Na^+-K^+ pump molecule, or altered regulation of the pump site, must account for its enhanced capacity during hypertension.

A clear interpretation of the role of the Na^+-K^+ pump in the pathogenesis of hypertension is difficult, however {157}. Comparison between SHR and WKY portal veins shows no difference in the electrogenic pump contribution to resting membrane potential {158}, implying that altered Na^+-K^+ electrogenesis is not ubiquitous to all vascular beds during chronic hypertension. Furthermore, more recent studies in SHR small mesenteric arteries have shown less ouabain-sensitive depolarization than in similar WKY arteries {159}. In the same preparations, the amplitude of ouabain-sensitive [22]Na efflux is similar in arteries from both rat strains {155}. Thus, although the stimulation of the Na^+-K^+ pump causes hyperpolarization and relaxation in many vascular muscle cell types, it is unclear if this counter-regulatory mechanism buffers arterial depolarization and contraction in hypertension.

SUMMARY

Arterial muscle membranes from many different rat models of hypertension show an increased permeability to Na^+, K^+, Ca^{2+}, and Cl^- ions. This observation has sparked the theory that arterial membrane alterations may represent a "universal defect" of hypertension. Due to the lack of evidence for an important influence of Cl^- flux on arterial reactivity, this chapter primarily reviewed vascular membrane mechanisms that regulate transmembrane Ca^{2+}, K^+, and Na^+ movements in hypertension. Arterial muscle membrane changes associated with high blood pressure may include altered membrane molecular components, as well as modified passive and active ion transport function. Further characterization of these membrane mechanisms will help us to comprehend the cellular basis of altered arterial muscle responsiveness in hypertension.

There is compelling laboratory and clinical evidence that Ca^{2+} influx is enhanced in arterial smooth muscle in hypertension. Remodeling of the phospholipid composition of the vascular plasma membrane to favor Ca^{2+} influx may contribute to arterial smooth muscle activation during hypertension. A depolarized membrane potential of in situ small arteries also may enhance voltage-dependent Ca^{2+} influx and arterial constriction in the intact circulation of hypertensive animals. In addition, other Ca^{2+} regulatory mechanisms may modify the level of $[Ca]_i$ and arterial contraction in hypertension. Evidence has been presented that active extrusion of Ca^{2+} from the arterial muscle cell is reduced in hypertension, thereby permitting increased $[Ca]_i$. A reduced activity of the Na^+-Ca^{2+} countertransporter also could impair Ca^{2+} extrusion, although a functional role for this exchange mechanism in small-resistance arteries has not been documented.

In response to the excitatory Ca^{2+} mechanisms of hypertension, the arterial muscle membrane likely activates other distinct, counter-regulatory processes to buffer further rises in $[Ca]_i$. Patch-clamp studies have demonstrated that a large-conductance, Ca^{2+}-sensitive K^+ channel [$I_{K(Ca)}$ channel] in the arterial muscle membrane is activated by acute or chronic increases in blood pressure. The enhanced open state of this channel would permit increased K^+ efflux, which may counteract pressure-induced excitation and constriction of arterial muscle during hypertension. Another putative compensatory mechanism for controlling arterial contraction during hypertension is the membrane Na^+-K^+ pump, which may show higher electrogenic activity during hypertension. However, despite the power of these membrane counter-regulatory mechanisms in controlling vascular smooth muscle responsiveness, they apparently only partially repress arterial excitation during hypertension, since elevated peripheral vascular resistance is found in this disease.

The vascular muscle membrane mechanisms discussed in this chapter likely represent only an incomplete list of the changes associated with the arterial smooth muscle membrane in hypertension. However, at our existing level of knowledge, these alterations in arterial membrane ion channels and ion transport mechanisms appear to be the most attractive to explain the increased arterial tone of hypertension. The future is bright with the anticipation that understanding the molecular basis of these vascular muscle changes ultimately will provide for the rational management of high blood pressure, and consequently the prevention of cardiac disorders associated with this disease.

ACKNOWLEDGMENTS

Supported by grants HL-HL40474 and PPG HL-29587 (to NJR), and HL-38645 and HL-38537 (to KH) from the National Institutes of Health.

REFERENCES

1. Tarazi RC, Levy MN: Cardiac responses to increased after-load. *Hypertension* 4(Suppl 2):II8–II18, 1982.
2. Schieken RM, Clark WR, Lauer RM: Left ventricular hypertrophy in children with blood pressures in the upper quintile of the distribution: The Muscatine Study. *Hypertension* 3:669–675, 1981.
3. Gonzales OA, Abboud FM: American Heart Association Annual Report, 1991.
4. Jones AW: Altered ion transport in vascular smooth muscle from spontaneously hypertensive rats. *Circ Res* 33:563–572, 1973.
5. Jones AW: Reactivity of ion fluxes in rat aorta during hypertension and circulatory control. *Fed Proc* 33:133–137, 1974.
6. Jones AW, Hart RG: Altered ion transport in aortic smooth muscle during deoxycorticosterone acetate hypertension in the rat. *Circ Res* 37:333–341, 1975.
7. Friedman SM, Friedman CL: Cell permeability, sodium transport, and the hypertensive process in the rat. *Circ Res* 39:433–441, 1976.
8. Garwitz ET, Jones AW: Aldosterone infusion into the rat and dose dependent changes in blood pressure and arterial ionic transport. *Hypertension* 4:374–381, 1982.
9. Garwitz ET, Jones AW: Altered arterial ion transport and its reversal in the aldosterone hypertensive rat. *Am J Physiol* 243:H929–H933, 1982.
10. Jones AW: Arterial tissue cations. In: Genest J, Kuchel O, Hamet P, Cantin M (eds) *Hypertension, Physiology and Treatment.* New York: McGraw-Hill, 1983, pp 488–497.
11. Rusch NJ, Hermsmeyer K: Vascular muscle calcium channels in hypertension. In: Coca A (ed) *Ionic Transport in Hypertension: New Perspectives.* Boca Raton, FL: CRC Press, 1993, pp 197–227.
12. Brayden JE, Nelson MT: Regulation of arterial tone by activation of calcium-dependent potassium channels. *Science* 256:532–535, 1992.
13. Berczi V, Stekiel WJ, Contney SC, Rusch NJ: Pressure-induced activation of membrane K^+ current in rat saphenous artery. *Hypertension* 19:725–729, 1992.
14. England SK, Wooldridge TA, Stekiel WJ, Rusch NJ: Enhanced single-channel K^+ current in arterial membranes from genetically hypertensive rats. *Am J Physiol* 264:H1337–H1345, 1993.
15. Folkow B: Physiological aspects of primary hypertension. *Physiol Rev* 62:347–504, 1982.
16. Kwan CY: Dysfunction of calcium handling by smooth muscle in hypertension. *Can J Physiol Pharmacol* 63:366–374, 1985.
17. Hermsmeyer K, Trapani A, Abel PW: Membrane-potential dependent tension in vascular muscle. In: Vanhoutte PM, Leusen I (eds) *Vasodilation.* New York: Raven Press, 1981, pp 273–284.
18. Hynes MR, Duling BR: Ca^{2+} sensitivity of isolated arterioles

from the hamster cheek pouch. *Am J Physiol* 260: H355–H361, 1991.

19. Postnov YV, Orlov SN: Cell membrane alteration as a source of primary hypertension. *J Hypertens* 2:1–6, 1984.

20. Bruner CA, Webb RC, Bohr DF: Vascular reactivity and membrane stabilizing effect of calcium in spontaneously hypertensive rats. In: Aoki K, Frohlich ED (eds) *Calcium in Essential Hypertension*. San Diego: Academic Press, 1989, pp 276–305.

21. Bohr DR: Cell membrane in hypertension. *NIPS* 4:85–88, 1989.

22. Bohr DR, Dominiczak AF, Webb RC: Pathophysiology of the vasculature in hypertension. *Hypertension* 18:III69–III75, 1991.

23. Rinaldi G, Bohr DR: Potassium-induced relaxation of arteries in hypertension: Modulation by extracellular calcium. *Am J Physiol* 256:H707–H712, 1989.

24. Bing RF, Heagerty AM, Swales JD: Membrane handling of calcium in essential hypertension. *J Hypertens* 5:S29–S35, 1987.

25. Tulenko TN, Bialecki R, Gleason MM, D'Angelo G: Ion channels, membrane lipids and cholesterol: A role for membrane lipid domains in arterial function. In: Colatsky TJ (ed) *Potassium Channels: Basic Function and Therapeutic Aspects*. New York: Alan R. Liss, 1990, pp 187–203.

26. Gleason MM, Medow MS, Tulenko TN: Excess membrane cholesterol alters calcium movements, cytosolic calcium levels, and membrane fluidity in arterial smooth muscle cells. *Circ Res* 69:216–227, 1991.

27. Cox RH, Tulenko TN: Altered excitation-contraction coupling in hypertension: Role of plasma membrane phospholipids and ion channels. In: Moreland RS (ed) *Regulation of Smooth Muscle Contraction*. New York: Plenum Press, 1991, pp 273–290.

28. Tsien RW: Calcium channels: Mechanism of selectivity, permeation, and block. *Ann Rev Biophys Chem* 16:265–290, 1987.

29. Bean BP: Pharmacology of calcium channels in cardiac muscle, vascular muscle and neurons. *Am J Hypertens* 4:406S–411S, 1991.

30. Bean BP, Sturek M, Puga A, Hermsmeyer K: Calcium channels in muscle cells isolated from rat mesenteric arteries: Modulation by dihydropyridine drugs. *Circ Res* 59:229–235, 1986.

31. Loirand G, Pacaud P, Mironneau C, Mironneau J: Evidence for two distinct calcium channels in rat vascular smooth muscle cells in short-term primary culture. *Pflügers Arch* 407:566–568, 1986.

32. Hermsmeyer K: Calcium alterations in resistance arteries in hypertension. In: Mulvany MJ, et al. (eds) *Resistance Arteries Structure and Function*. Amsterdam, Excerpta Medica, 1991, pp 322–324.

33. Yatani A, Seidel CL, Allen J, Brown AM: Whole-cell and single-channel calcium currents of isolated smooth muscle cells from saphenous vein. *Circ Res* 60:523–533, 1987.

34. Benham CD, Hess P, Tsien RW: Two types of calcium channels in single smooth muscle cells from rabbit ear artery studied with whole-cell and single-channel recordings. *Circ Res* 61:I10–I16, 1987.

35. Sturek M, Hermsmeyer K: Calcium and sodium channels in spontaneously contracting vascular muscle cells. *Science* 233:475–478, 1986.

36. Bean BP, Sturek M, Puga A, Hermsmeyer K: Nitrendipine block of channels in cardiac and vascular muscle. *J Cardiovasc Pharmacol* 9:517–524, 1987.

37. Oike M, Inoue Y, Kitamura K, Kuriyama, H: Dual action of

FRC8653, a novel dihydropyridine derivative, on the Ba^{2+} current recorded from the rabbit basilar artery. *Circ Res* 67:993–1006, 1990.

38. Ganitkevich VY, Isenberg G: Contribution of two types of calcium channels to membrane conductance of single myocytes from guinea-pig coronary artery. *J Physiol* 426:19–42, 1990.

39. Matsuda JJ, Volk KA, Shibata EF: Calcium currents in isolated rabbit arterial smooth muscle myocytes. *J Physiol* 427:657–680, 1990.

40. Hermsmeyer K, Sturek M, Rusch NJ: Nitrendipine inhibition of calcium current in rat vascular muscle cells. *J Cardiovasc Pharmacol* 12:S100–S103, 1988.

41. Nelson MT, Worley JF: Dihydropyridine inhibition of single calcium channels and contraction in rabbit mesenteric artery depends on voltage. *J Physiol* 412:65–90, 1989.

42. Hermsmeyer K, Sturek M, Rusch NJ: Calcium channel modulation by dihydropyridines in vascular muscle. *Ann NY Acad Sci* 522:25–31, 1988.

43. Worley JF, Quayle JM, Standen NB, Nelson MT: Regulation of single calcium channels in cerebral arteries by voltage, serotonin and dihydropyridines. *Am J Physiol* 261:H1951–H1960, 1991.

44. Noon JP, Rice PJ, Baldessarini RJ: Calcium leakage as a cause of high resting tension in vascular smooth muscle from the spontaneously hypertensive rat. *Proc Natl Acad Sci USA* 75:1605–1607, 1978.

45. Fitzpatrick DF, Szentivanyi A: The relationship between increased myogenic tone and hyporesponsiveness in vascular smooth muscle of spontaneously hypertensive rats. *Clin Exp Hypertens* 2:1023–1037, 1980.

46. Bruner CA, Webb RC: Increased vascular reactivity to Bay K 8644 in genetic hypertension. *Pharmacology* 41:24–35, 1990.

47. Aoki K, Asano M: Effects of Bay K 8644 and nifedipine on femoral arteries of spontaneously hypertensive rats. *Br J Pharmac* 88:221–230, 1986.

48. Aoki K, Asano M: Increased responsiveness to calcium agonist BAY K 8644 and calcium antagonist nifedipine in femoral arteries of spontaneously hypertensive rats. *J Cardiovasc Pharmacol* 10:S62–S64, 1987.

49. MacKay MJ, Cheung DW: Increased reactivity in the mesenteric artery of spontaneously hypertensive rats to phorbol ester. *Biochem Biophys Res Commun* 145:1105–1111, 1987.

50. Thompson LP, Bruner CA, Lamb FS, King CM, Webb RC: Calcium influx and vascular reactivity in systemic hypertension. *Am J Cardiol* 59:29A–34A, 1987.

51. Bolzon BJ, Cheung DW: Isolation and characterization of single vascular smooth muscle cells from spontaneously hypertensive rats. *Hypertension* 14:137–144, 1989.

52. Storm DS, Turla MB, Todd KM, Webb RC: Calcium and contractile responses to phorbol esters and the calcium channel agonist, Bay K 8644, in arteries from hypertensive rats. *Am J Hypertens* 3:245S–248S, 1990.

53. Rusch NJ, De Lucena RG, Wooldridge TA, England SK, Cowley AW: A Ca^{2+}-dependent K^+ current is enhanced in arterial membranes of hypertensive rats. *Hypertension* 19:301–307, 1992.

54. Mulvany MJ, Nyborg N: An increased calcium sensitivity of mesenteric resistance vessels in young and adult spontaneously hypertensive rats. *Br J Pharmacol* 71:585–596, 1980.

55. Tomobe Y, Ishikawa T, Yanagisawa M, Kimura S, Masaki T, Goto K: Mechanisms of altered sensitivity to endothelin 1 between aortic smooth muscle of spontaneously hyperten-

sive and Wistar-Kyoto rats. *J Pharmacol Exp Ther* 257:
555–561, 1991.

56. Van de Voorde J, Vanheel B, Leusen I: Endothelium-dependent relaxation and hyperpolarization in aorta from control and renal hypertensive rats. *Circ Res* 70:1–8, 1992.

57. Stekiel WJ: Electrophysiological mechanisms of force development by vascular smooth muscle membrane in hypertension. In: Lee EMKW (ed) *Blood Vessel Changes in Hypertension: Structure and Function.* Boca Raton, FL: CRC Press, 1989, pp 127–170.

58. Hermsmeyer K: Electrogenesis of increased norepinephrine sensitivity of arterial vascular muscle in hypertension. *Circ Res* 38:362–367, 1976.

59. Abel PW, Trapani A, Matsuki N, Ingram MJ, Ingram FD, Hermsmeyer K: Unaltered membrane properties of arterial muscle in Dahl strain genetic hypertension. *Am J Physiol* 241:H224–H227, 1981.

60. Hermsmeyer K: Electrogenic ion pumps and other determinants of membrane potential in vascular muscle (the 1982 Bowditch Lecture). *Physiologist* 25:454–465, 1982.

61. Stekiel WJ, Contney SJ, Lombard JH: Small vessel membrane potential, sympathetic input, and electrogenic pump rate in SHR. *Am J Physiol* 250:C547–C556, 1986.

62. Longhurst PA, Rice PJ, Taylor DA, Fleming WW: Sensitivity of caudal arteries and the mesenteric vascular bed to norepinephrine in DOCA-salt hypertension. *Hypertension* 12:133–142, 1988.

63. Lamb FS, Webb RC: Regenerative electrical activity and arterial contraction in hypertensive rats. *Hypertension* 13:70–76, 1989.

64. Stekiel WJ, Contney SJ, Lombard JH: Sympathetic neural control of vascular muscle in reduced renal mass hypertension. *Hypertension* 17:1185–1191, 1991.

65. Rusch NJ, Stekiel WJ: Ionic channels of vascular smooth muscle in hypertension. In: Cox RH (ed) *Cellular and Molecular Mechanisms of Hypertension.* New York: Plenum Press, 1991, pp 1–7.

66. Stekiel WJ, Contney SJ, Rusch NJ: Altered β-receptor control of in situ membrane potential in hypertensive rats. Hypertension 21:1005–1009, 1993.

67. Gebremedhin D, Fenoy FJ, Harder DR, Roman RJ: Enhanced vascular tone in the renal vasculature of spontaneously hypertensive rats. *Hypertension* 16:648–654, 1990.

68. Robinson BF, Dobbs RJ, Bayley S: Response of forearm resistance vessels to verapamil and sodium nitroprusside in normotensive and hypertensive men: Evidence for a functional abnormality of vascular smooth muscle in primary hypertension. *Clin Sci* 63:33–42, 1982.

69. Hulthen UL, Bolli P, Amann FW, Kiowski W, Bühler FR: Enhanced vasodilatation in essential hypertension by calcium channel blockade with verapamil. *Hypertension* 4(Suppl): II26–II31, 1982.

70. Ishii H, Itoh K, Nose T: Different antihypertensive effects of nifedipine in conscious experimental hypertensive and normotensive rats. *Eur J Pharmacol* 64:21–29, 1980.

71. Garthoff S: Calcium antagonist nifedipine normalizes high blood pressure and prevents mortality in salt-loaded DS substrain of DAHL rats. *Eur J Pharmacol* 74:111–112, 1981.

72. Kubo T, Fujie K, Yamashita M, Misu Y: Antihypertensive effects of nifedipine on conscious normotensive and hypertensive rats. *J Pharm Dyn* 4:294–300, 1981.

73. Thievant P, Baranes J, Le Hegarat M, Clostre F, DeFeudis FV: Effects of diltiazem on renovascular-hypertensive and on normotensive rats. *Gen Pharmacol* 13:165–167, 1982.

74. Pedersen OL, Mikkelsen E, Jespersen LT: Treatment with verapamil reduces blood pressure and tends to normalize vascular responsiveness and ion transport in the spontaneously hypertensive rat. *J Cardiovasc Pharmacol* 4:S294–S297, 1982.

75. Narita H, Nagao T, Yabana H, Yamaguchi I: Hypotensive and diuretic actions of diltiazem in spontaneously hypertensive and Wistar Kyoto rats. *J Pharmacol Exp Ther* 227:472–477, 1983.

76. Takata Y, Hutchinson JS: Exaggerated hypotensive responses to calcium antagonists in spontaneously hypertensive rats. *Clin Exp Hypertens* A5:827–847, 1983.

77. Pedersen OL, Christensen NJ, Ramsch KD: Comparison of acute effects of nifedipine in normotensive and hypertensive man. *J Cardiovasc Pharmacol* 2:357–366, 1980.

78. Maeda K, Takasugi T, Tsukano Y, Tanaka Y, Shiota K: Clinical study of the hypotensive effect of diltiazem hydrochloride. *Int J Clin Pharmacol Ther* 19:47–55, 1981.

79. Aoki K, Kawaguchi Y, Sato K, Kondo S, Yamamoto M: Clinical and pharmacological properties of calcium antagonists in essential hypertension in humans and spontaneously hypertensive rats. *J Cardiovasc Pharmacol* 4:S298–S302, 1982.

80. Muiesan G, Agabiti-Rosei E, Castellano M, Alicandri Cl, Fariello R, Beschi M, Romanelli G: Antihypertensive and humoral effects of verapamil and nifedipine in essential hypertension. *J Cardiovasc Pharmacol* 4:S325–S329, 1982.

81. Lewis GRJ: Long-term results with verapamil in essential hypertension and its influence on serum lipids. *Am J Cardiol* 57:35D–38D, 1986.

82. Frishman W, Charlap S, Kimmel B, Saltzberg S, Stroh J, Weinberg P, Monuszko E, Wiezner J, Dorsa F, Pollack S, Strom J: Thrice daily administration of oral verapamil in the treatment of essential hypertension. *Arch Intern Med* 146:561–656, 1984.

83. Rusch NJ, Hermsmeyer K: Calcium currents are altered in the vascular muscle cell membrane of spontaneously hypertensive rats. *Circ Res* 63:997–1002, 1988.

84. Keung EC: Calcium current is increased in isolated adult myocytes from hypertrophied rat myocardium. *Circ Res* 64:753–763, 1989.

85. Ives HE: Ion transport defects and hypertension. Where is the link? *Hypertension* 14:590–596, 1989.

86. Wei J, Janis RA, Daniel EE: Calcium accumulation and enzymatic activities of subcellular fractions from aortas and ventricles of genetically hypertensive rats. *Circ Res* 39:133–140, 1976.

87. Kwan C, Belbech L, Daniel EE: Abnormal biochemistry of vascular smooth muscle plasma membrane as an important factor in the initiation and maintenance of hypertension in rats. *Blood Vessels* 16:259–268, 1978.

88. Kwan C, Belbeck L, Daniel EE: Abnormal biochemistry of vascular smooth muscle plasma membrane isolated from hypertensive rats. *Molecular Pharm* 17:137–140, 1980.

89. Kwan C, Daniel EE: Biochemical abnormalities of venous plasma membrane fraction isolated from spontaneously hypertensive rats. *Eur J Pharm* 75:321–324, 1981.

90. Sunano S, Shimada T, Moriyama K, Shimamura K: Relaxation of mesenteric artery of stroke prone spontaneously hypertensive rats by calcium removal. *Clin Exp Pharm Physiol* 17:413–425, 1990.

91. Sunano S, Moriyama K, Shimamura K: The relaxation and Ca-pump inhibition in mesenteric artery of normotensive and stroke-prone spontaneously hypertensive rats. *Microvasc Res* 42:117–124, 1991.

92. Devynck M, Pernollet M, Nunez A, Meyer P: Analysis of

calcium handling in erythrocyte membranes of genetically hypertensive rats. *Hypertension* 3:397–403, 1981.

93. Orlov SN, Pokudin NI, Postnov VY: Calmodulin-dependent calcium transport in erythrocytes of spontaneously hypertensive rats. *Pflügers Arch* 397:54–56, 1983.
94. Vezzoli G, Elli AA, Tripodi G, Bianchi G, Carafoli E: Calcium ATPase in erythrocytes of spontaneously hypertensive rats of the Milan strain. *J Hypertens* 5:645–648, 1985.
95. Resink T, Tkachuk VA, Erne P, Buhler FR: Platelet membrane calmodulin-stimulated calcium-adenosine triphosphate. Altered activity in essential hypertension. *Hypertension* 8:159–166, 1986.
96. Carafoli E: Calcium pump of the plasma membrane. *Physiol Rev* 71:129–153, 1991.
97. Hermsmeyer K, Harder DH: Membrane ATPase mechanism of the K⁺ return relaxation in stroke-prone SHR and WKY arterial muscles. *Am J Physiol* 250:C557–C562, 1986.
98. Blaustein MP, Ashida T, Goldman WF, Wier WG, Hamlyn JM: Sodium/calcium exchange in vascular smooth muscle: A link between sodium metabolism and hypertension. *Ann NY Acad Sci* 488:199–216, 1986.
99. Thompson LE, Rinaldi GJ, Bohr DF: Decreased activity of the sodium-calcium exchanger in tail artery of stroke-prone spontaneously hypertensive rats. *Blood Vessels* 27:197–201, 1990.
100. Mulvany MJ, Aalkjaer C, Petersen TT: Intracellular sodium, membrane potential, and contractility of rat mesenteric small arteries. *Circ Res* 54:740–749, 1984.
101. Petersen TT, Mulvany MJ: Effect of sodium gradient on the rate of relaxation of rat mesenteric small arteries from potassium contractures. *Blood Vessels* 21:279–284, 1984.
102. Sada T, Koike H, Ikeda M, Sato K, Ozaki H, Karaki H: Cytosolic free calcium of aorta of hypertensive rats. *Hypertension* 16:245–251, 1990.
103. Papageorgiou P, Morgan KG: Intracellular free Ca²⁺ is elevated in hypertrophic aortic muscle from hypertensive rats. *Am J Physiol* 260:H507–H515, 1991.
104. Hermsmeyer K: Calcium antagonist effects on vascular muscle membrane potentials and intracellular Ca²⁺. In: Rubin RP, Weiss G, Putney JW (eds) *Calcium in Biological Systems*. New York: Plenum Press, 1985, pp 423–430.
105. Storm DS, Stuenkel EL, Webb RC: Calcium channel activation in arterioles from genetically hypertensive rats. *Hypertension* 20:380–388, 1992.
106. Stull JT, Gallagher PJ, Herring BP, Kamm KE: Vascular smooth muscle contractile elements. *Hypertension* 17:723–732, 1991.
107. Mecca TE, Webb RC: Vascular responses to serotonin in steroid hypertensive rats. *Hypertension* 6:887–892, 1984.
108. Aqel MB, Sharma RV, Bhalla RC: Increased norepinephrine sensitive intracellular pool in the caudal artery of spontaneously hypertensive rats. *J Hyperten* 5:249–253, 1987.
109. Bruschi G, Bruschi ME, Capelli P, Regolisti G, Borghetti A: Increased sensitivity to protein kinase C activation in aortas of spontaneously hypertensive rats. *J Hyperten* 6:S248–S251, 1988.
110. Turla MB, Webb RC: Augmented phosphoinositide metabolism in aortas from genetically hypertensive rats. *Am J Physiol* 258:H173–H178, 1990.
111. Rinaldi G, Bohr DF: Potassium-induced relaxation of arteries in hypertension: Modulation by extracellular calcium. *Am J Physiol* 256:H707–H712, 1989.
112. Soloviev AI, Bershtein SA: The contractile apparatus in vascular smooth muscle cells of spontaneously hypertensive rats possess increased calcium sensitivity: The possible role

of protein kinase C. *J Hyperten* 10:131–136, 1992.
113. McMahon EF, Paul RJ: Calcium sensitivity of isometric force in intact and chemically skinned aortas during the development of aldosterone-salt hypertension in the rat. *Circ Res* 56:427–435, 1985.
114. Nghiem CX, Rapp JP: Responses to calcium of chemically skinned vascular smooth muscle from spontaneously hypertensive rats. *Clin Exp Hyper Theory Pract* A5(6):849–856, 1983.
115. Desilets M, Driska SP, Baumgarten CM: Current fluctuations and oscillations in smooth muscle cells from hog carotid artery. *Circ Res* 65:708–722, 1989.
116. Trieschmann U, Isenberg G: Ca²⁺-activated K⁺ channels contribute to the resting potential of vascular myocytes. Ca²⁺-sensitivity is increased by intracellular Mg²⁺-ions. *Pflügers Arch* 414:S183–S184, 1989.
117. Cook NS: *Potassium Channels: Structure, Classification, Function and Therapeutic Potential*. Chichester: Ellis Horwood, 1990.
118. Longman SD, Hamilton TC: Potassium channel activator drugs: Mechanism of action, pharmacological properties, and therapeutic potential. *Med Res Rev* 12:73–148, 1992.
119. Bolton TB, Lang RJ, Takewaki T, Benham CD: Patch and whole-cell voltage clamp of single mammalian visceral and vascular smooth muscle cells. *Experientia* 41:887–894, 1985.
120. Bolton TB, Lang RJ, Takewaki T, Benham CD: Patch and whole-cell voltage clamp studies on single smooth muscle cells. *J Cardiovasc Pharmacol* 8:S20–S24, 1986.
121. Benham CD, Bolton TB, Lang RJ, Takewaki T: Calcium-activated potassium channels in single smooth muscle cells of rabbit jejunum and guinea pig mesenteric artery. *J Physiol* 371:45–67, 1986.
122. Inoue R, Okabe K, Kitamura K, Kuriyama H: A newly identified Ca²⁺ dependent K⁺ channel in the smooth muscle membrane of single cells dispersed from the rabbit portal vein. *Pflügers Arch* 406:138–143, 1986.
123. Beech DJ, Bolton TB, Castle NA, Strong PN: Characterization of a toxin from scorpion (*Leirus quinquestriatus*) venom that blocks in vitro both large (Bₖ) K⁺-channels in rabbit vascular smooth muscle and intermediate (Iₖ) conductance Ca²⁺-activated K⁺ channels in human red cells. *J Physiol Proc Suppl* 287:32P, 1987.
124. Cook NS, Hof RP: Cardiovascular effects of apamin and BRL 34915 in rats and rabbits. *Br J Pharmacol* 93:121–131, 1988.
125. Stuenkel EL: Single potassium channels recorded from vascular smooth muscle cells. *Am J Physiol* 257:H760–H769, 1989.
126. Shoemaker RL, Worrell RT: Ca²⁺-sensitive K⁺ channel in aortic smooth muscle of rats. *Proc Soc Exp Biol Med* 196:325–332, 1991.
127. Beech DJ, Bolton TB: Properties of the cromakalim-induced potassium conductance in smooth muscle cells isolated from the rabbit portal vein. *Br J Pharmacol* 98:851–864, 1989.
128. Okabe KK, Kitamura K, Kuriyama H: Features of 4-aminopyridine sensitive outward current observed in single smooth muscle cells from the rabbit pulmonary artery. *Pflügers Arch* 409:561–568, 1987.
129. Edwards FR, Hirst GDS: Inward rectification in submucosal arterioles of guinea-pig ileum. *J Physiol* 404:437–454, 1988.
130. Edwards RR, Hirst GDS, Silverberg GD: Inward rectification in rat cerebral arterioles; involvement of potassium ions in autoregulation. *J Physiol* 404:455–466, 1988.
131. Brayden JE: Electrophysiological correlates of vasodilation: A primary role for ATP-sensitive potassium channels. In:

Sperelakis N, Kuriyama H (eds) *Ion Channels of Vascular Smooth Muscle Cells and Endothelial Cells.* New York: Elsevier Science, 1991, pp 163–172.

132. Daut J, Maier-Rudolph W, von Beckerath N, Mehrke G, Günther K, Goedel-Meinen L: Hypoxic dilation of coronary arteries is mediated by ATP-sensitive potassium channels. *Science* 247:1341–1344, 1990.

133. Standen NB, Quayle JM, Davies NW, Brayden JE, Huang Y, Nelson MT: Hyperpolarizing vasodilators activate ATP-sensitive K+ channels in arterial smooth muscle. *Science* 245:177–180, 1989.

134. Singer JJ, Walsh JV: Large-conductance Ca^{2+}-activated K$^+$ channels in freshly dissociated smooth muscle cells. *Membr Biochem* 6:83–110, 1986.

135. Toro L, Stefani E: Ca^{2+} and K$^+$ current in cultured vascular smooth muscle cells from rat aorta. *Pflügers Arch* 408:417–419, 1987.

136. Latorre R, Oberhauser A, Labarca P, Alvarez O: Varieties of calcium-activated potassium channels. *Annu Rev Physiol* 51:385–399, 1989.

137. McManus OB: Calcium-activated potassium channels: Regulation by calcium. *J Bioenerg Biomembr* 23:537–560, 1991.

138. Walsh JV, Singer JJ: Identification and characterization of major ionic currents in isolated smooth muscle cells using the voltage-clamp technique. *Pflügers Arch* 408:83–97, 1987.

139. Smith JM, Jones AW: Calcium antagonists inhibit elevated potassium efflux from aorta of aldosterone-salt hypertensive rats. *Hypertension* 15:78–83, 1990.

140. Thompson LP, Bruner CA, Lamb FS, King CM, Webb RC: Calcium influx and vascular reactivity in systemic hypertension. *Am J Cardiol* 59:29A–34A, 1987.

141. Skou JC: The Na-K pump. *NIPS* 7:95–100, 1992.

142. Haddy FJ: Potassium and blood vessels. *Life Sci* 16:1489–1498, 1975.

143. Lang S, Blaustein MP: The role of the sodium pump in the control of vascular tone in the rat. *Circ Res* 46:463–470, 1980.

144. Haddy FJ: Abnormalities of membrane transport in hypertension. *Hypertension* 5:66–72, 1983.

145. Pamnani MB, Harder DR, Huot SJ, Bryant HJ, Kutyna FA, Haddy FJ: Vascular smooth muscle membrane potential and a ouabain-like humoral factor in one-kidney, one-clip hypertension in rats. *Clin Sci* 63:S31–S33, 1982.

146. Rinaldi G, Bohr DF: Potassium-induced relaxation of arteries in hypertension: Modulation by extracellular calcium. *Am J Physiol* 256:H707–H712, 1989.

147. Pamnani MB, Clough DL, Haddy FJ: Na$^+$-K$^+$ pump activity in tail arteries of spontaneously hypertensive rats. *Jpn Heart J* 20:S228–S230, 1979.

148. Abel PW, Hermsmeyer K: Sympathetic cross-innervation of SHR and genetic controls suggests a trophic influence on vascular muscle membranes. *Circ Res* 49:1311–1318, 1981.

149. Hermsmeyer K: Vascular muscle membrane cation mechanisms and total peripheral resistance. *Hypertension* 10(Suppl I):I20–I22, 1987.

150. Bukoski RD, Seidel CL, Allen JC: Differences in K$^+$-induced relaxation of canine femoral and renal arteries. *Am J Physiol* 245:H598–H603, 1983.

151. McCarron JG, Halpern W: Impaired potassium-induced dilation in hypertensive rat cerebral arteries does not reflect altered Na$^+$, K$^+$-ATPase dilation. *Circ Res* 67:1035–1039, 1990.

152. Webb RC, Bohr DF: Potassium-induced relaxation as an indicator of Na$^+$-K$^+$ ATPase activity in vascular smooth muscle. *Blood Vessels* 15:198–207, 1978.

153. Webb RC, Bohr DF: Potassium relaxation of vascular smooth muscle from spontaneously hypertensive rats. *Blood Vessels* 16:71–79, 1978.

154. Myers JH, Lamb FS, Webb RC: Contractile responses to ouabain and potassium-free solution in vascular tissue from renal hypertensive rats. *J Hyperten* 5:161–171, 1987.

155. Aalkjaer C, Kjeldsen K, Norgaard A, Clausen T, Mulvany MJ: Ouabain binding and Na$^+$ content in resistance vessels and skeletal muscles of spontaneously hypertensive rats and K$^+$-depleted rats. *Hypertension* 7:277–286, 1985.

156. Wong SK, Westfall DP, Menear D, Fleming WW: Sodium-potassium pump sites, as assessed by [^{3}H]-ouabain binding, in aorta and caudal artery of normotensive and spontaneously hypertensive rats. *Blood Vessels* 21:211–222, 1984.

157. Aalkjaer C, Mulvany MJ: Sodium and calcium metabolism in resistance vessels in hypertension. In: Kwan C-Y (ed) *Membrane Abnormalities in Hypertension*, Vol 1. CRC Press, Boca Raton, FL: 1989, pp 31–57.

158. Hermsmeyer K, Walton S: Specificity of altered electrogenesis of membrane potential in hypertension. *Circ Res* 40:I153–I156, 1977.

159. Stekiel WJ, Contney SJ, Lombard JH: Small vessel membrane potential, sympathetic input, and electrogenic pump rate in SHR. *Am J Physiol* 250:C547–C556, 1986.

CHAPTER 54

Contractile Proteins of Smooth Muscle

GARY J. KARGACIN & MICHAEL P. WALSH

INTRODUCTION

The mechanism of contraction of smooth muscle is generally believed to be fundamentally the same as that of
skeletal and cardiac muscles, i.e., contraction occurs according to the crossbridge cycling/sliding filament model,
whereby thick and thin filaments slide relative to one
another, without a change in length of the filaments, at the
expense of ATP hydrolysis {1,2}. This conclusion has
come largely from ultrastructural studies of a variety of
different smooth muscles {3} and has been supported
more recently by the direct observation of actin filaments
moving on myosin substrates {e.g., 4,5}. At the molecular
level, the contractile apparatus of smooth muscle consists
of the contractile proteins (actin and myosin, which are
organized into thin and thick filaments, respectively) and
associated regulatory proteins (tropomyosin, myosin light-
chain kinase, calmodulin, myosin light-chain phosphatase,
caldesmon, and calponin). The contents of actin, myosin,
and tropomyosin in various smooth muscle tissues have
been discussed by Hartshorne {6}. In general, smooth
muscles contain less myosin and more actin and tropomyosin than do skeletal muscles (table 54-1).

Electron microscopic studies suggest the existence of
mini-sarcomere structures, which are postulated to form
the basic contractile units of smooth muscle {3}. It is
important to note, however, that not all the available
evidence is supportive of the existence of mini-sarcomeres
and, as will be discussed later, there is also evidence that
smooth muscle cells may be more globally organized into
contractile and noncontractile regions. Considerable attention, therefore, continues to be devoted to elucidation of
the mechanism of smooth muscle contraction, in particular,
the role of Ca^{2+} in triggering contraction. The reader is
referred to recent review articles that supplement the information provided in this chapter {6,7–11} (see Chapter
55).

In general, the regulation of motile processes can be
divided into two main groups: actin- or thin-filament-linked
regulation and myosin- or thick-filament-linked regulation,
depending upon whether the regulatory mechanism is
physically associated with the thin or thick filament {12}.
The best-characterized thin-filament-linked regulatory
mechanism is the troponin-tropomyosin system exem-

plified by vertebrate striated muscle {13,14}. The best-
characterized thick-filament-linked regulatory mechanisms
are myosin light-chain phosphorylation-dephosphorylation (e.g., smooth muscle) {6}, direct Ca^{2+} binding
to myosin (e.g., molluscan muscle) {15}, and myosin
heavy-chain phosphorylation-dephosphorylation (e.g.,
Acanthamoeba, *Dictyostelium*) {16,17}. Much of our
understanding of how smooth muscle contraction is controlled by Ca^{2+} has come from biochemical experimentation with in vitro systems reconstituted from the purified
contractile and regulatory proteins (fig. 54-1). Avian
gizzard smooth muscle has been the source most commonly used for the isolation of these proteins due to its
ready availability in large quantities. However, a significant amount of work has also been done with proteins
isolated from vascular smooth muscles, and the indications
are very strong that the fundamental properties and principles deduced from study of the avian gizzard proteins are
equally applicable to mammalian vascular smooth muscle.
Differences that do exist appear to be subtle ones.

It is the purpose of the remainder of this chapter to
discuss the important properties of the contractile and regulatory proteins of smooth muscle, leading to an analysis
of our current understanding of how smooth muscle contraction is controlled.

ACTIN

Thin filaments are composed primarily of actin arranged in
a double helix of actin monomers, similar to the structural
organization of the thin filaments of striated muscle. One
complete turn of the helix occurs every 74 nm, corresponding to ~13 actin monomers, and the width of the
thin filament is 6–8 nm {25}. Decoration of actin filaments
with heavy meromyosin or myosin subfragment-1 (S_1; see
below) established the polarity of the filaments {26}. The
length of thin filaments in vivo is uncertain, but they are
probably at least as long as skeletal muscle thin filaments
(ca. 1 μm). Recent estimates of actin filament lengths from
hypercontracted gizzard smooth muscle cell fragments
suggest that the filaments may be 4–5 μm in length {27}.
One end of the actin filament disappears into amorphous
structures called *dense bodies*, which are either free in the

N. Sperelakis (ed.), Physiology and Pathophysiology of the Heart, Third Edition.
© *1995 Kluwer Academic Publishers. ISBN 0-7923-2612-1. All rights reserved.*

Table 54-1. Muscle content of actin, tropomyosin, and myosin

Muscle type	Molar ratio			Tissue concentration (mM)		
	Actin	Tropomyosin	Myosin	Actin	Tropomyosin	Myosin
Arterial smooth	28.6	4.8	1	1.6	0.27	0.056
Nonarterial smooth	15.5	2.7	1	0.87	0.15	0.056
Skeletal	4	0.6	1	0.7	0.1	0.18

cytosol or associated with the plasma membrane. The cytoplasmic dense bodies contain α-actinin; the membrane dense plaques contain both α-actinin and vinculin. The cytosolic dense bodies are thus believed to be analogous to the Z lines of striated muscles. The other ends of the actin filaments interdigitate with myosin filaments; this is seen most clearly in electron micrographs of longitudinal sections of smooth muscle that has been treated with saponin (detergent) to remove soluble proteins {3}. Decoration with myosin S_1 has demonstrated that the thin filaments insert into the dense bodies with the expected orientation, i.e., the arrowheads point away from the dense bodies, indicating the correct actin polarity for force development {28}. The membrane-associated dense bodies presumably provide the ultimate anchorage of the contractile network at the level of the plasma membrane.

Actin is structurally a highly conserved molecule {29}, consistent with its widespread involvement in contractile and motile events. Major advances have been made recently in determination of the structure of actin at atomic detail {29}. Actin has a monomer molecular weight of 42 kDa (374 or 375 amino acids) and exists in several variants, which differ little in amino acid sequence. Two actin types exist in smooth muscle: smooth α and smooth γ, which differ by only three amino acids, all at the amino terminus {30}. The α variant is predominant in vascular smooth muscles, the γ variant in enteric smooth muscles, and approximately equal amounts of α and γ actins are found in other smooth muscles, e.g., uterus {30,31}. Most smooth muscles also contain cytoplasmic α and β actins; for example, the ratio of smooth α to cytoplasmic β actin in aorta is 3:1 {31}.

Actin isoform expression in smooth muscle has been shown to change during development {32}, in culture {33,34}, and in response to substances such as interleukin 1β {35}. In microvascular pericytes, which contain both smooth muscle and nonmuscle actin isoforms {36}, the isoforms appear to be sorted into cellular domains {37,38}. At present there is no evidence that a similar sorting of actin isoforms into cellular domains occurs in adult smooth muscle cells in vivo {39}. Localization of actin isoforms with isoactin-specific antibodies failed to reveal a segregation of actin isoforms in thin filaments isolated from swine stomach smooth muscle but instead indicated that the isoforms were copolymerized into a single population of thin filaments {39,40}.

Actin has three particularly important properties: (a) the ability to polymerize to form long filaments (conver-

sion of monomeric G actin to polymeric F actin); (b) the ability to bind myosin and activate its MgATPase activity; and (c) the ability to bind tropomyosin and regulatory proteins, e.g., troponin in striated muscles and myosin light-chain kinase, caldesmon, and calponin in smooth muscles. G actin binds one mole of ATP/mole, which is hydrolyzed as the G actin polymerizes to form F actin. Actin also contains one mole of bound divalent cation/mole; this is probably Mg^{2+} in vivo.

TROPOMYOSIN

Tropomyosin is present in smooth muscle at a molar ratio to actin monomers of 1:7 and is thought to be located in the grooves between the two strands of the actin double helix, as it is in skeletal muscle {41,42}. Smooth muscle tropomyosin exists in two isoforms, α and β (α having a higher mobility on SDS-polyacrylamide gel electrophoresis), which differ in amino acid sequence from α and β tropomyosins of skeletal muscle {43}. Most smooth muscles contain roughly equal quantities of α and β isoforms {31}. The two skeletal and the two smooth muscle isoforms of tropomyosin all contain 284 amino acids and have molecular weights of ca. 33 kDa, but differ substantially on electrophoresis. For example, the α and β smooth muscle tropomyosins exhibit apparent molecular weights of 36 and 42 kDa, respectively, on SDS-polyacrylamide gel electrophoresis (fig. 54-1, lane Tm). Both homodimers ($α_2$ and $β_2$) and the heterodimer (αβ) have been detected in chicken gizzard in the ratio 1:1:2 {44}, although Strasburg and Greaser {45} did not observe the heterodimer. All these isoforms and platelet tropomyosin have been sequenced {46}. Amino-acid sequence comparisons indicate that gizzard α tropomyosin most closely resembles skeletal β tropomyosin. For this reason, Sanders and Smillie {46} have proposed that smooth muscle α and β tropomyosins be renamed β and γ, respectively.

Tropomyosin is a dimer composed of two elongated, α-helical polypeptides coiled around each other, with a total length of 41–42 nm, a width of 2 nm, and a helical pitch of 13.7 nm {46,47}. Other smooth muscles (rabbit and pig uterus, hog carotid artery, and calf aorta) contain a single tropomyosin subunit species {43,48,49}. Tropomyosin displays a tendency to form polymers by head-to-tail aggregation, which may reflect its organization on the actin filament. One strand of tropomyosin molecules is associated with each of the two actin strands in the thin

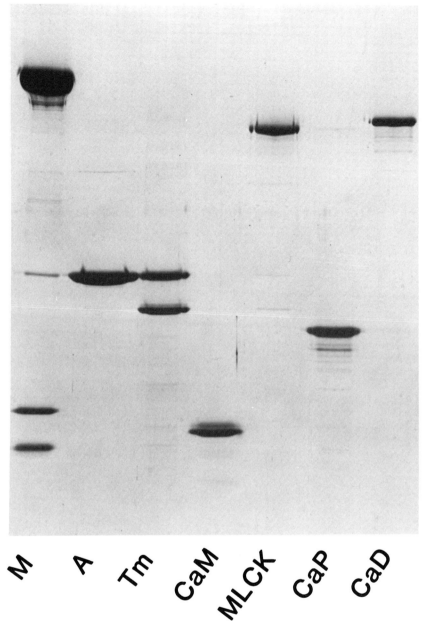

Fig. 54-1. Sodium dodecyl sulfate-polyacrylamide gel electrophoresis of chicken-gizzard contractile and regulatory proteins. Proteins were isolated by procedures referred to below and analyzed by electrophoresis in a 0.1% SDS, 7.5–20% polyacrylamide gradient slab gel that was stained with Coomassie Brilliant Blue. M = myosin (composed of heavy chains, M_r 205 kDa, and light chains, M_r 20 and 17 kDa) {18}; A = actin (M_r 42 kDa) {19}; Tm = tropomyosin (composed of α and β subunits of apparent M_r 36 and 42 kDa, respectively) {20}; CaM = calmodulin (M_r 16.7 kDa) {21}; MLCK = myosin light-chain kinase (M_r 136 kDa) {22}; CaP = calponin (M_r 34 kDa) {23}; CaD = caldesmon (M_r 140 kDa) {24}.

filament. Skeletal and smooth muscle tropomyosins both exhibit the same sevenfold repeating sequence, presumably corresponding to the seven actin-binding sites; one tropomyosin dimer spans seven actin monomers in the thin

filament, consistent with the calculated stoichiometry in vivo.

The function of smooth muscle tropomyosin has not yet been clearly established, although there is general agreement that it has a significant potentiating effect on the actin-activated myosin MgATPase {50,51}. It has been suggested that tropomyosin may play an important role in conjunction with caldesmon in regulating actin-myosin interaction in smooth muscle (see below). X-ray diffraction data indicate that tropomyosin on smooth muscle thin filaments moves further into the groove of the actin double helix upon activation of the muscle {25,52}. This is reminiscent of the situation with skeletal muscle tropomyosin/troponin and occurs despite the absence of troponin from smooth muscle.

MYOSIN

Smooth muscle myosin is a hexamer composed of two heavy chains (M_r 205 kDa) and two pairs of light chains (M_r 20 and 17 kDa); (fig. 54-1, lane M) to give a native molecular weight of ca. 484 kDa. Electron microscopy of rotary-shadowed myosin reveals the long rodlike tail and two-headed structure, similar to striated muscle and nonmuscle myosins {e.g., 53}. Smooth muscle myosin molecules have a tendency to aggregate into filamentous structures via interactions of parts of their tail regions (the LMM region; see below). The globular heads and part of the tail (HMM region) protrude away from the body of the thick filament, constituting the crossbridge to the thin (actin) filament. Mammalian smooth muscle myosin filaments are ~15–18 nm in diameter and 2.2 μm long. The filamentous structure of smooth muscle myosin in situ has not been firmly established, and both a bipolar filament arrangement with a central bare zone (devoid of crossbridges) and tapered ends, and a side-polar arrangement in which the crossbridges on one side of the filament have opposite polarity to those on the other side of the filament, have been proposed {3,54–56}.

Fragmentation of smooth muscle myosin with a variety of proteases has revealed much information about the domain structure of the molecule (fig. 54-2). The globular heads are composed of the amino-terminal ends of the heavy chains and both pairs of light chains, and each contains an actin-binding site and a site of ATP hydrolysis. Myosin can be cleaved by α-chymotrypsin into light meromyosin (LMM; composed of the last two thirds of the tail) and heavy meromyosin (HMM; composed of the two globular heads and one third of the tail) {57}. There is compelling evidence that myosin filaments exist in vivo in both the contracted and relaxed smooth muscle {58}. HMM can be cleaved with papain to S_1 (free myosin heads), which retain actin binding and the ATPase site {57}. HMM and S_1 have been widely used in kinetic studies due to their solubility properties. These fragments of myosin have also been very useful in studying the regulation of the actin-activated myosin MgATPase, in particular, the role of phosphorylation (see below). One drawback of these investigations, however, was the fact that the 20-kDa light chain of myosin (LC_{20}) is labile to proteolysis by α-chymotrypsin. This problem was overcome by Ikebe and Hartshorne {59}, who described the preparation of HMM and S_1, both with intact LC_{20}, by digestion of gizzard myosin with *Staphylococcus aureus* V8 protease.

It was first shown in 1973 {60} that skeletal muscle myosin could be phosphorylated, but the function of this phosphorylation reaction has still not been clearly elucidated. Subsequently, phosphorylation of smooth muscle myosin was demonstrated {61}, and this reaction is widely believed to be central to the regulation of smooth muscle

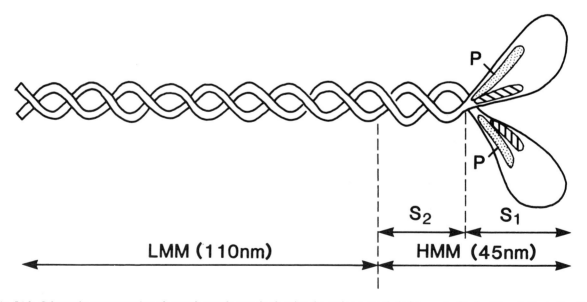

Fig. 54-2. Schematic representation of smooth-muscle myosin showing the major proteolytic fragments. Dashed lines indicate the sites of proteolytic cleavage. The 17- and 20-kDa light chains are shown in association with the globular heads, although their precise locations within the heads are unknown. The 20-kDa light chain can be phosphorylated as indicated (P).

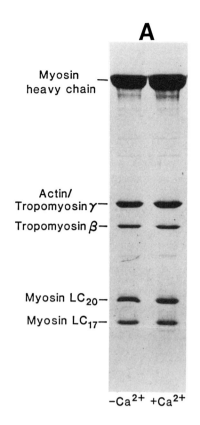

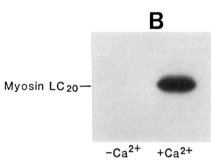

Fig. 54-3. Specific Ca^{2+}-dependent phosphorylation of gizzard myosin in vitro. Myosin (1 μM) was incubated at 30°C in 25 mM Tris-HCl (pH 7.5), 60 mM KCl, 10 mM MgCl$_2$, 1 mM [γ-^{32}P]ATP in the presence of actin (6 μM), tropomyosin (2 μM), CaM (0.1 μM), and MLCK (74 nM), and either 0.1 mM CaCl$_2$ or 1 mM EGTA. Reactions were initiated by the addition of ATP and quenched at t = 5 minutes by the addition of an equal volume of boiling SDS gel sample buffer. Proteins were separated by 0.1% SDS, 7.5–20% polyacrylamide gradient slab gel electrophoresis. The gel was stained with Coomassie Brilliant Blue (**A**) and autoradiographed (**B**). Only the region of the autoradiogram corresponding to myosin LC$_{20}$ is shown since no other protein bands were radiolabeled. All proteins were isolated from chicken gizzard by methods referred to in the legend to fig. 54-1.

contraction (see below). Phosphorylation of smooth muscle myosin has been thoroughly characterized both in vitro and in vivo, and is catalyzed by Ca^{2+}/calmodulin-dependent myosin light-chain kinase (see below). Specific phosphorylation of Ser[19] occurs on each of the two 20-kDa light chains of gizzard myosin. From a functional standpoint, considerable work has been done to determine the effects of myosin phosphorylation. Commonly, in vitro contractile systems are reconstituted from purified actin, myosin, tropomyosin, myosin light-chain kinase (MLCK), and calmodulin (CaM; fig. 54-3A). In the presence of MgATP and Ca^{2+}, myosin LC$_{20}$ is specifically phosphorylated (fig. 54-3B). In the absence of Ca^{2+}, under otherwise identical conditions, no myosin LC$_{20}$ phosphorylation is observed (fig. 54-3B). It is also possible to measure the actin-activated myosin MgATPase activity in such a reconstituted system and to observe the occurrence of superprecipitation (the increased turbidity of actomyosin upon activation). These two parameters are recognized as biochemical correlates of contraction in the intact muscle and can easily be measured in this very well-defined system. Results of a typical experiment are shown in table 54-2. In the presence of Ca^{2+}, myosin phosphorylation occurs (to ~2 mole P$_i$/mole myosin or ~1 mole P$_i$/mole LC$_{20}$), and substantial activation of the myosin MgATPase by actin and superprecipitation are observed. On the other hand, in the absence of Ca^{2+} little or no phosphorylation of myosin occurs and no actin activation of the myosin MgATPase or superprecipitation is observed. Myosin in the absence of actin exhibits a low MgATPase activity that is unaffected by phosphorylation (table 54-2). Smooth-muscle myosin, like its skeletal muscle counterpart, exhibits other ATPase activities: CaATPase at high [Ca^{2+}] (e.g., 10 mM), in which CaATP^{2-} is the substrate; and K$^+$/EDTA-ATPase in the presence of K$^+$ and the absence of divalent cations, in which KATP^{3-} is the substrate. While of no physiological significance, these ATPase activities, as well as the MgATPase in the absence of actin, are useful parameters for studying alterations in myosin structure induced by, e.g., phosphorylation.

Studies of the kinetics of phosphorylation of smooth muscle myosin by MLCK have led to contradictory conclusions about the mechanism of myosin phosphorylation. Some researchers favor a mechanism whereby the two heads of a myosin molecule are randomly phosphorylated {63–65}, whereas others maintain that phosphorylation is negatively cooperative and therefore occurs by an ordered mechanism {18,66,67}. Similarly, controversy exists as to whether or not both heads of myosin need to be phosphorylated before actin activation of the myosin MgATPase is observed {see 65 for discussion}. Some of the observed discrepancies in experimental results may be due to variations in ionic conditions and the filamentous state of myosin. The direct correlation between the level of myosin phosphorylation and the velocity of shortening of living arterial muscle {68} does not appear to be consistent with a negatively cooperative phosphorylation mechanism in which the MgATPase of only doubly phosphorylated myosin is activated by actin. Persechini et al. {69} presented evidence in favor of a random phosphory-

Table 54-2. Phosphorylation-induced activation of smooth muscle actomyosin MgATPase activity and superprecipitation

	MgATPase rate (nmoles P_i/mg myosin · min)		Myosin phosphorylation (moles P_i/mole myosin)		Superprecipitation	
	$+Ca^{2+}$	$-Ca^{2+}$	$+Ca^{2+}$	$-Ca^{2+}$	$+Ca^{2+}$	$-Ca^{2+}$
Reconstituted system	91.6	3.0	2.0	0.0	+	−
Myosin alone	3.1	3.1	2.0	0.0	+	−

Reaction conditions were as described in the legend to fig. 54-3. The reconstituted system contained all protein components, and a measure of the myosin MgATPase was also determined in the absence of actin and tropomyosin. Aliquots of reaction mixtures were withdrawn at t = 1, 2, 3, 4, 5, 6, and 7 minutes for quantification of ATP hydrolysis {59} and myosin phosphorylation {62}. ATPase rates were determined by linear regression analysis of the linear time courses of ATP hydrolysis. Superprecipitation was assessed by visual inspection: + denotes strong turbidity; − denotes complete clarity.

lation mechanism in intact bovine tracheal smooth muscle strips. It seems likely, therefore, that myosin phosphorylation occurs in vivo by a random mechanism and both singly and doubly phosphorylated myosins are active. This would be consistent with several studies with skinned fibers (see below) in which low levels of myosin phosphorylation were sufficient to induce maximal tension development.

Attention has been drawn to the possibility of phosphorylation of myosin at an additional site, also catalyzed by MLCK. Using high concentrations of kinase at low ionic strength, Ikebe and Hartshorne {70} observed phosphorylation of isolated gizzard myosin at two distinct sites, both located on LC_{20}. These were subsequently identified as ser^{19} (the preferred site) and thr^{18} {71}. Second-site phosphorylation caused a marked enhancement of the actin-activated MgATPase. The possibility that two-site phosphorylation of smooth muscle myosin may have physiological significance was suggested by the work of Haeberle and Trockman {72}, who observed the formation of both monophosphorylated and diphosphorylated forms of LC_{20} upon stimulation of glycerinated porcine carotid artery. Charge variants of LC_{20} have frequently been detected in experiments with intact and skinned smooth muscle fibers, some of which may be due to variable extents of phosphorylation {73,74}.

Both the heavy and light chains of smooth muscle myosin are expressed as several different isoforms {see 39 for review}. As has been the case with actin, it has proven difficult to find a functional correlate of myosin isoform expression in smooth muscle. A possible link between isoform expression and actomyosin ATPase activity similar to that observed in the slow- and fast-twitch forms of striated muscle has been suggested {75}. Kelley et al. {5} found that native smooth muscle myosin heavy chains are homodimeric but, in an in-vitro motility assay, the rate of movement of actin filaments by myosin attached to glass substrates did not depend on which smooth muscle myosin isoform was used.

CALMODULIN

Calmodulin was discovered in 1970 independently by Cheung {76} and Kakiuchi et al. {77} and was later identified as a high-affinity Ca^{2+}-binding protein {78}. It is now recognized that CaM belongs to a family of Ca^{2+}-binding proteins that includes troponin C of striated muscles, parvalbumins of fast-twitch skeletal muscles, brain S-100 protein, the intestinal vitamin D-dependent Ca^{2+}-binding protein, and many others {79}. Initially CaM was known as a Ca^{2+}-dependent activator of cyclic nucleotide phosphodiesterase, but it has since been shown to regulate a wide variety of enzymatic activities and physiological processes {see 80,81 for reviews}. These include the enzyme MLCK of smooth muscle {82}. Consistent with its diverse regulatory functions, CaM is ubiquitous in distribution and structurally highly conserved.

Ca^{2+} regulatory proteins like CaM respond to transient increases in cytosolic free $[Ca^{2+}]$ that result from cell activation by extracellular signals, e.g., hormones, neurotransmitters, growth factors, or membrane depolarization. CaM possesses four structurally homologous Ca^{2+}-binding sites with dissociation constants in the micromolar range {83}. The sarcoplasmic free $[Ca^{2+}]$ ($[Ca^{2+}]_i$) in the resting smooth muscle cell is ca. 0.1–0.2 µM {84–86} and rises to ca. 0.5–0.7 µM upon stimulation {85}. In the presence of MLCK, the affinity of CaM for Ca^{2+} is increased significantly {87}. As a result of the rise in $[Ca^{2+}]_i$, the kinase is activated in the stimulated, but not in the unstimulated, cell. The binding of Ca^{2+} to CaM induces a substantial conformational change, including the induction of greater α-helical content {88} and exposure of a hydrophobic region(s), which has been implicated in binding of CaM to various target enzymes {89}. The mechanism of Ca^{2+}-dependent activation of target enzymes by CaM is exemplified by MLCK as follows:

$$CaM$$
$$4Ca^{2+} \searrow \downarrow$$
$$Ca_4^{2+} \cdot CaM$$
$$\downarrow$$
$$Ca_4^{2+} \cdot CaM^*$$
$$\text{MLCK} \searrow$$
$$\text{(inactive}$$
$$\text{apoenzyme)}$$
$$Ca_4^{2+} \cdot CaM^* \cdot MLCK$$
$$\downarrow$$
$$Ca_4^{2+} \cdot CaM^* \cdot MLCK^*$$
$$\text{(active ternary complex)}$$

where * denotes the active conformation of the protein.

A great deal of information is now available about the structure of CaM. The amino acid sequences of several CaMs have been determined {90} and the three-dimensional structure was elucidated by x-ray crystallography {91}. The tertiary structure resembles a dumb-bell shape, with each globular end containing two Ca^{2+}-binding sites, the two ends being connected by an eight-turn, solvent-exposed central α-helix. Side chains within this helical region, as well as in both hydrophobic pockets formed within the globular domains, have been implicated in interaction with target enzymes {92–94}. Site-directed mutagenesis of CaM {e.g., 95} and MLCK {e.g., 96}, and NMR {97} and x-ray crystallography {98} of CaM complexed with synthetic peptides corresponding to the CaM-binding domain of MLCK have shed considerable light on the interactions between these two proteins {99}.

MYOSIN LIGHT-CHAIN KINASE

Myosin light-chain kinase catalyzes the transfer of the terminal phosphoryl group of $MgATP^{2-}$ to ser^{19} on each of the two 20-kDa light chains of myosin. The enzyme has been isolated from a variety of smooth muscle tissues and characterized {100}. The amino acid sequences of MLCK of chicken gizzard (107 kDa) {101}, rabbit uterine (126 kDa) {102}, and bovine stomach (129 kDa) smooth muscles {103} have been deduced from the corresponding cDNA sequences. These sequences are highly conserved except for an unusual region of repeated amino acids rich in lys, pro, ala, and thr located near the amino terminus of the mammalian enzymes. The apoenzyme, which is the inactive form of the kinase, consists of a single polypeptide chain. The holoenzyme, which is the active form of the enzyme, is a complex of the kinase polypeptide with CaM (1:1) containing bound Ca^{2+} (3–4 moles Ca^{2+}/mole CaM).

MLCK exhibits a high degree of substrate specificity: It phosphorylates only myosin and its proteolytic fragments (HMM and S_1) or the isolated LC_{20}. This high degree of specificity indicates rigid structural requirements in the substrate. The complete amino acid sequence of LC_{20} of chicken gizzard has been determined by direct protein sequencing {104,105} and was deduced from the cDNA sequence {106}. The amino acid sequences of porcine aortic LC_{20} {107} and human umbilical arterial LC_{20} {108} are identical to the gizzard protein except for the following substitutions: leu for met at position 60 in the porcine protein, tyr for ile at position 80, and ser for ala at position 113 in the human protein. The amino-terminal sequence of LC_{20} is Acetyl-ser-ser-lys-arg-ala-lys-ala-lys-thr-thr-lys^{11}-lys^{12}-arg^{13}-pro-gln-arg-ala-thr-SER^{19}-asn-val-phe-ala^{23}-, where the phosphorylated serine residue is shown in capitals. When the amino acid sequences around the phosphorylated serine residue of the regulatory light chains of rabbit and chicken-skeletal and chicken-gizzard myosins are compared, obvious sequence homologies are apparent, particularly at the carboxy-terminal side of the phosphorylated serine {see 109 for discussion}. Structure-function studies using synthetic peptides indicated that the four basic residues lys^{11}, lys^{12}, arg^{13}, and arg^{16} had a strong influence on the kinetics of phosphorylation {110,111}. Furthermore, relocation of arg^{16} to position 15 caused a complete switch in specificity of phosphorylation from ser^{19} to thr^{18}. Residues at the carboxy-terminal side of ser^{19} also contribute to the kinetics of phosphorylation {112}. Ala^{23} was not essential, but the hydrophobic residues phe^{22} and val^{21} had a strong influence on the V_{max} of phosphorylation of synthetic peptides. The synthetic peptide corresponding to residues 11–19 of chicken-gizzard myosin LC_{20} exhibited a very low V_{max} (0.032 μmoles P_i/min·mg compared with 36.2 μmoles P_i/min·mg for the intact light chain) and a relatively low apparent K_m (16.9 μM compared with 8.6 μM for the intact light chain). This peptide acts as a relatively potent inhibitor of MLCK with $K_i = 10$ μM {112}.

The importance of arg^{13}-arg^{16} for phosphorylation-dependent activation of smooth muscle actomyosin MgATPase activity was shown by replacing LC_{20} in gizzard HMM by various truncated forms of LC_{20} obtained by digestion with lysylendopeptidase or trypsin {113}. HMM containing LC_{20} beginning at lys^6 or lys^{12}, like HMM containing intact LC_{20}, exhibited actin-activated MgATPase activity, which was strongly dependent on phosphorylation. On the other hand, the actin-activated MgATPase activity of HMM containing LC_{20} beginning at arg^{13} was not significantly increased by phosphorylation (1.8 moles P_i/mole HMM).

MLCK is a particularly interesting enzyme from the point of view of structure-function relations. It has an active site, a CaM-binding site, sites of phosphorylation by various protein kinases, and an actin-binding site. The domain structure of the kinase is depicted in fig. 54-4. The catalytic domain is defined as gly^{526}-arg^{762} by homology with other protein kinases {114}. This domain begins with the consensus ATP-binding sequence, gly-Xaa-gly-Xaa-gly-Xaa$_{16-28}$-lys {115}. The deduced amino acid sequence

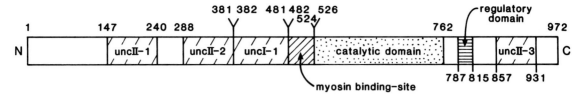

Fig. 54-4. Domain structure of smooth muscle MLCK. The numbering is derived from the full-length sequence of the chicken gizzard enzyme {101}. The amino and carboxy termini are indicated by N and C, respectively. The regulatory domain includes the pseudosubstrate domain and the CaM-binding domain.

{101} contains two classes of structural motifs (~100 amino acids long), referred to as *unc*-I and *unc*-II, which are found in the unc-22 gene product (twitchin) of the nematode *C. elegans* {116} and the giant skeletal muscle protein titin {117}. The smooth muscle kinase contains a single *unc*-I and three *unc*-II repeat motifs. These motifs are not found in MLCK of mammalian skeletal muscle or *D. discoideum*. Their function is unknown.

Partial proteolysis of smooth muscle MLCK with a variety of proteases, and structural and functional characterization of the resultant fragments, has shed a great deal of light on the structure-function relations of this enzyme {118}. The CaM-binding site, which has a predicted basic amphiphilic α-helical structure {119}, has the following sequence: ala^{796}-arg-arg-lys-trp-gln-lys-thr-gly-his-ala-val-arg-ala-ile-gly-arg-leu^{813}. This synthetic peptide binds to CaM in a Ca^{2+}-dependent manner and inhibits activation of MLCK by competing with the enzyme for binding to CaM {120,121}. Site-directed mutagenesis within this domain of MLCK indicates that CaM binding to the kinase involves an interplay of specific hydrophobic and electrostatic interactions {96,122}.

The region between the *unc*-I and the catalytic domains glu^{482}-arg^{524} has been identified as the myosin light-chain binding site {123,124}. This sequence is rich in acidic residues, suggesting that electrostatic interactions with basic amino acids flanking the phosphorylated ser^{19} in LC$_{20}$ play an important role in substrate binding.

The mechanism of regulation of MLCK has also been elucidated by limited proteolysis. Digestion with trypsin initially yields a 64-kDa fragment, thr^{283}-arg^{808}, which is inactive and cannot be activated by Ca^{2+}/CaM. Further tryptic digestion generates a 61-kDa peptide, thr^{283}-lys^{779}, which is constitutively active, i.e., it does not require Ca^{2+}/CaM for activity {125}. Examination of the amino acid sequence of MLCK reveals a domain (ser^{787}-val^{807}) with sequence homology to the region of LC$_{20}$ around ser^{19}:

```
        787
MLCK:   ser-lys-asp-arg-met-lys-lys-tyr-met-ala-arg-arg-lys-
        1
LC20:   ser-ser-lys-arg-ala-lys-ala-lys-thr-thr-lys-lys-arg-
                                                        807
MLCK:   trp-gln-lys-thr-gly-his-ala-val
        19                          21
LC20:   pro-gln-arg-ala-thr-ser-asn-val
```

This sequence within the kinase is referred to as the *pseudosubstrate prototope* {126} and its identification led

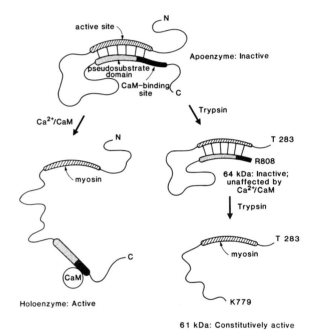

Fig. 54-5. Mechanism of activation of MLCK by Ca^{2+}/calmodulin or partial proteolysis. The pseudosubstrate domain (ser^{787}-val^{807}) and the CaM-binding domain (ala^{796}-leu^{813}) overlap in the region ala^{796}-val^{807}. Taken from Walsh {9} with the permission of The National Research Council of Canada.

to understanding the mechanism of regulation of the enzyme (fig. 54-5). The apoenzyme of MLCK is folded so that this pseudosubstrate domain is bound within the substrate-binding domain, glu^{482}-arg^{524}. This would prevent access to the myosin substrate and thereby explains why the apoenzyme is inactive. As indicated above, the CaM-binding site (arg^{796}-leu^{813}) overlaps the pseudosubstrate domain (ser^{787}-val^{807}). Binding of Ca^{2+}/CaM changes the conformation of the kinase and removes the pseudosubstrate domain from the myosin binding site, allowing myosin binding and catalysis to occur. The tryptic digestion experiments can be explained as follows (fig. 54-5). The 64-kDa fragment of MLCK contains the pseudosubstrate domain but has lost part of the CaM-binding site. This peptide is inactive since the pseudosubstrate domain is bound within the myosin-binding site, and it cannot be activated by Ca^{2+}/CaM since it is incapable of binding Ca^{2+}/CaM {125}. Further digestion with trypsin results in removal of the pseudosubstrate sequence and expression of constitutive activity since the catalytic domain is retained intact. This mechanism is supported by several studies with synthetic peptides {121,126,127} and site-directed mutagenesis {128}, including the observation that replacement of part of the pseudosubstrate sequence with the LC_{20} substrate sequence resulted in autophosphorylation in the absence of Ca^{2+}/CaM {129}. It is important to note, however, that substitution of several basic residues within the pseudosubstrate domain with ala or glu {130,131}, or reversal of a segment of the pseudosubstrate sequence {132}, failed to produce a constitutively active enzyme. Knighton et al. {133} have shown, however, that these apparent discrepancies may be explained by the fact that residues amino terminal to the pseudosubstrate sequence, specifically leu^{774}-leu^{786}, markedly enhance the potency of the synthetic peptide as a competitive inhibitor of MLCK.

The first high-resolution crystal structure of a protein kinase, cyclic AMP-dependent protein kinase, complexed with bound pseudosubstrate inhibitor peptide, was recently reported {134,135}. This enabled modeling of the catalytic core of smooth muscle MLCK and revealed that the pseudosubstrate sequence could be readily fit within the substrate binding site {133}. The intrasteric model for regulation of MLCK (fig. 54-5) by binding of the pseudosubstrate domain to the myosin binding site is therefore feasible from a structural standpoint.

MYOSIN LIGHT-CHAIN PHOSPHATASE

The implication that myosin phosphorylation plays a central role in the regulation of smooth muscle contraction led to the isolation and characterization of myosin light-chain phosphatases (MLCPs) from a variety of smooth muscle tissues. Pato and Adelstein {136} initially isolated two phosphatases from turkey gizzard: SMP-I consisted of three subunits of M_r 60 kDa, 55 kDa, and 38 kDa (the catalytic subunit) present in equimolar amounts and was independent of Mg^{2+} and relatively nonspecific; SMP-II consisted of a single polypeptide chain of M_r 43 kDa, required Mg^{2+} for activity, and appeared to be specific for LC_{20}. However, neither SMP-I nor SMP-II dephosphorylated intact myosin, suggesting that these phosphatases do not function in vivo in the dephosphorylation of myosin. Interestingly, the free catalytic subunit of SMP-I dephosphorylated HMM. This raised the intriguing possibility that subunit association-dissociation may be a physiological mechanism for controlling phosphatase activity by altering its substrate specificity {137}. Two other phosphatases, both of which were capable of dephosphorylating intact myosin, were also identified in turkey gizzard: SMP-III and SMP-IV. SMP-III exhibited a native molecular weight of 390 kDa and migrated as a single band of 40 kDa on SDS-PAGE {138}. The activity of SMP-III was unaffected by Ca^{2+} but activated by Mn^{2+}. This enzyme could not be classified, according to the criteria of Ingebritsen and Cohen {139}, as a type 1, 2A, 2B, or 2C protein serine/threonine phosphatase. SMP-IV was found to consist of two subunits of M_r 58 kDa and 40 kDa, with a native M_r determined by gel filtration of 150 kDa {140}. SMP-IV also could not be classified as a type 1 or 2 protein phosphatase. Phosphatases similar to SMP-I, -II, and -IV have been isolated from rabbit uterine smooth muscle {141}.

SMP-III and SMP-IV bind tightly to myosin ($K_{binding}$ = $3.8 \times 10^5 M^{-1}$ and $3.6 \times 10^5 M^{-1}$, respectively) and significantly more tightly to thiophosphorylated myosin ($K_{binding}$ = $1.1 \times 10^7 M^{-1}$ and $8.0 \times 10^6 M^{-1}$, respectively), consistent with their postulated role in the dephosphorylation of myosin in vivo {142}. No binding of SMP-III or SMP-IV to actin was detected. It appears likely, therefore, that myosin phosphatases in vivo are associated with the thick filament. Consistent with this conclusion, Ikebe and coworkers {143} recently isolated a myosin-associated phosphatase from chicken gizzard. This enzyme is a tetramer of 34-kDa subunits. Although its properties are not fully characteristic of a type 1 phosphatase, it most closely resembles this family of phosphatases. These investigators suggest that the native enzyme contains an additional myosin-binding subunit that is lost during purification. Alessi et al. {144} have described the major avian smooth muscle MLCP as a trimer of a 37 kDa catalytic subunit and 130- and 20-kDa regulatory subunits, which are presumably involved in binding to myosin.

REGULATION OF SMOOTH-MUSCLE CONTRACTION

Myosin phosphorylation-dephosphorylation

It was originally demonstrated by Sobieszek {61} that phosphorylation of smooth muscle myosin is required for actin activation of its MgATPase activity, which led to formulation of the phosphorylation theory of the regulation of smooth muscle contraction (fig. 54-6). According to this theory, stimulation of the smooth muscle cell induces an elevation of $[Ca^{2+}]_i$, the activating Ca^{2+} originating from intracellular stores [the sarcoplasmic reticulum (SR)], and the extracellular space {9}. The relative importance of these two sources of activating Ca^{2+} depends on the nature of the stimulus and the smooth muscle cell type. The $[Ca^{2+}]$ rises transiently from $0.12-0.27 \mu M$ in the resting cell to $0.5-0.7 \mu M$ in the stimulated cell {84–86}. This modest increase in $[Ca^{2+}]_i$ results in Ca^{2+} binding to CaM to form the complex $Ca_4^{2+} \cdot CaM$. The binding of Ca^{2+} to CaM induces a conformational change in CaM that involves exposure of a hydrophobic site(s). In its altered conformation, CaM can bind with high affinity (K_d ~ 1 nM) to the inactive apoenzyme MLCK to form the active holoenzyme, $Ca_4^{2+} \cdot CaM \cdot MLCK$. The activated kinase catalyzes the transfer of the terminal phosphoryl group of ATP to ser^{19} on each of the two 20-kDa light chains of myosin. Phosphorylated myosin can interact with actin and hydrolyze ATP at a fast rate, which provides the energy for rapid crossbridge cycling and the development of tension. Relaxation would occur most simply when Ca^{2+} is removed from the sarcoplasm by the action of Ca^{2+}-transport ATPases in the SR and sarcolemmal

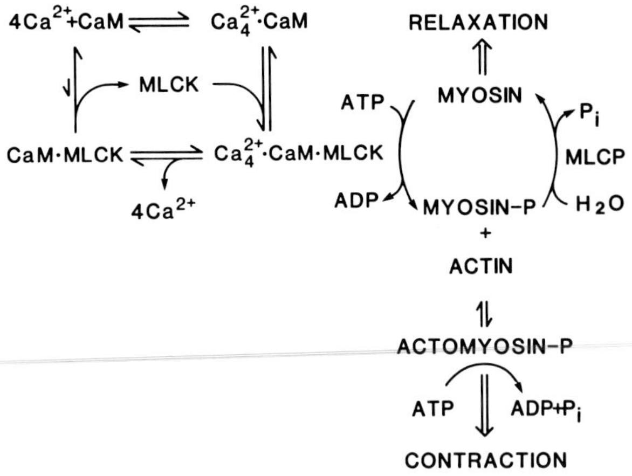

$$4Ca^{2+} + CaM \rightleftharpoons Ca_4^{2+} \cdot CaM$$

Fig. 54-6. Myosin phosphorylation-dephosphorylation as the primary mechanism in the regulation of smooth muscle contraction. CaM = calmodulin; MLCK = myosin light-chain kinase; MLCP = myosin light-chain phosphatase; myosin-P = phosphorylated myosin; actomyosin-P = acto-phosphorylated myosin; P_i = inorganic phosphate. Taken from Walsh {9} with the permission of The National Research Council of Canada.

Table 54-3. Actin activation of the MgATPase of thiophosphorylated smooth muscle myosin does not require Ca^{2+}

Actin	Ca^{2+}	MgATPase rate (nmoles P_i/mg myosin · min)
−	+	8.7
+	+	121.9
+	−	105.0

Myosin was thiophosphorylated (to ~2 moles/mole myosin) and then purified as previously described {147}. ATPase reaction conditions were as follows: 25 mM Tris-HCl (pH 7.5), 60 mM KCl, 10 mM $MgCl_2$, 0.1 mM $CaCl_2$ or 1 mM EGTA, 1 mM [γ-^{32}P] ATP, 1 μM thiophosphorylated myosin, 6 μM actin, 2 μM tropomyosin, 0.6 μM CaM, 93.5 nM MLCK, 30°C.

membranes and the sarcolemmal Na^+-Ca^{2+} exchanger {145}. This leads to dissociation of Ca^{2+} from the $Ca_4^{2+} \cdot CaM \cdot MLCK$ complex and inactivation of the kinase. As a consequence, myosin phosphorylation stops, and myosin, which had been phosphorylated during the activation phase of the contractile cycle, is dephosphorylated by MLCP. Actin and myosin dissociate and the muscle relaxes.

A substantial body of evidence has been accumulated from biochemical and physiological experimentation that supports this phosphorylation theory. Several types of experimental systems have been used: systems reconstituted from purified contractile and regulatory proteins; systems composed of crude actomyosin or myofibrillar preparations that contain associated regulatory and other proteins; in vitro motile systems in which movement of myosin-coated beads over an actin cable network, or movement of fluorescently labeled actin filaments over immobilized myosin, is recorded; skinned (demembranated) or permeabilized smooth muscle fibers and single cells; and intact smooth muscle fibers and single cells. As mentioned previously, several investigators have observed a positive correlation between myosin phosphorylation and the actin-activated MgATPase of smooth muscle myosin, superprecipitation, and tension development in skinned and intact smooth muscle fibers.

The ATP analog, adenosine 5'-0-(3-thiotriphosphate), abbreviated ATPγS, has been particularly useful in evaluating the phosphorylation theory. This nucleotide is useful because it is commonly a good substrate of protein kinases, but the thiophosphorylated protein is a poor substrate for phosphatases. Thus ATPγS is a good substrate of smooth muscle MLCK, permitting Ca^{2+}/CaM-dependent thiophosphorylation of smooth muscle myosin,

whereas thiophosphorylated myosin is quite resistant to phosphatase action. Thiophosphorylation of gizzard myosin resulted in loss of Ca^{2+} sensitivity of the actin-activated myosin MgATPase in a system reconstituted from the purified proteins {146} (table 54-3). Furthermore, incubation of skinned smooth muscle fibers with ATPγS in the presence of Ca^{2+} led to thiophosphorylation of myosin and induced Ca^{2+}-insensitive activation of tension upon subsequent addition of ATP {148,149} (necessary since ATPγS will not support actomyosin ATPase activity). Nucleotides that are poor substrates of MLCK (ITP, GTP, UTP, and CTP) are poor relative to ATP in inducing Ca^{2+}-sensitive superprecipitation of gizzard actomyosin or tension development in skinned smooth muscle fibers {150}. Although CTP is a poor substrate of MLCK, it is hydrolysed by acto-phosphorylated myosin. Following thiophosphorylation of myosin, addition of CTP to skinned fibers in the absence of Ca^{2+} induced rapid force development {151}.

It was very important to establish the reversibility of the effect of myosin phosphorylation on actin activation of the myosin MgATPase. Sellers et al. {152} used purified MLCK and MLCP to achieve the reversible phosphorylation of myosin and measured the actin-activated myosin MgATPase activity at each stage of the procedure. The actin-activated ATPase rate of unphosphorylated myosin (4 nmoles P_i/mg myosin · min) rose to 51 nmoles/mg myosin · min when myosin was phosphorylated to the extent of 2 moles P_i/mole myosin. Subsequent dephosphorylation with MLCP decreased the ATPase rate to 5 nmoles/mg myosin · min. Rephosphorylation with MLCK increased the rate again to 46 nmoles/mg myosin · min. Other groups have observed similar correlations between myosin phosphorylation and actin-activated myosin MgATPase activity or superprecipitation with the aid of myosin phosphatases {153,154}. Such approaches have been extended to skinned fibers. For example, myosin phosphatases have been used to dephosphorylate myosin and to induce relaxation in skinned fibers of hog carotid artery {155}, chicken gizzard {156}, and rat uterine smooth muscle {157}. The relaxant effect of addition of the catalytic subunit of type 2A protein phosphatase to skinned uterine fibers was prevented by prior addition to the bathing medium of either thiophosphorylated LC_{20} or

MLCK. Thiophosphorylation of myosin in the skinned fibers prevented the phosphatase-induced relaxation {157}.

Several pharmacological agents, including phenothiazine {158} and naphthalenesulfonamide {159} derivatives, have been synthesized that bind with high affinity to CaM in a Ca^{2+}-dependent manner. These and other agents inhibit MLCK activity by binding to CaM and preventing its interaction with the kinase. They also inhibit the Ca^{2+}-dependent actin-activated MgATPase activity of gizzard actomyosin {160–162}. Furthermore, a variety of CaM antagonists inhibited tension development in skinned intestinal and arterial muscle fibers {163,164}, intact arterial strips {165–167}, and bovine tracheal smooth muscle {168}, and induced relaxation of skinned taenia coli {169} and rabbit aortic strips {170,171}. The compound ML-9, a selective inhibitor of MLCK, inhibited K^{+}-induced contractions of rabbit mesenteric arterial strips and relaxed saponin-skinned fibers induced to contract by Ca^{2+} {172}.

Another approach used to evaluate the phosphorylation theory involved the generation of a Ca^{2+}-independent form of MLCK. Mild proteolysis of Ca^{2+}/CaM-dependent MLCK (130 kDa) with α-chymotrypsin yielded a stable, active fragment of 78.5 kDa that no longer required Ca^{2+} or CaM for activity {173}, i.e., similar to the constitutively active tryptic fragment of MLCK described earlier. This enabled us to phosphorylate myosin in the absence of Ca^{2+} and thereby to distinguish between the effects of myosin phosphorylation and those of other potential Ca^{2+}-dependent regulatory mechanisms that may be involved in the control of actin-myosin interactions. The isolated Ca^{2+}-independent kinase was used in experiments with smooth muscle actomyosin {151,173} and skinned fiber preparations {151,174} to determine the effects of myosin phosphorylation, achieved in the absence of Ca^{2+}, on the actin-activated myosin MgATPase and tension development. The crude gizzard actomyosin preparation, which contained MLCK and CaM, exhibited Ca^{2+}-sensitive actomyosin MgATPase activity (75.9% Ca^{2+} sensitivity), as expected. When myosin in this crude actomyosin preparation was phosphorylated by the Ca^{2+}-independent MLCK in the absence of Ca^{2+}, the Ca^{2+} sensitivity of the ATPase was essentially abolished (5.2% Ca^{2+} sensitivity). Myosin phosphorylation was therefore sufficient to induce actin activation of the MgATPase activity in a crude actomyosin preparation.

In skinned fiber experiments, incubation of fiber bundles with Ca^{2+}-independent MLCK and ATP in the absence of Ca^{2+} elicited tension development, which was reversed upon washout of the kinase. Tension development was shown to be accompanied by specific phosphorylation of the 20-kDa light chain of myosin, and relaxation was accompanied by dephosphorylation of the myosin {174}. The amount of tension developed following myosin phosphorylation in the absence of Ca^{2+} was comparable to that observed in the presence of Ca^{2+}. Maximum tension development could therefore be accounted for solely by myosin phosphorylation. Similar results were obtained using isolated, skinned chicken gizzard smooth muscle cells {175}. Mrwa et al. {176} compared the contractions of skinned smooth muscle elicited by Ca^{2+} and the Ca^{2+}-independent MLCK in the absence of Ca^{2+} in terms of isometric force, immediate elastic recoil, unloaded shortening velocity, shortening under a constant load, and ATPase activity. They concluded that the contraction induced by Ca^{2+}-independent kinase in the absence of Ca^{2+} is kinetically similar, though not identical, to a contraction induced by Ca^{2+}.

The Ca^{2+}-independent kinase also utilizes ATPγS as a substrate in vitro. Myosin thiophosphorylation could therefore be achieved in skinned fibers in the absence of Ca^{2+}, and this resulted in contraction of the fibers upon subsequent addition of ATP, again in the absence of Ca^{2+} {174}. On the other hand, treatment of skinned fibers with Ca^{2+}-independent MLCK and CTP in the absence of Ca^{2+} failed to induce force development. However, if myosin in the skinned fibers was first thiophosphorylated with ATPγS and Ca^{2+}-independent MLCK in the absence of Ca^{2+}, subsequent addition of CTP, still in the absence of Ca^{2+}, resulted in rapid maximal force development {151}.

Microinjection of constitutively active MLCK into isolated toad stomach smooth muscle cells induced specific phosphorylation of myosin LC_{20} {177} and contraction {178}.

Synthetic peptide inhibitors of MLCK, which are more specific than the pharmacological agents referred to earlier, have also proven useful in evaluating the functional significance of myosin phosphorylation. RS20, a peptide corresponding to the CaM-binding domain of MLCK (arg^{797}-ser^{815}), behaves as a CaM antagonist {120}. SM-1, a peptide corresponding to the pseudosubstrate domain of the kinase (ser^{787}-arg^{808}), acts as a competitive inhibitor with respect to the myosin substrate {121}. RS20 was found to completely relax skinned guinea-pig taenia coli maximally contracted by Ca^{2+}; this relaxation was accompanied by LC_{20} dephosphorylation {179}. These effects were reversed by the addition of CaM, as predicted. Microinjection of RS20 or SM-1 into single toad stomach cells blocked K^{+} contractions in a concentration-dependent manner {177,178}. Furthermore, both peptides inhibited Ca^{2+}-induced shortening of skinned single toad stomach cells {177}.

Phosphatase inhibitors have received a great deal of utilization in recent years as experimental tools to evaluate the physiological significance of protein phosphorylation-dephosphorylation reactions. Okadaic acid has been shown to induce contraction of several intact smooth muscle fiber preparations, e.g., human umbilical artery, rabbit aorta, guinea-pig taenia caecum {180}, and lamb trachea {181}. These contractions were independent of extracellular Ca^{2+} and did not involve mobilization of Ca^{2+} from internal stores {182}. Okadaic acid also induced contraction of saponin- {182} and Triton-skinned taenia coli {183}. MLCP was inhibited by okadaic acid in such experiments, and a low level of basal MLCK activity {184} was sufficient to induce myosin LC_{20} phosphorylation and force development. A distinct phosphatase inhibitor, calyculin A, has similar effects as okadaic acid on smooth muscle {182}.

The in vitro motility assay originally developed by Sheetz and Spudich {185} is a useful model of unloaded shortening velocity in the intact muscle. The original method involved microscopic examination of the directed movement of myosin-coated polymer beads along actin cables exposed by dissection of the fresh-water alga *Nitella axillaris*. Beads coated with smooth muscle myosin moved along the actin cables only when the myosin was phosphorylated {186,187}. The velocity of movement {0.2 μm/s) was one-tenth that of beads coated with skeletal muscle myosin, consistent with the slower shortening velocity of smooth compared with skeletal muscle. Furthermore, as expected, movement of beads coated with skeletal muscle myosin was independent of phosphorylation. The motility assay has been modified recently to examine the movement of fluorescently labeled actin filaments over myosin molecules adhering to a glass surface {188} or a nitrocellulose membrane {189}. Results obtained with this system confirm the requirement of phosphorylation of smooth-muscle myosin for movement. The overall conclusion reached from these diverse experimental approaches is that myosin phosphorylation is the key event in actin activation of the myosin MgATPase and initiation of tension development in smooth muscle.

Much attention has been devoted towards an understanding of the molecular mechanism whereby myosin phosphorylation leads to actin activation of the myosin MgATPase. Suzuki et al. {190} originally demonstrated that phosphorylation converted myosin from a form with a sedimentation coefficient of 10S to a 6S component, and suggested the 10S form to be a dimer. However, several subsequent studies established that this phosphorylation-induced change in sedimentation coefficient is due to a conformational change in monomeric myosin, rather than dimer formation {53,191,192}. Electron microscopy has revealed that the tail in 10S myosin is bent in two places (about one third and two thirds of the way down the tail from the head-tail junction) and folded so that the distal bend comes in close proximity to the neck region. On the other hand, the tail in 6S myosin is elongated and therefore resembles skeletal muscle myosin {53,192,193}. An important correlation between the transition of smooth-muscle myosin from the 10S to the 6S form and conversion of myosin from an inactive to an active state was demonstrated by Ikebe et al. {194}. Studies of this conformational transition of smooth muscle myosin and HMM have led to the suggestion that phosphorylation induces an important conformational change in the neck region of the molecule {195}. While these studies have been conducted with monomeric myosin, it is likely that similar changes occur in the neck region of myosin molecules assembled into filaments, in which form myosin is thought to exist in both contracting and relaxed smooth muscle {58}. The intramolecular interactions that lead to the 10S-6S transition in vitro are believed to reflect intermolecular interactions within myosin filaments. Phosphorylation would then affect interactions between neighboring myosin molecules in the thick filament, causing conformational changes that would then permit filament sliding and the development of tension. Recent studies with chimeric regulatory light chains composed of Ca^{2+}-binding domains derived from chicken skeletal and smooth muscle myosins indicate

that the third of the four domains in the light chain is responsible for controlling actin-myosin interaction {196}.

Other possible regulatory mechanisms

While it is now quite firmly established that myosin phosphorylation represents the primary Ca^{2+}-mediated mechanism for the regulation of smooth muscle contraction, a significant body of evidence has accumulated indicating the existence of additional secondary control systems. Several examples of dissociation between force, LC_{20} phosphorylation, sarcoplasmic free $[Ca^{2+}]$, and crossbridge cycling rates have been reported {197–206}, suggesting the existence of a regulatory mechanism(s) for smooth muscle contraction in addition to myosin phosphorylation-dephosphorylation. For example, while myosin phosphorylation has generally been found to be a prerequisite for the development of tension, and a correlation between the level of myosin phosphorylation and the maximum velocity of shortening (crossbridge cycling rate) has been frequently observed {e.g., 68,207}, several studies with intact and skinned fibers indicate that developed tension can be maintained in a variety of smooth muscle tissues during prolonged stimulation, in spite of the fact that myosin becomes dephosphorylated (reviewed in {208}). This maintenance of tension without myosin phosphorylation, the so-called latch state, is Ca^{2+} dependent and is characterized by a relatively low rate of ATP hydrolysis, i.e., noncycling or slowly cycling crossbridges. The latch state is believed to permit the conservation of energy during prolonged tonic contractions and appears to have a greater sensitivity to Ca^{2+} than does myosin phosphorylation {209}. Prior phosphorylation of myosin with consequent development of tension is required for expression of the latch state.

The mechanism of Ca^{2+}-dependent phosphorylation of myosin depicted in fig. 54-6 suggests that this could be simply an on-off switch for contraction. On the other hand, a certain degree of flexibility could be achieved by altering the activation state of MLCK through precise control of $[Ca^{2+}]_i$ within the activating range (~0.1–0.7 μM). This is achieved, for example, by agents that elevate cyclic nucleotide levels, resulting in relaxation of vascular smooth muscle {210}. Most of the effects of cyclic AMP are mediated by cyclic AMP-dependent protein kinase {211} and of cyclic GMP by cyclic GMP-dependent protein kinase {212}. However, cyclic AMP can activate cyclic GMP-dependent protein kinase and cyclic GMP can activate cyclic AMP-dependent protein kinase, although 10 times higher concentrations of the "opposite" cyclic nucleotide are required in each case {213}. Lincoln and coworkers {214} have made a very strong case for cyclic AMP activation of cyclic GMP-dependent protein kinase inducing vascular smooth muscle relaxation. This probably results from a reduction in $[Ca^{2+}]_i$, but the mechanism has not been elucidated. It may involve phosphorylation of phospholamban and release of inhibition of the SR Ca^{2+} pump {215}, activation of a plasma membrane Ca^{2+} pump {216}, or activation of K^+ channels, inducing hyperpolarization and decreasing Ca^{2+} influx {217}. Tang et al. {218} recently showed that isoproterenol inhibited carbachol-induced contraction of bovine tracheal smooth muscle strips by decreasing $[Ca^{2+}]_i$ and thereby LC_{20} phosphorylation. Interestingly, however, isoproterenol treatment of KCl-contracted muscle resulted in diminished LC_{20} phosphorylation and force without any change in $[Ca^{2+}]_i$, suggesting a different cellular mechanism in this case.

Additional flexibility in the contractile regulatory system could be achieved by regulating any one of the molecular steps downstream of the Ca^{2+} signal (fig. 54-6), and several such regulatory mechanisms have been proposed: (a) phosphorylation of MLCK resulting in decreased sensitivity to Ca^{2+}/CaM; (b) inhibition of MLCP through a receptor-activated, G protein-coupled pathway involving generation of arachidonic acid; (c) protein kinase C via an as-yet undefined pathway; (d) direct regulation of cross-bridge cycling by thin filament-associated proteins (caldesmon and calponin). Current knowledge of these putative modulatory mechanisms will be discussed in turn.

PHOSPHORYLATION OF MLCK

It has been known for a long time that smooth muscle MLCK is a substrate in vitro of cyclic AMP-dependent protein kinase [219]. Phosphorylation occurred at two sites in the apoenzyme: site A (ser[815]) and site B (ser[828]), which are close to the CaM-binding site (ala[796]-lys[813]). Only site B was phosphorylated in the presence of bound CaM [220]. Site B phosphorylation had no observable effect on MLCK activity, whereas site A phosphorylation decreased the affinity of the kinase for CaM up to 20-fold. These observations led to the suggestion that catecholamine-induced phosphorylation of MLCK may cause inactivation of the enzyme, leading to myosin dephosphorylation and relaxation of the muscle. Detailed analysis of phosphorylation of MLCK in bovine tracheal smooth muscle, however, did not support such a physiological regulatory mechanism [221]. Ser[815] of the kinase was phosphorylated only in response to KCl or carbachol treatment, both of which *contracted* the muscle. Isoproterenol relaxed tracheal smooth muscle strips stimulated with carbachol, but did not change the extent of ser[815] phosphorylation.

MLCK is also phosphorylated at site A in vitro by protein kinase C (PKC) [222,223], and Ca^{2+}/CaM-dependent protein kinase II (CaM kinase II) [224,225]. Phosphorylation of site A by PKC does not occur, however, in intact tracheal strips treated with phorbol ester [221]. On the other hand, as noted above, site A phosphorylation does occur in response to agents that induce an increase in $[Ca^{2+}]_i$, suggesting that a Ca^{2+}-dependent kinase is involved. Pretreatment of tracheal smooth muscle cells with KN-62, a specific inhibitor of CaM kinase II, did not affect the increase in $[Ca^{2+}]_i$ induced by ionomycin, but did inhibit phosphorylation of MLCK at site A [226]. Stull and coworkers [226] have suggested, therefore, that the Ca^{2+}-dependent phosphorylation of ser[815] of MLCK by CaM kinase II decreases the Ca^{2+} sensitivity of myosin light-chain phosphorylation in smooth muscle by increasing K_{CaM}, the concentration of Ca^{2+}/CaM required for half-maximal activation of MLCK.

INHIBITION OF MYOSIN LIGHT-CHAIN PHOSPHATASE

Several examples of agonist-induced sensitization of the contractile response of smooth muscles to Ca^{2+} have been reported {e.g., 227–229}. Muscle strips permeabilized with *S. aureus* α-toxin have been particularly useful experimental systems for investigating the mechanism of this Ca^{2+} sensitization. α-Toxin creates small holes in the plasma membrane that allow entry and exit of molecules <4 kDa, thereby enabling the clamping of $[Ca^{2+}]_i$ and the addition of small molecules such as GTPγS, while retaining intracellular proteins. Another advantage of α-toxin-permeabilized muscle is that it retains receptor coupling, i.e., Ca^{2+} sensitization in response to a variety of alpha-adrenergic, muscarinic, and eicosanoid agonists is maintained {228}. The Ca^{2+} sensitization process involves a GTP-binding protein {230} (possibly *rho* p21 {231}) and an increase in LC_{20} phosphorylation {230}: Addition of GTPγS to α-toxin-permeabilized strips increased both force and LC_{20} phosphorylation at a fixed, submaximal $[Ca^{2+}]$. The increased LC_{20} phosphorylation is due to inhibition of MLCP {232}, and recent evidence suggests that arachidonic acid relays the message from the plasma membrane to the myofilaments {233}: Arachidonic acid increased force and LC_{20} phosphorylation in α-toxin-permeabilized rabbit femoral artery at a fixed, submaximal $[Ca^{2+}]$, and slowed both relaxation and LC_{20} dephosphorylation upon removal of Ca^{2+}. Furthermore, arachidonic acid inhibited the HMM phosphatase activity of a purified smooth muscle MLCP by inducing dissociation of the oligomeric enzyme into subunits {233}.

The pathway for agonist-induced Ca^{2+} sensitization, as far as it has been elucidated to date, therefore, is as follows:

$$
\begin{array}{c}
\text{Agonist} \\
\downarrow \\
\text{Receptor} \\
\downarrow \\
\text{GTP-binding protein} \\
\downarrow \\
\uparrow \text{Phospholipase A}_2 \\
\downarrow \\
\uparrow \text{Arachidonic acid} \\
\downarrow \\
\downarrow \text{MLCP} \\
\downarrow \\
\uparrow \text{LC}_{20} \text{ phosphorylation} \\
\downarrow \\
\text{Contraction} \\
\text{(without a change in } [Ca^{2+}]_i)
\end{array}
$$

LC_{20} phosphorylation occurs upon inhibition of MLCP due to a low level of Ca^{2+}-independent MLCK activity expressed in the tissue {184}. This has been estimated at 3% of the MLCK activity in the presence of maximal

[Ca^{2+}] and CaM. It is unlikely that this activity is due to MLCK itself, since the Ca^{2+}-independent activity of the purified enzyme is <0.1% of the maximal Ca^{2+}/CaM-stimulated activity {184}. CaM kinase II can also phosphorylate myosin specifically at ser^{19} of LC$_{20}$ {234}. Since this enzyme can be rendered Ca^{2+} independent by autophosphorylation, it may account for the MLCK activity detected at low [Ca^{2+}]$_i$.

PROTEIN KINASE C

Numerous extracellular signals (peptide hormones, muscarinic cholinergic agents, neurotransmitters, growth factors, etc.) trigger membrane polyphosphoinositide turnover via activation of phosphoinositide-specific phospholipase C {235}, which catalyzes hydrolysis of membrane phosphoinositides, particularly phosphatidylinositol 4,5-bisphosphate, to generate two second messengers: 1,2-diacylglycerol (DG) and inositol 1,4,5-trisphosphate (IP$_3$) {236,237}. IP$_3$ induces Ca^{2+} release from the SR of smooth muscle {238}, and DG, which remains membrane bound due to its lipophilic character, activates the Ca^{2+}- and phospholipid-dependent protein kinase (PKC) {239}.

The possible involvement of PKC in the regulation of smooth muscle contraction originated with two main observations: (a) tumor-promoting phorbol esters (which bind to and activate PKC) induced slowly developing, sustained contractions of smooth muscle {e.g., 240,241}; and (b) gizzard myosin was phosphorylated in vitro by PKC at ser^1, ser^2, and thr^9 of LC$_{20}$ {242,243}. This phosphorylation alone did not affect the enzymatic properties of unphosphorylated myosin, but reduced the actin-activated ATPase activity of myosin phosphorylated by MLCK by ~50% {244}. This effect, however, would not appear to be consistent with the observed phorbol ester-induced *contractions* referred to above, and indeed studies with intact smooth muscle fibers do not support a physiological role for PKC-catalyzed myosin phosphorylation. For example, treatment of smooth muscle strips with agonists such as carbachol or phenylephrine, which induce phosphoinositide turnover and DG production, did not result in myosin phosphorylation at the PKC-specific sites, but only at the MLCK-specific sites (ser^{19} with a little thr^{18} phosphorylation) {245,246}.

In some instances, phorbol ester-induced contractions result from an increase in [Ca^{2+}]$_i$ with consequent phosphorylation of LC$_{20}$ on ser^{19} and activation of the muscle {e.g., 247}. In other cases, however, phorbol ester-induced contractions do not involve changes in [Ca^{2+}]$_i$ or the level of myosin phosphorylation {e.g., 240}.

PKC exhibits broad substrate specificity and at least three other proteins involved in the contractile machinery are phosphorylated in vitro: MLCK {222,223}, calponin {248}, and caldesmon {249}. PKC-catalyzed phosphorylation of MLCK occurs at site A (see above) but does not appear to occur in intact muscle {221}. The properties of calponin and cladesmon are discussed below.

Analysis of putative physiological roles of PKC is com-plicated by the fact that this enzyme exists as at least 10 isoenzymes, which differ in substrate specificity and regulatory properties {239,250}. In particular, PKC isoenzymes can be divided into two groups: Group A PKCs (α, β$_I$, β$_{II}$, and γ) require Ca^{2+}, phospholipid and diacylglycerol for activity, whereas group B PKCs (δ, ε, ζ, η, θ, and λ) are Ca^{2+} independent. To date, α, β, ε, and ζ PKC isoenzyme expression has been identified in smooth muscle {251–253}. The possibility that Ca^{2+}-independent isoenzyme(s) of PKC may play a role in smooth muscle contraction was suggested by studies with permeabilized single cells of the ferret aorta {254,255}. For example, addition of PKM (the constitutively active catalytic fragment of PKC produced by trypsin digestion) to the skinned cells at pCa 7 elicited a sustained increase in force that was reversible upon addition of a pseudosubstrate inhibitor peptide corresponding to PKC (19–31) {255}. More detailed discussions of PKC in relation to smooth muscle contraction can be found in recent reviews {252,256}.

THIN FILAMENT-ASSOCIATED REGULATORY PROTEINS

Biochemical methods have suggested the existence of a thin-filament-linked mechanism of regulation of ac-tomyosin MgATPase activity in a variety of smooth muscle tissues. Early studies of Ca^{2+}-mediated regulation of smooth muscle contraction provided indirect evidence for a thin-filament-linked regulatory mechanism similar to vertebrate striated-muscle troponin/tropomyosin {e.g., 257}. As discussed earlier, it is well established that smooth muscle contains tropomyosin, but further characterization has led to the conclusion that troponin is not present in vertebrate smooth muscles. Nevertheless, application of the myosin competition test {12} confirmed the existence of thin-filament-linked regulation in vertebrate smooth muscle {258}. In principle, this test involves hybridization of thin filaments of the muscle of interest (in this case, vertebrate smooth muscle) present in a crude actomyosin preparation with purified, and therefore unregulated, skeletal muscle myosin. If the resultant hybrid actomyosin MgATPase is Ca^{2+} sensitive, this indicates the existence of thin-filament-linked regulation in the muscle of interest. As noted above, Marston et al. {258} obtained a positive result when they applied the myosin competition test to vertebrate smooth muscle. Since this result was controversial {259}, we reexamined this question and confirmed Marston's conclusion (table 54-4).

Thin filaments were isolated from chicken gizzard using mild extraction conditions in order to retain actin-associated regulatory proteins. The protein composition of the resultant native thin filaments is shown in fig. 54-7. The major components, as expected, are actin and tro-pomyosin. In addition, proteins of M$_r$ 34 and 140 kDa are apparent; these were identified by Western blotting as calponin and caldesmon, respectively {248,260}. These and similar studies suggested that the actin-binding proteins, caldesmon and calponin, may be involved in regulating actin-myosin interactions and therefore the contractile

Table 54-4. Identification of thin filament-linked regulation in vertebrate smooth muscle using the myosin competition test

	MgATPase rate (nmoles P_i/mg myosin · min)		Ca^{2+} sensitivity (%)
	$+Ca^{2+}$	$-Ca^{2+}$	
Gizzard actomyosin + skeletal myosin	255.8	120.8	52.8
Gizzard actin + tropomyosin + skeletal myosin	308.7	313.2	0

Chicken gizzard actomyosin (1 mg/ml) and rabbit skeletal-muscle myosin (1 mg/ml) were incubated separately and together in 0.6 M KCl, 10 mM imidazole-HCl (pH 7.0), and 5 mM $MgCl_2$ with gentle stirring for 6 hours at 4°C to dissociate actin and myosin, and associated proteins. Samples were then dialyzed overnight against two changes (21 each) of 60 mM KCl, 10 mM imidazole-HCl (pH 7.0), 5 mM $MgCl_2$, 10 mM NaN_3, and 0.5 mM dithiothreitol to allow hybridization of skeletal myosin with gizzard actin and associated proteins. MgATPase activities were measured as previously described {260} in the presence and absence of Ca^{2+}. MgATPase rates have been corrected for the ATPase rates of the individual components: gizzard actomyosin = 6.0 ($+Ca^{2+}$) and 0.0 ($-Ca^{2+}$) nmoles P_i/mg actomyosin · min; skeletal myosin = 5.2 ($+Ca^{2+}$) and 4.9 ($-Ca^{2+}$) nmoles P_i/mg myosin · min. Taken from Walsh {9} with permission of The National Research Council of Canada.

state of smooth muscle. Structural and functional characterization of these proteins has lent support to this hypothesis.

CALDESMON

Caldesmon was first described in 1981 as a major protein component of chicken-gizzard smooth muscle that interacts with CaM in a Ca^{2+}-dependent manner {261}. The isolated protein was also found to interact with F actin {261}, tropomyosin {262}, and myosin {263}, these interactions being Ca^{2+} independent. Subcellular localization studies and analysis of isolated smooth muscle thin filaments support the notion that caldesmon is associated with actin in vivo. Caldesmon has been identified in and isolated from a wide range of muscle and nonmuscle tissues and cultured cells {see 9 for review}. The content of caldesmon in different smooth muscle tissues is quite variable. The tissue concentration of caldesmon in chicken gizzard was determined to be ~11 µM {264}. Haeberle et al. {265}, using a quantitative immunoblotting procedure, demonstrated that tonic vascular smooth muscles have the lowest caldesmon content (1 mole caldesmon per 205 moles actin), whereas phasic smooth muscles have the highest (1 mole caldesmon per 22–28 moles actin). The demonstration of immunologically crossreactive caldesmons in a variety of tissues from diverse species suggests a degree of structural conservation consistent with an important functional role.

Immunological methods have revealed the existence of two main classes of caldesmon: One class has a subunit molecular weight (determined by SDS-PAGE) of 120–150 kDa and the other class 70–80 kDa. The lower molecular weight forms of caldesmon have been observed in some, but not all, tissues examined and are particularly abundant in cultured cells {266}. The predominant, often exclusive, form of caldesmon expressed in smooth muscle cells is the high molecular weight form. In addition to being immunologically crossreactive, the two classes of isoforms of caldesmon exhibit similar functional properties, e.g., Ca^{2+}-dependent binding to CaM, Ca^{2+}-independent binding to actin, and inhibition of actomyosin MgATPase activity {267} (see below).

In some tissues, e.g., chicken gizzard and hog stomach, the high molecular weight isoform of caldesmon appears as two closely spaced bands on SDS-polyacrylamide gels {268–270}; these represent distinct isoforms that have been cloned and sequenced {271,272}. Native caldesmon is probably monomeric, but the isolated protein is susceptible to dimer and higher oligomer formation due to crosslinking via interchain disulfide bridges {273}. Caldesmon is a highly asymmetric molecule, as revealed by sucrose density gradient centrifugation (sedimentation coefficient = 2.7 S), gel filtration (Stokes radius = 91 Å) {268}, and low-angle rotary shadowing {269}, and the smooth muscle protein has monomer dimensions of 74 nm × 1.9 nm {274}.

Clues to the physiological function of caldesmon are provided by a series of binding studies. The stoichiometry of Ca^{2+}-dependent binding of CaM to caldesmon is 1 CaM : 1 caldesmon {261} with K_d in the micromolar range {267,275}, although Wang et al. {276} have suggested the presence of two CaM-binding sites on caldesmon. Caldesmon binding to F actin is Ca^{2+} independent and saturable, with maximal binding of 1 caldesmon to 6–10 actin monomers {24,268,277}. Isolated caldesmon binds to high-affinity sites on actin with K_d in the range of 0.05–1 µM {see 9 for references}. Most interestingly, in the presence of micromolar concentrations of Ca^{2+}, CaM and F actin compete for binding to caldesmon, whereas at lower levels of Ca^{2+} caldesmon binds exclusively to F actin {24,261,268}. The possibility was therefore suggested that caldesmon can flip-flop between actin and CaM as a function of $[Ca^{2+}]_i$, a phenomenon that may be related to its physiological function(s) (see below). However, the amount of CaM required to dissociate caldesmon from actin in the presence of Ca^{2+} is incompatible with the physiological concentrations of actin, caldesmon, and CaM. It is likely, therefore, that caldesmon remains associated with the actin filament in situ, even in the presence of Ca^{2+}. Furthermore, Lehman {278} has shown that chicken-gizzard thin filaments isolated either in the presence or absence of Ca^{2+} contain identical amounts of caldesmon.

The domain structure of caldesmon has been investigated by characterization of proteolytic fragments and deletion mutants (fig. 54-8). Specific chemical cleavage at the two cysteine residues in caldesmon with 2-nitro-5-thiocyanobenzoic acid generates an amino-terminal frag-

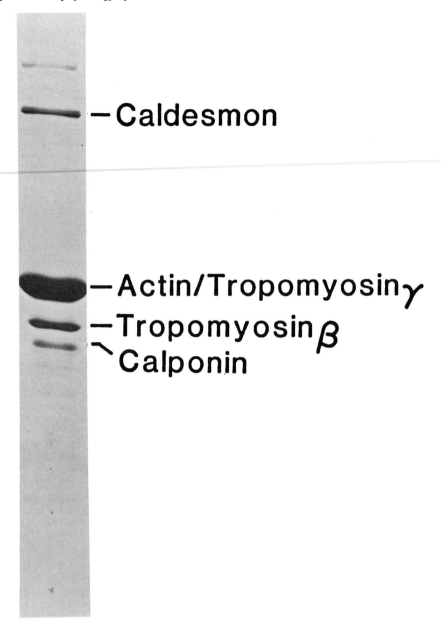

Fig. 54-7. Sodium dodecyl sulfate-polyacrylamide gel electrophoresis of native thin filaments prepared from chicken-gizzard smooth muscle. The protein components were identified by Western blotting.

ment (1–153) that binds myosin {279}. Chymotryptic digestion yields a carboxy-terminal fragment (451–756) that binds actin, tropomyosin, and Ca^{2+}/CaM, and inhibits the actin-activated myosin MgATPase {see 267 for references}. Actin and CaM binding are both retained by a CNBr peptide (659–756), which partially inhibits the actomyosin ATPase {280}. Analysis of deletion mutants has identified a strong actin-binding site (597–629) and a weaker binding site at the carboxy terminus (710–756)

{281}. An additional weak actin-binding site (483–578) appears to be present {282}. The CaM-binding domain has been narrowed down to seven amino acids (659–665): WEKGNVF {281–283}. A synthetic peptide (651–667) containing this sequence bound CaM in a Ca^{2+}-dependent manner and competed with caldesmon for Ca^{2+}/CaM binding {284}. This peptide also bound to F actin and was displaced by Ca^{2+}/CaM. It did not, however, affect the actomyosin ATPase. Addition of the peptide to saponin-

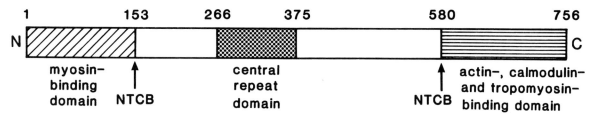

Fig. 54-8. Domain structure of smooth-muscle caldesmon. The numbering is derived from the full-length sequence of one of the chicken gizzard isoforms {272}. The amino and carboxy termini are indicated by N and C, respectively. The sites of cleavage by 2-nitro-5-thiocyanobenzoic acid (NTCB) are indicated.

permeabilized single ferret aortic cells induced contraction at pCa 7.0, which was inhibited at higher [Ca^{2+}] (>pCa 6.6) and by pretreatment with CaM {285}. These observations suggest that caldesmon plays an important inhibitory role in the regulation of smooth muscle tone. Two tropomyosin-binding sites have been identified in caldesmon: 564–620 and 621–756 {283}.

Examination of the amino acid sequence of caldesmon reveals a motif (13–15 residues long) located near the middle of the molecule that is repeated several times. The two high molecular weight isoforms of chicken-gizzard caldesmon differ in that one lacks one of these repeat motifs and is, therefore, 15 residues shorter. The two isoforms contain 9 and 10 repeat motifs, respectively. The function of this central repeat domain is unknown, although it may serve as a spacer between the myosin and actin-binding sites. Secondary structure predictions suggest it has a very high α-helical content, and this is supported by circular dichroic spectral analysis and hydrodynamic measurements of a fragment of caldesmon containing this domain {286}. Of particular interest is the fact that this domain is missing from the low molecular weight forms of caldesmon that are expressed predominantly in non muscle tissues and cultured cells {283}. Otherwise, the high and low molecular weight caldesmons are very similar.

Indirect immunofluorescence microscopy has revealed a periodic distribution of caldesmon along the stress fibers of cultured cells {266}. This coincides with the distribution of tropomyosin and is complementary to that of α-actinin. Caldesmon may, therefore, be associated with a contractile unit composed additionally of actin, myosin, tropomyosin, MLCK, and MLCP {266}, consistent with a functional role for caldesmon in the regulation of actin-myosin interaction. In support of such a notion, Small et al. {287} distinguished two structurally distinct actin-containing domains in smooth muscle: an actomyosin domain, made up of continuous longitudinal arrays of actin and myosin filaments, and an actin-intermediate filament domain, which forms longitudinal fibrils containing actin, filamin, desmin, and α-actinin-rich dense bodies, but which are free of myosin. Caldesmon was found to be located exclusively in the actomyosin domain by immunocytochemistry of ultrathin sections of smooth muscle. Electron microscopic studies led Craig and coworkers {288,289} to suggest that caldesmon is bound along the

actin double helix in register with tropomyosin, each caldesmon molecule spanning 14 actin monomers. However, the binding properties of caldesmon fragments suggest that the molecule is anchored to the actin filament via its carboxy terminus. The rest of the very elongated molecule could then protrude from the actin filament and interact with other molecular components such as myosin. Caldesmon binds to the S$_2$ domain of smooth muscle myosin with a stoichiometry of 1:1 and K$_d$ = 1 µM {263, 290}. The myosin-binding site in caldesmon is located near the amino terminus {279}, i.e., at the opposite end of the molecule to the actin-binding site. Of particular interest is the ability of caldesmon to crosslink actin and myosin filaments {263,291} (discussed below).

Many of the experimental results summarized above suggest, albeit indirectly, that caldesmon may function in regulating actin-myosin interaction, i.e., the contractile state of smooth muscle. This question has been addressed in several laboratories using well-characterized in vitro systems reconstituted from purified contractile and regulatory proteins. Sobue et al. {292} initially demonstrated that isolated caldesmon inhibited superprecipitation of desensitized chicken gizzard actomyosin, an effect that could be overcome by Ca^{2+}/CaM. We later showed that caldesmon inhibited the actin-activated myosin MgATPase activity of a system reconstituted from purified actin, myosin, tropomyosin, CaM, and MLCK without affecting myosin phosphorylation {293}. Maximal inhibition of the actin-activated myosin MgATPase correlated with maximal binding of caldesmon to actin, i.e., ~1 caldesmon per 7 actin monomers {277}. Consistent with these observations, addition of caldesmon to skinned chicken gizzard smooth muscle fibers induced relaxation without altering the level of myosin phosphorylation {294}.

Kinetic studies of the effects of caldesmon on the actomyosin ATPase and binding of actin to myosin subfragments generally indicate that caldesmon inhibits the ATPase by competing with myosin for actin binding {295–297}. This is consistent with identification of the amino terminus of actin as the caldesmon-binding site {298,299}; this is also the region of actin that binds the myosin head {300}. However, Marston and coworkers have provided evidence suggesting that caldesmon inhibits a catalytic step in the ATPase cycle {301,302}. The carboxy-terminal actin-binding domain retains the ability of the intact protein to inhibit the actomyosin ATPase {303}, and a deletion mutant lacking the carboxy-terminal 178 residues does not bind to actin or inhibit actomyosin ATPase activity {304}. Horiuchi et al. {305}, using the inhibitory carboxy-terminal fragment of caldesmon, observed a marked decrease in K_{ATPase} and $K_{binding}$ but no effect on V_{max} of the acto-HMM ATPase in the absence of tropomyosin, but did observe a two- to threefold decrease in V_{max}, in addition to lowering of the K_{ATPase} and $K_{binding}$, in the presence of tropomyosin.

Regulation of smooth muscle contraction by caldesmon has also been studied using the in vitro motility assay. Caldesmon completely inhibited the movement of actin filaments over immobilized, phosphorylated smooth muscle myosin {306}. The amount of caldesmon required for inhibition of actin filament movement was reduced in the presence of tropomyosin. Haeberle et al. {307} observed inhibition of actin filament movement over immobilized, thiophosphorylated smooth muscle myosin only under conditions favoring crosslinking of caldesmon via disulfide bridges.

The possibility that caldesmon may be regulated by phosphorylation-dephosphorylation was first suggested by the observation that partially purified caldesmon could be phosphorylated by a Ca^{2+}/CaM-dependent protein kinase and dephosphorylated by a protein phosphatase, both present in chicken gizzard {293,308}. The kinase was later identified as CaM kinase II {309–311} and the phosphatase as a type 2A protein phosphatase (SMP-I) {311a}. Phosphorylation of caldesmon by this kinase prevented inhibition of the actin-activated myosin MgATPase {308,312}, although others did not observe this effect of phosphorylation {313}. This discrepancy probably results from differences in the extent of phosphorylation of sites located in the carboxy-terminal actin-binding domain: Caldesmon is phosphorylated by CaM kinase II at three sites in the amino-terminal domain (ser[26], ser[59], and ser[73]) and at five sites in the carboxy-terminal domain (thr[469], ser[475], ser[587], ser[620], and ser[726]) {314}. The preferred site of phosphorylation is ser[73], followed by ser[26], ser[726], and ser[587]. Phosphorylation by CaM kinase II blocks the interaction of caldesmon with myosin {279}, presumably as a result of the introduction of negative charges into the amino-terminal myosin-binding domain.

Three other protein serine/threonine kinases have been shown to phosphorylate smooth muscle caldesmon in vitro: PKC {249}, cdc2 kinase {315}, and casein kinase II {316}. PKC phosphorylates two sites (ser[587] and ser[726]), both located in the carboxy-terminal domain, and results in reduced inhibition of acto-HMM and actomyosin ATPase activities due to a reduction in the affinity of caldesmon for actin {317,318}. cdc2 kinase phosphorylates five sites in smooth muscle caldesmon (ser[582], ser[667], thr[673], thr[696], and ser[702]) and inhibits actin binding {315,319}. Casein kinase II phosphorylates ser[73] and thr[83] of caldesmon and results in loss of myosin binding {319a}.

Caldesmon phosphorylation has been observed in a variety of intact smooth muscle strips in response to several contractile stimuli, including carbachol, K^+ depolarization, phorbol esters, histamine, ouabain, norepinephrine, angiotensin II, and endothelin-1 {320–324}. The sites phosphorylated in intact canine aortic smooth muscle treated with phorbol ester were identified as two serine residues, both located in the carboxy-terminal domain of caldesmon {325}. One corresponds to ser[702] of chicken gizzard caldesmon, whereas the other is unique to mammalian caldesmon and is located four residues from the carboxy terminus. Each of these serine residues is immediately amino terminal to a proline, suggesting that the kinase is a proline-directed kinase, i.e., a member of the cdc2 or mitogen-activated protein kinase (MAP kinase) family. MAP kinase was recently identified in chicken gizzard and vascular smooth muscle tissues by Western blotting {326,327}, and a purified MAP kinase (sea star p44[mpk]) phosphorylated serine and threonine residues in the carboxy-terminal domain of caldesmon, but only slightly attenuated its interaction with actin {326}.

The evidence therefore is strongly supportive of a physiological role(s) for caldesmon phosphorylation, probably involving different kinases with different site specificities and having different functional effects.

Based on the properties of caldesmon described above, two physiological functions have been proposed for this protein: (a) regulation of the contractile state of smooth muscle through its ability to inhibit actomyosin ATPase activity, and (b) an organizational role through its ability to crosslink actin and myosin filaments. Latch bridges (slowly or noncycling crossbridges), which are often observed during prolonged contractions of smooth muscle, may involve the crosslinking of actin and myosin via caldesmon {263,279,291,328}. These functions of caldesmon could be regulated by phosphorylation by various kinases, which affect the interactions between caldesmon and actin, or caldesmon and myosin.

CALPONIN

Calponin was first described by Takahashi et al. {329} as a 34-kDa protein that binds to actin in a Ca^{2+}-independent manner and to CaM in a Ca^{2+}-dependent manner. The protein has been purified from avian gizzards {248,329, 330}, bovine {331} and sheep aorta {332}, and porcine {330} and toad stomach {333}, and has been identified by Western blotting in several other bovine {334} and human smooth muscle tissues {335}. Calponin expression is essentially restricted to smooth muscle tissues {336}. The tissue content of calponin is approximately the same as that of tropomyosin {329} and confocal immunofluorescence microscopy confirmed that the subcellular localization of calponin correlates with that of tropomyosin and actin {333}.

Calponin exists as several isoforms as shown by two-dimensional gel electrophoresis {335}. The amino acid sequences of two chicken-gizzard calponin isoforms have been deduced from the cDNA sequences {337}. These isoforms, α and β, have 292 and 252 amino acids, respectively. Their sequences are identical, except that calponin β lacks a 40-residue sequence corresponding to α(217–256). The α and β isoforms are very basic, having pI 9.91 and 9.95 {337}. The carboxy-terminal region of calponin α contains three 29- to 31-amino acid repeats; the β isoform contains only two of these repeats. Regions of the calponin sequence are homologous to regions of other proteins of known sequence {330,337}; SM22α (a smooth muscle protein of unknown function), the mp20 gene product of *Drosophila* (a putative Ca^{2+}-binding protein present in every muscle tissue except the asynchronous oscillatory flight muscles), caldesmon, calpactin I, *ras* p21, α-actinin, and the candidate *unc-87* gene of *C. elegans*. The significance of these homologous sequences, however, is not evident.

Calponin binds to purified tropomyosin {338} as well as to actin and Ca^{2+}/CaM. However, it is not clear that calponin-tropomyosin interactions occur in situ. For example, the interaction between calponin and tropomyosin is disrupted at ionic strengths >100 mM KCl, i.e., below physiological ionic strength {330}. The K_d of actin for calponin is 4.6×10^{-8} M and is not affected significantly by the presence of tropomyosin {339}. Furthermore, as discussed below, phosphorylated calponin retains the ability to bind to immobilized tropomyosin at low ionic strength, but does not bind to actin or actin/tropomyosin. The physiological significance of the interaction between calponin and Ca^{2+}/CaM is also uncertain. As discussed below, the interaction between calponin and actin appears to have functional importance.

Several properties of calponin discussed above suggest that it may be involved in regulation of actin-myosin interaction in smooth muscle: (a) It binds to actin with high affinity; (b) it is localized on the thin filaments in situ; (c) it is weakly immunoreactive with troponin T {340}; and (d) it is present at the same molar concentration as tropomyosin, i.e., 1 calponin to 7 actin monomers. To address this hypothesis directly we examined the effects of calponin on the in vitro contractile system composed of the purified contractile and regulatory proteins (actin, myosin, tropomyosin, CaM, and MLCK) reconstituted at physiologically relevant molar ratios {248}. As shown in table 54-5, calponin had no effect on myosin phosphorylation, but caused a marked inhibition (~75%) of the actin-activated myosin MgATPase. This inhibition of the ATPase was independent of tropomyosin but was reversed by increasing the concentration of actin/tropomyosin, suggesting that the inhibitory effect was due to interaction of calponin with the thin filament rather than a direct effect on myosin {248}. Consistent with this conclusion, calponin did not interact with phosphorylated or dephosphorylated smooth muscle myosin {248}, and had no effect on the CaATPase or K^+/EDTA-ATPase activities of skeletal-muscle myosin in the absence of actin {341}.

Calponin-induced inhibition of the actomyosin ATPase has now been observed by several investigators {332,342–344}, and calponin was also shown to inhibit actin filament movement over immobilized skeletal muscle HMM or phosphorylated smooth muscle myosin, independent of the presence of tropomyosin {306}. Horiuchi and Chacko {343}, using smooth muscle acto-phosphorylated HMM, demonstrated that calponin affects a catalytic step in the ATPase cycle but has only a slight effect on the affinity of HMM for actin. A similar conclusion was reached by Nishida et al. {345} using smooth-muscle acto-thiophosphorylated myosin. Using chemically modified actin and actin crosslinked to myosin S1, we showed that the mechanism of inhibition of the actomyosin ATPase is different from that of troponin/tropomyosin or caldesmon in that it does not involve either the amino-terminal acidic region of actin or the area around lys[61] of actin, and does not fit a simple steric blocking model {346}.

Characterization of fragments of calponin generated by limited proteolysis and chemical cleavage suggests that the actin-binding domain lies within calponin α(145–182), the CaM-binding domain within α(61–144), and the tropomyosin-binding domain within α(7–144) {330,347, 348}. More refined definition of the functional domains of calponin will require site-directed mutagenesis.

Since it is unlikely that calponin functions to inhibit the actomyosin ATPase constitutively, it is reasonable to speculate that its inhibitory action is regulated in some way. Four possible mechanisms of regulation of calponin function have been considered: (a) direct binding of Ca^{2+} to calponin; (b) dissociation of calponin from actin by Ca^{2+}/CaM; (c) binding of GTP to calponin; and (d) phosphorylation of calponin. Our results suggest that of these possibilities only phosphorylation is consistent with a physiological regulatory mechanism.

With regard to the binding of Ca^{2+} to calponin, this has been demonstrated by UV difference spectroscopy {349} and $^{45}CaCl_2$ gel overlay {248}, although the estimated K_d for Ca^{2+} (7 μM) is high. Nevertheless, we investigated the effect of Ca^{2+} on calponin-mediated inhibition of the actomyosin ATPase {248}. Prephosphorylated myosin was mixed with actin with or without calponin, and in the presence or absence of Ca^{2+} (table 54-6). Calponin inhibited the actomyosin ATPase to a similar extent in the presence and absence of Ca^{2+}. Similar results were obtained using pre-thiophosphorylated myosin (table 54-6). We concluded, therefore, that calponin-mediated inhibition of the actomyosin ATPase is not regulated by the direct binding of Ca^{2+} to calponin.

The possibility that the binding of Ca^{2+}/CaM may

Table 54-5. Inhibition of the actin-activated myosin MgATPase by calponin

Ca^{2+}	Calponin	Actin-activated myosin MgATPase (nmoles P_i/mg myosin · min)	Myosin phosphorylation (moles P_i/mole myosin)
−	−	7.5	0.15
+	−	112.0	1.77
+	+	27.8	1.70

Actomyosin ATPase rates and myosin phosphorylation levels were measured at 30°C in a reconstituted contractile system composed of 1 μM myosin, 6 μM actin, 2 μM tropomyosin, 1 μM CaM, and 74 nM MLCK in 25 mM Tris-HCl (pH 7.5), 10 mM $MgCl_2$, 60 mM KCl, and 1 mM [γ-^{32}P]ATP in the absence or presence of 2 μM calponin and in the presence of 0.1 mM $CaCl_2$ or 1 mM EGTA.

Table 54-6. Calponin-mediated inhibition of the actomyosin ATPase is independent of Ca^{2+}

Assay system	Ca^{2+}	Calponin	ATPase rate (nmoles P_i/mg myosin · min)
Acto-phosphorylated myosin[a]	−	−	91.4
	+	−	114.7
	−	+	25.5
	+	+	40.4
Acto-thiophosphorylated myosin[b]	−	−	62.3
	+	−	66.5
	−	+	23.0
	+	+	24.2

[a] Myosin (1 μM) was phosphorylated by incubation at 30°C for 8 minutes in the presence of 1 μM CaM, 74 nM MLCK, and 2 μM tropomyosin in 25 mM Tris-HCl (pH 7.5), 10 mM $MgCl_2$, 60 mM KCl, 0.1 mM $CaCl_2$, and 1 mM [γ-^{32}P]ATP. The following additions were then made simultaneously: 6 μM actin ± 5 μM calponin in the presence of 0.1 mM $CaCl_2$ or 1 mM EGTA (final concentrations) and samples were withdrawn at 1-minute intervals (up to 5 minutes) for determination of the ATPase rates.
[b] Myosin was thiophosphorylated under identical conditions except for the replacement of radiolabeled ATP with unlabeled ATPγS. At the time of addition of actin ± calponin with Ca^{2+} or EGTA, 1 mM [γ-^{32}P]ATP was also added and ATPase rates were measured as described above.

Table 54-7. Effect of calmodulin on calponin-induced inhibition of the actomyosin ATPase

Calponin (μM)	Calmodulin (μM)	ATPase rate (nmoles P_i/mg myosin · min)	Myosin phosphorylation (moles P_i/mole myosin)
0	0.6	126.5	1.9
2	0.6	46.8	2.0
2	30	57.2	2.0

Reaction conditions were follows: 25 mM Tris-HCl (pH 7.5), 60 mM KCl, 10 mM $MgCl_2$, 0.1 mM $CaCl_2$, 1 mM [γ-^{32}P]ATP, 1 μM myosin, 6 μM actin, 2 μM tropomyosin, 0.6 or 30 μM CaM, and 74 nM MLCK ± 2 μM calponin. ATPase rates {59} and myosin phosphorylation levels {62} were measured as previously described.

regulate calponin-mediated inhibition of the actomyosin ATPase was examined as shown in table 54-7. A 15-fold molar excess of CaM over calponin caused only a very slight reversal of inhibition of the smooth muscle actin-activated myosin MgATPase. Furthermore, very high molar ratios of Ca^{2+}/CaM to calponin are required to dissociate calponin from F actin (half-maximal release of calponin from actin occurred at ~10 moles CaM to 1 mole calponin). At physiologically relevant molar ratios of CaM to calponin, therefore, the association of calponin with the thin filament and ATPase inhibition will be unaffected by Ca^{2+}/CaM.

As indicated earlier, a region within the calponin sequence (residues 18–42) exhibits some, albeit weak, similarity to residues 24–50 of the GTP-binding protein, *ras* p21, a region involved in binding to target proteins. Some weak similarity was also observed between the sequences around asp[119] and ala[146] of *ras* p21 (which are important for binding of the guanosine moiety of GTP {350}) and the sequences around asp[104] and ala[131] of calponin {337}. This raised the possibility that GTP may bind to and regulate calponin. However, we were unable to detect any binding of [^{35}S]GTPγS to purified calponin under conditions that showed significant binding to a preparation of bovine brain G proteins (predominantly G_i) {351}. Furthermore, GTP (at concentrations up to 5 mM) had no effect on the interaction between calponin and actin (Winder and Walsh, unpublished observation).

The fact that protein phosphorylation is the most common method of regulation of protein function by posttranslational modification {352} prompted us to investigate the possibility that calponin may be phosphorylated and dephosphorylated, and its capacity to inhibit the actomyosin ATPase may be altered as a result. Of several protein kinases tested, we found only two that phosphorylated calponin in vitro: PKC and CaM kinase II {248}. Phosphopeptide mapping suggests that the same sites are phosphorylated by the two kinases and the principal site of phosphorylation is ser[175] {352a}. We also identified and isolated a type 2A protein phosphatase (SMP-I), which is capable of rapidly dephosphorylating calponin {353}. The data in table 54-8 confirm inhibition of the actomyosin ATPase by purified calponin (which is unphosphorylated) and indicate that this inhibitory effect is lost following phosphorylation and restored upon dephosphorylation. Chicken gizzard smooth muscle, therefore, contains all the enzymatic machinery necessary to catalyze the reversible phosphorylation of calponin, and phosphorylation and dephosphorylation correlate with defined activity changes.

As indicated earlier, calponin interacts with actin, tropomyosin, and Ca^{2+}/CaM. The fact that phosphorylation of calponin resulted in loss of inhibition of the actomyosin ATPase provided a means to identify which of these protein-protein interactions is responsible for

Table 54-8. Effects of phosphorylation and dephosphorylation of calponin on inhibition of the actin-activated myosin MgATPase

Calponin	MgATPase rate (nmoles P_i/mg myosin · min)
None	124.1
Untreated	25.1
Phosphorylated	140.9
Phosphorylated and dephosphorylated	38.0

The actin-activated MgATPase activity of thiophosphorylated myosin was assayed as described in table 54-6 in the presence of 0.1 mM $CaCl_2$, and in the absence and presence of 2 μM calponin (untreated, phosphorylated to 1.7 moles P_i/mole by protein kinase C, and dephosphorylated to 0.05 moles P_i/mole).

calponin's inhibitory effect on the ATPase. Phosphorylated calponin retained the ability to bind to immobilized tropomyosin and Ca^{2+}/CaM; however, it no longer interacted with F actin or a complex of F actin and tropomyosin {248}. These results indicate that the calponin-actin interaction is responsible for inhibition of the actomyosin MgATPase. Loss of inhibition upon phosphorylation of calponin, therefore, is readily explained by loss of binding of calponin to actin as a result of phosphate incorporation, particularly at ser[175].

While these in vitro experiments are strongly supportive of regulation of calponin function by phosphorylation, it is important to verify that calponin phosphorylation occurs in intact muscle and its level of phosphorylation undergoes changes during a contraction-relaxation cycle. Barany et al. {354} and Gimona et al. {355} have reported that calponin is not phosphorylated in intact resting or stimulated smooth muscle. However, we have observed calponin phosphorylation in canine tracheal and colonic smooth muscles {356} and toad stomach smooth muscle {352a}. Canine tracheal strips were metabolically labeled with $^{32}P_i$ and stimulated with carbachol to induce contraction and subsequently relaxed by removal of extracellular Ca^{2+}. Levels of calponin phosphorylation were determined

at various times during this protocol following one- and two-dimensional gel electrophoresis. Calponin phosphorylation increased to three times the basal level 1 minute after carbachol stimulation and decreased to 1.9 and 1.2 times basal at 5 and 15 minutes, respectively. Calponin phosphorylation was 1.1, 1.3, and 0.8 times basal at 2, 5, and 15 minutes after removal of extracellular Ca^{2+} (Pohl, Winder, Walsh, and Gerthoffer, submitted for publication). Calponin phosphorylation, therefore, increased transiently in response to carbachol with a time course similar to the changes in shortening velocity {357}.

On the basis of the binding properties of calponin, its inhibition of actomyosin ATPase activity, the effects of phosphorylation, and the results of phosphorylation in intact muscle, we have proposed a model to explain the physiological role of calponin (fig. 54-9). At resting levels of sarcoplasmic free Ca^{2+}, MLCK, and CaM kinase II are essentially inactive so that myosin and calponin will be dephosphorylated. In this condition, myosin heads are dissociated from actin, calponin is bound to the actin filament, and the muscle is relaxed. Stimulation of the smooth muscle cell results in a transient increase in $[Ca^{2+}]_i$, which will trigger activation of MLCK, CaM kinase II, and, if the stimulus causes diacylglycerol production,

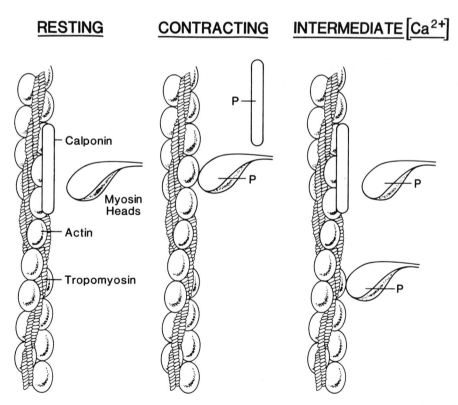

Fig. 54-9. A model of the postulated physiological role of calponin in regulation of smooth-muscle actin-myosin interaction. Calponin is shown spanning three actin monomers only because this is the maximum binding stoichiometry determined in vitro; the calponin content in situ is 1 mole/7 actin monomers. Only the S_1 regions of myosin are included for simplicity. P denotes phosphorylation. Taken from Walsh {9} with the permission of The National Research Council of Canada.

PKC. Calponin will be phosphorylated, causing it to dissociate from the thin filament, and myosin will also be phosphorylated, activating crossbridge cycling and the development of force. At these extremes of sarcoplasmic free $[Ca^{2+}]_i$, calponin serves no particular function, except perhaps to inhibit a low crossbridge cycling rate, which may otherwise exist under resting conditions. It is well established, however, that $[Ca^{2+}]_i$ peaks shortly after stimulation and then declines to an intermediate steady-state level during prolonged stimulation {e.g., 85,197,358}. We suggest that calponin comes into play in this situation. At an intermediate free $[Ca^{2+}]$, CaM kinase II and PKC, which are less sensitive to Ca^{2+} than is MLCK {359–361}, will be predominantly inactive, whereas MLCK will remain predominantly in the active state. Calponin dephosphorylation by SMP-I then induces its reassociation with the thin filaments. Even though myosin remains phosphorylated, the crossbridge cycling rate (equivalent to the actin-activated myosin MgATPase) will be inhibited due to the presence of dephosphorylated calponin bound to actin. The crossbridge cycling rate can therefore be set at any level between resting and maximally activated by precise adjustment of free $[Ca^{2+}]_i$, which will determine the ratio of phosphorylated/dephosphorylated calponin and phosphorylated/dephosphorylated myosin.

Calponin and caldesmon share several properties: (a) both bind to actin and tropomyosin in a Ca^{2+}-independent manner and to CaM in a Ca^{2+}-dependent manner; (b) both are located on thin filaments in situ; (c) both inhibit the actin-activated myosin MgATPase activity in a reconstituted contractile system; and (d) their inhibitory effects are regulated by phosphorylation. Several investigators have addressed the possibility that calponin and caldesmon may interact physically and/or functionally. Vancompernolle et al. {330} reported the binding of caldesmon to immobilized calponin, but this interaction was disrupted at low ionic strength (70 mM KCl) and is therefore unlikely to be of physiological significance. By studying the combined effects of calponin and caldesmon on actin-activated thiophosphorylated smooth muscle or skeletal muscle myosin MgATPase, respectively, Abe et al. {342} and Makuch et al. {344} concluded that the inhibitory effects of calponin and caldesmon were unaffected by each other's presence. Using smooth muscle acto-thiophosphorylated myosin, we observed that calponin was ~twofold more potent than caldesmon in inhibition of the ATPase {341}. Given the higher tissue concentration of calponin (1 mole/7 moles actin {329}) than caldesmon (1 mole/22–28 moles actin at most {265}), it appears that calponin is a more effective regulator of the actomyosin ATPase than is caldesmon. On balance, then, we favor the possibility that calponin is a bona fide thin filament-associated regulatory protein, whereas caldesmon serves a structural or organizational role: Through its ability to crosslink actin and myosin filaments, caldesmon may organize the contractile filaments into a three-dimensional network in which the actin and myosin filaments have the proper orientation and spatial distribution for effective force development in response to appropriate stimuli {362}.

STRUCTURAL PROTEINS

A discussion of the contractile and regulatory proteins of smooth muscle is incomplete without consideration of several structural proteins that are thought to play cytoskeletal roles in the organization and coordination of the contractile structures. For a more complete review of cytoskeletal and structural proteins in muscle and nonmuscle cells, the reader is referred to two recent reviews by Small et al. {363} and Luna and Hitt {364}.

Desmin and vimentin

In addition to thin (actin) and thick (myosin) filaments, smooth muscle cells contain a third type of filament, intermediate or 10-nm filaments {365}, which constitute a major part of the cytoskeleton. Intermediate filaments are relatively flexible, with a hollow core and an external diameter in cross section of 10 nm, and they represent 15–25% of the total structural protein. They are resistant to solubilization with high salt or nondenaturing detergents. However, they can be solubilized in denaturing solutions, such as high urea concentrations, but show a strong tendency to renature, forming 10-nm filaments when the denaturant is removed. The intermediate filament protein of smooth muscle, desmin, exhibits a molecular weight of 53–55 kDa {366–368}. Desmin is generally present in vertebrate smooth, cardiac, and skeletal muscles, and is apparently invariant within species but exhibits interspecies differences {369,370}. Avian desmin exists in phosphorylated and nonphosphorylated forms, but the significance of this phosphorylation is unknown {371}. Vimentin, a 57-kDa intermediate filament protein found in cultured cells, has also been identified in muscle. In smooth-muscle cells in culture, Absher et al. {33} noted that the expression of desmin decreased with time and the expression of vimentin increased. Nanaev {372} noted that desmin and vimentin were expressed to different extents in smooth muscle cells of different fetal blood vessels. The expression of desmin and vimentin also appears to depend on species, the type of smooth muscle, and pathological state. Indeed, vascular smooth muscle, unlike other smooth muscles, exhibits a preponderance of intermediate filaments composed of vimentin rather than desmin {373,374}.

The function of intermediate filaments in cells is not well understood {375}. They are believed to play a structural role in smooth muscle by forming a continuous network throughout the cell that maintains the general cell shape. Intermediate filaments are also associated with the cytoplasmic dense bodies in smooth muscle cells {365,376, 377} and may serve to anchor the contractile apparatus to the cytoskeleton and surface membrane. If they are removed from detergent-extracted smooth-muscle cells by limited proteolysis, however, the cells remain capable of contracting in the presence of ATP {366}. Furthermore, intermediate filaments are without effect on the ATPase activity and regulatory properties of smooth-muscle actomyosin.

Filamin

Filamin is a major component of smooth muscle, being present to the extent of 30–40% of the myosin content {378}. It has a subunit molecular weight of 250 kDa and exists in solution as an asymmetric dimer of 500 kDa {379} in which the two subunits, each ~80 nm long, are joined end to end. The filamin dimer is a potent crosslinker of actin filaments and causes gelation of F-actin solutions at molar ratios of filamin to actin of less than 1:200 {380}. Filamin can be cleaved by a Ca^{2+}-activated protease to a 240-kDa polypeptide, which retains the ability to bind to actin but cannot form dimers or crosslink actin filaments {381,382}. It appears, therefore, that the free ends of the filamin dimer contain the actin-binding sites and the dimer interface includes the 10-kDa peptide removed by proteolysis. The self-assembly site is near the carboxy terminus of each monomer, and the actin-binding site is near the amino terminus and is homologous to the actin-binding site of α-actinin {383}.

Filamin appears to be generally codistributed with desmin in avian smooth muscle cells {384,385}, except at the cell membrane, where filamin but not desmin is present. Filamin may play a role in the organization of actin filaments in the smooth muscle contractile apparatus by crosslinking sets of actin filaments to maintain them in parallel register, while leaving sufficient space for the interdigitation of myosin filaments. It should be noted, however, that cross sections of smooth muscle cells fixed in rigor or in a relaxed state show a different relative distribution of thick and thin filaments. In rigor, a tight bundling of thin filaments around thick filaments is apparent, whereas in relaxed muscle the thin filaments appear to be bundled into groups with myosin filaments between these groups {386}. If filamin or other thin filament proteins are involved in maintaining actin filaments in parallel register, it would be of interest to know if their interaction with actin changes as a muscle cell goes from rigor to a relaxed state.

α-Actinin, vinculin, and other proteins

α-Actinin was first described in skeletal muscle and has since been identified in smooth and cardiac muscles, and a variety of nonmuscle tissues. The native molecule is composed of two polypeptide chains (M_r 100 kDa each) and appears as a rod-shaped molecule (35 × 5 nm) in the electron microscope {387}. Crosslinking of actin filaments by α-actinin to form parallel and random arrays has been observed by electron microscopy. Parallel pairs of actin filaments are separated by 40–50 nm, suggesting the α-actinin molecules contain an actin-binding site at each end {388}. Tropomyosin is capable of displacing α-actinin from actin filaments {389}. Immunocytochemistry has revealed the localization of α-actinin in the cytoplasmic and membrane-associated dense bodies, suggesting that it may serve as attachment points for actin filaments. A similar argument is made in skeletal muscle, where α-actinin is confined to the Z discs.

Vinculin (M_r 130 kDa) exists as an approximately globular monomer in solution and is widely distributed in vertebrate tissues. It is concentrated where actin filament bundles are closely associated with plasma membranes, e.g., the membrane-associated dense bodies of smooth muscle cells {390}. Vinculin is not, however, found in the cytoplasmic dense bodies. It may function in the linkage of actin filaments to the sarcolemma, although its ability to bind directly to actin is controversial {27,388,391}. Metavinculin (M_r 130 kDa), dystrophin (M_r 427 kDa), and talin (M_r 215 kDa) have been found in smooth muscle cells associated with the plasma membrane {363,364,392} and probably serve to link the contractile structures to the plasma membrane, but their precise functions are largely unknown.

LONG-RANGE STRUCTURAL ORDER IN SMOOTH MUSCLE CELLS

In early histological studies (reviewed in {384,393}; see also reviews by Cooke {394} and Bagby {395} for other discussions of smooth-muscle organization), a striated pattern in smooth-muscle cells was noted but appears not to have been studied further. Recently, a number of authors have again suggested that there may be long-range order to the way in which the contractile and cytoskeletal structures in smooth muscle are organized. Fisher and Bagby {396} and Warshaw et al. {397} observed the "corkscrewing" of isolated smooth muscle cells during contraction and inferred from this that the attachment sites for the contractile apparatus in smooth muscle cells were helically arranged.

In permeabilized smooth muscle cells stimulated to contract, Bennett et al. {393} found that a series of bands along the cell axis were labeled by an antibody specific for phosphorylated smooth muscle light chains. This suggested that there were contractile zones in smooth muscle cells located at intervals along the length of the cell. Analysis of the motion of dense bodies in contracting permeabilized smooth muscle cells {398} also suggested that there were contractile zones located at approximately 6-μm intervals along the cell axis. In permeabilized gizzard smooth muscle cells that were firmly bound to a glass substrate, Draeger et al. {385} noted that the actin and myosin filaments formed regularly spaced nodes along the cell axis when the cells were exposed to MgATP. The nodes were spaced at approximately 20-μm intervals. Additional evidence for long-range structural order in smooth-muscle cells can be inferred from studies of the distribution of other membrane-associated cytoskeletal proteins. Draeger et al. {384,385} observed a regular (4- to 5-μm) spacing of vinculin-, talin-, and filamin-containing structures along the plasma membrane of gizzard smooth muscle cells. It should be noted, however, that both actin {333,385} and myosin {385} filaments appear to be distributed more or less uniformly throughout the cytoplasm of smooth muscle cells, and there does not appear to be any periodicity to the distribution of the thin filament-associated proteins, tropomyosin and calponin {333}. The latter results do not rule out the possibility that long-range order exists in smooth muscle cells, but rather suggest that cytoskeletal structures and the constraints they impose on the movement of actin- and myosin-containing filaments might be the most important determinants of this order. This would be in contrast to the highly ordered arrangement of the contractile filaments themselves in striated muscle. Additional experimental work will be required to explore these issues.

CONCLUSIONS

Detailed knowledge of the structure and function of isolated contractile proteins, combined with ultrastructural, kinetic, biochemical, and physiological studies, has led at least to reasonable hypotheses concerning how smooth muscle contracts and how this process is regulated. What emerges is the concept that smooth muscle contraction occurs via a sliding filament mechanism similar to that in striated muscles, although this is by no means proven beyond doubt. From the point of view of control, it is well established that contractile regulation is achieved by fluctuations in the concentration of sarcoplasmic free Ca^{2+}, and most investigators find that the mechanism whereby Ca^{2+} regulates smooth muscle contraction is via the reversible phosphorylation of myosin. Several aspects of this control system remain the subject of extensive investigation, e.g., the effects of phosphorylation on myosin conformation; the potential physiological significance of phosphorylation at more than one site on the myosin light chain by MLCK; the importance of other kinases, particularly PKC and CaM kinase II; and characterization of myosin light-chain phosphatases and their regulation.

Our understanding of the structure-function relations of smooth muscle contractile and regulatory proteins is increasing exponentially, in large part from the application of molecular cloning and site-directed mutagenesis. The recent elucidation of the high-resolution crystal structure of cyclic AMP-dependent protein kinase is a milestone that greatly enhances detailed understanding of the mechanism and regulation of this kinase and, since the primary structures of many kinases are homologous, sheds considerable light on the mechanisms of action and regulation of other kinases, including MLCK and PKC. Attempts are underway to crystallize these and other protein kinases. X-ray crystallography is being very effectively complemented by multidimensional NMR, which is now capable of determining the solution structure of proteins and protein-peptide complexes up to ~20 kDa. Further refinements in this techology will undoubtedly lead to clear definitions of substrate-binding sites and regulatory sites in protein kinases.

The complexity of PKC isoenzyme expression continues to be an important question of very broad significance. Why are there so many PKC isoenzymes? How do they differ in tissue and subcellular localization, translocation upon stimulation of the cell, substrate specificity, and regulation? In the context of smooth muscle specifically, which isoenzymes are expressed and what are their physiological substrates and functions?

It is becoming increasingly apparent that myosin phosphorylation-dephosphorylation is not the only mechanism for regulating smooth muscle contraction. There is substantial physiological and biochemical evidence for the existence of secondary control systems that can modulate the contractile state of the smooth muscle, e.g., the latch state in which developed tension is maintained in a Ca^{2+}-dependent fashion while myosin is dephosphorylated. It is clear that considerable attention will continue to be devoted to elucidating the biochemical basis and physiological importance of such secondary regulatory mechanisms. In this regard, the functional role of caldesmon and calponin, and their regulation, will require further definition. The mechanism of Ca^{2+}-sensitizing effects of a variety of contractile agonists, which involves a G protein and arachidonic acid production, will be the focus of considerable attention in the immediate future.

Many of the mechanical properties of smooth muscle are undoubtedly a consequence of the structure and organization of the cytoskeleton. Increasing attention is being directed towards thorough characterization of the cytoskeletal proteins: intermediate filament proteins and actin-binding proteins that presumably function in the spatial organization of the contractile machinery. As yet we know relatively little of the contribution these components make to the contractile properties of the muscle cell. Ultimately, it may turn out that the differences in mechanical properties observed in different smooth muscle tissues may be a function of the cytoskeletal proteins rather than the contractile proteins themselves.

The answers to these and many other questions will come from innovative application of a host of experimental approaches and techniques of molecular biology, biochemistry, biophysics, and physiology.

ACKNOWLEDGMENTS

The authors' research is supported by grants from the Medical Research Council of Canada, the National Institutes of Health (U.S.A.), the Alberta Heart and Stroke Foundation, and the Alberta Heritage Foundation for Medical Research (AHFMR). GJK is an AHFMR Scholar and MPW is an AHFMR Medical Scientist. We are very grateful to Gerry Garnett for secretarial support.

REFERENCES

1. Cooke R: The mechanism of muscle contraction. *CRC Crit Rev Biochem* 21:53–118, 1986.
2. Huxley HE: Sliding filaments and molecular motile systems. *J Biol Chem* 265:8347–8350, 1990.
3. Somlyo AV: Ultrastructure of vascular smooth muscle. In: Bohr DF, Somlyo AP, Sparks HV (eds) *Handbook of Physiology*, Section 2: *The Cardiovascular System. II: Vascular Smooth Muscle*. Bethesda, MD: American Physiological Society, 1980, pp 33–67.

4. Okagaki T, Higashi-Fujime S, Ishikawa R, Takano-Ohmuro H, Kohama K: In vitro movement of actin filaments on gizzard smooth muscle myosin: Requirement of phosphorylation of myosin light chain and effects of tropomyosin and caldesmon. *J Biochem (Tokyo)* 109:858–866, 1991.

5. Kelley CA, Sellers JR, Goldsmith PK, Adelstein RS: Smooth muscle myosin is composed of homodimeric heavy chains. *J Biol Chem* 267:2127–2130, 1992.

6. Hartshorne DJ: Biochemistry of the contractile process in smooth muscle. In: Johnson LR (ed) *Physiology of the Gastrointestinal Tract*, 2nd ed. New York: Raven Press, 1987, pp 423–482.

7. Gerthoffer WT: Regulation of the contractile element on airway smooth muscle. *Am J Physiol* 261:L15–L28, 1991.

8. Stull JT, Gallagher PJ, Herring BP, Kamm KE: Vascular smooth muscle contractile elements: Cellular regulation. *Hypertension* 17:723–732, 1991.

9. Walsh MP: Calcium-dependent mechanisms of regulation of smooth muscle contraction. *Biochem Cell Biol* 69:771–800, 1991.

10. Hartshorne DJ, Kawamura T: Regulation of contraction-relaxation in smooth muscle. *News Physiol Sci* 7:59–64, 1992.

11. Rembold CM: Regulation of contraction and relaxation in arterial smooth muscle. *Hypertension* 20:129–137, 1992.

12. Lehman W, Szent-Györgyi AG: Regulation of muscular contraction. *J Gen Physiol* 66:1–30, 1975.

13. Perry SV: The regulation of contractile activity in muscle. *Biochem Soc Trans* 7:593–617, 1979.

14. Weber A, Murray JM: Molecular control mechanisms in muscle contraction. *Physiol Rev* 53:612–673, 1973.

15. Kendrick-Jones J, Lehman W, Szent-Györgyi AG: Regulation in molluscan muscles. *J Mol Biol* 54:313–326, 1970.

16. Maruta H, Korn ED: Proteolytic separation of the actin-activatable ATPase site from the phosphorylation site on the heavy chain of *Acanthamoeba* myosin IA. *J Biol Chem* 256:503–506, 1981.

17. Kuczmarski ER, Spudich JA: Regulation of myosin self-assembly. Phosphorylation of *Dictyostelium* heavy chain inhibits formation of thick filaments. *Proc Natl Acad Sci USA* 77:7292–7296, 1980.

18. Persechini A, Hartshorne DJ: Phosphorylation of smooth muscle myosin: Evidence for cooperativity between the myosin heads. *Science* 213:1383–1385, 1981.

19. Ngai PK, Gröschel-Stewart U, Walsh MP: Comparison of the effects of smooth and skeletal muscle actins on smooth muscle actomyosin Mg^{2+}-ATPase. *Biochem Int* 12:89–93, 1986.

20. Bretscher A: Smooth muscle caldesmon. Rapid purification and F-actin cross-linking properties. *J Biol Chem* 259:12873–12880, 1984.

21. Walsh MP, Valentine KA, Ngai PK, Carruthers CA, Hollenberg MD: Ca^{2+}-dependent hydrophobic-interaction chromatography. Isolation of a novel Ca^{2+}-binding protein and protein kinase C from bovine brain. *Biochem J* 224:117–127, 1984.

22. Ngai PK, Carruthers CA, Walsh MP: Isolation of the native form of chicken gizzard MLCK. *Biochem J* 218:863–870, 1984.

23. Winder SJ, Walsh MP: Smooth muscle calponin. Inhibition of actomyosin MgATPase and regulation by phosphorylation. *J Biol Chem* 265:10148–10155, 1990.

24. Clark T, Ngai PK, Sutherland C, Gröschel-Stewart U, Walsh MP: Vascular smooth muscle caldesmon. *J Biol Chem* 261:8028–8035, 1986.

25. Vibert PJ, Haselgrove JC, Lowy J, Poulsen FR: Structural changes in actin-containing filaments of muscle. *J Mol Biol* 71:757–767, 1972.

26. Ishikawa H, Bischoff R, Holzer H: Formation of arrowhead complexes with heavy meromyosin in a variety of cell types. *J Cell Biol* 43:312–328, 1969.

27. Small JV, Herzog M, Barth M, Draeger A: Supercontracted state of vertebrate smooth muscle cell fragments reveals myofilament lengths. *J Cell Biol* 111:2451–2461, 1990.

28. Bond M, Somlyo AV: Dense bodies and actin polarity in vertebrate smooth muscle. *J Cell Biol* 95:403–413, 1982.

29. Kabsch W, Vandekerckhove J: Structure and function of actin. *Annu Rev Biophys Biomol Struct* 21:49–76, 1992.

30. Vandekerckhove J, Weber K: The complete amino acid sequence of actins from bovine aorta, bovine heart, bovine fast skeletal muscle and rabbit slow skeletal muscle. *Differentiation* 14:123–133, 1979.

31. Fatigati V, Murphy RA: Actin and tropomyosin variants in smooth muscles. Dependence on tissue type. *J Biol Chem* 259:14383–14388, 1984.

32. Eddinger TJ, Murphy RA: Developmental changes in actin and myosin heavy chain isoform expression in smooth muscle. *Arch Biochem Biophys* 284:232–237, 1991.

33. Absher M, Woodcock-Mitchell J, Mitchell J, Baldor L, Low R, Warshaw D: Characterization of vascular smooth muscle cell phenotype in long-term culture. *In Vitro Cell Dev Biol* 25:183–192, 1989.

34. Glukhova MA, Kabakov AE, Frid MG, Ornatsky OI, Belkin AM, Mukhin DN, Orekhov AN, Koteliansky VE, Smirnov VN: Modulation of human smooth muscle phenotype: A study of muscle-specific variants of vinculin, caldesmon, and actin expression. *Proc Natl Acad Sci USA* 85:9542–9546, 1988.

35. Trinkle LA, Beasley D, Moreland RS: Interleukin-1β alters actin expression and inhibits contraction of rat thoracic aorta. *Am J Physiol* 262:C828–C833, 1992.

36. Herman IM, D'Amore PA: Microvascular pericytes contain muscle and nonmuscle actins. *J Cell Biol* 101:43–52, 1985.

37. DeNofrio D, Hoock TC, Herman IM: Functional sorting of actin isoforms in microvascular pericytes. *J Cell Biol* 109:191–202, 1989.

38. Hoock TC, Newcomb PM, Herman IM: β actin and its mRNA are localized at the plasma membrane and the regions of moving cytoplasm during the cellular response to injury. *J Cell Biol* 112:653–664, 1991.

39. Murphy RA: Do the cytoplasmic and muscle-specific isoforms of actin and myosin heavy and light chains serve different functions in smooth muscle? *Jpn J Pharmacol* 58:67P–74P, 1992.

40. Drew JS, Moos C, Murphy RA: Localization of isoactins in isolated smooth muscle thin filaments by double gold immunolabeling. *Am J Physiol* 260:C1332–C1340, 1991.

41. Hanson J, Lednev V, O'Brien EJ, Bennett PM: Structure of the actin-containing filaments in vertebrate skeletal muscle. *Cold Spring Harbor Symp Quant Biol* 37:311–318, 1972.

42. Huxley HE: Structural changes in the actin and myosin containing filaments during contraction. *Cold Spring Harbor Symp Quant Biol* 37:361–376, 1972.

43. Cummins P, Perry SV: Chemical and immunochemical characteristics of tropomyosins from striated and smooth muscles. *Biochem J* 141:43–49, 1973.

44. Dabrowska R, Nowak E, Drabikowski W: Comparative studies of chicken gizzard and rabbit skeletal tropomyosin. *Comp Biochem Physiol* 65B:75–83, 1980.

45. Strasburg GM, Greaser ML: The native subunit pattern of tropomyosin. *FEBS Lett* 72:11–14, 1976.

46. Sanders C, Smillie LB: Amino acid sequence of chicken

gizzard β-tropomyosin: Comparison of the chicken gizzard, rabbit skeletal and equine platelet tropomyosins. *J Biol Chem* 260:7264–7275, 1985.

47. McLachlan AD, Stewart M: The 14-fold periodicity in α-tropomyosin and the interaction with actin. *J Mol Biol* 103:271–298, 1976.

48. Murphy RA, Herlihy JT, Megerman J: Force-generating capacity and contractile protein content of arterial smooth muscle. *J Gen Physiol* 64:691–705, 1974.

49. Fine RE, Blitz AL: A chemical comparison of tropomyosins from muscle and non-muscle tissues. *J Mol Biol* 95:447–454, 1975.

50. Sobieszek A, Small JV: Regulation of the actin-myosin interaction in vertebrate smooth muscle: Activation via a MLCK and the effect of tropomyosin. *J Mol Biol* 112:559–576, 1977.

51. Miyata H, Chacko S: Role of tropomyosin in smooth muscle contraction: Effect of tropomyosin binding to actin on actin activation of myosin ATPase. *Biochemistry* 25:2725–2729, 1986.

52. Parry DAD, Squire JM: Structural role of tropomyosin in muscle regulation: Analysis of the X-ray diffraction patterns from relaxed and contracting muscles. *J Mol Biol* 75:33–55, 1973.

53. Craig R, Smith R, Kendrick-Jones J: Light chain phosphorylation controls the conformation of vertebrate non-muscle and smooth muscle myosin molecules. *Nature* 302:436–439, 1983.

54. Cooke PH, Kargacin G, Craig R, Fogarty K, Fay FS, Hagen S: Molecular structure and organization of filaments in single skinned smooth muscle cells. In: Siegman MJ, Somlyo AP, Stephens NL (eds) *Regulation and Contraction of Smooth Muscle.* New York: Alan R. Liss, 1987, pp 1–25.

55. Cooke PH, Fay FS, Craig R: Myosin filaments isolated from skinned amphibian smooth muscle cells are side-polar. *J Muscle Res Cell Motil* 10:206–220, 1989.

56. Cross RA, Engel A: Scanning transmission electron microscopic mass determination of in vitro self-assembled smooth muscle myosin filaments. *J Mol Biol* 222:455–458, 1991.

57. Seidel JC: Fragmentation of gizzard myosin by α-chymotrypsin and papain, the effects on ATPase activity, and the interaction with actin. *J Biol Chem* 255:4355–4361, 1980.

58. Somlyo AV, Butler TM, Bond M, Somlyo AP: Myosin filaments have nonphosphorylated light chains in relaxed smooth muscle. *Nature* 294:567–569, 1981.

59. Ikebe M, Hartshorne DJ: Proteolysis of smooth muscle myosin by *Staphylococcus aureus* protease: Preparation of heavy meromyosin and subfragment 1 with intact 20,000-dalton light chains. *Biochemistry* 24:2380–2387, 1985.

60. Perrie WT, Smillie LB, Perry SV: A phosphorylated light-chain component of myosin from skeletal muscle. *Biochem J* 135:151–164, 1973.

61. Sobieszek A: Vertebrate smooth muscle myosin: Enzymatic and structural properties. In: Stephens NL (ed) *The Biochemistry of Smooth Muscle.* Baltimore, MD: University Park Press, 1977, pp 413–443.

62. Walsh MP, Hinkins S, Dabrowska R, Hartshorne DJ: Smooth muscle myosin light chain kinase. *Methods Enzymol* 99:279–288, 1983.

63. Chacko S: Effect of phosphorylation, Ca^{2+} and tropomyosin on actin-activated ATPase activity of mammalian smooth muscle myosin. *Biochemistry* 20:702–707, 1981.

64. Chacko S, Rosenfeld A: Regulation of actin-activated ATP hydrolysis by arterial myosin. *Proc Natl Acad Sci USA* 79:292–296, 1982.

65. Trybus KM, Lowey S: Mechanism of smooth muscle myosin phosphorylation. *J Biol Chem* 260:15988–15995, 1985.

66. Ikebe M, Ogihara S, Tonomura Y: Non-linear dependence of actin activated Mg^{2+}ATPase activity on the extent of phosphorylation of gizzard myosin and H meromyosin. *J Biochem (Tokyo)* 91:1809–1812, 1982.

67. Sellers JR, Chock PB, Adelstein RS: The apparently negatively cooperative phosphorylation of smooth muscle myosin at low ionic strength is related to its filamentous state. *J Biol Chem* 258:14181–14188, 1983.

68. Aksoy MO, Murphy RA, Kamm KE: Role of Ca^{2+} and myosin light chain phosphorylation in regulation of smooth muscle. *Am J Physiol* 242:C109–C116, 1982.

69. Persechini A, Kamm KE, Stull JT: Different phosphorylated forms of myosin in contracting tracheal smooth muscle. *J Biol Chem* 261:6293–6299, 1986.

70. Ikebe M, Hartshorne DJ: Phosphorylation of smooth muscle myosin at two distinct sites by myosin light chain kinase. *J Biol Chem* 260:10027–10031, 1985.

71. Ikebe M, Hartshorne DJ, Elzinga M: Identification, phosphorylation, and dephosphorylation of a second site for myosin light chain kinase on the 20,000-dalton light chain of smooth muscle myosin. *J Biol Chem* 261:36–39, 1986.

72. Haeberle JR, Trockman BA: Two-site phosphorylation of the 20,000 dalton myosin light chain of glycerinated porcine carotid artery smooth muscle. *Biophys J* 49:389a, 1986.

73. Ledvora RF, Bárány K, Vander Meulen DL, Barron JT, Bárány M: Stretch-induced phosphorylation of the 20,000-dalton light chain of myosin in arterial smooth muscle. *J Biol Chem* 258:14080–14083, 1983.

74. Gagelmann M, Rüegg JC, DiSalvo J: Phosphorylation of the myosin light chains and satellite proteins in detergent-skinned arterial smooth muscle. *Biochem Biophys Res Commun* 120:933–938, 1984.

75. Paul RJ, Hewett TE, Martin AF: Myosin heavy chain isoforms and smooth muscle function. In: Moreland RS (ed) *Regulation of Smooth Muscle Contraction.* New York: Plenum Press, 1991, pp 139–145.

76. Cheung WY: Cyclic 3′,5′-nucleotide phosphodiesterase. Demonstration of an activator. *Biochem Biophys Res Commun* 38:533–538, 1970.

77. Kakiuchi S, Yamazaki R, Nakajima H: Properties of a heat-stable phosphodiesterase activating factor isolated from brain extracts. Studies on cyclic 3′,5′-nucleotide phosphodiesterase II. *Proc Jpn Acad* 46:587–592, 1970.

78. Teo TS, Wang TH, Wang JH: Purification and properties of the protein activator of bovine heart cyclic adenosine 3′,5′-monophosphate phosphodiesterase. *J Biol Chem* 248:588–595, 1973.

79. Kretsinger RH: Structure and evolution of calcium-modulated proteins. *CRC Crit Rev Biochem* 8:119–174, 1980.

80. Cheung WY: Calmodulin plays a pivotal role in cellular regulation. *Science* 207:19–27, 1980.

81. Walsh MP, Hartshorne DJ: Calmodulin. In: Stephens NL (ed) *Biochemistry of Smooth Muscle,* Vol II. Boca Raton, FL: CRC Press, 1983, pp 1–84.

82. Dabrowska R, Sherry JMF, Aromatorio DK, Hartshorne DJ: Modulator protein as a component of the myosin light chain kinase from chicken gizzard. *Biochemistry* 17:253–258, 1978.

83. Potter JD, Strang-Brown P, Walker PL, Iida S: Ca^{2+} binding to calmodulin. *Methods Enzymol* 102:135–143, 1983.

84. DeFeo TT, Morgan KG: Calcium-force relationship as detected with aequorin in two different vascular smooth muscles of the ferret. *J Physiol* 369:269–282, 1985.

85. Williams DA, Fay FS: Calcium transients and resting levels in isolated smooth muscle cells as monitored with quin-2. *Am J Physiol* 250:C779–C791, 1986.

86. Williams DA, Becker PL, Fay FS: Regional changes in calcium underlying contraction of single smooth muscle cells. *Science* 235:1644–1648, 1987.

87. Olwin BB, Edelman AM, Krebs EG, Storm DR: Quantitation of energy coupling between Ca^{2+}, calmodulin, skeletal muscle myosin light chain kinase, and kinase substrates. *J Biol Chem* 259:10949–10955, 1984.

88. Klee CB: Conformational transition accompanying the binding of Ca^{2+} to the protein activator of 3′,5′-cyclic adenosine monophosphate phosphodiesterase. *Biochemistry* 16:1017–1024, 1977.

89. LaPorte DC, Wierman BM, Storm DR: Calcium-induced exposure of a hydrophobic surface on calmodulin. *Biochemistry* 19:3814–3819, 1980.

90. Burgess WH, Schleicher M, Van Eldik LJ, Watterson DM: Comparative studies of calmodulin. In: Cheung WY (ed) *Calcium and Cell Function*, Vol IV. New York: Academic Press, 1983, pp 209–261.

91. Babu YS, Sack JS, Greenhough TJ, Bugg CE, Means AR, Cook WJ: Three-dimensional structure of calmodulin. *Nature* 315:37–40, 1985.

92. Means AR, Van Berkum MFA, Bagchi IC, Lu KP, Rasmussen CD: Regulatory functions of calmodulin. *Pharmac Ther* 50:255–270, 1991.

93. Ikura M, Kay LE, Krinks M, Bax A: Triple-resonance multidimensional NMR study of calmodulin complexed with the binding domain of skeletal muscle MLCK: Indication of a conformational change in the central helix. *Biochemistry* 30:5498–5504, 1991.

94. Roth SM, Schneider DM, Strobel LA, Van Berkum MFA, Means AR, Wand AJ: Characterization of the secondary structure of calmodulin in complex with a calmodulin-binding domain peptide. *Biochemistry* 31:1443–1451, 1992.

95. Van Berkum MFA, Means AR: Three amino acid substitutions in domain I of calmodulin prevent the activation of chicken smooth muscle myosin light chain kinase. *J Biol Chem* 266:21488–21495, 1991.

96. Bagchi IC, Huang Q, Means AR: Identification of amino acids essential for calmodulin binding and activation of smooth muscle myosin light chain kinase. *J Biol Chem* 267:3024–3029, 1992.

97. Ikura M, Clore GM, Gronenborn AM, Zhu G, Klee CB, Bax A: Solution structure of a calmodulin-target peptide complex by multidimensional NMR. *Science* 256:632–638, 1992.

98. Meador WE, Means AR, Quiocho FA: Target enzyme recognition by calmodulin: 2.4 Å structure of a calmodulin-peptide complex. *Science* 257:1251–1255, 1992.

99. Kretsinger RH: Calmodulin and myosin light chain kinase: How helices are bent. *Science* 258:50–51, 1992.

100. Kemp BE, Stull JT: Myosin light chain kinases. In: Kemp BE (ed) *Peptides and Protein Phosphorylation*. Boca Raton, FL: CRC Press, 1990, pp 115–133.

101. Olson NJ, Pearson RB, Needleman DS, Hurwitz MY, Kemp BE, Means AR: Regulatory and structural motifs of chicken gizzard myosin light chain kinase. *Proc Natl Acad Sci USA* 87:2284–2288, 1990.

102. Gallagher PJ, Herring BP, Griffin SA, Stull JT: Molecular characterization of a mammalian smooth muscle myosin light chain kinase. *J Biol Chem* 266:23936–23944, 1991.

103. Kobayashi H, Inoue A, Mikawa T, Kuwayama H, Hotta Y, Masaki T, Ebashi S: Isolation of cDNA for bovine stomach 155 kDa protein exhibiting myosin light chain kinase activity.

104. Maita T, Chen JI, Matsuda G: Amino-acid sequence of the 20,000-molecular-weight light chain of chicken gizzard-muscle myosin. *Eur J Biochem* 117:417–424, 1981.

105. Pearson RB, Jakes R, John M, Kendrick-Jones J, Kemp BE: Phosphorylation site sequence of smooth muscle myosin light chain ($M_r = 20,000$). *FEBS Lett* 168:108–112, 1984.

106. Messer NG, Kendrick-Jones J: Molecular cloning and sequencing of the chicken smooth muscle myosin regulatory light chain. *FEBS Lett* 234:49–52, 1988.

107. Watanabe M, Hasegawa Y, Katoh T, Morita F: Amino acid sequence of the 20-kDa regulatory light chain of porcine aorta media smooth muscle myosin. *J Biochem (Tokyo)* 112:431–432, 1992.

108. Kumar CC, Mohan SR, Zavodny PJ, Narula SK, Leibowitz PJ: Characterization and differential expression of human vascular smooth muscle myosin light chain 2 isoform in nonmuscle cells. *Biochemistry* 28:4027–4035, 1989.

109. Walsh MP: Calcium regulation of smooth muscle contraction. In: Marmé D (ed) *Calcium and Cell Physiology*. Berlin: Springer-Verlag, 1985, pp 170–203.

110. Kemp BE, Pearson RB, House C: Role of basic residues in the phosphorylation of synthetic peptides by myosin light chain kinase. *Proc Natl Acad Sci USA* 80:7471–7475, 1983.

111. Kemp BE, Pearson RB: Spatial requirements for location of basic residues in peptide substrates for smooth muscle myosin light chain kinase. *J Biol Chem* 260:3355–3359, 1985.

112. Pearson RB, Misconi LY, Kemp BE: Smooth muscle myosin kinase requires residues on the COOH-terminal side of the phosphorylation site. *J Biol Chem* 261:25–27, 1986.

113. Ikebe M, Morita J: Identification of the sequence of the regulatory light chain required for the phosphorylation-dependent regulation of actomyosin. *J Biol Chem* 266:21339–21342, 1991.

114. Hanks SK, Quinn AM, Hunter T: The protein kinase family: Conserved features and deduced phylogeny of the catalytic domains. *Science* 241:42–52, 1988.

115. Kamps MP, Taylor SS, Sefton BM: Direct evidence that oncogenic tyrosine kinases and cyclic AMP-dependent protein kinase have homologous ATP-binding sites. *Nature* 310:589–592, 1984.

116. Benian GM, Kiff JE, Neckleman N, Moerman DG, Waterston RH: Sequence of an unusually large protein implicated in regulation of myosin activity in *C. elegans*. *Nature* 342:45–50, 1989.

117. Labeit S, Barlow DP, Gautel M, Gibson T, Holt J, Hsieh C-L, Francke U, Leonard K, Wardale J, Whiting A, Trinick J: A regular pattern of two types of 100-residue motif in the sequence of titin. *Nature* 345:273–276, 1990.

118. Pearson RB, Ito M, Morrice NA, Smith AJ, Condron R, Wettenhall REH, Kemp BE, Hartshorne DJ: Proteolytic cleavage sites in smooth muscle myosin-light-chain kinase and their relation to structural and regulatory domains. *Eur J Biochem* 200:723–730, 1991.

119. O'Neil KT, DeGrado WF: How calmodulin binds its targets: Sequence independent recognition of amphiphilic α-helices. *Trends Biochem Sci* 15:59–64, 1990.

120. Lukas TJ, Burgess WH, Prendergast FG, Lau W, Watterson DM: Calmodulin binding domains: Characterization of a phosphorylation and calmodulin binding site from myosin light chain kinase. *Biochemistry* 25:1458–1464, 1986.

121. Kemp BE, Pearson RB, Guerriero V Jr, Bagchi IC, Means AR: The calmodulin binding domain of chicken smooth muscle myosin light chain kinase contains a pseudosubstrate sequence. *J Biol Chem* 262:2542–2548, 1987.

122. Bagchi IC, Kemp BE, Means AR: Myosin light chain kinase structure function analysis using bacterial expression. *J Biol Chem* 264:15843–15849, 1989.

123. Herring BP, Stull JT, Gallagher PJ: Domain characterization of rabbit skeletal muscle myosin light chain kinase. *J Biol Chem* 265:1724–1730, 1990.

124. Herring BP, Fitzsimmons DP, Stull JT, Gallagher PJ: Acidic residues comprise part of the myosin light chain-binding site on skeletal muscle myosin light chain kinase. *J Biol Chem* 265:16588–16591, 1990.

125. Ikebe M, Stepinska M, Kemp BE, Means AR, Hartshorne DJ: Proteolysis of smooth muscle myosin light chain kinase. Formation of inactive and calmodulin-independent fragments. *J Biol Chem* 262:13828–13834, 1987.

126. Pearson RB, Wettenhall REH, Means AR, Hartshorne DJ, Kemp BE: Autoregulation of enzymes by pseudosubstrate prototopes: Myosin light chain kinase. *Science* 241:970–973, 1988.

127. Ikebe M, Reardon S, Fay FS: Primary structure required for the inhibition of smooth muscle myosin light chain kinase. *FEBS Lett* 312:245–248, 1992.

128. Ito M, Guerriero V Jr, Chen X, Hartshorne DJ: Definition of the inhibitory domain of smooth muscle myosin light chain kinase by site-directed mutagenesis. *Biochemistry* 30:3498–3503, 1991.

129. Bagchi IC, Kemp BE, Means AR: Intrasteric regulation of myosin light chain kinase: The pseudosubstrate prototype binds to the active site. *Mol Endocrinol* 6:621–626, 1992.

130. Herring BP: Basic residues are important for Ca^{2+}/calmodulin-binding and activation but not autoinhibition of rabbit skeletal muscle myosin light chain kinase. *J Biol Chem* 266:11838–11841, 1991.

131. Fitzsimmons DP, Herring BP, Stull JT, Gallagher PJ: Identification of basic residues involved in activation and calmodulin binding of rabbit smooth muscle myosin light chain kinase. *J Biol Chem* 267:23903–23909, 1992.

132. Shoemaker MO, Lau W, Shattuck RL, Kwiatkowski AP, Matrisian PE, Guerra-Santos L, Wilson E, Lukas TJ, Van Eldik LJ, Watterson DM: Use of DNA sequence and mutant analyses and antisense oligodeoxynucleotides to examine the molecular basis of nonmuscle myosin light chain kinase autoinhibition, calmodulin recognition, and activity. *J Cell Biol* 111:1107–1125, 1990.

133. Knighton DR, Pearson RB, Sowadski JM, Means AR, Ten Eyck LF, Taylor SS, Kemp BE: Structural basis of the intrasteric regulation of myosin light chain kinases. *Science* 258:130–135, 1992.

134. Knighton DR, Zheng J, Ten Eyck LF, Ashford VA, Xuong N-H, Taylor SS, Sowadski JM: Crystal structure of the catalytic subunit of cAMP-dependent protein kinase. *Science* 253:407–414, 1991.

135. Knighton DR, Zheng J, Ten Eyck LF, Ashford VA, Xuong N-H, Taylor SS, Sowadski JM: Structure of a peptide inhibitor bound to the catalytic subunit of cyclic adenosine monophosphate-dependent protein kinase. *Science* 253:414–420, 1991.

136. Pato MD, Adelstein RS: Dephosphorylation of the 20,000-dalton light chain of myosin by two different phosphatases from smooth muscle. *J Biol Chem* 255:6535–6538, 1980.

137. Pato MD, Kerc E: Limited proteolytic digestion and dissociation of smooth muscle phosphatase-I modifies its substrate specificity. *J Biol Chem* 261:3770–3774, 1986.

138. Tulloch AG, Pato MD: Turkey gizzard smooth muscle myosin phosphatase-III is a novel protein phosphatase. *J Biol Chem* 266:20168–20174, 1991.

139. Ingebritsen TS, Cohen P: Protein phosphatases: Properties and role in cellular regulation. *Science* 221:331–338, 1983.

140. Pato MD, Kerc E: Purification and characterization of a smooth muscle myosin phosphatase from turkey gizzards. *J Biol Chem* 260:12359–12366, 1985.

141. Pato MD, Kerc E: Comparison of the properties of the protein phosphatases from avian and mammalian smooth muscles: Purification and characterization of rabbit uterine smooth muscle phosphatases. *Arch Biochem Biophys* 276:116–124, 1990.

142. Sellers JR, Pato MD: The binding of smooth muscle myosin light chain kinase and phosphatases to actin and myosin. *J Biol Chem* 259:7740–7746, 1984.

143. Mitsui T, Inagaki M, Ikebe M: Purification and characterization of smooth muscle myosin-associated phosphatase from chicken gizzards. *J Biol Chem* 267:16727–16735, 1992.

144. Alessi DR, MacDougall LK, Sola MM, Ikebe M, Cohen P: *Eur J Biochem* 210:1023–1035, 1992.

145. Casteels R, Wuytack F, Himpens B, Raeymaekers L: Regulatory systems for the cytoplasmic calcium concentration in smooth muscle. *Biomed Biochim Acta* 45:S147–S152, 1986.

146. Sherry JMF, Gorecka A, Aksoy MO, Dabrowska R, Hartshorne DJ: Roles of calcium and phosphorylation in the regulation of the activity of gizzard myosin. *Biochemistry* 17:4411–4418, 1978.

147. Wang C, Ngai PK, Walsh MP, Wang JH: Ca^{2+}- and calmodulin-dependent stimulation of smooth muscle actomyosin Mg^{2+}-ATPase by fodrin. *Biochemistry* 26:1110–1117, 1987.

148. Cassidy PS, Hoar PE, Kerrick WGL: Irreversible thiophosphorylation and activation of tension in functionally skinned rabbit ileum strips by [^{35}S]ATPγS. *J Biol Chem* 254:11148–11153, 1979.

149. Hoar PE, Kerrick WGL, Cassidy PS: Chicken gizzard: Relation between calcium-activated phosphorylation and contraction. *Science* 204:503–506, 1979.

150. Cassidy PS, Kerrick WGL: Superprecipitation of gizzard actomyosin, and tension in gizzard muscle skinned fibers in the presence of nucleotides other than ATP. *Biochim Biophys Acta* 705:63–69, 1982.

151. Walsh MP, Bridenbaugh R, Kerrick WGL, Hartshorne DJ: Gizzard Ca^{2+}-independent myosin light chain kinase: Evidence in favor of the phosphorylation theory. *Fed Proc* 42:45–50, 1983.

152. Sellers JR, Pato MD, Adelstein RS: Reversible phosphorylation of smooth muscle myosin, heavy meromyosin, and platelet myosin. *J Biol Chem* 256:13137–13142, 1981.

153. Onishi H, Umeda J, Uchiwa H, Watanabe S: Purification of gizzard myosin light-chain phosphatase, and reversible changes in the ATPase and superprecipitation activities of actomyosin in the presence of purified preparations of myosin light-chain phosphatase and kinase. *J Biochem (Tokyo)* 91:265–271, 1982.

154. DiSalvo J, Gifford D, Bialojan C, Rüegg JC: An aortic spontaneously active phosphatase dephosphorylates myosin and inhibits actin-myosin interaction. *Biochem Biophys Res Commun* 111:906–911, 1983.

155. Rüegg JC, DiSalvo J, Paul RJ: Soluble relaxation factor from vascular smooth muscle: A myosin light chain phosphatase. *Biochem Biophys Res Commun* 106:1126–1133, 1982.

156. Hoar PE, Pato MD, Kerrick WGL: Myosin light chain phosphatase. Effect on the activation and relaxation of gizzard smooth muscle skinned fibers. *J Biol Chem* 260:8760–8764, 1985.

157. Haeberle JR, Hathaway DR, DePaoli-Roach AA: Dephosphorylation of myosin by the catalytic subunit of a type-2 phosphatase produces relaxation of chemically skinned uterine smooth muscle. *J Biol Chem* 260:9965–9968, 1985.

158. Levin RM, Weiss B: Selective binding of antipsychotics and other psychoactive agents to the calcium-dependent activator of cyclic nucleotide phosphodiesterase. *J Pharmacol Exp Ther* 208:454–459, 1979.

159. Hidaka H, Asano M, Tanaka T: Activity-structure relationship of calmodulin antagonists. Naphthalenesulfonamide derivatives. *Mol Pharmacol* 20:571–578, 1981.

160. Hidaka H, Naka M, Yamaki T: Effect of novel specific myosin light chain kinase inhibitors on Ca^{2+}-activated Mg^{2+}-ATPase of chicken gizzard actomyosin. *Biochem Biophys Res Commun* 90:694–699, 1979.

161. Hidaka H, Yamaki T, Naka M, Tanaka T, Hayashi H, Kobayashi R: Calcium-regulated modulator protein interacting agents inhibit smooth muscle calcium-stimulated protein kinase and ATPase. *Mol Pharmacol* 17:66–72, 1980.

162. Sheterline P: Trifluoperazine can distinguish between myosin light chain kinase-linked and troponin C-linked control of actomyosin interaction by Ca^{2+}. *Biochem Biophys Res Commun* 93:194–200, 1980.

163. Kerrick WGL, Hoar PE, Cassidy PS: Calcium-activated tension: The role of myosin light chain phosphorylation. *Fed Proc* 39:1558–1563, 1980.

164. Sparrow MP, Mrwa U, Hofmann F, Rüegg JC: Calmodulin is essential for smooth muscle contraction. *FEBS Lett* 125: 141–145, 1981.

165. Barron JT, Bárány M, Bárány K, Storti RV: Reversible phosphorylation and dephosphorylation of the 20,000-dalton light chain of myosin during the contraction-relaxation-contraction cycle of arterial smooth muscle. *J Biol Chem* 255:6238–6244, 1980.

166. Kanamori M, Naka M, Asano M, Hidaka H: Effects of N-(6-aminohexyl)-5-chloro-1-naphthalenesulfonamide and other calmodulin antagonists (calmodulin interacting agents) on calcium-induced contraction of rabbit aortic strips. *J Pharmacol Exp Ther* 217:494–499, 1981.

167. Asano M, Suzuki Y, Hidaka H: Effects of various calmodulin antagonists on contraction of rabbit aortic strips. *J Pharmacol Exp Ther* 220:191–196, 1982.

168. Silver PJ, Stull JT: Effects of the calmodulin antagonist, fluphenazine, on phosphorylation of myosin and phosphorylase in intact smooth muscle. *Mol Pharmacol* 23:665–670, 1983.

169. Crosby ND, Diamond J: Effects of phenothiazines on calcium induced contractions of chemically skinned smooth muscle. *Proc West Pharmacol Soc* 23:335–338, 1980.

170. Hidaka H, Asano M, Iwadare S, Matsumoto I, Totsuka T, Aoki M: A novel vascular relaxing agent, N-(6-aminohexyl)-5-chloro-1-naphthalenesulfonamide which affects vascular smooth muscle actomyosin. *J Pharmacol Exp Ther* 207:8–15, 1978.

171. Hidaka H, Yamaki T, Totsuka T, Asano M: Selective inhibitors of Ca^{2+}-binding modulator of phosphodiesterase produce vascular relaxation and inhibit actin-myosin interaction. *Mol Pharmacol* 15:49–59, 1979.

172. Saitoh M, Ishikawa T, Matsushima S, Naka M, Hidaka H: Selective inhibition of catalytic activity of smooth muscle myosin light chain kinase. *J Biol Chem* 262:7796–7801, 1987.

173. Walsh MP, Dabrowska R, Hinkins S, Hartshorne DJ: Calcium-independent myosin light chain kinase of smooth muscle. Preparation by limited chymotryptic digestion of the Ca^{2+}-dependent enzyme, purification and characterization. *Biochemistry* 21:1919–1925, 1982.

174. Walsh MP, Bridenbaugh R, Hartshorne DJ, Kerrick WGL: Phosphorylation-dependent activated tension in skinned gizzard muscle fibers in the absence of Ca^{2+}. *J Biol Chem* 257:5987–5990, 1982.

175. Cande WZ, Tooth PJ, Kendrick-Jones J: Regulation of contraction and thick filament assembly-disassembly in glycerinated vertebrate smooth muscle cells. *J Cell Biol* 97:1062–1071, 1983.

176. Mrwa U, Güth K, Rüegg JC, Paul RJ, Boström S, Barsotti R, Hartshorne D: Mechanical and biochemical characterization of the contraction elicited by a calcium-independent myosin light chain kinase in chemically skinned smooth muscle. *Experientia* 41:1002–1005, 1985.

177. Kargacin GJ, Ikebe M, Fay FS: Peptide modulators of myosin light chain kinase affect smooth muscle cell contraction. *Am J Physiol* 259:C315–C324, 1990.

178. Itoh T, Ikebe M, Kargacin GJ, Hartshorne DJ, Kemp BE, Fay FS: Effects of modulators of MLCK activity in single smooth muscle cells. *Nature* 338:164–167, 1989.

179. Rüegg JC, Zeugner C, Strauss JD, Paul RJ, Kemp B, Chem M, Li A-Y, Hartshorne DJ: A calmodulin-binding peptide relaxes skinned muscle from guinea-pig taenia coli. *Pflügers Arch* 414:282–285, 1989.

180. Shibata S, Ishida Y, Kitano H, Ohizumi Y, Habon J, Tsukitani Y, Kikuchi H: Contractile effects of okadaic acid, a novel ionophore-like substance from black sponge, on isolated smooth muscles under the condition of Ca deficiency. *J Pharmacol Exp Ther* 223:135–143, 1982.

181. Obara K, Takai A, Rüegg JC, DeLanerolle P: Okadaic acid, a phosphatase inhibitor, produces a Ca^{2+} and calmodulin-independent contraction of smooth muscle. *Pflügers Arch* 414:134–138, 1989.

182. Hartshorne DJ, Ishihara H, Karaki H, Ozaki H, Sato K, Hori M, Watabe S: Okadaic acid and calyculin A: Effects on smooth muscle systems. *Adv Prot Phosphatases* 5:219–231, 1989.

183. Takai A, Bialojan C, Troschka M, Rüegg JC: Smooth muscle myosin phosphatase inhibition and force enhancement by black sponge toxin. *FEBS Lett* 217:81–84, 1987.

184. Gong MC, Cohen P, Kitazawa T, Ikebe M, Masuo M, Somlyo AP, Somlyo AV: Myosin light chain phosphatase activities and the effects of phosphatase inhibitors in tonic and phasic smooth muscle. *J Biol Chem* 267:14662–14668, 1992.

185. Sheetz MP, Spudich JA: Movement of myosin-coated fluorescent beads on actin cables in vitro. *Nature* 303:31–35, 1983.

186. Sellers JR, Spudich JA, Sheetz MP: Light chain phosphorylation regulates the movement of smooth muscle myosin on actin filaments. *J Cell Biol* 101:1897–1902, 1985.

187. Umemoto S, Bengur AR, Sellers JR: Effect of multiple phosphorylations of smooth muscle and cytoplasmic myosins on movement in an in vitro motility assay. *J Biol Chem* 264:1431–1436, 1989.

188. Umemoto S, Sellers JR: Characterization of in vitro motility assays using smooth muscle and cytoplasmic myosins. *J Biol Chem* 265:14864–14869, 1990.

189. Warshaw DM, Desrosiers JM, Work SS, Trybus KM: Smooth muscle myosin cross-bridge interactions modulate actin filament sliding velocity in vitro. *J Cell Biol* 111: 453–463, 1990.

190. Suzuki H, Onishi H, Takahashi K, Watanabe S: Structure and function of chicken gizzard myosin. *J Biochem (Tokyo)* 84:1529–1542, 1978.

191. Suzuki H, Kamata T, Onishi H, Watanabe S: Adenosine triphosphate-induced reversible change in the conformation of chicken gizzard myosin and heavy meromyosin. *J Biochem (Tokyo)* 91:1699–1705, 1982.

192. Trybus KM, Huiatt TW, Lowey S: A bent monomeric conformation of myosin from smooth muscle. *Proc Natl Acad Sci USA* 79:6151–6155, 1982.

193. Onishi H, Wakabayashi T: Electron microscopic studies of myosin molecules from chicken gizzard muscle I: The formation of the intramolecular loop in the myosin tail. *J Biochem (Tokyo)* 92:871–879, 1982.

194. Ikebe M, Hinkins S, Hartshorne DJ: Correlation of enzymatic properties and conformation of smooth muscle myosin. *Biochemistry* 22:4580–4587, 1983.

195. Ikebe M, Hartshorne DJ: Conformation-dependent proteolysis of smooth-muscle myosin. *J Biol Chem* 259:11639–11642, 1984.

196. Rowe T, Kendrick-Jones J: Chimeric myosin regulatory light chains identify the subdomain responsible for regulatory function. *EMBO J* 11:4715–4722, 1992.

197. Morgan JP, Morgan KG: Vascular smooth muscle: The first recorded Ca^{2+} transients. *Pflügers Arch* 395:75–77, 1982.

198. Gerthoffer WT: Dissociation of myosin phosphorylation and active tension during muscarinic stimulation of tracheal smooth muscle. *J Pharmacol Exp Ther* 240:8–15, 1987.

199. Moreland S, Moreland RS, Singer HA: Apparent dissociation between myosin light chain phosphorylation and maximal velocity of shortening in KCl depolarized swine carotid artery: Effect of temperature and KCl concentration. *Pflügers Arch* 408:139–145, 1986.

200. Siegman MJ, Butler TM, Mooers SU, Michalek A: Ca^{2+} can affect V_{max} without changes in myosin light chain phosphorylation in smooth muscle. *Pflügers Arch* 401:385–390, 1984.

201. Wagner J, Rüegg JC: Skinned smooth muscle: Calcium-calmodulin activation independent of myosin phosphorylation. *Pflügers Arch* 407:569–571, 1986.

202. Tansey MG, Hori M, Karaki H, Kamm KE, Stull JT: Okadaic acid uncouples myosin light chain phosphorylation and tension in smooth muscle. *FEBS Lett* 270:219–221, 1990.

203. Ashizawa N, Kobayashi F, Tanaka Y, Nakayama K: Relaxing action of okadaic acid, a black sponge toxin, on the arterial smooth muscle. *Biochem Biophys Res Commun* 162:971–976, 1989.

204. Kühn H, Tewes A, Gagelmann M, Güth K, Arner A, Rüegg JC: Temporal relationship between force, ATPase activity, and myosin phosphorylation during a contraction/relaxation cycle in a skinned smooth muscle. *Pflügers Arch* 416:512–518, 1990.

205. Fisher W, Pfitzer G: Rapid myosin phosphorylation transients in phasic contractions in chicken gizzard smooth muscle. *FEBS Lett* 258:59–62, 1989.

206. Kenney RE, Hoar PE, Kerrick WGL: The relationship between ATPase activity, isometric force, and myosin light-chain phosphorylation and thiophosphorylation in skinned smooth muscle fiber bundles from chicken gizzard. *J Biol Chem* 265:8642–8649, 1990.

207. Dillon PF, Aksoy MO, Driska SP, Murphy RA: Myosin phosphorylation and the crossbridge cycle in arterial smooth muscle. *Science* 211:495–497, 1981.

208. Hai C-M, Murphy RA: Ca^{2+}, crossbridge phosphorylation, and contraction. *Annu Rev Physiol* 51:285–298, 1989.

209. Chatterjee M, Murphy RA: Calcium-dependent stress maintenance without myosin phosphorylation in skinned smooth muscle. *Science* 221:464–466, 1983.

210. McDaniel NL, Rembold CM, Richard HL, Murphy RA: cAMP relaxes arterial smooth muscle predominantly by decreasing cell $[Ca^{2+}]$. *J Physiol* 439:147–160, 1991.

211. Taylor SS, Buechler JA, Yonemoto W: cAMP-dependent protein kinase: Framework for a diverse family of regulatory enzymes. *Annu Rev Biochem* 59:971–1005, 1990.

212. Hofmann F, Dostmann W, Keilbach A, Landgraf W, Ruth P: Structure and physiological role of cGMP-dependent protein kinase. *Biochim Biophys Acta* 1135:51–60, 1992.

213. Shabb JB, Corbin JD: Cyclic nucleotide-binding domains in proteins having diverse functions. *J Biol Chem* 267:5723–5726, 1992.

214. Lincoln TM, Cornwell TL, Taylor AE: cGMP-dependent protein kinase mediates the reduction of Ca^{2+} by cAMP in vascular smooth muscle cells. *Am J Physiol* 258:C399–C407, 1990.

215. Raeymaekers L, Hofmann F, Casteels R: Cyclic GMP-dependent protein kinase phosphorylates phospholamban in isolated sarcoplasmic reticulum from cardiac and smooth muscle. *Biochem J* 252:269–273, 1988.

216. Furakawa K, Tawada Y, Shigekawa M: Regulation of the plasma membrane Ca^{2+} pump by cyclic nucleotides in cultured vascular smooth muscle cells. *J Biol Chem* 263:8058–8065, 1988.

217. Thornbury KD, Ward SM, Dalziel HH, Carl A, Westfall DP, Sanders KM: Nitric oxide and nitrosocysteine mimic nonadrenergic, noncholinergic hyperpolarization in canine proximal colon. *Am J Physiol* 261:G553–G557, 1991.

218. Tang D-C, Stull JT, Kubota Y, Kamm KE: Regulation of the Ca^{2+} dependence of smooth muscle contraction. *J Biol Chem* 267:11839–11845, 1992.

219. Adelstein RS, Conti MA, Hathaway DR, Klee CB: Phosphorylation of smooth muscle myosin light chain kinase by the catalytic subunit of adenosine 3′,5′-monophosphate-dependent protein kinase. *J Biol Chem* 253:8347–8350, 1978.

220. Conti MA, Adelstein RS: The relationship between calmodulin binding and phosphorylation of smooth muscle myosin kinase by the catalytic subunit of 3′,5′-cAMP-dependent protein kinase. *J Biol Chem* 256:3178–3181, 1981.

221. Stull JT, Hsu L-C, Tansey MG, Kamm KE: Myosin light chain kinase phosphorylation in tracheal smooth muscle. *J Biol Chem* 265:16683–16690, 1990.

222. Ikebe M, Inagaki M, Kanamaru K, Hidaka H: Phosphorylation of smooth muscle myosin light chain kinase by Ca^{2+}-activated phospholipid-dependent protein kinase. *J Biol Chem* 260:4547–4550, 1985.

223. Nishikawa M, Shirakawa S, Adelstein RS: Phosphorylation of smooth muscle myosin light chain kinase by protein kinase C. Comparative study of the phosphorylated sites. *J Biol Chem* 260:8978–8983, 1985.

224. Hashimoto Y, Soderling TR: Phosphorylation of smooth muscle myosin light chain kinase by Ca^{2+}/calmodulin-dependent protein kinase II: Comparative study of the phosphorylation sites. *Arch Biochem Biophys* 278:41–45, 1990.

225. Ikebe M, Reardon S: Phosphorylation of smooth myosin light chain kinase by smooth muscle Ca^{2+}/calmodulin-dependent multifunctional protein kinase. *J Biol Chem* 265:8975–8978, 1990.

226. Tansey MG, Word RA, Hidaka H, Singer HA, Schworer CM, Kamm KE, Stull JT: Phosphorylation of myosin light chain kinase by the multifunctional calmodulin-dependent protein kinase II in smooth muscle cells. *J Biol Chem* 267:12511–12516, 1992.

227. Nishimura J, Kolber M, van Breemen C: Norepinephrine and GTP-γ-S increase myofilament Ca^{2+} sensitivity in α-toxin permeabilized arterial smooth muscle. *Biochem Biophys Res Commun* 157:677–683, 1988.

228. Kitazawa T, Kobayashi S, Horiuti K, Somlyo AV, Somlyo AP: Receptor-coupled, permeabilized smooth muscle. Role of the phosphatidylinositol cascade, G-proteins, and modu-

lation of the contractile response to Ca^{2+}. *J Biol Chem* 264:5339–5342, 1989.

229. Rembold CM: Modulation of the [Ca^{2+}] sensitivity of myosin phosphorylation in intact swine arterial smooth muscle. *J Physiol* 429:77–94, 1990.

230. Kitazawa T, Gaylinn BD, Denney GH, Somlyo AP: G-protein-mediated Ca^{2+} sensitization of smooth muscle contraction through myosin light chain phosphorylation. *J Biol Chem* 266:1708–1715, 1991.

231. Hirata K, Kikuchi A, Sasaki T, Kuroda S, Kaibuchi K, Matsuura Y, Seki H, Saida K, Takai Y: Involvement of *rho* p21 in the GTP-enhanced calcium ion sensitivity of smooth muscle contraction. *J Biol Chem* 267:8719–8722, 1992.

232. Kitazawa T, Masuo M, Somlyo AP: G protein-mediated inhibition of myosin light-chain phosphatase in vascular smooth muscle. *Proc Natl Acad Sci USA* 88:9307–9310, 1991.

233. Gong MC, Fuglsang A, Alessi D, Kobayashi S, Cohen P, Somlyo AV, Somlyo AP: Arachidonic acid inhibits myosin light chain phosphatase and sensitizes smooth muscle to calcium. *J Biol Chem* 267:21492–21498, 1992.

234. Edelman AM, Lin W-H, Osterhout DJ, Bennett MK, Kennedy MB, Krebs EG: Phosphorylation of smooth muscle myosin by type II Ca^{2+}/calmodulin-dependent protein kinase. *Mol Cell Biochem* 97:87–98, 1990.

235. Rhee SG, Suh P-G, Ryu S-H, Lee SY: Studies of inositol phospholipid-specific phospholipase C. *Science* 244:546–550, 1989.

236. Berridge MJ: Inositol trisphosphate and diacylglycerol as second messengers. *Biochem J* 220:345–360, 1984.

237. Berridge MJ: Inositol trisphosphate and diacylglycerol: Two interacting second messengers. *Annu Rev Biochem* 56:159–193, 1987.

238. Somlyo AP, Somlyo AV: Flash photolysis studies of excitation-contraction coupling, regulation and contraction in smooth muscle. *Annu Rev Biochem* 52:857–874, 1990.

239. Nishizuka Y: Intracellular signaling by hydrolysis of phospholipids and activation of protein kinase C. *Science* 258:607–614, 1992.

240. Jiang MJ, Morgan KG: Intracellular calcium levels in phorbol ester-induced contractions of vascular smooth muscle. *Am J Physiol* 253:H1365–H1371, 1987.

241. Singer HA, Baker KM: Calcium dependence of phorbol 12,13-dibutyrate-induced force and myosin light chain phosphorylation in arterial smooth muscle. *J Pharmacol Exp Ther* 243:814–821, 1987.

242. Bengur AR, Robinson EA, Appella E, Sellers JR: Sequence of the sites phosphorylated by protein kinase C in the smooth muscle myosin light chain. *J Biol Chem* 262:7613–7617, 1987.

243. Ikebe M, Hartshorne DJ, Elzinga M: Phosphorylation of the 20,000-dalton light chain of smooth muscle myosin by the calcium-activated, phospholipid-dependent protein kinase. Phosphorylation sites and effects of phosphorylation. *J Biol Chem* 262:9569–9573, 1987.

244. Nishikawa M, Hidaka H, Adelstein RS: Phosphorylation of smooth muscle heavy meromyosin by calcium-activated, phospholipid-dependent protein kinase. *J Biol Chem* 258:14069–14072, 1983.

245. Kamm KE, Hsu L-G, Kubota Y, Stull JT: Phosphorylation of smooth muscle myosin heavy and light chains. Effects of phorbol dibutyrate and agonists. *J Biol Chem* 264:21223–21229, 1989.

246. Singer HA, Oren JW, Benscoter HA: Myosin light chain phosphorylation in ^{32}P-labeled rabbit aorta stimulated by phorbol 12,13-dibutyrate and phenylephrine. *J Biol Chem* 264:21215–21222, 1989.

247. Rembold CM, Murphy RA: [Ca^{2+}]-dependent myosin phosphorylation in phorbol diester stimulated smooth muscle contraction. *Am J Physiol* 255:C719–C723, 1988.

248. Winder SJ, Walsh MP: Smooth muscle calponin. Inhibition of actomyosin MgATPase and regulation by phosphorylation. *J Biol Chem* 265:10148–10155, 1990.

249. Umekawa H, Hidaka H: Phosphorylation of caldesmon by protein kinase C. *Biochem Biophys Res Commun* 132:56–62, 1985.

250. Huang K-P: The mechanism of protein kinase C activation. *Trends Pharmacol Sci* 12:425–432, 1989.

251. Karibe H, Oishi K, Uchida MK: Involvement of protein kinase C in Ca^{2+}-independent contraction of rat uterine smooth muscle. *Biochem Biophys Res Commun* 179:487–494, 1991.

252. Andrea JE, Walsh MP: Protein kinase C of smooth muscle. *Hypertension* 20:585–595, 1992.

253. Khalil RA, Lajoie C, Resnick MS, Morgan KG: Ca^{2+}-independent isoforms of protein kinase C differentially translocate in smooth muscle. *Am J Physiol* 263:C714–C719, 1992.

254. Brozovich FV, Walsh MP, Morgan KG: Regulation of force in skinned, single cells of ferret aortic smooth muscle. *Pflügers Arch* 416:742–749, 1990.

255. Collins EM, Walsh MP, Morgan KG: Contraction of single vascular smooth muscle cells by phenylephrine at constant [Ca^{2+}]$_i$. *Am J Physiol* 262:H754–H762, 1992.

256. Khalil RA, Morgan KG: Protein kinase C: A second E-C coupling pathway in vascular smooth muscle? *News Physiol Sci* 7:10–15, 1992.

257. Carsten ME: Uterine smooth muscle: Troponin. *Arch Biochem Biophys* 147:353–357, 1971.

258. Marston SB, Trevett RM, Walters M: Calcium ion-regulated thin filaments from vascular smooth muscle. *Biochem J* 185:355–365, 1980.

259. Bremel RD: Myosin linked calcium regulation in vertebrate smooth muscle. *Nature* 252:405–407, 1974.

260. Ngai PK, Scott-Woo GC, Lim MS, Sutherland C, Walsh MP: Activation of smooth muscle myosin Mg^{2+}-ATPase by native thin filaments and actin-tropomyosin. *J Biol Chem* 262:5352–5359, 1987.

261. Sobue K, Muramoto Y, Fujita M, Kakiuchi S: Purification of a calmodulin-binding protein from chicken gizzard that interacts with F-actin. *Proc Natl Acad Sci USA* 78:5652–5655, 1981.

262. Graceffa P: Evidence for interaction between smooth muscle tropomyosin and caldesmon. *FEBS Lett* 218:139–142, 1987.

263. Ikebe M, Reardon S: Binding of caldesmon to smooth muscle myosin. *J Biol Chem* 263:3055–3058, 1988.

264. Ngai PK, Walsh MP: Detection of caldesmon in muscle and non-muscle tissues of the chicken using polyclonal antibodies. *Biochem Biophys Res Commun* 127:533–539, 1985.

265. Haeberle JR, Hathaway DR, Smith CL: Caldesmon content of mammalian smooth muscles. *J Muscle Res Cell Motil* 13:81–89, 1992.

266. Bretscher A, Lynch W: Identification and localization of immunoreactive forms of caldesmon in smooth and non-muscle cells: A comparison with the distributions of tropomyosin and α-actinin. *J Cell Biol* 100:1656–1663, 1985.

267. Sobue K, Sellers JR: Caldesmon, a novel regulatory protein in smooth muscle and nonmuscle actomyosin systems. *J Biol Chem* 266:12115–12118, 1991.

268. Bretscher A: Smooth muscle caldesmon. Rapid purification

and F-actin cross-linking properties. *J Biol Chem* 259: 12873–12880, 1984.

269. Fürst DO, Cross RA, DeMey J, Small JV: Caldesmon is an elongated, flexible molecule localized in the actomyosin domains of smooth muscle. *EMBO J* 5:251–257, 1986.

270. Dingus J, Hwo S, Bryan J: Identification by monoclonal antibodies and characterization of human platelet caldesmon. *J Cell Biol* 102:1748–1757, 1986.

271. Hayashi K, Kanda K, Kimizuka F, Kato I, Sobue K: Primary structure and functional expression of *h*-caldesmon complementary DNA. *Biochem Biophys Res Commun* 164: 503–511, 1989.

272. Bryan J, Imai M, Lee R, Moore P, Cook RG, Lin W-G: Cloning and expression of a smooth muscle caldesmon. *J Biol Chem* 264:13873–13879, 1989.

273. Lynch WP, Riseman VM, Bretscher A: Smooth muscle caldesmon is an extended flexible monomeric protein in solution that can readily undergo reversible intra- and intermolecular sulfhydryl cross-linking. *J Biol Chem* 262: 7429–7437, 1987.

274. Graceffa P, Wang C-LA, Stafford WF: Caldesmon. Molecular weight and subunit composition by analytical ultracentrifugation. *J Biol Chem* 263:14196–14202, 1988.

275. Marston SB, Redwood CS: The molecular anatomy of caldesmon. *Biochem J* 279:1–16, 1991.

276. Wang C-LA, Wang L-WC, Lu RC: Caldesmon has two calmodulin-binding domains. *Biochem Biophys Res Commun* 162:746–752, 1989.

277. Velaz L, Hemric ME, Benson CE, Chalovich JM: The binding of caldesmon to actin and its effect on the ATPase activity of soluble myosin subfragments in the presence and absence of tropomyosin. *J Biol Chem* 264:9602–9610, 1989.

278. Lehman W: Caldesmon association with smooth muscle thin filaments isolated in the presence and absence of calcium. *Biochim Biophys Acta* 885:88–90, 1986.

279. Sutherland C, Walsh MP: Phosphorylation of caldesmon prevents its interaction with smooth muscle myosin. *J Biol Chem* 264:578–583, 1989.

280. Bartegi A, Fattoum A, Derancourt J, Kassab R: Characterization of the carboxyl-terminal 10-kDa cyanogen bromide fragment of caldesmon as an actin-calmodulin binding region. *J Biol Chem* 265:15231–15238, 1990.

281. Wang C-LA, Wang L-WC, Xu S, Lu RC, Saavedra-Alanis V, Bryan J: Localization of the calmodulin- and the actin-binding sites of caldesmon. *J Biol Chem* 266:9166–9172, 1991.

282. Mornet D, Audemard E, Derancourt J: Identification of a 15 kilodalton actin binding region on gizzard caldesmon probed by chemical cross-linking. *Bicohem Biophys Res Commun* 154:564–571, 1988.

283. Hayashi K, Fujio Y, Kato I, Sobue K: Structural and functional relationships between *h*- and *l*-caldesmons. *J Biol Chem* 266:355–361, 1991.

284. Zhan Q, Wong SS, Wang C-LA: A calmodulin-binding peptide of caldesmon. *J Biol Chem* 266:21810–21814, 1991.

285. Katsuyama H, Wang C-LA, Morgan KG: Regulation of vascular smooth muscle tone by caldesmon. *J Biol Chem* 267:14555–14558, 1992.

286. Wang C-LA, Chalovich JM, Graceffa P, Lu RC, Mabuchi K, Stafford WF: A long helix from the central region of smooth muscle caldesmon. *J Biol Chem* 266:13958–13963, 1991.

287. Small JV, Fürst DO, De Mey J: Localization of filamin in smooth muscle. *J Cell Biol* 102:210–220, 1986.

288. Lehman W, Craig R, Lui J, Moody C: Caldesmon and the structure of smooth muscle thin filaments: Immunolocaliza-

tion of caldesmon on thin filaments. *J Muscle Res Cell Motil* 10:101–112, 1989.

289. Moody C, Lehman W, Craig R: Caldesmon and the structure of smooth muscle thin filaments: Electron microscopy of isolated thin filaments. *J Muscle Res Cell Motil* 11: 176–185, 1990.

290. Hemric ME, Chalovich JM: Characterization of caldesmon binding to myosin. *J Biol Chem* 265:19672–19678, 1990.

291. Marston S, Pinter K, Bennett P: Caldesmon binds to smooth muscle myosin and myosin rod and crosslinks thick filaments to actin filaments. *J Muscle Res Cell Motil* 13:206–218, 1992.

292. Sobue K, Morimoto K, Inui M, Kanda K, Kakiuchi S: Control of actin-myosin interaction of gizzard smooth muscle by calmodulin and caldesmon-linked flip-flop mechanism. *Biomed Res* 3:188–196, 1982.

293. Ngai PK, Walsh MP: Inhibition of smooth muscle actin-activated myosin Mg^{2+}-ATPase activity by caldesmon. *J Biol Chem* 259:13656–13659, 1984.

294. Szpacenko A, Wagner J, Dabrowska R, Rüegg JC: Caldesmon-induced inhibition of ATPase activity of actomyosin and contraction of skinned fibres of chicken gizzard smooth muscle. *FEBS Lett* 192:9–12, 1985.

295. Horiuchi KY, Chacko S: Caldesmon inhibits the cooperative turning-on of the smooth muscle heavy meromyosin by tropomyosin-actin. *Biochemistry* 28:9111–9116, 1989.

296. Velaz L, Ingraham RH, Chalovich JM: Dissociation of the effect of caldesmon on the ATPase activity and on the binding of smooth muscle heavy meromyosin to actin by partial digestion of caldesmon. *J Biol Chem* 265:2929–2934, 1990.

297. Hemric ME, Chalovich JM: Effect of caldesmon on the ATPase activity and the binding of smooth and skeletal myosin subfragments to actin. *J Biol Chem* 263:1878–1885, 1988.

298. Bartegi A, Fattoum A, Khassab R: Cross-linking of smooth muscle caldesmon to the NH_2-terminal region of skeletal F-actin. *J Biol Chem* 265:2231–2237, 1990.

299. Adams S, DasGupta G, Chalovich JM, Reisler E: Immunochemical evidence for the binding of caldesmon to the NH_2-terminal segment of actin. *J Biol Chem* 265:19652–19657, 1990.

300. Sutoh K: Identification of myosin-binding sites on the actin sequence. *Biochemistry* 21:3654–3661, 1982.

301. Marston S: Aorta caldesmon inhibits actin activation of thiophosphorylated heavy meromyosin Mg^{2+}-ATPase activity by slowing the rate of product release. *FEBS Lett* 238:147–150, 1988.

302. Marston SB, Redwood CS: Inhibition of actin-tropomyosin activation of myosin MgATPase activity by the smooth muscle regulatory protein caldesmon. *J Biol Chem* 267: 16796–16800, 1992.

303. Szpacenko A, Dabrowska R: Functional domain of caldesmon. *FEBS Lett* 202:182–186, 1986.

304. Redwood CS, Marston SB, Bryan J, Cross RA, Kendrick-Jones J: The functional properties of full length and mutant chicken gizzard smooth muscle caldesmon expressed in *Escherichia coli*. *FEBS Lett* 270:53–56, 1990.

305. Horiuchi KY, Samuel M, Chacko S: Mechanism for the inhibition of acto-heavy meromyosin ATPase by the actin/ calmodulin binding domain of caldesmon. *Biochemistry* 30:712–717, 1991.

306. Shirinsky VP, Biryukov KG, Hettasch JM, Sellers JR: Inhibition of the relative movement of actin and myosin by caldesmon and calponin. *J Biol Chem* 267:15886–15892, 1992.

307. Haeberle JR, Trybus KM, Hemric ME, Warshaw DM:

The effects of smooth muscle caldesmon on actin filament motility. *J Biol Chem* 267:23001–23006, 1992.

308. Ngai PK, Walsh MP: The effects of phosphorylation of smooth muscle caldesmon. *Biochem J* 244:417–425, 1987.

309. Abougou J-C, Hagiwara M, Hachiya T, Terasawa M, Hidaka H, Hartshorne DJ: Phosphorylation of caldesmon. *FEBS Lett* 257:408–410, 1989.

310. Ikebe M, Reardon S, Scott-Woo GC, Zhou Z, Koda Y: Purification and characterization of calmodulin-dependent multifunctional protein kinase from smooth muscle: Isolation of caldesmon kinase. *Biochemistry* 29:11242–11248, 1990.

311. Scott-Woo GC, Sutherland C, Walsh MP: Kinase activity associated with caldesmon is Ca^{2+}/calmodulin-dependent kinase II. *Biochem J* 268:367–370, 1990.

311a. Pato MD, Sutherland C, Winder SJ, Walsh MP: Smooth muscle caldesmon phosphatase is SMP-I, a type 2A protein phosphatase. *Biochem J* 293:35–41, 1993.

312. Ngai PK, Walsh MP: Properties of caldesmon isolated from chicken gizzard. *Biochem J* 230:695–707, 1985.

313. Lash JA, Sellers JR, Hathaway DR: The effects of caldesmon on smooth muscle heavy actomeromyosin ATPase activity and binding of heavy meromyosin to actin. *J Biol Chem* 261:16155–16160, 1986.

314. Ikebe M, Reardon S: Phosphorylation of smooth muscle caldesmon by calmodulin-dependent protein kinase II. Identification of the phosphorylation sites. *J Biol Chem* 265:17607–17612, 1990.

315. Mak AS, Watson MH, Litwin CME, Wang JH: Phosphorylation of caldesmon by cdc2 kinase. *J Biol Chem* 266:6678–6681, 1991.

316. Wawrzynow A, Collins JH, Bogatcheva NV, Vorotnikov AV, Gusev NB: Identification of the site phosphorylated by casein kinase II in smooth muscle caldesmon. *FEBS Lett* 289:213–216, 1991.

317. Tanaka T, Ohta H, Kanda K, Tanaka T, Hidaka H, Sobue K: Phosphorylation of high-M_r caldesmon by protein kinase C modulates the regulatory function of this protein on the interaction between actin and myosin. *Eur J Biochem* 188:495–500, 1990.

318. Ikebe M, Hornick T: Determination of the phosphorylation site of smooth muscle caldesmon by protein kinase C. *Arch Biochem Biophys* 288:538–542, 1991.

319. Mak AS, Carpenter M, Smillie LB, Wang JH: Phosphorylation of caldesmon by p34^{cdc2} kinase. Identification of phosphorylation sites. *J Biol Chem* 266:19971–19975, 1991.

319a. Sutherland C, Renaux BS, McKay DJ, Walsh MP: Phospharylation of caldesmon by smooth-muscle casein Kinase II. *J Muscle Res Cell Matil*, in press.

320. Park S, Rasmussen H: Carbachol-induced protein phosphorylation changes in bovine tracheal smooth muscle. *J Biol Chem* 261:15734–15739, 1986.

321. Adam LP, Haeberle JR, Hathaway DR: Phosphorylation of caldesmon in arterial smooth muscle. *J Biol Chem* 264:7698–7703, 1989.

322. Adam LP, Milio L, Brengle B, Hathaway DR: Myosin light chain and caldesmon phosphorylation in arterial muscle stimulated with endothelin-1. *J Mol Cell Cardiol* 22:1017–1023, 1990.

323. Bárány M, Polyák E, Bárány K: Protein phosphorylation during the contraction-relaxation-contration cycle of arterial smooth muscle. *Arch Biochem Biophys* 294:571–578, 1992.

324. Bárány K, Polyák E, Bárány M: Protein phosphorylation in arterial muscle contracted by high concentration of phorbol dibutyrate in the presence and absence of Ca^{2+}. *Biochim Biophys Acta* 1134:223–241, 1992.

325. Adam LP, Gapinski CJ, Hathaway DR: Phosphorylation sequences in h-caldemon from phorbol ester-stimulated canine aortas. *FEBS Lett* 302:223–226, 1992.

326. Childs TJ, Watson MH, Sanghera JS, Campbell DL, Pelech SL, Mak AS: Phosphorylation of smooth muscle caldesmon by mitogen-activated protein (MAP) kinase and expression of MAP kinase in differentiated smooth muscle cells. *J Biol Chem* 267:22853–22859, 1992.

327. Adam LP, Hathaway DR: Identification of mitogen activated protein kinase (MAPK) in vascular smooth muscle. *J Mol Cell Cardiol* 24(Suppl III):S42a, 1992.

328. Walsh MP, Sutherland C: A model for caldesmon in latch-bridge formation in smooth muscle. *Adv Exp Med Biol* 255:337–346, 1989.

329. Takahashi K, Hiwada K, Kokubu T: Isolation and characterization of a 34,000-dalton calmodulin- and F-actin-binding protein from chicken gizzard smooth muscle. *Biochem Biophys Res Commun* 141:20–26, 1986.

330. Vancompernolle K, Gimona M, Herzog M, Van Damme J, Vandekerckhove J, Small V: Isolation and sequence of a tropomyosin-binding fragment of turkey gizzard calponin. *FEBS Lett* 274:146–150, 1990.

331. Abe M, Takahashi K, Hiwada K: Simplified co-purification of vascular smooth muscle calponin and caldesmon. *J Biochem (Tokyo)* 107:507–509, 1990.

332. Marston SB: Properties of calponin isolated from sheep aorta thin filaments. *FEBS Lett* 292:179–182, 1991.

333. Winder SJ, Kargacin GJ, Bonet-Kerrache AA, Pato MD, Walsh MP: Calponin: Localization and regulation of smooth muscle actomyosin MgATPase. *Jpn J Pharmacol* 58:29P–34P, 1992.

334. Takahashi K, Hiwada K, Kokubu T: Occurrence of anti-gizzard p34K antibody cross-reactive components in bovine smooth muscles and non-smooth muscle tissues. *Life Sci* 41:291–296, 1987.

335. Draeger A, Gimona M, Stuckert A, Celis JE, Small JV: Calponin. Developmental isoforms and a low molecular weight variant. *FEBS Lett* 291:24–28, 1991.

336. Gimona M, Herzog M, Vandekerckhove J, Small JV: Smooth muscle specific expression of calponin. *FEBS Lett* 274:159–162, 1990.

337. Takahashi K, Nadal-Ginard B: Molecular cloning and sequence analysis of smooth muscle calponin. *J Biol Chem* 266:13284–13288, 1991.

338. Takahashi K, Abe M, Hiwada K, Kokubu T: A novel troponin T-like protein (calponin) in vascular smooth muscle: Interaction with tropomyosin paracrystals. *J Hypertens* 6:S40–S43, 1988.

339. Winder SJ, Sutherland C, Walsh MP: Biochemical and functional characterization of smooth muscle calponin. In: Moreland RS (ed) *Regulation of Smooth Muscle Contraction*. New York: Plenum Press, 1991, pp 37–52.

340. Takahashi K, Hiwada K, Kokubu T: Vascular smooth muscle calponin. A novel troponin T-like protein. *Hypertension* 11:620–626, 1988.

341. Winder SJ, Sutherland C, Walsh MP: A comparison of the effects of calponin on smooth and skeletal muscle actomyosin systems in the presence and absence of caldesmon. *Biochem J* 288:733–739, 1992.

342. Abe M, Takahashi K, Hiwada K: Effect of calponin on actin-activated myosin ATPase activity. *J Biochem (Tokyo)* 108:835–838, 1990.

343. Horiuchi KY, Chacko S: The mechanism for the inhibition of actin-activated ATPase of smooth muscle heavy meromyosin by calponin. *Biochem Biophys Res Commun* 176:1487–1493, 1991.

344. Makuch R, Birukov K, Shirinsky V, Dabrowska R: Functional interrelationship between calponin and caldesmon. *Biochem J* 280:33–38, 1991.
345. Nishida W, Abe M, Takahashi K, Hiwada K: Do thin filaments of smooth muscle contain calponin? A new method for the preparation. *FEBS Lett* 268:165–168, 1990.
346. Miki M, Walsh MP, Hartshorne DJ: The mechanism of inhibition of the actin-activated myosin MgATPase by calponin. *Biochem Biophys Res Commun* 187:867–871, 1992.
347. Winder SJ, Walsh MP: Structural and functional characterization of calponin fragments. *Biochem Int* 22:335–341, 1990.
348. Mezgueldi M, Fattoum A, Derancourt J, Kassab R: Mapping of the functional domains in the amino-terminal region of calponin. *J Biol Chem* 267:15943–15951, 1992.
349. Takahashi K, Hiwada K, Kokubu T: Vascular smooth muscle calponin; a novel calcium- and calmodulin-binding troponin T-like protein. *Hypertension* 10:360a, 1987.
350. Pai EF, Kabsch W, Krengel U, Holmes KC, John J, Wittinghoffer A: Structure of the guanine-nucleotide-binding domain of the Ha-*ras* oncogene product p21 in the triphosphate conformation. *Nature* 341:209–214, 1989.
351. Winder SJ, Walsh MP: Calponin. In: Chock PB (ed) *Current Topics in Cellular Regulation*, in press.
352. Krebs EG: The phosphorylation of proteins: A major mechanism for biological regulation. *Biochem Soc Trans* 13:813–820, 1985.
352a. Winder SJ, Allen BG, Fraser ED, Kang H-M, Kargacin GJ, Walsh MP: Calponin phospharylation in vitro and in intact muscle. Biochem J 296:827–836, 1993.
353. Winder SJ, Pato MD, Walsh MP: Purification and characterization of calponin phosphatase from smooth muscle. Effect of dephosphorylation on calponin function. *Biochem J* 286:197–203, 1992.
354. Bárány M, Rokolya A, Bárány K: Absence of calponin phosphorylation in contracting or resting arterial smooth muscle. *FEBS Lett* 279:65–68, 1991.
355. Gimona M, Sparrow MP, Strasser P, Herzog M, Small JV: Calponin and SM22 isoforms in avian and mammalian smooth muscle. Absence of phosphorylation in vivo. *Eur J Biochem* 205:1067–1075, 1992.
356. Pohl J, Walsh MP, Gerthoffer WT: Calponin and caldesmon phosphorylation in canine tracheal smooth muscle. *Biophys J* 59:136a, 1991.
357. Gerthoffer WT: Calcium dependence of myosin phosphorylation and airway smooth muscle contraction and relaxation. *Am J Physiol* 250:C597–C604, 1986.
358. Takuwa Y, Takuwa N, Rasmussen H: Measurement of cytoplasmic free Ca^{2+} concentration in bovine tracheal smooth muscle using aequorin. *Am J Physiol* 263:C817–C827, 1987.
359. Stull JT, Nunnally MH, Michnoff CH: Calmodulin-dependent protein kinases. *Enzymes* 17:113–166, 1986.
360. Huang K-P, Huang FL, Nakabayashi H, Yoshida Y: Biochemical characterization of rat brain protein kinase C isozymes. *J Biol Chem* 263:14839–14845, 1988.
361. Marais RM, Parker PJ: Purification and characterization of bovine brain protein kinase C isotypes α, β, and γ. *Eur J Biochem* 182:129–137, 1989.
362. Walsh MP: Smooth muscle caldesmon. *Prog Clin Biol Res* 327:127–140, 1990.
363. Small JV, Fürst DO, Thornell L: The cytoskeletal lattice of muscle cells. *Eur J Biochem* 208:559–572, 1992.
364. Luna EJ, Hitt AL: Cytoskeleton-plasma membrane interactions. *Science* 258:955–964, 1992.
365. Cooke PH, Chase RH: Potassium chloride-insoluble myofilaments in vertebrate smooth muscle cells. *Exp Cell Res* 66:417–425, 1971.
366. Small JV, Sobieszek A: Studies on the function and composition of the 10 nm (100-Å) filaments of vertebrate smooth muscle. *J Cell Sci* 23:243–268, 1977.
367. Lazarides E, Hubbard BD: Immunological characterisation of the subunit of the 100 Å filaments from muscle cells. *Proc Natl Acad Sci USA* 73:4344–4348, 1976.
368. Hubbard BD, Lazarides E: The co-purification of actin and desmin from chicken smooth muscle and their co-polymerization in vitro to intermediate filaments. *J Cell Biol* 80:166–182, 1979.
369. Lazarides E, Balzer DR: Specificity of desmin to avian and mammalian muscle cells. *Cell* 14:429–438, 1978.
370. O'Shea JM, Robson RM, Huiatt TW, Hartzer MK, Stromer MH: Purified desmin from adult mammalian skeletal muscle: A peptide mapping comparison with desmins from adult mammalian and avian smooth muscle. *Biochem Biophys Res Commun* 89:972–980, 1979.
371. O'Connor CM, Balzer DR, Lazarides E: Phosphorylation of subunit proteins of intermediate filaments from chicken muscle and non-muscle cells. *Proc Natl Acad Sci USA* 76:819–823, 1979.
372. Nanaev AK, Shirinsky VP, Birukov KG: Immunofluorescent study of heterogeneity in smooth muscle cells of human fetal vessels using antibodies to myosin, desmin, and vimentin. *Cell Tissue Res* 266:535–540, 1991.
373. Frank ED, Warren L: Aortic smooth muscle cells contain vimentin instead of desmin. *Proc Natl Acad Sci USA* 78:3020–3024, 1981.
374. Gabbiani G, Schmid E, Winter S, Chaponnier C, De Chastonay C, Vandekerckhove J, Weber K, Franke WW: Vascular smooth muscle cells differ from other smooth muscle cells: Predominance of vimentin filaments and a specific α-type actin. *Proc Natl Acad Sci USA* 78:298–302, 1981.
375. Geiger B: Intermediate filaments: Looking for a function. *Nature* 329:392–393, 1987.
376. Tsukita S, Tsukita S, Ishikawa H: Association of actin and 10 nm filaments with the dense body in smooth muscle cells of the chicken gizzard. *Cell Tissue Res* 229:233–242, 1983.
377. Yamaguchi M, Robson RM, Stromer MH, Huiatt TW: Effect of calpain II on turkey gizzard muscle and structural dissection of cytoplasmic dense bodies by low ionic strength extraction. *Prog Clin Biol Res* 327:637–649, 1990.
378. Wang K, Ash JF, Singer SJ: Filamin, a new high molecular weight protein found in smooth muscle and nonmuscle cells. *Proc Natl Acad Sci USA* 72:4483–4486, 1975.
379. Wang K: Filamin, a new high-molecular-weight protein found in smooth muscle and non-muscle cells. Purification and properties of chicken gizzard filamin. *Biochemistry* 16:1857–1865, 1977.
380. Nunnally MH, Powell LD, Craig SW: Reconstitution and regulation of actin gel-sol transformation with purified filamin and villin. *J Biol Chem* 256:2083–2086, 1981.
381. Davies PJA, Wallach D, Willingham M, Pastan I, Lewis MS: Self-association of chicken gizzard filamin and heavy merofilamin. *Biochemistry* 19:1366–1372, 1980.
382. Davies PJA, Wallach D, Willingham MC, Pastan I, Yamaguchi M, Robson RM: Filamin-actin interaction. *J Biol Chem* 253:4036–4042, 1978.
383. Hock RS, Davis G, Speicher DW: Purification of human smooth muscle filamin and characterization of structural domains and functional sites. *Biochemistry* 29:9441–9451, 1990.

384. Draeger A, Stelzer EHK, Herzog M, Small JV: Unique geometry of actin-membrane anchorage sites in avian gizzard smooth muscle cells. *J Cell Sci* 94:703–711, 1989.
385. Draeger A, Amos WB, Ikebe M, Small JV: The cytoskeletal and contractile apparatus of smooth muscle: Contraction bands and segmentation of the contractile apparatus. *J Cell Biol* 111:2463–2473, 1990.
386. Kargacin GJ, Fay FS: Physiological and structural properties of saponin-skinned single smooth muscle cells: *J Gen Physiol* 90:49–73, 1987.
387. Suzuki A, Goll DE, Singh I, Allan RE, Robson RM, Stromer MH: Some properties of purified skeletal muscle α-actinin. *J Biol Chem* 251:6860–6870, 1976.
388. Jockusch BM, Isenberg G: Interaction of α-actinin and vinculin with actin: Opposite effects on filament network formation. *Proc Natl Acad Sci USA* 78:3005–3009, 1981.
389. Goll DE, Suzuki A, Temple J, Holmes GR: Studies on purified α-actinin. I. Effect of temperature and tropomyosin on the α-actinin/F-actin interaction. *J Mol Biol* 67:469–488, 1972.
390. Geiger B, Tokuyasu KT, Dutton AH, Singer SJ: Vinculin, an intracellular protein localized at specialized sites where microfilament bundles terminate at cell membranes. *Proc Natl Acad Sci USA* 77:4127–4131, 1980.
391. Wilkins JA, Lin S: A re-examination of the interaction of vinculin with actin. *J Cell Biol* 102:1085–1092, 1986.
392. D'Angelo Siciliano J, Craig SW: Properties of smooth muscle meta-vinculin. *J Cell Biol* 104:473–482, 1987.
393. Bennett JP, Cross RA, Kendrick-Jones J, Weeds AG: Spatial pattern of myosin phosphorylation in contracting smooth muscle cells: Evidence for contractile zones. *J Cell Biol* 107:2623–2629, 1988.
394. Cooke P: Organization of contractile fibers in smooth muscle. In: Dowben RM, Shay JW (eds) *Cell and Muscle Motility*, Vol 3. New York: Plenum Press, 1983, pp 57–77.
395. Bagby R: Toward a comprehensive three-dimensional model of the contractile system of vertebrate smooth muscle cells. *Int Rev Cytol* 105:67–128, 1986.
396. Fisher BA, Bagby RM: Reorientation of myofilaments during contraction of a vertebrate smooth muscle. *Am J Physiol* 232:C5–C14, 1977.
397. Warshaw DM, McBride WJ, Work SS: Corkscrew-like shortening in single smooth muscle cells. *Science* 236: 1457–1459, 1987.
398. Kargacin GJ, Cooke PH, Abramson SB, Fay FS: Periodic organization of the contractile apparatus in smooth muscle revealed by the motion of dense bodies in single cells. *J Cell Biol* 108:1465–1475, 1989.

CHAPTER 55

Mechanical Properties and Regulation of Vascular Smooth Muscle Contraction

STEVEN P. DRISKA

INTRODUCTION AND SCOPE

An understanding of vascular smooth muscle contraction is important to cardiologists and cardiac researchers because ultimately vascular smooth muscle determines both the amount of work the heart must do (by altering total peripheral resistance) and the amount of oxygen and substrates available to do it (by regulating coronary perfusion). With this relationship in mind this chapter will present a description of our present knowledge of the contractile process in vascular smooth muscle based on biochemical, biophysical, physiological, and mechanical studies. Since other chapters in this book cover the ultrastructure (Chapter 42), electrophysiology (Chapter 45), and metabolism and energetics (Chapter 56), these subjects will not be covered in any detail and will serve to delimit the boundaries of this chapter. The biochemistry of contractile proteins will be discussed only in relation to more highly organized systems. For more details the reader is referred to the chapter in this book on smooth muscle contractile proteins.

Mechanical responses of vascular smooth muscle and the regulatory processes involved have been studied in a variety of preparations, ranging from living animals to intact, excised cylindrical arteries, to helical or circular strips of the arterial media, to intact single smooth muscle cells. At the subcellular level, various protein preparations from smooth muscle have been studied, and usually MgATPase activity or superprecipitation (defined later) is taken as the manifestation of the actin-myosin interaction responsible for muscular contraction. Since the last edition of this book, much progress has been made in characterizing the "in vitro motility assay," a technique in which movement caused by smooth muscle proteins can be visualized in the light microscope. Somewhere between these approaches is that of skinned preparations. In these preparations, the plasma membrane has been damaged or destroyed by mechanical methods, detergents, bacterial toxins, or freezing, yet the array of myofilaments presumably remains intact because the preparations can develop measurable active force when they are bathed in appropriate solutions. A major contribution of these preparations has been in bridging the large gap between the biochemistry of isolated proteins and the physiology of

intact muscle. They have done this by demonstrating the applicability of biochemical findings to more organized systems capable of transducing chemical energy into mechanical work.

While the primary focus of this article is vascular smooth muscle, much of our knowledge, particularly in biochemistry, comes from the study of nonvascular smooth muscle, especially chicken gizzard. With the implicit understanding that there might be species and tissue differences, these findings from nonvascular smooth muscles will be assumed to apply to vascular smooth muscle as well.

MECHANICAL PROPERTIES

This section of the chapter will describe the most widely used preparations for studying mechanical properties of vascular smooth muscle (VSM), the underlying assumptions for each, which properties are measured and which are calculated, and the general utility of each for studying different aspects of vascular function. Then a brief summary of findings obtained from such preparations will be presented. The order of coverage will be from the most physiological to the least physiological.

Isolated arteries in vitro

Studies on excised arteries in vitro have been important in building an understanding of how smooth muscle functions when forming part of the wall of a pressurized tube. In these studies an artery is dissected from its location, cannulated at both ends, stretched to its in vivo length, and immersed in a suitable bathing solution. The longitudinal (axial) length is set and the axial force can be measured. The blood vessel is pressurized with either a gas or a saline solution, which may be flowing through it or static. The pressure within the vessel is measured, with the outside of the blood vessel being at atmospheric pressure. (Actually the difference, or transmural pressure, is measured.) The pressure can be set at any level by the apparatus, and pressure becomes the independent variable. The diameter of the vessel is a dependent variable and is measured by caliper devices or optical methods (for the external

N. Sperelakis (ed.), Physiology and Pathophysiology of the Heart, Third Edition.
© 1995 Kluwer Academic Publishers. ISBN 0-7923-2612-1. All rights reserved.

diameter) or radiological methods (for the internal diameter). Knowledge of the wall thickness at a known length and diameter allows the wall thickness to be computed at any tissue length and diameter, because the arterial wall itself has been shown to be essentially incompressible {1}. This then allows the computation of internal diameter from external diameter measurements and vice versa. It is important to point out that the diameter cannot be set at a specified value like the length of a muscle can be in a one-dimensional experiment. To achieve a given diameter, the pressure and/or level of activation have to be varied, and, if a constant diameter is to the maintained, a feedback system has to be used to vary the pressure. The orientation of the smooth muscle cells is usually assumed to be circumferential in these preparations; this means that the diameter, radius, and circumference are all approximately proportional to the average smooth muscle cell length. Complications arising from the fact that the wall has a finite thickness and the influence of this on cell-length homogeneity have been discussed {2}.

By application of the Law of Laplace for cylinders, $T = Pr$, the circumferential tension per unit length of artery can be computed. Here T is tension, P is transmural pressure, and r is the internal radius. This characteristic (T) is independent of wall thickness and has units of force/length, typically given in either dynes/cm or Newtons/m. Frequently it is desirable to estimate the stress arising from the distending pressure, which tends to stretch circumferentially oriented smooth muscle cells. This is the circumferential or tangential stress, which has units of force/wall cross-sectional area (typically dynes/cm^2 or Newtons/m^2). This can be compared to the stress developed by strips of smooth muscle. The average circumferential stress can be estimated by assuming that the wall is made of a uniform material and is isotropic and thin in relation to the radius of the cylinder. In this case, the circumferential stress is given by

$$S = P \, r/h,$$

where S is stress and h is wall thickness. Since these assumptions are generally not good ones, particularly that of a thin wall, a more refined approach can be taken that allows the calculation of circumferential stress throughout the thickness of the wall as a function of the radius, r {3}. Here stress is calculated by the formula

$$S = P \, (1 + r_o^2/r^2)/[(r_o/r_i)^2 - 1],$$

with r_i and r_o being the inner and outer radii, respectively. This formula has been used to compute circumferential stress as a function of radius within the wall and to compare it to the average stress in fig. 55-1. This is useful in illustrating the profile of stress within the arterial wall (fig. 55-1), but it still assumes the wall to be uniform, isotropic, and linearly elastic. Doyle and Dobrin {4} derived a similar result from finite deformation theory. They suggested that the higher circumferential stresses calculated for the inner layers of the arterial wall were responsible for the greater occurrence of elastic lamellae they observed in the inner layers of the carotid artery. The arterial wall is made of different structures (primarily endothelial cells, smooth muscle cells, elastin, and collagen), which differ in stiffness and radial location, and have nonrandom orientations, so the analytical treatment in fig. 55-1 is an oversimplification. Clearly a more com-

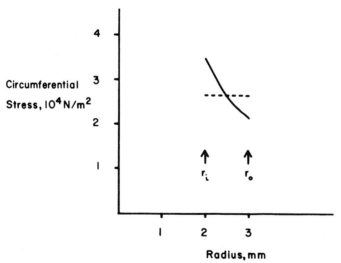

Fig. 55-1. Circumferential stress as a function of radial position in the wall of a pressurized artery. Stress was computed by the equation

$$S = P(1 + r_o^2/r^2)/[(r_o/r_i)^2 - 1]$$

for a relatively thick-walled vessel with an inner radius of 2 mm and a wall thickness of 1 mm. The transmural pressure used for calculation was 1.33×10^4 N/m^2 (100 mmHg). The dashed line indicates the average circumferential stress, given by

$$S = Pr_i/h,$$

where h is wall thickness. The stress is highest near the lumen and decreases towards the outside. In thin-walled vessels the dependence of stress on radial location is not as steep.

plete mathematical model of an artery needs to consider the nonlinear stiffness of given elements, their orientation, and the radius at which they are located.

In studies with intact excised arteries, it is common to measure the diameter over a wide range of transmural pressures and to repeat this process under varying degrees of smooth muscle activation. Changes in diameter and length are usually expressed as strains, strain being the length change divided by a reference length. From a number of such measurements it is possible to compute values of circumferential and longitudinal elastic moduli. (The elastic modulus is the change in stress divided by the change in strain.) The circumferential incremental Young's modulus is given by

$$E = \frac{\Delta P_i \, 2 \, d_e \, d_i^2 \, (1 - \sigma^2)}{\Delta d_e \, (d_e^2 - d_i^2)},$$

where d_e and d_i refer to the exterior and internal diameters, respectively, ΔP_i is the change in pressure, and Δd_e is the change in external diameter. Sigma (σ) is the Poisson ratio, which is 0.5 for an incompressible isotropic material undergoing small deformations. The Poisson ratio describes the ratio of strains in perpendicular directions when three-dimensional solids are deformed. This equation was popularized by Bergel {5} and applies when a blood vessel is held at constant length. In studies such as these, the value of E usually increases with pressure, meaning the vessel wall is becoming stiffer, i.e., less extensible with inflation. This is generally understood to be a result of more stress being borne by collagen, which is the stiffest element of the wall. One of the most interesting findings to come from these studies was that contraction of vascular smooth muscle was found to *decrease* the elastic modulus when the elastic moduli of stimulated and control arteries were compared at the same pressures. This is because in the constricted arteries less of the load was borne by the stiff collagen. However, when they were compared at the same diameter (and hence the same strain), the arteries with stimulated VSM were stiffer {6}.

Dobrin and Rovick {6} calculated circumferential stress as a function of arterial diameter for both passive and norepinephrine-stimulated arteries. The difference between the two stresses at a given diameter was taken as the active circumferential stress. They obtained a maximum value of $0.88 \times 10^5 \, N/m^2$ for the whole wall or $2.73 \times 10^5 \, N/m^2$ for the estimated smooth muscle component. This is in reasonable agreement, considering the low muscle content of the canine carotid artery {7}, with the active stress development found in many VSM strip preparations (summarized in Doyle and Dobrin {4}). This finding gives an idea of the loads applied to vascular smooth muscle in arteries compared to loads imposed in one-dimensional studies of VSM strips. The maximum active stress was found to be developed at a diameter that corresponded to that found with relaxed smooth muscle at a pressure of 150 mmHg' {8}. Maximum shortening is usually found when arteries are stimulated at pressures ranging from 50 to 175 mmHg (summarized in Dobrin {9}). Excitation of vascular smooth muscle in very distended arteries leads to decreased active stress development {8}, presumably analogous to the results of over-

stretching smooth muscle. When arteries are removed from their in vivo location, they retract approximately 30% {9}, indicating that they had been under longitudinal (axial) stress. Interaction of this axial stress with circumferential stress leads to complicated analytical relationships between stresses and strains in different directions. The arterial wall is not isotropic, meaning that its properties, such as stiffness, are different in different directions, and this makes the interactions between stresses in different axes more important. Dobrin and Doyle {10} analyzed the error arising from the assumption of isotropic mechanical properties and concluded from their data on canine carotid arteries that the error in the calculated circumferential elastic modulus was small between 75 and 135 mmHg pressure, and larger at both higher and lower pressures. The dynamic elastic properties have been studied with sinusoidal volume changes and, in general, the dynamic elastic moduli are 1.5- to 2-fold greater than the static values for the same artery (summarized in Dobrin {9}).

The study of three-dimensional mechanical properties of arteries and changes with aging or hypertension has provided valuable insights into these conditions. Cox {11} found that the value of the passive incremental elastic modulus was greater in carotid arteries of older rats when the vessels were compared ar the same value of strain. Larger values of maximum active stress development and also of maximum active constriction were found with carotid arteries from DOCA {12}, Goldblatt {12}, and spontaneously hypertensive {13} rats compared to the appropriate controls.

Studies on excised arteries have made important contributions to our understanding of vascular function, but like studies using other techniques, they have limitations. Their major strength is that they provide information about the internal diameter as the final dependent variable under the effect of physiological forces (i.e., distending pressure). Thus in this sense it is the best preparation to study to learn how arteries work. There are some limitations, however. It is always assumed that the outside pressure is zero or atmospheric. Clearly, this is not always the case in many situations, particulary for arteries within the ventricular wall. Secondly it is sometimes just assumed that the VSM is circularly oriented and that circumferential stress can be equated with VSM cell stress. In most cases the arterial wall has been considered to be isotropic, meaning that it has the same elastic modulus in all directions, which is not true.

More refined theoretical treatments of anisotropy allow better calculations of circumferential moduli {14}. Even when anisotropy is considered, the wall is viewed as being uniform in the radial direction (yet it has long been known to be a layered structure). Often calculations require the use of Poisson's ratio, which is 0.5 for isotropic materials undergoing small deformations. However, in many experiments the deformations are much larger and Poisson's ratio would be less than 0.5, even for an isotropic material. Most of these problems are due to the application of classical physical methods to soft biological tissues that undergo much larger deformations than the steel wires or tubes on which classical theories were based.

There has been some use of finite deformation analysis, and this is encouraging because it is more appropriate when strains are as large as those that occur with blood vessels {15}. The final limitation is that most studies use static pressures. The arterial wall has viscoelastic propertie, so a pressure-diameter tracing depends on the rate of change of pressure and the direction of change. Investigators usually inflate and deflate the arteries until reproducible responses are obtained, but the dynamic relationship of arterial diameter to the pulse pressure is required for complete physiological relevance. In spite of these limitations, the study of excised arteries has made major contributions to the knowledge of vascular function. It has been possible to extend some of these studies on large arteries to resistance vessels and terminal arterioles {16,17}. The mechanical properties of arteries have been the subject of a thorough review {9}.

Ring and strip preparations

The most commonly studied vascular smooth muscle preparation is the smooth muscle strip. These are either circularly oriented or (especially in the case of smaller vessels) helically oriented. Great care must be taken with helical strips because arterial diameter, strip width, and helix angle are all interrelated. Herlihy {18} has pointed out that the different helix angle could compromise comparisons between arteries of different diameters, even if strip width is the same, because stress development is a function of the helix angle. These preparations may or may not have the adventitial and intimal layers removed. The presence or absence of endothelial cells of the intimal layer is a major determinant of pharmacological responsiveness {19}. With these preparations length changes and forces are measured in just one direction, which is hoped to be the axis of the smooth muscle cells. Ring preparations have more in common with strip preparations than with intact arteries because, as with strips, force and length changes are imposed and measured in only one dimension. Rings are often everted so that the adventitia forms the inside and agonists, nutrients, and O_2 can reach the smooth muscle cells more easily. However, this manipulation may damage the muscle, and it imposes a large amount of stretch on the muscle cells nearest the endothelial cells.

In contrast to studies on intact arteries where diameter (and hence smooth muscle length) is dependent on transmural pressure and muscle activation, muscle length is the independent variable with muscle strips and rings. By analogy with striated muscle research, the length-isometric force and force-velocity relationships are most commonly studied. This approach has been quite fruitful for understanding how vascular smooth muscle functions, but it tells less about how arteries function. For cardiovascular relevance it would be most important to know the final length of the muscle after shortening against a nonconstant load, but this is seldom determined for vascular muscle, even though researchers in *airway* smooth muscle have recognized that the most important physiological response of smooth muscle is the length to which it shortens under

given conditions {20}. This would be analogous to knowing the inside diameter of an artery after stimulation at some pressure. Some studies of nonvascular smooth muscle have addressed this question, namely, whether the length-isometric tension curve is the same as the length-tension curve obtained by measuring the final length obtained after contraction against constant loads. The length-tension curves were found to be essentially the same regardless of the method used up to a length of 0.8 L_o. At greater lengths, a shortening defect was found, meaning that the muscle did not shorten as much as expected from the isometric length-tension curve {21}.

Length-tension cruve

The elegant correlation of mechanical and morphological data that forms the basis for the sliding-filament model of striated muscle contraction {22} is lacking in smooth muscle. However, the sliding-filament model is generally accepted, even though the precise dimensions of a smooth muscle sarcomere are not known. The thick filaments are slightly longer in smooth muscle, being 2.2 microns in smooth muscle versus 1.5 microns in striated muscle {23}. The thick filaments of striated muscle are bipolar, with myosin crossbridges oriented so as to pull thin filaments toward the center of the thick filament. In smooth muscle, it appears that the thick filaments are face polar or side polar {24}, meaning that the myosin thick filament would be able to cause sliding of thin filaments in the same direction along the whole side of the thick filament, while on the other side of the thick filament, thin filaments would be pulled in the opposite direction. Such a structure would allow a great deal more shortening than the bipolar thick filaments of striated muscle.

The thin filament length in smooth muscle is not known because of numerous technical difficulties, although there is some evidence that thin filament lengths may be longer than in skeletal muscle, averaging about 4.5 microns in supercontracted, permeable chicken gizzard cells {25}. This is intriguing because, as detiled below, long thin filaments could be partially responsible for the high force/ low velocity nature of smooth muscle contraction. Filament counts from electron micrographs of transverse sections of smooth muscles show a much higher ratio of thin to thick filaments, ranging from 12:1 to 18:1, than occurs in striated muscle. These filament counts are in good agreement with the amounts and ratios of myosin and actin in smooth muscles {26}, but because thick filaments are not in good lateral registration this has to be regarded as a random sampling process. Therefore, these data are consistent with a spectrum of sarcomere models ranging from one in which the thin-to-thick filament length ratio is the same as in skeletal muscle, but there are more thin filaments interacting with each thick filament, to the opposite extreme in which only two thin filaments interact with each end of the thick filament, but the thin filaments are much longer. These extremes are shown in fig. 55–2. The idea that long thin filaments could explain the high force generation and economy of smooth muscle has been

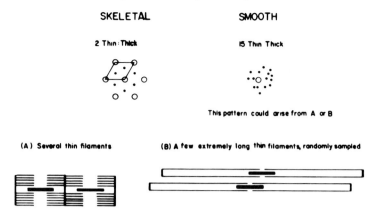

Fig. 55-2. Possible explanations of filament counts in electron micrographs of cross sections of smooth muscle. In the overlap region of vertebrate skeletal muscle (**left**), the area encompassed by the parallelogram contains a total of one thick filament and two thin filaments. The smooth muscle does not show as much order (**right**), and there are generally 12–18 thin filament profiles per thick filament profile. Because thick filaments in smooth muscle are not in good lateral registration, the plane of section might pass through the thick filament of one sarcomere, but only intersect thin filaments in adjacent sarcomeres. This makes sectioning a random sampling process, and the high number of thin filament profiles could arise from large numbers of thin filaments (**A**, lower left) or a smaller number of extremely long thin filaments (**B**, lower right). Both models represent extreme cases that are consistent with the 15:1 filament count and contain equal amounts of myosin and actin. In B the thin filaments are 8.25 microns long, giving rise to a 16.5-micron sarcomere; in A the sarcomere length is 2.9 microns. Both models use a 2.2-micron thick filament.

proposed {23,27}. Calculations of how long the thin filaments would have to be (for a 15:1 filament count) show that the hypothetical thin-filament length would be 8.25 microns (from tip to Z-line equivalent), making a 16.5-micron sarcomere. If the proteins of *skeletal* muscle were arranged in this type of sarcomere, only 18% as much myosin would be needed. The muscle would develop 47% more force and it would shorten only 12% as fast. While the true situation can be anywhere on this spectrum, the long sarcomere model has many attractive features in explaining mechanical data, and it maximizes the fraction of the limited number of thick filaments present that can develop force in parallel. At present all these models must be considered as possibilities when interpreting mechanical properties. The polarity of thin filaments emerging from opposite sides of dense bodies is like that of skeletal muscle near the Z line, providing support for a similar role for dense bodies and Z lines {28}.

The previous paragraph has explained the inability to describe a sarcomere length in smooth muscle, but it is still possible to compare the length-tension curves of skeletal and smooth muscle if the muscle length is expressed in relation to the optimum length for force development, L_o. (In skeletal muscle, L_o would correspond to sarcomere lengths of 2.0–2.2 microns.) All muscles develop a certain amount of passive tension (arising from elastic and connective tissue) when stretched. This passive tension, sometimes called the parallel elastic component (PEC), is particularly prominent in vascular smooth muscle, and it must be subtracted from the total tension of the stimulated muscle to obtain the active tension. The active tension is attributed to force generation by myosin crossbridges, and the accuracy of its measurement depends on the ability

to measure and subtract passive tension accurately. The length-passive tension curve is usually estimated by relaxing the tissue with drugs or calcium chelators, or it may be determined by imposing rapid shortening steps (quick releases) that discharge any force developed by the crossbridges before they can recover, revealing the passive tension due to elastic structures at the new length.

The active tension curve typical of vascular smooth muscle (fig. 55-3) shows an optimum length with decreasing forces developed at both longer and shorter lengths. Usually a smooth curve is obtained; sharp corners (like those found with single skeletal fibers) are not obtained, but this is not surprising in view of the complexity of most preparations relative to the single fiber studied with special instrumentation {22}. There has been one report of a plateau on the length-tension curve of smooth muscle {29}, but this was found with an invertebrate smooth muscle, the anterior byssus retractor of *Mytilus edulis*. Little data are available on force development in highly stretched VSM because tissues often are damaged by extreme stretching, and the high passive tensions subject the active tension measurements to large error. However, the decline of active force is steeper at lengths greater than L_o than it is at muscle lengths less than L_o. At short muscle lengths, smooth muscle retains its ability to develop force better than skeletal muscle. The common assertion that smooth muscle can shorten much more than striated muscle may be an exaggeration; Murphy {30} has pointed out that published length-tension curves of skinned skeletal fibers are similar to those of smooth muscle tissues, implying that the limited shortening capacity of skeletal muscle is more a consequence of length-dependent activation, rather than myofibrillar geometry. Recently,

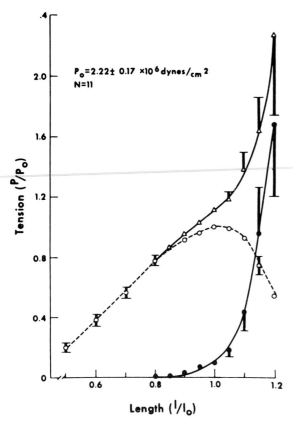

$P_o = 2.22 \pm 0.17 \times 10^6 \, dynes/cm^2$
$N = 11$

Fig. 55-3. Length-tension curve of hog carotid artery smooth muscle strips. Muscle length is expressed as a fraction of L_o, the optimum length for active force generation; tension is expressed as a fraction of P_o, the maximum active force. Closed circles: passive force estimated by quick release of the muscle from a longer length; triangles: isometric force during stimulation with K^+; open circles; active tension (the total tension in the stimulated muscle minus the passive tension at that length). Error bars represent ± 1 SE. From Herlihy and Murphy {175} by permission of the American Heart Association.

Price et al. have shown that the length-tension curve obtained in VSM depends on the level of activation. They found that the length-tension curve shifted to the right when lower concentrations of norepinephrine were used as a stimulus {31}.

If one compares the values of F_o (the maximum active force developed per unit cross-sectional area) obtained for skeletal and vascular smooth muscle, it is found that the smooth muscle can develop as much or more force. This is particularly surprising because the smooth muscle contains only about one fourth as much myosin {26}. The ability of vascular smooth muscle tissues to develop this much force has been shown to be a cellular property, and not the result of a complicated tissue architecture that confers a mechanical advantage to cells {32–34}. Thus, the length-tension curve and the high force development of vascular smooth muscle are a property of the individual cells. This

finding is corroborated by direct evidence from studies on single smooth muscle cells of amphibian stomach {35}. Force development by single cells from this tissue, when expressed relative to cross-sectional area, shows the same high value seen in smooth muscle strips {35}.

Application of the length-tension curve obtained from smooth muscle strips to intact arteries leads to some complications. As a first approximation, the mean circumference (average of inner and outer) can be equated to the muscle length. As the muscle contracts, however, there has to be a greater extent of contraction by the inner layer, since the wall thickening displaces mass towards the lumen. For example, in the case of an artery with a r_i/r_o ratio of 0.7, constriction leading to a decrease of r_o to 80% of its initial value causes r_i to decrease to 52% of its initial value. Circumferences are of course proportional to radii. This implies that there could be slippage between layers. The point to be made here is that the shortening capacity of vascular smooth muscle is adequate to cause pronounced constriction, but it is not possible to define equivalent muscle cell length or strip length at a given radius precisely. Even if all muscle cells in the artery had exactly the same length at some radius, cell-length inhomogeneity would appear at other radii {2}.

Force-velocity curve

The force-velocity relationship in vascular smooth muscle is qualitatively similar to that seen in skeletal muscle in that both are fit reasonably well by the hyperbolic equation of A.V. Hill:

$$(F + a)(V + b) = (F_o + a)b.$$

Values of V_{max}, the maximum shortening velocity, can be extrapolated from a linearization of the equation and expressed in muscle lengths/second. At 37°C these values are much lower in vascular smooth muscle (0.02–0.7 L_o/sec) than in skeletal muscle (typically 1–10 L_o/sec). There are some difficulties involved in measuring V_{max} in smooth muscle. Foremost among these is the finding that shortening velocities obtained with a given load are time dependent, i.e., the velocity depends on how long the muscle has been stimulated isometrically before it is allowed to shorten isotonically {36–40}.

In these experiments muscles are usually stimulated isometrically as tension develops and then rapidly released to shorten against selected constant loads. Surprisingly, the highest values of V_{max} (the unloaded shortening velocity) are measured before isometric tension is fully developed. This phenomenon will be discussed at length later, but its importance here is that it suggests that values of V_{max} in the literature may be underestimates.

Another complication with V_{max} measurements made by the method of isotonic quick releases is the transiently high shortening velocity observed following quick releases. It is not clear if this is a manifestation of crossbridge kinetics {40} or a damped series elastic component {41}. In either case, these initial rates are about six times greater than steady-state shortening velocities and could lead to overestimates of the true V_{max}. In afterloaded isotonic contractions, load (force) is an independent variable and velocity is the dependent variable. The opposite approach is sometimes taken, with velocity being the independent variable by imposing constant velocity shortenings on the muscle and measuring the force the muscle can exert under these conditions.

The maximum shortening velocity can also be estimated by a procedure known as the *slack test method*. In this method, a stimulated muscle is rapidly shortened to various lengths where force drops to zero. Force remains at zero while the muscle shortens to remove the slack and then force is redeveloped. The length changes are then plotted against the time for which the muscle remained slack, and the slope of this line is the unloaded shortening velocity. This technique has been used with various smooth muscle, and a similar decline in shortening velocity with time of stimulation has been found {42,43}.

The maximum shortening velocities of isolated VSM cells are about three times greater than reported shortening velocities for muscle strips from the same tissue {44}. A similar result had been reported earlier for *Bufo marinus* stomach muscle {45}. It was also found that the extent of shortening in these intact cells did not depend on the extracellular Ca^{2+} concentration, suggesting that there is no restoring force that would limit shortening or slow the shortening velocity {44}. These findings suggest that the shortening of isolated cells is truly unloaded shortening,

while in the whole tissue some extracellular component is imposing a load on the smooth muscle cells. If this suggestion is true, then measuring unloaded shortening velocity may only be possible with isolated cells {44}.

Series elastic component

The *contractile component* (CC) of muscle behaves like it is transmitting force to an external load through a spring, the *series elastic component* (SEC). In the early analog models of muscle, the anatomical feature responsible for the SEC was not known, and it was treated as something independent of the myofilaments that constitute the contractile component. Later studies on skeletal muscle led to the more modern view that much of the SEC is in the myosin crossbridge itself.

One way of measuring the SEC is to rapidly shorten a muscle during the peak of an isometric tetanus so that all force is discharged. With a very stiff SEC, very little shortening is required. A plot of length and force during this procedure defines the characteristics of the SEC. For skeletal muscles, rapid shortening by 3% totally discharges tension {46}, and using faster length changes with single fibers, a shortening of less than 1% is needed {47,48}. The force-length relationship is not linear at low values of force, so the linear region is often extrapolated to zero force. This intercept represents about 0.5% shortening

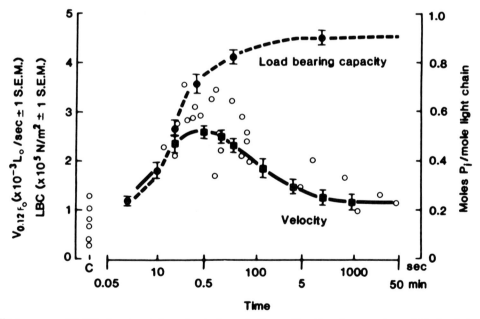

Fig. 55-4. Time courses of LC20 phosphorylation, shortening velocity, and load-bearing capacity on K^+ stimulation of hog carotid artery strips. Open circles: LC20 phosphorylation; filled squares: shortening velocity against a load that was 12% of the maximum active isometric force; filled circles load-bearing capacity. Load-bearing capacity is the peak force measured when a quick stretch of $0.025 L_o$ was applied at a rate of $0.1 L_o$ per second, and it provides a better estimate of the number of attached crossbridges than does isometric force measurement. Erro bars represent ± 1 SE; phosphorylation data are single points, and C denotes control, unstimulated muscle strips. Note the logarithmic time base. From Dillon et al. {38}, with permission of the American Association for the Advancement of Science.

with single fibers {47,48} and about 1.5% with whole muscle {46}. When similar experiments are performed with vascular smooth muscle strips, shortening of 2–3% was adequate to totally discharge force, and the linear extrapolation had an intercept of 1.5% shortening {49}.

Unfortunately the estimates of the series elasticity depend on the quality of the instrumentation and the speed with which the releases can be performed; series elasticities of 5–10% of muscle length have been reported in the past.

In summary it appears that isometrically contracting vascular smooth muscle is almost as stiff as skeletal muscle. The series elastic component has an important influence on measurement of isotonic shortening velocities because it has been reported to be responsible for transiently high shortening velocities after a release {41}. This undesirable influence of the SEC on shortening velocities could be avoided by using afterloaded isotonic contractions, but with this method shortening under different isotonic loads starts at different times after stimulation, a real disadvantage because of the dependence of shortening velocities on the duration of stimulation {38,39}.

Estimation of cellular mechanical properties in multicellular preparations

Until about 1986 it had not been possible to use single vascular smooth muscle cells for mechanical studies, although this was possible with the larger cells from amphibian stomach {35}. This meant that vascular smooth muscle cellular properties had to be inferred from mechanical measurements made on complex multicellular tissues, and because of this it was vitally important to know whether any mechanical advantages are conferred on cells as a result of tissue structure. The high force development of vascular smooth muscle tissues in spite of their limited myosin content {26}, coupled with recurring suggestions that a mechanical advantage for muscle cells exists in the arterial wall (see Driska et al. {34}), led to an examination of this possibility.

Two lines of evidence have ruled out the existence of mechanical advantages in the tissues examined. First, it was found that the force development of vascular smooth muscle strips did not depend on how long a segment of the strip was chosen for force measurement, i.e., force did not depend on how many cells long the preparation was {32}. The second type of experiment measured either the change in cell length or distance between features in the same cell in response to known changes in tissue length. In the absence of mechanical advantages, 10% shortening of the tissue would lead to a 10% reduction in mean cell length or distance between distinguishable cellular features. A 20% reduction in mean cell length would indicate a 2:1 mechanical advantage. Data of this type for hog carotid artery {33,34}, guinea pig taenia coli {50}, and rabbit bladder {21} strips, and rings of small arteries {51} indicated that the cells do not have a mechanical advantage and that cellular estimates of shortening velocity and active stress development made by proper normalization of tissue measurements are valid.

CONTRACTILE PROPERTIES OF SINGLE SMOOTH MUSCLE CELLS

Single cells can be dispersed from vascular smooth muscle by enzymatic digestion with collagenase and elastase {52–55} or papain {56}. A modification of the papain method that is suitable for nonvascular smooth muscle has also been published {57}. The size of the cells obtained depends on the method and tissue used, but the cells obtained by papain digestion of the swine carotid artery {56} are relaxed, Ca^{2+} tolerant, and surprisingly long (mean length 240 microns), which has made these cells useful for electrophysiological studies {58} and shortening velocity measurements {44}.

The maximum shortening velocities of isolated VSM cells are about three times greater than shortening velocities for muscle strips from the same tissue {44}, a finding that is similar to earlier results with *Bufo marinus* stomach muscle {45}. It was also found that the extent of shortening in these intact arterial cells did not depend on the extracellular Ca^{2+} concentration, suggesting that there is no restoring force that would limit shortening or slow the shortening velocity {44}. These findings suggest that the shortening of isolated cells is truly unloaded shortening, while in the whole tissue some extracellular component is imposing a load on the smooth muscle cells. If this suggestion is true, then measuring unloaded shortening velocity may only be possible with isolated cells {44}.

Certain mechanical measurements on isolated cells, such as the extent and velocity of shortening, can be made fairly easily. However, it is necessary to fasten cells to a force transducer for studies of force development or shortening against external loads, and this has only been achieved recently with vascular smooth muscle cells {55,59}, but these cell preparations were partially shortened. As a result, normalization of force to cross-sectional area could not provide meaningful comparisons to stresses developed by smooth muscle strips. Force velocity curves of *Bufo* stomach muscle cells have been obtained {60}.

Much has been learned about stomach muscle cells from the toad *Bufo marinus*, and even though these cells are neither vascular nor mammalian, the studies have produced data that are highly relevant to vascular tissue. The large size of these cells allows them to be tied around a microprobe and still have a portion of the cell left to generate force. The conclusions presented in the proceeding section receive strong support from the fact that the active stress development for single *Bufo* cells is as high as that estimated from vascular smooth muscle tissue measurements {35}, although force development by isolated VSM cells has not been as great {55}. A surprising finding is that the length-tension curve for a single cell seems to be rather poorly defined, having an ascending, but not descending, limb {61}. The investigators could show that a decrease in cell length resulted in less force, but they could not show that stretching the cell led to less force. This may have been due to the protocol used. These cells retain their cholinergic receptors and have been very useful in studies of pharmacology and electrophysiology.

Another interesting finding is that after direct electrical stimulation there is a measurable latency before force develops {35}, and the clear demonstration of it in a preparation free of agonist diffusion delays establishes this as a characteristic that all theories of regulation and excitation-contraction coupling must explain. Isolated cells are also useful in the measurement of intracellular {Ca^{2+}} with aequorin or fluorescent dyes {62}.

Mechanical properties of skinned preparations

Various techniques have been applied to decrease or eliminate the permeability barrier of the plasma membrane of vascular smooth muscle strip preparations and to allow direct activation of the contractile machinery by Ca^{2+}. Usually isometric tension is the measured response and in some cases ATPase activity can be measured. A major contribution of these preparations is that they serve as a bridge between muscle protein biochemistry and muscle mechanics. Sophisticated mechanical studies have not generally been performed with these preparations because force development usually declines with each contraction-relaxation cycle, and many such cycles would be necessary for a force-velocity curve. However, the ability of these preparations to answer key questions has led investigators to make the technical advances that have improved the performance of these preparations. For example, Chatterjee and Murphy obtained force development that was about 92% of that obtained by the tissue before skinning {63}. Also, the problem of declining force development in successive contractions is not as severe as it once was. Another important technical development is the finding that certain mechanical measurements (like the slack test) can be made during the same, prolonged contraction by using multiple force or length steps.

Methods of skinning vsm strips

The small size of VSM cells precludes true mechanical skinning of the sarcolemma, so the membrane is usually made permeable by dissolution with detergents {64} or glycerol {65}, physical trauma by grinding {66} or freeze-glycerination {67}, or through the action of specific agents such as staphylococcal alpha toxin {68} or ionophore A-23187 {69}. Nonionic detergents like Triton X-100 attack all membranes, but saponin treatment has been reported to disrupt the plasma membrane, but not the sarcoplasmic reticulum {70}. The freeze-glycerination technique is thought to involve membrane cracking, rather than dissolution {67}. Saida and Nonomura have reported that the divalent cation ionophore A-23187 can be used to reversibly skin smooth muscle, allowing anions such as ATP to enter, with resealing of the membrane occurring on removal of the agent {69}.

The procedure using staphyococcal alpha toxin, first introduced to smooth muscle research in 1979 by Cassidy et al. {68}, was not widely used until the late 1980s, and now has become the method of choice when one wants to make cells permeable to small ions without loss of cellular protein. This toxin is a protein whose subunits assemble

and incorporate into the plasma membrane to form 2-nm pores. The toxin does not enter the cell or the intracellular membranes. A general problem with agents that form channels is that because the membrane has not been solubilized, cell surface proteins remain, and substantial ecto-ATPase activity has been measured in many of these alpha-toxin treated preparations. (Ecto-ATPase refers to a membrane-bound ATPase on the extracellular surface of the plasma membrane, whose function is presumably to degrade any extracellular ATP present after being released as a neurotransmitter or cotransmitter.) The ecto-ATPase activity is high enough that one cannot be confident that the exogenous ATP added to the bathing solution reaches the myofilaments. If one desires to introduce large molecules (proteins, antibodies, etc.) into the cell, the membrane must be made more permeable. With mild saponin treatment, the cell can be made permeable while still retaining receptors and coupling mechanisms.

Two important criteria for skinned preparations are the active stress development and extracellular space measurements made with small solutes. Ideal preparations develop as much stress as the native tissue and allow small solutes to equilibrate through the entire volume of the tissue. However, larger solutes, such as proteins, antibodies, and perhaps even some drugs, may not reach their intended sites on the myofilaments.

Results with skinned preparations

Skinned preparations of smooth muscle have been used to demonstrate the Ca^{2+}-dependence of force generation {63–71}, ATPase {67,72}, and myosin light chain phosphorylation {63,66,68}. Kerrick and coworkers have made extensive use of skinned preparations in their studies on the role of myosin light-chain phosphorylation in the regulation of contraction. They found that when the myosin light chains in the preparations were irreversibly thiophosphorylated by ATP-γS, the force development was no longer dependent on Ca^{2+} {66}. This agreed with biochemical studies wherein ATPγS had the same effect on actomyosin MgATPase activity {73}. Skinned preparations have also been used to demonstrate Mg^{2+}-dependence of force development {65,70} and that relaxation induced by vanadate occurs at a step following light-chain phosphorylation {67}.

One practical disadvantage of skinned preparations is the amount of time required for a contraction-relaxation cycle, but it has been found that the relaxation rate can be increased by inorganic phosphate {74}. Using skinned preparations it has also been possible to demonstrate relaxation by the cyclic AMP-dependent protein kinase {75}. This enzyme has many substrates, but here it was presumably acting by phosphorylating myosin light chain kinase, which decreases the myosin kinase activity, leading to decreased levels of phosphorylated light chain and relaxation. An important result with skinned preparations is the demonstration of contraction in the absence of Ca^{2+} after addition of modified exogenous myosin light-chain kinase. The enzyme had been subjected to mild proteolysis so as to make its kinase activity independent of Ca^{2+} {76}. Furthermore, similar (but not identical) forces and shortening velocities were measured in Ca^{2+}-activated contractions and in contractions induced by the Ca^{2+}-independent MLCK in the absence of Ca^{2+} {77}.

Addition of various phosphoprotein phosphatases that are active against phosphorylated light chains causes dephosphorylation and relaxation of skinned smooth muscle preparations {78,79}. A very intriguing finding was that the addition of phosphatase to fibers contracting in submaximal Ca^{2+} concentrations caused dephosphorylation and, surprisingly, a slight *increase* in force. However, when added to fibers that had been made to contract, in the absence of Ca^{2+}, by previous addition of modified Ca^{2+}-independent MLCK, the phosphatase caused relaxation. The authors interpreted these results to mean that Ca^{2+} inhibits the deactivation of tension {79}. One interesting question addressed by some of these studies is whether the Ca^{2+} dependence of the various responses (force, shortening velocity, or ATP usage) is the same. Under conditions where isometric force development by chemically skinned guinea pig taenia coli and swine carotid artery strips was maximal, increasing the Ca^{2+}-calmodulin concentration increased unloaded shortening velocity about 50% {80}. With chemically skinned rat portal vein smooth muscle, increasing {Ca^{2+}} from pCa 6.0 to 4.5 causes practically no increases in isometric force development but increases the ATP usage significantly {71}. These findings suggest that more Ca^{2+} is required to saturate the processes regulating the rate of crossbridge cycling (and thereby the ATPase and shortening velocity) than is required to saturate the mechanisms regulating force maintenance.

ACTIN-MYOSIN MOTILITY ASSAY

In this assay the movement generated by actin-myosin interaction is visualized by fluorescence microscopy. It was first used to study the movement of myosin-coated beads on actin cables from the alga *Nitella* {81}. It is now more common to immobilize the myosin on a coverslip, and to observe the movement of fluorescently labeled actin filaments across the myosin surface in response to different conditions {82}. The bathing solution contains ATP, buffers, and appropriate salts, and may contain additional test proteins.

In practice, myosin is purified and modified if desired, and spread over a coverslip. Native thin filaments can be used, or actin can be purified from the tissue of choice. The toxic mushroom peptide. phalloidin is used to keep actin in the polymerized form (F-actin), and the phalloidin is usually labeled with rhodamine, enabling the actin filaments to be visualized by epifluorescence. Addition of ATP to the solution on the coverslip initiates movement. The velocity of sliding of individual filaments (in microns/sec) is usually calculated from videotapes of the experiments. This velocity is generally believed to represent the unloaded shortening velocity of a half-sarcomere. The only resistance to movement comes from any viscous resistance and any attachments of the actin filament to other myosin molecules.

Filament sliding velocities can help decide which models of smooth muscle sarcomere length are reasonable. In a striated muscle where filament lengths and sarcomere structure are known, the velocity of sliding can be converted to muscle shortening velocity in lengths/sec. The measured filament sliding velocity corresponds to the half-sarcomere shortening velocity of a muscle, so doubling the measured sliding velocity and dividing by the sarcomere length gives the corresponding shortening velocity in lengths/sec. However, as mentioned previously, filament lengths and sarcomere dimensions are not known in smooth muscle.

The measured filament sliding velocities are important because they can put bounds on the possible range of sarcomere sizes as follows: Smooth muscle myosin (gizzard) can make filaments slide at an average rate of about 0.8 microns/sec {83} at 25°C, meaning a full sarcomere could produce a shortening velocity of twice this, 1.6 microns/sec. If the sarcomere is long, for example, 10 microns, the normalized shortening velocity of the sarcomere (and the cell) would be 0.16 lengths/sec; if the sarcomere is shorter, for example, 3.2 microns, the same filament sliding velocity would correspond to a higher shortening velocity of 0.5 lengths/sec. At 37°C, an individual arterial cell can shorten at a rate of 0.28 cell lengths/sec [44]; if the filaments were sliding by one another at 0.8 microns/sec and the sarcomere was shortening at 1.6 microns/sec, a cell shortening velocity of 0.28 lengths/sec could be attained with sarcomere lengths up to 5.7 microns. Thus, the measured sliding velocities of smooth muscle myosin are high enough that it may be possible for smooth muscle to function with a filament arrangement (long sarcomere) that sacrifices cell shortening velocity in favor of force generation.

Force and stiffness cannot be directly measured with the motility assay, although very recently Sheetz et al. have used "optical tweezers" to estimate how much force a single kinesin molecule can generate {84}, and such an approach may become more widely available in the future.

One potential weaknesses of the method is that sometimes the direction in which an actin filament is sliding suddenly reverses {85}. It is not clear if this is a weakness of the method or a serendipitous finding that gives some insights into the nature of the crossbridge interaction. If the ionic strength is too high, the actin-myosin interaction is weak, and actin filaments diffuse off the myosin-coated surface and are lost. Sometimes agents like methyl cellulose are added to increase solution viscosity and to limit Brownian motion. This allows the filaments to stay near the myosincoated surface without diffusing too far away.

Advantages of the motility assay include that it actually measures movement, the distinctive feature of a muscle. The technique is especially suited for molecular genetic approaches to the study of contractile and regulatory proteins, in that it allows the effects of a mutation on motility to be studied. It provides an additional, more physiological system to the measurement of MgATPase, and is easier to quantitate than superprecipitation.

The technique has been used to answer questions about which portions of the myosin molecule are necessary. For example, it was found that myosin does not need to be in a filamentous form, but simply can be coated onto the surface as a monomer. Furthermore, heavy meromyosin (HMM), a proteolytic fragment of skeletal myosin that cannot form filaments but has both ATPase sites, can move actin filaments {86}. Even more surprisingly, myosin subfragment-1 (SF-1), a smaller fragment that consists of only the single globular ATPase portion of myosin, can also move actin in this assay {86}.

Phosphorylation of myosin is necessary for sliding to occur. If mixtures of unphosphorylated and phosphorylated smooth muscle myosin are coated on a surface, the thin filament sliding rate is dependent on the nature of the myosin mixture in an interesting way. In these experiments, completely thiophosphorylated myosin was used, and if more than about 50% of the myosin was thiophosphorylated, the maximum velocity was measured. But when the fraction of myosin thiophosphorylated dropped below about 40%, the sliding rate dropped abruptly {87}. It appeared that unphosphorylated myosin bound actin, but did not cause sliding, and the authors of this study attributed the slowing of the sliding by the addition of unphosphorylated myosin to be due to actin binding and causing a load. Experiments with chemically modified forms of myosin that bind actin but do not undergo the crossbridge cycle could produce similar behavior {87}. When mixtures of smooth and skeletal muscle myosin are coated on a surface, the actin sliding rate is a gradual function of the myosin composition, with smooth muscle myosin slowing the rate of sliding {87}. The sliding velocity of actin across both skeletal and smooth muscle myosin-coated surfaces is decreased by calponin or caldesmon {83}.

BIOCHEMISTRY OF THE CONTRACTILE PROTEINS

Contractile protein composition of smooth muscle

Like skeletal muscle, smooth muscle contains the structural proteins myosin, actin, and tropomyosin. It also contains smaller but significant amounts of other structural proteins (alpha-actinin, desmin or vimentin, vinculin and filamin), some of which are present in skeletal muscles. The chief qualitative difference from skeletal muscle is that it does not contain stoichiometrically significant amounts of the regulatory protein troponin {88–90}. Smooth muscle has been reported to contain a different type of thin filament regulatory protein called leiotonin {91,92}, but its role as a regulatory protein has not been widely accepted. More recently, vascular smooth muscle has been shown to contain three other proteins in sufficient quantities to function as structural proteins: caldesmon

{93}, calponin {94–96}, and a very basic 26,000 Da subunit, probably identical to a protein of known sequence but unkown function, SM22 {97}. It seems likely that the active components of the leiotonin preparations may have been calponin, SM22, or caldesmon (described below). All vertebrate muscle also contain enzymes known as myosin light chain kinase (MLCK) and myosin light chain phosphatase (MLCP), and in smooth muscle these enzymes appear to have an important role in the regulation of contraction.

Stoichiometry

Before considering specific properties of each of the purified proteins, it is appropriate to consider the amounts present in the cell. The most striking quantitative feature of the protein composition of smooth muscle is the abundance of actin and the scarcity of myosin relative to skeletal muscle {26}. The actin/myosin weight ratio in smooth muscle is about 10 times higher than in skeletal muscle, reflecting both a lower myosin content and a higher actin content {26}. These findings agree well with morphological measurements made with the electron microscope. The rather high tropomyosin content of smooth muscle, which had led to some confusion in the early biochemical literature, was seen to be consistent with the high actin content, implying a thin-filament structure like that of skeletal muscle, with one tropomyosin molecule spanning about seven actin monomers. Surveys of the contractile protein contents of several mammalian smooth muscles have revealed a dichotomy between two groups of tissues, those that have very high amounts of actin and those that have less (but still much more than skeletal muscles) {98}. The tissues in the first group (arteries) seem to develop more force than those in the other group (veins and other nonvascular smooth muscle), although some anomalous examples have been found. The higher amounts of actin present in smooth-muscle tissue carry over into myofibril and actomyosin preparations, and the preparation of myosin free from contaminating actin is more difficult than it is with skeletal muscle.

SPECIFIC PROTEINS

Myosin

Myosin is the major protein comprising the thick filaments of muscle and possesses the ATPase activity that converts the chemical energy of ATP hydrolysis to mechanical work. Its native molecular weight is about 470,000 Da, being composed of two heavy chains of 200,000 Da each and two of each of two classes of light chains, 20,000 and 17,000 Da. The 20,000-Da light chain can be phosphorylated by myosin light chain kinase, and this will be discussed in a subsequent section. Like myosin from other muscles, the smooth muscle protein binds Ca^{2+}, and this may possibly be involved in regulation.

Actin

Actin is a globular protein with a molecular weight of about 42,000 Da consisting of one polypeptide chain. Actin polymerizes to form a long double-helical structure known as F-actin, and this constitutes the backbone of the thin filaments in muscle. Actin activates the MgATPase activity of myosin in vitro, and this is the basis for the increased energy usage in contracting muscle. Actin is present in larger quantities (on a weight basis) than any other cellular protein in vascular smooth muscle, there being about 30 mg/g tissue in the hog carotid artery {26}. Actins from all types of muscle are quite similar, but not identical. Isoelectric focusing reveals that there are three isoforms in smooth muscle, termed *alpha*, *beta*, and *gamma* {99}, with the alpha subunit being most similar to skeletal actin.

Tropomyosin

Tropomyosin is a rod-shaped protein whose secondary structure is nearly 100% alpha helix. In striated muscle it is thought that the long tropomyosin molecules, which bind the regulatory protein troponin, lie in the grooves formed by the actin double helix and serve to control a block of six to seven actins by moving further into or out of the groove in response to Ca^{2+} binding by troponin. The absence of troponin in vertebrate smooth muscle means that this cannot be the role of tropomyosin here, but it is often thought to have a structural role in maintaining thin-filament rigidity. In biochemical studies, tropomyosin has been shown to be an activator of actomyosin ATPase in systems containing purified myosin light-chain kinase and phosphatase {100}, and it doubles the sliding rate of actin filaments in the in vitro motility assay {101}.

Troponin

Troponin is not found in Ca^{2+}-sensitive actomyosin preparations from smooth muscle {89,90} or thin-filament preparations {89}, nor could it be prepared from smooth muscle using skeletal muscle techniques. Most investigators believe it is not present, in spite of earlier {102} and recurring {103} reports of troponin or troponin-like components. The concept of thin-filament regulation has been further broadened by reports of the phosphorylation of thin filament components {104}. Wider acceptance of these results awaits further purification and characterization of the active components, which may prove to be calponin, caldesmon, or SM22. These topics are covered in more detail in Chapter 54.

Caldesmon

Caldesmon is a protein that binds to actin, myosin, and calmodulin and can inhibit actomyosin MgATPase activity in vitro. Sobue and Sellers {93} initially named the protein and suggested it might be involved in the regulation of contraction because in vitro, when Ca^{2+} concentrations increase (and more Ca^{2+} binds to calmodulin), the Ca^{2+}-calmodulin complex binds to caldesmon, displacing it from

the thin filaments. This first idea has been discounted because the affinity of Ca^{2+}-calmodulin for caldesmon does not seem to be high enough to cause displacement.

Caldesmon is present in 2 forms, *l*- and *h*-caldesmon, in smooth muscle and nonmuscle cells. Because of its particular amino acid composition, caldesmon's mobility on SDS gels is much less than expected, giving apparent molecular weights of 120 kDa or so, but the correct molecular weight has been found to be about 93 kDa {105,106}. Caldesmon has actin- and calmodulin-binding regions near the C terminus and a myosin binding region near its N terminus. This has led to the suggestion that caldesmon helps to maintain the organization of the contractile apparatus, acting as a flexible tether, keeping actin and myosin filaments reasonably close, but allowing them to slide by one another easily {107}. More recently, a peptide nearly identical to the C terminus of caldesmon has been shown to induce contraction of permeable cells under Ca^{2+}-free conditions, a result interpreted as the displacement of an inhibitory region of the native caldesmon from thin-filament binding sites by the exogenous, noninhibitory peptide {108}.

Caldesmon's ability to inhibit actomyosin MgATPase activity can be suppressed by phosphorylation of caldesmon by either protein kinase C or an endogenous kinase ("caldesmon kinase"), very tightly bound to caldesmon {109,110}. In fact, it was first thought that caldesmon was itself a kinase that autophosphorylated itself {111,112}. Subsequent work led to the conclusion that the kinase is a separate molecule, very similar to Ca^{2+}-calmodulin dependent protein kinase II, and is tightly bound to caldesmon {113}. Several workers unsuccessfully tried to show caldesmon phosphorylation in more intact systems, like intact arterial smooth muscle strips, but finally Adam et al. {114} found a slow increase in caldesmon phosphorylation from 0.45 to 1.0 mol/mol when swine arterial muscle was stimulated.

The issue of caldesmon phosphorylation has become more interesting since Adam et al. {115} reported that the sites on caldesmon that are phosphorylated by protein kinase C in vitro are not the sites phosphorylated in vivo when muscle strips are stimulated with phorbol esters. They found that the caldesmon sites phosphorylated in vivo were those typical of MAP (microtubule-associated protein) kinases. The interpretation was that the common practice of using phorbol esters to activate protein kinase C led to unexpected results. Apparently the phorbol esters activated protein kinase C, which triggered a kinase cascade, eventually resulting in the phosphorylation of caldesmon by some other kinase.

Calponin

Calponin is a protein with an apparent molecular weight of 34,000 Da that had been overlooked until its discovery by Takahashi in 1986 {94,116}. This is surprising because calponin is abundant, about half as much as tropomyosin, on a weight basis. The similarity of tropomyosin's subunit molecular weight to calponin and the fact that tropomyosin is a dimer and calponin is a monomer means that calponin is approximately equimolar to tropomyosin, suggesting that calponin may be a structural protein of the contractile apparatus. Calponin is a very basic protein, present as two isoforms with isoelectric points near pH 9. The cDNA has been cloned and the sequence of the two calponin isoforms has been deduced {117}. The smaller, beta, isoform is identical to the larger, alpha, isoform except for a 40-residue deletion near the carboxyl terminus. The calculated molecular weights are 22,333 and 28,127, although this difference is not apparent on SDS gels.

Interest in calponin grew when Winder and Walsh {96} showed that calponin inhibited actomyosin MgATPase activity in vitro, and that this inhibition could be removed by phosphorylation of calponin with either protein kinase C or the Ca^{2+}-calmodulin dependent protein kinase II. They suggested that reversible phosphorylation of calponin may be part of the regulatory mechanism in smooth muscle. The removal of inhibition by phosphorylation via kinases known to be activated during contraction, as well as other findings (see Chapter 54 for details), makes it very likely that calponin phosphorylation takes place in vivo, and several laboratories have tried to determine if it does take place. However, there is conflicting evidence, with two laboratories finding no calponin phosphorylation in swine carotid artery {118}, chicken gizzard, and guinea pig taenia coli {119}. Several preliminary reports of varying extents of phosphorylation have been presented, but none has yet established the stoichiometry conclusively {120–123}.

Myosin light-chain kinase (MLCK)

Myosin light-chain kinases are present in all types of muscle, where they catalyze the ATP-dependent phosphorylation of a specific serine residue in one of the light chains. Smooth muscle is the type of muscle where this phosphorylation seems to have its most clear-cut role, allowing actin activation of myosin MgATPase activity {124}. The enzyme has a catalytic subunit with a molecular weight of 100,000–140,000 Da and calmodulin, the ubiquitous 17,000-Da Ca^{2+}-binding protein {125,126}, is the regulatory subunit. The enzyme is activated when the Ca^{2+}-calmodulin complex binds to the catalytic subunit {127}. In vitro, the 140,000-Da subunit can be phosphorylated by the well-known cyclic AMP-dependent protein kinase, reducing the MLCK activity at a constant level of Ca^{2+}-calmodulin {128}. This would tend to relax smooth muscle and has attracted much attention as a possible mechanism for beta-adrenergic relaxation. However, the phosphorylation of MLCK at the site decreasing MLCK activity does not take place when Ca^{2+}-calmodulin is bound (as it would be expected to be in a contracting muscle) {128}. Therefore, it seems that this mechanism could reduce vascular reactivity in a relaxed blood vessel but not relax a constricted blood vessel, and the weight of the available evidence indicates that MLCK is not phosphorylated by the cAMP-dependent kinase. Interestingly, MLCK does seem to be phosphorylated by a different kinase, the Ca^{2+}-calmodulin dependent protein kinase II (sometimes called the *multifunctional* kinase).

Recent evidence {129,130} suggests that this may occur as a normal part of the activation process, which would decrease the MLCK activity, lower the extent of myosin light chain phosphorylation, and probably would lower the energy usage by the muscle during prolonged contraction.

The MLCK catalytic subunit is subject to proteolysis, losing first the ability to be inhibited by phosphorylation, then its Ca^{2+} requirement, and finally its activity. The first MLCK preparations studied had lower molecular weights (83,000) and were not Ca^{2+} dependent {131}, probably due to this fact.

Myosin light-chain phosphatase (MLCP)

The myosin light-chain phosphatases in muscle are difficult to purify without denaturation, so comparatively less is known about them. Originally it was thought that a specific enzyme dephosphorylated the phosphorylated myosin light chain; now it is realized that most phosphatases have rather broad specificity, and that more than one enzyme may dephosphorylate myosin, and it may have additional substrates. The enzyme removes the phosphate group from the phosphorylated 20,000 Da light chain. The dynamic balance of the reactions catalyzed by MLCK and MLCP determines the fraction of the light chains that are phosphorylated, so knowledge about this enzyme is just as important as knowledge about the kinase. Several different enzymes have been studied in turkey gizzard {132}. None is thought to be Ca^{2+} dependent, but Mg^{2+} modulation of phosphatase activity has been reported {133}. More recently it has been found that arachidonic acid can dissociate one of the protein phosphatases, decreasing its activity towards the phosphorylated light chain, which results in higher levels of phosphorylation at a given Ca^{2+}-calmodulin concentration {134}. In addition, a G-protein-linked mechanism of phosphatase inhibition has been reported {135,136}.

REGULATION OF THE CONTRACTILE SYSTEM BY Ca^{2+}

Myosin light-chain phosphorylation: Biochemistry

One of the most important questions in smooth muscle research is the nature of the regulatory systems governing contraction. The lack of troponin {88–90} meant that a different system must exist, and an obvious alternative was the myosin-linked system found in mollusks {88}. These molluscan muscles lack troponin, and Ca^{2+} causes contraction through binding to the myosin molecule. However, the regulatory system in VSM is more complicated than the simple molluscan system, even though myosin Ca^{2+} binding might be involved. It is now widely accepted that myosin light-chain phosphorylation is the dominant regulatory system, and many believe it is the only regulatory system. The myosin phosphorylation hypothesis, described below, was developed from in vitro experiments and has been strengthened by tests of it in living smooth muscle strips.

In 1975, Adelstein and Conti reported that phosphorylation increased the actin-activated MgATPase activity of myosin made from blood platelets {137}. Soon several laboratories reported that smooth muscle myosin light chain was phosphorylated in a Ca^{2+}-dependent manner and that this phosphorylation roughly paralleled the MgATPase activity in its Ca^{2+} dependence {100,138,139}. Subsequently it was shown that phosphorylation of smooth muscle myosin was required for appreciable actin-activated MgATPase activity {124}. Numerous lines of biochemical evidence led to the hypothesis that contraction is regulated by Ca^{2+} only through the Ca^{2+} dependence of the phosphorylation step {73}. This hypothesis predicts that if myosin can be maintained permanently phosphorylated, actin activation will no longer be Ca^{2+} dependent. Using different tissues and techniques, it was found that fully phosphorylated guinea pig vas deferens myosin was activated by actin in the absence of Ca^{2+} but further activated in its presence {100}; however, chicken gizzard myosin, when irreversibly thiophosphorylated, is activated no more by actin in the presence of Ca^{2+} than in its absence {73}. The results with chicken gizzard were consistent with the hypothesis that Ca^{2+} regulates contraction only through activation of the kinase and that phosphorylation is both necessary and sufficient for full activation. The vas deferens results, while also pointing to the necessity (but not sufficiency) of phosphorylation for full activation, also suggested the existence of a second site for the action of Ca^{2+}. While this might be an example of a true species of tissue difference, it is also possible that during protein preparation certain aspects of a Ca^{2+}-regulatory mechanism are lost or artifactually generated.

Later reports indicated that the relationship between myosin phosphorylation and ATPase activity might not be as simple as it was once thought to be. Because myosin is a hexamer, having two 200,000-Da heavy chains and two each of 17,000- and 20,000-Da light chains, a given myosin molecule can have zero, one, or two of its 20,000-Da light chains (LC20) phosphorylated. Each of the two 200,000-Da heavy chains has an ATPase site, and thus the question arises of whether phosphorylation of one light chain can activate the associated heavy chain's ATPase site, or whether both light chains must be phosphorylated before either of the ATPase sites are activated. A plot of MgATPase activity versus moles P/mole LC20 is not a straight line intercepting the origin (as it would be if the ATPase sites were independent), but rather a concave-up curve {140}. Persechini and Hartshorne {140} suggested that their results meant phosphorylation was an ordered process, with one light chain being preferentially phosphorylated, resulting in only about 10% of the activity of the doubly phosphorylated myosin. Addition of the second phosphate group was suggested to lead to a dramatic increase in ATPase, as both ATPase sites became maximally activated. However, results with intact muscle favor a random phosphorylation model, with phosphorylation of both heads required {141}.

Additional complications and subtleties of myosin light-chain phosphorylation have emerged. Besides serine-19 (the normal site), MLCK can also catalyze phosphorylation of threonine-18 in gizzard myosin {142}. Furthermore, another kinase present in smooth muscle, protein kinase C, can phosphorylate myosin light chains in vitro at two other sites near the N-terminus, decreasing the actin-activated MgATPase activity of heavy meromyosin (HMM) previously phosphorylated at serine-19 by MLCK {143}. Phosphorylation of light chains by protein kinase C does not, however, lower the sliding rate of actin filaments in the in vitro motility assay {101}. The physiological occurrence and significance of these findings is not clear because even when phorbol esters are used to deliberately induce phosphorylation of myosin by protein kinase C, much of the incorporated phosphate is attributable to phosphorylation by MLCK {144,145}. It is important to point out that most measurements of light chain phosphorylation in smooth muscle, whether done with ^{32}P incorporation or by change in the isoelectric point, could not identify which enzyme (protein kinase C or MLCK) phosphorylated the protein. Only peptide-mapping studies {144} could demonstrate which site on the light chain was phosphorylated.

Studies on the role of myosin light-chain phosphorylation in the regulation of contraction of intact smooth muscle

The hypothesis that smooth muscle contraction is regulated exclusively by myosin light-chain phosphorylation (LCP) makes several testable predictions: (a) On stimulation or relaxation, changes in LCP should precede or coincide with the mechanical response; (b) there should be low levels of phosphorylated LC20 in resting muscle; and (c) the magnitude of the mechanical response, whether force, shortening velocity, or stiffness, should be proportional to the extent of phosphorylation, although this proportionality need not be linear. Numerous workers have demonstrated that phosphorylation takes place on stimulation of intact smooth muscle {146–150} and that it coincides with or precedes the mechanical response. These findings support the hypothesis that phosphorylation is involved as a regulatory system in vivo, and light-chain phosphorylation has even been demonstrated in arteries of living animals {151}. However, changes in phosphorylation cannot always be detected on contraction of various smooth muscles, e.g., pig aortic strips {150}, and under some (unphysiological) experimental conditions "skinned" preparations can be induced to contract without measurable myosin light-chain phosphorylation.

Furthermore, it is not immediately apparent (but see the description of kinetic models below) how to explain all the mechanical responses in terms of phosphorylation, because it reaches its peak level before isometric force does and then declines during the time that force increases to its peak values {38,39,147,152,153}. During prolonged stimulation of the hog carotid, force is well maintained, while phosphorylation falls to near-resting values {38, 39,147}. This means that any proportionality between force and phosphorylation would have to have a time-dependent proportionality constant. With other smooth muscles, there can be a simple proportionality between LCP and mechanical output under some conditions but

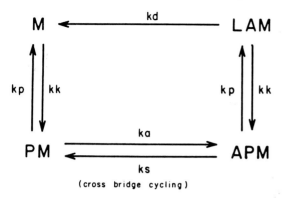

Fig. 55-5. Simplest model for regulation of contraction by phosphorylation. Myosin is depicted as being in one of four states: (1) detached, unphosphorylated (M); (2) detached, phosphorylated (PM); (3) phosphorylated and attached to the actin filament (APM); and (4) dephosphorylated while attached to actin (LAM), in other words, a latchbridge. States 3 and 4 are considered to be high-force states, so that force in the simulations represents the sum of states 3 and 4. The only Ca^{2+}-dependent step is assumed to be the reaction catalyzed by MLCK(kk). Other symbols: Phosphatase activity=kp; attachment rate=ka; crossbridge cycling rate=ks; and latchbridge dissociation rate=kd. From Driska {160}, with permission.

not others {154,155}. By measurements of shortening velocities after varying periods of isometric stimulation, it was found that velocity of shortening had a similar time course to light-chain phosphorylation {38,39}, as shown in fig. 55-4. This led to the suggestion that shortening velocity (but not isometric force) was regulated by light-chain phosphorylation.

To explain the decrease in shortening velocities during prolonged stimulation, it was proposed that phosphorylated crossbridges cycled rapidly and that attached crossbridges could be dephosphorylated, forming a so-called latchbridge that cycled very slowly if at all {38}. Evidence had been presented earlier for attached, noncycling crossbridges in smooth muscle {156}. Latchbridges were originally hypothesized to maintain force economically, but constitute an internal load that decreased the shortening velocities attained by phosphorylated cycling crossbridges. Also, the number of attached crossbridges was thought to be regulated by some other Ca^{2+}-dependent mechanism. Some support for the latchbridge hypothesis can be drawn from studies that show the rate of energy consumption decreases with time during isometric contraction {143,153}. However, the notion that the crossbridge cycle is slowed by an internal load has been criticized on energetic grounds because it predicts decreased efficiency of work production, an effect not observed {157}. The latchbridge hypothesis has attracted much attention, but it is currently based on rather indirect evidence. The latchbridge mechanism, if correct, would allow a vascular smooth muscle to shorten rapidly when stimulated, but then the crossbridge cycling rate would fall, decreasing the energy usage required to maintain tension. This would be

well suited to the role of vascular smooth muscle, allowing it to maintain the diameter of a blood vessel economically for long periods of time.

Studies on the regulation of skinned preparations by light-chain phosphorylation

One of the strongest arguments for the hypothesis that only phosphorylation regulates contraction comes from studies on skinned smooth muscle preparations. The ATP analog ATP-γS is a substrate for the light-chain kinase, but once the light chain is thiophosphorylated it is a poor substrate for the phosphatase. After treatment of skinned preparations with ATP-γS, force development no longer requires Ca^{2+} {66}. Uncertainties about whether thiophosphorylated light chain is functionally the same as phosphorylated light chain were answered by the demonstration that phosphorylation by ATP and a modified MLCK, which no longer required Ca^{2+} for activity, could remove the Ca^{2+} requirement for force development {76,77}. This seems to be strong evidence for the primacy of phosphorylation as the regulatory mechanism in this skinned preparation. Unfortunately, mechanical responses of the skinned preparations are not as completely characterized as those of intact tissue, but some data are available {77}.

Some studies {66,68,76} with skinned preparations have often been criticized because the amount of phophate incorporated into the light chain from ATP was not as great as expected, increasing from 0.01 mole P/mole LC20 to 0.20 mole P/mole LC20 when the [Ca^{2+}] was increased from 10^{-8} M to 1.6×10^{-4} M in gizzard preparations {66}. With rabbit ileum, the increase was even less, from 0.00 to 0.05 {68}. When these preparations were incubated with ATP-γS, however, the incorporation of thiophosphate in the light chain increased from 0.10 to 0.80 mole thiophosphate/mole LC20 for gizzard, and from 0.04 to 0.75 for ileum, over the same range of Ca^{2+} concentrations. Force development was the same in both cases, even though much higher levels of thiophosphorylation were achieved than of phosphorylation.

Taken at face value, these data were difficult to reconcile with a model that has force production regulated by phosphorylation. The disagreement between those studies and those supporting the latchbridge hypothesis and its postulation of a second site for Ca^{2+} action might have been simply due to a species or tissue difference. Alternatively, certain aspects of the regulatory mechanism of living muscle might have been lost on membrane disruption. Fortunately this impasse was partially relieved by the discovery of a high level of myosin light-chain phosphatase activity in swine carotid arterial smooth muscle {158,159}. This led to the reinterpretation of older evidence in terms of a new kinetic model, which proved to be very enlightening.

Early work on light-chain phosphorylation implicity assumed that dephosphorylation of crossbridges occurred much less frequently than ATP hydrolysis by myosin, i.e., it was assumed that phosphorylated light chains stayed phosphorylated for many crossbridge cycles. This is because the phosphorylation-dephosphorylation process appeared to be an energetically wasteful "futile cycle." For teleological reasons, it was assumed that dephosphorylation rates would not be very high. Our measurement of the dephosphorylation rates during relaxation of smooth muscle indicated that the phosphatase activity is quite high {158,159}. Since the enzyme is thought to be constitutively active (although the phosphatase activity may prove to be modulated somewhat), the phosphatase is active in contracting muscles when the steady-state phosphorylation can be quite high. Under these conditions both the phosphorylation and dephosphorylation reactions are occurring at high rates. One can compute that under these conditions the crossbridge might complete as few as three cycles before being dephosphorylated. This situation is very different than assumed in the early studies on phosphorylation as a regulatory mechanism, and because of this, the earlier experiments were reexamined in this light using a kinetic model of crossbridge regulation by myosin light-chain phosphorylation.

The mathematical model of crossbridge regulation used to examine the importance of kinase and phosphatase rates is shown in fig. 55-5. This model was used for simulations in our lab {160,161} and by others, particularly Hai and Murphy {162–167}. In the model, phosphorylation is the only regulatory mechanism, and an attached phosphorylated crossbridge can be dephosphorylated to form a latchbridge. If phosphorylation and dephosphorylation are infrequent compared to ATP hydrolysis by myosin, then force will be directly proportional to the level of light-

chain phosphorylation. This system becomes interesting when the myosin light-chain kinase and phosphatase activities are higher, and when the latchbridge maintains force for a long time, i.e., dissociates very slowly.

Figure 55-6 shows that under these conditions force is no longer a linear function of the level of phosphorylation, and maximum force can be obtained with low levels of phosphorylation (about 30% phosphorylation in the figure). Furthermore, the model {160} can explain the observed higher Ca^{2+} requirement for phosphorylation than for force {152}. These findings showed that many of the experimental observations originally thought to be evidence for a second regulatory system could, in fact, be explained by the kinetics of light-chain phosphorylation and dephosphorylation interacting with crossbridge attachment and detachment {160,168}. The theoretical work suggested that it may not even be necessary to postulate the existence of regulatory mechanisms besides light-chain phosphorylation. Opinions differ on whether a second mechanism needs to be postulated, but is seems that kinetic models of light-chain phosphorylation cannot explain all the observed physiology {168}, and the discovery of the putative regulatory protein calponin {94–96} has focused attention once again on additional mechanisms.

Ca^{2+} SENSITIZATION

The use of permeable preparations has uncovered the ability of VSM to change its sensitivity to the cytoplasmic $[Ca^{2+}]$. In these preparations, the $[Ca^{2+}]$ is heavily buf-

Percent Force

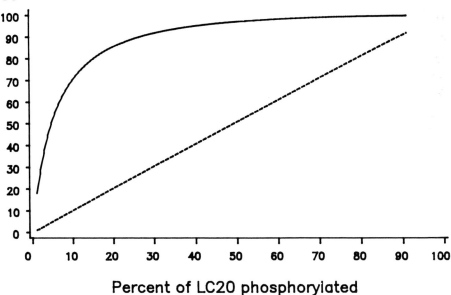

Percent of LC20 phosphorylated

Fig. 55-6. Theoretical force-phosphorylation relationships from simulations in two different cases where myosin light-chain phosphorylation is the only regulatory mechanism. The dashed straight line represents a case where latchbridges dissociate rapidly, and the solid curved line represents the case if latchbridges dissociate very slowly. Note that in the latter case, the force-phosphorylation relationship is not linear and high forces can be developed with little phosphorylation; e.g., about 85% of the maximum force can be developed with only 20% phosphorylation.

fered with EGTA, and agonists can cause a contraction, at a constant $[Ca^{2+}]$, by sensitizing the contractile system to Ca^{2+}. Under some situations the sensitization can occur by changing the balance between MLCK and phosphatases, so that the extent of myosin light-chain phosphorylation changes {135,169–171}. Somlyo's laboratory has shown that a G-protein-linked mechanism can inhibit the phosphatase activity {135,136} and additionally the phosphatase can be inhibited by arachidonic acid {134}. Inhibition of phosphatase would of course increase the level of myosin light-chain phosphorylation. Furthermore, Stull's lab has shown that myosin light-chain kinase can itself be phosphorylated, during a contraction, by Ca^{2+}-calmodulin-dependent protein kinase II, decreasing the MLCK activity and resulting in lower myosin light-chain phosphorylation {130}, which may partially explain the decline in phosphorylation during long contractions {172}. In other situations, thin-filament-linked mechanisms might change the availability of thin filament sites for crossbridge interaction, possibly by a mechanism involving phosphorylation of the thin-filament proteins calponin and caldesmon, as suggested by others {172,173}. In this latter

scenario, putative second regulatory mechanisms would be functioning in series with the myosin light-chain phosphorylation mechanism to modulate contraction.

These notions can be represented schematically as shown in fig. 55-7. In addition to the mechanisms described above, any mechanisms that change crossbridge attachment and detachment kinetics relative to phosphorylation and dephosphorylation kinetics could also change the mechanical output for a given level of myosin light-chain phosphorylation.

REGULATORY MECHANISMS: A SUMMARY

There is at present no uniformly accepted view of the mechanisms regulating smooth muscle contraction. All researchers agree that the regulatory system is different than the troponin system of skeletal muscle, and most researchers feel that myosin light-chain phosphorylation is involved as at least part of the system, but there is little uniform agreement beyond this. Myosin light-chain phosphorylation appears to be the only regulatory mechanism

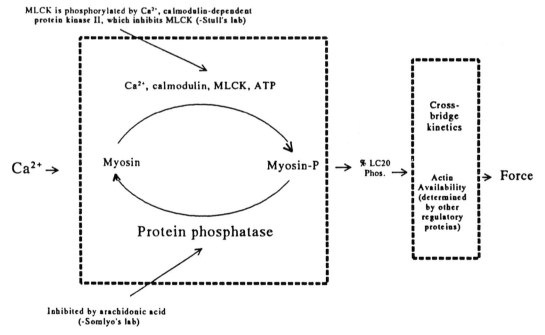

Fig. 55-7. Schematic depiction of regulatory systems operating in parallel and series. The relationship of the extent of myosin light-chain phosphorylation (% LC20 Phos.) to the intracellular $[Ca^{2+}]$ depends on the balance of the myosin light-chain kinase (MLCK) activity and the protein phosphatase activity. Stull's laboratory {130,172} has shown that the MLCK activity, at constant $[Ca^{2+}]$, can be decreased when MLCK is phosphorylated by the Ca^{2+}-calmodulin dependent protein kinase II. Somlyo's laboratory has shown that the protein phosphatase activity can be inhibited by both a G-protein dependent mechanism {135,136} and by an additional mechanism that involves a direct effect of arachidonic acid {134}. The following two types of mechanisms could operate in series with the myosin phosphorylation mechanism. First, the amount of force developed in response to a certain steady-state level of phosphorylation depends on the kinetics of phosphorylation and dephosphorylation relative to the kinetics of crossbridge attachment and detachment {160}, as illustrated in the previous figure. Second, any thin-filament-linked mechanisms that limit the availability of actin-myosin attachment sites (such as phosphorylation of caldesmon or calponin) could operate in series, determining the force output at a constant level of myosin light-chain phosphorylation.

in some isolated protein preparations and in some skinned fiber preparations, but additional mechanisms may operate in other protein preparations and in living smooth muscle tissues. Possible mechanisms include Ca^{2+} binding by myosin and phosphorylation of thin-filament components, including caldesmon and calponin.

A chapter such as this should provide some basis for the reader to see beyond all the disagreements towards some unified view of smooth muscle regulatory mechanisms. One approach, then, is to allow for the possibility that not all smooth muscles are identical in their regulatory mechanisms, just as they are not identical in many other respects. The diversity of smooth muscles has often been emphasized, and smooth muscle cells in chicken gizzard need not be regulated the same way as those in cow aorta. Another possible explanation is that under different experimental conditions, particularly experimental temperatures (phosphatases show extreme temperature dependence), different mechanisms are masked or unmasked as a different step in the crossbridge cycle becomes rate limiting for ATPase activity. This could be a result of the loss or even artifactual generation of regulatory mechanisms during the preparative procedures involved with each model system. If this possibility is accepted, it leads to the conclusion that the best preparations to study are the most physiological ones. Since myosin light-chain phosphorylation can be demonstrated on stimulation of strips of intact smooth muscle, the physiological *occurrence* of phosphorylation on contraction is established {146–149,153}, and biochemical work has demonstrated that it can act in a regulatory role {73,100,124,153}.

Mechanical studies in some tissues pointed to a role for phosphorylation in regulating the velocity of shortening rather than contractile force {38,39}, suggesting that another regulatory mechanism was needed to explain regulation of force in the living tissue {38,39,147,152}. The other proposed mechanisms (leiotonin, myosin Ca^{2+} binding, caldesmon, calponin, or thin-filament phosphorylation) that apparently regulate ATPase under other conditions might serve this purpose. However, in other living tissues, phosphorylation seems to correlate equally well with force and velocity {154,174}. It now seems that regulation by phosphorylation has to be analyzed in a more sophisticated way that considers the kinetics of phosphorylation and dephosphorylation in relation to kinetic steps in the crossbridge cycle {160,162}. Viewed in this way, some of the apparent differences in regulatory systems between smooth muscles may simply be a manifestation of differences in the kinetics of phosphorylation-dephosphorylation relative to crossbridge cycling. Furthermore, thin-filament regulatory mechanisms may operate in series with thick-filament regulatory systems so that even at constant levels of myosin light-chain phosphorylation, different levels of force can be attained.

The field of smooth muscle regulation is a very active one, and current research should soon resolve some of the apparent confusion. Progress is needed because a more complete understanding of the mechanisms regulating vascular smooth muscle contraction is of great importance.

REFERENCES

1. Carew TE, Vaishnav RN, Patel DJ: Compressibility of the arterial wall. *Circ Res* 23:61–68, 1968.
2. Murphy RA: Mechanics of vascular smooth muscle. In: Bohr DF, Somlyo AP, Sparks HV, Geiger SR (eds) *Handbook of Physiology. Sect 2: The Cardiovascular System. Vol II: Vascular Smooth Muscle.* Bethesda, MD American Physiological Society, 1980, pp 325–351.
3. Middleman S: *Transport Phenomena in the Cardiovascular System.* New York: Wiley-Interscience, 1972.
4. Doyle JM, Dobrin PB: Stress gradients in the walls of large arteries. *J Biomech* 6:631–639, 1973.
5. Bergel DH: The static elastic properties of the arterial wall. *J Physiol (Lond)* 156:445–457, 1961.
6. Dobrin PB, Rovick AA: Influence of vascular smooth muscle on contractile mechanics and elasticity of arteries. *Am J Physiol* 217:1644–1651, 1969.
7. Bunce DFM: *Atlas of Arterial Histology.* St. Louis, MO: Warren H. Green, 1974.
8. Dobrin PB: Influence of initial length on length-tension relationship of vascular smooth muscle. *Am J Physiol* 225:664–670, 1973.
9. Dobrin PB: Mechanical properties of arteries. *Physiol Rev* 58:397–460, 1978.
10. Dobrin PB, Doyle JM: Vascular smooth muscle and the anisotropy of dog carotid artery. *Circ Res* 27:105–119, 1970.
11. Cox RH: Effects of age on the mechanical properties of rat carotid artery. *Am J Physiol* 233:H256–H263, 1977.
12. Cox RH: Alterations in active and passive mechanics of rat carotid artery with experimental hypertension. *Am J Physiol* 237:H597–H605, 1979.
13. Cox RH: Comparison of arterial wall mechanics in normotensive and spontaneously hypertensive rats. *Am J Physiol* 237:H159–H167, 1979.
14. Hudetz AG: Incremental elastic modulus for orthotropic incompressible arteries. *J Biomech* 12:651–655, 1979.
15. Doyle JM, Dobrin PB: Finite deformation analysis of the relaxed and contracted dog carotid artery. *Microvasc Res* 3:400–415, 1971.
16. Duling BR, Gore RW, Dacey RG Jr, Damon DN: Methods for isolation, cannulation, and in vitro study of single microvessels. *Am J Physiol* 241:H108–H116, 1981.
17. Halpern W, Mongeon SA, Root DT: Stress, tension, and myogenic aspects of small isolated extraparenchymal rat arteries. In: Stephens NL (ed) *Smooth Muscle Contraction.* New York: Dekker, 1984, pp 427–456.
18. Herlihy JT: Helically cut vascular strip preparation: Geometrical considerations. *Am J Physiol* 238:H107–H109, 1980.
19. Furchgott RF: Role of endothelium in responses of vascular smooth muscle. *Circ Res* 53:557–573, 1983.
20. Jiang H, Rao K, Halayko AJ, Kepron W, Stephens NL: Bronchial smooth muscle mechanics of a canine model of allergic airway hyperresponsiveness. *J Appl Physiol* 72:39–45, 1992.
21. Uvelius B: Isometric and isotonic length-tension relations and variations in cell length in longitudinal smooth muscle from rabbit urinary bladder. *Acta Physiol Scand* 97:1–12, 1976.
22. Gordon AM, Huxley AF, Julian FJ: The variation in isometric tension with sarcomere length in vertebrate muscle fibres. *J Physiol* 184:170–192, 1966.
23. Ashton FT, Somlyo AV, Somlyo AP: The contractile apparatus of vascular smooth muscle: Intermediate high

voltage stereo electron microscopy. *J Mol Biol* 98:17–29, 1975.

24. Cooke PH, Fay FS, Craig R: Myosin filaments isolated from skinned amphibian smooth muscle cells are side-polar. *J Muscle Res Cell Motil* 10:206–220, 1989.

25. Small JV, Herzog M, Barth M, Draeger A: Supercontracted state of vertebrate smooth muscle cell fragments reveals myofilament lengths. *J Cell Biol* 111:2451–2461, 1990.

26. Murphy RA, Herlihy JT, Megerman J: Force-generating capacity and contractile protein content of arterial smooth muscle. *J Gen Physiol* 64:691–705, 1974.

27. Paul RJ: Chemical energetics of vascular smooth muscle. In: Bohr DF, Somlyo AP, Sparks HV, Geiger SR (eds) *Handbook of Physiology. Sect 2: The Cardiovascular System. Vol II: Vascular Smooth Muscle.* Bethesda, MD American Physiological Society, 1980, pp 201–235.

28. Somlyo AV, Bond M, Butler TM, Berner PF, Ashton FT, Holtzer HV, Somlyo AP: The contractile apparatus of smooth muscle: An update. In: Stephens NL (ed) *Smooth Muscle Contraction.* New York: Dekker, 1984, pp 1–20.

29. Cornelius F, Lowy J: Tension-length behaviour of a molluscan smooth muscle related to filament organisation. *Acta Physiol Scand* 102:167–180, 1978.

30. Murphy RA: Contractile system function in mammalian smooth muscle. *Blood Vessels* 13:1–23, 1976.

31. Price JM, Davis DL, Baker CH: Dependence of the length-tension relationship on agonist concentration in vascular smooth muscle. *Proc Soc Exp Biol Med* 182:494–504, 1986.

32. Driska SP, Murphy RA: Estimate of cellular force generation in an arterial smooth muscle with a high actin: myosin ratio. *Blood Vessels* 15:26–32, 1978.

33. Murphy RA, Driska SP, Cohen DM: Variations in actin to myosin ratios and cellular force generation in vertebrate smooth muscles. In: Casteels R, Godfraind T, Ruegg JC (eds) *Excitation-Contraction Coupling in Smooth Muscle.* Amsterdam: Elsevier/ North-Holland Biomedical Press, 1977, pp 417–424.

34. Driska SP, Damon DN, Murphy RA: Estimates of cellular mechanics in an arterial smooth muscle. *Biophys J* 24: 525–540, 1978.

35. Fay FS: Isometric contractile properties of single isolated smooth muscle cells. *Nature* 265:553–556, 1977.

36. Hellstrand P, Johansson B: The force-velocity relation in phasic contractions of venous smooth muscle. *Acta Physiol Scand* 93:157–166, 1975.

37. Uvelius B: Shortening velocity, active force and homogeneity of contraction during electrically evoked twitches in smooth muscle from rabbit urinary bladder. *Acta Physiol Scand* 106:481–486, 1979.

38. Dillon PF, Aksoy MO, Driska SP, Murphy RA: Myosin phosphorylation and the cross-bridge cycle in arterial smooth muscle. *Science* 211:495–497, 1981.

39. Dillon PF, Murphy RA: Tonic force maintenance with reduced shortening velocity in arterial smooth muscle. *Am J Physiol* 242:C102–C108, 1982.

40. Hellstrand P, Johansson B: Analysis of the length response to a force step in smooth muscle from rabbit urinary bladder. *Acta Physiol Scand* 106:221–238, 1979.

41. Mulvany MJ: The undamped and damped series elastic components of a vascular smooth muscle. *Biophys J* 26: 401–413, 1979.

42. Gunst SJ: Effect of length history on contractile behavior of canine tracheal smooth muscle. *Am J Physiol* 250: C146–C154, 1986.

43. Krisanda JM, Paul RJ: Energetics of isometric contraction in porcine carotid artery. *Am J Physiol* 246:C510–C519, 1984.

44. Dougherty TJ, Driska SP: Unusual [Ca^{2+}] dependence of vascular smooth muscle cell shortening velocity. *Am J Physiol* 260:C449–C456, 1991.

45. Bagby RM: Time course of isotonic contraction in single cells and muscle strips from *Bufo marinus* stomach. *Am J Physiol* 227:789–793, 1974.

46. Bressler BH, Clinch NF: The compliance of contracting skeletal muscle. *J Physiol* 237:477–493, 1974.

47. Ford LE, Huxley AF, Simmons RM: Tension responses to sudden length change in stimulated frog muscle fibres near slack length. *J Physiol* 269:441–515, 1977.

48. Cecchi G, Griffiths PJ, Taylor S: Muscular contraction: Kinetics of crossbridge attachment studied by high-frequency stiffness measurements. *Science* 217:70–72, 1982.

49. Paul RJ, Peterson JW: Smooth muscle energetics. In: Casteels R, Godfraind T, Ruegg JC (eds) *Excitation-Contraction Coupling in Smooth Muscle.* Amsterdam: Elsevier/North-Holland, 1977, pp 455–462.

50. Cooke PH, Fay FS: Correlation between fiber length, ultra-structure, and the length-tension relationship of mammalian smooth muscle. *J Cell Biol* 52:105–116, 1972.

51. Mulvany MJ, Warshaw DM: The active tension-length curve of vascular smooth muscle related to its cellular components. *J Gen Physiol* 74:85–104, 1979.

52. Van Dijk AM, Laird JD: Characterization of single isolated vascular smooth muscle cells from bovine coronary artery. *Blood Vessels* 21:267–278, 1984.

53. VanDijk AM, Wieringa PA, Van der Meer M, Laird JD: Mechanics of resting isolated single vascular smooth muscle cells from bovine coronary artery. *Am J Physiol* 246: C277–C287, 1984.

54. DeFeo TT, Morgan KG: Responses of enzymatically isolated mammalian vascular smooth muscle cells to pharmacological and electrical stimuli. *Pflügers Arch* 404:100–102, 1985.

55. Warshaw DM, Szarek JL, Hubbard MS, Evans JN: Pharmacology and force development of single freshly isolated bovine carotid artery smooth muscle cells. *Circ Res* 58: 399–406, 1986.

56. Driska SP, Porter R: Isolation of smooth muscle cells from swine carotid artery by digestion with papain. *Am J Physiol* 251:C474–C481, 1986.

57. Clapp LH, Gurney AM: Outward currents in rabbit pulmonary artery cells dissociated with a new technique. *Exp Physiol* 76:677–693, 1991.

58. Desilets M, Driska SP, Baumgarten CM: Current fluctuations and oscillations in smooth muscle cells from hog carotid artery: Role of the sarcoplasmic reticulum. *Circ Res* 65:708–722, 1989.

59. Brozovich FV, Walsh MP, Morgan KG: Regulation of force in skinned, single cells of ferret aortic smooth muscle. *Pflügers Arch* 416:742–749.

60. Warshaw DM: Force: velocity relationship in single isolated toad stomach smooth muscle cells. *J Gen Physiol* 89: 771–789, 1987.

61. Harris DE, Warshaw DM: Length vs. active force relationship in single isolated smooth muscle cells. *Am J Physiol Cell Physiol* 260:C1104–C1112, 1991.

62. Williams DA, Becker PL, Fay FS: Regional changes in calcium underlying contraction of single smooth muscle cells. *Science* 235:1644–1648, 1987.

63. Chatterjee M, Murphy RA: Calcium-dependent stress maintenance without myosin phosphorylation in skinned smooth muscle. *Science* 221:464–466, 1983.

64. Gordon AR: Contraction of detergent-treated smooth muscle. *Proc Natl Acad Sci USA* 75:3527–3530, 1978.
65. Filo RS, Bohr DF, Ruegg JC: Glycerinated skeletal and smooth muscle: Calcium and magnesium dependence. *Science* 147:1581–1583, 1965.
66. Hoar PE, Kerrick WG, Cassidy PS: Chicken gizzard: Relation between calcium-activated phosphorylation and contraction. *Science* 204:503–506, 1979.
67. Peterson JW: Vanadate ion inhibits actomyosin interaction in chemically skinned vascular smooth muscle. *Biochem Biophys Res Commun* 95:1846–1853, 1980.
68. Cassidy P, Hoar PE, Kerrick WG: Irreversible thiophosphorylation and activation of tension in functionally skinned rabbit ileum strips by [^{35}S]ATP gamma S. *J Biol Chem* 254:11148–11153, 1979.
69. Saida K: A method of skinning smooth muscle fibers with A23187. *Biomed Res* 2:134–142, 1981.
70. Saida K, Nonomura Y: Characteristics of Ca^{2+}- and Mg^{2+}-induced tension development in chemically skinned smooth muscle fibers. *J Gen Physiol* 72:1–14, 1978.
71. Arner A, Hellstrand P: Activation of contraction and ATPase activity in intact and chemically skinned smooth muscle of rat poral vein. Dependence on Ca^{2+} and muscle length. *Circ Res* 53:695–702, 1983.
72. Guth K, Junge J: Low Ca^{2+} impedes cross-bridge detachment in chemically skinned taenia coli. *Nature* 300:775–776, 1982.
73. Sherry JM, Gorecka A, Aksoy MO, Dabrowska R, Hartshorne DJ: Roles of calcium and phosphorylation in the regulation of the activity of gizzard myosin. *Biochemistry* 17:4411–4418, 1978.
74. Schneider M, Sparrow M, Ruegg JC: Inorganic phosphate promotes relaxation of chemically skinned smooth muscle of guinea-pig taenia coli. *Experientia* 37:980–982, 1981.
75. Ruegg JC, Paul RJ: Vascular smooth muscle. Calmodulin and cyclic AMP-dependent protein kinase after calcium sensitivity in porcine carotid skinned fibers. *Circ Res* 50:394–399, 1982.
76. Walsh MP, Bridenbaugh R, Hartshorne DJ, Kerrick WGL: Phosphorylation-dependent activated tension in skinned gizzard muscle fibers in the absence of Ca^{2+}. *J Biol Chem* 257:5987–5990, 1982.
77. Mrwa U, Guth K, Ruegg JC, Paul RJ, Bostrom S, Barsotti R, Hartshorne D: Mechanical and biochemical characterization of the contraction elicited by a calcium-independent myosin light chain kinase in chemically skinned smooth muscle. *Experientia* 41:1002–1006, 1985.
78. Haeberle JR, Hathaway DR, Depaoli Roach AA: Dephosphorylation of myosin by the catalytic subunit of a type-2 phosphatase produces relaxation of chemically skinned uterine smooth muscle. *J Biol Chem* 260:9965–9968, 1985.
79. Hoar PE, Pato MD, Kerrick WG: Myosin light chain phosphatase. Effect on the activation and relaxation of gizzard smooth muscle skinned fibers. *J Biol Chem* 260:8760–8764, 1985.
80. Paul RJ, Doerman G, Zeugner C, Ruegg JC: The dependence of unloaded shortening velocity on Ca^{2+}, calmodulin, and duration of contraction in "chemically skinned" smooth muscle. *Circ Res* 53:342–351, 1983.
81. Sheetz MP, Spudich JA: Movement of myosin-coated fluorescent beads on actin cables in vitro. *Nature* 303:31–35, 1983.
82. Kron SJ, Spudich JA: Fluorescent actin filaments move on myosin fixed to a glass surface. *Proc Natl Acad Sci USA* 83:6272–6276, 1986.
83. Shirinsky VP, Biryukov KG, Hettasch JM, Sellers JR: Inhibition of the relative movement of actin and myosin by caldesmon and calponin. *J Biol Chem* 267:15886–15892, 1992.
84. Kuo SC, Sheetz MP: Force of single kinesin molecules measured with optical tweezers. *Science* 260:232–234, 1993.
85. Sellers JR, Kachar B: Polarity and velocity of sliding filaments: Control of direction by actin and of speed by myosin. *Science* 249:406–408, 1990.
86. Toyoshima YY, Kron SJ, McNally EM, Niebling KR, Toyoshima C, Spudich JA: Myosin subfragment-1 is sufficient to move actin filaments in vitro. *Nature* 328:536–539, 1987.
87. Warshaw DM, Desrosiers JM, Work SS, Trybus KM: Smooth muscle myosin cross-bridge interactions modulate actin filament sliding velocity in vitro. *J Cell Biol* 111:453–463, 1990.
88. Bremel RD: Myosin linked calcium regulation in vertebrate smooth muscle. *Nature* 252:405–407. 1974.
89. Driska S, Hartshorne DJ: The contractile proteins of smooth muscle. Properties and components of a Ca^{2+}-sensitive actomyosin from chicken gizzard. *Arch Biochem Biophys* 167:203–212, 1975.
90. Sobieszek A, Bremel RD: Preparation and properties of vertebrate smooth-muscle myofibrils and actomyosin. *Eur J Biochem* 55:49–60, 1975.
91. Mikawa T, Toyo-oka, T, Nonomura Y, Ebashi S: Essential factor of gizzard "troponin" fraction. A new type of regulatory protein. *J Biochem* 81:273–275, 1977.
92. Ebashi S, Mikawa T, Hirata M, Toyo-oka T, Nonomura Y: Regulatory proteins of smooth muscle. In: Casteels R, Godfraind T, Ruegg JC (eds) *Excitation-Contraction Coupling in Smooth Muscle*. Amsterdam: Elsevier/North-Holland, 1977, pp 325–334.
93. Sobue K, Sellers JR: Caldesmon, a novel regulatory protein in smooth muscle and nonmuscle actomyosin systems. *J Biol Chem* 266:12115–12118, 1991.
94. Takahashi K, Hiwada K, Kokubu T: Isolation and characterization of a 34,000-dalton calmodulin- and F-actin-binding protein from chicken gizzard smooth muscle. *Biochem Biophys Res Commun* 141:20–26, 1986.
95. Takahashi K, Hiwada K, Kokubu T: Vascular smooth muscle calponin. A novel troponin T-like protein. *Hypertension* 11:620–626, 1988.
96. Winder SJ, Walsh MP: Smooth muscle calponin. Inhibition of actomyosin MgATPase and regulation by phosphorylation. *J Biol Chem* 265:10148–10155, 1990.
97. Pearlstone JR, Weber M, Lees-Miller JP, Carpenter MR, Smillie LB: Amino acid sequence of chicken gizzard smooth muscle SM22α. *J Biol Chem* 262:5985–5991, 1987.
98. Cohen DM, Murphy RA: Differences in cellular contractile protein contents among porcine smooth muscles: Evidence for variation in the contractile system. *J Gen Physiol* 72:369–380, 1978.
99. Izant JG, Lazarides E: Invariance and heterogeneity in the major structural and regulatory proteins of chick muscle cells revealed by two-dimensional gel electrophoresis. *Proc Natl Acad Sci USA* 74:1450–1454, 1977.
100. Chacko S, Conti MA, Adelstein RS: Effect of phosphorylation of smooth muscle myosin on actin activation and Ca^{2+} regulation. *Proc Nat Acad Sci USA* 74:129–133, 1977.
101. Okagaki T, Higashi-Fujime S, Ishikawa R, Takano-Ohmuro H, Kohama K: In vitro movement of actin filaments on gizzard smooth muscle myosin: Requirement of phosphorylation of myosin light chain and effects of tropomyosin and caldesmon. *J Biochem (Tokyo)* 109:858–866, 1991.

102. Carsten ME: Uterine smooth muscle: Troponin. *Arch Biochem Biophys* 147:353–357, 1971.
103. Marston SB, Trevett RM, Walters M: Calcium ion-regulated thin filaments from vascular smooth muscle. *Biochem J* 185:355–365, 1980.
104. Walters M, Marston SB: Phosphorylation of the calcium ion-regulated thin filaments from vascular smooth muscle. A new regulatory mechanism? *Biochem J* 197:127–139, 1981.
105. Graceffa P, Wang C-LA, Stafford WF: Caldesmon. Molecular weight and subunit composition by analytical ultracentrifugation. *J Biol Chem* 263:14196–14202, 1988.
106. Graceffa P, Jancsó A, Mabuchi K: Modification of acdic residues normalizes sodium dodecyl sulfate-polyacrylamide gel electrophoresis of caldesmon and other proteins that migrate anomalously. *Arch Biochem Biophys* 297:46–51, 1992.
107. Haeberle JR, Trybus KM, Hemric ME, Warshaw DM: The effects of smooth muscle caldesmon on actin filament motility. *J Biol Chem* 267:23001–23006, 1992.
108. Katsuyama H, Wang C-LA, Morgan KG: Regulation of vascular smooth muscle tone by caldesmon. *J Biol Chem* 267:14555–14558, 1992.
109. Sutherland C, Walsh MP: Phosphorylation of caldesmon prevents its interaction with smooth muscle myosin. *J Biol Chem* 264:578–583, 1989.
110. Ngai PK, Walsh MP: The effects of phosphorylation of smooth-muscle caldesmon. *Biochem J* 244:417–425, 1987.
111. Scott-Woo GC, Walsh MP: Characterization of the autophosphorylation of chicken gizzard caldesmon. *Biochem J* 255:817–824, 1988.
112. Scott-Woo GC, Walsh MP: Autophosphorylation of smooth-muscle caldesmon. *Biochem J* 252:463–472, 1988.
113. Scott-Woo GC, Sutherland C, Walsh MP: Kinase activity associated with caldesmon is Ca^{2+}/calmodulin-dependent kinase II. *Biochem J* 268:367–370, 1990.
114. Adam LP, Haeberle JR, Hathaway DR: Phosphorylation of caldesmon in arterial smooth muscle. *J Biol Chem* 264:7698–7703, 1989.
115. Adam LP, Gapinski CJ, Hathaway DR: Phosphorylation sequences in h-caldesmon from phorbol ester-stimulated canine aortas. *FEBS Lett* 302:223–226, 1992.
116. Takahashi K, Hiwada K, Kokubu T: Vascular smooth muscle calponin. A novel troponin T-like protein. *Hypertension* 11:620–626, 1988.
117. Takahashi K, Nadal-Ginard B: Molecular cloning and sequence analysis of smooth muscle calponin. *J Biol Chem* 266:13284–13288, 1991.
118. Barany M, Rokolya A, Barany K: Absence of calponin phosphorylation in contracting or resting arterial smooth muscle. *FEBS Lett* 279:65–68, 1991.
119. Gimona M, Sparrow MP, Strasser P, Herzog M, Small JV: Calponin and SM 22 isoforms in avian and mammalian smooth muscle—Absence of phosphorylation in vivo. *Eur J Biochem* 205:1067–1075, 1992.
120. Pohl J, Walsh MP, Gerthoffer WT: Calponin and caldesmon phosphorylation in canine tracheal smooth muscle. *Biophys J* 59:58, 1991.
121. Winder SJ, Allen BG, Fraser ED, Kang H-M, Kargacin GJ, Walsh MP: Calponin phosphorylation in vitro and in intact muscle. *Biophys J* 64:A31, 1993.
122. Driska SP, Cummings JJ Jr: Calponin is partially phosphorylated in arterial smooth muscle strips. *Biophys J* 64:A31, 1993.
123. Rokolya A, Moreland RS: Calponin phosphorylation during endothelin-1 induced contraction of intact swine carotid artery. *Biophys J* 64:A31, 1993.
124. Gorecka A, Aksoy MO, Hartshorne DJ: The effect of phosphorylation of gizzard myosin on actin activation. *Biochem Biophys Res Commun* 71:325–331, 1976.
125. Dabrowska R, Aromatorio D, Sherry JM, Hartshorne DJ: Composition of the myosin light chain kinase from chicken gizzard. *Biochem Biophys Res Commun* 78:1263–1272, 1977.
126. Dabrowska R, Sherry JM, Aromatorio DK, Hartshorne DJ: Modulator protein as a component of the myosin light chain kinase from chicken gizzard. *Biochemistry* 17:253–258, 1978.
127. Adelstein RS, Klee CB: Purification and characterization of smooth muscle myosin light chain kinase. *J Biol Chem* 256:7501–7509, 1981.
128. Conti MA, Adelstein RS: The relationship between calmodulin binding and phosphorylation of smooth muscle myosin kinase by the catalytic subunit of $3':5'$ cAMP-dependent protein kinase. *J Biol Chem* 256:3178–3181, 1981.
129. Stull JT, Hsu L-C, Tansey MG, Kamm KE: Myosin light chain kinase phosphorylation in tracheal smooth muscle. *J Biol Chem* 265:16683–16690, 1990.
130. Tansey MG, Word RA, Hidaka H, Singer HA, Schworer CM, Kamm KE, Stull JT: Phosphorylation of myosin light chain kinase by the multifunctional calmodulin-dependent protein kinase II in smooth muscle cell. *J Biol Chem* 267:12511–12516, 1992.
131. Daniel JL, Adelstein RS: Isolation and properties of platelet myosin light chain kinase. *Biochemistry* 15:2370–2377, 1976.
132. Pato MD, Adelstein RS: Dephosphorylation of the 20,000-dalton light chain of myosin by two different phosphatases from smooth muscle. *J Biol Chem* 255:6535–6538, 1980.
133. Moreland RS, Ford GD: The influence of Mg^{2+} on the phosphorylation and dephosphorylation of myosin by an actomyosin preparation from vascular smooth muscle. *Biochem Biophys Res Commun* 106:652–659, 1982
134. Cui Gong M, Fuglsang A, Alessi D, Kobayashi S, Cohen P, Somlyo AV, Somlyo AP: Arachidonic acid inhibits myosin light chain phosphatase and sensitizes smooth muscle to calcium. *J Biol Chem* 267:21492–21498, 1992.
135. Kitazawa T, Gaylinn BD, Denney GH, Somlyo AP: G-protein-mediated Ca^{2+} sensitization of smooth muscle contraction through myosin light chain phosphorylation. *J Biol Chem* 266:1708–1715, 1991.
136. Kitazawa T, Masuo M, Somlyo AP: G protein-mediated inhibition of myosin light-chain phosphatase in vascular smooth muscle. *Proc Natl Acad Sci USA* 88:9307–9310, 1991.
137. Adelstein RS, Conti MA: Phosphorylation of platelet moysin increases actin-activated myosin ATPase activity, *Nature* 256:597–598, 1975.
138. Aksoy MO, Williams D, Sharkey EM, Hartshorne DJ: A relationship between Ca^{2+} sensitivity and phosphorylation of gizzard actomyosin. *Biochem Biophys Res Commun* 69:35–41, 1976.
139. Sobieszek A: Vertebrate smooth muscle myosin: Enzymatic and structural properties. In: Stephens NL (ed) *The Biochemistry of Smooth Muscle.* Baltimore MD: University Park Press, 1977, pp. 413–443.
140. Persechini A, Hartshorne DJ: Phosphorylation of smooth muscle myosin: Evidence for cooperativity between the myosin heads. *Science* 213:1383–1385, 1981.
141. Persechini A, Kamm KE, Stull JT: Different phosphorylated forms of myosin in contracting tracheal smooth muscle. *J Biol Chem* 261:6293–6299, 1986.
142. Ikebe M, Hartshorne DJ, Elzinga M: Identification, phosphorylation, and dephosphorylation of a second site for myosin light chain kinase on the 20,000-dalton light

chain of smooth muscle myosin. *J Biol Chem* 261:36–39, 1986.

143. Nishikawa M, Hidaka H, Adelstein RS: Phosphorylation of smooth muscle heavy meromyosin by calcium-activated, phospholipid-dependent protein kinase. The effect on actin-activated MgATPase activity. *J Biol Chem* 258:14069–14072, 1983.

144. Bárány K, Polyák E, Bárány M: Protein phosphorylation in arterial muscle contracted by high concentration of phorbol dibutyrate in the presence and absence of Ca^{2+}. *Biochim Biophys Acta Mol Cell Res* 1134:233–241, 1992.

145. Rokolya A, Bárány M, Bárány K: Modification of myosin light chain phosphorylation in sustained arterial muscle contraction by phorbol dibutyrate. *Biochim Biophys Acta Bio-Energetics* 1057:276–280, 1991.

146. Janis RA, Moats Staats BM, Gualtieri RT: Protein phosphorylation during spontaneous contraction of smooth muscle. *Biochem Biophys Res Commun* 96:265–270, 1980.

147. Driska SP, Aksoy MO, Murphy RA: Myosin light chain phosphorylation associated with contraction in arterial smooth muscle. *Am J Physiol* 240:C222–C233, 1981.

148. Barron JT, Barany M, Barany K: Phosphorylation of the 20,000 dalton light chain of myosin of intact arterial smooth muscle in rest and contraction. *J Biol Chem* 254:4954–4956, 1979.

149. de Lanerolle P, Stull JT: Myosin phosphorylation during contraction and relaxation of tracheal smooth muscle. *J Biol Chem* 255:9993–10000, 1980.

150. Murray KJ, England PJ: Contraction in intact pig aortic strips is not always associated with phosphorylation of myosin light chains. *Biochem J* 192:967–970, 1980.

151. Moreland S, Antes LM, McMullen DM, Sleph PG, Grover GJ: Myosin light-chain phosphorylation and vascular resistance in canine anterior tibial arteries in situ. *Pflügers Arch* 417:180–184, 1990.

152. Aksoy MO, Murphy RA, Kamm KE: Role of Ca^{2+} and myosin light chain phosphorylation in regulation of smooth muscle. *Am J Physiol* 242:C109–C116, 1982.

153. Butler TM, Siegman MJ: Chemical energetics of contraction in mammalian smooth muscle. *Fed Proc* 41:204–208, 1982.

154. Haeberle JR, Hott JW, Hathaway DR: Regulation of isometric force and isotonic shortening velocity by phosphorylation of the 20,000 dalton myosin light chain of rat uterine smooth muscle. *Pflügers Arch* 403:215–219, 1985.

155. Gerthoffer WT: Calcium dependence of myosin phosphorylation and airway smooth muscle contraction and relaxation. *Am J Physiol* 250:C597–C604, 1986.

156. Siegman MJ, Butler TM, Mooers SU, Davies RE: Calcium-dependent resistance to stretch and stress relaxation in resting smooth muscles. *Am J Physiol* 231:1501–1508, 1976.

157. Butler TM, Siegman MJ, Mooers SU: Slowing of cross-bridge cycling in smooth muscle without evidence of an internal load. *Am J Physiol* 251:C945–C950, 1986.

158. Driska SP: High myosin light chain phosphatase activity in arterial smooth muscle: Implications for regulatory mech-anisms involving light chain phosphorylation. *Biophys J* 49:70, 1986.

159. Driska SP, Stein PG, Porter R: Myosin dephosphorylation during rapid relaxation of hog carotid artery smooth muscle. *Am J Physiol* 256:C315–C321, 1989.

160. Driska SP: High myosin light chain phosphatase activity in arterial smooth muscle: Can it explain the latch phenomenon? *Prog Clin Biol Res* 245:387–398, 1987.

161. Driska SP: Mechanical properties and regulation of vascular smooth muscle contraction. In: Sperelakis N (ed) *Physiology and Pathophysiology of the Heart*, 2nd ed. Boston: Kluwer Academic, 1988, pp. 879–898.

162. Hai CM, Murphy RA: Cross-bridge phosphorylation and regulation of latch state in smooth muscle. *Am J Physiol* 254:C99–106, 1988.

163. Hai CM, Murphy RA: Regulation of shortening velocity by corss-bridge phosphorylation in smooth muscle. *Am J Physiol* 255:C86–C94, 1988.

164. Hai C-M, Murphy RA: Ca^{2+}, crossbridge phosphorylation, and contraction. *Annu Rev Physiol* 51:285–298, 1989.

165. Hai C-M, Murphy RA: Cross-bridge dephosphorylation and relaxation of vascular smooth muscle. *Am J Physiol* 256:C282–C287, 1989.

166. Ratz PH, Hai C-M, Murphy, RA: Dependence of stress on cross-bridge phosphorylation in vascular smooth muscle. *Am J Physiol* 256:C96–C100, 1989.

167. Hai C-M, Murphy RA: Adenosine 5'-triphosphate consumption by smooth muscle as predicted by the coupled four-state crossbridge model. *Biophys J* 61:530–541, 1992.

168. Driska SP: Myosin light chain phosphorylation — Is it the whole story? *J Muscle Res Cell Motil* 11:429–443, 1990.

169. Himpens B, Kitazawa T, Somlyo AP: Agonist-dependent modulation of Ca^{2+} sensitivity in rabbit pulmonary artery smooth muscle. *Pflügers Arch* 417:21–28, 1990.

170. Kitazawa T, Somlyo AP: Desensitization and muscarinic resensitization of force and myosin light chain phosphorylation to cytoplasmic Ca^{2+} in smooth muscle. *Biochem Biophys Res Commun* 172:1291–1297, 1990.

171. Himpens B, Matthijs G, Somlyo AP: Desensitization to cytoplasmic Ca^{2+} and Ca^{2+} sensitivities of guinea-pig ileum and rabbit pulmonary artery smooth muscle. *J Physiol (Lond)* 413:489–503, 1989.

172. Stull JT, Gallagher PJ, Herring BP, Kamm KE: Vascular smooth muscle contractile elements: Cellular regulation. *Hypertension* 17:723–732, 1991.

173. Nishimura J, Moreland S, Ahn HY, Kawase T, Moreland RS, van Breemen C: Endothelin increases myofilament Ca^{2+} sensitivity in α-toxin-permeabilized rabbit mesenteric artery. *Circ Res* 71:951–959, 1992.

174. Merkel L, Gerthoffer WT, Torphy TJ: Dissociation between myosin phosphorylation and shortening velocity in canine trachea. *Am J Physiol Cell Physiol* 258:C524–C532, 1990.

175. Herlihy JT, Murphy RA: Length-tension relationship of smooth muscle of the hog carotid artery. *Circ Res* 33:275–283, 1973.

CHAPTER 56

Metabolism and Energetics of Vascular Smooth Muscle

CHRISTOPHER D. HARDIN & RICHARD J. PAUL

INTRODUCTION

The metabolism and energetics of vascular smooth muscle contractility have been comprehensively reviewed {1–11}. We will therefore not attempt to be encyclopedic but rather focus on what is widely accepted regarding the energy metabolism of vascular smooth muscle and the demands imposed upon that metabolism by contractile activity.

Since the appearance of the first edition, there has been substantial growth in the experimental base on which our understanding of smooth muscle behavior is formulated. Much attention has been given to the role of myosin light chain phosphorylation, not only as a mediator of the activation of actin-myosin interaction by calcium, but also in terms of its potential role as a modulator of the mechanical, energetic, and kinetic properties of smooth muscle {12,13}. The body of evidence indicating a functional compartmentation of energy metabolism in smooth muscle has grown considerably {14–16}. Application of nuclear magnetic resonance (NMR) to smooth muscle studies has provided a means for studying metabolism directly in living preparations. These studies have added many new dimensions to our understanding of smooth muscle mechanochemistry. We have incorporated the results of these recent studies in this updated review. The latter sections will focus on several issues that are currently unresolved and topics of some debate.

MUSCLE ENERGETICS: SMOOTH VERSUS SKELETAL MUSCLE

Amphibian skeletal muscles and vascular smooth muscles represent two extreme modes of how chemical energy stored in the form of the terminal phosphate bond of adenosine triphosphate (ATP) might be provided to the contractile proteins of muscles to supply the motive power needed to drive muscular contraction (cf. Kushmerick {17} for a skeletal muscle summary). During contraction at 0°C, amphibian skeletal muscle utilizes ATP approximately 100 times faster than its aerobic metabolism can resynthesize ATP. During a brief isometric tetanus, therefore, the available preformed high-energy phosphate compounds decline rapidly, limiting the ability of the muscle to maintain the developed force. After some period of time aerobic resynthesis of ATP is activated, and, on a time scale greatly longer than the sustained contractile period itself, the original phosphagen content is restored. To support the brief but intense period of ATP hydrolysis associated with contraction before the onset of aerobic recovery metabolism, skeletal muscles possess a large pool of preformed high-energy phosphate compounds, most notably phosphocreatine (PCr, 15–25 µmol/g fresh muscle). ATP, the substrate used directly by the contractile proteins, is substantially lower (3–5 µmol/g). ADP generated by the actomyosin ATPase is immediately rephosphorylated to ATP via the creatine kinase reaction.

Vascular smooth muscle (VSM) operates on the opposite tack. The initiation of contractile activity is associated with virtually no measurable decline in the available ATP + PCr content {18,19}, since the rates of ATP utilization by the contractile apparatus can be matched by aerobic resynthesis. Only if aerobic and glycolytic metabolisms are blocked can a net decline in the tissue content of ATP and PCr be noted. This leads then to two distinct strategies to study the energetics of vascular smooth muscle contraction, both of which are represented in the literature.

One method relies on measuring steady-state metabolic rates (that is, the rate at which ATP is being resynthesized) to estimate the usage of ATP. This method depends upon the assumption (verifiable, in most instances) that during the measurement period, the intracellular ATP + PCr pool is constant. Thus ATP utilization and production rates are equal. This method is, of course, subject to the limitation that, on short time scales, such may not be the case. An alternative method is to block all ATP resynthesis (using combinations of oxygen- and substrate-free environments and/or various metabolic poisons) and to measure directly the decline in intracellular ATP + PCr. This method is also subject to inherent limitations. The use of metabolic poisons, in general, raises the issue of how representative these measurements are of the normal tissue (cf. Daemers-Lambert {20}). The most common method for measuring the phosphagen content involves freeze clamping and analysis of tissue extracts. One is limited to one data point per tissue; thus this

N. Sperelakis (ed.), Physiology and Pathophysiology of the Heart, Third Edition.

technique requires statistical comparisons among a large population of tissues. This limitation has been overcome through the use of nondestructive NMR techniques since each tissue serves as its own control. In addition, ^{31}P-NMR provides a myriad of other information relevant to cell metabolism and energetics such as cytosolic pH and free [Mg^{2+}]. The advantage of this strategy, however, is that it is not dependent on the steady-state assumption and can be applied, in principle, to arbitrarily short time periods. Limiting the time resolution of the method, however, is the extremely low ATPase rate manifest in vascular smooth muscle, even when taken in comparison to the small pool size of preformed high-energy phosphates.

Both approaches have been used in the study of smooth muscle energetics, and, for the most part, the resulting data have proven complementary so that methodological limitations alone do not seem to play an important role in our understanding of the results.

These two energy-provision strategies appear to have evolved to meet the specific physiologic demands placed upon the various muscle types. Vascular smooth muscle's role in situ is to maintain blood vessel tone over long periods of time and to adjust tone gradually in response to changing conditions of the cardiovascular system. To do so economically, smooth muscle actomyosin possesses an extraordinarily low inherent ATPase and yet is capable of developing and maintaining forces quantitatively comparable to or greater than that of skeletal muscles. It has been estimated that only 3–5% of the total human basal metabolism is consumed by the vasculature and only about one fifth of that is required to maintain circulatory regulation {4}. While the total vascular mass is about 10 times greater than that of the heart itself, it consumes less than one half as much energy in fulfilling its role in distribution of cardiac output. The strategies for energy provision in smooth muscle differ in many ways from those in striated muscle since the rates of energy turnover in these two muscle types are so dramatically different.

HIGH-ENERGY PHOSPHATE CONTENT

Rather than presenting an exhaustive compilation of data, we will instead focus on the most typical values of various parameters, with the observed ranges indicated when possible. We would like to add the caveat that differences amongst smooth muscle can be as great as between smooth and striated muscle. Thus we will try to be cautious in our generalizations, while still attempting to elucidate underlying patterns.

Table 56-1 summarizes the content of high-energy phosphates found in quiescent mammalian muscles. The most notable feature is simply that vascular smooth muscle has, in general, the lowest content of preformed high-energy stores, in some cases less than one fiftieth of the preformed energy stores available to skeletal muscles. NMR measurements of the PCr/ATP ratio in smooth muscle generally confirm the measurements of the ratio determined chemically {21,22}. However, GTP and ATP cannot be resolved from each other by NMR and as much

Table 56-1. High-energy phosphate content of resting mammalian muscles

	ATP	PCr	Total ~P
Vascular smooth muscle	0.3–1	0.3–1	0.5–2
Other smooth muscles	1–2	1–3	2–5
Skeletal muscle	~5	10–15	15–25

All values in µmol/g wet tissue. The ranges have been estimated from tables of specific values contained in the reviews cited {1–11} and from refs. {17} and {44–47}. ATP = adenosine triphosphate; PCr = phosphocreatine; ~P = high-energy phosphagen.

as 12–15% of the total nucleoside triphosphate peak may be GTP, with the remainder being ATP based on measurements in uterus and bladder smooth muscle {21}. Since the PCr/ATP ratio determined by NMR generally agrees with that determined by biochemical analysis, virtually all of the ATP appears to be unbound, as in skeletal muscle.

At room temperature, while generating the maximum isometric tension, mammalian skeletal muscles would consume their available preformed high-energy phosphates in about 2–3 seconds. Smooth muscles, on the other hand, would not substantially deplete their supplies for 2–3 minutes. Daemers-Lambert and Roland {23} found no change in the ATP + PCr content of isolated oxygenated bovine carotid arteries after 30 minutes of maximal activation with potassium chloride, whereas similar experiments with metabolically inhibited iodoacetate-treated arteries led to a complete depletion of high-energy phosphates. On a much shorter time scale, Krisanda and Paul {24} did not detect any change in the ATP or PCr content of well-oxygenated hog carotid arteries in times as short as 30 seconds following activation of isometric tension development. Recent NMR data {25,26} substantiate the ability of vascular smooth muscle to maintain phosphagen stores for prolonged periods (>12 hours) under depolarizing conditions when supplied with substrate. Clearly, in the case of vascular smooth muscle, the aerobic capacity to resynthesize ATP is sufficient to rapidly achieve a balance with the ATPases associated with activation, development, and maintenance of contractile activity.

RESPIRATION

As discussed above, it has been observed that the metabolic capacity of vascular smooth muscle is sufficient to resynthesize ATP at least as rapidly as ATP is utilized by the contractile machinery. The biochemical pathways for ATP synthesis appear to be similar to those found in mammalian skeletal muscles. However, the regulation of those pathways may differ considerably. Early studies of the respiratory quotient {27,28} indicated that the primary substrate for energy metabolism is carbohydrate. Exogenous glucose would seem to be the most likely candidate as a preferred energy source. This is, however, contradicted by a fair amount of data indicating that little glucose is converted to CO_2 in studies employing isotopically labeled glucose {29}. Glycogen phosphorylase activity, one rate-limiting step for glycogenolysis, is well coordinated with contractility {30,31}. However, the breakdown of glycogen ceases after 15–30 minutes of stimulation in porcine carotid artery {32,33}, with approximately 50% of the initial content remaining. The rate-limiting step under these conditions appears to be the activity of the glycogen debrancher enzyme. This pattern can be altered by glycogen loading conditions. When glycogen is loaded for more than 6 hours in hog carotid artery, glycogen breaks down over several hours until glycogen levels reach ∼1–2 μmol/g blot weight of glucosyl units {34}, an amount reached in ∼30 minutes of contraction when arteries are not glycogen loaded. The diminished rate of glycogenolysis has only minor effects on the ability to maintain isometric force {33}, though the rate of force development is enhanced and rate of relaxation is apparently inhibited. Furthermore, glucose utilization (glycolysis) appears not to be correlated with glycogenolysis, suggesting some form of compartmentalization of carbohydrate catabolism in smooth muscle ({29,32} and see below).

The capacity of VSM to utilize a wide variety of substrates is present {35}. The necessary enzymes of glycolysis, the Krebs cycle, and the respiratory transport chain have been demonstrated in VSM {36–38}. Data from

Odyssey and Chase {39} suggest that fatty acids may predominate as the long-term oxidative substrate; however, the overall picture of oxidative substrate utilization is far from complete. Certainly when fatty acids are available, glycogen-sparing effects have been observed in hog carotid artery {40}. The interactions of carbohydrate and fatty acid metabolism in smooth muscle need further investigation.

Mitochondria isolated from vascular smooth muscle and characterized with respect to P/O ratio, respiratory control ratio, and substrate utilization appear not to differ substantially from the mitochondria of other mammalian tissues {41,42}. Recent experiments on intact VSM indicate that the P/O ratio in situ approaches its theoretical maximal value {43}.

The resting respiratory rates of mammalian smooth and skeletal muscles show relatively similar values. For both red and white skeletal muscles, basal respiratory rates are in the range 150–300 nmol O_2/min/g tissue {17,44–46}, while the smooth muscles range from 50 to 200 nmol O_2/min/g tissue {1–7}. This suggests that in the absence of an activated actomyosin ATPase and consequent contractile activity, the basal energy cost of housekeeping processes in mammalian muscle types is similar. A major difference arises, however, upon activation of contractile activity. In continuously twitching or tetanized mammalian skeletal muscle, for example, steady-state O_2 consumption rate increases by factors typically 25- to 50-fold {17,46}, as

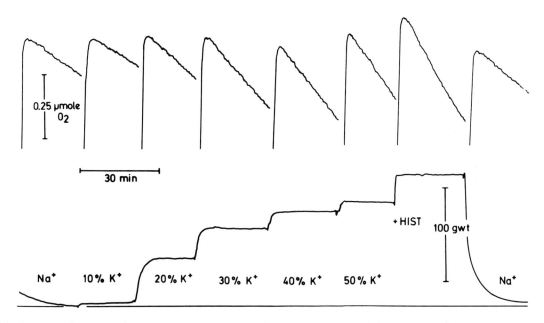

Fig. 56-1. **Top panel:** Records of O_2 concentration measured by O_2 electrode in a closed chamber containing a segment of hog carotid artery. The rapid vertical rises in the O_2 records correspond to changes of the bathing medium that both restored O_2 concentration to approximately the initial value and accomplished the change in ionic composition of the bathing physiologic saline solution. The downward slope of each trace is proportional to the O_2 consumption rate of the arterial segment in the chamber (cf. Paul et al. {51}) during the mechanical state directly below. **Bottom panel:** Record of the isometric tension development of the arterial segment in response to the indicated increase in the percentage substitution of Na^+ by K^+ in the bathing solution. Na^+ indicates normal saline (Krebs–Henseleit). Hist indicates the addition of 10^{-5} M histamine to the already K^+-depolarized artery segment.

does the recovery O_2 consumption rate following tetani of moderate (<15 seconds) duration {47}. In isometrically contracted vascular smooth muscle, the O_2 consumption rate increases typically no more than twofold {1–7}. The much lower maximum oxygen consumption rate of VSM is, of course, consistent with the above-mentioned differences in the inherent actomyosin ATPases, the pool size of preformed high-energy phosphates, and the different energy provision strategies between the two muscle types.

A consistent finding in studies of isolated vascular smooth muscle is that the increases in the rate of aerobic metabolism are very tightly correlated with the levels of maintained isometric tension under a wide variety of conditions {48–55}. This is illustrated in fig. 56-1 for studies using strips of hog carotid artery {53} stimulated to develop and maintain varying levels of isometric tension in response to graded isosmotic increases in the ratio of K^+ to Na^+ in the bathing saline. The upper panel shows continuous recordings of the oxygen tension determined polarographically by oxygen electrode in the bathing solution. The slopes of the oxygen concentration records are proportional to the rates of oxygen consumption by the arterial segment. It is evident from fig. 56-1 that the steady-state rate of O_2 consumption increases progressively as isometric tension increases and returns to the initial resting value when contractile activity ceases. The results of identical experiments with five artery segments are plotted in fig. 56-2 (open circles), demonstrating the tight linear correlation between suprabasal O_2 consumption rate and the level of maintained isometric tension.

In most cases, the quantitative correlation between isometric tension maintenance and increased O_2 consumption rate has been found not to change substantially over long periods of time (up to 12 hours in vitro), nor to vary *significantly* with the mode of stimulation of the blood vessel, whether ionic, pharmacological, or electrical {1–7,48–55}. Data illustrating this relative invariance are shown in fig. 56-2. Additional data beyond those discussed above are shown for experiments with hog carotid arteries in which isometric tension was varied by maintaining a constant elevated ratio of K^+ to Na^+ in the bathing solution, but varying the extracellular Ca^{2+} concentration {53}. Over the range of $[Ca^{2+}]$ from 0.1 to 1.0 mM, graded isometric tension responses similar to those shown in the lower panel of fig. 56-1 were obtained. The steady-state rates of O_2 consumption following this alternative mode of activating graded isometric contractions are shown in fig. 56-2 in experiments with five artery samples (filled circles). Clearly, in this case at least, the response of aerobic metabolism to increasing isometric tension maintenance was essentially invariant to the particulars of how the muscle was activated to produce tension. Similar comparative data obtained in studies with bovine mesenteric vein {49–51} display a likewise invariant dependence of steady-state suprabasal O_2 metabolism on graded isometric contractions produced by varying the concentration of three pharmacological stimulants: epinephrine, norepinephrine, and histamine (fig. 56-3).

While linearity between O_2 consumption rate and force ordinarily holds, increases in O_2 greater than that predicted

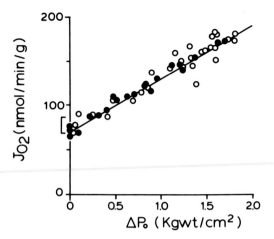

Fig. 56-2. Observed rates of O_2 consumption (J_{O_2}) are plotted against maintained isometric force (ΔP_o) in five hog carotid artery samples in response to varying levels of K^+ for Na^+ substitution in the bathing medium, as described by fig. 56-1 (open circles). In five other artery samples, maximal activation was maintained by 50% K^+-substituted saline, but extracellular $[Ca^{2+}]$ was varied (after depletion using Ca^{2+}-free saline and 0.5 mM EGTA) between 0.1 and 1 mM. Again, O_2 consumption rate is plotted against the maintained isometric force under these conditions (filled circles). The linear relation between force and O_2 consumption is identical for the two sets of activating conditions. The mean (± SD) resting rate of O_2 consumption for the 10 artery segments is shown by the bracker near the J_{O_2} axis. The fact that the linear regression through the force-dependent J_{O_2} data passes near the resting J_{O_2} value is suggestive that basal J_{O_2} was not substantially altered during isometric contraction.

can be evoked at high forces. This usually requires high levels of stimulation and unphysiologically high levels of Ca^{2+} {56–58}. The point of divergence from linearity plays an important role in differentiating between current theories of regulation of contractility as well as interpretation of smooth muscle energetics; this will be discussed further in subsequent sections.

In comparing various vascular smooth muscles from a variety of species, the increases in O_2 consumption rate above basal levels to maintain the maximum level of isometric force is in the range of 50–100 nmol O_2/min/g tissue {1–7}. Because the generally observed close correlation between isometric tension maintenance and suprabasal aerobic metabolism, it is generally believed that the ATP hydrolyzed by vascular smooth muscle actomyosin is rapidly resynthesized through primarily oxidative pathways.

The mechanisms responsible for the control of smooth muscle oxidative phosphorylation that match mitochondrial ATP supply to ATP demand may depend both on the specific smooth muscle and on the metabolic state of a given smooth muscle. ^{31}P-NMR has provided a means to monitor the high-energy phosphate content in a single preparation during manipulations that affect the rate of oxidative phosphorylation. Using ^{31}P-NMR, PCr was

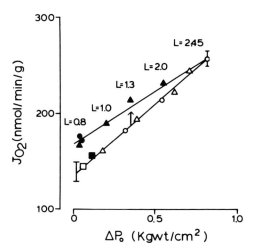

Fig. 56-3. O_2 consumption rate (J_{O_2}) is plotted against active isometric force (ΔP_o) for an experiment with a single segment of bovine mesenteric vein. The bar indicates the mean ($\pm$ SD) basal J_{O_2} measured periodically during the experiment. At a segment length L = 2.45 cm, the tissue was progressively activated with increasing concentrations of epinephrine ($\bigcirc$), then relaxed in normal saline. The alpha-adrenergic-blocker dihydroergotamine was applied ($\square$) and supramaximal epinephrine was readded ($\blacksquare$). The contractile effect of epinephrine was about 90% inhibited, as was the metabolic effect. This is taken to indicate that stimulus artifact effects of beta-adrenergic actions on the metabolic response were essentially negligible. The venous segment was then progressively activated with increasing concentrations of histamine ($\triangle$), describing the same linear correlation between J_{O_2} and ΔP_o as epinephrine. The muscle was then shortened in the presence of supramaximal histamine in four steps, allowing a measurement of J_{O_2} at each progressively smaller level of isometric tension maintenance ($\blacktriangle$) until, at L = 0.8 cm, active isometric tension was nearly fully abolished. At this zero active force length J_{O_2} remained somewhat elevated above the basal J_{O_2} level. This tension-independent activation energy was the same for both histamine and epinephrine ($\bullet$). again suggesting that specific pharmacologic actions of the drugs used on aerobic metabolism were negligible. The vertical arrow between the two lines shown indicates an hypothetical isotonic contraction of the preparation from a state approximately one-half maximally activated at length L = 2.45 cm to a fully activated state at L = 1.30 cm against a constant load of 0.36 kg wt/cm², as discussed in the text.

found to decrease substantially during a contraction in the gut smooth muscle taenia coli from guinea pig {59} and rabbit {22}, and in bladder smooth muscle from rabbit {21}. In many gut smooth muscles, control of oxidative phosphorylation may occur by similar mechanisms as in skeletal muscle, i.e., involving changes in the levels of high-energy phosphates (e.g., ADP, phosphorylation potential, etc.). However, in many vascular smooth muscle preparations, under many conditions, no observable change in PCr occurs during a contraction with an increase in oxygen consumption. In hog carotid artery, no change in the total high-energy phosphates (PCr + ATP), measured biochemically, was observable during a contraction that resulted in a doubling of oxygen consumption {18}.

In sheep aorta, during a depolarizing contraction with glucose as substrate, no change in PCr or ATP was observed using ^{31}P-NMR despite a stimulation of oxidative metabolism {19}. Hence, in many vascular smooth muscles, the control of oxidative metabolism appears to occur without a change in the levels of high-energy phosphates and hence without any change in the free [ADP].

Most measurements of respiratory control in vascular smooth muscle utilize tissues having glucose as the sole exogenous metabolic substrate. However, based on studies in cardiac muscle {60}, it is known that the nature of the available substrate may affect the relative role of changes in high-energy phosphates in respiratory control. In sheep aorta, when the glycolytic inhibitor 2-deoxyglucose was substituted for glucose in the bathing media, oxygen consumption was stimulated while PCr decreased and free [ADP] increased {19}. The effect was not directly the result of inhibition of glycolysis, since contractions with no substrate (no glucose) in the bathing solution induced no change in high-energy phosphates despite the stimulation of oxygen consumption. 2-deoxyglucose acts as a phosphate sink, thereby driving down PCr and ATP and resulting in an increased free [ADP]. Thus sheep aorta, and perhaps other vascular smooth muscles, can accomplish a control of oxidative phosphorylation by at least two classes of mechanisms, one dependent and the other independent of changes in the levels of high-energy phosphates. The metabolic state of the cell may play a key role in determining which class of mechanism(s) predominates in the control of oxidative phosphorylation.

AEROBIC GLYCOLYSIS

In well-oxygenated resting mammalian skeletal muscles, the steady production of lactic acid is rather small, ranging in the literature from 5 to 50 nmol lactate/min/g tissue {17,44,45}, as compared to a resting O_2 consumption rate of 150–300 nmol/min/g tissue. In general, the contribution of aerobic glycolysis to total ATP production rate in the resting muscle does not exceed 5%, and the bulk of the glucose or glycogen utilized is metabolized aerobically. In the early phase of skeletal muscular activity, before the onset of recovery metabolism, lactate production may increase substantially. Over longer term tetani, however, or averaged over the full period of recovery metabolism (several minutes), lactate production increases by factors only 2–4 times over the basal production rate. O_2 consumption rates, on the other hand, increase by factors typically 20- to 30-fold so that the energetics of both steady-state and/or recovery metabolism in support of mechanical activity in mammalian skeletal muscles is almost entirely oxidative.

In vascular smooth muscle, the situation is somewhat different. It has been known for some time that vascular smooth muscles maintain unusually high levels of lactic acid production {28}, even in well-oxygenated in vitro preparations. In earlier reports it was speculated that this reflected some sort of tissue damage. Most recent studies, obtained under conditions suitable to maintain healthy smooth muscle tissue in vitro, consistently report high levels of aerobic glycolysis (cf. Lundholm et al. {61} for a review). Substantial levels of aerobic glycolysis have been reported for a wide variety of smooth muscle types, including uterine, intestinal, and tracheal smooth muscles {1–7,61,62}.

For blood vessels with basal O_2 consumption rates in the range of 50–200 nmol O_2/min/g, typical resting aerobic lactic acid production rates are in the range of 100–250 nmol lactate/min/g, with a steady-state ratio of 1–2 moles lactate produced per mole O_2 consumed being most common. In terms of ATP production, this is a highly inefficient system. If glucose were the sole substrate, it can be calculated that this molar ratio of 1–2 means that 75–85% of the glucose equivalents utilized are metabolized only to lactic acid. The 15–25% of the remaining glucose, if completely oxidized, nonetheless would provide the bulk of the total ATP production (70–80%) due to the much higher ATP production per glucose molecule of oxidative metabolism.

In the earliest study examining in detail the role of aerobic glycolysis in the support of mechanical activity in vascular smooth muscle, Peterson and Paul {50} found that both O_2 consumption and lactic acid production rates increased linearly in response to increasing isometric tension development and energy demand. The proportion of ATP produced oxidatively and glycolytically remained approximately constant (that is, 25–30% of the total ATP production was ascribable to aerobic glycolysis and concomitant lactic acid production), regardless of the level of mechanical activity. In addition, this was found to be the case whether isometric force was varied by varying the level of pharmacological activation or by varying the length of the muscle at fixed supramaximal pharmacological activation.

These observations led to a fairly simple sort of picture in which the ATP produced by oxidative and glycolytic metabolism entered continuously into a pool of available ATP, which was then drawn upon more or less uniformly by the various intracellular ATPases, as needed. The observed fixed stoichiometry between oxidative and glycolytic metabolism was then, hypothetically at least, due to some undefined metabolic regulatory features {61}. More recent studies, however, beginning with that of Glück and Paul {52}, indicate that this naive picture is incorrect. In particular, evidence has accumulated that lactic acid production in VSM is a metabolic feature specifically coupled to the support of particular cellular activities. Precisely what activities are involved and how this coupling is effected are currently matters of some debate and are dealt with in more detail in the next section. It has become increasingly clear over the past several years that oxidative metabolism and aerobic glycolysis can vary independently, and often in opposing directions, depending on the conditions (for review see Paul et al. {2,9,14}).

COMPARTMENTATION OF CARBOHYDRATE METABOLISM IN VSM

As just described, vascular smooth muscle manifests a high degree of lactic acid production, even in well-oxygenated in vitro preparations. On the surface, this inefficiency of carbohydrate metabolism might be viewed as a metabolic defect. However, a growing body of evidence leads to the conclusion that oxidative metabolism and glycolytic metabolism may operate independently and, at times, support different classes of cell functions. Thus the apparent inefficiency of smooth muscle lactate production may really be a consequence of a compartmentalized metabolism-function coupling. In this section we will briefly summarize some of the results that have help define the roles for glycolysis and oxidative metabolism in smooth muscle.

Some of the first studies demonstrating separate regulation, and possible separate roles for glycolysis and oxidative phosphorylation, were those of Paul et al. {63}, who found in hog coronary arteries that addition of K^+ stimulates aerobic glycolysis (i.e., at constant external Na^+), while ouabain and K^+-free or Na^+-free bathing medium depress aerobic glycolysis. Ouabain, moreover, increases isometric force in these vessels, which is correlated with an increase in J_{O_2} concomitant with the decrease in J_{lac}. On the other hand, there are experimental conditions under which force and J_{O_2} decrease, whereas J_{lac} and the Na^+ pump are elevated. For example, in porcine coronary arteries {30}, isoproterenol relaxes a KCl-induced contracture, and J_{O_2} shows a parallel decrease, whereas J_{lac}, and presumably the Na^+ pump {64}, remain elevated. Similarly, readmission of K^+ to tissues incubated in K^+-free medium stimulates aerobic glycolysis while decreasing force and J_{O_2} in porcine vessels {65,67}, presumably due to stimulation of Na^+-K^+ transport. On this basis, it was then proposed that the energy production of aerobic glycolysis is somehow specifically coupled to the Na^+-K^+ transport system of vascular smooth muscles. A coupling between glycolysis and the Na^+ pump based on similar data has also been suggested for rat aorta {66}. In further support of this hypothesis, Campbell and Paul {67} have shown in porcine carotid artery over a wide range of K^+-transport rates that glycolytic ATP production varied approximately stoichiometrically with K^+ transport. These results indicate that glycolytic support of the Na/K pump may be stoichiometric over much of the physiological range.

In hog carotid arteries, Peterson observed a similar dissociation of lactic acid production from the energy cost of isometric tension maintenance with high-K^+ activation. With maintained activation via high-K^+ depolarization (50% K^+ for Na^+ substitution), varying the level of isometric tension development by altering the concentration of extracellular Ca^{2+} exerted no consistent effect on aerobic glycolysis, which simply remained at or near the resting level {53}. Adding histamine to the already K^+-depolarized artery segment, however, led to a sharp increase in aerobic glycolysis {54} to nearly the same value as that reported for histamine activation alone {52}.

During progressive removal and replacement of extracellular Ca^{2+} in arteries supramaximally stimulated with high K^+ plus added histamine, the level of aerobic glycolysis correlated linearly with the Ca^{2+}-activated stable isometric force. On this basis, it was suggested that the energy production of aerobic glycolysis may be coupled to intracellular or plasma membrane Ca^{2+} pumps that are responsible for the sequestration and homeostasis of intracellular $[Ca^{2+}]$. This was proposed, at least in part, since one well-known action of the H_2 receptor for histamine is predominantly vasodilatory, suggesting that histamine can activate intracellular Ca^{2+} sequestration or transmembrane extrusion (cf. Peterson {54}). A similar coupling between the energy requirements of the Ca^{2+} pump and glycolysis has been proposed by Lundholm and colleagues {6}.

The proposed coupling between glycolytically produced ATP and Ca-pump activity has been recently investigated in some detail. Since glycolysis was presumed to support membrane ATP-requiring processes, and since glycolytic enzymes had been shown to be associated with the plasma membrane in other tissues {68–72}, glycolytic support of membrane ATP-requiring processes should be demonstrable in an isolated plasma membrane preparation. In an isolated plasma membrane preparation from smooth muscle, glycolytic substrates and cofactors were sufficient to support calcium pump activity as measured by Ca^{2+} uptake of inside-out membrane vesicles {73}. These results demonstrate both that the glycolytic enzyme pathway is associated with the plasma membrane and that the membrane-associated glycolysis could support one of the membrane ion pumps. In the plasmalemmal vesicle preparation, glycolysis could support the calcium pump independent of the total [ATP] measured in the vesicle suspension {74}. In addition, at low total [ATP], glycolysis supported a greater extent of Ca^{2+} uptake than ATP added exogenously at matched ATP production rates. Therefore, glycolytically produced ATP is preferentially utilized by the smooth muscle calcium pump. The conclusions from these studies appear to extrapolate to the intact smooth muscle. In a porcine carotid artery preparation with glycogen stores depleted, the concentration of norepinephrine required for half-maximal contraction was decreased when glucose was removed from the bathing media {75}. In addition, after intracellular stores of calcium were depleted by precontractions in the absence of extracellular calcium, readmission of 2.5 mM calcium to the medium resulted in a higher tension transient in the absence of glucose compared to in the presence of glucose. Therefore, glycolytically produced ATP appears to be necessary for normal calcium homeostasis based on experiments using isolated and intact smooth muscle systems.

These two proposals that glycolysis may preferentially support the Na pump and that glycolysis may preferentially support the Ca pump may not be at all mutually exclusive. Indeed, both proposals may be reconciled with the view that the glycolytic ATP production may fuel multiple ATP-requiring processes localized at the plasma membrane. For example, in the plasma membrane vesicle preparation from smooth muscle, ATP produced by other plasma membrane-associated kinases were able to support

calcium pump function comparably to membrane-associated glycolysis {74}. Both pyruvate kinase and creatine kinase fueled the calcium pump independent of changes in the [ATP] in suspension and to a similar extent as the membrane associated glycolytic enzyme system. Therefore, all of the membrane-associated kinases preferentially support the calcium pump compared to ATP exogenously provided. A specific coupling between each kinase and the calcium pump is unlikely. Rather, all membrane-associated kinases may contribute to a pool of ATP that fuels membrane-associated ATP-requiring processes in a preferential manner compared to ATP produced away from the membrane.

The correlation between oxidative metabolism and isometric force, and that between aerobic glycolysis and the energy requirements of membrane ion pumps, underlie the hypothesis that energy metabolism is functionally compartmentalized. The ability of oxidative metabolism and aerobic glycolysis to vary independently has been demonstrated for a variety of other smooth muscle preparations {76–80} and suggests that this functional compartmentation of energy metabolism may reflect a biochemical compartmentation of enzyme cascades. Glycolytic enzymes are localized to the plasma membrane in smooth muscle, and the glycolytically produced ATP preferentially supports membrane associated ATPases such as ion pumps. ATP produced by oxidative phosphorylation appears to support contractile function. A colocalization of ATP supply with ATP demand my underlie both the preferential nature of locally produced ATP in supporting local ATPases but also the separate regulation and roles of the two ATP-producing systems of glycolysis and oxidative phosphorylation.

Although glucose utilization (glycolysis) may be functionally compartmentalized from oxidative metabolism, under many conditions glycogen metabolism (glycogenolysis) appears to correlate with contractile activity and hence oxidative metabolism {33}. Indeed, glycogen phosphorylase activity is well correlated with contractility {30,31}. A consequence of these observations may be that the pathways for glucose metabolism and for glycogen metabolism may be separate under many conditions. Work by Lynch and Paul {29} demonstrated that when glucose was labeled uniformly with ^{14}C, the lactate produced had almost exactly the same specific activity, despite a decline in the total tissue glycogen content. If the glycogen was unlabeled, then a dilution of the specific activity in the lactate would be expected if the pathways for glucose utilization and for glycogen utilization freely mixed. These experiments suggested that there may be separate pools of glycolytic and glycogenolytic intermediates in smooth muscle. Further studies demonstrated two pools of one glycolytic intermediate, glucose-6-phosphate {81}.

Recent work using ^{13}C-NMR provides further support of the idea that the pathways for glycolysis and glycogenolysis may be separable. ^{13}C-NMR techniques offer some distinct advantages over classical radioisotope techniques. Although NMR is not as sensitive as radiotracer methodologies, ^{13}C-NMR offers additional information. Using

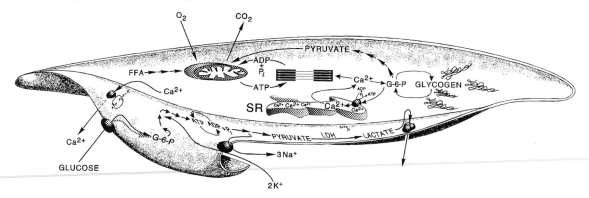

Fig. 56-4. Model of smooth muscle indicating the proposed compartmentation of metabolism and function. Energy-requiring processes associated with membrane function, such as the Na, K pump or Ca pump, are supplied with ATP by a membrane-associated glycolytic cascade. Glucose is the primary substrate for this pathway with lactate the major end product. There is evidence that suggests a similar colocalization of membrane ion pumps and glycolytic enzymes may also be found for internal membrane structures as the sarcoplasmic reticulum (SR). In contrast, the energy requirements for actin-myosin interaction appear to be supported primarily by mitochondrial oxidative phosphorylation. Free fatty acids (FFA) appear to be the major substrate, but a separate glycolytic enzyme cascade, utilizing glycogen but not glucose, also plays a role in this compartment.

^{13}C-NMR one can determine what compound is labeled and at what position the compound is labeled. Therefore, tagging glycolytic and glycogenolytic substrates at different positions allows investigations of the precise metabolic fates of the substrates. By labeling smooth muscle glycogen stores at a different position than glucose in the bathing medium, it was determined there was a simultaneous yet separable flux for glycolysis and glycogenolysis {82}. Although both glucose and glycogen were labeled (at different positions in the molecule), lactate was produced solely from glucose despite complete utilization of labeled glycogen stores. The label from glycogen disappeared from the NMR spectrum, presumably because the end product was labile. The labile product was likely to have been CO_2 produced by oxidation of the pyruvate produced by glycogenolysis. Thus the pyruvate produced from glycogenolysis was utilized by oxidative phosphorylation, whereas the pyruvate produced by glycolysis was catabolized to lactate. These two pathways share nine common enzymes and 10 common intermediates, yet the intermediates do not freely mix. Based on these data, and the observed coupling between the Na^+ pump and J_{lac}, we suggested a model (fig. 56-4) in which membrane-bound glycolytic enzymes in close opposition to the Na^+,K^+-ATPase formed one compartment, whereas glycogenolysis and the respiratory machinery were more closely associated with the contractile filaments. Indeed, glycolytic enzymes have been recently localized to the contractile apparatus in smooth muscle {83}. The lack of mixing of the intermediates of glycolysis and glycogenolysis may be the result of the two pathways having different locations in the smooth muscle cell.

An important feature of the organization of metabolism in vascular smooth muscle is that the compartmentation of ATP and of intermediates of carbohydrate metabolism is not absolute. When intact artery preparations are con-

tracted while oxidative metabolism is completely inhibited by NaCN, lactate is produced from both glucose and glycogen {82}. This result is consistent with a mixing of glycolytic intermediates during at least one step in the reaction sequence when the rate of mitochondrial utilization of pyruvate (derived from glycogen) was inhibited. The compartmentation of ATP pools also does not appear to be absolute. When the Na/K pump rate of intact hog carotid arteries was progressively stimulated above a typical physiological rate, glycolytically produced ATP ceased being the sole ATP source for the Na/K pump, as oxidatively produced ATP progressively accounted for a greater share of the ATP provision for the pump {67}. These observations fit well into a model of compartmentation of small metabolites and may be the result of a local balance between production and consumption; that is, for example, with a close juxtaposition of ATP-producing and -consuming enzymes, the local reaction rate may normally dominate the rate of diffusion away from the ATPase. However, when there exists a mismatch between local production and consumption, diffusion away from the production locus will become more pronounced. Hence the compartmentation observable in smooth muscle does not appear to rely on strict diffusion limitations; rather, it depends on a local balance of reaction and diffusion rates.

This reaction/diffusion model for the coupling of colocalized producing and consuming enzymes in smooth muscle may be a reflection of a more general feature of cell energetics. In cardiac muscle, for example, there is growing evidence for a specific role for glycolysis in the supply of ATP to ATP-responsive potassium channels {84}.

CHEMICAL ENERGY UTILIZATION
AND CONTRACTILE ACTIVITY

Resting vascular smooth muscle consumes ATP at a rate typically 0.5–1.0 μmol ATP/min/g tissue. The bulk of this ATP requirement is met, typically 70–90%, from oxidative metabolism and 10–30% from aerobic glycolysis {4}. Upon maximal activation at muscle lengths near optimal for isometric force development, the total steady-state ATP utilization rate increases by a factor of two or so in isolated VSM preparations. The difference between the initial resting metabolic rate and the maximally activated metabolic rate reflects the sum of all energy-consuming processes activated in parallel with or consequent to the mechanical activation. An underlying assumption in this method of measuring contractile energetics is, of course, that the energy requirements of basal processes remain more or less constant during the period of mechanical activity. Most evidence, albeit indirect, indicates this to be the case for pharmacological or ionic methods of stimulation {51–54} (figs. 56-2 and 56-3).

The increased ATP utilization rate upon mechanical activation can be conceptualized, at least, as occurring in three separate parts: (a) actomyosin ATPase in support of mechanical activity, (b) ATP-dependent processes that play some role in initiating and maintaining the activation processes underlying mechanical activity, and (c) all other ATPases activated through the particular means of stimulation chosen. In the more recent studies of smooth muscle energetics, some effort has been made to sort out the quantitative subdivision of the total increase in ATPase into these three categories. In many cases, the third category (which is roughly equivalent to a stimulus artifact) appears to make only a small to negligible contribution to the overall increase in tissue metabolism {51, 52,54} (cf. also fig. 56-3). The first category is most frequently approximated by the *tension-dependent* metabolism, which is measured by determining how suprabasal energy metabolism changes as the actomyosin interaction (i.e., force development) is varied. During such measurements, the level of stimulation (that is, in essence, the variable components of categories 2 and 3) is held fixed. If, at constant supramaximal stimulation, for example, the muscle is lengthened or shortened to lengths where tension development is abolished, the tension-dependent ATPase by definition goes to zero and the remaining suprabasal metabolism is called the *tension-independent* metabolism. This division assumed that changes in length per se do not affect the level of stimulation or their energy dependence. There is some evidence that length can influence activation parameters {85}.

An example of energy partition from measurements of O_2 consumption performed with a single segment of bovine mesenteric vein {86} is shown in fig. 56-3, which additionally illustrates the invariance of such measurements to the particular pharmacological agonist used. Upon supramaximal activation with epinephrine (10^{-6} M) at the optimal length for force generation (L = 2.45 cm for this sample), the O_2 consumption rate increased by 110 nmol min/g over the initial resting O_2 consumption rate

of about 140 nmol O_2/min/g. Progressive stepwise shortening of the muscle from this length with supramaximal histamine as a stimulant caused a decline in isometric tension maintenance as expected from the force-length relationship. This, in turn, led to a linearly correlated decline in the suprabasal O_2 consumption rate (upper line). When the muscle had freely shortened to L = 0.8 cm so that no isometric tension was evident, the O_2 consumption rate remained elevated over the basal rate by about 25 nmol O_2/min/g. This value, the tension-independent metabolism, is about 20% of the total suprabasal ATPase at maximum isometric tension and was not dependent on whether epinephrine or histamine was used to affect the stimulation. Simultaneous measurements of suprabasal aerobic glycolysis {50,87} gave similar values for the tension-independent component of aerobic glycolysis in bovine mesenteric vein.

Figure 56-3 also provides an opportunity to demonstrate the economy of circulatory regulation by vascular smooth muscle. Suppose the vessel segment of fig. 56-3 were at a vessel radius equivalent to the segment length L = 2.45 cm and partially activated so as to maintain that vessel caliber against a blood pressure equivalent to a wall tension of 0.36 kg wt/cm². Maintaining the pressure in the vessel constant, but maximally activating the vascular smooth muscle, would, for the particular sample of fig. 56-3, cause the vessel to shorten to a length of approximately L = 1.30 cm (as indicated by the vertical arrow). For the cylindrical blood vessel, this length change is equivalent to a reduction in caliber of about 45%. Using Pouiselle's Law to compute the change in flow resistance of the vessel, this amounts to a 12-fold increase in flow resistance. In terms of energy cost, however, the increased energy metabolism necessary to support the muscular activity for this circulatory regulation is less than 15% of the resting basal metabolism. Apparently, the energy cost of regulating peripheral circulation is very low.

The tension-independent metabolism discussed above reflects terms in both categories 2 and 3, as well as the possibility of some residual activated ATP hydrolysis by actomyosin, which nonetheless makes no contribution to tension development. Such a situation could arise, for example, through the generation of internally opposing forces that result in no net external force. That such an "internal load" might be the case is indicated by studies of vascular smooth muscle mechanics {88,89}. Huxley and Simmons {88} proposed that muscle stiffness is a direct measure of the number of actin-myosin crossbridges formed at any instant during mechanical activity. A comparison of resting stiffness (due to inert structural components) with the stiffness found at the extremes of length where active tension development is abolished could indicate the extent to which actin and myosin still interact. In studies of this sort with several arterial preparations, Pfitzer and Peterson {90} found that during the rise of isometric tension following stimulation, arterial wall stiffness increased in direct proportion to the isometric force developed. The same linear proportionality also applied between stable isometric force and stiffness when isometric force was varied by varying the extracellular [Ca^{2+}] in the high-

K^+ bathing medium {91}. These observations suggest that isometric tension and actomyosin interaction in VSM are indeed directly related. In hog carotid artery segments, maximally activated and at their freely shortened length so that no isometric tension was measurable, stiffness was elevated by some 10–15% above the purely passive stiffness, and this component required Ca^{2+} in the bathing medium {Peterson, unpublished observation}. This is indicative that at least a fraction of the tension-independent ATPase could be attributable to an actomyosin ATPase.

Measurements of the steady-state suprabasal energy metabolism and estimates of the actomyosin ATPase of vascular smooth muscles, determined as the tension-dependent ATPase, are presented in table 56-2. Comparisons of the contractile ATPase of the intact preparation determined in this way with that of the ATPase of purified isolated VSM actomyosin, while approximate at best, are in reasonable agreement {4,92,93}. From studies of the above sorts, two principal conclusions arise: (a) Despite the ability to develop forces comparable to or even greater than skeletal and cardiac muscles, the in situ activated ATPase of vascular smooth muscle actomyosin is extremely small. (b) The investment of energy in processes necessary to maintain the activation of contractile activity is substantial, on the order of 15–30% of the energy requirement of the actomyosin itself at maximal tension development. It is interesting to note this percentage holds for both smooth and skeletal muscle, which indicates that in absolute terms the energy cost of activation or tension-independent processes is considerably higher in striated than smooth muscle.

The extraordinary economy of tension maintenance in vascular smooth muscle and the detailed nature of the activation processes mentioned above are areas of intense interest in VSM physiology. An additional discussion of *activation energetics* is given in a subsequent section. The very low *tension cost* (or, alternatively, the high *holding economy*) of vascular smooth muscle appears to reside primarily in the molecular properties of the actomyosin itself, although structural and geometric factors may also play some part {92–96}. Barany {97} first described an inherent correlation between the ATPase activities of various myosins and the contractile velocities of the muscles from which the myosins originated. Vascular smooth muscle appears to be the slowest of all mammalian muscles in terms of its shortening velocity {96}, and this mechanical property appears to be a direct reflection of how slowly the actomyosin crossbridges hydrolyze ATP in going through their repetitive cycle of interaction with actin filaments. From comparisons of the actomyosin content of vascular smooth muscles and the observed rates of the tension-dependent metabolism, it has been estimated that the VSM myosin crossbridge goes through its cycle of interaction with actin filaments in about 0.75–1.5 seconds {92–95}. This is an extraordinarily slow rate of interaction when compared to skeletal muscle crossbridges, which are estimated to cycle at rates more like 100–150 times per second.

If the smooth muscle myosin crossbridge spends a large fraction of this very long cycle time in contact with the actin filament in the force-generating configuration, then the high holding economy of the tissue is not difficult to appreciate. A schematic representation of this model of the actomyosin crossbridge cycle is shown in fig. 56-5. The steady-state rate of a single myosin crossbridge is the sum of the time required to make one full pass through states 2, 3, 4, 5, and back to state 2. State 4, however, generates isometric tension so that the average tension maintained by a large number of crossbridges interacting asynchronously is proportional to the time spent in state 4 as a fraction of the total cycle time. Marston and Taylor {98}, in using purified myosins from four different types of

*Table 56-2. Supra*basal energy metabolism of isometrically contracted VSM

Preparation	(1) Total suprabasal metabolism µmol ATP/min/g kg wt/cm^2 force	(2) Tension-dependent metabolism µmol ATP/min/g kg wt/cm^2 force	(3) Tension-independent metabolism µmol ATP/min/g	Stimulus	Ref
Bovine mesenteric vein	1.64	1.28	0.20	Epi, NE, Hist	49–51
Hog carotid artery	0.68	0.43	0.27	Hist	52
	0.81	0.46	0.23	K^+	52
	0.40			K^+	53
	0.51			K^+ + Hist	54
Bovine mesenteric artery	1.22	1.12	0.11	Epi	6
	0.66			K^+	
Rat aorta	1.97			K^+	55
Bovine carotid artery	0.82			Electrical	23

In column (1), total *supra*basal metabolism has been divided by the observed isometric tension with the mode of stimulation indicated. Column (2) is that part of the total suprabasal metabolism that vanishes when isometric tension is abolished (but stimulation maintained), normalized to the isometric force. Column (2) is frequently taken as representative of the actomyosin ATPase, to the extent that force represents the quantity of activated actomyosin. Column (3) is the steady-state suprabasal metabolism required to maintain activation. Epi = epinephrine; NE = norepinephrine; Hist = histamine.

vertebrate muscles (including gizzard smooth muscle), have found that the time required for ATP to dissociate the smooth muscle crossbridge from actin (state 4–5 in fig. 56-5) is by far the slowest, but not nearly slow enough to fully account for the very high holding economy of smooth muscle relative to the other muscle types. Precisely what features of smooth muscle myosin are responsible for these inherent differences in the enzymatic activities and kinetics of otherwise apparently quite similar molecules is currently not understood.

SOME UNRESOLVED ISSUES

Holding economy and activation energetics

A picture of the actomyosin crossbridge cycle in which the overall cycle time of the crossbridge determines the actomyosin ATPase, while the fraction of the cycle time spent in the tension-generating state determines the force developed, yields, in a relatively direct way, the holding economy of the system. In this very simplified model, however, any factors (biochemical, mechanical, or otherwise) that alter the fraction of the full cycle time that the crossbridge spends in the tension-generating state could alter the observed holding economy of the tissue (cf. fig. 56-5).

Murphy and colleagues {99–108} reported such a phenomenon in vascular smooth muscle and have termed it the *latch state*. They determined the shortening velocity of hog carotid artery as a function of time during the development and maintenance of isometric tension. The maximum rate at which the muscle is capable of shortening, which is often taken as a direct index of the speed of the individual crossbridge cycle rate, became progressively slower over a period of 5–20 minutes following the activation of mechanical activity. Driska et al. {102} and Aksoy et al. {103} have found a similar decrease in myosin light chain phosphorylation with the duration of stimulation, despite the near constant maintenance of isometric force. This temporal correlation is suggestive of the possibility that myosin phosphorylation, in addition to its postulated role as a regulator of the smooth muscle actomyosin interaction (cf. Hartshorne {109} for a review), acts as a modulator of the speed of the smooth muscle actomyosin crossbridge cycle. In their model, phosphorylated myosin crossbridges are dissociated from actin filaments much more rapidly than dephosphorylated myosin crossbridges. This model is illustrated schematically by the dashed lines in fig. 56-5. If this is the case, one would expect the holding economy of highly phosphorylated VSM myosin to be less than that of active but dephosphorylated VSM myosin.

Recent evidence on hog carotid artery supports this hypothesis. Krisanda and Paul {24} measured both suprabasal J_{O_2} and unloaded shortening velocity at various points during the development and maintenance of isometric force. As shown in fig. 56-6, both parameters displayed similar, though not superimposable, biphasic

responses. Each of these parameters can be used to estimate the crossbridge cycle rate, and their decline with time of stimulation is similar to that of myosin light chain phosphorylation. The holding economy as well as velocity in these experiments differed from their maximum value by two- to threefold. Thus, even if extrapolated to account for the maximum possible differences in myosin phosphorylation, this mechanism is unlikely to account for the 100- to 2000-fold difference in holding economy between striated and smooth muscle. It is of interest to note that Butler and Siegman {5} also reported that the rate of phosphagen breakdown and velocity in rabbit taenia coli also showed a similar dependence on the duration of stimulation. However, they concluded that this behavior was unlikely to be dependent on myosin light chain phosphorylation.

While myosin phosphorylation, J_{ATP}, and V_{max} do show similar time courses, the question is whether these relations are correlative or causal. An underlying assumption is that this transient in J_{ATP} is related to actin-myosin interaction and not a transient in energy utilization ascribable to activation processes. Such processes would differ from that underlying the steady-state tension-independent metabolism, as described in the section, *Chemical energy utilization and contractile activity*. This energy utilization is a durable component, persisting throughout contractile activity and apparently associated more closely with the maintenance of the activated state of the muscle than with the actual actomyosin ATPase that generates contractile activity. Most frequently, these energy costs are ascribed to processes such as ATP-dependent Ca^{2+} translocation, other altered energy-dependent ion fluxes, protein phosphorylation-dephosphorylation cycles, and other miscellaneous processes {4}.

It has now been repeatedly observed using a variety of methodologies in vascular smooth muscles {2,6,23,24}, other smooth muscles {5}, as well as fast mammalian skeletal muscles {17} that the initiation and development of isometric tension is energetically far more costly than the steady-state maintenance of isometric tension (even when including the above-mentioned steady-state activation energy).

It is possible that this excess energy utilization is related to some form of intrinsic internal work performed by the actomyosin systems in stretching internal elastic elements during the development of isometric force, a term that might be essentially similar in all muscle types. For both the taenia coli {5} and hog carotid artery {24}, this has proven unlikely. Energy utilization has been measured during the redevelopment of isometric force following a fast shortening step that discharged all maintained isometric force. In both cases, the redevelopment of isometric force required no measurable excess energy utilization beyond the observed force maintenance state. This argues that only the activation of tension development from the resting state requires excess high-energy phosphate utilization. Evidence supporting the assumption that this transient excess in J_{ATP} is related to actin-myosin interaction was provided by Krisanda and Paul {24}. They showed that this transient was significantly reduced when

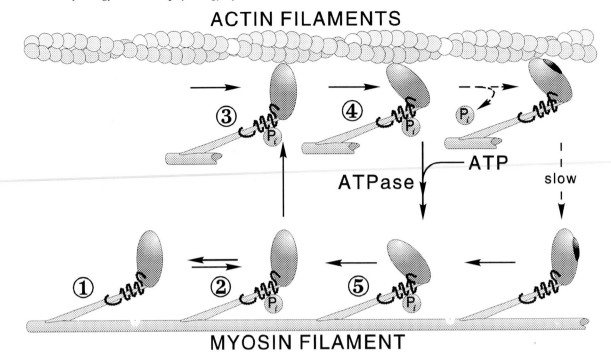

Fig. 56-5. A schematic model of the smooth muscle myosin crossbridge interaction with actin filaments is depicted. The transition from state 1 to state 2 represents the Ca^{2+}-calmodulin-dependent phosphorylation-dephosphorylation activation mechanism proposed for smooth muscle regulation. The cycle of interaction (states 2–5) hydrolyzes 1 ATP molecule and generates 1 quantum of tension with each pass. Only the angulated attached myosin crossbridge (state 4), however, generates isometric force. The inherent speed of the cycle is much slower in smooth than in striated muscle, with the ATP-dependent dissociation step (state 4–5) apparently being slowest. The dashed lines indicate formation of a proposed dephosphorylated actomyosin cross-bridge {105,106}, which then dissociates only very slowly and may be responsible for the very high holding economy of vascular smooth muscle.

the muscle was activated at lengths at which little active force was developed.

Whereas isometric force increases monotonically to a maintained maximal value after stimulation, many processes decline from maximal values during the steady phase of force maintenance. These include J_{ATP}, Vmax, myosin phosphorylation — as we have seen — phosphorylase *a* activity {110,111}, and importantly, intracellular Ca^{2+} concentration {112}. An understanding of the role of Ca^{2+} is clearly central. At high extracellular Ca^{2+} concentrations (5–7.5 mM), both Vmax and energy utilization are increased to a greater degree than isometric force {8,113}. Under these nonphysiological conditions, the linear relation between force and J_{O_2} was not invariant, and the tension cost increased at these high Ca^{2+} levels. The implication of these studies was that crossbridge number and cycle rate could be independently regulated.

A variable and regulatable holding economy in vascular smooth muscle was reported by Peterson {54}, who showed that the addition of histamine to hog carotid arteries already stimulated with high K^+ leads to an approximate 25% increase in the tension cost of stable isometric force, even when compared at the identical levels of isometric

tension. Data from Aksoy et al. {103} indicate that in the steady phase of isometric contraction, myosin light chain phosphorylation with high K^+ as activator is only about 18% of the total myosin. With histamine as activator, however, the more-or-less stable level of myosin phosphorylation is around 45%. If the "latch" model is correct, these extra, more rapidly cycling, crossbridges due to histamine activation could be the source of the excess tension cost in Peterson's experiments.

While the change in V_{max} correlated well with myosin phosphorylation in porcine carotid artery {103}, changes in energy utilization and V_{max} at high Ca^{2+} were not correlated with myosin phosphorylation in guinea pig taenia coli {5}. What is certain is that crossbridge number and cycle rate can be independently modulated in both striated and smooth muscle. Thus the simple notion that muscle stiffness, ATPase, and force development are all simply more or less equivalent measures of the number of activated myosin crossbridges is no longer tenable.

Energetics of work-producing contractions: Efficiency

ATP utilization under conditions in which the muscle is producing work is of particular interest to those concerned

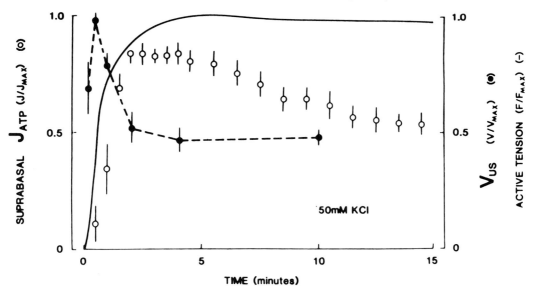

Fig. 56-6. The time course of suprabasal J_{ATP} (O), active isometric force (solid line) and unloaded shortening velocity (V_{us}, ●) in hog carotid artery following stimulation by increasing media KCl by 50 mM. Adapted from Paul {2} and Krisanda and Paul {24}, with permission.

with muscle energetics. Under conditions of maximum work production, the rate of ATP breakdown is greater in skeletal muscle by up to threefold over the isometric rate {17}. The increase in energy utilization in work-producing contractions over that observed under isometric conditions is often referred to as the *Fenn effect*. Similar studies on taenia coli {114} also show that the ATP breakdown increases by as much as 2.7 times over the isometric rate when actively shortening at loads less than isometric. In vascular tissue, on the other hand, the rate of ATP utilization estimated from measurements of O_2 consumption was not significantly different from the isometric rate when allowed to contract against a load {48} or in isovelocity contractions {115}. More recent experiments of phosphagen breakdown during contractions under conditions of maximal power output in hog carotid artery {116} indicate an increase in J_{ATP} of about threefold over the isometric rate.

The efficiency of muscle during work-producing contractions, i.e., the work produced per unit free energy change, is an energetic parameter closely tied to our understanding of the mechanism of mechano-chemical transduction. Although the tension cost in smooth muscle is substantially less than that of skeletal muscle, this does not appear to be the case in terms of efficiency. Butler et al. {113} reported that for working contractions in rabbit taenia coli, about 4 kJ of work were produced per mole of high-energy phosphagen breakdown. Krisanda and Paul {116} reported similar findings for hog carotid artery. Estimates of the free energy of ATP hydrolysis range from 35 to 50 kJ/mol, which yield an efficiency of about 10% for work production in smooth muscle. This is about four- to fivefold lower than in skeletal muscle {17}. In both of

these studies, a Fenn effect, as in skeletal muscle, was reported.

The effects of calcium on the efficiency of hog carotid artery were reported {117} for contractions in which work was performed after the attainment of a steady state. At low calcium concentration (0.15 mM), unloaded shortening velocity isometric force were lower than that observed at 2.5 mM, as previously reported. No Fenn effect was found at the low calcium concentration. However, and perhaps more important, little change in the efficiency was seen in comparison to the contraction at 2.5 mM calcium or when compared to contractions elicited by both KCl and histamine, conditions designed to maximize the intracellular calcium levels.

It is of interest, in terms of mechanisms of regulation, to know whether the lower velocities and force at low calcium were caused by an "internal load" {89} or were related to a direct effect of calcium on crossbridge cycle rate. Efficiency would be anticipated to be decreased by the presence of a constant internal load. These results thus suggest that the decrease in velocity observed at low extracellular concentrations is not likely to be due to the presence of such an "internal load." This would appear to rule out models in which slowly or noncycling dephosphorylated "latch" bridges were thought to pose such a load. Butler et al. {118} also presented data that indicated that under conditions designed to optimize the effect of an internal load, no change in efficiency was detected in rabbit taenia coli. Thus it is likely that the low efficiency of smooth muscle and the dependence of unloaded shortening velocity on calcium, potentially mediated through myosin light chain phosphorylation, are not due to the presence of an internal load. Clearly, more work needs to be done before the role of these effectors on smooth muscle efficiency can be stated with certainly. It is interesting to note that this is an example of how muscle energetics can play a unique role in distinguishing between various theories of the regulation of smooth muscle contractility.

Energetic consequences and tests of "latch" models

The concept of a modulable crossbridge cycle rate was embodied in terms of a kinetic model proposed by Driska {119} and Hai and Murphy {104}. These four-state models permitted quantitative tests of the validity of this type of latch model. In these models, phosphorylation of

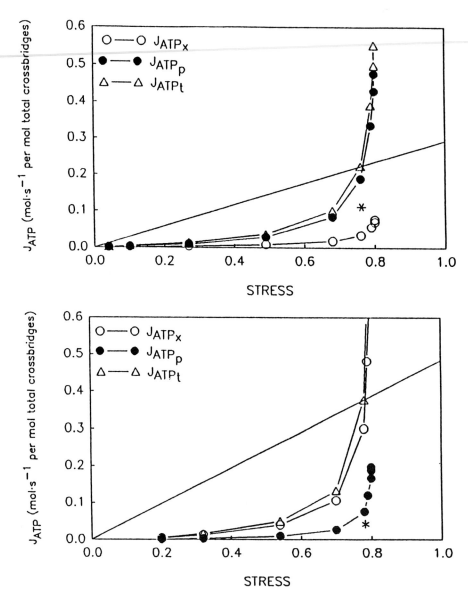

Fig. 56-7. Steady-state rate of ATP utilization as a function of stress. J_{ATP_x}, attributable to crossbridge, J_{ATP_p}, attributable to myosin light chain phosphorylation/dephosphorylation, J_{ATP_t}, J_{ATP_t}, and total ATPase rate. **Upper panel:** Relations predicted from the kinetic constants used by Hai and Murphy {104}. **Lower panel:** Relations predicted from the kinetic constants used by Paul {121} designed to minimize J_{ATP_p} relative to J_{ATP_x}. Both sets of kinetic constants can predict the observed relations for the time dependence of stress and myosin light-chain phosphorylation. Lines represent a linear relation between J_{ATP_t} and stress, plotted through the point (*) for which time course data were used to derive the kinetic constants. These model predictions can be compared to the experimental values given in figs. 56-2 and 56-3. Adapted from Paul {121}, with permission.

myosin light chains (MLC-Pi) is necessary for actin-myosin interaction. A novel aspect is that dephosphorylation of an attached crossbridge was proposed to decrease the rate of detachment, leading to the formation of a "latch" bridge. This model can fit the available data on the time courses of MLC-Pi and isometric force {104} as well as predicting a near-linear dependence of velocity on MLC-Pi {105}, an observation consistent with some, but not all {120}, studies of smooth muscle mechanics. The high economy of tension maintenance and relatively lower efficiency of smooth muscle, described in the previous sections, could also be explained by these kinetic models. The high economy was partly ascribable to the lower cycling of crossbridges in the latch state, whereas the relatively lower efficiency had a rather different and controversial explanation {106}. Hai and Murphy's model {107} predicted that the ATPase associated with the "futile" cycle of myosin light chain phosphorylation/dephosphorylation was the major (85%) fraction of ATP utilization by smooth muscle during contractile activity. Consequently, the work per total ATP hydrolysis might be expected to be lower than skeletal muscle {107}.

This latter consequence of their model conflicted with the more traditional view of smooth muscle energetics (discussed above) in which most (~80%) of the contractile energy utilization was assigned to crossbridge ATPase. This assignment is based on the dependence of energy utilization on muscle length and is subject to the limitations discussed above. In particular, if myosin light chain phosphorylation/dephosphorylation ATP utilization is a type of activation energy, is it dependent on length? However, recent studies of heat production in skinned Fibers {122} would suggest that this futile cycle accounts for less than 15% of the total energy usage.

A more readily testable prediction of this model was the dependence of the rate of contractile ATP utilization as a function of the steady-state level of isometric force generated. The kinetic model of Hai and Murphy {104} was tested by Paul {121,122} and, as shown in fig. 56-7, the predicted relations were highly nonlinear and not compatible with the data shown in fig. 56-2. Using other kinetic constants, Paul reported that several different models could fit the force and MLC-Pi time course data, including those with a lower fraction of myosin light chain phosphorylation/dephosphorylation ATP utilization. However, all were quite nonlinear in terms of the relation between ATP utilization and force. A model with a high crossbridge attachment/detachment rate ratios (fig. 56-5 K4/K3), without invoking latch, could fit both sets of data.

In a more recent studies, Hai and Murphy {108} combined the original four-state model with the Huxley model {123}, which incorporates crossbridge position and permits explicit velocity dependencies to be predicted. In this model, about 50% of total ATP utilization was attributable to myosin light chain phosphorylation/dephosphorylation. Though the relation between ATP utilization and force is curvilinear, there is a region in which ATP utilization is quasilinear with force. In this model ATP utilization would be approximately proportional to MLC-Pi. As force is maximized with MLC-Pi at about 30%, it is possible to

significantly increase ATP utilization at nearly constant levels of force by increasing MLC-Pi. This may explain the observed nonlinearities at high levels of Ca^{2+} {56–58} discussed above. At present, the available data may not permit differentiation between these alternate hypotheses on the basis of energetics. Thus the role of myosin phosphorylation in modulating smooth muscle velocity and energy utilization will likely continue to be the focus of considerable activity in the foreseeable future.

ACKNOWLEDGMENTS

The authors would like to express their indebtedness to Dr. John W. Peterson for his major contributions to the previous editions of this chapter.

REFERENCES

1. Hellstrand P, Paul RJ: Vascular smooth muscle: Relations between energy metabolism and mechanics. In: Crass MF, Barnes CD (eds) *Vascular Smooth Muscle*. New York: Academic Press, 1982, pp 1–35.
2. Paul RJ: Smooth muscle: Mechanochemical energy conversion relations between metabolism and contractility. In: Johnson LR (ed) *Physiology of the Gastrointestinal Tract*, 2nd ed. New York: Raven Press, 1987, pp 483–506.
3. Butler TM, Davies RE: High-energy phosphates in smooth muscle. In: Bohr DF, Somlyo AP, Sparks HV, Geiger SR (eds) *Handbook of Physiology. Section 2: The Cardiovascular System. Vol 2: Vascular Smooth Muscle*. Bethesda, MD: American Physiological Society, 1980, pp 237–252.
4. Paul RJ: Chemical energetics of vascular smooth muscle. In: Bohr DF, Somlyo AP, Sparks HV, Geiger SR (eds) *Handbook of Physiology. Section 2: The Cardiovascular System. Vol 2: Vascular Smooth Muscle*. Bethesda, MD: American Physiological Society, 1980, pp 201–235.
5. Butler TM, Siegman MJ: High-energy phosphate metabolism in vascular smooth muscle. *Ann Rev Physiol* 47: 629–643, 1985.
6. Lundholm L, Petterson G, Andersson RGG, Mohme-Lundholm E: Regulation of the carbohydrate metabolism of smooth muscle: Some current problems. *CRC Biochem Smooth Muscle* 11:85–108, 1983.
7. Paul RJ, Hellstrand P, Krisanda JM: Relations among oxygen consumption, phosphagen and contractility in vascular smooth muscle. In: Stephens NL (ed) *Smooth Muscle Contraction*. New York: Raven Press, 1982, pp 245–257.
8. Paul RJ, Krisanda JM, Lynch RM: Vascular smooth muscle energetics. *J Cardiovasc Pharmacol* 6:S320–S327, 1984.
9. Paul RJ: Smooth muscle energetics. *Ann Rev Physiol* 51: 331–349, 1989.
10. Paul RJ, Elzinga G, Yamada K (eds) *Muscle Energetics*. New York: Alan R. Liss, 1989, pp 1–627.
11. Paul RJ, Strauss JD, Krisanda JM: The effects of calcium on smooth muscle mechanics and energetics. In: Siegman MJ, et al. (ed) *Regulation and Contraction in Smooth Muscle*. New York: Alan R. Liss, 1987, pp 319–332.
12. de Lanerolle P, Paul RJ: Myosin phosphorylation/dephosphorylation and the regulation of airway smooth muscle contractility. *Am J Physiol* 261:L1–L14, 1991.
13. Murphy RA: Section Editor: Special Topic: Contraction in Smooth Muscle Cells. *Ann Rev Physiol* 51:275–350, 1989.

14. Lynch RM, Paul RJ: Functional compartmentation of carbohydrate metabolism. In: Jones D (ed) *Microcompartmentation*. Boca Raton, FL: CRC Press, 1988, pp 17–35.

15. Ishida Y, Paul RJ: Evidence for compartmentation of high energy phosphagens in smooth muscle. In: Paul RJ, Elzinga G, Yamada K (eds) *Muscle Energetics*. New York: Alan R. Liss, 1989, pp 417–428.

16. Paul RJ, Hardin CD, Campbell J, Raeymaekers L: Compartmentation of metabolism and function in smooth muscle. In: Paul RJ, Elzinga G, Yamada K (eds) *Muscle Energetics*. New York: Alan R. Liss, 1989, pp 381–390.

17. Kushmerick MJ: Energetics of muscle Contraction. In: Peachey LD (ed) *Handbook of Physiology. Section 10: Skeletal Muscle*. Bethesda, MD: American Physiological Society, 1983, pp 189–236.

18. Krisanda JM, Paul RJ: High energy phosphate and metabolite content during isometric contraction in porcine carotid artery. *Am J Physiol* 244:C385–C390, 1983.

19. Hardin CD, Wiseman RW, Kushmerick MJ: Vascular oxidative metabolism under different metabolic conditions. *Biochim Biophys Acta* 1133:133–141, 1992.

20. Daemers-Lambert C: Accion du fluoronitrobenzene sur le metabolisme phosphore due muscle lisse arteriel pendant la stimulation electrique (carotide de bovide). *Angiologica* 6:1–12, 1969.

21. Kushmerick MJ, Dillon PF, Meyer RA, Brown TR, Krisanda JM, Sweeney HL: ^{31}P-NMR spectroscopy, chemical analysis, and free Mg^{2+} of rabbit bladder and uterine smooth muscle. *J Biol Chem* 261:14420–14429, 1986.

22. Hellstrand P, Vogel HJ: Phosphagens and intracellular pH in intact rabbit smooth muscle studied by ^{31}P-NMR. *Am J Physiol* 248:C320–C329, 1985.

23. Daemers-Lambert C, Roland J: Metabolisme des esters phosphores pendant le development et le maintien de la tension phasique du muscle lisse arterial (carotides de bovide). *Angiologica* 4:69–87, 1967.

24. Krisanda JM, Paul RJ: Energetics of isometric contraction in porcine carotid artery. *Am J Physiol* 246:C510–C519, 1984.

25. Fisher MJ, Dillon PF: Phenylphosphonate: A ^{31}P-NMR indicator of extracellular pH and volume in the isolated perfused rabbit bladder. *Circ Res* 60:472–477, 1987.

26. Hardin CD, Wiseman RW, Kushmerick MJ: Tension responses of sheep aorta to simultaneous decreases in phosphocreatine, inorganic phosphate, and ATP. *J Physiol (Lond)* 458:139–150, 1992.

27. Kosan RL, Burron AC: Oxygen consumption of arterial smooth muscle as a function of active tone and passive stretch. *Circ Res* 18:79–88, 1966.

28. Kirk JE, Effersoe PG, Chiang SP: The rate of respiration and glycolysis by human and dog aortic tissue. *J Gerontol* 9:10–35, 1954.

29. Lynch RM, Paul RJ: Compartmentation of glycolysis and glycogenolysis in vascular smooth muscle. *Science* 222: 1344–1346, 1983.

30. Paul RJ: The effects of isoproterenol and ouabain on oxygen consumption, lactate production and the activation of phosphorylase in coronary arterial smooth muscle. *Circ Res* 52:683–690, 1983.

31. Namm DH: The activation of glycogen phosphorylase in arterial smooth muscle. *J Pharmacol Exp Ther* 178:299–310, 1971.

32. Lynch RM, Paul RJ: Compartmentation of carbohydrate metabolism in vascular smooth muscle: Effects of different energy loading conditions. *Am J Physiol* 252:C328–C334, 1987.

33. Lynch RM, Kuettner CP, Paul RJ: Glycogen metabolism during tension generation and maintenance in vascular smooth muscle. *Am J Physiol* 257:C736–C742, 1989.

34. Hardin CD, Kushmerick MJ: ^{13}C-NMR assessment of the dynamics and order of vascular glycogen synthesis and mobilization. *J Mol Cell Cardiol*. 24:S25, 1992.

35. Chace KV, Odessey R: The utilization by rabbit aorta of carbohydrates, fatty acids, ketone bodies, and amino acids as substrates for energy production. *Circ Res* 48:850–858, 1981.

36. Zemplenyi T: Enzymes of the arterial wall. *J Atheroscler Res* 2:2–24, 1962.

37. Zemplenyi T, Lojda Z, Mrhova O: Enzymes of the vascular wall in experimental atherosclerosis in the rabbit. In: Sandler M, Bourne GH (eds) *Atherosclerosis and its Origin*. New York: Academic Press, 1963, pp 459–513.

38. Kirk JE: Intermediary metabolism of human arterial tissue and its changes with age and atherosclerosis. In: Sandler M, Bourne GH (eds) *Atherosclerosis and its Origin*. New York: Academic Press, 1963, pp 67–117.

39. Odyssey R, Chase KU: Utilization of endogenous lipid, glycogen and protein by rabbit aorta. *Am J Physiol* 243: H128–H132, 1982.

40. Barron JT, Kopp SJ, Tow JP, Parrillo JE: Differential effects of fatty acids on glycolysis and glycogen metabolism in vascular smooth muscle. *Biochim Biophys Acta* 1093: 125–134, 1991.

41. Vallieres J, Scarpa A, Somlyo AP: Subcellular fractions of smooth muscle. 1. Isolation, substrate utilization and Ca^{2+} transport by main pulmonary artery and mesenteric vein mitochondria. *Arch Biochem Biophys* 170:659–669, 1975.

42. Wrogemmn K, Stephens NL: Oxidative phosphorylation in smooth muscle. In: Stephens NL (ed) *The Biochemistry of Smooth Muscle*. Baltimore, MD: University Park Press, 1977, pp 41–50.

43. Hellstrand P, Paul RJ: Phosphagen content, breakdown during contraction and oxygen consumption in rat portal vein. *Am J Physiol* 744:C250–C258, 1983.

44. Chapman JB, Gibbs CL, Loiselle DS: Myothermic, polargraphic, and fluorometric data from mammalian muscles. *Fed Proc* 41:176–184, 1982.

45. Cerretelli P, Di Prampero PE, Piiper J: Energy balance of anaerobic work in the dog gastrocnemius muscle. *Am J Physiol* 217:581–585, 1969.

46. Stainsby WN, Barclay JK: Relation of load, rest length, work and shortening to oxygen uptake by in situ dog semitendinosus. *Am J Physiol* 221:1238–1242, 1971.

47. Crow MT, Kushmerick MJ: Chemical energetics of slow- and fast-twitch muscles of the mouse. *J Gen Physiol* 79: 147–166, 1982.

48. Hellstrand P: Oxygen consumption and lactate production of the rat portal vein in relation to its contractile activity. *Acta Physiol Scand* 100:91–106, 1977.

49. Paul RJ, Peterson JW, Caplan SR: Oxygen consumption rate in vascular smooth muscle: Relation to isometric tension. *Biochim Biophys Acta* 305:474–480, 1973.

50. Peterson JW, Paul RJ: Aerobic glycolysis in vascular smooth muscle: Relation to isometric tension. *Biochim Biophys Acta* 357:167–176, 1974.

51. Paul RJ, Peterson JW, Caplan SR: A nonequilibrium thermodynamic description of vascular smooth muscle mechanochemistry. 1. The rate of oxygen consumption: A measure of the driving chemical reaction. *J Mechanochem Cell Motil* 3:19–32, 1974.

52. Glück E, Paul RJ: The aerobic glycolysis of porcine carotid

artery and its relation to isometric force. *Pflügers Arch* 370:9–18, 1977.

53. Peterson JW, Glück E: Energy cost of membrane depolarization in hog carotid artery. *Circ Res* 50:839–847, 1982.
54. Peterson JW: Effect of histamine on the energy metabolism of K$^+$-depolarized hog carotid artery. *Circ Res* 50:848–855, 1982.
55. Arner A, Hellstrand P: Energy turnover and mechanical properties of resting and contracting aortas and portal veins from normotensive and spontaneously hypertensive rats. *Circ Res* 48:539–548, 1981.
56. Arner A, Hellstrand P: Activation of contraction and ATPase activity in intact and chemically skinned smooth muscle of rat portal vein. *Circ Res* 53:695–702, 1983.
57. Siegman MJ, Butler TM, Mooers SU, Michner A: Ca^{2+} can affect Vmax without changes in myosin light chain phosphorylation in smooth muscle. *Pflügers Arch* 401: 385–390, 1984.
58. Krisanda JM, Paul RJ: Dependence of force, velocity and O$_2$ consumption on [Ca^{2+}]o in porcine coronary artery. *Am J Physiol* 255:C393–C400, 1988.
59. Vermue NA, Nicolay K: Energetics of smooth muscle taenia caecum of guinea-pig: A ^{31}P-NMR study. *FEBS Lett* 156: 293–297, 1983.
60. Ugurbil K, Kingsley-Hickman PB, Sako EY, Zimmer S, Mohanakrishnan CP, Robitaille PML, Thoma WJ, Johnson A, Foker JE, From AHL: ^{31}P-NMR studies of the kinetics and regulation of oxidative phosphorylation in the intact myocardium. *Ann NY Acad Sci* 508:265–286, 1987.
61. Lundholm L, Andersson RGG, Arnqvist HJ, Mohme-Lundholm E: Glycolysis and glycogenolysis in smooth muscle. In: Stephens NL (ed) *The Biochemistry of Smooth Muscle*. Baltimore, MD: University Park Press, 1977, pp 159–207.
62. Kroeger EA: Regulation of metabolism by cyclic adenosine 3',5'-monophosphate and ion-pumping in smooth muscle. In: Stephens NL (ed) *The Biochemistry of Smooth Muscle*. Baltimore, MD: University Park Press, 1977, pp 315–327.
63. Paul RJ, Bauer M, Pease W: Vascular smooth muscle: Aerobic glycolysis linked to sodium and potassium transport processes. *Science* 206:1414–1416, 1979.
64. Scheid CR, Honeyman TW, Fay FS: Mechanisms of β-adrenergic relaxation of smooth muscle. *Nature* 277:32–36, 1979.
65. Paul RJ: Aerobic glycolysis and ion transport in vascular smooth muscle. *Am J Physiol* 244:C399–C409, 1983.
66. Kutchai H, Geddis LM: Regulation of glycolysis in rat aorta. *Am J Physiol* 247:C107–C114, 1984.
67. Campbell JD, Paul RJ: The nature of fuel provision for the Na$^+$-K$^+$-ATPase in vascular smooth muscle. *J Physiol* 447: 67–82, 1992.
68. Caswell AH, Corbett AM: Interaction of glyceraldehyde-3-phosphate dehydrogenase with isolated microsomal subfractions of skeletal muscle. *J Biol Chem* 260:6892–6898, 1985.
69. Daum G, Keller K, Lange K: Association of glycolytic enzymes with the cytoplasmic side of the plasma membrane of glioma cells. *Biochem J* 939:277–281, 1988.
70. Jenkins JD, Madden DP, Steck TL: Association of phosphofructokinase and aldolase with the membrane of the intact erythrocyte. *J Biol Chem* 259:9374–9378, 1984.
71. Mercer RW, Dunham PB: Membrane-bound ATP fuels the Na/K pump: Studies on membrane-bound glycolytic enzymes on inside-out vesicles from human red cell membranes. *J Gen Physiol* 78:547–568, 1981.
72. Pierce GN, Philipson KD: Binding of glycolytic enzymes to cardiac sarcolemmal and sarcoplasmic reticular membranes. *J Biol Chem* 260:6862–6870, 1985.
73. Paul RJ, Hardin CD, Raeymaekers L, Wuytack F, Casteels R: An endogenous glycolytic cascade can preferentially support Ca^{2+}-uptake in smooth muscle plasma membrane vesicles. *FASEB J* 3:2299–2301, 1989.
74. Hardin CD, Raeymaekers F, Paul RJ: Comparison of endogenous and exogenous sources of ATP in supporting Ca^{2+}-uptake in isolated smooth muscle plasma membrane vesicles (PMV). *J Gen Physiol* 99:21–40, 1992.
75. Zhang C, Paul RJ: A specific dependence on glucose of excitation-contraction (E-C) coupling and relaxation in porcine carotid arteries. *J Mol Cell Cardiol* 24:S24, 1992.
76. Casteels R, Wuytack F: Aerobic and anaerobic metabolism in smooth muscle cells of taenia coli in relation to active ion transport. *J Physiol (Lond)* 250:203–220, 1975.
77. Davidheiser S, Joseph J, Davies RE: Separation of aerobic glycolysis from oxidative metabolism and contractility in rat anococcygeus muscle. *Am J Physiol* 247 (*Cell Physiol* 16): C335–C341, 1984.
78. Hellstrand P, Jorup C, Lydrup ML: O$_2$ consumption, aerobic glycolysis and tissue phosphagen content during activation of the Na$^+$/K$^+$ pump in rat portal vein. *Pflügers Arch* 401:119–124, 1984.
79. Paul RJ, Hellstrand P: Dissociation of phosphorylase a activation and contractile activity in rat portal vein. *Acta Physiol Scand* 121:23–30, 1984.
80. Kroeger EA: Effect of ionic environment on oxygen uptake and lactate production of myometrium. *Am J Physiol* 230: 158–162, 1976.
81. Lynch RM, Paul RJ: Compartmentation of carbohydrate metabolism in vascular smooth muscle: Evidence for at least two functionally independent pools of glucose-6-phosphate. *Biochim Biophys Acta* 887:315–318; 1986.
82. Hardin CD, Kushmerick MJ: Simultaneous and separable flux of pathways for glucose and glycogen utilization in vascular smooth muscle studied by ^{13}C-NMR. *J Mol Cell Cardiol*, in press, 1994.
83. Hardin CD, Paul RJ: Localization of two glycolytic enzymes in guinea pig taenia coli. *Biochim Biophys Acta* 1134: 256–259, 1992.
84. Weiss JN, Lamp ST: Glycolysis preferentially inhibits ATP-sensitive K$^+$ channels in isolated guinea pig cardiac myocytes. *Science* 238:67–69, 1987.
85. Price JM, Davis DL, Knauss EB: Length dependent sensitivity at lengths greater than Lmax in vascular smooth muscle. *Am J Physiol* 245:H379–H384, 1983.
86. Peterson JW: *Rates of Metabolism and Mechanical Activity in Vascular Smooth Muscle*. PhD thesis, Harvard University, University Microfilm no. 7424959, 1974.
87. Paul RJ, Peterson JW: Smooth muscle energetics. In: Casteels R, Godfraind T, Rüegg JC (eds) *Excitation-Contraction Coupling in Smooth Muscle*. Amsterdam: Elsevier/North-Holland Biomedical, 1977, pp 455–462.
88. Huxley AF, Simmons RM: Proposed mechanism of force generation in striated muscle. *Nature* 233:533–538, 1971.
89. Harris DE, Warshaw DM: Slowing of velocity during isotonic shortening in single isolated smooth muscle cells: Evidence for an internal load. *J Gen Physiol* 96:581–601, 1990.
90. Pfitzer G, Peterson JW: Stiffness of the arterial wall in response to potassium and pharmacological activation. In: Reinis Z, Pokorny J, Linhart J, Hild R, Schirger A (eds) *Adaptability of Vascular Wall*. Prague: Avicenum Czechoslovak Medical, 1980, pp 125–127.
91. Peterson JW: Relation to stiffness, energy metabolism, and

isometric tension in a vascular smooth muscle. In: Vanhoutte PM, Leusen I (eds) *Mechanisms of Vasodilatation*. Basel: S. Karger, 1978, pp 79–88.

92. Paul RJ, Glück E, Rüegg JC: Cross bridge ATP utilization in arterial smooth muscle. *Pflügers Arch* 361:297–299, 1976.

93. Rüegg JC: Smooth muscle tone. *Physiol Rev* 51:201–248, 1971.

94. Paul RJ, Rüegg JC: Biochemistry of vascular smooth muscle: Energy metabolism and proteins of the contractile apparatus. In: Kaley G, Altura BM (eds) *Microcirculation*, Vol 2. Baltimore, MD: University Park Press, 1978, pp 41–82.

95. Mrwa U, Paul RJ, Kreye VAW, Rüegg JC: The contractile mechanism of vascular smooth muscle. In: *Smooth Muscle Pharmacology and Physiology*. Paris: Inserm, 1976, pp 319–326.

96. Murphy RA: Mechanics of vascular smooth muscle. In: Bohr DF, Somlyo AP, Sparks HV, Geiger SR (eds) *The Handbook of Physiology. Section 2: The Cardiovascular System. Vol 2: Vascular Smooth Muscle*. Bethesda, MD: American Physiological Society, 1980, pp 325–351.

97. Barany M: ATPase activity of myosin correlated with speed of muscle shortening. *J Gen Physiol* 50:197–218, 1967.

98. Marston SB, Taylor EW: Comparison of the myosin and actomyosin ATPase mechanisms of the four types of vertebrate muscles. *J Mol Biol* 139:573–600, 1980.

99. Dillon PF, Aksoy MO, Driska SP, Murphy RA: Myosin phosphorylation and the crossbridge cycle in arterial muscle. *Science* 211:495–497, 1981.

100. Murphy RA, Aksoy MO, Dillon PF, Gerthoffer WT, Kamm KE: The role of myosin light chain phosphorylation in regulation of the crossbridge cycle. *Fed Proc* 42:51–56, 1983.

101. Dillon PF, Murphy RA: Tonic force maintenance with reduced shortening velocity in arterial smooth muscle. *Am J Physiol* 242:C102–C108, 1982.

102. Driska SP, Aksoy MO, Murphy RA: Myosin light chain phosphorylation associated with contraction in arterial smooth muscle. *Am J Physiol* 240:C222–C233, 1981.

103. Aksoy MO, Murphy RA, Kamm KE: Role of Ca^{2+} and myosin light chain phosphorylation in regulation of smooth muscle. *Am J Physiol* 242:C109–C116, 1982.

104. Hai CM, Murphy RA: Cross-bridge phosphorylation and regulation of latch state in smooth muscle. *Am J Physiol* 254:C99–C106, 1988.

105. Hai CM, Murphy RA: Regulation of shortening velocity by cross-bridge phosphorylation in smooth muscle. *Am J Physiol* 255:C86–C94, 1988.

106. Hai CM, Murphy RA: Ca^{2+}, crossbridge phosphorylation, and contraction. *Ann Rev Physiol* 51:285–298, 1989.

107. Hai CM, Murphy RA: Crossbridge phosphorylation and the energetics of contraction in swine carotid media. In: Paul RJ, Elzinga G, Yamada K (eds) *Muscle Energetics*. New York: Alan R. Liss, 1989, pp 253–264.

108. Hai CM, Murphy RA: ATP consumption by smooth muscle as predicted by the coupled four-state model. *Biophys J* 61:530–541, 1992.

109. Hartshorne DJ: Biochemistry of the contractile process in smooth muscle. In: Johnson LR (ed) *Physiology of the Gastrointestinal Tract*, 2nd ed. New York: Raven Press, 1987, pp 423–482.

110. Galvas PE, Kuetner C, Paul RJ, DiSalvo J: Temporal relationships among isometric force, phosphorylase and protein kinase activities in vascular smooth muscle. *Proc Soc Exp Biol Med* 178:254–260, 1985.

111. Silver PJ, Stull JT: Regulation of myosin light chain and phosphorylase phosphorylation in tracheal smooth muscle. *J Biol Chem* 257:6145–6150, 1982.

112. Morgan JP, Morgan KG: Stimulus-specific patterns of intra-cellular calcium levels in smooth muscle of ferret portal vein. *J Physiol (Lond)* 351:155–167, 1984.

113. Butler TM, Siegman MJ, Mooers SU: Chemical energy usage during stimulation and stretch of mammalian smooth muscle. *Pflügers Arch* 401:391–395, 1984.

114. Butler TM, Siegman MJ, Mooers SU: Chemical energy usage during shortening and work production in mammalian smooth muscle. *Am J Physiol* 244:C234–C242, 1983.

115. Paul RJ, Peterson JW: The mechanochemistry of smooth muscle. In: Stephens NL (ed) *The Biochemistry of Smooth Muscle*. Baltimore, MD: University Park Press, 1977, pp 15–39.

116. Krisanda JM, Paul RJ: The Fenn effect in vascular smooth muscle: Phosphagen breakdown during maximum power output in porcine carorid artery. *Biophys J* 45:346a, 1984.

117. Krisanda JM, Paul RJ: The effect of changes in active work production on the efficiency of porcine carorid artery. *Fed Proc* 45:766, 1986.

118. Butler TM, Siegman MJ, Mooers SU: Slowing of cross-bridge cycling rate in mammalian smooth muscle occurs without evidence of an increase in internal load. In: Siegman MJ, Srephens NL, Somlyo AP (eds) *Smooth Muscle Contraction*. New York: Alan R. Liss, 1987, pp 289–302.

119. Driska SP: High myosin light chain phosphatase activity in arterial smooth muscle: Can it explain latch phenomenon? In: Siegman MJ, et al. (eds) *Regulation and Contraction in Smooth Muscle*. New York: Alan R. Liss, 1987, pp 387–398.

120. Butler TM, Siegman MJ: High-energy phosphate metabolism in vascular smooth muscle. *Ann Rev Physiol* 47:629–643, 1985.

121. Paul RJ: Smooth muscle energetics and theories of cross-bridge regulation. *Am J Physiol* 258:C369–C395, 1990.

122. Paul RJ, Wendt IR, Walker JS, Gibbs CL: Smooth muscle energetics: Testing theories of crossbridge regulation. In: Sperelakis N, Woods JD (eds) *Frontiers in Smooth Muscle Research*. New York: Alan R. Liss, 1990, pp 29–38.

123. Huxley AF: Muscle structure and theories of contraction. *Prog Biophys Biophys Commun* 7:255–318, 1957.

CHAPTER 57

Control of the Coronary Circulation

MARK W. GORMAN, MIAO-XIANG HE, & HARVEY V. SPARKS, JR.

INTRODUCTION

Normal function of the heart depends on an adequate coronary blood flow. Myocardial metabolism and coronary flow are mutually interactive so that any increase in the metabolism of the normal heart is matched by an increase in coronary blood flow, and any significant restriction of flow results in the reduction of myocardial metabolism and cardiac performance. In this chapter we discuss the determinants of coronary blood flow, which include myocardial metabolism, humoral influences, and neural control. We will not discuss the role of physical factors in determining coronary blood flow because that is the subject of Chapter 58. In addition, we discuss certain pathophysiologic conditions, such as vascular responses to cardiac hypertrophy and myocardial ischemia, and the significance of coronary collateral vessels.

METABOLIC CONTROL OF CORONARY BLOOD FLOW

Myocardial metabolism normally exerts the single most important influence on coronary vascular resistance. There is a positive monotonic relationship between the extent of coronary vasodilation and myocardial oxygen consumption {2}. This means that oxygen delivery to the myocardium is closely matched to oxygen use. Despite the general importance of this relationship, significant alterations in coronary blood flow are possible at a given myocardial oxygen consumption. That is, although metabolism exerts a dominant influence on myocardial perfusion, changes in blood gases, neurogenic control mechanisms, and humoral mechanisms can exert a modulating effect on this relationship {1}.

There are three commonly observed manifestations of metabolic control of coronary blood flow. The first is the reactive hyperemia that results from a brief period of occlusion of a coronary artery. The second is autoregulation of coronary blood flow, the tendency of blood flow to remain constant despite altered perfusion pressure. The third is functional hyperemia, or the increase in coronary blood flow associated with increased myocardial metabolism. Although earlier investigators often made the

implicit assumption that the mechanisms responsible for all three of these phenomena were the same, it is now apparent that different mechanisms are involved. Therefore, we will consider these phenomena separately and evaluate the relative importance of each of the postulated mechanisms.

Reactive hyperemia

When a major coronary vessel is occluded for a brief period of time, its release is followed by a dramatic increase in blood flow. The peak increase occurs within a few seconds after the release of the occlusion. The amplitude of this peak depends on the duration of the occlusion, up to approximately 15 seconds. Longer occlusions cause no further increase in the peak response {3–5}, but the duration of the hyperemic response increases with the length of occlusion. The total excess flow that occurs during reactive hyperemia is greater than the flow "debt" incurred during the period of occlusion. Reactive hyperemia occurs in denervated and isolated hearts; thus it is generally agreed that the mechanisms responsible must reside within the heart itself. These mechanisms can be divided into two general categories, myogenic and metabolic. The myogenic hypothesis states that resistance vessels distal to an occlusion dilate in response to the reduction in wall stress {6}. The metabolic hypothesis states that a reduction in blood flow resulting from occlusion of a major vessel causes release of vasodilator substances either from myocardial cells or from the vessel wall itself {1}.

Vasoactive substances released from endothelial cells, such as nitric oxide (NO), could theoretically be classified as either myogenic or metabolic factors. In this review we will classify them as metabolic factors. In the case of NO this seems reasonable because NO formation inhibits myogenic vasoconstriction {7}. Myogenic responses as defined here, then, arise from vascular smooth muscle cells themselves.

It has proved difficult to identify the portion of reactive hyperemia caused by a myogenic response as opposed to the release of various vasodilator metabolites. A number of ingenious experiments have been performed in an effort to dissect these two phenomena. Eikens and Wilcken

N. Sperelakis (ed.), Physiology and Pathophysiology of the Heart, Third Edition.

{8,9} demonstrated that extremely short periods of occlusion (<1 second) resulted in reactive hyperemia. They stated that the metabolic insult caused by such short periods of occlusion would be unlikely to result in release of metabolic vasodilators and concluded that their experiments supported the myogenic hypothesis. Later studies by Greenfield's group {10} showed that the magnitude of reactive hyperemia depended on the placement of a brief occlusion within the cardiac cycle. They found that diastolic coronary artery occlusions of duration greater than 100 ms resulted in reactive hyperemia. The magnitude of the hyperemia was dependent upon the duration of the occlusion, and the onset of the response was delayed until postocclusion systole. These investigators took this as evidence that a metabolic phenomenon is responsible for the vasodilation because it seemed to be dependent on the increased metabolism that occurs during systole. In conclusion, the available data do not allow us to state with any degree of certainty what fraction of reactive hyperemia, following a very brief occlusion, is the result of a myogenic mechanism. In the absence of any specific blocker of a myogenic response, it would appear to be impossible to fully dissect these two phenomena.

Occlusions of longer duration appear to have a metabolic component. The evidence for this is that longer occlusions result in a reactive hyperemia of greater duration {3–5} and the release of several vasodilator metabolites {1}. Once the occlusion is released, the vasodilator substances cause an increased blood flow until they are metabolized, taken back up into cells, or washed out. Vessel wall PO_2 represents a variant of this hypothesis in which oxygen, a constrictor, is removed, resulting in vasodilation. There are several tests of the role of a particular vasodilator substance. If the vasodilator has a causal role, it should be present in the vicinity of the vascular smooth muscle in a concentration capable of resulting in vasodilation. Furthermore, agents capable of blocking the vasodilator's action should reduce reactive hyperemia, and agents capable of altering the vasodilator's concentration around the vascular smooth muscle should cause an appropriate change in the hyperemic response.

Potassium is released into the coronary venous effluent following a brief occlusion {11,12}. Furthermore, the time course of the return of potassium release to control levels is similar to the return of vascular resistance. This has led to the suggestion that potassium is responsible for at least a portion of reactive hyperemia. There are two arguments against this conclusion. First, Bunger and coworkers {13}, using the crystalloid-perfused guinea pig heart, were unable to block reactive hyperemia with ouabain, which blocked the vasodilator response to potassium. Second, Sparks and coworkers {12} calculated the increase in interstitial potassium concentration resulting from a 15-second occlusion and concluded that the increase was not sufficient to cause more than a very small portion of the vasodilator response observed. Thus, it appears that potassium is released but plays a minor role in causing reactive hyperemia.

Occlusion of a coronary artery results in a fall of tissue and microvascular PO_2 {14,15,113}. The question is: When does PO_2 fall far enough to cause relaxation of vascular smooth muscle? It now appears clear that vascular smooth muscle is sensitive to changes in PO_2 in the range likely to occur in the resistance vessel wall {16–18}. Part of this response is endothelial cell dependent {114}. One mechanism by which changes in vascular wall PO_2 may exert an influence is the release of prostaglandins {19}. Another mechanism is through the opening of ATP-sensitive potassium channels in vascular smooth muscle {40,42}. Even if PO_2 falls to a level that results in dilation during occlusion, it is unlikely to be responsible for the dilation following the occlusion. Once flow is restored, effluent PO_2 quickly rises to a value far higher than control {20}. This suggests that microvascular wall PO_2 is also elevated by the increased flow delivery of oxygen. Once microvascular wall PO_2 is elevated there would no longer be a stimulus for the continued vasodilation.

As mentioned above, vessel wall hypoxia results in release of prostaglandins. A number of studies have demonstrated that myocardial ischemia also results in release of prostaglandins into the venous effluent {21,22}. This suggests a causal role for prostaglandins in reactive hyperemia. However, the use of compounds such as indomethacin, which decrease the production of prostaglandins via the cyclooxygenase pathway, has not yielded uniform results. Alexander and coworkers {21} employed indomethacin and observed a reduction in hyperemia flow following a 20-second occlusion. However, these results could not be confirmed by three other groups {23–25}.

A number of investigators have demonstrated that coronary occlusion results in a rise in tissue adenosine content {26–29}. In addition, tissue adenosine content remains elevated after release of occlusion and returns to the control value with a time course very similar to that of the blood flow {29}. It is very likely that this increase in tissue content is at least partly the result of an increase in interstitial adenosine because adenosine can also be recovered from the venous effluent following coronary occlusion {26,28}. Most studies show that administration of theophylline or aminophylline, adenosine receptor antagonists, results in a reduction of reactive hyperemia by approximately 30% {25,30,31, but see 32,33}. In addition, infusion of the catalytic subunit of adenosine deaminase causes a reduction in reactive hyperemia by about 30% {34}. Theophylline in combination with adenosine deaminase causes no further decrease in reactive hyperemia. This result suggests that other factors are responsible for the remaining two thirds of the reactive hyperemic response {34}.

A major additional contributor to reactive hyperemia is nitric oxide (NO), presumably released from endothelial cells or possibly from nerves. At least two mechanisms could be responsible for NO formation during reactive hyperemia. The increased flow following release of the occlusion increases the shear stress to which endothelial cells are exposed, which should increase NO release {35}. Hypoxia also promotes NO formation {36}, and this mechanism may be at work prior to release of the occlusion. Both increased shear stress and hypoxia may stimulate endothelial NO synthesis by increasing intracellular calcium concentration {37}.

Inhibitors of NO synthesis reduce reactive hyperemia flow repayment by 26–34% {38,39}. These results may underestimate the true contribution of NO. Flow repayment in isolated guinea pig hearts was reduced 26% by L-NAME (nitro-L-arginine methyl ester, an inhibitor of NO synthase), even though inhibition of NO release was far from complete {38}. When oxyhemoglobin (an NO scavenger) was added together with L-NAME, flow repayment was reduced by 50%. The hyperemia reduction by L-NAME also provokes a compensatory increase in adenosine release, which would tend to minimize the flow reduction {38}. Simultaneous inhibition of NO synthesis and blockade of adenosine receptors reduces flow repayment by 57% in dog hearts {39}. Thus, the combined effects of adenosine and NO release account for more than half of the reactive hyperemic response.

Another potential contributor to reactive hyperemia is the opening of ATP-sensitive potassium channels (K_{ATP}^+) in vascular smooth muscle. These channels are opened by a decrease in intracellular [ATP], and are sensitized by increases in intracellular [ADP] {40}. This results in hyperpolarization of vascular smooth muscle cells and subsequent vasodilation. Glibenclamide prevents the opening of these channels, and reduces flow debt repayment following 30-sececond occlusions in dog hearts from 200% to 50% {41}. The reduction of reactive vasodilation in isolated guinea pig hearts is even larger {42}. Glibenclamide also inhibits adenosine-induced vasodilation {42,43}. This complication makes it difficult to assign a percentage to the contribution of K_{ATP}^+ channels in reactive hyperemia, but that percentage could be substantial. These channels may also be a part of the pathway through which other metabolites exert their influence.

K_{ATP}^+ channels are very important in the control of resting coronary vasomotor tone. Intracoronary infusions of high concentrations of glibenclamide severely reduce resting coronary flow both in vitro and in vivo, resulting in myocardial ischemia {44,45}. In dog hearts, glibenclamide produced an oscillating pattern of coronary flow {44}. The oscillations were decreased or abolished by the adenosine antagonist 8-phenyltheophylline. Thus the vasoconstriction (and ischemia) produced by closing K_{ATP}^+ channels stimulated adenosine release, which increased flow. Increased flow removed the stimulus for adenosine release, which allowed the flow to decrease again and initiate the oscillatory flow pattern.

Adenine nucleotides are also released into the venous effluent during reactive hyperemia. In the isolated guinea pig heart these nucleotides are released primarily by endothelial cells, and their total concentration (ATP + ADP + AMP) is similar to the adenosine concentration {46}. The amount of each individual nucleotide released is not known, but ATP and ADP can be quickly metabolized to AMP and adenosine by nucleotidases on extracellular membranes {122}. ATP causes vasodilation independently from adenosine, however, and although this vasodilation is endothelial cell dependent {47}, it is not mediated by NO in the guinea pig heart {48}. The lack of a specific

antagonist for ATP-induced vasodilation makes it difficult to fully assess its role. However, the nucleotide release rates in guinea pig hearts during reactive hyperemia suggest that ATP or other nucleotides deinitely contribute to the vasodilation without conversion to adenosine. Some of the released nucleotides apparently do contribute to reactive hyperemia in dog hearts by being converted to adenosine. α,β-methylene adenosine diphosphate (AOPCP, an inhibitor of ecto-5′-nucleotidase) reduces reactive hyperemia and the associated adenosine release {49}. Free radical formation during reactive hyperemia limits this extracellular adenosine formation somewhat by inhibiting ecto-5′-nucleotidase {49}.

In summary, it is obvious that several factors contribute to reactive hyperemia. Adenosine and NO are major components, accounting together for more than half of the response. ATP is also likely to be important, along with a myogenic component. K_{ATP}^+ channels in vascular smooth muscle also contribute to the response. It remains to be determined whether these channels are an independent contributor or whether they mediate the vasodilation initiated by other factors.

Autoregulation

Autoregulation of blood flow is defined as the tendency of flow to remain constant despite alterations in perfusion pressure. When perfusion pressure is suddenly changed, flow tends to follow the change in perfusion pressure. Over a period of seconds, however, flow then returns toward the previous value. The range of perfusion pressure over which flow remains relatively constant is 70–145 mmHg {50,51}.

When perfusion pressure drops below 70 mmHg, flow begins to fall linearly until it stops at a perfusion pressure well above zero. (See the section on ischemia for a discussion of the assumption that the descending limb of the autoregulation curve represents a region of perfusion pressures in which the coronary resistance vessels are maximally dilated.) Studies with microspheres have demonstrated that both the subepicardium and subendocardium exhibit autoregulation {52,53}. The mechanism of autoregulation is unknown. There are three generic theories: myogenic, tissue pressure, and metabolic. As in the case of reactive hyperemia, there is no direct evidence in favor of the myogenic mechanism. On the other hand, there are no experiments that rule it out. The tissue pressure hypothesis states that as perfusion pressure is lowered, extravascular compression decreases and resistance vessels dilate. Once again there is no direct evidence supporting this hypothesis. Many investigators have assumed that coronary autoregulation is the result of a metabolic mechanism. However, there are few studies that have tested the roles of specific vasodilator metabolites. Cyclooxygenase inhibitors do not affect autoregulation {54}. This would appear to rule out the participation of prostaglandins. In addition, Bunger and coworkers {13} found no evidence to support a role for potassium in coronary autoregulation. Reduced vessel wall PO_2 should accompany any fall in oxygen delivery resulting from reduced perfusion pressure {15}. However, there are no direct tests of the role of vessel wall PO_2 in autoregulation. Dole and Nuno {55} examined coronary autoregulation over a range of myocardial metabolic rates. They concluded that autoregulatory gain is enhanced by low venous PO_2 and attenuated by high venous PO_2. This supports the hypothesis that the mediator responsible for steady-state autoregulation is sensitive to the ratio of myocardial O_2 supply to demand (e.g., a metabolic factor).

Other results suggest a minimal role for PO_2-linked metabolites in steady-state autoregulation. By varying arterial PO_2 and PCO_2 at constant perfusion pressure and constant myocardial oxygen consumption, Broten et al. have developed equations that predict the expected flow changes resulting from changes in venous PO_2 and PCO_2 {56}. During autoregulation in dog hearts, the venous blood gas changes (assumed to represent tissue PO_2 and PCO_2) can account for only 23% of the changes in coronary vascular conductance {57}. This would include both direct effects of O_2 and CO_2 on vascular smooth muscle and any metbolites whose concentration is determined by O_2 or CO_2. Since many vasodilator metabolites (such as adenosine) are thought to be linked to tissue PO_2, this suggests that a large fraction of autoregulation is either not metabolic in origin, or is due to metabolites not linked to PO_2.

Schrader and coworkers {28} showed that reduction of perfusion pressure from normal levels resulted in elevation of tissue and coronary effluent adenosine content in isolated hearts. However, in vivo tests of the hypothesis that adenosine mediates autoregulation have been negative {58,59}. Adenosine deaminase does not alter the autoregulation curve in the same hearts in which it reduces reactive hyperemia {59}. Elevation of perfusion pressure above normal produced no changes in tissue or effluent adenosine content {28}. Furthermore, adenosine deaminase does not reduce resting coronary blood flow {34,59,108}. Negative results with adenosine deaminase must be carefully evaluated. If an investigator finds no effect of adenosine deaminase and concludes that adenosine does not mediate a particular response, the assumption is that enough adenosine deaminase activity is present to significantly lower interstitial adenosine. This assumption is usually buttressed by a calculation in which a turnover rate for adenosine in the interstitium is assumed. If the true rate is much higher than assumed, insufficient adenosine deaminase may have been present {116}. With this caveat, it appears that adenosine has little to do with mediating coronary vasodilation at rest or during autoregulation.

Nitric oxide can be ruled out as a mediator of coronary autoregulation. Inhibition of NO synthesis improves autoregulation in isolated guinea pig hearts {7}. This probably occurs because endothelial NO synthesis is stimulated by increased shear stress at higher pressure and flows, and vice versa.

One of the most interesting recent observations is that in the subepicardial microvasculature (vessels <100 μm) of dog hearts, vasodilation in response to reduced perfusion pressure is blocked by glibenclamide {60}. This suggests that coronary autoregulation is mediated by K_{ATP}^+ channels in vascular smooth muscle. The stimulus regulating these channels is uncertain. At first glance it seems unlikely that vascular smooth muscle ATP concentration decreases during moderate reductions in perfusion pressure. Smooth muscle PO_2 is influenced more strongly by arterial PO_2 than by tissue PO_2, and smooth muscle also has a high capacity for anaerobic glycolysis {15}. However, the fact that glibenclamide reduces resting coronary blood flow suggests that K_{ATP}^+ channels are tonically active. If this is the case, then any reduction in smooth muscle PO_2 may produce small but effective changes in K_{ATP}^+ channel opening. It has been estimated that less than 1% of these channels in vascular smooth muscle need to open in order to produce vasodilation {40}. The detailed control of these channels under in vivo conditions remains to be elucidated. However, it is possible that K_{ATP}^+ channels are the most important contributor to coronary autoregulation. In order to test this hypothesis further, the effect of K_{ATP}^+ channel blockade needs to be explored in whole organs, and for increases in perfusion pressure as well as decreases.

Functional hyperemia

Increased myocardial metabolism is normally matched by an increase in coronary blood flow and oxygen delivery. The relationship can be modulated by a number of stimuli; for example, sympathetic vasoconstrictor neural activity {61}, angiotensin {62,63}, antidiuretic hormone {64}, alterations in PCO_2 {65–68}, and vasoactive drugs {69}. Any modulation in coronary blood flow at a given metabolic rate leads to a change in oxygen extractions. For example, adrenergic vasoconstriction causes lower oxygen delivery and higher extraction of oxygen for a given myocardial oxygen consumption {61}.

The coupling of coronary vascular conductance to metabolism is easily observable in isolated hearts and so is not causally dependent upon nerves or hormones. Most investigators believe that increased metabolism is associated with release of a vasodilator substance from myocardial cells. It is postulated that this vasodilator elicits relaxation of coronary smooth muscle and thus increases flow to match the increase in metabolism. However, there is strong evidence favoring the participation of at least two vasodilator mechanisms, and it is probable that there are also other mechanisms that remain to be discovered. Several vasodilator systems that may be important in other contexts do not seem to be responsible for functional hyperemia. We doubt that vessel wall PO_2 falls during functional hyperemia. This is because coronary sinus PO_2 does not ordinarily change and because oxygen delivery to the resistance vessels is dramatically increased by the elevated blood flow {15}. Case and associates {65–67} have revived the hypothesis that an increase in vessel wall PCO_2 may be responsible for functional hyperemia. This idea is attractive because an increase in production of CO_2 should accompany an increase in oxygen metabolism. However, very large changes in arterial PCO_2 are necessary to elicit relatively modest changes in coronary vascular conductance. Given the very small changes that occur in coronary sinus PCO_2, it is unlikely that there is a sufficient hypercapnic stimulus to result in the observed functional hyperemia {68}. Changes in arterial PCO_2 may have indirect effects on the relationship between myocardial blood flow and oxygen consumption. For example, it appears that elevated hydrogen ion concentration causes coronary vascular smooth muscle relaxation {70} and enhances its sensitivity to adenosine {70,71}. Also, elevation in PCO_2 or hydrogen ion concentration results in unloading of oxygen from hemoglobin.

Feigl and coworkers have applied their model of PO_2 and PCO_2-linked changes in coronary vascular conductance to pacing-induced functional hyperemia {56}. Coronary sinus PO_2 decreased and PCO_2 increased in this situation. They concluded that 40% of the hyperemia can be explained by the combined changes in PO_2 and PCO_2 (which includes metabolites linked to O_2 and CO_2).

Functional hyperemia occurs in the presence of indomethacin, and this argues against a causal role for prostaglandin release {2,68}. In addition, the lack of changes in the hydrogen ion concentration {72,73} and osmolarity {11} of the coronary sinus effluent would seem to rule out these two potential vasodilator influences.

Potassium is elevated transiently when myocardial metabolism increases. The increase is sufficient to cause approximately one third of the initial increase in vascular conductance associated with increased heart rate {12}. If oxygenation of the myocardium is normal, however, potassium release quickly declines {74,75}. Thus, although potassium is a coronary vasodilator, it cannot be responsible for steady-state increases in coronary blood flow associated with increased metabolism.

Adenosine is the most venerable candidate for the cause of functional hyperemia in the heart. The adenosine hypothesis {1} states that increased metabolism is associated with an increase in adenosine release from myocardial cells. This release raises the interstitial concentration of adenosine, which in turn results in dilation of resistance vessels. The quantitatively most significant source of adenosine is probably the myocyte cytosol {76–81}. Two enzymes are responsible for adenosine formation in the cytosol. These enzymes are soluble (cytosolic) 5'-nucleotidase {84,118} and S-adenosylhomocysteine hydrolase (SAH) {78}. Under basal consitions in the isolated guinea pig heart, much of the adenosine released is formed by SAH. During periods of high adenosine release, however, the vast majority of adenosine is formed by the

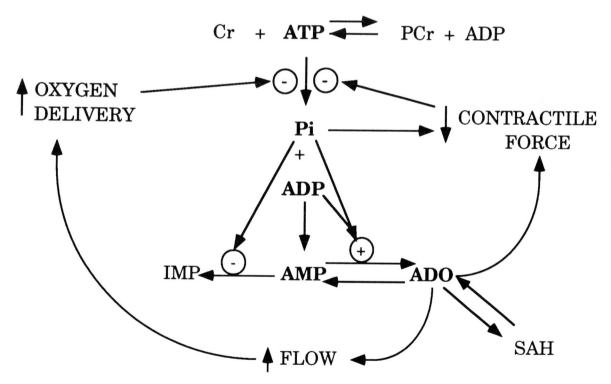

Fig. 57-1. Proposed feedback loop by which net hydrolysis of ATP (provoked by oxygen supply/demand imbalance) is minized. In most physiological situations ATP concentration will not change due to the creatine kinase reaction, and net hydrolysis of phosphocreatine (PCr) is the source of increased Pi and ADP. Increased adenosine (ADO) formation increases O_2 supply via increased flow, and deceases O_2 demand by decreasing contractile force. The impetus for increased adenosine formation is increased intracellular [AMP], [Pi], and [ADP]. Pi also decreases contractile force and helps to increase [AMP] by inhibiting IMP formation.

activity of 5'-nucleotidase {82}. Interstitial adenosine may also come from endothelial cells {118,119} and nerve terminals in the form of ATP {120}, which is broken down to adenosine by ectoenzymes {121}. These sources are probably of marginal quantitative significance at rest {119, 122} and of little or no importance when metabolism is elevated {119,122,123}. Increased adenosine formation is most closely related to a fall in the ratio of O_2 supply to demand, but can be influenced by other factors {123,124}.

A fall in the oxygen supply/demand ratio is linked to increased adenosine formation by an increase in substrate (AMP) concentration {83} and probably by an increase in 5'-nucleotidase activity as well {82} (fig. 57.1). Increased adenosine release correlates well with decreases in venous PO_2 and the adenine nucleotide phosphorylation potential ([ATP]/[ADP][Pi]) {87–90}, but neither of these variables is likely to directly influence enzyme activity. Two components of the phosphorylation potential, Pi and

ADP, may contribute to activation of 5'-nucleotidase {84, 85}. Since Pi, ADP, and AMP concentrations usually change in tandem, determination of their individual influences on adenosine formation is difficult. Recent experiments in our laboratory with PCr depletion and with 2-deoxyglucose infusion have lowered Pi concentrations during hypoxia or catecholamine infusion {86}. In both cases adenosine release was reduced while AMP and ADP were not. These results suggest that Pi is an important regulator of adenosine formation. Pi also improves the oxygen supply/demand ratio by reducing contractile force. Further studies of cytosolic 5'-nucleotidases and adenosine kinase are needed in order to clarify the regulation of adenosine formation.

There are four lines of evidence that lend support to the idea that adenosine is responsible for functional hyperemia. First, adenosine is a potent vasodilator. Second, metabolic machinery capable of rapid formation and de-

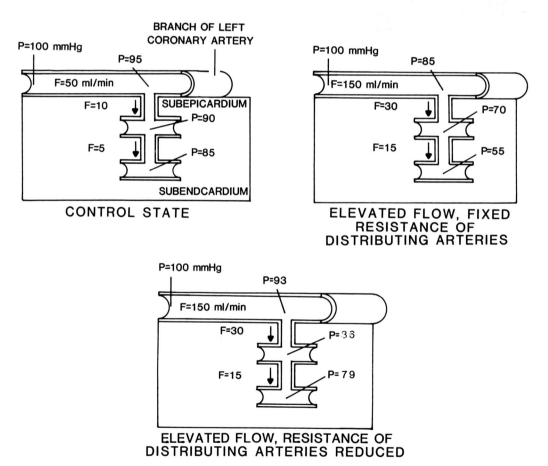

Fig. 57-2. Role of distributing artery dilation in maintaining subendocardial perfusion pressure during high-flow conditions. Distributing arteries in this schematic include a main branch of the left coronary artery and two transverse vessels that feed subepicardial and then subendocardial vessels. The pressure drop under control conditions is assumed to be 5 mmHg in each of the distributing arteries. When aortic pressure is 100 mmHg, this results in a subendocardial perfusion pressure of 85 mmHg. If flow is tripled without distributing artery dilation (upper right panel), the pressure drop triples across each segment and subendocardial perfusion pressure falls to 55 mmHg. In the bottom panel, flow is high but the distributing arteries have reduced their resistance by up to 50% (an 18% diameter increase). This prevents most of the fall in subendocardial perfusion pressure.

struction of adenosine is present in the myocardium. Third, a number of studies have demonstrated that most stimuli that result in increased myocardial metabolism also result in increased adenosine release into venous effluent, pericardial fluid, or epicardial transudate fluid {69,91–94}. In addition, most of these stimuli cause an increase in tissue content of adenosine {95,96}. Furthermore, adenosine deaminase lowers flow relative to oxygen consumption in canine hearts stimulated with norepinephrine {97}. However, there are other lines of evidence that confuse the issue. First, aminophylline and 8-phenyltheophylline, methylxanthines that antagonize the vasodilator action of adenosine, do not reduce functional hyperemia in preparations where they do reduce reactive hyperemia {98,99}. Second, it is possible to raise myocardial metabolism and coronary blood flow without increasing adenosine release when cardiac pacing is the stimulus {100}. Third, adenosine release in response to the administration of norepinephrine is phasic {101}. When norepinephrine is administered to an isolated guinea pig heart, adenosine release peaks within the first minute and then rapidly falls to a much lower level, while myocardial oxygen consumption and coronary conductance remain elevated and constant. Fourth, if perfusion pressure is increased above the usual level in isolated guinea pig hearts, isoproterenol infusion leads to functional hyperemia without the usual adenosine release {90}.

Some synthesis of these disparate results concerning adenosine seems possible. It is helpful to separate in vivo experiments from isolated heart experiments. In isolated buffer-perfused heart preparations, myocardial oxygenation seems adequate at rest but is probably inadequate during functional hyperemia. Decreases in high-energy phosphate concentrations occur in isolated hearts during functional hyperemia, which occurs only transiently, if at all, in vivo {87,102,103}. This oxygen supply/demand imbalance in isolated hearts stimulates adenosine formation, and the interstitial fluid concentration reaches highly vasoactive levels {104,105}. Adenosine can therefore initiate functional hyperemia in isolated hearts. During steady-state functional hyperemia, however, the interstitial adenosine concentration falls substantially and probably cannot account for all of steady-state hyperemia {104}. Some additional vasodilator mechanism must be present in the steady state.

The case for adenosine is less convincing in vivo. Indices of interstitial adenosine concentration in vivo suggest that it increases during functional hyperemia {93,106, 107}, but the high resting adenosine concentrations obtained with these methods are hard to reconcile with low resting flows and the inability of adenosine deaminase or adenosine antagonists to lower resting flow {99,108}. These experiments are therefore difficult to interpret. The best in vivo evidence in favor of adenosine is the reduction of functional hyperemia by adenosine deaminase during norepinephrine infusion {97}. Opposing this are the negative results with 8-phenyltheophylline and adenosine deaminase in conscious dogs {99}. Here again, myocardial oxygenation may be the key. Norepinephrine infusion produces functional hyeremia, but it exposes the coronary

vasculature to much higher norepinephrine concentrations than would exist under normal conditions of sympathetic stimulation. This results in more alpha-adrenergic vasoconstriction (and less flow) than would normally exist at a given level of myocardial oxygen consumption {61}. The lowering of the O_2 supply/demand ratio results in adenosine formation and a contribution to the hyperemia. In conscious dogs the O_2 supply/demand ratio may be higher during treadmill exercise, with no resulting adenosine formation. The tentative conclusion we reach is that adenosine contributes to functional hyperemia when oxygenation is compromised, such as in isolated hearts or during norepinephrine infusion in vivo. Under physiological conditions in conscious animals, adenosine does not seem to be necessary. Both in vivo and in vitro studies suggest that even when adenosine contributes to functional hyperemia it does so primarily in the early stages {101,104,109}. Its contribution in the steady state is much smaller or nonexistent. There must be at least one additional vasodilator mechanism at work that is especially important under physiological conditions.

Preliminary studies using glibenclamide to block K^+_{ATP} channels suggest a possible role for these channels in functional hyperemia. Glibenclamide reduced coronary blood flow by only 15% during treadmill exercise in conscious dogs {110}, but by 30% during isoproterenol infusion in anesthetized dogs {111}. A reduction in resting flow may contribute to these results. Since the increased flow during functional hyperemia prevents a fall in PO_2 at the arteriolar level {112}, the stimulus for opening these channels is unclear. Further studies of K^+_{ATP} channels are needed during functional hyperemia.

The role of nitric oxide in functional hyperemia at the microvascular level is uncertain. At the very least, though, NO plays an important role in steady-state functional hyperemia by dilating conduit vessels {115,125,126}. Dilation of distributing arteries including transmural vessels (in which flow induced dilation has not yet been described) is absolutely necessary for functional hyperemia to occur. This is illustrated in fig. 57-2, where hypothetical pressures and flows are indicated for rest and functional hyperemia. The hypothetical effect of the absence of distributing artery dilation on arterial pressures during functional hyperemia is shown. (See legend for details of calculations.) In the absence of distributing artery dilation, inlet pressure for the subendocardial microcirculation branching from the transmural vessel is 55 mmHg during functional hyperemia. This leaves very little pressure gradient for flow through the microcirculation. With dilation of distributing arteries, most of this pressure drop can be avoided. Another important point is that a fall in perfusion pressure, as occurs with functional hyperemia, will be accompanied by decreased transmural pressure (as in the second panel). This decrease will result in a reduction in diameter (an increase in distributing artery resistance) unless there is a compensatory reduction in vascular smooth muscle tone. This emphasizes the need for flow-induced dilation of distributing arteries to prevent an undue fall in microvascular pressures. It is worth considering whether what appears to be spasm during coronary

Table 57-1.

| | Myogenic | Adenosine | Nitric oxide | K^+_{ATP} channels | K^+ | ATP | PGs | Vessel wall | |
								PO_2	PCO_2
Resting flow	(+)	−	+	+ +	−	?	−	+	+
Reactive hyperemia	+	+ +	+ +	+ +		+	−	+	+
Autoregulation	(+ +)	+	−	(+ +)	−	?	−	−	−
Functional hyperemia	−	(±)	+	(+)	±	?	−	−	(−)
Ischemia	?	+ +	?	+ +	+	?	+	+	(±)

The contributions of various mechanisms to the control of the coronary circulation in several situations. PGs = prostaglandins; + + = major contribution; + = some contribution; ± = contributes to the initiation of the response but not in the steady state; − = little or no contribution; ? = contribution unknown. Parentheses indicate that the opinion is based on little information or is controversial. The ATP category includes potential contributions by ADP and AMP. PO_2 and PCO_2 refer to partial pressures at the vessel wall and their direct effects on vascular smooth muscle. See the text for more detailed discussions.

angiography could be a collapse of distributing arteries in the presence of increased flow (caused by the contrast medium) in vessels incapable of flow-induced dilation because of intimal lesions.

Table 57-1 summarizes our conclusions about the contributions of various local control mechanisms to coronary flow regulation under resting conditions and during reactive hyperemia, autoregulation, functional hyperemia, and ischemia.

NEURAL CONTROL OF CORONARY BLOOD FLOW

Both divisions of the autonomic nervous stystem innervate the coronary vessels {127–131}. Furthermore, coronary vascular smooth muscle cells have both alpha- and beta-adrenergic receptors {129,130,164,165}, as well as muscarinic cholinergic receptors {1}. Thus, the basic innervation of the coronary system allows for the full range of potential autonomic influence.

Sympathetic control

Stimulation of sympathetic efferents to the heart causes transient coronary vasoconstriction followed by a steady-state vasodilation {132–135}. The steady-state increase in flow is proportional to the increase in myocardial metabolism. This increase in flow can be prevented by agents that selectively block β_1 receptors, which are thought to reside primarily on myocardial cells {132,133,135,136}, but which also exist on coronary vascular smooth muscle {137,138}. With sympathetic activation in the presence of an alpha blocker, the initial vasoconstriction is abolished and the increase in steady-state flow is higher for any given level of myocardial metabolism {61,140–142}. Sympathetic activation in the presence of beta blockade results in coronary vasoconstriction, which can be blocked by various alpha-receptor blockers {132,133,136}. It appears that sympathetic stimulation results in a direct alpha-receptor-mediated constrictor effect, which competes with an indirect, metabolic vasodilator influence resulting from

stimulation of myocardial $beta_1$ receptors. It is also likely that $beta_1$ receptors of coronary smooth muscle are activated and that this contributes a vasodilator influence. However, the data suggest that the effect is minor when compared to the influence of direct alpha-mediated constriction and indirect β_1-mediated metabolic vasodilation {136}.

Sympathetic nerve stimulation reduces coronary sinus oxygen content to approximately half the value obtained when coronary alpha receptors are blocked {61,143–145}. Although this represents a rather dramatic vasoconstrictor influence in the face of increased metabolic need, there is no evidence that this results in impaired function of normal myocardium.

Exercise is accompanied by dramatic increases in coronary blood flow. However, blockade of coronary alpha receptors demonstrates that, even under these conditions, flow is somewhat limited by competing sympathetic alpha-receptor activation {141,142,166}. This constrictor influence may result from circulating catecholamines rather than direct neural effects {178}. Despite limiting flow, alpha tone during exercise does not cause any decrement in ventricular performance of the normal myocardium {141,142}.

The significance of coronary alpha tone under resting conditions remains controversial. The presence of basal alpha tone is implied by the observation that alpha blockade attenuates the decrease in coronary resistance resulting from activation of pulmonary stretch receptors {163} or the carotid sinus nerve {159,161,169}. Conscious, resting dogs have been given alpha blockers that are specific for postsynaptic, vasoconstrictor alpha receptors {170}. When administered in doses that caused similar reductions in cardiac preload and afterload, the drugs elicited significant reductions in late diastolic coronary resistance. When myocardial perfusion was compared between normal and sympathectomized regions of the heart in conscious dogs, data for {171} and against {172} resting alpha tone were obtained.

Coronary arteries may be innervated by sympathetic nerves containing neuropeptide Y {173}. Neuropeptide Y is released along with norepinephrine into coronary sinus blood draining human hearts during systemic hypoxia plus exercise {174}. This raises the possibility that a portion of the coronary constriction observed during sympathetic stimulation could be due to neuropeptide Y.

A number of studies have suggested that alpha receptors may be responsible for spasm of large coronary arteries {146–149}. This coincides with studies of isolated vessels that show there is a relatively higher population of alpha receptors in large coronary arteries than in small coronary arteries {150–153}. Interestingly, in vivo studies suggest that alpha-receptor-mediated vasoconstriction in large coronary vessels is not proportionately greater than that observed in the total coronary bed {175–177}.

Alpha-mediated coronary vasoconstriction is attracting increasing clinical interest as a possible mechanism for Pinzmetal's variant angina, as well as typical angina pectoris and myocardial infarction {146–148}. Patients with ischemic heart disease have been shown to be more suseptible to alpha-adrenergic-mediated increases in coronary resistance in response to the cold pressor test {180–182}. Conversely, when coronary alpha receptors have been blocked in patients with chronic stable angina, S-T segment depression during exercise is significantly reduced {183,184}. These observations suggest that alpha blockade improves oxygen delivery to the ischemic myocardium; this concept is supported by data from canine studies showing that blockade of coronary alpha receptors enhances coronary blood flow independent of changes in oxygen consumption {185,186}. Furthermore, there are now a number of papers suggesting that poststenotic coronary vasoconstriction occurs in response to increased sympathetic discharge and that this occurs via α_2 receptors {187}, (see section on myocardial ischemia). On the other hand, Nathan and Feigl have recently shown that the presence of alpha-adrenoreceptor tone promotes perfusion of the subendocardium by preventing a subepicardial steal during acute ischemia {188}.

Parasympathetic control

Stimulation of the vagus nerve, in paced hearts, causes a reduction in end-diastolic resistance. This reduction of resistance is blocked by atropine {154,155} and has led to the conclusion that parasympathetic cholinergic nerves innervate coronary resistance vessels. Reflex parasympathetic coronary vasodilation is elicited by activation of carotid body chemoreceptors, carotid body baroreceptors, and left ventricular receptors (see *Reflex control of the coronary circulation*). A careful study by Feigl {156} has failed to demonstrate sympathetic cholinergic vasodilation in the heart. This result was substantiated in a later study by Brown {157}.

Shepherd and VanHoutte postulate that acetylcholine reduces norepinephrine release from coronary artery sympathetic nerve endings, thereby lowering β_1 adrenoreceptor tone and causing coronary spasm {138}. This is most likely to happen when the coronary vascular smooth muscle is hypoxic and has lost its responsiveness to β_1 agonists. Reduced NO release by endothelial cells would also predispose to this effect, since the direct effect of

ACh on coronary vascular smooth muscle is constriction. Young et al. {189} suggest that in conscious calves nicotine causes coronary vasoconstriction via parasympathetic cholinergic nerves. Observations such as those in the above papers raise the distinct possibility that ACh can be a coronary vasoconstrictor in some pathophysiologic conditions.

Reflex control of the coronary circulation

Bilateral carotid artery occlusion results in coronary blood flow changes that are similar to those observed during stellate ganglion stimulation; i.e., there is an increase in coronary blood flow, which can be enhanced by alpha blockade {61}. Bilateral carotid artery hypotension results in increased coronary resistance in the presence of propranolol and vagotomy {144,158}. This increase in resistance can be prevented by sympathectomy or by alpha blockade. Electrical stimulation of the carotid sinus nerve reduces coronary vascular resistance as a result of inhibition of alpha-adredergic tone {159,161} and parasympathetic coronary vasodilation {160}. However, it is difficult to equate nerve stimulation with carotid sinus pressures that stimulate baroreceptors. Step increments in the carotid sinus pressure of beta-blocked, anesthetized dogs also increase coronary flow; atropine blocked most of the reflex coronary hyperemia, and the addition of an alpha blocker eliminated the remaining response {169}. Thus it appears that there is alpha-adrenergic vasoconstrictor coronary tone that is enhanced by carotid occlusion and abolished by increased baroreceptor nerve firing.

In addition, baroreceptor activation elicits a significant parasympathetic, cholinergic coronary dilation. When carotid body chemoreceptors are stimulated by nicotine, cyanide, or hypoxic-hypercapnic blood, parasympathetic cholinergic vasodilation occurs in the coronary bed of anesthetized dogs {160,162,169}. In unanesthetized dogs there is a two-step coronary response to intracoronary nicotine {163}. First, chemoreceptor stimulation elicits a direct parasympathetic coronary dilation, which was described above. Second, chemoreceptor stimulation reflexly increases the depth of ventilation; subsequent activation of pulmonary stretch receptors triggers coronary vasodilation by inhibition of sympathetic coronary vasoconstrictor tone.

In addition to the early period of coronary dilation, intracarotid nicotine results in a later period of coronary, alpha-mediated vasoconstriction {168}. This constrictor effect is less prominent in the left coronary artery (versus right coronary), probably because it is being masked by the metabolic hyperemia resulting from the chemoreceptor-induced increase in left ventricular afterload. The Bezold–Jarisch reflex results from excitation of cardiac receptors in response to intracoronary injections of veratridine. Feigl has demonstrated that the coronary effect of the Bezold–Jarish reflex is a parasympathetic vasodilation {190}. The colonic distension results in reflex coronary vasoconstriction {191}.

Activation of cardiac sensory nerves can result in coronary vasodilation. A study by Franco–Cereceda {192} indicates that calcitonin gene-related peptide (CGRP) is a more likely cause of the vasodilation thatn substance P.

CARDIAC HYPERTROPHY

Cardiac hypertrophy is often a compensatory response to an increase in cardiac work load, which leads to abnormally elevated systolic wall stress {193}. As the ventricle hypertrophies, the systolic wall stress decreases in proportion to the increased wall thickness. The systolic wall stress of an appropriately hypertrophied heart returns to normal or near-normal values, and compensated hypertrophy is generally of long duration {194–196}. Despite the appropriateness of the hypertrophied heart to the increased work load, left ventricular hypertrophy clinically defined by echocardiography or electrocardiogram is associated with increased mortality and higher risk of cardiac failure {197,198}. This may be linked to changes in the coronary circulation. In addition to clinical studies, various animal models of hypertrophy have been developed. Due to the prevalence of arterial hypertension in humans, this review will focus on pressure overload-induced hypertrophy in the adult left ventricle.

Most studies indicate that resting coronary blood flow and oxygen consumption per unit myocardial mass are within normal limits in hypertrophied left ventricle {199–205}. Thus, flow and oxygen consumption increase in proportion to the increase in myocardial mass. However, right ventricular hypertrophy is associated with an increased resting flow per gram of myocardium {206–211}. An uncompensated increase in right ventricular wall stress may account for the augmented perfusion {208,209}. Clinical and experimental evidence indicates that although coronary flow in hypertrophied hearts may be normal under resting conditions, regional ischemia may occur under stress, even in the absence of coronary artery disease. This is manifested clinically as angina pectoris {212–217}, electrocardiographic abnormalities {214,218, 219}, and fibrosis or infarction in subendocardium and papillary muscles {213,220–223}. Animal studies have found lactate production in hypertrophied hearts during pacing and catecholamine infusion, suggesting that regional myocardial ischemia occurred even though the total coronary flow was increased to the same extent as in normal hearts {212,224–226}.

Myocardial underperfusion under stress may result from a failure of vascular proliferation to keep pace with myocyte growth during hypertrophy. This is supported by findings of increased minimum coronary vascular resistance during reactive hyperemia or maximal pharmacologic vasodilation {198,202,210,227–231}. The cardiac concentration of cyclic GMP kinase, an index of vascularization, is decreased in hypertrophied hearts {232}. This hypothesis is further supported by animal studies showing decreased capillary density in hypertrophied hearts, and a failure of coronary artery luminal diameter to increase in proportion to the degree of hypertrophy {233–239}. Pressure overload hypertrophy leads to a greater increase in myocyte diameter in papillary muscle and subendocardium, re-

sulting in a greater decrease in capillary density in these deeper layers {240–242}. These anatomic changes may contribute to the increased minimum coronary vascular resistance.

Hypertensive changes in the coronary vasculature may also contribute to increased minimum vascular resistance in hypertrophied hearts. Although hypertrophy without increased pressure leads to increased minimum vascular resistance {210,243}, increased arterial pressure without hypertrophy (as in the right ventricle of some models of left ventricular hypertrophy) produces the same result {199,244}. Also, minimum coronary vascular resistance in patients with hypertensive hypertrophy becomes normal after treatment with hydralazine despite the continued presence of hypertrophy {203}. An additional source of increased vascular resistance in hypertrophied hearts may be an increased extravascular component {200,245–247}.

An additional abnormality in hypertrophied hearts is a reduction in the coronary reserve, defined as the difference between baseline and maximal flows. This phenomenon occurs primarily in severe hypertrophy {215,245–247}. It may result from the increase in minimum vascular resistance described above, or from an encroachment on the vasodilator reserve in order to maintain normal resting flows {250}. Elevated resting flow appears to be the cause in hypertrophy induced by volume overload {217,248}. Hypertrophy induced by exercise training or chronic thyroxine treatment does not reduce the coronary flow reserve {249,250}.

The transmural distribution of flow can also be abnormal in hypertrophied hearts, even under resting conditions, if the hypertrophy is severe {228,230,231,254}, Unlike the normal heart, where the highest flow occurs in the subendocardium, in hearts hypertrophied secondary to ascending aortic constriction, the highest flow occurred in the midwall of the left ventricle {230,231}. The subendocardial/subepicardial flow ratio was lower than normal. Since subendocardial flow was able to increase during exercise or pharmacologic vasodilation {228,231}, the change in flow distribution may result from redistribution of wall stress such that the highest systolic stresses occur in the midwall of hypertrophied hearts {230}. In less severely hypertrophied hearts, the coronary flow distribution at rest is normal {198–200}. However, a decrease in the subendocardial/subepicardial flow ratio occurs in hypertrophied hearts subjected to pacing tachycardia {200,228,255}, exercise {243,256}, catecholamine infusion {257}, adenosine infusion {210,211}, or reactive hyperemia {258,259}. This is associated in some cases with subendocardial dysfunction {260,261} and could contribute to the increased vulnerability of the hypertrophied subendocardium to ischemia.

Marcus and colleagues have used a Doppler probe to obtain measurements of coronary rective hyperemia in patients with cardiac hypertrophy at the time of cardiac surgery. The response of the left anterior descending coronary artery to transient occlusion was significantly reduced in patients with left ventricular hypertrophy secondary to mitral regurgitation {227} or to aortic senosis {215}. Relief of aortic obstruction did not improve the coronary response; therefore, extravascular compressive forces were not responsible for the perfusion abnormality associated with aortic stenosis {248}. Right ventricular hypertrophy, secondary to atrial septal defects, was associated with a hyperemic response of one half of that observed in control patients {262}. Argon clearance has also been used to measure coronary flow in patients with left ventricular hypertrophy secondary to aortic stenosis, or mitral or aortic regurgitation {263,264}. Coronary reserve was substantially reduced in these patients. When Strauer examined coronary reserve in patients with various degrees of hyperension and hypertrophy, he found abnormalities, even if the hypertrophy was relatively modest (30% increased left ventricular mass) {214}. Taken together, these observations suggest that reduced coronary reserve in patients with cardiac hypertrophy contributes to angina and heart failure.

ISCHEMIA

Responses to acute ischemia

When stenosis of a major coronary artery occurs, two compensatory events limit the potential fall in myocardial

blood flow beyond the stenosis. First, vessels distal to the stenosis dilate {4} in response to the fall in transmural pressure and increased metabolic vasodilator release (see discussion of autoregulation above). Second, flow from other major arteries reaches the region beyond the stenosis via preexisting collateral vessels linking arteries and arterioles of the two regions. The contribution of collateral flow to the potentially ischemic region depends on the species and on other unknown factors {265–267}. Some species such as dog have a higher number of preexisting collaterals than other species, such as pig and humans {265,266}. However, there appears to be a considerable variation in the number of collateral vessels within a given species, and the reason for this variation is not known {267,268}.

When stenosis of a coronary artery reaches a critical level, the combination of autoregulatory dilation of resistance vessels and collateral flow is no longer sufficient to provide a normal resting flow. At this point, flow to the subendocardium begins to fall {269,270}. The greater vulnerability of the subendocardium appears to be related to the higher intramyocardial forces that act on vessels supplying this region (see Chapter 58). The subendocardium uses more of its vasodilator capacity under normal circumstances. For this reason, less vasodilator reserve

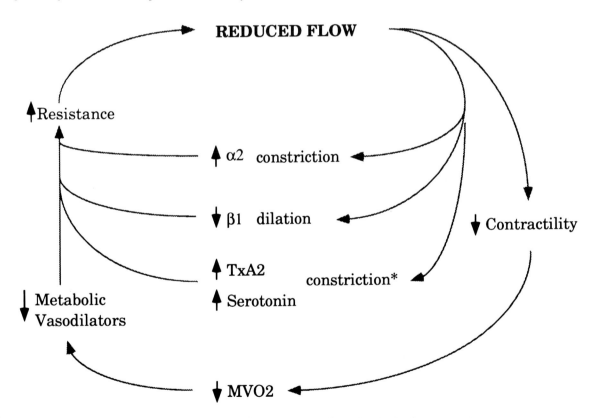

Fig. 57-3. Proposed positive feedback relationship initiated by myocardial ischemia. Both vasoconstrictor release and decreased myocardial metabolism cause vasoconstriction and a further drop in blood flow. This leads to the observed increase in vasodilator reserve with time distal to a stenosis. *Thromboxane A2 (TxA2) and serotonin will cause vasoconstriction in areas where the endothelium is damaged.

remains to compensate for a fall in perfusion pressure caused by the stenosis. A reduction in ventricular contractile force occurs very soon after coronary blood flow is decreased {271–274}. Ultimately, ventricular contraction in the ischemic region becomes so weak that paradoxical bulging occurs during ventricular systole because of the increase in intracavitary pressure {271,274}.

Vascular smooth muscle tone during ischemia

When ischemia is severe there is abundant release of metabolic vasodilators (adenosine, K^+, H^+, prostaglandins), which can account for decreased vascular resistance in the ischemic area. During less severe ischemia, an interesting interaction occurs between vascular smooth muscle tone and contractile force. As a coronary arterial stenosis is made progressively more severe, one might expect that blood flow and tension development would begin to fall only after the coronary vasodilator reserve is exhausted. However, flow and tension begin to fall well before maximal vasodilation occurs. This has been demonstrated most convincingly in experiments in which adenosine is infused distal to a flow-limiting coronary stenosis and in which pressure distal to the stenosis is held constant {275,279–281,291}. Although the amount of vasodilator reserve is greater in the subepicardium than in the subendocardium, measurements of the distribution of flow with radioactive microspheres have demonstrated that under certain experimental conditions, vasodilator reserve remains after significant flow and segment shortening reduction in both regions {281,284}. As the stenosis is made more severe, vasodilator reserve disappears in the subendocardium and diminishes in the subepicardium. The unused vasodilator reserve is not merely a pharmacologic phenomenon, since dilation can also be elicited by increasing metabolism via norepinephrine infusion or by increasing heart rate {145,282,291}.

The reasons for this unused vasodilator reserve in the face of reduced flow and tension are not fully understood. Figure 57-3 summarizes two major hypotheses. Both have the potential to become positive feedback loops that can accentuate the decline in flow distal to a stenosis. As depicted in the three inner loops, reduced flow may trigger the release of coronary vasoconstrictor substances. Norepinephrine is one potential vasoconstrictor released within ischemic myocardium. The net effect of norepinephrine release on vascular resistance depends on the balance between alpha-adrenergic vasoconstriction and metabolic coronary vasodilation. High doses of norepinephrine infused into moderately ischemic myocardium result in a net metabolic vasodilation {145,291}, but in similar preparations sympathetic nerve stimulation causes a net vasoconstriction mediated by α_2 receptors {285}. In addition, hypoxia within the ischemic region may prevent the direct vasodilator effect of norepinephrine mediated by coronary arterial β_1 receptors {138}. Finally, aggregating platelets release substances such as thromboxane A_2 and serotonin, which can cause vasoconstriction in areas where the endothelium has been damaged {139}.

An alternative explanation for unused vasodilator

reserve in ischemic myocardium, diagrammed in the outer loop of fig. 57-3, is that the reduction in contractile force reduces oxygen demand, and the resulting improvement in the O_2 supply/demand ratio reduces the release of metabolic vasodilators. For example, the high initial release of at least one putative metabolic vasodilator, adenosine, is not maintained at the peak level during prolonged ischemia {294}. According to this hypothesis, the heart does not maximally dilate during moderate flow reductions because the O_2 supply/demand ratio in most of the myocardium may be almost normal {290,291,295}. Although this is an attractive hypothesis, it is difficult to test because of the lack of a definitive measure of oxygen demand during reduced flow. The observation that metabolic stimulation of the ischemic myocardium produces vasodilation is consistent with this hypothesis {145,282}. One recent study of moderate ischemia supports the hypothesis that the noncontracting myocardium has a normal energy supply/demand balance {297}. In ischemic subendocardium distal to a stenosis, phosphocreatine concentration fell initially but recovered to normal levels after 1 hour. Contractile function remained depressed during this recovery of phosphocreatine.

The initial depression of contractile force during moderate ischemia may be mediated by cardiac myocyte K_{ATP}^+ channels. Adenosine release may be the stimulus that opens these channels {298}. (If the ischemia is severe enough a decrease in myocyte [ATP] will also contribute.) However, if the energy supply/demand returns to normal as suggested by the recovery of phosphocreatine, why does contractile function remain depressed? Adenosine release declines during continued ischemia, and the recovery of phosphocreatine suggests that myocyte [ATP] must also be near normal. The answer to these questions will require further study. This shutdown of contractile function during moderate ischemia may permit the survival of underperfused but viable myocardium following a decrease in flow or an increase in oxygen demand.

Prolonged ischemia

When a coronary artery stenosis is maintained for several hours, the distal coronary blood flow declines slowly. In some cases this can be due to platelet aggregation at the stenosis site, which increases the resistance of the stenosis {276}. Additional mechanisms must be present, however, since vascular resistance distal the stenosis also increases {288–292}. Again, the search for a vasoconstrictor substance released within the ischemic area has been unsuccessful {291}. Another possibility is that this flow decline represents a slower version of the metabolic shutdown proposed in fig. 57-3. Two other mechanisms that contribute to the increasing resistance during prolonged ischemia are cell swelling and the formation of leukocyte plugs in the microvessels. Pretreatment with either hypertonic mannitol or hyaluronidase prevent the cell swelling and increased resistance associated with prolonged ischemia in some experimental models {277, 288,293,296,301,302}.

Granulocytes have been shown to accumulate within

ischemic myocardium, and the degree of accumulation correlates negatively with blood flow changes during 3 hours of ischemia {283}. In addition, myocardial perfusion with granulocyte-depleted blood prevents a decrease in flow during 60 minutes of ischemia as well as capillary plugging following reperfusion (the "no-reflow" phenomenon) {278,299,300}. It seems likely that the dominant mechanism behind this slow increase in vascular resistance during prolonged ischemia depends on the initial degree of ischemia. If the initial ischemia is moderate, an increase in vascular smooth muscle tone is apparent, but during severe ischemia, cell swelling and leukocyte plugs are more likely to be the source of increasing vascular resistance.

COLLATERAL BLOOD FLOW

Collateral blood vessels are anastamoses between coronary arteries that can provide an alternative source of blood supply to myocardium jeopardized by occlusion or stenosis of the original vessel. Increased collateral flow provides a measure of immediate compensation when stenosis occurs. Furthermore, development of new collateral vessels can begin within 1–6 hours, depending on the degree of occlusion {265,303–305}. As a consequence, the blood pressure and flow distal to the occlusion begin to increase and continue to do so until the basal needs of the surviving subserved tissue are met. If an occlusion is released after full collateral development, the collateral vessels become nonfunctional within 24 hours {306}. If the same coronary artery is reoccluded between 3 and 90 days, full collateral flow is reestablished with 1 hour without myocardial damage. Although there has been considerable doubt concerning the functional role of collaterals in human hearts {307}, recent studies have confirmed the substantial potential of collaterals in minimizing myocardial infart size and cell death, and in improving the clinical outcome of ischemic heart disease {308,309}.

It has been suggested that collateral vessel development occurs from preexisting microscopic vascular connections between major coronary arteries. Schaper and colleagues have provided support for this idea {265}. They propose that local release of vasodilators dilates the connecting microscropic collateral vessels and increases the pressure and wall stress on the thin walled vessels. This stress results in wall damage, which includes cellular infiltration and breaks in the wall. Reparative processes then occur in which there is proliferation of endothelium and smooth muscle as well as progressive growth of the vessel. Thus there is a transition from the thin-walled, microscopic collateral vessel to large, thick-walled, large-lumen vessels. In some species such as the dog, collaterals also develop from small epicardial arteries {265}.

The exact determinants of the development of collateral vessels are not clear. Collateral development does not occur in response to exercise without preexisting ischemia {310–312} and is directed only toward ischemic areas {313}. Ischemia and/or a pressure gradient (and the resulting flow) across the collateral network are now considered to be the triggers of collateral growth {314,315}.

Evidence for DNA synthesis in all mesoderm-derived cells of hearts with progressive coronary occlusion {316} suggests that ischemic myocardium produces a chemical signal that triggers the events leading to DNA synthesis and to mitosis in collateral vessels. This chemical messenger may be the family of heparin-binding growth factors (HBGF) {317}. Under normal conditions, the receptors for HBGF are downregulated, and ischemia may lead to their upregulation {318,319}. Although heparin alone does not initiate angiogenesis, it increases the binding of the endothelial cell growth factor to endothelial receptors {320} and protects fibroblast growth factor from inactivation {321}. Animal studies using heparin indicate that it has the potential to accelerate collateral vessel development {322}. Other angiogenic factors have also been identified {323}. Angiogenesis is regulated by a number of different, sometimes redundant signals, and the same is likely to be true of coronary collateral vessel development.

ACKNOWLEDGMENTS

Preparation of this chapter was supported by U.S. Public Health Service grant HL-24232.

REFERENCES

1. Berne RM, Rubio R: Coronary circulation. In: Berne RM, Sperelakis N, Geiger SR (eds) *Handbook of Physiology.* Vol 1, Sect 2: *The Cardiovascular System.* Besthesda, MD: American Physiological Society, 1979, pp 873–952.
2. Harlan DM, Rooke TW, Belloni FL, Sparks HV: Effect of indomethacin on coronary vascular response to increased myocardial oxygen consumption. *Am J Physiol* 235:H372–H378, 1978.
3. Coffman JD, Gregg DE: Reactive hyperemia characteristics of the myocardium. *Am J Physiol* 199:1143–1149, 1960.
4. Khouri EM, Gregg ED, Lowensohn HS: Flow in the major branches of the left coronary artery during experimental coronary insufficiency in the anesthetized dog. *Circ Res* 23:99–109, 1968.
5. Olsson RA, Gregg DE: Myocardial reactive hyperemia in the unanesthetized dog. *Am J Physiol* 208:224–230, 1965.
6. Johnson PC: The myogenic response. In: Bohr DF, Somlyo SR, Sparks HV (eds) *Handbook of Physiology* Vol 2, Sect 2: *The Cardiovascular System.* Bethesda, MD: American Physiological Society, 1980, pp 409–422.
7. Ueeda M, Silvia SK, Olsson RA: Nitric oxide modulates coronary autoregulation in the guinea pig. *Circ Res* 70:1296–1303, 1992.
8. Eikens E, Wilcken DEL: Myocardial reactive hyperemia and coronary vascular reactivity in the dog. *Circ Res* 33:267–274, 1973.
9. Eikens E, Wilcken DEL: Reactive hyperemia in the dog heart: Effects of temporarily restricting arterial inflow and of coronary occlusions lasting one and two cardiac cycle. *Circ Res* 35:702–712, 1974.
10. Schwartz GG, McHale PA, Greenfield JG: Hyperemic response of the coronary circulation to brief diastolic occlusion in the conscious dog. *Circ Res* 50:28–37, 1982.

11. Scott JB, Radawski D: Role of hyperosmolarity in the genesis of active and reactive hyperemia. *Circ Res* 28(Suppl 1):126–32, 1971.

12. Murray PA, Belloni FL, Sparks HV: The role of potassium in the metabolic control of coronary vascular resistance of the dog. *Circ Res* 44:767–780, 1979.

13. Bunger R, Haddy FJ, Querengasser A, Gerlach E: Studies on potassium induced coronary dilation in the isolated guinea pig heart. *Pflügers Arch* 63:27–31, 1976.

14. Winbury MM, Howe BB, Weiss HR: Effect of nitroglycerin and dipyridamole on epicardial and endocardial oxygen tension: Further evidence for redistribution of myocardial blood flow. *J Pharmacol Exp Ther* 176:184–199, 1971.

15. Sparks HV: Effect of local metabolic factors on vascular smooth muscle. In: Bohr DF, Somlyo SR, Sparks HV (eds) *Handbook of Physiology*. Vol 2, Sect 2: *The Cardiovascular System*. Bethesda, MD: American Physiological Society, 1980, pp 475–513.

16. Chang AE, Detar R: Oxygen and vascular smooth muscle revisited. *Am J Physiol* 238:H716–H728, 1980.

17. Coburn RF, Polegmakers F, Gondrie P, Abboud R: Myocardial myoglobin oxygen tension. *Am J Physiol* 224:870–876, 1973.

18. Jackson WF, Duling BR: The oxygen sensitivity of hamster cheek pouch arterioles. *Circ Res* 53:515–525, 1983.

19. Kalsner S: Intrinsic prostaglandin release: A mediator of anoxia-induced relaxation in an isolated coronary artery preparation. *Blood Vessels* 13:155–166, 1976.

20. McNeil TA: Venous oxygen saturation and blood flow during reactive hyperemia in the human forearm. *J Physiol (Lond)* 134:195–201, 1956.

21. Alexander RW, Kent KM, Pisano JJ, Keiser HR, Cooper T: Regulation of postocclusive hyperemia by endogenously synthesized prostaglandins in the dog heart. *J Clin Invest* 55:1174–1181, 1975.

22. Needleman P, Iskoson PC: Intrinsic prostaglandin biosynthesis in blood vessels. In: Bohr DF, Somlyo SR, Sparks HV (eds) *Handbook of Physiology*. Vol 2, Sect 2: *The Cardiovascular System*. Bethesda, MD: American Physological Society, 1980, pp 613–633.

23. Owen TL, Ehrhart IC, Weidner WJ, Scott JB, Haddy FJ: Effects of indomethacin on local blood flow regulation in canine heart and kidney. *Proc Soc Exp Biol Med* 149:871–876, 1975.

24. Hintze TH, Kaley G: Prostaglandins and the control of blood flow in the canine myocardium. *Circ Res* 40:313–320, 1977.

25. Giles RW, Wilcken DEL: Reactive hyperemia in the dog heart: Interrelations between adenosine, ATP, and aminophylline and the effect of indomethacin. *Cardiovasc Res* 11:113–121, 1977.

26. Rubio R, Berne RM, Katori M: Release of adenosine in reactive hyperemia of the dog heart. *Am J Physiol* 216:56–62, 1969.

27. Olsson RA: Changes in content of purine nucleotide in canine myocardium during coronary occlusion. *Circ Res* 26:301–306, 1970.

28. Schrader J, Haddy FJ, Gerlach E: Release of adenosine, inosine, and hypoxanthine from the isolated guinea pig heart during hypoxia, flow-autoregulation and reactive hyperemia. *Pflügers Arch* 369:1–6, 1977.

29. Olsson RA, Snow JA, Gentry MK: Adenosine metabolism in canine myocardial reactive hyperemia. *Circ Res* 42:358–362, 1978.

30. Curnish RR, Berne RM, Rubio R: Effect of aminophylline on myocardial reactive hyperemia. *Proc Soc Exp Biol Med* 141:593–598, 1972.

31. Schutz W, Zimpfer M, Raberger G: Effect of aminophylline on coronary reactive hyperemia following brief and long occlusion periods. *Cardiovasc Res* 11:507–511, 1977.

32. Juhran W, Voss EM, Dietmann K, Schaumann W: Pharmacologic effects on coronary reactive hyperemia in conscious dogs. *Naunyn Schmiedbergs Arch Pharmacol* 269:32–47, 1971.

33. Bittar N, Pauly TJ: Myocardial reactive hyperemia responses in the dog after aminophylline and lidoflazine. *Am J Physiol* 220:812–815, 1971.

34. Saito D, Seinhart CR, Nixon DG, Olsson RA: Intracoronary adenosine deaminase reduces canine myocardial reactive hyperemia. *Circ Res* 49:1262–1267, 1981.

35. Buga GM, Gold ME, Fukuro JM, Ignarro LJ: Shear stress-induced release of nitric oxide from endothelial cells grown on beads. *Hypertension* 17:187–193, 1991.

36. Pohl U, Busse R: Hypoxia stimulates te release of endothelial-derived relaxant factor (EDRF). *Am J Physiol* 256:H1595–H1600, 1989.

37. Bassenge E: Endothelial regulation of coronary tone. In: Ryan US, Rubanyi GM (eds) *Endothelial Regulation of Vascular Tone*. New York: Marcel Dekker, 1992, pp 225–264.

38. Kostic MM, Schrader J: Role of nitric oxide in reactive hyperemia of the guinea pig heart. *Circ Res* 70:208–212, 1922.

39. Yamabe H, Okumura K, Ishizaka H, Tsuchiya T, Yasue H: Role of endothelium-derived nitric oxide in myocardial reactive hyperemia. *Am J Physiol* 263:H8–H14, 1992.

40. Nichols CG, Lederer WJ: Adenosine triphosphate-sensitive potassium channels in the cardiovascular system. *Am J Physiol* 261:H1675–H1686, 1991.

41. Aversano T, Ouyang P, Silverman H: Blockade of the ATP-sensitive potassium channel modulates reactive hyperemia in the canine coronary circulation. *Circ Res* 69:618–622, 1991.

42. Daut J, Maier-Rudolph W, von Beckerath N, Mehrke G, Gunther K, Goedel-Meinen L: Hypoxic dilation of coronary arteries is mediated by ATP-sensitive potassium channels. *Science* 247:1341–1343, 1990.

43. Belloni FL, Hintze TH: Glibenclamide attenuates adenosine-induced bradycardia and coronary vasodilatation. *Am J Physiol* 261:H720–H727, 1991.

44. Samaha FF, Heineman FW, Fleming CI, Balaban RS: ATP-sensitive potassium channel is essential to maintain basal coronary vascular tone in ivio. *Am J Physiol* 262:C1220–C1227, 1992.

45. Imamura Y, Tomoike H, Narishige T, Takahashi T, Kasuya H, Takeshita A: Glibenclamide decreases basal coronary blood flow in anesthetized dogs. *Am J Physiol* 263:H399–H404, 1992.

46. Borst MM, Schrader J: Adenine nucleotide release from isolated perfused guinea pig hearts and extracellular formation of adenosine. *Circ Res* 68:797–806, 1991.

47. DeMey JG, VanHoutte PM: Role of the intima in cholinergic and purinergic relaxation of isolated canine fermoral arteries. *J Physiol* 316:347–355, 1981.

48. Brown IP, Thompson CI, Belloni FL: Mechanisms of coronary vasodilatation produced by ATP in guinea-pig isolated perfused heart. *Br J Pharmacol* 105:211–215, 1992.

49. Kitikaze M, Hori M, Takashima S, Iwai K, Sato H, Inoue M, Kitabatake A, Kamada T: Sureroxide dismutase enhances ischemia-induced reactive hyperemia flow and adenosine release in dogs. *Circ Res* 71:558–566, 1992.

50. Mosher P, Ross J, McFate PA, Shaw RF: Control of coronary blood flow by an autoregulatory mechanism. *Circ Res* 14:250–259, 1964.

51. Shaw RF, Mosher P, Ross J, Joseph JI, Lee ASJ: Physiologic principles of coronary perfusion. *J Thorac Cardiovas Surg* 44:608–616, 1962.
52. Rouleau J, Boerboom LE, Surjadhana A, Hoffman JIE: The role of autoregulation and tissue diastolic pressures in the transmural distribution of left ventricular blood flow in anesthetized dogs. *Circ Res* 45:804–815, 1979.
53. Boatwright RB, Downey HF, Bashour FA, Crystal GJ: Transmural variation in autoregulation of coronary blood flow in hyperperfused canine myocardium. *Circ Res* 47:599–609, 1980.
54. Rubio R, Berne RM: Regulation of coronary blood flow. *Prog Cardiovasc Dis* 18:105–122, 1975.
55. Dole WP, Nuno DW: Myocardial oxygen tension determines the degree and pressure range of coronary autoregulation. *Circ Res* 59:202–215, 1986.
56. Broten TP, Romson JL, Fullerton DA, Van Winkle D, Feigl EO: Synergistic action of myocardial oxygen and carbon dioxide in controlling coronary blood flow. *Circ Res* 68:531–542, 1991.
57. Broten TP, Feigl EO: Role of myocardial oxygen and carbon dioxide in coronary autoregulation. *Am J Physiol* 262:H1231–H1237, 1992.
58. Hanley FL, Grattan MT, Stevens MB, Hoffman JIE: Role of adenosine in coronary autoregulation. *Am J Physiol* 250:H558–H566, 1986.
59. Dole WP, Yamada N, Bishop VS, Olsson RA: Role of adenosine in coronary blood flow regulation after reductions in perfusion pressure. *Circ Res* 56:517–524, 1985.
60. Komaru T, Lamping KG, Eastham CL, Dellsperger KC: Role of ATP-sensitive potassium channels in coronary microvascular autoregulatory responses. *Circ Res* 69:1146–1151, 1991.
61. Mohrman DE, Feigel EO: Competition between sympathetic vasoconstriction and metabolic vasodilation in the canine coronary circulation. *Circ Res* 42:79–86, 1977.
62. Britton S, Di Valvo J: Effects of angiotensin I and angiotensin II on hindlimb and coronary vascular resistance. *Am J Physiol* 225:1226–1231, 1973.
63. Cohen MV, Kirk ES: Differential response of large and small coronary arteries to nitroglycerin and angiotensin: Autoregulation and tachyphylaxis. *Circ Res* 33:445–453, 1973.
64. Green HD, Kepchar JH: Control of peripheral resistance in major systemic vascular beds. *Physiol Rev* 39:617–686, 1959.
65. Case RB, Felix A, Wachter M, Kyriakidis G, Castellana F: Relative effect of CO_2 on canine coronary vascular resistance. *Circ Res* 42:410–418, 1978.
66. Case RB, Greenberg H: The response of canine coronary vascular resistance to local alterations in coronary arterial pCO_2. *Circ Res* 39:558–566, 1976.
67. Case RB, Greenberg H, Moskowitz R: Alterations in coronary sinus pO_2 and O_2 saturation resulting from pCO_2 changes. *Cardiovasc Res* 9:167–177, 1975.
68. Rooke, T, Sparks HV: Arterial CO_2, myocardial O_2 consumption, and coronary blood flow in the dog. *Circ Res* 47:217–225, 1980.
69. Wiedmeier VT, Spell LH: Effects of catecholamines, histamine and nitroglycerin on flow, oxygen consumption and coronary blood flow during stellate ganglia stimulation. *Circ Res* 45:708–718, 1979.
70. Raberger G, Weissel M, Kraupp O: The dependence of the effects of intracoronary administered adenosine and of coronary conductance on the arterial pH, pCO_2, and buffer capacity in dogs. *Naunyn-Schmiedebergs Arch Pharmacol* 271:301–310, 1971.
71. Merrill GF, Haddy FJ, Dabney JM: Adenosine, theophylline, and perfusate pH in the isolated, perfused guinea pig heart. *Circ Res* 42:225–229, 1978.
72. Kittle CF, Aoki H, Brown E: The role of pH and CO_2 in the distribution of blood flow. *Surgery* 57:139–154, 1965.
73. Tarnow J, Bruckner JB, Eberlein HJ, Gethmann JW, Hess W, Patschke D, Wilde J: Blood pH and $PaCO_2$ as chemical factors in myocardial blood flow control. *Basic Res Cardiol* 70:685–696, 1975.
74. Gilmore JP, Nizolek JA, Jacob RJ: Further characterization of myocardial K^+ loss induced by changing contraction frequency. *Am J Physiol* 221:465–469, 1971.
75. Sybers HD, Helmer RP, Murphy QR: Effects of hypoxia on myocardial potassium balance. *Am J Physiol* 220:2047–2050, 1971.
76. Frick GP, Lowenstein JM: Studies of 5'-nucleotidase in the perfused rat heart: Including measurements of the enzyme in perfused skeletal muscle and liver. *J Biol Chem* 251:6372–6378, 1976.
77. Schutz W, Shrader J, Gerlach E: Different sites of adenosine formation in the heart. *Am J Physiol* 240:H963–H970, 1981.
78. Schrader J, Schutz W, Bardenheuer H: Role of S-adenosyl-homocysteine hydrolase in adenosine metabolism in mammalian heart. *Biochem J* 196:65–70, 1981.
79. Olsson RA, Saito D, Steinhart CR: Compartmentalization of the adenosine pool of dog and rat hearts. *Circ Res* 50:617–626, 1982.
80. Schrader J, Gerlach E: Compartmentation of cardiac adenine nucleotides and formation of adenosine. *Pflügers Arch* 367:129–135, 1976.
81. Belloni FL, Rubio R, Berne RM: Intracellular adenosine in isolated rat liver cells. *Pflügers Arch* 400:106–108, 1984.
82. Lloyd HGE, Deussen A, Wuppermann H, Schrader J: The transmethylation pathway as a source for adenosine in the isolated guinea pig heart. *Biochem J* 252:489–494, 1988.
83. Bunger R, Soboll S: Cytosolic adenylates and adenosine in perfused working heart. *Eur J Biochem* 159:203–213, 1986.
84. Darvish A, Britton SL, Metting P: Adenosine production by dog heart cytosolic 5'-nucleotidase is regulated by adenine nucleotides. *FASEB J* 5:A1104, 1991.
85. Skladanowski AC, Newby AC: Partial purification and properties of an AMP-specific soluble 5'-nucleotidase from pigeon heart. *Biochem J* 268:117–122, 1990.
86. He M-X, Gorman MW, Romig GD, Sparks HV: Linear relation between adenosine release and inorganic phosphate in isolated hearts. *FASEB J*, 1993, in press.
87. He M-X, Wangler RD, Dillon PF, Romig GD, Sparks HV: Phosphorylation potential and adenosine release during norepinephrine infusion in guinea pig heart. *Am J Physiol* 253:H1184–H1191, 1987.
88. He M-X, Gorman MW, Romig GD, Meyer RA, Sparks HV: Adenosine formation and energy status during hypoperfusion and 2-deoxyglucose infusion. *Am J Physiol* 260:H917–H926, 1991.
89. He M-X, Gorman MW, Romig GD, Sparks HV: Adenosine formation and myocardial energy status during graded hypoxia. *J Mol Cell Cardiol* 24:79–89, 1992.
90. Deussen A, Schrader J: Cardiac adenosine production is linked to myocardial PO_2. *J Mol Cell Cardiol* 23:495–504, 1991.
91. Miller WL, Belardinelli L, Bacchus A, Foley DH, Rubio R, Berne RM: Canine myocardial adenosine and lactate production, oxygen consumption and coronary blood flow during stellate ganglia stimulation. *Circ Res* 45:708–718, 1979.
92. Watkinson WP, Foley DH, Rubio R, Berne RM: Myocardial adenosine formation with increased cardiac performance in the dog. *Am J Physiol* 236:H13–H21, 1979.

93. Knabb RM, Ely SW, Bacchus AN, Rubio R, Berne RM: Consistent parallel relationships among myocardial oxygen consumption, coronary blood flow, and pericardial infusate adenosine concentration with various interventions and beta blockade in the dog. *Circ Res* 53:33–41, 1983.

94. Degenring FH: Cardiac nucleotides and coronary flow during changes of cardiac inotropy. *Basic Res Cardiol* 71: 291–296, 1976.

95. Foley DH, Herlihy JT, Thompson CI, Rubio R, Berne RM: Increased adenosine formation by rat myocardium with acute aortic constriction. *J Mol Cell Cardiol* 10:293–300, 1978.

96. McKenzie JE, McCoy FP, Bockman EL: Myocardial adenosine and coronary resistance during increased cardiac performance. *Am J Physiol* 239:H509–H515, 1980.

97. Downey HF, Merrill GF, Yonekura S, Watanabe N, Jones CE: Adenosine deaminase attenuates norepinephrine-induced coronary functional hyperemia. *Am J Physiol* 254: H417–H424, 1988.

98. Jones CE, Hurst TW, Randall JR: Effect of aminophylline on coronary functional hyperemia and myocardial adenosine. *Am J Physiol* 243:H480–H487, 1982.

99. Bache RJ, Dai X-Z, Schwarta JS, Homans DC: Role of adenosine in coronary vasodilation during exercise. *Circ Res* 62:846–853, 1988.

100. Manfredi JP, Sparks HV: Adenosine's role in coronary vasodilation induced by atrial pacing and norepinephrine. *Am J Physiol* 243:H536–H545, 1982.

101. DeWitt DF, Wangler RD, Thompson CI, Sparks HV: Phasic release of adenosine during steady state metabolic stimulation in the isolated guinea pig heart. *Circ Res* 53:636–643, 1983.

102. Gorman MW, Ning X-H, He M-X, Portman MA, Sparks HV: Adenosine release and high energy phosphates in intact dog hearts during norepinephrine infusion. *Circ Res* 70: 1146–1151, 1992.

103. Katz LA, Swain JA, Portman MA, Balaban RS: Relation between phosphate metabolites and oxygen consumption of heart in vivo. *Am J Physiol* 256:H265–H274, 1989.

104. Gorman MW, Wangler RD, Bassingthwaighte JB, Mohrman DE, Wang CY, Sparks HV: Interstitial adenosine concentration during norepinephrine infusion in the isolated guinea pig heart. *Am J Physiol* 260:H917–H926, 1991.

105. Headrick JP, Matherne GP, Berr SS, Han DC, Berne RM: Metabolic correlates of adenosine formation in stimulated guinea pig heart. *Am J Physiol* 260:H165–H172, 1991.

106. Van Wylen DGL, Willis J, Sadi H, Wiess J, Lasley R, Mentzer RM: Cardiac microdialysis to estimate interstitial adenosine and coronary blood flow. *Am J Physiol* 258: H1642–H1649, 1990.

107. Gidday JM, Kaiser DM, Rubio R, Berne RM: Heterogeneity and sampling volume dependence of epicardial adenosine concentrations. *J Mol Cell Cardiol* 24:351–364, 1992.

108. Kroll K, Feigl EO: Adenosine is unimportant in controlling coronary blood flow in unstressed dog hearts. *Am J Physiol* 249:H1176–H1187, 1985.

109. Deussen A, Walter C, Borst M, Schrader J: Transmural gradient of adenosine in canine heart during functional hyperemia. *Am J Physiol* 260:H671–H680, 1991.

110. Zhang J, Somers MJ, Cobb FR: Inhibition of ATP-sensitive potassium channels reduces basal vasomotor tone but not stimulated vascular responses in the coronary vasculature. *Circulation* 86(Suppl I):I484, 1992.

111. Narishige T, Egashira K, Akatsuka Y, Takeshita A: ATP-sensitive K^+ channel mediates coronary vasodilation associated with beta-1 adrenoceptor stimulation. *Circulation* 86(Suppl I):I485, 1992.

112. Gorczynski RJ, Duling BR: Role of oxygen in arteriolar functional vasodilation in hamster striated muscle. *Am J Physiol* 235:H505–H515, 1978.

113. Weiss HR: Effect of coronary artery occlusion in regional arterial and venous O_2 saturation, O_2 extraction, blood flow, and O_2 consumption in the dog heart. *Circ Res* 47:400–407, 1980.

114. Busse R, Pohl V, Kellner C, Klenim V: Endothelial cells are involved in the vasodilatory response to hypoxia. *Pflügers Arch* 397:78–80, 1983.

115. Hintze TH, Vatner SF: Reactive dilation of large coronary arteries in conscious dogs. *Circ Res* 54:50–57, 1984.

116. Sparks HV, Gorman MW: Adenosine in the local regulation of blood flow: Current controversies. In: Gerlach E, Schrader J, Berne R (eds) *Topics and Perspectives in Adenosine Research.* Berlin: Springer-Verlag, 1987, pp 406–415.

117. Lowenstein JM, Yu MK, Naito Y: Regulation of adenosine metabolism by 5'-nucleotidase. In: Berne RM, Rall TW, Rubio R (eds) *Regulatory Function of Adenosine.* Boston: Martinus Nijhoff, 1983, pp 117–129.

118. Nees S, Gerlach E: Adenine nucleotide and adenosine metabolism in cultured coronary endothelial cells: Formation and release of adenine compounds and possible functional implications. In: Berne RM, Rall TW, Rubio R (eds) *Regulatory Function of Adenosine.* Boston: Martinus Nijhoff, 1983, pp 347–355.

119. Kroll K, Schrader J, Piper HM, Henrich M: Release of adenosine and cyclic AMP from coronary endothelium in isolated guinea pig hearts: Relation to coronary flow. *Circ Res* 60:659–665, 1987.

120. Burnstock G: Purinergic nerves. *Pharmacol Rev* 24:509–581, 1972.

121. Pearson JD, Carlton JS, Gordon JL: Metabolism of adenine nucleotides by ectoenzymes of vascular endothelial and smooth muscle cells in culture. *Biochem J* 190:421–429, 1980.

122. Fredholm BB, Hedquivist P, Lindstrom K, Wennmalm M: Release of nucleosides and nucleotides from rabbit heart by sympathetic nerve stimulation. *Acta Physiol Scand* 116: 285–295, 1982.

123. Sparks HV, Bardenheuer H: Regulation of adenosine formation by the heart. *Circ Res* 58:193–201, 1986.

124. Bardenheuer H, Schrader J: Relationship between myocardial oxygen consumption, coronary flow and adenosine release in the improved isolated working heart preparation of guinea pigs. *Circ Res* 51:263–271, 1983.

125. Pohl V, Holtz J, Busse R, Bassenge E: Crucial role of endothelium in the vasodilator response to increased flow in vivo. *Hypertension* 8:37–44, 1986.

126. Kaiser L, Sparks HV: Mediation of flow dependent arterial dilation by endothelial cells. *Circ Shock* 18:109–114, 1986.

127. Randall WC, Armour JA: Gross and microscopic anatomy of the cardiac innervation. In: Randall WC (ed) *Neural Regulation of the Heart.* New York: Oxford University, 1977, pp 13–41.

128. Armour JA, Randall WC: Functional anatomy of canine cardiac fibers. *Acta Anat* 91:510–528, 1975.

129. Denn MJ, Stone HL: Autonomic innervation of dog coronary arteries. *J Appl Physiol* 41:30–35, 1976.

130. Dolezel S, Gerova J, Gero J, Sladek T, Vasku J: Adrenergic innervation of the coronary arteries and the myocardium. *Acta Anat* 100:306–316, 1978.

131. Schenk EA, Badawi AE: Dual innervation of arteries and arterioles: Histochemical study. *Z Zellforsch Mikrosk Anat* 91:170–177, 1968.

132. McRaven DR, Mark AL, Abboud FM, Mayer HE: Re-

sponses of coronary vessels to adrenergic stimuli. *J Clin Invest* 50:773–778, 1971.

133. Ek L, Ablad B: Effects of three beta adrenergic receptor blockers on myocardial oxygen consumption in the dog. *Eur J Pharmacol* 14:19–28, 1971.

134. Uchida Y, Murao S: Sustained decrease in coronary blood flow and excitation of cardiac sensory fibers following sympathetic stimulation. *Jpn Heart J* 16:265–279, 1975.

135. Mark AL, Abboud FM, Schmid PG, Heistad DD, Mayer HE: Differences in direct effects of adrenergic stimuli on coronary, cutaneous and muscular vessels. *J Clin Invest* 51:279–287, 1972.

136. Hamilton FN, Feigl EO: Coronary vascular sympathetic beta-receptor innervation. *Am J Physiol* 230:1569–1576, 1976.

137. Trivella MG, Broten TP, Feigl EO: β-receptor subtypes in the canine coronary circulation. *Am J Physiol* 259:H1575–H1585, 1990.

138. Shepherd JT, VanHoutte PM: Spasm of the coronary arteries: Causes and consequences (the scientist's viewpoint). *Mayo Clin Proc* 60:33–46, 1985.

139. Shepherd JT, Katusic ZS, Vedernikov Y, Vanhoutte PM: Mechanisms of coronary vasospasm: Role of endothelium. *J Mol Cell Cardiol* 23(Suppl I):125–131, 1991.

140. Imai S, Otorii T, Takeda K, Katano Y: Coronary vasodilation and adrenergic receptors in the dog heart and coronary. *Jpn J Pharmacol* 25:423–432, 1975.

141. Murray PA, Vatner SF: Adrenoreceptor attenuation of the coronary vascular response to severe exercise in the conscious dog. *Circ Res* 45:654–660, 1979.

142. Heydrickx GR, Muylaert P, Pannier JL: Alpha-adrenergic control of oxygen delivery to myocardium during exercise in conscious dogs. *Am J Physiol* 242:H805–H809, 1982.

143. Feigl EO: Control of myocardial oxygen tension by sympathetic coronary vasoconstriction in the dog. *Circ Res* 37:88–95, 1975.

144. Powell JR, Feigl EO: Carotid sinus reflex coronary vasoconstriction during controlled myocardial oxygen metabolism in the dog. *Circ Res* 44:44–51, 1979.

145. Buffington CW, Feigl EO: Adrenergic coronary vasoconstriction in the presence of coronary stenosis in the dog. *Circ Res* 48:416–423, 1981.

146. Yasue H, Touyama M, Shimamoto M, Kato H, Tanaka S, Akiyama F: Role of autonomic nervous system in the pathogenesis of Prinzmetal's variant form of angina. *Circulation* 50:534–539, 1974.

147. Yasue H, Touyama M, Kato H, Tanaka S, Akiyama F: Prinzmetal's variant form of angina as a manifestation of alpha adrenergic receptor-mediated coronary artery spasm: Documentation by coronary arteriography. *Am Heart J* 91:148–155, 1976.

148. Levene DL, Freeman MR: Alpha-adrenergic mediated coronary artery spasm. *JAMA* 236:1018–1022, 1976.

149. Hillis LD, Braunwald E: Coronary artery spasm. *N Engl J Med* 299:695–702, 1978.

150. Zuberbuhler RC, Bohr DF: Responses of coronary smooth muscle to catecholamines. *Circ Res* 16:431–440, 1965.

151. Mekata H, Niu H: Electrical and mechanical responses of coronary artery smooth muscle to catecholamines. *Jpn J Physiol* 19:599–608, 1969.

152. Andersson R, Holmberg S, Svedmyr N, Aberg G: Adrenergic alpha- and beta-receptors in coronary vessels in man: An in vitro study. *Acta Med Scand* 191:241–244, 1972.

153. Bayer B-L, Mentz P, Forster W: Characterization of the adrenoceptors in coronary arteries of pigs. *Eur J Pharmacol* 29:58–69, 1974.

154. Feigl EO: Parasympathetic control of coronary blood flow in dogs. *Circ Res* 15:509–519, 1969.

155. Tiedt N, Religa A: Vagal control of coronary blood flow in dogs. *Basic Res Cardiol* 74:267–276, 1979.

156. Feigl EO: Sympathetic control of coronary circulation. *Circ Res* 20:262–271, 1967.

157. Brown AM: Motor innervation of the coronary arteries of the cat. *J Physiol (Lond)* 198:311–328, 1968.

158. Feigl EO: Carotid sinus reflex control of coronary blood flow. *Circ Res* 23:262–271, 1968.

159. Vatner SF, Franklin D, Van Critters RL, Braunwald E: Effects of carotid sinus nerve stimulation on the coronary circulation of the conscious dog. *Circ Res* 27:11–21, 1970.

160. Hackett JG, Abboud FM, Mark AL, Schmid PG, Heistad DD: Coronary vascular responses to stimulation of chemoreceptors and baroreceptors: Evidence for reflex activation of vagal cholinergic innervation. *Circ Res* 31:8–17, 1972.

161. Religa Z, Trzebski A, Religa A, Glowienko A: Effect of the stimulation of afferent fibers in Hering's nerve on the blood flow and resistance in the coronary vessels of the dogs. *Pol Med J* 11:632–641, 1972.

162. Hashimoto K, Igakashi S, Uei I, Kumakura S: Carotid chemoreceptor reflex effects on coronary flow and heart rate. *Am J Physiol* 206:536–540, 1964.

163. Vatner SF, McRitchie RJ: Interaction of the chemoreflex and the pulmonary inflation reflex in the regulation of coronary circulation in conscious dogs. *Circ Res* 37:664–673, 1975.

164. Moreland R, Bohr DF: Adrenergic control of coronary arteries. *Fed Proc* 43:2857–2861, 1984.

165. Cohn RA, Shepherd JT, Vanhoutte PM: Effects of the adrenergic transmitter on epicardial coronary arteries. *Fed Proc* 43:2862–2866, 1984.

166. Gerwirtz PA, Stone HL: Coronary blood flow and myocardial oxygen consumption after alpha adrenergic blockade during submaximal exercise. *J Pharmacol Exp Therap* 217:92–98, 1981.

167. Ito BR, Feigl EO: Carotid chemoreceptor reflex parasympathetic coronary vasodilation in the dog. *Am J Physiol* 249:H1167–H1175, 1985.

168. Murray PA, Lavallee M, Vatner SF: Alpha adrenergic-mediated reduction in coronary blood flow secondary to carotid chemoreceptor reflex activation in conscious dogs. *Circ Res* 54:96–106, 1984.

169. Ito BR, Feigl EO: Carotid baroreceptor refles coronary vasodilation in the dog. *Circ Res* 56:486–495, 1985.

170. Vatner SF: Alpha-adrenergic tone in the coronary circulation of the conscious dog. *Fed Proc* 43:2867–2872, 1985.

171. Holtz J, Mayer E, Bassenge E: Demonstration of alpha adrenergic coronary control in different layers of the canine myocardium by regional myocardial sympathectomy. *Pflügers Arch* 372:187–194, 1977.

172. Chilian WM, Boatwright RB, Shoji T, Griggs DM: Evidence against significant resting sympathetic coronary vasoconstrictor tone in the conscious dos. *Circ Res* 49:866–876, 1981.

173. Corr LA, Aberdeen JA, Milner P, Lincoln J, Burnstock G: Sympathetic and nonsympathetic neuropeptide Y-containing nerves in the rat myocardium and coronary arteries. *Circ Res* 66:1602–1609, 1990.

174. Kaijser L, Pernow J, Berglund B, Lundberg JM: Neuropeptide Y is released together with noradrenaline from the human heart during exercise and hypoxia. *Clin Physiol* 10:179–188, 1990.

175. Buffington CW, Feigl EO: Effect of coronary artery pressure on transmural distribution of adrenergic coronary vasocon-

striction in the dog. *Circ Res* 53:613–621, 1983.

176. Kelley KO, Feigl EO: Segmental alpha receptor-mediated vasoconstriction in the canine coronary circulation. *Circ Res* 43:908–916, 1978.

177. Johannsen UJ, Mark AL, Marcus ML: Responsiveness to cardiac sympathetic nerve stimulation during maximal coronary dilation produced by adenosine. *Circ Res* 50:510–517, 1982.

178. Chilian WMK, Harrison DG, Haws CW, Snyder WD, Marcus ML: Adrenergic coronary tone during submaximal exercise in the dog is produced by circulating catecholamines: Evidence for adrenergic denervation supersensitivity in the myocardium but not in coronary vessels. *Circ Res* 58:68–82, 1986.

179. Maseri A, L'Abbate A, Baroldi G, Chierchia M, Marzilli M, Ballestra AM, Severi S, Parodi O, Biagini A, Distante A, Pesola A: Coronary vasospasm as a possible cause of myocardial infarction. A conclusion derived from a study of "pre-infarction" angina. *N Engl J Med* 299:1271–1277, 1978.

180. Mudge GH Jr, Grossman W, Mills RM Jr, Lesch M, Braunwald E: Reflex increase in coronary vascular resistance in patients with ischemic heart disease. *N Engl J Med* 295:1333–1337, 1976.

181. Mudge GH Jr, Goldberg S, Gunther S, Mann T, Grossman W: Comparison of metabolic and vasoconstrictor stimuli on coronary vascular resistance in man. *Circulation* 59:544–550, 1979.

182. Malacoff RF, Mudge GH Jr, Holman BL, Idoine J, Bifolck L, Cohn PF: Effect of the cold pressor test on regional myocardial blood flow in patients with coronary artery disease. *Am Heart J* 106:78–84, 1983.

183. Berkenboom GM, Abramowicz M, Vandermoten P, Degre SG: Role of alpha-adrenergic coronary tone in exercise-induced angina pectoris. *Am J Cardiol* 57:195–198, 1986.

184. Sheridan DJ, Thomas P, Culling W, Collins P: Antianginal and hemodynamic effects of alpha1 receptor blockade. *J Cardiovasc Pharmacol* 8(Suppl 2):S144–S150, 1986.

185. Liang IYS, Jones CE: Alpha$_1$-adrenergic blockade increases coronary blood flow during coronary hypoperfusion. *Am J Physiol* 249:H1070–H1071, 1985.

186. Jones CE, Liang IYS, Maulsby MR: Cardiac and coronary effects of prazosin and phenoxybenzamine during coronary hypoperfusion. *J Pharmacol Exp Ther* 236:204–211, 1986.

187. Heusch G, Schipke J, Thamer V: Sympathetic mechanisms in poststenotic myocardial ischemia. *J Cardiovasc Pharmacol* 8(Suppl):S33–40, 1986.

188. Nathan HJ, Feigl EO: Adrenergic vasoconstriction lessens transmural steal during coronary hypoperfusion. *Am J Physiol* 250 (*Heart Circ Physiol* 19):H645–H653, 1986.

189. Young MA, Knight DR, Vatner SF: Parassympathetic coronary vasoconstriction induced by nicotine in conscious calves. *Circ Res* 62:891–895, 1988.

190. Feigl EO: Parasympatheitc control of coronary blood flow in dogs. *Circ Res* 25:509–519, 1975.

191. Cevese A, Mary DA, Poltronieri R, Schena F, Vacca G: Efferent limb of the coronary vasoconstrictor reflex elicited by distension of the descending colon in anesthetized dogs. *Cardioscience (Italy)* 3:35–40, 1992.

192. Franco-Cereceda A: Calcitonin gene-related peptide and tachykinins in relation to local sensory control of cardiac contractility and coronary vascular tone. *Acta Physiol Scand* (Suppl 569):1–63, 1988.

193. Meerson FZ: The myocardium in hyperfunction, hypertrophy and heart failure. *Circ Res* 25(Suppl II):1–8, 1969.

194. Hood WP, Rackley CE, Rolette E: Wall stress in the normal and hypertrophied left ventricle. *Am J Cardiol* 22:550–558, 1968.

195. Gunther S, Grossman W: Determinants of ventricular function in pressure overload hypertrophy in man. *Circulation* 59:679–688, 1979.

196. Strauer BE: Myocardial oxygen consumption in chronic heart disease: Role of wall stress, hypertrophy and coronary reserve. *Am J Cardiol* 44:730–740, 1979.

197. Kannel WB: Prevalence and natural history of electrocardiographic left ventricular hypertrophy. *Am J Med* 75:4–11, 1983.

198. Cooper RS, Simmons BE, Castaner A, Santhanam V, Ghali J, Mar M: Left ventricular hypertrophy is associated with worse survival independent of ventricular function and number of coronary arteries severely narrowed. *Am J Cardiol* 65:441–445, 1990.

199. O'Keefe DD, Hoffman JIE, Cheitlin R, O'Neill MJ, Allard JR, Shapkin E: Coronary blood flow in experimental canine left ventricular hypertrophy. *Circ Res* 43:43–51, 1978.

200. Mueller TM, Marcus ML, Kerber RE, Young JA, Barnes RW, Abboud FM: Effect of renal hypertension and left ventricular hypertrophy on the coronary circulation in dogs. *Circ Res* 42:543–549, 1978.

201. Malik AB, Abe T, O'Kane H, Geha AS: Cardiac function, coronary flow, and oxygen consumption in stable left ventricular hypertrophy. *Am J Physiol* 225:186–191, 1973.

202. Wangler RD, Peters KG, Marcus ML, Tomanek RJ: Effects of duration and severity of arterial hypertension and cardiac hypertrophy on coronary vasodilator reserve. *Circ Res* 51:10–18, 1982.

203. Tomanek RJ, Wangler RD, Bauer CA: Prevention of coronary vasodilator reserve decrement in spontaneously hypertensive rats. *Hypertension* 7:533–540, 1985.

204. Peters KG, Wangler RD, Tomanek RJ, Marcus ML: Effects of long-term cardiac hypertrophy on coronary vasodilator reserve in SHR rats. *Am J Cardiol* 54:1342–1348, 1984.

205. Bing RJ, Hammond MN, Handelman JC, et al.: The measurement of coronary blood flow, oxygen consumption, and efficiency of the left ventricle in man. *Am Heart J* 38:1–17, 1949.

206. Archie JP, Fixler DE, Ullyot DJ, Buckberg GD, Hofrman JIE: Regional myocardial blood flow in lambs with concentric right ventricular hypertrophy. *Circ Res* 34:143–154, 1974.

207. Murray PA, Baig H, Fishbein MC, Vatner SF: Effects of experimental right ventricular hypertrophy on myocardial blood flow in conscious dogs. *J Clin Invest* 64:421–427, 1979.

208. Wyse RKA, Jones M, Welham KC, deLeval MR: Cardiac peformance and myocardial blood flow in pigs with compensated right ventricular hypertrophy. *Cardiovasc Res* 18:733–745, 1984.

209. Manohar M, Thurmon JC, Tranquill WJJ, Devous MD, Theodorakis MC, Shawley RV, Feller DL, Benson JB: Regional myocardial blood flow and coronary vascular reserve in unanesthetized young calves with severe concentric right ventricular hypertrophy. *Circ Res* 48:785–796, 1982.

210. Murray PA, Vatner SF: Reduction of maximal coronary vasodilator capacity in conscious dogs with severe right ventricular hypertrophy. *Circ Res* 48:27–33, 1981.

211. Murray PA, Vatner SF: Fractional contributions of the right and left coronary arteries to perfusion of normal and hypertrophied right ventricles of conscious dogs. *Circ Res* 47:190–200, 1980.

212. Fallen EL, Elliott WC, Gorlin R: Mechanisms of angina in aortic stenosis. *Circulation* 36:480–488, 1967.

213. Goodwin JF: Hypertrophic diseases of the myocardium. *Prog Cadiovasc Dis* 16:199–238, 1973.
214. Strauer BE: *Hypertensive Heart Disease*. New York: Springer-Verlag, 1980.
215. Marcus ML, Doty DB, Hiratzka LF, Wright C, Eastham C: Decreased coronary reserve. A mechanism of angina in patients with aortic stenosis and normal coronary arteries. *Engl J Med* 307:1362–1366, 1982.
216. Pichard AD, Gorlin R, Smith H, Ambrose J, Meller J: Coronary flow studies in patients with left ventricular hypertrophy of the hypertensive type. Evidence for an impaired coronary vascular reserve. *Am J Cardiol* 47:547–553, 1981.
217. Pichard AD, Smith H, Holt, et al.: Coronary vascular reserve in left ventricular hypertrophy secondary to chronic aortic regurgitation. *Am J Cardiol* 51:315–320, 1983.
218. Harris CN, Aronow WS, Parker DP, Kaplan MA: Treadmill stress in left ventricular hypertrophy. *Chest* 63:353–357, 1979.
219. Wrobewski EM, Pearl FJ, Hammer WJ, et al.: False-positive stress test due to undeteced left ventricular hypertrophy. *Am J Epidemiol* 115:412–17, 1982.
220. Moller JH, Nakeb A, Edwards JE: Infarction of the papillary muscle and mitral insufficiency associated with congenital aortic stenosis. *Circulation* 34:87–91, 1966.
221. Buchner F: Qualitative morphology of heart failure: Light and electron microscopic characteristics of acute and chronic heart failure. *Methods Arch Exp Pathol* 5:60–120, 1971.
222. Hittinger L, Shannon RP, Bishop SP, Gelpi RJ, Vatner SF: Subendocardial exhaustion of blood flow reserve and increased fibrosis in conscious dogs with heart failure. *Circ Res* 65:971–80, 1989.
223. Siri FM, Nordin C, Factor M, Sonnenblick E, Aronson R: Compensatory hypertrophy and failure in gradual pressure overloaded guinea pig heart. *Am J Physiol* 257:H1016–H1024, 1989.
224. Klocke F: Coronary blood flow in man. *Prog Cardiovasc Dis* 19:117–166, 1976.
225. Pasternac A, Nobej J, Streulens Y, et al.: Pathophysiology of chest pain in patients with cardiomyopathies and normal coronary arteries. *Circulation* 65:778–789, 1982.
226. Thormann J, Schlepper M: Comparison of myocardial flow, hemodynamic changes, and lactate metabolism during isoproterenol stress in patients with coronary heart disease and severe aortic stenosis. *Clin Cardiol* 2:437–445, 1979.
227. Marcus ML, Wright C, Doty D, Eastham L, Laughlin D, Krumm P, Fastenow C, Brody M: Measurements of coronary velocity and reactive hyperemia in the coronary circulation of humans. *Circ Res* 49:877–891, 1981.
228. Bache RJ, Vrobel TR, Arentzen CE, Ring WS: Effect of maximal coronary vasodilation on transmural myocardial perfusion during tachycardia in dogs with left ventricular hypertrophy. *Circ Res* 49:742–750, 1981.
229. Bache RJ, Aretzen CE, Simon AB, Vrobel RT: Abnormalities in myocardial perfusion during tachycardia in dogs with left ventricular hypertrophy. Metabolic evidence for myocardial ischemia. *Circulation* 69:409–417, 1984.
230. Rembert JC, Kleinman LH, Fedor JM, Wechsler AS, Greenfield JC Jr: Myocardial blood flow districution in concentric left ventricular hypertrophy. *J Clin Invest* 62:379–386, 1978.
231. Bache RJ, Vrobel TR, Ring WS, Emery RW, Anderson RW: Regional myocardial blood flow during exercise in dogs with chronic left ventricular hypertrophy. *Circ Res* 48:76–87, 1981.
232. Ecker T, Gobel C, Hullin R, Rettig R, Seitz G, Hofmann F:

Decreased cardiac concentration of cGMP kinase in hypertensive animals. An index for cardiac vascularization? *Circ Res* 65:1361–1369, 1989.
233. Lewis BS, Gotsman MS: Relation between coronary artery size and left ventricular wall mass. *Br Heart J* 35:1150–1153, 1973.
234. Roberts CS, Roberts WC: Cross-sectional area of the proximal portions of the three major epicardial coronary arteries in 98 necropsy patients with different coronary events. *Circulation* 62:953–959, 1980.
235. Stack RS, Rembert JC, Schirmer B, et al.: Ralation of left ventricular mass to geometry of the proximal coronary arteries of the dog. *Am J Cardiol* 51:1728–31, 1983.
236. Shipley RA, Shipley LJ, Wearn JT: The capillary supply in normal and hypertrophied hearts of rabbits. *J Exp Med* 65:29–42, 1937.
237. Roberts JT, Wearn TJ: Quantitative changes in the capillary muscle relationships in human heart during growth and hypertrophy. *Am Heart J* 21:617–633, 1941.
238. Rakusan K, Moravec J, Hatt PY: Regional capillary supply in the normal and hypertrophied rat heart. *Microvasc Res* 20:319–326, 1980.
239. Turek Z, Takusan K: Log normal distribution of intercapillary distance in normal and hypertrophic rat heart as estimated by the method of concentric circles. *Pflügers Arch* 391:17–21, 1981.
240. Breisch EA, White FC, Bloor CM: Myocardial characteristics of pressure overload hypertrophy. *Lab Invest* 51:333–342, 1984.
241. Honig CR, Gayeski TEJ: Capillary reserve and tissue O_2 transport in normal and hypertrophied hearts. In: Tarzi RC, Dunber JB Jr (eds) *Cardiac Hypertrophy in Hypertension*. New York: Raven Press, 1983, p 249.
242. Dowell RT: Hemodynamic factors and vascular density as potential determinants of blood flow in hypertrophied rat heart. *Proc Soc Exp Biol Med* 154:423–426, 1977.
243. Alyono D, Anderson RW, Parrish DG, Dia XZ, Bache RJ: Alterations of myocardial blood flow associated with experimental canine left ventricular hypertrophy secondary to valvular aortic stenosis. *Circ Res* 58:47–57, 1986.
244. Wicker P, Tarazi RC: Right ventricular coronary flow in arterial hypertension. *Am Heart J* 110:845–850, 1985.
245. Opherk D, Mall G, Zebe H, et al.: Reduction of coronary reserve: A mechanism for angina pectoris in patients with arterial hypertension and normal coronary arteries. *Circulation* 69:1–7, 1984.
246. Thormann J, Schlepper M, Neuss H: Coronary hemodynamics in simulated paroxysms of ventricular tachycardia. *Cardiology* 69:326–342, 1982.
247. Harrison DG, Barnes DH, Hiratzka LF, Eastham CL, Kerber RE, Marcus ML: The effect of cardiac hypertrophy on the coronary collateral circulation. *Circulation* 71:1135–1145, 1985.
248. Doty DB, Eatham CL, Hiratzka, LF, Wright CB, Marcus ML: Determination of coronary reserve in patients with supravalvular aortic stenosis. *Circulation* 66(Suppl I):I186–I192, 1982.
249. Yamamoto J, Tsuchiay M, Saito M, Ikeda M: Cardiac contractile and coronary flow reserves in deoxycorticosterone acetate-salt hypertensive rats. *Hypertension* 7:569–577, 1985.
250. Kobabyashi K, Tarazi RC, Lovenberg W, Rakusan K: Coronary blood flow in genetic cardiac hypertrophy. *Am J Cardiol* 53:1360–1364, 1984.
251. Nitenberg A, Foult J, Antony I, Blanchet F, Rahali M: Coronary flow and resistance reserve in patients with chronic

aortic regurgitation, angina pectoris and normal coronary arteries. *J Am Coll Cardiol* 11:478–486, 1988.

252. Cohen MV: Coronary vascular reserve in the greyhound with left ventricular hypertrophy. *Cardiovasc Res* 20:182–194, 1986.

253. Chilian WM, Wangler RD, Peters KG, et al.: Throxine-induced left ventricular hypertrophy in the rat. *Circ Res* 57:591–598, 1985.

254. Enzig S, Leonard JJ, Tripp MR, et al.: Changes in regional myocardial blood flow and variable development of hypertrophy after aortic banding in puppies. *Cardiovasc Res* 15:711–719, 1981.

255. White FC, Sanders M, Peterson T, et al.: Ischemic myocardial injury after exercise stress in the pressure-overloaded heart. *Am J Pathol* 97:473–481, 1979.

256. Bache RJ, Dai X-Z, Alyono D, Vrobel TR, Homans DC: Myocardial blood flow during exercise in dogs with left ventricular hypertrophy produced by aortic banding and perinephritic hypertension. *Circulation* 76:835–842, 1987.

257. Manohar M, Visgard GE, Bullard V, et al.: Blood flow in the hypertrophied right ventricular myocardium of unanesthetized ponies. *Am J Physiol* 240:H881–H888, 1981.

258. Sharon MS, Bache RJ: Reactive hyperemia following total and subtotal coronary occlusion in the awake dog. *Basic Res Cardiol* 77:656–667, 1982.

259. Mittmann U, Bruckner UB, Keller EH, et al.: Myocardial flow reserve in experimental cardiac hypertrophy. *Basic Res Cardiol* 75:199–206, 1980.

260. Nakano K, Corin WJ, Spaan JF Jr, et al.: Abnormal subendocardial blood flow in pressure overload hypertrophy is associated with pacing-induced subendocardial dysfunction. *Circ Res* 675:1555–1564, 1989.

261. Hittinger L, Shannon RP, Kohin S, Manders WT, Kelly P, Vatner SF: Exercise-induced subendocardial dysfunction in dogs with left ventricular hypertrophy. *Circ Res* 66:329–343, 1990.

262. Doty D, Wright C, Eastham C, Marcus ML: Coronary reserve in atrial septal defect. *Circulation* 62:111–115, 1980.

263. Tauchert M, Hilger HH: In: Schaper W (ed) *The Patho-Physiology of Myocardial Perfusion*. Amsterdam: Elsevier, 1979, pp 141–167.

264. Strauer BE: Ventricular function and coronary hemodynamics in hypertensive heart disease. *Am J Cardiol* 44:999–1006, 1979.

265. Schaper W: *The Collateral Circulation of the Heart*. Amsterdam: North Holland, 1971.

266. Gregg DE: The natural history of collateral development. *Circ Res* 35:335–344, 1974.

267. Schwarz F, Wagner HO, Sesto M, Hofmann M, Schaper W, Kubler W: Native collaterals in the development of collateral circulation after chronic coronary stenosis in mongrel dogs. *Circulation* 66:303–308, 1982.

268. Schwarz F, Flameng W, Ensslen R, Sesto M, Thormann J: Effect of coronary collaterals on left ventricular functions at rest and during stress. *Am Heart J* 95:570–577, 1978.

269. Kelly DT, Pitt B: Regional changes in intramyocardial pressure following myocardial ischemia. In: Bloor CM, Olsson RA (eds) *Current Topics in Coronary Research*, Vol 39. New York: Plenum, 1973, pp 115–130.

270. Bache RJ, Cobb FR, Greenfield JC: Myocardial blood flow distribution during ischemia-induced coronary vasodilation in the unanesthetized dog. *J Clin Invest* 54:1462–1472, 1974.

271. Tennant R, Wiggers CJ: The effect of coronary occlusion on myocardial contraction. *Am J Physiol* 112:351–361, 1935.

272. Katz AM: Effects of ischemia on the contractile process of heart muscle. *Am J Cardiol* 32:456–560, 1973.

273. Hillis LD, Braunwald E: Myocardial ischemia. *N Engl J Med* 296:971–978, 1977.

274. Theroux P, Franklin D, Ross J, Kemper WS: Regional myocardial function during acute coronary artery occlusion and its modification by pharmacologic agents in the dog. *Circ Res* 35:896–908, 1974.

275. Aversano T, Becker LC: Persistence of coronary vasodilator reserve despite functionally significant flow reduction. *Am J Physiol* 248:H403–H411, 1985.

276. Folts JD, Gallagher K, Rowe GG: Blood flow reductions in stenosed canine coronary arteries: Vasospasm or platelet aggregation? *Circulation* 65:248–255, 1982.

277. Powers ER, DiBona DR, Powell J Jr: Myocardial cell volume and coronary resistance during diminished coronary perfusion. *Am J Physiol* 247:H467–H477, 1984.

278. Engler RL, Dahlgren MD, Morris DD, Peterson MA, Schmid-Schonbein GW: Role of leukocytes in response to acute myocardial ischemia and reflow in dogs. *Am J Physiol* 251:H314–H322, 1986.

279. Pantely GA, Bristow JD, Swenson LJ, Ladley HD, Johnson WB, Anselone CG: Incomplete coronary vasodilation during myocardial ischemia in swine. *Am J Physiol* 249:H638–H647, 1985.

280. Gallagher KP, Folts JD, Shebuski RJ, Rankin JHG, Rowe GG: Subepicardial vasodilator reserve in the presence of critical coronary stenosis in dogs. *Am J Cardiol* 46:67–73, 1980.

281. Canty JM Jr, Klocke FJ: Reduced regional myocardial perfusion in the presence of pharmacologic vasodilator reserve. *Circulation* 71:370–377, 1985.

282. Grover GJ, Weiss HR: Effect of pacing on oxygen supply-to-consumption ratio in ischemic myocardium. *Am J Physiol* 249:H249–H254, 1985.

283. Engler RL, Dahlgren MD, Peterson MA, Dobbs A, Schmid-Schonbein GW: Accumulation of polymorphonuclear leukocytes during 3-h experimental myocardial ischemia. *Am J Physiol* 251:H93–H100, 1986.

284. Grattan MT, Hanley FL, Stevens MB, Hoffman JIE: Transmural coronary flow reserve patterns in dogs. *Am J Physiol* 250:H276–H283, 1986.

285. Heusch G, Deussen A: The effects of cardiac sympathetic nerve stimulation on perfusion of stenotic coronary arteries in the dog. *Circ Res* 53:8–15, 1983.

286. Cuttino JT Jr, Bartrun RJ Jr, Hollenberg NK, Abrams HL: Collateral vessel formation: Isolation of a transferable factor promoting a vascular response. *Basic Res Cardiol* 70:568–573, 1975.

287. Golenhofen K, Mandrek K, Schaper W, et al.: Mechanical activity of isolated canine coronary arteries after coronary occlusion. *Basic Res Cardiol* 76:480–484, 1981.

288. Frame LH, Powell WJ: Progressive perfusion impairment during prolonged low flow myocardial ischemia in dogs. *Circ Res* 39:269–276, 1976.

289. Guyton RA, McClenathan JH, Michaelis LL: Evolution of regional ischemia distal to a proximal coronary stenosis: Self-propagation of ischemia. *Am J Cardiol* 40:381–392, 1977.

290. Sparks HV, Gorman MW: Ischemic vasodilation or ischemic vasoconstriction? In: Vanhoutte PM, Leusen I (eds) *Vasodilation*. New York: Raven Press, 1981, pp 193–204.

291. Gorman MW, Sparks HV: Progressive coronary vasoconstriction during relative ischemic in canine myocardium. *Circ Res* 51:411–420, 1982.

292. Harris TR, Overholser KA, Stiles RG: Concurrent increases in resistance and transport after coronary obstruction in dogs. *Am J Physiol* 240:H262–H273, 1981.

293. Willerson JT, Powell WJ, Guiney TE, Stark JJ, Sanders CA, Leaf A: Improvement in myocardial function and coronary blood flow in ischemic myocardium after mannitol. *J Clin Invest* 51:2989–2998, 1972.

294. Wangler RD, DeWitt DF, Sparks HV: Effect of β-blockade on nucleoside release from the hypoperfused isolated heart. *Am J Physiol* 247:H330–H336.

295. Klocke FJ, Canty JM Jr, Arani DT, Krawczyk JA: Adjustments in regional coronary perfusion accompanying reductions in regional coronary arterial pressure. *Can J Cardiol* (Suppl A):200A–204A, 1986.

296. Willerson JT, Watson JT, Hutton I, Templeton GH, Fixler DE: Reduced myocardial reflow and increased coronary vascular resistance following prolonged myocardial ischemia in the dog. *Circ Res* 36:771–781, 1975.

297. Arai AE, Pantely GA, Anselone CG, Bristow J, Bristow JD: Active down regulation of myocardial energy requirements during prolonged moderate ischemia in swine. *Circ Res* 69:1458–1469, 1991.

298. Kirsch GE, Codina J, Birnbaumer L, Brown AM: Coupling of ATP-sensitive K⁺ channels to A1 receptors by G proteins in rat ventricular myocytes. *Am J Physiol* 259:H820–H826, 1990.

299. Parker PE, Bashour FA, Downey HF, Kechejian SJ, Williams AF: Coronary hemodynamics during reperfusion following acute coronary ligation in dogs. *Am Heart J* 90:593–5599, 1975.

300. Kloner RA, Ganote CE, Jennings RB: The "no-reflow" phenomenon after temporary coronary occlusion in the dog. *J Clin Invest* 54:1496–1507, 1974.

301. Parker PE, Bashour FA, Downey HF, Bouvros IS: Coronary reperfusion: Effects of hyperosmotic manitol. *Am Heart J* 97:745–752, 1979.

302. Sunnergren KP, Rovetto MJ: Hyaluronidase reversal of increased coronary vascular resistance in ischemic rat hearts. *Am J Physiol* 245:H183–H188, 1983.

303. Marcus ML, Kerber RE, Ehrhardt J, Abboud FM: Effects of time on volume and distribution of coronary collateral flow. *Am J Physiol* 230:279–285, 1976.

304. Jugdutt BI, Becker LC, Hutchins GM: Early changes in collateral blood flow during myocardial infarction in conscious dogs. *Am J Physiol* 237:H371–H380, 1979.

305. Schaper W, Pasyk S: Influence of collateral flow on the ischemia tolerance of the heart following acute and subacute coronary occlusion. *Circulation* 53(Suppl 1):157–162, 1976.

306. Khouri EM, Gregg DE, McGranahan GM: Regression and reappearance of coronary collaterals. *Am J Physiol* 220:655–661, 1971.

307. Hansen J: Coronary collateral circulation: Clinical significance on survival in patients with coronary artery occlusion. *Am Heart J* 117:290–295, 1989.

308. Topol EJ, Ellis SG: Coronary collaterals revisited: Accessory pathway to myocardial preservation during infarction. *Circulation* 83:1084–1086, 1991.

309. Hirai T, Fujita M, Nakajima H, Asanoi H, Yamanishi K, Ohno A, Sasayama S: Importance of collateral circulation for prevention of left ventricular aneurysm formation in acute myocardial infarction. *Circulation* 79:791–796, 1989.

310. Eckstein RW: Effect of exercise and coronary artery narrowing on coronary collateral circulation. *Circ Res* 5:230–235, 1957.

311. Sanders M, White FC, Peterson TM, Bloor CM: Effects of endurance exercise on coronary collateral blood flow in miniature swine. *Am J Physiol* 234:H614–H619, 1978.

312. Scheel KW, Ingram LA, Wilson JL: Effects of exercise on the coronary and collateral vasculature of beagles with and without coronary occlusion. *Circ Res* 48:523–530, 1981.

313. Scheel KW, Rodriguez RJ, Ingram LA: Directional coronary collateral growth with chronic circumflex occlusion in the dog. *Circ Res* 40:384–390, 1977.

314. Pasyk S, Schaper W, Schaper J, Pasyk K, Miskiewica G, Steinseifer B: DNA synthesis in coronary collaterals after coronary artery occlusion in conscious dog. *Am J Physiol* 242:H1031–H1037, 1982.

315. D'Amore PA, Rhompson RW: Mechanisms of angiogenesis. *Annu Rve Physiol* 49:453–464, 1987.

316. Schaper W, De Brabander M, Lewi P: DNA-synthesis and mitoses in coronary collateral vessels of the dog. *Circ Res* 28:671–679, 1971.

317. Quinkler W, Maasberg M, Bernotat-Danielowski S, Luthe N, Sharma HS, Schaper W: Isolation of heparin binding growth factors from bovine, porcine, and canine hearts. *Eur J Biochem* 181:67–73, 1989.

318. Schaper W, Gorge G, Winkler B, Schaper J: The collateral circulation of the heart. *Prog Cardiovasc Dis* 31:57–77, 1988.

319. Lee PL, Johnson DE, Cousens LS, Fried VA, Williams LT: Purification and complementary DNA cloning of a receptor for basic fibroblast growth factor. *Science* 245:57–60, 1989.

320. Schreiber AB, Kenney J, Kowalski WJ, Friesel R, Mehlman T, Maciag T: Interaction of endothelial cell growth factor with heparin. *Proc Natl Acad Sci USA* 32:6138–6142, 1985.

321. Gospodarowicz D, Cheng J: Heparin protects basic and acidic FGF form inactivation. *J Cell Physiol* 128:475–484, 1986.

322. Fujita M, Mikuniya A, Takahashi M, Gaddis R, Hartley J, McKown D, Franklin D: Acceleration of coronary collateral development by heparin in conscious dogs. *Jpn Circ J* 51:395–402, 1987.

323. Folkman J, Klagsburn M: Angiogenic factors. *Science* 235:442–447, 1987.

CHAPTER 58

Extravascular Coronary Resistance

JAMES M. DOWNEY

INTRODUCTION

Two phenomena determine the heart's resistance to coronary blood flow — the caliber of the resistance vessels as determined by smooth muscle in the walls of the coronary vessels and deformation of those vessels by the mechanical motion of the beating heart. Smooth muscle in the coronary bed is controlled by cardiac nerves and local metabolic processes in the heart. This smooth muscle is the effector for a rapid and efficient control system that ensures that the heart receives an appropriate blood flow under a wide variety of blood pressures and contractile states. An in-depth discussion of that control can be found elsewhere in this book.

The second process is not part of any purposeful control system, but it represents a necessary evil with which the heart must contend. *As the ventricle contracts to develop pressure in its lumen, forces are created within the myocardium, deforming the coronary vessels and increasing their resistance to flow.* It is convenient to refer to this mechanical impediment to flow as the *extravascular resistance*, since its origins are not related to smooth muscle activity within the blood vessels. This deformation is repetitive, with the heartbeat appearing and disappearing with a frequency much faster than the time constant of the vascular smooth muscle. The normal heart easily compensates for these periodic deficits in blood flow by adjusting the vascular smooth muscle tone so that the time-averaged coronary flow to any region of the heart remains in the proper range to ensure adequate nutrition. The magnitude of the extravascular resistance is quite large. Under normal hemodynamic conditions a third to a half of the coronary resistance is extravascular in origin {59}. In the presence of heart disease, the vascular smooth muscle reserve may become exhausted and thus incapable of sufficiently compensating for the extravascular component. This occurs in the presence of the additional resistance associated with a stenosed coronary artery {50} or a reduced driving pressure, as occurs with valve dysfunction {11} or hypotension {20}. Once coronary tone has reached the limits of its ability to dilate, the extravascular resistance becomes the major determinant of regional perfusion in the myocardium. Because this occurs commonly in ischemic heart disease in humans, a great deal of

investigation has been directed toward fully understanding the phenomenon of the extravascular resistance. In these patients coronary flow can be optimized if it is managed in a manner that keeps the extravascular resistance to a minimum. This chapter will attempt to summarize what is currently known concerning the extravascular resistance.

A HISTORICAL PERSPECTIVE

In 1687 J. Baptista Scaramucci suggested that the deep coronary vessels were squeezed empty in systole {62}. It is interesting that he correctly proposed both that systole should inhibit coronary perfusion and that the effect is most pronounced in the deep layers of the heart. It was not until the first half of the 19th century, however, that techniques for measuring blood flow became sophisticated enough to allow investigation of this phenomenon. Rebatel, in 1872, used a bristle-type flow meter to measure blood flow velocity in the right coronary artery of the horse {55}. He correctly noted that peak velocity occurred during systole, as occurs in the peripheral vascular bed. He also noted, however, that a second peak occurred in diastole. He attributes this second peak to the release of vascular compression during systole. Even though Rebatel's records were crude, his interpretation of an inhibitory effect of systole on coronary perfusion is compatible with our present understanding of the phenomenon.

Not all investigators believed that the extravascular effects were inhibitory. In 1938 Porter suggested that the heart's motion was actually aiding the propulsion of blood through the coronary arteries by a milking or muscle pump action {54}. Because a similar pump effect had been described in the peripheral circulation, such a concept seemed a priori to be true. This theory was supported by the observation that coronary sinus outflow came forth in spurts coincident with contraction. This pulsatile outflow persisted even when the coronary circulation was perfused from a nonpulsatile source. Porter's massaging theory was hotly debated over the ensuing years. Most of the debate centered around the phasic nature of the coronary flow and whether flow persisted during the systolic period. Unfortunately, the lack of an accurate blood-flow mea-

N. Sperelakis (ed.), Physiology and Pathophysiology of the Heart, Third Edition.

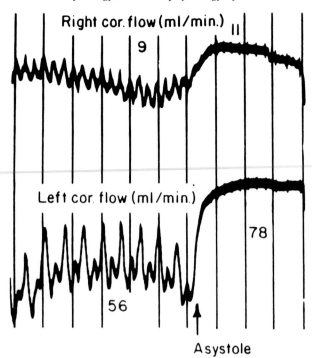

Fig. 58-1. Inhibitory nature of cardiac contraction to coronary perfusion was demonstrated by Sabiston and Gregg when they arrested the heart with maintained coronary perfusion pressure. Note that asystole is accompanied by an abrupt and sustained increase in both right and left coronary blood flow. From Sabiston and Gregg {59}, with permission.

suring device greatly confounded this work. Anrep et al. {1} presented evidence that little or no forward flow occurred during the systolic period, while Hochrein et al. {32} and Wiggers and Cotton {76} presented evidence that systolic flow was considerable. In 1940, Gregg and Green developed an orifice-plate flow meter, which had sufficient fidelity to measure phasic coronary flow {27}. This device revealed that coronary flow was greatly reduced but did not entirely stop during systole. The massaging theory began to fall out of favor with most scientists in light of the phasic coronary flow data, although Wiggers {75} revived the theory briefly by again, like Porter, examining venous flow patterns.

The massaging theory was laid to rest once and for all in 1957 by the classic experiment of Sabiston and Gregg {59}. The coronary blood vessels were perfused from an elevated reservoir, and the transient flow response to either a vagal asystole or sudden fibrillation was noted. In every case there was a dramatic increase in blood flow, as shown in fig. 58-1. The data were clear: *Removal of the coordinated heartbeat also lowered the coronary resistance to flow.* Figure 58-1 indicates that coronary resistance during a normal diastole is higher than that achieved with a steady-state asystole, but this appears to be an artifact of their flow meter. Katz and Feigl {38}, using modern high-

fidelity flow meters, found that the diastolic resistance at heart rates as high as 200 beats/min was not different from that during an asystole.

TRANSMURAL DISTRIBUTION OF EXTRAVASCULAR RESISTANCE

It has long been recognized that the subendocardium is a favored site for myocardial infarction in patients with diseased coronary arteries. The vulnerability of the sub-endocardium is now believed to directly result from a greater degree of extravascular resistance, which diverts flow away from that region. Although the transmural distribution of the total blood flow across the wall of the normal heart has been found to be uniform {23}, Griggs and Nakamura {28} discovered that partial occlusion of the coronary arteries consistently resulted in a preferential reduction of the subendocardial blood flow. They also noted that the stenosis caused a greater percentage of the coronary inflow to occur during systole and, therefore, concluded that flow delivered during the systolic period must have been distributed away from the subendocardium by the extravascular factors. In a study by Buckberg et al.

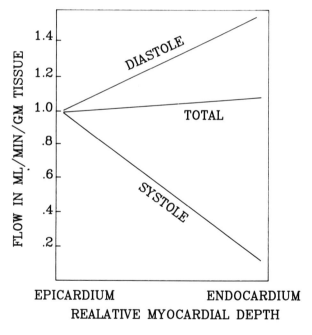

Fig. 58-2. Transmural distribution of the systolic coronary blood flow was revealed when coronary flow was measured while perfusing the coronary arteries with a pressure that fell to zero during each diastole (bottom line). The middle line indicates the distribution of flow observed when the coronary arteries were continuously perfused with aortic pressure. The upper line indicates the distribution of flow that must have occurred during diastole to compensate for the systolic gradient. Note that flow at the subepicardium shows little variation between systole and diastole. Adapted from Downey and Kirk {18}, with permission.

{11}, the partitioning of flow between systole and diastole was preferentially weighted toward systole by changing the phasic profile of the coronary perfusion pressure with valve lesions. Again, they found that such maneuvers distributed flow away from the subendocardium and that the severity of the subendocardial blood flow deficit was quantitatively related to the degree of encroachment on the diastolic perfusion pressure.

Downey et al. {17} carried the above line of reasoning one step further. By perfusing the coronary arteries with ventricular pressure, which falls to near zero during diastole, forward flow during diastole was eliminated. Blood-flow tracers injected during such conditions revealed what was believed to be the systolic distribution of the coronary blood flow. As can be seen in fig. 58-2, perfusion during systole assumes a steep gradient across the heart wall, with flow to the deeper layers approaching zero. This experiment was repeated in a technically elegant study by Hess and Bache {30}. They used chronically instrumented awake dogs and obtained essentially the same result.

The relative magnitude of the extravascular resistance at each depth was revealed when the Sabiston and Gregg experiment shown in fig. 58-1 was repeated by Russell et al. {58}, but this time with regional blood-flow measurements using microspheres. Figure 58-3 reveals that arresting

the heart had virtually no effect on flow to the sub-epicardial quarter of the left ventricle, while it doubled flow to the subendocardial quarter. The effect on flow in the midwall was intermediate between those two extremes. These data indicate that *cardiac contraction doubles the resistance in the subendocardial region, while it has virtually no effect on resistance at the subepicardium.*

ORIGIN OF THE EXTRAVASCULAR RESISTANCE

The extravascular resistance clearly results from mechanical deformation of the coronary vasculature. Although it is not difficult to appreciate that the contracting heart muscle can compress the coronary blood vessels and inhibit flow, it would be helpful if this process could be quantified. To do that would require a knowledge of the fundamental processes involved. Three possible mechanisms can be proposed. The first involves *shear strains* in the heart wall. Note that the term *strain* refers to the actual deformation of the tissue and is to be differentiated from *stress*, which is the force giving rise to those deformations. Adjacent muscle fibers may contract in such a way that they slide past one another, creating a region of shear between them. Any blood vessel passing through this region would then

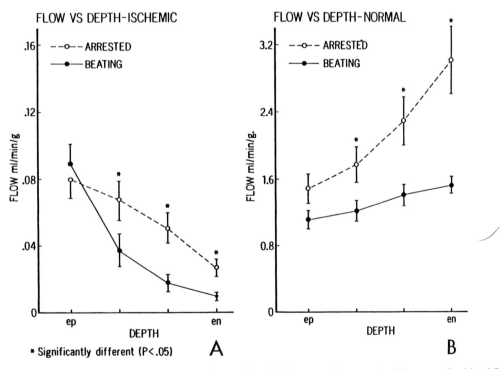

Fig. 58-3. Transmural distribution of the extravascular resistance in a dog heart can be appreciated by measuring blood flow prior to (solid line) and after (dotted line) arresting the heart. Coronary perfusion pressure was maintained throughout. The **left panel** represents collateral flow in the field of a ligated branch, while the **right panel** represents flow in a region with patent coronary arteries. The left panel reveals that extravascular factors account for about half of the resistance to the subendocardial region of the beating heart, while little effect is seen in the subepicardial regions. The right panel shows that collateral flow is nonuniformly distributed in the beating heart but that extravascular factors still account for about half of the subendocardium's resistance, even though the region is completely akinetic. Again little effect is seen at the subepicardium. From Russell et al. {58}, with permission.

be kinked at the interface, thereby increasing its resistance to flow or perhaps even totally pinching it off. It is likely that some shear strains do exist in the heart. Streeter et al. {70} have shown that muscle-fiber orientation changes as one passes from the epicardium toward the endocardium by about 120°. Some shear must exist between these nonparallel fibers. Feigl and Fry {24} confirmed the presence of this shear, but it is difficult to extrapolate those data to the present problem.

The second mechanism might be related to *traction forces* on the blood vessels. Increasing the length of a tube will increase its resistance. It would also tend to decrease the tube's diameter so that both the length effect and the diameter effect would tend to augment resistance by Poiseuille's equation when a tube is stretched. Since the ventricular wall thickens during systole, any vessels running perpendicular to the epicardial surface will experience an increased length at this time and an increased resistance.

The third possibility is that compressive stress within the myocardium is responsible for deforming the coronary blood vessels. Since the ventricular wall is comprised of soft tissue, compressive stresses in the subendocardium must at least equal the pressure in the ventricular lumen and could theoretically even exceed it. Attempts to measure the intramyocardial pressure indicate that it is substantial (see *Intramyocardial pressure* below). Experimental evidence shows that either shortening or pressure development can account for the extravascular resistance. Both shear and traction are a consequence of strains in the heart wall resulting from myocardial fiber shortening. On the other hand, stresses can occur in the absence of any strain.

The contribution of strains was examined by comparing the distribution of the systolic blood flow across the wall of the isovolumetrically beating heart to that of the normally ejecting heart {19}. In the isovolumetric state, pressure development is near normal but stains are minimal. Yet flow was diverted away from the subendocardium as effectively by isovolumetric contractions as by normal ejecting beats. Conversely, several studies have examined the coronary hemodynamics in the empty beating heart, which should have experienced the opposite, i.e., maximal strains but zero pressure in the ventricular lumen. Krams et al. {44} found that the systolic flow impediment in the empty beating cat heart was no different from that when the heart developed pressure. Furthermore, systole continued to divert flow away from the subendocardium when the dog heart was allowed to contract against zero afterload {74}. Flow was also diverted away from the subendocardium of rabbit hearts maintained in a prolonged systole and a vented ventricular chamber {25}. Finally, when shortening was prevented by depressing a segment with barbiturate but pressure development was normal, systole still inhibited coronary flow {65}. Thus *either shortening or pressure development appears to be a requirement for elevating the extravascular resistance.* That makes it unlikely that strains or shear per se account for the extravascular resistance but rather suggest that intramyocardial stresses are responsible.

VASCULAR WATERFALL

If the compressive stresses in the tissue are greater than the perfusion pressure, then the blood vessels are obliged to collapse and flow will cease to that region. However, what happens to vessels in regions where pressure is elevated above venous pressure but does not reach a magnitude equal to perfusion pressure? This condition has been extensively studied in the lung {53} and elsewhere {31}, and it has been found that the blood vessels respond to elevated tissue pressure by formng *waterfalls*.

The waterfall theory as presented by Holt {34,35} says that when the pressure surrounding a collapsible tube is between the inflow and the outflow pressures, there must be a point along the tube's length where the pressure inside the vessel falls below that outside the vessel. The vessel is obliged to collapse at the point where surround pressure exceeds that within. If the region completely collapsed, however, flow would cease, causing the pressure drop along the proximal segment of the tube to fall to zero. This would allow the full inflow pressure to be transmitted to the region of collapse, which would then reopen the tube.

An equilibrium will finally be achieved where the tube forms a short region of partial collapse as near to the outflow end as possible. The orfice formed at the region of collapse will adjust its dimensions so that it will abruptly drop the pressure inside the vessel from tissue pressure to venous pressure. Because only a very small portion of the vessel is involved in the partial collapse , the resistance of the patent upstream portion closely approximates the overall resistance of the vessel in the absence of any surrounding pressure when the vessel is fully patent. Since the pressure gradient across the upstream resistance is known — arterial pressure minus tissue pressure — flow can be calculated by the following equation:

$$Q = \frac{(\text{perfusion pressure} - \text{back pressure})}{\text{resistance}}.$$

Resistance in the equation is the resistance to flow as measured when tissue pressure is zero. Back pressure is either the tissue pressure (if arterial pressure > tissue pressure > venous pressure) or venous pressure (if tissue pressure < venous pressure).

In essence, *whenever local tissue pressure exceeds venous pressure, tissue pressure is simply substituted for venous pressure to determine the driving pressure.* Resistance in the equation is not altered. An important feature of the waterfall theory is that flow is inhibited in proportion to the magnitude of the tissue pressure.

IS THE CORONARY EXTRAVASCULAR RESISTANCE DUE TO WATERFALL FORMATION?

Compressive stresses in the contracting myocardium may be causing the formation of vascular waterfalls in the coronary veins. What makes this theory so attractive are the many reports that systolic intramyocardial pressure is high in the subendocardial region and falls off in the

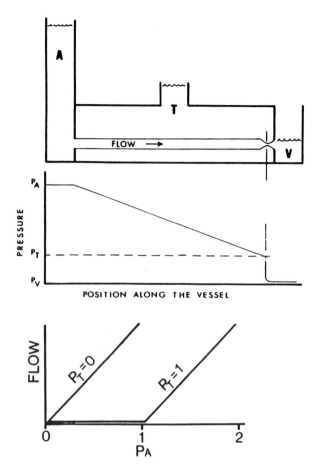

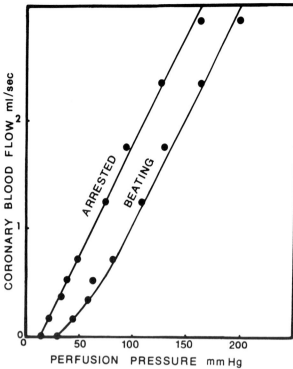

Fig. 58-5. The pressure-flow relationship for a canine coronary artery. Peak ventricular pressure remained constant at 100 mmHg. Note that beating shifts the curve to the right in a parallel fashion in the range of perfusion pressures above peak ventricular pressure. From Downey and Kirk {19}, with permission.

Fig. 58-4. The *upper panel* shows a simple model of the vascular waterfall. If the tissue pressure surrounding the vessel, T, is between arterial pressure, A, and venous pressure, V, then a region of partial collapse will form at the outflow end. The **middle panel** shows the pressure gradient along the length of the vessel. Note that pressure abruptly drops from T to V in the region of the partial collapse. The **bottom panel** shows the pressure flow curves for the vessel when T = 0 and when T = 1. Note that increasing T shifts the curve to the right but does not change the slope. From Downey and Kirk {18}, with permission.

epicardial regions. Thus the formation of vascular waterfalls could easily explain the gradient in transmural blood flow that systole imposes on the heart, since the flow impediment should be in proportion to the tissue pressure. One method of testing whether waterfalls form in the heart is to examine the pressure-flow relationship in the beating heart. The pressure-flow characteristics between a vascular waterfall system and a simple resistance are very different. Figure 58-4G-4 shows the pressure-flow curve for a vascular waterfall. Since the resistance of the blood vessel upstream of the collapsed region is not affected by changes in the surrounding pressure, the slope of the pressure-flow curve is independent of the surround pressure; changes in the surround pressure only shift the pressure-axis intercept.

Conversely, changes in resistance have no effect on the pressure-axis intercept — they only affect the slope of the line. Figure 58-5 shows that when the pressure flow curve of the coronary artery of a beating heart was compared with that for the same heart in an arrested state, the slopes were identical and only shifted in parallel fashion {18}. This indicates the *the heart beat does not affect the resistance, only the pressure-axis intercept.* The conclusion again was that only waterfall phenomena are associated with ventricular-pressure development. It should be noted that the two curves in fig. 58-5 are only parallel in the region of pressures above peak ventricular pressure. The convergence at low pressures can be explained by the complete collapse of vessels in those regions experiencing a compression in excess of perfusion pressure. (This phenomenon is examined in detail below in *Intramyocardial pressure*). Satoh et al. {61} examined nonbeating hearts in which pressures in the ventricular lumen could be varied and steady-state pressure-flow curves determined. They again found clear evidence of waterfall hemodynamics.

CRITICISMS TO THE WATERFALL THEORY

The waterfall hypothesis was first challenged by Spaan et al. {68}. Their criticism revolves around the magnitude of the capacitance of the coronary arteries. These investigators propose a large capacitance in the coronary circulation. Capacitance refers to the ratio of intravascular volume to intravascular pressure and is basically proportional to the elasticity in the vessel walls. When intramyocardial pressure rises, the difference between the pressure inside the coronary arteries and that outside of them is diminished, and thus the intravascular volume must also decrease since there is a dynamic equilibrium between stretch of the vessel wall, transmural pressure, and contained volume. Some of the expelled blood flows toward the veins, but much of that within the arterial vessels is regurgitated toward the coronary ostium. Thus, *much of the apparent increase in resistance during systole is actually the result of a hidden backflow of blood discharged from capacitance sites.* This *intramyocardial pump* theory nicely explains the phase reversal between the coronary arteries and veins as well. But if intramyocardial capacitance were sufficiently large, it could also prevent waterfall formation.

Since the capacitance vessels have intramyocardial pressure as their surround pressure, that compression will initially be transmitted through the vessel wall to the contained blood with the onset of each beat. The pressure within the vessel cannot fall to a value below the tissue pressure and allow waterfall formation until that capacitance site has emptied itself of blood. The capacitance would have to empty through the proximal and distal resistances, and the time constant for that emptying was thought to be about 3 seconds. The effect would be to force some blood retrograde into the arterial side, causing a reduction in inflow at the coronary ostium throughout systole, even though flow through the capillaries had not actually changed.

During the subsequent diastole the arterial flow would be abnormally high as the capacitance sites refilled, giving the appearance of reduced coronary resistance. Furthermore, if the time constant is as large as they reported, 3 seconds, then only a small percentage of the contained blood would empty with a single beat and the pressures within the vessels would never fall to a value low enough to allow waterfall formation. Most importantly, although phasic flow at the coronary ostium would be reduced by contraction of the ventricle, nutritional flow at the capillary level would continue unaffected throughout the cardiac cycle.

The critical point then hinges on the magnitude of the capacitive time constant. If it is much shorter than the duration of systole, then the pressure within the vessels would be quickly dissipated and waterfalls would be allowed to form. Spaan et al. {68} first arrived at their estimate of coronary capacitance by occluding the coronary artery and measuring the time constant at which pressure decayed. Several studies have since addressed the coronary capacitance since this time. When the coronary artery was presented with either a sine wave {13}

or a step function {14,21,43,46}, a much shorter time constant of less than 100 ms was determined. That time constant would allow waterfalls to form early in the systolic period. This author suggests that complete collapse of most of the coronary vessels causes blood trapped distal to an occluded coronary artery to bleed out very slowly, falsely indicating that the time constant was much longer than it actually was.

It should be noted that *if waterfall formation was being prevented by a long capacitive time constant, then the effect of the heartbeat on coronary blood flow would not be to inhibit flow, only make it appear pulsatile.* If that were the case, it would be hard to reconcile the fact that asystole is associated with a sustained decrease in coronary resistance {59} or that systole diverts blood flow away from the subendocardium {11,17}. Spaan also noted that the intramyocardial pump model failed to account for the subendocardial flow diversion and subsequently introduced the nonlinear intramyocardial pump model, in which he included a pressure-dependent vascular resistance {66}. Empirical data predicting vascular dimensions at differing transmural pressures revealed data similar to that assumed by the waterfall theory, that is, collapse as surround pressure exceeds lumenal pressure. This hybrid model is virtually identical to the waterfall-based model that we described, incorporating capacitance elements {46}.

TIME-VARYING ELASTANCE

More recently, Krams et al. have introduced the time-varying elastance theory to explain the extravascular resistance. As will be seen below, a radially oriented stress in equilibrium with the luminal pressure is thought to be the predominant compressive stress in the ventricle. Yet Krams et al. {44} and others {25,74} have seen that the extravascular resistance continues unabated when the heart contracts against zero pressure in the ventricle. During contraction of heart muscle, the muscle fibers behave as if they were passive elastic elements whose elasticity suddenly was reduced. The force of the contraction is then simply proportional to the decrease in elastance. This has been a very useful and accurate method for describing myocardial mechanics.

Krams et al. {44} proposed that the change in elastance of the myocardial fibers is also transmitted to the blood vessels, causing a similar change in the elastance of the vessel wall. The sudden change in elastance would cause a decrease in the caliber of the vessels and thus increase their resistance. The time-varying elastance theory is attractive since it explains why systole impedes blood flow in the absence of pressure in the ventricle. It is difficult experimentally, however, to separate changes in vascular capacitance from those in surround pressure, especially when the latter is not known. Furthermore, the time-varying elastance concept does not require an actual understanding of the mechanism of interaction but rather describes the resulting effect in empirical terms. Thus, by adjusting the instantaneous elastance, a near-perfect fit to almost any data could be achieved. To further complicate the theory, Resar et al. {57} found that there was no simple relationship between the elastance of the myocardial fibers and that of the vessels. Whether the coronary vessels actually do behave as linear elastic elements whose stiffness varies throughout the cardiac cycle awaits confirmation. Some ramifications of the time-varying elastance theory are difficult to reconcile with known observations. For example, the shift in the pressure flow curve seen with sudden asystole (fig. 58-5) would not be expected, but rather a counterclockwise rotation, since only resistance would be varying. Secondly, since there is no gradient of ventricular muscle contractility across the heart wall, it is difficult to explain the transmural gradient of flow away from the subendocardium during systole.

INTRAMYOCARDIAL PRESSURE

Since current evidence strongly supports the concept that extravascular resistance is the result of vascular waterfalls forming in response to intramyocardial pressure, what then is the magnitude of this pressure? Many investigators have attempted to measure it over the years. Most of these experiments involve inserting some pressure-sensitive element directly into the beating myocardium. Johnson and DiPalma {36} were the first to try this approach. They implanted segments of carotid artery into the ventricular wall and estimated the surrounding pressure by perfusing the segments at various pressures. They concluded that intramyocardial pressure during systole reached a peak of about twice ventricular pressure in the subendocardium but had very low values near the subepicardium. This basic protocol has been repeated using needles {40,45,73}, open catheters {9,26}, and catheter-tipped manometers {4–7,69}. Most of these investigators arrived at a similar result: Subendocardial pressure appreciably exceeded the pressure in the ventricular lumen. This point has been a matter of considerable controversy, however.

Brandi and McGregor {9} demonstrated that the pressure experienced by a bleb of saline injected into the heart wall is a proportional to its size. Furthermore, when they extrapolated their data to a bleb with zero volume, the extrapolated subendocardial pressure was equal to ventricular pressure. They suggested that there is an inescapable artifact associated with the direct measurements in that the transducer locally deforms the myocardium (perhaps stretching the fibers so that they are operating farther up the Starling curve) such that abnormally high forces are developed against the transducer. Three reports support the concept the subendocardial pressure does not exceed ventricular pressure. Heineman and Grayson {29} attempted to measure intramyocardial pressure using a micropipette and a Servonulling device. The size of the pipette tip was an order of magnitude smaller than any previous device tried. All of the pressures seen with the micropipette were equal to or less than ventricular pressure.

Downey and Kirk {18} measured the pressure-flow relationship in maximally dilated canine coronary arteries. They derived a model based on multiple parallel vessels at various depths in the heart, each exhibiting waterfall behavior. That model predicted that inflow should be a linear function of pressure when perfusion pressure is above the highest tissue pressure present in the heart wall. The model predicted that the curve would have a break point, below which it would become a nonlinear function of perfusion pressure. This curved portion would represent the range of perfusion pressures below the peak tissue pressure. Analysis of actual curves showed that the predicted break point was clearly present and that it occurred at perfusion pressures not different from peak ventricular pressure.

In a subsequent study, blood flow to the maximally dilated subendocardium was measured with microspheres under a wide variety of hemodynamic conditions {51}. It was found that a waterfall-type model accurately predicted regional blood flow to the subendocardium when a value for intramyocardial pressure equal to ventricular pressure was used in the calculation. When a value of twice ventricular pressure was employed, the correlation between predicted and actual blood flow was poor. While the controversy over the magnitude of the intramyocardial pressure is far from resolved, it is this author's opinion that *current evidence favors the concept that intramyocardial pressure approaches but does not exceed the pressure in the ventricular lumen.*

When considering the nature of the intramyocardial pressure, it is useful to analyze the compressive forces in the ventricular wall. First of all, the term *intramyocardial pressure* is a misnomer. The coronary deformation is undoubtedly the result of compressive stresses rather than hydrostatic pressure. Pressure is a scaler quantity that denotes a force that is equal in all directions, while a stress is a vector quantity representing a force within the material in a single direction. In the ventricle, widely differing stresses coexist; in the circumferential direction, a tensile stress results from the Laplace relationship {49}. A tensile stress is negative, trying to pull the material apart. If a deep cut were made in the epicardial surface, the cut would tend to pull apart during each systole, illustrating that the stress in that orientation is tensile and not compressive. Although the circumferential stress may exceed ventricular pressure in magnitude, this stress — being tensile — would not be expected to collpase coronary vessels but to pull them open.

A second stress is oriented in the radial direction, perpendicular to the epicardial surface {49}. This stress is compressive and represents the accumulative inward force of each muscle layer pressing inward on the muscle layer below it. It ranges from a value of zero at the epicardial surface, where no superior layers are present, to its highest value at the endocardial surface, where it represents the sum total of the forces from all layers. Since the ventricular wall is in equilibrium with the blood in the lumen of the ventricle, the sum of these forces must, in turn, be equal to luminal pressure. The radial stress, unlike the circumferential stress, is compressive. If a cut could be made in the ventricle at midwall depth and parallel to the epicardial surface, the radial stress would force the tissue in the vicinity of the cut back together, rather than pull it open. Similarly, any blood vessels passing at right angles to this stress would tend to be collapsed by it. The radial stress nicely explains why systole continues to inhibit flow when a region of the heart is made akinetic with barbiturates {47,65,72}. This phenomenon is difficult to explain by the time-varying elastance concept {44}.

Although the two stresses presented above are obligatory, it is not impossible to envision other compressive stresses in the ventricle, which may be of even greater magnitude. These could be the result of the complex geometry of the muscle fibers. Indeed such stresses have been formally proposed {40} but have yet to be proven. Such a stress could easily explain why systole continues to divert flow from the subendocardium, even when the ventricle contracts against zero afterload. In fact, Baird et al. {6} indeed saw that systolic intramyocardial pressure was quite substantial while the ventricle was vented. *All that can be said at present is that a radially oriented compressive stress ranging from near zero at the epicardial surface to near lumenal pressure at the endocardial surface is obligatory in the beating ventricle and that this stress alone could explain the gradient extravascular resistance seen across the heart wall.* Nevertheless, the possibility that some heretofore unidentified stress, perhaps associated with fiber shortening, can under certain conditions contribute to coronary vessel collapse also seems likely.

CORONARY RESISTANCE IN THE ABSENCE OF CARDIAC CONTRACTION

In the above discussion it was proposed that compression in the ventricular wall caused the formation of vascular waterfalls. In the simple model presented it was assumed that the coronary vessels, in the absence of any compression, would behave as simple linear resistors. That is not quite the case, however, and the effect of this deviation on the watefall theory must be explored at this point. In 1978, Bellamy described a study in which the pressure-flow relationship was determined for the coronary artery during diastole, a time when extravascular compression is thought to be negligible {8}. He found a linear relationship between the instantaneous flow and the instantaneous pressure. The most striking feature of these plots, however, was that they had a projected zero flow intercept of 40–50 mmHg. One dog that had an unusually slow heart rate even showed complete cessation of flow in late diastole. Furthermore, it was found that the zero-flow intercept was a function of coronary tone. When the coronary arteries were dilated, either pharmacologically or by reactive hyperemia, the intercept fell to 15–20 mmHg.

This apparent waterfall behavior is obviously not due to tissue pressure, since all evidence shows that intramyocardial pressure is quite low during diastole. Rather, it seems to be associated with forces in the blood vessel wall itself. The fact that the pressure-flow curves are linear indicates that a critical-closing type of behavior associated with vascular tone is occurring, similar to that described by Permutt and Riley {53}. Here forces originating within the vessel wall cause a region of partial collapse that acts as a regulator, constantly adjusting its lumen size to maintain a pressure equilibrium. This represents a fundamentally different process that the critical closing hypothesis forwarded by Burton {12} several decades ago, in which the vessel is either patent or completely collapsed. The fact that the collapsing forces originate within the vessel walls further complicates our understanding. Because of the Laplace relationship, the pressure required to open the vessel should be an inverse function of its radius, making it difficult to understand how such seemingly perfect regulation of the back pressure to flow could occur.

Physiologists, disturbed that such a fundamental aspect of hemodynamics had gone unnoticed all these years, have recently speculated that this phenomenon may be an artifact. Since Bellamy's measurements had been taken during the falling-pressure phase of a long diastole, it has been suggested that the pressure-flow curve is altered by vascular capacitance. Because pressure is falling, some back flow must occur as the capacitance in the coronary arteries empties. Since this back flow is mixed with a forward flow to the microcirculation, it is in essence concealed. The net effect is a shift in the pressure-flow curve towards higher pressures {21}.

Capacitance deep in the microcirculation, having a long time constant, could also serve as an apparent back pressure to arterial inflow by maintaining pressure in the region of the capillaries for several seconds after perfusion pressure was changed {67}. Several recent studies indicate that capacitance does cause the zero flow-pressure measurement to be artifactually high, but capacitance alone cannot fully account for the phenomenon. Kirkeeide et al. {41} caused the aortic pressure to oscillate by rapidly pumping blood into and out of the aorta. Under these conditions some diastoles found the aortic pressure rising instead of falling. If the perfusion pressure was rising, then the concealed back flow will be negative and in the same direction as the microcirculatory flow, and the curves will be shifted to abnormally lower pressures. The difference between curves plotted with a rising perfusion pressure and those with a falling perfusion pressure should reveal the magnitude of the artifact. It was found to be less than 10 mmHg. Attempts to measure the magnitude of the small-vessel capacitance by perturbations in the arterial pressure indicate that its time constant is in the range of milliseconds, not seconds {13,22,46}, which argues against the capacitance artifact proposed by Spann {67}.

Finally, collateral flow has been offered as a source of error in these studies. If the pressure in only one coronary branch is manipulated, collateral anastomosis will provide an apparent back pressure to flow. Although there is a contribution from collateral flow, it is also small and only raised the zero-flow intercept pressure about 10 mmHg {48}. More important contributions from collateral flow alter the shape of the curve, making it appear straighter than it actually is {48}. That artifact does not apply to those studies in which the entire coronary bed was manipulated {46}.

An important ramification of the nonzero intercept of the diastolic pressure-flow relationship is that classical

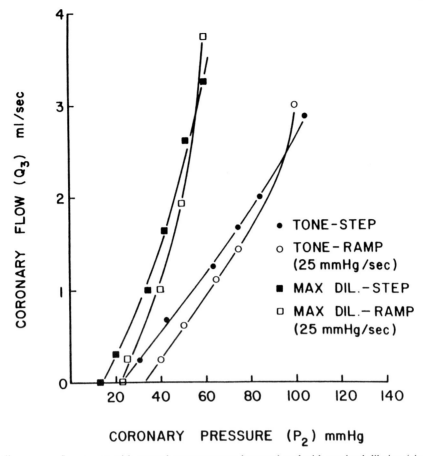

Fig. 58-6. Diastolic pressure-flow curves with normal coronary tone (squares) and with maximal dilation (circles). Open symbols are measurements made by the falling pressure method during a long diastole and contain a capacitance artifact. The solid symbols depict the measurements from the same hearts made by the pressure step method, which is thought to be free of capacitance artefact. Note that even when the contribution from capacitance is eliminated, the zero flow intercepts are above the right atrial pressure. From Lee et al. {46}, with permission.

resistance measurements have little utility in the coronary bed. Resistance, as traditionally calculated by observed perfusion pressure divided by observed flow, was thought to reflect the state of smooth muscle tone in a vascular bed. Such measurements are clearly pressure dependent for any given state of smooth muscle tone in both the beating heart (fig. 58-5) and the arrested heart (fig. 58-6). Thus it is not possible to equate a change in the traditionally calculated resistance — even if that calculation is made in late disatole — with changes in vascular tone if those measurements were made at different perfusion pressures.

The evidence, then, supports the concept that there is a waterfall associated with the coronary vasculature that provides an effective back pressure of 20–30 mmHg when tone is present and 10–20 mmHg when tone is absent. Unfortunately the exact mechanism for this phenomenon is not understood. It is presumed (but not yet proven) that compression outside the blood vessel will be additive to the waterfalls originating within the vessel wall. Certainly,

though, the extravascular forces are much greater than the vascular forces and, therefore, predominate in the beating heart.

EXTRAVASCULAR RESISTANCE IN THE BEATING HEART

In ischemic heart disease atherosclerosis causes the caliber of the large coronary arteries to become narrowed. Autoregulation will attempt to restore the flow by widely dilating the arteriolar bed. Since coronary tone is low to absent during myocardial ischemia, vasospasm not withstanding, the mechanical factors become the primary determinants of regional perfusion under those conditions. Because numerous studies indicate that the severity of ischemic injury is reciprocally related to the residual flow, effective patient management would require that steps be taken to minimize the extravascular resistance in the

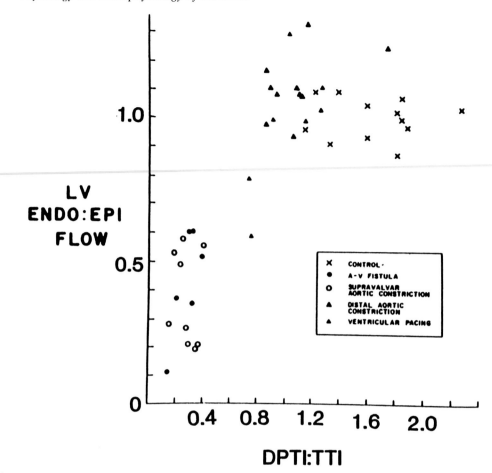

Fig. 58-7. Subendocardial ischemia is detected when the ratio of coronary flow to the subendocardium versus that to the subepicardium falls below 1. Subendocardial ischemia predictably occurs whenever the DPTI:TTI ratio falls below 0.8, regardless of the cause. From Buckberg et al. {33}, with permission.

beating heart. A clear understanding of its determinants would be essential.

By far the largest single determinant of the extravascular resistance is ventricular pressure. Most reports agree that intramyocardial pressure, irrespective of whether it was found to equal or exceed ventricular pressure, is proportional to ventricular pressure. Furthermore, because the perfusion pressure to the coronary vessels during systole is not likely to exceed left ventricular pressure, cessation of flow is predicted for the subendocardium, regardless of whether subendocardial compression just equals or actually exceeds ventricular pressure. This limits subendocardial flow to the diastolic period. That is not the case for midwall or subepicardial regions, but because the subendocardium is clearly the most vulnerable region of the heart to ischemia, it is worthwhile to consider it separately.

Buckberg et al. {11} recognized this fact and proposed a novel supply versus demand theory. The driving pressure (supply) for subendocardial flow per beat is in proportional

to the diastolic pressure time area (DPTI), that is, the area between ventricular pressure tracing (assumed to be the back pressure to flow) and the aortic pressure tracing during the diastolic period. Furthermore, they proposed that the metabolic requirements per beat were determined by the area under the ventricular pressure curve — the tension time index (TTI), as submitted by Sarnoff et al. {60}. They then proposed that *the ratio of DPTI to TTI described the supply-demand status of the subendocardium.* Indeed, whenever this ratio fell below about 0.7 in animal experiments, subendocardial ischemia occurred (see fig. 58-7).

The results of this and subsequent studies suggest that the DPTI-TTI ratio is an effective indicator of the adequacy of myocardial perfusion in the ischemic patient. Conditions that reduce this ratio include tachycardia, which reduces the percent of the cardiac cycle spent in diastole; aortic stenosis, which causes ventricular systolic pressure and, thus, demand to increase but diastolic perfusion pressure to fall; or aortic regurgitation, which causes a rapid runoff of aortic diastolic pressure and thus reduces the DPTI. Conversely, maneuvers that augment the DPTI-TTI ratio should be beneficial; these include counterpulsation with an intraaortic balloon pump {71}, which reduces afterload and augments diastolic aortic pressure. This index is also useful for predicting the hemodynamics across a stenotic coronary artery, as Griggs and Nakamura demonstrated {28}. In this case the reduced pressure distal to the lesion is simply substituted for the aortic pressure in the equation.

EXTRAVASCULAR COMPRESSION DURING DIASTOLE

Time-averaged blood flow is uniformly distributed across the wall of the normal heart {23}. *Because the subendocardium is underperfused during systole, it must be compensated by a reverse gradient of flow during diastole.* Intramyocardial pressure is quite low during diastole, and the reverse gradient is due to a gradient in vascular resistance across the wall of the heart. When perfusion pressure is normal, this compensatory gradient is the result of local autoregulation adjusting resistance in each region to achieve an adequate overall perfusion {50}. Studies by Downey et al. {15}, however, indicated that flow gradient favoring the subepicardium in diastole persists, even when autoregulation is abolished and the coronary arteries are maximally dilated. That finding indicates that there is also a greater vascular density in the subendocardium.

Baird et al. {5} have suggested that the reverse gradient in diastolic flow is the reflection of a corresponding gradient in diastolic compression. They found that diastolic compression, as revealed by a catheter-tip manometer, ranged from 6 mmHg at the subendocardium to 12 mmHg at the subepicardium. They reasoned that since subendocardial compression was half that in the subepicardium, flow to the subepicardial layers should be twice as great. The mechanics describing flow through collapsible tubes, however, would not support such reasoning, since the driving pressure for flow is the difference between arterial pressure and local tissue pressure. Assuming a coronary perfusion pressure of 100 mmHg, the driving pressure for flow at the subendocardium would be 100 − 6; or 94 mmHg. The driving pressure for flow at the subepicardium would be 88 mmHg. This would cause less than a 10% difference in flow, not 50%, as originally proposed. Furthermore, studies by Archie {3}, in which the pressure intercepts of regional pressure-flow curves were examined in arrested hearts, fail to confirm a gradient in back pressure across the heart wall. This small gradient of compression, then, is probably completely masked by critical closing phenomenon within the vessel wall.

One would expect an elevated diastolic pressure, as is in the case with the failing heart, to be transmitted through the myocardium and to impede diastolic perfusion. Kjekshus {42} was the first to attempt to describe this effect. Subendocardial ischemia was clearly created by elevating diastolic pressure to 18 mmHg by volume loading. More recently, Archie {3} has attempted to quantify the diastolic intramyocardial pressure by direct examination of regional pressure-flow curves in arrested hearts. Since waterfall theory predicts that the pressure-flow curve will intercept the pressure axis at a pressure equal to the surrounding pressure, he interpreted the projected intercept from each region to reflect intramyocardial pressure. He found that the full lumenal pressure was experienced in the subendocardial region and that this quickly fell to about half the lumenal value in the midwall and epicardium. It is noteworthy that appreciable impediment to flow persisted in the outer layers, rather than falling to zero, as appears to be the case in systole. A possible explanation was that a large portion of the circumferential stress in the passive diastolic state is carried by the visceral pericardium, rather than being dissipated in the ventricular wall.

The DPTI-TTI ratio, as presented by Buckberg et al. {11}, assumes the compressional component to the subendocardium through diastole to be lumenal pressure {33}, which is supported by Archie's findings. This concept was further supported by the study of Munch and Downey {51}, in which subendocardial blood flow with maximally dilated coronaries was correlated with predictions from DPTI calculations under conditions of elevated diastolic pressure, and the correlation was found to be excellent. Thus, we must conclude that *elevated diastolic ventricular pressure does inhibit subendocardial perfusion and that the degree of inhibition will be approximately by the same percentage as diastolic ventricular pressure is to coronary perfusion pressure.*

CONTRACTILITY AND THE EXTRAVASCULAR RESISTANCE

The contribution of contractile state to the extravascular resistance is controversial. If, indeed, the radial equilibrium stress is the primary source of compression in the heart wall, then contractility would not be expected to greatly influence it. The radial stress is only determined by pressure in the ventricular lumen. On the other hand, if the predominant component of compression is due to stress resulting from interaction between contracting muscle fibers, as is assumed in the time-varying elastance theory {44}, then it should be very sensitive to the contractile state.

Snyder et al. {65} approached this problem by examining the effect of changes in contractility on the magnitude of the extravascular resistance. A small coronary branch was cannulated and perfused at constant flow, the branch was maximally dilated with an infusion of adenosine, and contractility was either increased or decreased by injection of isoproterenol or pentobarbital directly into the perfusate. Because only a small portion of the ventricle received the inotropically active agent, overall ventricular dynamics, and thus, ventricular pressure, were not altered. Since perfusion rate was held constant, changes in the extravascular resistance were reflected by changes in perfusion pressure. Only very small changes in perfusion pressure accompanied the con-

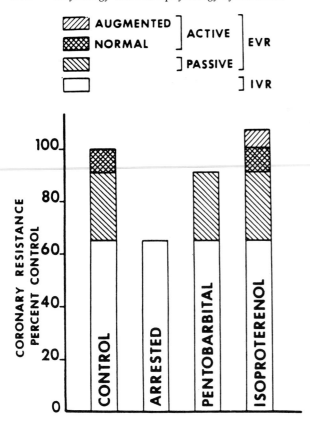

Fig. 58-8. The contribution of contractility to the extravascular resistance. When active shortening was prevented in the segment with pentobarbital, the coronary resistance decreased only by the amount indicated by crosshatching. Similarly, when shortening was greatly augmented with isoproterenol, resistance increased only by the small amount, indicated by the upper segment of the far right bar. Pressure development in the ventricle seems to be the major determinant of the extravascular resistance. IVR = intravascular resistance; EVR = extravascular resistance. From Snyder et al. {65}, with permission.

tractility changes. Yet vagal asystole revealed that almost half of the resistance in this preparation was extravascular in origin (see fig. 58-8).

The Snyder et al. study was repeated by Trimble and Downey {72}, this time using a constant-pressure perfusion and measuring regional flow changes with microspheres. Regional-flow data revealed that about a 20% decrease in the midwall flow had occurred following isoproterenol, but with little change in subendocardial flow, even when perfusion pressure was much higher than peak ventricular pressure. The interpretation again was that the massive increases in contractility had caused relatively little change in compression at the subendocardium and that compressional increases were limited to the midwall. Rendering the region akinetic with pentobarbital, however, caused subendocardial flow to increase, indicating that compression had been reduced in that region. The same kind of

study was simultaneously reported by Marzilli et al. {47}. Although Trimble and Downey reported no significant changes in subendocardial flow in response to changes in regional contractility with perfusion pressure equal to aortic pressure, Marzilli et al. reported much larger changes. In that study, abolition of contractility reduced subendocardial flow by 43%. The only real difference in the two models is that Marzilli et al. waited 5 minutes for the animals to equilibrate to the inotropic intervention before injecting the microspheres for flow measurement. Trimble and Downey injected the microspheres within 60 seconds of the intervention. Other than the possible involvement of some time-related stress-relaxation phenomenon, no explanation for the divergent data is apparent.

The importance of contractile state becomes apparent when the ventricle is vented. Under those conditions systole continues to inhibit coronary flow, even though the radially oriented equilibrium stress must clearly be absent {44}. Furthermore, the selective inhibition of flow to the subendocardium persists {74} just as it was when the ventricle developed pressure. It is this author's opinion that two separate stresses probably coexist in the ventricle, one related to shortening, and thus linked to contractile state, and the other being the radial equilibrium stress. They both have similar magnitudes and distributions. Thus in the normally beating heart either may predominate at any moment and contribute to the vascular deformation. When a segment is rendered akinetic the radial equilibrium stress predominates and maintains the compression. Similarly, when contraction occurs with an empty ventricle, the stress linked to the contractile state predominates.

EXTRAVASCULAR RESISTANCE AND THE COLLATERAL CIRCULATION

The coronary arteries are interconnected by numerous anastomoses that comprise a collateral circulation. If a major branch becomes occluded, flow does not completely stop in the region supplied by that artery, but continues at a reduced rate. This residual flow is delivered by the collateral vessels and, in the dog, averages about 20% of normal flow. This flow is clinically important in that it can oppose infarction during a coronary occlusion to a significant degree. The higher the collateral flow, the smaller the resulting infarct {56}. Anrep and Hausler {2} reported one of the earliest techniques for estimating this flow. They ligated a major coronary artery and inserted a catheter into the distal segment of that artery. It was noted that oxygenated arterial blood would flow from this catheter when it was vented to the atmosphere. This retrograde flow represented arterial blood that had entered the main coronary truck via collateral channels. Normally, this blood would have been forced through the microcirculation subtended by that artery, but instead it took the low–resistance pathway retrograde through the catheter. Microsphere measurements confirm that none of this flow enters the microcirculation during the collection of retrograde flow {39,78}. *Though the retrograde flow technique has been used an indicator of collateral flow for* many years {37,64}, there is still much disagreement as to what it really represents. The pressure gradient across the collateral vasculature during retrograde flow collection is aortic pressure minus atmospheric pressure. When the arterial segment is not vented, the driving pressure across the collateral vessels is obviously smaller — aortic pressure minus peripheral coronary pressure. Peripheral coronary pressure averages about 24 mmHg in the dog {46}. By this reasoning, retrograde flow should overestimate collateral flow. The retrograde flow procedure actually gives an estimate of the collateral resistance rather than the true collateral flow.

Wyatt et al. {77} examined the linearity of coronary collateral resistance and found that they closely approximated a fixed resistance running between the major arterial branches. Collateral flow ceased, however, when pressure in the ischemic artery was within 20% of aortic pressure. It was concluded that 80% of aortic pressure simply represented the pressure at the origin of the collateral vessels in the donor bed, but an alternative explanation may exist. Eng and Kirk propose that waterfall behavior exists in the collateral bed as well and that flow does not occur in them until a sufficient gradient exists to open them {22}.

In a recent study Messina {48} examined collateral flow with microspheres as a function of the pressure gradient between pressure in the circumflex artery and that in the left main coronary artery. Collateral flow seemed to cease abruptly when the gradient was less than 60 mmHg. Thus, *it is likely that a waterfall exists in the collateral vessels as well.* The factors that contribute to this behavior have yet to be clearly identified.

Are the collateral vessels affected by mechanical compression? Yes and no. Brown et al. {10} suggested that the collateral vessels may not be patent during systole, since retrograde flow was not affected by selective changes in systolic pressure. It has since been shown, though, that when aortic pressure is constant, the prolonged diastole of cardiac arrest does not increase retrograde flow, as would have been predicted, but rather usually depresses it {16}.

The key to those two apparently discrepant findings resides in the observation that *increasing diastolic volume increases the collateral resistance* {16,37}. Thus, in the Brown et al. experiment, when afterload (the systolic phase of the aortic pressure) was raised, the heart compensated by increasing its diastolic volume through the Frank–Starling mechanism. Thus, the increased pressure gradient was countered by an increased collateral resistance, and flow remained essentially constant. Collateral segments, at least in the dog, do not appear to get compressed during systole. The dog's collateral vessels may escape compression as a result of their epicardial location {63}. In the human, intramural collaterals have been described {63}, and this location may cause them to be more sensitive to compression. No data are available on this latter point.

To say that the collateral vasculature is unaffected by contraction of the heart is not to say that collateral flow is unaffected by systole, however. The vessels that the collateral channels supply are very much affected by cardiac contraction. Even though the collateral-dependent segment may be akinetic due to ischemic depression, ventricular pressure will be transmitted through that portion of the ventricle so that waterfalls would still be expected to form. It has been shown that *systolic compression impedes collateral flow to the inner layers of an ischemic segment to an equal or greater degree than occurs in a normally perfused region* {58}. The left panel of fig. 58-3 shows the distribution of blood flow to a collateral dependent region before and after arresting the heart with maintained coronary perfusion pressure. Note how flow increases markedly in the deep layers when the heart is arrested, even though the region was akinetic. For that reason, *the percentage of the cardiac cycle spent in systole, as well as the diastolic volume, becomes an important determinant of collateral flow.*

It should be noted that, unlike the case in the normally perfused heart, the inhibition to perfusion experienced during systole in collateral-dependent tissue is not compensated by a reverse gradient of flow in diastole. The collateral flow to myocardium distal to an arterial occlusion will always be distributed so that the subendocardium will receive only about one third of that received by the subepicardium {58}. This gradient of flow is thought to be primarily responsible for the subendocardium's proclivity for infarction. For an in-depth discussion of the subendocardium's vulnerability to ischemia, the reader is referred to the chapter on myocardial infarction elsewhere in this volume.

REFERENCES

1. Anrep GV, Cruickshank EWH, Downing AC, Subba RA: The coronary flow in relation to the cardiac cycle. *Heart* 14:111–113, 1927.
2. Anrep GV, Hausler H: The coronary circulation. I. The effect of changes of the blood pressure and the output of the heart. *J Physiol* 65:357–373, 1928.
3. Archie JP: Transmural distribution of intrinsic and transmitted left ventricular diastolic intramyocardial pressure in dogs. *Cardiovasc Res* 12:255–262, 1987.
4. Armour JA, Randall WC: Canine left ventircular intramyocardial pressures. *Am J Physiol* 220:1833–1839, 1971.
5. Baird RJ, Adeseshiah M, Okumori M: The gradient in regional myocardial tissue pressure in the left ventricule during diastole: Its relationship to regional flow distribution. *J Surg Res* 20:11–16, 1976.
6. Baird RJ, Dudka F, Okumori M, de la Roche A, Goldbrock MM, Hill T, MacGregor DC: Surgical aspects of regional myocardial blood flow and myocardial pressure. *J Thorac Cardiovasc Surg* 69:17–29, 1975.
7. Baird RJ, Manktelow RT, Shah PA, Ameli EM: Intramyocardial pressure: A study of its regional variations and its relationship to intraventricular pressure. *J Thorac Cardiovasc Surg* 59:810–823, 1970.
8. Bellamy RF: Diastolic coronary artery pressure-flow relations in the dog. *Circ Res* 43:93–101, 1978.
9. Brandi G, MacGregor M: Intramural pressure in the left ventricle of the dog. *Cardiovasc Res* 3:472–475, 1969.
10. Brown G, Gundel WD, Gott VL, Covell JW: Coronary collateral flow following acute coronary occlusion: A diastolic phenomenon. *Cardiovasc Res* 8:621–631, 1974.

11. Buckberg GD, Fixler DE, Archie JP, Hoffman JIE: Experimental subendocardial ischemia in dogs with normal coronary arteries. *Circ Res* 30:67–81, 1972.
12. Burton AC: On the physical equilbrium of small blood vessels. *Am J Physiol* 164:319–329, 1950.
13. Canty JM, Klocke FJ, Mates RE: Pressure and tone dependence of coronary diastolic input impedance. *Am J Physiol* 248:H700–H711, 1985.
14. Dole WP, Bishop VS: Influence of autoregulation and capacitance on diastolic coronary artery pressure-flow relationships in the dog. *Circ Res* 51:261–270, 1982.
15. Downey HF, Bashour FA, Boatwright RB, Parker PE, Kechejian SK: Uniformity of transmural perfusion in anesthetized dogs with maximally dilated coronary circulation. *Circ Res* 37:111–117, 1975.
16. Downey JM, Chagrasulis RW: The effect of cardiac contraction on collateral resistance. *Circ Res* 34:286–292, 1976.
17. Downey JM, Downey HF, Kirk ES: Effects of myocardial strains on coronary blood flow. *Circ Res* 34:286–292, 1974.
18. Downey JM, Kirk ES: Distribution of the coronary blood flow across the canine heart wall during systole. *Circ Res* 34:251–257, 1974.
19. Downey JM, Kirk ES: Inhibition of coronary blood flow by a vascular waterfall mechanism. *Circ Res* 36:753–760, 1975.
20. Downey JM, Kirk ES, Cowan D, Sonnenblick EH, Urschel CW: The adequacy of coronary blood flow during acute hypotension. *Circ Shock* 3:83–91, 1975.
21. Eng C, Jentzen JH, Kirk ES: Coronary capacitive effects on the high estimates of coronary critical closing pressure (abstract). *Circulation* 62:974, 1980.
22. Eng C, Kirk ES: Flow into ischemic myocardium and across coronary collateral vessels is modulated by a waterfall mechanism. *Circ Res* 55:10–17, 1984.
23. Feigl EO: Coronary physiology. *Physiol Rev* 63:1–205, 1983.
24. Feigl EO, Fry DL: Intamural myocardial shear during the cardiac cycle. *Circ Res* 14:536–540, 1964.
25. Goto M, Flynn A, Doucette J, Jansen C, Stork M, Coggins D, Muehrcke D, Husseini W, Hoffman J: Cardiac contraction affects deep myocardial vessels predominantly. *Am J Physiol* 261:H1417–H1429, 1991.
26. Gregg DE, Eckstein RW: Measurements of intramyocardial pressure. *Am J Physiol* 132:781–790, 1941.
27. Gregg DE, Green HD: Registration and intrepretation of normal phasic inflow into a left coronary artery by an improved differential manometric method. *Am J Physiol* 130:114–125, 1940.
28. Griggs DM, Nakamura Y: Effect of coronary constriction on myocardial distribution of iodoantipyrine. *Am J Physiol* 215:1082–1088, 1968.
29. Heineman F, Grayson J: Transmural distribution of intramyocardial pressure measured by a micropipette technique. *Am J Physiol* 249:H1216–H1223, 1985.
30. Hess DS, Bache RJ: Transmural distribution of myocardial blood flow during systole in the awake dog. *Circ Res* 38:5–10, 1976.
31. Hinshaw LB, Brake CM, Iampietro PF, Emerson TE: Effect of increased venous pressure on renal hemodynamics. *Am J Physiol* 204:119–123, 1963.
32. Hochrein M, Keller J, Mancke R: Die durchstromyung der koronararterien. *Arch Exp Path Pharmakol* 151:146–160, 1930.
33. Hoffman JIE: Determinanets and prediction of transmural myocardial perfusion. *Circulation* 58:381–391, 1978.
34. Holt JP: Collapse factor in the measurement of venous pressure: Flow of fluids through collapsible tubes. *Am J Physiol* 134:292–299, 1941.
35. Holt JP: Flow through collapsible tubes and through in situ veins. *IEEE Trans Biomed Eng* 16:274–283, 1969.
36. Johnson JR, DiPalma JR: Intramyocardial pressure and its relation to aortic pressure. *Am J Physiol* 125:234–243, 1939.
37. Kattus AA, Gregg DE: Some determinants of coronary collateral flow in the open-chest dog. *Circ Res* 7:628–642, 1959.
38. Katz SA, Feigl EO: Systole has little effect on diastolic coronary artery blood flow. *Circ Res* 62:443–451, 1988.
39. Kirk ES: Equivalence of retrograde blood flow and collateral flow following acute coronary occlusion in the dog. *Circulation* 52:66, 1980.
40. Kirk ES, Honig CR: Experimental and theoretical analysis of myocardial tissue pressure. *Am J Physiol* 207:261–267, 1964.
41. Kirkeeide R, Purshmann S, Schaper W: Diastolic coronary pressure flow relationship by induced long-wave pressure oscillations. *Basic Res Cardiol* 76:564–569, 1981.
42. Kjekshus JK: Mechanism for flow distribution in normal and ischemic myocardium during increased ventricular preload in the dog. *Circ Res* 33:489–499, 1973.
43. Klocke FJ, Weinstein IR, Ellis AK, Kraus DR, Mates RE, Canty JM, Anbar RD, Romanowski RR, Walllmeyer KW, Echt MP: Zero flow pressure and pressure flow relationships during long diastoles in the canine coronary bed before and during long diastoles in the canine coronary bed before and during maximal vasodilation. *Clin Invest* 68:970–980, 1981.
44. Krams R, Sipkema P, Westerhof N: Varying elastance concept may explain coronary systolic flow impediment. *Am J Physiol* 257:H1471–H1479, 1989.
45. Laszt VL, Muller A: Der myokardial druick. *Physiol Pharmacol Acta* 16:88–106, 1958.
46. Lee J, Chambers DE, Akizuki S, Downey JM: The role of vascular capacitance in the coronary arteries. *Circ Res* 55:751–762, 1984.
47. Marzilli M, Goldstein S, Sabbah HN, Lee TS, Stein P: Modulating effect of regional myocardial performance on local myocardial perfusion in the dog. *Circ Res* 45:634–640, 1979.
48. Messina LM, Hanley FL, Uhlig PH, Baer RW, Gratten MT, Hoffman JIE: Effects of pressure gradients between branches of the left coronary artery on the pressure axis intercept and the shape of the steady state circumflex pressure-flow relations in the dog. *Circ Res* 56:11–19, 1985.
49. Mirksy I: Left ventricular stresses in the intact human heart. *Biophy J* 9:189–208, 1969.
50. Moir TW: Subendocardial distribution of coronary blood flow and the effect of antiangial drugs. *Circ Res* 30:621–627, 1972.
51. Munch DF, Downey JM: Prediction of regional myocardial blood flow in dogs. *Am J Physiol* 239:H308–H315, 1980.
52. Permutt S, Brombergr-Barnea B, Bane HN: Alveolar pressure, pulmonary venous pressure and vascular waterfall. *Med Thorac* 19:239–260, 1962.
53. Permutt S, Riley RL: Hemodynamics of collapsible vessels with tone: Vascular waterfall. *J Appl Physiol* 18:924–932, 1963.
54. Porter WT: The influence of the heartbeat on the flow of blood through the walls of the heart. *Am J Physiol* 1:145–163, 1898.
55. Rebatel F: Recherches Experimentales sur la Circulation dans les Arteres Coronaires. *Paris, (quoted by Porter)*, 1872.
56. Reimer KA, Jennings RB: The wavefront phenomenon of myocardial ischemic cell death. II. Transmural progression of necrosis within the framework of ischemic bed size (myocardium at risk) and collateral flow. *Lab Invest* 40:633–640, 1979.
57. Resar L, Livingston JZ, Halperin HR, Sipkema P, Krams R, Yin FC: Effect of wall stretch on coronary hemodynamics in isolated canine interventricular septum. *Am J Physiol* 259:

H1869–H1880, 1990.

58. Russell RE, Chagrasulis RW, Downey JM: Inhibitory effect of cardiac contraction on coronary collateral blood flow. *Am J Physiol* 233:H541–H546, 1977.

59. Sabiston DC Jr, Gregg DE: Effect of cardiac contraction on coronary blood flow. *Circulation* 15:14–20, 1957.

60. Sarnoff SJ, Braunwald E, Welch GH, Case RB, Stainsby WE, Marcruz R: Hemodynamic determinants of oxygen consumption of the heart with special reference to the tension-time index. *Am J Physiol* 1⌃2:148–156, 1958.

61. Satoh S, Watanabe J, Keitoku M, Itoh N, Maruyama Y, Takishima T: Influences of pressure surrounding the heart and intracardiac pressure on the diastolic coronary pressure-flow relation in excised canine heart. *Circ Res* 63:788–797, 1988.

62. Scaramucci JB: Diario Parmense. *1687 (quoted by Porter)*, 1898.

63. Schaper W: Collateral Circulation of the Heart. *New York: Elsevier*, 1971.

64. Scheel KE, Rodriguez RJ, Ingram LA: Directional coronary collateral growth with chronic circumflex occlusion in the dog. *Circ Res* 40:384–390, 1977.

65. Snyder R, Downey JM, Kirk ES: The active and passive components of extravascular coronary resistance. *Cardiovasc Res* 9:161–166, 1975.

66. Spaan JAE: Interaction between contraction and coronary flow. In: *Coronary Blood Flow*. Boston: Kluwer, 1991, pp 163–192.

67. Spaan JAE: Coronary diastolic pressure-flow relation and zero flow pressure explained on the basis of intramyocardial compliance. *Circ Res* 56:293–309, 1985.

68. Spaan JAE, Breuls NPW, Laird JD: Diastolic-systolic coronary flow differences are caused by intramyocardial

pump action in the anesthetized dog. *Circ Res* 49:584–593, 1981.

69. Stein PD, Marzilli M, Sabbah HN, Lee T: Systolic and diastolic pressure gradients within the left ventricular wall. *Am J Physiol* 238:H625–H630, 1980.

70. Streeter D Jr, Spotnitz H, Patel D, Ross J Jr: Fiber orientation in the canine left ventricle during diastole and systole. *Circ Res* 21:65–74, 1969.

71. Swank M, Singh HM, Flemma FJ, Mullen DC, Lepley D: Effect of intraaortic balloon pumping on nutrient coronary flow in normal and ischemic myocardium. *Cardiovasc Surg* 76:538–544, 1978.

72. Trimble J, Downey JM: Contribution of myocardial contractility to myocardial perfusion. *Am J Physiol* 236:H121–H126, 1979.

73. Van Der Meer JJ, Reneman RS, Schneider H, Weibendink J: Technique for estimation of intramyocardial pressure in acute and chronic experiments. *Cardiovasc Res* 4:132–140, 1970.

74. Van Winkle DM, Swafford AN Jr, Downey JM: Subendocardial compression in beating dog hearts is independent of pressure in the ventricular lumen. *Am J Physiol* 261:H500–H505, 1991.

75. Wiggers CJ: The interplay of coronary vascular resistance and myocardial compression in regulating coronary flow. *Circ Res* 2:271–279, 1954.

76. Wiggers CJ, Cotton FS: Studies on the coronary circultion. *Am J Physiol* 106:597–610, 1933.

77. Wyatt D, Lee J, Downey JM: Determination of collateral flow by a load line analysis. *Circ Res* 50:663–670, 1982.

78. Yoshida S, Akizuki S, Gowski D, Downey JM: Discrepancy between microsphere and diffusable tracer estimates of perfusion to ischemic myocardium. *Am J Physiol* 249:H255–H264, 1985.

CHAPTER 59

Myocardial Infarction

TETSUJI MIURA

MYOCARDIAL INFARCTION IN HUMANS

Myocardial infarction refers to the death of myocardium in a region of the heart in which blood flow is insufficient to sustain cell viability. The underlying pathology of acute myocardial infarction in humans most commonly is due to atherosclerotic stenosis of the coronary arteries. The exact process by which the coronary blood flow is interrupted, however, is still unclear. Although thrombous formation over the coronary stenosis appears a final common mechanism of the blood flow interruption, the sequence of events leading to the thrombotic occlusion has not been completely understood. Coronary thrombi, especially those overlying ruptured plaque, are frequently found in autopsies of transmural infarctions {1}. Recent angiographic studies demonstrated that there is an occluding coronary thrombosis in approximately 90% of patients with acute transmural myocardial infarction at the earliest hours following the onset of symptoms, and the angiographic morphology of the infarct-related coronary artery suggests rupture of atheromatous plaques in most cases {2}. Another aspect of this problem is that coronary spasm commonly occurs just distal to a fixed obstructive lesion {3}. The pathological explanation of this finding may be that the tunica media of the mildly sclerotic artery remains normal or even hypertrophic {4,5}, while the severely sclerotic artery has an atrophic tunica media {4,6}. Platelets aggregating over the coronary stenosis may contribute to the coronary spasm by releasing thromboxane A2 and other vasoconstricting substances {7}. Therefore, the exact sequence of events that bring about a rapid coronary obstruction remains unresolved. Regardless of the sequence of events, clinical experience of the last decade reveals that perfusion can be restored in a large number of these patients by early intervention with thrombolytic agents.

The clinical manifestation of a myocardial infarction is variable and depends on the extent and the location of myocardial necrosis, and on the presence or absence of concurrent diseases such as diabetes mellitus. Most commonly, symptoms start with anterior chest pain or tightness of sudden onset, which is thought to be mediated by nerve endings in ischemic, but not necrotic, myocardium {8}. When a large portion of the myocardium becomes ischemic, or when advanced AV block occurs due to ischemia of the conduction system, symptoms of acute left ventricular failure predominate. Nausea and vomiting, presumably a vagal reflex, and Wenckebach-type second-degree AV block are commonly observed in patients with inferior infarction. Myocardial infarction can even be painless, particularly in patients with diabetes mellitus, and approximately 25% of nonfatal myocardial infarctions are unrecognized by the patient and are discovered only on subsequent unrelated ECG recordings or autopsies {9,10}.

Another important clinical feature of acute myocardial infarction is circadian periodicity in the incidence. The recent MILIS study {11} demonstrated that both myocardial infarction and transient myocardial ischemic events have a circadian peak of onset at about 9 a.m. This phenomenon is not well explained, but might be related to circadian rhythm of the endocrine systems, such as elevation of plasma catecholamines and cortisol in the morning. Nevertheless, this phenomenon also alludes complexity in the process leading to complete occlusion of coronary artery by thrombus.

NATURAL HISTORY OF INFARCTION

Spatial frame of infarction — Myocardium at risk

Interarterial connections in the coronary system occur almost exclusively at the large vessel level and in the dog can easily be seen between the epicardial arteries {12}. Capillaries from adjacent arterial branches have been shown to form end-capillary loops at the interface between the two perfusion fields without any apparent anastomoses {13}. Based on this anatomy, acute occlusion of a coronary artery actually results in a sharp border between the ischemic tissue surrounding it. This sharp border has been demonstrated as an abrupt transition of regional blood flow {14}, metabolites such as creatine phosphate and ATP {15}, and NADH fluorescence {16}. Overlap between adjacent branches was recently examined with the diffusible tracer ^{133}Xe, and it was revealed that less than 3% of the field of the anterior descending artery of the dog's heart communicates with the other branches {17}.

N. Sperelakis (ed.), Physiology and Pathophysiology of the Heart, Third Edition.

When a coronary artery is occluded in an experimental setting, the infarction will develop only within the field of the occluded artery, and none of the adjacent well-perfused tissue will be involved. The field of the occluded coronary artery is, therefore, often called the *region at risk* {18}. The concept of the region at risk is useful in studies that try to quantitate infarct size, since infarct size is often expressed as a percentage of the region at risk of infarction. Unfortunately, some confusion exists as to how to actually measure the field of the occluded artery. One authority has attempted to differentiate such measurements into two categories: those that yield an anatomic region at risk and those yielding a physiologic region at risk {19}. An anatomic region at risk would be marked by postmortem methods involving either barium angiography {20} or simultaneous infusion of different colored dyes down adjacent coronary branches {18}. Both simultaneously delineate the tissue served by each coronary branch. On the other hand, a physiologic region at risk is visualized by injection of a blood-flow tracer in vivo, such as microsphere autoradiography {21,22} or dye injection {23}. These methods would take the effect of collateral flow into account and define the region with an actual flow deficit under coronary occlusion. Differences between the two techniques would result from collateral contributions in the latter method. Whether these two regions are actually different or not depends on whether the coronary collateral vessels only interconnect the large arterial branches. If that is truly the case, then anatomic and physiologic regions at risk should be one and the same. In fact, when the region at risk was measured by microsphere autoradiography and by postmortem double-dye infusion in the same dog heart, the sizes of the two regions were

essentially identical {24}. While the dog heart is known to have well-developed collateral channels {12}, many species, such as the rabbit, the pig {16}, and the baboon {25}, have very sparse collateral connections. Significant differences between anatomic and physiologic regions at risk should be even less likely in those species, although it has not been investigated.

The size of the infarct is linearly related to the size of the region at risk in the setting of experimental coronary artery occlusion {26}, as is shown in fig. 59-1. Although virtually all studies have observed such a linearly {18,20, 26,27}, there are inconsistent findings concerning the zero-infact intercept for this relationship in the dog heart. Several studies using a conscious dog model reported that no infarction would occur when the region at risk was less than 20% of left ventricular mass {26,28}. On the other hand, other studies, such as the one shown in fig. 59-1 {26,29,30}, have failed to find a significant zero-infarct intercept. The reason for this discrepancy remains unclear. Anesthetic agents or methods used to mark the region at risk (barium gelatin angiogram, postmortem double-dye infusion, radiomicrosphere autoradiogram) do not seem to explain the difference in the literature {18,20,28,29,31,32}.

The existence (or absence) of zero-infarct intercept in a certain model of infarcts is an important issue when we assess the effects of cardioprotective drugs on infarct size. If there actually is not a significant zero-infarct intercept, then the percentage of the risk zone that infarcted would be independent of the size of the region at risk. That would greatly simplify the quantitation of infarct size and alteration of infarct size by drugs. On the other hand, if the model has a significant zero-infarct intercept, it must be analyzed for critical assessment of the drugs' effect,

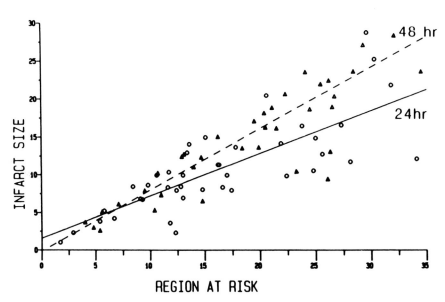

Fig. 59-1. Relationship between the size of the region at risk and the size of the infarct after 48 hours of coronary occlusion. The region at risk and infarct were visualized by radiomicrosphere autoradiography and triphenyltetrazolium staining, respectively. Reprinted from Miura et al. {26}, with permission.

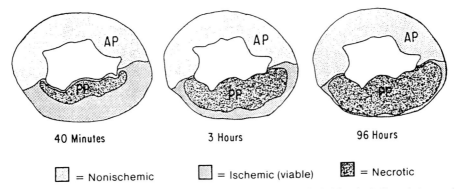

Fig. 59-2. Progression of myocardial infarction after the left circumflex artery was occluded for the indicated time period. In the left two panels the heart was reperfused for 96 hours, and the right panel depicts a permanent occlusion. Infarction, therefore, moves as a wavefront from the endocardium across the wall toward the epicardium. PP = posterior papillary muscle. Reprinted from Reimer and Jennings {18}, with permission.

whether the drugs indeed alter the infarct size-risk region relationship. This author suspect that lack of this caution regarding infarct analysis may be responsible for some of the discrepancy regarding infarct size alteration by several drugs in the literature.

Time frame of infarction — Wavefront phenomenon

Reimer and Jennings {18,33} demonstrated in the canine model that myocardial necrosis following coronary occlusion begins at the endocardium and then progresses across the wall toward the epicardium. They termed this the *wavefront of infarction*. A coronary branch was temporarily occluded in their model and then reperfused for 4 days. Twenty-eight percent of the region at risk infarcted after 40 minutes of infarction, 70% after 3 hours of occlusion, 72% after 6 hours of occlusion, and 79% with a permanent occlusion, as shown in fig. 59-2. Therefore, the wavefront of infarction is complete between 3 and 6 hours after coronary occlusion. A similar wavefront phenomenon is observed in the rabbit heart as well {34}, although the infarct in this species first appears in the midmyocardium and progress towards both subendocardial and subepicardial myocardium. This slight difference in the wavefront phenomenon in the rabbit is presumably due to larger contribution of intraluminal oxygen diffusion in thinner ventricles of this species than in the thick ventricle of the dog heart {34}. The extent to which this wavefront extends appears to be dependent on collateral blood flow, myocardial oxygen consumption, and perhaps other factors, will be discussed below.

Why does the infarction always begin at the subendocardium in the dog heart? Three possible mechanisms that could explain the subendocardium's proclivity for infarction have been considered. These include (a) reduced collateral flow in that region, (b) increased metabolic demand in that region, and (c) an abnormally low ischemic tolerance in that region. In the dog, collateral channels supply the region at risk with about 20% of its preocclusion blood flow. This flow is very nonuniformly distributed

across the ventricular wall and favors the subepicardial regions. Radiomicrospheres reveal that the subendocardium receives only about one third to one half of subepicardial blood flow in the region at risk {15,35}. This transmural gradient of collateral blood flow is the result of extravascular compression of the coronary vessels by the contracting heart {35}. For a more detailed discussion of this phenomenon, the reader is referred to Chapter 58 of this book.

Several investigators {36,37} have tried to measure tissue P_{O_2} as an estimate of the rate of oxygen consumption across the heart wall. Since blood flow has been shown to be uniformly distributed across the heart wall {38}, it was assumed that regions with an elevated oxygen consumption should exhibit a lower venous, and hence tissue, P_{O_2}. Myocardial P_{O_2} values measured by platinum polarographic electrodes inserted into the myocardium are in the range of 10–15 mmHg in the subendocardium and 20–25 mmHg in the subepicardium {36,37}. Although this difference appears small, it could have a profound effect on oxygen extraction, because these values are on the steep portion of the hemoglobin dissociation curve. Gamble et al. confirmed a reduced subendocardial P_{O_2} by a microoximetry technique {39}. In their method, cardiac tissue is rapidly frozen, and a thin slice of the frozen tissue is viewed under a microscope, a small vein identified, and the hemoglobin content in the red cells in the vein are measured by a monochrometer and detector in the microscope. Weiss et al. employed both microoximetry and regional blood flow measurement by radiomicrospheres and reported that the endocardial to epicardial oxygen consumption ratio was 1.3:1 {40}. In the study by Holtz et al. {41}, using a similar method, the ratio was 1.6:1. A significantly higher rate of oxygen utilization for the subendocardium appears to be firmly established.

Dunn and Griggs {42} demonstrated a greater metabolic activity in the ischemic subendocardium by a different approach. They occluded the entire coronary circulation, producing total ischemia, and after a short time they rapidly froze the heart and measured the regional distribution of lactate. The concentration of lactate was much higher in the subendocardium than the subepicardium. In this case the gradient could not have been the result of a blood flow gradient because coronary flow was completely eliminated. These regional differences in lactate were not observed when the experiment was repeated in a nonworking (fibrillating) heart, suggesting that the elevated metabolism of the subendocardial fibers probably reflects an elevated workload for the fibers in that region during contraction {43}.

Does the subendocardium have a lower tolerance for ischemia? This possibility was suggested by Lowe et al. {44}. They incubated slices of ventricle in vitro so that both blood flow and workload were zero in all regions. Nevertheless, ATP was still depleted more rapidly in the subendocardium. Aslo, ultrastructural changes associated with cell death were first seen in the subendocardium. Thus evidence for all three theories is convincing, and it is indeed likely that the proclivity for infarction at the subendocardium is multifactorial.

The wavefront phenomenon occurs in human heart as well. The study by Lee et al. {45} measured the infarct and the region at risk in autopsy specemens of acute myocardial infarction (3- to 16-day-old infarcts). The infarcts that ranged from 50% to 88% of the region at risk were subepicardial, which was very similar to the canine model. The actual rate at which the wavefront phenomenon progresses in the human heart is still an unanswered question.

Influence of collateral blood flow

The region at risk in the dog heart receives a residual blood flow of about 20% of the preocclusion flow. It is now established that collateral blood flow is the primary determinant of the percentage of the region at risk that will infarct {26,31}. Figure 59-3 illustrates the relationship between the normalized collateral flow to the ischemic subepicardium and the percentage of the region at risk that infarcted. A correlation coefficient of -0.9 indicates that about 80% of the variations in the extent to which the region at risk infarcted in this population can be attributed to variation in collateral flow. Open symbols are data from the authors' study {26} and closed symbols are from a study by Reimer and Jennings {18}. In spite of wide differences in methodology between the two studies, the relationship between the extent of infarction and the collateral blood flow was remarkably reproducible. What is also remarkable about fig. 59-3 is the wide range of collateral flows seen in the dog population. This variability creates a similar variability in the extent to which the region at risk infarcts.

Collateral flow in fig. 59-3 was normalized by dividing the absolute residual flow (proportional to oxygen supply) by the flow to the nonischemic region (proportional to oxygen demand) and multiplying by 100. We found that the correlation coefficient using the normalized collateral flow was significantly higher than that obtained when the absolute collateral flow was used {26,46}. There is a

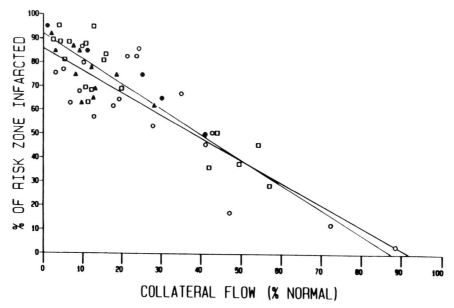

Fig. 59-3. The relationship between collateral blood flow to the ischemic subepicardium and percentage of the region at risk infarcted. Open circles and open squares represent dogs experiencing 24- and 48-hour coronary occlusion, respectively. The regression lines for these groups were not significantly different. Closed symbols represent experiments by Reimer and Jennings {48}. The triangles represent animals experiencing 96 hours of permanent coronary occlusion, while circles represent those reperfused at 6 hours. Reprinted from Miura et al. {26}, with permission.

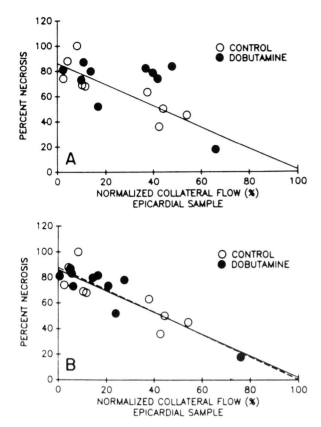

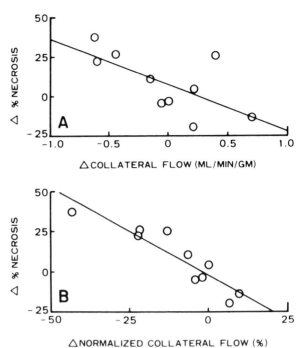

Fig. 59-4. The effect of dobutamine infusion on infarct size in the permanent coronary occlusion model. The **A:** Percentage of risk region infarcted versus collateral flow just before the dobutamine infusion (solid circle). **B:** The same infarct size data are plotted using the collateral flow during the dobutamine infusion. Solid lines are regression lines for control data (open circles). When collateral flow before dobutamine infusion was used (A), the relationship between percent necrosis and collateral flow was not significant. However, when collateral flow during dobutamine infusion was used (B), the relationship became highly significant and the regression line from the dobutamine group (dotted line) was virtually superimposed on the control regression line. Reprinted from Miura et al. {46}, with permission.

Fig. 59-5. Relationship between the modification of infarct size by dobutamine and the change in collateral flow induced by dobutamine. The percentage of risk zone, which would have infarcted in absence of dobutamine, was calculated by inserting collateral flow before dobutamine into the control regression equation. **A:** The difference between the actual and predicted infarct size is significantly correlated with the change in collateral flow induced by dobutamine infusion (r = −0.67). **B:** The correlation became better when normalized collateral flow was used (r = −0.92). Reprinted from Miura et al. {46}, with permission.

theoretical basis for this normalization procedure. The severity of ischemic injury has been thought to reflect the balance between oxygen supply and the demand for oxygen in the myocardium. Therefore, fig. 59-3 can be interpreted in the light of the coronary supply-demand ratio. The fact that better fit was achieved when both demand and supply were taken into account indicates that infarct size is influenced by oxygen demand as well. Although this many seem obvious a priori, the reader should be reminded that although tension development is the primary determinant of oxygen consumption in well-perfused myocardium {47}, ischemic myocardium is noncontractile.

In a recent study from this laboratory {46}, both collateral flow and oxygen demand were modified by do-butamine infusion begun shortly after coronary artery occlusion (fig. 59-4). The extent of infarction correlated poorly with collateral-flow measurements made just prior to drug infusion (Upper panel of fig. 59-4), but the relationship between the extent of infarction and collateral flow was identical to the control data when the collateral flow measured during dobutamine infusion was employed (lower panel of fig. 59-4). Furthermore, change in collateral blood flow induced by dobutamine correlated tightly with alteration of infarct size, which was calculated as the difference between actual infarct size and the size predicted from the collateral flow before dobutamine infusion (fig. 59-5). These findings indicate that the infarct size-collateral flow relationship shown in fig. 59-3 holds in each dog heart.

This linear relationship between collateral flow and infarct size is observed in a reperfusion setting as well. Early reperfusion simply has the effect of shifting the line in a parallel fashion downward {48,49}.

How much collateral flow is necessary for maintaining the myocardial viability? This flow value cannot be directly determined in vivo, but indirect estimation was possible in

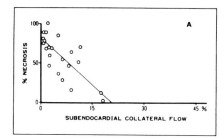 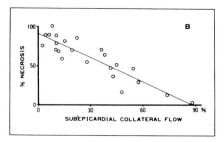

Fig. 59-6. The relationship between percentage of risk region infarcted and collateral blood flow. Collateral flow was measured by radiomicrospheres at 2–8 minutes after coronary occlusion, and infarct size was determined by tetrazolium staining at 24 or 48 hours of ischemia. **A:** Percent infarction versus subendocardial collateral blood flow; y = 81.15 − 3.96x, r = −0.77, p < 0.01. The zero infarct intercept was 20.5%, and the 95% confidence interval was between 10.4% and 37.5%. **B:** Percent infarct versus subepicardial collateral blood flow; y = 90.23 − 1.03x, r = −9.0, p < 0.01. Reprinted from Miura and Downey {50}, with permission.

the dog heart. Figure 59-6 shows the relationship between subendocardial or subepicardial collateral blood flow and infarct size {50}. Because there is a transmural gradient of collateral flow in the ischemic region away from the sub-endcardium, the X-intercept of the regression line in panel A of fig. 59-6 represents the critical flow for the salvage of ischemic myocardium at the most vulnerable site of infarction {50}. This intercept was 20.5% (95% confidence interval was between 10.4% and 37.5%). Unfortunately, the critical flow of 20.5% (of nonischemic region flow) does not necessarily mean that the ischemic myocytes can survive for days with this level, but it may rather be a minimum level for viability during early hours following coronary artery occlusion. Collateral blood flow is known to increase during the first hours after coronary occlusion {51,52}, and such an increase in the collateral flow is more marked in the tissue that has survived 24 hours later {53}.

It was mentioned above that some investigators find that the extent to which the region at risk infarcts varies with the size of the risk zone. That, of course, would be expected if the residual flow to the ischemic region was related to the size of the field of the occluded artery. Jugdutt et al. {20} reported an inverse relationship between the size of the region at risk and the collateral blood flow in dogs. Reimer et al. {54} measured the collateral blood flow in small and large ischemic zones on the same hearts. They found that collateral blood flow to the smaller ischemic zone was consistently higher than that in the corresponding large ischemic zone. When data from all dogs were pooled, however, the correlation between ischemic-zone size and collateral flow was not significant. We have confirmed the observation of Reimer et al. by using the ^{133}Xe washout technique for collateral flow determination {55}. Collateral blood flow seems to be inversely related to ischemic zone size in any given dog heart, but this relationship is masked by a large individual variation of collateral development in the canine population at large.

Myocardial oxygen consumption

The exact role of myocardial oxygen consumption as a determinant of infarct size is still not well defined. Muller

et al. have claimed that cardiac workload at the time of coronary occlusion is an important determinant of infarct size {56}. Using anesthetized dogs, they occluded two coronary branches on the same heart, one after another, followed by 90 minutes of reperfusion so that two infarcts were compared in each heart {56}. Oxygen demand, estimated from ventricular hemodynamics, was modified by dobutamine infusion and pacing during the second occlusion. A higher extent of infarction occurred in oc-clusions with increased oxygen demand. When oxygen demand was changed 45 minutes after occlusion, however, the infarct size was not modified in that model {57}. Contrary, the AMPIM study {31} reported that no sig-nificant correlation was found between rate-pressure product, an index of myocardial oxygen consumption, and infarct size in anesthetized canine models, although modest, but significant correlation was detected in con-scious dog models having lower rate-pressure products. Rate-pressure products at the time of coronary occlusion were not a determinant of infarct size in our rabbit model was well, which received coronary occlusion under anesthesia and then recovered from anesthesia after reper-fusion {58}. There is no clear explanation available for the different results between the study by Muller et al. {56}, the AMPIM study {31}, and ours {58}.

Latency of the transition from reversible to irreversible ischemic myocardial injury

It has been well known that there is transition from reversible ischemic myocardial injury to irreversible injury (i.e., myocardial cell death), but the timing of that tran-sition remains unclear. To get some insight into this issue, we analyzed the relationship between infarct size and the duration of ischemia in the rabbit heart. The rabbit was chosen as a model because coronary collaterals are poorly developed and supply less than 5% of normal flow in this species {34}. If the dog heart were used, large individual variation of collateral blood flow would have obscured the relationship between infarct size and ischemia duration. As shown in fig. 59-7, a "dose-response"-like relationship was observed between the ischemia duration and the per-centage of area at risk infarcted. Probit analysis of this

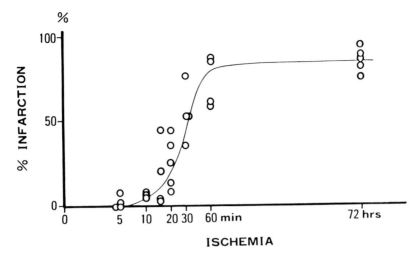

Fig. 59-7. Relationship between percentage of risk region infarcted and the duration of ischemia (log scale). Reprinted from Miura et al. {34}, with permission.

relationship predicted that 50% of myocardial cells are killed after 34 minutes of ischemia in this species. A very similar infarct size-ischemia duration relationship was reported in the pig heart {59}, which also lacks developed collaterals, but has a thicker ventricle and slower heart rate than in the rabbit. Therefore, the transition from reversible to irreversible myocyte injury may occur in the pig heart after about 40 minutes.

Histology and ultrastructure of infarction

Because the morphology of ischemic myocardium is markedly different between reperfused myocardium and that without reperfusion, it is convenient to consider these two conditions separately.

NONREPERFUSED INFARCTION

Under the electron microscope, morphological changes can be observed as early 15 minutes after ischemia. Those changes include disappearance of the mitochondrial dark granules with a more electron-lucent appearance in the matrix, destruction of mitochondrial cristae, swelling of nuclei with clumping and margination of chromatin, the appearance of numerous large amorphous densities in the mitchondria, and disruption of the sarcolemma {60,61}. The breaks in the sarcolemma are usually associated with subsarcolemmal blebs, and their appearance temporarily correlates with disappearance of vinculin, which is a component of the cytoskeletal attachment complex linking the sarcolemma and the Z-line of underlying myofibrills {62}. The degradation of the vinculin may be resonsible for fragility of the ischemic myocytes, allowing disruption of the sarcolemma as a consequence of cell swelling, Nevertheless, disruption of the sarcolemma and the amorphous densities in the mitochondria are believed to be diagnostic of irreversible ischmic injury {60,61}. Even

when these ultrastructural changes are fully developed, light microscopy can be unremarkable.

The role of myocardial lysosomes in infarction remains unclear. Lysosomes are morphologically intact during the first hour of ischemia {62}. However, some of the lysosomal enzymes are detectable in the nonsedimentable fraction of tissue homogenates as early as 15 minutes after the onset of ischemia {63}. Whether the close temporal relation of lysosomal enzyme release and disruption of the mitochondria or sarcolemmal changes mentioned above represent a cause-and-effect relationship remains unknown.

The microvasculature is also damaged after coronary occlusion, and after a certain period of ischemia, blood flow fails to recover in some regions. This has been termed the *no-reflow phenomenon* {64}. Whether microvascular injury precedes the myocyte damage is an interesting and obviously important question. Kloner et al. {65} examined the ultrastructural changes in the microvasculature and myocytes after 20–180 minutes of coronary occlusion. Myocyte damage was apparent after 20–40 minutes of ischemia, while microvascular injury, such as swollen endothelium with red-cell stasis, reduced pinocytotic vesicles, and endothelial blebs were not prominent until 60–90 minutes after coronary occlusion. Biopsies from the no-reflow region also revealed severe ultrastructural damage in the myocytes {64}. These findings suggest that myocyte destruction precedes structural destruction of the microvasculature. Tillmans and Kubler {66}, using an in-vivo microscopic technique, observed that after 15–20 minutes of ischemia capillary branches became plugged with red cells and leukocytes, while the capillaries downstream could be filled with fluorescent dextran, suggesting persistent plasma flow. Therefore, functional disturbances of microvasculature may well precede the structural changes and contribute to myocardial cell death, especially in situations where the primary obstruction is temporary, e.g., coronary spasm or spontaneous recanalization.

Under the light microscope, hematoxylin-eosin-stained histology reveals an increase in eosinophilia or hyper-eosinophilia of myocytes (coagulative necrosis). The most significant findings with infarction are granularity and disorganization of myofibrils, and separation of muscle fibers due to intercellular edema. Such changes may be noted in the center of the infarct as early as 2 hours postocclusion {67}, but the whole infarcted area will not be delineated until 12–24 hours postocclusion. The mechanism that produces coagulative necrosis is poorly understood. A hypothesis is that the proteins are somehow rendered insoluble by the ischemic process — much as proteins are coagulated by heat or formaldehyde. This would delay proteolysis by lysosomal enzymes and thus preserve the dense eosinophilic coagulate for several days {68}. These coagulated cells are eventually either liquefied by proteases or removed by fragmentation and phagocytosis by invading leukocytes.

In the nonreperfused setting, neutrophils are not observed within the infarct in the first several hours of coronary occlusion {67}. By 24–48 hours, neutrophils infiltrate deep into the infarct, and an acute inflammatory reaction predominates over the following 4–7 days. As for this neutrophil chemotaxis in the infarcted myocardium, activation of the complement system appears to play an important role, as in other inflammatory reactions. Earlier studies identified fixation of complements (Clq, C3, C5) in the infarcted region by using histochemical methods {69,70} and radiolabeled Clq {71}. Furthermore, Rossen et al. {72} found that exogenous Clq injected into the peripheral vein appeared in cardiac lymph in appreciable amounts and that there is a approximately 31,000-Da protein in myocardial mitochondria, which can react with Clq. Based on these findings, they have proposed that the 31,000-Dal proteins (and possibly other subcelluar constituents) are released from the myocytes during ischemia, bind with Clq in extracellular space, and activate complement cascade in infarcting myocardium {72}.

The infiltration of neutrophils is followed by an increased infiltration of lymphocytes and macrophages, which often contain lipofuscin pigments associated with scar formation. These progress from the periphery of the infarct toward the center. This chronic inflammatory reaction gradually subsides around the 14th day. Fibrosis follows and is generally complete within 6–8 weeks {73}.

REPERFUSED INFARCTS

Three major morphological differences are apparent between reperfused and nonreperfused infarcts. These include the rate of myocardial destruction, the formation of contraction bands, and the presence of intramyocardial hemorrhage. In myocardium that has suffered a severe ischemic insult, reperfusion causes very rapid changes in the ultrastructure, including massive swelling of the myocytes, sarcolemmal blebs, vacuolization within the myocytes, destruction of mitochondria, and the appearance of contraction bands {61,62,74,75}. In a study by Whalen et al. {76}, cell water increased by 21% during the first 2

minutes of reperfusion following a 40-minute ischemic insult. However, lysosomes appear to still be intact even after 20 minutes of reperfusion {75}.

The destruction of the myocardium is so rapid and complete with reperfusion that degenerative changes, including diffuse granularity, disorganization of the myofibrils, and contraction bands, can be noted by light microscopy 20 minutes following reperfusion. Yet, virtually no pathological findings can be detected after 60 minutes of continuous ischemia without reperfusion {67}. Contraction-band necrosis is characteristic of both reperfused myocardium and the calcium-paradox phenomenon {77}. For that reason, the contraction band has been believed to be associated with a massive influx of calcium, which probably enters either by structural defects in the sarcolemma or an increase in its permeability {78}. Recently, Vander Heide et al. {79} indicated that ATP generation by mitochondria is important in the formation of contraction bands. They found that contraction band formation in calcium paradox was significantly reduced when the heart was pretreated with amytal, a mitochondria inhibitor, or potassium cyanide. Whether mitochondria play the same role in contraction band formation due to ischemia/reperfusion remains unclear.

Massive intramyocardial hemorrhage is another feature of reperfused infarcts. This phenomenon has also been observed in autopsied human hearts that have received coronary thrombolytic therapy {80}. Fishbein et al. {81} reperfused the coronary artery for 30 minutes after 5.5 hours of occlusion in the dog. The area of vascular injury estimated by extravasation of colloidal carbon was consistently smaller than the area of infarction, and intramyocardial hemorrhage always was confined to the subendocardial necrotized region. In a study by Roberts et al. {82}, the presence of myocardial hemorrhage in hearts reperfused after 4 hours of coronary occlusion did not affect late collagen formation estimated as hydroxproline content. Thus hemorrhage may not be a particularly deleterious event in the infarcting heart.

While nonreperfused infarcts are only slowly invaded by neutrophils, reperfused infarcts exhibit margination of neutrophils along the blood vessels as early as 20 minutes after reperfusion, and extravascular neutrophils were noted in infarcting tissue at 50 minutes postreperfusion {67}. As for this accelerated neutrophil infiltration, two mechanisms appear important. First, hyperemia following the onset of reperfusion would supply large numbers of neutrohils to the reperfused region. Secondly, reperfusion washes out tissue adenosine, which may facilitate free radical production of neutrophils. Free radical production in neutrophils are under inhibitory control of the adenosine A2 receptors {83}. Accordingly, washout of adenosine from reperfused regions would allow neutrophils to generate free radicals, which per se are chemotactic {84}, resulting in further recruitment of neutrophils.

Infarct healing is also modified by reperfusion. Recently, we found that the proportion of organized infarct is a function of time and also infarct size in both nonreperfused and reperfused infarcts in the rabbit, as shown in fig. 59-8 {85}. What is remarkable about fig. 59-8 is that

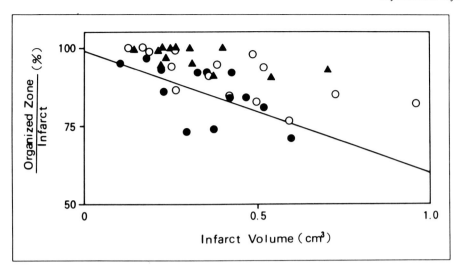

Fig. 59-8. Relationship between the ratio of organized to total infarct (%O/I) at 7 days after ischemia and the absolute size of the myocardial infarct. Closed circles: nonreperfused infarcts, y = 99.3 − 38.9x, r = −0.61. Open circles: 60 minutes ischemia/ reperfused infarcts, y = 100.8 − 23.7x, r = − 0.70. Closed triangles: 30 minutes ischemia/repefused infarcts, y = 101.5 − 15.0x, r = −0.63; all p < 0.05. The relationships between infarct size and %O/I in the 60-minute ischemia/reperfusion and the 30-min ischemia/reperfusion groups were shifted significantly upward compared with those with nonreperfused infarcts (p < 0.05, analysis of covariance). The solid line represents the regression line for the nonreperfused infarcts. Reprinted from Miura et al. {85}, with permission.

the relationship between infarct size and the percentage of infarct healed was significantly shifted upwards in reperfused infarcts, indicating acceleration of healing by reperfusion. Furthermore, this effect was observed even when reperfusion was done too late to significantly limit infarct size {85}. Rapid tissue destruction of necrotic tissues, earlier infiltration of neutrophils, and more supply of humoral factors important for tissue healing (such as plasma fibronectin) might be important in accelerating infarct repair following reperfusion.

BIOCHEMICAL EVENTS IN INFARCTION TISSUE

It is still not known exactly which biochemical event kills the ischemic myocyte. Once a coronary artery is occluded, numerous biochemical changes occur in many aspects of the heart's metabolism. These changes are still poorly understood, but attention has been focused on several specific metabolic species, including the high-energy phosphates, intracellular calcium, phospholipase, long-chain acyl CoA, long-chain acyl carnitine, and free radicals. Their role in ischemia will be discussed below.

High-energy phosphates and purines

The myocardial level of high-energy phosphates, i.e., ATP, ADP, and creatine phosphate (CP), declines following coronary occlusion, since the production of ATP is suppressed by the lack of oxygen. Within a minute of the onset of ischemia, anaerobic glycolysis becomes the

predominant pathway for ATP production. However, as the duration of ischemia is prolonged, anaerobic glycolysis per se is supressed. Glyceraldehyde phosphate dehydrogenase, a key enzyme of glycolysis, is inhibited by NADH and proton accumulated in the sarcoplasm {86,87}. Glycolysis is suppressed also at the level of fructose-6-phosphate (F-6-P), since phosphorylation of F-6-P to fructose-1,6-diphosphate requires ATP and cell acidosis inhibits phosphofructokinase {86}.

Not only ATP production, but also the major pathways of ATP consumption, are also altered during myocardial ischemia. The rate at which high-energy phosphates are degraded is dependent on myocardial oxygen consumption {88,89}, and rapid arrest of the contraction after ischemia preserves myocardial ATP levels {90}. Thus significant loss of ATP during the initial seconds of ischemia is probably explained by myosin ATPase. In addition to myosin ATPase of the myofibrills, there are a number of ATPases that would consume ATP until ATP levels fall below a certain level: Na,K-ATPase of sarcolemma, Ca^{2+}-ATPases of sarcoplasmic reticulum, and mitochondrial ATPase. Recent studies indicates that mitochondrial ATPase is a major pathway for ATP breakdown during ischemia {91,92}. The mitochondrial ATPase activity derives from the ATP synthetase, which generates ATP during oxidative phosphorylation. When the proton gradient across the mitochondrial membranes is lost, however, this enzyme catalyzes the reverse reaction and breaks down ATP to ADP and inorganic phosphate. Inhibition of the mitochondrial ATPase by oligomycin significantly slows down ATP degradation during ischemia

{91,92}, indicating this ATPase is indeed responsible for the ischemia-induced ATP depletion.

Not only high-energy phosphates, but also the total adenine nucleotide pool (AMP + ADP + ATP), also declines during ischemia {88}. Their degradation products — adenosine, inosine, hypoxanthine, and xanthine — accumulate in the ischemic myocardium, with inosine being the major product. There are two known pathways for AMP to inosine. The major pathway is the hydoxylation of AMP by 5'-nucleotidase to adenosine, which is then deaminated by adenosine deaminase to inosine {93}. There are two isozymes of 5'-nucleotidase i.e., membrane-associated 5'-nucleotidase (ecto) and intracellular 5'-nucleotidase {94,95}. Which of these isozymes has the major role in adenosine production in ischemic myocardium is still controversial {93,95}. Adenosine can pass through the sarcolemma and is taken up by a variety of cell types, regardless of their degree of ATP depletion {96,97}. Adenosine deaminase is present in endothelial cells as well as in cardiac myocytes {38,98}. Thus both the adenosine in myocytes and that taken up in the endothelial cells are possible sources of inosine in ischemic myocardium.

Another pathway from AMP to inosine is via deamination of AMP by AMP deaminase to IMP, which is then hydroxylated to inosine by 5'-nucleotidase. This pathway appears to be minor in myocardium, but predominates in ischemic skeletal muscle {99}. Inosine in the endothelial cell would be degraded by purine phosphorylase to hypoxanthine {100}, which would be oxidized to xanthine by xanthine oxidase {101}.

Whether ATP depletion in ischemic myocardium is the primary cause of cell death is unanswered. Many important cellular functions such as the sarcolemma's Na-K pump, the sarcoplasmic reticulum's Ca pump, and the myofibrillar sliding-filament system are all ATP-dependent processes. Obviously, many vital functions would be severely curtailed if the myocyte's ATP were depleted. Circumstantial evidence suggests that cell death occurs when ATP falls below a critical level. For example, an inverse relationship has been demonstrated between ATP content and the amount of necrosis in ischemic myocardium {102}. The degree of functional recovery from global ischemia and the tissue content of ATP are also correlated {103}. However, the quantitative relationship between ATP and cell viability is difficult to elucidate, because ischemic tissue samples are heterogeneous and quantitation of cell viability in a biopsy is difficult. Both Reimer et al. {89} and Schaper et al. {61} have suggested that 20–40% of the control level may be the minimal amount of ATP required to sustain cell viability. Jennings et al. reported that ATP in late, but still reversibly injured, ischemic myocardium was about 2.0 μM/g wet weight, which was about 40% of ATP in the nonischemic myocardium {104}.

Calcium metabolism

An uncontrolled rise of cytosolic calcium has been hypothesized to be a primary cause of cell death, not only in ischemic injury, but in other forms of cellular injury as well {105,106}. ATP depletion during oxygen deprivation will disturb Ca^{2+} levels because intracellular Ca^{2+} is maintained by many ATP-dependent mechanisms. These include Ca-ATPases in the sarcolemma and the sarcoplasmic reticulum and the mitochondrial Ca pump. As a result, sarcoplasmic Ca^{2+} level would rise. This assumption has been difficult to prove because of methodological difficulty in measurement of intracellular Ca^{2+} level. However, an intensive effort over the last decade has provided evidence that the sarcoplasmic Ca^{2+} level indeed is significantly elevated during myocardial ischemia. In a study by Steenbergen et al. {107} using nuclear magnetic resonance (NMR) and the magnetic resonance probe, 5F-BAPTA, a time-averaged intracellular Ca^{2+} level was estimated as being approximately 540 nM under control condition in beating isolated rat hearts. The Ca^{2+} level was elevated up to 3 μM after 15 minutes of ischemia. A similar observation using magnetic resonance was reported by Marban et al. {108}. Furthermore, a study Kihara et al. using aequorin as a Ca^{2+} indicator showed that both diastolic and systolic levels of sarcoplasmic Ca^{2+} increases during early ischemia {108}.

The mechanism of the elevation of sarcoplasmic Ca^{2+} during ischemia is not well understood. One possible mechanism is, as mentioned above, that factors maintaining Ca^{2+} homeostasis by ATPases are disturbed by ischemia-induced ATP depletion, resulting in Ca^{2+} release from sarcoplasmic reticulum and mitochondria, and Ca^{2+} influx across sarcolemma. Another possible route of Ca^{2+} entry is Na^+-Ca^{2+} exchange. In the normal heart Ca^{2+} is removed by the exchanger because the steep Na^+ gradient forms exchange of Na for intracelluler Ca^{2+}. The intracellular Na^+ level is known to be elevated during ischemia, and two mechanisms are likely to be involved: enhanced Na^+-H^+ exchange in response to proton accumulation and suppression of the Na^+/K^+ pump due to lack of ATP {110}. This elevated of intracellular Na^+ level would promote Ca^{2+} influx via Na^+-Ca^{2+} exchange.

Tho role of Na^+-Ca^{2+} exchange appears even more important in Ca^{2+} influx during reperfusion {110,111}. Reperfusion rapidly normalize extracellular pH, which would both accelerate Na^+-H^+ exchange and abolish any suppression of the Na^+-Ca^{2+} exchange due to acidosis. This hypothesis is supported by observations that pretreatment with amiloride, a Na^+-H^+ exchange inhibitor, significantly attenuated Ca gain in the myocardium and contractile dysfunction during reperfusion {111} and that reperfusion with acidic perfusate significantly improved postischemic contractile recovery {112}.

When cytosolic Ca^{2+} reaches critical levels, it triggers several injurious processes. First, it will further accelerate ATP degradation by activation of Ca^{2+}-dependent ATPases. Secondly, mitochondrial function is impaired by Ca^{2+} overload {113}. Calcium activates membrane phospholipase {114} and perhaps endogenous proteases {115–117}, which could weaken the cytoskeleton or sarcolemma {62}. Although these proposed mechanisms are very attractive, few critical tests of these theories are actually available and further study is indicated.

In support of the calcium theory is the observation suggesting that calcium channel blockers may protect the heart against ischemic injury. Calcium channel blockers reportedly preserve mitochondrial function, mechanical function, myocardial calcium content, ATP content, and viability of isolated cardiac myocytes during oxygen deprivation {107,115,116}. As reviewed by Kloner and Braunwald {118}, a number of animal studies reported limitation of infarct size by calcium channel blockers. Unfortunately, however, the most of the positive studies suffers from several methodological problems. First, infarct size was analyzed relatively early (<24 hours) after the onset of ischemia using tetrazolium staining. Accordingly, the apparent limitation of infarct size by calcium blockers might represent simply a delay in necrosis of the cells that have been "condemned" to die {119}. Another problem is that the effect of calcium channel blockers may have been overestimated in some studies because of fortuitous inclusion of animals with high collateral flow in the treated groups. This possibility cannot be excluded, since many of those studies did not analyze the collateral blood flow-infarct size relationship. These problems were rectified in recent studies that employed chronic animal models, determined infarct size by histology, and took major determinants of infarct size (i.e., size of area at risk and collateral blood flow) into account {31,48,120}. In these studies, verapamil failed to limit infarct size or showed very modest protection after very brief ischemic insults. Insufficient data are available to fully define the conditions amenable to calcium channels blockers, but it is clear that they must be given early in ischemia and blood flow must also be restored quickly.

Phospholipase

Activation of membrane phospholipase has also been proposed as yet another mechanism responsible for ischemic injury. Myocardial phospholipase activity, predominantly A1 and A2, has been found in sarcolemma, sarcoplasmic reticulum, mitochondria, and lysosomes {121–123}. Activation of endogenous phospholipase most likely results from Ca^{2+} overload {93,121–123}. Degradation of phospholipid in membranes may change their permeability {124} and further disrupt ionic homeostasis. Steenbergen and Jennings {125} analyzed lysophospholipid production by phospholipase in ischemic myocardium in vitro. Structural destruction of membranes was evident after 150 minutes of ischemia. At that time lysophosphatidyl choline was only slightly increased, but lysophosphatidyl ethanolamine had not changed and total lysophospholipids were less than 1% of total phospholipids. Incubation of the tissue in 1.25 mM Ca^{2+} did not increase the lysophospholipid content. The lysophospholipids, however, were increased markedly after 5 hours of ischemia. Their finding indicates that phospholipid degradation by phospholipase probably does not occur until long after the cells are irreversibly injured.

Long-chain acyl CoA and long-chain acyl carnitine

A reduced oxygen supply results in accumulation of mitochondrial NADH and $FADH_2$. NADH and $FADH_2$ not only inhibit beta oxidation of fatty acids, but also increase the intracellular concentration of intermediates of beta oxidation, i.e., long-chain acyl CoA and long-chain acyl carnitine {126}. These compounds are known to be detrimental to cellular function. Long-chain acyl CoA inhibits adenine nucleotide translocase, acyl-CoA synthetase, and triglyceride lipase {127,128}. Long-chain acyl carnitine inhibits Na-K ATPase and sarcoplasmic reticulum Ca^{2+} ATPase {128}. In high concentration, it even inhibits mitochondrial respiration {129}. Furthermore, long-chain acyl CoA and long-chain acyl carnitine are active detergents {128}, and these compounds may even cause structural damage in ischemic myocytes, especially in the mitochondria. Ninety five percent of the cell's CoA is in the mitochondrial matrix, and a large fraction of long-chain acyl carnitine is also found in the mitochondrial fraction from ischemic myocardium {128}. Although the biochemical data concerning lipid metabolism is incriminating, few studies have actually tested these theories in animal models of ischemic injury. Ichihara and Neely {130} failed to detect any detrimental effects of exogenous fatty acids or long-chain acyl CoA and carnitine esters during ischemia.

Free radicals

The biological role of free radicals, highly reactive molecules that possess unpaired electrons in their outer shell, has been investigated intensively for the last decades in many pathophysiological processes, including myocardial infarction {84,131,132}. Of particular interest are the oxygen-derived free radicals, superoxide and the hydroxyl radical. Multiple pathways for their production have been identified in ischemic myocardium, and their generation is thought to be considerable when oxygen is reintroduced into the ischemic myocardium via reperfusing blood.

There are four possible sources of free radicals in ischemia/reperfused myocardium: (a) invading neutrophils, (b) oxidation of purine by cardiac xanthine oxidase, (c) degradation of catecholamine by monoamine oxidase, and (d) mitochondrial electron transport. Activated neutrophils are known to produce large quantities of oxygen free radicals via NADPH oxidase as part of their bactericidal activity {132}. As mentioned in *Reperfused infarcts* above, reperfusion may facilitate accumulation and free radical generation of neutrophils by washing out adenosine from infarcting myocardium.

Xanthine oxidase is another possible source of free radicals. This enzyme oxidizes the purines xanthine and hypoxanthine to urate. About 20% of this enzyme exists as an oxidase form, which can transfer leftover electrons directly to oxygen, thus producing oxygen free radicals {133,134}. A considerable amount of xanthine oxidase is present in both the dog {133} and rat heart {134}. However, xanthine oxidase in the human heart is negligiable {135,136}, which makes the significance of this enzyme as a free radical source in the human heart doubtful.

Catecholamine degradation is the third possible source of free radicals. Excess electrons produced by the oxidation of catecholamines by monoamine oxidase are accepted by molecular oxygen, producing hydrogen peroxide and

Table 59-1. Studies on the effect of SOD on infarct size

Study	Free radical scavenger	Species	Col flow as covariate	Ischemia duration	Reperfusion duration	Infarct diagnosis
Positive studies						
Ambrosio et al. {141}	SOD	Dog	No	90 min	48 hr	Gross
Werns et al. {142}	SOD	Dog	Yes	90 min	6, 24 hr	TTC
Naslund et al. {143}	SOD	Pig	N/A	60 min	5 hr	TTC
Chambers et al. {133}	SOD + CAT	Dog	No	60 min	4 hr	TTC
Jolly et al. {144}	SOD + CAT	Dog	No	90 min	20 hr	TTC
Werns et al. {145}	SOD	Dog	No	90 min	6 hr	TTC
Downey et al. {134}	SOD + CAT	Rabbit	N/A	45 min	4 hr	TTC
Tamura et al. {146}	PEG-SOD	Dog	Yes	90 min	6 hr, 96 hr	TTC
Negative studies						
Uraizee et al. {147}	SOD	Dog	Yes	40 min	96 hr	HIST
Gallagher et al. {148}	SOD + CAT	Dog	No	180 min	24 hr	TTC
Nejima et al. {149}	SOD	Dog	Yes	90 min	7 days	HIST
Patel et al. {150}	SOD	Dog	Yes	120 min	4, 48 hr	TTC
Shirato et al. {151}	SOD	Rabbit	N/A	45 min	3, 24, 72 hr	TTC
Miura et al. {152}	SOD + CAT	Rabbit	N/A	45 min	72 hr	HIST
Klein et al. {153}	SOD	Pig	N/A	45 min	24 hr	NBT
Miura et al. {154}	SOD	Rabbit	N/A	20, 30, 60 min	72 hr	HIST
Przyklenk et al. {155}	SOD + CAT	Dog	Yes	120 min	4 hr	TTC
Richard et al. {156}	SOD + CAT	Dog	Yes	90 min	96 hr	HIST
Tanaka et al. {157}	PEG-SOD	Dog	Yes	90 min	96 hjr	HIST
Ooiwa et al. {158}	PEG-SOD	Rabbit	N/A	30 min	72 hr	HIST

SOD = superoxide dismutase; CAT = catalase; PEG-SOD = SOD conjugated to polyethylene glycol; Col flow = collateral blood flow; N/A = not applicable to this species; TTC = triphenyl tetrazolium; HIST = conventional histology; NBT = nitroblue tetrazolium staining.

hydroxy radicals {137}. Mitochondria are yet another possible source of free radicals. Under normal conditions, about 1% of the electron flow in the mitochondria ends up as superoxide {138}. This radical is removed by the endogenous scavengers, glutathione and superoxide dismutase. An increase in this superoxide leak might be a consequence of ischemic damage to the mitochondria, but this has not yet been demonstrated.

Although intensive studies have been performed regarding the possible contribution of free radicals to myocardial necrosis following reperfusion, it is still unsettled whether free radicals upon reperfusion indeed kills myocardial cells. This is in marked contrast with the established role of free radicals in the pathogenesis of myocardial stunning {139} and reperfusion arrhythmias {140}. To test whether oxygen free radicals contribute to necrosis, most of the studies have taken the approach of assessing alteration of infarct size by administration of specific free-radical scavengers before ischemia/reperfusion. Table 59-1 summarizes the results of such studies using superoxide dismutase (SOD), a specific free-radical scavenger {133,134,141–158}. There is a trend toward negative studies when infarct size is determined by histology and the relationship between collateral flow and infarct size in the experimental mode is incorporated in the assessment of the drug's effect. However, none of the methodological or species differences in the model alone cannot explain all the discrepancies between the studies to date. Therefore, it must be admitted that the existence of lethal myocardial injury due to free radicals upon reperfusion is still incon-

clusive at the present time. Whatever the case, none of the above approaches has produced an effective anti-infarct drug.

ISCHEMIC PRECONDITIONING

A surprising phenomenon that has been disclosed recently is that a brief period of ischemia can be protective against a subsequent ischemic insult. This phenomenon, called *preconditioning*, was first reported by Murry et al. {159}. They observed that myocardial infarct size after 40 minutes of ischemia was reduced to about 25% of the control value when the myocardium was preexposed to four cycles of 5 minutes of ischemia each separated by 5 minutes of reperfusion. This observation was confirmed in various models of myocardial infarction {160–162}, and intensive research for the last several years has resulted in a rapid expansion of our knowledge on this subject. Preconditioning is now known to protect myocardium against ischemia-induced arrhythmias {163}, reperfusion arrhythmias {164,165}, and perhaps even myocardial stunning {166}. In the following, however, the discussion will focus on infarct size limitation by preconditioning.

The preconditioning effect represents enhanced myocardial resistance to ischemic necrosis and is not the result of increased collateral blood flow. This was indicated by two lines of evidence. First, preconditioning significantly shifted the collateral flow-infarct size relationship in the dog heart towards smaller infarct sizes {159}. Secondly,

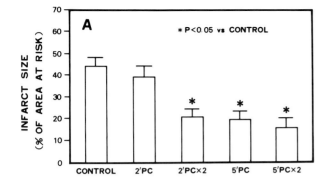

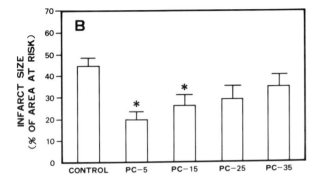

Fig. 59-9. Determinants of the infarct size-limiting effect of ischemic preconditioning. Myocardial infarction was induced by 30-minute coronary occlusion, which was followed by 72-hour reperfusion. **A:** Duration of preconditioning ischemia (2 minutes vs. 5 minutes) and number of preconditioning cycles (single episode vs. two cycles of preconditioning). Control = untreated controls; 2'PC = preconditioning with 2-minute ischemia followed by 5 minute reperfusion; 2'PCX2 = two cycles of 2-minute ischemia/5-minute reperfusion; 5'PC = preconditioning with 5-minute ischemia followed by 5 minute reperfusion; 5'PCX2 = two cycles of 5-minute ischemia/5-minute reperfusion. **B:** Decay of the infarct size-limiting effect of 5-minute preconditioning ischemia. Interval between the preconditioning ischemia (5 minutes) and the sustained 30-minute coronary occlusion was 5 minutes in PC-5, 15 minutes in PC-15, 25 minutes in PC-25, and 35 minutes in PC-35. Mean ± SEM. Reprinted from Miura and Iimura {167}, with permission.

infarct size is unequivocally limited by preconditioning in pig {161} and rabbit {162} hearts, both of which lack significant native coronary collaterals.

There are interesting features of the preconditioning effect. Figure 59-9 presents a summary of data from our studies using a rabbit ischemia/reperfusion model {167}. As shown in fig. 59-9, preconditioning with 5 minutes of ischemia limited infarct size to less than 50% of the control value, but preconditioning with 2 minutes of ischemia failed to significantly alter the infarct size. This indicates that there is a sharp threshold for protection between 2 and 5 minutes of ischemia. However, when preconditioning

with 2 minutes of ischemia was repeated two or four times, it then conferred the same protection as 5 minutes of ischemia. On the other hand, the infarct size-limiting effect of 5 minutes of preconditioning was not potentiated by its repetition. This finding is consistent with a study by Li et al. {160}, in which the extent of infarct size limitation was similar between preconditioning with a single, six, or 12 episodes of 5-minute ischemia in the dog heart.

Resistance to infarction afforded by preconditioning is not very longstanding. In the rabbit heart, protection by 5 minutes of ischemia spontaneously decays within 35 minutes following the preconditioning (panel B of fig. 59-7), although Van Winkle reported a slightly longer duration of protection {168}. The preconditioning effect reportedly disappeared somewhere between 30 and 60 minutes in the pig heart {169}, and it was diminished by half after 120 minutes in the dog heart {170}. Thus, preconditioning appears to protect myocardium from infarction for no longer than an hour.

There have been several proposed mechanisms for preconditioning. Firstly, the contribution of myocardial stunning to preconditioning has been an attractive hypothesis. Preconditioning stuns myocardium, and the resulting reduced contractile function lead to explain the reduced ATP demand in the preconditioned myocardium {184}. However, recent studies do not support this hypothesis. Murry et al. observed that myocardial stunning by 15 minutes of ischemia remained stable for 120 minutes in the dog heart, but protection against infarction conferred by preconditioning with 15 minutes of ischemia was substantially lost after 120 minutes {170}. Secondly, in a study from our laboratory {162} myocardial stunning in the rabbit was significantly less after preconditioning with two cycles of 2-minute ischemia than after a single or two cycles of 5-minute preconditioning. However, all three of the preconditioning protocols limited the infarct size to the same extent {162}. These findings indicate that myocardial stunning is not the mechanism for preconditioning.

The currently most attractive hypothesis was first proposed by Downey et al. {171,172}. They found that pretreatment with adenosine receptor antagonists (8-sulphophenyl-theophylline and PD115199) completely blocked infarct size limitation by preconditioning (fig. 59-10). Furthermore, R-phenylisopropyl-adenosine (R-PIA), an A1 receptor agonist, significantly limits infarct size (fig. 59-11). These findings were confirmed in our chronic rabbit model as well {173}. Furthermore, we recently demonstrated that preconditioning is markedly potentiated by dipyridamole, an adenosine nucleoside transport inhibitor, and that potentiation of preconditioning by dipyridamole was significantly attenuated by 8-phenyl-theophylline, an adenosine receptor antagonist {174} (fig. 59-12). These findings strongly indicate that endogenous adenosine accumulating during preconditioning ischemia mediates preconditioning. The adenosine hypothesis appears applicable to dog and pig hearts as well {175,176}. However, in the rat adenosine receptor antagonists have failed to abolish the preconditioning effect against infarction {155}, or ischemia-induced arrhythmias {177}, and reperfusion arrhythmias (Ishimito, Miura, and Iimura,

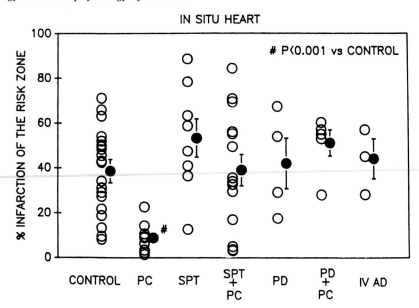

Fig. 59-10. Effect of adenosine receptor antagonists on infarct size-limiting effect of preconditioning in the rabbit. Infarct was induced by 30-minute coronary occlusion, and preconditioning (PC) was performed with 5-minute ischemia/10-minute reperfusion. Infarct size and the size of risk region were determined by tetrazolium staining and fluorescent particles, respectively. Administration of SPT or PD115199 prior to preconditioning completely blocked the preconditioning effect. SPT = 8-sulphophenyltheophylline; PD = PD 115199. Reprinted from Liu et al. {171}, with permission.

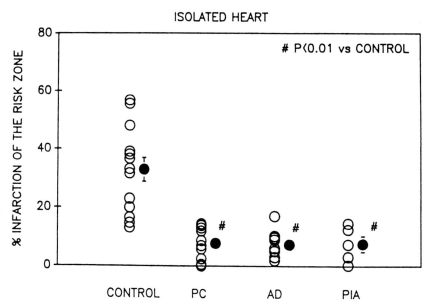

Fig. 59-11. Effect of adenosine and PIA on infarct size in isolated blood-perfused rabbit heart. Infarct was induced by 30-minute coronary occlusion, and preconditioning (PC) was performed with 5-minute ischemia/10-minute reperfusion. Infusion of adenosine (AD; 1.5 mg/5 min) and PIA (27 μg/5 min) before coronary occlusion limited infarct size to the same extent as preconditioning. Reprinted from Liu et al. {171}, with permission.

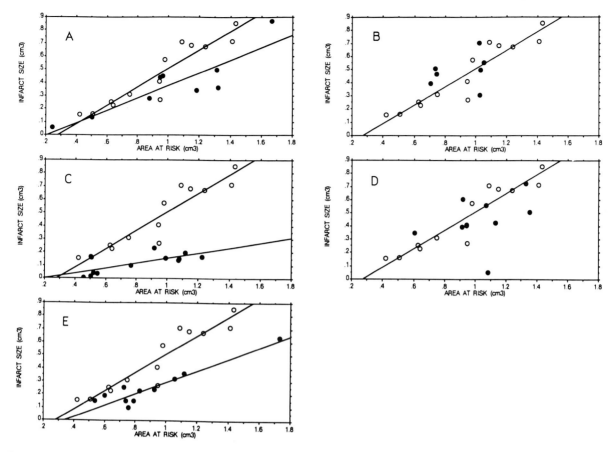

Fig. 59-12. Relationship between infarct size and size of area at risk in the rabbit. Myocardial infarction was induced by 30-minute ischemia, and the size of the infarct and size of area at risk were determined by histology and fluorescent particles, respectively, after 72-hour reperfusion. **A:** Control group (o) versus a group preconditioned with 2-minute ischemia/5-minute reperfusion (●). The difference in the slope between these two groups did not reach statistical significance. **B:** Control group (o) versus a dipyridamole group (●), which was given 0.25 mg/kg of dipyridamole at 22 minutes prior to the 30-minute ischemia. **C:** Control group (o) versus a DIP-2′PC group (●), which received dipyridamole 15 minutes prior to the 2-minute preconditioning. The regression line of the DIP-2′PC group was significantly less stepp than the control regression line. **D:** Control group (o) versus PT/DIP-2′PC group (●), which was given 8-phenyltheophylline and dipyridamole prior to the 2-minute preconditioning. The slope of the regression line in the PT/DIP-2′PC group was smaller than in the control group but larger than in the DIP-2′PC group (p < 0.01 for either comparison). Reprinted from Miura et al. {174}, with permission.

unpublished). The reason for this discrepant results between the species is unknown.

Of two subtypes of adenosine receptors (i.e., A1 or A2), current evidence suggests that the A1 receptor is responsible for preconditioning. Limitation of infarct size was achieved by an A1 agonist, R-PIA, but not the A2 agonist, CGS21680 {172}. Furthermore, Thornton et al. recently found that rabbits could not be preconditioned when their Gi proteins, which link A1 receptors with the intracellular signaling systems, were inactivated by pertussis toxin {178}.

If preconditioning is mediated by A1 receptors, which effector of the A1 receptor mediates the actual protection? One of the candidates is the ATP-sensitive K channel, which is thought to be opened by A1 receptor activation

through pertussis toxin-sensitive Gi proteins {179}. Gross and Auchampach {180} tested this hypothesis and found that blockers of ATP-sensitive K channels (glibenclamide and 5-hydroxydecanoate) abolished the preconditioning effect in the dog. A role of the ATP-sensitive K channel was further supported by a recent report that the infarct size-limiting effect of R-PIA was also blocked by pretreatment with glibenclamide {181}. However, Thornton and Downey {182} could not detect blockade of the preconditioning effect in the rabbit heart. These different results regarding the effect of glibenclamide on preconditioning suggest species differences in the mechanism of preconditioning. Other possible intracellular effectors of the A1 receptors have not been systematically studied with regard to their possible involvement in preconditioning.

Inhibition of mitochondrial ATPase by preconditioning is also an intriguing hypothesis. During ischemia a natural protein inhibitor of this ATPase is known to be induced in large mammals, including rabbits and dogs {183}. If the inhibitor persists after preconditioning ischemia, it could explain reduction of ATP demand in preconditioned myocardium {184}. However, this possible role of mitochondrial ATPase in preconditioning is not supported by recent studies reporting that preconditioning limited infarct size in the rat heart {177,185}, which has an insignificant level of mitochondrial ATPase activity.

Although several other mechanisms, including oxygen free radicals and cardioprotective stress proteins, have been proposed for preconditioning, results reported by recent investigations {186,187} do not support these theories.

CONCLUSIONS

In conclusion, myocardial infarction is a result of a complex sequence of events following coronary artery occlusion. Over the last decade, many investigations have rapidly expanded our knowledge of this phenomenon and have provided valuable insights into the pathophysiology of the ischemic myocardium. In addition, laboratory investigations have provided some clues (for example, preconditioning) to novel approaches to protecting the ischemic myocardium from necrosis. However, there is still a large gap between experimental and clinical findings regarding myocardial infarction. Coronary thrombolysis is currently the only established method for limiting myocardial infarct size in the clinical setting. To diminish the gap and to establish new interventions for this leading cause of mortality and morbidity, mutual collaboration between basic and clinical sciences is required now more than ever.

ACKNOWLEDGMENTS

The author wishes to thank Dr. James M. Downey for his invaluable advice and encouragement. Secretarial assistance by Ms. Hideko Kumasaka and Ms. Ikuko Miura is also greatly appreciated.

REFERENCES

1. Olive PB: Pathophysiology of acute myocardial infarction. *Ann Intern Med* 94:236–250, 1981.
2. Wilson RF, Holida MD, White CW: Quantitative angiographic morphology of coronary stenoses leading to myocardial infarction or unstable angina. *Circulation* 73:286–293, 1986.
3. Bertrand ME, LaBlanche JM, Tilmant PY, Tieuleux FA, Delforge MR, Carte AG, Asseman P, Berzin B, Libersa C, Laurent JM: Frequency of provoked coronary arterial spasm in 1089 consecutive patients undergoing coronary arteriography. *Circulation* 65:1299–1306, 1982.
4. Leary T: Experimental atherosclerosis in the rabbit compared with human atherosclerosis. *Arch Pathol* 17:453–492, 1934.
5. Leary T: Coronary spasm as a possible factor in producing sudden death. *Am Heart J* 10:338–344, 1935.
6. Horn H, Finkelstein LE: Arteriosclerosis of the coronary arteries and the mechanism of their occlusion. *Am Heart J* 19:655–682, 1940.
7. Mueller HS, Rao PS, Greenberg MA, Buttrick PM, Sussman II, Levite HA, Grose RM, Perez-Davila V, Strain JE, Spaet TH: Systemic and transcardiac platelet activity in acute myocardial infarction in man: Resistance to prostacyclin. *Circulation* 72:1336–1345, 1985.
8. Maliani A, Lombardi F: Consideration of the fundamental mechanisms eliciting cardiac pain. *Am Heart J* 103:575–578, 1982.
9. Margolis JR, Kannel WB, Feinleib M, Dawber TR, MacNamara PM: Clinical features of unrecognized myocardial infarction — silent and symptomatic. Eighteen year follow up: The Framingham Study. *Am J Cardiol* 32:1–7, 1973.
10. Sullivan W, Vlodaver Z, Tuna N, Long L, Edward JE: Correlation of electrocardiographic and pathologic findings in healed myocardial infarction. *Am J Cardiol* 42:724–732, 1978.
11. Muller JE, Tofler GH, Stone PH: Circadian variation and triggers of onset of acute cardiovascular disease. *Circulation* 79:733–743, 1989.
12. Schaper W: *The Collateral Circulation of the Heart.* Amsterdam: North-Holland, 1971.
13. Okun EM, Factor SM, Kirk ES: End-capillary loops in the heart: An explanation for discrete myocardial infarctions without border zones. *Science* 206:565–567, 1979.
14. Hirzel HO, Sonnenblick EH, Kirks ES: Absence of a lateral border zone of intermediate creatine phosphokinase depletion surrounding a central infarct 24 hours after acute coronary occlusion in the dog. *Circ Res* 41:673–683, 1977.
15. Yellon DM, Hearse DJ, Crome R, Grannel J, Wyse RKH: Characterization of the lateral interface between normal and ischemic tissue during acute myocardial infarction. *Am J Cardiol* 47:1233–1239, 1981.
16. Harken AH, Simson MB, Haselgrove, Wetstein L, Harden WR, Barlow CH: Early ischemia after complete coronary ligation in the rabbit, dog, pig, and monkey. *Am J Physiol* 241:H202–H210, 1981.
17. Downey JM, Yoshida S, Harpen MD: A functional estimate of the overlap between adjacent coronary circulations in the dog. *Basic Res Cardiol* 81:336–341, 1986.
18. Reimer KA, Jennings RB: The "wavefront phenomenon" of myocardial ischemic cell death. II. Transmural progression of necrosis within the framework of ischemic bed size (myocardial at risk) and collateral flow. *Lab Invest* 40:633–644, 1979.
19. Reimer KA, Jennings RB: Can we really quantitate myocardial cell injury? In: Hearse DJ, Yellon DM (eds) *Therapeutic Approaches to Myocardial Infarct Size Limitation.* New York: Raven Press, 1984, pp 163–184.
20. Jugdutt BI, Hutchins GM, Bulkley BH, Becker LC: Myocardial infarction in the conscious dog: Three-dimensional mapping of infarct, collateral flow and region at risk. *Circulation* 60:1141–1150, 1979.
21. Chambers DE, Yellon DM, Hearse DJ, Downey JM: Effects of flurbiprofen in altering myocardial infarc's in dogs: Reduction or delay? *Am J Cardiol* 51:884–890, 1983.
22. DeBoer LW, Strauss HW, Kloner RA, Rude RE, Davis RF, Maroko PF, Braunwald E: Autoradiographic method for measuring the ischemic myocardium at risk: Effects of verapamil on infarct size after experimental coronary artery occlusion. *Proc Natl Acad Sci USA* 77:6119–6123, 1980.

23. Darsee JR, Kloner KA, Braunwald E: Demonstration of lateral and epicardial border zone salvage by flurbiprofen using an in vivo method for assessing myocardium at risk. *Circulation* 61:29–35, 1981.

24. Yoshida S, Downey JM, Chambers DE, Hearse DJ: Nifedipine limits infarct size in closed chest coronary embolized dogs. *Basic Res Cardiol* 80:76–87, 1985.

25. Crozatier B, Ross J, Franklin D, Bloor CM, White FC, Tomoike H, McKown DP: Myocardial infarction in the baboon: Regional function and the collateral circulation. *Am J Physiol* 235:H413–H421, 1978.

26. Miura T, Yellon DM, Hearse DJ, Downey JM: The determinations of infarct size during permanent occlusion of a coronary artery in the closed chest dog. *J Am Coll Cardiol* 9:647–654, 1987.

27. Lowe JE, Reimer KA, Jennings RB: Experimental infarct size as a function of the amount of myocardium at risk. *Am J Pathol* 90:363–379, 1978.

28. Koyanagi S, Estham CL, Harrison DG, Marcus ML: Transmural variation in the relationship between myocardial infarct size and risk area. *Am J Physiol* 242:H867–H874, 1982.

29. Nakamura M, Tomoike H, Sakai K, Ootsubo H, Kikuchi Y: Linear relationship between perfusion area and infarct size. *Basic Res Cardiol* 76:438–442, 1981.

30. Melin JA, Becker LC: Salvage of ischemic myocardium by prostacyclin during experimental myocardial infarction. *J Am Col Cardiol* 2:279–286, 1983.

31. Reimer KA, Jennings RA, Cobb FR, Murdock RH, Greenfield JC, Becker LC, Bulkley BH, Hutchins GM, Schwartz RP, Bailey KR, Passamani ER: Animal models for protection ischemic myocardium: Results of the NHLBI cooperative study. Comparison of unconscious and conscious dog models. *Circ Res* 56:651–665, 1985.

32. Jugdutt BI: Different relations between infarct size and occluded bed size in barbiturate-anesthetized versus conscious dog. *J Am Coll Cardiol* 6:1035–1046, 1985.

33. Reimer KA, Lowe JE, Rasmussen MM, Jennings RB: The wavefront phenomenon of ischemic cell death. I. Myocardial infarct size versus duration of coronary occlusion in dogs. *Circulation* 56:786–794, 1977.

34. Miura T, Downey JM, Ooiwa H, Ogawa S, Adachi T, Noto T, Shizukuda Y, Iimura O: Progression of myocardial infarction in a collateral flow deficient species. *Jpn Heart J* 30:695–708, 1989.

35. Russell RE, Chagrasulis RW, Downey JM: Inhibitory effect of cardiac contraction on coronary collateral blood flow. *Am J Physiol* 233:H541–H546, 1977.

36. Moss AJ: Intramyocardial oxygen tension. *Cardiovasc Res* 2:314–318, 1968.

37. Windbury MM, Howe BB, Wiess HR: Effect of nitroglycerine and dipyridamole on epicardial and endocardial oxygen tension — future evidence for redistribution of myocardial blood flow. *J Pharmacol Exp Ther* 76:184–199, 1977.

38. Feigl EO: Coronary physiology. *Physiol Rev* 63:1–205, 1983.

39. Gamble WJ, Lafarge CG, Fyler DC, Weisul J, Monroe RG: Regional coronary venous oxygen saturation and myocardial oxygen tension following abrupt changes in ventricular pressure in the isolated dog heart. *Circ Res* 34:672–681, 1974.

40. Weiss HR, Naubauer JA, Lipp JA, Sinha AKL: Quantitative determination of regional oxygen consumption in the dog heart. *Circ Res* 42:394–401, 1978.

41. Holtz J, Grunwald WA, Manz R, Restorff WV, Bassenge E: Intracapillary hemoglobin oxygen saturation and oxygen consumption in different layers of left ventricular myocardium. *Pflügers Arch* 370:253–258, 1977.

42. Dunn RB, Griggs DM Jr: Transmural gradients in ventricular tissue metabolites produced by stopping coronary blood flow in the dog. *Circ Res* 37:438–445, 1975.

43. Dunn RB, Hickey KM, Griggs DM Jr: Effect of loading conditions on transmural lactate gradient in the ischemic left ventricule (abstract). *Physiologist* 18:200, 1975.

44. Lowe JE, Cummings RG, Adams DH, Hull-Ryde EA: Evidence that ischemic cell death begins in the subendocardium independent of variations in collateral flow or wall tension. *Circularion* 68:190–202, 1983.

45. Lee JT, Ideker RE, Reimer KA: Myocardial infarct size and location in relation to the coronary vascular bed at risk in man. *Circulation* 64:526–631, 1981.

46. Miura T, Yoshida S, Iimura O, Downey JM: Dobutamine modifies myocardial infarct size through supply-demand balance. *Am J Physiol* 254:H855–H861, 1988.

47. Suga H, Hayashi T, Shirahata M: Ventricular systolic pressure volume are as predictor of cardiac oxygen consumption. *Am J Physiol* 240:H320–H325, 1981.

48. Reimer KA, Jennings RB: Verapamil in two reperfusion models of myocardial infarction: Protection of severely ischemic myocardium without limitation of infarct size. *Lab Invest* 51:655–666, 1984.

49. Matsuki T, Shirato C, Cohen MV, Downey JM: Oxypurinol limits myocardial infarct size without pre-treatment. *Can J Cardiol* 6:123–129, 1990.

50. Miura T, Downey JM: Critical collateral blood flow level for salvage of ischemic myocardium. *Can J Cardiol* 5:201–205, 1989.

51. Jugdutt BI, Becker LC, Hutchins GM: Early changes in collateral blood flow during myocardial infarction in conscious dogs. *Am J Physiol* 237:H371–H380, 1979.

52. Marcus ML, Kerber RE, Ehrhardt J, Abboud FM: Effect on time on volume and distribution of coronary collateral flow. *Am J Physiol* 230:279–85, 1976.

53. Hirzel HO, Nelson GR, Sonnenblick EH, Kirk ES: Redistribution of myocardial blood flow from necrotic to surviving myocardium following coronary occlusion in the dog. *Circ Res* 39:214–222, 1976.

54. Reimer KA, Idecker RE, Jennings RB: Effect of coronary occlusion site on ischemic bed size and collateral blood flow in dogs. *Cardiovasc Res* 15:668–674, 1981.

55. Miura T, Downey JM: Collateral perfusion of ischemic myocardium is inversely related with the size of the ischemic zone. *Basic Res Cardiol* 83:128–136, 1988.

56. Muller KD, Sass S, Gottwik MG, Schaper W: Effect of myocardial oxygen consumption on infarct size in experimental coronary artery occlusion. *Basic Res Cardiol* 77:170–181, 1982.

57. Muller KD, Klein H, Schaper W: Changes in myocardial oxygen consumption 45 minutes after experimental coronary occlusion do not alter infarct size. *Cardiovasc Res* 14:710–718, 1980.

58. Miura T, Ogawa T, Iwamoto T, Shimamoto K, Iimura O: Dipyridamole potentiates the myocardial infarct size-limiting effect of ischemic preconditioning. *Circulation* 86:979–985, 1992.

59. Horneffer PJ, Healy B, Gott VL, Gardner TJ: The rapid evolution of a myocardial infarction in an end-artery preparation. *Circulation* 76(Suppl V):V39–V42, 1987.

60. Jennings RB, Ganote CE: Structural changes in myocardium during acute myocardial ischemia. *Circ Res* 34–35(Suppl III):III156–III168, 1974.

61. Schaper J, Mulch J, Winkler B, Schaper W: Ultrastructural, functional, and biochemical criteria for estimation of reversibility of ischemic injury: A study on the effects of global ischemia on the isolated dog heart. *J Mol Cell Cardiol* 11:521–541, 1979.

62. Steenbergen C, Hill ML, Jennings RB: Cytoskeletal damage during myocardial ischemia: Changes in vinculin immunofluorescence staining during total in vitro ischemia in canine heart. *Circ Res* 60:476–486, 1987.

63. Decker RS, Wildenthal K: Sequential lysosomal alterations during cardiac ischemia. II. Ultrastructural and cytochemical changes. *Lab Invest* 38:662–673, 1978.

64. Wildenthal K, Decker RS, Pool AR, Griffin EE, Dingle JT: Sequential lysosomal alterations during cardiac ischemia. I. Biochemical and immunohistochemical changes. *Lab Invest* 38:656–661, 1978.

65. Kloner RA, Rude RE, Carlson N, Maroko PR, DeBoer LWV, Braunwald E: Ultrastructural evidence of microvascular damage and myocardial cell injury after coronary artery occlusion: Which comes first? *Circulation* 62:945–952, 1980.

66. Tillmanns H, Kubler W: What happens in the microcirculation? In: Hearse DJ, Yellon DM (eds) *Therapeutic Approaches to Myocardial Infarct Size Limitation*. New York: Raven Press, 1984, pp 107–124.

67. Sommers HM, Jennings RB: Experimental acute myocardial infarction. Histologic and histochemical studies of early myocardial infarcts induced by temporary or permanent occlusion of a coronary artery. *Lab Invest* 13:1491–1503, 1964.

68. Robbins SL, Cotran RSS: *Pathologic Basis of Disease*. Philadelphia: WB Saunders, 1979.

69. Pinckard RN, O'Rourke RA, Crawford MH, Grover FS, McManus LM, Ghidoni JJ, Storrs SB, Olson MS: Complement localization and mediation of ischemic injury in baboon myocardium. *J Clin Invest* 66:1050–1056, 1980.

70. McManus LM, Kolb WP, Crawford WH, O'Rourke RA, Grover FL, Pinckard RN: Complement localization in ischemic baboon myocardium. *Lab Invest* 48:436–477, 1983.

71. Rossen RD, Swain JL, Michael LH, Weakley S, Giannini E, Entman ML: Selective accumulation of the first component of complement and leukocytes in ischemic canine heart muscle. A possible initiator of an extra myocardial mechanism of ischemic injury. *Circ Res* 57:119–130, 1985.

72. Rossen RD, Michael LH, Kagiyama A, Savage HE, Hanson G, Reisberg MA, Moake JN, Kim SH, Self D, Weakley S, Giannini E, Entman ML: Mechanism of complement activation after coronary artery occlusion: Evidence that myocardial ischemia in dogs causes release of constituents of myocardial subcellular origin that complex with human Clq in vivo. *Circ Res* 62:572–584, 1988.

73. Fishbein MC, Maclean D, Maroko PR: The histopathologic evaluation of myocardial infarction. *Chest* 73:843–849, 1978.

74. Schaper J, Schaper W: Reperfusion of ischemic myocardium: Ultrastructural and histochemical aspects. *J Am Coll Cardiol* 1:1037–1046, 1983.

75. Kloner RA, Ganote CE, Whalen DA Jr, Jennings RB: Effect of a transient period of ischemia on myocardial cells. II. Fine structure during the first few minutes of reflow. *Am J Pathol* 74:399–422, 1974.

76. Whalen DA, Hamilton DG, Ganote CE, Jennings RB. The effect of a transient period of ischemia on myocardial cells. I: Effects on cell volume regulation. *Am J Pathol* 74: 381–398, 1974.

77. Hearse DJ, Humphrey SM, Bullock GR: The oxygen paradox and the calcium paradox: Two facets of the same problem? *J Mol Cell Cardiol* 10:641–668, 1978.

78. Shine KI, Douglas AM, Ricchiati NV: Calcium, strontium, and barium movements during ischemia and reperfusion in rabbit ventricle. Implication for myocardial preservation. *Circ Res* 43:712–324, 1974.

79. Vander Heide RS, Angelo JP, Altschuld RA, Ganote CE: Energy dependence of contraction band formation in perfused hearts and isolated adult myocytes. *Am J Pathol* 125:55–68, 1986.

80. Bulkley, BH: Pathology of coronary atherosclerotic heart disease. In: Hurst JW (ed) *The Heart*, 6th ed. New York: McGraw-Hill, 1986, pp 839–856.

81. Fishbein MC, Y-Rit J, Lando U, Kanmatsuse K, Mercier JC, Ganz W: The relationship of vascular injury and myocardial hemorrhage to necrosis after reperfusion. *Circulation* 62:1274–1279, 1980.

82. Roberts CS, Schoen F, Kloner RA: Effect of coronary reperfusion on myocardial hemorrhage and infarct healing. *Am J Cardiol* 52:610–614, 1983.

83. Cronstein BNR, Levin RI, Belanoff J, Weissmann G, Hirshhorn R: Adenosine: An endogenous inhibitor of neutrophil-mediated injury to endothelial cells. *J Clin Invest* 78:760–770, 1986.

84. McCord JM: Oxygen-derived free radicals in postischemic tissue injury. *N Engl J Med* 312:159–163, 1985.

85. Miura T, Shizukuda Y, Ogawa S, Ishimoto R, Iimura O: Effects of early and later reperfusion on healing speed of experimental myocardial infarct. *Can J Cardiol* 7:146–154, 1991.

86. Neely JR, Whitmer JT, Rovetto MJ: Inhibition of glycolysis in hearts during ischemic perfusion. In: *Recent Advances in Studies on Cardiac Structure and Metabolism*, Vol 1. Baltimore, MD: University Park Press, 1969, pp 243–248.

87. Mochizuki S, Neely JR: Control of glyceraldehyde-3-phosphate dehydrogenase in cardiac muscle. *J Mol Cell Cardiol* 11:221–236, 1979.

88. Jennings RB, Reimer KA, Hill ML, Mayer SE: Total ischemia in dog hearts, in vitro. 1. Comparison of high energy phosphate production, ultilization, and depletion, and of adenine nucleotide catabolism in total ischemia in vitro vs. severe ischemia in vivo. *Circ Res* 49:892–900, 1981.

89. Reimer KA, Jennings RB, Hill ML: Total myocardial ischemia, in vitro. 2. High energy phosphate depletion and associated defects in energy metabolism, Cell volume regulation, and sarcolemmal integrity. *Circ Res* 49:910–911, 1981.

90. Hearse DJ, Braimbridge MV, Jynge P: Basic concepts. In: Protection of the Ischemic Myocardium: *Cardioplegia*. New York: Raven Press, 1981, pp 151–166.

91. Rouslin W, Erickson JL, Solaro RJ: Effects of oligomycin and acidosis on rates of ATP depletion in ischemic heart muscle. *Am J Physiol* 250:H503–H508, 1986.

92. Jennings RB, Reimer KA, Steenbergen C: Effect of inhibition of the mitochondrial ATPase on net myocardial ATP in total ischemia. *J Mol Cell Cardiol* 23:1383–1395, 1991.

93. Jennings RB, Steenbergen C: Nucleotide metabolism and cellular damage in myocardial ischemia. *Ann Rev Physiol* 47:727–749, 1985.

94. Rubio R, Berne RM, Dobson Jr JG: Sites of adenosine production in cardiac and skeletal muscle. *Am J Physiol* 225:938–953, 1973.

95. Shutz W, Schrader J, Gerlach E: Different sites of adenosine formation in the heart. *Am J Physiol* 240:H963–H970, 1981.

96. Liu MS, Feinberg H: Incorporation of adenosine-8-14C and

inosine-8-14C into rabbit heart adenine nucleotides. *Am J Physiol* 220:1242–1248, 1971.

97. Plagemann PGW, Wohlhueter RM: Nuleotide transport in mammalian cells and interaction with intracellular metabolism. Rall TW, Rubio R (eds) *Regulatory Function of Adenosine*. The Hague: Martinus Nijhoff, 1983, pp 179–201.

98. Berne RM: The role of adenosine in the regulation of coronary blood flow. *Circ Res* 47:807–813, 1980.

99. Berne RM, Rubio R, Dobson JG Jr, Curnish RR: Adenosine and adenine nucleotides as possible mediators of cardiac and skeletal muscle blood flow regulation. *Circ Res* 28(Suppl I):I115–I119, 1971.

100. Rubio VR, Wiedmeier T, Berne RM: Nucleoside phosphorylase: Localization and role in the myocardial distribution of purines. *Am J Physiol* 222:550–555, 1972.

101. Jarasch ED, Bruder G, Heid HW: Significance of xanthine oxidase in capillary endothelial cells. *Acta Physiologica Scabdinavica* 126(Suppl 548):39–46, 1986.

102. Jennings RB, Hawkins HK, Lowe JE, Hill ML, Klotman S, Reimer KA: Relation between high energy phosphate and lethal injury in myocardial ischemia in the dog. *Am J Pathol* 92:187–214, 1987.

103. Hearse DJ, Braimbridge MV, Jynge P: Models and markers for the investigation of myocardial tissue damage. In: *Protection of the Ischemic Myocardium: Cardioplegia*. New York: Raven Press, 1981, pp 50–94.

104. Jennings RB, Schaper J, Hill ML, Steenbergen C, Reimer KA: Efect of reperfusion late in the phase of reversible ischemic injury. Changes in cell volume, electrolytes, metabolites, and ultrastructure. *Circ Res* 56:262–278, 1985.

105. Farber JL: Biology of disease. Membrane injury and calcium homeostasis in the pathogenesis of coagulative necrosis. *Lab Invest* 47:114–123, 1982.

106. Cheung JY, Bonventre JV, Mails CD, Leaf A: Calcium and ischemic injury. *N Engl J Med* 314:1670–1976, 1986.

107. Steenbergen C, Murphy E, Watts JA, London RE: Correlation between cytosolic free calcium, contracture, ATP, and irreversible ischemic injury in perfused rat heart. *Circ Res* 66:135–146, 1990.

108. Marban E, Kitakaze M, Koretsune Y, Yue DT, Chacko VP, Pike M: Quantification of $[Ca^{2+}]_i$ in perfused hearts. Critical evaluation of the 5F-BAPTA and nuclear magnetic resonance method as applied to the study of ischemia and reperfusion. *Circ Res* 66:1255–1267, 1990.

109. Kihara Y, Grossman W, Morgan JP: Direct measurement of changes in intracellular calcium transients during hypoxia, ischemia, and reperfusion of the intact mammalian heart. *Circ Res* 65:1029–1044, 1989.

110. Lazdunski M, Frelin C, Vigne P: The sodium/hydrogen exchange system in cardiac cells: Its biochemical and pharmacological properties and its role in regulating internal concentrations of sodium and internal pH. *J Mol Cell Cardiol* 17:1029–1042, 1985.

111. Tani M, Neely JR: Role of intracellular Na^+ and Ca^{2+} overload and depressed recovery of ventricular function of reperfused ischemic rat hearts. Possible involvement of H^+-Na^+ and Na^+-Ca^{2+} exchange. *Circ Res* 65:1045–1056, 1989.

112. Kitakaze M, Weisfeldt ML, Marban E: Acidosis during early reperfusion prevents myocardial stunning in perfused hearts. *J Clin Invest* 82:920–927, 1988.

113. Nayler WG: The role of calcium in the ischemic myocardium. *Am J Pathol* 102:262–270, 1981.

114. Jennings RB, Reimer KA: Lethal, myocardial ischemic injury. *Am J Pathol* 102:241–255, 1981.

115. Jennings RB, Steenbergen C, Kinney RB, Hill ML, Reimer KA: Comparison of the effect of ischemia and anoxia on

sarcolemma of the dog heart. *Eur Heart J* 4(Suppl H): 123–137, 1983.

116. Jennings RB, Reimer KA, Steenbergen C: Myocardial ischemic and reperfusion: Role of calcium. In: Parratt JR (ed) *Control and Manipulation of Calcium Movement*. New York: Raven Press, 1984.

117. Reddy MK, Etlinger JD, Rabinowitz M, Fischman DA, Zak R: Removal of Z-lines and alpha actin from isolated myofibrils by a calcium-activated neutral protease. *J Biol Chem* 250:4278–4284, 1975.

118. Kloner RA, Braunwald E: Effects of calcium antagonists on infarcting myocardium. *Am J Cardiol* 59:84B–94B, 1987.

119. Hearse DJ, Yellon DM: Why are we still in doubt about infarct size limitation? The experimentalist's viewpoint. In: Hearse DJ, Yellon DM (eds) *Therapeutic Approaches to Myocardial Infarct Size Limitation*. New York: Raven Press, 1984, pp 18–41.

120. Adachi T, Miura T, Noto T, Ooiwa H, Ogawa T, Tsuchida A, Iwamoto T, Goto M, Iimura O: Does verapamil limit myocardial infarct size in a heart deficient in xanthine oxidase? *Clin Exp Pharmacol Physiol* 17:769–779, 1990.

121. Franson RC, Pang DC, Towle DW, Weglicki WB: Phospholipase A activity of highly enriched preparations of cardiac sarcolemma from hamster and dog. *J Mol Cell Cardiol* 10:921–930, 1978.

122. Franson RC, Waite M, Weglicki WB: Phospholipase A activity of lysosomes of rat myocardial tissue. *Biochemistry* 11:472–476, 1972.

123. Weglicki WB, Waite BM, Sisson P, Shohet SB: Myocardial phospholipase A of microsomal and mitochondrial fractions. *Biochem Biophys Acta* 231:512–519, 1971.

124. Chien KR, Reeves JP, Buja M, Bonte F, Parkey RW, Willerson JT: Temporal and topographical correlations with Tc-99m-PPi accumulation and an in vitro sarcolemmal Ca^{2+} permeability defect. *Circ Res* 48:711–719, 1981.

125. Steenbergen C, Jennings RB: Relationship between lysophospholipid accumulation and plasma membrane injury during total in vitro ischemia in dog heart. *J Mol Cell Cardiol* 16:605–621, 1984.

126. Vary TC, Reibel DK, Neely JR: Control of energy metabolism of heart muscle. *Ann Rev Physiol* 43:419–430, 1981.

127. Bricknell OL, Opie LH: Effects of substrates on tissue metabolic changes in the isolated rat heart during underperfusion and on release of lactate dehydrogenase and arrhythmias during reperfusion. *Circ Res* 43:102–114, 1978.

128. Neely JR, Feuvray D: Metabolic products and myocardial ischemia. *Am J Pathol* 102:282–291, 1981.

129. Pitts BJR, Tate CA, Van Winkle WB, Wood JM, Entman ML: Palmitylcarnitine inhibition of the calcium pump in cardiac sarcoplasmic reticulum: A possible role in myocardial ischemia. *Life Sci* 23:391–402, 1978.

130. Ichihara K, Neely JR: Recovery of ventricular function in reperfused ischemic rat hearts exposed to fatty acids. *Am J Physiol* 249:H492–H497, 1985.

131. Freeman BA, Crapo JD: Biology of disease. Free radicals and tissue injury. *Lab Invest* 47:412–426, 1982.

132. Klebanoff SJ: Oxygen metabolism and the toxic properties of phagocytes. *Ann Intern Med* 93:480–489, 1980.

133. Chambers DE, Parks DA, Patterson G, Roy R, McCord JM, Yoshida S, Parmley LF, Downey JM: Xantine oxidase as a source of free radical damage in myocardial ischemia. *J Mol Cell Cardiol* 17:145–152, 1985.

134. Downey JM, Miura T, Eddy LJ, Chambers DE, Hearse DJ, Yellon DM: Xanthine oxidase is a source of free radical in the ischemic rat heart but not the rabbit. *J Mol Cell Cardiol* 19:1053–1060, 1987.

135. Eddy LJ, Stewart JR, Jones HP, Engerson TD, McCord

JM, Downey J: Free radical producing enzyme xanthine oxidase, is undetectable in human heart. *Am J Physiol* 253:H709–H711, 1987.

136. Janssen M, de Jong JW, Bos E: Free-radical production by isolated perfused human hearts subjected to ischemia (abstract). *Circulation* 86(Suppl I):I88, 1992.

137. Cohen G: Oxygen radicals, hydrogen peroxide, and Parkinson's disease. In: Autor A (ed) *Pathology of oxygen.* New York: Academic Press, 1982.

138. Bovaris A, Chance B: The mitochondrial generation of hydrogen peroxide. *Biochem J* 134:707–716, 1973.

139. Bolli R: Mechanism of myocardial "stunning." *Circulation* 82:723–738, 1990.

140. Hearse DJ: Free radicals, membrane injury, and electrophysiological disorders. In: Zipes DP, Jalife J (eds) *Cardiac Electrophysiology. From cell to bedside.* Philadelphia: WB Saunders, 1990, pp 442–447.

141. Ambrosio G, Becker LC, Hutchens GM, Weisman HF, Weisfeldt ML: Reduction in experimental infarct size by recombinant human superoxide dismutase: Insights into the pathophysiology of reperfusion injury. *Circulation* 74:1424–1433, 1986.

142. Werns SW, Simpson PK, Mickelson JK, Shea MJ, Pitt B, Lucchesi BR: Sustained limitation by superoxide dismutase of canine myocardial injury due to regional ischemia followed by reperfusion. *J Cardiovasc Pharmacol* 11:36–44, 1988.

143. Naslund U, Haggmark S, Johansson G, Marklund SL, Reiz S, Ogberg A: Superoxide dismutase and catalase reduce infarct size in a porcine myocardial ischemia/reperfusion model. *J Mol Cell Cardiol* 11:1077–1084, 1986.

144. Jolly SR, Kane WJ, Bailie MB, Abrams GD, Lucchesi BR: Canine myocardial reperfusion injury: Its reduction by combined administration of superoxide dismutase and catalase. *Circ Res* 54:277–285, 1984.

145. Werns SW, Shea MJ, Driscoll EM, Cohen C, Abrams GD, Pitt B, Lucchesi BR: The independent effect of oxygen radical scavengers on canine infarct size reduction by superoxide dismuase and not catalase. *Circ Res* 56:895–898, 1985.

146. Tamura Y, Chi L, Driscoll EM, Hoff PT, Freeman BA, Gallagher KP, Lucchesi BR: Superoxide dismutase conjugated to polyethylene glycol provides sustained protection against myocardial ischemia/reperfusion injury in canine heart. *Circ Res* 63:944–959, 1988.

147. Uraizee A, Reimer KA, Murry CE, Jennings RB: Failure of superoxide dismutase to limit size of myocardial infarction after 40 minutes of ischemia and 4 days of reperfusion in dogs. *Circulation* 75:1237–1248, 1987.

148. Gallagher KP, Buda AJ, Pace D, Gerren RA, Shlafer M: Failure of superoxide dismutase and catalase to alter size of infarction in conscious dogs after 3 hours of occlusion followed by reperfusion. *Circulation* 73:1065–1076, 1986.

149. Nejima J, Knight DR, Fallon JT, Uemura N, Manders WT, Canfield DR, Cohen MV, Vatner SF: Superoxide dismutase reduces reperfusion arrhythmias but fails to salvage regional function or myocardium at risk in conscious dogs. *Circulation* 79:143–153, 1989.

150. Patel B, Jeouldi MO, O'Neill PG, Roberts R, Bolli R: Human superoxide dismutase fails to limit infarct size after 2 hours ischemia and reperfusion (abstract). *Circulation* 78:II373, 1988.

151. Shirato C, Miura T, Ooiwa H, Toyofuku T, Wilborn WH, Downey JM: Tetrazolium artifactually indicates superoxide dismutase-induced salvage in reperfused rabbit heart. *J Mol Cell Cardiol* 21:1187–1193, 1989.

152. Miura T, Hotta D, Downey JM, Iimura O: Effect of supero-

xide dismutase plus catalase on myocardial infarct size in rabbits. *Can J Cardiol* 4:407–411, 1988.

153. Klein HH, Pich S, Lindert S, Buchwald A, Nebendahl K, Kreuzer H: Intracoronary superoxide dismutase for the treatment of "reperfusion injury." A blinded randamized placebo-controlled trial in ischemic, reperfused porcine hearts. *Basic Res Cardiol* 83:141–148, 1988.

154. Miura T, Ogawa S, Ooiwa H, Adachi T, Noto T, Shizukuda Y, Iimura O: Human superoxide dismutase failed to limit the size of myocardial infarct after 20-, 30-, or 60-minute ischemia and 72-hour reperfusion in the rabbit. *Jpn Circ J* 53:786–794, 1989.

155. Przyklenk K, Kloner RA: Reperfusion injury by oxygen free radicals? Effect of superoxide dismutase plus catalase given at the time of reperfusion, on myocardial infarct size, contractile function, coronary vasculature, and regional myocardial blood flow. *Circ Res* 64:86–96, 1989.

156. Richard VJ, Murry CE, Jennings RB, Reimer KA: Therapy to reduce free radicals during early reperfusion does not limit the size of myocardial infarcts caused by 90 minutes of ischemia in dogs. *Circulation* 78:473–480, 1988.

157. Tanaka M, Stoler RC, FitzHarris GP, Jennings RE, Reimer KA: Evidence against the "early protection-delayed death" hypothesis of superoxide dismutase therapy in experimental myocardial infarction. Polyethylene glycol-superoxide dismuase plus catalase does not limit myocardial infarct size in dogs. *Circ Res* 67:636–644, 1990.

158. Ooiwa H, Stanley A, Felaneous-Bylund AC, Wilborn W, Downey JM: Superoxide dismutase conjugated to polyethylene glycol fails to limit myocardial infarct size after 30 min ischemia followed by 72 h of reperfusion in the rabbit. *J Mol Cell Cardiol* 23:119–125, 1991.

159. Murry CE, Jennings RB, Reimer KA: Preconditioning with ischemia: A delay in lethal injury in ischemic myocardium. *Circulation* 74:1124–1136, 1986.

160. Li GC, Vasquez JA, Gallagher KP, Lucchesi BR: Myocardial protection with preconditioning. *Circulation* 82:609–619, 1990.

161. Schott RJ, Rohmann S, Braun ER, Schaper W: Ischemic preconditioning reduces infarct size in swine myocardium. *Circ Res* 66:1133–1142, 1990.

162. Miura T, Goto M, Urabe K, Endoh A, Shimamoto K, Iimura O: Does myocardial stunning contribute to infarct size limitation by ischemic preconditioning? *Circulation* 84:2504–2512, 1991.

163. Vegh A, Szekeres L, Parratt JR: Protective effects of preconditioning of the ischemic myocardium involve cyclo-oxygenase products. *Cardiovasc Res* 24:1020–1023, 1990.

164. Shiki K, Hearse DJ: Preconditioning of ischemic myocardium: Reperfusion-induced arrhythmia. *Am J Physiol* 253:H1470–H1476, 1987.

165. Harger JM, Hale SL, Kloner RA: Effect of preconditioning ischemia on reperfusion arrhythmias after coronary artery occlusion and reperfusion in the rat. *Circ Res* 68:61–68, 1991.

166. Urabe K, Miura T, Iwamoto T, Ogawa T, Endoh A, Iimura O: Preconditioning attenuates myocardial stunning via adenosine receptor activation (abstract). *Circulation* 86(Suppl I):I24, 1992.

167. Miura T, Iimura O: Infarct size limitation by preconditioning: Its phenomenological features and the key role of adenosine. *Cardiovasc Res* 27:36–42, 1993.

168. Van Winkle DM, Thornton J, Downey JM: The natural history of preconditioning: Cardioprotection depends on duration of transient ischemia and time to subsequent ischemia. *Coron Artery Dis* 2:613–619, 1991.

169. Schwartz ER, Mohri M, Sack S, Arras M: Duration of

infarct size limiting effect of ischemic preconditioning in the pig (abstract). *Circulation* 84(Suppl II):II432, 1991.

170. Murry CE, Richard VJ, Jennings RB, Reimer KA: Myocardial protection is lost before contractile function recovers from ischemic preconditioning. *Am J Physiol* 260:H796–H804, 1991.

171. Liu GS, Thornton J, Van Winkle D, Stanley AWH, Olsson RA, Downey JM: Protection against infarction afforded by preconditioning is mediated by A1 adenosine receptors in rabbit heart. *Circulation* 84:350–356, 1991.

172. Thornton JD, Liu GS, Olsson RA, Downey JM: Intravenous pretreatment with A1-selective adenosine analogues protects the heart against infarction. *Circulation* 85:659–665, 1992.

173. Tsuchida A, Miura T, Miki T, Shimamoto K, Iimura O: Role of adenosine receptor activation in infarct size limitation by preconditioning. *Cardiovasc Res* 26:456–461, 1992.

174. Miura T, Ogawa T, Iwamoto T, Shimamoto K, Iimura O: Dipyridamole potentiates the myocardial infarct size-limiting effect of ischemic preconditioning. *Circulation* 86:979–985, 1992.

175. Kitakaze M, Hori M, Takashima S, Sato H, Kamada T: Augumentation of adenosine production during ischemia as a possible mechanism of myocardical protection in ischemic preconditioning (abstract). *Circulation* 84(Suppl II):II306, 1991.

176. Schwartz ER, Mohri M, Sack S, Arras M: The role of adenosine and its A1 receptor in ischemic preconditioning (abstract). *Circulation* 84(Suppl II):II191, 1991.

177. Li Y, Kloner RA: Ischemic "preconditioning" is not mediated by adenosine receptors in the rat heart (abstract). *Circulation* 86(Suppl I):I24, 1992.

178. Thornton J, Downey JM: Gi proteins are involved in preconditioning's protective effect (abstract). *Circulation* 84(Suppl II):II192, 1991.

179. Kirsch GE, Codiana J, Birnbaumer L, Brown AM: Coupling of ATP-sensitive K channels to A1 receptors by G proteins in rat ventricular myocytes. *Am J Physiol* 259:H820–H826, 1990.

180. Gross GJ, Auchampach JA: Blockade of ATP-sensitive potassium channels prevents myocardial preconditioning in dogs. *Circ Res* 70:222–233, 1992.

181. Grover GJ, Sleph PG, Dzwonczyk S: Role of myocardial ATP-sensitive potassium channels in mediating preconditioning in the dog heart and their possible interaction with adenosine A1-receptors. *Circulation* 86:1310–1316, 1992.

182. Thornton J, Downey JM: Blockade of ATP-sensitive potassium channels does not prevent preconditioning in rabbit heart (abstract). *Circulation* 84(Suppl II):II432, 1991.

183. Rouslin W, Pullman ME: Protonic inhibition of the mitochondrial adenosine 5′-triphosphatase in ischemic cardiac muscle. Reversible binding of the ATPase inhibitor protein to the mitochondrial ATPase during ischemia. *J Mol Cell Cardiol* 19:661–668, 1987.

184. Murry CE, Richard VJ, Reimer KA, Jennings RB: Ischemic preconditioning slows energy metabolism and delays ultrastructural damage during a sustained ischemic episode. *Circ Res* 66:913–931, 1990.

185. Yellon DM, Alkhulaifi AM, Browne EE, Pugsley WB: Ischaemic preconditioning limits infarct size in the rat heart. *Cardiovasc Res* 26:983–987, 1992.

186. Iwamoto T, Miura T, Adachi T, Noto T, Ogawa T, Tsuchida A, Iimura O: Myocardial infarct size-limiting effect of ischemic preconditioning was not attenuated by oxygen free-radical scavengers in the rabbit. *Circulation* 83:1015–1022, 1991.

187. Thornton J, Striplin S, Liu GC, Swafford A, Stanley AW, Van Winkle DM, Downey JM: Inhibition of protein synthesis does not block myocardial protection afforded by preconditioning. *Am J Physiol* 259:H1822–H1825, 1990.

Index